MENTAL HEALTH NURSING

UNIT IV **TRAVELERS ACROSS THE LIFESPAN** *571*

CHAPTER 24 **The Pediatric Traveler**
Sarah N. Lechner *573*

CHAPTER 25 **The Adult Traveler**
Elizabeth Nolan Arnold *617*

CHAPTER 26 **The Elderly Traveler**
Charlotte Eliopoulos *645*

CHAPTER 27 **Loss Along the Journey**
Miriam Jacik *661*

UNIT V **THE WOUNDED TRAVELER** *689*

CHAPTER 28 **The Journey Threatened by Stress and Anxiety Disorders**
Lisa Robinson *691*

CHAPTER 29 **The Journey Controlled by Thought Disorders**
Patricia D. Sullivan and Verna Benner Carson *725*

CHAPTER 30 **The Journey Colored by Mood Disorders**
Wendy Miller Resnick and Verna Benner Carson *759*

CHAPTER 31 **The Journey Anesthetized by Substance Abuse**
Elizabeth Nolan Arnold *793*

CHAPTER 32 **The Journey Troubled by Behavioral Disorders**
Pamela E. Marcus and Tommie Springham *841*

CHAPTER 33 **The Journey Compartmentalized by Dissociative Disorders**
Linda Stafford *863*

CHAPTER 34 **The Journey Undermined by Psychosexual Disorders**
Suzanne S. Stuntz, Anne Falk, Melinda Hiken, and Verna Benner Carson *879*

CHAPTER 35 **The Journey Challenged by Eating Disorders**
Willa A. Decker and Margaret Freeman *909*

CHAPTER 36 **The Journey Scarred by Suicide**
Pamela E. Marcus, Evelyn W. Lloyd, and Alix C. Rey *927*

CHAPTER 37 **The Journey Embedded in Psychophysiological Disorders**
Sue Ann Thomas and Frances B. Wimbush *949*

CHAPTER 38 **The Journey Clouded by Cognitive Disorders**
Elizabeth Nolan Arnold *977*

UNIT VI **THE JOURNEY AND SOCIETY** *1021*

CHAPTER 39 **The Journey Marked by Homelessness**
Daria Virvan *1023*

CHAPTER 40 **The Journey Marked by Violence**
Verna Benner Carson *1039*

CHAPTER 41 **The Journey Marked by Rape**
Patricia Sullivan *1085*

CHAPTER 42 **The Journey Marked by AIDS**
Verna Benner Carson *1103*

CHAPTER 43 **The Journey Through Community Mental Health Care**
Verna Benner Carson *1127*

CHAPTER 44 **The Journey Through Home Mental Health Care**
Verna Benner Carson *1151*

UNIT VII **IMPROVING THE JOURNEY** *1171*

CHAPTER 45 **Total Quality Management**
Mattie Lowery *1173*

CHAPTER 46 **Research and the Future of Practice**
Elizabeth Nolan Arnold, Tom Phillips, and Karen Babich *1193*

Appendix I Standardized Rating Scales *1207*

Appendix II *DSM-IV* Classification *1229*

Answers to *Check Your Reading* Questions *1239*

Index *1279*

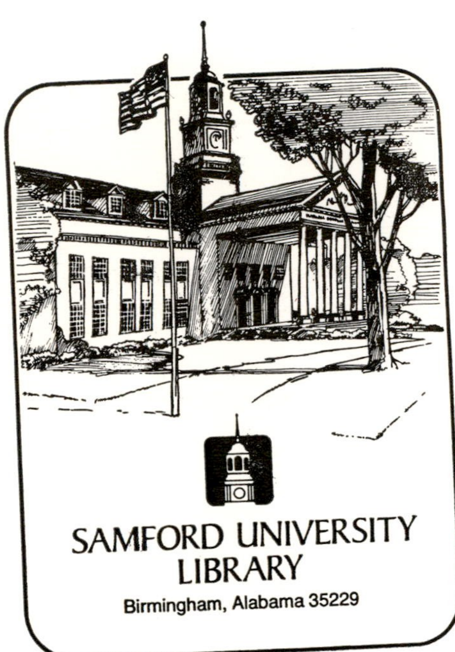

MENTAL HEALTH NURSING
THE NURSE-PATIENT JOURNEY

Verna Benner Carson, PhD, RN, CS-P
Associate Professor
School of Nursing
University of Maryland at Baltimore
Consulting Director
Psychiatric Home Care Program
Bay Area Health Care
Baltimore, Maryland

Elizabeth Nolan Arnold, PhD, RN, CS-P
Associate Professor
School of Nursing
University of Maryland at Baltimore
Baltimore, Maryland
Nurse-Psychotherapist
Family Counseling and Consulting Associates
Kensington, Maryland

W.B. SAUNDERS COMPANY
A Division of Harcourt Brace & Company
Philadelphia London Toronto Montreal Sydney Tokyo

W.B. SAUNDERS COMPANY
A Division of Harcourt Brace & Company

The Curtis Center
Independence Square West
Philadelphia, Pennsylvania 19106

Library of Congress Cataloging-in-Publication Data

Mental health nursing: the nurse-patient journey / [edited by] Verna Benner Carson, Elizabeth Nolan Arnold.—1st ed.

p. cm.

ISBN 0-7216-3520-2

1. Psychiatric nursing. I. Carson, Verna Benner. II. Arnold, Elizabeth Nolan.
[DNLM: 1. Psychiatric Nursing. 2. Nurse-Patient Relations. 3. Psychotherapy—methods. WY 160 M5493 1996]
RC440.M3546 1996 610.73′68—dc20

DNLM/DLC 95-17713

Mental Health Nursing: The Nurse-Patient Journey ISBN 0-7216-3520-2

Printed in the United States of America.

Last digit is the print number: 9 8 7 6 5 4 3 2 1

This book is dedicated to the Lord,
who renews our strength,
allows us to soar like eagles,
run and not grow weary,
and walk and not be faint.

He has blessed us with the love of
wonderful husbands:
John Carson and George Arnold
and precious children:
Adam, Johnny, and Robbie Carson,
and Mary Beth, Brian, Karen, Julie, and Christy Arnold.
They are the wind beneath our wings.

CONTRIBUTORS

Ellen A. Andruzzi, MSN, RN, CS-P
Bradenton, Florida

Elizabeth Nolan Arnold, PhD, RN, CS-P
Associate Professor
School of Nursing
University of Maryland at Baltimore
Baltimore, Maryland
Nurse-Psychotherapist
Family Counseling and Consulting Associates
Kensington, Maryland

Karen S. Babich, PhD, RN, FAAN
Director
Office of Science Policy and Program Planning
National Institute of Mental Health
Department of Health and Human Services
Rockville, Maryland

Verna Benner Carson, PhD, RN, CS-P
Associate Professor
School of Nursing
University of Maryland at Baltimore
Consulting Director
Psychiatric Home Care Program
Bay Area Health Care
Baltimore, Maryland

Nancy E. Conrad, EdD, RN
Assistant Professor
Widener University
Chester, Pennsylvania
Critical Thinking Exercises

Marcia Cooley, PhD, RN, CS-P
Assistant Professor
School of Nursing
University of Maryland
Baltimore, Maryland

Willa A. Decker, MS, RN
Assistant Professor
The University of Texas–Houston Health Science Center SON
Houston, Texas

Charlotte Eliopoulos, RNC, MPH
Author, Consultant, Educator in Geriatrics and Long-Term Care
President, Health Education Network
Glen Arm, Maryland

Anne Falk, MS, RN
Owings Mills, Maryland

Edna M. Fordyce, EdD, RN, CS-P
Associate Professor
Department of Nursing
Towson State University
Towson, Maryland

Margaret Freeman BS, MEd
Counselor
Houston Community College
Houston, Texas

Judy S. Fuhrmann, MS, RN, CS-P
Assistant Professor of Nursing
John Tyler Community College
Chester, Virginia
Clinical Nurse Specialist in Adult Psychiatric and Mental Health Nursing
Private Practice
Midlothian, Virginia

Melinda Hiken, MS, RN
Johns Hopkins Hospital
Department of Psychiatry
Baltimore, Maryland

Miriam Jacik, MSN, MSPsy
Adjunct faculty member
Continuing Education Department
Penn State University
State College, Pennsylvania
Clinical Manager
Psychiatric Home Care Services
Bay Area Health Care
Baltimore, Maryland

Suzanne Sayle Jimerson, MS, RN, CS-P
Assistant Professor
Adjunct Faculty
Northeastern University School of Nursing
Boston, Massachusetts
Professional Staff
Westwood Pembroke Health System
Boston, Massachusetts

Mary Ellen Lashley, PhD, RN, CRNP, CS
Associate Professor
Department of Nursing
Towson State University
Towson, Maryland

Sarah N. Lechner, MSN
Clinical Instructor
Yale Child Study Center
Yale University School of Medicine
New Haven, Connecticut
Clinical Nurse Specialist
Children's Psychiatric Inpatient Service
Yale New Haven Hospital
New Haven, Connecticut

Richard A. Lehne, PhD
Formerly
Lecturer, University of Arizona College of Nursing and University of Virginia College of Nursing
Research Assistant Professor

Department of Pharmacology
University of Virginia
School of Medicine
Charlottesville, Virginia

Evelyn W. Lloyd, MS, RN
Psychotherapist
Howard County Hospital
Columbia, Maryland

Mattie Lowery, MA, BSN
Assistant Vice President for Nursing Operation
The Union Memorial Hospital
Baltimore, Maryland

Pamela E. Marcus, MS, RN, CS-P
Clinical Specialist, Lecturer
Nurse Psychotherapist
Private Practice
Upper Marlboro, Maryland

Maureen McCarthy, MBA, PhD, MA, MS
Adjunct Professor
Old Dominion University
Norfolk, Virginia
Troy State University
Virginia Region
Norfolk, Virginia
Community Relations Coordinator
Chesapeake Community Services Board
Chesapeake, Virginia

Susan H. McCrone, PhD, RN, CS-P
Associate Professor
School of Nursing
University of Maryland at Baltimore
Baltimore, Maryland

Barbara J. Michaels, EdD, RN, LMFT
Instructor
El Centro College
Private Practice (Marriage and Family)
Dallas, Texas
Case Studies

Rebecca A. Newcomer, MS, RN, CS-P
Clinical Specialist–Psychiatric
Washington County Mental Health Center
Hagerstown, Maryland

Emily Sondak Nudelman, MS, RN, CS-P
Adjunct Faculty
School of Nursing
University of North Carolina at Greensboro
Greensboro, North Carolina
Clinical Nurse Specialist
Psychotherapist
Triad Psychiatric and Counseling Center
Greensboro, North Carolina

Thomas P. Phillips, PhD, RN, FAAN
Chief
Nursing Education and Practice Branch
Division of Nursing
Bureau of Health Professions,
Health Resources and Services Administration
Department of Health and Human Services
Rockville, Maryland

Pamela Price-Hoskins, MA, PhD, RN
Chief, Clinical Support Services
Laureate Psychiatric Clinic and Hospital
Tulsa, Oklahoma

Elizabeth Anne DeSalvo Rankin, PhD, RNC, NBCCH
Associate Professor, Psychiatric/Mental Health Nursing
Director
Division of Business & Industry
Office of Professional Development and Services
School of Nursing
University of Maryland at Baltimore
Baltimore, Maryland
Associate Trainer
American Hypnosis Training Academy
Silver Spring, Maryland

Wendy Miller Resnick, RN, MS, CS
Director
Support Services
Depression & Related Affective Disorders Association
In cooperation with The Johns Hopkins University School of Medicine
Baltimore, Maryland

Alix C. Rey, MD
Howard County Hospital
Department of Psychiatry
Columbia, Maryland

Lisa Robinson, PhD, RN, CS-P, FAAN
Professor
School of Nursing
University of Maryland at Baltimore
Baltimore, Maryland

Doris Scott, PhD, MS, BS
Assistant Professor
School of Nursing
University of Maryland at Baltimore
Baltimore, Maryland

Nancy C. Shoemaker, MS, RN
Quality Improvement Manager
Bay Area Health Care
Baltimore, Maryland

Tommie Springham, MS, RN, CS-P
Psychotherapist
Private practice
Silver Spring, Maryland
Baltimore, Maryland

Linda Stafford, PhD, RN
Assistant Professor
University of Texas–Houston Health Sciences Center
Houston, Texas

Suzanne S. Stuntz, BSN, RN
Senior Clinical Nurse
Nurse Therapist Day Hospital
Johns Hopkins Hospital
Baltimore, Maryland

Patricia D. Sullivan, MS, RN
Nurse Manager
Adult Psychiatry
Johns Hopkins Hospital
Baltimore, Maryland

Sue Ann Thomas, PhD, RN, CS-P
Director
New Life Directions
Ellicott City, Maryland

Daria Virvan, MSN, RN
Nurse–Psychotherapist
Town Center Psychiatric Associates
Rockville, Maryland
Therapia Psychotherapy Services
Bethesda, Maryland

Norma J. Walgrove, MSN, RN
Instructor
University of Maryland at Baltimore
Baltimore, Maryland
Nurse-Psychotherapist
Metro Maryland Counseling Center
Timonium, Maryland

Maureen Walsh, MS, RN, NP
Acupuncture Practitioner
Traditional Acupuncture and
Counseling Associates, Inc.
Crafton, Maryland

Frances B. Wimbush, PhD, RN
Assistant Professor
College of Nursing
University of Delaware
Newark, Delaware

Susan F. Woolsey, MS, RN, CS
Assistant Professor, retired
University of Maryland at Baltimore
School of Nursing
University of Maryland at Baltimore
School of Medicine
Baltimore, Maryland

JoAnn Zerwekh, EdD, RN, FNP
Faculty
University of Phoenix
Tucson, Arizona
Executive Director
Nursing Education Consultants
Dallas, Texas
Case Studies

REVIEWERS

Deanah I. Alexander, MSN, RNCS
School of Nursing
West Texas A&M University
Canyon, Texas

Janet A. Ambrogne, MSN, RN
Doctoral Student, School of Nursing
Medical College of Georgia
Augusta, Georgia

Judith A. Anderson, MSN, RN
School of Nursing
Medical College of Ohio
Toledo, Ohio

Wilda K. Arnold, EdD, BSN, RN
College of Nursing
Texas Women's University
Dallas, Texas

Verolyn Barnes Bolander, MS, RN
School of Nursing
University of Texas Medical Branch
Galveston, Texas

Sharon L. Carlson, BSN, MS, RN
School of Nursing
Otterbein College
Westerville, Ohio

Martha M. Colvin, PhD, RN, CNS
School of Nursing
Georgia College
Milledgeville, Georgia

Carol A. Distasio, RNC, MS, MPH
Bay Area Health Care
Baltimore, Maryland

Linda Erwin, MSN, RN
College of Nursing
Deaconess College
St. Louis, Missouri

Pamela Billings Farley, PhD, RN
School of Nursing
Berea College
Berea, Kentucky

Patricia H. Foster, EdD, RN
School of Nursing
University of North Florida
Jacksonville, Florida

Gloria M. Francis, PhD, RN, FAAN
School of Nursing
Virginia Commonwealth University
Richmond, Virginia

Jeanne Gelman, MSN, MA, RN
School of Nursing
Widener University
Chester, Pennsylvania

Amy L. Govoni, MSN, RNCS
Department of Nursing
Cleveland State University
Cleveland, Ohio

Carolyn Anne Green, EdD, MSN, RN
School of Nursing
Solano Community College
Suisun City, California

Heidi Koenig Hart, MS, RNC
School of Nursing
Walla Walla College
Portland, Oregon

Emily Wurster Hitchens, EdD, RN
School of Nursing
Seattle Pacific University
Seattle, Washington

Leta Martin Holder, EdD, MSN, RN
School of Nursing
Georgia College
Milledgeville, Georgia

Kathleen H. Hughes, MN, RNC
School of Nursing
St. Luke's College
Kansas City, Missouri

Susan R. Jacob, MSN, RN
School of Nursing
Memphis State University
Memphis, Tennessee

Kathleen Kadner, PhD, RN
College of Nursing
University of New Mexico
Albuquerque, New Mexico

Eileen W. Keefe, MS, RNC
School of Nursing, Baccalaureate Program
Louisiana State University Medical Center
New Orleans, Louisiana

Janet M. Mayorga, PhD, RNC
College of Nursing
University of Texas
El Paso, Texas

Lenora J. McClean, EdD, RN
School of Nursing
State University of New York
Stony Brook, New York

O. JoAnn McElravy, MS, RN
School of Nursing
University of Rhode Island
Kingston, Rhode Island

Frederica W. O'Connor, PhD, RN
School of Nursing
University of Washington
Seattle, Washington

Sharon Lynne Phillips, MSN, RN
Department of Nursing
Youngstown State University
Youngstown, Ohio

Michael J. Rice, PhD, RN
Intercollegiate Center for Nursing Education
Spokane, Washington

Betty W. Ross, PhD, RNCS
School of Nursing
Fairleigh Dickinson University
Teaneck, New Jersey

Emily Catherine Schlenker, MS, RN, FAIS
School of Nursing
Tennessee State University
Nashville, Tennessee

Sandra Schuler, MSN, RN
School of Nursing
Montgomery College
Takoma Park, Maryland

James C. Sorensen, EdD, MPN, RN
School of Nursing
Incarnate Word College
San Antonio, Texas

Carolyn Peoples Veiga, MSN, RN
Department of Nursing
Bowie State University
Bowie, Maryland

Claire Vernaleken, MSN, MA, RN
Counseling Psychology
Bloomfield College
Bloomfield, New Jersey

Sandra L. Warner, PhD, RNCS
College of Nursing
University of Texas Health Sciences Center
San Antonio, Texas

Charlotte J. Warren, RNCS, LPC, PhD
School of Nursing
Georgia State University
Atlanta, Georgia

Barbara A. Wehling, MSN, RN
Department of Nursing
Webster University
Webster Groves, Missouri

Jean E. Wold, MN, RN
School of Nursing
California State University
Chico, California

Susan Klasson Zareski, MN, RNC
Assistant Director of Nursing
El Camino College
Torrance, California

PREFACE

OUR VISION FOR THE BOOK

As we planned *Mental Health Nursing: The Nurse-Patient Journey*, we envisioned that it would forge new ground for psychiatric nursing. We wanted it to have a holistic focus that would make it unlike most other textbooks of mental health nursing. Although the content itself would be familiar to those knowledgeable about psychiatric nursing, our hope was that our method of presentation and the way in which we would link concepts would make it seem as if we had discovered a new path. We have *not* discovered a new path. What we *have* done is reframe what is known in a way that is more human, more meaningful, and more true to what is nursing.

We believe that psychiatric nursing is exciting, intriguing, and fascinating. The heart of psychiatric nursing is the human drama that unfolds differently and uniquely in each life and in each relationship. Most texts do not convey this unfolding drama, but instead convey a more mechanistic approach to psychiatric nursing. We have attempted to remedy this situation not only with a style of writing that seeks to hold your attention but also with the use of the *stories*. These stories, which open most chapters and often build throughout the chapters, are designed to take the abstract concepts of psychiatric nursing and breathe life into them. Our use of the metaphor of the "journey" to depict the process of psychiatric nursing also conveys a sense of the uniqueness of each person's walk through life and the uniqueness of each relationship formed on that walk. These approaches utilize the best from both existential and humanistic models and serve as major threads throughout *Mental Health Nursing*.

An important aspect of the existential component of our approach is that it encourages you to examine the patient's perceptions and the meanings that the patient assigns to events. At the heart of all illness is the quest for meaning, and one of the hallmarks of mental health is the ability to ascribe meaning to life's experiences. Another important aspect of the existential component of our approach is that it examines *your* ability to derive personal meaning and significance from every encounter with a patient. This focus on meaning is what makes a relationship empowering and life giving.

Our commitment to a holistic approach stems from our theistic world view, from which we derive our beliefs about people, the world, the existence and nature of God, and how we should interact with one another. A theistic world view holds forth a belief in the existence of God—more specifically, the existence of one God who has created us as complex and wonderful, with freedom to choose and the capacity for caring and compassion toward others. Although not everyone operates from a theistic world view, we all have our own world views, which consist of beliefs about the nature of reality, time, relationships, ourselves, others, and the existence and nature of an ultimate other.

Every book—including every textbook of psychiatric nursing—is written from the world view of its authors. Seldom, however, do the authors explicitly state that foundational world view for the reader. The danger of that practice is that it makes it difficult for you, the reader, to discern what is true from what is the author's personal position on an issue. We therefore believe that it is important for you to recognize the foundational world view from which we operate. Please be assured that we are not espousing a particular religion or faith. Instead, we are inviting you to look at the world—and at the world of psychiatric nursing—in a way that we believe most comprehensively addresses the needs of people in emotional pain.

Truly, people are more than the sum of their parts. In *Mental Health Nursing*, we therefore look at the total person, not just feelings and thoughts, but the interaction of those feelings and thoughts with biological, social, cultural, and spiritual aspects of the person. This holistic approach, a major thread in *Mental Health Nursing*, can be seen throughout the book in our reviews of etiological factors, in our applications of the nursing process, and in our descriptions of the impact of therapies on body, mind, and spirit. We believe in approaching and supporting people from their strengths, not just in diagnosing and responding to areas that need growth. This attitude conveys the belief that each person has worth, has value, and makes a difference in this world.

Two other features that distinguish our approach include the frequent use of a writing style that addresses *you* directly, and the use of the word *patient* instead of *client*. Addressing you personally underscores our intention to invite you to accompany us on the journey of mental health nursing. This is a personal journey—one that will have unique meaning for each person who reads these pages. As fellow sojourners, we invite you to fully engage in the journey. We believe that this engagement will be easier to the extent that we write to you as an individual rather than a distant, uninvolved third person.

Our use of the word *patient* flows from our belief that *patient* is a word that accurately portrays the longsuffering nature of many people who cope with psychiatric illnesses. The word *client*, used in many other nursing textbooks, fails to convey that meaning.

THE STRUCTURE OF THE BOOK

Mental Health Nursing: The Nurse-Patient Journey is organized into seven units:

Unit I. Background for the Journey
Unit II. The Nature of the Journey
Unit III. Facilitating the Journey
Unit IV. Travelers Across the Lifespan
Unit V. The Wounded Traveler
Unit VI. The Journey and Society
Unit VII. Improving the Journey

Unit I. Background for the Journey includes chapters on the beliefs of the authors, the history of mental health nursing, the mental health system, roles and practice settings for mental health nurses, legal and ethical issues in mental health nursing, and theories that guide the journey of mental health nursing.

Unit II. The Nature of the Journey includes a state-of-the-art chapter covering the neurobiological influences on mental health and mental illness. In another chapter, we focus on self-concept, not only from the patient's perspective but also from your perspective, as we look at how patients and nurses reciprocally influence one another. Next is a chapter unique to this textbook, dealing with the attributes and strengths that enable some people to be triumphant survivors in life's journey. The next two chapters deal with therapeutic communication skills and the development of therapeutic relationships. In the next chapter we review the nursing process and present an overview of its application to psychiatric nursing. Then, in a separate chapter, we take a closer look at the assessment step of the nursing process and its use in psychiatric nursing. The last chapter in this unit deals with the impact of culture on mental health, mental illness, and mental health care.

Unit III. Facilitating the Journey covers the therapeutic approaches used in mental health nursing. This unit therefore includes separate chapters on each of the traditional approaches: crisis intervention, individual therapy, group therapy, behavioral therapy, milieu therapy, and family therapy. In addition, we include a chapter dealing with mind-body-spirit therapies, including the use of therapies that stem from an Eastern approach to health and well-being. A separate chapter on patient and family education is also included because we believe in the power of knowledge in facilitating change in the lives of patients and their loved ones. Last, we offer an in-depth chapter on psychopharmacology.

Unit IV. Travelers Across the Lifespan gives an overview of normal developmental tasks and crises from childhood to old age and also explores age-related mental health issues. Chapter 25, "The Adult Traveler," is a distinctive feature of this textbook. The years covering adulthood, where we generally spend most of our lives, are frequently ignored completely or glossed over in textbooks of psychiatric nursing. To remedy that deficiency, we have presented in this chapter an in-depth look at the many challenges and issues that confront the developing adult. Another chapter takes a close look at the unique mental health issues affecting the elderly. The last chapter in this unit covers loss and its impact not only on the journey of the psychiatric patient but also on your own journey as well.

Unit V. The Wounded Traveler is the largest unit in the book. In it you will learn about specific mental illnesses and gain a window into the lives of the patients whose journeys are affected by them. The unit includes chapters on stress and anxiety disorders, schizophrenia, mood disorders, substance abuse, behavioral disorders, dissociative disorders, psychosexual disorders, eating disorders, and psychophysiological disorders. We have also included separate chapters on suicide and cognitive disorders.

Unit VI. The Journey and Society includes comprehensive coverage of homelessness, violence, rape, and AIDS. A separate chapter dealing with community mental health care also is included. The last chapter in this unit is a distinctive feature of this textbook; it focuses on home mental health care, which is on the cutting edge of psychiatric nursing.

The last unit, *Unit VII. Improving the Journey*, looks at total quality management, a subject that is important for all of us if we are to continue to improve the systems of care that serve our patients. The last chapter in the book addresses research and the future of practice. It invites you to continue your journey in mental health nursing through research, clinical activities, and contributions to the literature of mental health nursing.

THE STRUCTURE OF THE CHAPTERS

The chapters of *Mental Health Nursing* follow a consistent structure and include a number of highlighted features to help you focus on and learn content that will be critical to your education in psychiatric nursing.

Each chapter begins with a *quotation* chosen to spark your interest in the subject covered in the chapter. Next, *Learning Objectives* give you a "preorganizing" framework with which to approach your reading of the chapter. A list of *Key Terminology* follows, introducing important terms that will be defined within the body of the chapter and that are essential to your understanding of the content of the chapter.

After a brief introduction to the chapter, we then typically introduce a *story* drawn from literature, from the psychiatric literature, or written just for this book. The purpose of this story is to help bring to life the human drama that is mental health nursing and to give you a context for, and a reinforcement of, key content from the chapter. Frequently, we build upon these stories throughout the chapter. Additional glimpses into the lives of patients appear as *Case Examples* throughout the book.

Most chapters covering specific psychiatric disorders, and some other chapters as well, include an application of the *Nursing Process*. We use the six-step nursing process specified in *A Statement on Psychiatric-Mental Health Clinical Nursing Practice and Standards of Psychiatric-Mental Health Clinical Nursing Practice*. The six steps are: assessment, diagnosis, outcome identification, planning, implementation, and evaluation.

Many chapters include special boxes called *Medical Diagnoses and Related Nursing Diagnoses*. These boxes present diagnostic criteria for selected disorders from the American Psychiatric Association's *Diagnostic and Statistical Manual of Mental Disorders*, Fourth Edition *(DSM-IV)*. Then they suggest related NANDA nursing diagnoses that frequently accompany the psychiatric diagnoses. For each NANDA diagnosis, we provide a definition and an example of how a two-part diagnosis might be written for a specific patient.

Many of the chapters also include highlighted educational material called *Need to Know* boxes ("What Patients Need to Know," "What Families Need to Know," etc. . .) for you to share with patients and their families. This material is written in question-and-answer form in everyday language especially for use by patients and families.

Throughout the chapters, you will find *Check Your Reading questions* to help you review the content, clarify your thinking, and reinforce your learning as you progress through the chapter. Suggested answers to these questions appear at the end of the book.

Many of the chapters, particularly those covering specific mental disorders, conclude with *Case Studies*. These Case Studies present a brief case history, then demonstrate the application of the six-step nursing process to the case.

At the end of each chapter, after some brief conclusions, you'll find *Key Points to Remember*. These list-style summaries of key points made in the chapter will facilitate your review of the content and help you focus on the critical points of each chapter. After the Key Points, we provide suggested *Learning Activities*, most of which are experiential. Completing these activities is a way of making the content of the chapter more meaningful to you. Next, you'll find a *Critical Thinking Exercise*, designed to assist you in thinking creatively and flexibly about situations, and in looking beyond the obvious in your problem-solving. The chapters conclude with references and a list of *Suggested Readings* that we believe would be particularly helpful to you if you are interested in further exploration of the chapter's content.

At the end of *Mental Health Nursing: The Nurse-Patient Journey*, you'll find two appendices. In Appendix I, we've included a selection of standardized rating scales for psychiatric nursing. Incorporation of these tools into your assessment of patients with mental health problems will help you develop concrete outcomes for care and allow you to spot trends in the patient's progress in treatment. In Appendix II we reprint the complete *DSM-IV* classification of mental disorders.

We are privileged to be able to journey with you for a time in your study of mental health nursing. As you read this book and undertake that journey with us, we hope and pray that our vision of a shared journey will take hold in your own heart, and that you will offer that vision to patients throughout your nursing career.

Verna Benner Carson
Elizabeth Nolan Arnold

ACKNOWLEDGMENTS

The two years that preceded the publication of *Mental Health Nursing: The Nurse-Patient Journey* constituted one of the most difficult times in our lives. Writing a textbook should probably be a full-time occupation. However, we did not write the book in that way. Instead, we also maintained our full-time commitments to the University of Maryland School of Nursing and all of our outside commitments. Neither of us would recommend that approach as a prescription for good mental health!

However, as difficult as this time period was for us, it was also an incredibly blessed time. The blessings came as we tackled the project, received wonderful material from contributors, and produced chapters of which we both felt proud. Blessings also came from the support that we received from so many people, the most important of whom were our family members. They were unwavering in their backing of this creative effort. They accepted us as less-than-perfect wives, mothers, daughters, and sisters; tolerated our distractibility; lived with our constant fatigue; pitched in with meals, clean-up, and general errands; and shared our moments of joy. Our husbands, John and George, served as our in-house computer experts, found ways to make the job of word-processing easier, and saved us from many potential word-processing disasters. They encouraged us when it seemed as if the book would never be completed and urged us not to give up or become discouraged. Everyone should have such a wonderful cheerleading squad.

In addition to the support from our families, we were blessed with the help of others. The most visible help came from our roster of contributing authors, whose work formed the foundation of the book. Reviewers offered invaluable critiques that sharpened our writing skills and alerted us to material that needed to be clarified, expanded, or deleted. Nursing students helped us with literature searches and the copying of countless articles. They saved us hundreds of hours in the library and allowed us to focus on the reading and writing necessary to complete the manuscript. Barbara Michaels and JoAnn Zerwekh collaborated to produce the clinically accurate, true-to-life Case Studies that conclude many of the book's chapters. Nancy Conrad wrote the thought-provoking Critical Thinking Exercises at the end of each chapter, and Marjorie Fraser wrote the suggested answers to the book's Check Your Reading questions.

The staff members of W.B. Saunders Company were indispensable throughout the entire process and deserve a special word of thanks. Both of us have worked on other projects with Ilze Rader, Senior Editor at Saunders, and we appreciate not only her editorial expertise but also her calm and support. Marie Thomas, Ilze's assistant, quietly does much behind-the-scenes work that makes us look good. Our developmental editor, Lee Henderson, did a superb job in helping us to shape and mold the manuscript into the polished book that you now hold. Throughout the process, Lee was called on to be a man of many talents. When we needed praise to keep us going, he extolled us. When we were running out of energy, he coaxed us. When we were discouraged, he prayed for us. Regardless of where we were, he never lost sight of the vision for our book, and he kept us true to that vision.

Thanks also to our production team at W.B. Saunders Company. Blair Davis-Doerre and Ellen Thomas copy-edited the entire manuscript, helping us present the material with clarity, consistency, and precision, and ably fielding unexpected additions and changes. Michael Carcel managed the book's production, working with other members of the production team, with the typesetter, and with the printer to ensure that the quality of the book's manufacturing matched the quality of its contents. Ox & Company was responsible for the book's inspired graphic design, and Louis Fuiano designed the book's cover. Gene Floersch and Kathy Jaeger took our rough ideas for illustrations and turned them into finished figures that beautifully illustrate and amplify the text. Rita Martello coordinated the book's illustrations, ensuring that they were sized ideally and reproduced faithfully in the printed book.

Last, we would like to thank the many patients who allowed us to accompany them on their journeys. It is from these shared experiences that we developed the vision for the book.

Verna Benner Carson
Elizabeth Nolan Arnold

CONTENTS

UNIT I BACKGROUND FOR THE JOURNEY 1

CHAPTER 1 **Points of Departure:** Beliefs That Shape the Journey
Verna Benner Carson 3

An Invitation to the Journey 3
A Perspective for the Journey 4
Issues You Will Face on the Journey 7

CHAPTER 2 **The Wisdom of Past Travelers:** A History of Mental Health Nursing
Edna M. Fordyce, Mary Ellen Lashley, and Verna Benner Carson 11

Early Travelers 14
18th, 19th, and 20th Century Travelers 14
Changing Settings for Mental Health Care 19
The First and Second World Wars 21
Legislation 21
Psychobiological Treatment 23
Deinstitutionalization 23
Interpersonal Relationships 23
Nursing Professionalization 25
Family Advocacy 26
The "Decade of the Brain" 27
A Chronology of Significant Events in the History of Mental Health Nursing 27

CHAPTER 3 **Highways for the Journey:** The Mental Health System
Ellen A. Andruzzi and Verna Benner Carson 33

Diagnostic and Classification Systems 36
DSM-IV 36
ICD-9-CM 36
Public Policy and Judicial Decisions 37
Social Changes 42
Funding and Reimbursement 43
Treatment Settings 46

CHAPTER 4 **Alternate Routes for the Journey:** Practice Roles and Settings
Verna Benner Carson 51

Core Practice Roles 53
Practice Paths 58
Professional Performance Standards and Roles 60
Stress and Burnout 64

CHAPTER 5 **Rules of the Road:** Legal and Ethical Issues in Mental Health Nursing
Pamela Price-Hoskins 71

Principles of Ethics 72
Ethical Decision-Making 75
Ethical Dilemmas 77
Legal Parameters 81
Rights of Patients 83
Three Important Processes Affecting the Therapeutic Relationship 85

CHAPTER 6 **Guideposts for the Journey:** Theories Guiding Mental Health Nursing
Emily Sondak Nudelman and Elizabeth Nolan Arnold 91

What is a Theory? 93
Theories From Disciplines Other Than Nursing 94
Nursing Theories 95

UNIT II **THE NATURE OF THE JOURNEY** 125

CHAPTER 7 **Physical Dimensions of the Journey:** Neurobiological Influences
Susan H. McCrone 127
History of Biological Psychiatry *128*
Neuroanatomy *130*
Neurophysiology *137*
Emergence of Neurobiological Laboratory Tests *140*
Implications of Biological Psychiatry for the Cause of Mental Illness *142*

CHAPTER 8 **Shared Attributes of Every Traveler:** The Mosaic of Self-Concept
Judy S. Fuhrmann and Verna Benner Carson 151
The Journey Toward Self-Understanding *154*
The Journey Toward Mental Health or Mental Illness *166*

CHAPTER 9 **Unique Attributes of Successful Travelers:** Personal Strengths for the Journey
Norma J. Walgrove 175
Attributes of Successful Travelers *177*
Developing Your Patients' Personal Strengths *179*
Developing Your Own Personal Strengths *186*

CHAPTER 10 **Points of Intersection:** Therapeutic Communication
Elizabeth Nolan Arnold 191
Functional Nature of Communication *192*
Characteristics of Effective Communication *195*
Types of Communication *197*
Therapeutic Communication *202*

CHAPTER 11 **A Pathway for Healing:** Therapeutic Relationships
Elizabeth Nolan Arnold 231
Interpersonal Relationships *232*
Interpersonal Relationships and Mental Health *232*
Interpersonal Relationships and Mental Illness *232*
Interpersonal Relationships and Psychiatric Treatment *233*
Social Relationships Versus Therapeutic Relationships *233*
Therapeutic Relationships *234*
Definition *234*
Use of Self *236*
Importance of Self-Awareness *236*
Frameworks to Guide Therapeutic Relationships *237*
Conceptual Components *239*
Structuring Therapeutic Relationships *246*

CHAPTER 12 **A Map for the Journey:** The Nursing Process
Elizabeth Anne DeSalvo Rankin 265
Assessment *268*
Diagnosis *268*
Outcome Identification *272*
Planning *272*
Implementation *273*
Evaluation *274*
Documentation *276*

CHAPTER 13 **Getting to Know the Traveler:** Mental Health Assessment
Nancy C. Shoemaker 283
Structured Data Collection *285*
Attention to the Art of Nursing *285*
Self-Awareness *286*
Consideration of Patient Perceptions *286*
Beginning the Assessment *287*
Using Standardized Rating Scales *288*
Standards of Mental Health Assessment *288*
Conducting the Assessment *289*

CHAPTER 14 **Travelers From Many Lands:** The Impact of Culture
Maureen McCarthy 303
Understanding Culture-Related Terms *305*
Major Cultural Variables Affecting Mental Health Care *309*
Specific Cultural Groups *312*
Communication for Cultural Understanding *322*

UNIT III **FACILITATING THE JOURNEY** 327

CHAPTER 15 **Crisis Intervention**
Elizabeth Nolan Arnold 329
Theoretical Perspectives 331
Nature of Crisis 334
Crisis Intervention 345
Generic Crisis Intervention in Disasters 359
Psychiatric Emergency Services 361
Caring for Yourself 361

CHAPTER 16 **Individual Therapy**
Suzanne Sayle Jimerson 367
History of Psychotherapy 368
Psychoanalytical Psychotherapy 368
Long-Term Therapy to Short-Term Therapy 370
Short-Term Psychotherapy 371

CHAPTER 17 **Group Psychotherapy**
Elizabeth Nolan Arnold 385
Historical Development 386
Characteristics 390
Structural Components 392
Development 396
Conceptual Components 399
Common Communication Problems 408
Groups for Special Populations 409
Groups for the Elderly 413
Activity Groups 415
Psychoeducation Groups 415
Human Relations Groups 416
Ethical and Legal Issues 416

CHAPTER 18 **Behavioral Therapy**
Susan F. Woolsey and Elizabeth Nolan Arnold 421
Theoretical Perspectives 422
Principles of Application 424
Treatment Applications Based on Behavioral Approaches 434
Behavioral Strategies in Self-Management 437
Behavioral Strategies in Preventive Psychiatry 439

CHAPTER 19 **Milieu Therapy**
Rebecca A. Newcomer 443
Historical Perspective 444
Components of Milieu Therapy 445
Settings for Milieu Therapy 449

CHAPTER 20 **Family Therapy**
Marcia Cooley 463
Understanding Families 464
Family Interventions 470
The Process of Family Therapy 473

CHAPTER 21 **Mind-Body-Spirit Therapies**
Maureen Walsh and Verna Benner Carson 487
Eastern Mind-Body-Spirit Therapies 488
Historical Development 488
An Eastern View of Healing 490
Specific Therapies 491
Western Mind-Body-Spirit Therapies 496
Hydrotherapy 496
Nutrition 496
Exercise 498
Prayer 498
Meditation 498
Religious Practices 498
Doing "Good Works" 498

CHAPTER 22 **Patient and Family Education**
Elizabeth Anne DeSalvo Rankin 503
Foundation for the Journey into Patient Education 504
Nursing Process 509
Educating Patients About Mental Illness 515
The Biopsychosocial-Spiritual Model 515
Variables That Limit Learning 516
Choices in Educational Content 516

CHAPTER 23 **Psychopharmacology**
Richard A. Lehne and Doris Scott 523
Mechanisms by Which Central Nervous System Drugs Act 524
Antipsychotic Agents 526
Antidepressants 535

Lithium and Other Drugs for Bipolar Disorder *545*

Antianxiety Agents *549*

UNIT IV **TRAVELERS ACROSS THE LIFESPAN** 571

CHAPTER 24 **The Pediatric Traveler**
Sarah N. Lechner 573

The Beginning of the Journey: Considerations in Working With Children and Adolescents *574*

- The Child as Sojourner *574*
- Normal Development *574*
- The Family *576*
- The Outside World *577*
- Racial, Ethnic, and Cultural Differences *578*

Joining the Journey: The Therapeutic Relationship *578*

- Transference *578*
- Countertransference *578*
- Coping Mechanisms *579*
- Epidemiology and Risk Factors *579*

CHAPTER 25 **The Adult Traveler**
Elizabeth Nolan Arnold 617

Basic Assumptions About Adulthood *618*

Theoretical Perspectives on Adult Development *619*

The Adult Traveler in Early and Middle Adulthood *622*

Mental Health Issues in Normal Adulthood *626*

Nursing Diagnoses Appropriate to Normal Adulthood *628*

Accommodating to Social Changes: Implications for Adult Development *628*

Promoting the Mental Health of the Adult Traveler *633*

CHAPTER 26 **The Elderly Traveler**
Charlotte Eliopoulos 645

Facts About the Older Population *646*

Developmental Tasks of Aging *648*

Normal Mental Health in Late Life *648*

Psychiatric Disorders in the Elderly *649*

Promoting Mental Health in Later Life *652*

CHAPTER 27 **Loss Along the Journey**
Miriam Jacik 661

Definition of and Research on Loss and Grief *662*

Loss *664*

Grief *668*

Moving Beyond Loss and Grief *676*

UNIT V **THE WOUNDED TRAVELER** 689

CHAPTER 28 **The Journey Threatened by Stress and Anxiety Disorders**
Lisa Robinson 691

Theories of Anxiety *693*

- Psychobiological Theories *693*

Stress *694*

- The Immediate Stress Response *694*
- The Intermediate Stress Response *694*
- The Long-Term Stress Response *694*
- The Relationship Between Anxiety and Stress *695*

Anxiety Disorders *698*

- Generalized Anxiety Disorder *698*
- Panic Disorder With and Without Agoraphobia *699*
- Obsessive-Compulsive Disorder *701*
- Posttraumatic Stress Disorder *702*
- Phobias *706*

CHAPTER 29 **The Journey Controlled by Thought Disorders**
Patricia D. Sullivan and Verna Benner Carson 725

Differentiating Normal Perceptions From Psychosis *726*

Definitions of Symptoms and Disease *728*

The Cause of Schizophrenia *731*

CHAPTER 30 **The Journey Colored by Mood Disorders**
Wendy Miller Resnick and Verna Benner Carson 759

Our Understanding of Mood Disorders *761*

Defining Mood Disorders *763*

Cause of Mood Disorders *767*

CHAPTER 31 **The Journey Anesthetized by Substance Use**
Elizabeth Nolan Arnold 793
- Historical Perspective *794*
- Definition *797*
- Theoretical Models *799*
- Common Properties of Psychoactive Substances *800*
- Trajectory of the Journey into Substance Use Disorders *802*
- Diagnostic Classifications *803*
- Vulnerable Populations and Substance Use Disorders *824*
- Substance Use Disorders and the Family *828*

CHAPTER 32 **The Journey Troubled by Behavioral Disorders**
Pamela E. Marcus and Tommie Springham 841
- A Healthy Personality *842*
- Personality Disorders Defined *842*
- Personality Development: A View from Psychology and Biology *842*
- Descriptions of Personality Disorders *844*
- Clusters of Behaviors *844*
- Nursing's Journey With Patients Having Personality Disorders *855*

CHAPTER 33 **The Journey Compartmentalized by Dissociative Disorders**
Linda Stafford 863
- The Concept of Dissociation *864*
- The Dissociation Continuum *864*
- The Detour of Pathological Dissociation *865*

CHAPTER 34 **The Journey Undermined by Psychosexual Disorders**
Suzanne S. Stuntz, Anne Falk, Melinda Hiken, and Verna Benner Carson 879
- Definitions *881*
- Sexual Development Across the Lifespan *881*
- Sexual Response Cycle *882*
- Sexual Dysfunctions *886*
- Sexual Disorders *890*
- Homosexuality *893*
- Other Sexual Problems *894*
- Your Response to Sexual Disorders and Other Sexual Issues *895*

CHAPTER 35 **The Journey Challenged by Eating Disorders**
Willa A. Decker and Margaret Freeman 909
- Historical Background *910*
- Causes *911*
- Relationship to Other Psychiatric Problems *914*

CHAPTER 36 **The Journey Scarred by Suicide**
Pamela E. Marcus, Evelyn W. Lloyd, and Alix C. Rey 927
- Definitions Related to Suicide *929*
- Epidemiology *929*
- Prevalence *930*
- Suicide as a Symptom of Psychiatric Illness *930*
- Causes *932*
- Dynamics *934*

CHAPTER 37 **The Journey Embedded in Psychophysiological Disorders**
Sue Ann Thomas and Frances B. Wimbush 949
- Historical Overview *951*
- Diagnosis *951*
- Chronic Low Back Pain *953*
- Chronic Pelvic Pain *954*
- Irritable Bowel Syndrome *956*
- Hypertension *957*
- Migraine *958*
- Temporomandibular Disorder *960*
- Somatoform Disorders *961*

CHAPTER 38 **The Journey Clouded by Cognitive Disorders**
Elizabeth Nolan Arnold 977
- Historical Perspectives on Cognitive Dysfunction *979*
- Brain Function and Cognitive Disorders *980*
- Acute Cognitive Disorders: Delirium *982*
- Chronic Cognitive Disorders: Dementia *989*

UNIT VI **THE JOURNEY AND SOCIETY** 1021

CHAPTER 39 **The Journey Marked by Homelessness**
Daria Virvan 1023

What Homelessness Is *1025*
Who the Homeless Are *1026*
Areas of Homelessness *1028*
Factors Leading to Homelessness *1029*
Attitudes Toward the Homeless *1031*

CHAPTER 40 **The Journey Marked by Violence**
Verna Benner Carson 1039
Family Violence, Abuse, and the Journey *1040*
Characteristics of the Journey Marked by Family Violence and Abuse *1043*
Causes of Family Violence and Abuse *1044*

CHAPTER 41 **The Journey Marked by Rape**
Patricia Sullivan 1085
The Role of Nurses in the Journey Marked by Rape *1086*
Definition of Rape and Related Terms *1087*
Demographics *1087*
Incidence *1088*
Types *1088*

CHAPTER 42 **The Journey Marked by AIDS**
Verna Benner Carson 1103
Psychological Problems Associated with AIDS *1104*
AIDS: The Disease *1106*
Psychological, Social, and Spiritual Implications *1107*
Psychiatric Implications *1111*
Caregivers of People with AIDS *1112*
Nursing and AIDS *1114*

CHAPTER 43 **The Journey Through Community Mental Health Care**
Verna Benner Carson 1127
The Advent of Community Mental Health Care *1128*
The Population Served *1131*
The Philosophy *1135*
The Services Provided *1135*
The Role of Nursing *1136*
The Success *1146*
Future Directions *1147*

CHAPTER 44 **The Journey Through Home Mental Health Care**
Verna Benner Carson 1151
Historical Background *1152*
Psychiatric Home Care Defined *1153*
Bay Area Health Care's Model *1154*
Medicare Criteria *1156*
The Criteria of Other Payers *1158*
Populations Served *1159*

UNIT VII **IMPROVING THE JOURNEY** 1171

CHAPTER 45 **Total Quality Management**
Mattie Lowery 1173
Total Quality Management as a Team Effort *1174*
From Quality Assurance to Total Quality Management *1175*
Concepts of Continuous Quality Improvement and Health Care *1178*
Role of Nursing in the Continuous Quality Improvement Process *1180*
Patient Satisfaction Versus Patient Needs *1187*

CHAPTER 46 **Research and the Future of Practice**
Elizabeth Nolan Arnold, Thomas P. Phillips, and Karen S. Babich 1193
Identifying the Problem *1194*
Developing Solutions *1195*

Appendix I Standardized Rating Scales 1207
Appendix II *DSM-IV* Classification 1229
Answers to *Check Your Reading* Questions 1239
Index 1279

UNIT I
BACKGROUND FOR THE JOURNEY

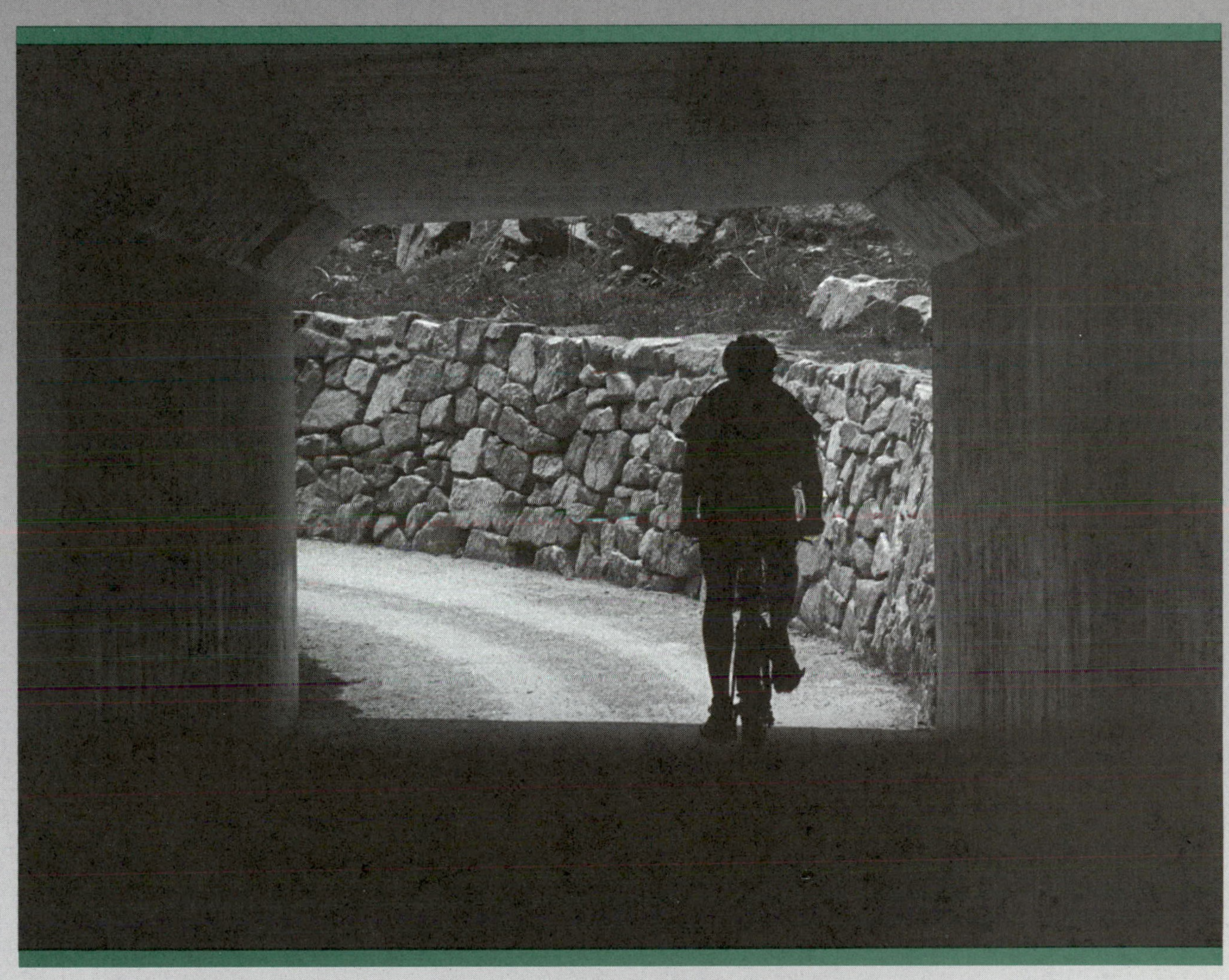

CHAPTER 1

POINTS OF DEPARTURE

BELIEFS THAT SHAPE THE JOURNEY

No stream rises higher than its source. What ever man might build could never express or reflect more than he was. It was no more than what he felt. He could record neither more nor less than he had learned of life when the buildings were built. . . . His philosophy, true or false, is there.

—Frank Lloyd Wright

LEARNING OBJECTIVES

After studying this chapter, you should be able to:

1. Talk about a holistic approach to psychiatric patients.
2. Define a world view and give at least two examples of different world views.
3. Discuss the characteristics of a theistic world view.
4. Discuss the relevance of philosophies or world views such as humanism, secularism, behaviorism, and existentialism to psychiatric nursing.
5. Discuss the metaphor of the "journey" as it relates to the nurse-patient relationship.
6. Talk about the issues that are likely to affect your journey as a student in psychiatric nursing.
7. Describe the Stallwood-Stoll model of human functioning.

KEY TERMINOLOGY

Behaviorism
Existentialism
Holism
Humanism
Monism
Pantheism
Polytheism
Secularism
Theism
World view

AN INVITATION TO THE JOURNEY

This chapter is a bit different than any you have encountered before—it is an open invitation to you to join Dr. Arnold, myself, and our contributors in the journey that is psychiatric nursing. As you begin your journey into psychiatric nursing, you may experience conflicting feelings—fear and curiousity; dread and anticipation; repulsion and compassion. Some of you will enjoy the journey and may continue on in psychiatric nursing. Others will decide that a different journey in nursing is more suited to your strengths. In any event, the experiences that you have in this specialty have the potential to transform you as well as your nursing practice. Psychiatric nursing is about a journey—the nurse-patient journey. Just as you have conflicting feelings about beginning the journey, the journey itself can be paradoxically joyful and sorrowful, happy and sad, exciting and frustrating, and extolling and humbling. It is never a boring journey; instead, it holds the promise of change for you as well as for the patient.

In psychiatric nursing we are privileged to accompany patients on parts of their lives' journeys. As fellow sojourners we are afforded glimpses into the private worlds of patients. Sometimes we are invited into those private worlds in an intimate way. Sometimes we are shocked by what we see and learn about in the patient's world, sometimes we are overcome with the magnitude of pain the patient has and is experiencing, and sometimes we want to run away. Other times we are drawn to offer whatever we can to ease the suffering and to assist the patient in living a fuller, happier, and more productive life. We believe that it is indeed a privilege to be able to work with psychiatric patients. Many times these are the least understood and most poorly treated of all patients in the health care system. Yet these patients have much to teach us about survival, about spiritual strength, about resiliency, and about the importance of being treated with respect, dignity, and compassion.

We have a shared vision for this textbook, and that vision is captured by the image of a journey. Life is a journey, psychiatric nursing is a journey, the nurse-patient relationship is a journey. We know that we are moving forward but we do not always know where we are going or where the next bend in the road will be. We know that each of our journeys is unique, yet there are times, for brief periods, when we walk with another.

A PERSPECTIVE FOR THE JOURNEY

In addition to our vision of the journey, we also desire to convey our beliefs about people and how people should be treated. These beliefs stem from our **world view,** which is a way of looking at the big picture of life and making sense out of it. A world view helps us to organize our experiences in a meaningful way and to draw conclusions about the significance of these experiences to our lives. We share this with you because it is important to be straightforward about foundational assumptions. However, it is not necessary for you to accept our world view to read and benefit from this textbook. Equally true, it is not necessary for patients to share in our world view to be cared for by us. We can and do respect individuals who hold different world views, and we strive to find areas of commonality.

▶ Check Your Reading

1. What is a world view?

Our Theistic World View

Sometimes a *world view* and *spirituality* are interchangeable terms, and for us this is true. We operate from a theistic world view. We believe (1) that a loving and benevolent creator God exists; (2) that we are created in God's image; (3) that God loves us; (4) that our actions toward each other should reflect God's love; (5) that hope of change always exists; and (6) that we are holistic beings—we have integrated physical, emotional and spiritual dimensions. **Theism** stresses forgiveness and treating people with kindness, patience, gentleness, and forbearance. These qualities are essential in psychiatric nursing where the symptoms that patients display are frequently viewed by society as repugnant and bizarre.

▶ Check Your Reading

2. What is a theistic world view?
3. What are the basic beliefs of a theistic world view?
4. What does a theistic world view stress regarding how we should treat others?

A Theistic View of People and Patients

We view patients as whole beings **(holism).** We think of patients as more than their symptoms; they are not just people who hear voices, who are very anxious, or who dress in bizarre ways, but patients are people who have rich life experiences to share with us who just happen to manifest a particular psychiatric symptom. Patients are just like us; in fact one of the most frightening awarenesses for a novice in psychiatric nursing is that we share many similarities with patients. It is always safer to believe that we are qualitatively different from the psychiatric patients for whom we care. Patients are wounded people, just as we are all wounded people—some of us more deeply and seriously than others (Nouwen, 1979). None of us gets through this life without some experiences of sadness, rejection, disappointment, isolation, loneliness, and confusion.

When we are wounded, we hurt all over. When something is wrong, it affects our whole being—mind, body, and soul. Therefore, it is imperative that when we attempt to understand and help, we get the whole picture. We need to know about patient's bodies—where do they feel tension or heaviness? How have they somatized their pain? We need to know about their minds—what are their thought processes? Are they confused, coherent, or scattered, or have they shut down their thinking? What have they done to survive and to make meaning out of their lives? We need to understand their feelings, which are essentially human expressions that give seasoning to experiences. Are they feeling sad, angry, rejected, or alone? Can they identify and express their feelings? We need to know about their social circle—who or what is their support? We need to know about their spirituality—what impact is their illness having on their spirit and their religious faith and practices? We need to know about their families—what part do families play in their healing? These understandings are all essential to piecing together the patient's story.

Another explanation we would like you to have is why we have chosen to use the word *patient* rather than *client* throughout the text. This choice is reflective of foundational beliefs about psychiatric patients. The term *client* is thought to denote a consumer of health care, a full participant in the health care process. It is a term that shifts the focus from psychiatric illness to mental health. But in truth the term *client* means someone who is dependent on another for protection. People whom we see in psychiatric hospitals usually refer to themselves as patients, as do people whom we see in their homes for psychiatric home care and those who come to see us privately. We have had the experience of being corrected by people who were referred to as clients. It is not uncommon for people to react negatively to the term *client* because it "cold" and "too businesslike." The term *patient*, on the other hand, means one who suffers and forbears (Levine, 1989). Somehow the term *patient* seems more accurate than *client* when describing the person in need of psychiatric services. Frequently, psychiatric patients have suffered not only their own private anguish and turmoil but also the stigma and rejection of society, upheaval and stress in their families, lack of understanding in their places of work, and sometimes the continuation of this suffering within the mental health system.

▶ Check Your Reading

5. What does a theistic world view tell us about people and patients?
6. Why do we need to know patients from a physical, social, emotional, and spiritual perspective?
7. What is the difference between the terms *patient* and *client*?

A Theistic Model of Human Beings

A model of human beings that best describes the interaction of body, mind, and spirit was developed by Jean Stallwood and Dr. Ruth Stoll (1975) and is shown in Figure 1–1. The model shows three concentric circles. The largest circle refers to the physical being, with five senses of seeing, hearing, touching, feeling, and smelling. The physical or body self is "world-conscious." The next circle is the psychosocial—that part of the person that gives one self-consciousness and personality through the emotions, the intellect, the moral sense, and the will. The innermost circle, the spirit, is the most difficult to comprehend because of its mystery and indefinable nature. The spirit is that part of the person that pervades all of the other dimensions. Within this spiritual center lies the potential for consciousness of and relatedness to God.

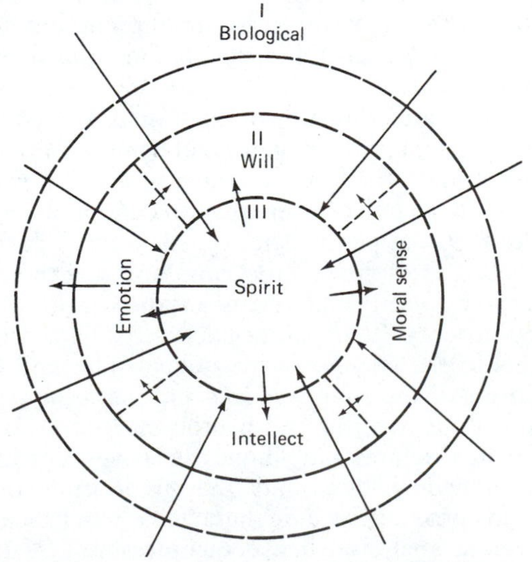

FIGURE 1–1
The Stallwood-Stoll model of human functioning. (Reprinted with the permission of Simon & Schuster from the Macmillan College text CLINICAL NURSING 3/e by Irene L. Beland and J. Y. Passos. Copyright ©1975 Macmillan Publishing Company.)

Because the human person is and functions as a dynamic whole and not three separate dimensions, each dimension influences and is influenced by the other two aspects of the person. This is shown on the model by the broken lines that make up the boundaries of the circles. These broken lines illustrate the flow between and among the three dimensions of a person. The model also depicts arrows flowing into and out of the three circles. This illustrates the mutually interactive nature of the person with outside influences such as social support, loving family and friends, the help of God, and material resources that strengthen the person. Therefore, when a person is feeling depressed, the experience includes not only sadness but also crying, sleeping and eating problems, slowed thinking, lack of energy, conflict in personal relationships, and a spiritual void expressed as hopelessness and despair about God's place in the person's life.

Any therapeutic approach that deals *only* with the mind, or *only* with the body is woefully inadequate. Going back to the example of the person who feels depressed, comprehensive treatment includes the use of an antidepressant, teaching about the causes and effects of depression, encouragement that hope exists because depression is treatable, attention to physical problems, involvement of the family and significant others in care, and discussion about ways to alleviate spiritual distress.

▶ Check Your Reading

8. What do the three concentric circles in the Stallwood and Stoll model of human beings represent?
9. To what does the innermost circle refer?
10. How does the model illustrate the interactive aspects of the dimensions of human beings?
11. What implications does the Stallwood and Stoll model have for psychiatric nursing?

A Theistic View of Brain Physiology

If you have heard that the 1990s are called the "Decade of the Brain," you might be wondering if we are discounting the importance of brain physiology in psychiatric illness in our holistic perspective. This could not be further from the truth. However, we *do not think* that understanding the brain holds the key to eradicating the pain of psychiatric illnesses. If this were the whole answer, then we could eliminate most of this textbook and focus exclusively on the brain. What we believe is that imbalances in brain physiology cause vulnerabilities or predispositions to certain psychiatric illnesses. In some people the physical imbalance is so overwhelming (such as is the case with an anecephalic infant) that we can do little cognitively, emotionally, spiritually, or physically to alter the outcome for that person. Examples of people in whom physiology dictates destiny, however, probably represent the minority.

Most of us have some physiological vulnerabilities with which we struggle, but we are certainly not defined by those characteristics. The determining factors that influence whether we develop an illness or not include things such as the presence or absence of a loving family, the presence or absence of significant others in our lives who supply us with love and affirmation, the adequacy and safety of our environment, and the adequacy of our diet to meet the demands for a healthy body and mind. Our understanding of the complex nature of human beings is so primitive that we cannot predict how much of one factor or another makes the difference between health and illness. What we do know is that people respond to love; that people can change, if only in small ways; and that the nurse-patient relationship makes a difference.

▶ **Check Your Reading**

12. How does a focus on brain physiology "fit in" with a theistic world view?

A Theistic Model of Intervention

As you review various approaches to caring for psychiatric patients, you will notice that most are not holistic. In general, few psychological approaches other than a nursing model, which is not specific to psychiatric illness, provide the nurse with a broad and comprehensive model for holistic intervention. One model, however, comes closest to the view that we hold: Lazarus's Multimodal Therapy (1981, 1985).

Lazarus postulates an approach that encompasses seven modalities and is captured by the acronym BASIC-ID. The letters stand for *b*ehaviors, *a*ffective processes, *s*ensations, *i*mages, *c*ognitions, *i*nterpersonal relationships, and *d*rugs. The only approach that Lazarus does not include is the spiritual.

In their work with chemically dependent patients, Brown and colleagues (1988) refined Lazarus's Multimodal Therapy to include the spiritual. The acronym for this modified approach is BASIC-IS. The "S" on the end of the acronym stands for spirituality. Brown and colleagues have found that effective intervention with the chemically dependent person must take into consideration spiritual concerns including values, sense of purpose and meaning in life, and relationship to the transcendant.

▶ **Check Your Reading**

13. What does a theistic world view suggest about our interventions with psychiatric patients?
14. What does the acronym BASIC-IS mean?

Other World Views

A theistic world view does not exclude consideration of ideas from other philosophies or world views. Many of the "isms" such as behaviorism, humanism, existentialism, and secularism are essentially nonreligious. Others such as monism, pantheism, and polytheism are religious. Although some of these world views have important contributions to make to our understandings of human behavior, "isms" generally have a narrow focus and are *ex*clusive rather than *in*clusive.

Behaviorism as a World View. **Behaviorism** suggests that people are no more and no less than the behaviors that they exhibit. Behaviorism focuses on changing behavior through controlled systems of reinforcers. The emphasis is on free will, choice, and personal meaning or the importance of feelings. In psychiatric nursing we study behavior; we believe that all behavior is meaningful, and we sometimes draw on techniques to change behavior. But we never lose sight of the fact that people are more than behavior.

Humanism as a World View. Let us look at **humanism,** a world view that extolls the value and importance of the human being. A humanist attempts to modify behavior and feelings by focusing on a person's innate goodness. The humanist believes that the person is always striving toward the good, that the power to change lies solely within the person, and that it is not necessary to recognize or draw upon God in the healing process. Humanism adds much of value to psychiatric nursing, and in this textbook we draw on humanist thinking. However, because humanism excludes the significance of the transcendant in human activity, it is not as comprehensive a world view as theism.

Existentialism as a World View. **Existentialism** focuses on the analysis of individual existence in a universe that is incomprehensible. The existentialist encourages the person to assume responsibility for freely made choices without any certain knowledge of what is right or wrong. We agree with some of the existentialist's notions—the importance of the person's story and how the person makes decisions when faced with choices. These are essential to understanding and assisting patients; thus, we have included "stories" as an existential thread throughout the text. But again, existentialism is not the whole story.

Secularism as a World View. **Secularism** is based on the belief that full understanding of the world comes through technical and scientific advances. Secularism in its purest form is, at the least, indifferent to religion; often, it overtly rejects religion, religious considerations, and spiritual issues.

Monism and Pantheism as World Views. **Monism** suggests that a basic oneness of being exists and that the transcendant force in the universe is not a personal God but rather a universal energy force. A monistic world view leads to a pantheistic world view. **Pantheism** suggests that everything is the same, and that there is no difference between what exists in the world and the universal energy. The pantheistic world view leads its followers to the conclusion that all peoples and things share in the divine energy source and that essentially all are God. Both monism and pantheism value relativism rather than absolutes and emphasize striving for balance within individual lives and the eradication of self. Pantheistic practices include therapeutic touch, acupuncture, chakra analysis, shiatsu (acupressure), Ayurvedic medicine, and polarity therapy. Monism and pantheism undergird much of Buddhism and Hinduism, although neither of these are monolithic belief systems.

Polytheism as a World View. **Polytheism** suggests that many gods exist in the universe. In polytheistic religions, sacrifices are frequently made to appease the gods or to appeal to the gods for special favors (Pacwa, 1992). Indigenous religions, as well as some forms of Buddhism and Hinduism, are polytheistic.

▶ **Check Your Reading**

15. Name two nonreligious world views.
16. Describe how humanism affects psychiatric nursing.
17. What contribution does behaviorism make to psychiatric nursing?
18. What does existentialism postulate that has significance for psychiatric nursing?
19. Describe monism, pantheism, and polytheism.
20. Contrast theism with monism, pantheism, and polytheism.

ISSUES YOU WILL FACE ON THE JOURNEY

The last area that we want to address in this chapter concerns your own journey as a psychiatric nursing student. Several specific issues face you as you first enter a psychiatric nursing rotation.

Anxiety About the New Situations You Will Encounter

It is not uncommon to feel stress and anxiety about new situations. You may have preconceived ideas about what a psychiatric hospital is like. Perhaps you have seen dramatizations on television or in the movies that have influenced your thinking. Perhaps you have a loved one with a psychiatric illness. Whatever the reasons, nursing students frequently approach the psychiatric experience with an increased stress level. The stress response can adversely affect your behavior. It is helpful to discuss this with your instructor and to seek suggestions to promote relaxation and adaptive thinking.

Threats to Your Role as a Nurse

Another issue confronted by psychiatric nursing students is role threat arising from several characteristics unique to psychiatric nursing. These include (1) a lack of professional attire; (2) a lack of structure; (3) decisions about whether or not to read the patient's chart; (4) the need for self-awareness; (5) fear of being injured and of injuring patients emotionally; (6) fear of rejection; (7) fear of identifying with patients; and (8) frustration over your inability to change patients.

Lack of Professional Attire. In a psychiatric setting, staff members generally wear street clothes rather than uniforms; they generally do not carry such professional equipment as stethoscopes or bandage scissors. Students often cannot tell the patients and staff apart and fear that they will be embarrassed by practicing newly formed interview and assessment skills on staff rather than on patients. Stripped of the security afforded by the outward symbols of the nursing role, students are left with the awareness that their main therapeutic tools are their communication and interpersonal skills, their ability to empathize, and their problem-solving abilities. Again, the result of this role threat is increased anxiety.

Lack of Structure. For students who are accustomed to the lock-step structure of a medical-surgical unit, the lack of structure—or rather the "different structure"—on a psychiatric unit can be quite disconcerting. The student wonders what to do with the time and feels guilty about not doing physical care. It is not readily apparent to the novice just how much energy can be expended in a meaningful relationship until the first time the student is intent on *really listening* to what the patient has to say. Students who get involved in the activities of the unit tend to "fit in" and to discover their place more quickly than students who wait on the sidelines to feel better. Students have shared that an article by J. A. Clement (1988) entitled "The myths and realities of psychiatric nursing, or I feel guilty when I just sit and talk" is helpful for dealing with the "different structure" of psychiatric nursing.

Decisions About Reading the Patient's Chart. Reading the patient's chart before meeting the patient is an issue that can be important to the nursing student. There are advantages to reading the chart prior to meeting the patient, but there are also advantages to reading the chart *after* meeting the patient. For the very anxious student, reading the chart is a concrete activity that lessens his or her anxiety and helps to structure the student's time. For less anxious students, meeting the patient without the benefit of chart knowledge allows them to get to know the patient free of bias. Most likely your instructor will assist you in making the chart-reading decision.

The Need for Self-Awareness. We described psychiatric nursing as a journey for you, and indeed it is. The journey into increased self-awareness is an exciting and rewarding but sometimes scary journey. To be an effective helper, each of us needs to know herself or himself—her or his thoughts, feelings, strengths and weaknesses; her or his values; and her or his reactions to people, places, and things. The goal of self-awareness is not to change all that we are—in fact, most students are affirmed in the communication and interpersonal skills they already possess—but rather, the goal is to know and understand ourselves so that we can effectively use the gift of who we are. Students approach the task of increasing self-awareness in many ways. Some find that keeping a journal is a wonderful process that allows them to freely express who they are without judgment. Others find meditation, prayer, periods of quiet solitude, sharing in groups or individual clinical supervision sessions, and completing process recordings (written verbatim accounts of their nurse-patient interactions) to be effective strategies to enhance self-awareness.

Fear of Injury and of Injuring Patients Emotionally. Many students begin the journey into psychiatric nursing feeling fearful that they will be harmed by patients or that they will say the "wrong" thing and cause harm to patients. The fear of physical harm at the hands of the "violent" patient has been greatly exaggerated by media portrayals of patients as wild and out of control. Likewise, the fear of causing irreparable harm to the patient by saying the wrong thing is very unlikely to happen. Although part of the focus of a psychiatric nursing course is to strengthen therapeutic communication skills, most patients are very attentive to nonverbal cues and are sensitive to the intent of the nursing student. If you are caring and concerned, most likely you will communicate this message even if your words somehow miss the mark. You might also have fears about your own ability to remain in control if a patient acts in an inappropriate way in front of you. Other students have reported the benefits of anticipating such incidents and thinking about acceptable responses beforehand.

Fear of Rejection by Patients. Another concern that students express as they journey into psychiatric nursing is that they will experience rejection by patients. It is not uncommon for psychiatric patients to be shy and wary with strangers. What appears to be rejecting behavior on the part of the patient may actually be the patient's fear of approaching new people. Although you may encounter patients who are shy or even hostile and withdrawn, many patients welcome the interest of the nursing student and are receptive to the student's overtures.

Fear of Identifying With Patients. As you journey into psychiatric nursing you may find that you encounter patients with problems, stresses, and conflicts very similar to your own. This may frighten you; you may find yourself thinking something like, "there but for the grace of God go I." When confronted with these feelings it will help you to talk to your instructor, who can assist you in looking at how you have effectively coped with your situation or who can help you in seeing the subtle differences between the patient's situation and your own.

Frustration Over Your Inability to Change Patients. You may find your journey frustrating because you are unable to complete goals that you have set for a particular nurse-patient interaction. Psychiatric nursing brings you face to face with the truth that you cannot change or be responsible for anyone else's behavior but your own. So if the patient is not cooperating, you can evaluate your own approach and modify it, but you cannot dictate or control the patient's choice of whether to respond to your approach. This is a hard lesson but one that has implications far beyond psychiatric nursing.

The Cost of Your Involvement

The last issue to look at concerning your own journey is the cost of your involvement. We ask you to provide holistic care; we ask you to be kind, empathetic, attentive, and reflective; we ask you to *care* about patients. What we are asking you to do has a cost attached to it. It is seldom acknowledged or mentioned. When you get involved and care about people, you feel their pain and sorrow. You get frustrated, sad, and sometimes angry. To stay healthy you have to find healthy outlets for the expression of those feelings. You need to talk about them in a supportive and accepting environment. You need to attend to your own spiritual needs, most importantly your relationship with God, as you understand God. You need to receive supervision to understand the dynamics of the nurse-patient relationship. In other words, you need to take care of yourself—body, mind, and spirit—just as you are teaching patients to take care of themselves. No one—and this is worth repeating—*no one* can continually give without receiving refreshment, nurturance, and inspiriting care. So take care of yourselves, not only during your journey into psychiatric nursing, but throughout your nursing career.

▶ Check Your Reading

21. Identify two of the issues that you will face as a nursing student entering a psychiatric nursing rotation for the first time.
22. Describe two of the situations characteristic of psychiatric nursing that may pose a threat to your role as a nurse.
23. Identify two common fears experiencd by nursing students entering a psychiatric nursing rotation for the first time.
24. Describe at least three strategies that you can use to cope with the anxiety that you might feel as a novice in psychiatric nursing.
25. What is meant by the "cost of involvement?"

CONCLUSIONS

Psychiatric nursing, like all of life, is a journey in which no guarantees exist about what lies ahead. We invite you to join us in the journey of psychiatric nursing—to be open to the possibilities that exist in this journey. We invite you to view your role with psychiatric patients as one involving a privileged position of sharing (if only for a brief period) in their journeys.

The psychiatric nursing journey, as well as the life journey, on which Dr. Arnold and I have embarked is undergirded by unwavering belief in a theistic world view—a world view that holds forth a creator God who considers us His beloved and calls us into relationship with Him. From this relationship and this world view, we are encouraged to respond to others with the same love that the Creator has poured forth on us. Our journey also has been affected by beliefs from several other world views, including humanism, existentialism, and behaviorism.

Your journey into psychiatric nursing is sure to be affected by multiple other issues, including your own feelings of uncertainty and fear; threats to your role as a nurse, including both the lack of professional attire and the lack of structure; indecision about issues such as whether or not to read the patient's chart; the focus on getting to know yourself better; fears of being injured and of causing injury, of being rejected by patients, and of identifying with patients; frustration over your inability to change patients; and, finally, an awareness that the cost of involvement can be high. We hope that you will counter these issues with a sense of your importance as an instrument of healing and with an awareness that you, stripped of the outward acoutrements of nursing, are a powerful force in the patient's attempts to construct a more healthy journey.

KEY POINTS TO REMEMBER

- Psychiatric nursing, like all of life, is a journey. We are privileged to accompany patients on parts of their journeys.
- Psychiatric patients, who are frequently the least understood and most poorly treated of all patients, have much to teach us about survival, spiritual strength, resiliency, and the importance of being treated with respect, dignity, and compassion.
- The underlying foundation for this textbook is a theistic world view. This world view includes (1) a belief in a loving and benevolent creator God; (2) a belief that we are created in God's image; (3) a belief that God loves us; (4) a belief that our actions toward each other should reflect God's love; (5) a belief that hope of change always exists; and (6) a belief that we are holistic beings—we have integrated physical, emotional, and spiritual dimensions.
- A theistic world view stresses forgiveness and treating people with kindness, patience, gentleness, and forbearance. These are qualities that are essential in psychiatric nursing.
- A theistic world view suggests that if psychiatric nurses are to make a difference in the lives of their patients, the focus of nursing interventions must be on all of the dimensions that make up the person—physical, emotional, social, and spiritual.
- Stallwood and Stoll identify a theistic model of human beings that demonstrates the interaction of all the dimensions that make up the person.
- A theistic world view is not inconsistent with a focus on the role of neurophysiology in psychiatric illness. However, brain physiology tells only part of the patient's story; the rest of the story draws from many other sources, including the patient's spirituality.
- A theistic model of intervention is holistic. It includes a focus on behaviors, affective processes, sensations, images, cognitions, interpersonal relationships, and spirituality.
- The term *patient* rather than *client* is used throughout the text because *patient* describes the long-suffering and forbearance of the person seeking psychiatric care.
- Several nonreligious world views exist, including behaviorism, humanism, secularism, and existentialism. In this textbook, we draw on behaviorism, humanism, and existentialism, realizing that they are not as comprehensive as theism.
- Three religious world views also exist: monism, pantheism, and polytheism. Monism purports that all in the universe is the same and that the divine is an impersonal energy force. Pantheism extends monism to state that because everything is one and all is the same, then we are all God. Polytheism holds forth a belief in many gods.
- Multiple issues will confront you as you begin your journey into psychiatric nursing. These issues include your own feelings of uncertainty and fear; threats to your role as a nurse, including both the lack of professional attire and the lack of structure; indecision about issues such as whether to read the patient's chart; the focus on getting to know yourself better; fears of being injured and of causing injury, of being rejected by patients, and of identifying with patients; frustration over your inability to change patients; and, finally, an awareness that the cost of involvement can be high.
- The cost of involvement can be offset by the knowledge that you are a powerful instrument of healing for the patient who is struggling to change his or her own story.

LEARNING ACTIVITIES

1. Read current journal articles on spirituality in nursing. See if you are able to determine the world view from which the authors are operating. Do you agree with the world view that is presented?
2. Think about your own world view. How do you view the "big picture" of life? Does God play a role in your world view? Does God play a role in your view of nursing? If so, what is His role?
3. Keep a journal about your own journey into nursing. Focus on the reasons you chose to pursue nursing as a career. What does your journey tell you about your own world view?
4. Think about clinical situations in which patients hold world views different from your own. How do you handle these situations?
5. Think about the issues that you will face as you journey into psychiatric nursing. What resources do you currently use to take care of yourself? What resources do you need to better care for yourself? What are your spiritual resources?

CRITICAL THINKING EXERCISE

All the students in Professor Smyth's psychiatric clinical laboratory have been asked to think about their life experiences and how they might affect their thoughts and beliefs about the importance of spirituality in psychiatric illness. Sarah's thoughts went to when she was 10 years old, to the day when her mother and brother were taken to the emergency department following an automobile accident with a drunk driver. Ever since that day she knew she wanted to be a nurse so that she could help others. Sarah was aware of the sadness that overcame her as she remembered how her brother's struggle to live had failed and how her mother continued to struggle with wanting to live. Sarah refused to go to church anymore. This learning experience was not going to be easy! Sarah had seen the inside of crisis centers all too often.

1. What assumptions can you make about Sarah's belief in God?
2. What evidence suggests that your assumptions are true?
3. What other information do you need to determine if your assumptions are valid?

Sarah was assigned to interview Mr. Jasline, a patient with a history of depression. After talking with him she discovered that he is also in the hospital for detoxification because of his chronic use of alcohol. Following the interview she discussed her feelings about Mr. Jasline with Professor Smyth.

1. How might Sarah's past experiences influence her practice?

2. What are possible responses that Sarah might have to Mr. Jaslin?

3. What conclusions can you draw from the above data?

REFERENCES

Brown H. P., Peterson, J. H., and Cunningham, O. (1988). A behavioral/cognitive spiritual model for a chemical dependency aftercare program. *Alcoholism Treatment Quarterly*, *5*(1/2), 153–159.

Clement, J. A. (1988). The myths and realities of psychiatric nursing, or I feel guilty when I just sit and talk. *Imprint*, February/March, 40–41.

Lazarus, A. A. (1981). *The practice of multimodal therapy*. New York: McGraw-Hill.

Lazarus, A. A. (1985). *Casebook of multimodal therapy*. New York: Guilford Press.

Levine, M. (1989). Beyond dilemma. *Seminars in Oncology Nursing*, *5*(2), 124–128.

Nouwen, H. J. M. (1979). *The wounded healer: Ministry in contemporary society*. New York: Doubleday.

Pacwa, M. (1992). *Catholics and the new age*. Ann Arbor, MI: Servant Publications.

Stallwood, J., and Stoll, R. (1975). Spiritual dimension of nursing practice. In I. L. Beland, and J. Y. Passos (Eds.), *Clinical nursing* (3rd ed.). New York: Macmillan.

SUGGESTED READINGS

Carson, V. B. (1993). Spirituality: generic or Christian. *Journal of Christian Nursing*, *10*(1), 24–27.

Sire, J. (1988). *The universe next door* (2nd ed.). Downers Grove, Il: Inter-Varsity Press.

Turner, S. (1990). Lean, green and meaningless. *Christianity Today*, September 24, 26–27.

CHAPTER 2

THE WISDOM OF PAST TRAVELERS

A HISTORY OF MENTAL HEALTH NURSING

Historians have always known that the past has importance. The past is somehow a part of the present and even the future. The past is a wise teacher.

—Fr. Charles, 1982

LEARNING OBJECTIVES

After studying this chapter, you should be able to:

1. Describe the contributions of the following people: Dorothea Dix, Linda Richards, Clifford Beers, Harriet Bailey, Euphemia "Effie" Taylor, Benjamin Rush, Phillippe Pinel, Adolph Meyer, Harry Stack Sullivan, Hildegard Peplau, William Tuke, and Dorothy Mereness.

2. Identify the influence of the following United States legislation: The Mental Health Act of 1946, the Hill-Burton Act, the Mental Retardation Facilities and Community Mental Health Centers Construction Act of 1963, the Community Mental Health Center Amendment of 1975, the Community Mental Health Systems Act, the Omnibus Budget Reconciliation Act, and the Americans with Disabilities Act of 1990.

3. Discuss the influence of World War I and World War II on the care of the mentally ill.

4. Identify important "firsts" in psychiatric nursing: the first psychiatric nurse, the opening of the McLean Training School for Nurses, the first psychiatric nursing textbook, the first psychiatric nursing journal, and the first psychiatric nursing professor.

5. Identify the historical significance of the following hospitals associated with the care of the mentally ill: Bethlehem Hospital, the Eastern Lunatic Asylum, Pennsylvania Hospital, and the McLean Asylum.

6. Discuss the impact of psychobiological therapies on the journey of psychiatric nursing.

7. Identify one effect of deinstitutionalization on the journey of psychiatric nursing.

8. Discuss the significance of the "Decade of the Brain" on the journey of psychiatric nursing.

KEY TERMINOLOGY

Almshouses
Asylums
Harriet Bailey
Clifford Beers
Bethlehem Hospital
Dorothea Dix
Dorothy Mereness
Adolph Meyer
Pennsylvania Hospital
Hildegard Peplau
Phillippe Pinel
Public mental hospitals
Retreats
Linda Richards
Benjamin Rush
Harry Stack Sullivan
Euphemia Taylor
William Tuke

The journey of the psychiatric nurses and the patients for whom they have cared has been arduous and rewarding, disheartening and encouraging, despairing and hopeful, buffeted and enhanced by societal forces and events, spanning centuries. In as much as a journey may involve many paths and many steps and may be influenced by numerous individuals as well as by predictable and unexpected events, so has been the journey of nurses who have chosen to care for patients suffering from mental illness.

Psychiatric nurses have met their patients in a diversity of settings and under an array of circumstances, some shamefully inadequate, neglectful, and harmful, some barely adequate, and in some fortunate instances, in environments that were appealing and comfortable places for the experience of recovery. Nurses caring for the mentally ill also have been either helped or hindered by colleagues in other nursing disciplines and by other health care providers. Like the patients for whom they have cared, mental health nurses have been misunderstood and ostracized.

Joyce Travelbee, a psychiatric nurse educator, observed that "an aura of mystery" continued to exist regarding the nature of psychiatric nursing (Travelbee, 1969, p. 21). She also noted that there was a "still prevalent belief . . . that psychiatric nurses are in some ways peculiar" and a belief that "the longer a nurse works with the mentally ill the more like 'them' she becomes" (p. 22). She characterized psychiatric nursing practice as "a searching, tiring, sometimes tedious but always interesting process" (p. 23).

In the following story, Dr. Edna Fordyce reflects on her own journey in psychiatric nursing.

EDNA FORDYCE'S STORY

My journey in psychiatric nursing began in 1953, when, as a junior nursing student in a diploma nursing program, I commenced my psychiatric affiliation at Rochester State Hospital in Rochester, Minnesota. This was the type of educational setting and curriculum experienced by most nursing students of that time. We spent three months on the campus of this hospital, living in a nurses' residence on the grounds, attending classes, and participating in the care of patients on the various wards of the hospital. Our schedule of classes and assignment to the hospital wards added up to a 40-hour week. The classes on mental illness and nursing care we attended were conducted by nurse instructors and physicians, most of them psychiatrists. One of our required textbooks was Helena Render's *Nurse-Patient Relationships in Psychiatry*, published in 1947. It is important to note that the modern pharmacological treatment of mental illness had not yet been instituted at that time; most of the medications in use today had not yet been discovered. And by comparison with today, little was understood about the causes and treatment of mental illness.

This experience was truly memorable and has influenced my life and career choices. I was challenged by the nursing responsibilities in which we participated. Nursing activities included daily personal care of the patients, playing table games with them on the units, and, when possible, taking them off the wards to activities or for walks on the hospital grounds. And yes, there were dances, an activity that was held twice weekly, to which we escorted patients and participated with them. For me, "dancing" meant skipping to the music alongside the patient partner rather than actually dancing.

Story by Edna Fordyce.

Assisting With Electroconvulsive Therapy

Every Monday, Wednesday, and Friday, 45 to 50 patients of the total 2000 who were hospitalized received the relatively new therapy of electroconvulsive therapy (ECT, sometimes referred to as "shock therapy"). I recall assisting in what seemed like the "herding" of these folks dressed in white gowns and blue-striped bathrobes through the network of hospital tunnels to receive their treatment. The treatment was given without the benefit of anesthesia, although the drug *curare* was administered before the treatment to lessen the risk of the fractures that could occur during the treatment. When the electric current was administered through electrodes placed on the patient's temples the patient experienced a *grand mal* seizure. Hospital staff, assisted by nursing students, held the patient on the bed until the seizure subsided. After the patients awakened, we gave them a glass of milk. When they were steady enough to walk without falling, they were once again "herded" through the hospital tunnels back to the nursing wards for bathing and dressing for the day. The red, sleepy faces with blood-tinged eyes remain in my memory even today.

Observing Prefrontal Lobotomies

I also observed the procedure of prefrontal lobotomy, which entailed the cutting of the prefrontal lobe tissues of the brain to calm the violent patient. I was assigned to care for some of these patients postoperatively. The superintendent of the hospital oversaw each procedure. This particular superintendent had a reputation for maintaining high standards of care for patients and was effective in obtaining state legislative support for the resources he requested such as more modern hospital buildings.

Memories of Overcrowding, Seclusion, and Green Lawns

Other memories of those days are still impressed in my consciousness. Paramount is the memory of the overcrowded state of the hospital wards. We had insufficient beds for everyone who was housed on each of the 16 wards. For example, one unit with a capacity for 45 patients housed over 90 patients. This overcrowding necessitated the use of cots at nighttime. After all the patients were bedded down for the night, we barely had room to pass through the cots to leave the ward after the completion of our assigned evening hours. Many hours of seclusion were among the daily experience for the most violent and psychotic patients. For others, this form of restraint was a periodic occurrence. I saw no other physical restraints utilized in the hospital. A few years prior to this time, a massive bonfire had been held in Minnesota to destroy mechanical restraints such as the canvas camisole restraints (straitjackets) so often associated with mental institutions. The hospital grounds were dominated by the long building of many wards, characteristic of the Kirkbride architectural plan and frequently the basis of hospital construction from 1854 to 1914 (Baxter and Hathcox, 1994). Several newer but smaller two-story buildings with four wards, semiprivate rooms, and well-lighted, spacious dayrooms also were present. The hospital also had its own farm; the fields and green lawn of the hospital grounds were maintained by patients and hospital employees.

Memories of Caring and Commitment

Overall I saw great kindness demonstrated toward patients by committed hospital staff from the various caregiving disciplines. Head nurses were responsible for each hospital ward. Many of them were registered nurses who had obtained their education from the training school that had previously existed at the hospital. This was a common type of educational program prior to World War II. Psychiatric aides, along with the nursing students, constituted the nursing staff under the supervision of the head nurse.

One head nurse, whom I greatly admired, was a model of commitment for everyone who knew her. She always assigned herself to be on duty for the special holidays of the year because on these days she needed to be with her "ladies." The ladies of whom this nurse, Esther Swenson, spoke were among the most disturbed, psychotically ill women hospitalized at this facility.

I am quite certain that neither Esther Swenson nor many of her nurse colleagues could have articulated a theory or framework for their nursing practice, as espoused in the contemporary textbooks. However, intuition, long hours spent with patients, and experience in responding to their behaviors, as well as their personal humanness, provided the basis for their practice of psychiatric nursing. The three months of my affiliation experience passed all too quickly, and soon I was to sadly bid farewell to a special nursing experience.

The reflections of George Sanatayana seem fitting as I reflect on these experiences as a nursing student: *"We must welcome the future remembering that soon it will be the past; and we must respect the past, remembering that once it was all that was humanly possible."*

Moving on—to a Psychiatric Unit in a General Hospital

After two years of general staff nursing, I ventured to assume a position in one of the new, although few, psychiatric units then existing in a general hospital. I was in charge of the insulin therapy room (insulin was administered to induce coma, with the intent of interrupting psychotic symptoms) and assisted with ECT. I was also the charge nurse assigned on designated shifts. Although these responsibilities were frightening, my confidence grew with experience. The year was 1956, and the new drug *chlorpromazine (Thorazine)* had just recently been released. My colleagues and I administered this medication with great hopes of alleviating the many symptoms (delusions and hallucinations) patients were experiencing. Other medications such as additional antipsychotic medications, antidepressants, and lithium, now so familiar, were not yet existent. The sedatives utilized then (such as phenobarbital) had only limited benefit in alleviating symptoms.

Returning to the State Hospital

After completing baccalaureate studies at the University of Minnesota (1960), I was fortunate to have the opportunity to return to the state hospital of my student psychiatric affiliation. This time, with a new bachelor's degree and a little experience, I was the new instructor of nursing for the diploma students from six schools of nursing having their 12-week psychiatric affiliation.

During these years, numerous new medications (both antipsychotics and antidepressants) were approved and administered. Also during this time, psychiatric admissions at the hospital became predominantly voluntary; previously, the majority of patients were admitted as "committed" or "involuntary." Largely because of the new medications, hospital wards now had a quieter and calmer atmosphere, and patients were more receptive to interactions and participation in hospital and ward activities.

On to Graduate School

When I undertook graduate study at the University of Washington from 1967 to 1968, my education was partially supported by federal funding that was then available for nurses seeking additional education. My hours of study were then devoted to the writings of notable psychiatric authors such as Harry Stack Sullivan and Viktor Frankl, as well as the emerging nurse theorists specializing in psychiatric nursing. Among these were Joyce Travelbee and Hildegard Peplau. Process recordings (verbatim accounts of nurse-patient interactions) were written, examined, and reviewed to enhance our relationship and supervision skills.

Teaching the Next Generation of Psychiatric Nurses

Since 1960, I have taught graduate and undergraduate students, and this has been a rewarding experience. Teaching has allowed me to participate in patient care in a variety of settings and to be involved in the changing forms of treatment for the mentally ill. Psychiatric nursing has also opened doors for me to participate in various activities such as mental health counseling in the community. It has also enabled me to contribute to my church "family" through the Stephen Ministry, a lay caregiving program that is in operation in many Christian denominations.

Just as Dr. Fordyce's story is unique and spans 40 years of momentous change within the profession, many stories exist of other individuals who have contributed to the specialty of psychiatric nursing. In this chapter, you will meet some of the individuals, read of important events, and learn about some of the settings for care that have existed through time. Our journey today has been made possible because of the efforts of a myriad of individuals. Their contributions, individually and as a group, have championed the cause of the mentally ill, gained more appropriate care for these often neglected patients, and increased the understanding upon which more effective care might be based. Their stories are woven with determination and perseverance, difficulties and triumphs.

However, before we can even look at these stories, we must review a time when there were no psychiatric nurses, psychiatric theory, or medical treatment, but yet there were still individuals who were mentally ill. Bailey, a psychiatric nurse and author, reported that "Mental disease is as old as the human race . . ." (1935, p. 1), and Alexander and Selesnick (1966, p. 3), historians of psychiatry, have observed that:

The mentally ill have always been with us . . . to be feared, marveled at, laughed at, pitied, or tortured, but all too seldom cured. Their existence shakes us to the core of our being, for they make us painfully aware that sanity is a fragile thing.

EARLY TRAVELERS

During the earliest times of history, behavior that was considered abnormal (frequently that of the mentally ill) was attributed to supernatural forces. Evil spirits or punishment from the gods, the devil, or demons was seen as the cause of diseases, including the mental diseases. Alexander and Selesnick (1966) report that witch doctors or medicine men were the first psychiatrists.

One of the prominent and perhaps most influential physicians of his own time and even to the present was *Hippocrates* (460–375 B.C.). According to the nurse historian Donahue (1985), Hippocrates was thought to have been a direct descendent of Asklepios, the chief healer of Greek mythology. Hippocrates prepared a classification of the mental disorders (Alexander and Selesnick, 1966). He also described body humors—yellow bile, black bile, phlegm, and blood—and attributed human behaviors to excesses of particular humors. For example, the excess of black bile was thought to be responsible for the disease of melancholia (depression).

Despite the writings and thinking of Hippocrates attributing illness causation to other factors, remnants of the early thinking regarding demonology recurred at various times. For instance, witch hunting occurred in Europe and in Colonial America. Those individuals thought to be witches and demons, mostly women, were hunted and killed in the most horrible manner. The cruel treatment of the mentally ill that occurred (e.g., beatings) was often intended to drive the evil spirits from the person and restore them to health (Deutsch, 1949).

▶ Check Your Reading

1. In early history, to what did people attribute the cause of mental illness?
2. Who were the earliest "psychiatrists"?
3. What did Hippocrates believe was the cause of depression?

18TH, 19TH, AND 20TH CENTURY TRAVELERS

Phillippe Pinel (1745–1826). "This gentle man taught compassionate treatment of the mentally ill by his own example" (Dolan et al, 1983, p. 122). Thus Dolan and her colleagues described the brave French psychiatrist **Phillippe Pinel,** M.D. In 1792, Dr. Pinel risked his own career in medicine, and perhaps his life, when as the chief of the Bicêtre mental hospital in Paris, he released patients from the incarcerating chains and other restraints that confined them. A famous painting depicts his similar actions at the women's asylum at Salpêtrière, also in Paris, France.

William Tuke (1732–1822). Meanwhile in England in the same year that Dr. Pinel removed the chains from patients at Bicêtre, **William Tuke,** a successful businessman, established the York **Retreat.** The York Retreat exemplified the humanitarian approach to the mentally ill, which was the basis of Pinel's actions. William Tuke and his fellow Quaker colleagues (the "Friends") believed that the tenets of the Quaker faith, which suggest treating people with kindness in a pleasant environment, could bring recovery to the ill. The York Retreat, first established by William Tuke, was administered by three generations of family members according to these basic beliefs. The pioneering efforts of Pinel and Tuke were precursors to the modern day milieu (environmental) therapy (see Chapter 18).

Benjamin Rush (1745–1813). In Colonial America, **Benjamin Rush,** M.D., was the first American to undertake the serious study of mental illness (Figure 2–1). Rush, along with Benjamin Franklin, was one of the signers of the Declaration of Independence. As well as being an inventor and physician, he was the author of the historic book on mental illness, *Diseases of the Mind*, which was published in 1812. Benjamin Rush attended patients at the Pennsylvania Hospital in Philadelphia for 30 years (Bailey, 1935).

Rush viewed the physician-patient relationship as a significant factor with curative benefits. Based on his view that mental illness was the result of faulty blood circulation in the brain, he devised methodologies of treatment such as the "tranquilizer chair" (Figure 2–2). The chair hung from the ceiling, and patients were restrained in the chair, with heads covered. This form of restraint, although innovative for its time, would not meet with current acceptable practices of medical care! Rush held a humane attitude toward the care of the mentally ill and, based on his many accomplishments, is credited as the "Father of American Psychiatry." Also among his treatment perspectives is evi-

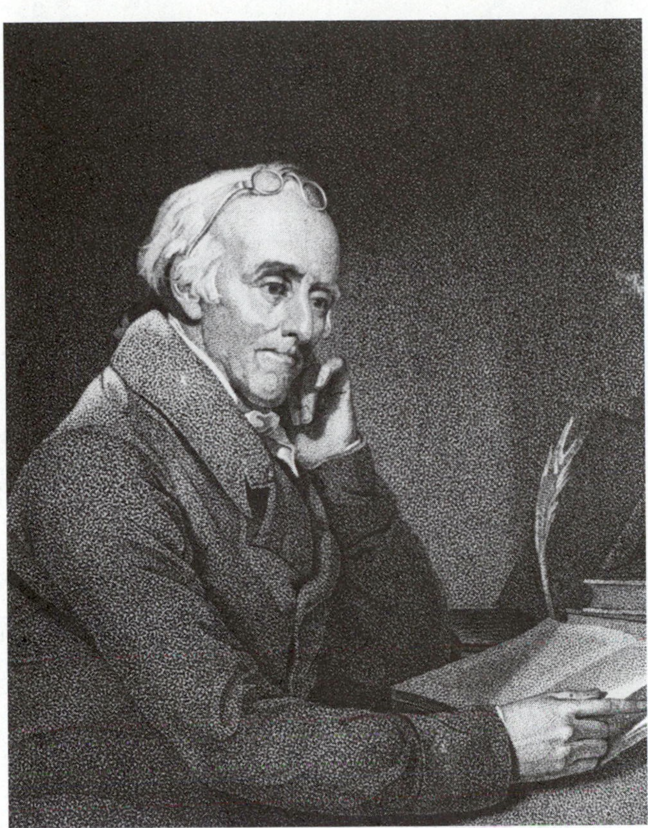

FIGURE 2-1
Benjamin Rush, M.D. (1745–1813). (Courtesy of the National Library of Medicine, Bethesda, MD.)

dence of the forerunner of what was later known as "attitude therapy." Rush advocated that gentleness was necessary for the depressed person and that firmness should be utilized when manic behavior was present.

Dorothea Lynde Dix (1802–1887). Dorothea Lynde Dix (Figure 2–3), a New England schoolteacher and crusader for reform in the care of the mentally ill, was first made aware of the dreadful conditions under which some mentally ill individuals existed when she was a volunteer Sunday School teacher at the East Cambridge jail in Massachusetts. There, criminals and "lunatics" were crowded together in dirty and cold prison conditions. Although initially without success, her first action was to obtain a means to provide some heat for this setting. Her Sunday visit in 1841 was the beginning of an extensive study of conditions throughout New England, which she undertook and about which she subsequently reported to the influential community leaders and legislatures of the respective states. Miss Dix's intention was that the "insane" persons of the community be cared for appropriately. For years she crusaded to obtain facilities for the care of the mentally ill. This eventually resulted in the establishment of at least 30 hospitals in the United States, Canada, Scotland, and Japan (Bailey, 1935; Tiffany, 1918). Among these hospitals was the first State Hospital in New Jersey (Trenton) and The Government Hospital for The Insane (now Saint Elizabeth's Hospital) in Washington, D.C.

At the outset of the Civil War (1861–1865), when she was nearly 60 years of age, Miss Dix arrived in Washington, D.C. to volunteer her services for nursing care and was appointed Superintendent of Female Nurses of the Union Army (1861). This appointment made Miss Dix "the first woman appointed to an administrative position in the federal government" (Flanigan, 1976, p. 13). One should remember that Miss Dix's efforts were ardently pursued and that they are all the more impressive because she experienced repeated episodes of illness that left her in a physically depleted condition and that had earlier necessitated that she abandon her career in teaching. The last several years of her life were spent in an apartment provided for her at the Trenton State Hospital in New Jersey (the first hospital she helped to establish). In concluding his biography of Miss Dix, Francis Tiffany (1918, p. 375) quotes from a letter by Dr. Charles H. Nichols, informing friends of her death:

> *Thus has died and been laid to rest in the most quiet, unostentious way the most useful and distinguished woman America has yet produced.*

The United States Postal Service issued the one-cent stamp of the Great Americans Series in 1983 in recognition of Miss Dix (Forester and Grandinetti, 1991; Figure 2–4).

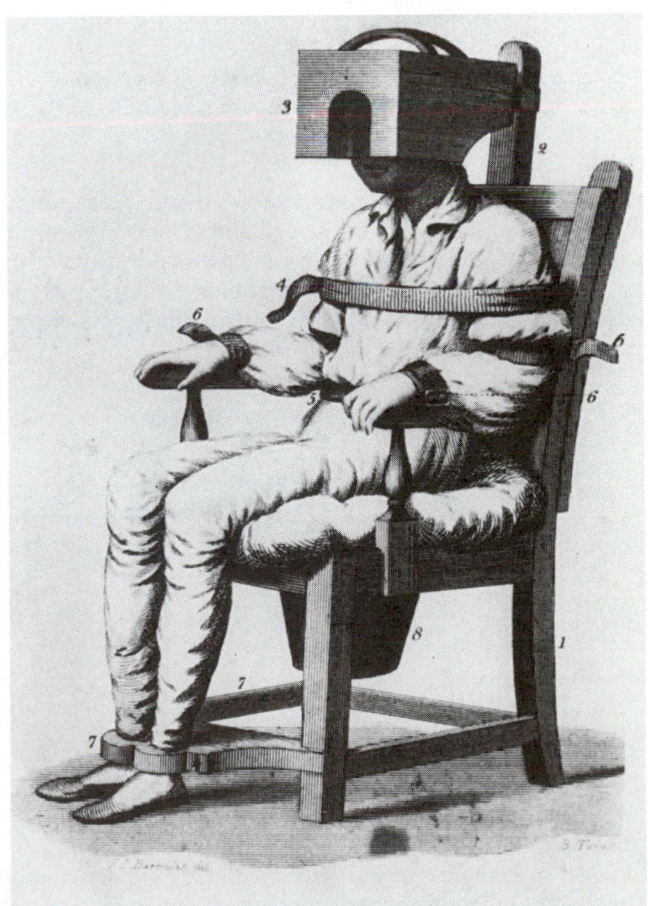

FIGURE 2-2
The "tranquilizer chair" devised by Benjamin Rush. (Courtesy of the National Library of Medicine, Bethesda, MD.)

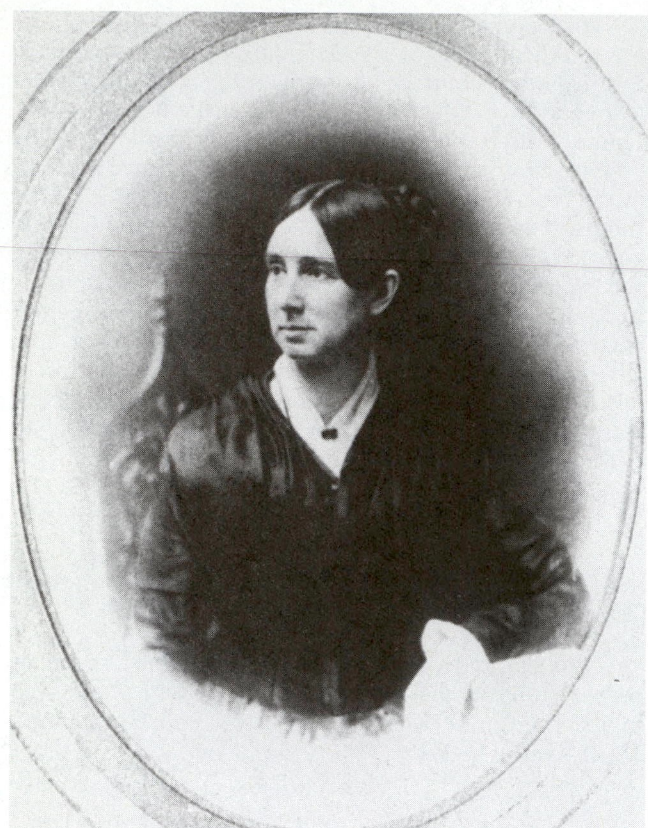

FIGURE 2–3
Dorothea Lynde Dix (1802–1887). (Courtesy of the National Library of Medicine, Bethesda, MD.)

Emil Kraepelin (1856–1926). Emil Kraepelin, M.D., was considered to have been one of most influential psychiatrists of his lifetime. From his observations, the first comprehensive descriptions of mental illnesses were developed. The descriptions Kraepelin developed of the mood disorders have been preserved and are still being studied and referred to at the present time. Dr. Kraepelin was Professor of Clinical Psychiatry in Munich, for 19 years.

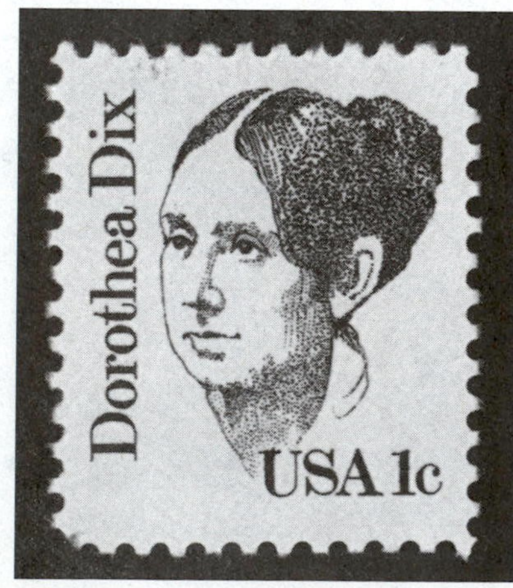

FIGURE 2–4
The Dorothea Dix one-cent stamp issued on September 23, 1983 by the U.S. Postal Service as part of its Great Americans Series.

Sigmund Freud (1856–1939). Sigmund Freud, M.D., a neurologist who studied with the notable neurologist Jean Martin Charcot, established a practice in Vienna. He originated a perspective of illness and treatment known as the psychoanalytical approach as well as a theory basis for understanding the formation and development of personality. After his visit to the United States in 1909, when he presented a series of lectures at Clark University in Massachusetts, his controversial ideas generated interest among American psychiatrists. In fact, Freud's influence is apparent today in the teaching and practice of psychiatry in the United States. Although the soundness of Freudian theory remains controversial, Freud's contributions are no less noteworthy.

Adolph Meyer (1866–1950). Adolph Meyer, M.D., was a professor of psychiatry at Johns Hopkins University in Baltimore. He is remembered for developing his biology of the whole personality or the "psychobiological" perspective of psychiatry. Meyer emphasized that psychiatry is a biological science and advocated that a comprehensive study of the individual's history including his or her life situation be undertaken. He enlisted the assistance of his wife, Mary Meyer, in a home visitation program to his patients. She is considered America's first psychiatric social worker. But perhaps her role was also the prototype of the modern community mental health nurse. As Director of the Henry Phipps Psychiatric Clinic at Johns Hopkins University, Meyer was a colleague of Euphemia "Effie" J. Taylor, the first Director of Nursing Services, among other significant persons.

Clifford Beers (1876–1943). Clifford Beers, a significant crusader for the mentally ill, wrote of his experiences as a patient. His first-person account of his mental illness and the circumstances he endured as a patient were to have an influence on many. The Mental Hygiene Movement was a direct outcome of his crusading efforts, which included his autobiography, *A Mind that Found Itself* (1908). Many influential persons of that day,

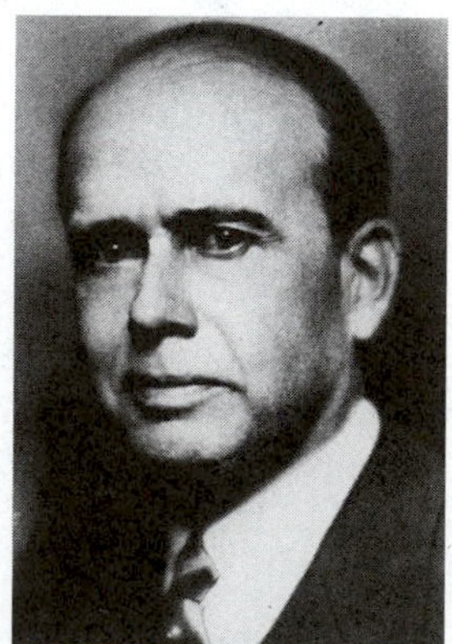

FIGURE 2–5
Clifford Beers (1876–1943). (Courtesy of the National Library of Medicine, Bethesda, MD.)

BOX 2–1 Clifford Beers: A Patient's Story

Clifford Beers (1876–1943) suffered from severe bipolar (manic-depressive) illness, with the first episode occurring during his college years. His story is sensitively portrayed in his 1908 publication, *A Mind That Found Itself.* In this autobiographical text, he describes with great insight and sobering detail his experience with mental illness. Mr. Beers describes his own life story as a "history of a mental civil war, which I fought single-handed on a battlefield that lay within the compass of my skull" (p. 1).

His story illustrates the painful isolation experienced by persons with mental illness. He notes that "for more than two years, I was without relatives or friends, in fact, without a world, except that one created by my own mind from the chaos that reigned within it" (p. 28). His story also depicts the cruelty imposed upon persons with mental illness in an era when little was known about the cause or treatment of such debilitating conditions. In one account, Mr. Beers describes a violent assault that he endured at the hands of his attendants while a patient at a mental institution (pp. 161, 164):

First I was knocked down. Then for several minutes I was kicked about the room—struck, kneed, and choked . . . I soon observed that the only patients who were not likely to be subjected to abuse were the very ones least in need of care and treatment.

Mr. Beers was instrumental in bringing into public view the problems within institutions for the mentally ill and the need for greater attention to the causes, treatment, and prevention of mental illness. The National Committee for Mental Hygiene was organized in 1909. Because of his pioneering efforts on behalf of the mentally ill, Clifford Beers became one of only a select few laypersons to be admitted for membership in the American Psychiatric Association as an honorary member. "The death of Clifford Beers, which occurred on July 9, 1943, brought to a close one of the most remarkable careers in modern philanthropy."

including Dr. Adolph Meyer (Box 2–1), provided Mr. Beers support and advisement in his endeavors.

Linda Richards (1891–1930). In September of 1872, **Linda Richards,** a young Bostonian woman, was admitted along with four other young women to the new Training School at the New England Hospital (the first American training school). Miss Richards (1911, pp. 10, 11) (Figure 2–6) described her student experiences as follows:

Our days were not eight hours; they were nearer twice eight. We rose at 5:30 A.M. and left the wards at 9 P.M. to go to our beds, which were in little rooms between the wards. Each nurse took care of her ward of six patients both day and night . . . . We wore no uniforms, the only stipulation being that our dresses should be washable.

Further, Miss Richards (1911, p. 11, 12) reported:

Every second week we were off duty one afternoon from two to five o'clock. We had no evenings out, no hours for study or recreation and no regular leave on Sunday. Only twice during the year was I given the opportunity to go to church.

We had no textbooks, nor did we have entrance or final examinations. Each nurse was quietly given her diploma as she completed her year of training.

After a rigorous year of study and clinical work, Miss Richards received a diploma from this one-year program. Because she was the first student to apply to and enter this new school and the first to graduate (on October 19, 1873), Linda Richards is designated as America's first trained nurse. She is also honored as the first psychiatric nurse in the United States.

In fact, more than any other nurse in the early 1900s, Linda Richards was able to assess patients in terms of their physical and emotional needs (Sills, 1973). After her graduation from the training school, Miss Richards became Night Superintendent at Bellevue Hospital in New York for one year. She then became Superintendent of the Boston Training School. Miss Richards established and directed the first training school for nurses in Japan (1885–1889). Upon her return to the United States, she

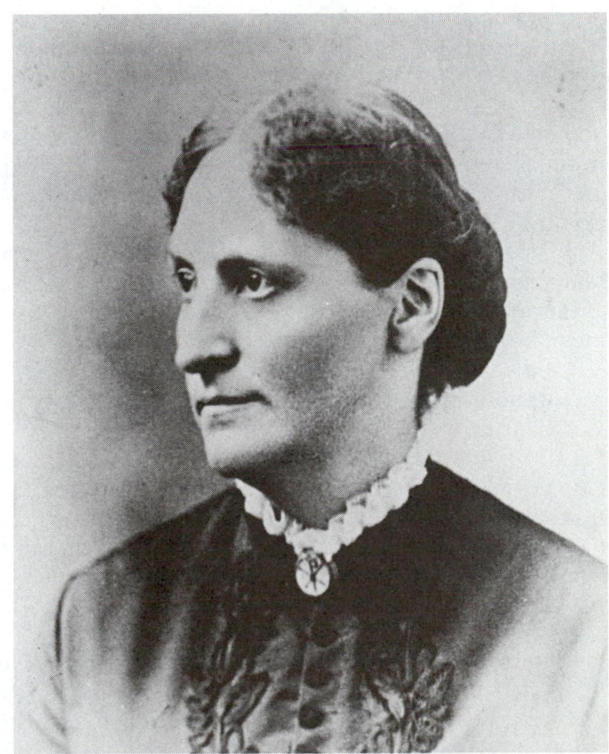

FIGURE 2–6
Linda Richards (1891–1930). (Courtesy of the National Library of Medicine, Bethesda, MD.)

became Superintendent of Nurses at the New England Hospital for Women and Children. She subsequently held similar positions at Brooklyn Homeopathic Hospital, Hartford Hospital, and the University of Pennsylvania Hospital (Dolan et al, 1983).

Along with Dr. Edward A. Cowles and Mary Palmer, Linda Richards planned the curriculum for the McLean Training School for Nurses established at the McLean Asylum (later the McLean Hospital) in 1882; the opening of the McLean Training School is considered by many to mark the beginning of modern psychiatric nursing (Sutton, 1986). During the latter years of her outstanding career, Miss Richards was Superintendent of Nurses at Tauton Insane Hospital (1899–1903), Worcester Hospital for the Insane (1903–1906), and the Michigan Insane Hospital (1906–1909). She reorganized or established training schools for nurses at these hospitals, believing that such educational programs were a necessity. She observed that better care for patients in the state hospitals could only be accomplished by better training for the nurses who worked there (Richards, 1911). Miss Richards contended that "It stands to reason that the mentally sick should be at least as well cared for as the physically sick" (p. 108). She believed that the two essential qualities for a good psychiatric nurse were patience and tact and that both of these qualities could be developed as the individual gained experience in the care of the mentally ill.

Former students of Miss Richards described her as kind, enthusiastic, just, and intelligent, with a sense of humor. She had a vigorous personality and was loved by the patients. Doona, a contemporary psychiatric nurse and author, observed that "Richards' kindness and gentleness in caring for the mentally ill proved what the new nursing could do" (1984, p. 56). When Sophia Palmer (first editor) and Mary E. P. Davis (first business manager), both former students of Linda Richards, established the *American Journal of Nursing* in 1900, they honored her by "presenting her with the first share of stock in the American Journal of Nursing Company" (Doona, 1984, p. 53).

Harriet Bailey (1875–1953). The first psychiatric nursing textbook, *Nursing Mental Diseases*, was authored by **Harriet Bailey,** B.S., R.N., a nurse educator and pioneer in psychiatric nursing (Church and Buckwalter, 1980). This textbook was published in 1920 by Macmillan as a clothbound book priced at $1.60. This publication was in print through the fourth edition done by Bailey in 1939. Church and Buckwalter report that the book went out of print in 1954, but this publication had been the standard textbook on mental nursing for 20 years. In the preface of the book, Miss Bailey stated that the text came about because colleagues had requested that she put her lecture notes together for reference use (Bailey, 1920). In the third edition (1935), the content had been noticeably expanded to 22 chapters, compared with 13 chapters in the original edition.

During her noteworthy career, Miss Bailey held the position of Assistant Superintendent of Nurses at the Henry Phipps Psychiatric Clinic of Johns Hopkins Hospital in Baltimore and Superintendent of Nurses at Manhattan State Hospital in New York, as well as other prominent responsibilities in nursing. As a psychiatric nurse educator and leader in nursing, Miss Bailey urged that the education of nurses include the teaching of mental health nursing. Church and Buckwalter credit Miss Bailey with being "one of psychiatric nursing's pioneers" and state that she "championed the cause of psychiatric nursing education above all others" in endeavoring to advance the respectability of psychiatric nursing (1980, p. 60).

Euphemia "Effie" Jane Taylor (1874–1970). Euphemia Jane Taylor directed the course in psychiatric nursing offered at the Johns Hopkins Hospital, where she was appointed as the first Director of Nursing Services at the Henry Phipps Psychiatric Clinic in 1913. Throughout her distinguished career, Miss Taylor (Figure 2–7) was a proponent for the inclusion of the content of psychiatric nursing in the nurses' educational program. Miss Taylor joined the faculty of the Yale School of Nursing in 1923 and assisted the first dean of the school, Annie W. Goodrich, in founding the new university school. (The Yale School of Nursing was the first autonomous university-based school of nursing having its own independent budget.) Miss Taylor succeeded Annie Goodrich, becoming the second Dean of the School of Nursing, a position she occupied for 10 years until 1944 when she

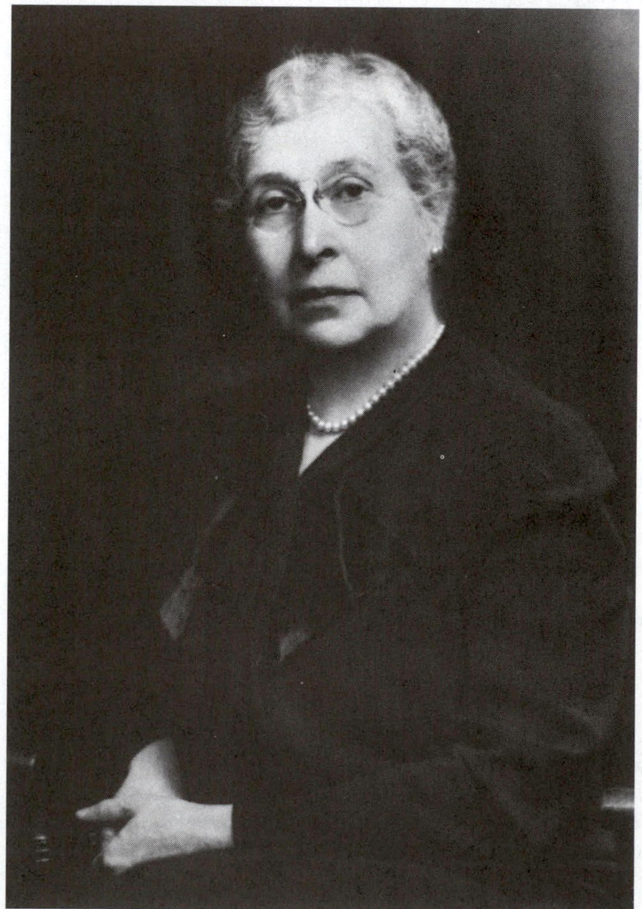

FIGURE 2–7
Euphemia "Effie" Jane Taylor (1874–1970). (Courtesy of the National Library of Medicine, Bethesda, MD.)

retired. Effie Taylor was the first psychiatric nurse to be designated Professor of Nursing when she was thus appointed in 1926. At that time, Annie Goodrich observed that Ms. Taylor possibly was the only professor of psychiatric nursing in the world (Dolan et al, 1983).

Miss Taylor was Superintendent of Nurses at the New Haven Hospital for 11 years. In 1937, Effie Taylor was elected President of the International Council of Nurses, a position she subsequently held for 10 years, including the crucial years during World War II. Buckwalter and Church (1979) observed that Effie Taylor "maintained a strong personal commitment to psychiatric nursing" (p. 125). At the American Nurses' Association (ANA) Convention on June 13, 1986, Effie J. Taylor was inducted into the ANA Nursing Hall of Fame as a "suffragette pioneer in the field of psychiatric nursing" (Convention Preview, 1986, p. 36). *"The history of Miss Taylor's many contributions to nursing provides an inspiring example of a humanitarian and nurse, who had a great impact on the development of her profession—nationally, internationally, and specifically in the field of psychiatric nursing"* (Buckwalter and Church, 1979, p. 131).

Harry Stack Sullivan (1892–1949). Harry Stack Sullivan, M.D., emphasized the significance of interpersonal relationships. He considered mental illness to be the result of disturbances in relationships beginning in early childhood or even infancy. His treatment approach focused on the restoration of effectiveness in communication and the growth of interpersonal relationships. His perspective, the Interpersonal Theory of Psychiatry, has made a significant contribution to the education and practice of many disciplines. Nurses found the components of this viewpoint applicable to nursing practice, and the basic tenets of this psychiatric perspective became a substantial framework for the subsequent focus on interpersonal relationships in nursing. Dr. **Hildegard E. Peplau's** classic publication, *Interpersonal Relations in Nursing* (1952), translated Dr. Sullivan's interpersonal perspective into a language that nurses could understand and utilize in their practice.

William Menninger (1899–1966). William Menninger, M.D., established a one-year postgraduate course in psychiatric nursing at the Menninger Hospital in Topeka, Kansas in 1932. Dr. Menninger recognized that psychiatric nursing was important in the patient's treatment and chances for recovery (Hall, 1967). Dr. Menninger was the 75th president of the American Psychiatric Association and served as Director of the Neuropsychiatric Consultants Division, Office of the Surgeon General during World War II.

▶ Check Your Reading

4. What is Phillippe Pinel credited with having done?
5. What did William Tuke do at the York Retreat?
6. Name America's first trained psychiatric nurse.
7. What is the name of the first psychiatric training school?
8. What was the title of the first psychiatric nursing textbook, and who wrote it?
9. Who was the first professor of psychiatric nursing?
10. What did Clifford Beers write?
11. What was the major contribution made to psychiatry by Emil Kraepelin?
12. Dorothy Lynde Dix was a crusader during which war?
13. Who is attributed with inventing the "tranquilizing chair?"
14. Dr. Harry Stack Sullivan is credited with a theory about what?
15. Dr. Hildegard Peplau wrote a psychiatric nursing textbook dealing with what topic?

CHANGING SETTINGS FOR MENTAL HEALTH CARE

The mentally ill have been "housed" or cared for in a variety of settings. Sister Charles Marie, a former dean of Catholic University's School of Nursing and a nursing historian, described the progression of settings in this way:

> *Originally hospitals functioned as shelters for the sick poor. In the latter part of the nineteenth century many state hospitals for the mentally ill were founded and poor farms were established. . . . Seriously ill mental patients who were judged dangerous to society were imprisoned, less harmful persons were allowed to roam about at will. Little thought was given to treatment, rehabilitation or prevention.*
>
> *(Frank, 1959, pp. 151,152)*

Throughout history, the settings for the care of the mentally ill have ranged from jails to **almshouses** to **asylums** and to private and **public mental hospitals.** The quality of the settings, including the hospitals, has varied greatly. One of the most famous hospitals—perhaps *infamous* is a better description—is the **Bethlehem Hospital** in London (Figure 2–8).

In the 16th century, King Henry VIII dedicated this facility as a lunatic asylum. By the 18th century, deterioration had reached a dreadful point, and the facility became known as the notorious "Bedlam" (Figure 2–9). The attendants, or keepers of the patients, were allowed to exhibit the boisterous patients for two pence (or one penny) a look. The more harmless patients were used to seek charity on the streets of London. In his writing of King Lear, Shakespeare referred to these individuals as the "Bedlam Beggars" (Bailey, 1935, p. 3).

In Colonial America, the prevailing attitude toward the mentally ill was anything but scientific. Many abuses were accorded to those whose illnesses were poorly understood. However, some had a more enlightened view toward the mentally ill. Through the efforts of Benjamin Franklin, patriot, inventor, and humanitarian statesman, the **Pennsylvania Hospital** in Philadelphia was founded. This hospital became the first general hospital to provide care for the mentally ill in the United States. In 1885 when the first two patients were admitted, one of them was identified as a "lunatic" (Noyes and Haydon, 1948, p. 360).

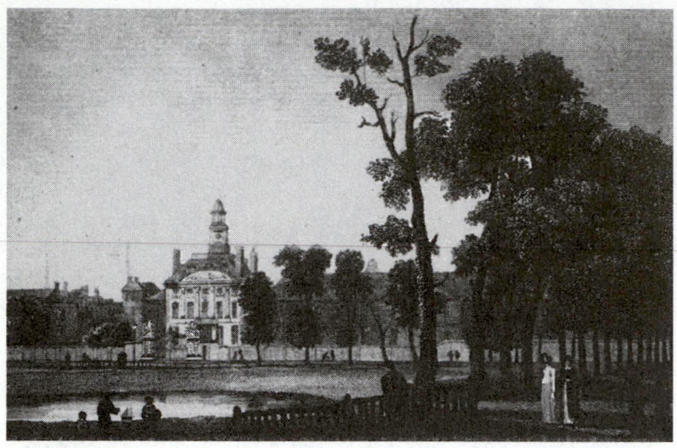

FIGURE 2–8
Bethlehem Hospital, London. (Courtesy of the National Library of Medicine, Bethesda, MD.)

Notable reformers such as Phillippe Pinel in France and William Tuke in England (both previously discussed) represented a humanitarian perspective. The influence of these men was not limited to Europe. Their ideas reached across the ocean and influenced a Baltimore businessman, Moses Sheppard (1775–1857). Mr. Sheppard, acquainted with the endeavors of Mr. Tuke, a fellow Quaker, in England, sought to provide for the mentally ill through his financial bequest, which was used to establish the Sheppard Asylum. The first patient was admitted to this asylum in 1891. The asylum further benefitted from a substantial bequest from the estate of Enoch Pratt. Mr. Pratt's donation carried with it a stipulation to the Board of Trustees that his name be incorporated into the name of the hospital. Therefore, the asylum's name was changed to the Sheppard and Enoch Pratt Hospital, which has carried on the humanitarian traditions of Moses Sheppard and Enoch Pratt for over 100 years (Forbush and Forbush, 1986; Figure 2–10).

As described earlier, the efforts of Dorothea Lynde Dix were instrumental in the establishment of numerous state mental hospitals during the 1880s. The care of the mentally ill remained within the purview of the state mental health systems until post World War II. At that time, legislation provided funding to include psychiatric units within general hospitals. This trend was furthered by a stipulation in the Community Mental Health Act of 1963 that stated that the services of a general hospital were considered to be incomplete if provisions were not made for the care of the mentally ill individual. More recently mobile treatment teams have provided care to the mentally ill, as have staff in Community Mental Health (CMH) Centers. For many, the patient's own home is becoming the preferred site for care as they receive psychiatric home care (see chapter 44). Day treatment hospitals and community rehabilitation programs are replacing inpatient hospitalization. Currently, the settings within the psychiatric care continuum provide the patient with many more alternatives for receiving care.

One of the most historic approaches for care has existed in Gheel, Belgium since 1851. In this community, mentally ill individuals reside in the family homes of residents of Gheel. They maintain some semblance of a "normal" life while seeing a psychiatrist on a regular basis.

Increasingly, nurses are venturing into private practice, either as solo practitioners or as members of a multidisciplinary group. In addition, psychiatric nurses are taking their skills into nontraditional settings such as schools, nursing homes, industry, and churches.

► Check Your Reading

16. Why is "Bedlam" famous?
17. What is the name of the hospital founded as a result of the efforts of Benjamin Franklin?
18. Why is Gheel, Belgium famous?
19. Name at least two alternative settings for psychiatric care outside of the inpatient unit.

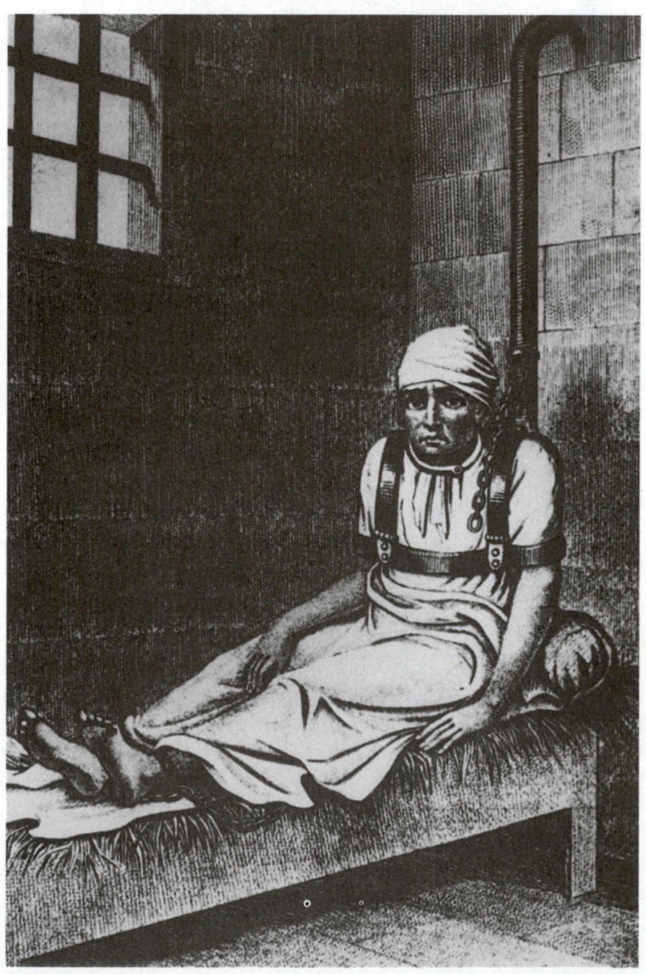

FIGURE 2–9
A patient, William Norris, in chains at "Bedlam," London's notorious Bethlehem Hospital. (Courtesy of the National Library of Medicine, Bethesda, MD.)

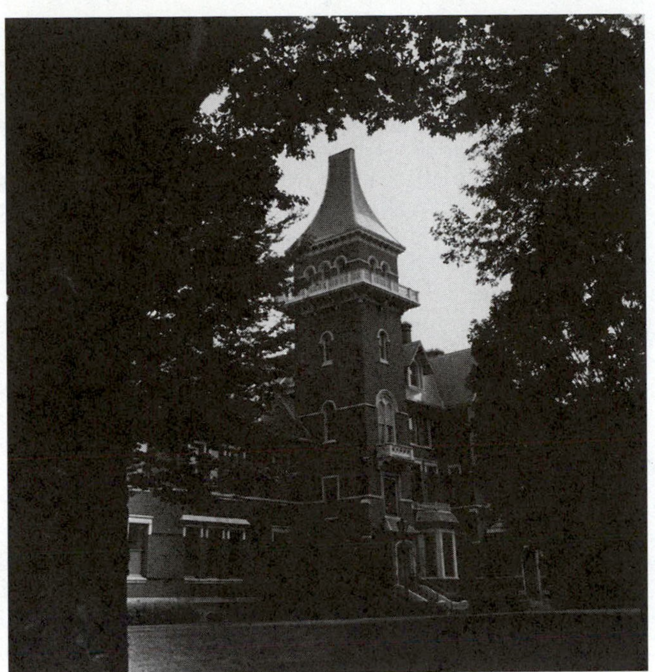

FIGURE 2–10
The Sheppard and Enoch Pratt Hospital, Towson, MD. (Photograph by Brian K. Glock. Courtesy of the Sheppard Pratt Health System, Towson, MD.)

THE INFLUENCE OF THE FIRST AND SECOND WORLD WARS ON MENTAL HEALTH CARE

Both World War I and World War II exposed the prevalence of mental illness, especially among the population of age for induction into military service. During World War I, between two and five percent of draftees were rejected because of psychiatric illness (Hall, 1967, p. 507). Many draftees who were inducted subsequently became ill during active duty in the armed forces. "Shell shock" was the term associated with the casualties of World War I. Later, during World War II, 14% of draftees were not eligible for military service because of psychiatric illness. The number of psychiatric casualties during World War II was even higher than those during World War I. Dr. Menninger reported the term "combat exhaustion" as a new mental illness associated with World War II (Hall, 1967, p. 510). Psychiatric services were overtaxed as casualties increased. Prominent psychiatrists of the time were enlisted to give leadership in the treatment of these patients. Dr. William C. Menninger, mentioned earlier, was one of those who served with distinction. He and others like him brought a special expertise to the treatment of mental illness throughout the military.

Meanwhile at home, conscientious objectors who declined active duty in the military served their equivalent of military service in some form of public service. Many of these individuals performed their service in the large public psychiatric hospitals. Their help was sorely needed because staffs in these facilities had been drastically diminished as personnel joined in wartime efforts in the military or in assembly plants. These newcomers to the psychiatric settings were exposed firsthand and for the first time to the dreadful conditions within these hospitals. They were horrified at the undesirable conditions of neglect, overcrowding, and the paucity of treatment (Sareyan, 1994). Not content to ignore or do nothing about these conditions, many put their observations in print in local newspapers and magazines. These writings, along with publications such as *The Shame of the States*, written by Albert Deutsch (1948), exposed the existing conditions and heightened the awareness of the public to what was phrased by one as "out of sight, out of mind" (Wright, 1947, p. 20). A novel, *The Snake Pit*, written by Mary Jane Ward (1946) and subsequently made into a motion picture by the same name, depicted similar deplorable conditions.

▶ Check Your Reading

20. What influence did World Wars I and II have on the treatment of mental illness?
21. What public service did conscientious objectors perform during wartime?
22. What was the impact of *The Shame of the States*, written by Albert Deutsch?

THE INFLUENCE OF LEGISLATION ON MENTAL HEALTH CARE

The National Mental Health Act of 1946. Following World War II, the National Mental Health Act (July, 1946) was enacted by the United States Congress with the purpose of improving the mental health of the nation's people. Several significant provisions of this legislation were realized as funds were established for the training of personnel in the four core disciplines, identified as psychiatry, nursing, clinical psychology, and social work. From this legislative action, the National Institute of Mental Health was also established, and funds were allocated for research into the causes and treatment of mental illness.

The Hill-Burton Bill of 1946. In 1946, the Hospital Survey and Construction Act, also called the Hill-Burton Bill, became law. This bill provided federal funding to the states for the purpose of surveying health needs and planning and constructing hospitals and other health centers. The federal government paid one third of the cost for the survey and construction; the states assumed responsibility for the other two thirds.

The National Mental Health Act of 1955. The Joint Commission on Mental Illness and Health was established as a result of The National Mental Health Act of 1955. The report of this study group, *Action for Mental Health*, was published in 1961. This study highlighted mental illness as a number one public health problem.

Kathleen Black and Mary F. Liston were nurses who served on the multidisciplinary commission (*Action for Mental Health*, 1961).

The Mental Retardation Facilities and Community Mental Health Centers Construction Act of 1963. With the enthusiastic support of President John F. Kennedy, this legislation became a reality. The purpose of this bill was to facilitate the treatment of persons with mental illness within their communities. To do so, it is necessary

- To save the patient from debilitating effects of institutionalization
- To return him or her to home and community life as soon as possible
- Thereafter, to maintain him or her in the community as long as possible

Therefore, aftercare and rehabilitation are essential parts of all service to mental patients, and the various methods of achieving rehabilitation should be integrated into all forms of services, among them day hospitals, night hospitals, aftercare clinics, public health nursing services, foster family care, convalescent nursing homes, rehabilitation centers, work services, and expatient groups (Action for Mental Health, 1961).

The funding for community mental health (CMH) programs was extended once again in 1970. At this time, Congress, in response to the Joint Commission on the Mental Health of Children, which cited inadequate services for young people, specifically earmarked money to serve youth. In addition, funding was added for drug and alcohol services.

The Community Mental Health Center Amendment of 1975 (PL 94-63). By 1975, the federal government amended its original 1963 law and specified that CMH centers must provide 12 services to qualify for federal monies. In addition to the original five services, specialized services for children and the elderly, screening, aftercare, transitional housing, drug abuse services, and alcoholism treatment were required.

In 1977, President Jimmy Carter mandated a major reassessment of Mental Health needs. He established a 20-member President's Commission on Mental Health, which included a nurse, Martha Mitchell, who was the Chairperson of the American Nurses' Association (ANA), Division on Psychiatric and Mental Health Nursing Practice. In 1978, the *Report to the President of the President's Commission on Mental Health* was published and focused on strengthening the CMH system as the foundation for the mental health system. This would involve improving community support systems, continuing the phasing out of large public hospitals, establishing a center with a focus on primary prevention within the National Institute of Mental Health (NIMH), and improving the delivery of services to underserved and high-risk populations. The report also advocated other major changes in the delivery of mental health care. These suggestions included establishing national health insurance that included coverage for mental health; encouraging private insurance carriers to include mental health coverage (including outpatient departments) in their packages; providing funding to increase the number of mental health professionals, especially those who work with children, the elderly, and minorities; developing advocacy programs for the chronic mentally ill (CMI); protecting the rights of all persons in need of mental health services; increasing support for research related to mental health and illness; providing public health education to increase the public's understanding of mental health and illness; and centralizing the evaluation efforts of governmental agencies.

The Community Mental Health Systems Act of 1980. In 1980, the Community Mental Health Systems Act was passed. It was designed to implement the recommendations of the President's Commission on Mental Health and to coordinate the two-tiered mental health system that had evolved since the original 1963 legislation that mandated the establishment of CMH centers. The most severely disabled of the CMI still resided within state institutions; those who are less disabled used the services of the CMH centers. Virtually no coordination existed between these two systems. Consequently, patients "fell through the cracks" so to speak because of the lack of continuity and communication between the two tiers.

Omnibus Budget Reconciliation Act of 1982. The programs authorized by this legislation were to be implemented in 1982, but before this could occur, a significant retrenchment by the federal government occurred in terms of its responsibilities in the area of mental health. The 97th Congress essentially repealed the 1980 Community Mental Health Systems Act with the passage of the Reagan administration's Omnibus Budget Reconciliation Act (PL 97-35). This bill moved the authority and administration of mental health programs from NIMH to the individual states. Each state received a block grant to cover alcohol abuse, drug abuse, and mental health services. As of 1984, federal funding for CMH and other mental health care delivery programs was terminated. CMH centers are now mandated to provide only five essential services: outpatient care, partial hospitalization, 24-hour hospitalization and emergency care, consultation and education, and screening services. The continued existence of CHM centers is dependent upon state support, private funding, and ability to earn revenue.

The decade of the 1990s promises no dramatic federal funding projects for the care of the mentally ill. Proposed health care reform does not even promise parity of mental health benefits with other health benefits. The political climate seems to support "smaller" rather than "bigger" when it comes to programs directed at meeting human needs. With so many programs competing for limited funds, the challenge of the mental health system is to try to do more with less.

The Americans with Disabilities Act of 1990. Most recently, the federal government mandated the elimination of discrimination against those with disabilities (which included those with a mental illness) with the passage of the Americans with Disabilities Act of 1990.

▶ **Check Your Reading**

23. What was the name of the bill passed in 1946? What impact did it have on issues of mental health?
24. For what purpose did the Hill-Burton Bill provide funding?
25. What was the purpose of the Community Mental Health Act of 1963?
26. What does the Americans with Disabilities Bill protect?

THE INFLUENCE OF PSYCHOBIOLOGICAL TREATMENT ON MENTAL HEALTH CARE

Throughout history, those involved in the treatment of mental illness and care of those afflicted with these illnesses have been attempting to use various somatic therapies, ranging from the tranquilizing chair to electroconvulsive therapy (ECT) to psychotropic drugs and to diet therapy. In 1938, as an alternative to the inducement of convulsion by drugs (e.g., Metrazol), two Italian psychiatrists, Dr. Ugo Cerletti and Dr. Lucio Bini, established electric shock therapy. Although at times this treatment, now termed ECT, has been criticized, it remains a valuable treatment for many individuals, particularly those suffering from depression.

The synthesis of chlorpromazine in December, 1950 by a French drug firm was one of the first cases of what would become the major treatment mode for mental illness worldwide. This medication was introduced in the United States in 1954 (The introduction of chlorpromazine, 1976; Swazey, 1974). A growing number of antipsychotic, antidepressant, antimania, and antianxiety medications have since been widely utilized to help reduce the need for hospitalization and to generally improve the quality of life for those afflicted with mental illnesses. This has made a tremendous impact on the nation. James Howe, a past president of the National Alliance for the Mentally Ill, observed that in the 16 years following the introduction of lithium, a drug used to control mood swings, this medication was credited with saving over 17 billion dollars. The continuing addition of new medications to treat the symptoms of serious mental illnesses have brought new hope and relief to the thousands who suffer from the painful consequences of mental illness.

▶ **Check Your Reading**

27. What was the name of the first antipsychotic drug introduced?
28. What is ECT?
29. What was the nationality of the doctors who invented ECT?
30. What is the effect of the drug lithium?

THE INFLUENCE OF DEINSTITUTIONALIZATION ON MENTAL HEALTH CARE

During the 1960s, an enthusiastic and extensive process of moving individuals from the **public mental hospitals** to the community was undertaken. This process of deinstitutionalization drastically reduced the numbers of patients who were hospitalized. For example, 552,150 patients were in the large public psychiatric hospitals in 1955 compared with only 109,939 patients in 1985 (Torrey, 1993). The state of Vermont was exemplary in the organized planning of the transition of individuals from the hospital to the community. In this state, their "pioneering rehabilitation program" was unusual because community support was present when the process of deinstitutionalization was put into effect (Harding et al, 1987). However, few other states can report such successful transitions. As a result, many of the mentally ill now live on the streets of our nation. Torrey (1993) reported that one third of the homeless are mentally ill. The *NAMI Advocate* reported in the March/April 1991 issue that "on any given day, the Los Angeles County Jail routinely houses 700 more people with mental illness than does the largest public mental hospital in the country, Pilgrim State in New York . . . Across America, one-third more mentally ill individuals reside in jails than in mental hospitals" (p. 1). Hatfield (1987) has observed that the family has become the prominent caregiver for the mentally ill. For an untold number of others, there simply are no caregivers.

▶ **Check Your Reading**

31. What has been the impact of deinstitutionalization on state mental hospitals?
32. What has been the impact of deinstitutionalization on communities?

THE INFLUENCE OF INTERPERSONAL RELATIONSHIPS ON MENTAL HEALTH CARE

As a result of the benefits derived from the new psychiatric medications given in the 1950s, many patients, for the first time, became able to engage in interpersonal relationships with psychiatrists, nurses, and others, which opened up new possibilities for their recovery. The responsibilities and activities of the psychiatric nurse were now expanded. The central focus of nursing literature, nursing conferences, and nursing education in the 1950s and 1960s increasingly became the nurse-patient relationship. Manfreda (1982, p. xi), a psychiatric nurse and author, said:

> *The development of interpersonal nursing marked an important milestone in American nursing. From the procedure oriented, to the more involved process of interaction, the emphasis shifted to the Nurse-Patient Relationship.*

Manfreda credited the contributions of anthropologists, psychiatrists, psychologists, and social scientists for their work establishing the roots of interpersonal nursing and wrote of the inspirational practice and writings of the nursing leaders in the 1930s. For example, she noted Helena Render's 1937 description of nurse-patient interaction recordings as a teaching method (Manfreda, 1982). Some of the other psychiatric nurses who also were authors included in Manfreda's historical discussion of the roots of interpersonal nursing were Olga Weiss, Elizabeth Bixler Torrey, Hildegard Peplau, Sister Kathleen Black, and Gwen Tudor Will.

Psychiatric nursing leaders emerged as authors of significant publications. A classic reference in psychiatric nursing was *Interpersonal Relations in Nursing* (1952) by Hildegard E. Peplau. O'Toole and Welt (1989) report that Dr. Peplau had completed her work on this book in 1948, but "it was not published until four years later because it was considered too revolutionary for a nurse to publish such a book without a physician as coauthor" (p. xviii). Box 2–2 tells Hildegard Peplau's story.

During the 1960s, other psychiatric nurses who were authors further contributed to the understanding of nurse-patient relationships. *The Dynamic Nurse-Patient Relationship: Function, Process and Principles* (1961) was authored by Ida Jean Orlando. Orlando's book, which focused on the needs of the patient and on the nurses' deliberative intervention (nursing process), became another classic publication. Joyce Travelbee, a student of Ida Orlando, later wrote another influential publication, *Interpersonal Aspects of Nursing*, first published in 1966. Another contribution to the literature was *Nurse-Patient Communication* by Garland K. Lewis (1973).

At the 1958 annual convention of the American Nurses' Association, the 16-mm film "Psychiatric Nursing: The Nurse-Patient Relationship" was premiered

BOX 2-2 Hildegard Peplau: A Pioneer Nursing Leader and Theorist in Psychiatric Nursing

Hildegard Peplau was born in 1909 in Reading, Pennsylvania. She began her nursing journey in the late 1920s as a student at the Pottstown Hospital School of Nursing in Pennsylvania. In her earliest professional years, she assumed positions in general and private duty nursing, operating room supervision and instruction, and college health. Dr. Peplau returned to school at Bennington College to pursue a bachelor's degree in interpersonal psychology. Her field experiences in her program of study and particularly her experiences at the Bellevue Hospital in New York City exposed her to many notable and influential psychiatric leaders of the time, including Dr. Lauretta Bender, Dr. Frieda Fromm-Reichman, and Dr. Harry Stack Sullivan. These significant experiences and relationships greatly influenced her thinking and outlook on psychiatric nursing.

During World War II, Dr. Peplau served in the Army Nurse Corps, both stateside and overseas. Here, she was once again introduced to many new and innovative psychiatric practices. Following World War II, Dr. Peplau studied at Teachers College, Columbia University, where she received her graduate degree in psychiatric nursing (and later her doctorate in education). The program in psychiatric nursing included lectures by prominent nurses including Mrs. Laura Fitzsimmons, then Psychiatric Nurse Consultant to the American Psychiatric Association. Field work included experiences at the New York State Psychiatric Institute, Columbia-Presbyterian Hospital, New York City. Her final examination was to demonstrate a wet sheet pack.

During these years of practice, Dr. Peplau observed many psychiatric nursing practices that today would be considered highly unusual. For example, nurses were considered to be custodians of patients. Families were excluded from the patient care experience and discouraged from visiting. Patients were considered to be hospital property and were often used to do the maintenance work within the hospital, including grounds-keeping, farming, and cooking. The most chronically ill patients were housed in back wards. Electric shock therapy (ECT), insulin therapy, lobotomy, and hydrotherapy were common treatments employed in the care of the mentally ill. Wards were often in a state of disrepair, with broken furniture, poor lighting, and chipped and peeling paint. Privileges were given to the more docile, agreeable, or entertaining patients. Such privileges included securing a desirable bed location near the radiator in winter or obtaining extra food. Restraints and seclusion rooms were commonly used to manage disruptive behavior.

During World War II, society evidenced a major change in attitude towards the mentally ill, as the number of psychiatric casualties from the war escalated. Dr. Peplau saw the passage of the Mental Health Act in 1946 as a major milestone for change in the practice of psychiatry. Dr. Peplau taught in the graduate program in psychiatric nursing at Teachers College (1948–1952) and later at Rutgers University in New Jersey (1954–1974). Funding through the Mental Health Act paid her salary. Dr. Peplau recalls that one nurse even called her "the kept woman of the government."

Changes in Dr. Peplau's professional practice mirrored changes in the field of psychiatric nursing. Her well known classic text *Interpersonal Relations in Nursing*, published in 1952, espouses her theory of nursing as a therapeutic, psychodynamic, interpersonal process and affirms the importance of the nurse-patient relationship as a therapeutic and educative instrument in the care of the mentally ill. In 1958, she initiated her own private practice in New York City and evolved her own approach to psychotherapy.

Dr. Peplau sees nursing as a rapidly changing profession, increasing in scope and complexity. While the biomedicalization of psychiatry, the emphasis on pharmacotherapy, and the proliferation of genetic and brain studies on mental illness causation are important advances, Dr. Peplau affirms that it is the human, interpersonal process that should be the major domain for nursing research, theory development, and practice. She states "Psychiatric problems are, in the main, problems of persons—not primarily of their biology or physiology" (Peplau, 1982; 1982a; Personal communication, 1991).

(*ANA in Review*, 1958, p. 2). The film was produced by the American Nurses' Association (ANA) and the National League for Nursing in cooperation with the Mental Health Education Unit of Smith, Kline and French Laboratories (1958) (who marketed the antipsychotic medication Thorazine [chlorpromazine]). The filming took place on the grounds of the New Jersey State Hospital at Greystone Park, with a nursing student portraying a withdrawn patient, "Trudy," who benefits from the nurse-patient relationship, as does the nurse working with Trudy. She learns from the recording and analysis of her nurse-patient interactions. The enduring worth of this fine production has been insured by its current availability on videotape.

Today, psychiatric nursing educators continue to assign to students the recording and subsequent analysis of their nurse-patient interactions. Thus, as noted by Manfreda (1982), the interpersonal aspects of nursing continue the perspective taught us by Miss Nightingale.

▶ Check Your Reading

33. What impact did the use of psychotropic medications have on the practice of psychiatric nursing?
34. What is the movie "Psychiatric Nursing: The Nurse-Patient Relationship" about?

THE INFLUENCE OF NURSING PROFESSIONALIZATION ON MENTAL HEALTH CARE

In 1892, Isabel Adams Hampton (later Isabel Hampton Robb) wrote about her vision for the professionalization of nursing. In Miss Hampton's textbook, *Nursing Ethics* (1901, pp. 35, 36), she wrote:

The trained nurse, then, is no longer to be regarded as a better trained, more useful, higher class servant, but as one who has knowledge and is worthy of respect, consideration and due recompense. . . . She is also essentially an instructor; part of her duties have to do with the prevention of disease and sickness, as well as the relief of suffering humanity... These are some of the essentials in nursing by which it has become to be regarded as a profession, but there still remains much to be desired, much to work for, in order to add to its dignity and usefulness. As the standard of education and requirements become a higher character and the training more efficient, the trained nurse will draw nearer to science and its demands and take a greater share as a social factor in solving the world's needs.

Although Mrs. Robb alludes to certain defining characteristics of a profession, for further definition it is valuable to examine the work of Abraham Flexner, who in 1915 identified the criteria by which a profession is to be judged. In the 80 years since Flexner wrote his criteria, other models have been proposed that also provide logical characteristics by which to evaluate a profession. However, Flexner's criteria are still relevant to current practice. Becker (1970) cites Flexner's criteria as including the following:

1. Professional activity is basically intellectual with great personal responsibility.
2. It is based on great knowledge, not routine activities.
3. It is practical rather than theoretical.
4. It has a technique that can be taught, which is the basis for professional education.
5. It is organized internally.
6. It is motivated by altruism, with members working for some aspect of the good of society.

Critically examining each of these criteria allows us to come to a conclusion about the status of all of nursing as a profession and also the status of psychiatric nursing as a professional specialty within nursing. Some of Flexner's criteria, for instance criteria 2 and 4, give rise to debate among nurses. For example, although nurses recognize that education is a requirement to be a nurse, the debate centers around how much preparation constitutes a professional level. Is the Associate Degree graduate a professional? What about the nurse who has earned a diploma? And, in psychiatric nursing those questions become even more critical because significant differences in the amount of time devoted to mental health and illness content exist across differing educational programs.

Few nurses would argue with the essential quality of the first criterion. Certainly in psychiatric nursing, nurses are confronted with situations that require a great deal of thinking and analysis. The answers to "why" a patient acts in a certain way or "what" will change that behavior can not be memorized, but must be reflected upon. Criterion 3 is accepted without question in nursing. Nursing has always defined itself as a practice profession, which means that theory is gained to enhance practice. Within psychiatric nursing, psychiatric nurse leaders are calling for those in the field to conduct research that is outcome oriented so that nurses can demonstrate the effectiveness of various nursing interventions (McBride, 1986). Criterion 5, which deals with internal organization is certainly true of both nursing as a whole and psychiatric nursing as a specialty. We have professional organizations that provide internal organization, the American Nurses' Association (ANA) provides organization to the profession as a whole, the National League for Nursing (NLN) provides internal organization to nursing education, and the Society for Education and Research in Psychiatric-Mental Health Nursing (SERPN) and the American Psychiatric Nurses Association (APNA) provide organization for the specialty of psychiatric nursing. We have standards of practice for the whole body of nursing as well as standards of practice for the specialty of psychiatric nursing. The ANA Statement on Psychiatric Nursing was first formulated in 1963, and in 1994, the Standards of Psychiatric and Mental Health Nursing Practice were revised. The ANA's Code of Ethics serves as another internal organizer and is applicable to the whole body of nursing practice.

The last criterion, which deals with altruistic motivation, is one that hardly needs defense in any nursing specialty. The whole thrust of nursing practice is to alleviate suffering of the individual, family, or larger group. Because most nurses will never become rich from

BOX 2-3 The National Alliance for the Mentally Ill: The Story of a Self-Help Organization

The National Alliance for the Mentally Ill (NAMI) is a national self-help organization devoted to providing support to the families of the mentally ill, promoting public education and research on mental illness, advocating on behalf of the mentally ill, and providing information and referral services. NAMI was organized by families affected by mental illness who wished to promote public understanding of the needs of the mentally ill and to improve social conditions for their mentally ill loved ones. In 1967, Charles and Harriet Shetler of Madison, Wisconsin, shattered by the diagnosis of schizophrenia in their 18-year-old son and feeling blamed by mental health professionals for his illness, began meeting with other families who had similar experiences. They sought mutual support and understanding from one another and fought for improved mental health services in their community. In 1979, Harriet Shetler and the members of her group began to pull together similar support groups throughout the nation. They invited persons from across the country to meet with them. From this meeting, it became evident that a united voice was needed to strengthen their position and to ultimately effect needed social change on a national level (McClory, 1986). From this initial assembly of self-help groups, the National Alliance movement began.

To a great extent, NAMI's strength and influence is derived from the personal experience with mental illness represented in its membership. The fundamental tenets of NAMI include the belief that mental illness is a biological disease process and not a result of dysfunctional family relationships. Rather than being viewed as the cause of mental illness, the family is seen as central to the support and treatment of the mentally ill member. In addition, laypersons are viewed as integral to the success and leadership of the organization (Hatfield, 1991). James Howe, past President of the National Alliance, is himself the father of a son suffering from chronic mental illness. NAMI has now grown to encompass more than 140,000 members and 1100 affiliate chapters nationwide (*NAMI Fact Sheet*, 1991).

The National Alliance for the Mentally Ill is a respected movement in the psychiatric community. In fact, Dr. E. Fuller Torrey, renowned psychiatrist, has proclaimed NAMI "the most important thing to happen for people with schizophrenia since antipsychotic drugs were introduced in the 1950's" (McClory, 1986, p. 19).

For more information about NAMI, write or call:

National Alliance for the Mentally Ill
200 North Glebe Road
Suite 1015
Arlington, VA 22203

1-800-950-NAMI

nursing remuneration, one must ask why else do nurses do what they do, if not to make a difference in society.

As a specialty within nursing, psychiatric nurses have a unique body of knowledge. This was first recognized with the establishment in 1943 of the first university program in psychiatric nursing at the Catholic University of America. In 1967, a clinical focus in psychiatric nursing was included for doctoral students at the Catholic University of America when the Doctorate in Nursing Science was initiated.

Earlier in this chapter, readers were reminded of the first psychiatric nursing textbook. Another publication worthy of mention is *Essentials of Psychiatric Nursing* (Taylor, 1994). This publication was first copyrighted in 1940 and has continued in print in 1994.

Among the current authors who are identified as nursing theorists are several psychiatric nurses; Joyce Fitzpatrick, Madeline Leininger, Betty M. Neuman, Ida Jean Orlando, Hildegard E. Peplau, Joyce Travelbee, Loretta T. Zderad, and Josephine G. Patterson are all credited with a theoretical contribution to nursing (Fordyce, 1988).

Specialized psychiatric nursing journals have made their appearance since 1963 with the initial publication of the *Journal of Psychiatric Nursing* (since 1981 it has been called *Journal of Psychosocial Nursing and Mental Health Services*) and *Perspectives of Psychiatric Care. Archives of Psychiatric Nursing* was introduced in 1987. (The first issue of the *American Psychiatric Nurses Association* was introduced in February, 1995.)

Another significant event in the specialty occurred with the development of the ANA Certification Program (1979). Two levels of certification were established, one for the generalist and one for the specialist.

▶ Check Your Reading

35. Where was the first university program in psychiatric nursing established?
36. Who wrote the first edition of *Essentials of Psychiatric Nursing?*
37. What are the two levels of certification established by the ANA Certification Program?

THE INFLUENCE OF FAMILY ADVOCACY ON MENTAL HEALTH CARE

The 1980s and 1990s have increasingly been characterized by the voices of consumers and families. The founding of the National Alliance of the Mentally Ill (NAMI) in 1979 brought families together for needed support. The membership of this remarkable organization has grown at an amazing rate, making it the fastest growing advocacy group in the United States. Its members have become effective crusaders for expanded resources and for improvements in existing resources for those who are mentally ill. They are also a valuable source of support for family members of the mentally ill (Jones, 1992; Box 2–3).

▶ Check Your Reading

38. What is NAMI?

THE "DECADE OF THE BRAIN"

By presidential proclamation, the 1990s have been designated the "Decade of the Brain." President George Bush signed the proclamation on July 17, 1990 upon the recommendation of the United States Congress, Joint Resolution 174. The joint cooperative efforts of public and federal government programs to study the brain with the hope of conquering brain diseases in the decade beginning with January 1, 1990 is the goal of this endeavor.

A former director of the National Institute of Mental Health, Lewis L. Judd, M.D., reported that because of the progress in neuroscience, 90% of the knowledge about the brain had been learned in the 10 years of 1980 to 1990 (Judd, 1990). The new tools of technology such as magnetic resonance imaging (MRI), positron emission tomography (PET), and computed tomography (CT) have provided researchers the "microscope" needed to view the brain structure and function. Brain abnormalities are being identified that are associated with several of the serious mental illnesses.

Lowery has urged that "psychiatric mental health nursing will need to take stock of itself—its practice, its education, and its research—if it is to successfully prepare for the changes in care of the mentally ill" (1992, p. 13). Lowery and other psychiatric nursing leaders are urging that, as attention is focused on the biochemical components of illness and treatment, interpersonal and psychosocial needs continue to receive the appropriate level of attention. Many challenges await psychiatric nurses now and in the future.

In *Healthy People 2000* (US Department of Health and Human Services, 1992) national health promotion and disease prevention objectives for the year 2000 that are associated with psychiatric nursing practice are a 10% reduction in suicide rates and an 18% reduction in adverse effects of stress. Additional objectives include a 15% reduction in homicide rates and a 10% decrease in assault injuries. Other goals address reducing the prevalence of mental disorders, increasing treatment for those with major depressive disorders, and increasing utilization of community support and employee mental health programs. It is also hoped that primary care providers will increase attention to the cognitive, emotional, and behavioral needs of their patients.

▶ Check Your Reading

39. What U.S. president declared the 1990s the "Decade of the Brain?"
40. What are the goals of *Healthy People 2000* that are appropriate for psychiatric nursing?
41. What do the acronyms *PET* and *MRI* mean?

CONCLUSIONS

The historical, social, political, and economic developments of the last century have carved the path and provided the inroads that have shaped the journey of psychiatric-mental health nursing practice. It is not surprising, then, that the future journey of psychiatric mental health nursing will be greatly influenced by the stories that are being lived out today by nursing leaders and practitioners, consumers, and all persons touched by mental illness. It is important for nurses to be involved in shaping the course of their destinies by developing an understanding of both the historical context in which their practice emerges and the present forces and future trends that are likely to shape and further define the position of psychiatric mental health nursing in the health care delivery system. The issues of homelessness, substance abuse, violence and human abuse, multiculturalism, and national health care reform will likely shape the course of psychiatric mental health nursing practice well into the next century. The psychiatric mental health nurse can be in an ideal position to address each of these issues through research, education, patient advocacy, and political action to insure that the path on which nursing journeys is well lit by knowledge, insight, and profound sensitivity for all persons who, in one way or another, have been touched by mental illness.

A CHRONOLOGY OF SIGNIFICANT EVENTS IN THE HISTORY OF MENTAL HEALTH NURSING

1751 Pennsylvania Hospital (Philadelphia) established through the efforts of Benjamin Franklin (this was the first hospital to make provisions for care of the "insane" as well as the physically ill)

1773 Eastern Lunatic Asylum in Williamsburg, Virginia established; this was the first public asylum (hospital) in the United States for persons of "insane or disordered minds"

1792 York Retreat in England founded by William Tuke

1792 Philippe Pinel in Paris, France removed the shackles from those held at the Bicêtre

1812 Publication of *Diseases of the Mind*, authored by Dr. Benjamin Rush, Philadelphia

1818 Founding of the McLean Asylum in Massachusetts

1841 Dorothea Lynde Dix volunteered at East Cambridge Jail as Sunday School teacher, thus embarking on a lifelong crusade for reform in the care of the mentally ill

1873 Linda Richards earns diploma as the first nurse to complete the one-year training program at New England Hospital

1881 First patient admitted to the Sheppard Asylum (Baltimore)

1882 Founding of the Training School for Nurses at the McLean Asylum, with the first graduates completing course of study in 1886

1900 Initial publication of the *American Journal of Nursing*

1908 Publication of *A Mind That Found Itself*, authored by Clifford W. Beers

1914–1918 World War I—psychiatric casualties of the war and shortage of nurses were evident

1920 Publication of *Nursing Mental Diseases*, authored by nurse educator Harriet Bailey

1926 Appointment of Effie J. Taylor as the first Professor of Psychiatric Nursing

1938 Introduction of electroconvulsive therapy (ECT), as devised by Dr. Cerletti and Dr. Bini in Italy

1939–1945 World War II, with a high toll of psychiatric casualties

1946 Publication of *The Shame of the States*, written by Albert Deutsch

National Mental Health Act passed by the U.S. Congress

Hill-Burton Bill passed by U.S. Congress

1949 National Institute of Mental Health established under the provisions of the National Mental Health Act of 1946

1947 Publication of *Nurse-Patient Relationships in Psychiatry*, authored by Helena Render

1952 Publication of *Interpersonal Relations in Nursing*, authored by Hildegard E. Peplau

1954 Advent of the utilization of the antipsychotic medication chlorpromazine (Thorazine), synthesized in France in 1950

1955 National Mental Health Study Act, which established the Joint Commission on Mental Illness and Health

1961 Publication of *Action for Mental Health*, final report of The Joint Commission on Mental Illness and Health

1963 Community Mental Health Centers Act passed by Congress

1963 Initial publication of the *Journal of Psychiatric Nursing*, Vols 1–4, 1963–1966; continued in 1967 as the *Journal of Psychiatric Nursing and Mental Health Services*

Initial publication of *Perspectives of Psychiatric Care*

1966 Enactment of the Medicare Bill

1973 *Standards of Psychiatric-Mental Health Nursing* published

Certification of Psychiatric-Mental Health Nurse Generalists established by the American Nurses' Association (ANA)

1979 American Nurses' Association established certification of psychiatric mental health nurse specialists

Founding of the National Alliance for the Mentally Ill (NAMI)

1982 Century Celebration of Psychiatric Nursing, Washington, D.C.

1987 Initial publication of *Archives of Psychiatric Nursing*

1990 Americans with Disabilities Act passed by the United States Congress

Presidential proclamation by George Bush declaring the 1990s the "Decade of the Brain"

KEY POINTS TO REMEMBER

- Hippocrates suggested that bodily humors were responsible for behaviors.
- In earliest recorded history, mental illness was attributed to the anger of the gods, the devil, or demon possession.
- Phillippe Pinel, a French psychiatrist, unchained mentally ill patients.
- William Tuke established the York Retreat in 1792. The York Retreat was a treatment facility for the mentally ill where kindness and a pleasant environment were viewed as essentials for healing.
- Benjamin Rush, the Father of American Psychiatry, published his book *Diseases of the Mind* in 1812. He advocated gentle and humane treatment for the mentally ill.
- Dorothea Lynde Dix crusaded for more humane treatment of the mentally ill by advocating that psychiatric hospitals be built from public funds.
- Emil Kraepelin developed the first comprehensive description of the mental disorders.
- Sigmund Freud developed his psychoanalytical theory of human behavior and the principles of psychoanalysis.
- Adolph Meyer, a professor at The Johns Hopkins University, was known for his psychobiological perspective.
- Clifford Beers, a former mental patient, wrote *A Mind That Found Itself*, a book that detailed his experiences as a patient.
- Linda Richards graduated in 1873 from the New England Training School and became America's First Trained Psychiatric Nurse.
- Harriet Bailey authored the first psychiatric nursing textbook, *Nursing Mental Diseases*, in 1920.
- Euphemia (Effie) J. Taylor was named the First Professor of Psychiatric Nursing at Yale University in 1926.
- Harry Stack Sullivan developed the Interpersonal Theory of Psychiatry.

- Hildegard Peplau took many of Sullivan's concepts and wrote them in a language that was understandable and useable to nurses in their practices.
- William Menninger started the first postgraduate school of psychiatric nursing in 1932.
- Over the course of centuries, as public opinion and knowledge about mental illness and the mentally ill waxed and waned, settings where the mentally ill have been cared for have ranged from almshouses, asylums, hospitals, community mental health (CMH) centers, mobile treatment teams, day hospitals, community rehabilitation centers, and private homes. The quality of these settings has also varied greatly.
- World Wars I and II focused attention on the large numbers of young men who were unable to serve in the military because of a preexisting psychiatric illness and the large numbers of young men who became psychiatrically disabled because of wartime conditions.
- Legislation, such as the National Mental Health Act, the Hill-Burton Bill, the Mental Retardation Facilities and Community Mental Health Centers Construction Act of 1963, the Community Mental Health Center Amendment in 1975, the Community Mental Health Systems Act, the Omnibus Budget Reconciliation Act, and the Americans with Disabilities Act of 1990 have all served to promote the delivery of care to the mentally ill, either through funding for education or research or through funding of construction for new facilities.
- Psychobiological therapies, including psychotropic drugs, have dramatically changed the practice of psychiatric nursing.
- Deinstitutionalization has reduced the number of chronically mentally ill patients residing in large state hospitals but has increased the numbers of patients who now live on the streets of our nation because of inadequate community resources to provide them with housing and care.
- Interpersonal relationships are a primary focus of psychiatric nursing practice.
- NAMI provides support for families who struggle to deal with a loved one who has a psychiatric illness.
- Research conducted during the Decade of the Brain will increase our understanding of the neurobiological influences on behavior and will shape the future journey of psychiatric nursing.

LEARNING ACTIVITIES

1. Interview several nurses to discover their stories. Why did they become nurses? What changes have they witnessed within the profession? In what direction do they see themselves journeying within the profession?

2. Go to the library and read at least one of the books mentioned in this chapter. Get a flavor of a particular historical time and place from the author's descriptions. (Suggested books: Clifford Beers, *A Mind That Found Itself;* Albert Deutsch, *Shame of the States;* Isabel Hampton, *Nursing Ethics;* A. Deutsch, *The Mentally Ill in America;* E. Tiffany, *The Life of Dorothea Lynde Dix;* or E. Fuller Torrey, *Nowhere to Go. The Tragic Odyssey of the Homeless Mentally Ill.*)

3. Set up a panel discussion with students portraying different historical figures. Have each character argue for the changes that she or he sees as essential to provide care for the mentally ill.

4. Begin to write your own story about why you chose nursing. As you journey through nursing as a student and later as a professional nurse, continue to make entries to your story. Over time you will be amazed at the patterns and themes as you weave the tapestry of your life's story.

5. Interview nurses from different educational backgrounds to determine what each believes about the qualifications of a professional. Ask each one if she or he sees herself or himself as a professional nurse. Ask for the reason behind the answer given.

CRITICAL THINKING EXERCISE

Ms. Fields, a junior nursing student, was writing a paper on the history of psychiatric nursing during her psychiatric-mental health nursing course. She decided to research the influence (if any) that Dr. Hildegard Peplau had on her current learning about psychiatric nursing. She began to write "Dr. Peplau was a pioneer in the development of psychiatric nursing. She wrote *Interpersonal Relations in Nursing* in 1952, in which she affirms the belief that nurses, through the use of the nurse-patient relationship can be therapeutic and educative instruments in the care of the mentally ill. Dr. Peplau believes that the human interpersonal process needs to be the major concern of the nurse's practice and that 'psychiatric problems . . . are problems of persons—not primarily of their biological or physiology' " (Peplau, 1952, 1991).

Ms. Fields continued to write: "Even though Dr. Peplau developed her theory on interpersonal relations in nursing in 1952, psychiatric nursing of today is still greatly influenced by Dr. Peplau's ideas. Although psychiatric nursing care has recently been influenced by the impact of biochemical and genetic knowledge, nursing must continue to recognize the importance of the interpersonal process."

1. As Ms. Fields wrote her paper on Dr. Peplau's influence on present day psychiatric nursing, what did she infer about Dr. Peplau's point of view?

2. What assumptions can we make about Ms. Fields' understanding of Dr. Peplau's point of view regarding present-day psychiatric nursing practice?

3. Does Ms. Fields present a precise, clear picture of Dr. Peplau's position?

1. What evidence does Ms. Fields present to support her assumptions about Dr. Peplau's point of view regarding psychiatric nursing?

2. What other information does Ms. Fields need to know to clarify her understanding of Dr. Peplau's ideas?

3. If you were to reason from Dr. Peplau's point of view about psychiatric nursing practice, what would you say about psychiatric nursing practice?

4. What other points of view might be considered when practicing psychiatric nursing?

REFERENCES

Action for mental health. Final Report of the Joint Commission on Mental Illness and Health 1961. New York: Basic Books Inc.

Alexander, F., and Selesnick, S. (1966). *The history of psychiatry.* New York: Harper & Row.

ANA in Review. (1958). Spring. Vol. VI, No. 1. New York: American Nurses' Association.

American Nurses' Association. (1994). *Standards of psychiatric and mental health nursing practice.* Kansas City: American Nurses' Association.

Bailey, H. (1920). *Nursing mental diseases.* New York: Macmillan.

Bailey, H. (1935). *Nursing mental diseases.* (3rd ed.). New York: Macmillan.

Baxter, W. E., and Hathcox, D. W. (1994). *America's care of the mentally ill: A photographic history.* Washington, D.C.: American Psychiatric Press.

Becker, H. (1970). *Sociological work: Method and substance.* Chicago: Adline.

Beers, C. (1908). *A mind that found itself.* New York: Doubleday.

Buckwalter, K. C., and Church, O. M. (1979). Euphemia Jane Taylor: An uncommon psychiatric nurse. *Perspectives in Psychiatric Care, XVIII,* (2), 62–66.

Convention Preview, Anaheim 86: Effie Taylor to Enter ANA Nursing Hall of Fame. (1986). *Journal of Psychosocial Nursing, 24* (5), May, 36.

Church, O. M. and Buckwalter, K. C. (1980). Harriet Bailey: A psychiatric nurse pioneer. *Perspectives in Psychiatric Care, 18* (2), March/April, 62–66.

Deutsch, A. (1948). *The shame of the states.* New York: Harcourt Brace & Company.

Deutsch, A. (1949). *The mentally ill in America.* (2nd ed.). New York: Columbia University Press.

Dolan, J., Fitzpatrick, M. L., and Herrmann, E. K. (1983). *Nursing in society: A historical perspective.* (15th ed.). Philadelphia: W. B. Saunders.

Donahue, M. P. (1985). *Nursing: the finest art.* St. Louis: C. V. Mosby.

Doona, M. E. (1984). At least as well cared for . . . Linda Richards and the mentally ill. *Image: The Journal of Nursing Scholarship, XVI,* (2), Spring, 51–56.

Fact sheet. (1991). National Alliance for the Mentally Ill, September.

Father Charles, quoted in Manfreda, M. L. (1982). *The roots of interpersonal nursing.* Cromwell: Cromwell Printing Company.

Flanigan, L. (1976). *One strong voice: The story of the American Nurses' Association.* Kansas City: American Nurses' Association.

Forbush, B., and Forbush, B. (1986). *Gatehouse: The evolution of the Sheppard and Enoch Pratt Hospital, 1853–1986.* Baltimore: The Sheppard and Enoch Pratt Hospital.

Fordyce, E. (1988). Theorists in nursing. In J. Flynn & P. Heffron (Eds.), *Nursing: From concept to practice* (2nd ed.). (pp 69–87). Norwalk: Appleton and Lange.

Forester, D. A., and Grandinetti, P. M. (1991). A distinguished history on postage stamps in nursing. *The American Philatelist,* 710–717.

Frank, C. M. (1959). *Foundations of nursing.* (2nd ed.). Philadelphia: W. B. Saunders.

Hall, B. H. (Ed.). (1967). *A psychiatrist for a troubled world.* New York: Viking Press.

Harding, C., Zubin, J., and Strauss, J. (1987). Chronicity in schizophrenia: Fact, partial fact, or artifact. *Hospital and Community Psychiatry, 38*(5), 479–491.

Hatfield, A. (1991). The national alliance for the mentally ill: A decade later. *Community Mental Health Journal, 27*(2), 95–103.

Hatfield, A., and Lefley, H. (Eds.). (1987). *Families of the mentally ill. Coping and adaptation.* New York: Guilford Press.

The introduction of chlorpromazine. (1976). *Hospital and Community Psychiatry, 27*(7), 505.

Jails: The new mental institutions. (1991). *NAMI Advocate, 12*(2), March/April, 1, 12.

Jones, S. (1992). The family as an advocate for the mentally ill. *Archives of Psychiatric Nursing, VI*(3), 145,146.

Judd, L. (1990). Putting mental health on the Nation's health agenda. NIMH Report. *Hospital and Community Psychiatry. 41*(2), February, 131, 132, 134.

Lewis, G. (1978). *Nurse-patient communication.* (3rd ed.). Dubuque: William C. Brown Company Publishers.

Lowery, B. (1992). Psychiatric nursing in the 1990's and beyond. *Journal of Psychosocial Nursing and Mental Health Services, 30*(1), 7–13.

Manfreda, M. L. (1982). *The roots of interpersonal nursing.* Cromwell: Cromwell Printing Company.

McBride, A. B. (1986). Present issues and future perspectives of psychosocial nursing theory and research. *Journal of Psychosocial Nursing, 24*(9), September, 27–32.

McClory, R. (1986). The history of NAMI. *Ways,* July, 16–19.

The nurse-patient relationship. [Film]. (1958.). Philadelphia: Smith Kline and French Company; (1990). Reissued on video for the American Psychiatric Nurses' Association. Thorofare, NJ, Charles B. Slack.

Noyes, A., and Haydon, E. (1948). *Textbook of psychiatric nursing* (4th ed.). New York: Macmillan.

Orlando, I. J. (1961). *The dynamic nurse patient relationship: Function, process and principles.* New York: Springer Publishing.

O'Toole, A. W., and Welt, S. R. (1989). *Interpersonal theory in nursing practice.* Selected works of Hildegard E. Peplau. New York: Springer Publishing.

Peplau, H. E. (1952). *Interpersonal relations in nursing.* New York: Putnam's.

Peplau, H. E. (1982a). Some reflections on earlier days in psychiatric nursing. *Journal of Psychiatric Nursing and Mental Health Services, 20*(8), August, 17–24.

Peplau, H. E. (1982b). Historical development of psychiatric nursing: A preliminary statement of some facts and trends. In S. Smoyak, and S. Rouslin (Eds.). *A collection of classics in psychiatric nursing literature.* (pp. 10–46). Thorofare: Charles B. Slack.

Public Law 487. (1946). The National Mental Health Act. 79th Congress, Second Session, July 3.

Public Law 182. (1955). Mental Health Study Act of 1955, July 28.

Public Law 88-164. (1963). Mental Retardation Facilities and Community Mental Health Centers Construction Act of 1963, October 31.

Public Law 94-63. (1975). The Community Mental Health Center Amendment.

Public Law 96-398. (1980). The Community Mental Health Systems Act.

Public Law 97-35. (1982). Omnibus Budget Reconciliation Act. 97th Congress.

Public Law 100-336. (1990). The Americans with Disabilities Act of 1990, 101st Congress, July 26.

Richards, L. (1911). *Reminiscences of America's first trained nurse (Linda Richards).* Boston: Whitcomb and Barrows.

Robb, I. H. (1901): *Nursing ethics.* (pp. 34,35). Cleveland: J. B. Savage, Cited in J. A. Dolan, M. L. Fitzpatrick, and E. K. Herrmann. (1983). *Nursing in society: A historical perspective.* (15th ed.) (p. 210). Philadelphia: W. B. Saunders.

Sareyan, A. (1994). *The turning point: how men of conscience brought about major change in the care of America's mentally ill.* Washington, D.C.: American Psychiatric Press.

Sills, G. M. (1973). Historical developments and issues in psychiatric mental health nursing. In M. M. Leininger (Ed.). *Contemporary issues in mental health nursing.* Boston: Little, Brown and Company.

Sutton, S. B. (1986). *Crossroads in psychiatry: A history of the McLean Hospital.* Washington, D.C.: American Psychiatric Press.

Swazey, J. P. (1974). *Chlorpromazine in psychiatry.* Boston: The Massachusetts Institute of Technology.

Taylor, C. M. (1990). *Mereness' essentials of psychiatric nursing.* (13th ed.). St. Louis: C. V. Mosby.

Taylor, C. M. (1994). *Essentials of psychiatric nursing.* (14th ed.). St. Louis: C. V. Mosby.

Tiffany, F. (1918). *Life of Dorothea Lynde Dix.* Boston: Houghton Mifflin.

Torrey, E. F. (1988). *Nowhere to go. The tragic odyssey of the homeless mentally ill.* New York: Harper & Row.

Torrey, E. F. (1993). The scandalous neglect of the mentally ill homeless. *National Forum, LXXIII*(1), 4–7, 12.

Travelbee, J. (1969). *Intervention in psychiatric nursing.* Philadelphia: F. A. Davis.

United States Department of Health and Human Services. (1992). *Healthy people 2000: National health promotion and disease prevention objectives.* Boston: Jones and Bartlett Publishers.

Ward, M. J. (1946; reprinted in 1964). *The snake pit.* New York: New American Library.

Wright, F. L. (1947). *Out of sight, out of mind.* Philadelphia: National Mental Health Foundation.

SUGGESTED READINGS

Bullough, V. L., Sentz, L., and Stein, A. P. (1992). *American nursing; A biographical dictionary. Vol. II.* New York: Garland Publishing.

Church, O. M. (1982). *That noble reform: The emergence of psychiatric nursing in the United States, 1881–1963.* [Doctoral dissertation]. Ann Arbor: University Microfilms International.

Flynn, L. M. (1993). Political impact of the family-consumer movement. *National Forum, LXXIII*(1), 8–12.

Smoyak, S. A., and Rouslin, S. (Eds.). (1982). *A collection of classics in psychiatric nursing literature.* Thorofare, NJ: Charles B. Slack.

Thompson, J. W. (1994). Trends in the development of psychiatric services. *Hospital and Community Psychiatry, 45*(10), 987–992.

Wilson, D. (1975). *Stranger and traveler: The story of Dorothea Dix, American reformer.* Boston: Little, Brown and Company.

CHAPTER 3

HIGHWAYS FOR THE JOURNEY

THE MENTAL HEALTH SYSTEM

U.S. Government policy toward severely mentally ill adults is undergoing as profound a reform as any in its 150 year history. Patient advocates are hopeful that a true sea change is underway; one that will guarantee a level of mental health security for all Americans, and treatment for the most severely mentally ill on a par with treatment for the "physically ill." They acknowledge, however, that as with past reforms, this will be no cure-all. And the current movement fits well the cyclical pattern that has long characterized the U.S. Government policy in this area.

—*P. Cody, 1993*

LEARNING OBJECTIVES

After studying this chapter, you should be able to:

1. Understand the significance of *DSM-IV* and *ICD-9-CM* on the practice of psychiatric nursing.

2. Appreciate the impact on the practice of psychiatric nursing of societal forces such as homelessness, the increasing numbers of aged Americans, unemployment, and the increasing numbers of young people who have both a psychiatric illness and a problem with substance abuse.

3. Talk about shifting federal policies toward the care of the mentally ill and the impact that these ever-changing policies have on the care of the mentally ill and on the practice of psychiatric nursing.

4. Understand how reimbursement policies affect the practice of psychiatric nursing.

5. Discuss the impact of institutional settings on the practice of psychiatric nursing.

KEY TERMINOLOGY

Deinstitutionalization
DSM-IV
Health maintenance organization
ICD-9
ICD-9-CM
Managed care
Medicaid
Medicare

The journey of every profession is shaped and transformed by the forces of history and happenings of the larger society. Psychiatric nursing is no different. Our journey has always reflected the changes that are happening in the world at large. Among the major influences on psychiatric nursing, as well as on the other mental health professions, over the past 50 years have been social changes, theoretical revisions and innovations, and the nation's economic conditions and political ideology (Shore, 1988). Another major influence is the stigma and misunderstanding that continues to surround the mentally ill. Many in the United States still believe that the mentally ill are somehow responsible for their illnesses; that if they were more determined, or had stronger character, or just tried harder, their problems would go away. This kind of ignorance about the nature of mental illness and the suffering it exacts on patients and loved ones allows those who are not afflicted (including those who control governmental purse strings) to feel justified in the meager and inconsistent support provided for programs to assist the mentally ill.

This chapter examines some of the external forces, which sometimes seem like intersecting highways, and their impact on the journey shared by psychiatric-mental health nurses and their patients. Specifically, we focus on the impact of the *Diagnostic and Statistical Manual-IV* ***(DSM-IV)*** and the *Clinical Modification of the World Health Organization's International Classification of Diseases—The Ninth Revision* ***(ICD-9-CM);*** public policy, including legislation and judicial precedent; social changes;

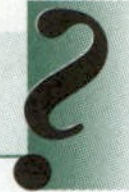

WHAT FAMILIES NEED TO KNOW **Myths and realities of serious mental illness**

Who is affected by serious mental illness?
The three serious types of mental disorders (schizophrenia, manic-depressive disorder, and major depression) affect up to 20% of the population. All three of these disorders are "brain" diseases that affect people of all ages, all races, and all socioeconomic groups. One family in 25 will be directly affected by a serious, chronic mental illness.

What causes serious mental illness?
Serious mental illness is organically based and cannot be cured at this time. However, these disorders are highly controllable with medication and support services. Poor parenting contributes, but is not the cause of serious mental illness.

Are seriously mentally ill people violent or mentally retarded?
People with serious mental illness can be violent but more frequently they are the *victims* of violence in our society. People with serious mental illness are not necessarily mentally retarded. Often, they are exceptionally gifted in many areas of intellectual development and creative expression.

What is a split personality?
By "split personality," most people are referring to a rare mental illness called multiple personality disorder. People with multiple personality disorder have two or more distinct personalities, often of different ages and genders. The mental illness known as schizophrenia is not the same thing as a "split personality." Schizophrenia is a disorder of a person's thought processes that interferes with the brain's ability to think clearly and logically.

What causes depression?
Serious depression—what mental health professionals call "major depression"—and manic-depressive disorder are considered "mood disorders" and are caused by chemical imbalances. These imbalances can be corrected dramatically by medication and support services.

Data from *Serious mental illnesses: Myths and realities.* Arlington, VA: National Alliance for the Mentally Ill, 1987.

reimbursement issues; and settings where psychiatric care is provided. It is important to recognize the mutually reciprocal relationships that exist among these diverse highways in the mental health system. For instance, social changes do not occur in isolation; they may occur in response to policy changes, and vice versa. Examining these forces separately is valuable for study purposes, but true understanding requires recognition of the complexity of these issues.

The following story is an account of one man's experience with the mental health system. The story illustrates how a policy change designed to save mental health dollars by downsizing hospitals had a ripple effect on a particular patient, Herman, and on several other agencies.

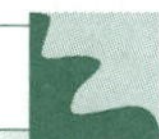

HERMAN'S STORY

In the autumn of 1992, Herman was one of 20 patients remaining at Greystone State Hospital in rural New England. He and the other patients were the only barrier remaining to the hospital's closure, and the state mental health bureaucracy was being pushed hard to find them placements and save millions of dollars a year.

On a Pathway to Nowhere

Herman was not a particularly difficult patient; he was something worse—an enigma. In his two years at Greystone, he had never assaulted a staff member or another patient or attempted to escape. Despite the fact that he shaved every morning, dressed in a suit on visiting days, and was sometimes mistaken for a doctor, he had never been issued a single pass to the hospital grounds.

Herman's admission to Greystone and his behavior inside it did not conform to any of the pathways in or out of a state mental hospital. He did not show symptoms of decompensated schizophrenia or any other major mental illness, so he could not be categorized, put on medication, taught better coping skills, and released. He had been committed because, while trying to kill himself, he had set his apartment building on fire and endangered many lives. His wife, who had left him some months before, told clinicians that he had sexually abused one daughter and beaten other children. He had no memory of the fire or his suicide attempt, and he showed no remorse, grief, or insight into it, despite repeated but gentle questioning by Greystone's clinicians. And so he was stuck at Greystone, categorized as a psychopath and a con artist who had failed to exhibit human responses that could have opened the pathway to his release.

A Dilemma With No Easy Answers

When Herman's characterization as a psychopath came face to face with the governor's directive to close Greystone, the state mental health director for the region came to our community care center. He was in a terrible bind. Herman's behavior was still impeccable, but a local forensic psychologist had recently interviewed him and confirmed the diagnosis: a dangerous psychopath. Yet Herman had to go, and soon. The state department of mental health wanted us to design a program for Herman so they could shut down Greystone without the risk of becoming the subject of a "60 Minutes" exposé depicting the state facility as being incompetent for releasing a dangerous psychopath.

The state administrators tried to transfer their quandary to us; now *we* were in a bind. We obviously could not supply as much security as a state hospital, yet we could not afford to offend the state administrators who were

Story from Murphy, M. J. (1993). Herman wept, or, the battle of narratives: A case study. *The Family Therapy Networker, 17*(3), 77–79.

the source of half of our operating budget. As the clinic director and I discussed the matter with state administrators, I realized that all of us—community mental health staff, state administrators, and Herman—were stuck together in a "narrative" that seemed to offer no easy answers.

Breakthrough

After much discussion, the director and I agreed to interview Herman for a place in our community support program. The state administrators wanted it to be a routine interview preliminary to discharge, but because our program was voluntary and we had to find out whether we could all get along and work together productively, we insisted on reserving judgment until we met Herman.

Two weeks later, I sat in my office waiting for Herman. As the community care center's forensic psychologist, I faced a crucial decision. Would I define the interview as a formal forensic evaluation, assessing Herman's dangerousness for later submission to the state? Or could it be an informal, confidential encounter in which we got to know each other as two people who might work closely together in the future?

At the last minute—as I greeted Herman in the waiting room—I decided to be informal. I told him about my choice as he settled himself into a chair in my office. He seemed pleased with my decision. I began gently urging him to tell me his story as I completed a family history.

About half an hour later, Herman was telling me about the Christmas holiday just before he tried to kill himself. His wife and family had left him, and he was working hard at restoring an apartment building he owned.

As he talked, I noticed a change in Herman's usually facile manner and self-possessed face. It was as if a sudden wind had blown in, darkening his features. "I really hoped that somehow they would come back and spend Christmas with me," he said, standing staunch in the growing gale. I leaned forward and rolled my chair a little closer to him. I don't remember exactly what I said, but it was something like, "It sounds like that really meant a lot to you."

Herman tried to contain his grief, but it overcame him. He wept, and we sat together for a couple of minutes. Then he collected himself. "Hmmm," he said, dabbing his eyes with a tissue. "Well I'll be damned. I don't know where that came from."

He may not have known where it came from but his tears sure made sense to me. He had shown himself to be a human being with feelings, capable of taking part in a relationship. I decided that Herman would do okay in our community support program. At the same time, I knew that by choosing to believe in a scenario of hope and recovery rather than one of pathology, I was taking a risk.

A Move to the Community

A week later, Herman left the state hospital. His wife and family obtained restraining orders against him, and we made agreements to notify the local police when Herman planned visits to the town where they lived. He moved into a supervised apartment shared with another patient and began making his way in the world. You might say that his tears had formed a river that carried him to a new definition of himself, but it was really a lot more complicated than that. His tears solved our agency's problem as well as his own.

Writing a New Story

I struggled to comprehend what had happened and began to understand that together Herman and I had created a new narrative, a new story. The new story, which unfolded as the weeks went on, depicted Herman as a man who had lost a great deal in his life; a man who, with his last shred of pride, had maintained himself in rigid isolation in the state hospital to avoid being categorized as a "mental patient." To break down and show his grief would have assuaged the anxieties of administrators, but for Herman it would have meant joining a club to which he did not choose to belong. He felt he had been unfairly imprisoned and had spent two long years in a marathon effort to maintain his integrity.

Later, I met with community support staff who were to deal with Herman every day. I presented them with the two narratives—Herman as a psychopath and Herman as a man choosing to grieve his losses in his own way—and suggested that while at any given moment either one might appear to have greater truth, they should not "marry" either one. Rather, they should allow Herman to define himself in his new situation to create a new story.

Herman returned weekly for therapy with me for a couple of months, and he now comes in about once every three weeks. He keeps himself busy, takes excellent care of his supervised apartment, and cooks elaborate meals for himself and his roommate, a patient with a lower level of daily functioning. He talks about getting a job someday. In four months, he has not attempted to contact his family or been in any trouble with the law.

As a humanistically oriented family therapist, I was intrigued to note that it was Herman's grief that provided the bridge to a new narrative. Had he not had the courage to show his feelings, our impasse would have continued indefinitely. What I had supplied was the open space within which a new narrative could be invented. My willful ignorance allowed us to encounter each other as two people who needed to define themselves anew.

As Herman gets more established, he is settling into a fairly rigid approach to life. No miracles have happened, but, to the relief of the state administrators, his new narrative is beginning to have real veracity, and most importantly, it is offering Herman a chance for a new life. Fortunately, Herman's narrative has a positive ending. This is not always the case when patients are caught in the changing world of mental health care.

DIAGNOSTIC AND CLASSIFICATION SYSTEMS AND THEIR IMPACT ON THE JOURNEY

You must be familiar with two diagnostic and classification systems in psychiatric nursing: the *ICD-9-CM* and the *DSM-IV.* It is important for you to understand both systems, because together they are used for compilation of statistics and for reimbursement of expenses (Figure 3–1).

DSM-IV

In the spring of 1994, the *Diagnostic and Statistical Manual of Mental Disorders-IV (DSM-IV)* was published; it represents the third revision in 15 years; the number of mental disorders included has increased from 106 to 300. The manual, touted by the American Psychiatric Association as scientific, actually intermingles science with social values. This intermingling resulted in political controversy during the two years prior to the publication of the manual. Gay men and lesbians effectively lobbied to have homosexuality dropped from the manual; Vietnam War veterans demonstrated to have Posttraumatic Stress Disorder included; and feminists waged a successful campaign to have Self-Defeating Personality Disorder removed (Kirk and Kutchins, 1994).

Whether the manual is scientific, knowledge and understanding of its contents are essential for psychiatric nurses as well as for other mental health professionals.

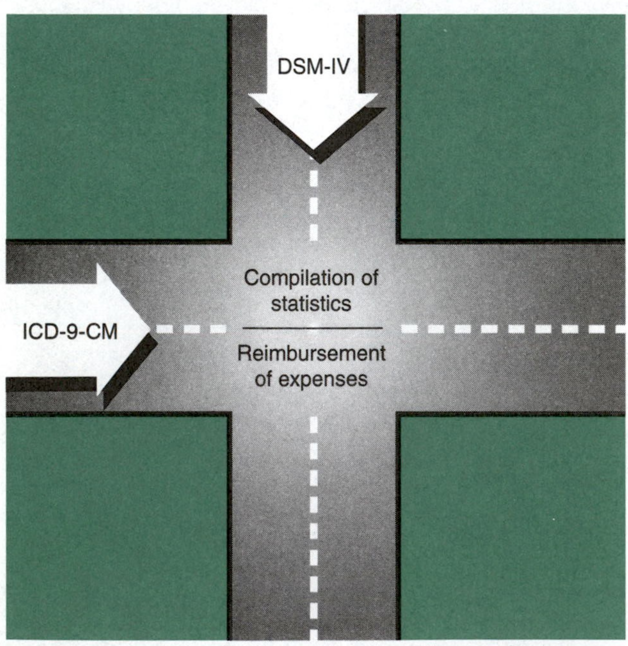

FIGURE 3–1
The *DSM-IV* and *ICD-9-CM* diagnostic and classification systems "intersect" for purposes of compilation of statistics and reimbursement of expenses.

Insurance companies use the *DSM-IV* to determine reimbursement for psychiatric services. Providers of psychiatric services must submit reimbursement claims that list an official diagnostic label accompanied by a DSM code number to be paid. The *DSM-IV* is the most cited book in psychiatry, and is used by courts, schools, social agencies, and college classrooms to establish diagnosis. The *DSM-IV* is the only diagnostic reference referred to in the Clinton health care reform proposal (Kirk and Kutchins, 1994).

The *DSM-IV* contains not only nomenclature but also the numerical codes for each of the disorders. The codes correspond with those in *ICD-9-CM* so as to facilitate the exchange of scientific data across international and language barriers. A complete *DSM-IV* classification list appears in Appendix II.

The *DSM-IV* retains the multiaxial assessment system that appeared in the previous edition. On Axis I the clinician reports "clinical disorders" and "other conditions that may be a focus of clinical attention." On Axis II the clinician reports personality disorders and mental retardation, and on Axis III he or she reports "general medical conditions." Axis IV is for reporting "psychosocial and environmental problems" (Box 3–1). On Axis V the clinician reports on a "global assessment of functioning."

The *DSM-IV* is the language of psychiatry, and if nurses are to communicate with other mental health care providers, they must be able to speak and understand this language. In addition, nurses are frequently involved in coding diagnoses on clinical records or insurance claims. For instance, in settings such as community mental health centers and in private practice, the nurse is responsible for making the diagnosis and entering it, along with the appropriate statistical code in the record. In institutions or other settings in which psychiatrists take responsibility for establishing the patient's diagnosis, the nurse may find the diagnosis recorded in the clinical record. See Figure 3–2 for an example of a completed multiaxial diagnosis.

ICD-9-CM

In 1978, the World Health Organization in Geneva published the *International Classification of Diseases—The Ninth Revision*, usually referred to as the *ICD-9.* This manual provides a classification of diseases for use in coding morbidity and mortality data for statistical purposes, and it is used in clinical situations to index hospital records by disease and procedure. However, in the United States, clinicians and others responsible for the care of patients found they needed a classification with more specificity than that provided by the *ICD-9.* Accordingly, the National Center for Health Statistics convened a steering committee in 1977. What resulted was the *ICD-9-CM*, the *Clinical Modification of the World Health Organization's International Classification of Diseases—The Ninth Revision.* In 1992, the World Health Organization published *ICD-10;* however, this is not in official use yet in the United States and may not be until

BOX 3-1 Examples of Axis IV Problems (Psychosocial and Environmental Problems)

- Problems with primary support group
  - Death of a family member
  - Health problems in family
  - Disruption of family by separation, divorce, or estrangement
  - Removal from the home
  - Remarriage of parent
  - Sexual or physical abuse
  - Parental overprotection
  - Neglect of child
  - Inadequate discipline
  - Discord with siblings
  - Birth of a sibling
- Problems related to the social environment
  - Death or loss of friend
  - Inadequate social support
  - Living alone
  - Difficulty with acculturation
  - Discrimination
  - Adjustment to life cycle transition (such as retirement)
- Educational problems
  - Illiteracy
  - Academic problems
  - Discord with teachers or classmates
  - Inadequate school environment
- Occupational problems
  - Unemployment
  - Threat of job loss
  - Stressful work schedule
  - Difficult work conditions
  - Job dissatisfaction
  - Job change
  - Discord with boss or coworkers
- Housing problems
  - Homelessness
  - Inadequate housing
  - Unsafe neighborhood
  - Discord with neighbors or landlord
- Economic problems
  - Extreme poverty
  - Inadequate finances
  - Insufficient welfare support
- Problems with access to health care services
  - Inadequate health care services
  - Transportation to health care facilities unavailable
  - Inadequate health insurance
- Problems related to interaction with legal system or crime
  - Arrest
  - Incarceration
  - Litigation
  - Victim of crime

From the American Psychiatric Association: *Diagnostic and Statistical Manual of Mental Disorders, Fourth Edition.* Washington, D.C., American Psychiatric Association, 1994, pp. 29, 30.

the late 1990s. The codes and terms provided in *DSM-IV* are fully compatible with both *ICD-9-CM* and *ICD-10*. The *ICD-9-CM* names of diseases and codes are used to designate Axis III in the multiaxial system of the *DSM-IV*.

▶ Check Your Reading

1. What is the *DSM-IV?*
2. Why does the psychiatric nurse need to understand and be able to use the *DSM-IV?*
3. What is the *ICD-9-CM?*
4. Why does the psychiatric nurse need to understand and be able to use the *ICD-9-CM?*
5. What is the multiaxial system of diagnosis?
6. Name the five axes and explain what each represents.

PUBLIC POLICY AND JUDICIAL DECISIONS AND THEIR IMPACT ON THE JOURNEY

Figure 3–3 summarizes the major changes in public policy and the major judicial decisions that have affected mental health care in the United States.

Public Policy

The National Mental Health Act (1946). Beginning in 1946 with the passage of the National Mental Health Act, the federal government took an active role in shaping the mental health delivery system. However, the government's role has shifted over time—both raising and dashing the hopes of those who are intimately involved with the issues of the mentally ill. Patients, families, psychiatrists, psychiatric nurses, and all other mental health providers anxiously watch the federal legislative process, especially the budgetary process. What Congress gives through the passage of one bill can be just as easily removed with the passage of another. Congress has passed laws that expanded the care of the mentally ill but then failed to adequately fund the programs that were mandated.

The Community Mental Health Act (1963). The passage of the Community Mental Health Act in 1963 launched a major shift in the delivery of care as well as in attitudes toward the mentally ill. Unfortunately, the promise of the 1963 legislation and the reality were quite different. In most states, little or no collaboration occurred between the large state hospitals, which were mandated to discharge patients, and the communities, which were mandated to place and care for these newly

Axis I: Clinical Disorders

Other Conditions That May Be a Focus of Clinical Attention

Diagnostic Code	*DSM-IV* Name
296.23	Major Depressive Disorder, Single Episode, Severe Without Psychotic Features

Axis II: Personality Disorders

Mental Retardation

Diagnostic Code	*DSM-IV* Name
301.6	Dependent Personality Disorder

Axis III: General Medical Conditions

ICD-9-CM Code	*ICD-9-CM* Name
382.9	Otitis Media, Recurrent

Axis IV: Psychosocial and Environmental Problems

Check:

- ☑ Problems with primary support group (specify): Victim of Child Abuse
- ☐ Problems related to social environment (specify): ____
- ☐ Educational problems (specify): ____
- ☐ Occupational problems (specify): ____
- ☐ Housing problems (specify): ____
- ☐ Economic problems (specify): ____
- ☐ Problems with access to health care services (specify): ____
- ☐ Problems related to interaction with the legal system/crime (specify): ____
- ☐ Other psychosocial and environmental problems (specify): ____

Axis V: Global Assessment of Functioning Scale: Score 53 ___ ___ ; Time Frame: Recurrent

FIGURE 3–2

Example of a completed multiaxial diagnosis. (Used with permission: American Psychiatric Association. *Diagnostic and Statistical Manual of Mental Disorders, Fourth Edition,* Washington, D.C., American Psychiatric Association, 1994, p. 34.)

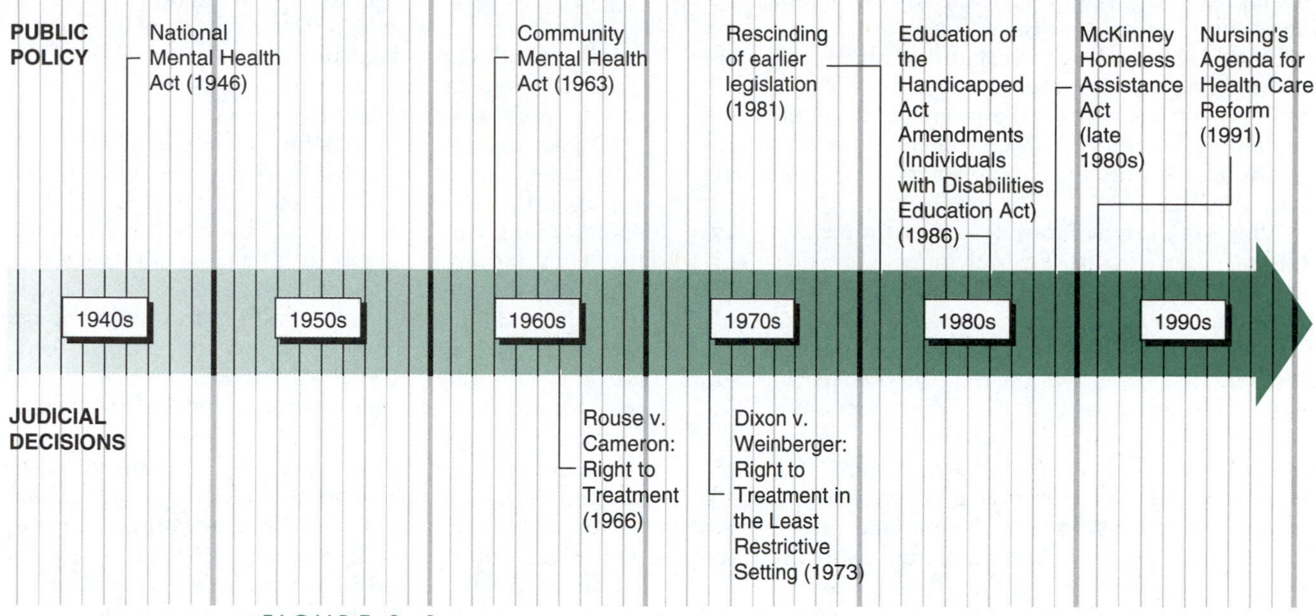

FIGURE 3–3
Major landmarks in public policy and judicial decisions affecting mental health care.

discharged patients. As described in the introductory story, Herman's journey was influenced by this public policy. The psychologist's dilemma was determining whether Herman could be cared for safely in a less restrictive setting. The process of moving patients like Herman from the large state hospitals, where many of them have resided for extended periods of time, into communities is referred to as **deinstitutionalization.** These patients were moved into community systems where the care was fragmented and inadequate. The planners of the 1963 legislation did not realize the magnitude of changes that were required to make community mental health a reality. Housing needed to be in place, and plans for vocational rehabilitation and leisure activities, access to either free or affordable medical care, and access to transportation were just some of the system components that were essential for success. These changes were material in nature; no concern was given to the need to change the attitudes of communities and to alleviate the fear and stigma attached to the mentally ill. Despite Congress's continued support of the community mental health movement through the 1970s serious implementation problems remained.

Rescinding of Earlier Legislation (1981). In 1981, the federal government began to reverse its position on the public approach to the mentally ill. At the request of President Reagan, Congress repealed the earlier community mental health legislation that had mandated 12 essential services. The mandated services were reduced to five, and no funds were to be used for inpatient care.

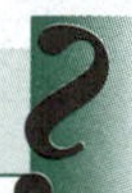

WHAT FAMILIES NEED TO KNOW **Stigma associated with mental illness**

What does "stigma" mean in regard to psychiatric patients?
Stigma means "damage to reputation." It is the covert and sometimes overt shame and ridicule our society places on mental illness.

Who suffers from the stigma of mental illness?
Stigma is destructive to families and patients who suffer from mental illness, and it often prevents people from seeking appropriate treatment. It also thwarts funding of research and services for the mentally ill and their families.

Why is so much stigma directed toward mentally ill people?
Some of the symptoms of serious mental illness such as auditory and visual hallucinations are frightening to the general public. It is natural for people to fear what they do not understand. In previous times, mental illnesses were thought to be caused by possession of evil spirits, and people with mental illness were placed in locked facilities. The public needs to be educated; unfortunately, this process of attitude change is often long and arduous.

What can I do to help reduce the stigma associated with mental illness?
Become educated about the causes of and current treatments for mental illness. Teach others with whom you come in contact what you have learned. Be an advocate. Education is the best way to bring the concept of mental illness out of the Dark Ages and to decrease discrimination.

This represented a major departure from the initial 1963 Community Mental Health Act.

Since 1980, with the fiscal and political support for the community mental health movement lost, homelessness, drug abuse, and violent crime have increased. Community Mental Health Centers continue to struggle with insufficient funding and a breakdown of community (Daw, 1993).

The McKinney Homeless Assistance Act (Late 1980s). The Stewart R. McKinney Homeless Assistance Act was passed in the late 1980s with the intent of solving the problem (largely caused by the Community Mental Health Act of 1963) of the homeless mentally ill. However, in 1992 an estimated 160,000 persons with mental illnesses were living on the streets. The 1992 report of the Federal Task Force on Homelessness and Severe Mental Illness offered "action steps" for implementation by various federal departments and agencies to improve the housing, income, health, and mental health status of these persons. The report fell short of making recommendations for prevention of homelessness among the domiciled mentally ill and for stabilizing mentally ill persons in permanent housing so that homelessness does not recur. Bassuk and Buckner (1992) observed that pulling the plug will not drain the sink so long as the faucet is left running.

The Task Force proposed a strategy for promoting systems integration but not for funding specialized housing. It only mentioned transitional facilities without describing how to expand the stock of affordable housing. Bassuk and Buckner (1992) surmise that the report reflected a deep sense of resignation about the severity of the ills within the mental health system and the limited nature of society's commitment to the neediest among us. They said that getting the homeless off the streets was a cosmetic expedient. What was required to solve the problem was a willingness to

- Care for the disenfranchised among us
- Include them in the community
- Provide the housing and community support they need
- Change ineffective systems

The Education of the Handicapped Act Amendments (1986). The Education of the Handicapped Act Amendments of 1986 (P.L.99-457) represents the most far-reaching public legislation ever enacted for disabled and developmentally vulnerable young children; it reflects public recognition of the needs of children whose mental health has long been neglected in most of the nation.

Included within the purview of early intervention are such elements as prevention, family focus, interdisciplinary cooperation, case management, and the use of multiple sources of funding. Never before had federal legislation been enacted with such remarkable potential for so many young children and their families. In 1989, each of the states was engaged in a five-year planning process with the intent of full implementation by 1991. As usual with most new federal initiatives, regulations were delayed, funding was inadequate for achieving all of the goals implicit in the law, and inter- and intrastate coordination was quite limited.

Later, the act was renamed the Individuals with Disabilities Education Act (IDEA), and the amendments are Part H. In 1991, Congress enacted P.L.102-119, reauthorizing Part H for 3 years. This new law prompted the states and professionals to develop innovative, cost-effective ways to serve children and families. As these new early intervention systems for children from birth to age three years emerged, it was important for service providers and consumers to meet, identify priorities and resources, collaborate and network, and facilitate plans for change.

However, the public policy is inconsistent even within laws passed by Congress. This is best exemplified by the 1990 Department of Defense Authorization Bill, which restricts payment by the department for a child's residential treatment to 150 days per calendar year, and in legislation that provides funding for nonresidential but not for residential forms of mental health services, e.g., the Children's and Communities Mental Health Systems Improvement Act of 1990 (Wells, 1991). These bills provide powerful illustrations of the impact of inadequate funding on the availability of services.

By 1993, all states were participating in the Education of the Handicapped Act Amendments of 1986 (P.L.99-457) at some level. Because federal funds were insufficient to cover the costs for all children from birth to age three years, flexibility was allowed for state programming. Usually this was determined by the amount of funding the state authorized to combine with the federal funds. Because of limited funding, some states do not serve all young children at risk (e.g., those born to mothers addicted to alcohol and drugs) but serve only those youngsters who have definitive diagnoses.

In addition to services for infants and toddlers, some states have statewide initiatives to develop community alternatives to residential treatment for adults. The goal of such programs is to redirect resources from institutional care to time-limited, patient-centered, and all-encompassing services.

Nursing's Agenda for Health Care Reform (1991). In 1991, nursing proactively developed an agenda for health care reform in anticipation of a public policy change. Krauss (1993) authored *Nursing's Plan to Provide Essential Mental Health Services.* The plan addressed needs in the following areas:

1. Primary care mental health services
2. Managed care
3. Universal access to basic mental health benefit packages
4. Structure and financing of the public mental health system for continuous care

What was meant by primary care mental health services? Millar (1995) describes it as broad in scope because it looks at the needs of the whole person, not separating people into mind-body dichotomies. It includes all services necessary for promotion of optimal mental health, prevention of mental illness, health maintenance, management of or referral of mental and general health problems, and rehabilitation. Millar emphasizes that some of primary mental health care, such as health promotion, illness prevention, and health maintenance, can be provided by the baccalaureate-prepared psychiatric-mental health nurse. They add that the role of the certified specialist in psychiatric-mental health nursing includes assessment, therapeutic interventions designed to enhance self-sufficiency, and progress toward optimal health. The role expands to include health promotion activities at the macrosystem level. Typical of such programs is the development of, or participation in, mobile services for the homeless; suicide prevention programs; rural mental health outreach coalitions; strategies to assist groups with predictable developmental crises; and other creative programming that is flexibly oriented to community needs.

Judicial Decisions

Judicial decisions have had significant impact on the practice of psychiatry. Specifically, decisions regarding the patient's right to treatment and the patient's right to treatment in the least restrictive setting are discussed.

Rouse v. Cameron: Right to Treatment (1966). A 1966 case (Rouse v. Cameron) in Washington, D.C. focused on the issue of a patient's right to receive adequate treatment. The court held that if patients were confined without treatment, this was tantamount to incarceration. The court affirmed that the purpose of involuntary hospitalization was treatment, not punishment. If the patient did not receive this treatment, the patient could be transferred, released, or even awarded damages for his or her period of confinement. The court stated that the hospital is not responsible for the success of the treatment, but that the hospital is responsible to demonstrate that an honest attempt to provide treatment was made (Birnbaum, 1960).

In 1972, a case decided in Alabama (Wyatt v. Stickney) extended this right to treatment to all mentally ill and mentally retarded individuals who were involuntarily hospitalized. The court defined criteria for adequate treatment in three areas:

1. Physical and psychological environments that are humane
2. Sufficient numbers of qualified staff who are able to administer adequate treatment
3. Individualized treatment plans (ITP)

The impact of the right to treatment decisions has had economic reverbations for the states. Adhering to the three criteria for adequate treatment is costly and has required states to reconsider how they allocate resources to the care of the mentally ill.

Dixon v. Weinberger: Right to Treatment in the Least Restrictive Setting (1973). The emphasis on personal freedom produced stringent standards for determination of dangerousness to self or others, which is the criteria for an involuntary admission. The cases behind this right have all asserted that if the patient can function in some setting other than a hospital setting, then the courts have a responsibility of placing him or her in such a setting. This was the ruling in a 1973 case (Dixon v. Weinberger). The judge placed responsibility on Washington, D.C. and on the federal government to identify patients who could be transferred to the community and to initiate this process, even if it involved creating alternative facilities.

Application of the humanitarian concept of the least restrictive environment while the person is in treatment has not been without problems. In fact, in some instances the result has been inhumane. Communities have not responded to this right to treatment in the least restrictive setting with adequate support, affordable housing, or meaningful treatment. For the chronically mentally ill who do not pose a threat to self or others yet who have woefully inadequate self-care and survival skills, this decision has often meant that they are vulnerable and living on the streets of our cities. Instances have been reported in which former inpatients died after being placed in group homes and foster homes that had inadequate safeguards. Bachrach suggests that instead of evaluating whether a setting is the least restrictive, we evaluate whether a setting is the "most therapeutic environment" (cited in Schulberg and Killilea, 1992).

Gladwell (1993) describes the plight of a 40-year-old man who has been jailed repeatedly, once for four and a half years, but has not been treated for bipolar disorder. The writer emphasizes that the Massachusetts law for involuntary commitment has a very narrow definition of dangerousness. The law requires that a patient who refuses treatment cannot be forced to accept it unless declared to be legally incompetent. Even with the record showing his attempts to kill his parents, he has been denied admission to inpatient care. Each time he appears in court, an attorney who values liberty over recovery from a serious illness, successfully defends his right to be jailed instead of hospitalized. Mr. M., the man in question, has a disorder that is treatable, but at the time of the writing of this report (May, 1993) he had not received treatment.

▶ Check Your Reading

7. What impact did the Community Mental Health Legislation of 1963 have on mental health delivery?
8. What happened in 1981 that impacted significantly on the community mental health movement?
9. What was the purpose of the Sherman R. McKinney Homeless Assistance Act? Did it achieve its intended purpose?
10. What are the areas addressed in nursing's agenda for health care reform?
11. What does "right to treatment" include?
12. What impact did the judicial decisions regarding "right to treatment in the least restrictive setting" have on the mental health care system?

SOCIAL CHANGES AND THEIR IMPACT ON THE JOURNEY

Figure 3–4 summarizes the major social changes that have affected mental health care in the United States.

The 1960s: A Decade of Change

A quick review of the past 40 years shows significant changes in society from decade to decade. The late 1960s and early 1970s were characterized by the coming of age of the "Baby Boomer" generation. This generation questioned values, structure, and religion; in fact, the whole fabric of American culture was the focus of their examination and rejection. They were an activist group who organized antiwar rallies and marches to challenge American involvement in the Vietnam War; took over draft offices and burned draft records; held peaceful sit-ins to protest rules and regulations of campus life; experimented with drugs in an effort to fill the spiritual void that was created when they discarded the religious beliefs of their parents; questioned sexual mores and supported sexual freedom; and questioned racial as well as gender discrimination. People had a sense that this generation could and would change the world. No doubt many of the issues that they challenged, such as sexual mores and drug use, have left a lasting impact on American society.

During this same time of social and political activism came the ground-breaking Community Mental Health Legislation of 1963. Mental health workers were caught up in the feeling that permeated the generation—that change was at hand and that people could make a difference. Great excitement and anticipation surrounded the community health movement.

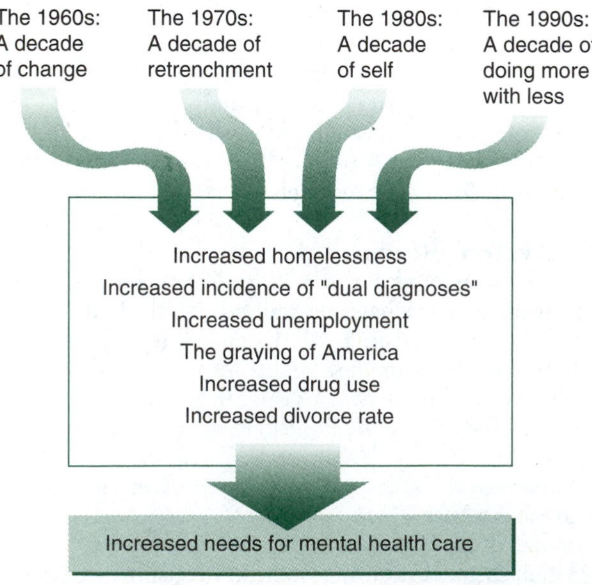

FIGURE 3–4
Influence of social changes on the need for mental health care.

The 1970s: A Decade of Retrenchment

Moving into the 1970s, the high expectations of the late 1960s and early 1970s gave way to resignation, disillusionment, and even depression. The protesters grew up; they married and began raising their own families. They no longer had the rallying points of the 1960s. The Vietnam War, a major focus for many youth, was over. The Civil Rights Movement had lost its impetus. The Equal Rights Amendment (ERA) movement, although still active, was losing ground.

Likewise, reality began to filter into the community mental health movement. The problems of insufficient funding and planning were increasingly apparent. Many patients discharged from state hospitals, as well as those who once would have been admitted to the large hospitals but were now being turned away, ended up living on the streets. The recognition that perhaps the problems of the mentally ill were bigger than we as a country were willing to tackle began to infiltrate public policy.

The 1980s: A Decade of Self

The 1980s ushered in a time of materialism and self-focus. Acquiring, owning, having, buying were the important words; serving, giving, taking care of, sacrificing, were not fashionable or popular ideas in American culture. This focus clearly had an impact on the care of the mentally ill. The clearest evidence of this is the 1981 Budget Reconciliation Act, which rescinded many of the earlier legislative mandates for financing community mental health treatment.

The 1990s: A Decade of Doing More With Less

In the 1990s Americans are faced with what seem to be overwhelming and intractable social problems. Many of these problems have their origins in the "value and moral revolution" of the 1960s, which rejected much of the Judeo-Christian heritage of the country but replaced it with something much less effective; the dead-end road of self-gratification. The results of the new value system include rampant drug use, homelessness in every major city in the United States, dissolution of families, more random violent crimes, growing incidence of acquired immunodeficiency syndrome and other sexually transmitted diseases, and a mental health system that is woefully inadequate to deal with the mental health fallout of these societal changes. The awareness of government's inability to "fix" things for us leaves us unsure of what direction to pursue for the solutions needed. One thing is clear—no human service program, including mental health programs, can expect massive infusions of money to solve problems. We all face the challenge of doing more with less and of finding creative solutions to devastating problems, one of which is the problem of homelessness.

Increased Homelessness

The ideals of the community mental health movement were based on the assumption that patients could live in the community with their families during treatment. Experience has shown that a large number of these patients had no families at all or none who would welcome them into their homes. As a result of this false assumption of the community mental health movement, many of the chronic mentally ill become homeless on the streets of our cities.

The increase in the homeless population has an impact on the journey of psychiatric nursing. Some nurses feel called to work with this population and in response to that call have either started "nurse-run" clinics to serve the homeless or have accepted positions with funded agencies whose focus is to serve this very needy population. (Refer to Chapter 39 for a comprehensive presentation of the problems of the homeless.)

An Increased Incidence of "Dual Diagnoses"

Another group that has required attention is the increasing number of young adults who have both chronic mental illnesses and substance abuse problems. Since the 1960s, drugs have become more easily obtained, and it is increasingly common for many young people to turn to illicit drugs to deal with the pain of their untreated mental illness. Many elude the grasp of the mental health service system or become patients only when in crisis (Pepper and Ryglewicz, 1984). These patients represent a major challenge to mental health providers because they do not respond well to established treatments and protocols. Nurses who provide care to these patients are called upon to exercise great patience and ingenuity. Frequently, an integrated approach using inpatient, partial, and outpatient treatment programs combined with attendance at a nearby college is an effective strategy for this group (Hoffman and Mastroianni, 1982).

Increased Unemployment

In 1992, Shore pointed out that during the recession of the 1990s, the increased numbers of unemployed Americans placed greater demands on the mental health system. This occurred at the same time that the ability or willingness to provide for these troubled Americans was curtailed. Shore urged mental health professionals, who certainly recognize the relationship of unemployment to mental health, to study it, discuss it, and apply their knowledge in practice; we see daily, first hand, the effects of job loss on human behavior, family functioning, and social and emotional well-being. Shore reminded us that persons who are usually stable experience intense emotional suffering when they lose their jobs. Imagine then, the difficulties experienced by persons with severe mental disorders when they try to find work in an economy with shrinking job opportunities. The stigma of mental illness often hampers their efforts in very tangible ways, even when the job market is favorable, further complicating their personal journey.

The "Graying of America"

In the last two decades, the population of people older than 65 years has increased more than twice as fast as that of people younger than 65. As people live longer, their use of health services, including mental health care services, increases as they contend with the demands and limitations imposed by chronic illnesses. It is estimated that over 80% of the elderly have chronic diseases, and at least 50% of that number suffer from physical and social limitations as a result of their chronic illnesses. A number of these individuals will face multiple hospitalizations to deal with exacerbations of chronic illness. Many psychiatric nurses have responded to the increase in the psychogeriatric population by specializing in the care of this group.

▶ Check Your Reading

13. Identify the social problem that is directly linked to the Community Mental Health Act of 1963.
14. What characterized the decade that spanned the mid-1960s through the mid-1970s? from the mid-1970s to the mid-1980s? from the mid-1980s to the present?
15. What impact has the drug problem had on the mental health system?
16. How has the "graying of America" affected the mental health system?
17. What does "dual diagnosis" mean?
18. What is the relationship between unemployment and mental health problems?

FUNDING AND REIMBURSEMENT AND THEIR IMPACT ON THE JOURNEY

Financing is perhaps the most pervasive problem facing the mental health field today (Williams, 1986), because it, more than any other factor, shapes our service delivery system and our journey. There is an ongoing need to treat those who are seriously mentally ill but also to provide treatment for those whose problems are less severe. Although these latter patients could be advocates for future service needs, the reality is that those with less severe problems may not have access to service that they can afford, because the restricted funding often means that only those with severe disorders can be treated.

Mental Health Care Before Insurance

Until the mid-20th century, mental health providers had few effective treatments for persons with mental illnesses. Those who developed acute symptoms either recovered "spontaneously" or went on to become chronically ill. The state hospitals were supported by tax funds requested by the executive branch of state government and appropriated by the state legislators. Much of the initial motivation for developing state hospitals in the 19th century was to reduce costs. The state hospitals were perceived to be cost effective, preferred treatment settings over smaller, more numerous county institutions (Baker, 1992).

As the population of the United States increased, so did the census in state mental hospitals. Few people had the means to pay for care in private psychiatric hospitals, so the majority of those who developed mental illnesses went to state hospitals. The financial support of these hospitals was rarely enough to support adequate care. Some had large enough appropriations to provide therapies such as occupational therapy, hydrotherapy, and electroconvulsive therapy to selected patients. Others could barely supply adequate diets and clean, comfortable surroundings.

The Advent of Medicare and Medicaid

When **Medicare** (federal insurance for those who are 65 years of age or older or for those who are judged to be disabled) and **Medicaid** (federal insurance for those who are judged to be in the lowest socioeconomic group) became available in 1965, government predicted that the quality of care in the psychiatric hospitals would improve. Medicare covered active treatment of patients older than age 65 for a limited time; it did not cover custodial care. Medicaid covered adult inpatient care under specified circumstances. State hospitals able to meet the standards set by the Health Care Financing Administration to receive Medicare and Medicaid reimbursements saw the Medicare and Medicaid programs as sources for additional funds. However, rather than use this influx of federal monies to improve care, states frequently responded with significant decreases in state appropriations.

The Current State of Funding and Reimbursement

Today in America, patients with severe, long-term mental illnesses must rely on tax-supported institutions and mental health centers for their care. Only a small percentage of such patients can afford the more desirable care provided by private hospitals. Mental health advocates urge governors and legislators to provide adequate funding for mental health care. They point out the serious problems that occur when mental health services are not readily accessible, such as homelessness, deterioration of the conditions of the patients, and the placement of mentally ill persons in jails and prisons.

Since 1981, the overall funding of human service agencies in the United States has been sharply curtailed. The separation of one human service agency or system from another, each operating as an independent entity, is also a significant problem. Each agency or system (education, mental health, substance abuse, and criminal justice) works hard to protect its turf in the competition for inadequate funds. With few exceptions, these systems seldom engage in joint planning or share resources and crossover funding streams. It is as if they each have a unique rather than a common destination in their journeys to assist the needy in our society. What is needed is a multilevel integration of services and a common road map.

The problem of funding adequate services for persons with serious mental illnesses was presented by Goldberg (1993). According to a report of the National Institute for Mental Health (NIMH) Advisory Council on the Cost and Treatment of Serious Mental Illness, approximately 5 million people—or 28% of the adult population—suffer from serious mental illness (April, 1993). A 1992 report of the U.S. Congress Office of Technology Assessment, *The Biology of Mental Disorders*, cited the total costs of serious mental illness for 1991 at $135 billion. According to the NIMH, this figure includes 20% of Social Security Insurance, $20 billion per year in direct treatment costs, and another $7 billion for long-term nursing care.

The U.S. Department of Veterans Affairs fills 40% of Veterans Administration hospital beds with veterans who have severe mental illnesses; the rest of the population fills 25% of all hospital beds. About one third of homeless single adults, and 10% to 15% of the incarcerated population, suffer from severe mental disorders.

Another change in funding patterns occurred in the early 1980s. The trend changed from categorical, i.e., for specific health conditions, to block grants, giving the states more authority over the distribution of federal funds. The placement of fund allocation decisions in the hands of state mental health authorities tilted the probable decision outcomes toward outmoded institutions that continued to be strongly supported in many states (Harshbarger and Demone, 1982).

In this same period, families, especially those who were members of the National Alliance for the Mentally Ill, made it clear what services were important to them and to their relatives with severe mental illnesses. Howe (1986) presents a list of community services needed by those with severe mental illness (Box 3–2).

In addition, Howe (1986) asserts that improved access to treatment, especially for treatment-resistant patients, requires a community commitment reflected in legislation. He decried "patient-resistant" treatment facilities where patients are slow to be admitted and quick to be discharged. Howe criticizes the limitations of most health insurance coverage for mental health services and underscores the dependence of severely mentally ill persons on public funding, not only for treatment but for income (Social Security Insurance), food stamps, vocational training and placement, and housing. He makes it clear that families must participate in ongoing advocacy efforts because very few possess the personal resources that long-term care of a loved one requires. Howe's suggestions were affirmed in a 1991 survey reported by Grosser and Vine. Families who were members of the Alliance for the Mentally Ill were interviewed, and they identified the tremendous burden placed upon them for

BOX 3-2 Community Services Needed by Patients With Severe Mental Illness

- Access to effective and cheap medication
- A permanent place to live with adequate food and support
- Access to periodic emergency inpatient treatment to deal with exacerbations of illness with minimal amount of red tape
- Meaningful and structured daytime activity
- Places to socialize and be accepted
- Access to medical and dental care
- Case management
- A system that recognizes the long-term nature of the illness and the need for continuous, long-term services and support
- Someone to care

various forms of care and support. In addition, these respondents ranked vocational and work programs as the highest priority in terms of needed nonresidential services.

Private Health Insurance. In 1994, approximately 153 million Americans had health insurance, but this insurance was absolutely tied to either having a job or being retired from a job that offered continued insurance benefits. Most individuals with insurance found that either they had no benefits for mental health, or that the mental health benefits were limited through a high copayment, high deductibles, an annual cap on the amount of money available, and a limit on inpatient stays and the number of outpatient visits (Krauss, 1993). As many as 37 million Americans were uninsured, and an estimated 50 million were underinsured. In response to inadequate coverage, some states passed "bare-bones" or "basic benefits" legislation requiring insurance companies to include certain benefits in all packages. These packages had high, discriminatory deductibles and, in some cases, absolutely no coverage for mental disorders (Krauss, 1993).

At the present time the United States is the only Western industrialized nation without a national health care plan. Health care is paid for in a variety of ways, such as:

- Out-of-pocket
- Private health insurance
- Medicaid—the federal and state plan for the poor
- Medicare—the federal plan for those over age 65
- Charity care

Health Maintenance Organizations. The emergence of **health maintenance organizations** (HMOs) has added a new twist to the delivery of mental health care. HMOs contract to provide care at a fixed yearly rate (capitation). Through **"managed care"** (an approach that involves close monitoring of utilization of health care benefits) the HMOs seek to provide preventive and remedial care at a lower cost than other types of health service organizations. Usually the HMOs severely limit mental health services, and the chronically mentally ill are frequently refused treatment. HMO members are forced to seek care for severe, long-term mental illnesses elsewhere, usually in the public sector.

Winslow (1995) reports that states have begun to seek to reduce Medicaid expenses by enrolling Medicaid recipients in HMOs. These people, now being wooed by HMOs that have such state contracts, have long turned to hospital emergency departments and to public health facilities for health care, and many do not understand how an HMO works.

For example, in Brooklyn, New York, the HMOs have not contracted with the city-owned Health and Hospitals Corporation, which provides care to 85% of the city's chronically mentally ill patients. Many of these patients do not understand that the HMO requires them to obtain a referral from their primary care physician for mental health services and that it requires them to go to a *contracted* facility for these services. Therefore, these patients continue to go to Health and Hospitals Corporation facilities and to go to them without referrals. The HMOs usually refuse to pay the Health and Hospitals Corporation hospitals, which are stuck with the bill. The HMOs still receive their per capita fee per enrollee, even though the patient did not receive care at a contracted facility. To complicate matters, little is known about how to finance or provide services to mentally ill people under managed care.

Mental Health Parity. Consumers, families, and advocates have lobbied for years to eliminate insurance discrimination against people seeking mental health care and to achieve parity with the coverage accorded other illnesses. In 1993, landmark legislation that required parity in insurance coverage for people seeking mental health care was passed in Maryland (SB-389). This law required that insurance companies and HMOs provide coverage for treatment of mental illness on the same terms and conditions as for any other illness. The legislation affected those employers with more than five employees (Raines, 1993a, 1993b).

Managed Care. Krauss (1993) quotes the definition of managed care provided by Hicks, Stallmeyer and Coleman:

> *Managed care spans a broad continuum of entities from the simple requirement of prior authorization for a service in an indemnity health insurance plan, to the assumption of all legal, financial and organizational risks for the provision of a set of comprehensive benefits to a defined population. . . . The goal of managed care is not simply to lower costs, but rather it is to ensure that maximum value is received from the resources used in the production and delivery of health care services in the population.*

Nursing supports the concept of managed care as a cost-effective monitoring system for the delivery of mental health services. Nursing also endorses the utilization of psychiatric-mental health nurses as highly qualified professional participants in both direct and indirect care roles within a managed care system. Krauss (1993) cautions the nursing profession to continuously monitor managed care systems to insure that the original objectives of cost-benefit and appropriate quality care are realized.

In response to the need to manage costs and to provide mental health services, some managed care companies have specialized in managing mental health care. They contract with insurers or employers to monitor the use of mental health benefits. They aim to minimize admissions to inpatient and residential treatment centers; to stimulate the utilization of alternative, less costly, forms of treatment; and to limit outpatient care to brief forms of therapy.

Direct Reimbursement for Advanced-Practice Psychiatric-Mental Health Nurses. The American Nurses' Association lobbied for many years for legislation that would authorize direct reimbursement to nurses who provide health care services to federal employees and their dependents. In the 99th Congress, legislation was enacted (P.L.99-2Sl) that authorized direct reimbursement for nonphysician providers, including registered nurses, in medically underserved areas. By November 5, 1990, direct reimbursement to advanced-practice nurses became policy.

Funding for Professional Training. Public support for the training of mental health personnel is also important (Knee, 1986). For nurses, the influence of public funding for advanced education can be seen in the figures for advanced degrees. In 1968, 40% of all those enrolled in specialty master's degree programs were in psychiatric nursing, and most were supported with federal traineeships. In 1978, with the significant decline in the availability of traineeships, less than 18% selected the field, and in 1988, only 7% of all nurses chose the specialty for their graduate degree. A survey by the American Nurses' Association in 1984 of 2000 psychiatric nursing specialists found that 78.5% of the respondents had received financial support from the National Institute of Mental Health (NIMH) for their graduate work. In 1989, fewer than 100 stipends were awarded to nurses (Pothier et al, 1990). The decline in available public funds means that fewer nurses with advanced preparation are in the field.

▶ Check Your Reading

19. What has happened to state funding of psychiatric care over the last 30 years?
20. What impact did Medicare and Medicaid have on the treatment of the mentally ill?
21. What is the purpose of health maintenance organizations? of managed care?
22. What impact has the decrease in available funds for training purposes had on the profession of psychiatric nursing?
23. What is mental health parity?

TREATMENT SETTINGS AND THEIR IMPACT ON THE JOURNEY

The basic functions of hospitals for the mentally ill are

- Restoration of patients to health so they can leave the hospital at the earliest possible moment short of success
- Sufficient functional improvement so patients can live as nearly normal lives as possible in the institutional setting

The effectiveness of hospitals in achieving these functions has always been dependent on the presence of adequate funding. As funding sources have expanded over the years to include commercial insurances as well as public funding, the nature of the settings for mental health care delivery has changed. The institutional setting has also had a direct impact on the nature of psychiatric nursing practice. For instance, in poorly funded state hospitals, the nurse's role may have been limited to custodial care with heavy use of restraints and seclusion. In institutions with adequate funding, nurses engage in many more therapeutic activities.

Private and Public Hospitals

As Lion and colleagues (1988) point out, the private and nonprofit psychiatric hospitals offer a wide range of services. These include the care of children, adolescents, adults, the elderly, and the medically ill. Not every hospital has every service available, but many do. They often provide a continuum of care from admission to residential aftercare. Some have adult day hospital and outpatient services as well. The diagnostic and treatment modalities, including psychotherapy, milieu, activity and cognitive therapies, electroconvulsive therapy, medications and cold wet packs, may be specialized or more eclectic. Many clinical settings work constructively with families and provide space for family support groups to meet. Often, the nurse-clinicians function as part of a treatment team. Both graduate nurse-generalists and certified specialists are employed as staff and in leadership positions. One result of reduced health benefits for mental disorders and of managed care has been a shorter length of stay than in the past. Nurses caring for patients in these hospitals find it necessary to rapidly assess the patient's needs and strengths, to develop an individual nursing care plan that is consistent with the treatment plan, and to start the discharge planning process as soon as the patient is admitted. The nurse, as part of the multidisciplinary team, must offer therapeutic care that effectively promotes relief of symptoms and strengthens healthy coping behavior in the patient.

Specialized Hospitals

The high incidence of chemical dependency (i.e., dependence on alcohol and on drugs such as cocaine, heroin, and other substances) has led to the establishment of hospitals for the treatment of persons with these disorders. These hospitals may be public or private. In addition, a few general hospitals have detoxification units for the care of patients who are acutely intoxicated and require a blend of skilled medical and psychiatric treatment for a limited period. Nurses are essential staff members in detoxification units and in hospitals for the treatment of chemical dependency. The treatment programs may rely on nurses to function as group and individual therapists, to work with family members of the dependent person, and to encourage attendance at self-help group meetings such as Alcoholics Anonymous and Narcotics Anonymous. Some of these specialized hospitals have rehabilitation programs; however, others may be limited by managed care rules and provide follow-up in outpatient programs. Some health insurance will not authorize payment for inpatient treatment until intensive outpatient treatment has been tried and evaluated for effectiveness. Many hospitals have developed treatment programs to fit this model.

Specialized Units Within Hospitals

Psychogeriatric Units. As America has begun to age and life expectancy has increased, many state as well as private psychiatric hospitals have responded by adding specialized units for the diagnosis and treatment of psychogeriatric patients. However, sometimes elderly patients in general hospitals for medical or surgical treatments exhibit problematic behaviors as a result of or in response to physical illnesses (Hall and Buckwalter, 1990). Psychiatric liaison nurses may be called to assist the staff to cope with the patient or to suggest that care be provided in the psychiatric unit or elsewhere.

Psychiatric Units Within General Hospitals. Many general hospitals include psychiatric care among the services offered. These units are designed for short-term, acute care. That is, patients are admitted, treated, and released rather quickly. Patients who require longer periods of hospitalization are generally transferred to a state facility. These units play an important role in the maintenance of patients with chronic mental illnesses within the community. These patients periodically experience exacerbations of their symptoms requiring a short-term stay for stabilization.

Forensic Units. Since the 1960s a significant increase in the number of incarcerated persons who suffer from severe mental illness has occurred. Gladwell (1993) points out that 30,000 seriously mentally ill Americans were locked up in local jails during this time period; patients with medical problems were treated like criminals. In some communities, the local mental health authority provided resources for some treatment. In others, no treatment was provided, and the patient stayed in jail until the court decided where the patient was to go. Nurses employed in these settings were challenged to use great ingenuity in their efforts to provide therapeutic care.

Some states have forensic psychiatry units or hospitals for accused persons who are found not guilty by reason of insanity but are deemed by the court to be too dangerous to others to be released. Most state and federal prison systems also have specialized sections for the care of prisoners who develop symptoms of mental illnesses after they have been convicted. Nurses are employed in both settings, and some have developed expertise at providing therapeutically effective care while maintaining a high level of security. Nurses in these settings must be informed about the applicable laws and do their part to ascertain that these laws are followed by nursing personnel.

Residential Treatment Centers

Children and adolescents with behavioral and emotional problems who can not be effectively managed in their homes are usually referred to residential treatment centers. The children placed in these centers are a highly vulnerable group whose needs often outstrip the system's ability to provide for their needs. Public policy favors placing children and adolescents for short durations—usually not long enough to see a cure. A continuum of care is needed but is not always provided. These children and their families often travel a difficult and painful journey. Nurses who work in such centers are called upon to enter into that journey in a way that connects with troubled children and families to give them affirmation and hope and to help them see alternatives (Wells, 1991).

Outpatient Settings and Community Mental Health Centers

All of the states have outpatient facilities for mental health treatment; some are attached to hospitals, and some are free standing. In addition, all of the states have mental health centers each serving approximately 250,000 people, with limited funding from the federal government.

Many of the persons with chronic mental illnesses also have a need for medical and dental care. Some centers employ Adult Nurse Practitioners to provide basic medical care. These nurses refer persons with more severe problems to physicians.

Nurses employed in community mental health centers often have administrative, case management, and therapeutic assignments. Many are expert at providing individual, group, and family therapy as well as managing a therapeutic milieu. In addition to contributing to the operation of community mental health centers, mental health nurses are also key providers of crisis intervention, including serving on hotlines for suicide prevention. The nurse's roles contribute to supporting the patient's journey within the community setting.

Since the mid-1970s, adult day hospitals, as a substitute for inpatient care, either have been included as part of some mental health centers or were operated by private group practices. Nurses are usually members of the staff of adult day hospitals, working as team members with psychiatrists and with ancillary therapists.

Home Care

Medicare authorized payment for psychiatric home care services in 1975. Although most home care agencies still do not offer psychiatric home care as one of their services, this is changing rapidly. With the shift to managed care and shorter and less frequent inpatient stays, patients are released into the community still very sick and needing intensive support. These needs are being met by psychiatric nurses who are leading the home care industry in developing innovative programs to meet the needs of psychiatrically homebound patients (Carson, 1994).

Private Practice

Since the mid-1970s, increasing numbers of certified specialists in psychiatric-mental health nursing have entered the private practice of psychotherapy. Some join group practices with other mental health professionals. Some engage in solo practice or in one of the therapies covered in Chapters 15 through 21. In the early years, nurses struggled for recognition as providers of psychiatric-mental health care that was covered by health insurance policies. A factor in this struggle was the question of including psychotherapies within the scope of nursing practice. In some states, the Boards of Nursing have regulations that specify that psychotherapies are within the scope of practice of qualified certified specialists. Nurses in several states have worked with legislators to pass laws that facilitate the recognition and acceptance of nurses as providers of health care for which their patients can be reimbursed by third-party payors.

▶ Check Your Reading

24. What is the purpose of inpatient psychiatric treatment?
25. What is a forensic unit?
26. Name two different types of specialty units for the treatment of psychiatric problems.
27. What is a residential treatment center and what does it offer?
28. What type of psychiatric nurse can be in private practice?
29. Describe the role of the psychiatric nurse in a community mental health center.
30. Name one change in the health care system that has encouraged the development of psychiatric home care programs.

CONCLUSIONS

The journey of psychiatric nursing is affected by the same external forces that affect all of society. This chapter reviewed the impact of the *Diagnostic and Statistical Manual-IV* (*DSM-IV*) and the *Clinical Modification of the International Classification of Diseases—The Ninth Revision* (*ICD-9-CM*) on psychiatric nursing. Additionally, public policy and judicial precedents are influential in molding the entire mental health care system, including psychiatric nursing. Legislation such as the Community Mental Health Act of 1963 shifted the focus of mental health care from large hospitals to community centers. Likewise, psychiatric nursing's journey shifted from hospital-based nursing, which was many times custodial in nature, to the community, where nursing practice assumed more independent and therapeutic functions. Legislation has resulted in unexpected and undesirable changes, such as the increase in the numbers of homeless mentally ill that resulted from inadequate planning and implementation of the 1963 legislation. Judicial precedents such as the Right to Treatment and the Right to Treatment in the Least Restrictive Setting have also had an impact on the journey of psychiatric nursing.

Social changes across the last four decades have shifted attitudes toward the care of the mentally ill. These changes have also resulted in increasing numbers of people requiring mental health care from a system with decreasing capacity to meet the needs of all who require assistance. Changes such as the dramatic increase in the homeless population, the proliferation of drug use and subsequent emergence of the dual diagnosis population, unemployment, and the "graying of America" have strained the mental health care system's ability to respond. Psychiatric nursing's journey is also affected by these changes as nurses have specialized in the care of these subpopulations.

Funding is the most pervasive problem facing the mental health system. Legislative effectiveness has been limited by inadequate funding. Likewise, inadequate funding has contributed to the social changes that have strained the mental health care system. Most Americans have inadequate mental health care coverage, and the public funding for these services has also been seriously curtailed. Medicare and Medicaid, which were anticipated to improve mental health care for those eligible for these insurances, have fallen short of the expected improvement. As states received funding from Medicare and Medicaid, they made subsequent cutbacks in the amount of support that they appropriated for mental health care. Those who have private or commercial insurances find that mental health coverage does not have equal parity with other medical conditions. Insurance companies impose caps on benefits and high deductibles or high copays. In this age of health maintenance organizations (HMOs) and Managed Care Companies, we are faced with the realities that HMOs frequently refuse to provide care for the chronic mentally ill and that Managed Care may not always mean quality care. Funding for mental health issues has also been reduced, with the available traineeships for advanced practice nurses all but disappearing.

Institutions where psychiatric care is delivered have changed dramatically over the last four decades. In the 1960s, most mental health care was provided in either large state hospitals or exclusive private facilities. This changed with the Community Mental Health Act of 1963 as increasing numbers of community mental health centers grew up all over the country. This change has continued with a proliferation of various types of community-based sites developing in response to legislation, judicial precedents, societal changes, and available funding. Currently, the mental health care landscape supports specialized hospitals, psychiatric units within general hospitals, specialized psychiatric units within hospitals, residential treatment centers, community mental health care centers, outpatient clinics, day treatment centers, home care, nurse-run private practices, as well as nurse-run clinics.

KEY POINTS TO REMEMBER

- The *DSM-IV* contains the diagnostic criteria for mental illnesses. Nurses must understand and be able to use the *DSM-IV* for reimbursement and for chart documentation.

- The *ICD-9-CM* is the *Clinical Modification of the World Health Organization's International Classification of Diseases—The Ninth Revision.* This manual provides a classification of diseases for use in coding morbidity and mortality data for statistical purposes, and it is used in clinical situations to index hospital records by disease and procedure.

- In 1946, with the passage of the National Mental Health Act, the federal government assumed an active role in regulating mental health care in the United States.

- The government's role mandated a major shift in the mental health care system when the Community Mental Health Act was passed in 1963, moving the care of the chronically mentally ill away from the large state hospitals to the community. However, the community mental health movement was underfunded.

- In 1981, the federal government reversed its position on community mental health and repealed earlier legislation that had mandated 12 services. The mandated services were reduced to five and no funds were allocated for inpatient care.

- Since 1980, with fiscal and political support for the community mental health movement lost, homelessness, drug abuse, and violent crime have increased.

- The Stewart R. McKinney Homeless Assistance Act was passed in the 1980s to deal with the growing problem of the homeless mentally ill. The legislation was never funded sufficiently to address the areas of change mandated by the law.

- The Education of the Handicapped Act Amendments of 1986 represented the most far-reaching public legislation ever enacted for disabled and developmentally vulnerable children. As with previous legislation, funding was inadequate for achieving the goals implicit in the law, and inter- and intrastate coordination was quite limited.

- Nursing developed its own agenda for health care reform, calling for primary care services, managed care, universal access to a basic mental health benefit package, and structure and financing of the public mental health system for continuous care.

- Judicial decisions such as the Right to Treatment and the Right to Treatment in the Least Restrictive Setting have affected the mental health delivery system as well as psychiatric nursing. The Right to Treatment decision mandates that (1) patients receive treatment in physical and psychological environments that are humane; (2) that care is provided by sufficient numbers of qualified staff; and (3) that patients have individualized treatment plans. The Right to Treatment in the Least Restrictive Setting has probably contributed to the homeless problem. Patients who do not present a clear danger to themselves or others but who are unable to adequately care for themselves have been released into the community without adequate support, affordable housing, or meaningful treatment.

- Certain social changes such as homelessness can be traced to legislative mandates such as the Community Mental Health Act of 1963. Homelessness, unemployment, increased drug use and the growing number of young people with dual diagnoses, and the "graying of America" have all contributed to the mental health problems in the United States.

- Funding is probably one of the most pervasive problems facing the mental health field today. Medicare, Medicaid, private health care insurance, out-of-pocket payment, and charity care are the reimbursement sources for mental health care. Most private insurers place severe restrictions on mental health coverage. Many HMOs refuse to treat the seriously and persistently mentally ill. Advanced-practice certified specialists in psychiatric-mental health services can receive direct reimbursement for psychiatric services.

- Institutions where psychiatric care is provided have changed, moving away from the large state hospitals as the primary providers of care. Private hospitals, general hospitals with specialized psychiatric units, specialized hospitals, residential treatment centers, and a wide variety of outpatient services have developed to provide care for the psychiatric patient. The role of the psychiatric nurse has changed along with the changing landscape of psychiatric institutions, with the nurse moving away from a custodial role to that of a direct provider of psychiatric services and sometimes the administrator of a psychiatric facility.

LEARNING ACTIVITIES

1. Call your state legislature and obtain copies of the Nurse Practice Act governing the practice of the Certified Nurse Specialist in Adult Psychiatric-Mental Health. What are the boundaries of the nurse's practice in your state?

2. Find out what legislation your state has passed that directly affects reimbursement for mental health services. Does your state's Medicaid program reimburse for mental health services? Does your state have "parity" legislation that mandates that mental health coverage be equal to other coverage?

3. Do some research into the continuum of psychiatric care in your state. Does your state have state and private psychiatric hospitals, community mental health centers, partial hospitalization programs, day treatment programs, psychosocial programs, mobile treatment, and psychiatric home care programs?

4. Find out when your local Alliance for the Mentally Ill (AMI) meets and attend one of their meetings. What impact has the Alliance had on the care of the mentally ill in your area? Consider joining or supporting them financially.

CRITICAL THINKING EXERCISES

Consider the following statement about the "right to treatment in the least restrictive setting" presented earlier in this chapter. In a 1973 case (Dixon v. Weinberger), it was ruled that if a patient can function in some setting other than a hospital setting, the courts have a responsibility to place him or her in such a setting. Schulberg and Killilea (1992) comment that the application of the humanitarian concept of the least restrictive environment has not been without problems, and at times, it has been inhumane. Communities have not responded with adequate support, affordable housing, or meaningful treatment. The chronically mental ill, who are not a threat to self or others but have inadequate self-care or survival skills are often vulnerable and end up living on city streets. Incidences of patient deaths in group homes and foster homes with inadequate safeguards have been reported.

1. What do you think is the main issue here?

2. What is the point of view of the authors, Schulberg and Killilea, concerning the 1973 ruling related to the right to treatment in the least restrictive setting?

3. What evidence supports Schulberg and Killilea's position?

4. Consider any biases.

Mr. Que, a nurse on the inpatient psychiatry unit, was informed by Mr. Zee, a patient on the unit for four hours, that he was leaving the hospital. Mr. Zee was admitted with a history of self-destructive behavior and a recent attempt to physically harm his wife. Mr. Que knows that according to the law the patient has a right to refuse treatment. However, he is aware that it is his professional responsibility to provide the patient with a safe environment.

1. What if Mr. Que decides to let the patient leave?

2. What else could happen as a result of Mr. Que's decision?

3. What is an alternative approach to Mr. Que's letting the patient leave?

REFERENCES

American Psychiatric Association (1994). *Diagnostic and statistical manual of mental disorders-IV.* Washington, D.C.

Baker, F. (1992). Effects of value systems on service delivery. In H.C. Schulberg and M. Killilea (Eds.), *The modern practice of community mental health* (pp. 246–264). San Francisco: Jossey-Bass.

Bassuk, E. L., and Buckner, T. C. (1992). Out of mind—out of sight, the homeless mentally ill. *American Journal of Orthopsychiatry. 62*(3), 330–331.

Birnbaum, M. (1960). The right to treatment. *American Bar Association Journal,* 499.

Carson, V. B. (1994). Doing psych, but talking med-surg language. *Caring Magazine, 13*(6),32–41.

Cody, P. (1993). U.S. policy toward the severely mentally ill: A search for humane treatment. *Family Therapy News, 24*(3), 3–6.

Daw, J. (1993). Community mental health centers face an uncertain future. *Family Therapy News, 24*(3), 9.

Gladwell, M. (1993). Justice on the edge of insanity. *The Washington Post, 116*(132) B1, B8, B9.

Goldberg, J. R. (1993). Research snapshot: Severe mental illness. *Family Therapy News, 24*(3) 2.

Greenblatt, M. S. (1955). Toward a therapeutic community. In M. S. Greenblatt, et al (Eds.), *From custodial to therapeutic patient care in mental hospitals* (p. 213). New York: Russell Sage.

Grosser, R. C., and Vine, P. (1991). Families as advocates for the mentally ill. *American Journal of Orthopsychiatry, 61*(2) 282–290.

Hall, G. R., and Buckwalter, K. C. (1990). From almshouses to dedicated unit: Care of the institutionalized elderly with behavioral problems. *Archives of Psychiatric Nursing, 4*(1), 3–11.

Harshbarger, D., and Demone, H. W. (1982). Impact of public policy on mental health services. In H. C. Schulberg and M. Killilea (Eds.), *The modern practice of community mental health* (pp. 230–245). San Francisco: Jossey-Bass.

Hoffman, F. L., and Mastroianni, X. (1992). The hospitalized young adult: New directions in psychiatric treatment. *American Journal of Orthopsychiatry, 62*(2), 297–301.

Howe, J. W. (1986). Financing of mental health services for severely mentally ill persons. In *Financing for mental health services and research: Current perspectives.* Atlanta: Emory University School of Medicine.

Kirk, S. A., and Kutchins, H. (1994). Is bad writing a mental disorder? *The New York Times,* June 20, 1994.

Knee, R. (1986). Speaking for the National Association of Social Workers. In *Financing for mental health services and research: Current perspectives* (pp. 89–91). Atlanta: Emory University School of Medicine.

Krauss, J. B. (1991). Put the community back in mental health. *Archives of Psychiatric Nursing, 5*(1), 1, 2.

Krauss, J. B. (1993). Executive summary. In *Health care reform: Essential health services.* Washington, D.C.: American Nurses Publishing.

Lion, J. R., et al (1988). *Modern Hospital Psychiatry.* New York: Norton.

Millar, T. P. (1995). An adaptive approach to primary prevention in child psychiatry. *Perspectives in Biology and Medicine, 38* (2), 256–273.

National Alliance for the Mentally Ill. (1987). *Serious mental illnesses: Myths and realities.* Arlington, VA: NAMI.

Pepper, B., Albert, N., and Ryglewicz, H. (1993). The multineed/multisystem client: A confluence of variables. *TIE-LINES, 10*(2), 1,2.

Pepper, B., and Ryglewicz, H. (1984). Who is the young adult chronic patient? *TIE-LINES, 1*(1), 1, 2.

Pothier, P. C., et al (1990). Dilemma and directions for psychiatric nursing in the 1990s. *Archives of Psychiatric Nursing, 4*(5), 284–291.

Raines, L. (1993a). Legislative report. In *Legislative update* (p. 1). Baltimore: Mental Health Association of Maryland.

Raines, L. (1993b). Parity passes. *Mental Health Report: Newsletter of the Mental Health Association of Prince George's County,* 1.

Schulberg, H. C., and Killilea, M. (1992). Community mental health in transition. In H. C. Schulberg & M. Killilea (Eds.), *The modern practice of community mental health* (pp. 40–84). San Francisco: Jossey-Bass.

Shore, M. F. (1988). Follow the leader. *Readings, A Journal of Reviews and Commentary in Mental Health.* American Orthopsychiatric Association, *3*(2), 13–15.

Shore, M. F. (1992). Mental health work in a free-fall economy. *American Journal of Orthopsychiatry, 62*(2), 162.

Wells, K. (1991). Long-term residential treatment for children. *American Journal of Orthopsychiatry, 61*(3), 324–326.

Williams, R. (1986). Community mental health centers. In *Financing for mental health services and research: Current perspectives* (pp. 92–94). Atlanta: Emory University School of Medicine.

Winslow, R. (1995). Welfare recipients are a hot commodity in managed care now. *Wall Street Journal,* April 12, 1, 8.

Wyatt v. Stickney, 344 F. Supp. 373, 375, (1972).

SUGGESTED READINGS

Baker, F. (1992). Effects of value systems on service delivery. In H.C. Schulberg and M. Killilea (Eds.), *The modern practice of community mental health* (pp. 246–264). San Francisco: Jossey-Bass.

Bassuk, E. L., and Buckner, T. C. (1992). Out of mind—out of sight, the homeless mentally ill. *American Journal of Orthopsychiatry, 62*(3), 330–331.

Grosser, R. C., and Vine, P. (1991). Families as advocates for the mentally ill. *American Journal of Orthopsychiatry, 61*(2) 282–290.

Hall, G. R., and Buckwalter, K. C. (1990). From almshouses to dedicated unit: Care of the institutionalized elderly with behavioral problems. *Archives of Psychiatric Nursing, 4*(1), 3–11.

CHAPTER 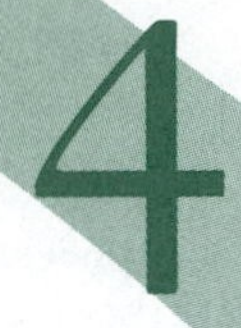

ALTERNATE ROUTES FOR THE JOURNEY
PRACTICE ROLES AND SETTINGS

Two roads diverged in a yellow wood,
And sorry I could not travel both
And be one traveler, long I stood
And looked down one as far as I could
To where it bent in the undergrowth;
Then took the other, as just as fair,
And having perhaps the better claim,
Because it was grassy and wanted wear,
Though as for that the passing there
Had worn them really about the same,
And both that morning equally lay
In leaves no step had trodden black.
Oh, I kept the first for another day!
Yet knowing how way leads on to way,
I doubted if I should ever come back.
I shall be telling this with a sigh
Somewhere ages and ages hence:
Two roads diverged in a wood, and I—
I took the one less traveled by,
And that has made all the difference.

—Robert Frost

LEARNING OBJECTIVES

After studying this chapter, you should be able to:

1. Discuss the scope and implications of the ANA Standards of Clinical Practice.
2. Discuss the ANA Standards of Professional Performance.
3. Differentiate direct and indirect care.
4. Define the term *advocate.*
5. Differentiate between the two levels of psychiatric-mental health clinical practice.
6. Define the term *peer review.*
7. Define the term *accountability* and discuss to whom the nurse is accountable.
8. Discuss the role of lobbying and networking in collaboration.
9. Define the terms *stress* and *burnout.*
10. Discuss the strategies to deal with burnout and restore spiritual balance.

KEY TERMINOLOGY

Acountability
Advocate
Burnout
Certified specialist
Collaboration
Continuing education
Direct care
Indirect care
Lobbying
Networking
Peer review
Performance standards
Practice standards
Preventive care
Primary care
Psychiatric consultation-liaison nurse
Psychiatric-mental health registered nurse
Psychiatric-mental health advanced practice nurse
Role
Secondary prevention
Self-care
Steward of resources
Stress
Tertiary prevention

Each of us traverses a different journey into nursing. Even though we may end up walking together on the same path, the decisions that lead each of us to choose first nursing and then a specialty within nursing are as varied and individual as each of us. It is true that all nurses share commonalities. We have a core of knowledge, skills, and values that link us in this profession. But there are just as many differences that separate us. This is true in the specialty of psychiatric nursing—we have a core of knowledge and skills regarding communication and interpersonal relationships, various treatment modalities, and the causes of psychiatric disorders. Beyond this core lies a tapestry of unique roles, interpretations of roles, and functions that clearly draw from but also expand on the core knowledge and skills. What draws us to particular specialties within nursing is the spiritual aspect of our nursing journey—the meaning that the specialty holds for us and whether we have a sense of vocation or calling to a particular specialty. This chapter examines the richness that exists in psychiatric nursing, the various roles that psychiatric nurses fill, the functions that they perform, the challenges that they face, and the stress inherent in their journeys. In the following story, you will get a glimpse into Dr. Lisa Robinson's psychiatric nursing journey.

LISA ROBINSON'S STORY

It is a good and an appropriate time to look back on the beginnings of psychiatric consultation-liaison nursing. While it pleases me that many people regard me as the "grandmother" of the specialty, I must admit that other nurses both wrote about their experiences and influenced my thinking at the same time that I began organizing my observations. I was a student nurse in the mid-1950s. (I use the words *student nurse* advisedly because at the time students were used differently than they are today. Clearly the hospital school of nursing staffed its units with students from whom they expected labor in return for training. The hospital was not the clinical laboratory that it has become in the last part of this century. Students were not expected to think about clinical problems or to intervene from a theory base. They were expected to read the procedure manual and, from its directives, to act in a rote but accurate manner.) I trained at a small community hospital where the nurses prided themselves on their reputation as good bedside nurses. They were gentle. They kept patients and utility rooms immaculate, and they dutifully stood if a physician entered the chart room.

Story by Lisa Robinson, Personal communication, 1991.

Childhood

I had entered that school of nursing because I knew the hospital well. I had spent the better part of my childhood there, undergoing two-stage plaster procedures annually to correct the polydactylism with which I was born. Indeed, when I was not in the hospital, but chanced to be driven by, I would secretly marvel at the myriad of stories that were being simultaneously played out behind the many windows that stood in rows across the building's facade. In play, I longed to be the nurse in the black stockings and blue and white dress with starched white bib and apron. Little did I imagine in those school-age years that a decade later my fantasies would become reality.

Student Experiences

As a student, I was told that certain things had to be done: like making square corners on beds, cleaning utility rooms, and seeing that patients' navels were cleaned with cotton swabs. When I spent time talking to patients, I was told that there were "more important things that needed doing." Instructors never asked what patients felt or thought. In fact, the mental lives of patients were denied. It was their lesions, their physical symptoms, and the therapeutic effects of their treatments that reflected clinical reality.

My favorite author was Catherine Norris, who published regularly in the *American Journal of Nursing.* I eagerly read each description of patient states and her interventions. In my clinical experiences, I was drawn to patients who were morose, angry, agitated, mute, or dying. It was a challenge to sit with them and communicate my desire to help. There was a special sense of accomplishment when they allowed me to share their senses of being.

Graduate School and a First "Real" Job

After graduation I worked and then returned for a master's degree in psychiatric nursing. In 1965, I was fortunate to be offered a job in a community hospital that had a small department of psychiatry. The departing nurse told me that supervisors from the general hospital might call me periodically for help with a problem patient. This was the genesis of my awareness of psychiatric consultation-liaison nursing as a formal model of practice. In the ensuing five years, I wrote my first paper on consulting work and was pleased and interested to compare my thoughts with those of a few others who also published their experiences: In that handful of writers was Betty Sue Johnson of Duke University. Also at that time, an important collection of papers from Yale University called *Social Interaction and Patient Care* was published. It was edited by two sociologists on faculty who were important to psychiatric consultation-liaison nursing because of their influence on the research topics of nurses enrolled in the graduate program in nursing at Yale. These two sociologists, James Skipper and Robert Leonard, helped to bring psychosocial issues of patient care under the scrutiny of research. They nurtured the minds of nurses who would, in their master's research, begin to develop theoretical links underlying the values that guide psychiatric consultation-liaison nursing. The compiled papers included a study by Rhetaugh Dumas and colleagues on the incidence of postoperative nausea and vomiting as it related to preoperative teaching. It also contained a paper by Esther Lucille Browne on the "humanness" of hospitalized patients. These and other papers focused on psychosocial aspects of the nurse's role, the importance of communication, the patient's view of his or her situation, and physician–nurse–patient relationships.

A Teaching Position

After earning my doctorate, I was invited to teach at the University of Maryland School of Nursing. The administration was open minded and supportive. Dean Marion Murphy did not flinch when I designed a course around those experiences that I had found so rewarding in clinical practice. In the early 1970s, more psychiatric nurses and educators began to consult on the general wards, and they too wrote. By the mid-1970s, there was a relatively large body of literature describing the functions of the psychiatric consultation-liaison nurse. There was no theory to speak of, other than what was borrowed from Caplan on consultation process, from the general psychiatric literature, and from the descriptive studies from Yale. In a decade of teaching and supervising clinical practica, I graduated a small cadre of psychiatric consultation-liaison nurses who found employment that allowed them to function successfully. Meanwhile, I was traveling a great deal, giving lectures and workshops on the specialty. My travels took me as far as the Rockies. I saw in the literature, however, that the specialty had spread even beyond those tall peaks.

A First Conference for the Specialty

In the mid-1980s, an enterprising young doctoral student at Rush University organized a conference in Chicago for psychiatric consultation-liaison nurses. The timing and location were ideal for several reasons. For one, Jane Bryant, a University of Maryland graduate, had, with another psychiatric consultation-liaison nurse (Peggy Dulaney), formed a loose network of specialists who were beginning the work of organizing their thoughts about the philosophy, objectives, and functions of the specialty. It was they who really structured the talent and energy of the group so that five years later the American Nurses' Association published our standards and our Scope of Practice statement. But it was at the Chicago conference that we all met face to face. There we began to construct the document that would guide future generations of psychiatric nurses who would become psychiatric consultation-liaison nurses. We debated in Chicago. We listened to Peggy Dulaney update our efforts in San Francisco. At the third annual conference, in Boston, Peggy told us that "for sure" the ANA was going to publish our work, thereby formalizing and giving credence to our informal specialty. It was finally in Charleston, South Carolina, at the fourth conference, that our now-expanded group heard the news. The ANA had approved our work, and it was on the way to the printer. At that conference, Peggy was recognized for her continuous efforts. She was elected the first chairperson of the group.

The Specialty Today

Today, shortly after the 9th conference in San Diego, we number about 1000 specialists. Most of us are master's-prepared psychiatric nurses. Our standards are bound and in hand. In 1994, we became a separate entity from the ANA and adopted a new name, the International Society for Psychiatric Consultative-Liaison Nurses (ISPCLN).

Some years ago, someone asked me how I started psychiatric consultation-liaison nursing. I did not have a ready answer but later ruminated about the question. I realized then that my interest and enthusiasm came from that little girl who liked to "play nurse" in her effort to identify with the "aggressor." Fifty years ago, there were no child life workers in pediatric wards. Ether, hissing autoclaves, well-meaning adults who restrained struggling, terrified children, and dark sleepless nights in unfamiliar cribs was the context out of which developed my drive to comfort and protect. Perhaps it was from my need to be secure that came the drive for psychiatric consultation-liaison nursing.

Lisa Robinson's story is unique and provides a glimpse into her particular journey into psychiatric nursing and specifically into the path of psychiatric consultation-liaison nursing. Just as in Robert Frost's poem, she chose a particular path, leaving others unexplored.

CORE PRACTICE ROLES

The practice roles of the psychiatric nurse have evolved over the years (review Chapter 2 for psychiatric nursing's historical journey) from custodians of those who were viewed as deviant to multifaceted roles that include many functions (Gregg, 1954; Church, 1987). The American Nurses Association (ANA) describes psychiatric-mental health nursing as:

> . . . the diagnosis and treatment of human responses to actual or potential mental health problems. Psychiatric-mental health nursing is a specialized area of nursing practice, employing theories of human behavior as its science and purposeful use of self as its art (Coalition of Psychiatric Nursing Organizations, 1994, p. 7).

Box 4–1 summarizes the "phenomena of concern" to psychiatric-mental health nursing.

The ANA recommends the baccalaureate degree as the entry-level educational preparation for psychiatric nursing. Psychiatric-mental health nursing demands knowledge of numerous theories drawing from a variety of sources, including biological, cultural, environmental, psychological, and sociological theories. In 1994, the ANA published revised Standards of Psychiatric-Mental Health Clinical Nursing Practice (Box 4–2).

The "Standards of Care" of the ANA Standards of Psychiatric-Mental Health Clinical Nursing Practice give rise to many of the roles of the psychiatric-mental health nurse. These **roles** include (Figure 4–1):

- Provider of direct and indirect care to patient and family
- Manager of the environment
- Teacher
- Coordinator of care
- Provider of a continuum of care
- Advocate for patients and their families
- Champion of preventive care
- Partner with the patient and family on their journey

Provider of Direct and Indirect Care to Patient and Family

The ANA (1976) differentiates between the direct and indirect care roles. **Direct care** involves the actions carried out by the nurse for a particular patient and family. **Indirect care** encompasses all the patient-related activities performed by someone other than the nurse. **Standards of Care** refer to specific behaviors expected of the nurse as care provider. Both the direct and indirect care roles require that the nurse uses the nursing process to:

- Collect data
- Formulate a nursing diagnosis
- Identify expected outcomes
- Implement care
- Evaluate the effectiveness of that care

The nurse provides direct and indirect care to patients and their families in diverse settings. For instance, the psychiatric nurse may work with patients in community mental health centers, in an inpatient psychiatric setting, in the patients' homes, in private practice, in schools, in industry, in general hospitals, or in nurse-run clinics. An example of a nurse-run clinic is Open Gates in Baltimore, Maryland. In 1993, the University of Maryland School of Nursing collaborated with the Episcopalian Diocese in Baltimore to open a clinic. This clinic is set up to serve neighborhood residents who are either uninsured or

BOX 4–1 The "Phenomena of Concern" to Psychiatric-Mental Health Nursing

Actual or potential mental health problems or patients pertaining to:

- The maintenance of optimal health and well-being and the prevention of psychobiological illness
- Self-care limitations or impaired functioning related to mental and emotional distress
- Deficits in the functioning of significant biological, emotional, and cognitive systems
- Emotional stress or crisis components of illness, pain, and disability
- Self-concept changes, developmental issues, and life process changes
- Problems related to emotions, such as anxiety, anger, sadness, loneliness, and grief
- Physical symptoms that occur along with altered psychological functioning
- Alterations in thinking, perceiving, symbolizing, communicating, and decision-making
- Difficulties in relating to others
- Behaviors and mental states that indicate the patient is a danger to self or others or has a severe disability
- Interpersonal, systemic, sociocultural, spiritual, or environmental circumstances or events that affect the mental and emotional well-being of the individual, family, or community
- Symptom management and side effects and toxicities associated with psychopharmacological intervention and other aspects of the treatment regimen

Reprinted with permission from *A Statement on Psychiatric-Mental Health Clinical Nursing Practice and Standards of Psychiatric-Mental Health Clinical Nursing Practice*,

BOX 4-2 ANA Standards of Psychiatric-Mental Health Clinical Nursing Practice

Standards of Care

Standard I. Assessment
The psychiatric-mental health nurse collects patient health data.

Standard II. Diagnosis
The psychiatric-mental health nurse analyzes the assessment data in determining diagnoses.

Standard III. Outcome Identification
The psychiatric-mental health nurse identifies expected outcomes individualized to the patient.

Standard IV. Planning
The psychiatric-mental health nurse develops a plan of care that prescribes interventions to attain expected outcomes.

Standard V. Implementation
The psychiatric-mental health nurse implements the interventions identified in the plan of care.

Standard Va. Counseling
The psychiatric-mental health nurse uses counseling interventions to assist patients in improving or regaining their previous coping abilities, fostering mental health and preventing mental illness and disability.

Standard Vb. Millieu Therapy
The psychiatric-mental health nurse provides, structures, and maintains a therapeutic environment in collaboration with the patient and other health care providers.

Standard Vc. Self-Care Activities
The psychiatric-mental health nurse structures interventions around the patient's activities of daily living to foster self-care and mental and physical well-being.

Standard Vd. Psychobiological Interventions
The psychiatric-mental health nurse uses knowledge of psychobiological interventions and applies clinical skills to restore the patient's health and prevent further disability.

Standard Ve. Health Teaching
The psychiatric-mental health nurse, through health teaching, assists patients in achieving satisfying, productive, and healthy patterns of living.

Standard Vf. Case Management
The psychiatric-mental health nurse provides case management to coordinate comprehensive health services and to ensure continuity of care.

Standard Vg. Health Promotion and Health Maintenance
The psychiatric-mental health nurse employs strategies and interventions to promote and maintain mental health and prevent mental illness.

Advanced Practice Interventions Vh–Vj

The following interventions (Vh–Vj) may be performed only by the certified specialist in psychiatric-mental health nursing.

Standard Vh. Psychotherapy
The certified specialist in psychiatric-mental health nursing uses individual, group, and family psychotherapy; child psychotherapy; and other therapies to assist patients in fostering mental health, preventing mental illness and disability, and improving or regaining previous health status and functional abilities.

Standard Vi. Prescription of Pharmacological Agents
The certified specialist uses prescription of pharmacological agents in accordance with the state nursing practice act, to treat symptoms of psychiatric illness and improve functional health status.

Standard Vj. Consultation
The certified specialist provides consultation to health care providers and others to influence the plans of care for patients and to enhance the abilities of others to provide psychiatric and mental health care and effect change in systems.

Standard VI. Evaluation
The psychiatric-mental health nurse evaluates the patient's progress in attaining expected outcomes.

Standards of Professional Performance

Standard I. Quality of Care
The psychiatric-mental health nurse systematically evaluates the quality of care and effectiveness of psychiatric-mental health nursing.

Standard II. Performance Appraisal
The psychiatric-mental health nurse evaluates own psychiatric-mental health nursing practice in relation to professional standards and relevant statutes and regulations.

Standard III. Education
The psychiatric-mental health nurse acquires and maintains current knowledge in nursing practice.

Standard IV. Collegiality
The psychiatric-mental health nurse contributes to the professional development of peers, colleagues, and others.

Standard V. Ethics
The psychiatric-mental health nurse's decisions and actions on behalf of patients are determined in an ethical manner.

Standard VI. Collaboration
The psychiatric-mental health nurse collaborates with the patient, significant others, and health care providers in providing care.

Standard VII. Research
The psychiatric-mental health nurse contributes to nursing and mental health through the use of research.

Standard VIII. Resource Utilization
The psychiatric-mental health nurse considers factors related to safety, effectiveness, and cost in planning and delivering patient care.

Reprinted with permission from *A Statement on Psychiatric-Mental Health Clinical Nursing Practice and Standards of Psychiatric-Mental Health Clinical Nursing Practice*, ©1994, American Nurses' Association, Washington, D.C.

underinsured. Many of those who make use of the services of Open Gates are considered the working poor. The mental health needs of the patients who use Open Gates are met by a psychiatric nurse faculty member who sees patients one day a week and provides psychotherapy. Another example of a setting where psychiatric nurses practice is found in Box 4–3, which describes the role of the psychiatric nurse in an Emergency Department setting.

Providing both direct and indirect care involves expertise regarding psychobiological therapies (such as electroconvulsive therapy, medications, diet, and exercise) and psychotherapeutic techniques (Schanding et al, 1982). Inherent in this role is the absolute requirement that the nurse keep abreast of the latest research regarding treatment strategies. In addition, the nurse must use delegation and supervision skills to ensure that the indirect care is delivered appropriately.

Standard Vh, focusing on the role of the nurse as psychotherapist, also involves the direct care role of the nurse but is written for the certified specialist in psychiatric-mental health nursing who has obtained additional education and extensive clinical experiences and who participates in ongoing clinical supervision.

BOX 4–3 The Role of the Psychiatric Nurse in an Emergency Department Setting

The psychiatric nurse works collaboratively with Emergency Department personnel to:

- Respond to psychiatric admissions after the Emergency Department physician has determined that there is need for a psychiatric evaluation
- Perform an immediate psychiatric evaluation including mental status examination
- Communicate findings with the on-call psychiatrist
- Collaborate with Emergency Department nurses to develop plan of care
- Remain available by telephone to Emergency Department staff

Modified from Dunn, J. (1989). Psychiatric intervention in the community hospital emergency room. *Journal of Nursing Administration, 19*, 36–40.

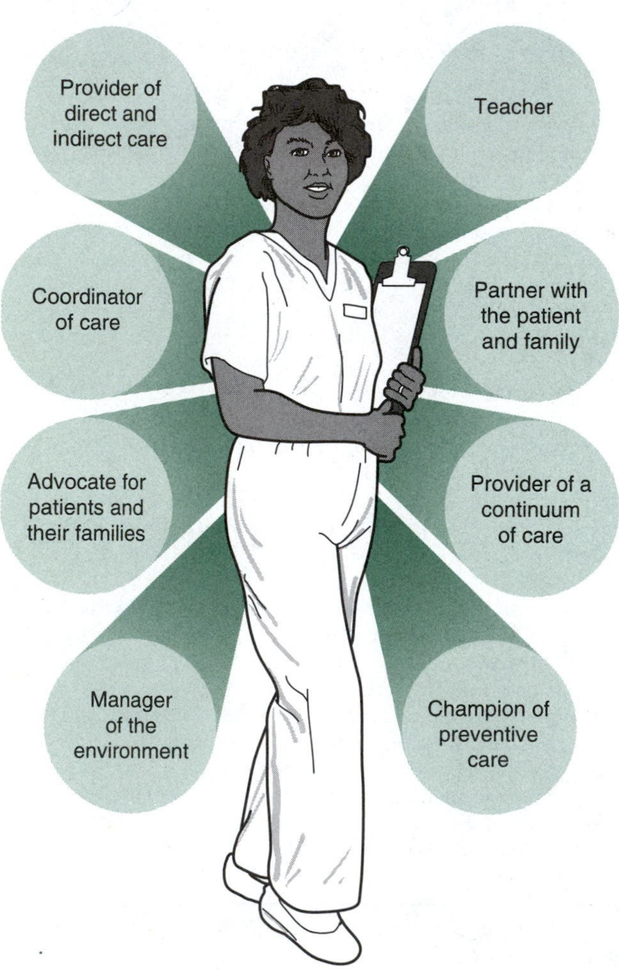

FIGURE 4–1
Roles of the psychiatric-mental health nurse stemming from the *Standards of Care* of the *ANA Standards of Psychiatric-Mental Health Clinical Nursing Practice.*

Manager of the Environment

The nurse is considered the guardian of the therapeutic environment (see Chapter 19 for a comprehensive presentation of the psychiatric-mental health nurse's role in managing the therapeutic milieu). The role of managing the environment recognizes the nurse's ability to negotiate environmental issues and to teach patients and families to do the same. This role draws on the nurse's ability to assess potentially stressful characteristics of the environment and to develop strategies to eliminate or improve these stressors. Managing the environment focuses on the global aspects of appearance, ambiance, and safety as well as the micro aspects of orienting new patients to the unit and assisting each patient to fit into the environment comfortably.

Teacher

The role of teacher is an essential one and is one of the primary intervention strategies of the nurse in improving mental health (see Chapter 22 for a comprehensive discussion of the psychiatric-mental health nurse's responsibilities involving patient and family education). Teaching focuses on **self-care** and assisting the patient and family to attain greater facility at living with the effects of mental illness. In the 1990s with the increased emphasis on self-determination of patients, involvement of patients and families in care, limited government funding to support community mental health programs, and the emergence of the intervention model of rehabilitation, teaching has assumed even greater importance.

Teaching is a skilled intervention that requires the nurse to consider appropriate teaching methods, the patient's style of learning, and the patient's ability to learn. Health teaching focuses on assisting the patient and family to understand and manage illness symptoms and medications; to improve relationships, communication skills, and problem-solving techniques; to develop coping strategies for dealing with stress; and to improve basic hygiene and activities of daily living (Slavinsky, 1984; Carson, 1994).

Coordinator of Care and Provider of a Continuum of Care

These two roles go hand in hand. The holistic perspective of the nurse provides the ability to recognize and appreciate not only the "here and now" needs of clients, but also the "round the clock" activities. This perspective is essential not only in an inpatient unit where multiple therapies and activities must be coordinated, but also in the community where the patient and family require a seamless transition into a continuum of care to prevent them from falling "through the cracks" of the health care system (Barratt, 1989; Carson, 1994). The nurse's role in facilitating progress within the health care system to progressively less restrictive settings is a role that cannot be understated (Slavinsky, 1984; Forker, 1988). The nurse may act as discharge planner in the inpatient unit coordinating various community referrals. At the time of discharge, a community mental health or psychiatric home care nurse may assume case management responsibilities to ensure that the inpatient referrals actually become a reality (see Chapter 44 for a further discussion of case management). This role involves:

- Advocating for the patient
- Networking with a variety of community resources
- Negotiating the most appropriate services for the patient
- Exercising tremendous patience and a stick-to-it attitude to provide continuity of care

Advocate for the Patient and Family

Being a patient **advocate** involves three roles:

- Educating patients about their rights and responsibilities
- Negotiating for mental health services
- Influencing legislation on local, state, national, and international levels

The advocacy role is especially important in reeducating people who continue to stigmatize and ostracize the mentally ill. Advocacy is a critical role in monitoring local, state, and national legislative trends. In the present time of limited resources, funds designated for treatment and rehabilitation of the mentally ill are particularly vulnerable to the legislative process.

It should be noted that even though the role of advocate is recognized by the nursing profession, courts, consumers, and administrators do not share this perception (Zerwekh and Claborn, 1994). Miller and coworkers (1983) conducted a study that indicated that consumers of health-related services consider the physician to be one who protects patient rights. Additionally, Miller and coworkers (1983) found that even though nurses were serving as mediators between patients and institutions, nurses were seldom able to effect change within the institution's structure. This lack of effectiveness seems to be directly related to the degree of power and authority allowed the nurse by a particular system.

Champion of Preventive Care

Being a champion of preventive care is a role that has implications for direct care to patients and families as well as to groups and communities. This role draws from the community concept of primary prevention. This concept precedes disease and is applied to a healthy population. As a champion of **preventive care,** the nurse supports a wellness focus as opposed to an illness focus. Such a focus (**primary care**) includes health promotion, illness prevention, and protection against disease. Within the scope of preventive care lie many of the independent functions of the psychiatric nurse, including:

- Providing information about mental health issues, such as facilitative communication skills, parenting, stress reduction, principles of mental health, and sex education
- Affecting societal changes that have an impact on mental health (e.g., improved living conditions, greater access to affordable housing, and better education)
- Making appropriate referrals before mental illness occurs
- Teaching patients in an inpatient setting strategies to prevent future hospitalizations
- Working with community and legislative groups on issues related to mental health

In addition to championing preventive care, the psychiatric nurse is also involved in both secondary and tertiary prevention. **Secondary prevention** involves those nursing activities directed at reducing actual illness by early detection and treatment of the problem. **Tertiary prevention** involves those nursing activities that focus on reducing the residual impairment or disability resulting from an illness.

Partner With the Patient and Family on Their Journey

The last role, entering into a partnership with the patient and family on their journey, is the role that synthesizes all the others. This role focuses the nurse on the patient and family's story, a story replete with personal struggles and victories. This role allows the nurse to glimpse the special meaning inherent in that story. Finally, this role allows the nurse to choose the personal gifts and professional skills that will assist the patient and family to divert the journey to one of greater health and improved functioning (McBride, 1990).

These roles are always integral to the functioning of the psychiatric-mental health nurse regardless of the specialty path that is chosen within the field. For instance, in Dr. Robinson's story, it is implicit that as a psychiatric consultation-liaison nurse she enacted all eight of the roles. As a **psychiatric consultation-liaison nurse,** she served as a mediator for patients with the primary staff who may have lacked the understanding of psychiatric issues to be able to intervene effectively with the patient. She provided direct patient care as she worked with individual patients who were hospitalized in both psychiatric and general hospital facilities. Her involvement in managing the environment was a direct function of her inpatient role as well as a function of her consultative role in assisting general hospital nurses to deal with the psychiatric patient. Teaching self-care was part of her direct work with patients and her consultative work with staff. Coordinating various aspects of care and providing a continuum of care are evident in her focus on the importance of psychiatric-mental health issues to the general hospital patient as well as to the designated psychiatric patient. Her role as a consultant involved advocating for the mental health needs of all patients, and her accompaniment of patients and families on their journeys is evident in her quote "... I was drawn to patients who were morose, angry, agitated, mute, or dying."

▶ Check Your Reading

1. Define direct care.
2. Define indirect care.
3. What does it mean to be the "manager of the environment"?
4. Give two examples of topics that might be taught by the nurse in his or her role as teacher.
5. What is a continuum of care?
6. What is involved in being a patient advocate?
7. Give two examples of psychiatric nursing functions that are part of preventive care.
8. Define primary, secondary, and tertiary care.
9. What does it mean to be a partner with the patient and family in their journey?

PRACTICE PATHS

Let's look at some other practice paths chosen by psychiatric-mental health nurses. The ANA delineates two levels of expertise within psychiatric-mental health clinical nursing practice: basic and advanced. The basic-level practitioner is the Psychiatric-Mental Health Registered Nurse. The advanced-level practitioner is the Psychiatric-Mental Health Advanced Practice Registered Nurse.

Basic Level: Psychiatric-Mental Health Registered Nurse

The title ***Psychiatric-Mental Health Registered Nurse*** describes the psychiatric-mental health nurse who is a licensed RN with a baccalaureate degree in nursing and demonstrated clinical skills, within the specialty, that exceed those of a beginning R.N. or a novice in the specialty. The designation *Psychiatric-Mental Health Registered Nurse* applies to those nurses who have met the formal certification criteria of the ANA. The letter "C," placed after the R.N. (i.e., R.N.,C.) indicates the basic-level certification status of the nurse.

The practice path chosen by the psychiatric-mental health registered nurse is characterized by direct care. In fact, these nurses provide most of the direct care to patients during inpatient psychiatric hospitalizations. The setting itself may be specialized to serve the needs of a particular type of psychiatric patient, e.g., the patient with schizophrenia, the severely and persistently mentally ill patient, or the patient with an eating disorder. Each of these types of patients requires from the nurse an integration of all eight roles discussed earlier. The "how" of each role differs with the patient and the setting. The following story from Art Worden illustrates the role of the psychiatric-mental health registered nurse who has chosen a path of psychogeriatrics. Art Worden's story illustrates both the general roles of the psychiatric nurse and the variation of those roles when applied to a specific patient population (Box 4–4).

Advanced Level: Psychiatric-Mental Health Advanced Practice Registered Nurse

The title ***Psychiatric-Mental Health Advanced Practice Registered Nurse*** describes registered nurses educated at the master's level, at a minimum, who are nationally certified as clinical specialists or nurse practitioners in psychiatric and mental health nursing. The preparation of these advanced practice nurses is distinguished by a depth of knowledge of theory and practice, supervised clinical practice, and competence in advanced clinical nursing skills. This nurse has the ability to function independently and to manage complex mental health problems. The doctorally prepared psychiatric-mental health registered nurse in advanced practice has both a Master's Degree in Nursing and a Doctorate in Nursing or a related field. Nurses with earned doctorates generally follow one of two traditions:

- Advanced development of the clinical aspect of psy-

BOX 4-4 Art Worden's Story

I chose geropsychiatry for several reasons. The geriatric population is obviously a population that requires more support than it has received in the past. Many of the elderly people who require help have outlived their support systems, and they find themselves alone at a time when they most need support. At this time in their lives, when they have ended careers, lost loved ones and friends, and are experiencing new obstacles to everyday living, they are in need of support, understanding, and advocacy. The job of helping people adjust to these changes and continue to live productive lives is both challenging and rewarding.

The aged who are chronically ill present an even greater challenge. They enter their later years with unresolved deficits, and as their social support falls away, they sometimes find that life is more difficult than they can manage. Many of the patients admitted to inpatient geropsychiatric units present with multiple medical conditions that may be the cause or the result of the psychiatrically manifested illness. This has forced me to remain current in medical-surgical practices and procedures.

Patient advocacy takes on an increasingly important role with elderly patients. I find that I spend a large part of my time acting as an advocate or teaching patients to be more assertive. Because so many elderly patients tend to be dependent, they may "fall through the cracks" and fail to receive needed services. This is one of the most important functions a nurse can perform in assisting the geriatric patient.

I really enjoy my job; I am challenged and rewarded every day. The best part of it is the way I get to know—I mean really know—so many interesting and enjoyable people.

chiatric nursing with a strong research focus (Doctor of Nursing Science—D.N.Sc.)

- Research and theory development in the science of psychiatric-mental health nursing (Doctor of Philosophy—Ph.D.)

The psychiatric-mental health registered nurse in advanced practice has been historically referred to as a clinical nurse specialist (CNS). The term *advanced practice registered nurse*, which may apply to a nurse anesthetist, clinical specialist, nurse midwife, or nurse practitioner, has emerged in response to the need for uniform titling within the nursing profession. The appropriate designation for advanced clinical practice in this specialty is that of the Certified Specialist in Psychiatric and Mental Health Nursing (R.N., C.S.). In the 1994 ANA *Standards of Psychiatric-Mental Health Clinical Nursing Practice*, the advanced practice nurse is referred to as a **certified specialist.**

The advanced practice registered nurse in psychiatric-mental health chooses practice paths that include the provision of direct patient care in the form of individual, family, and group psychotherapy, provided in diverse settings including private practices, homes, and clinics (Wille and Frederickson, 1981). The variety of settings in which the advanced practice R.N. provides services is mind-boggling and limited only by the entrepreneurial skills of the individual nurse coupled with the ability to sell the value of her or his clinical skills to an employer. For instance, certified specialists in psychiatric-mental health nursing work in outreach to the homeless, in psychiatric home care, in prison systems, and on college campuses. They are employed by industry to establish wellness programs. They work in nursing homes to develop and implement programs to manage demented behaviors of the elderly residents. They serve as community advisors regarding programs promoting mental health. They are employed in rehabilitation centers to assist in meeting the psychological problems of patients requiring intensive rehabilitation. They work in school systems from the elementary level through college to provide psychological care and to promote the mental health of young people (Campinha-Bacote, 1988; Farrant, 1988; Moffett, 1988; Adams, 1989; Tunmore, 1989; Yoest, 1989).

In addition to the practice path involving direct care, the certified specialist is involved in indirect care roles, including teaching, consulting, administering, and conducting research. The psychiatric consultation-liaison nurse provides all of these services within the general hospital setting (Dulaney and Crawford, 1988; Hicks, 1989).

In the last 20 years, increasing numbers of nurses are obtaining doctoral education in psychiatric and mental health nursing. Their practice paths continue to include the direct and indirect care roles. What exemplifies their practice is a high level of expertise and competence and the scope of influence they bring to bear on professional and community concerns.

A review of the journey of progression within psychiatric-mental health nursing illustrates the movement from novice, to advanced beginner, to competent nurse, to proficient practitioner, and finally to expert described by Benner (1984). The novice enters the profession armed with basic education providing a foundation in the therapies, nurse-patient relationships, and therapeutic communication. The initial experiences and supervision of the psychiatric nurse foster a progression to advanced beginner. At this stage, the nurse has coped with enough "real life" situations to begin to observe recurrent meaningful patterns in patient behavior as well as an awareness of personal skills and weaknesses in given patient situations. For instance, an advanced beginner could realistically identify the changes in a patient's verbal activity preceding an aggressive outburst. In Benner's (1984) classification system, the competent nurse parallels the basic level of certification of the psychiatric-mental health registered nurse.

The psychiatric-mental health registered nurse may continue the skill-honing process through additional clinical experience and supervision, continuing education, and graduate education and may move on to the next level of certification, which is that of the certified specialist in psychiatric-mental health nursing. The certified specialist equates to Benner's proficient nurse. At this level of expertise, the nurse is broadening the scope of practice to include attention to more general issues within the profession.

The highest level of expertise is achieved by the master's prepared nurse with experience and the doctorally prepared nurse, whose position is analogous to Benner's expert nurse. Although still involved in direct care, the focus of the doctorally prepared nurse is with the exapanding and strengthening of theory informing the profession and constituting the foundation of practice for the novice practitioner. This path from novice to expert in psychiatric and mental health nursing is an exciting journey (Figure 4–2).

▶ **Check Your Reading**

10. What are the two levels of expertise within psychiatric-mental health clinical practice?
11. What level of education is required at the basic level of practice?
12. What level of education is required at the advanced level of practice?
13. What practice role is fulfilled by the basic level psychiatric-mental health registered nurse?
14. Name three of the indirect care roles performed by the certified specialist.

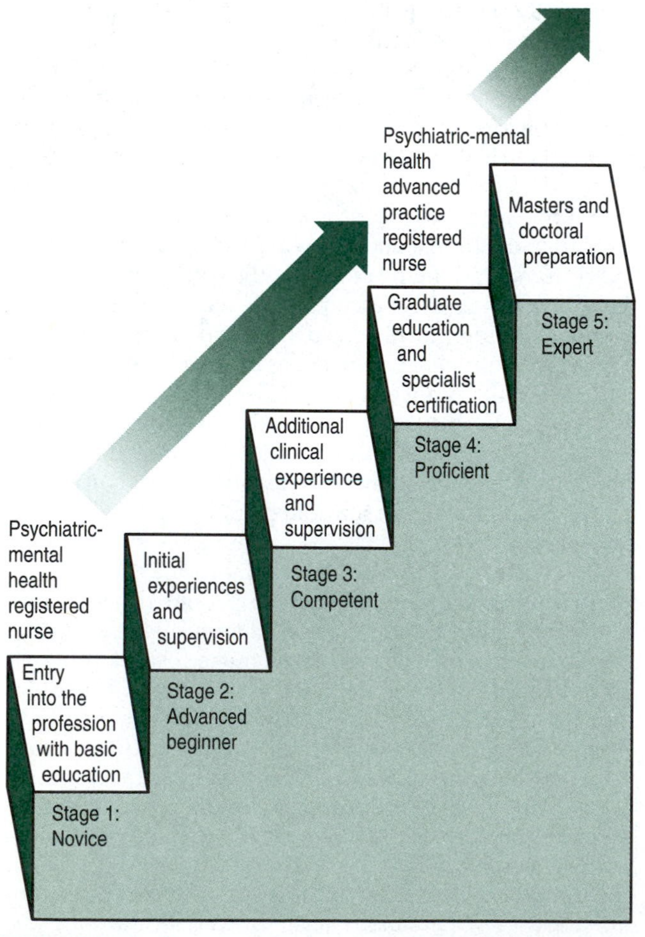

FIGURE 4–2
The journey from novice psychiatric nurse to expert psychiatric nurse.

PROFESSIONAL PERFORMANCE STANDARDS AND ROLES

In addition to the "Standards of Care" and related roles that directly affect the patient, the psychiatric-mental health nurse is expected to adhere to the "Standards of Professional Performance" set forth by the ANA (see Box 4–2). **Professional behavior standards** are statements of the expected role behaviors nurses take in caring for their patients. These standards give rise to the following roles (Figure 4–3):

- Bearer of professional standards
- Lifelong learner
- Community participant
- Ethical decision-maker
- Collaborator
- Researcher
- Steward of resources

Bearer of Professional Standards

As bearer of professional standards, each nurse is responsible for monitoring the quality of her or his own practice as well as the practice of other nurses. Nurses participate in self-evaluation as well as **peer review** and continuous quality improvement teams (see Chapter 45 for a comprehensive discussion of quality issues). This process of evaluation is imperative to maintain quality of care. As a result of the evaluation process, changes are implemented by individuals, units, and organizations to improve care.

Inherent in the evaluation process is the concept of **accountability.** Every nurse is accountable both personally and publicly for the quality of care that he or she delivers. In 1980, Hildegard Peplau wrote an article entitled "The Psychiatric Nurse—Accountable? To Whom? For What?" (Peplau, 1980). Peplau discusses the shift in accountability from personal to public. In the following quote (1980, p. 131), she stresses the importance of the accountability of the professional nurse to self.

The primary accountability of a professional is here—a matter of integrity—honesty in the moral sense, and purity of motives so that professional aims are pursued. Adherence should be to the purpose of the work with patients, which, stated generally, is to promote health-conducive behavior, and in the process, to aid the release and development of the patient's potential, while safeguarding all patient rights. To accomplish

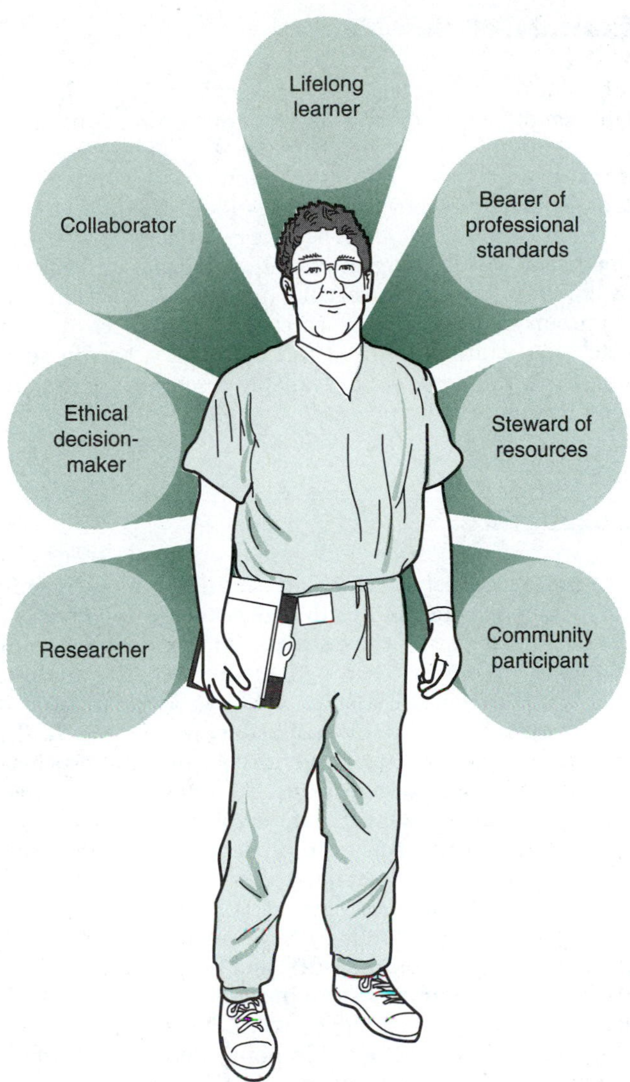

FIGURE 4–3
Roles of the psychiatric-mental health nurse stemming from the *Standards of Professional Performance* of the ANA *Standards of Psychiatric-Mental Health Clinical Nursing Practice.*

these purposes requires constant evaluation of one's practices, keeping up with and testing new theories, and periodically reviewing clinical data with peers for the possibility of inappropriate action based on faulty inferences.

Peplau continues to say that for nurses this review must address two issues:

- How does the individual nurse use time while at work?
- Does that nurse's use of time support the interests of patients?

Additionally, nurses are accountable to nurse colleagues in the work situation and in the profession at large. One of the most important kinds of peer review involves nurses' disclosure and assessment of clinical data from nurse-patient relationships in a supervisory review process in which nurse colleagues openly discuss and comment on each other's work. Peer review in psychiatric nursing is probably more important than in other nursing disciplines. This importance stems from the fact that the focus of psychiatric nursing is the understanding of human behavior, which always contains a certain amount of ambiguity. The peer review process assists the nurse in maintaining a therapeutic role with the patient and provides collegial support (Johnson et al, 1982; Pesut and Williams, 1990). Johnson et al (1982) identify a model for a professional support group in which members come together for practical help, sharing of experiences, information giving, and stimulation of new ideas. Figure 4–4 illustrates this model.

In a 1990 study by Pesut and Williams, psychiatric clinical specialists supported the need for continued clinical supervision post master's education. The respondents in this study identified the following characteristics as essential for the effective supervisor:

- Ability to share knowledge
- Ability to provide feedback
- Personal warmth
- Clinical competence
- Openness to self-examination
- Mentally healthy

Nurses are accountable beyond the work situation to be spokespersons for what nursing is and does. If psychi-

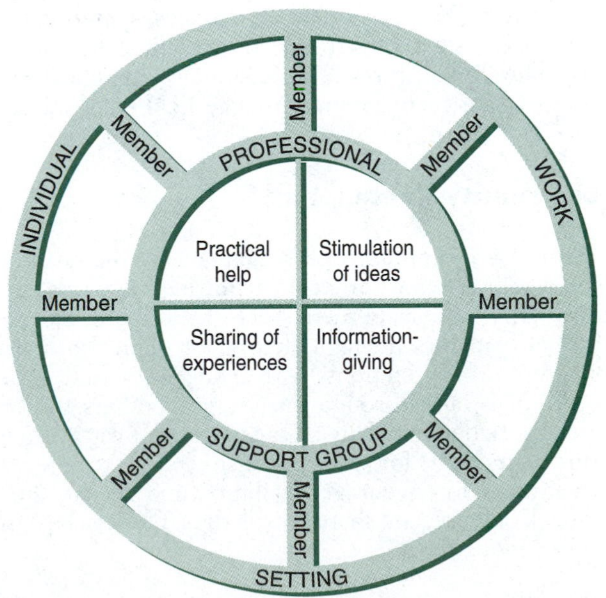

FIGURE 4–4
The model of a professional support group developed by Johnson and colleagues. (Modified from Johnson, R. M., Richardson, J. I., Von Endt, L., & Lindgren, K. S. (1982). The professional support group: A model for psychiatric clinical nurse specialists. *Journal of Psychiatric Nursing and Mental Health Services, 20*(2), 9–13.

atric nurses are unable to articulate the health problems that they treat, it is difficult to make a case for nursings' needs before legislators, third-party payers, administrators, other health professionals, and even nurses themselves.

Nurses are accountable to the public to ensure that "they get their moneys' worth" when nursing services are involved. This means that nurses monitor competencies within the profession; they communicate to the public the meaning of the credentialing process; and they monitor and report any abuses of patients that they observe.

Hospital accountability procedures can include a review of records to guarantee that each patient has a written individual treatment plan. It is only the nurse's personal accountability, however, that ensures that these plans are actually implemented.

Lastly, psychiatric nurses are accountable to the patients whom they serve. This accountability means that the nurse must disclose to the patient the purpose of nursing activities, the nature of what is to be done, the mutual responsibilities of nurse and patient, and the expected outcomes. Accountability does not mean that the nurse is responsible for the success of treatment, but rather for the nature of the effort directed toward meeting specified outcomes and for keeping the patient informed regarding the purpose of the work to be done.

Lifelong Learner

The nurse as lifelong learner is engaged in a process of continually expanding her or his base of knowledge, understanding of human behavior, and repertoire of interpersonal skills. **Continuing education,** through formal course work, seminars, in-services, symposia, and conferences, is a requisite for staying clinically competent. The nurse grows professionally as knowledge expands and is incorporated into the field of practice.

Community Participant

The nurse is a community participant and as such assumes responsibility to assist others in acquiring knowledge and skills. This responsibility is met through formal and informal teaching, through sharing of clinical observations and interpretations with colleagues and other professionals, and through encouraging others to continue to seek out knowledge. One of the best ways to keep enthusiasm high for the profession and to prevent stagnation is to encourage, facilitate, and reward those who seek out, use, and share knowledge. This can be done in a variety of ways:

- Through monetary incentives that defray the cost of education and seminars
- Through verbal affirmation
- Through recognition in a professional group
- Through merit pay increases

Ethical Decision-Maker

The nurse is responsible for providing care that is competent, sensitive, and holistic. Such a responsibility represents a sacred trust between the public and the nursing profession. This trust requires that nurses act morally and ethically in all situations. Boundaries are necessary within the nurse-patient relationship to protect the patient's well-being and safeguard against any patient exploitation, including sexual exploitation. The nurse is cognizant of situations in which ethical choices are not black and white but rather more complex, and in such situations, the nurse seeks available resources to assist in the decision-making process.

Collaborator

The nurse as collaborator recognizes that nursing is only one component of the health care team. As members of the health care team, nurses must work with other team members to ensure that patients receive the highest quality of care possible (Benfer, 1980). In psychiatry, every patient must have an individualized treatment plan (ITP) that reflects the collaborative efforts of nursing, psychiatry, social work, occupational therapy, recreational therapy, and any others who are involved in the patient's care. Table 4–1 identifies the other mental health team members and their respective roles.

Collaboration goes beyond the level of the individual patient and extends to issues involving programs, units, institutions, communities, and the United States as a whole. Collaboration subsumes the role of advocate described under core practice roles. Nursing is responsible to make its voice heard in policy debates that affect mental health care. Participating in the decision-making process is essential if nursing is to articulate its unique perspective regarding patient care issues. Nursing has a responsibility to be involved in the whole continuum of primary, secondary, and tertiary services related to mental health issues.

Successful collaboration may involve the development of networking and lobbying skills as well. **Networking** (Meisenhelder, 1982) includes developing a group of associates whose skills, talents, knowledge, and influence may enhance the nurse's own goals. For instance, a community mental health nurse's effectiveness as a case manager increases exponentially if he or she has developed a network of resources in the community that can be called on to assist a particular patient.

According to Meisenhelder (1982), networking occurs at three levels. The first is that of the grass roots level among staff nurses to promote cohesiveness, unity, and a base of emotional and professional support. The second occurs at the leadership level with the common goal of increasing the power of nurses in the health care system. The third is informational networking, which is absolutely essential for political activism.

Lobbying is a strategy used to influence policy decisions by influencing the policy makers (Bushy and

TABLE 4–1 Other Members of the Psychiatric Treatment Team

Psychiatrist
Physician who specializes in mental disorders. Responsible for diagnosis and treatment. The psychiatrist may be the team leader or administrator of the inpatient unit. This is especially true in facilities that are philosophically guided by the medical model of treatment

Clinical Psychologist
Professional whose training and education focused on mental health issues. Provides psychotherapy, plans and implements programs of behavior modification, conducts psychological testing, and conducts research

Psychiatric Social Worker
Social worker whose preparation involves a 2-year Master's Program with specialization on mental health issues and supervised clinical practice post Master's. Focuses on assisting the patient and family to cope more effectively, to identify appropriate community resources, to assist the patient to maintain or develop a support system, and to facilitate the patient's transition from inpatient to the community. The psychiatric social worker is also involved in providing psychotherapy and may engage in private practice

Occupational Therapist
Professional with a baccalaureate degree in occupational therapy. Uses creative and manual techniques to assist patients in working toward specific psychotherapeutic goals. Also, may work with patients to develop independent living skills to smooth the transition between hospital and community

Creative Arts Therapist
Uses a variety of modalities, including dance, art, poetry, and music, to assist the patient to relate in a more open and honest manner and to increase social interaction and self-esteem

Recreational Therapist
Plans and guides recreational activities to target the therapeutic needs of patients. Activities are designed to facilitate social interaction, healthy recreation, and interpersonal and intrapsychic experiences

Psychiatric Paraprofessional
Referred to as the psychiatric aide, technician, or attendant. Provides much of the direct care to hospitalized patients, especially in large public institutions. Usually receives on-the-job training directed at increasing interpersonal skills and sensitivities. The psychiatric paraprofessional plays an important role in maintaining the therapeutic environment of many inpatient units; therefore, it is essential that he or she be under the supervision of a professional nurse

Mental Health/Human Service Worker
Newest addition to the psychiatric team. Receives training at certificate, associate, and baccalaureate levels. The mental health/human service worker's popularity is increasing in light of the growing need for additional mental health workers, inability of the traditional professional services to meet the increasing demands for more personnel, proven effectiveness, and relative economy of employing such a worker.

Smith, 1990). Historically, nursing has not been seen as a powerful political force despite the potential for power inherent in the large numbers of nurses. Given the size of the profession, however, it is conceivable that group power could be exercised through organized lobbying efforts. The purpose of such efforts would be to influence public as well as legislators' opinions through careful analysis and persuasive communication of current issues (Dumas, 1994).

Researcher

The last performance standard of the ANA deals with the nurse as researcher. The inclusion of research as a performance standard speaks strongly to the need for continual striving to develop the profession further. We do not have all the answers. In fact, even with the plethora of published research, psychiatric nursing is in its infancy in defining effective interventions for specific psychiatric disorders. Jones (1987, p. 217) states that "... psychotherapy is a practice science, not a mystical art embodied in the therapist whose charisma is the motor of therapy." Even though individual skills play an important role in the administration of any scientific procedure, the principles for action are derived from a scientific base (Simpson, 1989).

The research standard covers levels of research participation from the nurse who participates in studies designed by other nurses or health professionals to the nurse who acts as principal investigator in conducting research. Nursing's involvement in research also includes incorporating new research findings into practice as well as monitoring the protection of human subjects.

Steward of Resources

Increasingly, nurses are becoming **stewards of resources,** being forced to examine ways to conserve resources. We are being called on to do more with less: less staff, less latitude in how long we can keep a patient in the hospital, less autonomy in deciding the length of patient treatment in outpatient settings, less freedom to choose the type of provider that we would like, and less freedom to continue old systems and processes without careful examination and perhaps restructuring. Questions such as the following are being directed to nurses on a daily basis:

- What is the best use of the patient's insurance benefits?
- How can we deliver quality care in a cost-effective manner?
- Who is both qualified and cost-effective to provide certain services?

Nurses must be good stewards of all the resources that they manage, including their own time and talents, the material resources of the agencies for which they work, and the insurance and personal resources of the patients and families for whom they care.

▶ **Check Your Reading**

15. Define peer review.
16. What does it mean to be accountable?
17. Why is continuing education important?
18. What is the nurse's responsibility as a community participant?
19. What is a collaborator?
20. Define networking.
21. Define lobbying.
22. Give two acceptable levels of research participation for the psychiatric-mental health nurse.
23. What does stewardship involve?

STRESS AND BURNOUT

Understanding Stress and Burnout

Without question, nursing is a stressful profession. **Stress** is part of both the direct and the indirect care roles. Faced daily with the pain and suffering of others, nurses are called on to give comfort, solace, and support even when their own resources for doing so are depleted. In addition to difficult client issues that cause the nurse stress, administrative issues, such as poor working conditions and unreasonable demands, siphon energy away from the nurse's primary focus, which is the care of the patient. Dawkins et al (1985) suggest three reasons for examining stress in nursing:

1. Stress is costly to the individual nurse, resulting in psychosomatic illnesses, impaired mental health, alcoholism, and drug abuse.
2. Stress is costly to the organization, resulting in absenteeism, tardiness, turnover, and sabotage of programs.
3. Stress interferes with nurses' ability to care for patients adequately.

Most of the research that exists on nursing stress focuses on nurses who work in settings in which physical health is the focus. It is equally important to examine the stressors that exist in psychiatric nursing (Pines and Maslach, 1978; Jones, 1987). Dawkins et al (1985) developed a 78-item Psychiatric Nurses' Occupational Stress Scale (PNOSS) and administered it to 43 nurses at one hospital. The findings of this study are of particular interest in that 50% of the high stressor items are produced by administrative/organizational issues. The most stressful item involved not being notified of changes before they took place. Negative characteristics of patients are viewed as relatively unstressful. Figure 4–5 illustrates some of the stressors encountered by psychiatric-mental health nurses.

Stress can lead to **burnout,** which is defined by Arnold (1989) as an exhaustion of physical and emotional strength. Muldary (1983) suggests that nurses are particularly vulnerable to burnout resulting in an "erosion of spirit and a general demoralization under conditions perceived as highly stressful" (p. 7).

Arnold (1989) discusses burnout as a spiritual issue for the nurse whose inner spirit is assaulted and whose life feels fragmented. Arnold (1989) suggests that there is a need to make whole and to draw life back into balance. The stress that is experienced catapults the nurse into a crisis of meaning. Malaise of the spirit is said to occur when the spirit is "pitted against a reality that cannot be changed" (Arnold, p. 326) or ordered in a meaningful way. Box 4–5 suggests questions to be used by the nurse to help maintain or restore balance and wholeness.

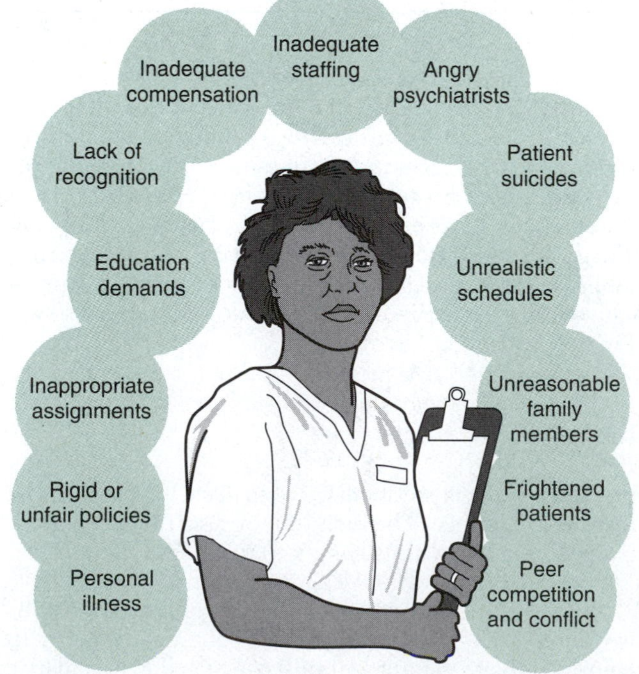

FIGURE 4–5
Some stressors encountered by psychiatric-mental health nurses.

BOX 4-5 Questions to Be Used by the Nurse to Help Maintain or Restore Balance and Wholeness

- How do my ordinary activities of daily life fit into my life goals?
- What is missing or what needs to be eliminated to help me achieve balanced wholeness?
- Why is it that I put so much stock in the words and ideas of others and have so little faith in the legitimacy of my own?
- Who defines me—myself or others?

Modified from Arnold, E. (1989). Burnout as a spiritual issue: rediscovering meaning in nursing practice. In V. B. Carson (Ed.), *Spiritual Dimensions of Nursing Practice*. Philadelphia: W. B. Saunders Company.

Strategies for Dealing With Stress and Burnout

Many strategies have been suggested for dealing with stress and ultimately burnout. Many of these strategies focus on changing the external environment in which nurses practice (Pines and Maslach, 1978); establishing an interpersonally supportive environment; and educating nurses about ways to deal with conflict, to negotiate, and to manage change (Cronin-Stubbs and Brophy, 1985).

Arnold (1989) suggests a model of dealing with burnout that addresses the inner processes of the nurse and gets at the core of burnout: a spiritual crisis of meaning (Figure 4–6). Incorporated into this model is an A-B-C mnemonic for the mutually dependent processes involved in restoring or maintaining a creatively balanced lifestyle.

Developing Awareness. The first step of the process is developing awareness. This involves naming the stressful event and owning one's personal contribution to the situation. By naming a stressful event, we take it from the realm of intangible and all-pervasive to the concrete and manageable. The step of admitting there is a problem is absolutely essential as a prelude to identifying solutions. It is beneficial to allow this awareness to place the problem within the scope of the whole fabric of our lives, to evaluate the significance of this problem or situation to self-perceptions and overall meaning.

Achieving Balance. The second aspect identified by Arnold (1989) is achieving balance. This involves the recognition that we cannot have all of our wants satisfied in the ways that we decide are best for us, and it is not possible to meet them all at the same time. Conflicting wants, needs, and responsibilities must be continually balanced. Priorities must be established. This is a process that ebbs and flows as the demands of life change.

Nurses are particularly vulnerable to the self-deceptive belief that they must be all things to all people, and in the process of living out this belief, they forget to be anything for themselves. In attempting to balance work, family, education, leisure, and spiritual activities, it is not unusual for the leisure and spiritual activities, those that directly nurture the self, to be put aside in favor of meeting the needs of others. Responsibilities have a way of becoming dictatorial, demanding more and more of the nurse's time and energy and leaving the nurse feeling physically exhausted, estranged from the people most significant in life, and spiritually depleted.

Countering the effects of imbalance requires diligence and alertness to the insidious ways that responsibilities have of getting out of control. Some responsibilities may need to be given up or delegated to others, or it may be possible to discover more energy-efficient and time-efficient ways of meeting responsibilities. It is essential to establish priorities and make decisions regarding time commitments. The nurse must have the courage to say "no" when feeling overburdened and the determination to set aside regular, planned time for the people most important in his or her life. Lastly the nurse needs to take time for spiritually renewing activities, such as taking a walk, reading a favorite book, praying, meditating, or spending time with a good friend.

Making Choices. The next step in the process of maintaining spiritual balance involves making choices: looking at alternatives and deciding *what is to be done* as well as *how to think* about circumstances. Choices such as whether to work a double shift or to study for an upcoming examination and to volunteer for one more hospital committee or to keep the commitment to attend a child's championship soccer game are the kinds of choices with which nurses are frequently confronted. It is important that we examine these choices carefully so as to avoid falling into a pattern of always choosing work over family or everything else over self.

Just as important as choosing to do or not to do particular tasks are the choices that we have regarding

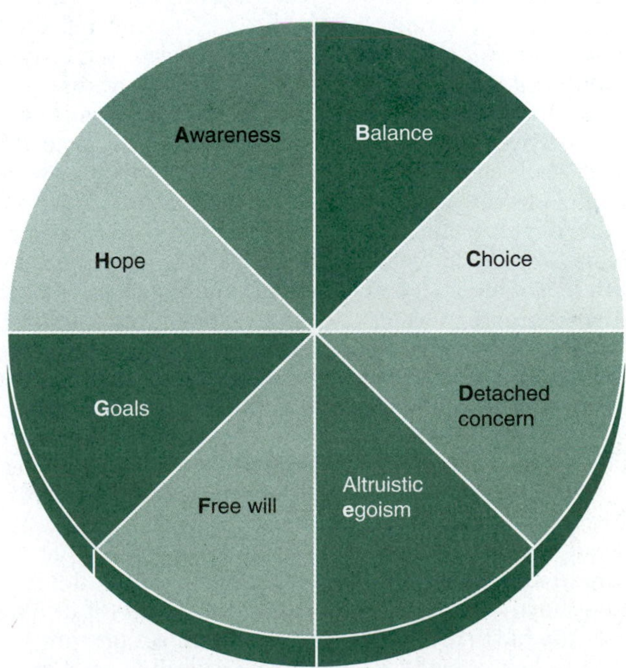

FIGURE 4–6
Arnold's model of dealing with burnout.

how we think about change and situations that are problematic. For instance, sometimes our choice might be to acknowledge that circumstances are beyond our ability to control and to use this experience to further our own growth. Another choice might be to confront the inner tension that is felt and to explore whether there is a way from our own experiences to make a difference for others. These two choices allow the nurse to find spiritual meaning in difficult situations. Another choice that exists for the nurse is to resist the possibilities for change that are inherent in the present circumstances and to focus on the negatives of the situation. This last choice keeps the nurse rooted in the present and mired in the circumstances of change that are so threatening.

Developing Detached Concern. The fourth step in achieving spiritual balance is the development of detached concern. This does not refer to distancing ourselves from others but rather detachment from our own ego involvement. Detached concern allows us to do our best at any given moment without excessive concern about how our performance affects the past or future. The nurse focuses on the here and now and is intent on making the most out of the present situation. Meaning is drawn from the present, and the nurse does not dwell on the past, avoiding "what could have been"; also the focus is not on the future, in wishful "if onlys."

Detached concern, with its present orientation, keeps us directed to the only aspect of life that we can truly control. Except in our minds, we can never go back, we can never redo what is done, and we can never predict what will be. We can, however, fully immerse our time and talents in the current situation. By shifting attention away from our own concerns, we are freer to engage in life.

The ability to achieve detached concern can be developed. One practical strategy involves the ability to laugh at ourselves and to avoid taking ourselves too seriously. Another strategy is the use of quiet reflective time, when we allow ourselves to appreciate the diverse implications of a situation. Contemplation allows us to see our overinvolvement in a situation and to recognize the places where our own ego and interests blind us to the total realities. Along with meditation, prayer may be helpful in allowing us to detach our egos from a situation. By turning a problem over to God or a Higher Power (as defined by the individual), the problem is viewed from a different vantage point, allowing the consideration of other options.

This attitude of detached concern carries with it a "letting go" of preconceived expectations about how life should unfold and how people should behave and instead embraces the possibilities inherent in every situation. This approach to life can be both frightening and freeing.

In psychiatric nursing, detached concern is of particular importance. Patients with psychiatric illnesses frequently say and do things that are hurtful to others. A nurse in close relationship with a patient is also subject to these hurtful behaviors and must have a way of dealing with the hurt that allows continued interaction with the patient. For instance, a patient who is dealing with anger at his family yells at his primary nurse, "Get out of my room, you're just like my wife, I don't want to hear your nagging voice." The nurse without detached concern feels angry and hurt and avoids further involvement with this patient. With detached concern, the nurse acknowledges the immediate visceral reaction to the patient's outburst but is able to avoid interpreting this behavior as a personal assault to self. Instead the nurse recognizes the outburst as an essential aspect of the patient's healing process and plans to use this to open up discussion with the patient at a later time.

Practicing Altruistic Egoism. This is the next necessary ingredient to achieving spiritual balance. Quite simply, this involves extending the altruistic caring that is so freely given to others to the care of ourselves. Periodically, we must stop and take stock of the activities we are engaging in just because we want to, not because we have to. If we have difficulty remembering the last time that we chose to do something for ourselves, it is only a matter of time until our reserve of comfort and empathy, so freely given to others, will be depleted. To take care of self is not self-indulgent; it is necessary. It is absolutely true that we cannot give to others what we do not possess ourselves. Just as healthy bodies require food, water, and rest, healthy spirits require nourishment and respite as well.

Exercising Free Will. The exercise of free will helps us to stick to deliberately chosen paths. It keeps us focused on our inner struggles and conflicts and helps us avoid quick solutions and escapes to difficult problems. Free will allows us to challenge the belief that we are merely buffeted along by the winds of life without any control over the outcome of our life. The exercise of free will is one of the major antidotes to the spiritual doldrums linked with burnout. Free will informs us that, regardless of the circumstances in which we find ourselves, we have the ability to make committed and deliberate choices; to live out our convictions despite obstacles and our own wavering certainty. It involves personal responsibility, persistence, and accountability.

Developing Goals. Without goals, we go through life without direction. Goals allow us to operate from a coherent foundation, organizing efforts and activities in a meaningful way. Setting goals is an active phase of productive living and a powerful strategy for preventing burnout. Goals must be realistic to be helpful. Goals that strive for perfection doom the nurse to failure before any action is undertaken.

Realistic goals require two steps. The first is a focus on our inner gifts that might help us to achieve our aims. During this step, it is often beneficial to seek feedback from a friend or advisor who can help us to look at our potential. The second step is to recognize that most goals are not achieved without the help and cooperation of others, including God (however defined). Input from others, such as friends, sharing groups, spiritual directors, mentors, or supervisors, often provides fresh insights and perspectives. The process of sharing also fosters a sense of community, which is supportive to goal achievement.

Fostering Hope. The last aspect of achieving spiritual balance and preventing burnout is fostering hope. This attribute allows us to experience the possibility of our own worth as we see ourselves fitting into the larger picture of life. Hope is an attitude-oriented as well as an action-oriented way of being. Attitudinally, hope involves expectations of ourselves, others, situations, and God. We always "hope for something better"—a raise, a resolution of an interpersonal conflict, relief from pain, healing, even a sunny day. These expectations, subject to change and revision, keep us moving forward. Expectations give direction to our actions and ways of interacting. The possibilities that we see act as guideposts for choices we make. Without hope, we are actors without a director. We lack an image of the possible endings in the drama of life in which we are participating. Without hope, it is difficult to see that what we do has meaning beyond ourselves.

▶ Check Your Reading

24. What is stress?
25. What is burnout?
26. What makes burnout a spiritual issue?
27. Name at least three of the strategies to deal with burnout.

CONCLUSIONS

In this chapter we have explored the richness of the roles, practice paths, and responsibilities of the psychiatric nurse. The journey that takes a nurse into psychiatric nursing, regardless of the specialization of that journey, is never dull or boring. It is a journey that deals with the drama of human destiny, the successes, the failures, but most importantly the process of life itself as it plays out. Psychiatric nurses perform a role in the unfolding story of every patient and family with whom they interact. These stories are forever changed because of the nurse's contribution. Serving as a health supportive resource, the nurse guides, assists, affirms, and even cajoles the patient and family in the choices that they make and the paths they choose.

This chapter examined the ANA professional practice and performance standards. These standards provide structure and direction to all that the psychiatric nurse does, including the eight roles:

- Direct caregiver to patient and family
- Manager of the environment
- Teacher
- Coordinator of care
- Provider of a continuum of care
- Advocate for patients and their families
- Champion of primary care
- Partner with the patient and family on their journey.

Different practice paths were examined with respect to the two levels of expertise within psychiatric-mental health clinical practice: the basic and the advanced levels. Within these practice paths, nurses focus on direct and indirect care roles. These roles also were examined. Last, stress and burnout were considered. Arnold's (1989) approach to burnout as a spiritual issue was presented, and strategies to deal with burnout were explicated.

KEY POINTS TO REMEMBER

- The progression into psychiatric nursing represents a spiritual journey for the nurse involved.
- The core practice roles include provider of direct and indirect care, manager of the environment, teacher, coordinator of care, provider of a continuum of care, advocate for the patient and family, champion of preventive care, and partner with the patient and family on their journey.
- The ANA published Standards of Practice for the Basic and Advanced Levels of Psychiatric-Mental Health Clinical Practice.
- The ANA delineates two levels of expertise within Psychiatric-Mental Health Nursing Practice.
- The Basic Level Psychiatric-Mental Health Registered Nurse possesses a baccalaureate degree, has demonstrated skills, and has met the certification requirements.
- The Advanced Level Psychiatric-Mental Health Registered Nurse possesses at least a Master's Degree, has demonstrated proficient skills, and has met the certification requirements.
- The ANA published Professional Performance Standards that give rise to specific roles.
- Nursing is a stressful career.
- Stress can lead to burnout, which is a spiritual issue about meaning.
- There are specific strategies for dealing with burnout and restoring spiritual balance. These include:

  Developing awareness
  Achieving balance
  Making choices
  Developing detached concern
  Practicing altruistic egoism
  Exercising free will
  Developing goals
  Fostering hope

LEARNING ACTIVITIES

1. Answer the questions posed in Box 4–5. Is your life in balance? If not, why not?

2. Observe the nurses in the settings where you are receiving your clinical experiences. What roles do you observe these psychiatric nurses fulfilling? What roles are not being met? Why do you think that there are some roles that are not being addressed by the nurses that you observe?

3. Call your State Nurses' Association to inquire about the lobbying practices of nurses in your state. What are they lobbying for? Is the lobbying done by individual nurses, the state organization, or a professional lobbyist hired by the state nurses' association?

4. As you obtain clinical experience, make note of what areas are "researchable" for the practice of psychiatric nursing.

CRITICAL THINKING EXERCISES

Miss Pebble, a nursing instructor, wants to increase her students' ability to develop critical thinking skills while they are in the psychiatric clinical experience. During postconference, she asks the students to think about the following:

1. What assumptions do you bring with you to the psychiatric setting about mental illness?
2. What experiences lead you to this point of view?
3. What implications will your assumptions have for your clinical practice—negative and positive?

Miss Pebble gave them the following word game:

1. What meaning do you assume the word *Insane* has?
2. Consider other meanings.
3. Do the alternate meanings (points of view) have implications for the student's inferences about what the patient is communicating?
4. What inference can be drawn about the teacher's beliefs about critical thinking?
5. What evidence suggests that the purpose for this exercise is clear; unclear?

REFERENCES

Adams, T. (1989). Growth of a specialty. *Nursing Times, 85*(40), 31–32.

American Nurses' Association (1976). *Statement on Psychiatric and Mental Health Nursing Practice.* Kansas City, MO: American Nurses' Association.

American Nurses' Association (1980). *A Social Policy Statement.* Kansas City, MO: American Nurses' Association.

Arnold, E. (1989). Burnout as a spiritual issue: Rediscovering meaning in nursing practice. In V. B. Carson (Ed.), *Spiritual Dimensions of Nursing Practice.* Philadelphia: W. B. Saunders Company.

Barratt, E. (1989). Community psychiatric nurses: Their self-perceived roles. *Journal of Advanced Nursing, 14,* 42–48.

Benfer, B. A. (1980). Defining the role and function of the psychiatric nurse as a member of the team. *Perspectives in Psychiatric Care, 18*(4), 166–177.

Benner, P. (1984). *From Novice to Expert.* Menlo Park, California: Addison-Wesley Company.

Bushy, A., and Smith, T. O. (1990). Lobbying: The hows and wherefores. *Nursing Management, 21*(4), 39–45.

Campinha-Bacote, J. (1988). Culturological assessment: An important factor in psychiatric consultation-liaison nursing. *Archives of Psychiatric Nursing, 2*(4), 244–250.

Carson, V. B. (1994). Doing Psych, but talking Med-Surg language. *Caring Magazine, 13*(6), 32–38, 40–41.

Church, O. M. (1987). From custody to community in Psychiatric Nursing. *Nursing Research, 36*(1), 48–55.

Coalition of Psychiatric Nursing Organizations (1994). *A Statement on Psychiatric-Mental Health Clinical Nursing Practice and Standards of Psychiatric-Mental Health Clinical Nursing Practice* (p. 8). Kansas City, MO: American Nurses' Association.

Cronin-Stubbs, D., and Brophy, E. B. (1985). Burnout: Can social support save the psych nurse? *Psychosocial Nursing and Mental Health Services, 23*(7), 8–13.

Dawkins, J. E., Depp, F. C., and Seltzer, N. E. (1985). Stress and the psychiatric nurse. *Journal of Psychiatric Nursing, 23*(11), 9–15.

Dulaney, P. E., and Crawford, G. W. (1988). Ten years in liaison nursing: Concepts, models and conventional wisdom. *Issues in Mental Health Nursing, 9,* 425–431.

Dumas, R. (1994). Psychiatric nursing in an era of change. *Psychosocial Nursing and Mental Health Services, 32*(1), 1–14.

Dunn, J. (1989). Psychiatric intervention in the community hospital emergency room. *Journal of Nursing Administration, 19*(10), 36–40.

Farrant, E. (1988). A skilled occupation? *Nursing Times, 84*(19), 38–40.

Forker, J. E. (1988). The community as site for psychiatric-mental health nursing clinical practicum. *Journal of Professional Nursing, 4*(6), 447–452.

Frost, R. (1971). *The Road Not Taken.* New York: Henry Holt & Company.

Girgenti, J. R., and Mathis, A. C. (1994). Putting psychiatric nursing standards into clinical practice. *Nursing Standards, 32*(6), 39–42.

Gregg, D. (1954). The psychiatric nurse's role. *American Journal of Nursing, 54*(6), 848.

Hicks, S. (1989). The psychiatric nurse in liaison psychiatry. *Australian and New Zealand Journal of Psychiatry, 23,* 89–96.

Johnson, R. M., Richardson, J. I., Von Endt, L., and Lindgren, K. S. (1982). The professional support group: A model for psychiatric clinical nurse specialists. *Journal of Psychiatric Nursing and Mental Health Services, 20*(2), 9–13.

Jones, J. G. (1987). Stress in psychiatric nursing. In R. Payne and J. Firth-Cozens (Eds.), *Stress in Health Professions.* New York: John Wiley & Sons Ltd.

McBride, A. B. (1990). Psychiatric nursing in the 1990's. *Archives of Psychiatric Nursing, 4*(1), 21–28.

Meisenhelder, J. (1982). Networking and nursing. *Image, 14*(3), 77–82.

Miller, B. K., Mansen, T. J., and Lee, H. (1983). Patient advocacy: Do nurses have the power and authority to act as a patient advocate? *Nursing Leadership, 6,* 56.

Moffett, M. J. (1988). Evolution of psychiatric community care. *Journal of Psychosocial Nursing, 26*(7), 17–21.

Muldary, T. (1983). *Burnout and Health Professionals: Manifestations and Management.* Norwalk, Connecticut: Appleton & Lange.

Peplau, H. E. (1980). The psychiatric nurse—accountable? to whom? for what? *Perspectives in Psychiatric Care, 18*(3), 128–134.

Pesut, D. J., and Williams, C. A. (1990). The nature of clinical supervision in psychiatric nursing: A survey of clinical specialists. *Archives of Psychiatric Nursing, 4*(3), 188–194.

Pines, A., and Maslach, C. (1978). Characteristics of staff burnout in mental health settings. *Hospital and Community Psychiatry, 29*(4), 233–237.

Schanding, D., Garber, R. L., and Siomopoulos, V. (1982). A small study on how the staff of an inpatient psychiatric unit spends its time. *Perspectives in Psychiatric Care, 20*(2), 91–93.

Simpson, K. (1989). Community psychiatric nursing—a research based profession? *Journal of Advanced Nursing, 14,* 274–280.

Slavinsky, A. T. (1984). Psychiatric Nursing in the year 2000: From a nonsystem of care to a caring system. *Image: The Journal of Nursing Scholarship, 16*(1), 17–20.

Smith, M., Buckwalter, K. C., and Albanese, M. (1990). Psychiatric nursing consultation: A different choice for nursing homes. *Journal of Psychosocial Nursing and Mental Health Services, 28*(3), 22–28.

Tunmore, R. (1989). Liaison psychiatric nursing in oncology. *Nursing Times, 85*(33), 54–56.

Wille, R., and Frederickson, K. C. (1981). Establishing a group private practice in nursing. *Nursing Outlook, September,* 522–524.

Yoest, M. A. (1989). The clinical nurse specialist on the psychiatric team. *Journal of Psychosocial Nursing, 27*(3), 27–32.

Zerwekh, J., & Claborn, J. C. (1994). *Nursing Today Transition and Trends.* Philadelphia: W. B. Saunders Company.

SUGGESTED READINGS

Carson, V. B. (1994). Doing Psych, but talking Med-Surg Language. *Caring Magazine, 13*(6), 32–38, 40–41.

Dumas, R. (1994). Psychiatric nursing in an era of change. *Psychosocial Nursing and Mental Health Services, 32*(1), 1–14.

Girgenti, J. R., and Mathis, A. C. (1994). Putting psychiatric nursing standards into clinical practice. *Nursing Standards, 32*(6), 39–42.

Peplau, H. E. (1980). The psychiatric nurse—accountable? to whom? for what? *Perspectives in Psychiatric Care, 18*(3), 128–134.

CHAPTER 5

RULES OF THE ROAD
LEGAL AND ETHICAL ISSUES IN MENTAL HEALTH NURSING

Do unto others as you would have them do unto you.

—The Golden Rule

What does the Lord require of you? To act justly and to love mercy and to walk humbly with your God.

—Micah 6:8b

LEARNING OBJECTIVES

After studying this chapter, you should be able to:

1. Define the terms associated with ethics.
2. Recognize the discomfort created by ethical dilemmas.
3. Analyze practice dilemmas and name the principles of ethics involved.
4. Claim your own hierarchy of ethical principles and evaluate ethical decisions in light of your choices.
5. Increase your self-understanding through the analysis of personal ethical choices.

KEY TERMINOLOGY

Accountability
Advocacy
Assault
Autonomy
Battery
Behavior control
Beneficence
Confidentiality
Conventional level
Covenant
Fidelity
Informed consent
Involuntary treatment
Justice
Love
Moral (ethical) dilemma
Moral distress
Moral uncertainty
No-suicide contract
Nonmaleficence
Paternalism
Personal boundaries
Postconventional level
Preconventional level
Therapeutic alliance
Veracity
Voluntary treatment

The world is full of ethical choices, choices in which none of the alternatives seems good. We make choices with a certain ethical uncertainty, and in the process we experience ethical distress. Questions arise such as: Did I do the right thing? Was I fair? Could I have been more loving in my actions? Whose rights are important in this issue? Do I have the right to decide? Does anyone have the right to make decisions for another person? Sometimes there is no right answer—only more questions.

The health care industry seems to have more than its share of ethical questions, possibly because of its intimate, life-and-death nature. Nurses routinely make choices that have moral significance, often unbeknownst to anyone except the nurse. In psychiatric nursing, in which the symptoms of the illnesses have an impact on a patient's safety, behavior, thinking, and relating, the ethical issues abound. Because of the choices that psychiatric nurses routinely make, it is necessary to learn about ethics and the law; the nurse's practice is to exemplify the introductory quotes, that is, to choose to act with justice, mercy, and consistent regard and respect for the other. The challenge is to discern what is just in a given situation and to determine how to balance justice, mercy, and love.

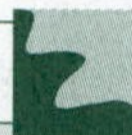

MRS. SWANSON'S STORY

Mrs. Swanson was 68 years old when she awoke in a psychiatric hospital, her first admission in her lifetime. Her thoughts raced. "I am so afraid," she thought. "Why are these people coming into my room? What do they want? Why are they asking me to leave my room and join the group? What group? Why do they speak English? They look like humans. How do they know my name? Maybe the spacemen who kidnapped me are holding me for ransom and are trying to find out what humans are like. I hope they don't hurt me. I'm not going to eat or drink anything. There is no way I am going to let them poison me. I guess I should be grateful that I am still alive, but I wonder what they plan to do with me. Maybe they will let me go home. Home!" Mrs. Swanson thought, as tears rolled down her cheeks. "What must my husband be thinking? He must be so frightened, wondering what could have happened to me. He must be looking everywhere for me. If only I could tell him I am okay. I hope he didn't see them jolt my body and throw me into the spacecraft. I hope he didn't see me leave him, our farm, and our animals behind. How long have I been held captive? I wish someone would give me answers.

"Another woman just entered the door, and she is asking me if she could turn on some lights. Why is she asking me? I'm her prisoner. But the woman is so kind, maybe I had better answer her. 'Please turn the light on,' I responded. The woman turned on a reading lamp. I looked around and saw that I was sitting in a comfortable rocking chair. There was a bed, a chest of drawers, a desk, and a clock. They must tell time like on Earth, or did it just look similar? I'll wait to see what happens at 12:59.

'I need to take your vital signs,' the young woman said, 'then how about a shower and breakfast?' I shrank back. Vital signs? Does she think I'm dead?

" 'Am I dead?' I asked.

" 'What do you think?' she asked.

"I considered. Maybe I am dead. But I thought I'd go to heaven. 'Is this heaven?'

" 'No,' she smiled, 'this is Memorial Hospital, and you are in the psychiatric unit.'

" 'Memorial in Hudson?'

" 'Yes. You seem surprised.'

" 'Oh, thank God!' I screamed, and began sobbing. Two other people ran into the room at that point, alerted by my scream. 'I'm home! The spacemen brought me back to earth! You're real! You really are human!"

I began shaking, and my chest started hurting. The woman quickly wrapped the blood pressure cuff around my arm and took a reading. I thought the shock of the kidnapping and space journey had taken its toll on my body. I was glad to be in the hospital where people would take care of me.

If you were taking Mrs. Swanson's journey, how would you want to be treated? Would you want your nurse to understand your concerns about eating and drinking? Would you expect to be forced to take medication? Would you want your nurse to support your view of reality? This chapter explores the ethical and legal boundaries that guide your journey as a caring professional in relationship with Mrs. Swanson and other psychiatric patients. In addition, patients' rights are addressed.

PRINCIPLES OF ETHICS TO GUIDE THE JOURNEY

As we are faced with **ethical dilemmas**, we ask ourselves:

- "How can I best care for my patient?"
- "Is my patient able to make good decisions?"
- "Do I have the right to make decisions for the patient?"

Answering these questions leads us to choices that, it is hoped, produce the least damage to human integrity. Underlying our choices are a number of ethical principles or the reasons given for the choices that we make. There are eight principles of ethics that guide helping relationships, as follows:

- Justice
- Love
- Beneficence
- Nonmaleficence
- Autonomy
- Paternalism
- Veracity
- Fidelity

From a theistic world view, justice and love subsume all the other principles. Not everyone who engages in ethical decision-making, however, does so from a theistic perspective, and the world view influences the preferred principles. For instance, a humanist might value the principle of autonomy over other principles. As you are confronted with ethical dilemmas, you are confronted with three tasks. First, you need to define your own world view. Second, you make decisions consistent with that world view. Third, you use professional judgment in the appropriate application of the selected principles to your decision-making.

▶ Check Your Reading

1. What are the two main ethical principles operating in a theistic world view?
2. Name the eight ethical principles.

Justice as a Guide on the Journey

Justice is the distributive principle concerned with the equitable treatment and fair handling of people. Although justice has always been important in ethical decisions, health care reform has brought the principle of justice into focus. Justice is concerned with making right or appropriate decisions about providing or withholding health care from individuals, families, or populations.

The question of what is just is difficult to answer. Is reward or health care given to those in need? To those who can pay for it? To those who have made contributions to society? To those who have the potential to make a contribution? Personal and societal values shape the application of justice, and people hold strong opinions. The 1994 referendum in California to deny health care, educational benefits, and other social benefits to illegal immigrants is an example of the difficulty in deciding what is just. The citizens of California voted that justice is not served by rewarding illegal immigrants with services which they did not earn or for which they did not pay. The courts in California immediately responded by blocking the enactment of the referendum, arguing that it is unjust to deprive any person, illegal alien or citizen, of the basic necessities of life.

Health care reform advocates *universal access* as the new norm for justice but only for basic services. There is no consensus, however, about what constitutes basic services. Some argue that coverage for mental health services is a basic service; some consider such coverage to be optional, additional, or a luxury service.

Considerations of justice are important not only for global issues such as health care reform, but also in the small everyday decisions that nurses face. For instance, if a nurse decides that one patient can have a second dinner, while another patient is denied dessert, the principle of justice is in operation. As with any just decisions, all onlookers evaluate the rightness or fairness of the decision. Just decisions are difficult to render but are required by the nurse. Because psychiatric patients are most often treated in groups, many patients determine the fairness of a decision. Many of these kinds of decisions are often made in consultation with the group of patients affected by the decision and by the person about whom the just action is being determined.

▶ Check Your Reading

3. Define justice.
4. Give one example in which justice is the issue in the care of the mentally ill.

Love as a Guide on the Journey

Love, when applied to ethical decision-making, has nothing to do with what the Greeks referred to as "eros," or desiring something for self, but rather "agape," meaning a self-giving and sacrificial attitude. Love in this context is different from friendship in that its survival does not depend on reciprocal admiration. Love is an overall moral principle, all-inclusive and exceptionless, that from a theistic world view governs all our actions. Love derives from a relationship with God that results in service to others.

Loving patients is exemplified when you are able to accept a patient unconditionally even though the patient behaves in ways that are undesirable. This does not mean that you accept the behaviors. In fact, the most loving action that you can take is to set limits on behaviors that threaten the patient or other people. An example of such love balanced with limit setting is shown in Case Example 5–1.

Case Example 5–1 Mimi's Story

All morning, Mimi screamed obscenities at anyone who even looked her way. Everyone, patients and staff included, was on edge. Jim, the nurse assigned to Mimi, approached her at a respectful distance and spoke to her. "Mimi," Jim said, "I can see you are upset this morning. We are all concerned about you and how you are feeling, but people are getting upset because of your screaming. I would like to help you calm down. I'd like to go to the quiet room together and stay with you while you try to calm down. If that doesn't help, then we can try a dose of the medication that the doctor ordered for you. I don't want people getting angry at you, so let's do something to improve the situation."

▶ Check Your Reading

5. Define love when it is applied to ethical dilemmas.
6. What is the relationship between justice and love as ethical principles?

Beneficence as a Guide on the Journey

Beneficence operates whenever you engage in making decisions for persons who are incompetent and do not have the faculties to decide for themselves. Whenever possible, families are included in the operation of beneficence for incompetent people.

Beneficence is active, even aggressive, in promoting good, preventing harm, and removing evil. For instance, when the symptoms of psychiatric illness place a patient at risk, it is your responsibility actively to thwart harmful actions that could lead to suicide or homicide. It is more difficult to deal with thoughts, feelings, attitudes, and negative self-talk that are also harmful but in a more subtle way. The application of beneficence in the subtle situations of harm requires more skillful confrontation.

Nonmaleficence as a Guide on the Journey

Nonmaleficence means that no harm or risk of harm may be inflicted on another. This principle focuses more on the provider than on the patient; you resist sarcasm, showing irritation, comparing one patient to another in a belittling way, displacing unpleasant feelings onto others, or using patients to meet your own needs. Nonmaleficence requires you to be self-aware, to manage personal behavior, thoughts, and feelings and to take responsibility for your actions. Further, this level of maturity and mental health is an excellent role model for others.

▶ **Check Your Reading**

7. Define beneficence.
8. Define nonmaleficence.
9. Give an example of violation of beneficence and nonmaleficence.

Autonomy as a Guide on the Journey

Autonomy means choosing freely and living with the consequences of the choice. This does not mean that persons live in isolation and alienation; autonomy is most powerful when operating in community (Danis and Churchhill, 1990). You encourage autonomy when you provide the patient with adequate information and the necessary support needed to make choices. Assisting persons to choose the right and the good may not generate the choice that you would have made. Supporting the person's choice, however, enables autonomy.

Supporting autonomy does not preclude the patient's right to change a choice. For example, a mother may decide not to sign a permit for psychotropic medication for an adolescent child. That choice may be difficult to make, given the recommendation of the treatment team. But after living with that choice for a week and seeing the continuing pain and aggressive behavior of her psychotic child, the mother may reconsider her choice.

You encourage autonomy by:

- Giving information
- Assisting the patient and family to sort through values, observations, facts, and alternatives
- Understanding the immense responsibility of autonomy
- Supporting patients and family in and through the process.

▶ **Check Your Reading**

10. What is autonomy?
11. What are some of the conflicts that arise when we respect the patient's autonomy?

Paternalism as a Guide on the Journey

Paternalism is based on the belief that the knowledge and education of the professional authorizes the professional to make decisions for the good of the patient, regardless of the patient's wishes. Paternalism derives from parental protection of and decisions for a child and indicates the nature of the relationship (Levenson, 1986–87.)

A patient who has made a serious suicide attempt provides an opportunity for paternalism (Whiteworth, 1982). The person who interrupts the attempt commits the first paternalistic act—interrupting the patient's decision. The patient does not want to be evaluated for possible psychiatric intervention; therefore, insistence that the person receive evaluation is the second paternalistic act. Telling the patient of the need for a short hospital stay and handing a pen to sign admission papers are paternalistic. If the person decides to go home or leave the hospital when staff think the patient is still in danger of suicide, paternalism also operates. Do staff members file involuntary commitment papers and hold the patient for a court hearing? Do staff members manipulate and coerce the patient to stay or to decide tomorrow? Do staff members talk relatives into refusing transportation or housing? These are all acts of paternalism. The purpose is to maintain the life of the person; the actions are consistently done on behalf of the person. Clinical judgment and team decision-making assist in knowing when to use paternalism, professional standards, legal requirements, and autonomy. Personal and professional conflicts, values, and judgment are inherent in ethical decision-making as this example shows.

Veracity as a Guide on the Journey

Veracity refers to telling the truth, an obligation that is sometimes difficult to meet in the health care setting (Lutzen, 1990). First, patients sometimes ask questions without concrete answers. They want guarantees that symptoms will go away, that they will get better, when there are no such guarantees. It is difficult at times to know what is the truth. A family might ask you if their daughter is in control of her behavior and intentionally aggressive. Or will that same daughter ever improve enough to be able to return to college? A young woman with a history of having been sexually abused may ask you if it is possible for her ever to be a good mother. These concerns call for support and excellent communication skills, but concrete answers are inappropriate. Sometimes veracity is an obligation that is difficult to enact.

Second, other kinds of questions have answers, but you may be uncomfortable answering because you fear that your response may threaten your relationship with the patient. Sometimes the question highlights behavior that you are ashamed of or do not want to acknowledge. The patient may ask: "Are you angry with me?" "Were you talking about me to that other nurse?" "Why are you afraid of me?" How would you handle these opportunities for veracity?

▶ **Check Your Reading**

12. Define paternalism.
13. Define veracity.
14. Give an example when paternalism is the preferred principle.
15. Give one example when patients ask for an answer and veracity is difficult to operationalize.

Fidelity as a Guide on the Journey

Fidelity is faithfulness to obligations, duties, or observances; it is keeping promises and is akin to veracity. Fidelity is vital in establishing trustworthy relationships with patients and staff members. Following through, being reliable, and telling the truth regardless of the personal consequences fit the standard of fidelity (Lutzen, 1990).

Fidelity begins with seemingly small incidents: "I'll be back in 15 minutes." "I will go for a walk with you right after dinner." "I will sit with you and your husband while you explain your need for your medication." Your work reality is filled with unexpected needs, changes in plans, and multiple priorities. Making commitments to a patient, family, or a group of patients necessitates follow-through or confidentiality with full understanding of that reality. There are times when a commitment or promise simply cannot be kept. When you use fidelity, you must tell the patient that the commitment cannot be kept and why (short of violating someone else's confidentiality) and make amends. Amends may be an apology, an acknowledgment of the other's disappointment, or setting up another time to fulfill the commitment.

Fidelity also includes the following:

- Carrying out physicians' prescriptions for patients
- Questioning and refusing to administer inappropriate or unsafe prescriptions
- Documenting on management reports why promises could not be kept
- Following through with consistency the treatment plan developed by the team or the nursing staff on other shifts

Teamwork depends on faithful following through, as if the commitment were personally made. This kind of team fidelity requires thoughtful consideration of the obligations placed on other staff when promises are made that other people will have to fulfill.

From the simple definitions and explanations of the eight ethical principles, one can see the overlap and potential conflict among ethical principles, for example, autonomy and beneficence or paternalism and veracity.

▶ Check Your Reading

16. What is fidelity?
17. How does fidelity play a part in team work on a unit?
18. Give one example of a situation in which it would be difficult to tell the patient the truth.

ETHICAL DECISION-MAKING THROUGHOUT THE JOURNEY

In addition to relying on principles to arrive at ethical decisions, we might use one of two different models of ethical decision-making. The first model developed by Kohlberg deals with justice; the second developed by Gilligan is based on care.

Lawrence Kohlberg's model of moral development focuses on three levels—preconventional, conventional, and postconventional (Kohlberg and Kramer, 1969). During the **preconventional level,** the child responds to rules of society and labels of good and bad. The child acts out of an absolute respect for authority rather than any respect for or understanding of morality. As the child continues to develop, he moves into satisfying his own needs rather than being concerned with the needs of others.

Kohlberg's second level, the **conventional level,** is characterized by conformity to the rules expected by family and culture with no thought to consequences. At first, the child is totally focused on meeting the "good boy/good girl" expectations to win approval from others. Later in the conventional level, the child focuses on following fixed rules, on respecting authority and law, and on maintaining the social order.

The third level proposed by Kohlberg, the **postconventional level,** occurs when the individual makes a conscious effort to define his or her own morality apart from outside authorities. The individual begins the postconventional level when he sees himself as a participant in the changing matrix of social obligations and responsibilities. As the individual's moral development continues, however, universal ethical principles, such as justice, human rights, and respect for the dignity of human life, become important as the individual's conscience serves as the final arbiter in ethical dilemmas.

Kohlberg's framework highlights justice as the guiding principle for decisions. Moral development is evaluated by the degree of autonomy and accountability of the individual making the judgment with the highest levels of morality attained by the individual who independently makes and lives with the consequences of the decision. A criticism of this framework is the emphasis on the individual alone. Because developmental research on Kohlberg's model has included mostly men, the framework is thought to reflect a male socialization in middle-American society.

In studies using Kohlberg's model, women consistently appear deficient in moral development. Generally, women exemplify the conventional "good girl" morality, whereas men usually achieve a higher level of moral development, even occasionally moving into the level of autonomous morality. This finding is not surprising to Kohlberg, who believed that men and women see moral problems in the same light. He concluded, however, that the deficient female moral development was a direct function of remaining in the home helping and pleasing others. Kohlberg believes that as women move into the workplace they will be confronted with the inadequacy of this moral perspective and progress like men toward the higher levels of moral decision-making in which rules are subordinated to universal principles of justice.

An alternative to the autonomy of the individual making ethical decisions is Gilligan's (1982) "perspective of care." Gilligan challenged Kohlberg's assumptions that justice and moral rights are the highest form of moral development. She studied young girls, college women, and housewives to determine how they frame ethical problems and discovered that females tend to focus on conflicting personal responsibilities rather than conflicting rights and justice. Women focus on their responsibilities within the context of family and community and require that other factors as well as justice be considered. The relationship of this framework is considered more "female" in orientation because of the emphasis on caring and mercy.

Gilligan reminds us that social conditioning is vital in determining the ways in which people conceptualize moral problems, the issues that they perceive as ethical conflicts, and the values that they use to resolve the conflicts. Girls and boys are socialized in different ways. Boys frequently engage in games with rigid rules that they use to resolve interpersonal conflicts. The first step in the process of individuation for a boy involves separating himself from others. A boy's skills at intimacy and relationships are developed later.

Girls engage in less competitive and less structured games with more flexible attitudes toward rules. Girls tend to deal with conflicts by stopping the games and finding alternative activities so as to preserve the relationships. Girls generally identify who they are simultaneously through their relationships.

Gilligan's perspective is useful to nursing because of the emphasis on obligation, sacrifice, and sensitivity about hurting others. She believes that a moral person is one who responds to need and demonstrates care and responsibility in relationships.

Figure 5–1 emphasizes the importance of social conditioning and social scripting for moral decision-making. The figure does not emphasize the difference in

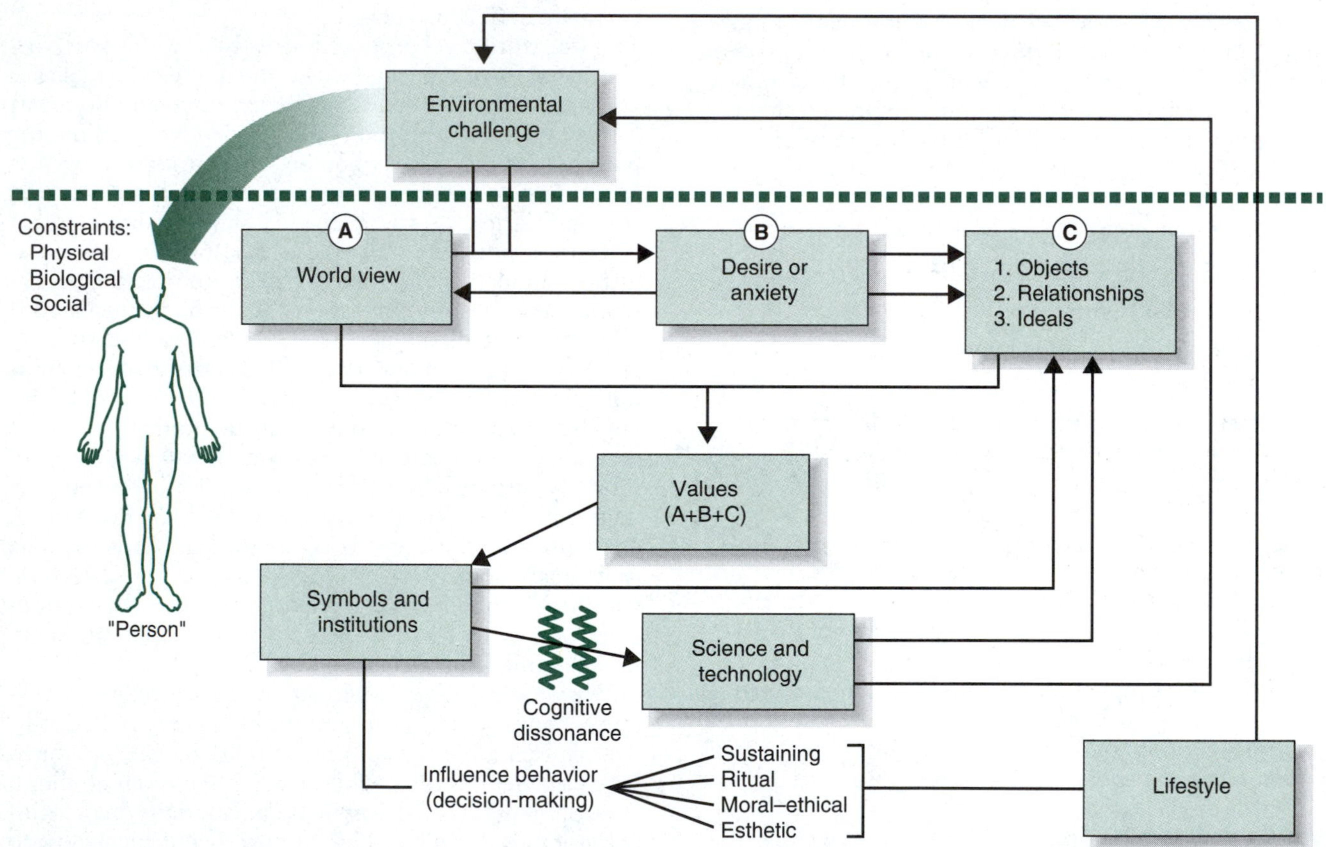

FIGURE 5–1

Social and environmental factors affecting our moral values. Whether we are a health care consumer or practitioner, we are subject to a variety of personal and environmental influences that condition and color the values we develop and the decisions we make. Below the *broken horizontal line* are the many personal factors we need to consider. Initially three elements, *A*, our fixed or process world view, *B*, our emerging desires and concerns, and *C*, our ideals, personal relationships, and experiences combine to create our personal values. These values are then given social expression in our laws, cultural values, and institutions. But science and technology also have an impact on our symbols and institutions, sometimes in a positive way, sometimes creating a disturbance or challenge (a cognitive dissonance). Filtered through our social institutions and symbols, our personal values are expressed in a particular lifestyle. The way we live as individuals then feeds back and impacts on our social and physical environment. The interaction between our personal lifestyles and the environment feeds back to us as individuals. As a result, we experience physical, biological, and social constraints. But the changing environment also has an impact on our world view and leads to new desires or anxieties. Because this network of interacting factors is constantly changing for each one of us, we should be aware of these factors and how they might affect our decisions in biomedical ethics *as well as other issues.* (From *Ethical decisions in medicine.* Brody, H. [1976]. Boston. Published by Little, Brown and Company.)

social conditioning experienced by boys and girls. As you look at the figure, however, keep in mind that world view *(box A)*; desires and anxieties *(box B)*; and objects, relations, and ideals *(box C)* differ for boys and girls.

Moral and ethical perspectives may be developed from two perspectives, justice and care. These principles are not really "male" or "female," and the view of them as such serves only to polarize the genders. Although neither perspective is totally adequate in making ethical decisions, most people emphasize one over the other and argue that one model is superior to the other. Truth is most likely found, however, in the tension between justice and care with neither being superior to the other. Both need to be considered when making ethical decisions. This explains why ethics in real life is not a simple, factual exercise; ethics requires complex judgment, clarity of thinking, and ownership of one's own values (Ketefian, 1989).

▶ Check Your Reading

19. What are the three levels of ethical decision-making as described by Kohlberg?
20. How does Gilligan's theory differ from that of Kohlberg?

ETHICAL DILEMMAS THROUGHOUT THE JOURNEY

There are multiple ethical dilemmas; they entail a broad spectrum from "is there something wrong in this situation?" to "what is the right thing to do?" Six ethical dilemmas in the practice of psychiatric-mental health nursing are presented for exploration.

Informed Consent

Informed consent is a choice:

- Based on understanding the situation, the outcomes, the alternatives, and the risks and benefits
- Made freely, without inducement, force, or any other kind of coercion
- Made by a competent person who fully comprehends all the information being given (Whitlock, 1989)

The opposite of informed consent is **assault** (threatening to touch or creating a fear of being touched) and **battery** (intentional touching without the person's permission).

How often are you expected to, or expect yourself to, assist a person who does not want assistance? From helping with bathing and toileting to secluding and restraining, nursing staff have multiple opportunities to be uncertain and experience dilemma and distress (Fowler, 1989) and to act anyway, on behalf of the patient.

The center of the informed consent dilemma is the patient's understanding. Multiple factors influence the patient's ability to process information and apply it to the real-life situation. With psychiatric patients, the factors are even more complex (Tarbuck, 1992).

The symptoms of psychiatric illnesses affect thought, perception, and mood. The disorders interfere with the patient's ability to hear (versus what they are told), process information, and interpret data. To compound the problems presented by the psychiatric illness, add the ordinary anxiety with which all persons deal daily, topped with the additional anxiety of the situation and its meaning; subtract the person's coping effectiveness; and weigh the patient's true understanding of the information presented.

Let's return to our opening story of Mrs. Swanson. Given her state of mind, was it possible for her to give informed consent? She was under the impression that she was a captive, possibly of a benevolent species. Would she have trusted her captors enough to think they were telling her the truth? She did not think she was ill, so why would she consent to take medication? If she did agree, would her consent have been valid? Similar considerations play a role whenever informed consent is obtained from patients diagnosed with psychiatric illnesses.

An article in *Time* (Willwerth, 1994) entitled "Madness in fine print" addressed the issue of informed consent in relation to enrolling schizophrenic patients, who have information processing deficits, in experimental research. Willwerth reported that ten different UCLA-VA experiments were under investigation for "ill-informed consent" (p. 62). The investigations focused on the manner in which investigators were informing study participants about the risks involved in their participation. Evidence indicated that some researchers deliberately withheld information about the high risk for psychotic relapse and used coercive techniques to enlist the participation of subjects.

Each person has a set of "meaning questions" that influence the decision. For instance, in the above-mentioned *Time* article, one patient, Harry Cummings, confronted the following meaning questions: "Will these drugs make me better? What if I don't participate, will my Veteran's benefits be cut off?" In the example of Mrs. Swanson in our beginning story, her meaning questions might include: "If I eat and drink what they give me, will I get to go home? If I cooperate, will I be able to see my husband again?" Other patients may be confronted with questions such as: "Does this mean I'm crazy? Am I being punished? Am I hopeless? Can I ever get well? Will I be able to get rid of these voices? What if I'm not strong enough to help myself? Will my spouse divorce me? Will I end up in a back ward or as a homeless person? What if I can't hold down a job? What if my insurance is cancelled?" and so on.

Meaning questions in fact must be answered honestly and weighed carefully to come to an informed decision. Unanswered questions, however, and answers that are meaningless to the patient complicate the patient's ability to make an informed decision. You can see why a professional might be tempted to make a paternalistic, even beneficent response and make the decision for the patient. It is easy for those of us who have the education, experience, and distance from the intimacy of the patient's life to convince ourselves that we are in an excellent position to give advice. It is generally not in the patient's best interest, however, to short-circuit the patient's decision-making process.

Why not give advice? If clinicians had only education, experience, and objectivity, one might be able to make a case for telling the patient what to do. There are factors, however, that create a subtly coercive environment when advice is given. When you are asked for advice, your expertise is acknowledged. You have the power to influence, and that power carries tremendous responsibility. You can never be absolutely sure that your advice is absolutely objective, free of your own biases. How can you know with certainty what will work in another person's life? Are you aware of all the latest research related to the patient's concerns or all the available options? What if you have a different perception of the patient's illness than the patient does?

The core issue involved with giving advice is power and the misuse of it. We must take care not to abuse the power we have in relationships with patients so that we block the patient's ability to choose freely. Patients may need someone to assist them to arrive at an attribution or meaning to a specific decision. Communication skills of listening, reflection, restatement, and so forth are invaluable to this process. In informed consent, the goal for the nurse is to assist the patient to weigh accurate information in light of the meaning of that decision and to choose fully, including the willingness to live with the consequences of the choice.

Informed consent is extremely complex. Yet, how much time is given to a patient and the family to make a choice and sign the paper? The point is, informed consent is not a goal or an end point; it is a process (Varricchio and Jassak, 1989). At any point, patients may change their minds, may ask more questions, may need someone to listen as the meaning of a decision or condition is explored. The nursing staff are invaluable in this process. The patient's status in the process of informed consent needs to be communicated to the multidisciplinary treatment team so that all those involved may be of assistance in supporting the patient's self-determination and autonomy.

▶ Check Your Reading

21. What are the requirements for informed consent?
22. Define informed consent.
23. What is the risk in giving the patient advice?

Use of Electroconvulsive Therapy

Many issues juxtapose when electroconvulsive therapy (ECT) is discussed: world view (see Chapter 1), body integrity, knowledge base, informed consent, and outcome of treatment, to name a few. If you believe that the brain is a complex memory bank, organized like files, the idea of blowing a ray of electricity through those files is absurd. Why disorganize those files? The person may never get all the information found and stored properly. How does ECT work? For what disorders is ECT used? Have you read the latest studies on the efficacy of ECT? Because the physician recommends ECT for a particular patient, under what circumstances would you communicate concern about that recommendation? To whom would you communicate concern? Case Example 5–2 demonstrates an ethical dilemma involving ECT.

Case Example 5–2 Wanda's Story

Wanda, 31 years old and mayor of her city, was admitted to a psychiatric hospital for psychotic depression after a serious suicide attempt. Immediately before her attempt, a friend with whom she was having an affair sent flowers to her office. She was horrified. What would her colleagues think? her husband and children? She was instantly overwhelmed with guilt over the violation of her marriage vows and impulsively ran her car off a bridge.

Wanda was admitted to an inpatient unit, severely depressed, experiencing psychotic ideation, and still expressing suicidal ideation. Robert, one of the psychiatric nurses on the unit, began to work with Wanda. They quickly established a therapeutic relationship in which they discussed the affair, guilt, conflict resolution, meaning of the relationship and her marriage, and her belief that she needed to seek forgiveness from God. In addition, Wanda was placed on fluoxetine (Prozac). Robert provided medication and illness teaching for Wanda.

The psychiatrist recommended ECT. Robert was shocked that this recommendation was offered to the patient because Wanda seemed to be responding. Wanda agreed to the ECT because of her continuing inability to function at home or in her job. Robert, having diagnosed Wanda's condition as "inability to function related to values conflict," questioned the psychiatrist about the recommendation for ECT and expressed reservations regarding Wanda's ability to provide informed consent. The psychiatrist assured Robert that Wanda had given informed consent; with this assurance, Robert supported Wanda's decision.

After the first ECT treatment, Wanda emerged from the psychosis. She had only a vague recollection of the hours of conversation with Robert. Her depression abated, she could think clearly and concentrate, and she wondered why she was in the hospital. Wanda had two more treatments and was functioning as mayor again within a week.

Several questions arise from this example. Was Wanda able to give informed consent for ECT? Because she was experiencing a psychotic depression, the ECT treatments were apparently the treatment of choice for Wanda. Since a positive outcome was achieved, is informed consent even relevant? Does the end justify the means?

Although a "cure" or definite positive outcome was achieved, what about caring for Wanda as a person? The issues for Wanda had not changed, although the psychotic depression was resolved. For the nurse, informed consent was the reason for his acquiescence. Wanda's autonomy and right to self-determination were honored, against the nurse's personal choice for Wanda. Beneficence and paternalism could have been the principles emphasized by the nurse, however, and a different process could have occurred. Had Robert continued to be concerned after talking with the psychiatrist, the next step probably would have been to get the latest research on ECT. If Robert was still not comfortable with the treatment plan, he could have talked to his supervisor, clinical specialist, clinical ethicist, or patient advocate to assist him to develop strategies to approach Wanda, her family, and the psychiatrist about ethical issues surrounding the treatment choice.

▶ Check Your Reading

24. Explain the reason Robert objected to Wanda receiving ECT.
25. What are the options open to a nurse faced with an ethical dilemma?

Use of Medication When the Patient Refuses

There are many factors creating **moral distress** (knowing the right action but perceiving constraints because of institutional policies, written or unwritten; Fowler, 1989). The patient who signs admission and treatment papers but refuses prescribed medication creates distress for the nurse. The patient is deemed capable of giving informed consent and therefore is capable of giving informed refusal. The patient's condition warrants a fair trial of a particular medication, and the nurse has considerable manipulation and persuasion powers (Lutzen, 1990) to talk the patient into taking the medication. For Mrs. Swanson in the opening story of the chapter, the nurse would have had to work hard to get the patient to take medication she might think is poison. What would help most, however, in alleviating the psychotic symptoms she seemed to exhibit?

When the nurse uses persuasion and manipulation to get the patient to take medication, paternalism is operating. The nurse is acting on what she believes is best for the patient, despite the patient's own assessment. Yet, it is not uncommon, after several doses of medication, that patients are quite often grateful for the nurse's cajoling and convincing. The patient is now functioning at a near-normal level and is no longer suffering the anguish of psychosis.

The opposite may also be true. Patients may agree to take medication while under constant surveillance. These patients may decide to "cheek" medication given by the nurse or quit taking medication immediately after discharge. Even though discharge criteria are met and the patient is functioning much better, paternalism was not useful in producing long-term benefit for the patient. Had beneficence been used, the patient's personhood would have been reaffirmed, and perhaps a greater willingness to take medications might have been achieved.

What is in the patient's best interest? Ultimately the patient decides. The nurse-patient relationship creates a context within which the patient's dilemma, and the nurse's dilemma in helping the patient, may be explored, and the best choice for the patient may emerge.

▶ Check Your Reading

26. When we use manipulation to convince a patient to take medication, what principle are we using?
27. What characteristics of psychiatric illnesses interfere with the patient's ability to recognize that he or she needs medication?

Ideals of Practice Versus Reality

In nursing school, as difficult and demanding as it is, students do not experience the "real world." Faculty intentionally simplify the students' learning environment by selecting out certain experiences, objectives, patients, and settings to facilitate students' learning. This approach serves students well because the complexity of the health care environment may actually overwhelm students and make learning even more difficult. The goal of academic preparation, by graduation, is to expose students to the full range of options in nursing and to enable mastery through application of all that the students have learned.

There are factors, however, that occur with graduation and licensure that cannot be introduced in nursing school:

- Legal accountability for one's own actions as well as for actions delegated to unlicensed assistive personnel
- Increase in the number and acuity of patients being served
- Awareness of the need for additional growth in knowledge base necessitated by choosing a particular setting and population with which to work
- Awareness of being a novice in nursing, with much to learn
- Recognition that newly acquired skills need refinement, art, and creativity
- Awareness of the need to work out relationships with team members representing various levels of expertise, years of socialization, values, and cultures
- The experience of ongoing work versus the short-term experience of semesters and changing environments

These are only a few of the variables that new graduates confront. Nursing education provides a foundation of knowledge and the tools to acquire the knowledge and skills that are still needed. There is no way, however, that new graduates enter the work world feeling totally prepared to handle any and all situations.

So what about the ideals of practice versus the reality? If you are practicing ethically, you need to understand that there is no "ideal," yet at the same time you must not tolerate abuses in the name of "reality." You need to practice with one foot firmly grounded in "what is" and the other foot in vision of "what ought to be" (Zoloth-Dorfman, 1994). For instance, Joan, the nurse in charge, recognized that today the needs of the patients are greater than the resources (time, staff, equipment, supplies, medications) available (what is); further, no more resources can be acquired from other sources. Therefore, "what ought to be" cannot be attained in the usual deployment and allocation of resources. Several options are available to Joan.

A viable option in this situation is to change what can be changed: allocation in the usual way. Joan can rearrange the schedule, stagger the use of equipment, assign staff in different ways, and cancel nonessential tests and treatments (those that can wait until next shift or next day). This option is an effort to resolve a **moral (ethical) dilemma** (an issue in which there is no right or best solution) and decrease **moral distress** (the psychic pain experienced when no answer is a good one). In the process of living out an option, Joan will probably encounter **moral uncertainty**. For instance, Mr. Kay is having an acute episode of psychosis with paranoid features. In an effort to redeploy resources, Joan assesses that Mr. Kay will probably react suspiciously to the change, not be willing to participate in the added group activities, and may escalate in response to the changed environmental stimulation. Should Joan:

- Give a PRN antipsychotic in anticipation of Mr. Kay's response?
- Deploy a staff member to be particularly alert to Mr. Kay's needs with the understanding that another patient will receive less individual attention?
- Assign Mr. Kay specific treatment activities that require his spending time away from the group?
- Do nothing special?

And what about individual consideration for each and every patient receiving professional services under the accountability of Joan today? Is there time, need, or purpose to include other members of the team to assist in solving the dilemma of fewer resources? By definition, moral uncertainty has no clear solution. There is no room for Joan to become overwhelmed and immobilized by the ethical issues. Joan is expected to think clearly, clarify her own hierarchy of ethical values, and act consistently on behalf of the patients served, in a timely, planned, calm manner. It is no surprise that the person with this level of ethical responsibility must be educated to make such decisions and is held legally accountable for doing so. **Accountability** is defined as taking full responsibility for one's actions.

▶ Check Your Reading

28. List three factors that new graduates confront when they leave the school environment.

29. What are some of the reality situations that confront the new graduate and highlight the conflict between the ideal and the real?

Good of the Group Versus the Freedom of the Individual

Society is organized in families and other groups. All persons function in and derive benefit from groups. Much of psychiatric-mental health treatment occurs in groups.

Democratic principles emphasize the importance of the individual within the context of the group: thus the nurse's mandate to weigh the rights of the individual against the good of the group. Quite often, the nurse and other members of the treatment team must struggle with two mutually exclusive principles: "the greatest good for the greatest number," contrasted with the "primacy of the individual." Many of our current social issues bring home this conflict: gun control, smoking, pollution, and domestic violence to name a few.

In the psychiatric-mental health arena, what is the right thing to do? Some mentally ill persons, not harmful to themselves or others, choose to live homeless. Sometimes they are arrested for violating society's rights through petty theft, loitering, and pandering. Sometimes they are victims of rape, theft, and murder because of the vulnerability of homelessness. Should they have to live with, and pay for, the consequences? Do they choose homelessness because they are sick and therefore not capable of choosing? If society decides that homelessness is not a choice, where is adequate housing provided? Who pays for the housing? Who forces the person to use the housing provided, and how is that enforced? Does forcing someone to sleep in shelter constitute false imprisonment? There are many questions and no easy answers.

In a small, relatively simple environment of an inpatient unit, how does the nurse respond to the aimless wandering of one patient into other patients' rooms (the individual's right to privacy)? How does the nurse respond when a patient screams angry obscenities, disturbing the patients in the group session next door (the individual's right to freedom of expression versus the group's right to a safe environment)? In a therapeutic milieu (environment), the nurse is responsible for managing the ambiance of the unit. So what does the nurse do? (See Chapter 19 for a comprehensive discussion of the nurse's role in maintaining a therapeutic environment.)

It is said that one person's rights end at the next person's nose. How far does that right extend? To olfactory cells in the nose? To one's ears? Language and vocabulary as well as volume and intensity? We do not tolerate physical aggression, but where does the line exist for verbal abuse, emotional abuse, or sexual abuse? Although society, families, churches, legislatures, and courts try to determine general guidelines, the nurse judges, decides, legislates, and acts every hour of the day. The decisions differ from nurse to nurse, setting to setting, situation to situation, and sometimes day to day.

The guiding principle in the struggle of individual versus group rights is this: How can both individual and group rights be affirmed, within the context of the individual's and group's responsibilities? The solutions require sensitivity, creativity, commitment, and support. The answers do not come easy. Often, both the individual and the group cannot be affirmed; a choice must be made and the consequences accepted. After such an experience, it helps to talk with a friend or spiritual advocate, or God. Clarification, illumination, and comfort may emerge (Fowler, 1989). Wisdom and choices may accrue. But there will never be a time when you always know the right thing to do.

▶ Check Your Reading

30. Identify one conflict in which the nurse must make a choice between the good of the individual and the good of the staff.
31. What is the guiding principle when a conflict between the individual's and group's needs occurs?

Behavior Control

Behavior control once meant only the manipulation of a person's behavior by design. Now, with the institutionalization of biofeedback, meditation, medication, and other variables, behavior control is more complex. The use of food, odors, and pleasurable stimuli; the installation of patient-controlled analgesia (PCA) units; and the installation of transcutaneous electrical nerve stimulation (TENS) units to alter mood, pain, and behavior, are opportunities to alter, and possibly to control, behavior.

The crux of the issue of behavior control is accountability. The person who controls the behavior is accountable for it. Right behind the issue of accountability is the question of control: Does a person have control (at least 51%) over one's behavior? At what point is one in control and accountable?

Coercive behavior controls are seclusion and restraint. If a patient cannot control himself or herself, staff exert control to prohibit harm to the self or others. In this case, behavior control is justified on the principles of beneficence over autonomy. The protection of self and others is emphasized over the freedom of movement. Chemical restraints (medications) may be viewed as less coercive to staff members but are actually the most restrictive form of restraints and involve the same ethical issues (Parker, 1993).

There are more subtle behavior controls, such as rewarding desirable behavior, punishing undesirable behavior, and allowing natural consequences to flow from the person's behavior. We have all been socialized through these processes. These forms of behavior control, however, are formally applied in school settings, with individuals who are developmentally delayed, and with the chronically mentally ill to name a few. These methods of reinforcement are considered ethically appropriate, even morally right (see Chapter 18 for complete discussion of behavior therapy).

Behavior control is an ethical issue when the person being manipulated or controlled is harmed physically, emotionally, spiritually, financially, or socially by the manipulation. For instance, the nursing staff expect all patients to be asleep before evening change of shifts so that fewer staff are required; the evening nurse medicates all patients with PRN sleeping medication or antihistamines, turns off the television, and sends everybody off to bed an hour before the night shift arrives.

A patient may decide to enter into a **no-suicide contract** with the therapist, choosing to forego suicide as an option, under the specifics of the contract. The therapist-nurse may have encouraged the decision and may have indicated that the therapeutic relationship would be terminated without the contract. The therapist-nurse has used the power of the relationship and will enforce consequences if the patient does not enter into the contract or breaks the contract. This is a form of behavior control. Is it unethical? The patient may believe so and question the therapist-nurse's fidelity.

There are multiple ethical issues, arising by the moment, in every relationship, in every setting. Ethical principles that clarify, guide, and comfort the nurse have been presented. For an expert practitioner, the ethical issues do not go away and may, in fact, be more poignant and more distressing than for a novice practitioner with much yet to learn.

▶ Check Your Reading

32. What is the most restrictive form of constraint?
33. What is the crux of the behavior control issue?
34. Name two types of coercive behavior controls.

LEGAL PARAMETERS FOR THE JOURNEY

In addition to ethics with its endless questions, there are legal restrictions and obligations with firm boundaries that influence the practice of psychiatric nursing. Some are mandated through laws from state to state; others are mandated by professional and consumer protection groups and acknowledged among professional groups and in courts as being the power of the law.

Voluntary Versus Involuntary Treatment

When persons are harmful to themselves or others or cannot take care of themselves properly, they are in need of help. If the person chooses treatment, enters into an active decision-making process with the treatment team, and works to achieve treatment goals, a positive treatment relationship and outcome are likely to result. The illness and ensuing dysfunctional behavior patterns, however, may keep the patient from participating fully in the recommendations made and the patient may need to grapple with meaning and purpose of illness as stated earlier. With either situation, the patient may voluntarily agree to accept treatment. This **voluntary treatment** must be based on informed consent.

Some persons, however, do not agree to enter into treatment, and the clinicians who have made the determination of need for treatment must make a decision: Is this person of imminent danger to self or others or unable to take care of fundamental human needs? If either answer is yes, the clinician has a legal obligation both to protect the person and society and to protect the person's right to freedom. This is the first step of **involuntary treatment,** sometimes called commitment. Although the specific protocol and time frame vary from state to state, the guidelines in Box 5–1 capture the legal requirements.

▶ Check Your Reading

35. Define voluntary treatment.
36. What is required before an involuntary admission can occur?

Nurse Practice Acts

Each state has defined nursing and nursing practice. Although these definitions are conceptual to allow for evolution in knowledge base and practice, they also establish boundaries within which the nurse must practice. Boards established in each state are delegated the responsibility of protecting the public from abuse of nursing practice. Most state practice acts specify the following information:

- Process to obtain licensure and practice within that state
- Defines the educational requirements for entry into practice
- Defines scope of practice for each level of nursing practice
- Process by which board of nursing members are selected
- Identifies situations in which disciplinary action is warranted
- Details appeal steps and if nurse believes disciplinary steps taken by board are not fair.

▶ Check Your Reading

37. Identify three types of information included in each state's nurse practice act.
38. What is the purpose of the nurse practice acts in each state?

Boundary Issues

Maintaining appropriate distance while offering oneself for a healing relationship requires considerable skill (see Chapter 11 for a thorough discussion of nurse-patient relationships). How close is too close? When is professional conduct actually alienating? There are at least two participants and several audiences to consider in addressing boundary issues: the patient; the nurse; and the profession's, institution's, and society's standards.

Patients often have "damage" to sense of self and where they believe their **personal boundaries** are. Some patients have no sense of boundaries because they have endured repeated personal violations. These patients often intrude into others' personal space by standing too close, moving too quickly toward others, touching inappropriately in the wrong place, or touching for too long at a time. What is an inappropriate statement or act to most people does not bother these patients at all. They have deficits in boundary awareness and boundary maintenance.

Boundaries may also be closed and rigid, and the person may need an unusually large amount of personal space. Actions or statements that are unusual but appropriate to most people may be highly intrusive to patients with rigid boundaries. Culture also has a profound influence on the awareness and maintenance of boundaries. For instance, some cultures talk loudly and stand close to one another, whereas other cultures have no physical contact (see Chapter 14).

Nursing staff may have the same deficits in boundary awareness and maintenance. People who migrate to health careers because of experience in a dysfunctional

BOX 5-1 Legal Requirements for Involuntary Detention

- When the accountable clinician decides to detain the patient, the papers to notify the court (or its designee) must be completed; the patient needs to know, and family needs to be notified if the patient agrees.
- The hospital/clinic/clinician may not hold a patient against his will for any length of time, unless the state has been notified. This allows the state or its designee to oversee the patient's rights, assure a hearing of the facts, and determine what is in the best interest of the patient and society.
- The state (via judge, court, hearing) determines if the patient may exercise his prerogative and refuse treatment or if the patient is to be held involuntarily (against his will) for treatment.
- A length of time is determined, after which the patient shall have the right to speak to the court or its designee. Again the court determines the patient's current status in relation to harm to self or others and ability to care for basic human needs. The patient may be required to remain in treatment involuntarily or may be released from treatment at that hearing.
- At any time before the hearing, the patient may decide to enter into treatment voluntarily or may get better and not have to be forced by the treatment team to continue in treatment. The court is simply notified of the change in patient health status or decision and the hearing cancelled.

BOX 5–2 Common Boundary Dilemmas

- The patient's door is closed; the psychiatric technician knocks and quickly opens the door, catching the patient stepping out of the shower.
- The psychiatric technician knocks and is told not to come in; the technician is obligated to document a personal evaluation of the patient's status (15-minute checks) and must see the patient. Since the patient answered, shall the technician document personal evaluation or insist on seeing the patient? What if the patient says, "I'm fine. I'm trying to take a nap"? What if the patient says, "Leave me alone! Why won't you trust me?" What if the patient says, "I'm not dressed."?
- Being attracted to a patient is not uncommon. How does the nurse deal with that? What if the patient asks her to meet him at the coffee shop on her break? What if the nurse gives her phone number to the patient and offers her support after discharge?
- What if the grandmotherly, nurturing nurse regularly touches, pats, and caresses her patients, giving them all the same amount of attention? Is there potential for boundary violation?

family often have boundary problems. They may be more *or* less tolerant with societal norms related to aggressive language, physical comforting, and signals of intimacy, for instance. In addition, the professions have made a distinction between professional and social relationships; these relationships may not exist in the same time frame, and they have specific principles that guide them (see Chapter 11). The purpose of this distinction is to protect the patient from abuse of power and exploitation in the relationship. In a professional relationship, the good of the patient is the central and sole concern; the needs of the helping person are met separate and apart from the helping relationship (Dzlech, 1993).

Ethically, nurses must be alert to the possibility of sexual, emotional, and financial exploitation, both for themselves and for the members of the health care team with whom they work (Tammelleo, 1991). Box 5–2 lists some common boundary dilemmas that occur in hospitals and other settings.

Boundary violations exist on a continuum. They may be as horrific as rape, intercourse without consent, or emotional battering. They may be as subtle as extra long hugs, accidental brushes against private parts, or the quiet assurance that the staff member is the only one who really understands and can help. Constant awareness, confrontation, and discussion among staff is absolutely necessary for staff to maintain professional, helpful relationships with patients.

Boundary violations may occur among staff as well. Therefore the same kind of monitoring and diligence is necessary to maintain open communication in the work group. The mildest influence of social relationships in the work group is pairing (see Chapter 17), which may considerably hinder the group's healthy function. Energy needed for patient care is siphoned off into social relationships.

▶ Check Your Reading

39. Give two examples of behaviors that a person with undefined or loose boundaries might display.
40. What characterizes an individual with rigid boundaries?

RIGHTS OF PATIENTS ON THE JOURNEY

People needing psychiatric-mental health services are similar to all people in every other respect: They have the right to life, liberty, and the pursuit of happiness. Because of the stigma of psychiatric illness, however, extra effort is made to ensure that the rights of psychiatric patients are safeguarded. The American Nurses' Association Code for Nurses is one document that codifies the rights of psychiatric patients. Other attempts to codify the rights of psychiatric patients include those put forth by the U.S. Mental Health Systems Act (1980), by Pelletier (1992), and by the American Hospital Association (1994).

American Nurses' Association Code for Nurses

Written in 1976, with subsequent interpretive statements (ANA, 1985), the ANA Code for Nurses establishes baseline expectations for all registered nurses without exception.

Item 1 of the Code states that: *The nurse provides services with respect for human dignity and the uniqueness of the patient, unrestricted by considerations of social or economic status, personal attributes, or the nature of health problems.* This item requires the nurse to act consistently on behalf of all patients. If ethically distressed, the nurse may refuse to provide a particular treatment or have the patient transferred to another nurse's care. These are not options, however, if the nurse is distressed over the patient's condition (such as AIDS), personal attributes (such as conviction of rape), or socioeconomic status (such as homelessness). Nurses are committed to caring for all people.

Item 2 of the Code states that: *The nurse safeguards the patient's right to privacy by judiciously protecting information of a confidential nature.* Confidentiality is a mandate of the profession, with legal consequences in the case of patients with AIDS or chemical dependency. Probably because the stigma of these illnesses is so great, these patients are specifically protected at a higher level of legal sanction. All patients, however, have the right to "tell their story" in their own way, to a person of their own choice. Psychiatric records are histories of intimate, sometimes damaging information; therefore, confidentiality includes medical and other written and electronic records. Telephone answering devices, cellular phones, computers, and facsimile machines must also be used with utmost caution.

Item 3 of the Code states that: *The nurse acts to safeguard the patient and the public when health care and safety are affected by the incompetent, unethical, or illegal practice of any person.* When a nurse suspects or confirms impaired practice in himself or another, he has an ethical obligation to act to safeguard individual patients and society as a whole. Within an organization, there are ethics and clinical practice committees that encourage and receive such information. The State Board of the profession to whom the clinician belongs is also an excellent source for assistance in dealing with a clinician who jeopardizes the safety and health of patients. The State Board is the next step when an organization refuses to accept or investigate a legitimate concern for practice.

Item 4 of the Code states that: *The nurse assumes responsibility and accountability for individual nursing judgments and actions.* The nurse, by virtue of legal license and ethical obligation, is held responsible for consistently acting on behalf of patients, including respecting the autonomy of patients.

Item 5 of the Code states that: *The nurse maintains competence in nursing.* An example earlier in this chapter illustrated the ethical dilemma that may occur when the nurse has not maintained a current knowledge base and clinical judgment in the specific area of practice. The example was outdated knowledge related to electroconvulsive therapy.

Item 6 of the Code states that: *The nurse exercises informed judgment and uses individual competence and qualifications as criteria in seeking consultation, accepting responsibilities, and delegating nursing activities to others.* Health care is expensive, chaotic, and rapidly changing. The nurse is expected to act on behalf of the patient by using all appropriate resources, including resources for the nurse. Assistive personnel are a wonderful resource when used appropriately. Willingness to take on new responsibilities is expected when the nurse has adequate knowledge and clinical judgment to perform the new responsibility. Anyone expecting the nurse to increase responsibility should also be aware of the ethical mandate to assist the nurse to demonstrate competency.

Item 7 of the Code states that: *The nurse participates in activities that contribute to the ongoing development of the profession's body of knowledge.* The nurse participates in the development of clinical protocols, testing new ways of practice, and writing nursing care plans.

Item 8 of the Code states that: *The nurse participates in the profession's efforts to implement and improve standards of nursing.* The nurse must be aware of the standards and any updates in order to implement and improve them. Membership in the State Nurses Association provides ready access to the latest information on standards development and implementation. Standards are implemented in a variety of ways. Nurses and institutions have different ways to implement standards. Sharing various methods of implementation helps everyone to improve standards. For instance, some agencies use case managers, others use clinical pathways, and others use standards of care. Some nurses focus on the nature of the nurse-patient relationship to encourage participation in treatment. Other nurses may identify and use the patient's internal motivators. Others may work on goals and encourage the patient to be actively pursuing these goals.

Item 9 of the Code states that: *The nurse participates in the profession's efforts to establish and maintain conditions of employment conducive to high-quality nursing care.* The environment within which a nurse practices influences the quality of care provided. For instance, one agency may be highly structured, and the nurses there work primarily with policies, procedures, and protocols. Another agency may have little structure and may expect the nurse to practice at a high standard regardless of education or experience. When conditions adversely affect the work of the practice environment, the nurse has an ethical responsibility to communicate and suggest solutions.

Item 10 of the Code states that: *The nurse participates in the profession's efforts to protect the public from misinformation and misrepresentation and to maintain the integrity of nursing.* Misinformation exists about various diseases and their effects, the vulnerability of the community to the effects of mental illness, and the contribution nursing makes to health care. A nurse's responsibility goes far beyond a particular practice setting and patient or family group. The obligation includes embracing the community's understanding of health and the myriad factors that influence it. For example, being involved in the local parent-teacher organization and being involved in the passage of legislation for public health endeavors are ways to influence community health. Failure to fulfill this obligation adversely affects society's relationship with nursing.

Item 11 of the Code states that: *The nurse collaborates with members of the health professions and other citizens in promoting community and national efforts to meet public health needs.* Nurses are aware of the necessity to address issues related to health and health care on the community, state (provincial), and national levels. The Code requires each nurse to participate in some way beyond his or her employment to help meet the health needs of the public.

Other Attempts to Codify the Rights of Psychiatric Patients

One attempt to codify the rights of psychiatric patients is the Bill of Rights for Patients included in the U.S. Mental Health Systems Act (1980) (Box 5–3). Another attempt to codify the rights of psychiatric patients more concretely, on a daily basis, was put forth by Pelletier (1992). A third attempt to codify those rights was developed by the American Hospital Association (1994) (Box 5–4).

▶ Check Your Reading

41. Name at least four rights of psychiatric patients.
42. What is the purpose of the ANA Code for Nurses?

BOX 5-3 Mental Health Systems Act Recommended Bill of Rights for Patients

- The right to appropriate treatment in settings and under conditions most supportive of and least restrictive to personal liberty
- The right to an individualized, written treatment plan
- The right to ongoing participation in the planning of services and the right to a reasonable explanation of general mental condition, treatment objective, adverse effects of treatment, reasons for treatment, and available alternatives
- The right to refuse treatment except when the patient is of imminent danger to self or others

THREE IMPORTANT PROCESSES AFFECTING THE THERAPEUTIC RELATIONSHIP

The three processes to be explored here strengthen the nurse's role in any setting; in addition, there are other significant processes. These were chosen because of their significance for the therapeutic relationship of psychiatric patients with nurses. The three processes are confidentiality, therapeutic alliance, and advocacy.

Confidentiality

A therapeutic relationship (see Chapter 11) absolutely requires that the nurse handle intimate communications with utmost respect, almost with awe. To trust another is a gift, which, for psychiatric patients, must be earned. **Confidentiality** of information is basic to the relationship (Stern, 1990). Ethical dilemmas develop, however. The patient asks you if you can keep a secret; another says you must promise not to tell after the information is already shared. With whom may the information be shared? Guidelines for maintaining confidentiality in psychiatric-mental health nursing are presented in Box 5-5.

The one exception to confidentiality relates to the Tarasoff Decision (*Tarasoff v. the Regents of the University of California*, 1976). In the Tarasoff case, a California court clearly established the therapist's duty to use reasonable care to protect a known, intended victim of a patient's threats. The court ruled that this duty might be discharged by either warning the prospective victim or taking other reasonable steps under the circumstances. Many state and some federal courts have agreed with the California ruling that a Tarasoff-type duty to warn exists for mental health care professionals. The extent of this duty to warn, however, and how it may be discharged varies from state to state.

▶ **Check Your Reading**

43. What does it mean to keep information confidential?
44. Name two of the conflicts that arise from the issue of confidentiality.
45. What is the implication of the Tarasoff decision?

Therapeutic Alliance

Although much has been said about boundary maintenance and prohibition of sexual or exploitative behavior, the other side of boundary maintenance, the **therapeutic alliance,** has not been mentioned in an ethical context. One is obliged to attempt to reach the patient, to make a connection that is healthy and encouraging, and to journey for a while with that person. There are days when you may treat that obligation as an unreasonable burden or an unrealistic expectation. The nurse who chooses to be in psychiatric-mental health nursing also chooses to be available to patients for healthy therapeutic relationships. Dealing with countertransference, cultural differences, and personality differences (See Chapters 10, 11, and 14) are necessary in nursing if you are to be available for patients.

Using the power inherent in the relationship for the sole and specific good of the patient is necessary. Is insistence on payment for service or not sharing one's phone number in the best interest of the patient; in the best interest of the nurse? Maybe both, but you are obliged to be brutally honest with yourself about real motives and desires. Psychiatric nurses find it useful to be in a supervisory relationship with a supportive, objective professional who has more experience and who can assist the nurse to look at these issues.

▶ **Check Your Reading**

46. What is a therapeutic alliance?

Advocacy

The primary role of **advocacy** is to protect the patient's rights and interests. Fortunately the entire team as well as society has a role to play in advocacy: What hurts one hurts all; what helps one is an encouragement to all. A strict advocacy role requires one to rise above a fear of reprisal and assertively speak for the patient or insist that the patient be heard. Anyone who assesses that the patient's rights may be in jeopardy is required to make that situation known. Many ways exist to communicate a concern that the patient has not been heard. Ethics committees exist for the purpose of advocacy for the patient in a complex environment. Administrators often have open-door policies in relation to ethical issues; many institutions have policies protecting an employee who speaks out on behalf of a patient.

Once the institution has heard and responded and a conclusion is reached, you have acted appropriately. This action is appropriate whether or not the decision is the one you would have made or the decision you

BOX 5-4 A Patient's Bill of Rights

Introduction

Effective health care requires collaboration between patients and physicians and other health care professionals. Open and honest communication, respect for personal and professional values, and sensitivity to differences are integral to optimal patient care. As the setting for the provision of health services, hospitals must provide a foundation for understanding and respecting the rights and responsibilities of patients, their families, physicians, and other caregivers. Hospitals must ensure a health care ethic that respects the role of patients in decision making about treatment choices and other aspects of their care. Hospitals must be sensitive to cultural, racial, linguistic, religious, age, gender, and other differences as well as the needs of persons with disabilities.

The American Hospital Association presents *A Patient's Bill of Rights* with the expectation that it will contribute to more effective patient care and be supported by the hospital on behalf of the institution, its medical staff, employees, and patients. The American Hospital Association encourages health care institutions to tailor this bill of rights to their patient community by translating and/or simplifying the language of this bill of rights as may be necessary to ensure that patients and their families understand their rights and responsibilities.

Bill of Rights*

1. The patient has the right to considerate and respectful care.
2. The patient has the right to and is encouraged to obtain from physicians and other direct caregivers relevant, current, and understandable information concerning diagnosis, treatment, and prognosis.

   Except in emergencies when the patient lacks decision-making capacity and the need for treatment is urgent, the patient is entitled to the opportunity to discuss and request information related to the specific procedures and/or treatments, the risks involved, the possible length of recuperation, and the medically reasonable alternatives and their accompanying risks and benefits.
3. Patients have the right to know the identity of physicians, nurses, and others involved in their care, as well as when those involved are students, residents, or other trainees. The patient also has the right to know the immediate and long-term financial implications of treatment choices, insofar as they are known.

   The patient has the right to make decisions about the plan of care prior to and during the course of treatment and to refuse a recommended treatment or plan of care to the extent permitted by law and hospital policy and to be informed of the medical consequences of this action. In case of such refusal, the patient is entitled to other appropriate care and services that the hospital provides or transfer to another hospital. The hospital should notify patients of any policy that might affect patient choice within the institution.
4. The patient has the right to have an advance directive (such as a living will, health care proxy, or durable power of attorney for health care) concerning treatment or designating a surrogate decision maker with the expectation that the hospital will honor the intent of that directive to the extent permitted by law and hospital policy.

   Health care institutions must advise patients of their rights under state law and hospital policy to make informed medical choices, ask if the patient has an advance directive, and include that information in patient records. The patient has the right to timely information about hospital policy that may limit its ability to implement fully a legally valid advance directive.
5. The patient has the right to every consideration of privacy. Case discussion, consultation, examination, and treatment should be conducted so as to protect each patient's privacy.
6. The patient has the right to expect that all communications and records pertaining to his/her care will be treated as confidential by the hospital, except in cases such as suspected abuse and public health hazards when reporting is permitted or required by law. The patient has the right to expect that the hospital will emphasize the confidentiality of this information when it releases it to any other parties entitled to review information in these records.
7. The patient has the right to review the records pertaining to his/her medical care and to have the information explained or interpreted as necessary, except when restricted by law.
8. The patient has the right to expect that, within its capacity and policies, a hospital will make reasonable response to the request of a patient for appropriate and medically indicated care and services. The hospital must provide evaluation, service, and/or referral as indicated by the urgency of the case. When medically appropriate and legally permissible, or when a patient has so requested, a patient may be transferred to another facility. The institution to which the patient is to be transferred must first have accepted the patient for transfer. The patient must also have the benefit of complete information and explanation concerning the need for, risks, benefits, and alternatives to such a transfer.
9. The patient has the right to ask and be informed of the existence of business relationships among the hospital, educational institutions, other health care providers, or payers that may influence the patient's treatment and care.
10. The patient has the right to consent to or decline to participate in proposed research studies or human experimentation affecting care and treatment or requiring direct patient involvement, and to have those studies fully explained prior to consent. A patient who declines to participate in research or experimentation is entitled to the most effective care that the hospital can otherwise provide.
11. The patient has the right to expect reasonable continuity of care when appropriate and to be informed by physicians and other caregivers of available and realistic patient care options when hospital care is no longer appropriate.
12. The patient has the right to be informed of hospital policies and practices that relate to patient care, treatment, and responsibilities. The patient has the right to be informed of available resources for resolving disputes, grievances, and conflicts, such as ethics committees, patient representatives, or other mechanisms available in the institution. The patient has the right to be informed of the hospital's charges for services and available payment methods.

*These rights can be exercised on the patient's behalf by a designated surrogate or proxy decision maker if the patient lacks decision-making capacity, is legally incompetent, or is a minor.

BOX 5-4 A Patient's Bill of Rights *continued*

The collaborative nature of health care requires that patients, or their families/surrogates, participate in their care. The effectiveness of care and patient satisfaction with the course of treatment depend, in part, on the patient fulfilling certain responsibilities. Patients are responsible for providing information about past illnesses, hospitalizations, medications, and other matters related to health status. To participate effectively in decision making, patients must be encouraged to take responsibility for requesting additional information or clarification about their health status or treatment when they do not fully understand information and instructions. Patients are also responsible for ensuring that the health care institution has a copy of their written advance directive if they have one. Patients are responsible for informing their physicians and other caregivers if they anticipate problems in following prescribed treatment.

Patients should also be aware of the hospital's obligation to be reasonably efficient and equitable in providing care to other patients and the community. The hospital's rules and regulations are designed to help the hospital meet this obligation. Patients and their families are responsible for making reasonable accommodations to the needs of the hospital, other patients, medical staff, and hospital employees. Patients are responsible for providing necessary information for insurance claims and for working with the hospital to make payment arrangements, when necessary.

A person's health depends on much more than health care services. Patients are responsible for recognizing the impact of their life-style on their personal health.

Conclusion

Hospitals have many functions to perform, including the enhancement of health status, health promotion, and the prevention and treatment of injury and disease; the immediate and ongoing care and rehabilitation of patients; the education of health professionals, patients, and the community; and research. All these activities must be conducted with an overriding concern for the values and dignity of patients.

BOX 5-5 Guidelines for Maintaining Confidentiality in Psychiatric-Mental Health Nursing

- Do not promise to keep a secret. Secrets are appropriate in a social relationship but not in a therapeutic one.
- Do promise to respect the person's confidence and to share it only with members of the team who need to know. For instance, share information with the direct care staff that the patient intends to commit suicide tonight. Share financial concerns and medication problems with the multidisciplinary team. Share with the supervisor a revelation that a team member was perceived to be making sexual advances toward the patient.
- Be careful to neither deny nor confirm someone's presence in the mental health system. This includes the patient's friends in the community who say, "Oh, Mary M., my best friend, is at your clinic. How is she doing?" Or the nurse's spouse may ask how a fellow coworker is faring on a unit at the hospital. A child may want a specific example, including defining characteristics, of how the nurse/parent helped somebody that day. Each of these is problematic in relationship to confidentiality.
- Be careful with medical and electronic records. Do not read the charts or listen to reports about persons for whom you will not be providing services. To do so in curiosity is not to be indulged as a professional.

thought the patient wanted made. The obligation continues beyond the walls of the organization, however, if you know some deception has occurred, and the patient's best interest was not at the heart of the decision.

Another important factor related to advocacy is relationship. Advocacy is difficult to do honestly and accurately in the absence of a trusting, helpful, therapeutic relationship. In any relationsip, each person has responsibilities and accountabilities. **Covenant** may be a more appropriate way to think about the obligation to protect a patient's rights and interests (Bernal, 1991), that is, placing the role of advocacy in the context of the relationship in which both persons have role responsibilities to each other.

Advocacy is one of many responsibilities, and you must ethically weigh the consequences of acting on one responsibility to the detriment of another. For instance, advocating for the patient's right to refuse medication may escalate the patient's symptoms of ambivalence and reinforce the patient's refusal even though the medication has had demonstrated effectiveness for this patient in the past.

Working in institutional settings with others caring for the same patients also makes advocacy difficult. There may be relatively little agreement among the 24-hour nursing staff, for instance, about the patient's insistence that he sleep nude. Institutional and hierarchical structure may create difficulty for the nurses who desire to be advocates (Bernal, 1991).

Advocacy is necessary, but all team members have an ethical obligation to protect the patient's wishes and desires. Only rarely must one act independently and in isolation.

▶ Check Your Reading

47. What is the purpose of advocacy?

CONCLUSIONS

Ethics is the way one thinks about and discusses moral problems. Ethical principles that guide nursing practice are justice, love, beneficence, nonmaleficence, autonomy, paternalism, veracity, and fidelity. Two theoretical frameworks are the primary models used to discuss ethics: Kohlberg's theory is an individual developmental model that, at its highest level, culminates in justice. Gilligan's "framework of care" is a model more comfortable for nurses that, at its highest level, culminates in mercy. The best ethical decisions, however, are probably made when both principles (justice and caring) are applied.

Common ethical dilemmas facing psychiatric-mental health nurses involve the application of ethics principles: informed consent, ECT with unsuitable patients, coercion in the use of medication, ideal practice contrasted with the realities of practice, or group and individual rights in conflict. Legal guidelines, including the process for involuntary admission, freedom from coercion, nursing practice acts, and boundary issues, are important in psychiatric nursing practice.

Patients, although ill, maintain their constitutional rights: They have the right to use the telephone and to have access to mail as well as access to personal property. Patients also have rights to privacy, care, and participation in treatment planning. In addition, the patient has the right to treatment in the least restrictive environment that will provide adequate therapeutic structure, support, and benefit. The nurse's role in ethics includes confidentiality, therapeutic alliance, and advocacy.

Throughout the chapter, more questions were posed than answers given. Such is the nature of ethics. To struggle with ethical uncertainty, to confront ethical dilemmas, and to live with ethical distress are part of the awesome responsibility of nursing.

KEY POINTS TO REMEMBER

- There are eight principles that guide ethical decision-making: justice, love, beneficence, nonmaleficence, autonomy, paternalism, fidelity, and veracity.
- Kohlberg postulated a theory of moral development that has three levels: the preconventional level, in which external rules determine right and wrong actions; the conventional level, in which family's and community's rules are accepted and used to determine right and wrong; and the postconventional level, in which the individual uses his or her own conscience to arrive at decisions. Justice is emphasized in Kohlberg's theory.
- Gilligan postulated a theory regarding the moral development of women. Gilligan believes that women approach moral issues from a perspective of care and mutually connected and responsible relationships. This perspective of care provides an alternative to Kohlberg's model.
- There are many ethical dilemmas facing the psychiatric nurse. Informed consent, the use of ECT with unsuitable patients, use of medication when the patient refuses, ideals of practice versus reality, the good of the individual versus the good of the group, and behavior control were among the ethical dilemmas presented.
- Legal parameters provide firmer boundaries for practice than those provided by ethical principles.
- Patients can voluntarily admit themselves to a psychiatric facility, or if they are a danger to self or others, they may be involuntarily admitted or committed to an inpatient facility.
- Nurse Practice Acts define the boundaries of practice within each state.
- Boundary issues are important between the nurse and the patient as well as among staff members.
- Psychiatric patients maintain all their civil liberties.
- The ANA Code for Nurses specifies baseline expectations for all registered nurses.
- There are three processes inherent in the nurse's ethical responsibilities, including confidentiality, therapeutic alliance, and advocacy.

LEARNING ACTIVITIES

1. Think about some clinical situations that have placed you in an ethical conflict. What were the conflicting issues? What principles did you use to resolve the conflict?
2. When you find yourself in difficult situations in which the answers are neither clear nor easy, what principles do you tend to rely on most of the time?
3. The principle of autonomy is an important one in American society because of the value we place on individual rights. Do we have the right to take our own life? Support your answer using ethical principles.
4. When you see or read about a homeless person who has a psychiatric illness what is your reaction as to your own or society's responsibility? What principles are you using in your response?
5. How does your own world view (e.g., theistic, pantheistic, humanistic, secular) affect your own ethical decision-making?

CRITICAL THINKING EXERCISES

Concerning the issue of universal coverage for health care, do you think that mental health coverage should be included? Would your opinion change if you or a loved one needed mental health services? If these services are not included among basic services, how do you think they should be paid for? Who should pay for them? How does the principle of justice apply to your answer?

Mr. Thomas, a student nurse in his second day of the psychiatric rotation, reads a nurse's note about a patient that he is about to be assigned to. It reads: Patient Mr. Z. was actively hallucinating and delusional all day. Refused nurse's attempts to talk to him.

1. What can the student infer from the note about his patient's behavior?
2. Does the note paint a clear and precise picture of the patient's behavior?
3. What are alternate ways of conceptualizing a note about Mr. Z. to bring more focus to an overall picture of his behavior?

Later in the day Mr. Z. becomes violent, and the student observes the staff forcibly subduing the patient while administering an injection of a major tranquilizer. The patient is yelling "You can't do this to me, I have rights."

In this situation

1. What are the patient's rights, and are they being violated?

2. What ethical principles might be in conflict in providing therapeutic care for Mr. Z?

3. What suggestions would you have about balancing Mr. Z's rights with those of the group?

4. What ethical principles would be involved?

REFERENCES

American Hospital Association (1994). *Values in Conflict: Resolving Ethical Issues in Health Care* (2nd ed.). Chicago: American Hospital Association.

American Nurses Association (1985). *Code for Nurses with Interpretation Statements.* Kansas City: American Nurses' Association.

Bernal, E. W. (1991). The nurse as patient advocate. *Hastings Center Report, 22*(4), 18–23.

Broskar, M. A. (1994). Ethical decision making in patient care, 85. *American Nurse,* March, 10.

Byrt, R. (1993). Moral minefield. *Nursing Times, 89*(8), 63–66.

Curtin, L. L. (1994). Morals: From Bobbit to Kevorkian. *Nursing Magazine, 25*(6), 42–43.

Danis, M., & Churchhill, L. R. (1990). Autonomy and the common weal. *Hastings Center Report, 21*(1), 25–31.

Dziech, B. W., & Hawkins, M. W. (1993). Personal boundaries: Demystifying the gray areas. *Employee Assistance,* September, 2–25.

Fowler, M. D. M. (1989). Ethical decision making in clinical practice. *Nursing Clinics of North America, 24*(4), 955–965.

Gilligan, C. (1982). *In a Different Voice.* Cambridge: Harvard.

Ketefian, S. (1989). Moral reasoning and ethical practice. *Annual Review of Nursing Research,* 7, 173–195.

Kohlberg, L., & Kramer, R. (1969). Continuities and discontinuities in childhood and moral judgment. *Human Development, 12*(2), 93–120.

Levenson, J. L. (1986–87). Psychiatric commitment and involuntary hospitalization: An ethical perspective. *Psychiatric Quarterly, 58*(2), 106–112.

Lutzen, K. (1990). Moral sensing and ideological conflict: Aspects of the therapeutic relationship in psychiatric nursing. *Scandinavian Journal of Caring Science, 4*(2), 69–76.

Mental Health Systems Act (1980). 96th Congress, Publication L. 96-398, Section 9501.

Myers, S. (1990). Seclusion: A last resort measure. *Perspectives in Psychiatric Care, 26*(3), 24–28.

Omery, A. (1989). Values, moral reasoning, and ethics. *Nursing Clinics of North America, 24*(2), 499–508.

Parker, J. G. (1993). Chemical restraints and the child psychiatric patient—a question of autonomy or veracity? Unpublished paper.

Pelletier, L. (1992). Becoming a client. In J. Haber, A. Leach, P. Hoskins, and B. Sidelea (Eds.), *Comprehensive psychiatric nursing.* St. Louis: C. V. Mosby.

Sabin, J. E. (1994). Managed care: A credo for ethical managed care in mental health practice. *Hospital and Community Psychiatry, 45*(9), 859–860.

Stern, S. B. (1990). Privileged communication: An ethical and legal right of psychiatric clients. *Perspectives in Psychiatric Care, 26*(4), 22–25.

Tammelleo, A. D. (1991). Sexual relationship with patient: License revocation. *Regan Report on Nursing Law, 32*(2), 4.

Tarasoff v. Regents of the University of California. 17 Cal., 3d. 425, 551. p. 2d 334, 1976.

Tarbuck, P. (1992). Mental health: Ethical standards and human rights. *Nursing Standard,* 7(6), 27–30.

Varricchio, C. G., & Jassak, P. F. (1989). Informed consent: An overview. *Seminars in Oncology Nursing, 5*(2), 95–98.

Whiteworth, R. A. (1982). The ethics of suicide intervention: Seen as a nursing problem. *Canadian Journal of Psychiatric Nursing, 23*(1), 12–14.

Whitlock, R. (1989). Ethical issues and the nurse. In J. B. Carson (Ed.), *Spiritual dimensions of nursing practice.* Philadelphia: W.B. Saunders Company.

Willwerth, W. (1994). Madness in fine print. *Time,* Nov. 7, 62.

Zoloth-Dorfman, L. (1994). First person plural: Community and method in ethics consultation. *Journal of Clinical Ethics, 5*(1), 49–54.

SUGGESTED READINGS

American Hospital Association (1994). *Values in Conflict: Resolving Ethical Issues in Health Care* (2nd ed.). Chicago: American Hospital Association.

Curtin, L. L. (1994). Morals: From Bobbit to Kevorkian. *Nursing Magazine, 25*(6), 42–43.

Dziech, B. W., & Hawkins, M. W. (1993). Personal boundaries: Demystifying the gray areas. *Employee Assistance,* September, 2–25.

Myers, S. (1990). Seclusion: A last resort measure. *Perspectives in Psychiatric Care, 26*(3), 24–28.

Sabin, J. E. (1994). Managed care: A credo for ethical managed care in mental health practice. *Hospital and Community Psychiatry, 45*(9), 859–860.

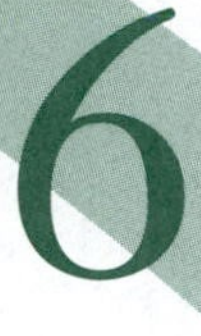

CHAPTER 6

GUIDEPOSTS FOR THE JOURNEY

THEORIES GUIDING MENTAL HEALTH NURSING

Not to know what has been transacted in former times is to be always a child. If no use is made of the labors of past ages, the world must remain always in the infancy of knowledge.

—Marcus Tullius Cicero

LEARNING OBJECTIVES

After studying this chapter, you should be able to:

1. Identify the nature and role of theories as guideposts for the journey.
2. Describe the historical contributions of classical Greek scholars to mental health nursing.
3. Identify the contributions of science and psychology to mental health nursing.
4. Specify the role of psychoanalytic theory in mental health nursing.
5. Compare and contrast ego developmental, humanistic, and existential models of psychology.
6. Describe selected tenets of behavioral theory.
7. Analyze the role of nursing theory in mental health nursing.

KEY TERMINOLOGY

Archetypes
Behavioral models
Collective unconscious
Conditioning
Dynamism
Ego
Ego psychology
Existential models
Humanistic psychology
Id
Metaparadigm
Nursing theory
Operant conditioning
Psychoanalysis
Psychology
Psychosocial crisis
Reinforcer
Self-efficacy
Self-reinforcement
Social learning theory
Superego
Theory
Unconscious

To provide quality professional care, as opposed to mere comfort, kindness, and concern, a framework for understanding personality and mental health is imperative. Psychiatric nurses practice from a comprehensive theory base, derived from the disciplines of philosophy, medicine, psychology, sociology, education, and, of course, nursing. Using the metaphor of the journey, theory serves as the essential guidepost to navigate the way while also pointing out the hidden roads a professional traveler might chance upon but not necessarily be able to recognize or share as an essential part of the journey. Theories direct the traveler by mapping out established routes to reach the desired destination.

The theories presented in this chapter do not represent an exhaustive study of all theoretical viewpoints used in mental health nursing. Rather the goal of this chapter is to provide the professional traveler with a representative kaleidoscope of the shifting points of view that have shaped current thinking about personality and have described the best ways to treat mental disorders. Beginning with those of the early Greek scholars, ideas about human behavior by many serious scholars from a variety of disciplines are discussed. Each of these theorists grappled with the essential nature of personality. They had to reexamine, question, and modify old assumptions to fit evolving paradigms about the nature of personality and corresponding modes of treating disorders of the mind. Each scholar's thoughts about the mind and human behavior help the psychiatric nurse discover the unifying elements between the past and present journeys in ways that directly affect clinical practice. Through each theorist's story of the mind-body-spirit connections present in every person's human journey, the authors hope that the richness of psychiatric-mental health nursing can be realized. For it is a specialty that is solid, important, and necessary to our scientific understanding of people with or without mental illness.

To suggest that theory development emerges solely from a scientific base and does not significantly reflect the reality of the theorist's journey would be erroneous and simplistic. Each theoretical model reflects not only the theorist's careful thinking about the phenomena described in the model but also his or her rich personal history. The story of each theoretical perspective commonly begins on a personal note, reflecting the author's formative life experiences as well as professional reflections. Theoretical models radiate a lustrous version of whole lives lived in the service of describing a human phenomenon as it is both objectively observed and subjectively experienced. These parallel perspectives provide an integrity to the structure and craftsmanship of each theoretical framework. Betty Neuman's Systems Model is no exception as she thoughtfully describes the influences in her life that led to the development of her theoretical framework for the discipline of nursing.

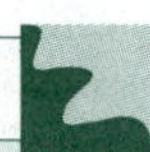

BETTY NEUMAN'S STORY

I believe the real roots of the Neuman Systems Model are embedded in my early childhood years. My view of the world was shaped by the simple events of farm life and the hardiness of my parents in responding to them. There was reverence, dignity, and respect for all life. For example, when a new animal was born, it was always given a name by my mother. When human needs arose in our rural community, my parents were always the first to offer food, clothing, or solace of various kinds. My mother, a self-taught midwife, delivered babies in the area. Although we had limited financial resources, we never felt poor. I was aware at an early age of the importance of God in my life and of having my needs met holistically. For instance, we would walk three miles and cross a river to go to church on Sundays. Neighborhood youth would visit on Sunday afternoons to play games and sing religious songs while my mother played the organ. Other joys were sharing home-baked bread and making toys. Because my parents were organic farmers, their farming more than met our physical needs. Lack of transportation and long distances precluded regular medical care, so much of our medicine was from herbs that my mother harvested from the woods, following directions passed down from Native Americans who had once lived in the area. In these early, formative years, creativity, caring, and self-reliance in problem-solving were automatic. With such a caring and trustworthy environment, our developmental needs were satisfied. An unconscious expectation was patterned for a holistic view of people, and environmental influences were seen as manageable. This background, in addition to a knowledge of systems theory and an avid interest in human behavior, formed an important base for the development of the Systems Model in 1970.

Story by Betty Neuman.

Impact of Early Professional Experiences

Another major factor was experiential. Obviously, my background in psychiatric nursing was important as a starting point for considering the relevant relationships in client data. But there were other important experiences that contributed to the development of the Neuman Systems Model. Through role-modeling the teaching and practice of mental health consultation for graduate students at UCLA from 1967 to 1973, I learned the value of working with other disciplines. I always requested, from the clinical agencies in Greater Los Angeles, the presence of the other health care disciplines involved with each case presentation, and I worked collaboratively with these disciplines to resolve issues in problem cases. This experience was invaluable. As a result of that collaboration, I found that the "total" data were available to help me consider the nature of patient variables, referred to in the Model as "interacting variables."

Consultation with interdisciplinary resources (visiting nurse associations, public health departments, teen posts, jails, and schools) had the effect of strengthening my belief in patients as holistic beings, subject to both internal and external forces. The importance of exploring all aspects of the patient's condition, of identifying the adequacy of resources (internal and external), and of supporting and integrating care with other disciplines to reinforce existing patient strengths became clear to me. Without a total knowledge of a patient's condition and without a blending of the efforts of many disciplines to resolve the patient's problem, the effectiveness of the nurse was reduced. I learned the importance of the influence of one variable on another. For example, it became clear that psychological difficulties could cause or contribute to physical problems, or vice versa. Without a spiritual commitment, motivation and hope for wellness are reduced. Making explicit the relationships among the variables in the Model was exciting and challenging. At the time, however, I had only intuitive knowledge and not a graphic model for describing these connections.

An Opportunity to Formulate Ideas

In 1970, there was an opportunity to formalize my ideas. I was assigned the task of developing and coordinating an entry-level graduate course related to four variables affecting mental health: physiological, psychological, sociocultural, and developmental. The purpose of the course was to provide students with a breadth of understanding before selection of a clinical specialty track focusing on one of these four variables. My persistent concern was how to make individual lectures interesting and meaningful for the students. The Model came into being in 1970 and was readily accepted by the teaching faculty as a tool for conveying their lecture content. The Model set the variables into a broader, holistic, systems perspective that allowed faculty to place their content within the broader human context of variable interactive relationships and possibilities. From this content, faculty made assumptions and generated hypotheses.

Refining the Model

Rae Jeanne Young, a close colleague and the course co-coordinator, had a definite impact on the Model; together, we struggled to clarify the Model's concepts with and for the students. The richness of student and faculty input enhanced the robustness of the Model. Evaluation over a two-year period proved the utility and value of the Neuman Systems Model, earlier referred to as "The Total Person Approach to Patient Problems" (see the list of publications in the May/June 1972 issue of *Nursing Research*). Unfortunately the course itself did not continue after I resigned from UCLA in 1973. The Betty Neuman Systems Model, however, has lived on over the years, gaining in strength as it continues to influence current applications in practice, education, and research.

Incorporating the Spiritual

In 1975, my first consultation for the Model occurred at Neumann College in Aston, Pennsylvania, as faculty engaged in curriculum revision. Although the original Model subsumed the spiritual variable under the sociocultural variable, I recall being excited about discussing with faculty the treatment of the spiritual concerns of patients. (The spiritual variable was not made explicit initially because in the secular environment at UCLA, it was not dealt with as a nursing concern.) Were I to redo the Model, I would place spirituality as a central, dominant variable, satisfying further my belief that all input *first* comes through to the mind and *then* to the body.

The Neuman Systems Model satisfies my lifelong quest for "caring" in considering all aspects of a patient's condition within the environment. To be holistic is to "care"; "to help each other live," which is my motto, is to care.

Betty Neuman's story speaks eloquently of how theory development in the human sciences is deeply rooted in its author's own human experience, not as a tangential appendage but as a unifying element at its core.

As we begin our examination of theories as guideposts for the journey, it is important to remember that no one theoretical framework can adequately describe the complexity of the human being or the multidimensional nature of behavior. Human beings represent unique and complex systems that defy precise definition or easy explanation. Given this qualification, each respective conceptual model represents the particular world view of its originator and highlights significant factors to explain human functioning. You will find it necessary to extract the critical concepts from all of the presented theories and to begin to synthesize them into a broader framework that has personal meaning. These theoretical understandings both govern and direct psychiatric mental health nursing practice.

WHAT IS A THEORY?

Basically a **theory** consists of concepts that represent "a concise summary of thoughts related to a phenomenon" (Meleis, 1991, p. 12). Each concept provides a symbolic shorthand for describing an abstract reality. For example, the concept of anxiety in Peplau's model symbolizes a fairly wide range of behaviors, spanning both physiological and psychological aspects of the phenomenon. When one hears the term *anxiety*, behaviors associated with anxiety are brought to mind as a gestalt, without much further explanation. Thus, *theories never represent absolute truths but rather portray an abstract representation of a phenomenon and a conceptual tool to describe it in an organized way.*

Theories develop within a historical context that necessarily builds on, but also challenges, classic ways of thinking about a subject. Changes in theoretical perspective usually represent a major *paradigm shift* in thinking. The new way of thinking creates an intellectual upheaval and a radical new interpretation of the *relative truths* that shape scientific thinking about a defined subject (Kuhn, 1970). For example, the behavioral approach to the treatment of mental illness represents a major deviation from Freudian thinking about the role of the unconscious in shaping behavior and as the focus of psychological treatment.

In some instances, theory fills a vacuum of thinking about a subject. For example, Florence Nightingale's *Notes on Nursing* provided the first serious documentation of nursing as a professional form of caring about other human beings. Wundt's establishment of the first School of Psychology performed a similar service for psychology.

The real strength of having a theoretical base for practice is that it provides a systematic way of ordering knowledge about a subject. This allows the knowledge to be shared with others in deepening a common understanding of the phenomenon under scrutiny. Moreover, nurses are reading from the same text in planning and implementing actual nursing care. Theoretical knowledge provides a framework for considering the nature of human behavior and the best ways to treat maladaptive functioning. It allows a researcher to classify observations about a phenomenon in a precise way. This process is a necessary prerequisite for generating hypotheses capable of being tested experimentally.

THEORIES FROM DISCIPLINES OTHER THAN NURSING

Contributions from the Early Greek Scholars

Great thinkers have been fascinated by uniquely human emotional, psychological, and cognitive processes since the earliest days of civilization. Tracing its roots to ancient times, before the common era (BCE), current understandings of psychiatric-mental health nursing emerged originally from the writings of ancient Greek scholars. Their masterful voices spoke of the *whole person*, consisting of mind, body, and spirit, both interrelated and irreducible. At the time, this was a revolutionary shift from a previous theory of the mind as influenced solely by magical spirits from external sources. These early Greek scholars comprehensively and lucidly challenged this long-standing but crippling world view of the mind and introduced humans' natural resources as a factor in affecting behavior. Along with Hippocrates, a physician contemporary of classical Greek philosophers, including Socrates, Plato, and Aristotle (Hall and Lindzey, 1970; Fancher, 1990), distinguished themselves as the original scholars of the mind.

Socrates

One of the first Greek scholars to explain the nature of the mind was Socrates (470–399 BCE). Socrates was the son of a sculptor of stone and a midwife. After reading the book of Anaxagoras, the first philosopher of Athens, he became obsessed with searching "his own mind and the minds of his fellow citizens in an attempt to discover the essence of man and of goodness" (Rader, 1969, p. 10). His pursuit of meaning took the form of question and answer, a dialectic carried on between two or more people or within oneself, as the primary method of investigation. The singular goal of the Socratic method was to discover the truth. The process involved collecting all available data and, through critical examination, determining not only the essential nature of the data, but also how they fit with other pieces of data. The contemporary cognitive processes of active listening and critical thinking are basically an outgrowth and extension of *Socratic questioning* (Paul, 1993). Socrates' famous statement, "An unexamined life is not worth living," is widely quoted today as a rationale for seeking self-awareness.

Unfortunately, Socrates managed to offend those in power with his outspoken new ideas and his critical spirit. His crime essentially was questioning the status quo of the current social order, and his defense was brilliant and forthright. For this, he received the death penalty (Taylor, 1933).

Plato

Plato (427–347 BCE) was a member of one of the finest families in Athens. The shock of the trial and subsequent execution of Socrates when Plato was 28 shaped his future career. He began to write his famous dialogues designed to complete the work of Socrates (Rader, 1969). Plato speculated that character and intelligence are inherited. He argued that the soul was imprinted with special knowledge and that these inherent notions would manifest themselves when a relevant external event or stimulus triggered them into awareness. Sigmund Freud (1914) credits Plato's book, *The Nature of Soul*, with anticipating his own ground-breaking work on dream interpretation.

Plato described the soul—or the *psyche* as the Greeks called it—as the center of will, self-motion, and knowing. Organized into three parts or kinds of operation—reason, passion, and appetite—Plato believed that the logical psyche, or rational soul, dominated the psyche. The role of the rational soul was to process information and solve problems and to permit the planning and implementation of decisions. Unchecked, human appetites threatened the balance of effective living, entrapping a person in intemperate behaviors. Ideally, reason prevailed over appetite, augmented by passion, as the "spirited" element. Plato viewed the spirited element of the soul as being "akin to our 'sense of honor,' manifested in indignation, which takes the side of reason against appetite but cannot be identified with reason, since it is found in children and animals and it may be rebuked by reason" (Plato, quoted in Rader, 1969, p. 682). Freud's later ideas about the structure of personality are recognizable byproducts of these earlier philosophical understandings.

Aristotle

Aristotle (384–322 BCE), born 15 years after the death of Socrates, was the son of a court physician of King Amyntas II of Macedonia. He pursued a career as a philosopher, initially as a member of Plato's school. Subsequently, he founded a school of his own, the Lyceum, which he presided over for 12 years (Jaeger, 1934). Similar to his teacher Plato, Aristotle identified the soul as the center of mental activity. He argued, however, that experience comes from the external world through the senses rather than as innate knowledge as proposed by Plato. Aristotle defined three aspects of the soul, which he characterized as vegetative, sensitive, and rational. To him, the most primitive was the vegetative soul. He envisioned the vegetative soul as being responsible for nourishment and reproductive functions. The sensitive soul was more sophisticated and was thought to control movement, sensation, memory, and imagination. Aristotle contended that the rational soul operated at a higher level. He believed that it was designed to orchestrate reasoning, consciousness, and ethics. The rational soul was exclusive to humankind. In contrast to Plato (who envisioned the soul as imprinted with special knowledge), Aristotle described this soul as a blank slate—a *tabula rasa*—to be filled and molded, based on the individual's experiences and subsequent reactions.

Aristotle proposed that an individual exercises judgment based on experience. This judgment consists of the impact of the physical sensations on the soul, with the mind acting as the agent of interpretation for the activities of life. By linking the soul with actions of the physical being, Aristotle made an important contribution to the study of psychology. He removed much of the mysticism previously associated with the soul and its function, thus opening the door for serious scientific investigation. In making a conceptual leap from undefinable causes to mind-body causality of mental disorders, Aristotle anticipated the psychosomatic interest of modern science in explaining human behavior. Because of Aristotle's innovative ideas, the Greek term *psyche*, which simply means the mind, is now part of the common vernacular.

Hippocrates

Hippocrates (460–377 BCE), a physician and contemporary of early Greek philosophers, suggested a link between body type and characteristic behaviors. He based his assumptions on an ancient Greek theory that the physical universe consists of four basic elements: air, earth, fire, and water. Revered as the "father of medicine," Hippocrates hypothesized that the body consists of four corresponding humors: blood, black bile, yellow bile, and phlegm. At a time when mental illness generally was interpreted as the presence of evil spirits or supernatural forces, Hippocrates placed it within the context of disease by claiming that imbalances in the body humors caused the symptoms of mental illness. For example, he asserted that excess black bile accounted for the development of depressive symptoms. Galen later proposed a general topology of physique and disposition, by suggesting that overabundance of any of these humors accounted for characteristic personality traits. The terms *sanguine* (hopeful), *melancholic* (sad), *choleric* (hot tempered), and *phlegmatic* (apathetic) continue to describe mood even though these ancient psychophysiological theories have long since been discarded (Leibert and Spiegler, 1982).

Hippocrates understood that health required the presence of certain positive physiological and environmental conditions. He recognized that the mind and body interact as a whole. In fact, he instructed his patients on how to harness the power of their minds to heal their bodies—a radical concept that is currently being reconsidered by many modern-day healers. The relevance of these early scholarly thoughts about consciousness and the structure of the mind to psychiatric nursing practice is summarized in Table 6–1.

Contributions From Early Scientists

René Descartes

Two unlikely scientists contributed in different ways to our current understanding of behavior. The first was René Descartes (1596–1650), a Renaissance scholar, who upheld the idea that mind and body were connected through a complicated mechanism between soul and brain as follows (Descartes, 1931, article 42):

> *Thus, when the soul desires to recollect something, this desire causes the gland, by inclining successively to different sides, to thrust the spirits towards different parts of the brain until it comes across the part where the traces left there by the object we wish to recollect are found.*

Although his ideas may sound somewhat naive today, they were revolutionary in Descartes' era, and, more important, they clearly demonstrate an initial understanding of the interactive role body, mind, and soul play in regulating behavior. The role of the unconscious, although implied rather than explicit, is explained as memory traces.

Charles Darwin

In 1871, Charles Darwin (1809–1892) startled Victorian society with a radically different explanation of the mind. He challenged previous philosophical views of humans (and the mind) as having an invariate existence by introducing a more naturalistic theory. Instead of viewing the human organism as a fixed object, Darwin was convinced that it should be considered as an adaptive organism, capable of change. He highlighted the importance of function and adaptation with his theory of evolution—or "survival of the fittest"—forever altering the way humankind viewed the process of growth and change (Fancher, 1990).

Darwin borrowed extensively from earlier schools of thinking. Despite the fact, however, that both Galileo and Descartes centuries before had pointed out similar observations, he receives the official credit for describing the first set of assumptions about the adaptation of an organism to its environment. In his book *The Origin of the Species* Darwin laid out an impressive thesis that within any given population, those best able to adapt to their environment have the greatest likelihood of surviving. He stressed the importance of direct observation in describing human behavior, pointing to its validity in studying animal behavior.

Darwin also received credit for focusing on individual differences as important determinants of behavior. He speculated that people with more highly adaptive gene pools were better physically equipped to survive. This became the genesis of his theory of evolution by natural selection.

According to Darwin, mental traits similarly conform to the principles of evolution. He argued that emotions were inherited and served an adaptive purpose. Furthermore, he placed great significance on the usefulness of physical gestures that accompany all emotional reactions. For example, the wide-eyed expression of surprise heightened one's visual field, permitting the person to see an item of interest more vividly. In this manner, Darwin connected emotional expression directly to a physiological response in the nervous system. He considered that humans were influenced both by conscious rational thought and by the unconscious, or instincts. Instincts were believed to be left over from an animalistic past.

Darwin believed that all life forms are basically motivated by two distinct drives: the will to survive and the desire to reproduce. Freud later elaborated on the idea

TABLE 6–1 **Relevance of the Ancient Greek Philosophers to Psychiatric Nursing Practice**

Philosopher	Central Tenets	Relevance to Psychiatric Nursing Practice
Socrates	Socratic questioning and dialogue between people can help them in their search for truth	Active listening helps to elicit the truth Critical thinking, in which nurse and patient examine a problem carefully, consider the presence of faulty assumptions, review the evidence and the ideas of everyone concerned, and draw conclusions based on the evidence, is an effective problem-solving strategy
Aristotle	The mind, body, and soul are interrelated and cannot be understood separately	Nurses take a holistic approach to patient care
Hippocrates	Mental disorders must be seen in the context of disease	Thorough knowledge of the biochemical factors involved in mental illness, the use of pharmacological interventions, and the use of dynamic approaches to mental illness are required in the treatment of mental disorders
	The mind has power to control the functions of the body	Through such interventions as imagery, biofeedback, and relaxation techniques, nurses can help patients achieve more control over the reactions of their bodies
Plato	Free will exists	Nurses empower patients, foster their self-control, and educate them about the power of positive thinking, self-reliance, and confidence
	Interpretation of one's reality varies with one's individual perceptions	Nurses assess patient perceptions and help patients to become aware of their perceived realities. Nurses also help patients to see how this version is influenced, enhanced, and undermined. Nurses can employ strategies to facilitate self-promoting perceptions
	Habits are repetitive positive and negative behaviors that become automatic	Nurses recognize that considerable effort is required to change behavior when modification is necessary. They recognize the importance of short-term and long-term goals

of unconscious instincts to develop his own thesis on the libido and thanatos as basic instinctual drives present in every human being. So in many ways, Darwin's work is considered a precursor of the psychoanalytic approach to the study of behavior, without which Freud's ideas might not have achieved such broad acceptance.

Darwin's theory of evolution has many far-reaching implications for nursing practice. Genetic makeup and adaptive functioning indicate that human physiology can predispose one to either successful or unsuccessful psychological functioning. An evolutionary perspective also challenges the nurse to consider the importance of individual differences in planning care. That conscious thought enters into expression of behavior, but is supplemented by unconscious instincts, provides the nurse with a clearer understanding of the nature of unconventional behaviors.

The Advent of Psychology as a Formal Discipline

The discipline of psychology emerged in the late 19th century, essentially as a by-product of philosophy and experimental physiology. By 1896, the field was well established as a respected academic science. Two forward thinkers—Wilhelm Wundt of Germany and William James of the United States—were largely responsible for this recognition. They are considered the "psychological popes of the old and new worlds" (Fancher, 1990, p. 239).

Wilhelm Wundt

Wilhelm Wundt is generally credited with establishing modern psychology as a science (Fancher, 1990). He graduated from the University of Tübingen Medical

School in Germany. Wundt disliked private medical practice, however, and instead chose to work as a physiologist in an academic setting. In 1879, Wundt opened an experimental laboratory in Leipzig, the first of its kind, to research the conscious experiences of adults. His research centered around examining the association between sensory nerve stimulation and subsequent motor nerve response. With the aid of an instrument known as the *thought meter*, he determined that stimulation did not lead to an immediate reaction. Rather a period of time elapsed in midsequence, and Wundt concluded from these studies that thoughts occurred at this juncture.

Wundt identified the central nervous system as the force behind thinking and attention—the process whereby thoughts take form. By isolating the connection between conscious thoughts and the central nervous system, Wundt had, in effect, begun the study of the interrelationship between physiology and mental functions. Wundt realized that his assumptions implied the mind possessed its own inborn creative sources. Furthermore, Wundt understood that the mental mechanisms it sheltered would extend beyond attention, into many alternative and diverse functions. For his method and overall contributions to the field, Wundt is identified as the "father of experimental psychology" (Fancher, 1990).

From his research, Wundt became aware that there was another aspect of mental functioning that was inaccessible by experimental or physiological means. This area was larger than individual consciousness and encompassed social consciousness. Ethnic, cultural, religious, and social dynamics fell into this realm of psychology and helped explain other important determinants of behavior and personality.

Underlining both subtypes (the physiological aspect of psychological functioning and the social implications) is the notion that exploration of conscious experiences is critical to understanding mental health behaviors. Introspection is an essential conduit for accessing these experiences and providing information about psychological processes. Wundt believed the processes of sensation and voluntary movement are of paramount importance. At this intersection, psychology and physiology meet. Wundt defined internal sensations as the psychological state that one experiences. Therefore, an internal sensation is a feeling or a mood. This reaction occurs within the individual—intrapsychically.

Wundt defined voluntary movement as the actual muscular action that is generated by a psychological impulse; in other words, the behavioral action taken as a direct consequence of the psychological state. Both feeling states (also known as affect and action) are identified as critical psychological expressions. Although Wundt's theory was later rejected as being too narrow, he retains his place in the history of psychology as its first experimental scientist. According to Murphy (1949 p. 159):

> *Before Wundt published his physiological psychology and established his laboratory, psychology was little more than a waif knocking now at the door of physiology, now at the door of ethics, now at the door of epistemology. In 1879, it set itself up as an experimental science with a local habitation and a name.*

By insisting on an empirical method for the study of behavior, Wundt created the important link between an experimental and a social psychology and established the legitimacy of psychology as a science.

William James

William James (1842–1910) is considered a pioneer of American psychology. He was an American philosopher who published the first textbook in psychology in 1890, a two-volume treatise on *Principles of Psychology.* Two years later, he revised his original work into *Psychology: The Briefer Course* for classroom use (Alport, 1892). James was born in New York City and raised in privileged circumstances as the eldest son of five children, in a family where education and intellectual pursuits were highly valued. Although financially secure, his father suffered from severe anxiety and struggled with feelings of insecurity, unfulfillment, and indecisiveness. Ultimately, his father resolved these issues independently.

The younger James (Fancher, 1990) was undoubtedly influenced by both his family atmosphere and their values. He cherished opportunities for learning but, like his father, was prone to emotional difficulties. In fact, James battled serious bouts of depression, anxiety, and ambivalent feelings about his self-worth during much of the first half of his life. James attended Harvard University and Harvard Medical School, concentrating his studies on physiology. Unfortunately, during James' course of study, family conflicts, coupled with his own failing physical health, led James to thoughts of suicide. Instead of killing himself, however, James opted to continue his education in physiology abroad.

In Germany, in 1867, James first encountered Wilhelm Wundt's article on physiological psychology—an article that was to change the course of his life and work. When James read about Wundt's work, he was struck by the interplay between physiology and psychology and began to incorporate those concepts into his own work.

James returned to Harvard, but he became despondent again. He felt pessimistic and anxiety-ridden, until a chance reading about free will, written by French philosopher Charles Renouvier (1815–1903), inspired him to empower himself. Renouvier defined free will in terms of self-control. He stated that by maintaining a thought, one exerts free will. Stimulated by his new sense of empowerment, James began to use free will to modify his thoughts and attitudes. Fascinated by the concept of free will, he read profusely on the subject and eventually came upon the work of a British philosopher, Alexander Bain (1818–1903). Bain wrote at length about habit and emphasized the importance of voluntary repetition as the means by which actions become habitual and thus automatic. As James successfully applied both Renouvier's and Bain's ideas in coping with his own personal crises, he was able to harness his personal creative power, and he began to believe in its efficacy. Motivated by his enhanced knowledge of free will and the successful resolution of his own crisis, William James formulated a new set of principles of psychological theory (Fancher, 1990).

The essence of James' theory is rooted in the ideas of the classical Greek scholars discussed earlier. Similarly to Socrates and Aristotle, James believed that the search for truth about human beings lies in having an open mind and a systematic reasoned approach to examining the meaning of human behavior. James, however, expanded their notion of the verification process beyond the dimensions of the individual soul to include its integral link with the larger schema of human experiences. He described the subjective life of a person as a "stream of thought consciousness. . . . It is nothing jointed, it flows. A 'river' or 'stream' are metaphors by which it is most naturally described" (James, 1950, p. 239). James viewed man as a choice maker and saw attention to the task as a necessary prerequisite for dispelling tangential interests and associations.

James understood that people are influenced by many factors in the formation of their free will actions, and he viewed free will as a correlate of full attention to difficult tasks. Through self-examination, James became aware of his own motivators. He surmised that human behavior was clearly associated with the interpretation of one's reality. James emphasized the significance of perceptions and presumed that a psychological belief in oneself fueled creative energy. He hypothesized that autonomy and determination are human resources that facilitate the implementation of free will.

As James pursued this line of inquiry, he considered the significance of behavior and how it might develop. He described habit as essential for a stable society. Although habits could be either good or bad, they provided predictability to behavior. James accepted Bain's sequence of habit formation as *voluntary repetition* (Fancher, 1990, p. 247), in which a person, acting on her or his own volition, repeats a behavior until eventually that behavior becomes permanently imprinted into the nervous system. In this way, the behavior becomes automatic. Once a habit is established, it is difficult to undo.

Many of the innovative ideas of James, a powerful writer, about the "science of mental life" are still valid today. His chapter on habit, with its practical maxims of maintaining focus, permitting no exceptions, and continuous practice, provided a pragmatic lead into our current understanding of how behavioral therapies work. The idea that one has free will and can make reasoned choices that affect feeling and behavior reaches into the heart of many behavioral cognitive approaches to change. His lectures on the nature of pragmatism, proposing it as a reality-based and action-oriented approach to behavioral decisions (James, 1907) is a recognizable forerunner of contemporary reality-based theories of therapeutic approaches to behavioral change.

James spearheaded the development of psychology as a professional discipline in the United States. He taught the first psychology courses at a university level and brought the message of this new discipline to the general

TABLE 6–2 **Relevance of the Early Psychologists to Psychiatric Nursing Practice**

Psychologist	Central Tenets	Relevance to Psychiatric Nursing Practice
Wilhem Wundt	There is an association between sensory nerve stimulation and motor response	Nurses take a holistic approach to patient care
	Neurological and physiological status affect mental status. There is a link between mood, behavior, and mental function	Nursing assessment and potential intervention must track this sequence to promote successful function
	Conscious thought occurs and originates in the central resources. Each person has innate creative resources	Nurses must assist patients in becoming aware of their thoughts and in benefiting from their inner resources
William James	Free will exists	Nurses empower patients, foster their self-control, and educate them about the power of positive thinking, self-reliance, and confidence
	Interpretaton of one's reality varies with one's individual perceptions	Nurses assess patient perceptions and help patients to become aware of their perceived realities. Nurses also help patients to see how this version is influenced, enhanced, and undermined. Nurses can employ strategies to facilitate self-promoting perceptions
	Habits are repetitive positive and negative behaviors that become automatic	Nurses recognize that considerable effort is required to change behavior when modification is necessary. They recognize the importance of short-term and long-term goals

population in the United States. Because he was able to apply so many of the concepts he wrote about from his own personal journey, his theory has an especially powerful ring of truth to it. Table 6–2 summarizes the relevance of these early psychologists to psychiatric nursing practice.

▶ Check Your Reading

1. How does theory reflect the personal journey of the theorist?
2. What are some of the contributions the early Greek scholars made to the development of psychology?
3. In what ways did Wundt and James mark the journey of psychology as a profession?

Psychodynamic Theories

Sigmund Freud

Sigmund Freud's (1856–1939) groundbreaking theory of personality structure and development and his insistence on psychological treatment of behavioral symptoms revolutionized thinking about mental health disorders. His discovery of unconscious motivation represented a monumental breakthrough in the treatment of emotionally disturbed people. Freud believed that the vast majority of mental disorders were not organic in origin but rather developed as the result of unresolved emotional conflicts in childhood. His psychodynamic formulations grew out of personal observations regarding his own behavior, his family, and friends as well as those of his patients.

Freud was born in Freiberg, Moravia (Czechoslovakia), in 1856. His father recognized his academic talents early and encouraged Freud to develop them. As a youngster, he was interested in history and humanities, with a tendency toward law. Freud's life, however, took a completely different direction as a result of a chance scientific reading he encountered just before completing high school. He found the article so compelling that he made a spontaneous decision to enroll in the University of Vienna's Medical School.

Although Freud never intended to enter private medical practice, he had no choice in the matter. As a Jew in an anti-Semitic environment, he was denied opportunities in academic settings. Consequently, Freud established a practice in neurology. He continued to pursue his research and publication, however, which earned him respect and attention—but also drew sharp criticism because of the radical nature of his ideas.

Among the patients Freud treated were *hysterics*—people who were suffering despite the absence of a physiological cause. Many physicians of the day refused to treat these patients, believing them to be malingerers or impostors. As a student of Jean-Martin Charcot (1825–1893), a famous French psychiatrist, Freud understood the genuineness of their symptoms and considered them worthy of his care. Freud learned from Charcot how to perform hypnosis, and although his results were mixed, his experiences provided the impetus to consider other psychological methods of treatment. Then Josef Breuer (1842–1925), a Viennese doctor and an old friend of Freud's, offered a supplemental treatment to hypnosis. Breuer had begun talking with a hysterical patient about her symptoms and their origin while she was under hypnosis. This strategy effectively cured her and became known as the cathartic method. Freud employed talk therapy (cathartic method) as a primary means of treating individuals with mental symptoms and later added the concept of free association with dramatic results in his patients. His writings spanned more than 40 years and included 23 volumes, which had an influence not only on the psychiatric community but also on the development of literature, art, and social ideologies (English and English, 1958; Strachey, 1964). For example, impressionist and surrealist art often contains unconscious symbolism as well as reality. In literature, fairy tales are said to reflect the unconscious, and the presence of the unconscious is also found in the *stream of consciousness* method of writing and in drawing.

Freud offered the psychiatric world a systematic way of looking at the structure and function of personality. Although psychiatry today has broadened, refined, and even refuted Freud's original ideas about individual behavior, the essence of his pioneering contributions remain as a powerful foundation for current thinking about human personality. Current psychiatric terminology, including the unconscious, defense mechanisms, repression, transference and countertransference, the concept of resistance, interpretation, and the stages of psychosocial development, initially were defined by Freud. Popular contemporary terms such as *anal retentive* personality, *Oedipus complex*, *tip of the iceberg*, *erogenous zones*, and *Freudian slips* (of the tongue) trace their origins to Freud. Among the many psychological concepts that still hold true today is Freud's most important: his insistence that all behavior is motivated, and much of it is not within the person's conscious awareness.

THE DYNAMICS OF THE PERSONALITY

Freud describes the dynamics of personality in terms of basic instincts and anxiety. Instincts arise internally, whereas anxiety, although also a state of tension, derives from external sources. Freud identified two basic drives or instincts in humans: *Libido* was defined as the pleasure principle in the life drive. *Thanatos*, derived from the Greek word meaning death, incorporated humans' destructive instincts. A person's libido seeks satisfaction through sex and satisfying hunger or thirst needs. Thanatos represents a person's aggressive drive to kill or be killed. The life instincts provide energy for human survival and reproduction. Self-destructive behaviors toward self or others are better explained by the instinctual energy associated with thanatos (Hall and Lindzey, 1970). The three structures of the mind, id, ego, and superego, use the psychic energy represented in humans' instinctual drives to regulate all living processes.

Freud believed in psychic determinism: All behavior, no matter how random it may appear, has an identifiable cause both created and interpreted by an individual's personal history and experiences. He held that the earlier unresolved conflicts a child had with significant adults continued to have an impact on the person's life until they could be brought into conscious awareness. Although current thinking challenges Freud's insistence that "remembering repressed traumatic situations is the ultimate goal" (Alexander, 1959, p. 322) of therapy, there is no question that helping patients talk about unresolved conflicts, past as well as present, is beneficial.

Anxiety, a concept described later in this chapter and discussed in Chapter 28, has the dual functions of warning a person of an approaching physical or psychological threat and motivating a person to take action. When anxiety reaches an intolerable point and cannot be resolved easily by the ego, the ego employs defense mechanisms to ward off the perceived danger the environment or person imposes. Although everyone uses ego defense mechanisms to some degree, the ego's persistent inability to master the situation, to harness difficult emotions, or to control dangerous impulses usually results in psychiatric symptoms. Freud identified three types of anxiety: objective anxiety, neurotic anxiety, and moral anxiety. With objective anxiety, the threat is real and external to the person experiencing it. Neurotic anxiety occurs when there is conflict between the id and ego, whereby the ego is unsuccessful in quelling the urges of the id. According to Freud, neurotic anxiety can present as free floating, phobic, or panic. Free-floating anxiety is a vague, nebulous dread without an objective stimulus. Phobic anxiety is characterized by a specific irrational fear about a displaced object, for example, fear of heights, fear of crowds, claustrophobia. Murder, suicide, and violence often are undesired outcomes of panic. Freud defines moral anxiety as anxiety emerging from conflicts between the ego and the superego, in which a person fears punishment by his or her conscience for actions taken.

THE STRUCTURE OF THE PERSONALITY

Freud originally identified a topographic theory of how the mind functions and described the landscape of the mind as having three distinct mental processes. He considered the *conscious* part of the mind to be the tip of the iceberg. It represented all of the material a person was aware of at any given moment in time. Just below the surface of awareness is the *preconscious.* Although the preconscious does not lie within a person's awareness, material contained in this layer of the mind can be retrieved rather easily through conscious effort. By contrast, the **unconscious** material consists of all of the repressed memories, passions, and unacceptable urges lying deep below the surface. The vast realm of the unconscious has a forceful, unseen effect on the conscious thoughts and behaviors of a person. Recognition of the contents of the unconscious usually cannot be retrieved by an individual through personal efforts. With the skillful intervention of a therapist, however, it is possible to bring unconscious material into conscious awareness.

Later, Freud taught that personality is composed of three major systems: the id, ego, and superego. Although they are distinct systems, the three work closely together. Generally, behavior is the result of this interaction. Rarely does one system function to the exclusion of the others. Ideally the three systems work as a team, under the rational administrative leadership of the ego. Because only so much energy is available to any person, the three systems often compete with one another for dominance. One system can overpower the effectiveness of the other two systems. For example, an overly responsible person governed by the superego may have great difficulty experiencing the fun and conviviality a person with a better balance of id might. The patient with antisocial disorder frequently experiences serious difficulty getting in touch with the superego and ego stability that most mature, responsible adults possess. Although not incompatible with Freud's earlier topographical model, his structural view of how the mind functions is not totally comparable either. Rather they represent two different approaches to the study of personality functioning (Marmer, 1994).

Id. At birth, an infant is all **id,** motivated by instinctual drives of hunger and thirst. As the mind's most primitive system, it is from the id that the ego and superego later evolve. The id is considered the source of all psychic energy, providing vital empowerment to both the ego and the superego. The validity of Freud's argument about the energy effect of the id is evidenced in the renewal of strength most people feel after a good vacation or recreational respite.

Freud believed that all inherited and instinctual psychological processes reside in the id. He considered it to be the "true psychic reality" because the id is aware only of emotional perceptions. It is not privy to the constraints of an objective reality. Consequently, the laws of logic do not apply to thoughts stimulated by the id. The *pleasure principle* is its guiding force.

Whenever tension is experienced, the id is driven to reduce this tension instantly in an attempt to return to a tension-free, or pleasurable, state. The pleasure principle has two methods of reducing tension: reflex action and primary process. *Reflex action,* as the name implies, is inherent and automatic. Gagging is a reflex. The human body has many such reflexes, such as crying and laughing, which successfully alleviate certain forms of tension.

Not all tension, however, can be reduced or removed through reflex action. This is particularly true of psychic or emotional tension, commonly called anxiety. Naturally, the remaining tension causes frustration. Freud labeled as *primary process* the energy discharge of mental impulses, occurring without delay and uninhibited by any reality factors. Through primary processes, the id attempts to diminish tension by creating an image of the object that would rectify the uncomfortable situation. For example, the mirages of water that people experience in the desert enable them to experience in their minds the reality of plentiful water. This mental image is known as wish-fulfillment. The id perceives the mental image of water to be synonymous with the actual fluid because it knows only subjective reality. Primary process is seen in the images of small children, with the ego rupture of feelings present in severe mental illness, with autistic thinking, and in dreams.

Wish-fulfillment cannot sustain the individual because one obviously cannot drink imaginary water. Therefore, primary process alone does not suffice to reduce tension. To successfully accommodate to changes in the journey external reality must be considered, which requires the development of secondary processes grounded in truth. Secondary psychological processes mark the emergence of the ego; they are associated with the preconscious and conscious elements of personality.

Ego. Freud conceptualized a higher level of functioning that he classified as *secondary psychological processes* and assigned to the ego. He viewed the **ego** as the "executive of personality because it controls the gateways to actions, selects the features of the environment to which it will respond, and decides what instincts will be satisfied, and in what manner (Hall and Lindzey, 1970, p. 34).

The ego has a regulatory function (the reality principle), which allows a person to delay gratification and to consider environmental factors that are either favorable or unfavorable to the discharge of mental impulses. It determines the response needed by an individual to negotiate with the objective world of reality. The essential difference between the ego and the id is that the id knows only subjective experience, whereas the ego can differentiate between subjective reality, memory images, and objective reality. Through secondary processes, an individual is able to recognize the reality factors of a situation and to make conscious decisions based on all of the evidence.

The ego is charged with the mission of self-preservation. Governed by the reality principle, it nevertheless derives from the id and is never entirely free from it. The reality principle puts the desires of the id on hold to tolerate the tension, until a satisfactory outlet for tension reduction is produced. Reality becomes the utmost priority but only by visualization of an object that can reduce tension. This kind of teamwork makes it possible to arrive at the ultimate goal of tension reduction, thereby gratifying the id as well.

Secondary process provides the energy to plan a course of action and to test this action, in an effort to determine the validity of the plan. The hungry man thinks about where he can eat dinner and then seeks that destination. This process is known as *reality testing* because the individual is attempting to factor in reality to implement a plan for tension reduction. It is the ego that coordinates the expression of self, with attention to the various demands from id, superego, and reality.

Superego. The superego is the last portion of personality to be developed. It represents the ideal rather than the real, seeking perfection, as opposed to pursuing pleasure or engaging reason. The **superego** represents the moral component of personality and incorporates the child's view of his or her parents' values and ideals. Consequently, it internalizes and absorbs these messages on morality and righteousness. The goals of the superego are to

- Curb the impulses of the id, especially the sexual and aggressive ones
- Influence the ego to endorse moralistic goals
- Strive for perfection (Hall and Lindzey, 1970)

Two subsystems operate in the superego: the conscience and the ego-ideal. The conscience corresponds to the child's version of what her parents have condemned. The child makes these interpretations, based on what led to punishment or disapproval. Memory images activated by a person's conscience create guilt associations and inhibit behavior or destroy its temptation permanently. Conversely, the ego-ideal internalizes what the parents consider morally good—the standards of virtue. When standards imposed by the superego are realized, a person feels the pride of achievement. Similar to the id, however, the superego is irrational and relies on the ego for reality testing.

Ordinarily, personality is successfully integrated under the supervision of the ego. The ego is capable of exerting this influence because it is most effective in tension reduction—which is to say it is fueled with the greatest amount of psychic energy. Difficulties in mentally healthy functioning occur when the ego fails to maintain control of the psychic energy, allowing the id or superego to prevail instead. Too much superego influence is just as detrimental to personal growth as is being controlled by id. Eric Berne later popularized Freud's concepts of id, ego, and superego in applying them to a theoretical framework of communication as child, adult, and parent.

DEVELOPMENTAL STAGES

Freud (1960, 1969; Hall and Lindzey, 1970; Smith and Vetter, 1982; Fancher, 1990) is believed to be the first theorist to propose developmental stages of personality. Freud described five psychosexual stages of development, ending in adolescence, but he emphasized the significance of early childhood experiences. According to Freud, personality is largely determined by the age of five. Each developmental stage makes a contribution to the development of a mature personality and involves focusing on a particular bodily zone (mouth, anus, genitals), referred to as an *erogenous zone.* Each erogenous zone represents a vital function, readily observable as a focus of attention in the behaviors of the child. Freud argued, however, that the pleasure associated with the erogenous zone exceeded that of mere need satisfaction. Freud referred to the first three stages of psychosexual development (oral, anal, and phallic) as pregenital stages to distinguish them from the genital stage, in which energy associated with egocentricity gets transformed into genuine love of others.

Freud's first stage of psychosexual development, referred to as the *oral stage,* occurs from birth through approximately the first year of life. During this time, the infant sucks to nourish himself or herself—not only as a vital function, but also to pacify or comfort the self. The infant puts everything in its mouth, even its own body parts. Because the process of eating for the infant also includes being held, there are psychological as well as physical satisfactions associated with the oral stage of personality development. Naiveté, in believing anything one is told; biting sarcasm; and belligerence are all examples of adult personality traits reflective of difficulties stemming from this stage (Hall and Lindzey, 1970). The way an alcoholic often drinks directly from the bottle mimics behaviors from this early stage of development.

Freud identifies his next stage of psychosexual development as the *anal stage*. Extending from 18 months until approximately age three, the anal stage focuses on voluntary regulation of excretion, emphasizing body control and mastery. For the first time, the child becomes aware that his instinctual impulses are controllable as the task of toilet training becomes an issue. Emotional trauma associated with toilet training can result in later emotional dysfunctions. Expulsive traits (such as temper tantrums and slovenliness) or retentive traits (such as withholding and stubbornness) may develop as a result. The term *anal retentive* is sometimes used to describe people with an excessive need to retain control and not let go of details.

The *phallic stage* usually lasts from age three through five years. The genitalia become the focal body point during this period, as the child discovers erotic pleasure when the genitals are touched. Autoerotic behavior and its associated pleasures coincide with the Oedipus complex, which Freud believed to be his greatest discovery (Hall and Lindzey, 1970). In this complex, named after the King of Thebes who murdered his father and married his mother, the young child feels attachment for the parent of the opposite sex and experiences hostility toward the parent of the same sex. Freud believed that a little boy suffered from castration anxiety, fearing that his father would cut off his penis. Resolution of the Oedipus complex allows a boy to identify with his father and later to develop attachment for women other than his mother. The counterpart of the Oedipus complex in little boys is the Electra complex in little girls. Once a little girl discovers she does not have a penis, she develops what Freud referred to as penis envy. She views her mother as a threat to her relationship with her father. To resolve the conflict, little girls play with their dolls and substitute the wish for a baby for the wish for a penis. The Electra complex is resolved by the little girl's identification with her mother, which frees her to achieve her own sexual identity. Freud's ideas about castration anxiety and penis envy seem outrageous in a modern age in which men and women are viewed as more equal, and a person is thought of as a whole person. His assertion that "anatomy is destiny" no longer has the ring of truth. Freud was quite correct, however, in assuming that a person's successful negotiation of future relationships with the opposite sex had their roots in the level of acceptance children feel early from opposite-sex and same-sex parents.

Freud does not pay much attention to the *latency stage* other than to say that it is a rather prolonged childhood period of quiescence. He considered it to be unremarkable from a psychodynamic perspective. Occurring between seven and thirteen years, the child's sexual impulses are repressed until adolescence, when hormonal changes reactivate them, and they burst forth with great intensity. Latency, however, is important from the perspective that the child is developing the skills needed to make the transition from a full home environment to one that includes the broader perspective of school and playmates. During the latency stage, children develop relationships with peers, allowing them to develop the self-confidence needed to compete and collaborate with others outside of the family unit. Usually the child in the latency stage shows great interest in peers of the same sex and little interest in peers of the opposite sex.

Freud's final stage of psychosexual maturity, the *genital stage*, begins in adolescence and extends into adulthood. In this stage, the adolescent redirects self-love into attachment to others. Successful passage through this period of development allows the transformation of the child with pleasure-seeking tendencies to assume deliberately the mantle of a "reality-oriented, socialized adult" (Hall and Lindzey, 1970, p. 53). Earlier stages of development are integrated into the personality with the final outcome incorporating elements from all of the previous stages. Healthy completion of these stages enables the mature adult to maintain tolerable levels of anxiety and to employ tension-reduction techniques proficiently. Individual personality is the outcome of this complex process. Table 6–3 contrasts Freud's psychosexual stages of development with Erik Erikson's psychosocial stages.

PSYCHOANALYTIC TECHNIQUES

Considered the "father of **psychoanalysis,**" Freud carefully laid out a method of treating behavioral symptoms by psychological rather than physical means. His thoughts about the value of talking about painful issues are the basis for most counseling practices today. Freud viewed the patient's remembrance of repressed memories as the goal of psychoanalytic therapy and the method by which this material is elicited by the analyst as catharsis and free association. The therapeutic goal of the cathartic method was to have the patient explore bothersome symptoms in depth. As the patients relived in their minds the nature of their symptoms and put them into words, they were able to draw out the emotionally laden memory associated with the symptom. This cathexis enabled the patient to experience an emotion that had been previously denied. Once a patient achieved insight about the origin and nature of the repressed feelings, the symptom lost its power.

Freud (1960, 1969) later refined his psychoanalytic technique to include free association. Free association requires full and honest, uncensored disclosure of thoughts and feelings as they come to mind. Freud understood that free association led the patient on a path to the pathological ideas that caused pain. He encouraged his patients to share everything, without evaluating the merit of their responses. By listening to people's associations, Freud came to the conclusion that talking about difficult emotional issues had the potential to heal the emotional wounds of mental illness.

Within the therapeutic relationship, Freud described a relatively rigid therapeutic intervention method in which the patient had to fit a certain mold of activity. He observed, however, that not all patients fitted the mold.

TABLE 6–3 Comparison Between Freud's Psychosexual Stages and Erikson's Psychosocial Stages

Age (Years)	Erikson's Psychosocial Stages	Primary Person Orientation	Strengths	Qualities	Freud's Psycho-sexual Stages	Jung's Psycho-social Orientation
0–2	Trust vs. mistrust	Mother	Hope	To receive, to give	Oral	Largely unconscious
2–4	Autonomy vs. shame/doubt	Father	Will power	To control, to let go	Anal	
4–6	Initiative vs. guilt	Basic family	Purpose	To make, to play act	Oedipal	Beginning ego consciousness
6–12	Industry vs. inferiority	Neighborhood, school	Competence	To make things, to put things together	Latency	
13–19	Identity vs. identity diffusion	Peer groups	Fidelity	To be one's self	Puberty	Individual consciousness
Young adult	Intimacy vs. isolation	Partners in marriage, friendship	Love	To share's one's self with another	Genital	Social adaptation, achievement
Adult	Generativity vs. self-absorption	Children, community	Care	To take care of, to create		Inner reflection, individuation
Old age	Integrity vs. despair	Humankind	Wisdom	To accept being, to accept not being		Self-knowledge of the meaning of one's existence

From Arnold, E., and Boggs, K. (1995). *Interpersonal relationships: Professional communication skills for nurses* (p. 13). Philadelphia: W. B. Saunders; adapted from Erikson, E. (1982). *The life cycle completed.* New York: W. W. Norton & Co.

During the course of therapy, certain patients developed emotional blocks that got in the way of full catharsis. Those patients who refused or were unable to comply with full catharsis were considered resistant. Freud held that this was because of *transference* distortions. Each analysand brings into the therapeutic situation certain beliefs and feelings associated with past experiences that can color or distort the way in which the person experiences the current reality. For example, a person may have had bad experiences with authority figures in the past and therefore relates to authority figures in the present as being inflexible or critical even when there is no evidence of the therapist having such characteristics. These unconscious distortions interfere with the work of the therapy and influence the ways in which the patient perceives the therapist.

Freud noticed also that the behaviors of the analysand and the therapist had a reciprocal effect on one another. When the therapist responds with feelings of his own, his behavior reflects the therapist's distortions of the situation. These perceptual distortions constitute *countertransference* reactions and also disrupt the flow of the therapy. Transference and countertransference reactions are discussed in more detail in Chapter 11.

RELEVANCE TO NURSING

Freud's theory has relevance to psychiatric nursing practice at many junctures. First, it offers a comprehensive explanation of complex human processes and suggests that many diverse sources stemming from the past affect personality. Freud's theory of the unconscious is particularly valuable as a baseline for considering the multidimensional nature of behavior. By becoming familiar with these diverse conscious and unconscious influences, a nurse can develop and begin to formulate a hypothesis about the root causes of patient suffering. The id, ego, and superego represent different, often conflicting, needs coexisting within each person's psyche. Understanding the structural nature of the mind allows the nurse to respond more appropriately when obvious conflicts emerge in the nurse-patient relationship.

Freud's conceptualizations of transference and countertransference find their way into many therapeutic interactions. A professional nurse requires constant self-awareness to avoid confusing his or her own intrapsychic conflicts with that of the patients.

Clinical interventions derived from psychodynamic thought are vast. Individual talk sessions with patients that emphasize attentive listening and focus on underlying themes are important tools of healing in psychiatric care. Although the current emphasis in treatment is on the here and now, sensitivity to understanding the meaning of a patient's conversation usually results in improved patient care.

Carl Jung

Carl Jung (1875–1961) was born in Switzerland, the only child of a minister and his wife. He initially entered the University of Basel, seeking a degree as a philogist, but became more interested in medicine and psychiatry. Consequently, he obtained a degree in medicine from the university and began working at a psychiatric clinic in Zurich.

Jung initially was impressed with Freud's work, and he viewed him as an important mentor. In turn, Freud admired the brilliance of Jung's thinking and shared many ideas with him. But in 1914, Jung broke all contact with Freud because of his opposition to Freud's insistence that sexual energy was the driving force in humans. Jung then developed his own method of psychoanalysis, referred to as *analytical psychology*, which had a strong emphasis on dream interpretation and self-disclosure (Jung, 1916, 1953).

Jung built on Freud's ideas, but he differed with Freud on several fundamental issues. Instead of viewing libido as the pleasure principle, Jung characterized it as psychic energy, "the total force which pulses through all the forms and activities of the psychic system and establishes a communication between them" (Jacobi, 1951).

THE STRUCTURE OF THE PERSONALITY

Like Freud, Jung believed in the unconscious. But he took the concept a step further to embrace a **collective unconscious,** which he defined as comprising a person's racial and cultural heritage and consisting of universal images held by all humans. He categorized the latter as **archetypes.** According to Jung, the collective unconscious was the foundation for the entire personality structure. Usually, it is unconscious, but it can rush uninvited into consciousness during a psychotic break, presenting as a primary process with chaotic material and distorted feelings that are frightening to the individual experiencing them. Jung defined a *personal unconscious,* consisting of memories that once were conscious but are no longer remembered. He agreed with Freud that *conscious awareness* was a much smaller part of the personality, frequently governed by elements of the unconscious until they were drawn into conscious awareness through therapy.

One of Jung's most important concepts was that of **archetypes.** Jung defines them as "a universal thought form (idea) which contains a large element of emotion" (Hall and Lindzey, 1970, p. 85). He contends that archetypes represent experiences that have existed for a long time in the collective unconscious. Their energy continues to have an influence on present generations. Examples of commonly recognized archetypes include the earth mother, birth, death, the magician, unity, and the wise old man.

Of particular importance in the study of personality are the archetypes that influence interpersonal behavior. Some become so important to the structure of personality that they evolve into systems of their own and have a dramatic influence on behavior. Four of the most important include persona, shadow, anima-animus, and the self (Fordham, 1953). Jung defined the *persona* as the social mask people wear to meet the varying demands of social situations. The persona can include physical appearance, gestures, and manner of verbal presentation, all designed to satisfy the social needs of a situation. When the persona represents the essential nature of a person, all is well. When it is at odds with a person's personality, a persona can restrict the full expression of self tremendously.

Jung observed a paradox about personality structure, in that within each person's psyche many different elements, some light and some dark, coexist. (Jung, 1973). For each path a person chooses, there is the one that was not chosen. Recognition of the shadow side of self is not a disavowal of choices made but rather a completion of all that was involved in making the choice so that the person recognizes that there was a choice and on what basis it was made (Moore, 1992). Jung defined the *shadow* as the inferior side of the psyche, the part that is disowned by an individual, only to reappear in dreams or to find itself personified in another person. For example, Adrienne develops a particular intense dislike for Jackie without really knowing why the feeling is so intense. Jung (1973) would suggest that the feelings occur because Adrienne's unconscious recognizes qualities in Jackie that she also possesses but does not want to acknowledge consciously. Becoming aware of one's shadow side permits more leverage in interpersonal relationships and offers an opportunity to integrate all qualities productively into one's personality.

Jung also proposed the existence of a worldwide shadow, accounting for much of the evil in the world that cannot be attributed to personal choice. According to Jung, every person is capable of both terrible wrongs and courageous right actions, given the right set of circumstances. To ignore or minimize the presence of evil in the world is a dangerous proposition, examples of which are found in the many people each year who are duped into giving away their life savings for falsely advertised good causes.

Jung insisted that division of psychological characteristics as being "male" or "female" was an artificial distortion of psychological reality that did both men and women a disservice. According to Jung, both men and women contain the opposite characteristics—aggressiveness in women, tenderness in men—as integral parts of their personality. He labeled these characteristics *anima* (emotional characteristics traditionally associated with women) and *animus* (rationalizing characteristics traditionally associated with men). Men and women are most human when they are able to acknowledge and act on the paradox of having both types of characteristics coexisting within a unified self.

Jung considered the self, which he envisioned as embodying a person's longing for unity and wholeness, as the personality's most important structural system. Symbolized in the form of a circle, with neither beginning nor end, the self represents the core of the personality. Jung described the two primary orientations of self as *extroversion*, in which a person enjoys full participation in the outer world, and *introversion*, in which a person is mainly oriented toward the inner world. The extrovert makes decisions spontaneously and is happiest in a crowd. Extroverts are uncomfortable with a lack of action. By contrast, the introvert needs time to reflect before making decisions and prefers the company of one or two people to being in large crowds.

Jung also identified four psychological functions that help account for the way a person processes information and makes decisions: thinking, feeling, sensing, and intuition. Although everyone has all four psychological functions available for use, Jung proposed that people use one more than the other three. He identified the one used most often as the superior function and the least differentiated as the inferior function. Evidence of the inferior function is found in dreams and fantasies (Hall and Lindzey, 1970). Jung's descriptions of the attitudes and four fundamental psychological functions formed the basis for the Meyers Briggs Temperament Scales used extensively today in career and marital counseling.

Jung believed that the goal of personality development was self-realization. This was to be accomplished through individuation, which he described as developing a strong sense of self as apart but always in connective harmony with community (transcendent function). The self could find fulfillment through symbolic meaning, achievement, and religious experiences (Jung, 1958). Personal accomplishments in work and relationships could be forms of self-expression leading to individuation. In the process of achieving selfhood, Jung believed that humans were transformed from purely biological creatures into spiritual individuals. Although his description of the collective unconscious could be interpreted as a somewhat pantheistic world view, Jung was a deeply spiritual man, and he believed that spirituality was a necessary part of mental health (Jung, 1933).

RELEVANCE TO NURSING

Many of Jung's concepts are relevant in the nursing care of mentally ill patients. He introduced the idea of humans' cultural heritage as being an important dimension of self. He spoke of the self as being central to unity and wholeness. Jung's insistence that men and women, although different, also possess characteristics that can aid in their understanding of one another is extremely helpful in promoting more satisfying gender roles. He offered an explanation for the common tendency to project our undesired characteristics onto others and to reject their existence in ourselves. Understanding the origin of our irrational thoughts about others and our biases can aid in a more compassionate approach toward patients.

Interpersonal Psychodynamic Theory: Harry Stack Sullivan

Sullivan's (1894–1949) interpersonal model evolved in opposition to psychoanalytic theory's strong emphasis on reducing personality to biological drives. Harry Stack Sullivan was trained in psychodynamic methodology and championed the interpersonal model (1954, 1972; Hall and Lindzey, 1970; Smith and Vetter, 1982). Although he recognized the Freudian concepts of psychic energy, anxiety reduction, and the unconscious, Sullivan rejected other fundamental aspects of Freud's theory. His theory is classified as a **psychodynamic** (interpersonal) one because it is based on human relationships. Sullivan proposes that personality cannot be studied apart from the social and cultural influences on behavior, and his theory draws on knowledge from anthropology and sociology in addition to psychology.

Sullivan viewed any unit of behavior that a person demonstrated in a relationship as a **dynamism,** which he defined as an energy transference. A dynamism could be one of fear, intimacy, hostility, or lust. Sullivan viewed personality as a tension system in which tensions emerged and had to be relieved. He identified two basic sources of tension: needs and anxiety.

Rather than looking at instinctual drives as the driving force behind behavior, Sullivan's theory centers around the concept of anxiety as an interpersonally determined experience. He viewed the pursuit of biological satisfaction and the pursuit of emotional security as the motivators for most behavior. Satisfaction needs encompass the fundamental biological demands necessary for survival, that is, the need for nourishment, rest, sex, freedom from loneliness, and so forth. These needs are present immediately and require the infant to interact with others. Presumably, as a result of these positive interactions, need fulfillment occurs. The developing human benefits concurrently from attachment to others and from the tenderness this provides (security needs).

Security needs are psychological. They refer to the need to avoid anxiety and to feel safe and accepted. Psychological security leads to a sense well-being and belonging, congruent with the social norms and value systems of a person's community. According to Sullivan, a person becomes mentally ill when the person's self-system compromises his or her capacity to meet his or her needs for physiological satisfaction or psychological security.

According to Sullivan, anxiety develops from real or imagined threats to the self. The degree of anxiety is proportional to the amount of threat it stimulates. Anxiety is to be avoided at all costs. It first develops in infancy when the there is a breakdown in the mother-child interaction.

THE SELF-SYSTEM

Sullivan portrayed the self-system as an important dynamism, which operates to prevent an individual from experiencing anxiety. In the process of becoming a mature human being, a person develops three personifications of the self-concept, as the "good me," the "bad me," and the "not me," to ward against anxiety. Ideally the good me, in which the person experiences the self as good and worthwhile, predominates in the personality structure. The good me evolves out of the child's security and knowledge of the mother's approval. The bad me develops from observations of behaviors that the mother does not like and serves as a deterrent against behaviors that would earn disapproval. The not me portion of self-concept relates to activities and behaviors that are so ego-alien, they must be disowned by an individual as not being a part of them. Sullivan believed that not me manifestations of behavior are present in psychosis and in delusional thinking.

Sullivan suggested that personality functioning was actually best determined through observation of particular modes of interpersonal behavior. He identified three cognitive processes:

- Protaxic thinking (instinctual perceptions)
- Parataxic thinking (cause-effect relationships are established)
- Syntaxic thinking (consistent with Freud's secondary processes)

In infancy, only the protaxic mode exists, but as the child develops and interacts with important interpersonal figures, thinking progresses to a higher level (Marmer, 1994). Ideally, therapy supports syntaxic thinking processes as a way of establishing the validity and organizing information obtained through lower modes of cognitive functioning.

Sullivan's interpersonal model disputes the notion that cognitive insight alone brings about therapeutic change. Instead, his model stresses the nature and quality of the interpersonal relationship as the primary basis for healing. Furthermore, Sullivan firmly believed that the social attempt to separate these phenomena defeats the point. According to Sullivan, the essence of personality lies at this juncture and is best understood in its relation to the current interpersonal encounter.

Although the interpersonal therapist will take a patient history as background data, the major thrust of therapeutic intervention takes place through a corrective emotional experience that examines components of the self-system used to defend the individual against the emergence of anxiety. Once the patient becomes aware of components in the self-system that are not working or are dissociated from memory, the process of therapy takes on a reeducation focus. By directly experiencing a healthy authentic relationship with a helping person, working through difficult interpersonal problems, and learning better communication strategies, the patient is better able to establish healthy relationships with other people. Each relationship between a professional helping person and a patient is founded on respect and equality.

RELEVANCE TO NURSING

Sullivan's theory is the foundation for Hildegard Peplau's theory of interpersonal relationship. His thought that therapy should basically be used as a forum to educate patients and to assist them in gaining personal insight is the basis for Peplau's use of the nurse as an "educative instrument." It was Sullivan who first used the term *participant observer*, meaning that professional helpers cannot be isolated from the therapeutic situation if they are to be effective. Sullivan would insist that the nurse must interact with the patient as an authentic human being. Mutuality, respect for the patient, unconditional acceptance, and empathy, proposed as essential characteristics in modern therapeutic relationships, were important aspects of Sullivan's theory of interpersonal therapy.

Sullivan also demonstrated that a psychotherapeutic environment is an invaluable treatment tool. His idea of a psychotherapeutic milieu evolved around an accepting atmosphere, which provided numerous opportunities for practicing interpersonal skills and developing relationships. Group psychotherapy, family therapy, and educational and skill training programs as well as unstructured periods can be incorporated into the design of a psychotherapeutic environment to facilitate healthy interactions. This method is now being used in virtually all residential and day hospital settings.

▶ Check Your Reading

4. In what ways might psychoanalytic theory principles influence an assessment of a psychiatric patient?
5. What do you consider Carl Jung's most important contributions to the study of personality?
6. In what ways does Sullivan's interpersonal theory challenge the ideas of the psychoanalytic model?

Ego Theory: Erik Erikson

Erik Erikson's original work on personality development (1950, 1982) forms the foundation for understanding psychological growth and development. He was born in Frankfurt, Germany, in 1902 (Smith and Vetter, 1982). Erikson's formal education ended with the completion of high school. Instead of attending college, he traveled throughout Europe, eventually landing in Vienna. He accepted a position at the day care center Anna Freud had created for the children of student psychoanalysts, and it was here that his fascination for observing and documenting of human development at different points in the life span began. Erikson studied under Sigmund Freud's instruction, completing his education in 1933. He soon became one of the first child psychoanalysts in the United States.

Erikson practiced **ego psychology** because he focused on the ego. His vision of the ego differs from Freud's original concept of a fixed object. In Erikson's theory, the ego is separate and liberated from the id, developing across the course of the complete life cycle. In fact, Erikson contended that ego development is influenced by family, social, and even environmental factors. He described his theory as based on the epigenetic principle, in which sequential maturation occurs according to a biological time pattern, and maintained that "eight basic strengths emerge as we go through life, each the outgrowth of a time-specific developmental confrontation" (Erikson, 1988, p. 74). In contrast to epigenesis in the embryo, however, " where a strength is not adequately developed according to the given sequence for its scheduled period of critical resolution, the supports of the environment may bring it into appropriate balance at a later period" (Erikson, 1988, p. 75). Thus, life cycle psychological theory has a more hopeful note for successful resolution of psychosocial tasks.

Erikson (1982) described the human life cycle as a series of eight ego developmental stages, spanning from birth to death. Each stage presents a **psychosocial crisis** whose goal is to integrate both physical maturation and societal demands. At each maturational juncture, the person either masters the psychosocial crisis effectively (and thus strengthens his or her ego), or the inverse occurs. Each step forward involves a disconnection with previous ways of thinking about the self and a loss of the comfort associated with the previous sense of self. Consequently, each psychosocial crisis creates anxiety. Although Erikson's stages of ego development follow the chronological pattern Freud proposed, they incorporate and focus on psychosocial factors to a much larger extent.

1. *Basic trust versus mistrust* occurs in infancy. Initially, the newborn is completely dependent on others to meet its needs. Gradually, the infant acquires limited control by relying on the five senses. General trust is learned when the infant's needs are tended to satisfactorily and consistently. Self-trust is formed when the infant is able to rely on his or her inputs. Conversely, the infant learns to mistrust a withholding, inconsistent world that thwarts self-reliance. Trust is a critical issue with Erikson, and he emphasizes its importance in therapeutic relationships. *The interpersonal strength is hope.*
2. *Autonomy versus shame and doubt* coincides with toddlerhood, which starts before a child reaches two years of age. During this stage, muscular development advances, allowing rudimentary language, ambulation, and bodily control. The child who is encouraged to take more responsibility for self is better able to feel and act independently. Shame and doubt emerge when parents inhibit their child's natural striving for independence by somehow undermining it. *The interpersonal strength is will.*
3. *Initiative versus guilt* takes place in early childhood. The central issue here revolves around the child's attempts to pursue and obtain a goal, to achieve a sense of purpose. This stage corresponds to Freud's Oedipus complex. Mastery requires the child to identify with the parent of the same sex and to adopt parental values to mold the superego. Guilt is experienced if the child's own directives are shunned. *The interpersonal strength is purpose.*
4. *Industry versus inferiority* occurs during latency. At this phase, interactions outside the family structure assume increasing significance. The child is challenged to comply with social values, establish friendships, and acquire new skills, all of which can lead to feelings of competency. Failure at this endeavor, however, leads to feelings of inferiority. *The interpersonal strength is competence.*
5. *Identity versus role confusion* is the crisis associated with adolescence. The struggle here is to find oneself in the midst of turmoil. Mastery involves integrating a sense of personal identity, based on sexual maturity, individuation from the family, meaningful peer relationships, and decisiveness about ambitions in life. *The interpersonal strength is fidelity.*
6. *Intimacy versus isolation* is the first of the three adult stages. It occurs as a person seeks mature love, closeness, and sharing with another. Mastery of this psychosocial stage results in a capacity for being in a sustained, intimate relationship. *The interpersonal strength is love.*
7. *Generativity versus stagnation* occurs during middle age—from 30 to 60 years old. The central issue in this stage is work and productivity. The emphasis here is on generativity; that is, a genuine regard for improving society by one's own efforts. This requires a concern for others. Stagnation is rooted in a lack of this concern, which leaves the individual void of meaningfulness and searching for that elusive quality. *The interpersonal strength is caring.*
8. *Ego integrity versus despair* entails a review of one's accomplishments. A positive evaluation leads to ego integrity, whereas a negative appraisal causes despair. Despair relates to feelings of loss and dissatisfaction with one's inability to uphold his or her values. *The interpersonal strength is wisdom.*

Erikson's stages of ego development are also discussed in Chapters 24 through 26. Erikson's contributions to the understanding of human development are significant. He expanded on previous theories of human development and included the influence of social and cultural factors as relevant antecedents and supports for personal growth. Erikson forced psychological attention on developmental crises in adulthood and the interactions needed to resolve them. Erikson's theory of ego development is a hopeful one in that people always carry within them the potential to rework a previous psychosocial stage in a more personally satisfying way.

RELEVANCE TO NURSING

Nurses use Erikson's model as an important part of patient assessment. Analysis of behavior patterns, using Erikson's framework, can identify age-appropriate or arrested development of normal interpersonal skills. A developmental framework helps the nurse know what types of interventions are most likely to be effective. For example, children in Erikson's initiative versus guilt stage of development respond best if they actively participate and ask many questions. Elderly patients respond to a life review strategy that focuses on the integrity of their life as a composite of experience. In the therapeutic encounter, individual responsibility and the capacity for improving one's functioning are addressed. Treatment approaches and intervention strategies can be tailored to support the patient's developmental level.

Humanistic Theories

Humanistic psychology arose in protest to the psychoanalytic school of thought, which proponents of humanistic psychology believed explicitly excluded human potential and the possibility of choosing life patterns supportive of personal growth. Humanistic frameworks emphasize a person's capacity for self-actualization. They seek to understand behavior from the patient's perspective, as he or she subjectively experiences it.

Abraham Maslow

Abraham Maslow (1908–1970) is considered the father of humanistic psychology. In 1962, he suggested that humanistic psychology represented the third force in psychology, the first two being psychoanalysis and behaviorism (Bugental, 1967). Maslow conceptualized human motivation as a hierarchy of dynamic processes (needs) that are critical for the development and growth of all humans. Central to his theory is the assumption that humans are active rather than passive participants in life, striving for self-actualization. Maslow (1968) focuses on human need fulfillment, which he describes in six incremental stages, beginning with physiological survival needs and ending with self-transcendent needs (Figure 6–1). Although these needs are present in all humans, the behaviors that emanate from them differ according to a person's unique biological makeup and environmental factors. Maslow describes humans' more basic needs as D-motives or deficiency needs, meaning that they are so basic to existence that they must be resolved to reduce the tension associated with them. Because they have the greatest strength, needs at a lower level must always be satisfied before a person turns his attention to higher-level needs. As an example, a homeless person is not going to be interested in joining a support group to get more in touch with his or her feelings and experience the joy of belonging when issues of basic survival remain unresolved. Maslow describes self-esteem and self-actualization as B-motives, or "being needs," reflective of growth motivation.

As basic deficiency needs are met, a person turns attention to personal growth needs to develop his or her human capacity to the fullest extent possible. Maslow's

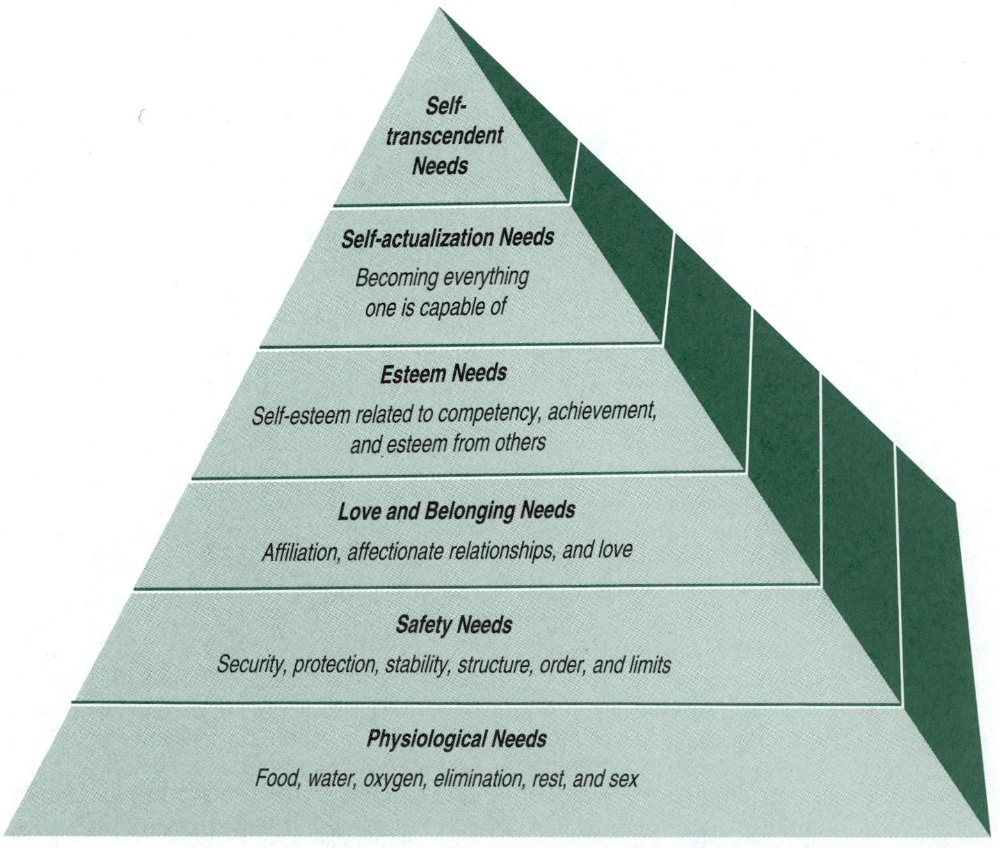

FIGURE 6–1
Maslow's hierarchy of needs. (Adapted from Maslow, A. H. (1972). *The farther reaches of human nature.* New York: Viking.)

TABLE 6–4 Behaviors Associated with a Self-Actualized Person

Characteristic	Behavior
Realistic orientation	Can see the world and the people in it accurately and without value orientations; not given to unrealistic wishful thinking
Spontaneity	Behavior marked by simplicity and naturalness
Acceptance of self and others	Has a positive self-concept and an uncritical acceptance of self and others
Close relationships with others	Values people and is valued by others; relationships are deep and meaningful
Autonomous thinking	Has strong convictions and is able to act on them; does not depend on the approval of others
Appreciation of life	Is glad to be alive and appreciates what life brings; enjoys life at its fullest
Creativity	Is able to solve problems in creative ways
Consideration of and respect for others	Respects and values individual differences

Adapted from Maslow, A. (1956). Self actualizing people: A study of psychological health. In C. Moustakas (Ed.), *The self: Explorations in personal growth*. New York: Harper & Row.

(1968) emphasis on being needs or growth needs is about human potential. He suggests looking at personal strengths rather than at their personality deficits. A person's striving for personal growth leads one to realize one's fullest expression of talents and personality assets, "the human being at his best" (Maslow, 1963). Self-actualized people develop a problem-centered approach to life, identify with mankind, and transcend their environment. They develop a philosophical outlook on life rather than being overwhelmed by every life event. Most important, they can distinguish the means from the end and act in an ethical manner that brings inner peace. According to Maslow, the self is the inner core of personality, holding some characteristics in common with others and possessing other characteristics not held by many others. Using a case study method, Maslow arrived at his description of self-actualized people by studying the behaviors of remarkable people such as Thomas Jefferson, Abraham Lincoln, Eleanor Roosevelt, and Albert Einstein as well as the behaviors of those he, Maslow, came into contact with and admired (Maslow, 1970). Behaviors associated with a self-actualized person are presented in Table 6–4. Maslow's theory of self-actualization has influenced the field of psychiatry in providing a rationale for the development of sensitivity and encounter groups, which help people get in touch with who they are in the moment and their human potential.

RELEVANCE TO NURSING

The value of Maslow's model in nursing practice is twofold. First, the emphasis on human potential and the patient's strengths is key to successful nurse-patient relationships. The second value lies in establishing what is most important in the sequencing of nursing actions in the nurse-patient relationship. For example, attempting to collect any but the most essential information when a patient is struggling with drug withdrawal is inappropriate. Following Maslow's model as a way of prioritizing actions, the nurse would meet the patient's physiological need for stabilizing vital signs and pain relief before collecting general information for a nursing database.

Carl Rogers

Carl Rogers is clearly one of the most prominent humanist psychologists. He was born in 1902 in Oak Park, Illinois, and grew up in a family environment that stressed hard work and religious commitment. After college and a stint in the seminary, he transferred to Columbia University, where he received his Ph.D. in 1931. His theory evolved from observations in his clinical work with psychiatric patients, but his work has been extended to the field of education as well as psychology.

Carl Rogers (1961, p. 200) defined the self as

> *the organized, consistent, conceptual gestalt composed of perceptions characteristic of the "I" or "me" and the perceptions of the relationships of the "I" or "me" to others and the various aspects of life together with the values attached to these perceptions.*

He developed a person-centered model of psychotherapy that emphasizes the uniqueness of the individual. First described in his classic text, *Counseling and Psychotherapy* (1942), Rogers believed that all humans have an innate potential to develop and make full use of their talents and personality characteristics. Rogers (1963) referred to this natural guidance system, unique to each individual, as the *actualizing* tendency. With the actualizing tendency as a natural guide for personal growth, people live their lives in ways that promote personal satisfaction as well as growth and development. When people disregard their actualizing tendency in favor of trying to please others and receive approval, they develop symptoms. They forget what they know to be true about themselves and consequently become confused, unable to evaluate behaviors that can lead to personal growth.

Rogers' person-centered model of psychotherapy is based on the premise that people have within themselves everything they need for self-understanding and for changing their attitudes and behaviors. A person-centered counseling approach is designed to reestablish the person's actualizing tendency as the natural guide for behavior. Certain conditions or attitudes of the therapist offered to the patient, such as unconditional positive regard, empathy, and congruence, are regarded as necessary and sufficient conditions for successful therapy results (Rogers, 1942). These therapist-offered conditions allow patients to experience their unique, true feelings in a safe, supportive interpersonal environment. Rogers speaks of congruence, which means that the therapist acts in an authentic manner, as the first critical condition for successfully helping people. The therapist allows the patient to see the therapist as he or she is in the relationship without needing to hide behind a role. The openness of the therapist is in direct opposition to the psychoanalytic approach, in which the person of the therapist is unavailable to the patient.

The second necessary condition for successful therapeutic outcome is unconditional acceptance and positive regard. Rogers describes unconditional positive regard as a therapist attitude, in which the therapist offers full acceptance of the patient just as he or she is, with no strings attached. By providing a climate of unconditional positive regard, patients are able to experience whatever feeling they have without fear of reprisal or disapproval. Empathetic understanding is the third critical attitude and occurs when the therapist is able to experience the feelings and personal meanings as if they were happening to the therapist and is able to communicate that understanding to the patient. By expressing thoughts out loud and having them understood, the patient is encouraged to trust in his or her own experience. A person who feels understood by others feels freer to self-disclose at a deeper level, and it becomes easier to listen more accurately to oneself.

RELEVANCE TO NURSING

Rogers' humanistic model encourages nurses to look at each patient as a unique human being, a person who feels, knows, and experiences life in a special way. His theory portrays people as being basically good with an inherent potential for self-actualization. Rogers' necessary conditions for a successful therapeutic outcome provide a valuable structure for understanding personal attitudes the nurse needs to have to facilitate change in the patient. Rogers' (1963) insistence that "man does not simply have the characteristics of a machine, he is not simply a being in the grip of unconscious motives, he is a person in the process of creating himself, a person who creates meaning in life" (p. 82) has a powerful influence on the conduct of the nurse-patient relationship. The attitudes of unconditional positive regard, empathetic understanding, and genuineness achieved through self-awareness are foundational concepts in effective nurse-patient relationships. A person-centered nursing approach recognizes the uniqueness of the individual and tries to engage the patient as an equal collaborator in the journey toward mental health.

Existential Theories

Yalom (1980) speaks of existential models of human behavioral therapy as an orphan looking for a home, as there is no single model associated with existentialism. Instead, existential theories attempt to define what it means to be fully human and to find meaning in existence. Focused on personal freedom, authenticity, anxiety, meaning, and death, existential models were heavily influenced by secular and religious philosophers such as Heidegger (1962), Kierkegaard (1957), and Tillich (1952). Martin Buber's (1970) description of an I-Thou relationship designed to enhance awareness and acceptance of the uniqueness of each human being is a natural outgrowth of these earlier writings. Buber believed that "relation is reciprocity" (p. 58). Whether or not the other person fully appreciates the deed is not as important as the person's extending the soul's creative power to another with his or her whole being. In that extension of self lies the possibility of a human connection capable of transforming the meaning of the experience between two people. Theoretical concepts related to the I-Thou relationship are found in Chapter 11.

Existential models essentially view mental illness as occurring when a person loses contact with his or her essential humanness and is unable to establish human relationships with others based on honesty. Basically, the person is living a lie, and the meaning of life centers around the anxiety needed to maintain an inauthentic way of being. These people suffer from feelings of intense isolation from others and a chronic sense of emptiness. They have lost faith in themselves and have difficulty learning from and accepting the natural limits of life circumstances.

Taking personal responsibility is key to existential therapy approaches. The existential therapist would argue against using a specific set of therapeutic strategies, preferring instead to develop a meaningful relationship in which both participants are fully present in the immediacy of the moment. Existential therapists encourage their patients to shed the lies that hide the reality of their existence and to develop human relationships that reflect and support their personal integrity.

Existential models view anxiety as an important wake-up call motivating people to take charge of their lives and to make needed changes. People are free to make decisions that enable them to find real meaning in their lives and to discard maladaptive or unsatisfying life patterns. They are the architects of their own destiny, free to choose the person they wish to become. If a person chooses to abdicate the responsibility for authentic living, the result is anxiety, depression, and guilt. Existentially based concepts are found in the theoretically based psychotherapies of Ludwig Binswanger, Rollo May, Viktor Frankl, William Glasser, and Irving Yalom. Two representative frameworks are presented here.

Viktor Frankl

Viktor Frankl was born in 1905, a Jewish man who spent three years in a concentration camp, losing his wife, mother, father, and brother during this tragic time. He observed that some people in the concentration camp were able to sustain their personal integrity and to emerge strengthened despite of losing all that they held dear and suffering intense emotional pain. Their sense of self-respect and personal integrity remained untouched. From this experience, Frankl developed *logotherapy* (logo, taken from the Greek word for meaning), a form of support designed to help people who have lost their reason for living to reclaim their sense of self-respect. Logotherapy is a future-oriented therapy, focused on one's need to find meaning and value in living as the most important life task. "Everyone has his own specific vocation or mission in life; everyone must carry out a concrete assignment that demands fulfillment. . . . Each man is questioned by life; and he can only respond by answering for his own life; to life he can only respond by being responsible" (Frankl, 1969, pp. 170–171).

Strategies proposed by Frankl include dereflection and paradoxical intention. *Dereflection* involves helping patients to refocus their attention away from anxiety-producing stimuli. For example, the therapist might encourage a man fearful of impotency to concentrate on his partner's pleasure rather than his performance. *Paradoxical intention* involves instructing a patient to exaggerate the behavior that is causing distress. For example, Frankl describes a case in which a bookkeeper experienced such anxiety when he tried to write legibly in his ledger that he was in danger of losing his job. Frankl encouraged him to deliberately write with an illegible scrawl. Ironically, he found he was unable to do this when it became a conscious act, and the symptoms that caused him so much distress vanished quickly. This technique has been used successfully with obsessive-compulsive behaviors found in individuals and families.

William Glasser

William Glasser, a psychiatrist, developed his model of reality therapy as an outgrowth of his work with patients in a variety of clinical settings. He proposes that "unhappiness is the result and not the cause of irresponsibility" (Glasser, 1976). Reality therapy is a highly pragmatic model that focuses on the here and now as the only reality to be considered. Glasser proposes that there is no way a person's past can be rewritten, so it is fruitless to consider it. Blaming personal failures on external circumstances, lack of opportunity, poor family relationships, or virtually any other circumstances is not acceptable. Instead the reality therapist encourages the patient to rewrite his or her life script and to consider definite plans based on the personal responsibility and self-discipline needed for a different outcome. The therapist becomes the therapeutic ally, but it is ultimately up to the patient to develop a functional understanding of reality. Strategies focus on what the patient does and not on what the patient feels. The approach is a positive one in which the therapist conveys the belief that the patient can influence his or her feelings and has the capability to develop a more successful pattern of living. Persistent refocusing on progress, taking the next step, and considering practical issues needed for successful resolution of difficult life problems help patients develop the positive attitudes needed for successful living.

▶ Check Your Reading

7. Why might Erikson's theory remain so relevant today?
8. How does humanistic theory enhance the personal journey of the patient?
9. In what ways do humanistic and existential models parallel and diverge from each other?

Behavioral Theories

Behavioral approaches to therapy initially were developed as a protest response to Freud's assumption that a person's destiny was carved in stone at an early age. By contrast, a behaviorist considers personality as what people do and not who they are. Behavioral models postulate that personality consists of learned behaviors. Consequently, personality is synonymous with behavior. If you change the behavior, you change the personality.

Behavioral models originated from lessons learned in experimental animal laboratories during the 19th century, first with Pavlov's dog experiments and later in the 20th century with Skinner's research on rat behavior. These behavioral theorists developed their observations of animal behavior into systematic applications of learning principles that could be applied to humans. Used in education as well as in psychiatric settings to manage problem behaviors, behavior modification, programmed learning, biofeedback, and token economies are commonly used techniques based on behavioral models. Behavioral models emphasize the ways in which observable behavioral responses are learned and can be modified in a particular environment. Three of the most influential behavioral theorists were Ivan Pavlov, James Watson, and B. F. Skinner. Their models focus on a belief that it is possible to influence behavior through a process referred to as conditioning. **Conditioning** involves pairing a behavior with a condition that reinforces or diminishes the behavior's occurrence.

Ivan Pavlov

Ivan Pavlov (1849–1936) was a Russian physiologist. He won the Nobel Prize for his outstanding contributions to the physiology of digestion, which he studied through his well-known dog experiments. From incidental observations of the dogs, he noticed that they were able to anticipate when food would be forthcoming, and they would begin to salivate even before actually experiencing the meal. Pavlov labeled this process *psychic secretions.* He hypothesized that the psychic component was a learned association between two events: the presence of experimental apparatus and the serving of meat.

Pavlov (1928) formalized his observations of behaviors in dogs in a theory of classical conditioning. He observed that the dog salivated naturally whenever it was presented with food but did not have a similar reaction to the sound of a tuning fork, an unconditioned stimulus (UCS). By repeatedly sounding the tuning fork when the dog was presented with food, the dog began to associate salivation with both the food and the tuning fork. Pavlov was able to "condition" the dog's response so that the dog continued to salivate when the tuning fork was rung without food being present.

In *classical conditioning*, a neutral stimulus (such as the bell tone) is repeatedly paired with a stimulus that innately elicits a response (such as food triggering salivation). Through this process, the neutral stimulus is transformed into a conditioned stimulus. The eliciting stimulus (in this case, the meat) is called the unconditioned stimulus. Repetitive pairing of the two causes the establishment of a predictable pattern, and subsequently learning occurs. Classical conditioning sometimes is referred to as *respondent conditioning* because the subject is basically a passive agent. Respondents are responses that result from specific, identifiable stimuli. They may be learned responses (as in the case of an animal wincing when a tone is heard that has been repeatedly paired with a shock) or unlearned (such as when a physical reflex is provoked and produced).

Pavlov introduced the term *reinforcement* in describing his dog's selective response to a given stimulus. Although he considered his scientific observations to represent physiological responses, rather than psychological, his ideas formed the foundation for the development of behavioral therapies and are widely used in educational settings.

James B. Watson

Watson (1919, 1928) was an American psychologist who developed the school of thought referred to as behaviorism. He was strongly influenced by Pavlov's conditioning principles and began to apply these principles to human beings. Watson placed a strong emphasis on the role of the social environment in shaping behavior. He is best known for his experiments with little Albert. The experiment consisted of standing behind the child, who liked animals, and making a loud noise with a hammer every time the child reached for the animal (a large white rat). After a number of repetitions, little Albert became afraid of the white rat and later of all furry animals and objects, without the presence of the loud noise.

B. F. Skinner

B. F. Skinner was part of a second wave of behavioral theorists who expanded the notion of stimulus-response behavioral approaches to learning to include the concept of reinforcement (Skinner, 1987; Hall and Lindzey, 1970; Smith and Vetter, 1982; Fancher, 1990). He was born in 1904 and earned his college degree as an English major, but he did not find satisfaction with literature. Although the literature described the way people functioned, it could not explain why they did so. Through his reading, however, Skinner happened on the writings of prominent behaviorists. Here he began to find potential answers to the questions that haunted him about the psychology of behavior. Skinner attended Harvard Graduate School in psychology and was recognized there as an outstanding student. At Harvard, Skinner concentrated his studies on behavioral change—specifically, *behavioral learning* and *modification.* In addition to his studies of rat behavior at the University, Skinner raised his second daughter for the first two and a half years in an air conditioned box, which he called a baby tender. The baby tender was marketed commercially, but needless to say it never caught on with the public.

Skinner is generally recognized as one of the prime movers behind the behavioral movement in mental health. Like Freud, he believed that all behavior is determined. But he differed with Freud about its origin. Skinner proposed that human behavior is supported by reinforcement contingencies and that it is possible to predict and control the behavior of others through an understanding the nature of humans' reinforcers. In taking this stand, he also distanced himself from Pavlovian thinking, which viewed behavioral change as a simple stimulus-response connection. Skinner added a second principle of learning that includes motivation and social reinforcement (Woodward, 1982) (Figure 6–2).

Skinner based his theory on his research with rats, in which he was able to elicit responses. Using the famous Skinner box, he demonstrated that if he reinforced a rat with food for pressing a level when a light would go on and did not reinforce the rat when the light was off, the rat "learned" to press the lever so that it would get the food. He labeled the light as a *discriminative stimulus*, meaning that it was the paired association of the reinforcer with behavior and not the stimulus itself that caused the rat to press the lever. The discriminative stimulus acts as a cue for the desired behavior. Examples in everyday life include the bell that signals students to leave class, traffic lights, and business bonuses. Behavior modification, a form of treatment used extensively with patients suffering from a wide range of disorders, such as retardation, sexual dysfunctions, enuresis, violence, and

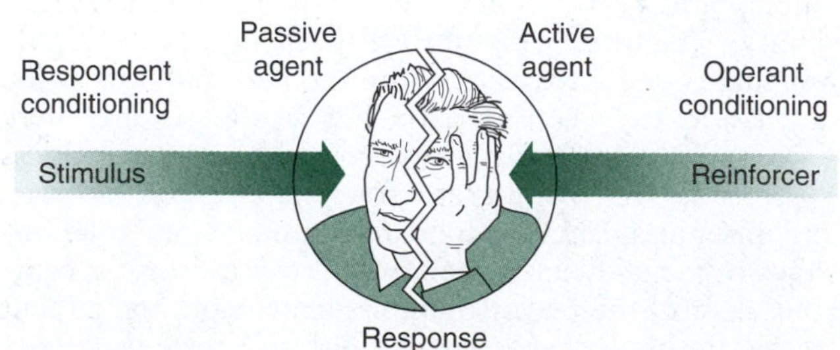

FIGURE 6–2
Respondent conditioning versus operant conditioning.

autism; chronically ill patients; and adolescents with behavior problems, emphasizes Skinner's basic premise that all behavioral responses, being learned, can also be unlearned.

Skinner labeled the most important segment of his theory **operant conditioning.** Operant conditioning refers to the manipulation of selected reinforcers to elicit and strengthen desired behavioral reinforcers. Reinforcers refer to the consequences of the behavior. Skinner believed that a person performs a behavior (discharges an operant) and receives a consequence (reinforcer) as a result of performing the behavior. The consequence makes it more or less probable that the person will repeat the behavior. If the consequence is positive, the chances of repetition increase. Negative consequences have a deterrent effect on behavior. For example, the use of Antabuse discourages people from drinking because it causes physical effects if the person tries to drink while on the medication. Absence of reinforcement also decreases behavior. Thus, if a person typically gets attention by making a joke and no one laughs at it, this particular behavior tends to decrease because it is not being reinforced. At the heart of Skinner's theory is the proposition that reinforcement ultimately determines the existence of behavior.

Skinner defines **reinforcers** as anything that increases the occurrence of a behavior. *The value of a reinforcer lies in its meaning to a particular individual.* A reinforcer for one person may not have any effect as a reinforcer on another. According to Skinner, there are two types of reinforcers: (1) primary reinforcers, which are of survival importance, such as food, water, and sex, and (2) secondary (conditioned) reinforcers, such as money, material goods, and praise.

Change is measured by counting the rate of occurrence related to a specific behavior. The clinician uses cumulative written records to assess an individual's rate of response. Beginning with a thorough analysis of target behaviors, the goal of behavioral therapy is to change the respondent's behavior by providing positive reinforcement (token, gift, or praise) if a behavior is accomplished or negative reinforcement (withdrawing sanctions or verbal disapproval) if the behavior ceases to exist. Complex behaviors usually need to be broken down into smaller steps. This allows for *shaping* behavior, which consists of progressively reinforcing the smaller steps needed to achieve a certain behavior.

RELEVANCE TO NURSING

Skinner's behavioral model provides a concrete method for modifying behaviors or replacing them. Behavior management and modification programs based on his principles have proved to be successful in altering targeted behaviors. Programmed learning and token economies represent extensions of Skinner's thoughts on learning. The efficacy of behavioral models is easier to test empirically because the data are straightforward. Behavioral methods are particularly effective with adolescent acting-out behaviors and many forms of chronic mental illness.

Albert Bandura

Albert Bandura attempted to rectify the oversimplification of a two-factored behavioral theory by developing a model based on social learning through imitation (1962, 1977). **Social learning theory** conceptualizes psychological functioning as an integration of both environmental conditions and personal attributes. This integration is ongoing and reciprocal. In 1977, Bandura wrote a book, *Social Learning Theory*, in which he postulated that people do alter their behavior in response to situational changes. He also proposed that people learn best by observation, by watching others perform, and by the subsequent modeling of behavior. Bandura based his conclusions on research findings that not all behavioral responses could be accounted for by connective cues between stimulus-response, or response reinforcement. Instead, he observed that behavioral change occurred in many instances as a result of external social discriminative cues that influenced behavior. For example, in many societies, aggressive behaviors are not modeled, or socially reinforced, for little girls as they are for little boys as being particularly desirable ways of acting.

Bandura believed that human behavior is best explained by considering it as a reciprocal interaction continuously occurring between the organism and behavioral, cognitive, and environmental influences. He proposed that people observe which behaviors are rewarded or punished and "vicariously" embrace the implications of the modeling stimuli they witness. In addition to external reinforcement, people engage in **self-reinforcement,** whereby an individual reinforces himself in the absence of an actual reinforcer. Bandura believes that symbolic, vicarious, and self-regulatory processes are instrumental in determining the precise behavioral action one assumes. For example, a student notices that another has completed his or her homework assignment. This knowledge stimulates the first student to complete his or her own work.

This vicarious learning is much more efficient because instead of repeatedly trying new behaviors and judging the effect of such actions, humans possess the ability to witness another's actions and outcomes. Through this experience, the person learns modes of behavior that can help him or her avoid potentially dangerous responses and speed up the acquisition of new or advantageous behaviors.

MODELING

Bandura considered modeling an important principle of learning. Modeling affects learning because of the information it provides the individual. Cognitive functions are the critical components in this process. The actual learning and the activation of the system occurs in a four-step process:

- Attentional processes
- Retention

- Motor reproduction
- Motivation

The quality of one's attentiveness to and accurate perception of an observed behavior has obvious implications for its success as a learning experience. The *attentional processes* circumscribe what is focused on in the observation. Certain factors affect the attentional process. These include personal attributes of the model, such as how charismatic and capable she is. The behavior itself influences attentiveness. The degree of relevancy it bears to the observing individual's life circumstance and the complexity of the behavior are two factors that play a part in the process.

The second process in the sequence is retention. *Retention* refers to the ability to recollect the information. Symbolic representation through imagery or language allows the experience to be coded in memory, thereby creating a method for the observer to continue benefiting from past observational experiences.

Motor reproduction is identified as the third phase. It is not necessarily achieved, however, immediately following retention. In fact, for most complex skills, practice is usually required before reactment can be perfected. Self-corrective measures can be used to make improvements, but sometimes confounding variables (such as physical limitations or incomplete data collection of the observation itself) permanently preclude the development of the desired behavior.

The last process is *motivation*. Social learning theory recognizes the fact that not all learned behavior is executed. Performance of the behavior at some future date is linked to the reinforcement it will produce. People favor development of behaviors that have no negative consequence.

SELF-EFFICACY THEORY

In addition to his contributions related to observational learning and modeling, Bandura (1977, 1978) proposed a theory of self-efficacy that also has relevance for psychiatric nursing. **Self-efficacy** refers to a person's belief or expectation that he or she has the capacity to effect a desired outcome through his or her own personal efforts. Bandura (1977) suggests that all psychotherapeutic strategies should have the common goal of "creating and strengthening expectations of personal efficacy" (p. 193). He submits that perceptions of self-efficacy affect motivation in rather profound ways and that people tend to avoid those situations that challenge their perceptions of self-efficacy. The stronger the belief that a person will be able to master a difficult situation, the more active the person's personal efforts are likely to be, and the more persistent he or she will be in achieving the goal.

RELEVANCE TO NURSING

Social learning theory has blended cognitive functioning with environmental factors, in an attempt to balance inner and outer resources and to offer a more comprehensive conception of human behavior. Nursing practice incorporates techniques from operant and classical conditioning to assist individuals in changing their own behavior or to use these principles for more effective parenting. Also the patient's education in relation to cognitive processes highlighted in this theory can be explained to enhance client understanding about skill development and motivation.

► Check Your Reading

10. What are some of the differences between behavioral and social learning models?
11. How would you differentiate between a respondent conditioning and an operant conditioning strategy?
12. What do you see as the value of behavioral models for psychiatric nursing?

Biological Theories

The advent of psychopharmacology presented a major challenge to the previous psychodynamic approaches to mental illness. Within the last four decades, clinicians have increasingly noted that psychoactive chemicals could significantly alter the symptoms of major thought disorders, depression, and anxiety disorder. Medications having differential effects on different neurotransmitters helped restore brain function, allowing patients with mental illness to continue their journey productively, with greater satisfaction and with far less emotional pain. The observations of clinicians working with mentally ill patients led to significant scientific research regarding the ways in which brain chemistry and physiology might explain these effects. The biopsychiatric treatment of mental illness refuted the idea of mental illness as being determined by social conflicts with significant others. Instead, the theoretical stance in a biochemical model of mental illness is that people have a natural predisposition that places them at particular risk for mental illness. Inborn chemical features of reactivity make an individual susceptible to particular disorders, given the appropriate level of stress.

A biological model of mental illness focuses on neurological, chemical, biological, and genetic issues. A biological perspective seeks to understand how the body and brain interact to create emotions, memories, and perceptual experiences. They argue that hereditary factors and biochemical influences in the brain govern how messages are transmitted within the body as well as how moods and motivation get activated. Biological models explain how these factors interact and contribute to human functioning. There have been tremendous breakthroughs in understanding and identifying the significant role that neurotransmitters and chemical imbalances play in mental health. Owing to the wealth of knowledge in this area and its importance in understanding the biological factors in mental illness, Chapter 7 is devoted to this topic.

The danger in accepting a purely biological theory of mental illness is that, when carried to an extreme, it suggests social control of behavior through modification of the brain's biochemistry and refutes the idea of personal responsibility for behavior. A biological model defines mental illness as an individual disorder. Such a theory ignores the measureless influences of social, environmental, cultural, economic, and educational factors that play a role in the development and treatment of mental illness.

Blending the Nonnursing Theories

Ideally, different theoretical perspectives complement one another and enrich the therapeutic journey. They address the complex nature of biopsychosocial and spiritual meaning and value in a person's life. No one theory adequately reveals the complexity of human behavior. A multidimensional view of each human being can provide the kinds of information needed, the method of assessment most applicable to an individual patient's problem, and the types of intervention most likely to achieve desired therapeutic outcomes. For example, medication may significantly reduce troublesome symptoms and allow a relationship to develop. The relationship may provide a patient with the capacity for insight, the most direct route to a more productive and satisfying life. Other patients with similar symptoms but lacking insight or simply wanting symptom relief might benefit from a behavioral approach.

Each psychological theory perspective emphasizes a particular psychological lens for making sense of human beings and their behavior. Consider depression as an example. A psychoanalytic perspective would explore depressive symptoms as being related to repression of earlier hostility and aggressive drives. Taken from a behavioral perspective, a clinician would focus on understanding the antecedent conditions for the development of symptoms and would prescribe behavioral strategies to eliminate the symptom. A social learning theorist might consider the depressive symptoms as representing *learned helplessness*. Interventions would teach the patient constructive ways to manage life differently. The clinician with a biological perspective would understand a person's depressive symptoms as a misfiring of neurotransmitters. This clinician would orchestrate a medical approach to symptom management by prescribing antidepressants or electroconvulsive therapy to correct the chemical imbalance. By contrast, a humanistic perspective would emphasize a person's individual strengths and human potential. Understanding a person's subjective experience of the depressive symptoms and their relationship to events in the present would be a primary focus of intervention. Psychodynamic approaches to the treatment of depression would focus on the relationship between nurse and patient, whereas an existential approach would emphasize personal responsibility for discovering the meaning of the person's current circumstances in light of the larger journey.

The decision to use a particular theoretical approach should reflect the individualized situation of the patient and the comfort of the clinician in applying a theoretical perspective. Woodward (1982) suggests that "theoretical differences and priority debates are a conspicuous characteristic of normal scientific practices rather than a deviation from them" (p. 408). Taken in this spirit, students are encouraged to select those concepts and ideas that enrich their discussion and application of theoretical and historical perspectives to the study and practice of psychiatric nursing.

NURSING THEORIES

Value of Theoretical Frameworks in Nursing

Although theory from other disciplines adopted and modified by nursing is critical to the understanding of psychiatric-mental health nursing, this knowledge is incomplete without specific attention paid to nursing theory. Donaldson and Crowley (1978) define a *discipline* as "a unique perspective, a distinct way of viewing all the phenomena, which ultimately defines the limits and nature of its inquiry" (p. 113). The discipline of nursing has a unique body of knowledge, specifically ordered to inform its members of the content and process needed for effective nursing. Governing this unique body of knowledge are theories of nursing representing a number of world views about the discipline of nursing and its particular domain of knowledge. General theories of nursing lay out the domain of the profession, establish the boundaries of nursing practice, provide a basis for research, and serve as a guide for curriculum development (Arnold and Boggs, 1995).

Psychiatric-mental health nursing is recognized as a subspecialty within the larger discipline of professional nursing. McCracken (1994) notes that "programs grounded in theory are more likely to be clinically consistent and organized" (p. 44). The theoretical foundations of professional and psychiatric nursing practice provide the nurse with confidence in his or her ideas and direct actions taken in therapeutic relationships. By blending theory with the nurse's own personal style (i.e., therapeutic use of self), nurses can implement the nursing process in creative ways that truly reflect both the art and the science of psychiatric nursing.

Meleis (1991) claims that, "the primary use of theory is to guide research" (p. 21). Certainly, this is a valid use of theory and particularly important in understanding a science of such complexity and inferred knowledge. Theories are as much designed to raise essential questions about phenomena as to answer them. Research opens up new opportunities for understandings never before considered. Through research and empirical testing of theoretical concepts, scholars verify theoretical knowledge, enrich current understandings with new findings, and refute past wisdom. Critical thinking about theoretical perspectives as well as reflective dialogue and debate among scholars about the validity of a theory cannot help but stimulate creativity, self-awareness, and development of cognitive competence.

Theory development in nursing has provided opportunities for nurses to describe, empirically test, and evaluate the nature of professional nursing practice. In an interview with Jacqueline Fawcett, Virginia Henderson notes that a profession is known by its literature. Theory development in nursing has provided opportunities for nurses to test empirically and describe the nature of nursing practice and its impact on patient outcomes in the professional literature. Moreover, graduate students in universities throughout the United States and abroad have provided ideas, struggled to understand the language and meaning of concepts, critiqued ideas, and developed important research studies to support the validity of nursing theory. Thus, nursing theories have a special integrity springing from the commitment and continuous refinement of major propositions and ideas by nursing's primary and contributing authors. Although difficult to prove pragmatically, there is little question that nursing theory has played an important role in helping nurses define their identity as members of a professional discipline.

What Is Nursing Theory?

Nursing theory represents the unique systematic study of nursing experience. Each theoretical perspective evolves from a broader structural base of nursing knowledge, beginning with a **metaparadigm,** or world view, of what constitutes the phenomena of concern in professional nursing. Nursing's metaparadigm consists of four elements: person, environment, health, and nursing. Nursing is included as a separate dimension so that the activities of professional nursing are identifiable as being quite distinct from those of other disciplines. These four elements of concern to nursing are found in each theorist's presentation, although the way in which they are described differ according to the theorist's orientation.

Nursing knowledge proceeds from the general to the more specific in a structural hierarchy which begins with a metaparadigm, develops into conceptual models, and completes its structural mission with the construction of theories that can be tested empirically. *Conceptual models* represent abstract word images of each theorist's thinking about the nature of person, environment, health, and nursing. Corresponding to the concepts (main ideas) in the model are assumptions, defined as the values, ideas, and principles of the theorist. Conceptual models cannot be tested empirically because they do not spell out the relationships between the different concepts. Conceptual models often contain single belief statements, referred to as postulates, which expand the meaning of a concept. Conceptual models in nursing sometimes are categorized as developmental, systems, interactionist, and more recently as caring as a way of describing their primary focus.

Nursing theories represent the most tangible and specific description of nursing knowledge. They can be tested empirically because they specifically define the relationships among concepts, assumptions, and postulates found in a particular nursing model. Key concepts of selected nursing theories are presented in Table 6–5. For a more complete explanation of the conceptual theory models in nursing practice, see the original works of the theorists and nursing theory texts identified in the references at the end of the chapter.

Early Nursing Theorists

"The journey from the days of Florence Nightingale to modern nursing has been long, hard, and bumpy" (Meleis, 1991, p. 49). It is only within the last 40 years that a body of knowledge distinctly labeled as *nursing*, linked to but separate from what nurses do, has been established and confirmed through research. Even more recently, nurses have declared professional nursing to be a distinct, autonomous health discipline and have insisted that their work be valued as skilled nursing care.

Theory development in nursing began with Florence Nightingale's observations in her classic work, *Notes on Nursing*, written in 1859 and published a year later. Modern nursing theory development in which a body of knowledge labeled distinctly as professional nursing did not emerge as a serious endeavor until the 1950s. Early theorists believed that until nurses could define the boundaries and activities of professional nursing, the profession would continue to be defined by others. Consequently, academic nursing leaders, such as Virginia Henderson, Dorothea Johnson, Hildegard Peplau, and Dorothy Orem, developed theoretical models designed to direct nursing practice and to establish the domain of a body of knowledge referred to as professional nursing. They provided a simple but clear linkage between abstract concepts and what nurses actually do. Since that time, other nursing theorists, such as Myra Levine, Martha Rogers, Imogene King, Sister Callista Roy, Madeline Leininger, Jean Watson, Betty Neuman, and Rosemarie Rizzo Parse (Meleis, 1991), have joined the ranks of serious nursing scholars in developing theories about the body of knowledge that is uniquely nursing.

Evolution of Theory Models in Psychiatric Nursing

The theoretical journey to psychiatric nursing as a subspecialty emerged as a reality in the 1950s first with Peplau's interpersonal relationship theory in 1952. The 1960s saw the proliferation of nursing theories and the development of several models with special applicability to psychiatric nursing (Paterson and Zderad, Orlando, Roy, Travelbee, and Wiedenbach). What these theoretical models had in common was a special focus on the nurse-patient relationship. They emphasized the relationship as a human experience with meanings that could be understood and validated. Within the relationship, the person of the nurse engages with a patient as a holistic being, "not as an additive summation, but rather as a gestalt" (Paterson and Zderad, 1988, p. 25). The nurse

TABLE 6–5 **Key Concepts of Selected Nursing Theories**

Theorist	View of the Person: Goal	View of the Person: Composition	View of Health	View of the Environment	View of Nursing: Nature	View of Nursing: Purpose
Peplau	Equilibrium	System with physiological, psychological, and social components	Forward movement of the personality	Significant others	Therapeutic interpersonal process	Helping people to meet needs and develop
Johnson	Balance	Behavioral system with seven subsystems	Equilibrium	External inputs	External force toward balance	Restoration, attainment, or maintenance of system stability
Orem	Constancy	Whole with physical, psychological, interpersonal, social aspects	Meeting self-care needs	External forces	Systems that address self-care requisites	Help people to meet self-care needs
Roy	Equilibrium	System with biopsychosocial components	Adaptation	External conditions	Manipulation of stimuli to foster coping	Promotion of adaptation
Rogers	Increased complexity of pattern	Indivisible energy field	Increasing innovativeness of patterning	Contiguous, continuously interacting energy field	Promotion of repatterning	Facilitating health potential
Zderad and Patterson	Self-awareness	Holistic being with meaning and choice	Choice and responsibility wholeness	Peak life events	Genuine encounter	Affirmation of validation of human experience
Neuman	System stability	Holistic being with physioiological, psychological, sociocultural, spiritual variables	Equilibrium	Internal and external stressors	Stress-reducing activities	Promotion of equilibrium
Watson	Sense of inner harmony	Integrated and inseparable spritual, mental, and physical spheres	Unity and harmony	Energy field external to the person	Transpersonal caring	Promoting harmony
Leininger	Individual/social well-being	Composite of individual, cultural, and social components	Improving human condition	Contextual factors (patient's culture)	Transcultural caring	Improving healthy conditions or lifeways
Parse	Process of becoming	Open being	Process of becoming	Energy field in continuous interaction with the person	Interpersonal processes	Improving quality of life

Adapted from Leddy, S., and Pepper, J. M. (1993). *Conceptual bases of professional nursing* (3rd ed.) (pp. 174–175). Philadelphia: J B Lippincott.

uses self as a primary therapeutic agent who walks with the patient, listens empathetically to the patient's report of his or her experience, and actively enters the patient's world as a fellow human traveler (Travelbee, 1961). Meleis (1991) notes: "Properties of interaction as validation (Wiedenbach), meeting (Orlando), being totally present and relating (Paterson and Zderad) are delineated and defined by this group of theorists."

"Caring" Models

Current models of relevance to psychiatric nursing have developed around a caring mode of involved interaction with patients (Marriner-Tomey, 1994). According to these theorists (Watson, Leininger, Neuman), the essence of nursing is caring. Benner and Wrubel (1989) characterize caring as the foundation of excellence in nursing practice. There is little argument that caring is critical to understanding psychiatric-mental health nursing.

In a caring relationship, Montgomery and Webster (1994) state that there is a deep subjective involvement with the patient that contains "existential or spiritual significance." Nurses, using a caring model, "value feelings, intuition, and other forms of subjective participation in the client's world" (p. 293), in addition to more scientific understandings of a mentally ill patient. The nurse assumes the role of *participant observer*, as originally spoken of by Sullivan in a psychological framework, and Peplau (1952) from the nursing perspective. Therapeutic distance is maintained from the symptoms of the patient rather than from the patient as a human being (Montgomery, 1993). Nursing interventions are designed to acknowledge the shared humanity of nurse and patient while supporting the natural healing resources within the patient in developing creative solutions to difficult problems of living.

"Relationship" Models

Although principles of communication and relationship lend themselves to implementation of all nursing frameworks, those that specifically focus on interpersonal relationships include Peplau, Travelbee, Orlando, Wiedenbach, Riehl-Sisca, Erickson and colleagues, Barnard, and Mercer (Marriner-Tomey, 1994). The nursing theory framework chosen for the study of the nurse-patient relationship in this book is that of Hildegard Peplau.

Hildegard Peplau

Hildegard Peplau was the first nurse to identify psychiatric nursing both as an essential element of general nursing and as a specialty area that embraces specific governing principles (Peplau, 1952). She was the first nurse theorist to describe the nurse-patient relationship as the foundation of nursing practice (Forchuk, 1991). In shifting the focus from what nurses do "to" patients to what nurses do "with" patients, Peplau (1989) engineered a major paradigm shift from a model focused on medical treatments to an interpersonal relational model of nursing practice. She identified ways in which the nurse makes specialized use of a professional relationship to identify and intervene therapeutically in psychosocial nursing problems.

Peplau (1987) viewed nursing as a developmental educative instrument designed to help individuals and communities use their capacities in living more productively. Her theory is mainly concerned with the processes by which the nurse helps patients make positive changes in their health care status and well-being. Observation, interpretation, and intervention form the essence of a nurse-patient relationship. Raw data must be interpreted and transformed into a meaningful explanation, acceptable in meaning to the nurse and patient.

A transformation process occurs as the nurse observes and listens to the patient and develops impressions and general ideas about the meaning of the patient's situation. These inferences are validated with the patient for accuracy. Illness is viewed as a unique opportunity for experiential learning, personal growth, and improved coping strategies for living (Peplau, 1982a, b).

The dynamic nursing approach proposed by Peplau is not that of a passive spectator observer. Peplau advocates being participant observers in therapeutic conversations. She insists that nurses must observe not only the behavior of the patient, but also their own. Data are collected by interacting directly with the client. Nurses have a keen awareness not only of their own role and what is appropriate, but also of the roles the patient may be projecting on them: friend, parent, protagonist, or sex object. Because none of these roles are useful in providing nursing care to patients, Peplau asserts that the social and personal needs of the nurse should not be a part of the nurse-patient conversation.

In Peplau's classic text, *Interpersonal Theory of Nursing*, developed around the concept of the nurse-patient relationship, the nurse-patient relationship is laid out as a dynamic learning experience in which personal-social growth can occur. Peplau (1952) outlines four developmental phases of the nurse-patient relationship: orientation, working (comprising identification and exploitation), and resolution. Chapter 11 details the developmental phases proposed in her theory.

When Peplau first presented her theory of *interpersonal nursing* in 1952, the model quickly became the accepted foundation of psychiatric nursing practice. A nurse herself, Peplau was determined to professionalize the practice of nursing. Her theory had its foundations in the analytic drive-reduction model described earlier. Peplau placed considerable emphasis, however, on the importance of the interpersonal relationship, which she identified as the communication process that occurs between patient and nurse. She believed that by analyzing the interpersonal interactions occurring within the nurse-patient relationship, the nurse could enhance a patient's personal growth. Every interaction with a patient presented another opportunity for the patient to experience a positive relationship and to gain personal insights.

There are four crucial elements inherent in Peplau's model:

- Mutuality
- Phasic relatedness
- Anxiety gradient
- Uniqueness

Mutuality is the reciprocal process that occurs between nurse and patient. Through meaningful, shared verbal encounters, the nurse and patient work together to achieve identified health goals. The nurse's clinical skill, creative capacity, and style have a powerful effect on the quality of the therapeutic experience and considerable influence on what the patient will learn. Likewise, because the nurse is a person involved in this reciprocal process, he or she also grows with each interaction.

Phasic relatedness refers to the contrived, purposeful, therapeutic relationship that the professional nurse has with a patient. There are sequential steps to phasic relatedness that range from initiation to termination. Specifically, these steps are known as orientation, identification, exploitation, and resolution. The nurse must have self-awareness to participate effectively in this process. The role involves using the actual relationship and its unique dynamics to help the patient in seeking interpersonal experiences that offer alternative outcomes. For example, the nurse can provide feedback and help patients improve their effectiveness in communication and coping. Thus, each interaction has the potential to be educative.

The anxiety gradient is a critical aspect in Peplau's theory. Anxiety is present in all relationships and manifests itself in the nurse-patient relationship as well. Peplau proposed that anxiety-producing events actually awaken past unmet needs. Peplau envisioned the nurse's role as aiding the patient in the management or alleviation of anxiety. This requires that the professional first address the current anxiety and assist the patient in coping with it effectively (based on deliberate problem-solving techniques), as opposed to automatic responsive behavior rooted in defense mechanisms.

Peplau outlined simple steps to accomplish this goal, the first of which is to support the patient in identifying and labeling his or her anxiety accurately. The sufferer may be unaware that he or she is experiencing anxiety. Anxiety, however, is observable. Thus, by assessing the patient for evidence of anxiety and asking if he or she feels uncomfortable, nervous, or anxious, the nurse fosters self-recognition, and can validate that feeling. Next, the patient is encouraged to identify strategies to relieve the experience of anxiety. This is achieved by questioning the patient about how he or she soothes the self to reduce the tension. Often, such inquiries necessitate repetitive questioning by the nurse until an adequate response is presented. This process empowers the patient by connecting successful stress-reducing techniques with anxiety. On completion of step two, the patient is ready to consider the facts and circumstances that provoke him or her. In other words, the patient attempts to determine the precipitating causes of anxiety. The primary aim, however, is to highlight the description of the anxious experience and provide the nurse with enough data to speculate about the cause. Again the nurse assists the patient to ascertain these data by asking probing questions about the particulars of these anxiety-producing situations. Successful completion of this step leads to the next one, which entails the patient gaining personal insight into the precipitating cause of anxiety.

Uniqueness is the final element in Peplau's model. The content and characteristics of the nurse-patient relationship are unique. Each interchange is an original that cannot be duplicated, although patterns may emerge, so that the process can be replicated in other settings. This uniqueness addresses the collaborative effort inherent in the relationship and the significance of each member. Both play an important role in ensuring that this relationship will be educational, growth producing, and successful.

Ida Orlando

Ida Orlando (Andrews, 1983) focuses on *patient participation* in the nursing process. According to her theory, the patient assumes a central role. The patient collaborates in the nursing assessment to identify patient assets and health needs. Once this is ascertained, the nurse and patient must distinguish between those needs that he or she can meet autonomously and those that require assistance.

The nurse's role is to offer any assistance necessary to meet the unfulfilled needs. Special attention, however, is paid to the patient's sense of adequacy or well-being, with effort directed at increasing patients' competencies, thereby strengthening their health. *Patient validation* in both assessment and evaluation is crucial. It is imperative that the patient validate the fact that these needs are actually being met to his or her satisfaction (Andrews, 1983). The patient can be viewed as an integral member of the health care team, involved in and responsible for the treatment plan and its implementation. Patient validation of its efficacy provides a valuable outcome standard to ensure the delivery of quality care.

► Check Your Reading

13. Why should nurses be concerned with nursing theory?
14. How would you describe the structure of nursing knowledge?
15. What is meant by a "caring" relationship in psychiatric nursing?
16. What do you see as Hildegard Peplau's contribution to psychiatric nursing?

CONCLUSIONS

In this chapter, we have examined a variety of mental health theories. No one theory adequately describes the richness or the uniqueness of a human being. No theory adequately identifies the multidimensional determinants or aspects of human behavior. Nevertheless, theoretical frameworks provide a systematic way of understanding and communicating about human personality and behavior.

The evolution of psychiatric nursing has its roots in the theories of ancient Greek scholars. Later, scientists such as Descartes and Darwin added to our understanding of the human mind by describing mind-body connections and identifying its developmental aspects. Freud is recognized as the father of psychoanalysis. In addition to describing the structure of the mind, he introduced the concept of talking about painful emotional issues as the means of resolving them. Jung added another dimension to the study of behavior by establishing the concept of shadow and the paradox of men and women each having characteristics typically associated with the opposite sex. Sullivan broadened early psychoanalytic thinking by proposing personality development as an interpersonal phenomenon, and Rogers took it a step further by describing a person-centered approach to psychotherapy. Existential models focus on the here and now relationship occurring between the therapist and patient. By contrast, behavioral models view personality as behavior that can be learned and unlearned, and biological models focus on the physical basis and function of neurotransmitters in mental illness.

All of these theories are relevant to the study of personality and human behavior. It is critical for nurses to integrate these concepts with the concepts held about nursing as a profession. Now that you have been exposed to an overview of some of the more important theorists of relevance to psychiatric nursing, it becomes your challenge to incorporate these concepts into a holistic framework to guide you on your clinical journey.

KEY POINTS TO REMEMBER

- Psychiatric nurses practice from a comprehensive theory base, derived from the disciplines of philosophy, medicine, psychology, sociology, education, and, of course, nursing.
- Theories never represent absolute truths but rather portray an abstract representation of a phenomenon and a conceptual tool to describe phenomena in an organized way.
- Theory consists of concepts that represent "a concise summary of thoughts related to a phenomenon." Each concept provides a symbolic shorthand for describing an abstract reality.
- Theories develop within a historical context that necessarily builds on but also challenges classic ways of thinking about a subject. Changes in theoretical perspective usually represent a major paradigm shift in thinking.
- Current understandings of psychiatric-mental health nursing emerged originally from the writings of ancient Greek scholars. Their masterful voices spoke of the "whole person," consisting of mind, body, and spirit, both interrelated and irreducible.
- Darwin highlighted the importance of function and adaptation with his theory of evolution—or "survival of the fittest"—forever altering the way humankind viewed the process of growth and change. He believed that those best able to adapt to their environment have the greatest likelihood of surviving.
- Wundt created the important link between an experimental and a social psychology and established the legitimacy of psychology as a science.
- James spearheaded the development of psychology as a professional discipline in the United States. He taught the first psychology courses at a university level and brought the message of this new discipline to the general American population.
- Freud believed that the vast majority of mental disorders were not organic in origin but rather developed as the result of unresolved emotional conflicts in childhood. All behavior, no matter how random it may appear, has an identifiable cause.
- Freud taught that personality is composed of three major systems: the id, ego, and superego.
- Jung developed the notion of the collective unconscious, consisting of man's cultural and ethnic heritage. Within the unconscious exist universal archetypes, the most important of which include persona, shadow, self, animus, and anima.
- Sullivan proposes that personality cannot be studied apart from the social and cultural influences on behavior.
- Erikson describes a theory based on the epigenetic principle and consisting of eight psychosocial developmental stages.
- Maslow's theory of self-actualization focuses on basic needs, which he describes as six incremental stages of personal growth needs.
- Rogers developed a person-centered model of psychotherapy that emphasizes the uniqueness of the individual.
- Existential models focus on taking responsibility, personal freedom, authenticity, anxiety, meaning, and death.
- Behavioral models consider personality as what people do and not who they are; they propose that personality consists of learned behaviors.
- Bandura proposed a social learning theory that conceptualizes psychological functioning as an integration of both environmental conditions and personal attributes.
- Biological models of mental illness focuses on neurological, chemical, biological, and genetic issues.
- Nursing theory represents the unique systematic study of nursing experience. The four elements that make up its metaparadigm are person, environment, health, and nursing.

LEARNING ACTIVITIES

1. To help you develop a personal philosophy of psychiatric nursing complete this exercise at the beginning of your psychiatric nursing rotation and refine it at the end. After reading this chapter, develop your own philosophical perspective on how you want to approach the study of psychiatric patients and their behavior. Include all of the ideas that you believe to be important in interacting with and treating psychiatric patients. Give a thoughtful, personal rationale for why you believe your approach is appropriate. Provide a short paragraph about the personal influences that have contributed

to your philosophical approach to psychiatric nursing. After completing the exercise, consider how difficult it was for you to develop your personal philosophy of psychiatric nursing. As you heard the philosophies of other students, did any of their ideas broaden or suggest new perspectives in your thinking?

2. To help you develop an appreciation for the process of Socratic questioning, think of a clinical situation or human dilemma in which the process of critical thinking, using a Socratic questioning method, might apply. Specify the nature of the problem in a concise problem statement. Identify the underlying assumptions and the stakeholders (anyone involved with the problem). Get their perceptions of the problem through asking questions about who, why, what, where, and how the problem exists. Develop a solution that is rational and meets the dimensions of the problem. Seek evidence for the beneficial effects of implementing the solution you choose, and identify the consequences (including negative ones) related to its implementation. Validate your conclusions with the stakeholders you identified. As you share your critical thinking problem with your classmates, ask for their reactions and further suggestions or modifications to your thinking.

3. To help you develop an appreciation for the meaning of a peak experience, respond to the following instructions by Maslow (1968, p.71):

I would like you to think of the most wonderful experience or experiences of your life; happiest moments, ecstatic moments, moments of rapture, perhaps from being in love, or from listening to music or suddenly "being hit" by a book or painting, or from some great creative moment. First list these. And then try to tell me how you feel in such acute moments, how you feel differently from the way you feel at other times, how you are at the moment a different person in some ways

Share your answer with the other students. Identify commonalities in the experience of special or peak moments. Identify common themes about differences in experience of feelings. How could you use this exercise in your practice of psychiatric nursing?

CRITICAL THINKING EXERCISE

Consider the following passage from this chapter:

Freud's theory has relevancy to psychiatric nursing at many junctures. First, it offers a comprehensive explanation of complex human processes and suggests that many diverse sources stemming from the past affect personality. Freud's theory of the unconscious is particularly valuable as a baseline for considering the multidimensional nature of behavior. By becoming familiar with these diverse conscious and unconscious influences, a nurse can develop and begin to formulate a hypothesis about the root causes of patient suffering.... Understanding the structural nature of the mind allows the nurse to respond more appropriately when obvious conflicts emerge in the nurse-patient relationship.

1. What is the point of view of the authors?

2. What assumption(s) are the authors making?

3. What inference(s) can you draw from the authors' statement about Freud?

While in the clinical area, the head nurse is overheard telling another nurse that she thinks that Freud was a male chauvinist and thinks that his ideas about women are not useful in today's world.

1. What assumptions can the student make about the two different statements about Freud?

2. What inferences can you draw about the head nurse's belief system?

3. What do you think are the reasons the head nurse made her statements about Freud?

4. How would you test your assumptions about the head nurse's reasons?

REFERENCES

Alexander, F. (1959). Current problems in dynamic psychotherapy in its relation to psychoanalysis. *American Journal of Psychiatry, 116;* 322.

Alport, G. (1985) (Ed.) *William James' psychology: The briefer course.* Notre Dame, Indiana: Notre Dame Press. (Originally published in 1892 by Henry Holt & Company.)

Andrews, C. M. (1983). Ida Orlando's model of nursing. In J. J. Fitzpatrick & A. L. Whall (Eds.), *Conceptual models of nursing: Analysis and application* (pp. 47–65). Maryland: Robert J. Brady Co.

Arnold, E., Boggs, K. (1995). *Interpersonal relationships: Communication skills for nurses.* Philadelphia: W. B. Saunders.

Bandura, A. (1962). Social learning through imitation. In M. R. Jones (Ed.), *Nebraska symposium on motivation.* Lincoln: University of Nebraska Press.

Bandura, A. (1977). *Social learning theory.* Englewood Cliffs, New Jersey: Prentice-Hall, Inc.

Bandura, A. (1978). Reflections on self efficacy. In S. Rachman (Ed.), *Advances in behavior research and therapy* (Vol. 1). Oxford: Pergamon Press.

Benner, P., and Wrubel, J. (1989). *The primacy of caring: Stress and coping in health and illness.* Menlo Park, CA: Addison-Wesley.

Buber, M. (1970). *I and thou.* W. Kaufmann, (Trans.) New York: Charles Scribner's Sons.

Bugental, J. (1965). *The search for authenticity.* New York: Holt, Rinehart & Winston.

Bugental, J. (1967). *Challenges of a humanistic psychology.* New York: Harper & Row.

Darwin, C. (1871). *The origin of the species.* New York: Appleton.

Darwin, C. (1873). *The expression of the emotions in man and animals.* New York: Appleton.

Decartes, R. (1931). *The passions of the soul* (G. T. R. Ross, Trans.). In *The philosophical works of Decartes* (Vol. 1). Cambridge: Cambridge University Press.

Donaldson, S.K., Crowley, D.M. (1978). The discipline of nursing. *Nursing Outlook, 26,* 113–120.

Encyclopedia Americana, International Edition (Vol. 2) (pp. 288–292). (1974). New York: Americana Corp.

English, H., & English, A. (1958). *Comprehensive dictionary of psychological and psychoanalytic terms.* New York: Longmans, Green & Co.

Erikson, E. H. (1950). *Childhood and society.* New York: W. W. Norton & Co.

Erikson, E. H. (1982). *The life cycle completed.* New York: W. W. Norton & Co.

Erikson, J. (1988). *Wisdom and the senses: The way of creativity.* New York: W. W. Norton & Co.

Fancher, R. E. (1990). *Pioneers of psychology.* New York: W. W. Norton & Co.

Field, W. E. (1979). *The psychotherapy of Hildegard E. Peplau.* New Brunfels, TX: PSF Publications.

Forchuk, C. (1991). A comparison of the works of Peplau and Orlando. *Archives of Psychiatric Nursing* 5(1), 38–45.

Forchuk, C., Beaton, S., Crawford, L., Ide, L., Voorber, N., and Bethune, J. (1989). Incorporating Peplau's theory and case management. *Journal of Psychosocial Nursing* 27 (2), 35–38.

Forchuk, C., and Brown, B. (1989). Establishing a nurse-client relationship. *Journal of Psychosocial Nursing* 27 (2), 30–34.

Fordham, F. (1953). *An introduction to Jung's psychology.* London: Penguin.

Frankl, V. (1969). *The will to meaning.* Cleveland: New American Library.

Freud, S. On the history of the psychoanalytic movement. In J. Strachey (Ed.), *The standard edition of the complete psychological works of Sigmund Freud* (Vol. 14). (Originally published in 1914.)

Freud, S. (1960). *The ego and the id.* (J. Strachey, Trans.). New York: W. W. Norton & Co.

Freud, S. (1961). *The interpretation of dreams.* (J. Strachey, Trans. and Ed.). New York: Scientific Editions.

Freud, S. (1969). *An outline of psycho-analysis.* (J. Strachey, Trans.). New York: W. W. Norton & Co.

Glasser, W. (1965). *Reality therapy.* New York: Harper & Row.

Hall, C. S., & Lindzey, G. (1970). *Theories of personality.* New York: John Wiley & Sons, Inc.

Heidegger, M. (1962). *Being and time.* New York: Harper & Row.

Jacobi, J. (1951). *The psychology of C. G. Jung* (Revised). New Haven: Yale University Press.

Jaeger, W. (1934). *Aristotle: Fundamentals of the history of his development.* Oxford: Clarendon Press.

James, W. (1907). *Pragmatism: A new name for some old ways of thinking.* Lectures II and VI. New York: Longmans, Green & Co.

James, W. (1950). *Principles of psychology* (Vol. 1). New York: Dover Publications.

Johnson, D. E. (1980). The behavioral system model for nursing. In J. P. Riehl and C. Roy (Eds.), *Conceptual models for nursing practice* (2nd ed.) (pp. 207–216). New York: Appleton-Century-Crofts.

Jung, C. G. (1916). *Analytical psychology.* New York: Moffatt, Yard.

Jung, C. G. (1933). *Modern man in search of a soul.* (W. S. Dell and C. F. Baynes, Trans.). New York: Harcourt Brace Javonovich.

Jung, C. G. (1953). *Collected works.* Vol. 7. *Two essays on analytical psychology.* In New York: Pantheon Press.

Jung, C. G. (1958). *Psyche and symbol.* Garden City, New York: Doubleday.

Jung, C. G. (1973). *Memories, dreams, reflections.* A. Jaffé (Ed.). (R. Winston and C. Winston, Trans.). New York: Pantheon Books.

Jung, C. G. (1975). *Letters.* G. Adler and A. Jaffé (Eds.). (R. F. C. Hull, Trans.). Bollington Series XCV:2. Princeton: Princeton University Press.

Kierkegaard, S. (1957). *The concept of dread.* Princeton: Princeton University Press.

Leibert, R., and Spiegler, M. (1982). *Personality: Strategies and issues.* Homewood, Illinois: The Dorsey Press.

Leininger, M. (1978). *Transcultural nursing: Concepts, theories and practices.* New York: John Wiley & Sons.

Levine, M. (1969; 1973). *Introduction to clinical nursing.* Philadelphia: F. A. Davis.

Marmer, S. (1994). Theories of the mind and psychopathology. In *The American Psychiatric Press textbook of psychiatry.* Washington, D. C.: American Psychiatric Association Press.

Marriner-Tomey, A. (1994). *Nursing theorists and their work* (2nd ed.). St. Louis: Mosby.

Maslow, A. H. (1963). Self-actualizing people. In G. B. Levitas (Ed.), *The world of psychology* (Vol. 2). New York: Braziller.

Maslow, A. H. (1968). *Toward a psychology of being.* (2nd ed.). Princeton: Van Nostrand.

Maslow, A. H. (1970). *Motivation and personality* (rev. ed.) New York: Harper & Row.

Maslow, A. H. (1972). *The farther reaches of human nature.* New York: Viking Press.

McCracken, A. (1994). Special care units: Meeting the needs of cognitively impaired persons. *Journal of Gerontological Nursing April,* 41–46.

Meleis, A. L. (1991). *Theoretical nursing: Development and progress,* (2nd Ed.). Philadelphia: J. B. Lippincott.

Montgomery, Webster, (1994).

Moore, T. (1992). *Care of the soul.* New York: Harper Collins.

Neuman, B. (1992). *The Neuman systems model* (2nd ed.). Norwalk, Connecticut: Appleton-Century-Crofts.

Neuman, B., and Young, R. (1972). A model for teaching total person approach to patient problems. *Nursing Research 21*(3), 264–269.

Nightingale, F. (1860). *Notes on nursing: What it is and what it is not.* Philadelphia: W. B. Saunders.

Paterson, J., and Zderad, L. (1988). *Humanistic nursing.* New York: National League for Nursing.

Paul, R. (1993). *Critical thinking* (2nd ed.). Santa Rosa, California: Critical Thinking Foundation.

Pavlov, I. P. (1928). *Lectures on conditioned reflexes.* (W. Horsley Gantt, Ed. and Trans.). New York: International Publishers.

Peplau, H. E. (1952). *Interpersonal relations in nursing.* New York: G. P. Putnam Sons.

Peplau, H. E. (1982a). Therapeutic concepts. In S. A. Smoyak and S. Rouslin (Eds.), *A collection of classics in psychiatric nursing literature* (pp. 91–108). Thorofare, New Jersey: Charles B. Slack. (Originally published in 1957.)

Peplau, H. E. (1982b). Interpersonal techniques: The crux of psychiatric nursing. In S. A. Smoyak and S. Rouslin (Eds.), *A collection of classics in psychiatric literature* (pp. 276–281). Thorofare, New Jersey: Charles B. Slack. (Originally published in 1962.)

Peplau, H. E. (1982c). Some reflections on earlier days in psychiatric nursing. *Journal of Psychosocial Nursing and Mental Health Services 20*(8), 17–24.

Peplau, H. E. (1987). Interpersonal constructs for nursing practice. *Nursing Education Today* 7, 201–208.

Peplau, H. E. (1989). Future directions in psychiatric nursing from the perspective of history. *Journal of Psychosocial Nursing 27*(2), 18–28.

Rader, M. (1969). *The enduring questions: Main problems of philosophy* (2nd ed.), New York: Holt, Rinehart & Winston.

Rogers, C. R. (1942). *Counseling and psychotherapy: Newer concepts in practice.* Boston: Houghton Mifflin Co.

Rogers, C. R. (1961). *On becoming a person.* Boston: Houghton Mifflin Co.

Rogers, C. R. (1963). Toward a science of the person. *Journal of Humanistic Psychology,* 72–92.

Rogers, M. (1970). *An introduction to the theoretical basis of nursing.* Philadelphia: F. A. Davis.

Skinner, B. F. (1935). Two types of conditioned reflex and a pseudotype. *Journal of General Psychiatry 12,* 66–77.

Skinner, B. F. (1957). *Verbal behavior.* Englewood Cliffs, New Jersey: Prentice Hall.

Skinner, B. F. (1987). Whatever happened to psychology as the science of behavior? *American Psychologist 42,* 780–786.

Smith, B. D., & Vetter, H. J. (1982). *Theoretical approaches to personality.* Engelwood Cliffs, New Jersey: Prentice Hall, Inc.

Strachey, J. (Ed.) (1964). *The standard edition of the complete psychological works of Sigmund Freud.* London: Hogarth Press.

Sullivan, H. S. (1954). *The psychiatric interview.* New York: W. W. Norton & Co.

Sullivan, H. S. (1972). *Personal psychopathology.* New York: W. W. Norton & Co.

Taylor, A. E. (1933). *Socrates.* New York: Appleton.

Tillich, P. (1952). *The courage to be.* New Haven: Yale University Press.

Watson, J. (1919). *Psychology from the standpoint of a behaviorist.* Philadelphia: J. B. Lippincott.

Watson, J. (1928). *The ways of behaviorism.* New York: Harper & Bros.

Woodward, W. (1982). The "discovery" of social behaviorism and social learning theory, 1870–1980. *American Psychologist 37*(4), 396–410.

Yalom, I. (1980). *Existential psychotherapy.* New York: Basic Books.

SUGGESTED READINGS

Erikson, E. H. (1950). *Childhood and society.* New York: W. W. Norton & Co.

Forchuk, C. (1991). A comparison of the works of Peplau and Orlando. *Archives of Psychiatric Nursing* 5(1), 38–45.

Forchuk, C., Beaton, S., Crawford, L., Ide, L., Voorberg, N., & Bethune, J. (1989). Incorporating Peplau's theory and case management. *Journal of Psychosocial Nursing* 27(2), 35–38.

Hall, C. S., and Lindzey, G. (1970). *Theories of personality.* New York: John Wiley & Sons, Inc.

Marriner-Tomey, A. (1994). *Nursing theorists and their work* (2nd ed.) St. Louis: Mosby.

Neuman, B. (1992). *The Neuman systems model* (2nd ed.). Norwalk, CT. Appleton-Century-Crofts.

Peplau, H. E. (1987). Interpersonal constructs for nursing practice. *Nursing Education Today* 7; 201–208.

Rogers, C. R. (1961). *On becoming a person.* Boston: Houghton Mifflin Co.

UNIT II
THE NATURE OF THE JOURNEY

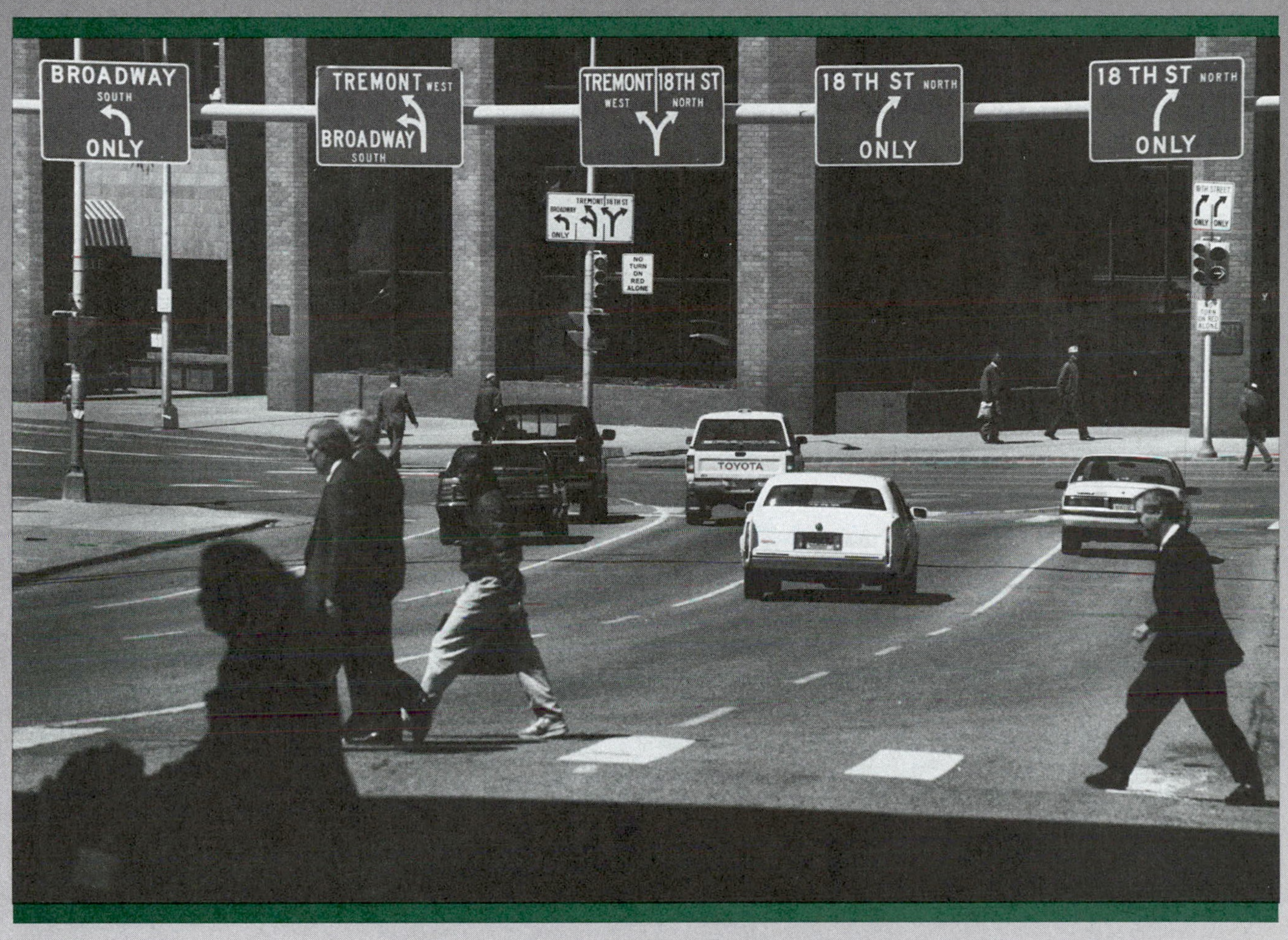

CHAPTER 7

PHYSICAL DIMENSIONS OF THE JOURNEY

NEUROBIOLOGICAL INFLUENCES

Men ought to know that from the brain, and from the brain only, arise our pleasures, joys, laughter and jests, as well as our sorrows, pains, griefs, and fears. Through it, in particular, we think, see, hear, and distinguish the ugly from the beautiful, the bad from the good, the pleasant from the unpleasant. . . . It is the same thing which makes us mad or delirious, inspires us with dread and fear, whether by night or by day, brings sleeplessness, inopportune mistakes, aimless anxieties, absentmindedness, and acts that are contrary to habit. These things that we suffer all come from the brain, when it is not healthy, but becomes abnormally hot, cold, moist, or dry, or suffers from any unnatural affection to which it is not accustomed. Madness comes from its moistness.

—Hippocrates

LEARNING OBJECTIVES

After studying this chapter, you should be able to:

1. Identify the significant contributors to the development of biological psychiatry.
2. Explain the cellular organization of the neuron.
3. Discuss the effect of membrane permeability on neuronal transmission.
4. Identify the major neurotransmitters and their effect on neuronal transmission.
5. Describe the gross structures of the brain.
6. Explain the importance of the neuroendocrine cascade.
7. Identify the laboratory tests used for diagnostic evaluation of psychiatric patients.
8. Discuss the importance of biological psychiatry on the understanding of the cause of selected mental illnesses.
9. Identify the implications of biological psychiatry for the practice of psychiatric nursing.

KEY TERMINOLOGY

Action potential
Basal ganglia
Brain imaging
Catecholamine hypothesis
Dizygotic
Dopamine hypothesis
GABA
Kindling
Limbic system
Monozygotic
Motor homunculus
Neuroendocrine system
Neuroscience
Neurotransmitters
Psychobiology
Sensitization
Somatosensory area
Ventricular system

The journey of exploration in the field of psychiatry to uncover the cause of mental illness has encompassed many decades and much mysticism. Hopes have been raised for the discovery of a distinct biological basis for the major mental illnesses only to have those hopes squelched by contradictory evidence. As technology continues to improve, more and more is uncovered about the biological factors that contribute to the development of mental illnesses.

This chapter will help you to understand the biological revolution in psychiatry. The chapter begins with a historical perspective and traces the development of knowledge to the present. The field of biological psychiatry is experiencing an explosion of knowledge; new advances are being made every day in the understanding of the cause and treatment of mental disorders. These advances have and will continue to have a significant impact on the practice of psychiatric nursing. Only by understanding the biological factors that affect the cause and treatment of mental illness will psychiatric nurses be able to treat patients like Mr. T.

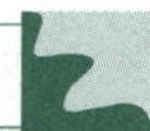

MR. T'S STORY

A 22-year-old male, Mr. T., was taken to a psychiatrist by his concerned parents. They complained that he had no interest in girls and dating and had just been fired from his third job this year. They feared that he would never leave home. They said that he had always been "a little different." The parents added that he had always had "spells" in which he seemed dizzy, looked over to one side, as if hallucinating, and chewed.

The patient presented in a stern, humorless manner. He was dressed and groomed appropriately but his speech was intense, circumstantial and included many details, clarifications, and qualifications. Although he denied any delusions or hallucinations, he exhibited an extreme preoccupation with religious, moral, and philosophical issues. When the hour was up, the patient continued to talk and resist the doctor's efforts to terminate the interview. In the following week, he called the office twice to expand on issues and sent three lengthy letters.

A physical examination showed no abnormalities. A neurological exam, routine laboratory data, EEG, and CT scan were all within normal limits.

Does this patient have a mental illness? Does he require medication? What assurances could you give his parents that this young man will ever leave home?

Story from Tomb, D. A., and Christensen, D. D. (1987). *Case Studies in Psychiatry for the House Officer.* Baltimore: Williams & Wilkins.

The following pages will provide you with information to understand better the nature of Mr. T.'s illness and some treatment options available once a diagnosis has been made.

For centuries, people have misunderstood the nature of mental illness. This has led them to react to it with embarrassment, shame, guilt, and fear. People have identified mental illness as God's punishment to sinners, as a spiritual torment caused by demonic possession, or as a moral defect caused by weakness of will. In earlier centuries, the mentally ill were burned at the stake or locked away because they were thought to be possessed. Others were chained in filthy cells for most of their lives.

The advocates for the mentally ill of the 1980s comforted themselves with the belief that the mentally ill now live in a more enlightened era. Although it is true that the mentally ill are no longer confined in chains, many people who suffer from mental illness are still the victims of subtler versions of social stigmatization, cruelty, and prejudice. This prejudice grows out of ignorance and misunderstanding derived from a failure to realize the impact of brain disease on the development of mental illness and the belief that one could overcome mental illness by simply trying harder.

Psychiatry now recognizes that serious mental illnesses are diseases in the same sense that cancer and hypertension are diseases. People who suffer from mental illness are afflicted with a disease of the brain, not from weak will, laziness, bad character, or poor parenting. The recognition that mental illnesses are diseases affecting the brain is the basis of the biological revolution in psychiatry. **Psychobiology** involves the study of the biochemical foundations of thought, mood, affect, emotion, and behavior. It takes into consideration both internal and external influences, such as genetic factors, biological contributions from other body systems, and the external environment across the lifespan of the given individual (Hill, 1991; McEnany, 1991; Bushness and DeForge, 1994).

In this chapter, we explore the history of biological psychiatry; review the basic cellular organization of the brain, neuroanatomy, neurophysiology, and neuroendocrinology; identify the most current diagnostic procedures; describe the etiological implications of psychobiology on some major mental illnesses; critique the literature on the biological revolution in psychiatry; and explain the implications that psychobiology may have on the practice of psychiatric nursing.

HISTORY OF BIOLOGICAL PSYCHIATRY

Early Roots of Biological Psychiatry

Although the biological model of psychiatry derives from Kraepelin and other psychiatrists and neurologists of the late 19th and early 20th centuries, in fact, its roots date back much further. The biological model represents the mainstream of medical traditions for understanding mental illness. From the time of the classical Greeks, mental illnesses were assumed to be caused by some type of aberration in body function. In classical times, Hippocrates believed that disturbed mental functioning was secondary to an imbalance in the four body humors (blood, phlegm, black bile, and yellow bile). For instance, depression (or melancholia) was thought to be caused by an excess of black bile.

Furthering the idea of a biological basis for mental illness, Asclepiades described phrenitis and mania noting physical aspects of each condition. He also recommended coarse biological treatments, such as placing patients with certain mental conditions in a room filled with light, perhaps an early precursor for light treatment of Seasonal Affective Disorders.

In the Dark Ages (400–1200 A.D.), ideas emerged regarding the classification of psychobiopathology. Descriptions were written about cyclic patterns of mood, melancholia, mania, psychotic behavior, epilepsy, and dementia.

During the Renaissance, many believed that mental disorders resulted from spiritual imbalances or witchcraft. Weyer (cited in Andreason, 1984) believed that psychopathology was caused by an interaction between the physical and spiritual domains of the individual.

Despite these early roots, the biological approach to psychiatry, which began in Europe, has been late in arriving to the United States. Indeed, for many of the early years in the United States, psychiatry was almost synonymous with psychoanalysis.

Biological Psychiatry in the Early 20th Century

In 1910, Sigmund Freud delivered a series of lectures at Clark University in Worcester, Massachusetts. Freudian psychoanalysis enchanted Americans and sparked a revolution in psychiatry that spanned the entire nation. By the 1940s, psychoanalysis dominated American thinking in psychiatry. Interestingly, Freud began his work hoping to understand and map the brain rather than the mind. His early training was as a researcher in the brain sciences, what is today called *neuroscience.* He studied with the leading brain and neurological researchers of his day, Brücke, Meynert, and Charcot.

Freud was prohibited from becoming involved in research because of his Jewish background and economic station. One of his earliest published works, however, was a treatise on aphasia, placing him clearly in the tradition of the brain research of his era. Once in practice, Freud abandoned the biological approach because he found that it had limited applicability to his patients.

Meanwhile, in Europe, neuroscientists, neurologists, and psychiatrists continued their work in describing and mapping the structure of the brain. Great neurologists such as Broca and Wernicke had proved that the brain contained specific areas that controlled different functions. They found that damage to different tiny areas within a larger specific area could cause different kinds of damaged language function. Injuries that occurred in the front (in *Broca's area*) left a person nearly mute but able to understand everything clearly, whereas damage further back (in *Wernicke's area*) left a person speaking fluent nonsense and able to understand nothing.

Golgi was developing new staining techniques so that brain cells could be better visualized under the microscope. Fiber tracts connecting different parts of the brain were being traced, and the effects of electrical stimulation were being studied.

While neurologists were mapping and staining, Emil Kraepelin was laying the foundations for the modern biological revolution in psychiatry. Kraepelin's contribution to psychiatry was to describe and identify specific types of major psychiatric illnesses. Through close observation and longitudinal study over the course of several years, he differentiated manic-depressive insanity from dementia praecox (later renamed schizophrenia by Eugene Bleuler). Kraepelin viewed these disorders as illnesses that were probably caused by some yet unrecognized physical factor. Most of the advances in biological psychiatry represent a series of footnotes to and amplifications of Kraepelin's textbooks (Andreason, 1984).

In the United States, however, Freudian psychoanalysis prevailed over Kraepelinian biological psychiatry. In addition, another school of thought, particularly American, the behavioral approach, was soon added. Shortly after Freud visited the United States, behaviorism was founded by John B. Watson. His most influential followers were Clark Hull and B. F. Skinner. While Freud hoped to map the functions of the brain and Kraepelin the abnormalities of the brain, the behaviorists hoped to map the general laws governing human behavior. They believed that the proper way to study how humans think and feel is through studying what they do. For the behaviorists, behavior, not ideas or emotions, was the proper focus of psychology.

Historically the psychodynamic theory arising from the work of Freud and the behavioral theory arising from the work of Watson have dominated American thinking. In contrast, European thinking, although influenced by psychodynamic and behavioral thinking, has been predominantly biological.

Era of Biological Psychiatry in America

By the 1980s in the United States, the emphasis in psychiatry was swinging from psychological models of mental illness toward a biological model. The biological model has been shaped by the growth of the neurosciences. **Neuroscience** encompasses a set of related disciplines that share the common goal of understanding the relationship between brain structure and function and human thoughts, feelings, and behavior. Some of these disciplines include:

- Neuroanatomy (the study of brain structure)
- Neurophysiology (the study of brain function)
- Neurochemistry (the study of chemical processes that control brain function)
- Neuroendocrinology (the study of the relationship between glandular function and brain function)
- Neuropharmacology (the study of the effects of drugs on the brain)

In the past decade, there have been a number of developments in biology that directly affect psychiatry. Two of the most important are advances in genetics and in the molecular biological studies of neuroreceptors. Advances in genetics may eventually lead to the identification of factors predisposing individuals to the development of some major mental illnesses. Advances in neuroreceptor research may lead to the development of more sophisticated and rational psychopharmacotherapies for psychiatric disorders.

Other areas of research directly affecting the revolution in biological psychiatry include:

- The development of **brain imaging** techniques, such as magnetic resonance imaging (MRI), positron emission tomography (PET) scan, and computed tomography brain scan (CT scan)
- The heightened understanding of the biological dimension of emotion
- Research supporting the role of neurochemicals in the formation and enactment of behavior
- A shift in knowledge about the brain's capacity to change and heal itself after birth (brain plasticity)
- The growth in the understanding of molecular genetics (Barondes, 1990)

During the past 20 years, the neurosciences have produced an explosion of knowledge about how the brain works. New, sophisticated ways of studying the brain in vivo have emerged that have led the way to the identification of abnormalities in brain structure or chemistry as contributing to the cause of many mental illnesses.

Let's return to the case of Mr. T.

In assessing his case, some important information might have been overlooked had the new ideas about linkages between neuroanatomy, neurophysiology, and behavioral symptoms not been understood. In interviewing Mr. T.'s parents, the psychiatrist learned that his mother's pregnancy had been complicated by toxemia and a difficult delivery. At 14 months, Mr. T. had been hospitalized with a high fever and seizures. In school, Mr. T. was often accused of not paying attention, and even his parents described him as a daydreamer.

Despite the normalcy of Mr. T.'s EEG, the psychiatrist recognized that this standard procedure often fails to detect a deep temporal lobe seizure focus in about 50% of patients. Diagnostic specificity of the EEG is enhanced by sleep deprivation and the use of sphenoidal or nasopharyngeal recording electrodes. Indeed, after completion of this additional procedure, Mr. T. was accurately diagnosed with temporal lobe epilepsy. If these additional diagnostic procedures—only recently recognized—had not been used, Mr. T. might have received a diagnosis of schizophrenia, which would have adversely affected the rest of his life.

Psychiatric nursing, especially in the United States, is moving from the study of the "troubled mind" to the "broken brain." The journey begins with one small step, the understanding of the brain.

▶ Check Your Reading

1. What is psychobiology?
2. Who first described light treatment for depression?
3. What did the behaviorists hope to map?
4. What does the term *neuroscience* encompass?
5. What new areas of research directly affect the biological revolution in psychiatry?

NEUROANATOMY

The Brain

Macrostructure

The brain is one component of the central nervous system that is encapsulated by the skull. The brain performs the functions that make us human, humane, and unique. It is the physical source of our ability to speak, to write, to think, to create, to love, to laugh, to despair, and to hate (Andreason, 1984). As our language indicates, we tend to speak and think as if we were controlled by something else. For example, when we fall in love, we "give someone our heart." When we display our feelings, we "wear our hearts on our sleeves." Similarly, when we become emotional, we "spill our guts." In fact, it is our brains that are intricately involved in all of these activities.

The most impressive feature of the brain is its size. It weighs approximately 3 lb in the average man; women's brains are somewhat smaller. Brain size is closely related to head size but has no relationship to intelligence. The brain looks like a large hunk of rather shapeless creamy pinkish fat. Its surface is covered with furrows (sulci), but beneath these furrows it looks rather uniform throughout. The surface is somewhat darker than the rest of the brain and is made up of unmyelinated (uninsulated) cells commonly called the *gray matter.* Most of the brain is made up of myelinated (insulated) cells commonly called the *white matter.* The glial cells surround the neurons to create the appearance of white matter. To complicate things a little, there are a few areas of gray matter embedded deep within the white matter.

The brain is divided into two globular halves, the left and right hemispheres. These appear to be more or less symmetrical and are attached to each other by a thin strip of white matter called the *corpus callosum.* Both hemispheres are attached to the spinal cord, which travels through the bony structure of the vertebrae and sends out small threads of nerve bundles that transmit messages to and from the brain. Afferent tracts of nerve bundles travel to the brain, and efferent tracts travel away from it.

The brain tissue is soft, delicate, and easily damaged. It is encased in the thick, bony skull and covered with a tough, fibrous sac (the dura mater, or "hard mother") filled with cerebrospinal fluid in which it is suspended and cushioned. Figure 7–1 shows the macrostructure of the brain.

SURFACE STRUCTURE

Each of the cerebral hemispheres has traditionally been divided into four "lobes," which are named for the bones of the skull that surround them: frontal, parietal, occipital,

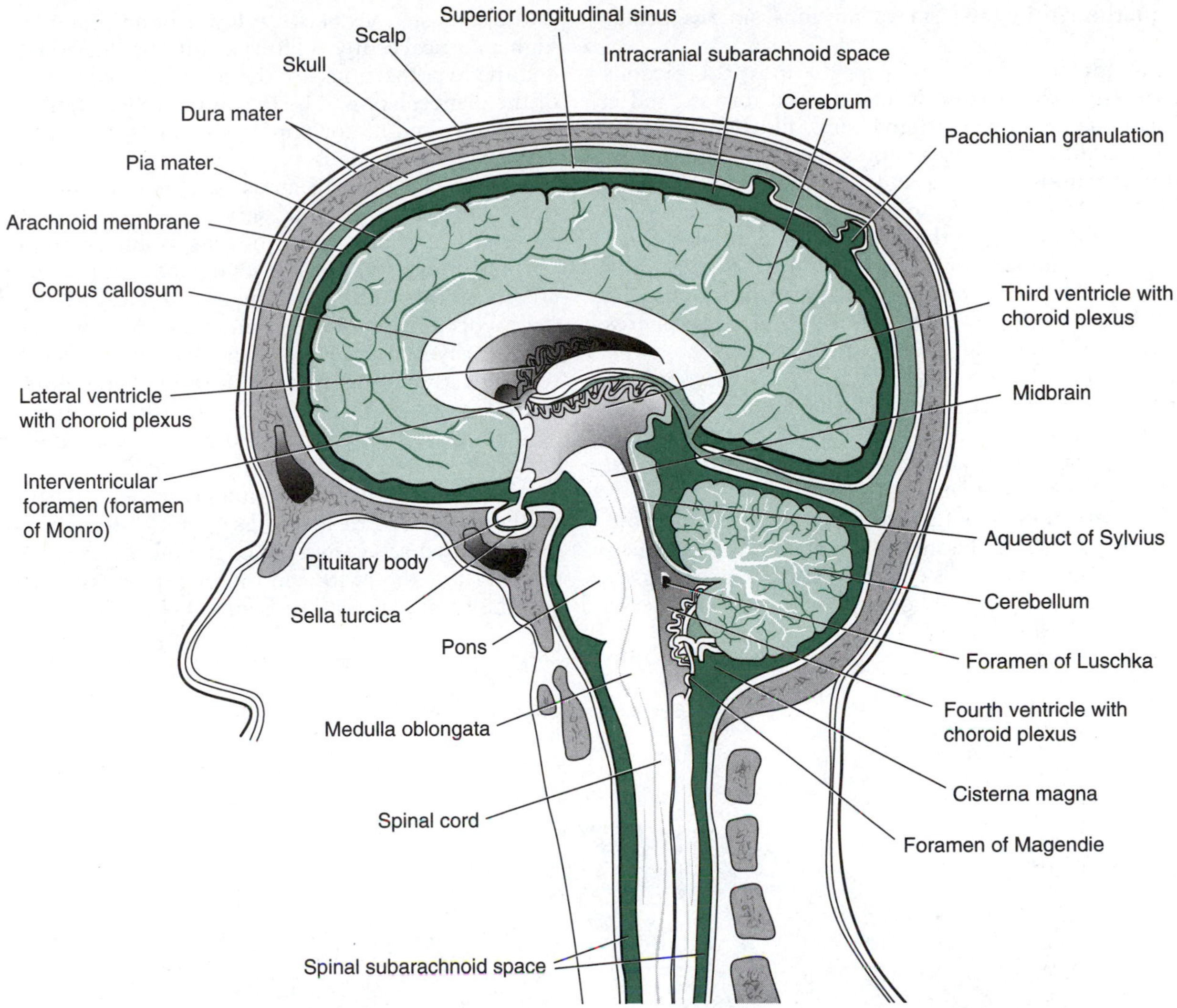

FIGURE 7–1
The macrostructure of the brain.

and temporal. See Figure 7–2 for a view of a hemisphere. The frontal lobe is the largest of the lobes, beginning at the front of the brain and reaching back to the central sulcus. The area between the central and precentral sulci helps control body movement and so is called the *motor area.* Penfield charted the relationship between parts of the cortex and specific muscle groups; his graphic depiction of this relationship is often called the **motor homunculus** (Figure 7–3). Motor control is highly lateralized. The left side of the brain governs the right side of the body, and the right side of the brain governs the left side of the body.

Broca discovered the localization of speech in the posterior frontal area. Broca's area is the part of the brain that contains information about details of grammar and provides information permitting people to organize words into fluent speech. The remainder of the frontal lobe modulates various aspects of thinking, feeling, imagining, and decision-making. The frontal lobe is the seat of intellectual functioning, with responsibility for judgment, reasoning, and abstract thought. It is also responsible for social consciousness and the inhibition of unacceptable behavior. This area was the target for the prefrontal lobotomies performed in the early days of psychiatry.

The parietal lobe is the region behind the central sulcus. Part of it is called the **somatosensory area.** This area is configured so that it almost perfectly parallels the motor strip in terms of the parts of the body it controls (see Figure 7–3). The somatosensory area receiving sensations from the arms and legs is adjacent to the motor strip that governs movement of these parts. Similar to the motor fibers, the sensory fibers govern the opposite side of the body. It receives information about various bodily sensations and synthesizes and elaborates sensory impulses. It also modulates spatial orientation.

The occipital lobe receives and sends out information. It contains the primary visual receptive area. The area is responsible for the storing of visual information and thus the interpretation of visual responses. Disruption in this area may lead to illusions and hallucinations.

The temporal lobe is perhaps the most conspicuous lobe of the brain because it juts out and forward and is demarcated by the deep sylvian fissure. The temporal lobe receives auditory impulses, stores memory patterns for symbolic sounds, receives and transmits gustatory impulses, and receives and transmits olfactory input. Wernicke's area is located in the temporal lobe. It is a storage center programmed to permit us to recognize and comprehend information presented in auditory form.

The activities that the two cerebral hemispheres perform are sometimes referred to as *higher cortical functions.* These hemispheres are called the *telencephalon,* or *endbrain,* because they are the most highly developed of the brain structures. The next sets of structures within the brain are the *diencephalon,* or *interbrain,* and the *basal ganglia,* or *lower nerve knots.*

Diencephalon structures cannot be seen from the outside of the brain because they are embedded deep within it. These structures consist of small masses of gray matter made up of the cell bodies of neurons. They serve as the relay stations between lower brain centers and the higher cortical centers. The thalamus, or "marriage bed," and the hypothalamus are the most important structures of the diencephalon. The thalamus is the major pathway for sensory and motor impulses to and from the cerebral hemispheres, and it is the modulator of emotions and behavior. The hypothalamus regulates hormonal function. The **basal ganglia** serve as regulators of body movement and integrators of sensory information.

The midbrain, pons (bridge), and medulla (marrow) are sometimes grouped together and called the *brain stem.* This portion of the brain is the most primitive and is primarily concerned with the capacity for survival. It regulates the heart beat, respiration, and other vital functions. It also receives information from the remainder of the body through the spinal cord and cranial nerves.

The cerebellum is sometimes considered a part of the midbrain. It is a relatively large and intensely foliated structure that serves as a major modulator of movement, working together with the motor regions of the cortex and the basal ganglia (see Figure 7–1).

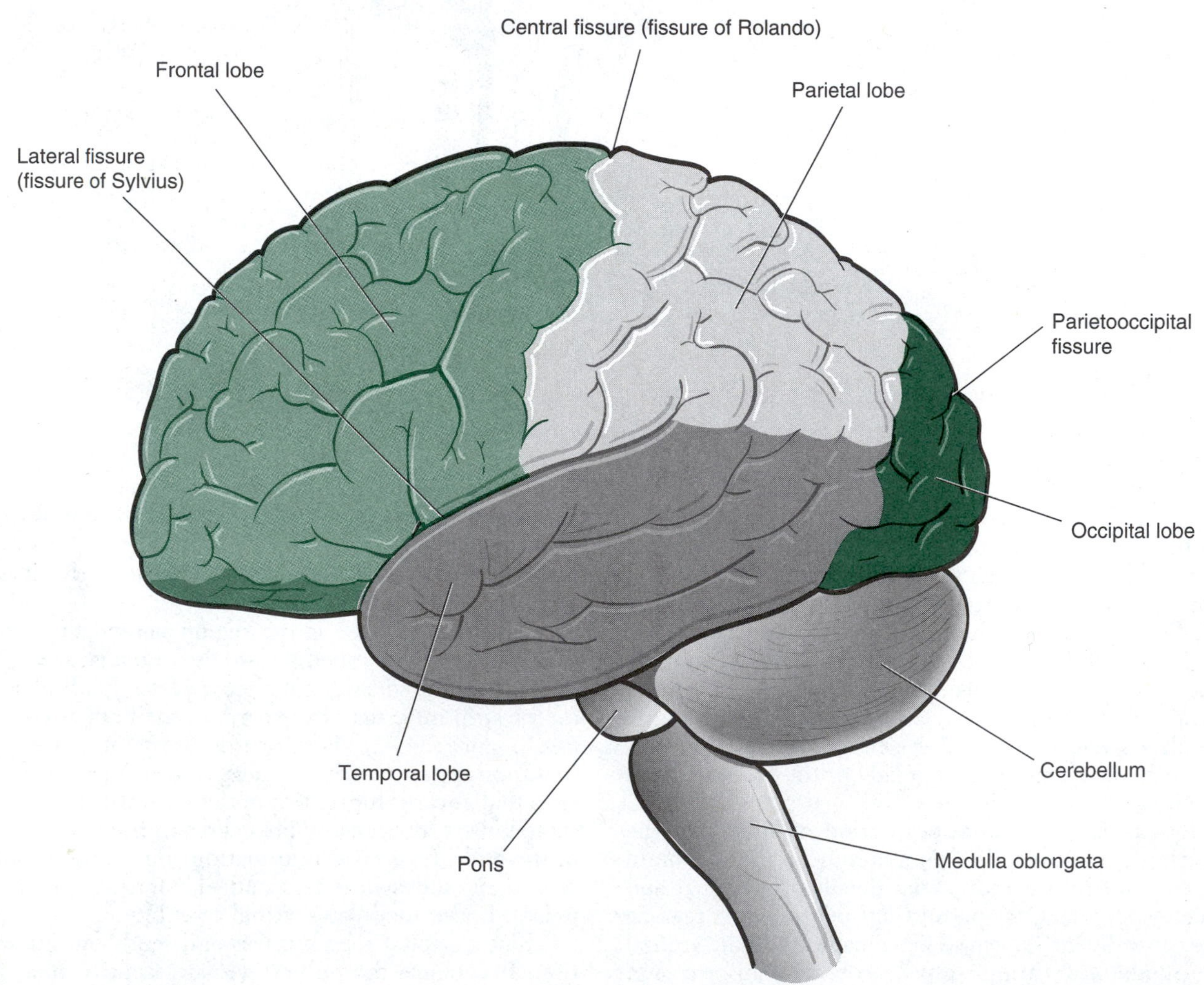

FIGURE 7–2
A hemisphere of the brain.

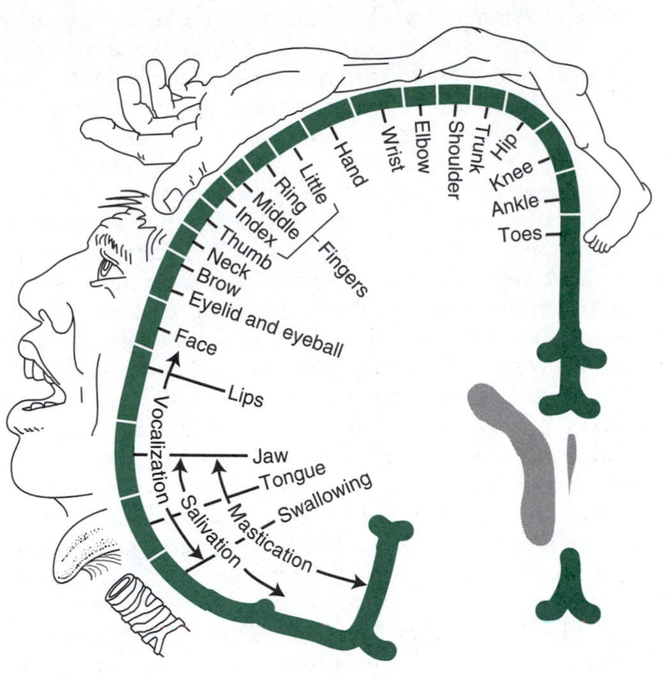

Precentral sulcus: The motor area

Postcentral sulcus: The sensory area

FIGURE 7–3
The motor homunculus and the somatosensory homunculus.

▶ Check Your Reading

6. What differentiates white matter from gray matter?
7. What structure connects the right hemisphere with the left?
8. Afferent tracts travel in which direction from the brain? In which direction do efferent tracts travel?
9. What are the functions of the frontal, parietal, occipital, and temporal lobes?
10. What function does the somatosensory area serve?
11. Disruption in the occipital lobe may lead to what?
12. What is the function of the structures of the diencephalon?
13. What is the role of the thalamus?
14. What does the hypothalamus regulate?
15. What does the brain stem regulate?
16. The cerebellum is involved with which function of the body?

INNER STRUCTURE

The Limbic System. Another brain system that appears in both the frontal and the temporal lobes but is not visible from the outer brain is the **limbic,** or "border" **system** (Figure 7–4). It is connected to a variety of gray matter centers that are deep inside the brain. The limbic system is an important modulator of emotions and may be one of the systems that plays a role in the development of mental illnesses. The cortical part of this system consists of the cingulate gyrus, which arches back around the corpus callosum, connects with the parahippocampal gyrus in the temporal lobe, and curves under to form the uncus (or hook). Subcortical portions include the septal region near the septum pellucidum (or translucent divider), the fornix, and the mammillary bodies.

The pineal gland, residing just below the posterior end of the corpus callosum, is thought to partially regulate the sleep-wake cycle. The paired mammillary bodies function in the processes of learning and memory. Toward the front are the two optic tracts that carry fibers from the nerve cells lining the back of the eyeball. These tracts cross, as do many other tracts in the brain. Their place of crossing is called the *optic chiasm.* Just above the optic tract is the olfactory tubercle, a cranial nerve collecting information about how things smell. In the middle of all of these structures is the thalamus. There are actually two thalami, one on each side of the brain, and they are usually fused in the midline by the massa intermedia. Arching above the thalamus is the fornix, part of the limbic system, and below it are the structures of the hypothalamus.

Depending on the cut of the brain, different structures are visible. In Figure 7–4, the corpus callosum is seen as clearly connecting both hemispheres. Tiny hollow areas appear, which are the frontal and temporal horns of the lateral ventricles. These are portions of the brain containing cerebrospinal fluid. The frontal horns are bounded on each side by the caudate (tail-like) nuclei, which are also part of the basal ganglia, as are the claustrum (cloister) and the putamen (stone). Because of their shape they have sometimes been called the *lenticular* (lenslike) nuclei and the *corpus striatum* (striped body). The large oval thalami appear in the midline, with the tiny, slitlike third ventricle lying between them.

The components and connections of the limbic system contain most of the elements that define individual personality, cognitive style, and patterns of behavior. Information from the external environment is collected through the hippocampus of the temporal lobe, frontal lobe, cingulate gyrus, and olfactory bulb. The thalamus and septal nuclei serve as transmitters to pass information from major structures, such as mammillary bodies, hypothalamus, amygdala, and hippocampus. Damage to the septal nuclei, mammillary bodies, amygdala, and hippocampus produces loss of the ability to learn new information and retain it in long-term memory. Other structures, such as the hypothalamus and pituitary, are regulators of hormonal functioning, governing activities such as thirst, sex drive, and appetite. It is believed that the cause of some types of mood disorders may lie in hyperarousal of the hypothalamic-pituitary-adrenal axis.

Other structures, such as the cingulate gyrus and the frontal lobe, are known to be involved in the ability to think creatively and make decisions. These structures also modulate the ability to start and stop various behaviors. Many neuroscientists believe that the key to understanding many aspects of mental illness may lie within the limbic system and its connections (Benes, 1993).

The Basal Ganglia. The basal ganglia lie within the primitive motor system, sometimes referred to as the *extrapyramidal system.* Within this system, the chain of command runs from certain regions in the frontal and parietal cortex, down through the caudate and putamen, to the globus pallidus, and on to the thalamus. Feedback loops occur throughout the system.

The basal ganglia are considered modulators of movement and integrators of sensory information. The basal ganglia share with the limbic system a particular neurotransmitter, dopamine, that is considered important in the development of schizophrenia. Some neuroscientists therefore believe that the study of the basal ganglia may improve the understanding of schizophrenia. Also, the structures of the basal ganglia tend to be selectively damaged in some important diseases. Huntington's chorea is characterized by a "broken" caudate nucleus. Parkinson's disease results from the death of nerve cells in the substantia nigra (black substance), a gray matter center that is part of the basal ganglia but located in the midbrain. Both of these diseases of the basal ganglia have symptoms similar to those of some common mental illnesses.

The Ventricular System. The ventricular system consists of four fluid-filled cavities buried deep within the brain. There are two lateral ventricles, one within each hemisphere. Each of the lateral ventricles has projections into the frontal lobe, the occipital lobe, and the temporal

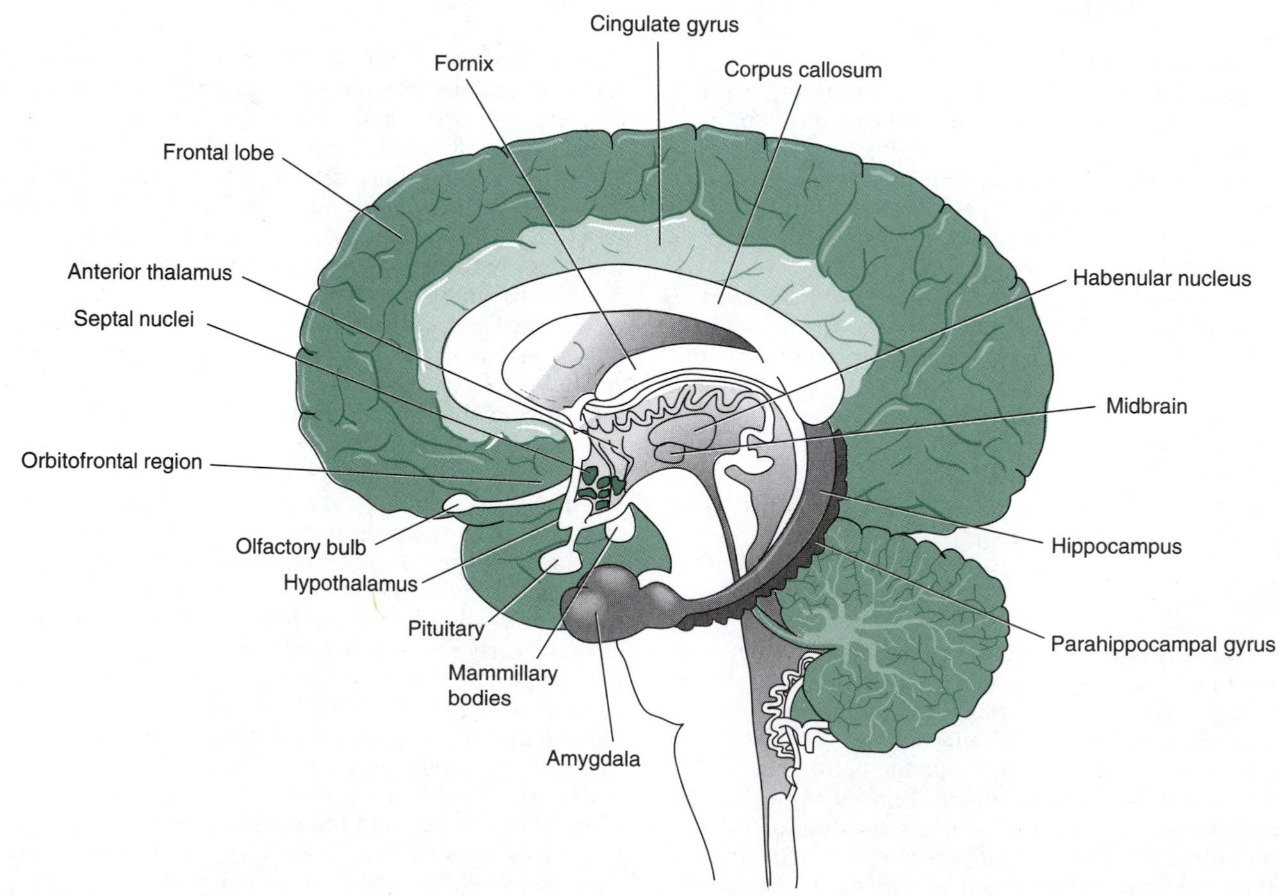

FIGURE 7–4
The structures of the limbic system.

lobe. The frontal and temporal horns of the lateral ventricles are connected to the much smaller midline third ventricle, which is surrounded on each side by the two thalami. The third ventricle extends down and is connected to an even smaller fourth ventricle, which then flows into a fluid-filled column that runs through the center of the spinal cord. The ventricular system is filled with cerebrospinal fluid (see Figure 7–1).

The ventricular system is of interest to neuroscientists for several reasons. First, when brain cells are damaged or die, the substance of the brain grows smaller, and the ventricles enlarge to fill the empty space within the skull; thus, ventricular enlargement provides a useful index of brain atrophy or shrinkage. Also, the ventricles are major landmarks that can be seen clearly with CT scans. Finally, ventricular enlargement has been noted in some patients with schizophrenia and dementia.

▶ **Check Your Reading**

17. What is the role of the limbic system?
18. What mental disorder may be associated with hyperarousal in the hypothalamic-pituitary-adrenal axis?
19. What mental disorder is associated with dysfunction of the basal ganglia?
20. Why is the ventricular system of interest to neuroscientists?

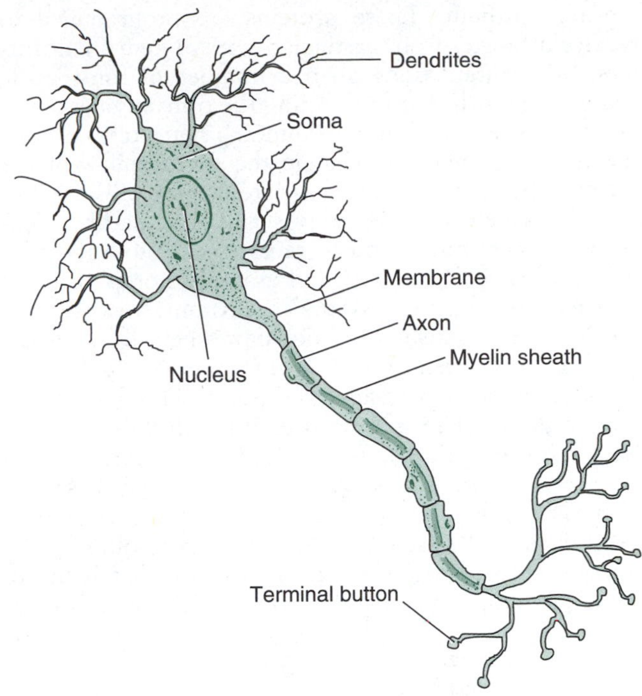

FIGURE 7–5
The structure of a neuron.

Microstructure

In the small-scale world of the brain, the building blocks are nerve cells: neurons and glial cells. Currently, neuroscientists believe that the neurons are responsible for formulating and transmitting all the messages of the brain. The glial (glue) cells are thought to be cementing, supporting, and nourishing structures for the neurons. The brain has been estimated to contain 10 trillion cells of which 90% are glial cells.

Neurons differ in shape and appearance depending on their purpose. Some neurons (afferent neurons) are specialized to receive messages, whereas others (efferent neurons) send out messages. Figure 7–5 shows the structure of a neuron. The main work center of the neuron is the cell body, which contains the nucleus of the cell. The cell body sends out tiny fingers of branching fibers called *dendrites* (treelike structures). This treelike web around the cell body enormously increases its ability to receive information, allowing other cells to communicate either to the cell body or to the dendrites.

In addition to the dendrites, the cell body sends out a long, tubular projection to communicate with other neurons. This projection—the axon (axis)—is usually myelinated. The axons are the "wires" of the nervous system. Although some axons are relatively short, others may be as long as 1 m. The myelinated sheath is composed of glial cells, called *Schwann cells*, that wrap themselves around the neuron. The space between the Schwann cells is called the *node of Ranvier*. This organization permits electrical impulses to travel from the cell body to the end of the nerve by skipping from node to node. The end of the axon branches out into as many as 1000 terminals.

The messages are sent down the axons through a process of electrical conduction. When an axon is at rest, it is filled with and surrounded by a fluid containing a high concentration of electrically charged substances, such as sodium (+), potassium (+), and chloride (–), called ions. When a message arrives at the axon telling it to fire, an event called an **action potential** occurs. The permeability of the membrane forming the axon changes, and this change causes positively charged sodium ions, which have been floating outside of the membrane, to flow in, thereby triggering a large positive charge inside the cell. The larger the axon, the faster the message can travel. Figure 7–6 shows a membrane potential.

When the electrical impulse traveling down the axon reaches its presynaptic terminal, it spreads out in hundreds of nerve terminals that communicate with the dendrites and cell bodies of other neurons. The communication point between the neurons is called the synapse (junction). Figure 7–7 shows an axon and a synapse.

Clustered at the end of the nerve terminal are hundreds of tiny sacs (synaptic vesicles) containing chemical substances called **neurotransmitters.** When an impulse reaches the presynaptic terminal, it is accompanied by the entry of calcium ions (Ca^+). These ions enhance the migration of synaptic vesicles toward the presynaptic membrane. Once the vesicles reach the presynaptic membrane and receive a strong positive charge, the sacs surrounding the packets of neurochemicals burst, and neurochemicals flow into the synaptic cleft. Released neurotransmitters in the synaptic cleft interact directly with receptor molecules in the postsynaptic membrane.

Research has indicated that the receptors are specific sites on the neuronal membrane that contain particular types of protein. These proteins are programmed to receive messages from particular types of neurotransmitters. Such interactions open a number of ion-specific channels, allowing or prohibiting the transmission of the nerve impulse. In addition to binding neurotransmitters, the receptors may also change the permeability of the membrane, they may communicate outside of the cell to send messages, and they may act as modulators. Neurotransmitters not bound to receptors are quickly inactivated by specific enzymes. For example, norepinephrine is inactivated by the enzyme monoamine oxidase, and dopamine is inactivated by dopamine beta-hydroxylase.

It is known that some drugs may increase or decrease the sensitivity of particular receptors. This may either explain the mechanism of action of the drugs or account for their side effects. For example, prolonged use of antipsychotic drugs may eventually lead to oversensitivity of receptors thereby causing tardive dyskinesia (a movement disorder characterized by involuntary rolling of the tongue or twitching of facial or other small muscles in some people). Other psychoactive drugs, such as diazepam (Valium), may bind to the modulating component in the **GABA** (gamma-aminobutyric acid) receptor, preventing it from functioning appropriately and giving GABA free rein as an inhibitor.

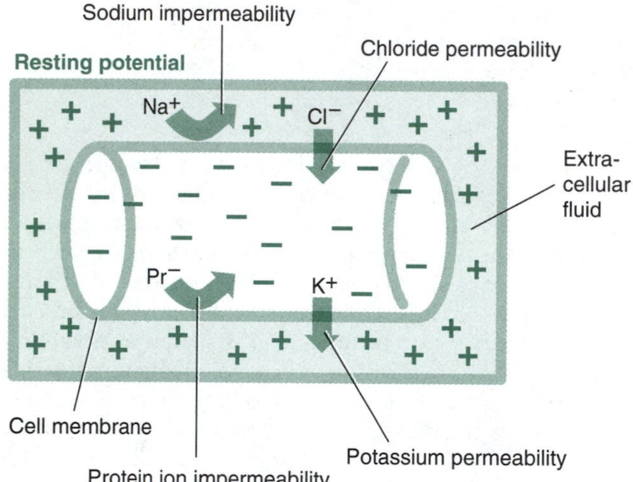

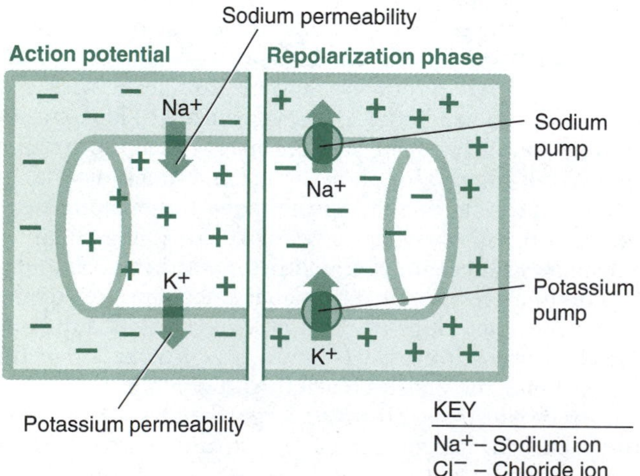

FIGURE 7–6
A membrane potential.

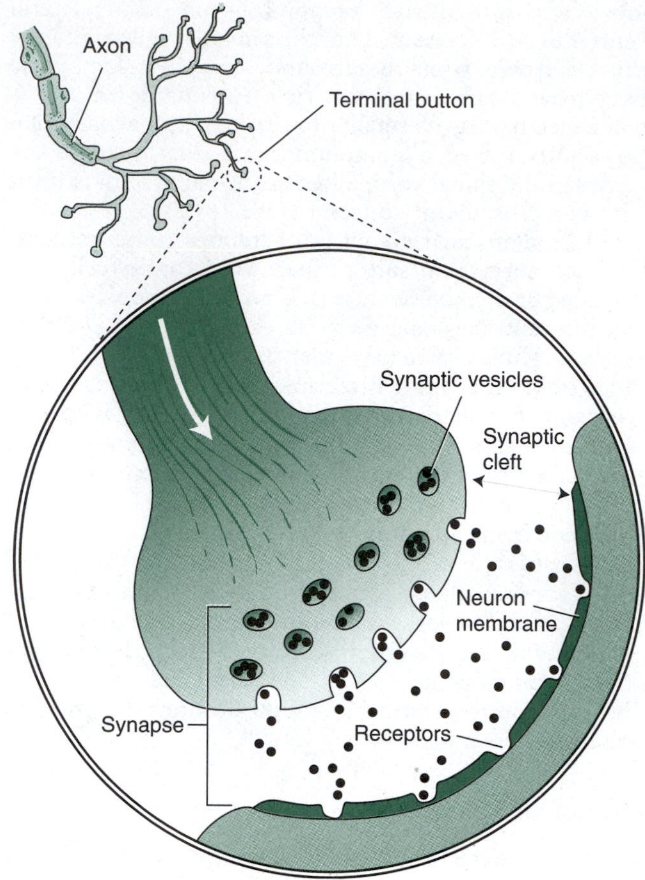

FIGURE 7–7
An axon and a synapse, shown enlarged.

Several secondary messenger systems in the postsynaptic structures also appear to be involved in neuronal transmission through ion systems. Much of the work in neuroscience during the past decade has been focused on the identification of neurotransmitters and their receptor sites and on the better understanding of these secondary messenger systems.

▶ **Check Your Reading**

21. What are the functions of the cell body, axon, and dendrites?
22. Describe the ionic changes that occur in the cell during an action potential.
23. What is the function of the neurotransmitter?

Neurotransmitters

Neurotransmitters of various types can carry different types of messages. Excitatory neurotransmitters open the sodium ion channels in the postsynaptic membrane, causing depolarization of the neuron and allowing transmission of the neuronal impulse. Inhibitory neurotransmitters open the chloride ion channels, causing hyperpolarization of the neuron and inhibition of the neuronal impulse. Although neurotransmitters were previously identified as excitatory or inhibitory, studies have indicated that the same neurotransmitters may play both roles in the body. Current research in neuroscience involves identifying and charting locations of neurotransmitters in the brain and learning how they interact with receptor sites in other neurons. Eight substances have been identified as neurotransmitters. These are classified into three main groups (Box 7–1).

Many neuroscientists believe that mental illness is caused by dysfunction in the brain leading to a breakdown in the neurotransmitter systems (Utas and Cotman, 1993). In this chapter, we will take a closer look at four important neurotransmitter systems: those for acetylcholine, dopamine, norepinephrine, and serotonin. Figure 7–8 shows three of these neurotransmitter systems.

Acetylcholine. Acetylcholine was the first substance recognized as a neurotransmitter within the central nervous system. Although it appears everywhere in the brain, it is found in particularly high concentrations in the basal ganglia and motor cortex. It is known that drugs used to treat schizophrenia and depression interact in some way with acetylcholine, primarily by inhibiting it. These interactions are called *anticholinergic side effects.*

Dopamine. Dopamine is the neurotransmitter that has been identified as elevated in some patients suffering from schizophrenia. Many of the drugs used to treat schizophrenia decrease dopamine transmission. (Dopamine pathways are located in three regions: the substantia nigra, the midbrain, and the hypothalamus.) The dopamine-containing cells of the midbrain project to the limbic cortex, a part of the brain thought to be disrupted in schizophrenia. The dopamine cells of the hypothalamus project to the pituitary, a system important in regulating emotional functions, such as the stress response and sexuality.

BOX 7-1 Neurotransmitters in the Brain

Cholinergic Neurotransmitters

Acetylcholine

Biogenic Amines

Dopamine
Norepinephrine
Serotonin
Histamine

Amino Acids

γ-Aminobutyric acid (GABA)
Glycine
Glutamate

Norepinephrine. Another important neurotransmitter system carries norepinephrine (also called noradrenaline). This system, also called the *noradrenergic system,* begins in a small area of the brain stem and projects from there in a broad, netlike manner up through the midbrain and over the entire cerebral cortex. Some research from neurochemical and pharmacological studies indicates a role for the depletion of norepinephrine in the cause of some types of depression.

Serotonin. Another system implicated in the etiology of depression is the serotonin (or serotoninergic) system. Similar to the norepinephrine system, the serotonin system begins in the midbrain and projects widely throughout the cerebral cortex. It also has input into the thalamus. Some investigators have postulated that there are two subtypes of depression: one caused by abnormalities in norepinephrine balance and the other by abnormalities in serotonin balance (Gold et al, 1988; Bushness, and De Forge, 1994). Current research also indicates a role for the effects of low serotonin levels on aggressive behavior.

▶ Check Your Reading

24. What is the effect called when some drugs used to treat depression and schizophrenia inhibit the acetylcholine system?
25. What neurotransmitter is involved with the development of schizophrenia?
26. What two neurotransmitters are implicated in the development of depression?

NEUROPHYSIOLOGY

To understand the brain more fully, you must know not only the anatomical structures, but also how various parts are related to one another to perform various functions or tasks. This is the scope of the branch of neuroscience called neurophysiology.

Sensory System

The sensory system is composed of many systems widely distributed throughout the brain. Physical sensations are localized in a region called the *somatosensory area,* located just behind the motor strip. The motor strip forms the rear border of the frontal cortex, and the somatosensory area forms the front border of the parietal cortex, which is devoted to integrating sensory information of various types. This area perfectly parallels the motor strip in relation to the body part controlled. Similar to the motor fibers, the sensory fibers are crossed, so that the left side of the brain feels what is happening on the right side of the body and vice versa.

This sensory area collects information about various bodily sensations, such as heat, cold, pain, and pressure or touch. The information sent to this part of the brain is collected by special receptor cells located

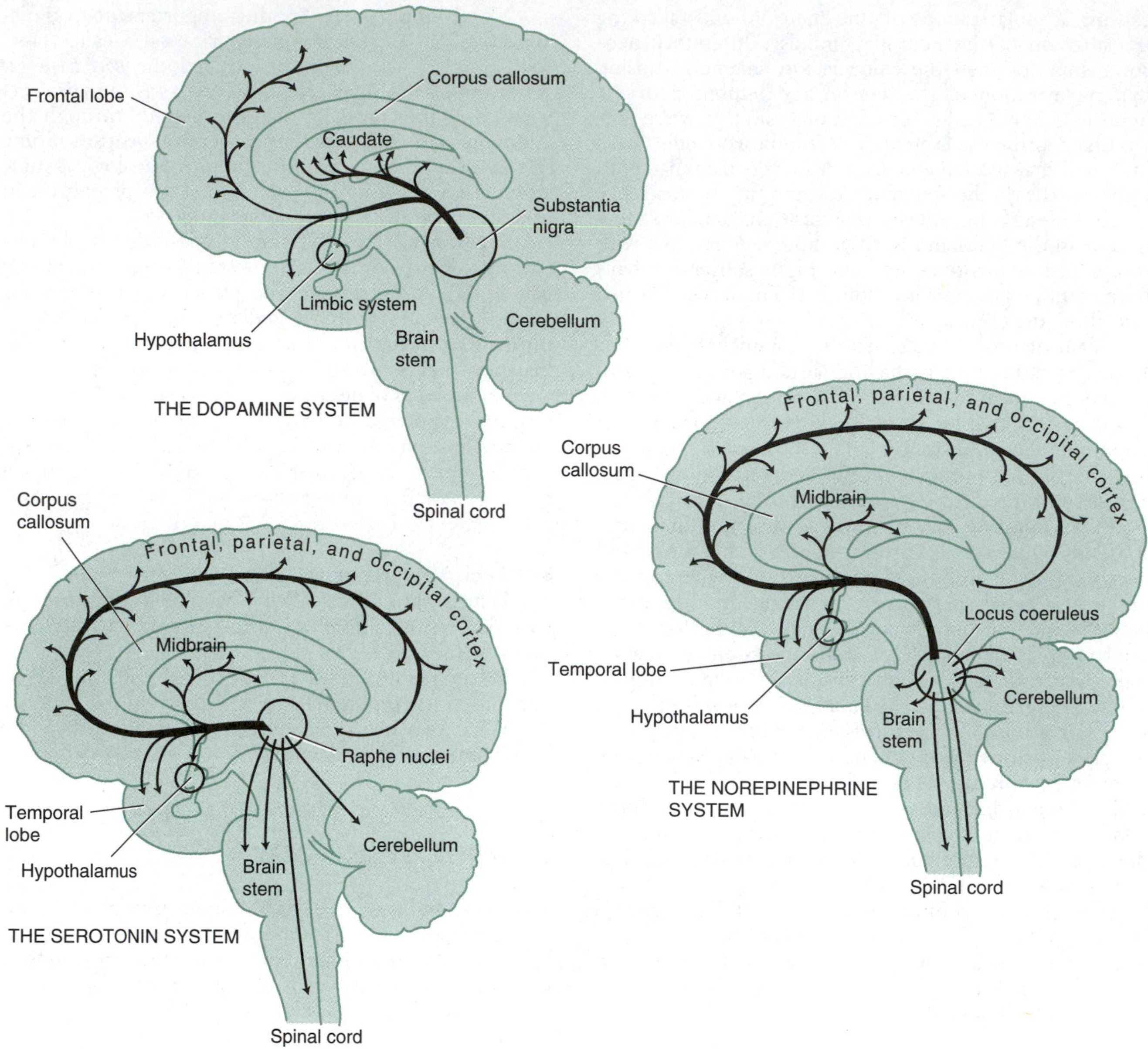

FIGURE 7–8
The dopamine, norepinephrine, and serotonin systems. (Redrawn from THE HUMAN BRAIN COLORING BOOK by Marian C. Diamond. Copyright © 1985 by Coloring Concepts, Inc. Reprinted by permission of HarperCollins Publishers, Inc.)

all over the body. These receptor cells are designed to measure changes in things such as temperature or pressure to the skin. The information they collect is sent on to the thalamus by way of the spinal cord and then on to the somatosensory cortex.

Language System

The language system is unique to the human mind. It is located almost totally in the left hemisphere in most people except in true left-handed individuals. The components of the language system include:

- Broca's area in the frontal lobe
- The auditory cortex and Wernicke's area in the temporal lobe
- The angular gyrus in the parietal lobe
- The visual area in the occipital lobe

The various areas are specialized regions connected by nerve-fiber pathways. Damage to any particular center or the connecting fiber tracts leads to different types of language abnormalities. For example, because Broca's area is the part of the brain that contains information about details of grammar and provides the information permitting people to organize words into fluent speech, damage to Broca's area leads to difficulty in speaking fluently. The angular gyrus is the language storehouse that contains the information that permits us to recognize language when it is presented in visual form, whereas Wernicke's area permits recognition of language in auditory form.

In some patients with mental illness, the language system appears to be affected. Abnormalities in the language system of some patients with schizophrenia is one example. For instance, some patients with schizophrenia use neologisms, private words or phrases coined by the speaker that have special meaning to the speaker and cannot be understood by others. In response to a query by the nurse, for example, the patient responds "ethiuel tanigram."

Memory System

The memory system is localized in many different parts of the brain and probably is not lateralized to only one hemisphere. Memory traces tend to be recorded bilaterally and in several places at the same time. In addition to the hippocampus, the mammillary bodies, the septal region of the limbic system, and part of the thalamus have been identified as structures involved in memory. When damage occurs on only one side, memory usually remains intact, but bilateral lesions lead to a complete memory deficit.

Neuroscientists have conceptualized memory as a two-stage process. Short-term memory is stored temporarily, then forgotten. Long-term memory actually involves learning. In some processes, short-term memory is consolidated and converted to a long-term memory. The hippocampus, mammillary bodies, anterior thalamus, and septal region are probably all centers involved in converting short-term memory to long-term memory.

Frontal System

The understanding of the function of the frontal lobes has been modified significantly. This system now appears to be an important coordinator of emotion, volition, judgment, and creativity. This system, similar to those of the limbic, memory, and language systems, has been noted as being affected by mental illness.

In 1936, the Portuguese psychiatrist and neurologist Egas Moniz advanced our understanding of the frontal lobes by developing techniques of psychosurgery. He speculated that cutting prefrontal fiber tracts in humans might be useful in relieving the agitation of psychotic patients, especially schizophrenics. In 1949, Moniz received a Nobel Prize for developing the technique of prefrontal lobotomy. Although used extensively in the 1950s, it was later realized that the procedure created severe personality deficits in addition to relieving severe agitation.

A more refined charting of the frontal system is now under way with the results indicating an important role in the manifestations of such major mental illnesses as schizophrenia and affective disorders. The frontal lobes contain the cingulate gyrus, which is part of the limbic system. They also receive input from the hypothalamus and the basal ganglia and send messages back to these structures. It is possible that different parts of the frontal system are specialized to perform particular types of volitional and emotional functions.

As stated earlier, research suggests the possibility of malfunction in the frontal lobe in patients diagnosed with schizophrenia. These patients often display bizarre, socially inappropriate behavior and act unpredictably or impulsively. They also tend to have difficulty initiating spontaneous behavior, either through speech or social interactions. Similar to patients with frontal lesions, they may have poor grooming or hygiene. It is difficult to determine, at this point in the process of research, whether these symptoms arise from abnormalities in the frontal system itself or whether they may be caused by a breakdown in communication between the frontal system and other systems.

▶ Check Your Reading

27. What type of information does the sensory area collect?
28. What difficulty does damage to Broca's area create?
29. Which area permits recognition of language in auditory form?
30. In what illnesses is frontal lobe dysfunction suggested?

Neuroendocrine System

The command center of the **neuroendocrine system** lies in the hypothalamus. While nuclei in the brain stem control muscular activities, such as breathing or heart rate, the hypothalamus serves as the mediator between the brain and the body by regulating the endocrine system.

The endocrine system is a group of glands scattered throughout the body. It includes the thyroid, the adrenals, the part of the pancreas that produces insulin, and the sexual glands (testes in males and ovaries in females). The hypothalamus communicates with these glands through hormones, chemical messengers traveling through the bloodstream. The hypothalamus receives continuous feedback from the organs of the endocrine system, which also produce hormones, and uses the feedback to monitor the pituitary. Feedback loops regulate the production of estrogen from the ovaries, androgen (testosterone) from the testes, corticosteroids from the adrenal glands, and thyroid from the thyroid gland. In addition to all of these functions, the hypothalamus with the pituitary as an intermediary is the center for the regulation of aggression, appetite, thirst, water balance, and growth rate. Figure 7–9 illustrates the neuroendocrine cascade.

Research during the last 5 to 10 years has suggested that patients with mood disorders may be suffering from an imbalance in the hypothalamic-pituitary-adrenal axis. Many of the symptoms of mood disorder are consistent with these types of neuroendocrine abnormalities because they involve changes in appetite, sleep regulation, and adaptability to stress and change.

▶ **Check Your Reading**

31. Where is the command center of the neuroendocrine system?
32. What changes occurring in depression are consistent with neuroendocrine abnormalities?

EMERGENCE OF NEUROBIOLOGICAL LABORATORY TESTS

Diagnostic evaluation in most areas of medicine involves three components: history, physical examination, and laboratory tests. Until fairly recently, psychiatrists tended to use only part one of the program of diagnosis. History taking was important, whereas physical examination was likely to elicit few findings (Andreason, 1984). Few laboratory tests were available to the psychiatrist.

Dramatic changes have occurred in the last decade and continue to occur in the diagnostic process in psychiatry. A number of laboratory tests have been developed to illuminate the physical processes underlying the patient's symptoms. Although none of the tests currently provide definitive proof of any particular diagnosis, they have increased the knowledge of physiological changes that accompany mental disorders. Tests include a variety of brain imaging techniques; blood, urine, and cerebrospinal fluid measures of neuroendocrine and neurotransmitter function; and sleep electroencephalography to evaluate the electrical activity of the brain.

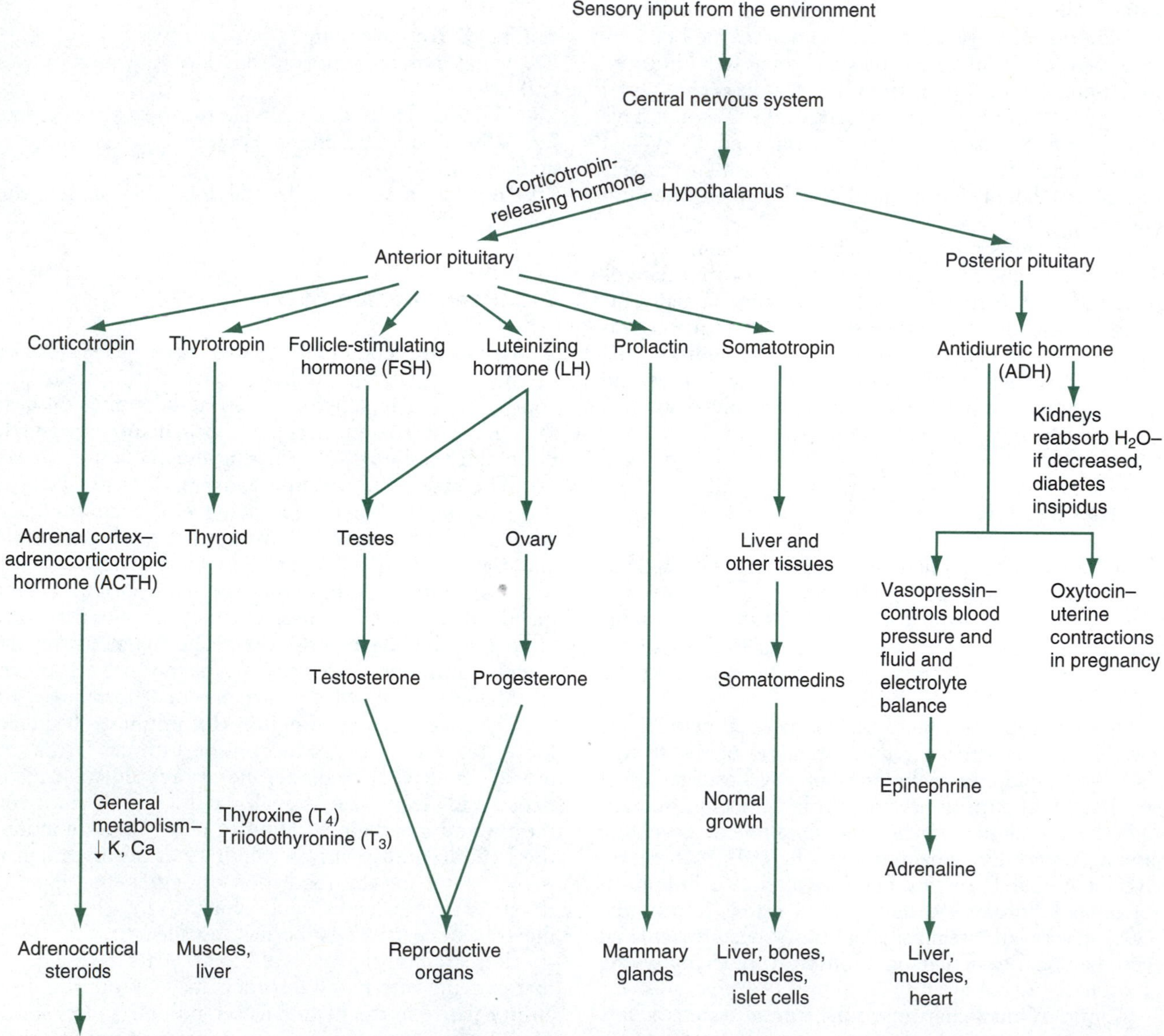

FIGURE 7–9
The neuroendocrine cascade.

Brain Imaging Tests

Computed Tomography

Methods for viewing the brain in vivo were revolutionized during the early 1970s through the introduction of a series of new brain imaging techniques. The most widely used technique is CT scanning. This technique involves sending an x-ray beam through a part of the body, such as the brain, to a set of detectors on the other side. Because the x-ray beam is diminished by the tissues that it passes through, the information collected by the detectors on the other side can be used to construct a picture of different parts of the brain. Its various parts differ in density, from bone being the most dense to fluids the least dense.

The scanner eventually reconstructs a computerized image of the brain by rotating around the body 1 degree at a time and collecting information on the detectors. The process continues until a full 360-degree rotation has been completed. Dense substances such as bone appear white, whereas less dense substances such as cerebrospinal fluid appear nearly black. Gray matter (unmyelinated nerves) would look lighter than white matter (myelinated nerves) because it contains less fat.

Radiologists and psychiatrists working together have developed a method of measuring ventricular size that corrects for overall brain size. This method is called *ventricular-brain ratio* (VBR). It has been found that ventricular enlargement is present in some patients suffering from schizophrenia. It does not, however, provide a tool for differential diagnosis because not all schizophrenic patients have this CT abnormality, whereas patients with other illnesses, such as mania or dementia, may also have abnormal CT scans (Begley et al, 1992). It does indicate that some types of schizophrenia may be due in part to abnormalities in the limbic system.

One exciting area of current research in biological psychiatry involves the correlation between structural brain pathology and various types of schizophrenic symptoms. Through this correlation, a more refined system of classification may be able to be developed. This could have further implications for the prescription of certain types of psychopharmacological drugs.

Magnetic Resonance Imaging

MRI is a technique used for diagnostic evaluations. It has two main advantages over the CT scan: It produces images of extremely high resolution with clear differentiation between small gray matter and white matter structures, and the scanning procedures involve essentially no risk because no radiation is used. Because body cells are rich in hydrogen, phosphorus, and other elements, they are sensitive to electromagnetic forces. The MRI is completed by placing the patient inside a huge circular magnet whose forces cause the hydrogen atoms of the body to move in response. When the force is turned off, the atoms move back to their original position, producing an electromagnetic signal. Different tissues in the body produce different signals. As with CT scanning, these signals are fed into a computer, which creates a picture of the body tissue based on black, gray, and white tiny dots. Although the CT scan cuts tend to be fixed at relatively arbitrary points, an MRI can produce many different views of the three-dimensional structure of the brain (Begley et al, 1992).

Positron Emission Tomography

The CT scan and MRI produce what are known as *static* images of the brain, which yield information on abnormalities of brain structure. Scientists have been developing techniques of *dynamic* brain imaging capable of providing information of brain function.

PET involves the introduction of radioactive substances taken up by the brain. This is accomplished through the injection of glucose labeled with the fluorine-18 positron. Because glucose is the fuel that provides brain cells with nourishment, it serves as a useful substance to differentially identify metabolism in the various parts of the brain. Radiation is emitted from those parts of the brain that are most active and therefore take up the largest amounts of isotopes. Information about the amounts of radiation taken up is then collected on a set of detectors surrounding the brain in a 360-degree circle. As with CT scanning, the brain is broken down into relatively small grids and sectioned in slices.

There are several drawbacks to this diagnostic method. Although a PET scan can accurately track brain function, it cannot resolve structures fewer than 0.5 in apart. This technique also remains expensive. During the past several years, PET scanning has been used to study brain function in patients with affective disorders, schizophrenia, and childhood autism. Through PET scanning, investigators have compared normal subjects with those patients with schizophrenia and autism and scientists have determined that patients suffering from autism and schizophrenia may have a *hypofrontal* pattern while at rest. (Begley et al, 1992). Further studies have tagged the use of neurotransmitters and psychoactive drugs in the brains of patients with mental illnesses.

SQUID Brain Mapping

The superconducting quantum interference device (SQUID) senses tiny changes in magnetic fields. When neurons fire, they create an electric current. These electrical fields induce magnetic fields, which indicate neuronal activity. In this way, brain action can be mapped through the depiction of magnetic fields. This device looks like a strange hair dryer. It has been used most extensively with normal volunteers in an attempt to delineate brain areas associated with the acquisition and utilization of different types of knowledge.

▶ Check Your Reading

33. What do CT scans use through the body to construct the image?
34. What is being correlated in examining schizophrenia?

35. What are the advantages of magnetic resonance imaging over CT scans?
36. What PET abnormalities have been found in some patients with schizophrenia and autism?
37. In what area of research has the SQUID been used?

Neurochemical Tests

In contrast to brain imaging techniques, neurochemical research tends to proceed by inference. Samples of blood, urine, and occasionally cerebrospinal fluid are analyzed to determine the levels of brain chemicals being circulated. Blood tests are also used to determine drug levels for titration with some psychoactive drugs, such as the antidepressants nortriptyline and desipramine, and drugs to treat bipolar disorder, such as lithium and carbamazepine (Tegretol).

Tests of Neuroendocrine Function

It has been noted for years that patients suffering from depression had symptoms similar to people with diseases of the thyroid and adrenal glands. Some of those symptoms included fatigue, change in appetite, and insomnia. Studies have identified that some patients with major depression have neuroendocrine abnormalities, specifically abnormalities of cortisol production (Sachar et al, 1973). The dexamethasone suppression test (DST) was designed to determine if the communication system between the brain and the adrenal glands is dysfunctional. The patient is given a tablet containing dexamethasone, a potent synthetic hormone similar to cortisol. As the blood level of this substance is elevated, the hypothalamus in normal individuals reads the plasma cortisol level as high. It stops sending corticotropic-releasing hormone to the pituitary gland, and, in turn, the pituitary gland stops sending adrenocorticotropic hormone to the adrenals. In so doing, taking the dexamethasone tablet suppresses the hypothalamic-pituitary-adrenal axis, and within 12 hours the blood levels of cortisol drop to low levels. This is considered normal suppression.

In some patients with major depression, their system fails to suppress the dexamethasone, and their plasma cortisol levels continue to be high. The DST is said to be abnormal. Although it is an important diagnostic tool, it identifies depression only in about 50% of the people with major depression because only half have abnormal suppression. Interestingly the DST tends to return to normal when the patient has recovered from the depression. It therefore provides a useful method of monitoring response to treatment.

Other challenge tests have been used to invoke panic disorders with lactate infusion; carbon dioxide inhalation; or the administration of yohimbine, caffeine, or isoproterenol.

Evaluation of MHPG Excretion

Another laboratory test being used more widely is the evaluation of MHPG excretion in urine. MHPG (methoxyhydroxyphenylglycol) is an important breakdown product of norepinephrine. In some people with depression, there is a deficit of norepinephrine in the brain. This leads to a generalized slowing and impairment of function that expresses itself as depressive symptoms. In studying the norepinephrine system of patients with depression, it was determined that they fell into one of three groups: those with relatively high MHPG excretion, those with low excretion, and those with intermediate levels of excretion. Those three groups responded differently to antidepressant medications. Those patients with low MHPG responded best to antidepressant drugs that stimulate the norepinephrine system, whereas those with high MHPG responded to antidepressant drugs that affect the serotonin system (Andreason, 1984).

Electroencephalography

Electroencephalography (EEG) has been used diagnostically in psychiatry for many years. A similarity has been noted in symptoms of patients with temporal lobe epilepsy and some psychiatric diagnoses. Specifically, when the abnormal focus is on the left side, patients tend to be obsessional, humorless, very concerned with religious ideas and have a low libido. These patients closely resemble patients with a diagnosis of obsessive-compulsive personality disorder. In addition, drugs such as carbamazepine, used to treat patients with epilepsy, are now being used to treat patients with depressive disorders.

During the last few decades, neuroscientists have begun to focus on the electrical activity of the brain during sleep. Laboratory studies of sleep in depression confirm that the depressed patient's subjective complaint of insomnia is supported by objective research indicating that sleep patterns are disturbed. This is apparent in non-REM abnormalities in the depressed patient, such as prolonged sleep latency, increased wakefulness, and early morning awakening. It has been suggested that depressed patients are in a chronic state of sleep arousal. They also tend to have a higher mean sleep temperature and flattened sleep curve (Gold et al, 1988).

▶ Check Your Reading

38. What neuroendocrine abnormality do people with major depression experience?
39. For what mental disorder are challenge tests being used?
40. What neurotransmitter does MHPG measure?
41. Patients with temporal lobe epilepsy resemble people with which psychiatric disorder?

IMPLICATIONS OF BIOLOGICAL PSYCHIATRY FOR THE CAUSE OF MENTAL ILLNESS

Despite the tremendous advances in biological psychiatry in the last few decades, the question still remains: What causes mental illness? In the past, the answer to the question was easy: The mentally ill were sinners in the hands of an angry God. There was no controversy because nearly everyone assumed that mental illness was a "spiritual disease," caused by supernatural forces, and that its victims were in some way responsible for their own suffering. Although these attitudes are changing, for many people with a mental illness the stigma still remains. Even today, mental illnesses tend to carry an aura of guilt and moral responsibility.

Confusion about the causes of mental illness has arisen because most people tend to assume that there must be a dichotomy between the mind and the body; hence a disease of the mind must be categorically different from a disease of the body. People cannot control their bodies but can control their mind or spirit. As indicated in the previous discussion of neuroanatomy and neurophysiology, this distinction between mind and body is indeed false. The word *mind* refers to those functions which reside in the brain. When one talks, thinks, or feels, electrical impulses pass through complicated, highly specialized electrical circuits making up the brain. These messages are modulated through chemical processes. Certainly one important etiological factor in the development of mental illness involves the disruption in the normal flow of circuits through the brain.

As with most diseases, mental illnesses are probably caused by multiple factors, some physical, some environmental, and some hereditary. At this point in time, the causes of mental illness are only partially understood. Various types of mental illness are associated with different brain abnormalities, including the loss of nerve cells and excesses and deficits in neurotransmitters between neurons. Sometimes the problems may be associated with the pattern of wiring or circuitry, sometimes poor communication in the command centers, and sometimes in the way the messages move along the wires. The tendency to develop these abnormalities may run in families and therefore be connected to heredity. It may also be due to a broad range of environmental factors, including infection, nourishment, injury, or stress.

Schizophrenia

The search for a cause of the syndrome of related symptoms classified as the disease schizophrenia is perhaps one of the highest priorities in modern psychiatry (Case Example 7–1). Schizophrenia probably produces more years of suffering than any other disease of humans (Andreason, 1984; Erlenmeyer-Kimling et al, 1993; Prager and Jeste, 1993; Torrey et al, 1993).

Case Example 7–1 Mark's Story

Mark is 41 years old, single, and unemployed. He was brought into the emergency room by the police for striking an elderly woman in his apartment building. Mark's chief complaint is "That ugly woman. She and the rest of them deserve more than that for what they put me through."

Mark has been continually ill since the age of 22. During his first year of law school, he had become more and more convinced that his classmates were making fun of him. When a girl that he had dated broke off a relationship with him, he believed that she had been "replaced" by a look-alike. He called the police and asked for their help in solving the "kidnapping." He was asked to leave law school and seek psychiatric help. Although he has been hospitalized 12 times, in the last five years, he has been hospitalized only once for three weeks. Despite the recommendation for continuance of medication on an outpatient basis, Mark stopped taking his medications shortly after leaving the hospital.

Mark maintains that his apartment is the center of a large communication system that involves all of the major television networks, his neighbors, and many "actors" in the neighborhood. There are secret cameras in his apartment that monitor all of his activities. He is not certain who controls the voice that visits him occasionally. He also hears harassing voices telling him which stocks to buy when he is going over his investments.

From Spitzer, R. L., Gibbon, M., Skodal, A. E., Williams, J. B., and First, M. B. (1989). *DSM III-R Casebook.* Washington, D.C.: American Psychiatric Press.

Neurochemical Factors

Changes in brain chemistry are clearly present in some types of schizophrenia. The most widely accepted theory concerning these neurochemical abnormalities is the **dopamine hypothesis** (Reynolds, 1989). According to this hypothesis, schizophrenia is due, in part, to overactive transmission of the neurotransmitter, dopamine, in the brain circuitry. As indicated in Figure 7–5, dopamine is an important messenger in many parts of the limbic system, responsible for the control of emotion and personality. The first evidence for support of this idea came from the development of antipsychotic drugs. These drugs blocked the dopamine receptors in the neuron, preventing them from accepting messages sent through the neurotransmitter, dopamine. Advances have delineated specific dopamine receptors whose blockade seems to improve the positive and negative symptoms of schizophrenia depending on which receptors are blocked. These receptors seem to occur in increased numbers in the basal ganglia and limbic systems of patients suffering from schizophrenia. These results suggest that schizophrenics have "overheated circuits" in their limbic systems because the neurons programmed to receive messages have a larger number of receptors and, therefore, are oversensitive. These receptors are blockaded by antipsychotic drugs (Reynolds, 1989).

Structural Factors

Some patients suffering from schizophrenia have also been noted to have brain abnormalities at the larger structural level. The abnormalities noted most consistently are ventricular enlargements. This is presumably due to brain shrinkage secondary to neuronal death. Ventricular enlargement suggests atrophy may be in deep subcortical gray matter, such as the thalamus, parts of the limbic system, or the basal ganglia. The rate of enlargement in schizophrenic patients ranges from 10% to 50% (Suddarth et al, 1990). In general, the structural abnormalities appear in patients who are more chronically ill and have more social and intellectual deterioration (negative symptoms). It has also been noted that these patients tend to have a poor adjustment even during early childhood, such as lack of interest in making friends or participating in school activities. Additionally, they are less likely to respond to traditional antipsychotic medications.

The evidence from neurochemical and structural studies suggests that schizophrenia is not a single disease but a group of related symptoms that are classified as a single syndrome. One type, referred to as "florid" or "positive" schizophrenia, is characterized by prominent "positive" symptoms, such as delusions and hallucinations. This type tends to respond well to traditional antipsychotic medication treatment. These individuals may suffer from "neurochemical" schizophrenia. Another type, characterized by predominant "negative" or defect symptoms, such as blunted affect and impoverished speech, may be due to diffuse structural damage to the brain as evidenced by ventricular enlargement. In some individuals, there has been improvement in these symptoms with clozapine, a newer antipsychotic drug.

Genetic Factors

People have recognized for centuries that the tendency to develop mental illness runs in families; in other words, mental illness may be influenced by genetic transmission. Early studies of the relatives of schizophrenics summarized by Slater (1968) indicated that although the disorder occurs in only about 1% of the population, parents of schizophrenics had the disease 3.8% of the time, siblings 8.7%, and children 12%. These data support the idea that the rate of schizophrenia is clearly higher in families of schizophrenic patients. Kallman (1946) examined comparative rates of psychiatric disorders in **monozygotic** (identical) twins versus same-sex **dizygotic** (fraternal) twins, both reared together and apart. He found a concordance rate of 86% for monozygotic twins raised either together or apart. Other studies have identified rates of 50% for monozygotic and 10% to 15% for dizygotic twins (Andreason, 1984).

Another hypothesis is that schizophrenia may be due to a viral illness occurring early in life and producing some type of mild encephalitis, or brain inflammation, that predisposes an individual to the development of schizophrenia. This idea has been supported in part by studies of viruslike agents found in the cerebrospinal fluid of some schizophrenics (Andreason, 1984). It has also received support by the observation that more schizophrenics are born during the winter months when viral diseases are more prevalent.

▶ Check Your Reading

42. The drug clozapine has been effective in the treatment of which type of schizophrenic symptoms?
43. There is a higher incidence of schizophrenia in which type of twins?
44. The viral theory of the cause of schizophrenia is supported by what evidence?

Mood Disorders

The story of the search for causes of mood disorders parallels quite closely the exploration of the cause of schizophrenia (Case Example 7–2). The classification of mood disorders includes depressive disorders as well as bipolar disorders. Depressive illness represents a major public health problem. It is estimated that 13% to 29% of the population has some depressive symptoms at any given time (Weissman and Myers, 1978).

Case Example 7–2 Mrs. B's Story

Mrs. B., a 45-year-old legal secretary and mother of two, is brought to a mental health clinic by her concerned husband. Mrs. B. was dressed in wrinkled and slightly soiled clothing. Her hair was carelessly combed and there was a faint body odor about her. Her face was drawn and expressionless. She said nothing unless asked a direct question. Even then, her answers were delayed, spoken slowly and softly, and of a droning and monotonous quality. Mr. B. related that this is the first time in their 26-year marriage that Mrs. B. has acted in this manner. He stated that his wife refuses to see anyone because she wants to rest but he never sees her sleeping. He said that he forces her to eat and became frightened yesterday when she stated that she wanted to die.

Neurochemical Factors

The drug research with mood disorders has led to the formulation of the **catecholamine hypothesis** of depression. This hypothesis states that depression is due, in part, to a deficiency of norepinephrine, one of the major catecholamine systems in the brain (Schildkraut, 1965). Because both monoamine oxidase inhibitors and tricyclic antidepressants increase the availability of norepinephrine at the synapse, investigators cited these drug actions as supporting the norepinephrine deficiency hypothesis of depression.

One early method for measuring norepinephrine was to evaluate the amount of MHPG (one of the breakdown products) in the urine of depressed patients. When urinary MHPG was examined, it was found that some depressed patients, especially those with severe melancholic depression or bipolar patients in the depressed phase, tended to have lower MHPG. This was not true, however, with all patients with a diagnosis of depression (Andreason, 1984).

More recent studies, employing the direct assay of norepinephrine and mass spectroscopic assay of MHPG, support the opposite conclusion—that in major depression, the locus coeruleus–norepinephrine system is activated. These studies report normal or increased levels of cerebrospinal fluid and plasma norepinephrine and increased cerebrospinal fluid and urinary MHPG in patients with major depression (Koslow et al, 1983; Roy et al, 1985; Bushness and DeForge, 1994).

In addition to catecholamines, three neurotransmitters have been studied in relation to mood disorders. The first is acetylcholine, which stimulates the locus coeruleus. Based on pharmacologic data, it has been postulated that patients with major depression possess a hyperresponsive cholinergic system (Janowsky et al, 1980). The second neurotransmitter is GABA, an inhibitory agent that restrains the firing of the locus coeruleus. Cerebrospinal fluid and plasma GABA levels tend to be low in depressed patients (Gerner and Hare, 1981). A third transmitter hypothesized to affect depression is serotonin. Similar to norepinephrine, serotonin transmission is also stimulated by antidepressant drugs. The principal breakdown product of serotonin is 5-hydroxyindoleacetic acid (5-HIAA). In a subgroup of depressed patients, approximately 45% have been found to have low 5-HIAA in their cerebrospinal fluid (Andreason, 1984).

These hypotheses combine to suggest the possibility that there may be subgroups of depressive illness. These developments then may lead to the differential prescription of antidepressant drugs based on neurochemical findings.

Neuroendocrine Factors

Investigation suggests that depressed patients may have another chemical imbalance in their brains. This imbalance involves the regulation of endocrine function through secretions from the hypothalamus to the pituitary gland. Some depressed patients produce large amounts of cortisol and are unable to suppress normally. These phenomena point to a defect in the hypothalamic-pituitary-adrenal axis. Challenge tests with insulin and thyrotropin-releasing hormone suggest that defects do not lie in target organs but are probably at the level of the hypothalamus or higher (Roy et al, 1987).

Genetic Factors

Family studies have consistently shown that the relatives of people suffering from mood disorders have a much higher rate of mania and depression than occurs in the general population. For example, about 20% of the parents of patients with depression also have depression, and the rate in brothers, sisters and children is even higher—possibly as high as 30%. The rate tends to be higher in female relatives than in male relatives. This parallels the higher incidence of depression diagnosed in females. Interestingly the spouses of people suffering from depression also have a relatively high rate of depression—about 20% (Andreason, 1984).

Twin studies also indicate that 65% of monozygotic twins have concordance for the illness as compared with only 14% of dizygotic twins (Kety, 1979).

Circadian Rhythm Hypothesis

Several features of mood disorders suggest abnormalities in circadian rhythms. These include the inherent cycles of depression, the pronounced abnormalities in rest-activity cycle, the length and timing of sleep stages, and the clinical responsiveness to experimental alterations in circadian organization. Changes in both non-REM and REM sleep in patients with mood disorder seem to reflect a pathological state of arousal (Avery et al, 1982).

In addition, a subcategory of mood disorders, seasonal affective disorder, has been identified that seems to point to the importance of circadian rhythms in the cause of depression. People with this syndrome have an apparent reaction to changes in environmental factors, such as climate, latitude, and light.

Kindling and Behavioral Sensitization Hypothesis

Another model that attempts to account for the cyclical pattern of mood disorders is the kindling-sensitization hypothesis (Post et al, 1981). Electrical **kindling** refers to the capacity for intermittent subdepolarization of electrical stimuli in the neuron to produce eventual depolarization and subsequent frank seizure activity. **Sensitization** refers to the effect of repeated stressors on behavioral outcomes. For instance, repeated exposure to inescapable shock may produce a progressive increase in behavioral and neurochemical abnormalities (Cassens et al, 1980). In this model, kindled limbic seizures or the sensitization of the limbic system may account for many features of mood disorders. This could then explain the predisposition for depression caused by stressful early childhood experiences, the gradual worsening of episodes over time, and the decreasing amount of time between depressive episodes (Post et al, 1981).

▶ Check Your Reading

45. Which factors in mood disorders point to changes in circadian rhythms?
46. What symptoms of mood disorders support a kindling-sensitization model?

Anxiety Disorders

Although it is clear that environmental factors play an important role in the production of anxiety disorders, research has also demonstrated that major biological mechanisms have etiological significance (Case Example 7–3).

Case Example 7–3 Jack's Story

A 27-year-old married electrician, Jack, came to his nurse practitioner complaining of dizziness, sweaty palms, heart palpitations, and ringing of the ears of more than 18 months' duration. Jack stated that he also experiences dry mouth and throat, periods of uncontrollable shaking, and a constant watchful feeling that interferes with his ability to concentrate. Jack complained that these feelings have remained almost constant for the last two years. He also has many worries, including the fear of a sudden death of his father, the fear of infidelity on the part of his wife, and the fear that he is not a good father. These fears appear to be unwarranted.

From Spitzer, R. L., Gibbon, M., Skodal, A. E., Williams, J. B., and First, M. B. (1989). *DSM-III-R Casebook*. Washington, D.C.: American Psychiatric Press.

Neurochemical Factors

The GABA system was mapped somewhat later than the acetylcholine, dopamine, serotonin, and norepinephrine systems. In contrast to the excitatory nature of the other classic neurotransmitters, investigators were aware that the GABA system probably worked to exert an inhibitory effect. It has been determined that one way antianxiety drugs work may be to enhance the effect of the GABA system in the brain, thereby assisting it in modulating or slowing down other brain systems that might be stimulating arousal or anxiety (Gurguis and Uhde, 1990; Brawman-Mintzer et al, 1994; Brown et al, 1994).

Scientists have also discovered a *benzodiazepine receptor* in the brain of the rat. Benzodiazepine receptors are widely distributed throughout the cerebral cortex, cerebellar cortex, amygdala, hippocampus, and dentate gyrus, suggesting that they have a diffuse and important modulating effect. GABA and benzodiazepine receptors tend to be located close to one another on neurons, implying that they may mutually facilitate one another.

A recent development in the treatment of one type of anxiety disorder, panic disorders, has been identified. Through the use of lactate infusion, investigators are able to produce a panic attack in about 90% of untreated patients who have complained of panic attacks in the past. This infusion did not produce panic attacks in a significant number of normal controls with no history of panic attacks (Pitts and McClure, 1967). Patients with panic disorder who had been pretreated with the antidepressant imipramine typically reported no panic attacks. This creates some question as to the relationship biochemically of panic disorder and depression. Patients with panic disorders tend to have a higher level of epinephrine, suggesting some abnormality in the catecholamine system.

Genetic Factors

Evidence is steadily accumulating that a predisposition to develop anxiety disorders may also be partly hereditary. Early studies, based on the review of patients' records and family histories, suggested that relatives of people with anxiety disorders have an illness rate of about 20% as compared with a general population rate of 5%. Female relatives are affected about twice as often as male relatives. Crowe (1984) summarized lifetime prevalence rates for first-degree relatives of a patient with a panic disorder as 61%.

Torgerson (1983) compared 32 monozygotic and 53 same-sex dizygotic twins in Norway and concluded that hereditary factors were significant in panic disorder but not in generalized anxiety disorder. This suggests that there may be a significant genetic component to a predisposition for panic disorders, but the data on anxiety disorders are still equivocal.

To capture the complexity of the issue and the enormity of the task of understanding mental illness, Guze (1989) suggests that we conceptualize cause based on a "biopsychosocial model that views the role of biological and genetic sciences in interplay with environment, learning and culture in growth and development of all forms of life, including human life" (p. 318).

▶ Check Your Reading

47. How do antianxiety drugs work within the system?
48. Patients with panic disorders share some biochemical similarities with what other type of illness?

CONCLUSIONS

Before the findings from this revolution in psychiatry can be incorporated into the practice of psychiatric nursing, nurses must have a basic understanding of the neurosciences. Because the education of nurses has always required a foundation in both the social and the natural sciences, nurses are in a unique position to expand their knowledge base of anatomy and physiology to incorporate the neurosciences. Although the neuroscience body of knowledge is relatively new to nurses, it differs from our previous understanding of mental disorders as arising from a psychodynamic or social interactionist model. The administration of somatic therapies that directly alter the brain and mind's function has always been within the purview of nursing. Now we have an opportunity to understand as well as contribute to the knowledge of how these therapies work.

The emphasis on biological psychiatric nursing will continue to be needed until we are as comfortable in understanding the physiodynamics of mental illness as we are with the psychodynamics. This blend will provide both a basis for examining old practices and a basis for developing new intervention strategies. This new perspective should help us to stretch our creativity and allow us to develop new nursing approaches to the treatment of mental illnesses.

KEY POINTS TO REMEMBER

- Psychobiology involves the study of the biochemical foundations of thought, mood, affect, emotion, and behavior.
- The term *neurosciences* encompasses a set of related disciplines that share the common goal of understanding the relationship

between brain structure and function and human thoughts, feelings, and behavior.

- New areas of brain research affecting the revolution in biological psychiatry include brain imaging, understanding the biological dimensions of emotion, the role of neurochemicals in the formation and enactment of behavior, shifting knowledge of brain plasticity after birth, and understanding molecular genetics.
- Myelination differentiates white matter from gray matter.
- The corpus callosum connects the right hemisphere with the left.
- Afferent tracts travel to the brain.
- Glial cells are the supporting, cementing, and nourishing structures for the neuron.
- The cell body is the work center of the neuron. The axons are the wires of the nervous system. The dendrites increase the ability of the neuron to receive information.
- During an action potential, the permeability of the membrane forming the axon changes, causing positively charged sodium ions to flow in.
- The function of the neurotransmitter is to send the message chemically.
- An anticholinergic effect occurs when some drugs used to treat depression and schizophrenia inhibit the acetylcholine system.
- It is believed that dopamine is involved in the development of schizophrenia.
- Norepinephrine and serotonin are implicated in the development of depression.
- Serotonin has been linked with aggressive behavior.
- The frontal lobe is the seat of intellectual functioning. The parietal lobe receives information about various bodily sensations and synthesizes and elaborates sensory impulses. The occipital lobe receives and sends out information. It contains the primary visual area. The temporal lobe receives auditory impulses, stores memory patterns for symbolic sounds, receives and transmits gustatory impulses, and receives and transmits olfactory input.
- Disruption in the occipital lobe may lead to illusions and hallucinations.
- Diencephalon structures serve as relay stations between the lower brain centers and the higher cortical centers.
- The thalamus is the major pathway for sensory and motor impulses to and from the cerebral hemispheres and the modulator of emotions and behavior.
- The hypothalamus regulates hormonal function.
- The brain stem regulates the activities of the heart, respiration, and other vital functions.
- The cerebellum is a major modulator of movement.
- The role of the limbic system is to modulate emotions.
- The pineal gland partially regulates the sleep-wake cycle.
- The paired mammillary bodies function in the process of learning and memory.
- Depression may be associated with hyperarousal in the hypothalamic-pituitary-adrenal axis.
- The basal ganglia function as modulators of movement and integrators of sensory information.
- Schizophrenia may be associated with basal ganglia dysfunction.
- Huntington's chorea and Parkinson's disease involve basal ganglia structures.
- The ventricular system is of interest to neuroscientists because ventricular enlargement provides a useful index of brain atrophy, and ventricles are major landmarks seen on CT scans. Ventricular enlargement has also been noted in some patients with schizophrenia and dementia.
- Damage to Broca's area leads to difficulty in speaking fluently.
- Wernicke's area permits recognition of language in auditory form.
- In schizophrenia, there is a possibility of frontal lobe dysfunction.
- The command center of the neuroendocrine system lies in the hypothalamus.
- Changes in appetite, sleep regulation, and adaptability to stress and change occurring in depression are consistent with neuroendocrine abnormalities.
- CT scans use X-ray beams through the body to construct an image.
- CT and MRI identify structure, whereas PET identifies function.
- Some patients with schizophrenia and autism have been found to have hypofrontality on PET scans.
- SQUID has been used with normal volunteers to delineate areas associated with the acquisition and utilization of different types of knowledge.
- Some people with major depression experience abnormalities of cortisol production.
- Patients with temporal lobe epilepsy resemble patients with obsessive-compulsive disorder.
- Patients with major depression may experience prolonged sleep latency, increased wakefulness, and early morning awakening.
- There is a higher incidence of schizophrenia in monozygotic twins.
- The viral theory of the cause of schizophrenia is supported by a viruslike agent found in the cerebrospinal fluid of some schizophrenics and the observation that more schizophrenics are born during the winter months, when viral diseases are more prevalent.
- Norepinephrine, serotonin, acetylcholine, and GABA have been studied in relation to mood disorders.
- The hypothalamic-pituitary-adrenal axis is implicated in the inability of the neuroendocrine system to suppress cortisol.
- Inherent cycles of depression, the pronounced abnormalities in rest-activity cycle, and the length and timing of sleep stages are all factors in mood disorders that point to changes in circadian rhythms.
- The gradual worsening of episodes over time and the decreasing amount of time between episodes are symptoms of mood disorders supporting a kindling-sensitization model of etiology.
- The benzodiazepine receptor facilitates the GABA system.

LEARNING ACTIVITIES

1. Draw and diagram an axon and a synapse.
2. Draw and diagram a neuron.
3. Make a chart showing the disorders of schizophrenia, depression, and anxiety. For each of the disorders, identify the major neurotransmitters involved, the area of the brain most implicated, and the results of the brain dysfunction.
4. As you proceed through your psychiatric clinical experience, formulate both a psychodynamic and a biological explanation for each of your patients' diagnoses. Once you have done that, go back to the formulation and show the interaction of environment, experience, and biology.
5. What role do you think that spirituality plays in biological psychiatry?

CRITICAL THINKING EXERCISES

Mr. Norman, an 18-year-old, was admitted to the crisis center after he was found running down the street naked at 2 o'clock in the morning. He was diagnosed as having an acute psychotic episode. Mr. Alder, a nurse who has 30 years of experience with psychiatric patients, tells his new graduate nurse, Mr. Newman, about the way the patient's family used to be informed about the treatment and causes of schizophrenia. He states that he was taught that families were to blame for causing the illness, particularly the mother who gave out mixed messages. Today we are taught that biology and chemistry play an important role in the development of major psychiatric disorders.

1. What inference can Mr. Newman draw about Mr. Alder's beliefs about nursing practice?
2. What are the consequences of attributing the etiology of mental illness to biological factors?

Mr. Alder approaches Mr. Norman's mother and father to give them information about their son's condition. He tells them about their son's drugs and their actions. He also tells them that it is important that they know about the illness so that they can support their son to reach his best level of functioning. Mr. Newman notices that Mr. Norman's parents are attentive and listening to Mr. Alder's instruction.

1. What information would the nurse want to include in discussing Mr. Norman's illness and care?
2. What is an alternative to the above approaches?

REFERENCES

Andreason, N. (1984). *The Broken Brain.* New York: Harper & Row.

Avery, D. H., Wildschiodtz, G., and Rafaelsen, O. J. (1982). Nocturnal temperature in affective disorder. *Journal of Affective Disorders, 4,* 61–71.

Barondes, S. H. (1990). Biological approach to psychiatry. *The Journal of Neuroscience, 10*(6), 1707–1710.

Begley, S., Wright, L., Church, V., and Hager, M. (1992). Mapping the brain. *Newsweek*

Benes, F. M. (1993). Neurobiological investigations in cingulate cortex of schizophrenic brain. *Schizophrenia Bulletin, 19*(3), 537–550.

Brawman-Mintzer, O., Lydiard, R. B., Crawford, M. M., Emmanuel, N., Payeur, R., Johnson, M., Knapp, R. G., and Ballenger, J. C. (1994). Somatic symptoms in generalized anxiety disorder with and without comorbid psychiatric disorders. *American Journal of Psychiatry, 151*(6), 930–933.

Brown, T. A., Barlow, D. H., and Liebowitz, M. R. (1994). The empirical basis of generalized anxiety disorder. *American Journal of Psychiatry, 151*(9), 1271–1281.

Bushness, F. K. L., and DeForge, V. (1994). Seasonal affective disorder. *Perspectives in Psychiatric Care, 30*(4), 21–25.

Cassens, G., Roffman, M., Kuruc, A., Orsulak, P. J., and Schildkraut, J. J. (1980). Alterations in brain norepinephrine metabolism induced by environmental stimuli previously paired with inescapable shock. *Science, 209,* 1138–1140.

Charlton, B. G. (1990). A critique of biological psychiatry. *Psychological Medicine, 20,* 3–6.

Crowe, R. (1984). The role of genetics in the etiology of panic disorder. *Psychiatric Update, 3,* 402–410.

Erlenmeyer-Kimling, L., Cornblatt, B. A., Rock, D., Roberts, S., Bell, M., and West, A. (1993). The New York high-risk project: Anhedonia, attentional deviance, and psychopathology. *Schizophrenia Bulletin, 19*(1), 141–152.

Gerner, R. H., and Hare, T. A. (1981). CSF GABA in normal subjects and patients with depression, schizophrenia, mania, and anorexia nervosa. *American Journal of Psychiatry, 138,* 1098–1101.

Gold, P. W., Goodwin, F. K., and Chrousos, G. P. (1988). Clinical and biochemical manifestations of depression. *New England Journal of Medicine, 319,* 348–353.

Gurguis, G. N., and Uhde, T. W. (1990). In J. R. Walker, G. R. Norton, and C. A. Ross (Eds.), *Panic Disorder and Agoraphobia: A Guide for the Practitioner.* Pacific Grove, California: Brooks/Cole Publishing.

Guze, S. B. (1989). Biological psychiatry: Is there any other kind? *Psychological Medicine, 19,* 315–323.

Hill, L. (1991). The neurophysiology of acute anxiety: A review of the literature. *CRNA: The Clinical Forum for Nurse Anesthetists,* 2(2), 52–61.

Janowsky, D. S., Risch, S. C., Parker, D., Huey, L., and Judd, L. (1980). Increased vulnerability to cholinergic stimulation in affective disorder patients. *Psychopharmacology Bulletin, 16,* 29–31.

Kallmann, E. (1946). The genetic theory of schizophrenia. *American Journal of Psychiatry, 103,* 309–322.

Kety, S. S. (1979). Disorders of the human brain. *Scientific American, 24*(3), 202–218.

Koslow, J. H., Maas, J. W., Bowden, C. L., Davis, J. M., Hanin, I., and Javaid, J. (1983). Cerebrospinal fluid and urinary biogenic amines and metabolites in depression and mania: A controlled univariate analysis. *Archives of General Psychiatry, 40,* 999–1010.

McEnany, G. W. (1991). Psychobiology and psychiatric nursing: A philosophical matrix. *Archives of Psychiatric Nursing, 5,* 255–261.

Pam, A. (1990). A critique of the status of biological psychiatry. *Psychological Medicine, 20,* 3–6.

Pitts, N. E., Jr., and McClure, J. N., Jr. (1967). Lactate metabolism in anxiety neurosis. *New England Journal of Medicine, 277,* 1329–1336.

Post, R. M., Ballenger, J. C., Uhde, R. W., Putman, F. W., and Bunney, W. E. (1981). Kindling and drug sensitization: Implications for the progressive development of psychopathology and treatment with carbamazepine. In M. Sandler (Ed.): *The Psychopharmacology of Anticonvulsants* (pp. 27–53). Oxford: Oxford University Press.

Prager, S., and Jeste, D. V. (1993). Sensory impairment in late-life schizophrenia. *Schizophrenia Bulletin, 19*(4), 755–772.

Reynolds, G. P. (1989). Beyond the dopamine hypothesis. *British Journal of Psychiatry, 155,* 305–316.

Roy, A., Pickar, P., Linnoila, M., and Potter, W. Z. (1985). Plasma norepinephrine level in affective disorders: Relationship to melancholia. *Archives of General Psychiatry, 42,* 1181–1185.

Roy, A., Pickar, P., Paul, S., Doran, A., Chrousos, G. P., and Gold, P. W. (1987). CSF corticotropin-releasing hormone in depressed patients and normal control subjects. *American Journal of Psychiatry, 144,* 641–645.

Sachar, E. J., Hellman, L., Roffwarg, H. P., Halpern, F. S., Fukushima, D. K., and Gallagher, T. F. (1973). Disrupted 24-hour pattern of cortisol secretion in psychotic depression. *Archives of General Psychiatry, 28,* 19–26.

Schildkraut, J. J. (1965). The catecholamine hypothesis of affective disorders: A review of supporting evidence. *American Journal of Psychiatry, 122,* 509–520.

Slater, E. (1968). A review of earlier evidence in genetic factors in schizophrenia. In D. Rosenthal and S. Kety (Eds.), *The Transmission of Schizophrenia* (pp. 15–26). Oxford: Pergamon Press.

Spitzer, R. L., Gibbon, M., Skodol, A. E., Williams, J., and First, M. (1989). *DSM III-R Casebook.* Washington, D.C.: American Psychiatric Press.

Stein, M. B., Walker, J. R., and Forde, D. R. (1994). Setting diagnostic thresholds for social phobia: Considerations from a community survey of social anxiety. *American Journal of Psychiatry, 151*(3), 408–413.

Suddarth, R. L., Christison, G. W., and Torry, E. F. (1990). Cerebral anatomical abnormalities in monozygotic twins discordant for schizophrenia. *New England Journal of Medicine, 322,* 789–794.

Torgerson, S. (1983). Genetic factors in anxiety disorders. *Archives of General Psychiatry, 40,* 1085–1089.

Torrey, E. F., Bowler, A. E., Rawlings, R., and Terrazas, A. (1993). Seasonality of schizophrenia and stillbirths. *Schizophrenia Bulletin, 19*(3), 557–562.

Utas, J., and Cotman, C. W. (1993). Excitatory amino acid receptors in schizophrenia. *Schizophrenia Bulletin, 19*(1) 105–117.

Weissman, M. M., and Myers, J. K. (1978). Rates and risks of depressive symptoms in a U.S. urban community. *Acta Psychiatrica Scandinavia, 57,* 219–231.

SUGGESTED READINGS

Bushness, F. K. L., and DeForge, V. (1994). Seasonal affective disorder. *Perspectives in Psychiatric Care, 30*(4), 21–25.

Guze, S. B. (1989). Biological psychiatry: Is there any other kind? *Psychological Medicine, 19,* 315–323.

Hill, L. (1991). The neurophysiology of acute anxiety: A review of the literature. *CRNA: The Clinical Forum for Nurse Anesthetists,* 2(2), 52–61.

Janowsky, D. S., Risch, S. C., Parker, D., Huey, L., and Judd, L. (1980). Increased vulnerability to cholinergic stimulation in affective disorder patients. *Psychopharmacology Bulletin, 16,* 29–31.

McEnany, G. W. (1991). Psychobiology and psychiatric nursing: A philosophical matrix. *Archives of Psychiatric Nursing, 5,* 255–261.

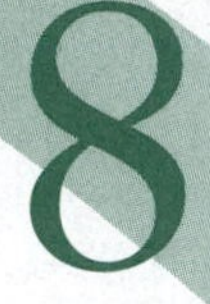

CHAPTER 8

SHARED ATTRIBUTES OF EVERY TRAVELER

THE MOSAIC OF SELF-CONCEPT

Man is empowered by God to hope and hopes fervently, until that for which he is hoping takes the cloak of oblivion from his eyes whereupon he will at last view his real self. And he who sees his real self sees the truth of real life for himself, for all humanity, and for all things.

—*Kahlil Gibran*

LEARNING OBJECTIVES

After studying this chapter, you should be able to:

1. Define self, self-concept, and all of the interrelated dimensions of self-concept
2. Describe the key factors that influence the development of the self and self-concept
3. Discuss the reciprocal relationship between basic human needs according to Maslow and the progression through the developmental stages according to Erikson
4. Explain how human beings are more alike than they are different and how sharing our humanness can affect another's self-concept

KEY TERMINOLOGY

Birth order
Body image
Cognitive processes
Developmental tasks
Emotional processes
Family constellation
Gender identity
God-consciousness
Hierarchy of needs
Ideal self
Meaning
Perceptual processes
Personal identity
Personality
Physical self
Psychological self
Purpose
Role conflict
Roles
Self
Self-awareness
Self-concept
Self-confidence
Self-efficacy
Self-esteem
Self-respect
Self-position
Sibling position
Social self
Spiritual self

Pat Benner (1984) states in her book *From Novice to Expert: Excellence and Power in Clinical Nursing Practice*, "Nursing students enter a new clinical area as novices; they have little understanding of the contextual meaning of the recently learned textbook terms. But, students are not the only novices: any nurse entering a clinical setting where she or he has no experience with the patient population may be limited to the novice level if the goals and tools of patient care are unfamiliar" (p. 21). In the following stories, you are introduced to Sarah and Glen, both nursing students, both novices as they enter into the realm of psychiatric nursing. Let's take a look at how Sarah and Glen view themselves, their strengths, their weaknesses, and their fears and anticipations about psychiatric nursing.

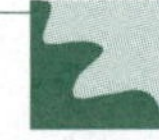

THE STORIES OF TWO STUDENT NURSES

Sarah and Glen, two senior nursing students, are sitting in their apartment attempting to complete a written assignment prior to their first clinical day in a psychiatric facility. The directive given in class was to "go home, think about who you are, and write down in a journal all that you know about yourself, your strengths, weaknesses, any special qualities, even how you see yourself physically. What is there about you that will affect how you relate to the patients that you will meet during the upcoming semester?" The following journals were written:

Sarah

"Who am I? I am Sarah Smith! I am 20 years old. I was born in Washington, D.C. I am 5′11″, weigh 120 pounds, and my parents think I'm too thin. But my own opinion is that I could lose a few pounds. I am a nursing student in my last semester of school. I should graduate in June if I can finish this psych thing and get through it as fast as possible. I'm more of a med-surg type of person and am scared to death of entering a psych facility. What will I do all day without IVs to check, shots to give, or treatments to do? I'm not much of a talker. I've always been a thinker and a doer. My mother always said, 'If you want something done, ask Sarah to do it.' My dad left when I was 3 years old. He was an alcoholic! This communication stuff really has me concerned; I'm just not good at it. My younger sister was always the talker-feeler person in our family, so I didn't have to be. I'll just have to see how this semester goes. Why do we have to write this stuff anyway? I hope I don't have to talk about religion."

Glen

"I am Glen. I am 19 years old, the younger brother of two older sisters. I was born in Minnesota, and I'm Irish Catholic. I can't wait to go to the psych hospital. I have been waiting for this experience since I decided to come to nursing school. Med-surg was OK, but I kept getting into a time crunch because I wanted to talk with my patients instead of doing all the tasks that were assigned—like bed-making, washing out my patients' elastic stockings, and the like. We always seemed to get into wonderful conversations about their feelings, and I just couldn't leave. The problem was, I was always late for post-conference, and I usually got a message from my instructor that I forgot to complete all of my assignments. I felt terrible! Maybe now that I'm going to psych I can finally listen to people's feelings and not worry about doing things. My parents always taught me that it's what people have to say that is important and that I've always been a good listener. God knows, I had enough practice listening to all of my sisters' problems. Oh! I almost forgot . . . I am 5′10″ tall, and I weigh 170 pounds. (I think I'm huggable!) I hope my patients like me! I wonder what psych patients are like? I wonder if I can do as well as I think I can?"

How are these two students going to do in their "psych rotation," as they call it? Will both succeed? Will one have an easier time than the other? Will their experiences be the same? What will they need to learn to have a meaningful experience? What will they need to do to have a positive experience? Will they have to learn the same things? What challenges will each face during this stage of growth and development as people and as professionals? Who are the patients that they will meet?

In the psychiatric arena, nurses are called upon to "use the self" therapeutically. This demands that the nurse know who she or he is personally and that she or he intertwine that personal self with the knowledge and skills required by the specialty to gain experience that will allow the professional self to develop. Becoming an expert is dependent less on time and more on experience and on the refinement of "head" knowledge through encounters with many practical situations that add depth, nuances, and shades of difference to theory (Benner 1984).

Expert nurses grow to the point that their perceptual abilities give direction to the nursing care that is delivered. "The expert nurse often describes her perceptual abilities as 'a gut feeling' or 'a sense of uneasiness' or 'a feeling that things are not quite right.' Experts dare not stop with vague hunches, but neither do they dare to ignore those hunches that could lead to early identification of problems and the search for confirming evidence" (Benner, 1984, p. xix).

Thus, the transition from student or novice to expert practitioner requires time, experience, and risk-taking. The nurse must understand that he or she may not have all of the answers in a situation or may not be totally sure of "all the right moves." Instead, the nurse must trust in his or her limited theory based abilities and be willing to share his or her humanness to facilitate connectedness with others.

Psychiatric nurses learn to trust that patients often know what is needed to remedy a situation. Furthermore, if patients are given the opportunity to put forth their story, they are frequently able to articulate the problem to the point where options become evident. For the nurse, the key to this process is to allow herself or himself the opportunity to "be present to the patient" even when the answers are not apparent.

To "connect" with another human being, one must clearly define the "self" that is being offered. In this chapter you explore the development of the self and concepts related to self. Questions are asked that will stimulate thinking about the self. Such thinking begins the "journey toward understanding each individual's uniqueness." Once the personal self is explored, the professional self that is "becoming" can emerge, so that caring, kindness, and commitment can be shared with peers and patients as each searches for meaning and understanding in his or her experiences.

Sarah and Glen are about to embark on an incredible journey into their self and the self of others. They may be surprised to find that they are more similar to their patients than they ever believed was possible.

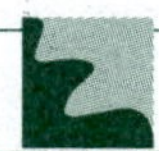

THE STORIES OF TWO PATIENTS

Ray

Ray came into the hospital because of depression. Although only 26, he felt older than his years. Although Ray was well groomed and attractive, his shoulders were bent, and his eyes were sad. He appeared to be burdened with the weight of many sorrows. Initially, he attributed his sadness to a work situation in which he had been passed over for a promotion. But as his story unfolded, it became apparent that the missed promotion was only his most recent disappointment:

"I am the oldest of three brothers. I used to tell myself that my family was loving and close. That's what we always told each other. But I have slowly come to realize that our only family bond was the well-kept secret that Mom is an alcoholic. My father avoided our home situation by working two jobs. I remember having to care for my younger brothers when my mother was too drunk and my dad was gone. I think that's why I am so responsible now—almost too responsible. I seldom laugh or see the lighter side of things. When I let myself think about it, I feel angry that somehow I got cheated out of being a kid. We never hugged in our family. I remember that when I went away to college, my mother gave me a hug. She felt like a board. I'm sure that I was just as stiff with her. Can you believe that I don't know how to hug? What do you do when someone kisses you on the cheek? Kiss them back or what? These may seem like dumb questions, but we just didn't kiss one another in my family.

I really never did fit in. Maybe it was because I was too busy acting grown up, but my parents never told me I was doing a good job, and my brothers resented me for being the boss. I wasn't much of an athlete, but I loved music. I learned to play the guitar, and I can sing pretty well. But when I was little, if you didn't hit a baseball, you were a loser. I remember some of the boys in my neighborhood calling me 'gay Ray.' That still hurts. The fact that I didn't get the promotion stirred up a lot of old and painful feelings for me."

Renae

Renae was seen in outpatient therapy to monitor her serum levels of lithium, a medication that she had been taking for several years. Renae had been diagnosed with bipolar disorder, characterized primarily by manic episodes. Renae's story reveals that, despite her illness, she had had a happy childhood:

"I am the middle sister. I have a pretty good relationship with both of my sisters. Oh yeah—we argue. Don't all sisters? But when I need someone to talk to, I usually go to one of them. We have an interesting family. Some people would say we have a high craziness factor. I prefer to think of us as flamboyant. I'm not the only manic-depressive. My older sister has the same thing, only she tends to get depressed. I prefer *my* symptoms— especially when I am not out of control. I have so many ideas. I write and draw and dance. The arts are really my thing. My mom gets mildly depressed, but she has never received treatment. I think my dad is mildly manic, although he denies it. But I know—I recognize the signs. What a trip, that my mother and father got hooked up together!

I had my first manic episode right after high school graduation. I really 'freaked out.' I got wilder throughout the summer. I messed with drugs and had sex with anyone. By the end of the summer, I was depressed and tried to kill myself by jumping from a tree. I ended up with a really bad fracture of my arm. I spent some time in a psych hospital and was released. But I had to get sick several more times before I was diagnosed with manic-depression and started taking lithium.

During the last 10 years, I would take my medication for a while, then I would begin to feel good and stop the medication. And I would always get sick again. When I get sick, my main symptom is wild sexual behavior. When I don't take my medication, I am 5′3″ tall and weigh 120 pounds; I weigh 160 pounds when I do take my medication. I want to understand my illness and put it into the larger picture, if you know what I mean. It was very humiliating to realize that I could never control my illness without lithium. I am beginning to think of my mania as both a gift and a burden. I think it is my illness that allows me to always want more, to see things in different ways and to have boundless energy. My imagination is great, but I have to be careful with whom I share it. When I tell people about my fantasies and they know my history, they panic and think I am getting manicky. They don't know that this is just who I am."

Which nursing student would be better suited to work with which patient? What are the commonalities involved between student and patient? What are the differences? What are the identifiable strengths within each of the students that fit with the patients' strengths? We examine these issues as we move through the chapter.

In the examples just cited, both students and patients have a great deal to offer each other, once the initial hesitancies are overcome. When students are anticipating their first psychiatric experiences, they often express fears about personal safety and concern about perceived inadequacies in communicating with patients. Questions such as "What if they are out of control?" and "What if I say something to set them off?" characterize the initial concerns. As the psychiatric experience progresses, the nature of the students' fears changes. The focus shifts to an awareness that similarities exist between the patients and themselves, and new fears emerge that are related to the students' own mental health such as "Could I end up like this?," "Am I all that different?," and "What makes me healthy and them sick?" Although these concerns may be frightening, their recognition that patients are not so different signals a transition in the students' thinking. This transition allows the students to understand the patients and begin to assume the "helper" role.

Patients also have fears, such as "sounding like I'm crazy," "being seen as weak and ineffective," and "finding no one to understand me." As students and patients begin to experience each other, the fears dissipate and the similarities of the human experience take hold.

▶ Check Your Reading

1. What is necessary for a novice nurse to become an expert?

2. To use the self therapeutically, what is required of the nurse?
3. Why is it important for nurses to know themselves?
4. What are two of the initial concerns of students beginning a psychiatric clinical experience?
5. What are two common fears of patients as they reveal themselves to nurses?

THE JOURNEY TOWARD SELF-UNDERSTANDING

In the students' journals at the beginning of the chapter, Sarah and Glen describe themselves as they begin their psychiatric nursing experience. Is their self-knowledge adequate? Is this all they need to know about themselves in order to be able to contribute to the growth of others?

Sarah and Glen's initial journal entries are certainly a beginning toward self-understanding, but as they progress they will need to question more deeply to discover more knowledge about self. Such questions as "Who am I, really? Do I know me? Does my physical appearance reflect the me that I want to express? What cultural influences have had an impact on me? What am I? What do I do? Which roles do I fulfill? Where am I spiritually? Who would I like to be? How do I feel about me? How do I feel about other people? What do I have to offer to others?" may be asked. These questions are asked by everyone at some point in time—in fact, they may be asked many times in the course of a lifetime. The answers, although not easy to find, are essential for the development and understanding of the self. Box 8–1 provides questions to encourage self-awareness in the nurse-patient relationship.

BOX 8-1 Questions to Encourage Self-Awareness in the Nurse-Patient Relationship

- Can I *be* in some way which will be perceived by the other person as trustworthy, dependable, or consistent in some deep sense?
- Can I be expressive enough as a person that what I am will be communicated unambiguously?
- Can I let myself experience positive attitudes toward this other person—attitudes of warmth, caring, liking, interest, respect?
- Can I be strong enough as a person to be separate from the other?
- Am I secure enough within myself to permit him his separateness?
- Can I let myself enter fully into the world of his feelings and personal meanings and see these as he does?
- Can I receive him as he is? Can I communicate this attitude?
- Can I act with sufficient sensitivity in the relationship that my behavior will not be perceived as a threat?
- Can I free him from the threat of external evaluation?
- Can I meet this other individual as a person who is in the process of *becoming*, or will I be bound by his past and by my past?

Reprinted from Rogers, C. R., Vol. 37, 1958. © ACA. Reprinted with permission. No further reproduction authorized without written permission of the American Counseling Association.

Like the students and patients described in this chapter each of us has a unique story to tell about who we are and how we became that person. In each story, there are similar threads that link us with every other human. These threads are the shared humanity that allows us to enter and understand another person's lived experiences.

We are all holistic beings with integrated biological, psychosocial, and spiritual natures. The experiences that influence our development differ from one to another. Regardless of how our experiences differ, each of us develops a self-concept and body image, attains certain levels of self-esteem, and assumes **roles** of our own and of others' choosing. These similarities are explored in the remainder of this chapter.

The Self and Self-Concept

Robinson states that the **self** is "the part of the human being that knows himself (herself) as 'I.' It is the thinking, knowing, feeling part of the human organism which deals with the world" (1974, p. 19). Miller and Keane (1987) describe the self as "the complete being of an individual comprising both physical and psychological characteristics and including both conscious and unconscious components.

To deal with reality both alone and within relationships, we must be able to view the self, reflect upon the self, and understand the self (Dufaulf, 1990; Jerome and Ferrard-McDuffie, 1992). As Peck puts it, "to know the world, we must not only examine it, but we must simultaneously examine the examiner" (1978, p. 51). For self-understanding to be consistent, self-examination must be a lifelong activity. To know who we are, we must possess self-knowledge and self-awareness. **Self-awareness** is made up of all of those things that we know about ourselves—where we invest our energies, where we devote our time, where we derive our satisfactions, where we meet our greatest frustrations, what we strive for, what we consider to be "us."

According to Arnold and Boggs (1995), **"Self-concept** is the term given to the part of the self that lies within conscious awareness—self-concept encompasses all that a person perceives, knows, values, feels, and holds to be true about his or her identity." The self-concept possesses a unified nature, yet is differentiated into a constellation of unique dimensions, each with its own diverse functions. Embedded into the self-concept are physical, psychological, social, and spiritual dimensions, which characterize the inner state of an individual and allow that individual to relate to the environment in a very unique way (Figure 8–1).

The **physical self** includes the development of a body image and an understanding of physiological functioning. The **psychological self** makes up our personal identity and forms the umbrella for **cognitive processes**, **perceptual processes**, and **emotional processes**. The **social self** is represented by the many different roles that we assume in presenting ourselves to others. The **spiritual self** allows us the opportunity to connect with God and to find **meaning** and **purpose** in our individual experiences. The **ideal self** is the "me I think I ought to be" or "the me that I would like to be." Whereas our ideas about who we actually are make up the self-concept or perceived self, our ideas about who we should be form our ideal self. **Self-esteem** can be defined as the individual's personal judgment of his or her own worth. The individual arrives at this judgment by analyzing how well he or she matches up to his or her own standards and how well his or her performance compares with that of others (Arnold and Boggs, 1995). Self-esteem is how we feel about what we know about our self; a person's self-esteem is the key to behavior. Self-esteem influences thinking processes, emotions, desires, values, and goals (Dugas, 1983). "Typically, we constantly compare our perceived self to our ideal self, and the wider the gap between the two, the lower our level of self esteem" (Sanford and Donovan, 1984, p. 8) (Figure 8–2).

Although the self-concept is a dynamic phenomenon able to respond creatively to novel situations encountered over the lifespan, it is also a stable and internally consistent representation of who we are. The stability of self-identity is essential in forming meaningful interpersonal relationships based on reciprocal trust.

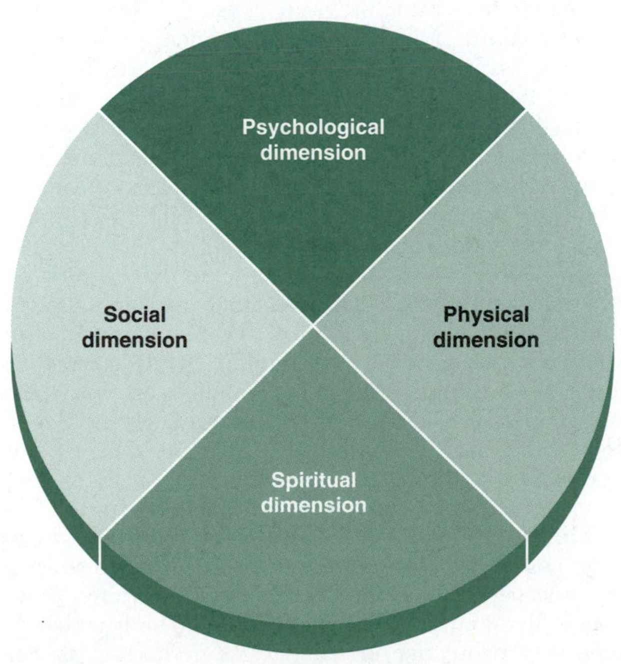

FIGURE 8–1
The four dimensions of self-concept.

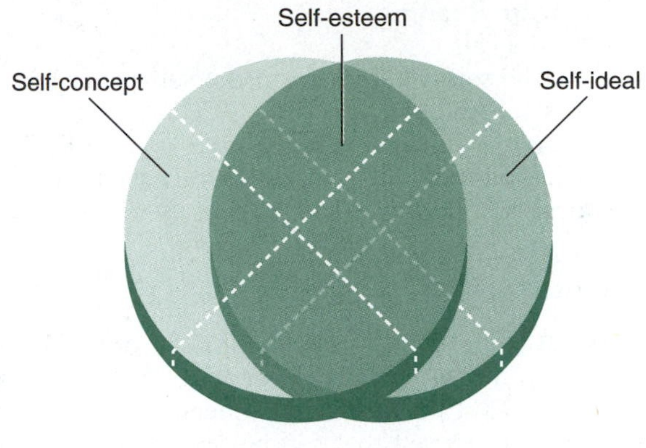

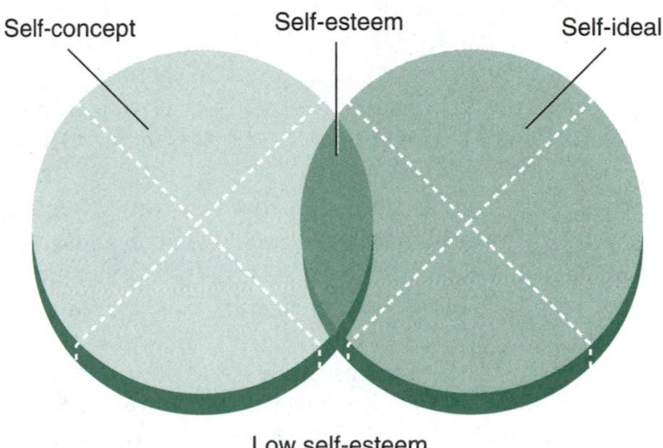

FIGURE 8–2
Relationship between self-concept, self-ideal, and self-esteem.

Development of the Self and Self-Concept

The self and the self-concept, with all of their interrelated components, begin to develop during infancy and continue to develop over the course of our lifetime. The awareness of self begins as vague physical sensations from inner and outer stimuli that soon become firmed up as we grow, develop, and begin to interact with others. Many of our experiences of self are named and defined by others. As we begin to learn language, we adopt the words that others have used to describe who we are and how well we do what we do. Therefore, much of our self-concept is made up of what we are told by significant others.

"People are not born with the beliefs and images that determine their self image. Children learn self-image by interacting with their environment, family, and reference groups" (Strassen, 1992, p. 38). Oftentimes, as we grow, we need to learn how to objectively evaluate what we have been told about ourselves with what we begin to see for ourselves so that we can see the real talents, abilities, and self-worth that we possess.

▶ Check Your Reading

6. Define the self.
7. How is the self different from the self-concept?
8. What is self-esteem?
9. What are the dimensions of the self-concept?
10. What happens to self-esteem when the self-concept and the ideal self are far apart?

The Physical Self

What do I look like? Does my body look like other human bodies of the same age and same gender? Am I pleasing to the eye? Do I need to be concerned about any particular part of myself that can be seen by others? Am I short? Am I taller than most people? Am I muscular? Am I thin? What do I need to do to look more desirable? The picture that each of us creates concerning our physical self is called **body image** (Rieser, 1992). Once we recognize the fact that we are separate physical beings—separate from our mothers and separate from the environment, we begin our journey of trying to find out if we're OK when compared with others.

Both our outward appearance and our inner workings, sensations, and sounds represent the necessary processes and sometimes "warning signals" concerning our physiology. The outward appearance of each human being is generally the same, a head, a trunk, and extremities. Physical differences are present in some people because of genetic or birth alterations, traumatic injury, or illness; however, the majority of individuals have the same general appearance.

The physical self represents the boundary between the inner self, or who we believe we are, and the environment around us. As we learn to dress, or hide our physical boundary from the world, we begin to choose costumes that reflect our feelings of security (Fisher, 1974). Fisher noted that research findings suggest "that the greater a person's uncertainty about the protection provided by his own body border, the more he will seek compensatory ways of reaffirming that border" (p. 22). "In other words, when an individual doubts his boundaries, he may try to reinforce them by making them more visually vivid through the use of attention-getting clothing" (1974, p. 23).

Similarities in the Physical Self. On a macroscopic level, the physical self functions in a similar fashion across individuals. Each of us has a heart that acts as a pump to send oxygenated blood to hungry tissues; each of us has a brain where thought is centered; and each of us has a digestive system that delivers nutrients to the rest of our organs and other body parts. However, on a microscopic level, differences exist in physiological functioningthat have a direct impact on self-concept and **personality**. For instance, an individual's ability to deal with stress is probably directly related to the levels of neurotransmitters found in the brain. Some research certainly supports this theory in relation to the schizophrenic patient or to the child with attention deficit disorder (see Chapter 7). Although the hormones, enzymes, and neurochemicals may differ in amount (i.e., too little in some, too many in others) and may fluctuate at different times in certain individuals, the basic inner life processes are "close in kind" when we are considered to be "healthy."

Differences in the Physical Self. In addition to recognizing that human bodies are similar, we learn that our own bodies are unique. We learn that some of us are athletic, some graceful, some move like the wind, and some are clumsy. We learn that we all come in different shapes, sizes, colors, and sexes, but the most significant factor is the way we view our physical selves. Each of us relates to others based on how we feel about what we see concerning our physical selves.

Culture and the Physical Self. Culture also influences how we feel about our physical selves. Depending on what a given culture values, individuals reflecting the desired norm feel good about the self, whereas those who are different from what is desired, feel inferior and unattractive. Fontaine (1991, p. 670) points out that the desired "ideal woman" has changed considerably from before the 19th century to the present:

> *In Western culture, prior to the nineteenth century, the female reproductive figure, plump with full breasts, was the erotic ideal—In 1966, the cultural ideal took a sudden turn to a thin, skeleton image—The current ideal woman is to be lean, strong, and graceful—The pressure continues to be on women to control and master their bodies. Self-discipline, compulsive exercising, and continuous dieting are equated with goodness and beauty.*

Fontaine goes on to state in her article that "men are less dependent on body size and shape as a primary definition of masculinity" (p. 669). However, men are increasingly affected by cultural pressures to "look good."

Reflect back on the students' journal entries at the beginning of the chapter. Do they contain any clues that body image is an issue with either student? Do you feel that Sarah is influenced by cultural pressures? Does it sound as if Glen is experiencing the same pressures, or does he seem to value different physical characteristics?

The Four "Body Spaces." Each physical self demands its own personal "body space," which is the amount of distance with which most people are comfortable in different social settings. Body space is also very much affected by culture. Four body spaces have been identified in the literature: intimate distance is considered to be 3 to 18 in; personal 1½ to 4 ft; social 4 to 12 ft; and public interaction more than 10 to 12 ft (Hall, cited in Dugas, 1983; Figure 8–3). Each of us has a personal preference related to the closeness that another is allowed without experiencing discomfort. Would Ray and Glen experience the same level of comfort while interacting within the intimate space range? What do you think might happen if Glen put his arm across Ray's shoulders? How about Sarah and Renae? Can you visualize the approximate distance between Ray and Sarah as they become engaged in conversation for the first time?

Developmental Stages and Body Consciousness. Body consciousness seems to be heightened during certain stages of development and during certain events. The toddler is conscious of body parts and body products, being very protective of what is his or hers. It is well known that body integrity and wholeness are very important issues during the toddler and preschool years

(Arnold and Boggs, 1995). For instance, when blood must be drawn from a toddler, it is imperative that it be done quickly and that an adhesive bandage be placed on the puncture site immediately so that the child does not think he or she will "deflate" or "lose all of the air from inside," as one toddler described it.

Adolescence is another developmental stage during which body image is of utmost concern. The adolescent undergoes dramatic changes as he or she moves toward physical maturity. An increase in height, weight, secondary sexual characteristics, acne, growing pains, and new body fluids are incredible changes that occur within a very short time. How important the adolescent considers his or her physical appearance to be can be evaluated by noting how many times during the day he or she showers, combs his or her hair, and stands in front of the mirror—necessary activities during the "identity stage," but activities that take up time and energy to the exclusion of other activities.

"It has been stated that adolescent girls report high levels of anxiety, insecurity, and self-consciousness about their bodies as they struggle with their developing identity. Much more so than boys, adolescent girls' positive or negative self-esteem is directly related to satisfaction or dissatisfaction with their physical appearance" (Fontaine, 1991, pp. 669, 670). Is it any wonder that anorexia nervosa and bulimia have become so prevalent recently?

Certain bodily changes occur naturally as part of the developmental process. Some of these changes are welcomed as a rite of passage; others can have a tremendous impact on self-concept. For example, consider six-year-old Megan who loses her first baby tooth and cannot wait to put it under her pillow for the "Tooth Fairy." Megan has undergone a distinct change in body image. Her smile is different, and she may have trouble eating. Yet she is excited. Loosing a tooth means "growing up," and, as such, Megan welcomes the loss. Contrast Megan's reaction with that of her 14-year-old brother, Josh, whose face is covered with acne and whose teeth have braces. He hates to smile and tells his mother, "I look like a geek." Both children have experienced body changes that are congruent with development, yet the impact on their self-concept is remarkably different.

Body image is also influenced by individual patterns of physical and emotional maturation. For instance, a child who skips a year of school because of exceptional intellectual ability may experience difficulty because physical and social skills lag behind. Likewise, a child who experiences physical growth at a rate greater than that of his or her emotional and social development is disadvantaged because a larger physique carries expectations of more mature behavior (Felker, 1974).

Aging causes heightened body awareness when we see the beginning of facial wrinkles, thinning or graying of hair, and the spontaneous eruption of "liver spots." Millions of dollars are spent attempting to "make it all go away" when the truth is that "it won't go away." We may be able to postpone the signs of aging, but, as time goes by, the changes are noticed. If we are able to incorporate the "changed body image" into our conscious acceptance, we can give up the masquerade, stop buying hair dye and wrinkle and thigh cream, and spend our money on things that can add *zest* to our lives as we age.

Other developmental or situational changes cause increased body consciousness and ultimately have an impact on body image. A preoccupation occurs with the "physical self" when our bodies function differently than usual. Consider the changes that occur with early pregnancy as the fetus develops and later in pregnancy, the woman's inability to physically maneuver the body. Some women are thrilled with their changing body image and prematurely wear maternity clothes as a way of announcing to the world, "I'm going to be a mother." In contrast, the pregnant unwed teenager may force her growing body into tight jeans in an effort to conceal her changing body from parents and peers.

How a person adapts to bodily changes depends upon his or her own meaning for himself or herself as well as the meaning that significant others impose. This ascribed meaning influences adaptation. For instance, Josh, the teenager with acne, feels bad about himself, but he finds it helpful that several of his friends also have acne. His parents are supportive and remind him that his acne will clear with time. On the other hand, the teenage girl who is hiding her pregnancy has a different set of circumstances. Her parents are rigid, and her boyfriend refuses to marry her. Her situation, with its body image changes,

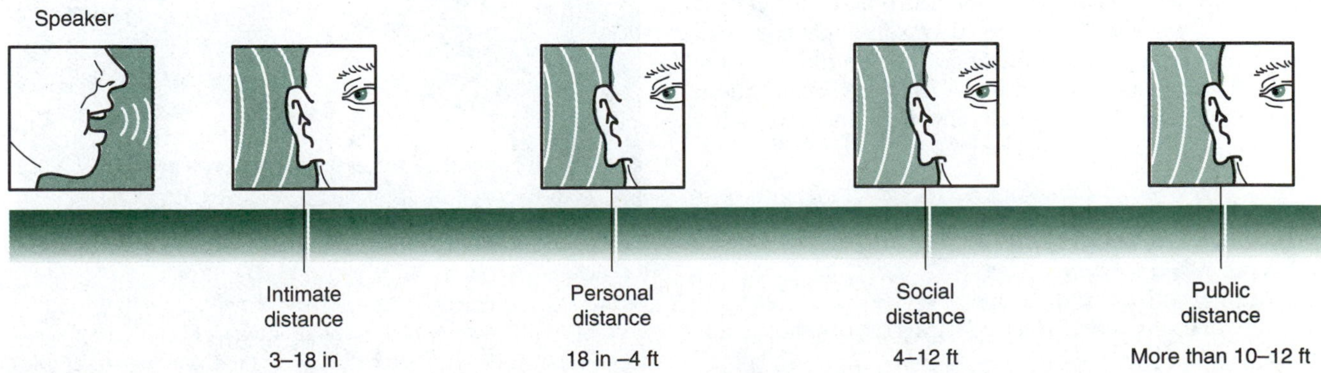

FIGURE 8–3
The four "body spaces."

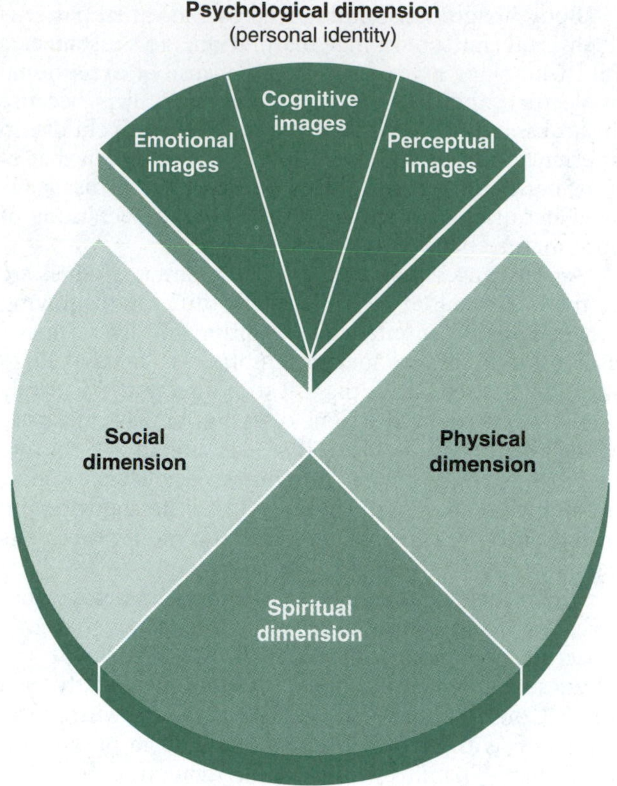

FIGURE 8–4
The three components of our psychological dimension, or "personal identity."

carries consequences that will have a lifetime impact on her self-concept.

As can be seen, many changes take place during the normal course of development that affect body image and, ultimately, the self-concept. Think about the anxieties that develop concerning body integrity, body function, and body image with the onset of illness, the need for surgery, or a sudden, traumatic injury. Even the medications can cause alterations in the physical self that disrupt the body image. Psychotropic drugs used to treat psychiatric illness often cause physical changes, as well as altered subjective sensations. Fluid retention, weight gain, posture and gait changes, and physical rigidity are side effects that often accompany psychotropic drugs. These side effects are so disturbing that some patients will discontinue their medication once their thinking clears. They often find themselves in a Catch-22 predicament: "What is worse, my real body and the illness, or relief from the illness and awful changes to my body?"

▶ Check Your Reading

11. Define body image.
12. What is body space?
13. Define the four body spaces.
14. Cite one influence that culture has on the physical self.
15. Give two examples of developmental processes that affect the physical self.

The Psychological Self

Personal identity is composed of perceptual, cognitive, and emotional images that we have of ourselves. Figure 8–4 illustrates the components of personal identity. Taken together, these images form a unified sense of who we are. This aspect of the self is viewed as the internal regulator of all self functions. It has both a conscious realm, that which we are aware of, and an unconscious realm, the mental data of which we are unaware. All data that are received by the senses are interpreted by our perceptual, cognitive, and emotional processes. Each of these processes is examined.

Perceptual Processes. Perception is the experience of sensing, interpreting, and comprehending the world in which we live. Perception is basically how we make sense of what we experience. Two people can interpret the same event in entirely different ways. The old adage of "is the glass half full or half empty" is an example of how one event can be seen in two different ways (Figure 8–5). In our initial stories, both Ray and Sarah came from families in which alcoholism was a problem. We can be assured that the alcoholism affected both of them, but we can be just as sure that they possess very unique perceptions of how it affected each of their lives.

How we perceive situations influences how we think and feel about ourselves, others, and the world that we inhabit. We each have an inner world, which consists of how we perceive reality. The external world also is present, where reality objectively exists. Our inner reality may be consistent with the external reality or it may be

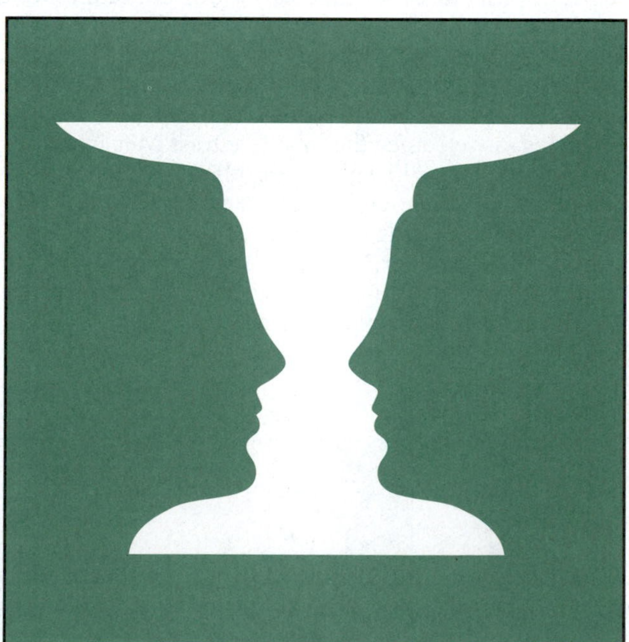

FIGURE 8–5
"Is the glass half empty or half full?" The answer depends on your perceptions. Likewise, whether you see two faces or a vase in this figure depends on your perception. (From the Westinghouse Learning Corporation Self-Instructional Unit 12. Perception, 1970.)

very different. When the inner reality is close to the external reality, the person is said to be "grounded in reality or reality oriented." When these realities are at great odds with each other, the person is said to have a "distorted perception of reality." A distorted perception of reality may occur in a limited area of the person's life, and, as such, the impact also may be limited. Or the distortion can affect all aspects of thinking and behavior, as noted in hallucinations and delusions. A person is said to have a mental illness when they lose a sense of reality and no longer interact with the real, objective world.

Development of Perceptual Processes. The earliest roots of our self-perception develop in our relationship with our parents and continue to be modified and formed by relationships and experiences with others. The infant incorporates an awareness of similarities and differences between the parents but also an awareness of their reactions to his or her behavior. Parents who show delight in their infant are laying the groundwork for a healthy self-identity in their child. On the other hand, parents who are stressed and unable to focus on the child's behavior communicate very different messages to the developing self of their child. These earliest parental experiences cannot be overly emphasized. Infants who experience a broad and positive array of interpersonal experiences with their parents are better equipped to develop a broad array of interpersonal skills and self-understandings. This foundation translates into a strong sense of self-worth as well as an openness to others.

Refer back to the patient and student stories. Both Ray and Renae experienced significant emotional problems. Ray's earliest experiences taught him that he was different and didn't fit in, whereas Renae learned that she was special, and she was able to view her illness as a biological rather than a personal deficiency in her self-identity. As a child, Sarah missed her father's affirmation but used that experience to become a responsible doer in her family. Glen, fortunate in his parent's approval and support, developed into a champion listener.

The perceptual dimension of self is not fixed or static and continues to develop over time and to increase in complexity. As the child's world expands to include experiences with siblings, friends, other adults, and teachers, the inner reality of the child grows to include the feedback received from these people. The richer and more varied a child's early experiences, the more developed the perceptual processes. Generally, the child's outward behavior is a direct reflection of self. As a result of continued reinforcement of behavior, the child develops a more consistent view of self, and behavior becomes more predictable.

Individuals who develop healthy perceptual abilities are able to view a situation in broad terms and to contemplate alternative explanations for events. Their inner reality represents a minimum of distortion with the external reality. They are able to evaluate new information and to conclude that former perceptions are no longer valid. They are able to view the effects of their behaviors and to revise attitudes and actions that seem inappropriate. Their behaviors reflect a healthy balance between dependence and independence. They are able to extend themselves to others as well as to reach out for assistance.

Other experiences, such as illness, affect one's developing perceptual abilities. Either physical, psychological, or spiritual suffering can limit one's abilities to perceive without significant distortions. Developmental changes such as older age can narrow perceptions due to physical and social limitations. Drugs, both prescribed and illicit, can also affect perceptual abilities.

The Impact of Perceptual Processes on Self-Concept. In healthy development, the self-concept corresponds closely with confirmed, factual perceptions. In less-than-healthy development, the self-concept is hemmed in by unresolved conflicts and misinformation. When confronted with new information, the individual is now unable to perceive it and integrate it into his or her self-concept without significant distortion. Once these false perceptions are established as true, they can become self-perpetuating (Bandura, 1977). For example, people who perceive themselves as unintelligent will seek out experiences and engage in behaviors that support this perception. This unhealthy process can be seen as a pattern used in relatively unimportant ways but also in very significant areas of life. For instance, Ray never received affirmation for being a delightful little boy, even though he had artistic and musical talent. Instead, he received the message that he was never good enough as a son, brother, or friend because he didn't fit in with other's expectations. He accepted their conclusions and distorted all experiences through his perceptual curtain of disapproval. Successes in other areas of his life were perceived as "just good luck" and were never fully integrated into his self-concept.

In contrast, Renae's self-perception reflected a high-spirited, creative, and fun-loving child. This perception was validated by parents, siblings, friends, and teachers. When she became ill, she was able to view her illness as a part of herself, but certainly not all of who she was. She was able to maintain her initial positive self-image.

This does not mean that perceptual processes cannot change and that the self-concept is destined to remain the same. Fortunately, distorted perceptual processes, although resistant to change, can be corrected through healthy interpersonal relationships. For example, when a nurse and patient each share their perceptions of a given situation, discrepancies can be explored in a nonjudgmental dialogue. This process allows the patient to validate his or her perceptions with the nurse's perceptions or to challenge, analyze, and explore the misperceptions.

▶ Check Your Reading

16. Define personal identity.
17. What is perception?
18. How do our perceptual processes develop?
19. In what way does perception relate to the self-concept?
20. What does it mean that someone is "reality oriented?"

Cognitive Processes. In the 16th century, René Descartes attempted to approach all philosophical inquiry with an attitude of doubt. His argument was "I can doubt everything except one thing, and that is the very fact that I doubt. But when I doubt I think; and when I think I must exist." He then concluded, "I think, therefore I am" (Hergenhahn, 1982). James Sire (1990) takes issue with the conclusions of Descartes and posits, "We think because we are—in fact because we are like God" (p. 18). Many theorists have attempted to understand not only the process of thinking but also the interrelationship between thinking and behavior. Thinking is an active and creative mental process stimulated by internal and external conscious data. The process involves creating mental images from the perceived data, drawing conclusions about these images and the meaning they hold for us, and organizing these images into thoughts that are useable and retrievable. One of our uniquely human capacities is that we can think about our own thinking and reflect on and evaluate the effectiveness of this process.

Some aspects of our cognitive abilities are physiologically dependent on our genetic inheritance and on our unique neurological functioning. However, the process of cognition is most commonly viewed as belonging to the psyche. The cognitive self includes not only the innate intelligence of the individual but also a constellation of all past remembered events, educational experiences, and thinking style. The self-concept of a healthy individual is reflected in clear, logical, and rational thinking. Conversely, disease, trauma, and drugs can significantly impair cognitive processes by interfering with brain function.

Development of Cognitive Processes. Although many learning theorists have attempted to explain the development of cognitive processes, Jean Piaget (1952, 1970) offers the most comprehensive developmental explanation. Piaget defines intelligence as a dynamic trait that is always related to an individual's adaptation to the environment under the existing circumstances (Hergenhahn, 1982). Piaget performed extensive observational studies of children, including his own. He concluded that children were equipped at birth to perform certain highly organized reflexes such as sucking, grasping, looking, and reaching. He focused not on the individual act, but on the potential to perform the act. He referred to this potential as a *schema.* The grasping schema refers to the child's ability to grasp things, and, as such, is a cognitive structure that makes all acts of grasping possible. The schemata that an individual possesses determine how the individual will be able to actively respond to and think about the physical environment. For the child to deal effectively with the environment, the schemata available to the child must change. The change in schemata occurs through the processes of *assimilation* and *accommodation.*

Assimilation refers to the way a person responds to the environment based on existing schemata. No cognitive growth occurs with assimilation because experiences are continually assimilated into existing cognitive structures. However, a second, equally important process, accommodation, provides for modification of existing cognitive structures. Ideally, every experience a person has involves both assimilation and accommodation. The modification that occurs can be equated with learning. Piaget postulated that the driving force behind intellectual growth was the individual's innate tendency to experience harmony between self and environment. He called this driving force *equilibration.* Seeking psychotherapy is an excellent example of an individual driven by equilibration. Let's look again at Ray. Because he was passed over for a promotion, he experienced a change in his perception of his environment that prohibited him from experiencing harmony. He tried to assimilate the disappointment into his previous cognitive structures but was unable to do so. He was also not able to arrive at a satisfactory way of thinking about the situation that would allow him to accommodate. He experienced *disequilibration* to such a degree that he sought outside assistance to help him deal with the cognitive and affective discord.

Piaget identified four stages of cognitive development. These include the sensorimotor stage, preoperational thinking, concrete operations, and formal operations. The stages are characterized by a progression from simple to complex and from concrete to abstract thinking. Table 8–1 provides the characteristics of each stage.

Influences on Cognitive Processes. Because cogni-

TABLE 8–1 The Stages of Cognitive Development According to Piaget

Stage	Characteristics
Sensorimotor (0–2 yr)	Development proceeds from activity to imagining and solving problems through the senses and movement
Preoperational (2–7 yr)	The child moves from knowing the world through sensation and movement to prelogical thinking and finding solutions to problems
Concrete operational (7–11 yr)	The child moves from prelogical thought to solving concrete problems through logic
Formal operation (11 yr–adulthood)	Logical thinking is expanded to include solving abstract and concrete problems

Data from Piaget, J. (1952). *The origin of intelligence in children.* New York: International Universities Press.

tive processes derive from both physiological and psychological structures, alteration in either can have an effect on cognitive functioning. Renae's manic episodes were directly related to changes in her brain physiology. These changes dramatically inhibited her ability to reason logically and to act rationally. Similar changes in cognitive functioning can result from hypoglycemia, pain, hormonal changes, and certain drugs. Likewise, strong emotions and psychological stress can result in a temporary diminution of cognitive abilities. Sensory deprivation, such as that which occurs in intensive care units, also can result in impaired cognitions.

The Evaluative Aspect of Cognitive Processes. Bandura (1977) defines an aspect of cognition that allows us to evaluate what we can do. He calls this quality **self-efficacy,** which he defined as our ability to perform certain tasks based on what we know. Our perceived self-efficacy may or may not correspond to reality. That is, we may believe we are more or less capable than the facts of our actual performance would indicate. Take the story of Ray, who believed he was a failure as a son and brother. Yet, to an objective outsider, Ray might appear to be exemplary in both areas because of his responsible behavior.

► Check Your Reading

21. How is intelligence defined by Piaget?
22. What are the stages of cognitive development according to Piaget?
23. Define assimilation, accomodation, and disequilibration.
24. What are two influences on the cognitive process?
25. Define self-efficacy and perceived self-efficacy.

Emotional Processes. The emotional or affective self consists of the spontaneous feelings that we experience in response to life. These reactions provide the "icing on the cake" and the "spice of life." Without feelings, we would go through the motions of living in a gray, dull mist without experiencing the emotional peaks and troughs that color all that we do. On the positive side, we would experience no sadness over loss, but we would also have no joy over gain. Life would be flat.

Feelings are spontaneous. We cannot control how we feel about a certain event, but we can control how we express those feelings. Much of the work of psychiatric nursing is to encourage patients to become aware of their feelings, to discover the meanings behind the feelings, and to make active choices about how they will respond. "Being in touch with our feelings is the only way we can ever become our highest self, the only way we can become open and free, and the only way we can become our own person" (Viscott, 1976, p. 22).

Incorporated into the emotional aspect of the self-concept is the self-esteem. As stated previously, self-esteem is the measure of how a person feels about what is seen and known about the self. According to Sanford and Donovan (1984) there are two categories of self-esteem: global self-esteem and specific self-esteem. "Global self-esteem is the measure of how much we like and approve of our perceived self as a whole. Specific self-esteem is the measure of how much we like and approve of a certain part of ourselves" (p. 9).

Look at Glen's journal. Glen sounds positive about his abilities as a listener, a student nurse who can enter into another's emotional world. His specific self-esteem in this area sounds strong. His abilities to complete task-oriented activities, however, do not get the same positive comments. He may feel less adequate in this particular realm of functioning, therefore feeling a lower specific self-esteem in this area. His overall global self-esteem sounds fairly high. Sarah is just the opposite—positive about her task-oriented abilities and shaky on her communication talents—but her overall global self-esteem sounds positive.

Two other concepts are related to self-esteem. "One is **self-confidence**, the feeling that one is a competent person with the ability to accomplish things. The other is **self-respect**, the feeling that what one is doing or has done is right according to the value system held" (Dugas, 1983, p. 662).

Virginia Satire, a noted author and family therapist in the 1970s, has successfully taken the abstract concept of self-esteem and solidified it into concrete terms to enhance understanding through visualization. Satire pictured the self-esteem of each of us as a "huge, black iron pot which stood on three legs." As she worked with families, she was able to get them to describe their level of self-esteem by referring to "low pot" or "high pot." As she stated in her book *Peoplemaking*, "a female family member may say, 'My pot is high today,' and all would know that she felt on top of things, full of energy and good spirits, and secure in the knowledge that she really mattered. Another family member might say, 'I feel low pot,' which meant that she felt tired, bored, or bruised, not particularly lovable" (1972, p. 21). Satire goes on to explain that "the crucial factor in what happens both inside people and between people is the picture of individual worth that each person carries around with him or her—their pot" (p. 21).

Sanford and Donovan (1984) have identified necessary requirements for the development of a solid foundation of self-esteem. Their research points out that in our early years we need to acquire the following traits to ensure positive feelings about the self.

- A sense of significance: "I count in this world."
- A sense of competence: "I can do it."
- A sense of connectedness to others balanced by a sense of separateness from them: "I can disagree with a loved one and still know we are connected."
- A sense of realism about ourselves and the world: "I have a good sense of what my capabilities and weaknesses are."
- A coherent set of ethics and values: "I have a set of standards that influences my behavior and from which I evaluate the behavior of others."

BOX 8-2 Characteristics of People with High Versus Low Self-Esteem

High Self-Esteem	Low Self-Esteem
Expect people to value them	Expect people to be critical of them
Are active self-agents	Are passive or obstructive self-agents
Have positive perceptions of their skills, appearance, sexuality, and behaviors	Have negative perceptions of their skills, appearance, sexuality, and behaviors
Perform equally well when being observed as when not watched	Perform less well when being observed
Are nondefensive and assertive in response to criticism	Are defensive and passive in response to criticism
Can accept compliments easily	Have difficulty accepting compliments
Evaluate their performance realistically	Have unrealistic expectations about their performance
Are relatively comfortable relating to authority figures	Are uncomfortable relating to authority figures
Express general satisfaction with life	Are dissatisfied with their lot in life
Have a strong social support system	Have a weak social support system
Have a primary internal locus of control	Rely on an external locus of control

From Arnold, E., and Boggs, K. (1995). *Interpersonal relationships: Professional communication skills for nurses* (2nd ed.). Philadelphia: W. B. Saunders, p. 67.

However, as important as it is to develop these requirements early in life, self-esteem continues to develop over a lifetime. This allows us to "make up" for some of the early deficiencies.

Self-esteem affects everything that we do in life. Positive self-esteem enables us to meet life's demands with a sense of confidence. Negative self-esteem leads us to doubt our abilities to perform; it gives us a sense that we do not have what it takes and never will. Because the development of self-esteem is a lifelong process, if any of the early requirements are lacking, they can be cultivated over time (Mixson, 1989; Husted et al, 1990; Klose and Tinius, 1992). In fact, we experience times in life when our ideals are in question or in transition, and our self-esteem will plummet or be shaky as a result. At other times, we may face challenges that demand a reevaluation of who we are and who we want to become. Self-esteem will fluctuate during these times as the self-concept becomes less than clear. These opportunities for growth have potentially positive outcomes, but the process can be quite painful and disorganizing. Again, let's look at what Sanford and Donovan (1984, p. 17) say:

> *Some women have low self-esteem because of something we call self-concept dislocation—which occurs when a major event in a person's life forces her to change the way she looks at and thinks about herself, sometimes radically. A woman who has recently had a mastectomy or gotten divorced will probably go through self-concept dislocation—it is not only triggered by unhappy experiences. Anytime a woman makes a major change in her life—whether by getting married, going back to school, having a baby, or changing jobs—her concept of herself will be forced to change, and she may have difficulty adjusting to the new image she has of herself.*

Men, too, must face similar periods (i.e., retirement, birth of first child, death of wife, divorce, job change, to name a few) during their development when they must adjust their self-concept and therefore experience fluctuating self-esteem. Box 8–2 contrasts people with high and low self-esteem.

▶ Check Your Reading

26. What is the difference between global and specific self-esteem?
27. Define self-confidence and self-respect.
28. What traits are necessary for the development of self-esteem?
29. What is the emotional self?
30. What is the effect of positive self-esteem on behavior, thinking, and goals?

The Social Self

One aspect of self is defined by the roles that we assume. This dimension of self, the social or public self, represents the ways that we are known by others (Baumeester, 1986). Some of these roles are gender related, such as male, female, daughter, son, mother, father, lover, or spouse. A role is defined as a socially expected behavior pattern associated with an individual's function in various social groups, such as student, friend, or boss, and are very much affected by the culture in which we are raised.

Family Role. Usually our first social group is that of our nuclear family—or family of origin. "Coming into a family is much like walking in on a party that has been going full blast for some time. There is no guarantee that we will be welcomed, that we will 'fit in' with what is already going on, or that we will even understand what is going on" (Sanford and Donovan, 1984). What is fairly certain, however, is that preformed expectations of where we fit in and how we fit in will be present.

Each role carries different expectations. Family roles always mean pairs, as you cannot take the role of a wife without a husband, or father without a son or daughter. Beliefs about what each role means can differ. It is important to find out what the various roles mean to each family member (Satire, 1972).

Each of us fills roles that are *ascribed*, such as family position or gender, and roles that we *assume* or choose. Toman (1969) studied the importance of **birth order**, or **sibling position**, within the family of origin and its implication for relationships outside the family system. For example, being the youngest sister of brothers would allow the female child to have vast experience with older brothers but no real day-to-day living experience with older sisters or younger siblings. As a result, it could be hypothesized that as an adult, she would tend to feel most comfortable when interacting with older men, like her brothers, but less comfortable when dealing with women.

Glen is the youngest brother of two older sisters. Would this give him an advantage over Sarah in working with Renae? Based on birth order experience, how do you think Sarah could relate to Ray? How can three children in the same family and from the same biological parents be so different in talents, abilities, behaviors, and total personalities? This is a question frequently asked by many. However, if one looks at what is going on within the family during the birth of each child, one can see some obvious answers. The parents are different ages as each child enters the family. The demands are different with the addition of each child. The challenge of integrating a new family member is different each time another sibling arrives.

How about the element of individual recognition that is consciously or unconsciously considered by each sibling: "What must I do differently than my brothers and sisters to be recognized?" The development of each child's own unique set of behavioral traits is an interesting phenomenon to observe. For example, one child may come forth as the "intellectual giant," one child will have no time for intellectual pursuits but will devote timeless energies to the "athletic role," and the third child will travel in the direction of the "artistic one." It is almost as though the child knows there is a unique place that must be found where individual abilities will be praised.

Gender Role. Gender identification is another factor that must be considered when examining roles. "**Gender identity**, or sex role, is the expectation of appropriate male and female behavior found in the attitudes and beliefs of a particular society" (Strassen, 1992, p. 3). Traditional socialization of women has involved teaching the female to focus on listening, nurturing, affiliating, and being sensitive to the needs of others. The sex role socialization for men has traditionally emphasized competition, aggressiveness, leadership, power, and task completion (Strassen, 1992).

In recent years, a considerable effort to move away from the traditional values and move toward gender equality is an obvious trend with a desired outcome. The male "take charge" attitude could be adopted by both men and women during situations in which aggressiveness and power were needed, and the feminine characteristics could come to the forefront in both sexes during situations that call for care, concern, and a more humanistic approach. In *Passages*, Sheehy (1974) explains that this blending of characteristics normally takes place after the midlife crisis. The ideal, however, would be that this dual nature could be expressed earlier in our lives.

Since the women's liberation movement began in the 1960s, women have experienced a devaluation of their roles as wives and mothers. Many women have moved into the workforce and now juggle many roles, trying to fulfill them all. Consequently, it is not uncommon for women to feel enormous pressure and **role conflict** when they cannot resolve the compelling demands on their time. Role conflict may occur at any time when different expectations place women in situations in which they have to choose one role function to the detriment of another.

Men also have experienced tremendous role confusion since the demand for "equality between the sexes" has emerged. Behaviors that were once discouraged are now "expected," such as gentleness, tenderness, sharing of feelings, and showing domestic talents, while at the same time, males are expected to maintain the masculine characteristics, especially in the work setting. Much work still remains to be done in the area of blending female and male characteristics.

Other Rules. Glen clearly stated in his journal entry that he experienced role conflict when he was faced with talking with his patients and tending to their emotional needs or pleasing his instructor and staff with the task-oriented patient care duties. Glen knew that both were important but that others could perform the tasks, while very few individuals might respond to the human side of the patient care situation. For Sarah, her previously held family role of doer will influence how she presents to her patients in the psychiatric setting. Sarah will need to learn how to sit and listen to stories rather than "do for her patients."

There are roles that we assume throughout life, some more willingly than others. Many people choose the roles of spouse and parent, while others choose the single life without children but meet their affiliative needs in aunt, uncle, mentor, or teacher roles.

Oftentimes people find that the circumstances of their life force them to assume roles that they really do not like and would not choose. For example, . . . "there is the sixteen-year-old son who becomes the 'man of the house' after his father's death. The child in this condition usually ends up with all the responsibilities and none of the privileges of the new role. To take on a new role, he leaves his real role behind, and this becomes a very lonely and unsure place to be" (Satire, 1972, p. 167). Other roles that people find themselves in that are not of their choosing are widow, single parent, divorcee, victim of violence, and psychiatric patient. No matter what the role, stereotypical expectations and stigma will be involved (Herd, 1994). As one patient wrote*:

We are human
Just as you
We like the same
Things you enjoy to do
Don't dismiss us
By turning up your nose
Your eyes may be open
But the mind is closed
Don't speak to us as though
We are unaware
If you let us respond
You'll find we are
Very much there
Mental illness is
Illness of the mind
Which is no excuse
To treat us unkind
Because one day
You may wake up
With thoughts unclear
like us. You'll want
someone to care

* Poem by Valerie Gough.

Some roles must be earned, such as those that accompany education and formal certification. Registered nurses, physicians, physical therapists, and occupational therapists must complete extensive academic and clinical education prior to sitting for licensure. Social workers, ministers, and counselors must complete an internship prior to actual practice to cultivate the skills necessary to fulfill their roles.

Roles carry with them expectations, prescribed functions, and boundaries. Sometimes the expectations, functions, and boundaries are flexible; other times they are very rigid. Some parents identify what they want their children's occupations and professions to be before they are born. The child has very little to say about the direction of his or her life. He or she just lives out the script that is written. On the other hand, some parents provide their children with many opportunities to examine vocational opportunities and support the child's independent choices. Judith Viorst (1986), in her book *Necessary Losses*, states that "studies show that children know exactly which role the parent unconsciously assigns to them. . . Perhaps we can measure a family's health by the freedom it gives us not to accept the assignments" (p. 253).

Reflect on Ray's story. In his family, the expectations of him as the oldest son were quite rigid. He was expected to carry out the responsibilities that had been abdicated by his parents. He shouldered functions that far exceeded his emotional maturity. In other families where roles are more fluid, a child might be expected to do extra work to help out if a parent were ill, but this would clearly be a temporary situation.

A common nursing diagnosis for people assigned to uncomfortable or inappropriate roles is Personal Identity Disturbance. Related diagnoses are as follows:

- Altered Family Processes
- Altered Parenting
- Anticipatory Grieving
- Decisional Conflict
- Dysfunctional Grieving
- Hopelessness
- Ineffective Individual Coping
- Parental Role Conflict
- Powerlessness
- Situational Low Self-Esteem
- Sleep Pattern Disturbance

Box 8–3 lists questions that you might ask a patient in an assessment interview centered on role relationships.

▶ Check Your Reading

31. Define role.
32. What is role conflict?
33. Of what importance is sibling position?
34. What is gender identity?
35. Give an example of an ascribed role. An assumed role.

The Spiritual Self

The spiritual self functions to help the individual connect with God, find meaning, and make sense from life's circumstances. Within the spiritual self reside beliefs about the universe, our place in it, and feelings of transcendence, joy, hopefulness, and love. The spiritual self is expressed through behaviors of selflessness, commitment, moral decisions, choice, self-discipline, honesty, and reverence for God, a higher power, or however this is defined by the person. The spiritual self allows the individual to interpret events from a broader perspective than self, taking in the "big picture" and allowing transcendence of the bonds of ego and personal desires. The spiritual self that strives for meaning seems to be a universal phenomenon, regardless of religious belief or conviction.

The Spiritual Self and World View. The aspect of spirituality that allows for **God-consciousness** varies across different world views. From a Judeo-Christian world view, spirituality is shaped by the belief in a personal God who is involved in the daily activities of His children. Such a belief might be expressed in behaviors of service, prayer, and stewardship, which are interpreted as God's will. Conversely, spirituality from an Eastern world perspective is shaped by a belief in an impersonal energy or life force that permeates the universe. This type of spirituality might be expressed in meditation, mystical experiences, and striving for peace, harmony, and a disappearance of self. For others, spirituality might be shaped by a belief that people control their own destiny. Such a spirituality might be expressed in humanistic values.

The Spiritual Self and Morality. The spiritual self is also the seat of morality. This aspect of the self is thought to develop out of the earliest interaction between the child and parents and significant others. Initially, a child feels that any behavior that makes her or him feel good must be good, and if it produces discomfort or sadness, it is bad. The child's main concern is his or her own pleasure. This state of affairs is very short lived. To fit into society, the child needs to learn which behaviors are acceptable and which are not. The parents have the task of defining what is good behavior and what is not. Regardless of whether parents do this consciously or unconsciously, directly or indirectly, they begin the process of shaping the child's behaviors, by giving affection for behaviors that are pleasing and withholding affection when the child's behavior is displeasing to them. Over time, the child learns that what is good pleases his parents, and what is bad displeases them. These early learnings provide not only the basis for personal integrity but also a structure for wrestling with moral dilemmas.

Development of the Spiritual Self. Although spiritual development has some parallels with psychosocial development, the milestones are not as clear cut or as predictable. In fact, it is not unusual for individuals to be spiritually unaware and suddenly experience an authentic spiritual event that transforms their lives. Generally speaking, though, a certain level of cognitive development and emotional maturity are requisite for dealing with the tough questions that accompany spiritual growth. Questions such as "Is there something beyond me that gives order to the universe?," "Where do I stand in relationship to God?," "Does my life have a purpose? If so, what is it? Is it discernible?," "Is my purpose in life related to God?," "Are there ethical principles that go beyond my immediate concerns that should guide my actions?," "Is there something beyond death? If so, what?," and "What is the meaning of suffering?," may be asked (Carson, 1989).

Spiritual Distress. Sometimes the distress that we see in people is misdiagnosed as psychological when it more correctly stems from a spiritual crisis of loss of faith or meaning. The road to spiritual maturity is certainly not an easy one; the answers to the questions are not readily available. Individual faith traditions hold out resources for truth. For the Christian, the scriptures are seen as God's word. For the Jew, the Torah is studied by scholars for understanding of God's word. For the Muslim, truth is found in the Koran. The truth is that much of spirituality resides in faith, which by definition is a belief in that which we cannot see. Ultimately, the spiritual aspect of the self views life as a mystery to be lived and not a problem to be solved (Arnold and Boggs, 1989).

The presence of a spiritual self allows the individual to transcend immediate circumstances with the realization that a truth exists that is larger than, but encompasses, self and serves to illuminate and give meaning to individual experiences. Spiritually developed people are less self-involved and more focused on meeting the needs of others through acts of kindness, charity, and service (Carson, 1989).

In Renae's story, her illness was interpreted as a "burden and a gift." This interpretation allowed her to view her illness as having a significance beyond her suffering. She saw in her illness possibilities that transcended her psychic pain and lack of control and moved her into the realm of creativity and artistic expression. Ray, on the other hand, was so tied to seeking approval that he was unable to view his failed promotion as anything but failure. Only through therapy did he allow his spiritual self free reign to begin to ask such questions as "What does this mean for my life?" and "Is there something more that I should be taking from this event other than my feelings of despair?"

BOX 8-3 Questions to Ask in an Assessment Interview Centered on Role Relationships

Family

"Can you tell me something about your family?"

"How would you describe your family unit, e.g., age, sex, health status of members?"

"Who assumes responsibility for decision-making?"

"What changes do you anticipate as a result of your illness (condition) in the way you function in your family?"

"Who do you see in your family as being most affected by your illness (condition)?"

"Who do you see in your family as being supportive of you?"

Work

"Can you tell me something about the work you do?"

"In general, how would you describe your satisfaction with your work?"

"Can you tell me something about how you get along with others on your job?"

"What are some of the concerns you have about your job at this time?"

Social

"How do you like other people to treat you?"

"To whom do you turn for support?"

"If _____ is not available to you, who else might provide social support for you?"

From Arnold, E., and Boggs, K. (1995). *Interpersonal relationships: Professional communication skills for nurses* (2nd ed.). Philadelphia: W. B. Saunders, p. 141.

▶ **Check Your Reading**

36. Define the spiritual self.
37. What is the universal aspect of the spiritual self?
38. In what way does a world view affect the spiritual self?
39. How does morality develop within the spiritual self?
40. What role does cognitive development have in the growth of the spiritual self?

BOX 8–4 Characteristics of a Self-Actualized Person

A quality of genuineness

A passion for living

Ability to get along well with others

A strong sense of personal worth

A view of life situations as an opportunity, not a threat

Ability to experience each moment fully

Moments of intense emotional meaning, "peak experience"

Full acceptance of self and others

Identification with fellow human beings

High sense of responsibility with a strong desire to serve humanity

Integrity of purpose

From Arnold, E., and Boggs, K. (1995). *Interpersonal relationships: Professional communication skills for nurses* (2nd ed.). Philadelphia: W. B. Saunders, p. 14.

THE JOURNEY TOWARD MENTAL HEALTH OR MENTAL ILLNESS

All individuals have the same basic needs that require satisfaction for physiological and psychological homeostasis to be maintained. As we saw in Chapter 6, Maslow (1970) pointed out these facts in his **"hierarchy of needs."** According to Maslow, each of us must meet basic needs before we are able to meet needs at a higher level of development. In Maslow's hierarchy of needs, physiological needs are the most basic and include requirements for food, water, and air. Safety needs come next, and they pertain to our need for a secure physical environment. Love and belonging needs include the desire for relationships and connectedness with other people. Esteem needs refer to the desire to be recognized as worthwhile and valuable, and self-actualization needs include the desire for self-fulfillment as individuals realize their potential (Box 8–4; see also Fig 6–1).

In addition to the commonality of needs, we know that individuals must also systematically pass through certain physical and psychological developmental levels for maturation to occur. Erikson (1963) identified the "Eight Stages of Man" that represent the developmental challenges faced by all (Table 8–2). (See Table 6–3 in Chapter 6.)

A reciprocal relationship seems to exist between basic needs and **developmental tasks.** Basic needs must be met, to a certain degree, for a person to deal with developmental tasks, and the developmental tasks must be dealt with and somewhat mastered for the basic needs to be met. If there is a deficiency in one area, there may be a deficiency in the other (Figure 8–6). Look at the issue of trust. If an infant's basic physiological needs are met, trust can develop. If the basic needs are not met in a timely fashion, trust will not develop as solidly as hoped. On the other hand, the child needs to interact with caregivers or basic needs may not be met positively.

Add to these stresses the normal life situations and life crises that confront us at various times plus biological factors, family position, environment, and cultural influences, and it can be seen that innumerable stimuli can cause "A THREAT TO SELF." With the challenges presented within the developmental levels, stress is evident, and anxiety is generated. If successful coping strategies are developed to reduce the anxiety, the stress will be decreased, and the individual will gain new ways of coping and interacting with the world. Adaptation will have taken place, and the individual, in time, will be successfully prepared to move on to the next developmental level and its inherent tasks.

On the other hand, if the individual cannot successfully maneuver and accomplish the developmental tasks or if basic needs are either not met at all or inadequately met, anxiety increases, along with the use of exaggerated coping mechanisms. The individual becomes less able to perceive objective reality and accomplish the task at hand. Disequilibrium ensues, resulting in maladaptive behavior (Figure 8–7).

If a person does not accomplish a major developmental task, he or she cannot successfully move on to the next challenge or phase without experiencing some degree of intrapsychic conflict. The individual may be able to go forward physically and intellectually, but certain aspects of the personality are put on "emotional hold"; further emotional development is arrested at a level short of maturity. The discomfort that results can range from slight to moderate to total personality disintegration, depending on the level of inadequate problem resolution. The behavior demonstrated by the individual will alert others that difficulties are present and that certain needs are not met.

As an individual meets basic needs, makes developmental adjustments, establishes familial and social roles, and faces crisis situations, he or she establishes his or her own unique coping styles. The individual who has frustrated needs, inadequate developmental adjustment, and inadequate means of dealing with crises also develops a coping style. As a pattern of coping develops, a characteristic way of relating to the world emerges.

TABLE 8–2 **Erikson's "Eight Stages of Man"**

Age	Stage	Primary Person Orientation	Strengths	Qualities
0–2 yr	Trust vs. mistrust	Mother	Hope	To receive, to give
2–4 yr	Autonomy vs. shame/doubt	Father	Will power	To control, to let go
4–6 yr	Initiative vs. guilt	Basic family	Purpose	To make, to play act
6–12 yr	Industry vs. inferiority	Neighborhood, school	Competence	To make things, to put things together
13–19 yr	Identity vs. identity diffusion	Peer groups	Fidelity	To be one's self
Young adult	Intimacy vs. isolation	Partners in marriage, friendship	Love	To share one's self with another
Adult	Generativity vs. self-absorption	Children, community	Care	To take care of, to create
Old age	Integrity vs. despair	Humankind	Wisdom	To accept being, to accept not being

Adapted from Erikson, E. (1982). *The life cycle completed.* New York, Norton.

Usually each of us has a mix of coping responses, some of which are growth producing and some of which are not. If a person has too many unhealthy styles, his or her life experiences will become limited, and his or her ability to meet his or her needs and cope with stresses may be lessened. This person is said to experience a disturbance in homeostasis as a result of a threat to self and an alteration in the perception of reality. The view of the world becomes distorted, and the individual may communicate inappropriately and inadequately. The psychic discomfort felt by the individual is demonstrated through various mental health problems, such as interpersonal conflicts, psychophysiological manifestations, psychotic disorders, or behaviors indicative of sensory deprivation.

However, if the individual is able to cope successfully with the threat to self, homeostasis is restored, the individual's self-concept, coping abilities and self-esteem are affirmed, and the individual journeys on better prepared to deal with the next stressful event. A positive self-concept, essential to mental health, develops from more than success at coping. In fact, a positive self-concept is developed from the cumulative effect of positive, growth-enhancing experiences with others where we are affirmed for who we are. Mentally healthy individuals possess self-concepts that reflect balance among all the dimensions of self. The balance established is unique to each person and endows the healthy self with a special integration and wholeness not found in anyone else. The totality of the self-concept is more than the sum of its parts and represents a remarkable organized system where dimensions are integrated and function in a reciprocal fashion.

Robinson (1983) says that mental health can be described as "a dynamic state in which thought, feeling, and behavior, that is age appropriate and congruent with the local and cultural norms, is demonstrated. It is characterized by the use of behaviors that alter stressors and promote problem resolution" (p. 74). The mentally healthy individual is able to select from among his or her talents, skills, thoughts, and feelings and utilize these components of self to work toward goal attainment.

Most of us usually fit somewhere between mental health and mental illness, depending on life challenges and coping abilities. If we look at the health-illness continuum and apply the same continuum to mental health and mental illness, it would look like Figure 8–8. The amount of difficulty an individual experiences in coping with daily living and the quality of relationships with self, others, the environment, and God determine where the person falls along the continuum. The placement is based on factors such as the type, number, frequency, and rigidity of the coping maneuvers or defense mechanisms needed to help the individual feel secure, availability of support systems, and innate resiliency.

Refer back to the story of Ray, the patient who was

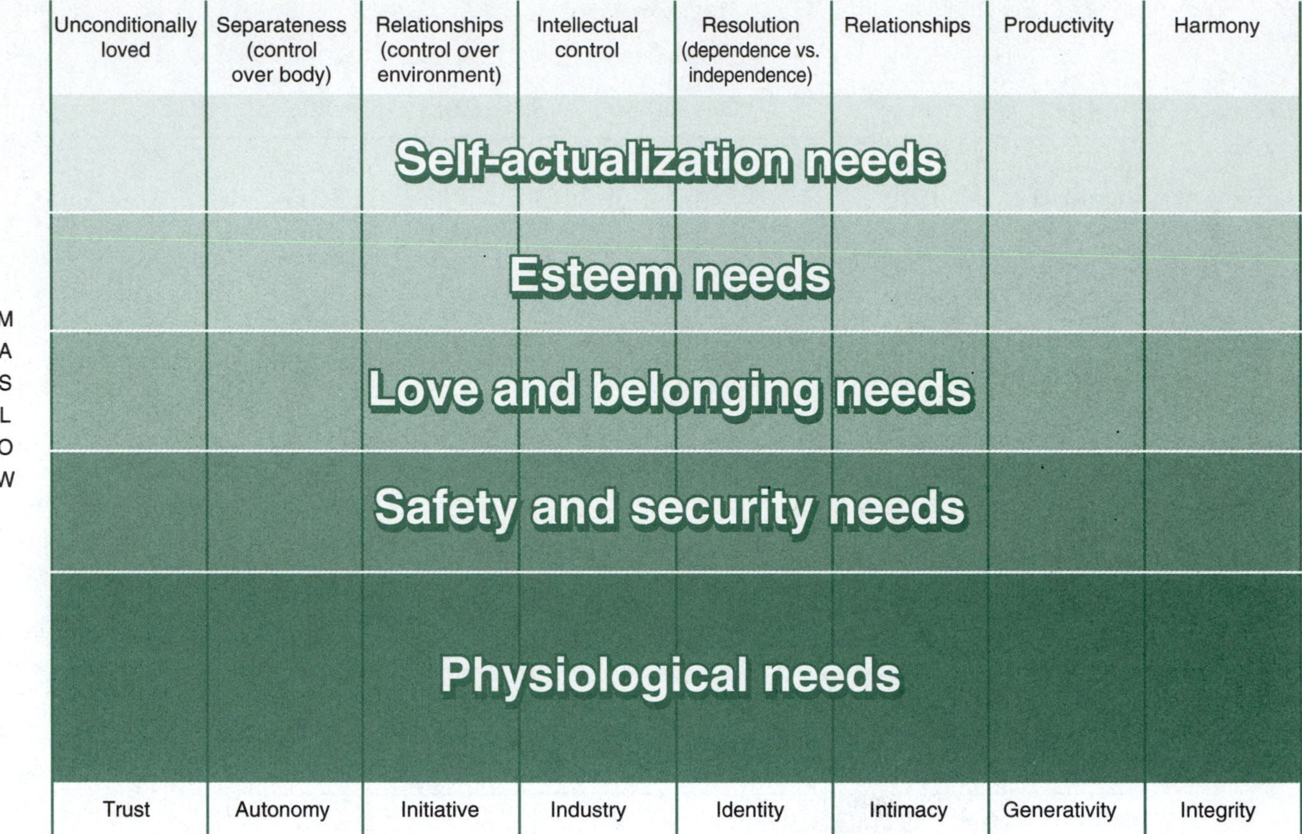

FIGURE 8–6
Relationship between Maslow's hierarchy of basic needs and Erikson's developmental tasks.

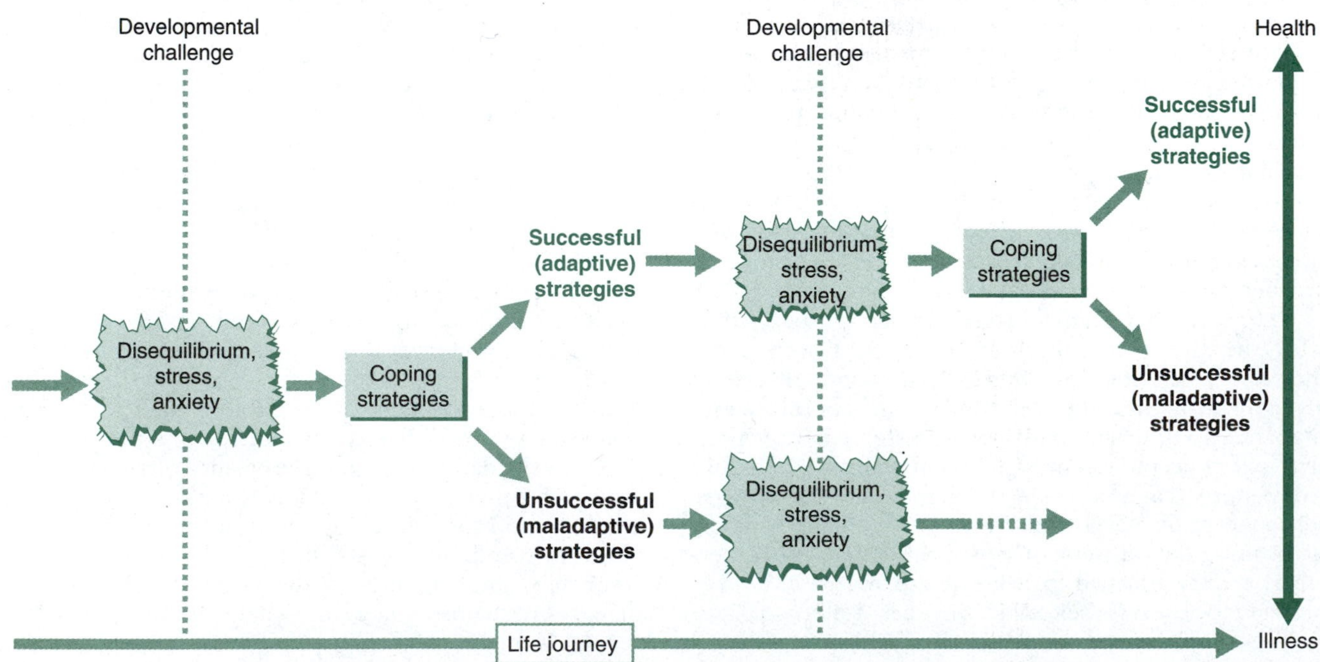

FIGURE 8–7
Relationship between successful coping and achievement of developmental tasks.

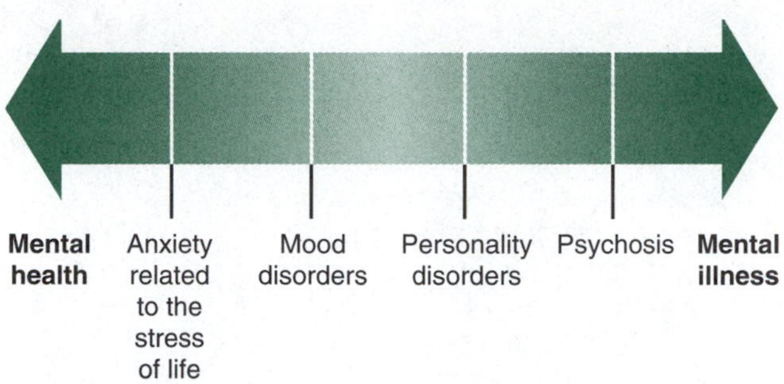

FIGURE 8–8
The continuum of mental health and mental illness.

depressed because he was passed over for a job promotion. His self system was threatened; he felt anxious and unsure of his place in his job. He tried to rationalize that he would get the next promotion. When this approach failed him, he sought professional assistance to alleviate his depression. When Ray felt depressed, the emotional, perceptual, and cognitive processes of his psychological self were certainly involved. In addition, his physical self suffered from sleeplessness and loss of appetite. His spiritual self questioned his worth and the meaning of his life, and his social self withdrew from interpersonal exchanges. Ray's response to stress was holistic, and Ray's experience highlights this in all aspects of the self.

Personality Development

As the self develops, a personality emerges that reflects an individual's automatic response to the outside world. Personality is composed of all the behavioral traits and attitudinal characteristics by which we are recognized as individuals. Personality reflects an enduring pattern of behavior that is considered to be both conscious and unconscious and reflects a means of adapting to a particular environment and its cultural, ethnic, and community standards.

To examine our personalities, we need to examine the customary ways in which we automatically perceive, think, feel, and react to the world. Sarah and Glen can ask themselves the following questions, which will shed light on their personalities. "Do I think in concrete terms or abstract terms? Do I deal with facts and specifics or do I like to look at the whole picture when facing a situation? Am I an auditory learner, a visual learner, or a 'doer' and then reflect on what I experienced in order to learn? Do I rely on my intuition or do I depend on logical deductions to choose my interaction with the world? Do I like to plan my activities and follow them to the letter or do I like to leave things open ended, praising myself for the ability to be flexible?"

These are questions that emerge when one looks at personality tendencies: "How do I primarily relate to the world? Do I get my major satisfactions from working with others or working and thinking alone? Do I feel more fully understood in a group of people or do I get more satisfaction by spending moments by myself?"

One of the formal investigative methods used to answer the above questions is by answering the Myers-Briggs Personality Inventory Rating Scale, or Myers-Briggs Type Indicator. Drawing from the initial work by Carl Jung (Chapter 9), a humanistic psychologist who made significant contributions to science and philosophy, Katharine Briggs and Isabel Briggs Myers developed a tool that could "show how we like to look at things and how we like to go about deciding things" (Cited in Myers and Myers, 1993, cover page). The Myers-Briggs Personality Inventory is used in business and education all over the world to investigate personality preferences. The results can identify whether an individual is primarily an INTROVERT or EXTROVERT, SENSOR or INTUITIVE by nature, a FEELER or a THINKER when it comes to making decisions, or a JUDGER or PERCEIVER, wanting things planned and organized or open ended and free floating.

The above categories are general but show an individual's preferred, and usually automatic, method of meeting the world. *Preferred* is the key word. The nonpreferred way of approaching the world can be developed within each individual so that a broader view of the world is seen and more breadth is added to an individual's usual way of looking at and dealing with the world. Under stress, the preferred and automatic interactions identified are again called into play. The authors state on the front of their Self-Scorable Myers-Briggs form that "knowing your own preferences and learning about other people's can help you understand where your special strengths are, what kinds of work might be enjoyed, and how people with different preferences can relate to each other and be valuable to society" (Myers and Myers, 1993, cover page).

A contrasting view of the Myers-Briggs is offered by Sire (1990), who suggests that as soon as we label ourselves and each other, we limit human possibilities. We begin to believe that *we are the label* rather than hold the view that the label describes an aspect of who we are. Sire suggests as an alternative to personality inventories such as the Myer-Briggs that we cultivate self-awareness to understand ourselves and relationship skills to understand others.

Sarah and Glen are facing a new challenge as they prepare to meet their patients. As a result, each will experience some degree of threat to self just because the experience is a new one. The way that each interprets the stress of this new experience will determine which coping mechanisms will be called into play. If they are able to remember past situations where success was the outcome, they should be able to face the challenge in a positive, growth-producing manner. If the threat becomes overwhelming, defensive behaviors will emerge, and the integration of new behaviors will not be possible. If each has the support of other students and understanding faculty, they should be able to look at the past self, the present self, and the ideal professional self and learn how to become willing and able to experience others.

When they meet their patients, Sarah and Glen will be asked to do what all psychiatric nurses are asked to do. They will be expected to assess their patients, identify problem areas that need to be addressed, and focus on their patients' strengths. The students will be asked to formulate goals and devise interventions that will be dependent on the nature of the problem and the patients' special characteristics and talents.

The most important tool that the students have will be their self, as expressed in its own unique way to therapeutically bring about change. The students will learn theories to back up their approaches and techniques for therapeutic communication. They will learn nursing diagnoses that are commonly seen in psychiatric disorders and will learn some general interventions that can be utilized in an attempt to establish trust, foster hope, and help patients feel as though they are supported and connected with another person.

If each of the students has the privilege of working with an expert nurse in the field of psychiatric nursing, they will be able to see where they are traveling as they journey toward the development of a professional image. One such expert nurse is Diane (see Diane's story). Once a student-novice, Diane is now a seasoned psychiatric nurse with many years of experience with different types of patients. Her journey illustrates how an expert nurse sees her role and her professional responsibilities, and how her professional self merges with her personal self. It is actually difficult to identify where Diane's personal self stops and her professional self begins because they have intertwined to form one being—one self.

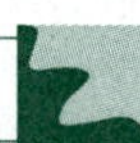

DIANE'S STORY

Someone asked me an interesting question the other day. The question was, "Why did you choose psychiatric nursing as your specialty?" As I reflected back on my career, I found that I was drawn to the human side of every patient care situation within which I became involved.

When I worked on a medical unit, I was touched by the loneliness and anxiety experienced by patients and their families as they faced the crisis of hospitalization and physical illness.

As I used highly technical skills in the trauma center to treat patients surrounded by machines, tubes, monitors and limited family contact, I realized the patients needed someone to help them understand the meaning of their experiences, regardless of their level of consciousness or their abilities to interact.

As I came in contact with individuals experiencing psychiatric difficulties, I realized that, just like the trauma patient surrounded by machines that interfered with human interaction, the psychiatric patient was armed with behaviors that kept others at a distance, therefore accentuating loneliness rather than allowing the interactions that would reinforce his or her humanness.

I learned in school that "we are all more alike than different." I knew that if I could understand the limits, losses, and changes experienced by individuals and their families and could break through the loneliness experienced, then hopefully I could provide an opportunity for "connectedness" and could help others realize that they could gain control over their situations.

Everything that I do now focuses on listening to stories about the human condition and what patients long forand attempting to get them involved in activities whereby they can realize their strengths as well as their problems. They can also learn how to relate to others so that they can gain control over their lives.

The core of mental illness, it seems to me, is loneliness and powerlessness. I feel that if I can help others relate in some way to the world around them, then I have intervened successfully.

Diane seems to know that the nurse is a person, not just that the person is a nurse. Sarah and Glen have much of their journey still before them. As they continue to journey, they will frequently return to many of the questions on which they reflected as they began their psychiatric clinical experience. Their selves will continue to change and expand as they encounter and process new experiences. They will find that just as life is a journey, so too is the discovery of our own self as well as the discovery of another's self.

▶ Check Your Reading

41. What is the importance to mental health of meeting basic needs?
42. What happens if an individual fails to accomplish a major developmental task?
43. What are the characteristics of mental illness?
44. What are the characteristics of mental health?
45. Define personality.

CONCLUSIONS

In this chapter you have examined the self, self-concept, and all the interrelated ideas that are part of the umbrella of the self. You met Sarah and Glen, two nursing students, getting ready to embark on a journey that included stops where they could view their own selves as well as the selves of psychiatric patients. You met Ray and Renae, two patients with different psychiatric problems. Ray expressed a self that was riddled with uncertainties and feelings of inferiority. Renae's self, despite struggling with a bipolar disorder, was strong and confident. You read about the factors that contribute to the development of the self. You were presented with an array of other concepts such as self-esteem, self-ideal, personality, and cognitive, psychological, spiritual, and social selves. Hopefully, you have gained a better understanding of what makes you "YOU," but also what makes me "ME." The process of becoming "I" or "YOU" is wonderfully complex. However, understanding the process is critically important for nurses who must know themselves as well as be able to know others.

KEY POINTS TO REMEMBER

- Knowing oneself is essential to using oneself therapeutically.
- Moving from novice nurse to expert nurse requires time as well as experience, through which theory gets refined through practice.
- The self is the part of the human being that knows himself or herself as "I"; it includes the thinking, knowing, feeling part of the individual that deals with the world; it involves physical as well as psychological characteristics and conscious and unconscious components.
- The self-concept is the conscious knowledge, perceptions, feelings, and thoughts that an individual has about the self.
- Self-esteem is the person's judgment of personal worth.
- Self-awareness is what the person knows about the self.
- The self-concept includes the physical, psychological, social, spiritual, and ideal self dimensions.
- The physical self includes body image or how a person views her or his physical appearance.
- The physical self represents the boundary between inner self and the external environment.
- The physical self is influenced by cultural norms.
- The physical self demands its own body space. Four body spaces are identified in the literature. They include intimate, personal, social, and public spaces.
- Development influences the physical self.
- Personal identity is composed of perceptual, cognitive, and emotional images that we have of ourselves.
- Perception is how we make sense out of what we experience.
- A person who is reality oriented is one whose inner reality is close to external reality.
- Perceptual processes are affected by early parental interactions.
- Perceptual processes influence the development of the self-concept.
- Piaget defines intelligence as a dynamic trait that is always related to an individual's adaptation to the environment under the existing circumstances.
- The cognitive self includes our innate intelligence, as well as all past remembered events, educational experiences, and thinking style.
- A schema is the potential to perform an act.
- Assimilation refers to the way a person responds to the environment based on existing schemata.
- Accommodation modifies the existing schemata.
- Equilibration is the driving force to maintain harmony between the self and the environment.
- Disequilibration is the experience of disharmony between the self and the environment.
- Piaget identified four stages of cognitive development, including the sensorimotor stage, preoperational thinking, concrete operations, and formal operations.
- Cognitive function is influenced by physiological as well as psychological factors.
- Self-efficacy is the aspect of cognition that allows us to evaluate what we can do.
- Self-esteem is part of the emotional or affective self.
- Self-esteem consists of global and specific self-esteem.
- Five traits are necessary for the development of self-esteem. These traits include (1) a sense of significance; (2) a sense of competence; (3) a sense of connectedness to others balanced by a sense of separateness from them; (4) a sense of realism about ourselves and the world; and (5) a coherent set of ethics and values.
- Self-esteem is the key to behavior, thinking, feeling, desires, values, and goals.
- The social self refers to the roles that we fill.
- A role is defined as a socially accepted behavior pattern associated with an individual's function in various social groups.
- Each role carries expectations.
- Roles can be ascribed or assumed.
- Sibling position influences roles in a family.
- Gender identity is an important factor when considering roles.
- The spiritual self allows us to develop God-consciousness and to make sense from life's circumstances.
- The spiritual self that strives for meaning seems to be a universal phenomenom.
- The spiritual self is shaped by different world views.
- The spiritual self is the seat of morality.
- Spiritual development may parallel psychosocial and cognitive development, but this is not always true.
- Frequently, spiritual distress is misinterpreted as psychological distress.
- Mental health depends on having basic needs met and on accomplishing developmental tasks.
- Personality refers to an enduring pattern of automatic responses to the world. It is a pattern of behavior that is both conscious and unconscious and is a means of adapting to a particular environment and its cultural, ethnic, and community standards.

LEARNING ACTIVITIES

1. Refer to the beginning of the chapter and reread the questions to which Sarah and Glen responded in their journals. Write your response to those same questions.
2. What are your unique characteristics?
3. What personal qualities will facilitate or hinder your experience in psychiatric nursing?
4. Reflect on a time when your self-concept was threatened.

How did you cope with that situation? How did it influence your self-esteem?

5. How has your family life influenced your perceptual abilities?

6. Can you identify any cultural factors that have affected your self-concept? your body image? roles that you have assumed?

7. How has your spiritual self influenced your decision to become a nurse?

8. What is your sibling position? How has your sibling position influenced your abilities to get along with others?

9. What factors have an impact on your cognitive abilities?

10. How close is your ideal self to your self-concept?

CRITICAL THINKING EXERCISE

Jules is a 24-year-old high school math teacher who was admitted to the psychiatric unit following his physical assault on and verbal threats to "finish off" teacher A. The verbal and physical assault followed an assembly during which teacher A won the best teacher of the year award. Jules believed that he deserved the award and asked his parents to attend the awards ceremony because he wanted to finally show his parents that he had done something that would make them proud of him. Jules is the third son of four boys of parents who are both biochemists. His mother is a laboratory researcher, and his father is a college professor. Both his older brothers have degrees in biochemistry and are employed at prestigious companies. His younger brother will graduate Yale next year with a 4.0 average. When his parents noticed that their son was not the recipient of the award and because they were very late for an important conference, they left the ceremony early, leaving a note of apology to their son about their reason for leaving.

1. Under what assumptions about his "concept of self" is Jules operating?

2. What inferences has Jules drawn about his parents' image of him?

3. To what conclusions has Jules come about his self-worth in relation to his siblings?

After four days, nurse Whyet talked to Jules about his actions. Her purpose was to assess his self-esteem. Ms. Whyet asked him what he liked about himself. His response was "My parents think I'm not as smart as the rest of my family. I feel like I'm never good enough." Nurse Whyet notices that he is very upset and attempts to make him feel better. She states, "Of course you're good enough. Being a math teacher is a very important job." Jules states, "I guess you're right."

1. What assumption can you make about Ms. Whyet's knowledge about the development of a concept of self?

2. What alternative responses might be used?

REFERENCES

Arnold, E., and Boggs, K. (1995). *Interpersonal relationships: Professional communication skills for nurses* (2nd Ed.). Philadelphia: W. B. Saunders.

Bandura, A. (1977). *Social learning theory.* Englewood Cliffs, NJ: Prentice-Hall.

Baumeester, R. (1986). *Public self and private self.* New York: Springer-Verlag.

Benner, P. (1984). *From novice to expert: Excellence and power in clinical nursing practice.* Menlo Park, CA: Addison-Wesley.

Carson, V. (1989). *Spiritual dimensions of nursing practice.* Philadelphia: W. B. Saunders.

Dufaulf, M. A. (1990). Personal and work resources as variables associated with role mastery in the novice nurse. *Journal of Continuing Education in Nursing, 21*(2), 78.

Dugas, B. (1983). *Introduction to patient care: A comprehensive approach to nursing* (4th ed.). Philadelphia: W. B. Saunders.

Erikson, E. (1963). *Childhood and society.* New York: Norton.

Felker, D. (1974). *Building positive self concepts.* Minneapolis: Burgess.

Fisher, S. (1974). *Body consciousness.* New York: Aronson.

Fontaine, K. L. (1991). The conspiracy of culture: Women's issues in body size. *Nursing Clinics of North America, 26* (3), 669–676.

Herd, F. Jr. (1994). Studying mental illness: A student's perspective—How stigma could impair familial functioning in a supportive role. *Journal of Psychosocial Nursing and Mental Health Services, 32*(6), 50, 51.

Hergenhahn, B. R. (1982). *An introduction to theories of learning* (2nd ed.). Engelwood Cliffs, NJ: Prentice-Hall.

Husted, G. L., Miller, M. C., and Wilczyski, E. M. (1990). 5 ways to build your self esteem. *Nursing 90, 20*(5), 152, 154.

Jerome, A. M., and Ferrard-McDuffie, H. R. (1992). Nurse self awareness in therapeutic relationships. *Pediatric Nursing, 18*(2), 153–156.

Klose, P., and Tinius, T. (1992). Confidence builders: A self esteem group at an inpatient psychiatric hospital. *Journal of Psychosocial Nursing and Mental Health Services, 30*(7), 5–9, 37, 38.

Maslow, A. (1970). *Motivation and personality* (2nd ed.). New York: Harper & Row.

Miller, B. F., and Keane, C. B. (1987). *Encyclopedia and dictionary of medicine, nursing, and allied health* (4th ed.). Philadelphia: W. B. Saunders.

Mixson, K. (1989). How to enhance our self esteem. *Advancing Clinical Care,* 4(6), 98.

Myers, P., and Myers, K. (1993). *Myers-Briggs type indicator.* Palo Alto, CA: Consulting Psychologists Press.

Peck, M. S. (1978). *The road less travelled.* New York: Simon and Schuster.

Piaget, J. (1952). *The origin of intelligence in children.* New York: International Universities Press.

Piaget, J. (1970). *Structuralism.* New York: Basic Books.

Rieser, P. A. (1992). Educational, psychological and social aspects of short stature. *Journal of Pediatric Health Care, 6*(5), 325–334.

Robinson, L. (1974). *Liaison nursing: Psychological approach to patient care.* Philadelphia: F. A. Davis.

Robinson, L. (1983). *Psychiatric nursing as a human experience.* Philadelphia: W. B. Saunders.

Sanford, L., and Donovan, M. E. (1984). *Women and self esteem.* New York: Penguin Books.

Satire, V. (1972). *Peoplemaking.* Palo Alto, CA: Science and Behavior Books.

Sheehy, C. (1974). *Passages: The predictable crises in adult life.* New York: Bantam Books.

Sire, J. (1990). *Discipleship mind.* Downers Grove, IL: Intervarsity Press.

Strassen, L. (1992). *The image of professional nursing.* Philadelphia: J. B. Lippincott.

Toman, W. (1969). *Family constellation.* New York: Springer Publishing.

Viorst, J. (1986). *Necessary losses.* New York: Ballantine Books.

Viscott, D. (1976). *The language of feelings.* New York: Pocket Books.

SUGGESTED READINGS

Dufaulf, M. A. (1990). Personal and work resources as variables associated with role mastery in the novice nurse. *Journal of Continuing Education in Nursing, 21*(2), 78.

Herd, F. Jr. (1994). Studying mental illness: A student's perspective—how stigma could impair familial functioning in a supportive role. *Journal of Psychosocial Nursing and Mental Health Services, 32*(6), 50, 51.

Jerome, A. M., and Ferrard-McDuffie, H. R. (1992). Nurse self awareness in therapeutic relationships. *Pediatric Nursing, 18*(2), 153–156.

Klose, P., and Tinius, T. (1992). Confidence builders: A self esteem group at an inpatient psychiatric hospital. *Journal of Psychosocial Nursing and Mental Health Services, 30*(7), 5–9, 37, 38.

CHAPTER 9

UNIQUE ATTRIBUTES OF SUCCESSFUL TRAVELERS

PERSONAL STRENGTHS FOR THE JOURNEY

One day at a time, with multiple setbacks, we rebuilt our lives... on the three cornerstones of recovery—hope, willingness, and responsible action.

—*P. E. Deegan*

LEARNING OBJECTIVES

After studying this chapter, you should be able to:

1. Describe at least four characteristics of a "triumphant survivor."

2. Explain the implications of control, challenge, and commitment as they relate to hardiness.

3. Describe the five themes of resilience.

4. List the six stages in the journey of recovery from loss and grief.

5. Note the five domains of empowerment and the interventions that nurses can perform to promote personal strengths.

6. Recognize the importance of hope, humor, social support, and spirituality for the patient and family on their journey toward survivorship.

7. Explain at least two strategies that develop personal strengths in the nurse who is caring for patients and families trying to overcome mental health problems and significant loss and grief.

KEY TERMINOLOGY

Despair
Empowerment
Equanimity
Existential aloneness
Grief
Hardiness
Loss
Meaningfulness
Mental Illness
Perseverance
Protest
Recovery
Reinvestment
Reorganization
Resilience
Searching
Self-reliance
Survivorship

Everyone can probably think of somebody they have known or heard about who readily overcame significant illness or loss. "What a survivor!" "How did that person do that?" and "I'm not sure I could do as well if that happened to me!" would be typical comments heard about him or her. Others under similar circumstances may not do as well. Why is it that some overcome difficulties, while others do not? What are the attributes that make the journey successful? Some persons manage to triumph over the odds. Others settle for less or lose interest in life, failing to "make a go of it." Why is it that some family members weather the turmoil of family crises without overwhelming emotional difficulty, while others find it difficult to function? Some survive; others do not or take longer to get on their feet again. What makes the difference?

This area has been the focus of popular and nursing literature, especially relative to survivorship and cancer patients. But, can it also be applied to patients and families experiencing mental health problems, as well as those dealing with loss and grief? Some think so because with current improvements in the treatment of mental illness, individuals are joining the mainstream of the community, sometimes for the first time. Their return demonstrates that they can be survivors too.

Do nurses play a part in this human drama? They do! Nurses deal with many survivors in their work settings, especially as the focus of health care shifts more and more to the community. However, for nurses to help patients and families to survive illness and loss, they need to understand the human spirit and the many psychosocial aspects affecting the lives of these individuals. Nurses must have the skills, sensitivity, and understanding to promote a successful journey for the lives of patients and families who are experiencing mental health problems or dealing with loss and grief.

This is the story of a real person, an actual survivor of a mental health problem. In addition, the attributes of survivorship, hardiness, and resilience are explored. Ways in which the nurse can promote personal strengths in patients and families are discussed by examining the stages in the journey of overcoming grief and loss. Some implications for coping with mental health problems are also noted. Interesting frameworks used in two mental health settings in which nurses practice and promote empowerment are presented. Ways in which nurses can further intervene and participate in the patient's journey of survivorship through the use of hope, humor, social support, and spirituality are also reviewed. The conclusion of this chapter explores strategies for nurses to develop their own personal strengths while they promote strengths in the patient and the family.

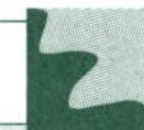

VICKIE'S STORY

Vickie is a survivor. Even in her darkest times, she expressed determination to get through her difficulties. A psychiatric nurse who has known Vickie for nearly 15 years remembers the front that Vickie once maintained—laughing and smiling even when she was discouraged. Vickie so hoped that people would like her.

Childhood

Vickie had a stormy childhood. At the age of 14 she was removed from an abusive home in the southern United States. At 18, she ran away from another abusive situation and showed up in Maryland on the doorstep of an aunt whom she barely knew. This extended family knew her only as "Bill's daughter." They had little to do with either of her parents. Vickie's life continued to be stormy. In the beginning she struggled, mostly on her own.

Young Adulthood

Vickie was no stranger to problems and crises. Her alcohol abuse and reliance on marijuana worsened behavior that was already rebellious. She remembers her 20s as a time fraught with attempts at self-destruction. Episodes of overdosing and cutting herself included an incident of slashing her own throat. In addition, Vickie could be verbally abusive to those who tried to get close to her. At times, she was absolutely convinced that no one liked her.

For 10 years Vickie remained unstable and struggled to survive. Because of her threatening and bizarre behavior, she was hospitalized repeatedly, diagnosed as schizophrenic, medicated with a variety of psychotropic medications, and monitored by the community mental health service.

Referral to "Way Station"

At one point, Vickie was referred by a community mental health nurse to a psychosocial program called Way Station, located in Frederick, Maryland. The agency provided supervised housing, among other mental health services. Vickie was admitted to the program. But she was not yet ready for the responsibility of behaving appropriately. Eventually the program leaders asked her to leave.

Vickie recalls that her "forced expulsion" greatly affected her. She thinks she was beginning to see life's possibilities but was unwilling to let others know that she wanted to change. Ultimately, she did negotiate her return to the program, but she first went south and tried to live with her parents again. The atmosphere was still not supportive, so she returned to Maryland.

Crisis

When Vickie was 28 years old and again a client of Way Station, she made a serious suicide attempt that left her comatose and in an intensive care unit for two weeks. During this time, Vickie again came in contact with community mental health nurses, as well as the hospital nurses. Together with the nurses at Way Station, these community nurses provided a continuity of caring.

In addition, the caring response from workers and other clients at Way Station began to have an effect on Vickie. She felt sad. Probably for the first time in her life she allowed herself to experience that feeling. She realized that she had hurt them by disregarding herself. She discovered that they really did care about her.

A New Diagnosis

It was at this time that Vickie's diagnosis was changed to multiple personality disorder. The health care team gradually reduced Vickie's medications, and today she manages with small doses of antianxiety and antidepressant agents. With psychotherapy, Vickie has been able to reconnect her feelings with her body and no longer "feels numb" or neutral. She had lived that way for too long, she says. "Now a big part of me loves living. I'm learning new ways and I want people to like me for who I really am," she exclaims.

Moving Away From Way Station

Gradually Vickie is moving away from Way Station. She no longer lives in supervised housing. At age 33 she manages her own home and lives with a friend. She is going to school to gain additional job skills and plans to seek a part-time job when she completes her résumé. "I get scared thinking about working full time, but I know how to climb out of the hole, and I don't have to feed those dark thoughts. I'll fake it till I make it!" she proclaims.

The local chapter of Civitan, a national civic organization, has invited Vickie to join their membership. "Because they think so much of me, they asked me to be secretary," she said with a big smile. "It's a way for me to give back." Civitan facilitates worthy community projects, and Way Station has benefited from the organization's fund-raising. This opportunity pleases Vickie. Her interest in doing for others is a characteristic of a "triumphant survivor."

Vickie has progressed from a life of rejection and chaos to one of acceptance and order. She continues to have her ups and downs, but her ability to survive has been due in part to her personal attributes and to the caring of many people during these years.

ATTRIBUTES OF SUCCESSFUL TRAVELERS

Survivorship

Stearns (1988), a professor of psychology, has written about **survivorship** after interviewing hundreds of clients who have experienced personal crises that involve major illness and traumatic losses. She concluded that certain characteristics describe "triumphant survivors" and provide them with a strength that supports them through tragedy and trauma.

Individuals who are typical of the survivors that Stearns describes manage to stay active through times of trouble, live each day moment by moment, and proceed with a sheer determination to get to the next step. Overcoming helplessness and getting beyond making a career out of suffering further typifies survivors. She found that some people initially feel entitled when disaster strikes. Those who get beyond that feeling of entitlement recognize that life does not give them special treatment just because of their circumstance. When they reach this point, recovery can begin and lives can be rebuilt, often in new ways.

Stearns (1988) points out that survivors who have connections with significant others gain strength from the relationships. Also, avoiding destructive or negative contacts while healing promotes recovery. She notes that survivors give careful consideration to who they spend time with. Developing a network of individuals and groups consisting of friends, family, and community connections provides a healthy social support system that upholds them during recovery.

Nurses practice in settings where they can encourage patients and families to overcome difficult times as they proceed toward survivorship. In this vein, Stearns (1988) points out that survivors look for encouragement wherever they are and demonstrate courage in a number of ways. Nurses can be alert to signs of courage. They can be sensitive to a patient's requests for help, notice his or her willingness to grow and change, and coach his or her curiosity about the meaning of each circumstance. Ultimately, survivors become involved in helping others. They get beyond being a victim or feeling helpless and take control of their future. Then, life can become "a story yet to be completed" (Stearns, 1993). "Triumphant survivors" make decisions that shape the years to come and promote their recovery. Nurses are capable of promoting a healthy future for patients and their families who are overcoming emotional/physical trauma and/or illness.

Likewise, Vickie encountered nurses in her community throughout her years of recovery. Nurses in the emergency department and mental health nurses at Way Station encouraged her to overcome despair and get on with life. As a survivor, Vickie has gone beyond the victim stage and taken responsibility for her future. As she has moved toward mental health, she has gradually been able to set appropriate boundaries for herself without relying on Way Station staff to direct her. Consequently, she exemplifies the traits of survivors in many ways.

Hardiness

Hardiness, as a personality characteristic, has been defined in the nursing literature as an "inherent health-promoting factor in a stress laden environment" (Bigbee, 1985, p. 55). Individuals who possess hardiness are thought to be able to resist illness when experiencing stressful life events. A composite of *control*, *commitment*, and *challenge* relates to the presence of hardiness (Kobasa, 1979). Three hypotheses that relate these concepts to persons under stress and have significant implications for the interventions that nurses perform with patients and families are the following (Kobasa, 1979):

- Those who have a greater sense of control over what occurs in their lives will remain healthier than will those who feel powerless in the face of external forces.
- Those who feel committed to the various areas of their lives will remain healthier than will those who are alienated.
- Those who view change as a challenge will remain healthier than those who view it as a threat.

Nurses can recognize individuals who may be at risk for illness when stress is experienced. Interventions for those who feel out of control, hopeless, and hostile can be planned to reduce tension, thereby controlling the effects of a stressful environment. Assisting patients to gain more control over their environment allows them to access "personal hardiness" and move toward "hardy health behaviors" (Tartasky, 1993, p. 228).

In *Surviving Mental Illness*, Hatfield (1993) reports that individuals who have experienced **recovery**, not a "cure" or the return to a premorbid state, claim a "kind of readaptation to the illness that allows life to go forward in a meaningful way" (p. 184). Survivors stress the benefit of encouragement from family and health care providers who emphasize their personal strengths. These positive strokes promote their sense of accomplishment and usefulness.

By devising strategies for themselves to control symptoms and promote stability, survivors are able to activate the control aspect of hardiness. Therefore, with a growing "acceptance of the illness, the maintenance of a hopeful attitude and the right kind of support," patients and families can be challenged to survive the odds (Hatfield, 1993, p. 184).

Although the information about hardiness and **mental illness** is limited, the caring nurse can access the "coping self that is responsive to positive stimuli and open to change" (Hatfield, 1993, p. 187). Hatfield goes on to point out that empathic listening and supportive psychotherapy can help a schizophrenic patient "process his or her experience of the disease and its consequences" (p. 187). Certainly, Vickie was counseled at length about her behavior, which moved her toward better control of herself.

Similarly, Lambert and Lambert (1987) believe that nurses can demonstrate commitment by helping patients examine themselves and experience the results of their behavior, challenging them to grow and seek new opportunities. Emphasizing personal strengths can promote self-esteem and enhance self-control. Therefore, nurses can promote the components of hardiness, i.e., control, commitment, and challenge.

It is apparent that the nurses and staff of Way Station challenged Vickie to see the value of having healthy control over herself. She can be trusted to care for herself. She has made a commitment to life and those who care about her. Even though she is sometimes fearful, she "loses the fear" and takes risks to go on, accepting the challenge of the moment and the future.

Resilience

The ability to bounce back following a crisis or significant loss is an interesting phenomenon. Kadner (1989) defines **resilience** as an "ability to recover from or adjust easily to misfortune or change" (p. 20). Wagnild and Young (1990) recognize resilience as the ability to be flexible and adaptable, a characteristic that is important for recovery. What makes it possible for some to come out of situations stronger, while others remain devastated for long periods of time or never rise above the sick or victim role?

Nurses can enhance resilience and promote survivorship by demonstrating an understanding of the ways in which patients and families conceptualize stressful life events. Awareness of several underlying themes that are representative of successful adjustment after significant loss can assist nursing interventions. Wagnild and Young (1990) describe these themes that constitute resilience as equanimity, perseverance, self-reliance, meaningfulness, and existential aloneness (p. 252).

Equanimity implies that viewing life "with a wide-angle lens," and accepting the sad times along with the happy, enables one to eventually experience major life events with a positive focus. One survivor claimed "You can't take yourself seriously and survive anything . . . learn to roll with the punches" (Wagnild and Young, 1990, p. 253).

But, more than that, it takes a persistence to keep on struggling in spite of hard times and discouragement. Sometimes **perseverance** means being "bull-headed and stubborn . . . simply going through the motions . . . it would take time to get over their losses" (p. 254).

Furthermore, those who exhibit resilience believe in themselves and their abilities. **Self-reliance** requires a search for resources within oneself to handle day-to-day activities. Major changes may need to occur, and strength to carry out changes comes from within. One woman who had to protest an unfair situation following her loss exclaimed, "I don't take things lying down if I can help it! That much I've learned" (Wagnild and Young, 1990, p. 254).

Those who find that life has a purpose and think what they have to offer is valuable can adjust to their loss by gaining meaning from their experience. **Meaningfulness** can revive an outlook on life and change a seemingly negative situation into a time of growth and opportunity. Another survivor, while reporting her conclusions, said "I'm so excited about some recent change, I can't wait to tell you" (Wagnild and Young, 1990, p. 254).

Recognizing that some experiences in life must be handled alone acknowledges an **existential aloneness.** Wagnild and Young (1990) describe this theme as a "realization that each person's life path is unique" (p. 254). Aloneness can be an opportunity for "creativity, comfort, and self-acceptance" (p. 254). A woman who was widowed expressed herself by saying "I'm me again, just me" (p. 254). In like manner, Vickie points out, "I value more and more the time that I can now spend alone."

These themes are typical of resilience found in patients and families who "bounce back" despite difficult life situations. The nurse can view this concept philosophically while relating to patients. By giving genuine support and allowing patients opportunities to ventilate feelings, strengths from within patients can be expressed and encouraged. Actively listening to patients as they explain their life story provides them a means to look at their situation in new ways. The nurse who reflects a confidence in their ability and resourcefulness is providing a worthwhile intervention.

Vickie has experienced resilience, as a result of others having a confidence in her to rise above her difficulties. With the encouragement of nurses and others who worked with her through the years, she has come to realize that she has a resource within her to "bounce back" when a setback or loss occurs.

▶ **Check Your Reading**

1. Name three attributes of successful travelers.
2. List three characteristics of what Stearns calls "triumphant survivors."
3. Name the three components of hardiness.
4. List the five themes that constitute resilience.

DEVELOPING YOUR PATIENTS' PERSONAL STRENGTHS

Helping Patients Overcome Loss and Grief

Recognizing survivorship as a journey of recovery that is accomplished in stages can provide nurses, patients, and families a perspective of the healing process that takes time and includes suffering. Onega (1991) raises questions about the concept of suffering and asks whether the suffering of those experiencing a serious mental or physical illness is the same phenomenon as experiencing **grief** associated with death and dying (p. 72). The possibility that the suffering is similar seems likely.

Bailey (1988) portrays six stages in the journey of grief. These stages have implications for other significant losses, including physical and mental illness. The stages are loss, protest, searching, despair, reorganization, and reinvestment.

Loss, the first stage, begins the recovery process. The reaction is similar whether it is the loss of a spouse or the shock of a personal crisis or illness that initiates this stage. Life is altered, changed, never to be the same. Loss has occurred regardless of its form. Curry and Stone (1992) elaborate and point out that shock, denial, and confusion are typical during this stage. Nurses need to recognize that individuals and families express these emotions and cope accordingly, primarily to protect themselves as they adjust to the pain of the loss. Emergency involuntary hospitalization for a mental illness can be an example of an event that triggers grief and loss of dreams, "face," and expectations for the individual and the family. Even though the events leading up to hospitalization may occur over time, the act of entering a treatment program abruptly symbolizes the reality of the loss of functioning that may or may not be readily recovered.

Once the shock of the loss, hospitalization, illness, or death subsides, **protest,** the second stage of recovery, sets in. Curry and Stone (1992) describe this stage as one of increasing anger, which becomes a kind of emotional or physical protest. Feelings of abandonment, anger, and rage are common and can be directed inward or toward others. Assisting patients to regain some sense of control via a "calm, nonjudgmental, exploring attitude is fundamental" (p. 183). Newly hospitalized psychiatric patients can be a challenge for nurses while they learn to accept responsibility for their behavior. During that process, staff may become scapegoats or targets of patients' anger. It is important that nurses not personalize the blaming and become defensive about the projected hostility.

> Vickie demonstrated protest frequently throughout the years of her recovery. Repeatedly, she lashed out angrily at staff who were caring for her because she believed the problem was theirs and that they did not care. In retrospect, she admits she was angry at herself for lacking the control and the skills to know how to manage her life effectively.

Seemingly the duration of anger has no timetable, but as Stearns (1988) mentioned, as long as individuals feel entitled to receive special attention, they remain somewhat static. Vickie was no exception. Eventually she began to realize that she needed to take responsibility for herself and she needed to stop expecting special attention.

The third stage of grief, **searching,** occurs when the patient begins to attempt to reestablish normalcy, sometimes futilely, perhaps endeavoring to recreate life as it used to be (Curry and Stone, 1992, p. 183). Young adult psychiatric patients may plead with their parents to allow them to return home, despite potentially violent episodes prior to involuntary admission. During this time nurses are effective by being supportive, encouraging verbalization of thoughts and feelings, and helping patients and families explore their options. Reassurance that mood swings are common as patients move toward survivorship, provides information and gives hope to patients and families that the grieving process is progressing.

As the reality of the loss or illness truly sets in, the patient and family experience **despair**. This stage emphasizes that there is no turning back. Grief and the depression associated with the loss are painful for everyone. Struggling through the despair stage is a difficult process because of the "agony, hopelessness and purposelessness of despair" that is inherent in the journey of grieving (Curry and Stone, 1992, p. 185).

Patient safety is of utmost concern to nurses during this time, as survivors may become acutely suicidal, requiring close monitoring. Also, maintenance of physical well-being is an important intervention because poor eating habits, a lack of exercise, and inadequate sleep may hinder progress during the despair stage. Gentle encouragement and redirection is a worthy consideration during this time, until the patient is more motivated to take care of himself or herself.

> As she went in and out of despair, Vickie had a variety of nurses in community settings monitoring her behavior. Emergency department nurses were eager to gain her trust when she was brought there. Inpatient psychiatric nurses were challenged to regularly assess her suicidal potential. As an outpatient she

expressed her needs to nurses, as well as to her therapist, psychiatrist, and other Way Station staff. All made an effort to stay in tune with her progress with the hope of encouraging her recovery.

Nurses can be available to provide patients and families emotional support in many settings. Curry and Stone (1992) point out that "patience and tolerance for tears and silence are necessary coping skills for nurses" (p. 187). Sustaining patients and families through the despair stage can be anxiety provoking. A common tendency for nurses who get anxious is to overfunction for survivors. For example, the nurse may take over tasks for patients that they are capable of doing for themselves to alleviate their pain or for the nurse's convenience. However, the opportunity for patients to do for themselves is eliminated. Sometimes it is the "little things" that make the difference: what to wear, how to spend time, what to have for lunch. If the nurse decides, the patients do not experience a sense of accomplishment that may move them through this stage. Limiting dependency, while promoting independence, is the balance that nurses need to maintain and to which they must be sensitive.

As recovery proceeds, survivors eventually reach a point when they begin **reorganization.** Curry and Stone (1992) describe this stage as a time when depression lifts and energy returns in spurts. Again, this is a transitional phase when relationships become altered, roles shift, and living standards and arrangements change. In the case of a bereaved wife depressed by the death of her husband, she may experience an improvement in her mood. She gains a semblance of life without her spouse and assumes new roles as her routine stabilizes. Similarly, parents of a young adult psychiatric patient may find themselves restructuring their lives as their child moves to a supervised living situation in the community. Members of the whole family will be adapting to new living arrangements. Their roles in relationship to the young adult will change. No longer are parents daily monitors of behavior.

Vickie has been in the process of reorganization. She is living life in a new way. She realizes that she has grown beyond despair and loss. As she prepares to leave Way Station, she recognizes her own ambivalence. "I want to leave, but I don't want to leave. It is a double-edged sword. It is painful either way, but I can handle my feelings now." Interactions with staff have focused on her strengths and promoted her survivorship, even when she might not have recognized it herself. Her volunteer work is evidence that she has begun to give to others, a step Stearns (1988) identified as being an important part of proceeding toward "triumphant survivorship."

Nurses can be instrumental in helping patients and families talk at length about the transitions and explore pitfalls in anticipation of the changes. Each stage can be a time for the nurse, the patient, and the family to discuss their ideas for future coping when confronted with a return of symptoms or stressful circumstances.

Vickie has arranged with staff and friends to alert her when her "red flags" occur, contracting with them to warn her of their recurrence, as she is not always aware. "I start cleaning feverishly, everything has to be perfect," she claims. Then they tell her it is time to "slow down" and look at what is making her anxious.

The last stage of recovery is a time of **reinvestment.** For the bereaved spouse, it may be moving on to new and significant relationships. For the psychiatric patient, it is also a time for growth and new goals. Investing in new and healthy activities that promote self-esteem and independence indicates a shift toward this end. Curry and Stone (1992) state that this phase may take considerable time. Actually there is no way to predict the duration of any stage for those surviving grief, loss, or the effects of a mental illness.

Nurses who work in the community have the opportunity to care for survivors who reach the stage of reinvestment. As occasions arise, nurses can offer patients the reassurance that recovery is a process, occurring over time with ups and downs as each stage is experienced. Naturally, progression is not smooth or orderly. Occasionally, setbacks occur and progress is delayed. Patients and families may proceed at different speeds. The nurse needs to be sensitive to each person's location in the process, as they may differ.

Along these same lines, Hatfield (1993) concludes that individuals with a major mental illness experience "a process by which the person is continually trying to maximize the fit between his or her needs and the environment" (p. 184). Efforts at healing may be ongoing, even though some patients seem to be on a plateau. Also, recovering patients can experience periods of organization followed by disorganization. For a time they may look worse, but changes may be taking place in "attitudes, perception, and meaning and these may eventually result in higher levels of growth" (p. 184).

Clearly, Vickie is reinvesting in life, excited about the future. She realizes that her "voices" can still intrude upon her thoughts, but now she is stronger and can make better choices about her behavior and activities. She is "losing the fear" and can laugh and smile because her feelings are genuine. She does not have to cover up the sadness that used to consume her. Leaving Way Station permanently will find her involved with a new life, new friends, new activities, and a new routine. A successful journey through the stages of recovery have enhanced her investment in the future.

Finally, the nurse who works creatively with survivors as they progress through the stages of recovery from grief and loss does well to remember the concepts of hardiness—commitment, control, and challenge (Kobasa, 1979). Regardless of the patient's problem, whether it be physical, emotional, or mental, these concepts can be beneficial when planning and carrying out nursing interventions.

For example, when the nurse involves the patient in the nursing process by mutually setting short- or long-term objectives, survivorship, hardiness, and resilience are enhanced. Helping patients to devise their own goals and consider how they can achieve them promotes commitment, not to mention self-control and challenge. In addition, progressing from one stage to the next gives a sense of movement that can imply that they are resilient or "bouncing back."

But what about those who have not yet reached a point in their journey where they can conceive of a positive future? Nurses can suggest that readiness will eventually occur. They can provide support for the efforts that patients make. Even if the patient is unable or unwilling to participate in planning, the nurse can be looking for strength in the family. The opportunity may give the nurse a way to access the hardiness and resilience of family members or significant others. They may be further along in their journey toward recovery and survivorship than is the patient.

Empowerment

The healing process of recovery takes place as patients become empowered to accept changes in themselves and their circumstances. Taking as much responsibility as they can handle comfortably and trusting those individuals involved in their care contributes to recovery. Such a philosophy has been the "ARTWorks paradigm" of the ALI/LifeSkills Program situated in the psychiatric treatment settings of the Washoe Medical Center in northeast Reno, Nevada. Acceptance, responsibility, and trust are the concepts basic to the paradigm that promotes **empowerment** of the patient (Bowler, 1991, p. 21).

The basic assumption of the Nevada program is that "people need not be ruled by their circumstances, but can choose how they experience their environment" (Bowler, 1991, p. 23). The paradigm is best summarized as follows (p. 22):

Acceptance of What Is
Responsibility for One's Experience of What Is
Trust in One's Self and the Ability of Others to Make Appropriate Choices in the Face of What Is

These concepts define the unit as a "healing health care environment" and the nurse a "healing agent" (p. 23). Nursing staff utilize the paradigm principle as they plan and carry out their practice. The nursing program there includes nurse-led classes, community meetings, and group therapy sessions. Nurses are encouraged to "develop diverse skills through case management and program facilitation" for a complex client population, including problems with addictions, as well as mental illness (p. 24).

Nurses were among those who helped Vickie take responsibility for both her dysfunctional and healthy behaviors. "When they let me fall out of their net, reality would hit. Then I had to take responsibility for myself and put my life back together." Gradually, Vickie established a different experience as she was given the opportunity to try out different behaviors. By allowing her to experiment with a variety of approaches toward accomplishing her goals, the nurses in Way Station empowered Vickie, much as the nurses in the Nevada program empower their clients (Figure 9–1).

Bowler (1991) points out that clients in the Nevada program devise their own treatment plans, grounded in the 12-step philosophy of recovery. In addition, staff and clients are encouraged to nurture themselves, along with others, thereby empowering those involved to love and care in a way that is liberating and enriching.

In light of this notion, Bowler (1991) believes that psychiatric-mental health nurses cannot "create an environment of personal transformation for clients unless they can also experience their own empowerment and commitment to a greater vision" (p. 21). She calls upon nurses to relinquish the "victim role" and avoid blaming "the system" or "the administration" for what is wrong and learn to care for themselves. Applying the principles of the ARTWorks paradigm helps nurses to create their own experience. The ALI/LifeSkills program teaches that (p. 23)

trust, acceptance, vision, forgiveness, apology, responsibility and action help individuals attain a better quality of life when applied in one's day-to-day affairs . . . as the satisfying practice environments are, in reality, within themselves.

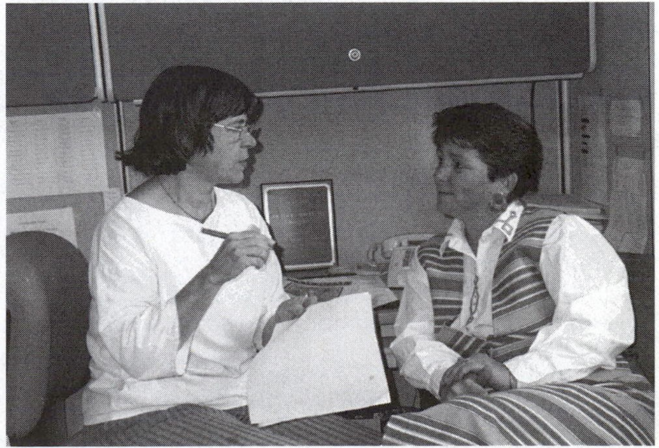

FIGURE 9–1
Francy and other Way Station nurses empowered Vickie to accomplish her goals.

Empowerment is envisioned somewhat differently in another Midwest community mental health center where a community support service serves clients who are primarily schizophrenic and manic depressive. Empowerment is a major theme of their work with a client-run drop-in center. Connelly et al (1993) analyzed four levels of empowerment experienced by these clients as process domains of participating, choosing, supporting, and negotiating. A fifth domain, personal significance, describes the effects of empowerment for the person.

Initially, *participation* exists when patients have "a place to be themselves" and to become involved, even if it means just being with others, drinking coffee, having a smoke. On the next level, *choosing*, the individual is free to choose among a variety of options, implying self-control and taking responsibility for one's behavior. *Supporting*, the third level of empowerment, includes caring, relating, accepting, coaching, and sharing. Friendship is a very important aspect of this level. Here, patients can help each other. *Negotiating*, the fourth level described, is a time for mutual respect and feelings of near equality and cooperation, as well as readiness to take a stand on issues (Connelly et al, 1993).

Through her journey of survivorship, Vickie has had opportunities to experience each of these domains. One cannot mistake her sense of empowerment and her feelings of *personal significance* now that she is on her own. Because she was given choices about treatment goals and options, she experienced the staff's support. "They were right beside me, even when I made a mistake. That became a tool to help me grow."

In yet another setting, "the ability to use one's self in the therapeutic process in the service of empowering the client" is described by Hammond (1988) as part of an empowerment treatment model, which she has developed as a therapist working with women. Her principles have implications for mental health nurses, as they promote survivorship. Some of Hammond's procedures and strategies include (pp. 75–80)

- Establishing mutual identification points—owning and expressing common or shared experiences with the client to facilitate joining, which can serve to model an example of survival
- Acting as a power agent—taking advantage of opportunities to influence other relevant systems in which the client participates, such as making telephone calls on the client's behalf and advocating whenever possible
- Validating strengths—identifying and relabeling behaviors to indicate the existence of strengths or competencies
- Self-disclosure—timely and appropriate self-revelations to serve as examples of skill-teaching
- Skill-teaching—such as in child management, assertiveness, relaxation, organization of support groups, and résumé-writing, to foster self-reliance, mastery, and competency

Hammond (1988) believes that these interventions contribute to her functioning as a role model for her clients. "Openness, the capacity to feel, the ability to be action-oriented, and the reorganization of self-identity from victimization to empowerment" are all important characteristics for the clinician (p. 80).

On the other hand, Keith (1991) encourages survivors, their families, and health care providers to "assume responsibility for creating their own balance" when striving for an environment of survivorship (p. 113). Responsibility to accept this condition provides an atmosphere in which success or failure can be owned by the participants. She stresses that if professionals think they must "fix it" for patients, they deny patients independence and the opportunity to determine their destiny, environment, and life. Like Stearns (1988), Keith believes that determination to take responsibility for self promotes recovery and that an active, aggressive, and sometimes defiant role in their own healing process needs to happen for patient recovery.

Nurses can be empowering facilitators by helping patients to see that "they are not their illness" (Keith, 1991, p. 114). Allowing individuals to express their feelings and validate their emotions gives them the opportunity to access resources within themselves and others to "fight the battle" (p. 114). When the healing process is allowed to proceed, hope can begin to be experienced.

Instilling Hope

Deegan (1988) describes hope as "the turning point which must be followed by a willingness to act . . . not . . . absence of pain or struggle . . . a transition from anguish to suffering . . . leading forward to a new future" (p. 14). On the other hand, Stotland (in Raleigh, 1992) defines hope as "an expectation of goal attainment modified by the importance of the goal and the probability of attaining it" (p. 443). When patients begin to anticipate that they can achieve a goal, hope comes into view. Therefore, "I'm willing to try . . . I am hopeful . . . I discover that I can do" become a part of the process of recovery, as explained by Deegan (p. 14).

But where does hope come from, especially when life is grim and hopeless? Raleigh (1992) claims that patients experiencing chronic illness report that the most common sources of hope are family, friends, and religious beliefs. A number of strategies to alleviate hopelessness include (p. 446)

- Getting busy doing something
- Praying or undertaking religious activities
- Thinking about other things
- Talking to others

Others helped "by visiting me . . . listening to me . . . talking to me" (p. 446). The findings in Raleigh's study are similar to Stearns' (1988) and to her work with those surviving loss and grief. Both authors proclaim the value of being active and having personal relationships, especially family and friends.

The informed nurse is in a position to encourage patients to seek visits from family and friends and become involved in meaningful activities. However, family and friends are not always available, either for reasons of location, inconvenience, or emotional distance. Quite often emotional cut-off exists when a family member is mentally ill, leaving the individual without that resource for hope. Nurses are sometimes in a position to be like temporary family for patients until they can become reunited or develop new social connections.

Vickie was without an emotionally close family in the earlier days of her journey; thus, nurses and staff at Way Station became her family. They spent time with her, talked to her, and listened to her. Their efforts encouraged her to see a caring that went beyond her problems, for they had confidence in her strengths and ability to survive.

In that vein, Keith (1991) describes hope as "a positive expectation, a leap of faith from despair . . . in the process of assuming responsibility" (p. 114). Certainly the Way Station staff were an important part of helping Vickie make that leap, assume responsibility for herself, and experience hope.

Raleigh (1992) reminds nurses that their companionship and willingness to listen fosters hopefulness. In addition to encouragement, nurses work with a patient to set realistic goals that are readily attainable, based on the patient's progress and current motivation. Creativity and imagination may be in order as nurses brainstorm with the patient about the next horizon. Accomplishment of "even little steps" provides patients with a sense of "I can do it."

In addition, Leete (1987), a survivor of schizophrenia, encourages families and professionals to maintain a hopeful attitude. Efforts to recover will seem futile to individuals trying to survive if the people around them are devastated too. Nurses must believe in each person's capacity to grow, focus on the healthy, adaptive aspects of the patient's personality and consider them partners in the recovery process (Hatfield, 1993). Again, positive feedback about strengths serves to enhance self-esteem and confidence as patients struggle toward a stronger sense of a self and survival. These actions, on the part of nurses, as well as other professionals, family, and friends, can instill hope for patients who want to make themselves "whole by learning the lessons our lives teach us, lovingly and with compassion and humor" (Keith, 1991, p. 114).

Using Humor

The road toward survivorship is a bumpy one. There are pits and potholes along the way. Humor can absorb some of the shock and grease the wheels of the vehicle that carries survivors.

Sumners (1988) describes the therapeutic use of humor in the recovery of substance abusers. Her ideas have implications for anyone recovering from a mental health problem who is persevering to survive their difficult experiences. In the process of recovery, humor is a valuable coping skill that nurses can encourage clients to use constructively and appropriately. More specifically,

Humor helps to cushion the pain of self-revelation, to initiate, reestablish, and maintain relationships, and to enable the individual to own and express a full range of emotions without damaging others (Sumners, 1988, p. 177).

Individuals overcoming substance abuse experience different types of humor throughout the stages of their recovery. During each stage, humor functions to alleviate stress and feelings of anger, anxiety, frustration, and tension. Extinguishing these feelings with substances can be one way to cope, but humor, an "emotion-focused coping strategy," is a healthier alternative (Sumners, 1988, p. 173).

It is of interest that the types and functions of humor utilized in recovery from substance abuse depend upon the stage of recovery. Drinking and transition, early recovery, and ongoing recovery are the recovery stages that Sumners (1988) describes. Table 9–1 illustrates the types of humor and their functions during these stages.

It is apparent that the type of humor used changes as a patient progresses toward recovery. Initially, he or she has negative feelings, expressed with sarcasm or ridicule. Exploring the underlying themes of the humor can reveal unexpressed feelings. Consequently, humor can be a way to safely let go of the feeling in a socially acceptable manner. Laughter, rather than the abused substance, releases the tension. Previously, numbing sensations with substance abuse served as a way of coping. However, humor is a more constructive way to deal with negative feelings.

As recovery progresses and social supports expand, addicted clients find that humor "breaks the ice" in social situations and reduces isolation especially as they become members of support groups or actively participate in the community. Circumstances that used to be threatening become less overwhelming, even humorous, as perspectives change and thinking shifts beyond self-centeredness (Sumners, 1988).

Nurses are in unique positions to utilize humor in their practice settings because of their consistent presence and rapport with patients and families. Warner (1984) points out that self-disclosure and humor are two interventions that can be a part of the dynamic process between nurse and patient and instrumental in changing social withdrawal to reintegration.

Humor therapy can include patient assignments to "find a joke you like, dislike, find offensive, find funny,

TABLE 9–1 The Types and Coping Functions of Humor Used in Each Stage of Recovery from Substance Abuse

Stage of Recovery	Types of Humor	Coping Functions
Drinking and transition	Attacking, sarcasm, tendentious wit, ridicule, jokes	Relief of anger, hostility, anxiety, aggression, expression of negative feelings
Early recovery	Jokes, self-disparaging, storytelling, practical jokes, puns, absurdity	Detachment, promotion of inclusion in group, social relationships, tension relief, problem solving, communication
Ongoing recovery	Irony, satire, jokes, intellectual play, stories	Acceptance of life's paradox, enhancement of feelings of relatedness to humanity, building and sustaining relationships

From *Issues in Mental Health Nursing, 9,* 169–179. Sumners, A. D. [1988]. Taylor & Francis, Inc., Washington, D.C. Reproduced with permission.

etc. . . .” (Warner, 1984, p. 19). The spontaneous behaviors that result can be most enlightening. Skilled psychiatric nurses can monitor the process positively in a group situation. In addition, they can encourage patients to share humorous life events, discuss individually funny excerpts from a group session or the unit, mirror humorous techniques along with positive or negative feedback that is “cushioned by humor” (p. 20).

At some point, Vickie began to see the futility of her addictive behaviors, perhaps as others humored her by sharing their similar experiences in trying to cope with substance abuse. Because of the numerous fun activities at Way Station, Vickie and others like her were able to have experiences that relieved the intensity of their past situations, brought them closer to those who shared similar fears, and created a new self-acceptance. An improved sense of well-being was apparent to those who participated in the fun.

In addition, Vickie came to realize that she was not the only one who had to deal with substance abuse and mental health problems. Others in the group had overcome addiction. People were there to guide her with a sense of humor. She could laugh at herself, as well as others, much like McKenzie (1982), who used “the tool of humor to laugh over situations that formerly made me tense” (p. 19).

Even though McKenzie was a survivor of schizophrenia rather than substance abuse, the functions of humor seemed similar and helped her cope with her illness and circumstances.

However, the nurse is urged to be cautious in the use of humor with the mentally ill. The possibility of misunderstanding can be a stumbling block to which nurses need to be sensitive. In any situation, humor can be used negatively, possibly in a sarcastic or a passive-aggressive manner that is not appropriate or therapeutic. However, refocusing on positive interpersonal communications can be a way of restoring relationships, should humor be used negatively.

Similarly, Vickie knows that laughter is an important element in the lives of the members of the psychosocial program at Way Station. Members and staff experience times that are lighthearted and even silly. An annual retreat for members and staff alike is an example of a time of laughter. Activities are geared to promote interaction that is appropriately self-disclosing and social. The sharing of games, skits, singing, and meals provides an equalizing effect that humanizes staff and creates an enjoyable atmosphere of closeness and fun. In this relaxed setting, survivors can discover their strengths and risk new ways of coping.

When the road to recovery is greased by the good humor of those who understand what survivors are dealing with, the journey can be more tolerable.

Engaging Social Support

Social support can be a cushion for both individuals and their families who are on the bumpy road of dealing with mental health problems, as well as loss and grief. Anthony (1993) emphasizes that “a common denominator of recovery is the presence of people who believe in and stand by . . . persons one can trust to ‘be there’ in times of need” (p. 18). Social support, which facilitates recovery, can originate from a variety of sources beyond family and friends, including acquaintances, clubs, sports, churches, and self-help groups.

Jennie Forehand, a Maryland legislator, pleaded with her audience at a Depression and Related Affective Disorders Association (DRADA) symposium at Johns Hopkins University to “never give up” on a family member who is struggling with mental health problems (Walgrove, 1994, p. 4). She pointed out that the agony she experienced when a member of her family was hospitalized for psychotic depression was typical for the families she had come to know as a result. Families endure the disruption of their lives along with the patient. Striking the balance between the family maintaining their own sense of self and providing the necessary support for the patient's recovery is a significant challenge.

Caplan (1974) explains support systems as "social aggregates that provide individuals with opportunities for feedback about themselves and for validations of their expectations about others" (pp. 4, 5). In addition, social support systems help individuals to deal with their emotions, give guidance, and promote competence. Nurses, in their working relationships with patients and families, have many opportunities to interact meaningfully in a manner that provides encouragement and support. Offering the belief that a patient is capable of accomplishing even small objectives promotes competence that can inspire them to press on to overcome other obstacles.

Vickie had such a relationship with her therapist at Way Station. "She never threw me away," she exclaimed, as she told of how people stood beside her, even when she made a mistake! She was allowed to choose her own goals toward recovery. Sometimes she didn't trust or disliked those trying to help her, but they still negotiated with her, offering her choices.

Deegan (1988), a clinical psychologist and a recovered mentally disabled person, claims that the love and support of others was paramount in her recovery. She recalls those who loved her and did not give up, even when she gave up. Although they were powerless to make her better, they did not abandon her. Some suffered with her. "They remained hopeful, despite the odds. Their love . . . was like a constant invitation . . . to be something more than all this self-pity and despair" (p. 14).

Fluctuations between dependence and independence in relationships are common experiences that patients recognize, as indicated by a female mental health client who was interviewed by the Canadian Mental Health Association (Hatfield, 1993, p. 138):

What you need is to have a lot of support, even at the beginning. You just need someone to help you get through the rough spots. . . . Here, they're pushing for you to be independent and on your own, but at the same time, they're supporting you. If something happens that you can't handle, they're here.

As mentioned, self-help groups provide a meaningful outlet for patients to gain self-esteem and confidence. In Hatfield (1993), Leete says, "we offer each other . . . support and encouragement, friendship . . . draw strength and hope . . . The realization that it can be done is one of the most useful aspects of any support group" (p. 126). Frese (1994) speaks about his experience of coping with schizophrenia and points out that "recovering persons benefit greatly from associating with others with similar disabilities" (p. 5).

The National Alliance for the Mentally Ill (NAMI) is a well-known resource for patients and families. Not only is the Alliance a self-help network, but it functions as a strong political organization that represents the interests of the mentally ill and their families. Local chapters throughout the country are available to provide support. (To locate a local NAMI affiliate, call 1-800-950-6264.)

Nurses working with mental health patients are in a position to refer individuals and their family members to an accessible and appropriate support group, such as NAMI. It behooves the caring nurse to be knowledgeable about local support and self-help groups so that referrals can connect patients with support groups that foster survivorship. To become more fully aware, the nurse might consider going to a meeting, as some groups welcome attendance by mental health professionals.

Addressing Spiritual Issues

Traveling the road of survivorship while dealing with issues of loss, grief, or other mental health problems is a lonely trek. When despair sets in, patients believe that no one cares. Questions like "Where is God?" "Why is this happening to me?" and "What is the purpose of this suffering?" surface, and nurses may feel at a loss about what to say.

Addressing spiritual issues when a patient is extremely anxious or possibly psychotic can create considerable anxiety for the inexperienced clinician. The anxiety of the spiritual crisis may be compounded by the patient's cognitive confusion because of an acute psychotic episode. In addition, mental health programs are not focused on meeting patients' spiritual needs (Miller, 1990). Consequently, spirituality, an important aspect of the personality, is often neglected and the needs of the whole person are not taken into consideration.

Accessing the spiritual nature of the mentally ill patient can provide an opportunity for his or her personal growth. The reach toward a greater and higher power can lift the individual out of the pit of despair and aloneness. Sullivan (1993) reported the words of one informant in a study of spirituality and the mentally challenged (p. 129):

It put the worries off on someone else. I feel that there is someone else out there that has the power to help. . . . This world can be a bit frightening when you just think about the reality of it. You feel just like an ant at a picnic. . . . It (spirituality) just makes you feel more secure.

Another informant in the above study expressed that there was a limit to the depths of despair as it related to periods of psychiatric hospitalizations (p. 129):

I knew that there was a way out and that God was always watching or taking care of me and that in the end result He had it in control—and so I didn't have to do anything stupid or desperate. . . . I might go through heck but He wasn't going to let me go to the bottom.

Sullivan (1993) found that the participants "spoke of their spirituality providing continual direction for them"

(p. 131). For example, another comment was "The faith that you have in God makes a lot of difference in how you feel about things around you" (p. 131). The spiritual dimension of the person is an important part of feeling like a whole person, a person who is connected in mind, body, and spirit.

How do nurses fit into this area of survivorship? Can their relationships contribute to positive change in the lives of patients and families? Nurses need to recognize that spiritual beliefs are a significant resource for coping and learning to live with pain, whether it be physical, emotional, or mental. "A dynamic spiritual belief system enables us to trust that somehow tomorrow will not be beyond our capacities" (Stoll, 1989, p. 194).

Nurses can strengthen the patient's and family's spirituality by supporting the "use of coping strategies such as prayer, music reminiscence, devotional reading, church attendance, physical exercise and journaling" (Stoll, 1989, p. 205). When the nurse and the patient share the same faith, they may have an occasion to share a time of prayer or a favorite scripture reading. Patients can be encouraged by the nurse's assurance of continued prayer on their behalf. Carson (1983) describes the calming influence of prayer with an agitated male patient who was placed in seclusion. Because of the trust and rapport that she shared with him, the patient was responsive to this intervention and benefited from the reassurance of God's love. Fortunately for the patient, an understanding nurse was available and was comfortable in addressing his spiritual need.

▶ Check Your Reading

5. List three of the six strategies for helping your patients to develop their personal strengths.
6. Name Bailey's six stages in the "journey of grief."
7. Define "empowerment."
8. Define "hope."
9. Describe how humor is typically used during each stage of recovery from substance abuse.
10. Explain the importance of social support for people with mental illness.
11. Describe appropriate ways in which a nurse can strengthen the spirituality of patients and their families.

DEVELOPING YOUR OWN PERSONAL STRENGTHS

Recognizing Attributes Typical of Nurses

Nurses also have characteristics of survivorship, hardiness, and resilience. These attributes propel them through the years of education and the juggling act of career and family. Determination and perseverance are predominant strengths that exemplify commitment. However, control can be an issue.

Nurses tend to be the eldest sibling or a big sister or big brother in the family (Toman, 1961). As the oldest, being in either authority or control can become the favored position. This stance can hinder the nurse-patient relationship. Without self-awareness, nurses, in their eagerness to be good caretakers, can overfunction for patients. Inadvertently, nursing interventions may stifle patients' efforts to accomplish actions on their own. This limits the patient's sense of control and diminishes the opportunity to develop commitment. It becomes the nurse's challenge to be sensitive to patients' needs by fostering their independence and encouraging responsibility.

Nurses who foster resilience in patients and families are often like cheerleaders who can genuinely encourage self-reliance and an attempt to find meaning, even in difficult circumstances. Taking the time to listen to the stories of patients' lives can help put events into perspective and make sense out of temporary chaos as they recover from illness or loss.

Again, the ability to empower patients means avoiding problems created by fostering helplessness. Individuals can learn to believe they are incapable or helpless if they are not readily involved in the decision-making process or are simply told what to do. Frequently, nurses find themselves in a position of giving advice rather than assisting patients to solve problems. Asking questions that provide the patient and family the opportunity to think about "what's next?" or "where do we go from here?" can stimulate their involvement.

The ability to maintain a nonanxious presence, despite an anxiety-provoking situation, is an important attribute that all nurses need to strive for. But sometimes nurses do become anxious and focus prematurely on rescuing patients from stress. When that happens, patients do not access their potential for growth during crisis and become dependent. Understanding the balance between allowing dependency while encouraging independence requires considerable sensitivity, patience, and skill. Managing these variables while dealing with one's own anxiety becomes a "juggling act" that nurses are well familiar with.

Dealing With Constraints Imposed by the Health Care System

Unfortunately, the inherent stress of the health care system places constraints upon the eager nurse who wants to be sensitive to the needs of individual patients. System dictates to do "more with less" frequently place nonprofessional staff in positions of spending more time with patients than the professional nurse. Meanwhile, professional nurses are expected to accept the ramifications of short staff, long shifts, and increased documentation. In addition, they are called upon to supervise staff and delegate patient care to others, while they themselves have limited opportunity to be with their patients. Finding ways to have quality time with patients requires creativity of time management.

The atmosphere created by the above constraints can lead to authoritarian management, serious tension, and morale problems that are conducive to acting-out behaviors by patients, as well as by staff. Morrison (1990) believes that when staff overly value being in control, violent behavior in psychiatric inpatient settings results.

Tensions mount because of "a rigid rule structure and strict adherence to a role that defines staff behaviors" (p. 36). Morrison (1990) also points out that nonprofessional nursing staff are more likely to need to be authoritarian, especially with patients, than are professional staff. Power struggles can then result between patients and staff, as well as between staff members themselves.

In retrospect, Vickie points out that she appreciated staff members' willingness to allow her to experience the consequences of her disruptive behavior. They did not allow themselves to become involved in a power struggle with her. Most likely her behavior was anxiety provoking for staff members, but they did not pressure her to comply. Instead, they set limits for her. Although the pain of her initial dismissal from the program at Way Station was anxiety provoking, she recognized that she returned more motivated to explore the available growth-producing activities, i.e., job training, symptom management, and leisure activities. Despite the rules, she felt the benefit of the staff's acceptance of "who she was," even though they were compelled to carry out a policy that made her uncomfortable. The calm manner in which they dealt with her promoted her recovery. She knew she could return and give it another try.

Managing a balance of control and autonomy can be a fragile strategy for the professional nurse manager. The integrity of patients and staff alike is involved if staff overreact to constraints that are too tight. Nurses need to contain their anxiety and think about what is best for those in their care and under their supervision. It can be especially challenging for the nurse manager when patients or staff members test limits and act out. When management begins to lose control, patient safety and progress are jeopardized, and dysfunctional behavior is enabled.

▶ Check Your Reading

12. Describe a danger of the nurse's being the eldest sibling or a big brother or big sister.
13. What management style can result from a health care system that requires you to "do more with less?"
14. What are the dangers of such a management style?

CONCLUSIONS

Promoting the attributes of the successful traveler is a challenge for the nurse. Like recovering from physical problems, the notion of survivorship can be applied to dealing with mental health issues, including grief and loss. Nurses can promote the traits of the "triumphant survivor" in patients and their families by fostering personal strengths that relate to hardiness (control, commitment, and challenge) and the themes of resilience (equanimity, self-reliance, existential aloneness, perseverance, and meaningfulness). By understanding the stages of grief (protest, searching, despair, reorganization, and reinvestment), the nurse can provide reassurance that recovery is a process of progress toward survivorship. Over time, resolution of a significant loss, whether it be the death of a family member, the effects of a mental or physical illness, or the disappointment of a major event, does occur.

Also, nurses can be involved in empowerment as they encourage patients to accept themselves, take responsibility for their own experience, and trust in themselves and others. A treatment setting that allows participating, choosing, supporting, and negotiating fosters that kind of atmosphere. And nurses who remember the importance of instilling hope, utilizing humor, accessing social support, and inspiring the spirit of the person promote survivorship. Interventions can be planned with these areas in mind.

The nurse who promotes survivorship is also a survivor. Caring for others in a meaningful way requires attributes of survivorship, hardiness, and resilience. Because nurses work in stressful environments, it is important that they have a clear sense of personal goals and needs to prevent the discouragement of burnout.

Finally, nurses promoting the successful journey of a mental health client, like Vickie, help to create pride and a feeling of accomplishment.

Vickie has maintained stability and sobriety for an extended period. She is looking forward to greater independence. She continues to complete and revise her goals for the future. "I did it," she exclaims. "I survived!"

One wonders whether she feels like "The Little Engine That Could." After pulling an especially heavy load, he was so happy when he came to the top of the hill. While climbing he kept saying, "I think I can, I think I can." When he made it to the top, he exclaimed, "I knew I could, I knew I could."

Nurses are partners with patients and families experiencing mental health problems, including loss and grief. They provide encouragement while patients and families struggle to reach the top of "their hill." When they look back and realize what they have survived, they can proudly tell the story of their journey to others, much the same as Vickie has. Then their journey can become a source of strength for others who are chugging along their own uphill road.

KEY POINTS TO REMEMBER

- Patients and families experiencing mental health problems, including loss and grief, can be survivors and can resume life with meaning, sometimes in new ways.
- The attributes of hardiness and resilience are characteristics of survivors who successfully travel life.

• Nurses can encourage hardiness and resilience by being sensitive to the balance of allowing appropriate dependency and promoting timely independence.

• Patients and families need to recognize that overcoming mental health problems, including loss and grief, is a process that can be worked through. Knowing the stages provides nurses a way of acknowledging progress.

• Nurses can be instrumental in the empowerment of patients and families to accept themselves as they are and to take responsibility to make healthy choices for themselves.

• Hope can be a turning point for those discouraged by mental health problems. Sometimes nurses can instill hope by the interventions they use.

• Humor, when used therapeutically, can be a shock absorber and can grease the journey of the successful traveler. Nurses can promote humor in the treatment setting that helps patients see themselves in humorous ways that reduce their anxiety.

• Social systems can be cushions that support individuals and families who are experiencing mental health problems. A substantial support system enhances recovery. Nurses are in positions to encourage the development and expansion of social support.

• Spirituality is a reach for the beyond, an attempt to connect with a power that is beyond oneself that can direct.

• Acknowledging the importance of spiritual beliefs facilitates the acceptance of the whole person (mind, body, and spirit) who is recovering and moving toward survivorship.

• Nurses can be successful travelers on their own journeys. Attributes of survivorship, hardiness, and resilience enhance their ability to be survivors too.

LEARNING ACTIVITIES

1. Ask an individual you admire who has lived through a major disappointment or loss what he or she did to survive the experience.

2. Visit a senior citizen center and interview a group of men and women. Ask them what has helped them to remain in control of their lives in spite of aging and health problems.

3. Get permission to attend a support group for the mentally ill (e.g., National Alliance for the Mentally Ill) or alcoholics (e.g., Alcoholics Anonymous); attend and listen to the members share their stories.

4. Talk to a senior member of your family and ask him or her what helped him or her the most to survive hard times in the past.

CRITICAL THINKING EXERCISES

Nick Gowen, a nurse cotherapist involved in his first outpatient group with multiple abusers, noticed the approach his cotherapist Jamie Johnson was using. Patient Mr. A., a cocaine abuser, told a story about how he wrecked the family car and when he got out of it, he looked back at it and it reminded him of a Crackerjack box. As he was telling the story, he joked and laughed about how only crackers jump from Crackerjack boxes. Mr. Gowen thought that the incident was very serious and told Mr. A. that this was no laughing matter. Mr. A. looked at Mr. Gowen and said, "Don't be a stick in the mud. It's a big joke that I'm still alive."

1. What inference can be made about Mr. Gowen's position regarding laughter in a therapeutic group?

2. Explore ways that Mr. A. could have perceived Mr. Gowen's comment.

3. What assumption(s) can the reader make about Mr. Gowen's comment?

As the group continued, Ms. Johnson looked at Mr. A. and stated, "Share with us your feelings about what is so funny about your accident." Mr. Gowen wondered why Ms. Johnson was allowing this discussion to continue since it was obvious that Mr. A. was in a state of denial about his responsibility for his drug abuse.

1. What assumption(s) can be made about Ms. Johnson's approach?

2. What can be inferred about what Ms. Johnson thinks about Mr. Gowen's comments?

3. What other information is needed to determine if your assumptions are valid?

REFERENCES

Anthony, W. A. (1993). Recovery from mental illness: The guiding vision of the mental health service system in the 1990's. *Psychosocial Rehabilitation Journal, 16*(4), 11–23.

Bailey, J. (1985). Strategies for coping with loss. In J. Abbott (Ed.). *Hospice resources manual for local churches* (pp. 30–36). New York: Pilgrim Press.

Bigbee, J. (1985). Hardiness: A new perspective in health promotion. *Nurse Practitioner, 10*(11), 51–56.

Bowler, J. B. (1991). Transformation into a healing health care environment: Recovering the possibilities of psychiatric nursing. *Perspectives in Psychiatric Care, 27*(2), 21–25.

Caplan, G. (1974). *Support systems and community mental health.* New York: Behavioral Publications.

Carson, V. B. (1983). Prayer in a psychiatric setting. In J. A. Shelly and S. D. John (Eds.), *Spiritual dimensions of mental health* (pp. 93–97). Downers Grove: Inter-Varsity Press.

Connelly, L. M., Keefe, B. S., Kleinbeck, S. V., Schneider, J. K., and Cobb, A. K. (1993). A place to be yourself: Empowerment from the client's perspective. *Image: Journal of Nursing Scholarship, 25*(4), 297–303.

Curry, L. C., and Stone, J. G. (1992). Moving on: Recovering from the death of a spouse. *Clinical Nurse Specialist, 6*(4), 180–190.

Deegan, P. E. (1988). Recovery: The lived experience of rehabilitation. *Psychosocial Rehabilitation Journal, 11*(4), 11–19.

Frese, F. J. (1994). Coping with schizophrenia requires effort. *The Menninger Letter, 2*(3), 4, 5.

Gibson, C. H. (1991). A concept analysis of empowerment. *Journal of Advanced Nursing, 16*, 354–361.

Hammond, V. W. (1988). Conscious subjectivity or use of one's self in therapeutic process. *Women and Therapy, 6*(4), 75–81.

Hatfield, A. B. (1993). *Surviving mental illness.* New York: Guilford Press.

Kadner, K. D. (1989). Resilience: Responding to adversity. *Journal of Psychosocial Nursing, 27*(7), 20–25.

Keith, S. J. (1991). Surviving survivorship: Creating a balance. *Journal of Psychosocial Oncology, 9*(3), 109–115.

Kobasa, S. (1979). Stressful life events, personality, and health: An inquiry into hardiness. *Journal of Personality and Social Psychology, 37*(1), 1–11.

Lambert, C. E., and Lambert, V. A. (1987). Hardiness: Its development and relevance to nursing. *Image: Journal of Nursing Scholarship, 19*(2), 92–95.

Leete, E. (1987). The treatment of schizophrenia: A patient's perspective. *Hospital and Community Psychiatry,* 38, 486–491.

McKenzie, C. (1982). Recovery. In H. Shelter and P. Straw (Eds.), *A new day: Voices across the land* (pp. 18–20). Arlington, VA: National Alliance for the Mentally Ill.

Miller, J. B. (1990). Mental illness and spiritual crisis: Implications for psychiatric rehabilitation. *Psychosocial Rehabilitation Journal, 14*(2), 29–47.

Morrison, E. F. (1990). The tradition of toughness: A study of nonprofessional nursing care in psychiatric settings. *Image: Journal of Nursing Scholarship, 22*(1), 32–38.

Onega, L. L. (1991). A theoretical framework for psychiatric nursing practice. *Journal of Advanced Nursing, 16,* 68–73.

Raleigh, E. D. (1992). Sources of hope in chronic illness. *Oncology Nursing Forum, 19*(3), 443–448.

Stearns, A. K. (1984). *Living through personal crisis.* Chicago: Thomas More Press.

Stearns, A. K. (1988). *Coming back: Rebuilding lives after crisis and loss.* New York: Random House.

Stearns, A. K. (1993). Coming back from crisis and loss: Traits of the "Triumphant Survivor." Lecture given at Taylor Manor Hospital, Ellicott City, Maryland, January 20, 1993.

Stoll, R. I. (1989). Spirituality and chronic illness. In V. B. Carson (Ed.), *Spiritual dimensions of nursing practice* (pp. 180–214). Philadelphia: W. B. Saunders.

Sullivan, W. P. (1993). It helps me to be a whole person: The role of spirituality among the mentally challenged. *Psychosocial Rehabilitation Journal, 16*(3), 124–134.

Sumners, A. D. (1988). Humor: Coping in recovery from addiction. *Issues in Mental Health Nursing,* 9, 169–179.

Tartasky, D. S. (1993). Hardiness: Conceptual and methodological issues. *Image: Journal of Nursing Scholarship, 25*(3), 225–229.

Tomau, W. (1961). *Family constellation.* New York: Springer.

Wagnild, G., and Young, H. M. (1990). Resilience among older women. *Image: Journal of Nursing Scholarship, 22*(4), 252–255.

Walgrove, N. J. (1994). A family member's perspective. In W. Resnick (Ed.), *Smooth sailing: Reviews of the 1994 Mood Disorders Symposium,* (pp. 4, 5). Baltimore: Depression and Related Affective Disorders Association.

Warner, S. L. (1984). Humor & self-disclosure within the milieu. *Journal of Psychosocial Nursing, 22*(4), 17–21.

SUGGESTED READINGS

Connelly, L. M., Keefe, B. S., Kleinbeck, S. V., Schneider, J. K., and Cobb, A. K. (1993). A place to be yourself: Empowerment from the client's perspective. *Image: Journal of Nursing Scholarship, 25*(4), 297–303.

Gibson, C. H. (1991). A concept analysis of empowerment. *Journal of Advanced Nursing, 16,* 354–361.

Hatfield, A. B. (1993). *Surviving mental illness.* New York: Guilford Press.

Lambert, C. E., and Lambert, V. A. (1987). Hardiness: Its development and relevance to nursing. *Image: Journal of Nursing Scholarship, 19*(2), 92–95.

Stearns, A. K. (1984). *Living through personal crisis.* Chicago: Thomas More Press.

CHAPTER 10

POINTS OF INTERSECTION THERAPEUTIC COMMUNICATION

Words do have a critical function . . . in identifying unconscious conflicts, tracing the evolution of false connections in the mind, clarifying what belongs to whom, and providing the relief of having put into words what could not be spoken about—helping to find sense when there had been confusion and/or nonsense.

—*P. Casement*

LEARNING OBJECTIVES

After studying this chapter, you should be able to:

1. Specify different conceptual definitions of communication.
2. Identify characteristics of effective communicators.
3. Define therapeutic communication as a specialized form of communication used in psychiatric nursing.
4. Identify four models of communication applicable to psychiatric nursing practice.
5. Compare and contrast the different types of communication.
6. Apply different types of listening responses: minimal encouraging, restatement, paraphrasing, reflection, silence, summarizing, and validation.
7. Specify the use of selected verbal interventions in psychiatric nursing: redirecting, reframing, confrontation, modeling, mirroring, humor, use of metaphors, coaching, and giving information.
8. Identify barriers to communication in the nurse-patient relationship.

KEY TERMINOLOGY

Circular communication models
Clarification
Closed-ended questions
Coaching
Cognitive behavioral communication models
Cognitive processing communication models
Context
Focused questions
Gestures
Global movements
Humor
Kinesics
Linear comunication models
Metacommunications
Metaphors
Minimum encouragers
Mirroring
Modeling
Neurolinguistic programming
Nonverbal communication
Open-ended questions
Paraphrasing
Physical appearance
Proxemics
Redirections
Reflecting
Reframing
Restating
Silence
Summarizing
Therapeutic (active) listening
Validation
Verbal communication

Within the context of every nurse-patient relationship, the nurse accompanies the patient as a professional guide on a time-limited, exploratory journey that ideally leads to the patient's discovery of the inner self and its potential for healing emotional wounds. Therapeutic conversations represent the points of interpersonal connection, through which patients are able to tell the story of their journey and the nurse is able to provide encouragement, support, and resourceful information. As patients speak of their immediate experience and the life events that led up to their current circumstances, they give voice to their fears, feelings, beliefs, hopes, desires, and private realities.

Mind, body, and spirit are inextricably linked in each person's narrative. Nonverbal actions and facial expressions accompanying the words accent or add meaning to the description of the journey by interjecting the ways in which the person holistically experiences his or her reality.

Psychiatric nurses help patients to clarify the meaning of the journey, both as interested professionals and as *participant observers* in the patients' personal worlds. Organizing the patient's communication cues into a coherent message so that both nurse and patient can follow the journey's unfolding allows each person's story to reveal itself in a broader context. The purpose of holding therapeutic conversations with mentally ill patients is to help them find new meanings in their experiences in which uncertainty, misunderstanding, and confusion previously reigned. This *forward movement*, as described by Peplau (1952), leads the patient toward mental health and a deeper sense of personal integrity.

The challenge for psychiatric nurses is to integrate an understanding of communication and psychiatric nursing principles with their own unique roles as counselors, coaches, facilitators, advocates, teachers, and resource persons for the mentally ill. Therapeutic communication strategies enhance the quality of the journey by providing a means of understanding the suffering of the patient and developing the most appropriate ways to assist the patient on selected pathways to healing. The accuracy of the nurse's understanding affects the quality of the assessment data and related nursing interventions. Through communication, the nurse uses imagination and intuition to help patients plan the most effective ways to facilitate the healing process (Gendron, 1994). With active listening responses, the nurse helps the patient, controlled by fear or false beliefs, to experience new connections with self and others. Although the words a nurse uses can empower the patient and provide social support needed for weathering physical, psychological, spiritual, and social crises, ultimately it is the nurse's actions, expressed with authenticity and genuine caring, that captures the patient's attention (Johnson, 1994). Therapeutic conversations are the means by which the nurse and patient holistically encounter each other as unique human beings engaged in a human journey toward optimal mental health.

This chapter introduces you to the multifaceted nature of communication, the characteristics of effective communicators, and the types of communication found in everyday conversation. It identifies therapeutic communication as a form of conversation specially adapted to the needs of the mentally ill patient and selected theories of communication as the basic framework for understanding the nature of therapeutic communication. Listening responses and verbal interventions are offered as the central behaviors through which each interpersonal journey with a patient takes place.

In the children's story, *Looking Through the Looking Glass*, Lewis Carroll effectively captures the multiple meanings words have for different people and the confusion people experience in trying to communicate with each other when the words carry different meanings.

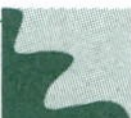

ALICE'S STORY

I don't know what you mean by 'glory,' " Alice said. Humpty Dumpty smiled contemptuously. "Of course you don't—till I tell you. I meant 'there's a nice knock-down argument for you!' " "But 'glory' doesn't mean 'a nice knock-down argument,'" Alice objected. "When I use a word," Humpty Dumpty said in a rather scornful tone, "it means just what I choose it to mean—neither more or less." "The question is," Alice said, "whether you can make words mean so many different things." "The question is," said Humpty Dumpty, "which is to be master, that's all." Alice was too much puzzled to say anything; so after a minute Humpty Dumpty began again. "They've a temper, some of them—particularly verbs; they're the proudest—adjectives you can do anything with, but not verbs; however, I can manage the whole lot of them! Impenetrability! That's what I would say!" "Would you tell me please," said Alice, "what that means?" "Now you talk like a reasonable child," said Humpty Dumpty, looking very pleased. "I meant by 'impenetrability' that we've had enough of that subject, and it would be just as well if you'd mention you didn't mean to stop here all the rest of your life." "That's a great deal to make one word mean," Alice said in a thoughtful voice.

From Carroll, L. (1909). *Through the looking glass* (pp. 103–104).

Like Humpty Dumpty, psychiatric patients often develop a language that is internally consistent and meaningful to them but is difficult for others to follow or understand. Like Alice, you need to decode the meaning of the patient's personalized vocabulary before communication can proceed. Box 10–1 describes the qualities of communication that make it a "point of intersection."

BOX 10-1 The Qualities of Communication that Make It a "Point of Intersection"

- A means of connecting
- A process of being with another
- A way of sharing meaning
- A measure of response-ability

FUNCTIONAL NATURE OF COMMUNICATION

A Means of Connecting

Communication is a complex interactional process that occurs between people and involves the cognitive, spiri-

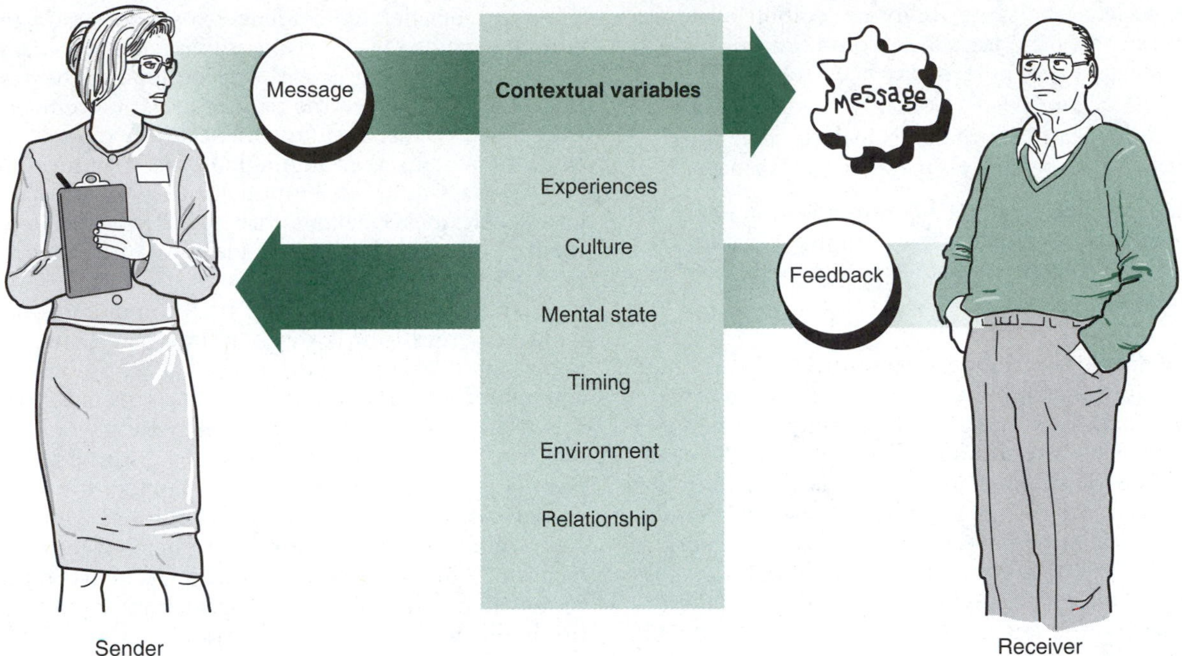

FIGURE 10–1
Contextual variables affecting communication.

tual, and emotional connections with others. This connection with others "encompasses short-term or fleeting encounters, as well as long-term associations" (Johnson, 1994, p. 6). It is considered to be central to the development of meaningful relationships and critical to a purposeful exchange of ideas.

Communication is a learned process. At an early age, children learn from their parents and significant others how to use communication as a means of connecting with others. Initially, they imitate the words of their elders without necessarily understanding their meaning. Later, they refine their communication style and expand the complexity of their language use as they begin to incorporate cultural and peer norms learned in the larger community.

Communication has both factual (content) and emotional (relationship) components that affect its use as a connective intersection in conversation. When people talk with one another about their personal experiences, they are not objectively relaying the actual experience, but rather how they perceive the experience as happening. Interpersonal contextual filters of previous life experience, religious beliefs, values, culture, and present circumstances color the meaning of each person's perceived experience. Successful communication requires "wholeness and integrity in the personal encounter, the achievement of engagement rather than detachment" (Carper, 1975, p. 156). To integrate the presence of contextual filters into a meaningful conversation, it is essential to develop a common interpretation. Placing a conversation within a context means that the interaction between the organism and the environment is taken into account in listening and in framing responses. Common contextual variables are presented in Figure 10–1.

Developing a common language allows you and the patient a comfortable mechanism for cocreating and sharing meaning. Because each person has his or her own unique way of organizing perceptions and communicating with others about the meaning of them, it is important to examine how people communicate and to explore those problems of communication that interfere with productive interpersonal relationships.

Mental illnesses create significant barriers to the development of a common language. They affect the meaning of words and behaviors. Consequently, it is more difficult to use communication as meaningful points of intersection in the usual sense with these patients. They frequently live in a fantasy world constructed of distorted and hidden meanings that defend them against being hurt, and their words serve as a barrier instead of a bridge to relationship. Research has shown that psychiatric patients have less interpersonal flexibility in their relationships, and communication tends to miss its mark as a point of intersection. They report their experiences in ways that do not readily produce shared meanings. Patients tend to generalize, embellish, delete, distort, omit data, or make shifts in their narratives so that it becomes difficult for others to follow their original experience. They do not communicate on a feeling level as easily as mentally healthy people (Topf and Dambacher, 1981).

Studies of the characteristic linguistic patterns in schizophrenic and manic-depressive populations (Fraser et al, 1986) and in psychotic versus neurotic communicators (Jeanneau and Bengt-Ake, 1993) report that psychotic patients tend to be less verbally expressive, to use fewer words to convey ideas, and to avoid speaking of emotionally charged issues. The psychotic patient does not seem to have the same ability to symbolize and use language as a primary format in communication. Such research suggests that nurses may need to:

- Vary communication formats to include modalities other than words—activities or nonverbal formats
- View the psychotic patient's communication deficit as a part of the disorder rather than simply a desire to avoid a relationship or a personal commentary on the nurse's competence

People with mental illness demonstrate a wide range of communication complications, from distorted perceptions to blocked or tangential speech, from highly personalized language to nonverbal, bizarre body movements. Some of these communication difficulties are profound, as in the case of autistic and severely retarded patients who cannot communicate at all through normal verbal channels. Other communication difficulties represent complicated responses and disturbances with information retrieval that make communication more difficult but not impossible. It is difficult to isolate all of the factors that make the interaction more complicated, but inevitably they represent a narrow range of communication behaviors characterized by a lack of clarity or recognizable interactive purpose. Other blocks include a lack of flexibility; overreaction; inappropriate laughter; and repetitive, tangential, vague, or negative messages.

Explanations for the cause of a mentally ill patient's communication difficulties vary along a continuum from strictly biological to explanatory interpretations based on their social origins. There seems to be little question that biological factors play a role in the development of the more serious forms of information processing and communication difficulties observed in the schizophrenic patient or the profoundly negative lens through which the depressed patient experiences and interacts with others. Biological theories suggest that intrinsic misfiring of neurotransmitters affecting feeling and thinking processes account for the disturbances in communication. By correcting the biochemical miscommunications between neurotransmitters through pharmacological agents, communication becomes a possibility. Pharmacological treatment of the biological component of mental illness varies depending on the severity of the symptoms and the individual preference of the patient. Common antipsychotic, antimanic, antidepressant, and antianxiety medications can reduce psychiatric symptoms and provide the potential for establishment of rapport in the nurse-patient relationship.

Psychosocial dynamic theories claim that communication is more than just a reflection of the biological organism. Communication has both social meaning and significance. A person's communication difficulties reflect a particular social and cultural pattern of relating that has been learned over a significant period of time. Psychodynamically oriented theorists believe that what happens to people particularly early in life as a result of important experiences with significant others in their lives has a profound impact on their later communication patterns. There is considerable evidence to support the value of communication as a psychiatric intervention, starting with Freud, whose greatest contribution may be describing the ways in which the patient's relating of his or her experiences create healing. Ross (1994) reports several research studies that highlight hope and meaning as powerful antidotes to emptiness, despair, helplessness, and hopelessness, feelings that are often associated with mental illness. Hope and meaning are transmitted through human connections.

Current experts propose that communication difficulty emerges from a dynamic interplay between biological and social factors (Gebbard, 1992). Both normal and abnormal communication patterns are a function of this process. Although there is increasingly robust evidence of a biological component in disturbed communication patterns, there is strong support for a second hypothesis that suggests an integration of biological and psychosocial factors in explaining unconventional behaviors. Communication (what happens between people) creates neurochemical and neuroanatomical changes in the brain, which, in turn, contribute to and moderate the development of mental illness. The *kindling* theory, whereby people remember prior unhealthy scenarios as if they were occurring in the present and experience similar symptoms without the stressor being present, is a good example of the powerful interplay between life events and biochemical brain changes. (See Chapter 7 for a complete discussion of the biological basis of behavior.) In the 1990s, when even the most biological interventions require communication, there seems to be little question that verbal connections between helping professionals and their patients play a significant role in reducing psychiatric symptoms. Whether biologically determined or socially learned, therapeutic communication remains the critical factor in the personal movement toward health and well-being of the psychiatric patient.

A Process of "Being With" Another

Reaching another human being through a therapeutic conversation involves not simply talking to the other about a problem or need, but actually *being with* the other in understanding and resolving the barriers to successful realization of the journey's potential. Weingarten (1992) notes: "Every conversation creates an opportunity for connection and disconnection; reflection and haste, dialogue and monologue; understanding and misunderstanding; collaboration and instruction; no change and change" (p. 45). Effective use of communication as the means of healing in therapeutic encounters involves staying with mentally ill patients as they search the unknown. It requires empathetically waiting with patients as difficult emotions threatening the journey emerge into view; providing the listening responses that allow the experience of the journey to take a concrete shape; and offering teaching, counsel, and support when needed. Handled appropriately, therapeutic conversations become the primary means by which information is transmitted, experiences are shared, and interpersonal bonds are formed. By bringing the contrasts and uniformities of life experience into sharper focus through words and actions, communication serves to illuminate the path to self in psychiatric nursing situations. Nurses use therapeutic communication principles and strategies as a counseling tool and as an educative instrument to facilitate the patient's forward movement toward health (Peplau, 1952).

A Way of Sharing Meaning

The need for each person to find meaning in life is both universal and profound (Ross, 1994). A human life journey is always a mystery to be unraveled, at once personal, but only discoverable through the sharing of it. First, there are the concrete facts, but then there is a second, equally important, reality, found in each life event's symbolic significance to the person. Each person's experience of the meaning of the journey and the qualities of the people involved are not bound by time, space, or circumstance. In the unconscious, memories of long ago reside next to immediate information and are interwoven with present meanings. Thus the journey's personalized meaning mirrors each person's human potential as they participate in an original life voyage (Cody, 1994).

Communication offers a shared place in time in which the meaning of the journey can be properly displayed. People meet and understand each other as unique human beings when they can "share meaning or co-create meaning, and they are able to coordinate their actions to reflect their mutual meaning-making. . . . In the process of co-creating or sharing meaning, individuals have the experience of knowing and being known by the other" (Weingarten, 1992, p. 47). Significant conversations become the integrative force that promotes self-esteem and creates the possibility of shared emotional connections between self and other. In the process of discussion, conversations help reunite parts of the self that have been disowned or misunderstood and activate personal resources.

A Measure of Response-Ability

Personal responsibility is identified as the cornerstone of mental health. Covey (1991) translates this into *response-ability*—the ability to take charge of one's life without blaming circumstances or others for one's life. Conscious choices made based on values, imagination, and self-determination can modify mental pathology in ways that are essential to mental health. The capacity to make meaningful responses about one's life has a direct relationship to being able to communicate effectively. Ruesch and colleagues (1957) note that:

> *To be understood, a person must be able to express himself clearly; to understand others, he must be capable of observing and evaluating behavior; to establish relationships, he must be able to respond; and to reach agreements, he must be able to combine all these activities in a continuing exchange of messages.*

Certain characteristics make effective communication more probable.

CHARACTERISTICS OF EFFECTIVE COMMUNICATION

Innate differences related to communication always exist between people, evidenced in their communication style, language usage, and cultural or personal interpretations of the meaning of a message. This is a given. Effective communicators, however, display certain characteristics that people who have trouble communicating do not exhibit. Effective communicators demonstrate self-awareness and awareness of the needs of others in the communication. They give simple, clear messages that are appropriate to the situation and responsive to the needs of others. Effective communicators recognize that timing is a critical element in successful communication. They validate frequently to make sure that the receiver has heard the message as the sender intended it.

Self-Awareness

Effective communicators work at becoming aware of their personal communication style and how it affects other people. They obtain this information from careful reflection and asking for feedback. Effective communicators use this self-knowledge as the basis for framing their ideas and responses. They realize that the therapeutic process advances when the content and manner of presentation are familiar and acceptable to the patient and stalls when the communication feels alien. As effective communicators develop personal knowledge of their biases, interpersonal strengths, and limitations, they seek the knowledge or experience that will offset their limitations, or they make proper referrals. Effective communicators continually make efforts to ensure that their personal attitudes and knowledge level contribute to, rather than detract from, conversations.

Awareness of the Needs of Others

Whether communication is a point of intersection or a missed connection to some extent reflects the nature of the relationship existing between the sender and receiver. "Each person's contribution to the production of meaning-making in the conversation is given equal attention" (Weingarten, 1992, p. 47). Effective communicators are sensitive to their listener's needs. They recognize that in the delivery of clear messages, the way the communication is delivered **(metacommunication)** is as important as the words themselves. Voice pitch and volume must meet the demands of the situation. Speaking in a well-modulated and easily understood manner, effective communicators try to project variety in their vocal tones. Their voices convey enthusiasm, and although they may not feel confident, effective communicators work hard to project an image of confidence and self-assurance. Other nonverbal factors that affect communication, such as body odor, facial expression, gestures, amount of space, and touch, are carefully orchestrated so that they do not detract from the sender's message. In every conversation, effective communicators reflect the principle that *therapeutic communication is always an interpersonal process, founded on mutual respect.* Messages always give evidence of confirming the other person and respecting their values.

Use of Simple, Clear Messages

Effective communicators use words that are clear and easy to understand. A clear message requires that the verbal and nonverbal components of the message support each other. Effective communicators avoid words with multiple or complex meanings and refrain from using technical jargon. Each message is simple yet detailed enough for full comprehension. It contains the core elements of meaning and sufficient detail to support the main ideas, with tangential and irrelevant details excluded. Sometimes, important messages get lost because the sender tries to make too many points in the same message.

Use of Appropriate Messages

Effective communicators carefully consider the message in terms of its accurate appraisal of a situation and the level of emotion accompanying it. Useful messages fit the situation, feelings, or circumstances they are describing. They make sense to the listener. When there is a poor fit between the message and the actual events, the listener strains to make sense of it. Unless it is something of interest, inappropriate data are dismissed, or the listener misunderstands it.

The degree of emotion complements the content of the message. It is almost impossible to respond to a simple message delivered with great emotional intensity when the message does not call for that level of emotion. Conversely, content messages that logically call for high emotion but fail to convey the emotional feeling one would normally expect simply do not affect the receiver with much personal resonance. Feelings that accompany the substance of the message ideally support the content; they neither override nor diminish its meaning.

Use of a Flexible Communication Style

Flexibility is essential to effective communication. The effective communicator adapts a fluid communication style, always taking into account the varying responses of the receiver to each part of the conversation. This requires a careful, continual assessment of what is occurring throughout each interaction. The sender must be able to judge his or her audience and be able to make immediate changes to meet individual needs in communication as they appear. Receivers of any message differ from one another in their educational level, preferred representational system, and what is needed for full comprehension. For example, some people require a great deal of verbal detail or written instructions and diagrams to understand a message fully. Others are put off by detail and just want the "bottom line." Such distinctions are significant. It is important to measure when to pursue a topic or train of thought and when to back off. Changing a phrase or action to one that fits the receiver's language and communication style can eliminate many communication obstacles.

Appropriate Timing

Effective communicators recognize that timing is a critical element in successful communication. Contact between people takes time. Conversations are never in haste. The conversation emerges as a collaborative effort with sensitivity to the other person's mood and current circumstances. For example, the sender realizes that the same message delivered when the receiver is tired, preoccupied with other matters, about to start a new project, or just finished meeting with someone else is received differently than in times of relative tranquility. Important messages are timed for the conversational moment when the sender has the receiver's full, undivided attention. Effective communicators offer complex conversation topics and explanations from their logical beginning rather than expecting the receiver to make cognitive connections and conceptual leaps. They involve the receiver in the process as well as the outcome of the conversation by offering frequent opportunities for reflection and for asking questions.

Asking for Validation

Effective communicators ask for validation frequently. **Validation** is a special form of feedback in which the sender asks the receiver for his or her personal reaction to the message to determine whether the message received is the same as the one that was sent. Effective communicators validate frequently, recognizing that if the message is distorted, it can create more problems than if the message was never sent. They never take it for granted that a message has been received as it was intended, just because it was appropriate or was delivered clearly and simply or within a trusting relationship. There are all sorts of reasons why a message is not received correctly—anxiety, anger, shame, cultural differences, prior life experience, feelings about the topic or sender, just to mention a few. Validation allows the sender to correct misperceptions, to rectify distortions, or to give more information to enhance understanding, all of which serve to create a "dialogically shared domain of meaning" (Anderson and Goolishian, 1990, p. 162).

▶ Check Your Reading

1. What are some of the different ways in which communication is defined?
2. What are the characteristics of effective communicators?
3. What is meant by the statement: A good psychosocial assessment depends on the skillful use of communication strategies?
4. Why is clear communication so important in psychiatric nursing?

TYPES OF COMMUNICATION

As noted earlier, people meet each other interpersonally and share the experiences that make up their human journey through communication. The points of intersection in a therapeutic conversation take place on many different levels. This is because people react to one another as a composite whole: cognitively, affectively, and behaviorally. They respond not only to the words that are actually spoken or written, but also to how a message is presented and the environmental circumstances under which it occurs. People observe nonverbal gestures and movements and assign meanings to them; they interpret messages and message delivery through the filters of their culture and their belief systems. Thus, communication is a fertile process, capable of providing a ready access to a deeper and broader way of being. A major nursing role is to motivate patients into exploring the vast potential of communication responses available to them and then to help them develop the proper communication tools needed to reflect on their experience in ways that enhance their development of critical life skills.

For the purposes of describing the richness of communication, it is divided in three distinct categories:

- Verbal communication
- Nonverbal communication
- Metacommunication

This separation is artificial in that the three elements occur simultaneously as part of an inclusive message. Verbal communication expresses the message's cognitive meaning in words. Metacommunication comments on its affective (emotional) meaning. Nonverbal communication gives clues about how the person is experiencing the transaction as a unified whole of mind, body, and spirit. Understanding the precise meaning of anyone's communication provides a clearer focus on what the experience means to the other person. In clinical settings, the art of communication also requires "a perceptual awareness that singles out relevant information from irrelevant, grasps a situation as a whole rather than as a series of tasks, and accomplishes this rapidly and without incremental deliberative analysis of isolated facts or bits of information" (Benner and Wrubel, 1982, p. 13).

Verbal Communication

Verbal communication refers to words, verbal and written, and most people consider it to be the primary means of sharing experience. People not only respond to the communication of others, but also they affect it through the words they use. Thus, words have an *action-oriented* function as well as an *information* role. They are used to organize and describe life experience. Words also allow people to choose, to make decisions, and to take action. Putting experiences and feelings into words helps create boundaries for them. People use words as an interpersonal bridge to explain themselves to others, for understanding the other person, and for problem solving. Figure 10–2 displays some of the many uses of words.

Message Confusion

The possibility of misunderstanding the meaning of a message or the intentions of the sender exists as a potential reality for several reasons. Because people carry internal images, consisting of memories, relationships, and perceptions of reality compatible with their beliefs about themselves, they are not always on the same wavelength about the meaning of a message. Message confusion created by stress, distraction, or cultural interpretations limits full comprehension, whereas cognitive disorders, psychosis, depressive negativity, or anxiety can more seriously modify the objective meaning of a message. To communicate effectively, both patient and nurse must be reading from the same sheet of music, and each must have a clear understanding of the other's intent.

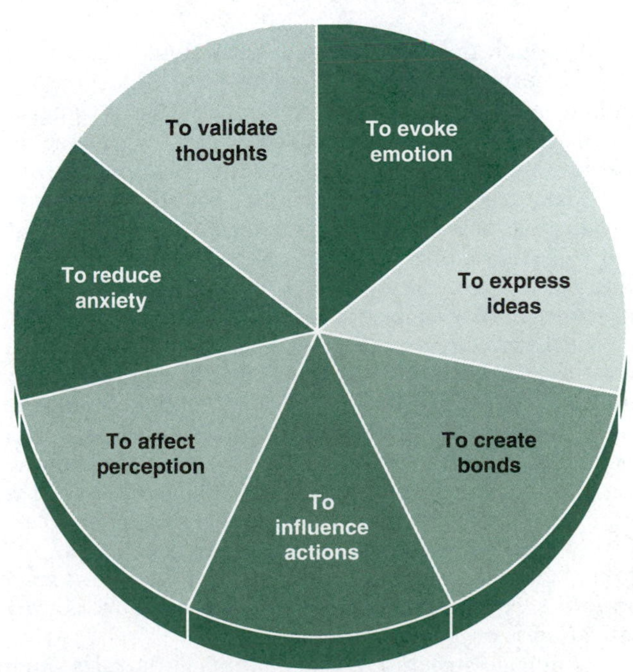

FIGURE 10–2
Some uses of words.

Part of the reason for word meaning confusion lies in the divergent forms, interpretations, and nuances words objectively symbolize in any given language. Apart from the influence of mental images and mood, previously described, misunderstandings about the meaning of words or the way in which a person uses them can occur between people of different ethnic, geographic, or economic backgrounds. Tannen (1995) suggests they also arise between genders.

Most languages have two levels of meaning related to words: denotation and connotation. *Denotation* refers to the objective meaning the culture assigns to the word. A culture may assign different spellings and completely different meanings to the same phonetic word: sight, site, or cite, for example. The culture may assign different meanings to the same word, depending on the social context in which the word is used. For example, the word *love* can be used as a noun to describe a feeling of intimacy between two people, "Our love is forever," or it can be used as verb to indicate a willingness to engage in an activity, "I would love to do that." Alice in Wonderland discovers the double meanings of phonetic words in her conversation with the duchess.

"If everyone minded their own business," said the Duchess in a hoarse growl, "the world would go round a great deal faster than it does." "Which would not be an advantage," said Alice, who felt very glad to have an opportunity of showing off a little of her knowledge. "Just think what work it would make with the day and night! You see the earth takes twenty four hours to turn round on its axis—" "Talking of axes," said the Duchess, "chop off her head!"

From Carroll, L. (1909). *Through the looking glass* (p. 96).

Although the words axis and axes sound alike, their literal meaning is quite different—as might be the outcome of their different interpretations in this vignette. Word use can change depending on the degree of relationship that exists between the communicators. Some languages, French for example, have different terms for personal pronouns that distinguish between intimate and more casual relationships. A person would use *vous* in most casual conversations but would use *tu* with an intimate family member as the word form for *you*.

Connotation refers to a more personalized use of the word that generally is not found in the dictionary. For example, the word "cool" carries an explicit denotative meaning related to temperature. Cool is also used in a more personalized way, e.g., "that's cool" to indicate something is worthwhile or pleasing. The latter use of the word demonstrates it connotative meaning. Said sarcastically, "that's really cool," the same term can mean the direct opposite. *There is a danger in assuming that word symbols have the same meaning to people.* This is why validation is always so important.

Language structure and communication rules often are not reflected in the conversations of the mentally ill for different reasons. This is partly because neurochemical and neuroanatomical changes in the brain can color their reality. Patients frequently use primitive concrete symbolic images that disguise the real meaning of their communication. They encode their messages in multilevel symbolic language and give ordinary words specialized meanings that are entirely consistent with their internal maps of reality but not readily understood by those unfamiliar with their personalized language. Some of the more universal symbols people use in talking about themselves include house or car for self, water or cave for the unconscious, fierce animals such as lions or tigers for aggression (Leuner et al, 1983).

Communication style also suffers. For example, psychotic patients often speak symbolically or have an empty way of relating that is hard to follow. Such patients tend to answer with single-word answers and tolerate lengthy silences. These silences can create an enormous pressure on you to become overactive. The fact is that you can communicate with a psychotic patient if you are willing to follow the patient's lead in pacing the conversation and can employ a variety of strategies. Your response has crucial consequences. It can create a climate of acceptance and a sincere desire to understand, or it can create pressure for the patient to "perform." The most constructive interactions are always those marked with personalism and sensitivity to the unique needs of a fellow traveler.

Nonverbal Communication

Language is only one of the symbolic ways people share their experiences. People also use a wide variety of nonverbal behaviors to enhance, disguise, negate, or modify their verbal messages. In fact, the meaning of communication is interpreted primarily through nonverbal rather than verbal communication. Mehrabian (1972) suggests that nonverbal means account for more than 90% of the message transmission between people (55% transmittal through body cues and another 38% through metacommunication). Only 7% of a person's message is actually transmitted through words. **Nonverbal communication** acts to modify spoken words in a variety of ways:

- By reinforcing or contradicting them
- By emphasizing or diminishing their importance
- By identifying or underlining the emotion associated with them

The expression of nonverbal behaviors can be conscious or unconscious. Some behaviors are within the person's control, for example, handshaking, smiling, and nodding one's head. Other behaviors are clearly not within the person's control; blushing, facial tics, shaking, sweating, and heart palpitations are primarily involuntary physiological responses that communicate meaning. Nonverbal communication behaviors that may or may not be fully under the control of the patient include physical appearance; use of eye contact; use of hand gestures; posture;

facial expressions; amount of distance tolerated between people; and peculiarities of dress or grooming, mannerisms, and body movements. People sometimes use nonverbal actions to direct another person's behavior or to stop the flow of conversation with behaviors such as stopping midsentence, avoiding eye contact, burping, or getting up and walking away.

Nonverbal communication behaviors can send several conflicting messages at the same time. For example, smiling while pulling back from the other person in an interaction or looking at one's watch can send mixed signals, even though the body posture and words may indicate attention. Usually a person, at best, is distracted by the incongruence and, at worst, entirely discounts the meaning of the verbal message as being invalid in light of the contradictory nonverbal behaviors. When the nonverbal component of the message contradicts the verbal, most people tend to pay more attention to the nonverbal behaviors because they are less likely to be under the voluntary control of the sender (Taylor et al, 1989). Unfortunately, nonverbal communication behaviors also are more likely to be misinterpreted. For example, a patient who walks away from you in the middle of a conversation may be experiencing anxiety with the closeness of the relationship rather than disinterest or discomfort with the topic. Validation of the meaning of nonverbal behaviors is always an essential component of an accurate interpretation.

Physical Appearance

From the first encounter with a patient, the nurse and patient form initial impressions of each other that have an impact on their subsequent communication. The professional demeanor of the nurse can instill confidence in the nurse's competency. Nonverbal behaviors of openness, presence, and attention in the form of eye contact and an interested, friendly facial expression invite the patient to participate in the relationship as much as the actual words.

A lot of information is available in the physical appearance of the patient. Observe the **physical appearance** of the patient, noting posture, body odor, makeup, clothing, skin tone, hygiene, and facial expression. Judgments about the meaning of appearance, however, sometimes do a person a disservice. Many people judge the worth of a person by his or her appearance. Some assessments may be prematurely stereotypical. For example, the presence of long hair or an earring may not really reveal a "hippie." A prim and proper costume may not totally represent a woman as being uptight and prudish. Poor hygiene can result from temporary physical as well as emotional discomfort. Alice in Wonderland painfully experiences having her physical appearance misunderstood as something other than what she knows she is. She tells the Pigeon:

> "But I'm not a serpent I tell you!" said Alice. "I'm a—I'm a—" "Well! What are you?" said the Pigeon. "I can see you're trying to invent something!"
>
> I—I'm a little girl," said Alice, rather doubtfully, as she remembered the number of changes she had gone through that day. "A likely story indeed!" said the Pigeon in a tone of the deepest contempt. "I've seen a good many little girls in my time, but never one with such a neck as that! No, No! You're a serpent and there is no use denying it"

From Carroll, L. (1881). *Alice's adventures in wonderland* (p. 89).

The truth is that Alice's physical appearance *had* undergone a change, which could lead to such a conclusion. Similar misperceptions are true of people's appearance in different phases of their lives, those who present with an uncommon physical appearance, and those who suffer sudden shock. People with preconceived ideas about how other people should look and act may judge uncommon physical appearances in much the same way as the Pigeon viewed Alice—and be equally wrong.

Some generalizations about personal appearance can prove valid. Poor hygiene, particularly when coupled with other symptoms of a psychotic disorder, is commonly found in schizophrenic patients. Too much makeup or too little attention to physical appearance may indicate poor self-esteem. Depressed patients frequently take little interest in their appearance and present with a dejected droop of the shoulders. Garish makeup and seductive clothing often accompany manic disorders. The skin tone of a person on drugs often appears pale, and the facial expression is blunted or wild looking. Without sleep or in cases of depression, a person loses normal color. Depressed patients sometimes have loose clothing or clothing that is too tight because of recent weight loss or gain. Self-awareness, an open mind about the meaning of physical appearance, and validation help prevent the possibility of an inaccurate assessment.

Body Language

Kinesics describes body language displayed through physical movements, gestures, and facial expression (Birdwhistell, 1970; Richmond et al, 1987). A patient's body language can be an important source of information because it is less under the control of the patient. Unfortunately, body language lends itself to misinterpretation because of culture, illness, or the mood of the person expressing it. For example, the facial expression of mentally ill patients frequently undergoes transformation reflective of their psychiatric disorder. Many schizophrenic patients present with a flat or blunted emotional expression. It is difficult to "read" the patient's facial expression. Although the schizophrenic patient's face cannot show any expression of feelings, this does not mean that he or she is not experiencing feelings. Rather the feelings are potentially overwhelming and unmanageable. Therefore, it is appropriate for you to suggest feelings and ask for validation when they normally would be expected.

Depressed patients frequently present with a sad expression, the mouth turned downward and a furrowed brow. By contrast, the facial expression of a person with an anxiety disorder presents a portrait of the patient as constricted and tense. Manic patients often have an animated facial expression, which changes to belligerence when angered.

Related to facial expression is the use of eye contact and involuntary eye movements. Eye contact is an interactive behavior that helps to regulate communication. Its primary use is to signal speaking and listening roles in a conversation. People use eye contact to indicate interest and attention. Dropping eye contact can signify that the conversation is over. Lack of eye contact can indicate low self-esteem or anxiety about a conversation topic. Frequently, psychiatric patients avoid eye contact, especially when speaking of emotionally disturbing topics. Cultural norms can dictate use of eye contact, so lack of eye contact does not necessarily suggest pathology. Verbal validation and careful observation of cultural norms can prevent unfortunate mistakes being made about the use of eye contact.

The expression in a person's eyes also conveys information. Eyes that are empty and lifeless are characteristic of schizophrenia. The eyes of the depressed person often reflect sadness. Excitement is read in the eyes of the manic patient. Rapid eye movements can signal a person out of control and often are the first warning sign of impending violence. Sometimes the only way to notice pain in cognitively impaired patients is through their facial expression, particularly their eyes.

Gestures

People have voluntary control over many of their **gestures,** referred to as emblems, illustrators, or regulators. *Emblems* are generalized gestures that have a distinct meaning to a social group: for example, V sign for victory, handshake, power fist, or hand slapping to signal a job well done. The precise meaning of the gesture may or may not be understood by those outside of the cultural group. Other gestures are referred to as *illustrators* and serve as nonverbal cues to expand what is being communicated verbally. Examples of illustrators include pointing, pounding the fist to emphasize a point, or using open hand motions to grab the receiver's attention. *Regulators* are nonverbal behaviors that provide the sender with information about the impact of the message, the receiver's feelings about the relationship, a desire to change the direction of the conversation, or a need to end it. Examples of regulators are looking at one's watch, yawning, leafing through a magazine when someone is speaking, leaning forward, sleeping, or turning away from the sender.

One set of gestures, not directly under the control of a patient, is referred to as *adaptors.* People experiencing anxiety often use stylized or ritualistic body movements, adaptors, to release tension. These behaviors are observed more frequently in mentally ill patients who lack full command of their anxiety or the way their body chooses to express it. Examples include facial tics, hand wringing, head scratching, twirling one's hair, head jerking, scratching, touching the nose when speaking, or stroking parts of the body. Careful observation of adaptors and when they occur can give you important clues about topics and situations that create anxiety for your patients.

Global Physical Movements

Global physical movements are another form of nonverbal communication. Many mentally ill patients have distinctive and bizarre body movements, which initially can be frightening to behold. Once you develop an understanding of their role in mediating anxiety, these bizarre movements become less troublesome. Pacing back and forth often is a strong indicator of increased anxiety, as are the rocking and head banging found in some severely retarded and seriously regressed mentally ill patients. Changes in body movements can signal discomfort with the situation or a more generalized negative or positive response to the environment. For example, the patient who uses eye contact for the first time after many sessions of looking away from you in other interactions may be indicating greater trust and comfort in talking with you.

Personal Space

Proxemics describes the study of personal physical space. The amount of personal physical space each person needs varies with the situation, with cultural norms, and with their internal psychological needs. Hall (1966), an anthropologist, extensively studied the amount of space people need in most situations. He identified four basic distances people use for interaction (see Figure 8–3). Most conversations between nurses and patients take place within a personal and social space of 3 to 6 feet.

The needs of the patient dictate the use of space to some extent. A patient in an acute stress state needs more interpersonal space and becomes frightened when staff move in too close. This is particularly true of the psychotic patient, who may misidentify nursing staff or misinterpret the intent of their actions. Usually the patient signals the amount of space needed through nonverbal behaviors. If the patient appears uneasy or moves away, closer contact usually is not desired. Shorter interactions and allowing enough space for comfort work better than pushing the issue.

It is not uncommon for a psychotic patient to move into a social distance with a nurse and appear to circle the nurse without speaking, moving in and out of the immediate area. Inviting the patient to sit down may be all that is needed. With more regressed patients, you can signal the invitation through nonverbal behaviors, such as smiling, using eye contact, and nodding when the patient sneaks a furtive look at you. Engaging the patient in a largely nonverbal game such as ping pong can permit access to the patient's space without appearing intrusive.

Maintaining Confidentiality

The nurse protects the psychological space of the patient through confidentiality. All communication between nurse and patient must be treated as privileged information. Only those directly involved with the patient's care should have access to this information. Patients, even those who appear to have limited comprehension, need to know what information will be shared with others. *Information about adult patients to third-party callers cannot be shared under any circumstances without the patient's consent.* Information about a minor, however, can be shared with the parent. If a patient is in danger of harming himself or herself or others because of a mental illness, you are legally obligated to make this fact known to the appropriate authorities. Examples include child abuse and when a patient threatens suicide or harm to others. Nurses need to make their patients aware that if the patient tells the nurse about any child abuse situation, and this includes abuse at the hands of someone other than the patient, legally the nurse must inform Child Protective Services. Knowing this beforehand prevents some of the sense of betrayal a patient can feel when you report an abuse case to the appropriate authorities.

In writing progress notes, you need to be aware that others will be reading the chart without having you available for interpretation. It is easy to write more of an interaction, to include personal data beyond that needed for general care of the patient, or to extend your interpretation of its meaning beyond the actual data. As professionals, nurses must be aware of their own biases and take special care in handling privileged information. This is an ethical and legal responsibility that demonstrates respect for the patient's integrity as a person.

Metacommunication

Watzlawick and colleagues (1967) suggest that one cannot not communicate. Even when words are not spoken, people communicate with one another. Metacommunication is communication about the communication or lack thereof. As an integral but implicit part of the message, it represents the interpersonal bridge between the verbal and nonverbal components of communication. Metacommunication relates to the sender's expectations, the influence of emotions, the level of attention, and the bias of attitudes and values. It is emotionally based and emphasizes the relationship aspect, rather than the content of the message. For example, a person may speak of wanting to have a deeper relationship with his wife and then in the same message describe her controlling behaviors and how uncomfortable they make him. Although part of the message addresses one desire, the other speaks to his concerns about moving closer. The metacommunication here is the emotional *ambivalence* expressed in this person's message. Another patient may not speak of any difficulty but signal his ambivalence nonverbally through missed joint appointments or by ignoring his wife's requests.

Metacommunication aids the receiver in accurately interpreting the emotional meaning of the content. Examples of metacommunication include the patient's speech patterns or vocalizations. The relationship aspects of the patient's message also are found in the timing of comments, tone of voice, silence, verbal inflections, and even manner of makeup and dress. Phrasing and emphasis can significantly modify the meaning of the message. Part of the analysis includes the manner in which the patient is interacting with the nurse. Usually, patients interact with the nurse, particularly after the relationship is well established, the same way they interact with significant others in the environment. Thus, understanding the meaning of the here-and-now interaction with the patient gives clues to patient responses in the larger environment.

Vocalizations are sounds and verbal inflections that are not words but tell the listener how to interpret the message. Sobbing and vocal tones that are abrasive, soft, or hesitant provide clues to the sender about the meaning of the message and the attitude of the communicator. Vocalizations are particularly useful in helping the nurse decode the meaning of a mixed message in which the verbal and nonverbal components do not match.

People with psychotic disorders sometimes use primitive vocalizations to cope with their anxiety. For example, the schizophrenic patient may laugh inappropriately with no visible stimulus in the environment. Understanding this tendency helps you to respond more effectively to the underlying dynamics (auditory hallucinations) of the patient's communication.

A patient's speech pattern yields important clues about diagnosis and source of anxiety. Many chronically ill patients demonstrate disordered language patterns. Their dysfunctional patterns are qualitatively different from more functional speech patterns, characterized by a lack of clarity, vague or irrelevant language, and loosely connected ideas that are hard to follow. Understanding the wide array of presentations associated with complex communication aids in formulating nursing diagnoses and appropriate nursing interventions. Common speech patterns found in the chronically mentally ill can fall into one or more of the categories shown in Table 10–1.

"Confirming" Communication

Confirmation is an abstract concept related to respect and interpersonal sensitivity. It is so important that it can make the difference between a message being heard or being perceived as hurtful. *Confirming communication is an essential characteristic of therapeutic interactions.* In the context of a caring nursing intervention, confirming responses acknowledge, respect, and respond to the personhood of the patient, as a fellow and unique human traveler. Buber (1957) speaks of using confirmation as the means of understanding and responding to the other person, in the full measure of who they are and what they are capable of becoming. Frankl (1963) views confirmation as recognizing and validating another's experience as real and meaningful. Confirming responses are those that accept the characteristics of the other as meaningful, support their intrinsic value, and help people find meaning in their present circumstances. So often, mentally ill patients feel a sense of depersonalization; they feel erased by society and, more painfully in many cases, by the family who is supposed to support and value their existence. In the role of surrogate, nurses can help patients develop depth and coherence to their sense of

TABLE 10–1 Common Speech Patterns Found in the Chronically Mentally Ill

Pattern	Definition	Found in
Poverty of speech	A tendency to speak very little, to use one-word answers or phrases	Schizophrenia, depression, and acute situational stress
Pressured speech	Rapid speech with little change in intonation between ideas	Manic-depressive disorders, crisis situations, and anxiety disorders
Flight of ideas	Rapid switching from one idea to another, with little connection between them	Manic-depressive disorders and crisis situations
Thought blocking	Sudden stopping in the middle of a sentence, especially when it involves an anxiety-provoking thought	Global anxiety in most mental disorders, schizophrenic responses to internal stimuli, and cognitive mental disorders
Halting speech	Slow speech with little change in vocal intonation between ideas	Depressive and cognitive disorders and mental retardation
Circumstantial speech	Speech in which the details presented in the message and main point of the conversation have little or no relation to one another	Disorders involving emotionally difficult content, schizophrenia, and cognitive mental disorders
Loose associations	Speech in which there is an absence of logical connections between thoughts and ideas	Schizophrenic disorders
Echolalia	Repeating or echoing the sender's comments	Schizophrenic disorders
Confabulation	Filling in the blanks, replacing data with fantasy	Cognitive mental disorders
Word salad	Words put together that do not go together or make sense	Schizophrenic disorders
Neologisms	Nonsensical linking together of sounds	Schizophrenic disorders
Double bind	Two conflicting elements linked together in the same message	Dysfunctional communication

self. Feeling valued as a person by you enables many patients to begin to value their own integrity as someone of worth and interest (Sieburg, 1975). Table 10–2: contrasts "confirming" and "disconfirming" responses.

THERAPEUTIC COMMUNICATION

Theoretical Models of Therapeutic Communication

Linear, circular, and cognitive processing models form a basic framework for exploring the more specialized forms of communication referred to as therapeutic communication.

Linear Models

Linear models of communication typically present as a simple, straightforward model involving a sender, a message, and a receiver, focusing on the structure of the communication process. The *sender* is defined as the person who transmits verbal and nonverbal messages. The *receiver* is the recipient of the message, the person who listens. The *message* is the content part of the communication, including the response feedback that may represent the transaction of a new message. Messages are transmitted from sender to receiver through sensory motor channels of communication. These channels of communication can include one or more of the following sensory channels as presented in Figure 10–3.

The sender *encodes* verbal messages. Encoding refers to the format the sender uses for the message content. Each person's encoding usually reflects the fundamental norms and values of their culture, their previous life experiences and current understanding of the situation, their feelings about the receiver, and a host of influences from the environment. In analyzing the meaning of a person's message, the helping person needs to take the context of the situation and the usual verbal style of the patient into consideration. The encoded message also contains feelings, emotions, and, sometimes, a more personalized symbolic context based on the sender's private interpretation of a situation.

When the receiver listens to a message, that person uses a cognitive process whereby the words are decoded into language symbols, mutually understood by all participants. *Decoding* involves taking the patient's words, looking for the key symbols hidden within them for the meaning of the message, and restating it in words relevant to the current patient situation. Sometimes, decoding can be accomplished easily with the use of listening responses to develop specific data rather than vague generalities. For example, asking the patient, "Could you give a specific example of . . . ?" can help make problems more accessible for mutual understanding. Other times the decoding of a message is difficult, as when the psychotic patient uses symbolic language. Decoding this patient's communication is an art. The best way to decipher the complexity of the psychotic patient's message is by identifying the underlying themes.

> Jeffrey Beber tells his nurse that he knows something that will terrify her if he reveals it to her. When pressed, he shares that there are evil people in the world who are going to take over the universe and create mass chaos. He's doing his part, he tells the nurse, by making ammunition and stor-

TABLE 10–2 Contrast Between "Confirming" and "Disconfirming" Responses

Characteristic of Response	Example
Confirming	
Connecting through direct acknowledgment	"Yes, I can understand how that could be a problem."
Disconfirming	
Erasing the person by not acknowledging the existence of a communication	Treating the patient's statement as if it never happened; not giving a verbal or nonverbal response
Confirming	
Supporting or validating personal meaning	"I can see that you are really trying to get the most out of your treatment program." "I can really understand why this is so important for you to grasp."
Disconfirming	
Discounting meaning	"Well, your problem is not at all uncommon; most people resolve it by . . . ."
Confirming	
Asking for clarification	"It sounds like you are really worried about. . . . Can you elaborate a little more on how this is affecting you?"
Disconfirming	
Responding with an irrelevant or tangential comment	"You can't do anything about . . . , so let's talk about happier times in your life."
Confirming	
Expression of personal feelings	"I know that was very difficult for you to reveal, and I'm glad you felt comfortable sharing it with me."
Disconfirming	
Impersonal expression of feeling	"Most alcoholics don't realize how much their family suffers from the consequences of their drinking."
Confirming	
Active listening	Listening with one's full presence, focus, and attention
Disconfirming	
Interrupting the flow of conversation	Cutting the patient off or changing the subject

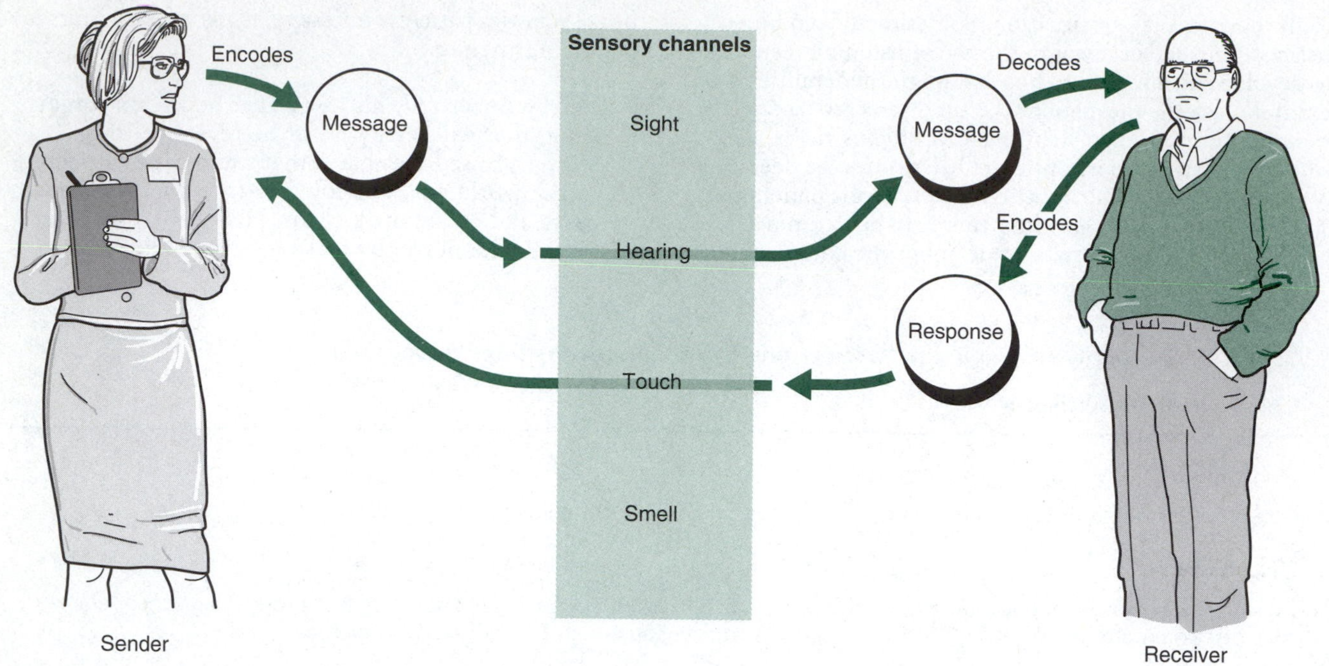

FIGURE 10–3
A linear model of communication, showing the channels of communication.

> ing it underground so that it can't be found but will be ready for instant use when the time comes. "Someday, if I just seem to disappear, it's because I know too much," confides Jeffrey with a worried look on his face.

For maximum effectiveness, the nurse uses themes that reflect only what the patient reveals or that relate to the symbolic comments initially made by the patient. In this example, the nurse might respond:

> Jeffrey, what you are telling me sounds very scary, and I can't help but wonder if you are not feeling particularly vulnerable right now, here on the unit. Is this something we might need to talk about?

Expecting the patient to speak in normal language is more useful than simply ignoring the patient's psychotic speech or trying to develop an understanding of its literal meaning through listening responses. Despite their fears, most mentally ill patients experience relief when the nurse is able to decode a symbolic message accurately. Usually the patient nods or says "yes" when the nurse is right. Occasionally an appropriate decoding leads to full discussion of the underlying theme.

It is as important to develop an understanding of the mentally ill patient's language as it is to connect with the culturally diverse patient through words. Ways to understand the culture of the mentally ill are based on the Berlin and Fowkes model (1993) more typically used as a communication format with culturally diverse patients. This model describes a communication process, identified by the acronym LEARN (***l***isten, ***e***xplain, ***a***cknowledge, ***r***ecommend, ***n***egotiate). First, *the nurse listens to the patient's perception of the problem.* Second, *the nurse explains his or her perception of the patient's dilemma.* Third, *the nurse acknowledges the similarities and differences between the two views,* which helps clarify the meaning of the problem. Fourth, *the nurse makes recommendations based on the mutual understanding of the problem.* Finally, *the nurse and patient negotiate a treatment plan that incorporates the important elements of the patient's culture in the implementation of the plan.* Developing a mutual understanding of the patient's message is the highest form of connecting with someone because of the effort involved in listening and empathetically understanding another's world.

Circular Models

Circular communication models broaden the process of communication to include internal and external factors that represent revolving communication patterns with feedback loops, affecting the communication of both parties. They are based on the premise that each person in any interaction is a unique biological, psychological, spiritual being with different life experiences, all of which influence the communication process. Communications reflect what the person is thinking and feeling as well as all of the environmental factors surrounding the communication.

One of the more well-known circular models is the transactional model, originally developed by Berne (1964). Berne postulates that the way an individual communicates duplicates earlier communication patterns and reflects one of three ego states: parent, adult, and child. The parent represents the authority figure and "should" messages. The adult ego state is the thinking reality aspect. The child represents the creative, fun, "want" messages. Each ego state is appropriate in certain situations and equally inappropriate in other situations. For example, to achieve an identified goal, the *parent* state provides the self-discipline to reach goals, the *adult* state would ask questions about the purpose of the actions taken, and the *child* would ask for time out for leisure to replenish the self. Knowing which ego state the situation calls for helps facilitate communication. As long as the communication flows between designated ego states, whether they be parent-child, parent-parent, or adult-adult, the communication represents a complementary transaction (Figure 10–4).

Dysfunctional communication (crossed transactions) occurs when one person communicates from a particular ego state, and the other responds from a different ego state. For example, the nurse responds to a patient as an adult. The patient, in return, responds from a child ego state, to the nurse as parent (see Figure 10–4). The equality needed in adult-to-adult communication is missing. This can be corrected by teaching patients to express their feelings with "I" statements, for example, "I feel angry because I didn't get my pass today," instead of withdrawing or acting out the feelings.

The advantages of using a transactional model are several. First, it is relatively easy to learn. Concrete examples and correction of missed transactions are readily available and easily understandable. Second, it is self-reinforcing. Once a person learns how to recognize the different ego states and to incorporate "I" statements, it is easy to manage and self-monitor one's communication. The transactional model places responsibility for communication on the patient. Another advantage of using the model is that it takes the emotionality out of the communication. Obviously, however, a transactional model of communication that requires cognitive processing and abstract thinking would not be a communication model of choice with cognitively impaired patients.

Cognitive Processing Models

Cognitive processing communication models assert that individuals develop their own models of the world based on a combination of sensory inputs and the way they are interpreted by the person. Two such models are referred to as neurolinguistic programming and cognitive models.

NEUROLINGUISTIC PROGRAMMING

Neurolinguistic programming models developed from the premise that people create internal representations of their reality and tend to categorize their experience according to a dominant sensory mode (visual, auditory, or kinesthetic). These models focus on the preferred ways in which people access and mentally process their messages. **Neurolinguistic programming,** originally developed by Bandler and Grinder (1975, 1982), is a communication model that uses observations of a person's

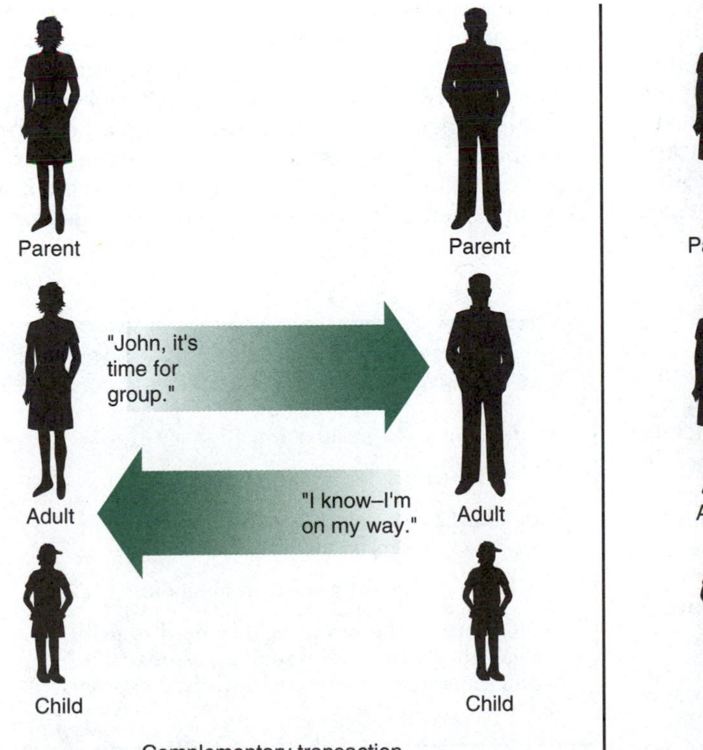

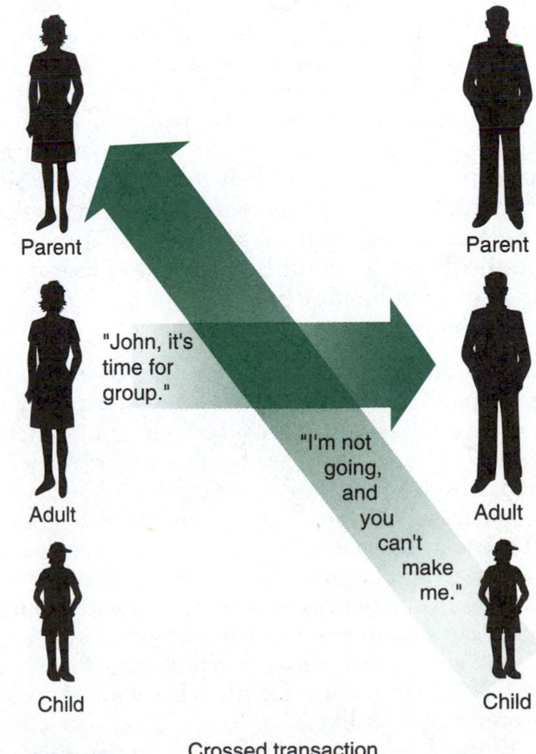

FIGURE 10–4
A circular model of communication, showing complementary and crossed transactions.

BOX 10-2 Verbs Commonly Associated With the Three Most Common Representational Systems of Neurolinguistic Programming

Visual	Auditory	Kinesthetic
Observe	Describe	Balance
Examine	Tell	Maneuver
Inspect	Report	Operate
Study	Listen	Steer
Survey	Hear	Adjust
Watch	Heed	Handle
Focus	Command	Finger
Appear	Instruct	Palpate
Notice	Persuade	Weigh
Picture	Recount	Manage
Looks like	Divulge	Engineer
Look at	Inform	Control
Overlook	Notify	Manipulate
Scan		
Recognize		
Note		
Identify		

verbal speech patterns and nonverbal behaviors to determine how people access their information. Knowledge of the patient's communication style helps you select the most appropriate channel to transmit important messages. According to this model, people use a variety of sensory motor modalities—visual, auditory, kinesthetic, touch, and smell—as a means of accessing and processing information. Most often, people favor one modality as their "primary" representational system. By tuning into the patient's speech—particularly the verbs—and eye movements, you can identify the patient's dominant representational style (Knowles, 1983). You can anchor your messages with the verbs likely to be received readily by the patient. Verbs commonly associated with the three most common representational systems (visual, auditory, and kinesthetic) are found in Box 10–2. To illustrate the application of neurolinguistic programming, consider the following application.

> Marsha Calhoun is scheduled for discharge from the day hospital next week. She has expressed anxiety about how she will be received by her family when she returns home. Specifically, she worries about her first day back home. The nurse can help Marsha become more specific about the problems she thinks will occur by using Marsha's preferred representational system in the way she frames her opening sentence. To match her response to the patient's representational system, the nurse might say:
>
> *If Marsha uses a visual representational system:* "I'd like you to picture for me what your first day at home will look like."
>
> *If Marsha uses an auditory representational system:* "Can you describe for me what you think your first day will be like?"
>
> *If Marsha uses a kinesthetic representational system:* "How do you plan to handle your first day home?"
>
> By framing the same question within Marsha's preferred sensory representational system, the message is more likely to be understood.

Neurolinguistic programming offers a theoretical framework for using reframing as a communication strategy. Emphasizing the positive aspects of a situation gives the patient a different perspective and more flexibility in resolving difficult situations. Reframing, discussed later in the chapter, is based on assumptions outlined in Box 10–3.

COGNITIVE BEHAVIORAL MODELS

Cognitive behavioral models of communication also focus on the importance of internal cognitive representations, but rather than having the emphasis on the sensory representation, the focus is on how the information is processed. According to this theoretical model, thinking moderates mood and behavior. For behavioral change to occur, the person's thinking must change. A person's belief system participates in and helps create the meaning of current sensory inputs.

Cognitive behavioral communication models hypothesize that one's normal cognitive processing is affected adversely by stress, creating flaws in thinking or cognition (Beck, 1987). Although a person in stress can perceive reality, the cognitive images are immediately linked to previous content stored in memory. Referred to as *cognitive distortions,* the cognitive image triggers emotional remembrances surrounding the thought. When this occurs, a person's normal ability to reason effectively diminishes, and a cycle of altered thinking and feeling results in maladaptive, self-defeating behaviors. Even one associated tangential aspect of a current image can trigger an irrational belief system and thereafter shape a person's perception and frame of reference for the current data. The current situation takes on added meanings that may

BOX 10-3 Assumptions That Form the Foundation of Reframing

All behavior has a positive intention.

All behavior is useful in some context.

People make the best choice they can for themselves at any given moment.

It is better to have choices than no choices.

People have all the resources they need to make the changes they want—the resources just may not be organized, sequenced, or contextualized appropriately.

From *Issues in Mental Health Nursing, 12:* 9–18. Pesut, D. (1991). Taylor & Francis, Inc., Washington, D.C. Reproduced with permission.

TABLE 10–3 **Common Cognitive Distortions**

Cognitive Distortion	Examples
Dichotomous thinking	
All or nothing	"I must do everything perfectly and completely at all times or else I am a failure." "I must have your approval. Without it, I am no good."
Black-or-white thinking	"Either you love me or you don't." "You are the best therapist who ever existed." "You are the worst possible therapist for me." "This is the worst possible thing that ever happened to me."
Magnification or minimization	
Polarized assessment	"I'm not going to get a good credit rating when they check my references." "I don't think much about my father's infidelity."
Absolute thinking	
Should, ought, never	"I should never be angry." "I ought to be more industrious, like my father." "I should know better than to trust men."

or may not have anything to do with the reality of the situation. Common cognitive distortions are presented in Table 10–3.

Beck and Emery (1985) believe that negative automatic thoughts and images occurring immediately after a psychological trauma are a critical dynamic in anxiety disorders and depression. The automatic cognitive processing assigns a meaning of danger to the current situation that is difficult to erase. Passivity usually follows, with internal feedback loops continuing to reinforce one another. Cognitive communication models basically are designed to help patients identify their automatic thoughts and change their negative self-statements into more positive self-statements. The process of reframing negative statements helps the patient restore an appropriate emotional tone and meaning to the current situation.

Cognitive therapists train their patients to notice and interrupt their negative thinking patterns. They encourage patients to observe the external circumstances that may have contributed to the arousal of their automatic thoughts. Patients are encouraged to evaluate the validity of their thoughts and to seek evidence that highlights a different interpersonal schema—one that is more in touch with the reality of the current circumstances. Where information is biased and represents inaccurate or incomplete data, the patient is persuaded to develop alternative explanations. By changing their internal dialogue, patients are able to shed their irrational beliefs. Nurses play an important role in helping patients develop their own mental probes to offset negative thematic content. Questions the patient can use as mental probes might include:

- "On what grounds am I making this judgment?"
- "Are there any alternative explanations for what happened?"
- "What is the worst that will happen if I am right?"
- "If what I think is true, how useful is it for me to continue this line of thinking—what purpose does it serve?"

Seligman (1991) asserts that "the most convincing way of disputing a negative belief is to show that it is factually incorrect" (p. 221). For example, you might ask patients who believe that they receive approval only when they are doing something for others to recall a situation in which they felt approved of without having to do anything for it. With encouragement such as "think back in your life, was there anyone who thought you were special?" most patients can come up with one situation. With even one such example, a negative belief stands in jeopardy.

As patients learn to recognize their self-defeating patterns and use self-talk to reduce their impact on self-concept, cognitive therapists lead them a step further. Cognitive models propose that patients get better as they are able to restructure their thinking from a blaming, self-doubting frame to a reclaiming framework, emphasizing personal strengths rather than deficiencies. Thus the therapist, employing a cognitive orientation, would focus on the following questions in helping patients redirect their thought patterns in a healthier manner:

- What do you want?
- How would you be different if you had it?
- What would you have to do to get it?
- What stops you from having it now?
- What resources do you have available to help you achieve your goal?
- How can you utilize the resources you have or could make available?
- What are you prepared to do to achieve your goal?

With these questions as a guide, the patient is able to reclaim the inner resources needed to fashion the direction of the journey in a more productive way. Because there is a strong interrelationship between perception, memory, cognition, and feelings in this model, what stimulates survivorship or reduces psychological vulnerability varies from person to person. This is where individualization of nursing actions comes into play.

Definition of Therapeutic Communication

Therapeutic communication is defined as a special form of communication that has a health-related purpose and develops as a continuous flow of interaction between nurse and patient, with input from both contributing to its nature and progression. Therapeutic communication principles derive from theoretical models of social communication. Table 10–4 summarizes important differences between social and therapeutic communication. The purpose of therapeutic communication is to allow the nurse to foster a meaningful connection with the patient (Havens, 1986). With each interaction, there should be a cognitive and emotional meeting between persons, one of whom is the patient and the other a helping professional—in this case the nurse. Therapeutic communication becomes a dialogue in which the nurse helps patients look at complex human data from different perspectives and then assists them in developing socially constructive responses to the irrational beliefs, thoughts, and feelings that imprison them.

Often, mental illness is associated with people continuing to do the same behaviors over and over but expecting a different outcome. The task of therapy often has to start with convincing the patient that this is not possible. Awareness of the need to change personal behavior if you want a different outcome and specific actions to support a different outcome are necessary prerequisites to change. Change does not happen in a vacuum. Here you play an important role in stimulating awareness of problem areas and needs. Moreover, it is important to convert each significant problem statement into a goal statement and then to support the patient's efforts in meeting the goal through constructive changes in behavior. Through therapeutic conversations with you, patients begin to adopt constructive communication strategies and attitudes in their interactions with others. Immediate feedback stimulates further growth, and the goal of achieving a different, more positive reality becomes possible.

Purpose of Therapeutic Communication

The primary purpose of therapeutic communication is to help patients discover the truth about themselves in ways that allow them to experience new possibilities in their lives and to alter ineffective life patterns (Wachtel, 1993). *The nurse's role in the communication process is to help patients transform vague, tangential, or distorted statements into clear, concrete, workable statements that have the same meaning to both participants and to use these mutually developed understandings as the basis for therapeutic intervention.* In the course of discussion, patients learn to make sense out of the ways in which they behave. The nurse enlists the patient as a collaborator in the process of self-discovery and uses words, actions, and knowledge to help patients develop more a more positive view of themselves and more adaptive ways of interacting in the world (Havens,

TABLE 10–4 **Important Differences Between Social and Therapeutic Communication**

Social Communication	Therapeutic Communication
Can occur at any time and is not time-limited	Occurs within designated time frames and terminates when therapeutic goals are achieved
Responsibility for the structure and conduct of the conversation is the responsibility of both parties	Responsibility for the structure and conduct of the conversation is ultimately the nurse's.
Communication is spontaneous and not necessarily goal directed	Communication is purposeful and directed toward mutually established goals
The needs and concerns of both partners can receive equal consideration	The focus of the conversation is always on the needs and concerns of the patient
The purpose is for both parties to achieve greater intimacy in the relationship	The purpose is for the patient to achieve greater self-understanding from the relationship
Self-disclosure of the details of private life is acceptable for both parties	Self-disclosure of the nurse's private life is limited and acceptable only under certain circumstances
Social decorum and adherence to the rules of etiquette are expected	Conversation does not always reflect adherence to the rules of social etiquette
Can continue spontaneously at any time, depending on the desires of the participants	Formally terminates with the end of the session or relationship

1986). Through interactions with you, patients learn to share feelings and ideas about the nature of their journey. In the process, the patient begins to feel accepted and more willing to look at difficult life issues from a different perspective.

Focus of Therapeutic Communication

The focus of therapeutic communication is on the patient as a person. A patient focus means that the nurse suspends all judgments about what the patient is revealing, and time spent with the patient should be free from distractions, both environmental and personal. Concerns that the patient presents for consideration or specific information you convey to the patient related to his or her health care represent the content of therapeutic dialogue. Concentrating on the patient's needs and concerns requires you to maintain those issues the patient needs to resolve for mental health and personal fulfillment as a consistent focal point. The health-related purpose of therapeutic communication provides the direction for people to develop more adaptive thoughts, feelings, and behaviors. Furnishing opportunities for patients to identify more reality-adapted opportunities for personal growth places patients in charge of their own health care.

Responsibility of Therapeutic Communication

The primary responsibility for the structure and conduct of the relationship lies with the nurse. It is the patient's role to do most of the talking. You are responsible for creating the type of interpersonal environment needed for full disclosure of difficult issues and feelings. This includes maintaining boundaries, making sure therapeutic conversations are purposeful and related to identified health-related goals, documenting important information, and developing relevant interdisciplinary care plans with other health team members.

Role of Self-Disclosure in Therapeutic Communication

Self-disclosure can be a highly effective communication tool, if it is used appropriately. Self-disclosure by the nurse of relevant but neutral personal experiences, observations, and feelings is an informational source that the patient can appreciate within a shared human encounter. Appropriate self-disclosure draws the participants together in a mutual experience, enhances trust, and provides a more equal relationship (Ivey, 1988). Certain guidelines, however, determine the suitability of self-disclosure.

For optimal effectiveness, *the nurse's self-disclosure must fit the demands of the situation and the needs of the patient.* Sharing personal information that is not directly related to the goals of the relationship serves to distract from rather than enhance goal achievement. Self-disclosures that are pertinent but suggestive of behaviors that are not achievable by the patient not only miss their mark, but also can increase anxiety. Similarly, data of an intensely personal experience, even though relevant, may make the patient uncomfortable. For example, sharing a rape experience or an abuse experience may not be appropriate, even though the patient initially brings up the topic. Because it is unlikely that the event no longer has meaning to the nurse, the event cannot help but stimulate feeling in the nurse during the retelling, and this is not helpful to the patient. With self-disclosure, the needs of the patient should be the focus of conversation. You also need to be sensitive to each patient's needs, readiness, vulnerability, and cultural background before sharing personal information.

The nurse's self-disclosure of personal feelings *about* the patient may be appropriate in certain circumstances. In general, this type of self-disclosure should be more about the behavior of the patient or clearly evidenced personal characteristics. Using *I* statements and verbs that express your feelings are particularly appropriate, for example, "I think you have made significant progress during your hospitalization, particularly with (give examples)." Statements such as "One of the things I like best about you is your dry sense of humor" or "Right now, I am feeling that you are trying to shut me out by closing your eyes and appearing to sleep," give patients information about the way their behavior affects others. Personal feelings of a deeper nature, either positive or negative, are not appropriate data for sharing. Evaluative self-disclosures such as "I'm very proud of you," "You're my favorite patient," or "I'm so disappointed that you couldn't stay sober over the weekend" are more closely related to the nurse's ego than the patient's behavior. They tend to diminish the patient and compromise your effectiveness.

Factors Affecting Therapeutic Communication

Environmental Factors

The *physical setting, timing,* and *selection of therapeutic approach* all can influence the sending and receiving of communication. Self-disclosure occurs most easily in a private setting. Usually, it is best to use the same room for each session, away from the mainstream of activity. If there are limited options in choosing the most appropriate place for an interaction, picking the quietest place within the large day room is the place to start. The patient's bedroom usually is not an appropriate place because this is the patient's personal space.

Different standing and seating positions make it easier or more difficult for patients to engage in conversation. Interactions taking place from a sideways sitting position rather than directly face to face are sometimes easier for the mentally ill patient to tolerate. Communicating from a position in which both participants are at eye level with each other is more effective than conducting the conversation from unequal physical stations (Argyle, 1975). If more than one person is to be involved, you as the nurse should decide whether the patient is to be the primary informant. Then the others are asked to hold their comments until they are asked for them. If the interview is a family-group experience, in which all participants can contribute equally, structure the session with this expectation. Major determinants will include the cognitive abilities of the patient and the purpose of the interview.

Time is an important variable in planning for a therapeutic interaction. Determining the amount of therapy that can be accomplished in the time available, checking on resources that may be required, and leaving enough time for summarizing the session are all important considerations. The initial interview will take longer because you and the patient are unfamiliar with each other. Timing of interventions parallels the development of the relationship and current circumstances.

Timing is important from two perspectives. First is the issue of allowing enough time for the person's message to show itself fully. You must approach your patients gently, allowing them to tell their story in their own manner. Second, in working with mentally ill patients, it is particularly important to avoid overloading the circuits because processing of information may take longer. Presenting one idea at a time and waiting until the patient demonstrates some readiness to hear messages, especially when significant change is required, become important.

Focusing on the interaction between the organism and his or her environment is another area of concern. Successful communication is dependent on your ability to learn your patients' language, to reflect accurately on the nature of their feelings, and to convey verbally words and ideas in a conversational format easily understood by the patient. You need to draw on a broad spectrum of verbal and nonverbal behaviors to respond effectively to the often disjointed conversations of mentally ill patients.

Conversational flexibility takes many forms because patients come from many walks of life and life experiences, ranging from well educated to functionally illiterate, from being socially adjusted to being socially inept, and from wealth to abject poverty. The patient's readiness, educational level, and ability to assimilate new information are also determinants in structuring the relationship and planning the most appropriate interventions.

Another important consideration is the patient's behavior. For example, the patient's mood may fluctuate within the same conversation, beginning with congeniality, moving into anger, and ending in tears. Pauses, silences, and even the pacing of messages can provide cues to the types of modifications you need to make in response to a patient's behavior. By carefully observing the patient, you can notice subtle changes, as when the patient's voice tightens, quavers, or catches with discussion of emotionally difficult material. These observations help you to know when to press for more information, when to back off because the patient is not ready to deal with the material, and when to make an observation about the patient's emotional expression.

Cultural Factors

Learning the patient's interpersonal language and style becomes even more difficult when nurse and patient are of two different cultures. Culture has a powerful effect on language, not only the words, but also on the structure and nuances of communication. Language has a basic structure and a strong linkage to the reality it seeks to explain, which sometimes is not readily translatable into another language. Words in different languages may mean the same thing, or they may mean something completely different. Communication rules about the communication (metacommunication) also differ. Grammar, vocal tone, verbal inflections, and body language may be understood by one culture as having one meaning and may have the opposite meaning in another culture. For example, eye contact in Western cultures signifies openness and connection. In some Eastern cultures and with Native American patients, direct eye contact is viewed as a sign of disrespect or aggression. For Mexican and African-American patients, averting the eyes is a normal behavior when a person is speaking, particularly if the person is receiving a reprimand. It does not signal lack of attention. Nodding the head and simultaneously smiling usually means agreement with the speaker's ideas in Western cultures, but it is simply a polite gesture having little connection with content agreement in Asian cultures. Hall (1966), in his multicultural research of space use, noted that Americans typically stand closer to each other than people from England or Germany, whereas Middle Eastern cultures typically permit even closer interpersonal contact.

The cultural impact on language expression varies within the culture as well as among cultures. The factors that make up a culture are highly complex and cannot be fully described in terms of cultural language commonalities and differences. This is because each person is unique. One person may choose to retain many parts of his or her original culture. Another may take on the aspects of the new culture or may integrate the new with the old. Others may reject or deny their cultural origins. A cultural assessment should include attention to the individual expression of cultural beliefs as well as to common expectations for cultural behaviors.

Beyond language, culture influences behavior in terms of a shared knowledge, belief system, and values that transcend location and time. Perceptions are culturally bound and dependent on whether or not they support the person's cultural world view of reality (Jackson and Meadows, 1991). A person's cultural heritage is traceable through its origins to ethnic roots, historical and political ideology, religion, family, social class, and occupation. Some cultures prescribe a limited range of behaviors and frames of reference for behavior. For example, Asian patients typically use a formal, contextual way of relating with strict formal codes of conduct and asymmetrical power relationships. Americans tend to relate with more equality in language style among men and women than those of Asian and Hispanic descent.

Cultural codes permeate family organization, roles, relationships, and behavioral expectations, affecting intrapersonal behavior and interpersonal relationships.

TABLE 10–5 **Culture-Bound Mental Illnesses**

Cultural Group	Culture-Bound Illness
Hispanic	*Susto* (soul loss): Caused by a severe fright. When the fright occurs, the spirit captures the soul of the victim. Symptoms include anorexia, apathy, depression, and withdrawal
African-American	*Voodoo illness:* Caused by a supernatural magical hex from which the person cannot escape. Symptoms include nausea, vomiting, diarrhea, or bizarre behavioral symptoms. Carried to an extreme, it can result in voodoo death
Asian	*Hsieh-ping:* A trance state created by the possession of the victim's body by dead relatives

Adapted from Campinha-Bacote, J. (1988). Culturological assessment: An important factor in psychiatric consultation-liaison nursing. *Archives of Psychiatric Nursing,* 2, 2410–2450.

Frequently, communication conflicts arise because of differences in fundamental cultural beliefs or because of cultural stereotyping, which increases during times of stress. Table 10–5 provides examples of culture-bound mental illnesses, and Chapter 14 provides detailed information regarding the role of culture in the nurse-patient journey.

Therapeutic use of cultural understandings can be an invaluable resource in the nurse-patient relationship. If the nurse can develop with the patient a mutually adaptive view of cultural differences in which it is possible for each party to retain important social values and to negotiate conflictual areas, the relationship blossoms into meaningful encounter. Although you may have the foundation for understanding the general features of a cultural group, this knowledge base may not be as extensive as that needed to understand a particular patient or the degree to which the culture influences the patient's behavior. Therefore, you need to ask about a person's cultural background as part of the psychosocial data collection. Inquiries into cultural differences should be balanced and nondiscriminatory. Kleinman, Eisenberg, and Good (1978, p. 256) suggest the following open-ended questions as being relevant to developing a person-oriented understanding of cultural influences. Of critical importance to effective communication and an understanding of patients are the reasons they attribute to the development of their mental illness and the types of treatment the person finds acceptable.

- What do you think has caused your problem?
- Why do you think it started when it did?
- What do you think your sickness does to you?
- How severe is your sickness?
- What kind of treatment do you think you should receive?
- What are the most important results you hope to achieve from these treatments?
- What are the chief problems your sickness has caused?
- What do you fear the most about your sickness?

▶ Check Your Reading

5. What are the characteristics of therapeutic communication?
6. In what ways do therapeutic conversations differ from social conversations?
7. How do linear, circular, and cognitive behavioral models differ from one another?
8. What are some of the different ways in which types of communication are identified?

Strategies for Therapeutic Communication

Therapeutic communication strategies consist of two distinct categories, both of which are equally necessary in conversations with patients: therapeutic listening and verbal and nonverbal intervention strategies. Therapeutic listening skills have been identified as the most important communication tool that nurses use with psychiatric patients. Verbal interventions develop from information obtained through active listening and include all of the words used in therapeutic conversations. Without nonverbal interventions to complement and support verbal interaction, the message is only half-heard. Nonverbal intervention strategies, such as touch and body language, ideally complete nurses' verbal interventions.

Therapeutic (Active) Listening

Kemper (1992) defines the process of **therapeutic (active) listening** as "an interpersonal, confirmation process involving all the senses in which the therapist attends with empathy to the patient's verbal and nonverbal messages to facilitate the understanding, synthesis and interpretation of the patient's situation" (p. 22). Therapeutic listening consists of an active interpersonal give-and-take response process. All of the active listening strategies presented in this chapter are designed to achieve the dual outcome of getting enough information for comprehensive understanding of the patient's real message and of affirming the personhood of the patient. Active listening responses are deliberately designed to expand, clarify, and verify the content of the message and the intentions of the sender.

CHARACTERISTICS OF ACTIVE LISTENING

Active Listening Is Purposeful. Often, defensive speech patterns, personalized use of vocabulary, distracting mannerisms, unrelated or irrelevant thoughts, or a lack of flow in the conversation can be frustrating. Patients often are not fully aware of how their behavior strikes others and how this, in turn, affects the responses they receive. Active listening responses are the most effective way to help patients stop using the habitual thoughts and actions that prevent them from getting the satisfaction from life they desire. A primary value of using them is that they help patients replace faulty thinking with a conscious awareness of how their personal history and sense of self influence their decisions and actions.

Active Listening Requires Disciplined Attention. It involves attending to auditory cues and careful observation of patient behaviors. Initial perceptions by the nurse become the foundation for decoding the meaning of the patient's message. Decoding the message requires you to put many pieces of data together internally in a unified whole. Your understanding of the message gets replayed for the patient through listening responses to check its accuracy (validation). If more information is required to complete understanding, you need to clarify the parts that are not understood, always taking into consideration the needs of the patient. Mentally ill patients require special attention to the underlying themes in their communication. Often their communication is as convoluted and concrete as what Alice in Wonderland experienced in her conversation with the March Hare and the Mad Hatter.

> The Hatter opened his eyes very wide on hearing this; but all he *said* was, "Why is a raven like a writing desk?" "Come, we shall have some fun now!" thought Alice. "I'm glad they've begun asking riddles—I believe I can guess that," she added aloud. "Do you mean that you think you can find out the answer to it?" said the March Hare. "Exactly so," said Alice. "Then you should say what you mean," the March Hare went on. "I do," Alice hastily replied; "at least I mean what I say—that's the same thing, you know." "Not the same thing a bit!" said the Hatter. "Why, you might just as well say that 'I see what I eat' is the same thing as 'I eat what I see'!"... And here the conversation dropped.

From Carroll, L. (1881). *Alice's adventures in wonderland* (p. 112).

Active Listening Is Focused. It requires more than simply hearing the content of a patient's message and responding to it. Hearing is a physiological process, whereas active listening involves all of the senses and has a distinctive psychological component. Focused listening is an interpersonal process of full concentration, dependent on a willingness to suspend judgment until such time as the deeper meaning of the sender's communication becomes readily apparent. It involves a three-step process:

1. Observing the patient's behaviors, hearing the patient's words, listening for themes, and recognizing relevant verbal and nonverbal communication patterns
2. Integrating all of this information into a logical whole
3. Reflecting back to the patient your interpretation of the message for validation

For example, you would make a mental note of whether the patient's facial expressions and body posture were appropriate to the emotions being expressed verbally. You might observe that certain elements of a situation are left out of the conversation. The cognitive integrating aspects of active listening come into play as you consider: "Does the patient's body language, facial expression, timing of comments, and vocal tones convey the same message as the words?" If not, what might be an alternative explanation, or what are the specific areas that need further exploration?

Active Listening Is Both a Personal and a Shared Interpersonal Experience. The process of active listening involves making sense of the sender's message and attaching meaning to it. Because what a person says is not always what the person means, the active listener is watchful for verbal and nonverbal messages, for what the person does not say as well as what the person says, and for congruence between the content and feeling dimensions of the message. In assessing the meaning of the patient's communication, also take into account his or her personal values, prejudices, beliefs, and life experiences. These factors influence how you assess the meaning of the patient's message and respond to it.

When the flow of conversation is only in one direction, it can get quite uncomfortable. Communication is a two-way process. Some patients have trouble giving information or need more prompting to achieve greater ease in communicating. If the flow of responses does not seem to happen easily, you can increase the sense of mutuality by giving a broader factual or general listening response than would be needed with a more verbal patient.

Active Listening Is a Process of Continual Dialogue. It goes beyond the formal statements of the patient to the heart of the patient's story; it is a not one-time exchange of a central idea. The human journey is a series of moving events and their associated feelings. Polster (1992, p. 151) suggests that listening to the patient's story becomes the means for connecting with the patient in a mutual understanding of the series of events constituting the patient's human journey:

> *Stories are the gathering of experiences; through their thematic development they transform otherwise unconnected events into a meaningful unity. When a patient told me, first, that his mother had died when he was 7 years old, and, second, that from then on his father periodically would mope, and, third, that he would repeat the words, "it can't work," he was connecting these experiences. Then, when he also said that he had made up his mind right then, at age 7, never to feel like a failure, he put down a marker acknowledging the continuity through his life.*

Feelings are normalized as you help the patient distinguish legitimate feelings from the pathological issues with which the patient entangles them. Patients speak of feeling relief in being able to say the unspeakable without the self-recrimination that comes from speaking about it only with oneself. Parts of the story, repressed in memory, are reconnected with each other in a dialogue that begins to make sense and to take on meaning. For many patients, being listened to as a person of value is a first-time gift of major importance and value. The restoration of relevant connections between events and feelings allows the patient to place them in perspective and enables the patient to move on with a different life story in which life events act as contributors rather than dictators of a sense of self.

Stories of the human journey invariably contain important information about the patient's self-concept, both in character and in circumstances. Often, patients omit crucial contextual information necessary to understand their story fully. For example, a patient may complain to you that he is working three jobs because he is afraid of the future. One of the jobs is in a clothing store in the evening, and this creates problems with family life. Although he listens to you and agrees that maybe decreasing the number of jobs would not really affect his income dramatically, what he neglects to reveal is that he really does not enjoy being home and he likes the financial benefit of getting his clothes at a reduced cost. When patients reconstruct their story for you, they often present it in terms of their emotions or as discrete events, but the facts and feelings are not linked together or considered by them as part of a larger communication pattern. They cannot identify what really matters to them about a situation or how this knowledge could be used to shape a different way of being and behaving. Noticing what patients omit from the conversation about their journey, for example, denial of feelings, can be as important as the descriptions themselves. As patients link events and feelings and thoughts about the events together in their minds, as they hear their stories reflected back to them, as they are encouraged to elaborate on their story, it is possible to draw different conclusions about their meaning in the present. Active listening responses are specifically designed to achieve these goals.

STRATEGIES FOR ACTIVE LISTENING

Active listening responses help bring the patient's story to life. The story of the journey is sometimes told in a voice filled with earnestness, passion, and authenticity; other times, the narrative slowly unfolds, sounding curiously limp and narrow. Within the story, you may hear the patient struggling with life issues similar to your own. This does not mean that you are mentally ill but simply that there are many common themes to everyone's human journey. Usually it is a complicated story, and if you listen well, it is possible to recognize and understand the patient's story as a richly complicated and intriguing account of a human being. Therapeutic conversations provide points of intersection through which patients can enlarge and better understand their self-reflections.

The process of active listening typically involves the use of several verbal listening responses, which are used to develop the full meaning of a patient's story. For example, nurses usually use questions, minimum encouragers, and clarification for data collection. Asking the patient to expand and elaborate on incomplete or inadequate data or to clarify conflicting responses encourages the patient to move into deeper content. Other listening responses test your understanding of the interaction and are designed to expand the patient's awareness of important material. Listening responses should directly relate to the patient's comments. Phrasing the listening response in the patient's vocabulary and at the patient's developmental level of understanding facilitates ease of dialogue and, consequently, greater understanding.

Using Minimum Encouragers

Minimum encouragers are defined as simple leads into a conversation that provide the patient with cues through body actions, vocalizations, or a short phrase, such as "go on" or "let's hear more," to continue talking. They prompt the patient to continue with the discussion without providing much information about what the nurse expects from the conversation. They demonstrate personal interest in what the patient is saying without biasing the patient's responses. For example, you might use eye contact to demonstrate that the patient has your full attention. Looking directly at someone when he or she is speaking conveys concentration. Maintaining eye contact decreases distraction from other thoughts.

Leaning forward also indicates interest. Vocalizations such as "um" and "ah" and nonverbal encouragers such as nodding and smiling result in increased information flow because they send a nonverbal message of approval that positively reinforces the speaker.

Using Questions

In social conversations, questions are simple inquiries. Questions assume a more complex role in therapeutic relationships as listening responses. What people think they hear may not be what the sender intended to convey. *If nurses are to understand their patients, they need to ask questions about what they are hearing and validate the accuracy of their inferences.* The nurse uses questions as a primary listening response to elicit more information, demonstrate empathy, and show respect for the patient's thoughts and feelings. Questions have an implicit value, in that they allow a patient, in providing answers, an opportunity to think things through out loud. As patients hear themselves speak, they develop different understandings, and new insights can emerge. Hearing immediate feedback coupled with the nurse's skillful use of questions to elicit deeper understanding and greater detail often helps patients solve their own problems with minimal verbal intervention from the nurse. Excessive use of questioning, however, can interrupt the flow of the conversation. As much as possible, the patient should take the lead in telling the story of their journey.

Three types of questions, open-ended, closed, and focused, help develop a patient's story. **Open-ended questions** are inquiries in which there are many possible directions the receiver can go, and the respondent constructs the answer in his or her own way. They are similar to those asked on an essay test and frequently begin with "what, how, when, why, can you tell me, or can you give me an example?" Open-ended questions give the patient the most latitude in answering them. For instance, you might ask the patient who claims to be depressed, "You say you are depressed. Can you tell me how your depression is affecting your daily life?" The value of an open-ended question is that the respondent may be bothered by something that would not be immediately obvious or known to the interviewer. Having the opportunity to answer the question as one chooses may more accurately reflect the patient's immediate concerns. Sometimes, it is appropriate to use a cluster of open-ended questions to get full details about a situation:

Nurse: You say you feel as if you aren't able to do your work. Can you give me an example of what you mean?

Patient: I just can't seem to concentrate, and I can't anticipate the next step.

Nurse: How does that seem to occur?

Patient: There are some days when I go into work and I just can't get anything done. I know what I want to do, but I just can't seem to get my brain in gear.

Nurse: What is it like when your brain isn't in gear?

Patient: I feel confused, and I start projects, but then something distracts me and I don't finish my work.

With this series of open-ended questions, the nurse is able to identify the patient's perspective of his current interpersonal difficulties in ways that would not be possible with a more directive line of questioning. Notice, however, that the nurse's use of questioning never advanced beyond the data presented by the patient.

By contrast, **closed-ended questions** are those that directly ask for a specific answer. They offer the receiver a narrow range of response options: yes or no, either this or that, for example. Close-ended questions are similar in format to multiple-choice tests, in which there is a limited scope of predetermined answers from which to choose. Although closed-ended questions are restrictive, they are quite useful in certain situations. For example, they can reinforce an implicit assumption:

Nurse: So, when you are with your drinking buddies, you really feel like you belong?

Closed-ended questions can be used to focus the patient on two conflicting parts of an ambiguous statement:

Nurse: I'm still not clear; are you saying that your parents are opposed to your giving up your job, or that they just don't care?"

A third type of questioning involves focused questions. **Focused questions** are partially open-ended questions that directly ask about specific parts of the data. Used to target certain information, focused questions are more limited than open-ended questions, but they require more than a simple yes or no, right or wrong answer. Focused questions are particularly useful in eliciting a specific feature about a broad area or content that the patient has initiated for discussion or when the patient presents insufficient detail. For example, instead of using a close-ended question to follow up on the patient response that he has trouble "anticipating the next step," the nurse might ask the patient: "What happens when you try to anticipate the next step?" or "Are there any situations in which anticipating the next step is easier (harder) than others?"

There are advantages to using all three types of questions. Open-ended questions encourage the most spontaneous answers. Closed-ended questions are useful when immediate information is needed in a situation or when the patient's responses characteristically are so tangential that no information is forthcoming. They sometimes provide a comfortable lead-in for patients who have trouble being verbally expressive. Focused questions bring forward details about more general information.

In general, questions should begin with items or issues that are nonthreatening and easy to answer. You might open the dialogue with a patient by asking, "How can I help you?" or "Can you tell me a little about what brought you into the hospital?" or simply "Where would you like to start?" Although questions are an important listening response strategy, they should be used judiciously and tactfully. Otherwise the dialogue can sound more like an inquisition to the patient.

Restating

Restating is a mirroring strategy in which you replay all or part of the patient's message, exactly as stated, for emphasis or clarity. First identified by Carl Rogers (1965), restatement makes no judgment about the other person's message. You simply repeat the patient's statement, "You're saying, I don't know what to do?" or a part of it, "a little confused?" Use restating to emphasize a part of the patient's dialogue or to interject doubt with a questioning tone, without moving away from the patient's statement. A restatement is introduced by the nurse as a tentative inquiry, often with an introductory phrase about the rationale for its use: "I just want to be sure that I understand, are you saying that . . . ?" It is important to use this strategy sparingly because overuse can lead to a stilted communication style that sounds like a parrot.

Paraphrasing

Paraphrasing is a communication strategy in which you take the patient's words and rephrase the message content into a similar statement of meaning. The purpose of the paraphrase is to broaden the scope of the patient's comment and to developed a shared meaning of the content. Paraphrased comments are a direct way of demonstrating your interest and attention. The rephrased response reflects the patient's meaning only in the context of what has just been said. Otherwise, it may take on an interpretation that extends beyond the patient's meaning. Effective paraphrased comments are expressed tentatively. Usually the paraphrased statement is shorter and more concise than the patient's original statement and echoes an underlying theme:

> *Patient:* I feel very isolated; I don't have any friends or anyone to hang with anymore.
>
> *Nurse:* Something has happened to the friendships you used to have?

Paraphrasing is particularly useful in helping patients clarify mixed or ambiguous messages:

> *Patient:* It just seems that Hal always sees what I don't do right instead of the many things I do for him. It's so discouraging because I really think I am a good wife.
>
> *Nurse:* It sounds like you think that Hal doesn't appreciate you.

In this example, the nurse captures the essence of the conflict between the patient and her husband in a single succinct statement.

Clarifying

Clarifying resembles paraphrasing in that you ask the patient to expand on a previous thought. It is different in that clarification is a listening response that directly asks for information not contained in the patient's statement. Clarification responses are framed in the form of a question that requests the patient to expand, simplify, or explain a message in a different way. Ideally, this listening response brings the patient's dialogue into sharper focus. Clarification is essential when the patient is rambling or the message is so vague that you cannot follow it. At such times, it can be appropriate to say "I'm sorry, I'm confused. Can you state your concern in another way (or give me an example of what you mean)?" Asking the patient to be more specific can help him or her move consciously forward into the next part of the story. This can be accomplished by the use of clarifying probes, which might include one or more of the following: "In what ways . . . ?"; "How do you mean . . . ?"; "Can you give me an example of what you mean by . . . ?"; "Can you explain more fully?"

Reflecting

Reflecting is a communication strategy used to help the patient focus on the feelings experienced in relation to a situation. Many people have difficulty expressing their feelings directly. Other people are aware of the feeling but cannot always attach it to the situation in which it originated.

Reflective statements tend to elicit a deeper awareness of the feelings. They help a patient hear not only his or her words, but also the feelings and anxiety behind them. For example, saying to a patient, "You've really had a tough time recently," can initiate a flood of conversation about the nature of the rough time. Reflective listening responses are particularly useful when there should be an emotion attached to the situation that is left out in the patient's reporting of a situation or as a lead-in to a deeper exploration of feeling. You can identify empathetically how you might feel in a similar situation and put your feelings into words. For example, you might say, "Most people in your situation would feel quite angry if this . . . (identify stressor[s] in situation) . . . happened to them."

When using reflection to facilitate communication, take note of the patient's nonverbal behavior. The patient's facial expression or body movements may suggest the underlying emotion as well as its impact on the patient. A well-timed reflection can reveal an emotion that has escaped the patient's notice. If a patient's emotional expression seems overly intense, it would not be prudent to focus on the emotion as a first-line intervention. If the patient seems unusually agitated, inquiry into the emotion may escalate the mood. It is better to continue with restatement and paraphrasing until the patient's emotional state evidenced through nonverbal behavior demonstrates a readiness to listen to the nurse's reflection. Likewise, it is important to address only the more obvious emotion attached to the situation. Otherwise the reflected statement can be viewed as intrusive.

Some communication experts suggest using a compound sentence to connect the feeling with the situation; for example, the nurse might say to an alcoholic patient who has resumed drinking, "You seem to feel guilty *because* you didn't keep your promise to stop drinking." When employing a compound sentence in a reflective listening response, value statements are never proper. Deep interpretations of feeling that go beyond the scope of an active listening response are not appropriate without having the advanced training needed to process their meaning. "You seem to feel guilty because you never really loved your wife" is an interpretative statement that goes beyond the facts.

Using Silence

Silence is a brief pause during which you do not speak. *With silence, only the words are missing; the feelings and felt connections remain present* (Renwick, 1992). The silent moment is a shared moment in time when the nurse is with the patient emotionally but not verbally. Silence is a listening response that allows the patient additional time in the interaction to think about what has been said without an intrusive comment. By waiting a few seconds rather than moving directly to the next question, the patient has more of a chance for further elaboration. Moreover, you have the opportunity to think before responding, and this may result in a more thoughtful response. Allowing more response time for elderly and culturally diverse patients respects their need for additional time to process information. You can use attending behaviors of eye contact, leaning forward, and smiling to convey interest and acceptance.

Silence is helpful in situations involving powerful emotions. For example, sitting with the patient who is in tears for a moment before verbally speaking acknowledges the depth of the emotion. The short silence can be followed by an empathetic statement, such as "This subject seems very painful to you; can you tell me about it?" or an open-ended question, such as "Can you tell me what the tears are about?"

Another use of silence is following an important point that you wish to emphasize. The momentary pause accentuates the key ideas and encourages the patient's notice of important ideas. Prolonged silences usually are uncomfortable for both nurse and patient. After more than a minute or so of silence, interject a neutral verbal comment, such as "You seem to be silent; I wonder what is going on with you right now," or a minimum encouraging lead-in, such as "A penny for your thoughts," may be enough to break the silence.

Summarizing

In general, most listening responses respond to a single message, but this is not so with summarizing. **Summarizing** is similar to paraphrasing in that it makes statements about content. The scope of the statement, however, is much broader. The essence of a part or all of an interview can be included. Summary statements can be used at the end of a therapeutic conversation to review important points or as a transition when it is necessary to move to another topic. For example, you might say, "It seems to me that what you are saying . . . ? Can we move on and talk about . . . ?" (Renwick, 1992, p. 34). Summarizing synthesizes the meanings of several messages and helps the patient link themes and feelings together:

> *Nurse:* So, it sounds as if you would find it difficult to apply for that job because you don't have a resume, you lack confidence about the interview, and you are afraid you will not be able to explain your hospitalization.

At the end of the summary, the nurse should give the patient an opportunity to validate or expand on the summary with a statement such as, "You have shared a lot with me today. Is there anything else you would like to add or change about my comments?"

Validating

It is not enough simply to use listening responses and to assume that communication has taken place. Validation is a form of perception checking through asking for feedback to verify that the patient and nurse have the same understanding of the message content, feelings, and what has transpired between them. The purpose of validation is to check the accuracy of the communication process and to provide the patient with an additional opportunity to correct any misperceptions:

> *Nurse:* I just want to be sure I heard you right. I think you are saying that you are afraid to go back into the community because you are afraid you will become homeless quickly. Have I heard you correctly?

or

> *Nurse:* You said you were looking forward to your mother's visit, yet you went off the ward when your mother was due to visit. My sense is that you didn't really want to see her, is that true?

Table 10–6 summarizes common strategies for active listening.

▶ Check Your Reading

9. What are the characteristics of active listening?
10. What criteria would you use to choose each of the following listening responses in therapeutic conversations: restatement, paraphrasing, reflection, clarification, silence, summarizing?
11. How would you use silence as a therapeutic listening response?

Verbal Interventions

Active listening skills used by the nurse, inquiring consistently and gently to increase the precision of the patient's description of a problem, are critical to a mutual discovery and understanding of the patient's journey. Usually, however, they are not enough to help patients restructure their behavior into more constructive, enduring patterns. Individual patients may feel supported by the nurse's communicating, through his or her behavior, in a variety of ways, "I have confidence in your ability to change your life," but again, more may be needed. Verbal interventions take a more proactive role in helping patients learn new behaviors. The therapeutic verbal strategies described next are useful in helping patients to

- Develop or enhance self-management skills
- Monitor their own behavior
- Empower patients to take successful charge of their own affairs
- Develop different attitudes to deal more constructively with conflict or distress

Criteria for using proactive verbal interventions are based on changes in the patient's behavior and consist of noting the patient's emotional state and his or her progression toward achieving treatment goals. When the patient demonstrates reduced involvement in the treatment process, movement toward identified goals seems stalled,

TABLE 10–6 **Common Strategies for Active Listening**

Strategy	Definition	Sample Statement
Restating	Repeating part or all of the patient's statement, often with an introductory phrase about the purpose of the restatement	"Let's see if I understand: [followed by the patient's statement]." "Are you saying that: [followed by the patient's statement]."
Reflecting	Identifying the feelings associated with the patient's statement	"It sounds as if you feel bad that your mother didn't visit." "You sound very discouraged."
Paraphrasing	Selectively rewording part of the patient's message to reflect your understanding	*Patient:* "I feel like I don't have a niche anywhere." *Nurse:* "It's hard to figure out where you fit in?"
Clarifying	Directly asking the patient for information not contained in the original message	"Can you give me an example of what you mean by. . . ." "In what ways . . . ?"
Using silence	Deliberately pausing briefly in the dialogue	
Summarizing	Making a statement that synthesizes the meanings of several messages	"Today we talked about . . . ." "So it sounds as if you would find it difficult to ask your parents for the money for several reasons . . . ."

the patient becomes resistant, or the patient seems to have exhausted his or her personal resources, you will have to use a more proactive approach. Nurses can use knowledge of the patient's behavior patterns to select the most appropriate intervention. Incorporating the patient's personal strengths as part of the process takes best advantage of the situation.

REINFORCING STRENGTHS

It is important to work from the patient's strengths and to minimize problem areas. People grow more from developing their strengths rather than developing an awareness of their weaknesses (Ivey, 1988). The patient's strengths can include personal characteristics, social support, situational opportunities, and community resources. Most important is the patient's ability to recognize and use what is available, both intrapersonally and interpersonally. Looking for each person's unique strengths is an important aspect of intervention. Even with the most compromised patient, there are strengths and personal assets that can be activated for use in the forward movement toward health. For example, cooperation with treatment, persistence in the face of adversity, a sense of humor, and intellect are all examples of positive assets that the patient can use to facilitate personal change.

Another way of using patient strengths is as an integral part of constructive feedback. Although people learn from negative feedback, constructive feedback is more likely to be received favorably if an acknowledgment of the patient's strengths accompanies it. For example, the nurse might say to the patient, "You will have to lose your privileges because we found that you are hoarding your medication, but the fact that you told your wife you had them tells us that a part of you wants to cooperate with your treatment. How do you think we might strengthen this part of you?" Including the patient's strengths in the feedback forces the patient to consider the healthier side of the personality as an ally in counteracting the more uncertain maladaptive aspects of behavior.

CONFRONTING

No matter how correct the communication strategies used by the nurse, at times patients may, because of their illness and feelings of low self-esteem, become hostile, verbally abusive, or seductive. When such a situation occurs, the nurse needs to set appropriate limits. It is fruitless to respond in kind. Instead you should continually return the focus to the goals of treatment. For example, you might say, "Jack, I'm not trying to give you a hard time, but I think it is important for us to both work towards the same goal. How do you think we might do that?" Or "Josette, your urine revealed alcohol and drug use. I'm worried that you won't be able to continue with the program if you have another such urine test. What do you think we should do?" Asking the patient to participate in developing the solution helps ensure mutuality and patient involvement, necessary components in achieving treatment goals.

SETTING LIMITS

Although you should encourage mentally ill patients to process difficult feelings of anger, guilt, fear, and depression, clear limits always must be placed on destructive or divisive self-expressions that threaten self or others. *Scapegoating, excessive self-blame or blaming of others, emotional withdrawal, and aggressive threats to self or others need to be addressed directly and contained if necessary* (Cotton et al, 1983).

There are a number of verbal interventions the nurse can use to contain difficult emotions that threaten to get out of control. First, patients need reassurance that the staff will decisively move to contain any self-destructive behaviors. It is helpful to identify, in a calm, matter-of-fact tone, the underlying emotions, fantasies, and fears that destructive self-expressions evoke. Interventions such as redirection, modeling, coaching, humor, metaphors, and constructive feedback can be effective when the patient's anxiety is high but not out of control. Chapter 15 describes more specific techniques for communicating with violent patients in psychiatric settings.

GIVING CONSTRUCTIVE FEEDBACK

Nurses use constructive feedback tactfully to help people change distorted patterns of thinking, feeling, and behavior. Without reality-based communication to clarify, expand, and reframe experience, the distorted thinking associated with mental illness continues unabated. For most mentally ill people, their basic communication experience with themselves and others has not been helpful. They have lost touch with who they are, and because of this, they experience a deep sense of isolation and separation from others. Needing to protect themselves from an alien interpersonal environment, mentally ill patients develop images that serve as the wellspring of their anxieties and fears. Over time, these inner images become their only source of informational feedback. Frequently, this information is incorrect or distorted by their dysfunctional thinking processes.

The purpose of feedback is to help mentally ill patients develop a realistic appraisal of their situation and the role they play in maintaining or changing it. Used therapeutically, feedback can strengthen a person's resource pool in meeting difficult challenges by suggesting alternative options. Feedback helps patients connect their feelings and behavioral actions with actual situations. Honest sharing of the nurse's thoughts can challenge the validity of recurring attitudes and thoughts that diminish the self-image of the patient. You might use feedback as a listening response in the form of a simple comment, such as "That was a helpful answer," "I really liked your response," "I think I have a better understanding now . . . ." Feedback can be used to correct misunderstandings or to provide facts about behaviors in need of change with a comment such as "It seems like whenever you go on pass, you get into a fight. Any ideas about how you might prevent this from occurring?"

Feedback may have to be conveyed with strong language and an outlining of immediate consequences when simpler feedback messages are not heard. The manner in which you deliver constructive feedback and the tact with which the patient's problems are addressed are critical. Nurses need to use a consistent, nonjudgmental approach spoken in a firm, even tone. Underlying most out of control communication are multiple, concurrent, and conflicting goals originating either within the patient or between the patient's goals and those of the health care team. Nurses should present *reasonable consequences and practical feedback to the patient that take into account not only the behavior of the patient, but also the context, intent, and alternative explanations for the situation.* It is important to find out the precise nature of the problem before proceeding with the feedback. Here are some sample statements: "I need to understand your concerns better. You are upset because . . . "; "I can see that you are upset. Before I respond, let me see if I have a full understanding of what you are upset about. You feel that . . . ." By using nondefensive language and gaining an understanding of the problem from the patient's perspective, you can tailor the feedback in the most clinically helpful way. Fox (1993) uses feedback as an acronym for identifying important elements of the process. According to this author, effective feedback:

- *F*ocuses on what is changeable
- *E*xtends and shares parts of each of you
- *E*licits feelings, reactions, suggestions, and questions
- *D*escribes rather than confines, judges, or interprets
- *B*uilds on honesty and openness
- *A*llows time and space for thorough consideration
- *C*oncentrates on and reinforces observable changes
- *K*nits secure relationships (p. 94)

REDIRECTING

Redirecting is a communication strategy in which you refocus the patient from a tangential train of thought to a more precise discussion of the topic at hand. The strategy is useful when:

- The patient has obvious self-destructive or divisive expressions of feeling and talking about the feelings does not reduce anxiety
- You and the patient are stuck with repetitive dialogue, with no forward movement toward identified goals

People tend to talk about those things that bring them pleasure and to avoid topics that cause discomfort. Others treat complex issues simplistically or stereotypically go over someone else's role in a situation without considering their own role in the scenario. Stories that begin with "Let me tell you about Sally" or "I really think that Harry has a serious mental problem; what do you think?" are tip-offs to therapeutic conversations that may need redirection. Often, patients are not consciously aware of these communication patterns. Without awareness, the patient is unable to change them. You may have a stronger awareness of central issues a patient needs to consider. By changing the conversational flow to the areas the patient needs to discuss, you can both broaden and deepen the patient's perspective on important life issues.

> Jennifer LaRue is a 55-year-old woman admitted to the psychiatric unit with a major depressive episode. For the past few sessions, she has been

talking about the verbal abuse she has suffered from her husband in great detail, including what she said, what he said, and how unhappy she is in the relationship. She talks about the impact of the abuse but not about her role in perpetuating her helplessness. Using a redirecting strategy, her nurse might say: "It sounds as if you have had a very bad time with your husband for a long time. My sense is that we have a relatively good picture of what happens and how it has contributed to your depression. I'm wondering now if we might look at some ways in which you could recapture your sense of self and feel like less of a victim."

The nurse in this situation does not negate the patient's feelings. By redirecting the patient from a focus on the problem to a stronger emphasis on finding the solution, the dialogue can progress toward health-related goal achievement. This strategy is particularly useful when the patient cannot shift from a blaming mode or ruminates about the past without connecting it to present circumstances.

In times of anxiety about upcoming events or around unexpressed feelings, for example, failing to talk about the recent death of a beloved family member, redirection may be the intervention of choice. One way this can be handled is to use a sensitive response that brings the patient back to the topic which requires discussion: "I can see that you would like to pursue this (identify tangential topic) . . . more, but I am afraid that we won't get to discuss some things that also are important to consider before your discharge next week." In the case of unexpressed feelings, you could say, "I notice you haven't mentioned your grandfather's death, and I know he is important to you. It would seem that this is something we should talk about."

Other situations requiring redirection occur when the patient offers so many details that you have trouble sorting them out. In this situation, you may use a listening response to help the patient focus on the more relevant details, such as "I'd like to stop you right here. You are giving me so much information that I'm having trouble sorting it out. Can we focus on . . . . first, and then consider some of the other areas?" Redirecting the conversation should not force the issue or corner the patient. Rather the strategy calls the patient's attention to feelings and issues that might not otherwise be available to them.

MODELING

Modeling is a communication strategy in which the nurse or the patient puts into words or acts out behaviors to help the patient see what a dialogue or behavior looks like in action. Modeling occurs as a conscious demonstration of a behavior through role-playing and direct verbal intervention or through your actions, which are designed to shape the patient's behavior, through imitation of your behavior. Typically the nurse models effective communication behaviors, such as acting in a thoughtful way rather than impulsively, appropriate self-disclosure, a reasoned approach to problem-solving, or respect for self and the rights of others, throughout the relationship.

Role-playing is an active, conscious form of modeling in which the patient practices desired patterns of behavior with you before employing them in real-life situations. This communication strategy is particularly useful with patients having social skill deficits. For example, saying no to unreasonable requests, asking for a favor or for an undesired behavior to stop, accepting or giving compliments and criticism, and requesting a reconsideration of a decision from an authority figure are behaviors favorably responsive to role playing. Practicing effective ways to respond to these behaviors may be a new experience for patients, who have never had role models to provide this type of teaching. The process gives the patient a chance to develop confidence and offers a unique opportunity for constructive feedback in a safe interpersonal environment.

Another form of role-playing for the patient who is reluctant to engage fully in the process is walking the patient through the steps verbally. For example, you might say to the patient: "I wonder if you could just talk me through how you are going to keep your temper in check the next time you feel really frustrated?" As the patient talks through the various steps, you can help the patient identify potential difficulties with the plan, reinforce positive behaviors, and develop more appropriate coping techniques. Writing them down as part of a "prevention plan" on a 3 × 5 card and placing the card in a prominent place has proven valuable for many patients.

Miller (1989) suggests that the nurse's empathetic modeling of appropriate feelings can help patients in denial of their feelings with beginning acceptance, as in her example of an incest victim:

> *Nurse:* If my father had sex with me, I would be very scared and ashamed.
>
> *Patient:* I love my father.
>
> *Nurse:* I would love my father and that would make it hurt even more that he had done that to me (p. 29).

Modeling of appropriate feelings must be done gently with respect for the feelings of the patient and the context of the situation. Even if the intervention does not produce immediate effects, naming the feelings makes them available for future consideration and acknowledges their existence as legitimate.

REFRAMING

Reframing is a communication strategy that offers a different interpretation of the patient's situation. By modifying the meaning of a situation, there are more options for changing behavior. Pesut (1991) states that "by definition, 'to reframe' means to change the conceptual, or emotional, setting of some event or thing or to place it in another frame that fits the facts of the same concrete situation equally well or even better (p. 10). This author offers such examples as withdrawal reframed as "taking care of oneself," passivity as "accepting things as they are," or insensitivity as "protecting oneself from hurt."

Reframing is a particularly useful tool in dealing with the patient's resistance (LaClave and Brack, 1989). The goal of reframing is to help the patient achieve a change in perspective by presenting an alternative explanation from a different viewpoint. Reframing allows difficult situations or circumstances to come together in a new way. The strategy carries the present situation forward into a different future. Out of the reframed experience comes the possibility of responding to it in a more constructive manner. Some authors refer to reframing as finding the positive elements in an otherwise negative situation (Erickson et al, 1983; O'Hanlon, 1984).

If patients can begin to look at their problems in terms of actions rather than as personality traits or deliberate attempts of others to diminish them, the possibility of change increases. The problem has boundaries and is workable because it can be examined outside of the personal realm. Watzlawick and colleagues (1974) suggested that by reframing "fighting" as "commitment" in therapy with couples, they could radically change a couple's interactions. Thinking of shyness or abusive behavior, for instance, as skill deficits rather than as fatal flaws encourages a different way of thinking about them and dramatically resets the direction of their resolution.

USING METAPHORS

Metaphors are figures of speech or verbal images that carry the meaning of feelings and emotions from one situation to another. Abstract words related to concepts, such as love, fear, and anger, often are difficult to image because patients cannot see their presence. A metaphor provides a tangible image that a person can visualize. For example, the patient may not agree with you that he is very angry, but the metaphor "you look like a bomb ready to explode at any moment" is immediately recognizable. Metaphors do not add *facts* to a description but add *depth* of meaning to the nature of a phenomenon, as expressed through its relationship to something else. Metaphors bring together two asymmetrical images that do not normally fit together. The unexpected positioning of the two images together forces the attention of both participants to the association between the abstract image and the concrete situation under review.

Metaphors offer creative insights, giving voice to that which has been silenced in a person's life. They join, separate, and recombine ideas to provide new wisdom. The title character in the movie *Forrest Gump* uses an interesting metaphor to talk about the role of uncertainty in our lives. Limited intellectually but gifted with a special form of wisdom, Forrest makes the most of every opportunity. His metaphor for the unknown quality of the life process given him by his mother is that "life is like a box of chocolates; you never know what you are going to get until you bite into it."

Common metaphors in psychiatric settings include building walls to keep people out; a diamond in the rough; the calm after the storm; and therapy is like peeling an onion, one layer comes off at a time. Through symbolic interpretation, a new potential emerges. Nurses use metaphors to identify better ways of handling things. For example, saying to the patient "If you give a man a fish, you feed him for a day, but if you teach him how to fish you feed him for life" describes the role of the nurse in helping the patient discover the best ways to resolve his or her problems. Gendron (1994) describes a useful metaphor for supporting the self-definition of a patient that seems particularly appropriate for the mentally ill: "She seemed to want to be in the driver's seat of her situation, but it was as if the weather was bad and she was unsure of the road. I translated this sense to my approach to care: She needed guidance, but also as much control as she could handle" (p. 27).

USING HUMOR

Humor is a resource both nurse and patient use to ease an overly intense moment, put situations into perspective, and share connected moments. Miller (1979) describes laughter as follows: "Laughter is a way to realize life as it is—irrational, lunatic, unpredictable, periodically very difficult and very easy, absolutely simple and extraordinarily complicated—an opportunity to fully enjoy and appreciate it as such" (p. 141).

Humor cuts through defensiveness. Typically, humor is contagious and can provide new insights. It allows people to see themselves more objectively and at a distance. Humorous comments or anecdotes change mood and reduce the impact of stressors (Martin and Lefcourt, 1983). Physiologically, humor can reduce muscle tension, stimulate the cardiovascular system, and enhance pulmonary function (Ferguson and Campinha-Bacote, 1989, p. 32). Shared jokes form bonds between people. Humor also assists with learning.

> Mrs. Jones, a 32-year-old, upper middle class, well-respected individual, brought her six-year-old son, Johnny, to the clinic for discipline problems. When Mrs. Jones and Johnny entered the room, Johnny said to the family therapist, "You're black." Mrs. Jones' mouth fell open and her eyes widened. The therapist smiled and said, "No, in fact I am brown!" Johnny remarked, "I am white." The therapist picked up a piece of white paper and said smiling, "This is white, you look a little pink to me!" The little boy laughed and said, "You're right!" Mrs. Jones smiled and laughed in apparent relief over the child's embarrassing remark. She remarked, "That's right Johnny!" Mrs. Jones relaxed after the therapist explained color differences to Johnny.

The surprise element in humor catches the imagination of the other person. Consider the dialogue between Alice and the Gryphon (Carroll, 1881, p. 161).

> "Ten hours the first day," said the Mock Turtle: "nine the next, and so on." "What a curious plan!" exclaimed Alice. "That's the reason they're called lessons," the Gryphon remarked: "because they lessen from day to day." This was quite a new idea to Alice.

There is a delightful cleverness to humor that makes one feel emotionally and intellectually connected with the other person in a shared experience. The experience of having shared a joke often lingers after the participants have left the original encounter, creating again a smile or renewed laughter.

"Laughing with is not the same as laughing at" (Warner, 1989, p. 21), and you need to be sensitive to the patient's possible interpretation of a humorous remark. Timing is important. Humor is valued more in a well-established relationship than in the beginning stages before trust is earned. Before using humor as a therapeutic strategy, you should be aware of the patient's normal response patterns and current mood. Humor requires a certain amount of flexible thinking, which not all patients possess. Patients with rigid, concrete thinking styles may not be able to see the humor in a situation without hints. Despite this, obsessional patients enjoy humor. When a patient is feeling vulnerable or tired, a humorous comment may feel insensitive or out of place. If the patient is incapable at the moment of appreciating a humorous remark, the comment may be hurtful rather than helpful. Humor should focus on events, circumstances, or situations and not on the personal characteristics of the person. Sarcasm or humor about another person is never appropriate.

Also, observe how the patient uses humor. A good sense of humor demonstrated by the patient may be a sign of increased mental health, and it offers an opportunity for the patient to affirm a positive characteristic in a humorous dialogue with you. Humor also can be used in a pathological way. When it becomes the primary form of communication or is used in a self-demeaning way, it needs to be discouraged. Humor in the patient can act as a defense against closeness or as a way of camouflaging poor self-esteem. When humor is used in this way, you need to call attention to the behavior without diminishing the patient:

> Bill Waters has been unable to find a job for the past three years. He blames his age, and says they don't want an old saw horse like him. When the nurse asks him about his job skills and his personal assets, he says, "my two daughters, they are both college graduates and have good jobs. They have my genes and they're my best asset." He laughs at his joke.

After acknowledging Bill's pride in his daughters, the nurse might respond *with a similar light tone:* "Bill, I'm sure your good genes are only one part of you. I bet you have other assets. How about letting me in on some of them."

MIRRORING

Mirroring is a communication strategy in which the nurse reflects through words behaviors observed in the patient that the patient might not otherwise notice. The nurse acts as a "verbal" mirror for the patient. For example, you might say, "When you talk about your wife and children, you look very sad." Your observation can stimulate the patient to put unconscious feelings into words. Another way of mirroring the patient's behavior is to share how the patient's behavior affects you. You might say, "I feel cut off when you start to talk about your family, as if there is a glass wall between us. I can see you, but it is difficult to feel that I have the full picture." When using mirroring as a communication strategy, it is important to stay within the framework of the data the patient presents, to make comments with a tentative observation, and to ask for validation. Comments on behaviors the patient potentially can accept allows the patient freedom to explore their meaning. Mirroring difficult emotions before the patient is ready to accept them, making value judgments, or providing interpretative statements is counterproductive. Even if you are correct, the patient can feel such discomfort that the beneficial value of the strategy gets lost.

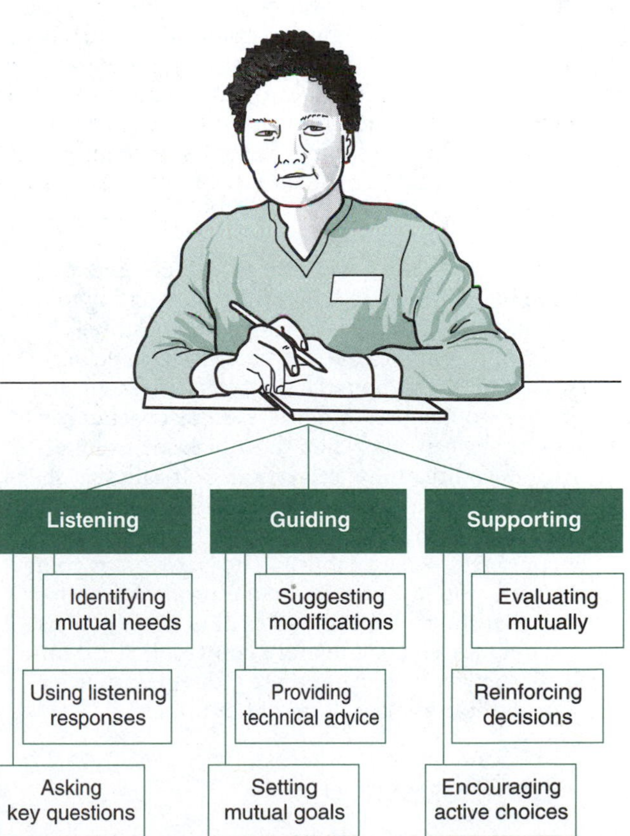

FIGURE 10–5
The psychiatric nurse's role in coaching patients. (Adapted from Arnold, E., and Boggs, K. [1995]. *Interpersonal relationships: Professional communication skills for nurses* [2nd ed.]. Philadelphia: W. B. Saunders, p. 395.)

COACHING

Peplau (1952) describes the functions of teacher, technical expert, and resource person as integral to the role of psychiatric nurse. From a communication perspective, the teaching role involves providing ongoing helpful guidance to the patient in planning, making decisions, and implementing actions that support goal achievement. **Coaching** is a strategy in which the nurse works with the patient informally, providing suggestions, monitoring, and evaluating behavioral change. Coaching consists of the behaviors identified in Figure 10–5. The process of coaching involves a careful review of progress, strengthening the patient's motivation, negotiating new objectives and alternative methods with patients, and assessing new developments in the patient's treatment needs. Because more than 50% of chronic mentally ill patients demonstrate significant deficits in the type of coping and social skills needed for successful independent living, coaching is extremely relevant as a nursing intervention (Gerhart, 1990). Some of the types of skills needed by chronically mentally ill patients involve grooming, budgeting, cooking meals, making and keeping appointments, and using public transportation. Higher functioning patients can benefit from coaching related to all aspects of interpersonal relationships with significant people in their environment. In coaching patients, it is helpful to develop small concrete assignments, the origin of which can come ideally from the patient, but also from you. These assignments teach patients that they are capable of intervening on their own behalf and that they need to work between therapeutic sessions to accomplish behavioral change. Successful accomplishment of small tasks reinforces mastery and self-esteem.

> Karen Jenkins has panic attacks "which seem to come out of nowhere." They are frightening to her; she feels like she is having a nervous breakdown or is going to die. Karen describes feeling sweaty; her heart pounds; she feels nauseated; and she has trouble breathing. Her nurse coaches her in actions she can take when the attack seems imminent: deep breathing, relaxation. Self-talk that she is experiencing a panic attack and will not die from it or have a nervous breakdown also helps. Karen is encouraged to keep a journal, noting what is going on just before the attack, the duration of the attack, and what she feels afterwards. All of these actions will help Karen assume more control, but it is unlikely she would develop these strategies on her own, without the coaching of her nurse.

OFFERING INFORMATION

Offering information can be a part of the coaching process, or it can be offered as a discrete block of data that serves as a resource to the patient. The goal of providing information is to help patients learn new things and, through knowledge, attain competency. When information is offered, the nurse should offer it in a way that respects the patient's personal choices and needs of the moment. Information is more likely to be retained if it is understandable and acceptable to the patient. Frequently the information is understandable, but unless it also takes into account the patient's beliefs, attitudes, and current life circumstances, it will fall on deaf ears. If the patient's attention is reduced because of anxiety, use shorter words and simpler sentence constructions. Repetition and contextual cues are simple strategies that can enable patients to move forward in the conversation. Using similar verbal expressions and analogies from the patient's experience also enhances shared meanings. For example, using a painting example to illustrate a point with an artist, an academic example with a professor, or a child care example with a mother facilitates conversation. Most patients also appreciate concrete examples rather than general information. Giving explicit behavioral directions so that the patient knows exactly what is expected can cut down on misunderstandings afterward. Box 10–4 identifies important elements of offering information to patients. The nurse may offer information about the availability, time, and location of support groups in the area, medication instructions, treatment options, discharge instructions, and what to do in case of emergency. Chapter 22 presents health teaching as a primary means of offering more extensive information.

BOX 10-4 Important Elements of Offering Information to Patients

- Assess what the patient already knows, patient readiness, and patient ability to learn.
- Use familiar terminology.
- Build on what the patient already knows.
- Present one idea at a time in a logical sequence.
- Provide concrete examples of abstract ideas.
- Repeat important ideas and concepts.
- Provide time for practice.
- Use return demonstrations and validation to evaluate comprehension.
- Provide positive reinforcement and corrective suggestions.
- Give the patient written instructions when needed.

► Check Your Reading

12. What are the differences between the following verbal intervention strategies: mirroring, redirecting, and reframing?
13. When is humor appropriate, and what criteria do you need to consider in using this strategy?
14. How would you use feedback as a verbal intervention strategy with a mentally ill patient?

Barriers to Therapeutic Communication

Barriers to communication can occur within the patient, within the nurse, or because of the environment in which the communication takes place.

Barriers Within the Patient

Not every patient is equally motivated, emotionally able, or intellectually equipped to participate in a conversation. Communication does not achieve its desired outcomes when the patient is not committed to making changes in behavior. Part of the nurse's assessment includes seeking answers to the following questions:

- Is the patient emotionally invested in wanting to make changes?
- Does the locus of control reside within the patient, or is it assigned to other people?

Before the work begins in earnest, you must help the patient work through resistance. Sometimes education works. Other times, weighing the benefits and losses for making the changes versus maintaining the status quo is helpful. In some way, you must enlist the patient's interest. When the topic under discussion has personal relevance, the patient is more inclined to pay close attention. Topics that have little meaning or a negative interpretation are likely to be discounted or to go unheard.

Motivation for change also relates to the intellectual and neurological status of the patient:

- Does the patient have the cognitive ability to hear and understand the meaning of the message?
- Does the patient have the capacity to pay attention for the required length of the conversation (hallucinations, delusions, attention deficits)?
- Is the patient able to think clearly and critically about the information presented?

In each instance, it is important to match the patient's cognitive abilities with the level of communication.

Internal sensory inputs, such as hallucinations, illusions, and delusions, may decrease the patient's ability to process information. They are mentioned in this chapter as a barrier to communication and are found in greater detail in other chapters because they appear with regularity in psychotic and some cognitive disorders. *Hallucinations* are sensory experiences that have no discernible external stimulus. Usually, they are vivid and intrusive. Frequently, they are threatening and frightening to the person experiencing them. Although hallucinations can reflect a stress response to actual events in the environment, they present as a diffuse riddle with such deep emotional overtones that you may not be able to decipher the message. Auditory hallucinations are more frequently associated with psychotic disorders; visual and tactile hallucinations more frequently develop with physiological disturbances, such as drug or alcohol toxicity or organic brain syndromes. Many times, you can tell that patients are experiencing hallucinations from their behavior. Patients may appear to be carrying on a conversation with someone who is not there, or they may clutch their head or look distracted. Some patients conceal their hallucinations because they are aware that they are not socially acceptable. Questions you can ask to determine the existence of hallucinations are: "Are you ever bothered by hearing voices that other people don't seem to hear?" or "Do you think you may see things that other people don't seem to see?" If the patient is having a hallucination, you might say, "Mr. Hendricks, I don't hear the voices (or see the situation as you describe it) but I can see that you are bothered by them."

Illusions are misperceptions of visual or auditory external stimuli. Examples of illusions include mistaking the identity of people or objects in the environment or misperceiving their environment as being someplace else. Cognitively impaired patients sometimes mistake their spouse for a stranger. They often think they are back in a different time or place and misidentify people in the current environment as people from the past.

> Francis Rogers thinks he is on Wall Street and has just made a terrible mistake with his law practice. He calls the nurse by his daughter's name, Sherry, and asks her to help him. A gentle reorientation, touch, and redirection often take care of the problem. The nurse might answer, touching his arm gently, "Mr. Rogers, my name is Judy and I am your nurse. We are at Jefferson Memorial Hospital, and we will take care that you don't make mistakes. Sherry is your daughter; can you tell me about her?"

Note that the nurse refocuses the conversation without discounting the patient's communication.

Delusions are fixed erroneous beliefs that cannot be corrected by logical argument (chiefly because they are emotionally, not intellectually, driven). They arise as a protective response to a perceived threat to the ego. Delusional patients cannot acknowledge that the delusion is not real or that it can represent an exaggeration of reality, even with evidence to the contrary. Decoding the underlying dynamics is a useful communication strategy.

> Natalie Quinn believes that she has a "magnetic field" surrounding her that is so strong others cannot survive when they get too close to her. She feels she must stay apart from others on the unit or she will destroy them. The nurse might respond to Natalie's delusion by getting to the underlying themes: "It must be quite frightening and very lonely to think that if people get close to you, you can destroy them."

With this or a similar comment, the nurse can help the patient focus on the emotional dynamics of her delusional thinking without a direct challenge to their validity.

Delusions are most frequently associated with paranoid and depressive disorders, dementia, and drug-induced psychosis.

Barriers Within the Nurse

When student nurses begin to interact with psychiatric patients, usually they experience anxiety about what they will say and how the patient is likely to respond. They worry about whether or not they will say the right thing and what will happen if they do not respond appropriately. This is normal, but generally these fears are groundless because the person behind the symptom almost always benefits from having a human encounter marked by respect and a genuine willingness to learn about the patient as a person. There is little chance of destroying the relationship or of hurting a patient if you strictly adhere to the boundaries of a professional relationship and implement the suggested strategies presented here with authenticity and caring.

The key to communicating successfully with patients is to be extremely patient, to seek ways of demonstrating through words and actions that the patient is a person of value, and to offer specific help with learning the most effective ways the patient can realize his or her fullest potential. From time to time, it may be necessary to detail the nature of the relationship and the nature of the nurse and patient roles in mutually achieving designated goals. Agreement about the boundaries of the relationship and safety against physical or emotional harm protect the integrity of the relationship. With these guidelines in mind, it is rather difficult to make a serious mistake. Small mistakes in communication (and these potentially occur with any communication) offer a unique opportunity for you and the patient to make critical judgments about their meaning and to resolve more complex communication problems in the patient's life. It is important to remember that (1) the patient responds to your communication as a whole, (2) communication takes place within the larger context of a caring relationship, and (3) communication is a process and not an event, so misunderstandings will arise and can be corrected. Often, it is the working through of misunderstandings that creates the strongest potential for healing. It is not as important to be a perfect communicator as it is to be a sensitive professional human guide who is committed to understanding and helping a human traveler who temporarily has lost his or her way.

Self-awareness of your own communication patterns is essential to the development of effective therapeutic communication. Should anxiety be a significant problem in the clinical setting, as when a student has previous personal or family experience with mental illness or aberrant behavior, it is important to discuss this with a trusted instructor or student support services and to resolve it outside of the clinical arena.

Communication is an art and as such requires practice and attention to detail. Some of the more common errors nurses make in communicating with their patients are presented in Table 10–7.

TABLE 10–7 **Common Errors That Nurses Make in Communicating With Patients**

Error	Description	Examples
Giving unsupported (false) reassurance	Using pseudocomforting phrases in an attempt to offer reassurance	"It will be okay" "Everything will work out"
Giving advice	Making a decision for a client; offering personal opinions; telling a client what he should do; using phrases such as "ought to," "should do"	"I feel you should" "If I were you I would . . ."
Making false inferences	Making an unsubstantiated assumption about what a client means. Interpreting his behavior without asking for validation. Jumping to conclusions	"What you really mean is you don't like your doctor" "Subconsciously you are blaming your husband for the accident"
Moralizing	Expressing own personal values about what is right and wrong, especially on a topic that concerns the client	"Abortion is wrong" "It is wrong to refuse to have that operation"
Value judgments	Conveying your approval or disapproval about the client's behavior or about what he has said. Using words such as "good," "bad," or "nice"	"That really wasn't a nice way to behave" "She's a good patient"
Using social responses	Polite superficial comments that do not focus on what the client is feeling or on what he is trying to say. Use of clichés	"Isn't that nice" "Hospital rules, you know" "Just do what the doctor says" "It's a beautiful day"

Modified from Arnold, E. and Boggs, K. (1995). *Interpersonal relationships: Professional communication skills for nurses* (2nd ed.). Philadelphia: W. B. Saunders, p. 225.

GIVING UNSUPPORTED (FALSE) REASSURANCE

Reassurance can be extremely helpful to patients in supporting their efforts and validating their perceptions of how to proceed with difficult tasks (Teasdale, 1989). When you offer reassurance without providing any relevant evidence to support it, however, the patient often perceives it as being invalid or questions whether you really are in touch with the reality of his or her situation. Consider the following example:

> William Ramsey is going for his first job interview. He has made good progress with his treatment at the day center, and he is due to be discharged next week. The nurse and Mr. Ramsey have practiced a mock interview and Mr. Ramsey has answered difficult questions well. Mr. Ramsey looks very apprehensive, and tells his nurse he is afraid he will "blow the interview." In an effort to be supportive, the nurse tells Mr. Ramsey, "Nonsense, you will do very well in the interview. Just have confidence. I know you'll do well."

A better response would be: "I can understand how you would be worried, but you did very well in our practice session, and if you can do the same thing in the interview, I think you will do quite well."

GIVING ADVICE

Giving advice is another communication pitfall. The patient's effectiveness outside of the clinical situation depends on his or her ability to use new learning in ways that are compatible with his or her personality. It is much more important to help patients develop their own resources than to offer advice, as tempting as that might be to speed up the process. People who are able to feel that their personal resources are relevant to the task at hand feel much more in charge. Asking the patient for input and demonstrating that their contributions are of value foster personal responsibility and self-direction. In addition, a major problem with giving advice is that you may feel resentful when the patient does not follow your "sound advice." This is because the advice may or may not fit the reality of the situation from the patient's perspective. It is important to differentiate giving advice from giving suggestions. *Giving advice tells the patient what to do:* "I would do this" or "You really need to do . . . if you want a successful outcome." *Giving suggestions points out resources or typical "next step" ideas the patient can try:* "Adding to what you have already said, another suggestion would be to . . ." or "Have you thought about possibly contacting the National Mental Health Alliance for a listing of support groups in your area?" With the latter examples, you build on the patient's statements and suggest the next step instead of telling the patient how the task should be done.

MAKING FALSE INFERENCES

Assuming the nature of feelings or making quick but false inferences about the data leaves patients feeling betrayed and misunderstood. An example is speaking about a behavior as if it is a personal characteristic. "Jack doesn't do his assigned chores on the unit" gets translated into "Jack is lazy or uncooperative." Assuming the nature of feelings occurs more often when you feel threatened, as when a patient makes a sexually provocative comment. A personalized response can be experienced by the patient as attacking: "You seem to have a lot of sexual feelings about me." A better response would be: "I am experiencing some of your comments as sexually tinged. I wonder if you are having some feelings that we should talk about." The second response invites the patient to own his or her feelings and to talk about them rather than to act on them. It identifies the patient as being responsible for his or her feelings. Moreover, the feelings may not be sexual at all but rather a protective distancing from the threatening closeness of a relationship with another human being. Even if the patient identifies the feelings as being sexual, you have the opportunity to provide information about what is and what is not appropriate in relationships and may help correct false perceptions the patient may have about his or her sexuality.

MORALIZING

Moralizing involves making a value judgment about behaviors or personal characteristics. We all have a tendency to value certain behaviors and to condemn others. Sometimes the behaviors are objectively good or evil, but it is easy to label them as such without critically questioning their validity or viewing them on a continuum, related to many other factors or circumstances in a person's life. For example, young people get into prostitution for a number of reasons, none of which may have anything to do with a desire to become a prostitute. Instead of looking at behavior as a single event or passing judgment on the character of a patient, you need to view behavior as active reflections of multidetermined factors. In the same situation, each of us might act differently. Given the right set of circumstances, each of us might draw the same conclusions as the patient. Words such as terrible, good, bad, worse, better, fine, and substandard are value-laden and of little use in a therapeutic setting.

Value judgments usually reflect your bias rather than a true appraisal of the situation. Trying to assess another person's motivations and the "goodness of intentions" without the other person's input gives incomplete data. Personal discomfort can direct you to select only certain behaviors to focus on. Elimination or exclusion of undesirable data does the patient a disservice and compromises treatment. Asking "why" instead of "what happened here" leads to the development of value judgments. Furthermore, because behavior generally is multidetermined, a patient may have little awareness of exactly why certain behaviors occurred. For example, if you ask the patient, "Why did you start drinking again when you know your wife has threatened to leave you if you do," the patient feels ashamed or defensive and fishes for excuses. A better lead-in would be, "Joe, your drinking has consequences; your wife has threatened to leave you if you drink again. Let's try to retrace your steps last week and see if we can find some triggers for your drinking." The latter statement focuses on behaviors and uses description. Evaluation of the other person or of his actions does not become the focus of the intervention. With descriptive statements, the facts are less likely to be disputed because they simply are statements of reality. Joe will have to take responsibility if he wants to achieve a different consequence. The link between cause and effect occurs, but the patient has more to work with because you have suggested an alternative solution.

USING SOCIAL RESPONSES

Limited use of social response behaviors is appropriate in the nurse-patient relationship, particularly during the orientation phase. They can be overused and distract from the therapeutic purpose of the relationship if not used sparingly during the working phase. Clichés and an inability to focus on content can suggest to the patient that you are not interested in what the patient is saying or lack the professional competence or confidence (or both) to use communication skills therapeutically.

Nursing Interventions to Minimize Barriers to Therapeutic Communication

To avoid barriers in communication, you can

- Do reality checks of your personal biases in communication. If you note bias, you can seek supervision to correct attitudes and perceptions that get in the way of the relationship
- Make statements of observations about behavior rather than inferences
- Reflect only what you observe and then only within the context of your competency level
- Focus listening responses and feedback on the sharing of ideas and feelings that the patient generates
- Focus feedback on behaviors rather than the person
- Use description rather than evaluation statements about the patient or his or her actions
- Frequently validate the accuracy of observations and interpretations of data

▶ Check Your Reading

15. How would you compare and contrast hallucinations, illusions, and delusions?
16. Describe how you would respond to a patient with each of the identified communication barriers.
17. What are some of the different ways in which you may create barriers in the communication process?
18. Identify some ways in which you could focus feedback on behaviors rather than on the person.

CONCLUSIONS

This chapter discusses the role of communication as points of intersection in the nurse-patient journey. Communication offers a means of connection with patients, a process of being with a patient, a way to share meaning, and a measure of responsibility. As psychiatry moves from a psychodynamic to a psychobiological model, there is a danger that the importance of communication as a means of healing will lessen. In addition, as mental health care delivery changes from a long-term to a brief therapy model with shorter hospital stays, higher acuity rates, and more frequent readmissions, communication patterns in psychiatric nursing will need to accommodate to them. Despite these changes, the therapeutic communication principles presented in this chapter are likely to be as relevant in the 21st century as they are today. They will continue to serve as the foundation for helping patients identify and challenge faulty assumptions, learn new behaviors, and imagine and explore new and different alternatives. Research in the 21st century will need to focus on ways to humanize an increasingly bureaucratic approach to mental health care, and the starting point for these studies is in the field of communication. In the decade of the brain, tomorrow's nurses must ensure that the psychodynamic aspects of psychiatric nursing remain prominent and well integrated with biological approaches to mental illness. For it is only through communicating with others that we can learn about and maintain our humanity as fellow travelers in a life journey of increasing unknowns.

KEY POINTS TO REMEMBER

- Reaching another human being through a therapeutic conversation involves not simply talking to the other about a problem, but actually *being with* the other in understanding and resolving barriers to the successful completion of the journey.
- There are several different types of communication: verbal communication, metacommunication, and nonverbal communication, which ideally all blend together as a logical composite to support the meaning of a message. Communication is a complex phenomenon that takes place on many different levels. People react to one another cognitively, affectively, and behaviorally.
- Effective communicators demonstrate certain characteristics, including self-awareness and awareness of the needs of others in the communication. They give simple, clear messages that are appropriate to the situation and responsive to patient needs. Effective communicators recognize that timing is a critical element in successful communication. They validate frequently to make sure that the receiver has heard the message as the sender intended it.
- Normal communication models—linear, circular, and cognitive processing models—form a basic framework for exploring the more specialized forms of communication referred to as therapeutic communication.
- Therapeutic communication is a special form of communi-

cation that has a health-related purpose and develops as a continuous flow of interaction between nurse and patient, with input from both contributing to its nature and progression. Therapeutic communication serves as the primary means through which all nursing interventions occur.

• Therapeutic listening skills, defined as "an interpersonal, confirmation process involving all the senses in which the therapist attends with empathy to the patient's verbal and nonverbal messages to facilitate the understanding, synthesis, and interpretation of the patient's situation," have been identified as the most important communication tool that the nurse uses with psychiatric patients.

• Active listening requires more than simply hearing the content of a patient's message and responding to it. Active listening is focused listening. The process of active listening involves making sense of the sender's message and attaching meaning to it.

• Active listening skills include the use of minimum encouragers, appropriate questions, restatement, paraphrasing, reflection, clarification, silence, summarizing, and validation.

• Verbal interventions take a more proactive role in helping patients learn new behaviors. They are designed to help patients (1) develop or enhance self-management skills, (2) monitor their own behavior, (3) empower them to take successful charge of their own affairs, and (4) develop different attitudes to deal more constructively with conflict or distress. Verbal interventions build on the patient's strengths. They include confronting, constructive feedback, redirecting, reframing, mirroring, modeling, use of metaphors, humor, coaching, and giving information.

LEARNING ACTIVITIES

1. Think of a situation in which you felt understood by another person. In a written paragraph or two, answer the following questions:

   a. What did you say in this situation?

   b. How did the other person respond to you?

   c. What was going on in the situation that helped you experience being understood?

   d. What made this interaction special for you?

   e. What were the underlying themes that contributed to your sense of being understood?

Discuss in class or with a small group commonalities and differences between your answers and those of your classmates. How would you use the information you learned in this exercise in your nursing practice?

2. Identify a situation in which a communication breakdown occurred. Describe the situation in enough detail so that it can be role played, (i.e., who was involved, the exact conversation as you remember it, the physical setting, and timing). In your narrative, use a third-person format to describe the events as they occurred, even if you were personally involved. Using the information in the chapter and class discussion, analyze the reasons for the communication breakdown. Discuss how this communication might be improved with some of the principles discussed in the chapter. Role-play with a partner: (a) the communication breakdown scenario and (b) use of active listening and verbal interventions to achieve a different outcome. Discuss in class or with a small group the different reactions of the participants. Consider how you could use this learning with psychiatric patients.

3. Using the acronym for feedback, identified on page 218, identify a situation in the clinical area in which feedback would be appropriate. Role-play this situation using the steps outlined in the chapter.

4. Identify the communication dynamics in each patient's behavior and role-play the verbal intervention strategies you would use in each of the following situations:

   a. Jon Verne is a 58-year-old retired banker with a history of treatment for alcoholism. Within the last two years he has started drinking again. His wife is an attorney who has threatened to divorce him if he doesn't stop drinking. He tells you that he has only started drinking again because he sees there is no hope for the marriage because his wife is verbally abusive and "obsessed about his drinking." He does not view his drinking as a problem.

   b. Polly Jackson is a 38-year-old housewife. She is very depressed and cannot see anything of value in her life. When pressed, she cannot think of any time in her life when she was happy. She has lost her appetite and has trouble sleeping. She says her life simply isn't worth living.

   c. Mary Turner is about to be discharged from day treatment. She will be starting a new job as a social work assistant, and she is both excited and anxious about her "new beginning."

   d. Jeremy Bolles is a new admission. He tells you that there are people out there seeking to destroy the United States. He warns you to be careful and tells you he will reveal more to you "when you are ready to hear it."

CRITICAL THINKING EXERCISES

Miss Miller, a student nurse, is writing a process recording concerning her patient Mr. Tallon. She knows that she must show her instructor that she understands the concept of therapeutic communication and give examples of how her responses were therapeutic. She begins to write: Mr. Tallon said that he was very upset about his wife's desire to obtain a divorce. When he spoke, his voice was emotionless, his hands folded, his eyes were downcast, and he smiled at me.

1. What inference can be drawn about the student's understanding of the communication process?

2. Is Miss Miller's description of Mr. Tallon clear?

3. What evidence leads you to this conclusion?

Miss Miller continues to write: After I talked with Mr. Tallon for 20 minutes, I decided to comment on the difference between what he said and how he acted. He responded, "You women are all alike; you always find fault with everything."

1. What assumptions is the patient making about Miss Miller?

2. What inference can the nurse draw about Mr. Tallon's response?

3. What might have happened if a different question(s) were asked?

REFERENCES

Anderson, H., and Goolishian, H. (1990). Beyond cybernetics: Comments on Atkinson and Heath's "Further thoughts on second-order family therapy." *Family Process, 29,* 1510–1563.

Argyle, M. (1975). *Bodily communication.* Madison, Connecticut: International Universities Press.

Arnold, E., and Boggs, K. (1995). *Interpersonal relationships: Professional communication skills for nurses.* Philadelphia: W. B. Saunders.

Bandler, R., and Grinder, J. (1975). *The structure of Magic I.* Palo Alto, California: Science and Behavior Books.

Bandler, R., and Grinder, J. (1982). *Reframing neurolinguistic programming and the transformation of meaning.* Moab, Utah: Real People Press.

Beck, A. (1987). Cognitive therapy. In J. Zeig (Ed.), *The evolution of psychotherapy.* New York: Brunner/Mazel.

Beck, A., and Emery, G. (1985). *Anxiety disorders and phobias: A cognitive perspective.* New York: Basic Books.

Benner, P., and Wrubel, J. (1982). Skilled clinical knowledge: The value of perceptual awareness. *Nurse Educator,* 7 (3), 11–17.

Berlin, E., and Fowkes, W. (1993). A teaching framework for cross-cultural health care. *Western Journal of Medicine, 139* (6), 9310–9338.

Berne, E. (1964). *Games people play.* New York: Grove Press.

Birdwhistell, R. (1970). *Kinesics and context.* Philadelphia: University of Pennsylvania Press.

Buber, M. (1957). Distance and relation. *Psychiatry, 20,* 97–104.

Campinha-Bacote, J. (1988). Culturological assessment: An important factor in psychiatric consultation-liaison nursing. *Archives of Psychiatric Nursing, 2* (4), 2410–2415.

Carper, B. (1975). *Fundamental patterns of knowing in nursing* [Dissertation]. New York: Teachers College, Columbia University.

Carroll, L. (1881). *Alice's adventures in wonderland.* Compiled and Arranged by C. Edens (1989) in the ultimate illustrated edition. New York: Bantam Books.

Carroll, L. (1909). *Through the looking glass and what Alice faced there.* New York: Dodge Publishing Co.

Casement, P. (1991). *Learning from the patient.* New York: The Guilford Press.

Cody, W. (1994). Meaning and mystery in nursing science and art. *Nursing Science Quarterly,* 7 (2), 48–51.

Cotton, P., Drake, R., Whitaker, B., and Potter, J. (1983). Dealing with suicide on a psychiatric in-patient unit. *Hospital and Community Psychiatry, 34* (1), 510–559.

Covey, S. (1991). *Principle-centered leadership.* New York: Simon and Schuster.

Crowther, D. (1991). Metacommunications: A missed opportunity? *Journal of Psychosocial Nursing, 29* (4), 13–16.

Diers, D. (1990). Response. *Journal of Professional Nursing, 6,* 240–241.

Emrich, K. (1989). Helping or hurting? Interacting in the psychiatric milieu. *Journal of Psychosocial Nursing, 27,* 12.

Erickson, H., Tomlin, E., and Swain, M. (1983). *Modeling and role modeling: A theory and paradigm for nursing.* Englewood Cliffs, New Jersey: Prentice-Hall.

Eriksson, K. (1992). Different forms of caring communication. *Nursing Science Quarterly, 5* (2), 93.

Ferguson, S., and Campinha-Bacote, J. (1989). Humor in nursing. *Journal of Psychosocial Nursing, 27* (4), 29–34.

Fox, R. (1993). *Elements of the helping process: A guide for clinicians.* New York: The Haworth Press.

Frankl, V. (1963). *Man's search for meaning: An introduction to logotherapy.* New York: Simon and Schuster. (Originally published in 1959.)

Fraser, W., King, K., Thomas, P., and Kendell, R. (1986). The diagnosis of schizophrenia by language analysis. *British Journal of Psychiatry, 148,* 2710–2718.

Gadow, S. (1989). Clinical subjectivity: Advocacy with silent patients. *Nursing Clinics of North America, 24* (4), 5310–5341.

Gebbard, G. (1992). Psychodynamic psychiatry in the decade of the brain. *American Journal of Psychiatry, 149* (8), 991–998.

Gendron, D. (1994). The tapestry of care. *Advances in Nursing Science, 17* (1), 25–30.

Gerhart, U. (1990). *Caring for the chronic mentally ill.* Itasca, Illinois: F. E. Peacock Publishers.

Hall, E. (1966). *The hidden dimension.* New York: Doubleday.

Havens, L. (1986). *Making contact: Uses of language in psychotherapy.* Cambridge, Massachusetts: Harvard University Press.

Ivey, A. (1988). *Intentional interviewing and counseling* (2nd ed.). Monterey, California: Brooks/Cole Publishing Co.

Jackson, A., and Meadows, F. (1991). Getting to the bottom to understand the top. *Journal of Counseling and Development, 70,* 72–76.

Jeanneau, M., and Bengt-Ake, A. (1993). Linguistic characteristics of neurotic, borderline, and psychotic personality organization. *Scandinavian Journal of Psychology, 34,* 610–675.

Johnson, J. (1994). A dilectical examination of nursing art. *Advances in Nursing Science, 17* (1), 1–14.

Kasch, C. C. (1984). The role of strategic communication in nursing theory and nursing research. *Advances in Nursing Science, 6,* 71–88.

Kemper, B. (1992). Therapeutic listening: Developing the concept. *Journal of Psychosocial Nursing, 30* (7), 21–23.

Kleinman, A., Eisenberg, L., and Good, B. (1978). Culture, illness and care. *Annals of Internal Medicine, 88,* 251–258.

Knowles, R. (1983). Building rapport through neurolinguistic programming. *American Journal of Nursing, 83* (7), 1011–1014.

LaClave, L., and Brack, G. (1989). Reframing to deal with patient resistance. *American Journal of Psychotherapy, 43* (1), 68–75.

Leuner, H., et al. (1983). *Guided affective imagery with children and adolescents.* New York: Plenum.

Magnan, M. A. (1989). Listening with care. *American Journal of Nursing, 89,* 219–221.

Marlowe, H., and Marcotte, A. (1984). Nonverbal decoding. *Journal of Psychosocial Nursing, 22* (4), 8–15.

Martin, R., and Lefcourt, H. (1983). Sense of humor as a moderator of the relation between stressors and mood. *Journal of Personality and Social Psychology, 45,* 1313–1324.

Mehrabian, A. (1972). *Non-verbal communication.* Chicago: Aldine Publishing Co.

Merrick, P. (1992). Communication: An all important process. *Image, 11* (3), 5.

Miller, J. (1979). *Breaking through: Freeing yourself from fear, helplessness, and depression.* New York: Thomas Y. Crowell, Publishers.

Miller, L. (1989). Modeling awareness of feelings: A needed tool in the therapeutic communication workbox. *Perspectives in Psychiatric Care, 25* (2), 210–229.

O'Hanlon, B. (1984). Framing interventions in therapy: Deframing and reframing. *Journal of Strategic and Systemic Therapies, 3* (2), 1–4.

Pasquali, E. (1990). Learning to laugh: Humor as therapy. *Journal of Psychosocial Nursing, 28* (3), 31–35.

Peplau, H. (1952). *Interpersonal relations in nursing.* New York: G. P. Putnam Sons.

Pesut, D. (1991). The art, science, and techniques of reframing in psychiatric mental health nursing. *Issues in Mental Health Nursing, 12,* 9–18.

Polster, E. (1992). The self in action: A Gestalt outlook. In J. Zeig (Ed.), *The evolution of psychotherapy: The second conference* (pp. 143–151). New York: Brunner/Mazel.

Renwick, P. (1992). Teaching the use of interpersonal skills. *Nursing Standard, 18* (7), 31–34.

Richmond, V., McCroskey, J., and Payne, S. (1987). *Nonverbal behavior in interpersonal relations.* Englewood Cliffs, New Jersey: Prentice-Hall.

Rogers, C. (1965). *Client-centered therapy.* Boston: Houghton-Mifflin.

Ross, L. (1994). Spiritual aspects of nursing. *Journal of Advanced Nursing, 19,* 439–447.

Ruesch, J., Brodsky, M., and Fisher, A. (1957). *Psychiatric care, psychiatry simplified for therapeutic action* (in collaboration with J. Fisher and J. Castor). New York: Grune & Stratton.

Seligman, M. (1991). *Learned optimism.* New York: Alfred A. Knopf.

Sieberg, E. (1969). Dysfunctional communication and interpersonal responsiveness in small groups. In *Dissertation abstracts index.* Denver: University of Denver.

Sieburg, E. (1975). *Interpersonal confirmation: A paradigm for conceptualization and measurement.* San Diego: United States International University.

Simon, J. (1988). Therapeutic humor: Who's fooling who? *Journal of Psychosocial Nursing and Mental Health Services, 26* (4), 8–12.

Stricker, G., and Fisher, M. (Eds.), (1990). *Self disclosure in the therapeutic relationship.* New York: Plenum.

Tannen, D. (1995). *Talking from 9 to 5: How women's and men's conversational styles affect who gets heard, who gets credit, and what gets done at work.* New York: Morrow.

Taylor, A., Meyer, A., Rosegrant, T., and Samples, B. T. (1989). *Communicating* (5th ed.). Englewood Cliffs, New Jersey: Prentice-Hall.

Teasdale, K. (1989). The concept of reassurance in nursing. *Journal of Advanced Nursing, 14,* 4410–4450.

Topf, M. (1988). Verbal interpersonal responsiveness. *Journal of Psychosocial Nursing, 26* (7), 8–16.

Topf, M., and Dambacher, B. (1981). Teaching interpersonal skills: A model for facilitating optimal interpersonal relations. *Journal of Psychiatric Nursing and Mental Health Services, 19* (12), 29–33.

Travelbee, J. (1963). What do we mean by rapport? *American Journal of Nursing, 63,* 70–72.

Wachtel, P. (1993). *Therapeutic communication.* New York: Guilford Press.

Warner, S. (1989). Humor and self-disclosure within the milieu. *Journal of Psychosocial Nursing, 22* (4), 110–121.

Watzlawick, P., Beavin, J. H., and Jackson, D. D. (1967). *Pragmatics of human communication.* New York: Norton.

Watzlawick, P., Weakland, J., and Fisch, R. (1974). *Change: Principles of problem formation and problem resolution.* New York: Norton.

Weingarten, K. (1992). A consideration of intimate and non-intimate interactions in therapy. *Family Process 31,* 410–459.

SUGGESTED READINGS

Emrich, K. (1989). Helping or hurting? Interacting in the psychiatric milieu. *Journal of Psychosocial Nursing, 27,* 12.

Eriksson, K. (1992). Different forms of caring communication. *Nursing Science Quarterly, 5* (2), 93.

French, H. P. (1979). Reassurance: A nursing skill. *Journal of Advanced Nursing, 4,* 6210–6234.

Magnan, M. A. (1989). Listening with care. *American Journal of Nursing 89,* 219–221.

Simon, J. (1988). Therapeutic humor: Who's fooling who? *Journal of Psychosocial Nursing and Mental Health Services, 26* (4), 8–12.

Topf, M. (1988). Verbal interpersonal responsiveness. *Journal of Psychosocial Nursing, 26* (7), 8–16.

Travelbee, J. (1963). What do we mean by rapport? *American Journal of Nursing, 63,* 70–72.

CHAPTER 11

A PATHWAY FOR HEALING
THERAPEUTIC RELATIONSHIPS

A nurse's job is not only to monitor and administer treatments physicians prescribe. It's to help patients navigate an alien culture, feel more safe, confront vulnerability, regain faith in the bodies that have failed them or die with some measure of peace... there are times when patients need affirmation, confidence building and reassurance more than they need drugs, tests and procedures.

—*S. Gordon*

LEARNING OBJECTIVES

After studying this chapter, you should be able to:

1. Identify the role of interpersonal relationships in mental health and mental illness.
2. Compare and contrast the structure and function of social versus therapeutic relationships.
3. Describe the theory, nature, and structural components of therapeutic relationships.
4. Identify the tasks associated with each phase of the therapeutic relationship: preinteraction, orientation, working, and termination.

KEY TERMINOLOGY

Acceptance
Advocacy
Authenticity
Boundaries
Caring
Empathy
Empowerment
Meaning
Mutuality
Orientation phase
Preinteraction phase
Self-awareness
Termination phase
Therapeutic relationship
Therapeutic use of self
Trust
Working phase

Chapter 11 is about nurse-patient relationships in mental health clinical settings. The chapter centers around the question: How does the nurse-patient relationship bring together the nurse and patient's humanness as fellow travelers in a healing encounter of benefit to the patient? The patient can refer to an individual, a family, or a community, although the model presented in this chapter specifically addresses relationships with individual patients. Clinical settings can include the patient's home, clinics, or partial or full hospitalization. The term *healing encounter* embraces all of the human nursing applications in which the nurse helps patients draw on their inner resources in purposeful ways. The nurse-patient relationship creates a time-limited space in which the potential exists for a healing encounter. Occurring as a stepping stone in the river of life, the relationship can bear the patient to a different and, it is hoped, more satisfying place. Together, nurse and patient awaken the deeper qualities of life's journey in a mutually meaningful, humanly connected encounter. Chapter 11 identifies the work of the therapeutic relationship, distinguishes between social and therapeutic relationships, and describes three theoretical frameworks that guide therapeutic relationships. Having knowledge of the essential elements and the phases of a therapeutic relationship helps the nurse understand the basic structure and process of the relationship in mental health settings.

Without question, the quality of a person's interpersonal relationships is an essential element of mental health. The basic work of psychiatric nursing is to help people develop a sense of self through a healing professional relationship. There is no single approach that is applicable to all persons' problems. Each journey is unique, requiring special interventions tailored to meet the individualized needs of the patient. The "person" of the nurse and how that nurse experiences the patient as a fellow human being is fundamental to a successful relationship. As Peplau (1952) notes, "The kind of person each nurse becomes makes a substantial difference in what the patient will learn as he is nursed throughout his experience with others" (p. xii).

As nurses engage in therapeutic relationships with

psychiatric patients, they need a framework to understand how the relationship unfolds and what successful relationships entail. Most experts on helping relationships (Peplau, 1952; Satir, 1985) agree that the therapeutic alliance established between professional and patient furnishes a healing pathway for patients to uncover feelings of unworthiness, shame, and misunderstanding. Peplau suggests that it is the primary means by which people discover the richness of who they are as human beings. If one accepts this premise, the therapeutic relationship in psychiatric nursing becomes not only the basis for all nursing interventions, but also a primary catalyst for patient change. Within the relationship, the nurse and patient generate a joint perspective of their role as travelers in unraveling the journey's meaning. Theoretical understandings of relationship principles and personal knowledge of the patient suggest the most appropriate nursing approaches needed for successful outcomes.

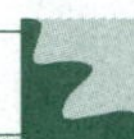

THE STORY OF THE LITTLE PRINCE

The tale of *The Little Prince* by Antoine de Saint-Exupéry illustrates the essential nature of the bonding required in a therapeutic relationship. In this children's tale, a flower and a fox instruct a young prince on the real meaning of relationship."I cannot play with you," the fox said. "I am not tamed. . . ."

"What does that mean—tame?" "It is an act too often neglected," said the fox. "It means to establish ties." "To establish ties?" "Just that," said the fox. "To me you are still nothing more than a little boy who is just like a hundred thousand other little boys. And I have no need of you. And you, on your part, have no need of me. To you, I am nothing more than a fox like a hundred thousand other foxes. But if you tame me, then we shall need each other. To me, you will be unique in all the world. To you, I shall be unique in all the world." "I'm beginning to understand," said the little prince . . . (p. 80).

The fox gazed at the little prince, for a long time. "Please tame me!" he said. "I want to, very much," the little prince replied. "But I have not much time. I have friends to discover, and a great many things to understand." "One only understands the things that one tames," said the fox. "Men have no more time to understand anything. They buy things all ready made at the shops. But there is no shop anywhere where one can buy friendship, and so men have no friends any more. If you want a friend, tame me. . . ." (pp. 80, 83–84).

Story from de Saint-Exupéry, A. (1943). *The little prince* (K. Woods, Trans.). New York: Harcourt Brace.

This chapter is about the process of "taming" in the nurse-patient relationship, an interpersonal process by which one human struggles to know and accept the other as "unique in all the world," a relational process by which human beings connect with each other in meaningful ways.

INTERPERSONAL RELATIONSHIPS

Interpersonal Relationships and Mental Health

Cashden (1982) notes that the self "is thoroughly and irreducibly interpersonal" (p. 125). Our humanity and how we experience our human existence are inextricably linked with and influenced by others. Meaningful human involvement is the means by which one learns about the self, finds value as a human being, and develops a coherent personality structure. Many authors (Barnard, 1985) believe that **meaning,** defined as a cognitive and emotive process of developing and maintaining certain reliable ideas or images about the order and significance of a person's life, is essential to human survival. Without relationships to validate and make sense of one's personal experience, a person finds the world untrustworthy and one's own place in it uncertain. Normal family, social, and work relationships typically furnish an interpersonal bridge between self and other, entered into for the purpose of discovering a valid, unifying way of experiencing the self and for explaining the significance of the journey.

Interpersonal Relationships and Mental Illness

Mental illness affects the self in ways that invariably compromise interpersonal relationships. Whether biologically determined or interpersonally motivated, the mentally ill patient has developed maladaptive communication styles and interpersonal defenses that seriously cripple interpersonal relationships (Hagerty et al, 1993). Although a person's way of handling unhealthy relationships may have been essential for survival at an earlier stage of life, usually it does not meet the demands of his or her current life script as a responsible adult.

Peplau (1952) believes that mental illness represents an opportunity for personal growth and insists that each person has within his or her humanness the capacity to overcome ineffective ways of relating with others. Through a different relationship experience with a trained professional who wants to understand the person behind the symptom and who knows how to elicit the best from that person, the possibility exists for experiencing relationships differently and for healing a ruptured or fragmented relationship.

Mental illness assaults personal meanings and thereby creates a profound disruption in the ability to make connections with others. Patients identify their state of being as characterized by a deep sense of loneliness and isolation. For them, relationships do not exist as supportive and nourishing. Patients often describe feeling like an outsider and worry that it may be impossible to free themselves from their sense of emptiness and despair.

The value of a therapeutic relationship in mental illness is that it provides the patient with an "experience of being understood and of being related to another human being" (O'Toole and Welt, 1989, p. 11). A therapeutic relationship offers the patient hope and the possibility of discovering that he or she has meaning, even if at the time it is to only one other person, the therapist. To find that you have been able to "establish ties" and to discover that the other person values you as a worthy human being "just as you are" confirms the self in permanent ways and models the behaviors needed to develop healthy interpersonal relationships.

Interpersonal Relationships and Psychiatric Treatment

Although the 1990s have been designated as the decade of the brain, and psychopharmacology has a critical role to play in moderating the symptoms of mental illness, healing of mental illness usually takes more than medicine (Gebbard, 1992). Interpersonal relationships play a major role in the assessment and treatment of psychiatric symptoms. The experience of having a mental illness and the personal meaning of its symptoms affect the whole person. Understanding the particular personal meanings that characterize each unique person's experience of his or her interpersonal world is just as important as discerning the physical and psychological origins of the illness. Through greater understanding of their illness and discovery of ways to engage with others fully in meaningful relationships, patients are able to experience healthier functioning, increased autonomy of thinking and action, and a stronger sense of self. Patient education, an increasingly important dimension of psychiatric treatment, is far more successful when it is delivered by a knowledgeable health professional within the context of a trusting relationship. Thus, the therapeutic relationship forms "both the context and the means through which change occurs" (Fox, 1993, p. 111).

Social Relationships Versus Therapeutic Relationships

Moving from the concept of a social relationship to a therapeutic relationship requires a thorough understanding of the similarities and differences between social and therapeutic relationships. Principles of relationships with psychiatric patients, regardless of diagnosis, originate with our understandings of what constitutes successful interpersonal relationships in everyday life. Personal relationships characterize and help direct our experiences of life. Supportive relationships strengthen, enrich, and sustain a person's conduct of life. By contrast, flawed relationships diminish a person's sense of self, leaving the person feeling lonely and helpless, without the needed resources for successful direction of his or her life.

Elements Common to Both

There are clear similarities between the qualities of successful relationships in everyday life and in psychiatric settings—acceptance, respect, genuineness, mutual appreciation, and honesty. As any relationship develops, each person typically reveals more of who he or she is as a person, regardless of specific content. Both social and therapeutic relationships require similar levels of courtesy and respect for the person. Both depend on a sense of "mutuality, trust and partnership in a common situation" (Friedman, 1985). Therapeutic relationships depend on many of the same conversational techniques to facilitate the discussion. Theoretical and conceptual perspectives, however, establish the parameters of therapeutic relationships and clearly distinguish therapeutic relationships from all other types of relations between people.

Elements That Differ

Where therapeutic relationships differ is in their (1) purpose, (2) focus, (3) responsibility, (4) degree of self-disclosure, and (5) level of personal involvement.

PURPOSE

Social relationships have a wide variety of purposes that usually take into consideration the needs of all involved parties. In a social relationship, both participants assume personal responsibility for its development, and the relationship can last indefinitely. The reasons a social relationship ceases to exist does not depend on set criteria. By contrast, a therapeutic relationship has defined boundaries and a time-limited nature. The essential qualities of the therapeutic relationship require a health-related purpose. The goals of a therapeutic relationship relate to resolving an identified health care need and enhancing skills for living a more productive, satisfying life for the patient. When the patient accomplishes the health-related goals of a therapeutic relationship, the relationship ends.

FOCUS

The personal focal point of the relationship is different with social and therapeutic relationships. Social relationships typically focus on the needs, concerns, and desires of both participants. When the needs of one of the participants supercede that of the other participant, it happens spontaneously and usually as a result of the particular dynamics in the relationship. By contrast, the focus of the therapeutic relationship is always on the patient's needs or concerns and directly linked to the reasons the patient sought treatment. *It becomes the ethical responsibility of the nurse to ensure that any personal needs, concerns, and desires of the nurse get handled outside the therapeutic relationship.*

RESPONSIBILITY

In contrast to a social relationship in which the role and functions of each participant vary with each relationship, therapeutic relationships depend on a particular definition of role function and responsibility. The responsibilities for the relationship differ because of the differences in purpose between social and therapeutic relationships (Friedman, 1985). In a therapeutic relationship, the nurse has a professional responsibility for the structure and conduct of the relationship. Therapeutic relationships are by their nature one-sided, with the helping person held fully responsible for ensuring that the relationship is a safe harbor for patients. Participants enter the relationship from different positions, one as a person in need of nursing intervention, the other as a helping person. Because of the purpose of the relationship, the patient cannot get to know or experience the helping person in the same way as in a social relationship, without destroying the relationship.

The nurse is responsible for maintaining proper boundaries in the relationship situation. In a therapeutic relationship, mutuality, trust, and partnership in a common situation are confined to the designated therapeutic sessions and related concerns. These interpersonal boundaries provide predictability and safety for patients. They provide a special place in time and space for patients to discuss the intimate details of their situation and to express private emotions both verbally and nonverbally without fear of having them misunderstood or acted on. Social contact with the patient cannot extend beyond the limits of the relationship and must relate only to helping the patient meet the health-related goals of the relationship.

DEGREE OF SELF-DISCLOSURE

Communication in a social relationship is spontaneous, whereas therapeutic relationships require that it be purposeful. In social relationships, both parties have an equal opportunity to know and fully experience the other. There are no constraints on the level of verbal intimacy other than what the particular situation imposes or participants choose to impose. A similar equality of self-disclosure and intimacy is not appropriate in therapeutic relationships. Nurses limit their self-disclosure in the relationship to information needed to advance the health-related goals of the relationship. Information of a common rather than private nature is preferred.

LEVEL OF PERSONAL INVOLVEMENT

In mental health settings, *the therapeutic relationship represents a personal relationship within a professional context.* The professional context provides the boundaries of the relationship. It is the nurse's capacity to make personal emotional connections with the patient that determines its success. The patient expects the nurse to be involved as a "participant observer in the relationship process without either withdrawing from the patient, absorbing the patient's anxiety, or overidentifying with the patient as a person" (Peplau, 1952). Conceptual threads—purpose, mutuality, authenticity, empathy, active listening, confidentiality, and respect for the dignity of the patient—serve to strengthen the entire process; they flow throughout each of the identifiable phases of the nurse-patient relationship. When the personal involvement of the nurse reflects all of these characteristics in connection with the goals of the relationship, the relationship blossoms.

The nurse must retain the capacity to gauge the amount of distance in the relationship and to apply corrections when needed, much as the navigator corrects when the ship strays off course. Some relationships that begin as therapeutic slip into an overinvolved relationship unless you continually reflect on the meaning and purpose of the relationship. Overinvolvement stifles the patient's autonomy. Unless the patient has the tools to take the responsibility for his or her journey, the patient remains in a dependent role. You then become an enabler of the pathology rather than a resource guide to mental health. An overinvolved relationship is most likely to occur when the patient is exceptionally needy or is able to strike a responsive cord in your own emotional needs. You can become so committed to the patient as a person that the commitment begins to override treatment considerations and professional responsibilities to self and others (Morse, 1991). Overinvolvement should be suspected when nurses think they are the only one with whom the patient can relate, or they treat certain patients differently from the majority. Underinvolvement is equally undesirable. If you do not become a *participant* as well as an observer in the relationship and experience the encounter only as an outside observer, the interpersonal ties that become the crux of intervention do not occur. Many mentally ill patients come from life situations marked by conflict, rejection by others, hostility, or neglect. They doubt their own worth, tend to be self-absorbed, and carry a heavy burden of constant anxiety. The therapeutic relationship becomes a corrective experience for the patient and greatly influences the patient's concept of himself or herself. It must be designed so that it gives the patient a sense of being valued by the nurse, and this can occur only through your psychological presence in the relationship. Table 11–1 summarizes some of the differences between a social and a therapeutic relationship.

THERAPEUTIC RELATIONSHIPS

Definition of Therapeutic Relationships

The pathway to achieving therapeutic outcomes is through the nurse-patient relationship. A **therapeutic relationship** represents a time-bound alliance between nurse and patient, consciously entered into and characterized by respect, acceptance, empathy, and genuineness. Usually, it exemplifies a significant emotional encounter for patients. Therapeutic relationships build on the premise that the resources for healing reside within the patient for the development of meaning. Thus, the personal strengths of a patient become the groundwork for generating a personally relevant treatment plan. Therapeutic relationships with the mentally ill can be complex because patients distrust them. You have to earn

TABLE 11–1 **Some Differences Between a Social and a Therapeutic Relationship**

Therapeutic Relationships	Social Relationships
Encounters and interactions have a definite health-related purpose	Encounters and interactions are spontaneous, with or without definite purpose
Goals of the relationship directly link to achievement of health-related outcomes	Goals of the relationship vary, and goal achievement may or may not be identifiable
Relationships are time limited and terminate when outcomes are achieved	Relationships can last indefinitely, and there are no set criteria for ending them
Focus of the relationship is always on the patient and health-related needs and concerns	Relationship ideally takes into consideration the needs of both participants
Nurse assumes responsibility for the structure and conduct of the relationship	Participants share responsibility for the structure and conduct of the relationship
Self-disclosure by the patient is encouraged; self-disclosure by the nurse is limited	Self-disclosure is spontaneous and expected of both participants
Mutuality and personal involvement in partnership are limited to meeting the identified goals of the relationship; physical intimacy is prohibited	Mutuality and personal involvement are limited only by the needs and desires of the participants and may include physical intimacy

the patient's trust before the patient is able to take advantage of the help offered.

Therapeutic relationships embrace both the art and the science of nursing practice. Over time, nurses develop a style and philosophy of relationship that reflect their personal values and beliefs about relationships and how they should interact with their patients. As with all other relationships, the unique nature and quality of the relationship depend on the particular qualities and commitment of its participants. The shifting demands of the interpersonal situation create challenges and opportunities for practicing new behaviors. How successfully you creatively adapt communication principles to meet the individualized needs of patients represents the *art* of psychiatric nursing. Application of theoretical knowledge to development of the relationship process and achievement of expected treatment outcomes constitutes the *science* of psychiatric nursing. Both perspectives are equal and integral elements of successful nurse-patient relationships.

Therapeutic relationships are made up of distinct individuals, each with their own motivations, strengths, limitations, unique characteristics, and shared moments. Nurse and patient enter the relationship with his or her own personalized perception of the world, his or her community, and self. These meanings greatly influence the meaning of the relationship, readiness to engage, and motivation to maintain the relationship. Within the context of the relationship, nurse and patient agree to work together for a designated period of time to promote the patient's health and well-being. Thoughts and feelings they have about the experiences they share while together form the content of the relationship. Attitudes of the participants, such as respect, empathy, authenticity, and mutuality will affect the relationship process. Therapeutic relationships provide a stable, safe place for self-exploration and mutual discussion because the focus, time, place, and responsibilities of the participants are laid out from the onset of the relationship and are carried through to its termination.

Typically, therapeutic relationships with mentally ill patients progress through distinct sequential phases, originally described by Peplau (1952) as orientation, working (identification and exploitation), and termination (resolution). Phases of the relationship typically overlap, and ideally they reinforce the patient's progressive movement toward health.

Not all therapeutic relationships progress as a straight linear advance toward a desired outcome. Instead the nurse and patient travel down a winding path, sometimes bumpy, sometimes smooth, at times uninteresting, and other times embellished by human drama. The desired outcomes are off in the distance, known but not always readily visible. As the relationship deepens, there is a gradual understanding of new and deeper meanings about self and other. More superficial interpersonal communications characterizing the initial phases of the relationship are not lost. The nurse integrates their meaning into the relationship as essential threads in the working knowledge of both participants. Although some therapeutic relationships extend over weeks or months, others take place over the span of an 8-hour work shift, and still others take place in a single 1-hour session.

The essence of a therapeutic relationship is the helping process. This helping process provides resources and assists people to get in touch with their personal resources and strengths as the means to help themselves. Note that the outcome for the relationship is not to change the person's personality but rather to enable people to get in touch with their personal strengths and to use them in the service of deeper satisfaction and improved functioning. This is consistent with Peplau's belief that "the nurse does not have the power to change the behavior of patients" (Peplau, 1992, p. 14).

Establishing and maintaining growth-producing relation-

ships requires time, effort, and constant attention. In a therapeutic relationship, each person takes a position toward the other and the experiences as they unfold. Attitudes begin to develop, some dealing with fundamental issues of valuing, that shape the goals and conduct of the relationship. To learn how each patient's values and life goals shape a person's perceptions of meaning, their interests, and their behaviors is an intricate task. Although nurses may have general knowledge of human behavior, each person stands as an individual personality, unique among human beings. Significant individual differences among patients prevail and must be known and accepted by the nurse. Each patient's unique characteristics are embedded in a social context that you must also grasp if the patient is to realize full growth potential. Careful study of the patient is not enough. You need to develop individualized strategies to help patients see value in themselves, value in their efforts, and value in relationship. Warmth and valuing in the nurse-patient relationship can radiate to other relationships. The special study and sensitive, human-reasoned approaches that need to occur in the relationship, however, do not occur rapidly, and they do not normally happen without you expending considerable energy in processing its dynamics.

▶ Check Your Reading

1. What does the process of "taming" have in common with the therapeutic relationship with mentally ill patients?
2. How do the fundamental characteristics of a therapeutic relationship make the relationship safe for patients?
3. What are the primary differences between a social and a therapeutic relationship?
4. How can the nurse make the therapeutic relationship a healing pathway for the patient to feel valued as a worthwhile human being?

Use of Self in Therapeutic Relationships

In contrast to many other forms of nursing practice, in which knowledge of technical equipment and psychomotor skills are measures of competence, the basic tools and competencies of the nurse in psychiatric nursing center around the therapeutic use of self. **Therapeutic use of self** refers to the nurse's presence, "a physical 'being there,' and psychological 'being with' a patient for the purpose of meeting the patient's health care needs" (Gardner, 1992, p. 191). Each therapeutic relationship necessarily reflects your personality, beliefs, and values. Use of self as a therapeutic tool comprises your whole person: psychological, physical, social, and spiritual elements, used purposefully with patients (Uys, 1980). It does not occur spontaneously but usually involves considerable forethought based on critical thinking principles. Based on a firm scientific foundation and threaded with a strong sense of compassion and commitment, therapeutic use of self is a deliberate application of self, employed in the interest of the patient.

Importance of Self-Awareness in Therapeutic Relationships

To use the self as a tool effectively, you should have a basic understanding of communication principles and an adequate knowledge base of common therapeutic disorders and interventions. Empathy for the humanity of others and a willingness to learn from the patient are other essential prerequisites. Equally important is **self-awareness** (Rogers, 1951). Your knowledge of personal response patterns, strengths, and limitations can influence the interaction in positive ways because you have more leverage in responding.

Lack of self-awareness can pose serious problems in relationships. Therapeutic relationships with mentally ill patients symbolize an act of trust—trust that you will continue the journey even in the face of serious obstacles. Behaviors occur that cross the line of socially acceptable behavior. They can be personally offensive and in deep conflict with your social value system. In no other setting are you so likely to become the immediate target of idealizing, hostile, critical, dependent, and rejecting behaviors than in therapeutic relationships with the seriously mentally ill. Although it is possible to recognize the behavior as part of the mental disorder intellectually, it is not always easy to have the same understanding and acceptance emotionally in a human-to-human relationship. These behaviors can seriously test your commitment and values.

Because most of us are socialized to avoid strong feelings, it often comes as a surprise to find that the work of the relationship with the patient sometimes emerges only after display of strong feeling or aberrant behavior. Without self-awareness, it becomes humanly impossible to accept the patient as a person regardless of his or her behavior. Yet this is exactly what needs to occur for healing. *The nurse must become the patient's therapeutic ally—confronting when necessary, confirming always, as a steadfast companion on the journey to mental health.* For, as Sullivan (1954) notes, ". . . no one has grave difficulties in living if he has a very good grasp on what is happening to him" (p. 24).

Another reason for self-awareness in relationships with the mentally ill lies in the roller coaster effect of patient emotions that unpredictably occur with regularity. It is easy to get drawn into the patient's drama—to empathize when one should confront or to challenge when the patient needs understanding. Yet there is a delicate balance between staying involved and preserving objectivity that is essential to maintain. Self-awareness helps you establish the needed caring objectivity. It helps you keep in focus that these feelings are not created by you personally but are being displaced onto you from events and relationships in the patient's past.

Self-awareness helps keep the relationship honest. The process of self-reflection compels nurses to get in touch with their own value positions so that they do not project them onto others or reject those who do not share similar values. True acceptance of patients "just as they are" depends on your awareness of your own attitudes and behaviors in the relationship. In the tale of *The Little Prince*, a king details the nature of self-awareness:

> "Then you shall judge yourself," the king answered. "That is the most difficult of all. It is much more difficult to judge oneself than to judge others. If you succeed in judging yourself rightly, than you are indeed a man of true wisdom" (de Saint-Exupéry, 1943).

The process of looking at one's own behaviors makes it easier to separate the patient's needs from one's own. It is human nature to want to have one's efforts acknowledged and to want confirmation that those efforts yielded positive results. Yet Jacobs (1978) notes that the helping person's confirmation must come "through the expression of him/herself in the service of the task" (p. 113) and not from direct approval by the patient. As a patient gets better, it is easy to feel elated with the patient's personal growth and the part you played in it. It is easy also to feel discouraged and angry when a patient does not comply with treatment, withholds information, or spurns your offers of help. Self-awareness helps you to sort out unconscious feelings of countertransference and reduces the possibility of behaviors such as overprotection, manipulation, domination, and sexual feelings from compromising the work of the relationship. A byproduct of self-awareness is self-confidence, which enhances your credibility as a helping person. Box 11–1 summarizes the primary benefits of self-awareness in the nurse-patient relationship.

Self-awareness actually begins unconsciously with a person's internal organization of life experience. In the course of everyday living, people develop working models of how they should act, how they expect other people to act, and what they consider as normal behavior. Rarely do people with major mental illness fit these working models. Their behaviors are erratic, unusual, and not easily understood. Self-awareness in the therapeutic relationship must develop from a conscious and continuous reflection on your behavior, its possible impact on the patient, and an understanding of how the patient's behavior influences you. Rogers (1958) poses 10 questions, outlined in Box 11–2, that you can use for self-reflection before beginning a patient-centered relationship. Each question directs you to look inward, to travel beyond technical competency to an understanding of the human connections between self and other.

BOX 11-1 Primary Benefits of Self-Awareness in the Nurse-Patient Relationship

- Can help you respond therapeutically to difficult patient behaviors
- Facilitates full acceptance of patients
- Helps establish needed caring objectivity
- Makes it easier to separate what belongs to the patient and what belongs to you
- Increases your self-confidence, which enhances the quality of interactions

Frameworks to Guide Therapeutic Relationships

Nurses need to have a theoretical framework to guide their practice and provide direction for their interventions built on strong scientific rationales and consistent with their values and beliefs. The richness of therapeutic relationships traces its roots to a blending of the psychological and nursing theory models, as described in Chapter 6. Of special note in understanding the nature and development of the nurse-patient relationship are three models of interpersonal process, which are briefly summarized next.

Nursing Frameworks: Hildegard Peplau

The uniqueness of psychiatric nursing is embedded in nursing theories, which provide its special perspective. Nursing theory creates a particular care context that differentiates psychiatric nursing practice from the practice of psychiatry, social work, and other allied health professionals. For example, nurses provide health teaching and monitor medication, two activities that solidly belong to the domain of nursing. The approach to a patient is holistic and based on a synthesis of medical, social, philosophical, and psychological principles drawn together through the concept of caring.

Peplau (1952) conceptualizes relationship as an alliance between a helping professional and a patient characterized by significant emotional bonds and connections. Essential to the development of the therapeutic relationship are certain caring behaviors, recognized as important to its development today as it was more than 40 years ago. Box 11–3 contains characteristics of caring behaviors in therapeutic relationships.

First, you need to have the professional knowledge and skills required to work with the mentally ill patient. Included in your tool box are pathophysiology and pharmacology related to the treatment of mental illness. When combined with assessment, communication, teaching, and ethical and legal principles, this knowledge provides you with the knowledge base required of psychiatric nurses. Peplau believes that the therapeutic relationship is founded on attentiveness to the patient's experience, with a respectful deference to the patient's understanding of his or her problem areas and personal strengths. *Positive connectedness* is viewed by Peplau as a critical dimension that goes beyond the mere exchange of information. There has to be an emotional attachment of genuine interest to the patient's story. In every as-

BOX 11-2 Questions for Self-Reflection Before Beginning a Patient-Centered Relationship

What are the personal and professional strengths that I bring to this relationship?

In what ways could my personal life circumstances potentially get in the way of establishing or maintaining this relationship? In what ways might they be helpful?

Can I understand that each patient's symptoms are a form of communication telling me something about his or her emotional pain?

Can I comprehend how difficult it is for a patient who is hurting to share his or her deepest pain or to recognize self-imposed psychosocial-spiritual alienation from self and others?

Can I grasp the characteristics of some patients with whom one intervention works and of those for whom another intervention works?

What criteria will I use to know when to support a vulnerable patient and when to confront self-destructive behavior?

How will I be able to maintain therapeutic neutrality and empathy in the face of intense emotions directed toward me and/or the patient's self-destructive behaviors?

How do I sustain optimism and hope when progress is slow or seemingly nonexistent with the chronically mentally ill patient?

How can I sincerely demonstrate confidence in my patients' capacity to develop a different meaningful way of life and to manage their own affairs?

BOX 11-3 Characteristics of Caring Behaviors Reported in Therapeutic Relationships

Professional knowledge and skills

Respectful deference to the patient

Attentiveness to the patient's experience

Positive connectedness

Assurance of human presence

pect of the relationship, you are a participant as well as an observer. The patient must have the assurance of human presence found in the form of your attitudes, behaviors, and words to support the content of the relationship. Otherwise the patient's situation can never be as fully explored as it should be in a therapeutic relationship.

The particular value of Peplau's model (1952) lies in her descriptions of the type of relationship desired in psychiatric nursing and in careful descriptions of the developmental stages of the therapeutic relationship (orientation, working [identification and exploitation], and resolution [termination] phases). These phases of relationship still serve as the matrix for understanding relationships in psychiatric nursing as well as most other areas of professional nursing.

Psychological Frameworks: Carl Rogers

Rogers's (1951) patient-centered model of therapeutic relationships is useful in several ways. He reframed earlier psychoanalytic frameworks that considered patients' early relationships with significant others as the central focus for discussion. His theory has a distinctly humanistic orientation (see Chapter 6). From the therapist's perspective, the model focuses on the patient as a person in the "here and now"; from the patient's perspective, it focuses on how the patient feels he or she is subjectively experienced by the helping person in the relationship. Rogers's insistence that people have within themselves all of the tools for realizing their highest potential is consistent with nursing's goal that the patient should reach his or her optimum level of psychosocial functioning and personal independence. Rogers views the patient as an active participant as well as a recipient of care. He suggests that patients automatically seek self-actualization of their potential, if given appropriate feedback and encouragement, which are provided in ways that are understood and acceptable to the patient. Rogers considers attitudes held by the professional as conditions that are "necessary and sufficient" for therapeutic change. He labels these as empathy, genuineness, unconditional acceptance, and positive regard.

Existential Frameworks: Martin Buber

Buber's (1970) model emphasizes the need for the nurse-patient relationship to be one of equal and respectful partnership. In an I-thou relationship, each participant experiences and values the other as a unique human being surrounded by a distinctive environmental background and possessing an original set of personal strengths, behaviors, and problems. The essence of an I-thou relationship is the mutual discovery of the other person's characteristic humanness. I-object relationships occur when the helping person acts in a prescribed way without considering the ways in which this person is different from others. Buber suggests that the essence of an I-thou relationship is just the opposite. Actions performed with the person and the experiencing of the other as a valued unique human being confirms his or her humanness in a meaningful way. Buber uses the term *confirming* communication to refer to comments that recognize the individuality of the person and the term *disconfirming* communication as comments that fail to acknowledge the unique existence of the other. Nurses can unintentionally disconfirm psychiatric patients by discounting their comments as unimportant, by not picking up on themes, and by assuming the patient cannot take responsibility. Nurses confirm their patients each time they make a special effort to acknowledge and respond to a patient's individualized needs. Even making it a point to call the patient by name confirms the unique individuality of a patient. (See Chapter 10 for examples of confirming and disconfirming responses.)

The specific helping skills you use with the patient differ with each relationship. The basic assumptions of a therapeutic relationship, however, are the same (Figure 11–1):

- It is an I-thou relationship.
- Certain conditions of unconditional acceptance and positive regard, genuineness, and empathy are necessary conditions for successful outcomes.
- The natural progression of the relationship will follow definable stages that are valid for all relationships.

To meet the goals of the relationship, you should consistently use a process of self-reflection, critical thinking, and values clarification in deciding the most appropriate interventions.

▶ Check Your Reading

5. What is the primary value of Peplau's interpersonal theory of nursing for psychiatric nursing?
6. How does Rogers view the patient and the patient's role in therapeutic relationships?
7. What is the essence of Buber's approach to relationships with patients?

Conceptual Components of Therapeutic Relationships

No matter how skilled the nurse is in applying communication principles, the nature of the nurse's personal involvement is most important and is most likely to be remembered as the critical factor in treatment. Casement (1991) suggests that the patient's emotional experience of the relationship between nurse and patient can be as important as the cognitive insights the patient gains about resolving his or her mental conflicts. Rieman (1986) identifies feeling valued as a unique human being, being listened to, and having one's thoughts and feelings understood by another human being as the most significant curative factors identified by patients in a phenomenological study of nurse-patient behaviors. The knowledgeable and caring nurse serves as an ally in helping patients identify personal strengths, community resources, and alternative strategies to resolve life problems. Of equal importance is the careful attention to respecting boundaries, caring, advocacy, unconditional acceptance, mutuality, authenticity, and trust.

Boundaries

Scott (1988) defines **boundaries** as "a dynamic line of demarcation separating an individual's internal (body, mind, and spirit) and external environments, and varying in permeability and flexibility" (p. 24). Boundaries mark a symbolic separation between people that makes it possible for them to experience their own reality in a unique way and to understand the nature of others. People with well-defined boundaries know who they are and what is important to them. They are clear about their boundaries, and others trust them because they know what they stand for. People with loose boundaries usually have difficulty separating their issues and needs from those of others. They tend to be people pleasers with deep underlying resentments. Rigid boundaries do not allow a person much flexibility to relate differently when a situation calls for a wider range of behavior.

Each person ultimately determines his or her own boundaries, influenced by personal preference, culture, time of day, attitudes of the people involved, and previous life experience. Boundaries surround social relationships with invisible lines drawn to define space, time, and type

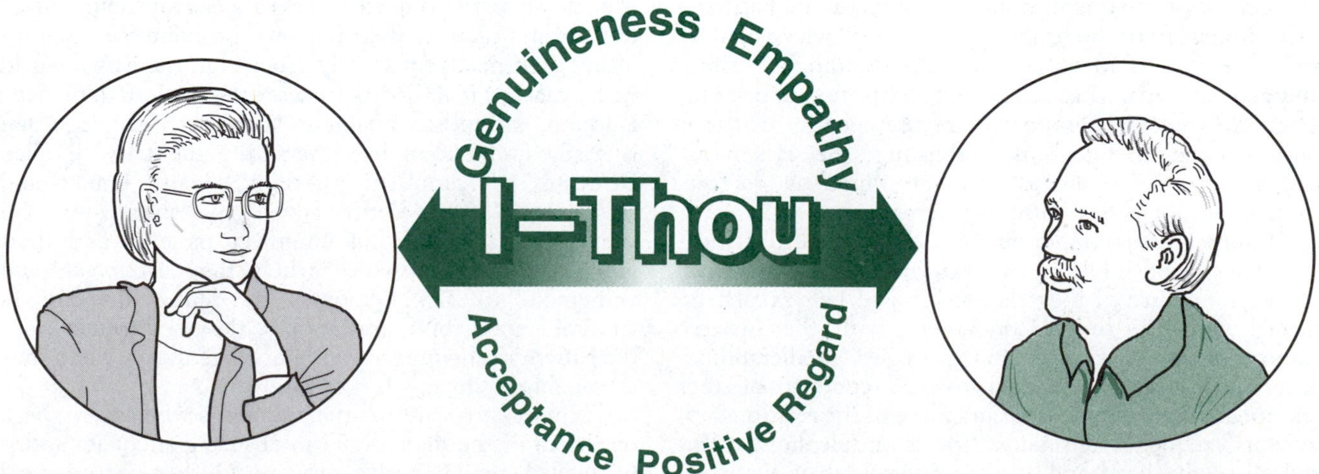

FIGURE 11–1
Buber's characteristics of a therapeutic relationship.

BOX 11-4 Guidelines for the Development of Appropriate Boundaries in Nurse-Patient Relationships

Do	Do Not
Establish set times for the relationship sessions	Give the patient private information about yourself
Begin and end sessions on time	Give or exchange personal phone numbers with a patient
Call the person by his or her given name	Give gifts (your presence and your interest are the best gifts)
Protect the patient's right to privacy and confidentiality	Arrange to see the patient at times or in places other than those dictated by treatment
Give patients full information about their disorder and medications	Discuss the correctness or value of the therapeutic interventions of other health team members with the patient
Safeguard the patient from becoming too vulnerable in the relationship	Bend the unit rules for a patient without careful consideration and without consultation with others involved in the patient's care
Provide security from harmful behaviors to self or others	Accept gifts from patients (an exception might be a small token made in occupational therapy)
Prewarn the patient about the end of sessions and the therapeutic relationship	Give information about adult patients to others not directly involved in their care, without their permission
	Make promises to a patient that you cannot keep

of appropriate interaction. They spell out the limits of behavior in relationships. For example, a flirtatious comment in a social situation may be appreciated, whereas the same behavior would be offensive in the work situation. Boundary violations found in everyday life include sexual harrassment, moving too close to a person, sharing confidential information, entering a person's room, going through a person's possessions, or taking advantage of someone's inability to say no to unreasonable demands.

Personal and interpersonal boundaries are an issue with mentally ill patients, who have either nebulous boundaries or fixed boundaries that do not allow other people to know them. Mentally healthy people usually are able to choose when and under what circumstances they take self-defining positions; those with mental illness do not feel they have this flexibility. Boundaries are particularly important for the seriously mentally ill, who feel they are vulnerable to attack and misunderstanding any time they actively engage in a relationship with another person. They are extremely important in therapeutic relationships because they aid in establishing the patient as separate from the nurse and the nurse as neither controlling nor controllable by the patient.

Interpersonal boundaries in a therapeutic relationship consist of internal and external parameters that define the nature of the relationship and help create its special space in time. Consistency with the surface parameters of a relationship provides predictability. External boundaries related to the conduct of the relationship include the time and place of the relationship sessions, frequency of sessions, limits on telephone calls, and all of the legal and ethical dimensions of a nurse-patient relationship. Internal boundaries require that you maintain a focus on the patient, giving that patient full attention and caring during the course of the interaction, while respecting the personal integrity of both participants. Patients appreciate interpersonal boundary limits that are realistic, negotiated in advance, and matter-of-factly enforced with adequate firmness and respect for their personal integrity. Well-established boundaries mutually understood by you and the patient allow you much more flexibility in relating therapeutically to patients. Box 11-4 presents guidelines for the development of appropriate boundaries in nurse-patient relationships.

Advocacy

Advocacy is a broad concept that Peplau (1952) recognized early as an essential role for the psychiatric nurse. Mentally ill patients need nurses to speak for them. Often, they cannot identify their personal problems or communicate their needs effectively. Locked in their own world with a marked inability to process information, to manage emotion, and mostly unable to speak with language that is easily understood by others, the mentally ill need advocates who can act on their behalf. Tanner and colleagues (1993) describe advocates, "as persons who stand along side of and empower patients and their families to have a voice when they are weak and vulnerable" (p. 278). Gadow (1989) defines **advocacy** as a moral responsibility of the nurse designed to maximize the patient's self-integrity and personal dignity when they are unable to do this for themselves.

Nurses advocate for their patients when they speak on behalf of the mentally ill in ensuring adequate access to needed mental health services. On a more personal level, you can note early signs of patient change and bring them to the attention of the appropriate person, including the patient. Coaching patients to define themselves and to articulate their needs step by step is a form of advocating for the full potential of the patient. You can make appropriate referrals and act as the patient's advisor in describing their needs to other health professionals. As a member of the multidisciplinary health care team, you can advocate for the patient with authority, authenticity, and compassion in presenting the patient's case to the other team members.

Caring

The therapeutic relationship between nurse and patient in mental health settings is first and foremost a significant human relationship, of which the hallmark is caring. **Caring** is an intangible interactive process with physical, psychosocial, and spiritual dimensions that finds expression through actions designed to promote the health and well-being of patients. Caring represents a gift of self based on a sound knowledge base and intuitive awareness of the patient's needs. In a study of patient perceptions of caring behaviors, Brown (1993) found that *patients valued personalized care, in which their individualized needs were addressed, above all else.* Caring behaviors need not be acknowledged by the other to qualify as caring. This is an important distinction because frequently the mentally ill or cognitively impaired patient cannot fully acknowledge, reciprocate, or even directly experience your caring in a consistent fashion. Caring behaviors have the ring of truth only when they specifically emerge out of the patient's need.

Caring behaviors can develop only in a climate of respect for the uniqueness of the other. Respect for each person represents a perspective of caring that many psychiatric patients have not experienced as a part of their journey before meeting the nurse. The interventions are simple. Patients experience caring by being treated as a person worthy of being taken seriously, by having their thoughts and feelings listened to with concentration, and by receiving competent attention to their needs from a professional person—with no strings attached.

Caring finds expression in many individual and nonspecified behaviors: through your knowledge, interest, patience, respect, and willingness to accept the patient just as the person is, holding to boundaries and being consistent, fair, and truthful. Caring behaviors require a knowledge of the other acquired through active listening, a giving of self with its attendant vulnerability and risk taking, arising from a commitment to ethical values and proper behaviors. Thus, "the caring attitude is conveyed to the patient, not by a single act, but through repeated encounters as events evolve in the daily life of the unit" (Benfer and Schroder, 1985, p. 459).

Complicating the issue of what caring means to the patient is the realization that the concept varies in different cultures. For example, a Vietnamese patient would view recognizing the family unit as his or her most important resource for sharing as a caring behavior, whereas a patient in the dominant culture would view sharing with the therapist as primary. Developing an openness and respect for feelings, values, and experiences of all patients regardless of race, color, creed, or medical condition are essential characteristics of caring behaviors.

In a therapeutic relationship, you model how to have a caring, nonexploitative relationship with another human being. The therapeutic relationship is a powerful, rich resource of healing possibilities. Within the relationship, you and the patient become cocreators of a human experience that, by its nature, seeks to help the participants become self-aware, self-responsible, and self-actualizing. Out of the relationship can come the impetus to develop new solutions and different ways of being in the world. Difficult emotions such as anger can be expressed and resolved collaboratively. Respect for the individual dignity and autonomy for each person consistently marks a caring encounter.

Mutuality

Mutuality involves inclusion and connection; it implies equal partnership in achieving a goal. The concept of mutuality offers many unique opportunities to validate and affirm another human being. Morse (1991) describes it as the infrastructure of a connected relationship. *A connected relationship is one in which "the nurse views the patient first as a person and second as a patient"* (p. 458). Trust, reciprocity, respect for the uniqueness of the other, and sharing of feelings are interwoven into an ontological experience between two individuals. (*Ontological* means "related to being," or relating.) Mutuality in a relationship exists in the special reality of the helping relationship and "is ever and again reconstituted in accordance with men's meetings with one another" (Rotenstreich, 1959b).

Both Rogers and Buber formally recognized the importance of mutuality in their theories about the nature of the therapeutic relationship. They emphasized that people can change and can take responsibility for themselves with appropriate support. According to Rogers, mutuality requires a search for common ground in understanding issues. The patient presents his or her perceptions of reality, whereas you can bring additional understandings to the situation.

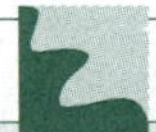

STEVEN'S STORY

One of Steven's goals is to get married. He has trouble meeting women and significant difficulty sustaining heterosexual relationships. Although he wants to achieve his goal, Steven is not taking any of the steps that might allow him to reach his goal. He doesn't want to participate in group therapy, which would help him with his social skills. Going to places or engaging in activities that would provide access to meeting women is not something he feels comfortable doing. In this situation, the nurse can refer to Steven's strengths as potential resources in achieving his goal, while pointing out that certain actions on Steven's part are essential to his successful goal achievement.

Buber defined the concept of mutuality as based on the premise that two people in a relationship recognize and respect the separateness, uniqueness, and need for self-growth of the other as well as in oneself. Thus, mutuality is not emotional fusion with a patient. It requires an acknowledgment of the independence of the other before entering as a sharing presence into the full reality of the other (Berry, 1985).

Mutuality helps to humanize a highly structured relationship by creating a shared experience of the patient's story and human potential. As a participant observer in a patient's human journey, the nurse is in a unique position to point out the patient's strengths as they emerge in the relationship. Strengths may be acknowledged directly in such statements as "I notice that you have a good sense of humor in our relationship, and I would encourage you to use it in other situations." Other situations allow the nurse to emphasize potential strengths indirectly. For example, when the patient asks for additional contact and there is no therapeutic reason to do so, you may want to give the patient the message that you have confidence in the patient's ability to handle things in your absence. Pointing out the patient's tangible strengths coupled with the statement, "if this is not an emergency, do you think we could discuss it with the attention it deserves in our next scheduled meeting," reinforces this confidence.

Mutuality in a joint discussion of ideas and feelings can challenge or validate the reality of the patient's experience, which helps to restore the balance needed to be mentally healthy. Most mental disorders tend to predispose a person to anxiety and depressed or aggressive moods, which compromise goal achievement. Feelings often get in the way of clear thinking, or faulty thinking disturbs the balance of emotions. Moreover the natural inclination of many patients is to persist in using maladaptive behaviors that result in unfavorable outcomes because they lack the self-confidence or have a reduced ability to perceive, compare, and develop alternative solutions. Yet to change an outcome, patients need to change the actions they have been using thus far. They must learn to develop different behaviors conducive to achieving a more favorable result. Teyber (1993, p. 29) suggests a useful approach with the following dialogue:

I would like for you and I to become partners. I cannot figure out what is wrong and tell you what to do on my own and you have not been able to solve your problems by yourself, so let's work on them together. You are the world's foremost expert on you, and I have skills and knowledge about problems such as yours to contribute. By working together we have the best chance of succeeding.

Ongoing feedback is an important aspect of mutuality that may be key to effecting change and promoting well-being in patients. As you observe changes in the patient's behavior, there is an unique opportunity to point out an erroneous perception or identify a distortion of the danger involved in choosing one alternative behavior over another. Hearing you identify changes in performance can produce a different shared evaluation of the meaning of events and motivations. Noting changes in the patient's self-confidence, ability to make decisions, and capacity to take responsibility for the progress in his or her own life validates the struggle in the patient's experience and, in some instances, serves as a new window of information. The patient may give you feedback about values that are critical to the patient's mental health but would not typically be considered. For example, you might think that making a commitment to weekly outpatient sessions would be a good idea for an Asian patient. In the Chinese culture, however, mental illness is a stigma, so ongoing outpatient intervention for mental illness would not fit with the patient's cultural perceptions of mental illness and how it should be treated. Box 11–5 presents strategies to enhance mutuality.

Unconditional Acceptance

It is easier to respect people whose ideas and values parallel our own. Much more difficult is full acceptance and respect for people whose ideas, feelings, and values are quite unlike those we hold as valid. Logically, people know that single characteristics, for example, sexual orientation, race, or religious beliefs, do not define the nature of a person. Yet many people, including nurses, base their evaluations of others on their individual characteristics, values, or ideological positions.

Rogers's view of unconditional **acceptance** is the capacity of the nurse to affirm the patient's humanity and to validate their life experience without questioning its validity or judging it in any way. This does not mean that you condone all patient behaviors or allow the patient to act out in ways that are damaging to self or others. It does mean that you must strive to understand all human behavior as a form of communication and the patient behind the behavior as communicating in the only way available at the time. With some behaviors, particularly those of a hostile or sexual nature, it is easy to become oversensitive. Behaviors that the nurse views as inappropriate, distasteful, or misguided are likely to be rejected and the people engaging in them treated badly. Noncompliance when you and the patient have agreed on certain actions can be frustrating. When you become emotionally involved with a patient's well-being, it is difficult not to take criticism personally. Areas of acceptance that are most difficult for novice nurses include differences in

BOX 11–5 Strategies to Enhance Mutuality

Search for common ground in understanding issues

Acknowledge the patient's autonomy

Use the relationship to create shared experiences of reality

Point out patient strengths

Comment on changes in patient behaviors

culture, lifestyle, sexual orientation, life decisions, values, and refusal or sabotage of services offered by the nurse.

Empowerment

The word *power* comes from the Latin word, *posse*, meaning "to be able." Empowerment requires that a patient take an active part in all phases of the nurse-patient relationship, in the assessment and planning phases as well as in the implementation phase. The organizing principle of empowerment is a shared vision, providing the focus for directed action toward a unified purpose (Schmieding, 1993).

Mental illness is a disease of the powerless. The mentally ill represent a disempowered segment of the population, often misunderstood, avoided, oppressed, or ridiculed as being inferior. Only those with special genius or preeminent talent escape its stigma. For example, mental health insurance benefits in no way parallel the benefits for physical illness. Yet the mentally ill may suffer as much as the patient with any other illness. Treatment, if available, may be just as effective as it would be for other chronic physical illness. A diagnosis of serious mental illness must be acknowledged on some job applications and may prevent a person from obtaining a job. The concept of empowerment has an important role in helping the mentally ill seek new ways of living, expand their personal horizons, and make a legitimate place for themselves in society.

Hawks (1992) defines **empowerment** as "the interpersonal process of providing the proper tools, resources and environment to build, develop, and increase the ability and effectiveness of others to set and reach goals for individual and social ends" (p. 609). Empowerment prepares patients through patient education and coaching and reinforces their efforts in developing more effective strategies for negotiating their environment through counseling. The counseling takes the form of pointing out strengths, supporting effective strategies, and working through feelings about the changes.

Strategies designed to help patients take maximum control of their lives are most representative of empowerment. Empowerment strategies need to link directly with the patient's goals. They should be both practical and action oriented. As patients take charge of their lives, their journey becomes more interesting and worth the effort. Of all the possible empowerment interventions, validation of the patient's efforts is most important. The chronically mentally ill usually have experienced little validation of their efforts and their choices. For the nurse to acknowledge their efforts, their choices and their personal strengths as being real and valuable is particularly reinforcing for these patients (Tobias, 1990).

In a qualitative research study of chronically mentally ill patients attending a patient-run drop-in center, Connelly and associates (1993) identified four attributes of empowerment as participating, choosing, supporting, and negotiating. The importance of this research is that it described empowerment from the patient's perspective. These patients reported that the simple act of participating was personally empowering. Developing choices gave them a sense of control over their lives. As patients share their experiences and help one another, the peer group provides empowerment through interpersonal safety. The final step in empowerment occurs when the patient is willing to take a stand on an issue he or she feels deeply about. Thus, empowerment is a concept in which "power is both taken and given" (p. 301).

Personal responsibility is key to the development of effective empowerment strategies. Empowerment cannot be given to another, but you can take every opportunity to encourage patients to become active participants in therapeutic activities, to make choices, and to be a mutual partner in the development of solutions to the patient's major conflicts. Through the role of advocate, you can empower patients to become active participants and informed decision makers in their own care (Curtin, 1979; Corcoran, 1988).

Empathy

Egan (1986) describes basic **empathy** as "listening carefully to the client and then communicating understanding of what the client is feeling and of the experiences and behaviors underlying those feelings" (p. 99). Although empathy shares some of the characteristics of sympathy in that they both evidence expression of compassionate understanding, they differ in their purpose and orientation. In contrast to sympathy, which stops at an expression of feeling, empathy represents a mutual interpersonal process in which the nurse is able to capture the inner struggle of the patient, bring together different aspects of the patient's situation in a meaningful way, and communicate that understanding in a way that is understood as truth by the patient. It is both an attitude and a communication strategy in which your role as participant observer is particularly relevant.

Empathy allows you to access the inner world of the patient experientially. It includes "a personal capacity, affective resonance and cognitive functioning. All are operative and complementarily interwoven in interpersonal functioning" (Fox, 1993, p. 43). Empathic comments enhance the patient's self-awareness and potential for personal growth. By paying close attention to key words and phrases, you can reflect them back to the patient with the same affect in which they were originally expressed. For example, following a patient's description of deep sadness related to the recent suicide of her son, you might empathetically comment, "I don't think there is anything more difficult in life than having to face the death of your child."

Egan (1986) categorizes advanced empathy as the ability of the helping person to go beyond the surface feelings and to articulate hidden feelings that are not emotionally available to the person. For example, you may realize that the patient who has nothing good to say about your intervention may actually be experiencing similar emotions about his own inability to interact with you. Understanding the patient from this perspective affects how you respond empathetically. Box 11–6 identifies nursing behaviors associated with the process of empathy.

BOX 11-6 Nursing Behaviors Associated with the Process of Empathy

Wanting to know and understand the patient as a person

Going beyond appearances and superficial assessments; listening actively to understand fully the patient's message, intent, and associated feelings

Asking the right questions and waiting for the meaning to reveal itself

Placing yourself momentarily in the patient's position and experiencing what it would be like to "walk in his shoes"

Stepping back and reflecting on what you are hearing, observing, and intuitively thinking about concerning what the patient is revealing to you; developing an appropriate response

Sharing your observations or reflecting your feelings with the patient

Authenticity

Authenticity, a critical element of mental health, refers to learning and accepting our own truth as unique human beings. Mental illness inevitably involves losing touch with oneself, completely or partially. Many people entering psychotherapy have never encountered themselves or known who they are or what they want from life. The aim of a therapeutic relationship is to help a person discover or recapture a genuine sense of self. The nurse models authenticity by *being* genuine. In therapeutic relationships, authenticity means being real with the patient, not hiding behind the mask of professionalism. Although intimate aspects of the helping person's life are not shared with the patient, what is brought into the relationship are your natural feelings and attitudes. Authenticity means, for example, that you feel free to tell a patient honestly and directly that you do not want to answer a personal or provocative question. If you are angry, anxious, hold a different value, or make a mistake, you share this information. A simple statement that does not carry with it a judgment about the other person, and a thinking statement that goes beyond the range of expected responses to the heart of the matter reflect authenticity.

Authenticity depends on self-knowledge and common sense about what is appropriate in any given situation. First, you need to develop self-awareness of personal biases and values. By maintaining constant attention to how personal feelings and values may be interacting with the relationship, you have more options. Rather than deny the existence of strong feelings, the authentic nurse integrates them into the conversation in meaningful ways. For example, Brandon (1983) describes an incident in which a suicidal patient asked him if he could see any reason why he should live. Brandon answered him honestly, that at the moment he could see why the person wanted to die and why he didn't feel he had much reason to live. Later, when the man recovered from his depression, he told Brandon how much his honesty had meant to him. Jourard (1968, p. 182) refers to authenticity as a multidimensional way of being that:

> *. . . calls for a courage and a willingness to let the world be what it is, to let the other be who he is, and to let oneself be who one is. It calls as well for a commitment to truth, as it changeably presents itself. It calls for a readiness to suspend concepts and beliefs about self, others, and world, and to perceive what is. It calls for a willingness to suspend imagination, wish, and fantasy, a readiness to inform and revise concepts with fresh inputs of perception.*

There is a caution about being straightforward. You need to present the truth with compassion and an awareness of the impact a genuine comment may have on the patient. Looking for receptive moments and delivering difficult comments with tact and respect for the patient's dignity provide a useful base for the mutual appreciation of honesty in the relationship. If you are blind to the needs of the other person, it is possible inadvertently to disregard important feelings or attitudes of a person. There is authenticity perhaps, but it is one-dimensional, demonstrated without caring, and not of the nature Jourard and others describe as valuable in helping relationships.

Trust

The concept of **trust** involves a patient's inner confidence that a helping person respects, understands, and responds fairly to that person. Before the actual therapeutic work can begin, the patient must be assured of a secure atmosphere and established measures to support the direction of the task. Trust lays the foundation of the nurse-patient relationship, as the patient strives to establish that the nurse is a trustworthy person (Forchuk, 1991). How nurses interpret their roles and present them to others affects the trust patients have in them.

Trust is a mutual process. It begins with your own confidence in your skills and includes the firm belief that the patient is capable of changing his or her behavior. People want to believe that the person treating them has the expertise to make their work together meaningful. Covey (1991) notes that "trustworthiness is more than integrity; it also connotes competence" (p. 171).

Trust of self anchors and necessarily precedes trust of others. Mental illness makes it more difficult for patients to trust their own reality. They lack confidence in their own behaviors, their feelings, or their competence in mastering difficult life situations. If people cannot trust themselves, it becomes almost impossible for them to trust others. Consequently the mentally ill patient may experience great difficulty in trusting your intentions and actions. It is not unusual for the patient to feel that the health care professional does not understand or care about the patient's perspective. (Sometimes, unfortunately, this is true). Such feelings, whether warranted or not, can lead to anger, suspicion, and adversarial relationships in clinical settings.

Trust must be earned. Helping patients to understand the limits as well as the possibilities in achieving treatment goals during therapeutic relationships is important. Describing the process of therapeutic relationships initially and referring back to those understandings when the relationship stalls facilitate a realistic appraisal of what is possible in the relationship. For example, some patients want instant change and good feelings to emerge from their relationships with the nurse. They figure that if they say it all, you will pick up the information and translate it into simple directives the patient can take, and all will be well. Patients need to understand that behaviors developed over years cannot be reversed in a single session or even within a short period of time.

The road to recovery is a winding one, characterized by detours and temporary setbacks. As with any chronic illness, resistance to change is to be expected. Working through misunderstandings and difficult places in the relationship is a necessary part of the working phase of a therapeutic relationship. This is as important for you to understand as it is for the patient. Otherwise, you may feel inadequate when the patient seems to "switch" from being in tune with your suggestions to becoming stalled or more critical of the help received in the relationship.

Some patients expect you to be a mind reader. They assume you know everything about them. These patients need help with understanding that within the therapeutic process, the primary task of the patient is to put into words difficult feelings and situations that both nurse and patient can process. The most effective nurse-patient relationships are those demonstrating nursing interventions individualized to the qualities of the patient and the demands of the therapeutic situation.

The patient needs to know that the relationship is a safe place in which to discuss important issues (Havens, 1989). Simple professional attitudes, for example, reliability, honesty, and consistency, help construct the relationship as a safe place for meaningful dialogue. *Reliability*, simply stated, is doing what you say you will do. It is the core element of a trusting relationship. Patients look for reliability in the principled actions of their nurses. They require the assurance that their nurse is committed to maintaining the established boundaries of a therapeutic relationship. In the therapeutic situation, the patient needs a helping professional and not a friend, even though there may be considerable pressure from the patient and strong inclination on your part to broaden the relationship. Here self-awareness and self-reflection become particularly important. The patient counts on you to make the distinction between social and therapeutic relationships, by not confusing sociability with social involvement in a therapeutic relationship. The patient expects you to be honest when mistakes occur and nonjudgmental about the patient's background and behaviors.

A related but often intangible intervention is consistency. Schultz and Videbeck (1994) identify consistency as a major building block of trust, symbolized in both structural and attitudinal reliability. *Structural consistency* means that you organize the relationship around the patient's health-related needs and do not deviate from helping the patient achieve identified goals. Knowing that the relationship structure is stable (i.e., meets at a regular time with a clear purpose) builds trust. Consistency also relates to behavioral attitudes, experienced intuitively by the patient but not always identified as an explicit part of the relationship.

Attitude consistency develops from self-awareness. It means that you strive to provide a consistent and equitable level of care for every patient, regardless of behavior and personal attributes. It is important to make all treatment decisions based on appropriate therapeutic rationale, rather than reflective of more personal reasons. Patients observe their nurse's behavior in their own relationship with a nurse, but they also look for uniform application of the same basic rules to all patients. If there are marked differences in the way the nurse responds to patients, the patient cannot help but wonder why and may make assumptions about the nature of those differences which may be damaging to the development of trust. The realization that some patients are more "special" or equal than others reduces trust. It is important to make clinical decisions about all patients in a consistent, fair way that is readily observable.

Consistency in approach with each individual patient also builds trust. Full acceptance of the patient and realistic limit setting are the essential elements of a consistent approach. Patients test your commitment by acting out in ways that are likely to cause you concern. Much of the time, acting-out behaviors are not deliberate actions but rather reflect underlying anxiety or a wish to avoid the feeling of anxiety. Acceptance validates a person's self-worth. Limit setting offers boundaries to the relationship and identifies acceptable behavior in ways that support rather than punish the patient's efforts. Consequences for behaviors that exceed the limits of the relationship or threaten to sabotage the goals of the relationship are outlined before their occurrence. This consistency in approach allows the patient to trust that the relationship is safe. Thorne and Robinson (1988) outline five steps for promoting reciprocal trust in the nurse-patient relationship (Box 11–7).

BOX 11-7 Steps for Promoting Reciprocal Trust in the Nurse-Patient Relationship

Listen with intent to what the patient is saying

Curb any preconceptions about the patient

Solicit the patient's perspective

Validate your conclusions

Identify specific patient competencies that can help the patient manage particular problems associated with chronic illness

From Thorne, S. E., and Robinson, C. A. (1988). Reciprocal trust in health care relationships. *Journal of Advanced Nursing, 13,* 782–789. Published by Blackwell Science Ltd.

► **Check Your Reading**

8. How do boundaries facilitate the goals of the therapeutic relationship?
9. In what ways are caring and mutuality related in the nurse-patient relationship?
10. How is authenticity integrated into a nurse-patient relationship?
11. Explain the meaning of the statement: Reciprocal trust is an essential characteristic of the nurse-patient relationship.
12. What role does consistency play in the development of trust?

BOX 11-8 Tasks of the Preinteraction Phase

- Establishing goals for the professional relationship
- Creating a supportive physical environment
- Working out the details of timing
- Coordinating the goals of the relationship with the expected outcomes of the treatment plan
- Sharing the goals for the relationship with the health care team

Structuring Therapeutic Relationships

The purposes of the relationship with a mentally ill patient and all nursing interventions associated with it are twofold: (1) to help patients develop more effective ways of coping with their situations and (2) to teach them more productive ways of interacting with the significant people in their lives. The nurse's role is to create the conditions in which a person can learn to use his or her own strengths and environmental resources in solving interpersonal problems and in meeting environmental demands. The relationship itself consists of three interrelated and overlapping phases. Although the progression through the sequential phases of the relationship is linear, patients return to previous phases during times of stress. Furthermore, all of the earlier developmental phases are incorporated into increasingly complex understandings of the meaning of the therapeutic relationship.

Preinteraction Phase

The preinteraction phase is the only part of the therapeutic relationship in which the patient is not actively involved. Box 11–8 identifies the relevant tasks of the **preinteraction phase.**

ESTABLISHING GOALS FOR THE PROFESSIONAL RELATIONSHIP

During the preinteraction phase, examine your professional goals. Professional goals are like guideposts that help you define essential role responsibilities and select the most appropriate communication strategies in each phase of the relationship (Arnold and Boggs, 1995). Identifying professional goals before the relationship begins alerts you to feelings that do not belong in a therapeutic relationship. If you do not establish professional goals for your behavior, the potential for responding automatically to the patient as an object, rather than as a complex and unique human being, increases. Although usually not shared with the patient, professional goals keep you clear about boundaries and expectations in the relationship.

CREATING A SUPPORTIVE PHYSICAL ENVIRONMENT

The goal of the preinteraction phase is to establish a safe harbor in which the patient can feel comfortable (Fox, 1993). If one thinks of the relationship as a safe harbor, everything about the physical setting must be structured to support the patient's experience of that harbor. The room or space in which the relationship takes place should be quiet, free from distraction, well ventilated, and conducive to noninterruptive interactions. Making sure that the furniture is comfortable and arranged to foster an I-thou discussion are important considerations. The nurse and patient should have enough space between them and be able to see each other's face.

WORKING OUT THE DETAILS OF TIMING

Checking room availability and coordinating times with the person responsible for scheduling the space is important. Not uncommonly, you and patient arrive at the designated room only to find that it is occupied. Establishing set times for the interaction reinforces the purpose of the relationship and lets the patient prepare appropriately. The room should have a readily visible clock, or you should have a watch to ensure appropriate time limits. Physical factors, such as your arriving on time and being emotionally available, are important. As the fox tells the little prince:

> "It would have been better to come back at the same hour," said the fox. "If for example, you come at four o'clock, I shall begin to be happy. I shall feel happier and happier as the hour advances. At four o'clock, I shall already be worrying and jumping about. I shall show you how happy I am! But if you come at just any time, I shall never know at what hour my heart is ready to greet you... one must observe the proper rites..." (de Saint-Exupéry, 1943, p. 84).

These simple interventions implicitly say to the patient: "This relationship is important enough to warrant a specific space and a special time for just you, on which you can count."

COORDINATING THE GOALS OF THE RELATIONSHIP WITH THE EXPECTED OUTCOMES OF THE TREATMENT PLAN

Before beginning a therapeutic relationship, you need to make sure that relationship goals fit into the patient's overall treatment plan. This consistency of approach directly relates to the individualized needs of a patient and treatment outcomes as a basis for planning care. Increasingly, nurses are expected to demonstrate that they are using interventions that support desired patient outcomes. Moreover, nurses often lose track of the effects they are having with a patient when they do not reflect on how their work articulates with the overall treatment goals and the efforts of other health team members. Careful integration of relationship goals with patient outcomes before, during, and after the implementation of the relationship can serve as an excellent source of tangible evidence of nursing care. These data can prove useful in helping nurses appreciate the results of their efforts.

SHARING THE GOALS FOR THE RELATIONSHIP WITH THE HEALTH CARE TEAM

In planning the structure of the safe harbor, nurses should take into account the interface of the planned relationship with the patient and those of other members of the interdisciplinary health care team. Patients are extremely sensitive to existing tensions and disagreements between their caregivers. They may have trouble responding to the overtures of one member of the health care team when they feel caught between conflicting attitudes and contradictory messages about their care. Or, in the case of acting-out patients, the tensions may be exploited unconsciously to the detriment of the relationship. Simple actions such as working out the timing of interactions so that they do not conflict with other patient activities recognize the interdisciplinary approach needed for successful patient outcomes. Sharing plans with other health team members reduces the possibility of misunderstandings between professionals and between patient and professional. Once all of the structural arrangements for the relationship are in place, the relationship with the patient can begin.

Orientation Phase: Assessment and Diagnosis

The orientation phase of the therapeutic relationship is particularly important because it sets the stage for all that follows. It begins with the establishment of the relationship as a safe harbor for self-disclosure and learning new behaviors and ends with the establishment of a therapeutic contract that specifically defines the nature of the actions needed for desired outcomes. Box 11–9 summarizes the tasks of the **orientation phase** of the relationship.

ESTABLISHING THE RELATIONSHIP AS A SAFE HARBOR

Desired outcomes for the orientation phase involve the instillation of hope and a commitment to continue with the relationship. During the orientation phase, the conceptual threads of trust, empathy, acceptance, and genuineness are particularly important in helping patients experience the relationship as a safe harbor. *The nurse who uses a respectful proactive approach, moves slowly, and demonstrates unswerving perseverance and commitment generally is most successful.* As Polster (1987) notes, "it is enough for the therapist in this extraordinary context to exercise ordinary kindness, simplicity, clearmindedness, good language, recognition of implication, and an enduring fascination for the life of the patient."

ENCOUNTERING THE PATIENT

The orientation phase of the nurse-patient relationship begins with the first encounter (Forchuk, 1992). Your introduction needs to be receptive and compassionate. Body movements, facial expression, and vocal tone are as important as the actual words. As with other beginnings, it is appropriate to use customary amenities: to shake hands and to give the patient your name. Asking the patient what he or she prefers to be called signals your desire to know this person as a unique individual. For example, "Hi, I'm Carole Monagle, and I will be your student nurse today. How do you like to be called?"

It is important to realize that when the nurse and patient encounter each other for the first time, they meet as strangers (Peplau, 1952). Neither really understands the other. There is an added dimension of discomfort for the mentally ill patient, who camouflages the self-concept for protection against interpersonal vulnerability. Chronically mentally ill patients who have experienced multiple or long hospitalizations usually require more time in the orientation phase (Forchuk, 1992). They do not seek the relationship unless they are particularly anxious or upset.

Understanding just how vulnerable the mentally ill patient feels in the beginning of a relationship wherein his or her responsibility is to self-disclose personal details of his or her life helps. Although many images, ideas, and affects make up the self-concept, the patient usually cannot consciously link these with his or her personal

BOX 11–9 Tasks of the Orientation Phase

- Establishing the relationship as a safe harbor
- Encountering the patient
- Establishing role responsibilities
- Developing rapport
- Collecting assessment data
- Validating assessment data
- Formulating appropriate diagnoses
- Developing a therapeutic contract

experience in a logical, coherent manner and, therefore, feels uncomfortable talking about them. Others feel so traumatized by past relationships that the idea of entering another relationship seems incomprehensible, particularly one that requires intimate disclosure. Psychotic patients may be so influenced by their symptoms that it is impossible to relate in a meaningful way until medication restores their ability to process information. For each of these patients, the idea of entering a relationship is extremely difficult. The small talk that predominates during the orientation phase allows you and the patient to experience each other as persons without forcing a dialogue that is frightening to the patient.

The primary goal of the orientation phase is to establish a working alliance with the patient and to gain enough relevant assessment data to begin the development of a care plan. First the trustworthiness of the travelers to make the journey together must be established. You need to convey a patient attitude and to signal a welcoming attitude without making demands on the patient for critical content. The fox instructs the Little Prince on the best way to begin the process of relationship:

> "What must I do to tame you?" asked the little prince. "You must be very patient," replied the fox. "First you will sit down at a little distance from me—like that—in the grass. I shall look at you out of the corner of my eye, and you will say nothing. Words are the source of misunderstandings. But you will sit a little closer to me, every day" (de Saint-Exupéry, 1943, p. 84).

The time needed to accomplish the goals of the relationship varies from patient to patient and from situation to situation.

ESTABLISHING ROLE RESPONSIBILITIES

You need to identify your role, the kind of information you will be seeking from the patient, and the time you will be spending with each new patient. The introduction is followed by formally establishing the parameters of the relationship. Although disconnected from the next statement for purposes of emphasis, the introduction and role responsibilities usually take place as one introductory statement. The purpose statement includes *what* your role is as a helping person, *when* and under what circumstances the relationship will take place, and *why* the relationship may prove beneficial. For example:

I will be meeting with you for an hour, beginning at 10:00, and asking you some questions about yourself. We can spend the time talking about things that are of interest and concern to you. People often find that when they talk about what is important to them, it helps to sort out things and develop better ways of handling problems. What you say to me of a personal nature will be kept confidential except if it might be harmful to yourself or others.

Discovering the patient's ideas about why he or she is seeking treatment and what the patient would like to gain from the relationship reinforces a sense of partnership. A good beginning is to ask open-ended questions about what brought the patient to the hospital (clinic) or made the patient seek treatment. Once the reason for seeking health care has been established, a second question—"what would you like to get out of our working together?"—provides information about the patient's expectations.

DEVELOPING RAPPORT

Even while introducing yourself to the patient, you begin to observe patterns of communication—does the patient seem interested, for example. Patients entering psychiatric treatment experience a wide spectrum of feelings, such as hopefulness, shame, anger, and extreme loneliness. The initial goal of the orientation phase is to put the patient at ease. The patient's comfort is crucial to the success of the therapeutic process and depends on your ability to create an accepting atmosphere that nurtures and supports the patient's self-revelations (Havens, 1989). Responding to patients as people first and as patients second enhances the possibility of establishing meaningful rapport in the orientation.

Although testing behaviors can occur at any time in the relationship, they emerge initially when the patient begins to experience the possibility of closeness. Testing behaviors are those actions and words that threaten to sabotage the relationship. These behaviors are purely defensive: They help the patient maintain a sense of personal integrity, which can neutralize a potentially precarious interpersonal situation. If nurses realize that the patient is basically trying to determine whether they are trustworthy and competent, they will not take testing behaviors personally, and there is a good possibility of developing a therapeutic alliance. Consider that the patient previously has used pathological defensive behaviors to protect against becoming too vulnerable. Character patterns developed over many years are not erased easily. A flexible approach is required to protect the relationship from the patient's destructive psychological patterns. For example, the psychotic patient may get up abruptly and leave the interview. With a dynamic understanding of the patient's illness, you might respond in a moderate tone, "This may not be a good time for us to talk, but I would like to talk with you. Would you mind if I came back a little later?" You might choose, by listening to the patient's signals, to use shorter interactions and perhaps a neutral object such as a magazine or game to make the patient feel more at ease.

Unacceptable testing behaviors, such as abusive verbal interactions, flagrant denial of boundaries, and serious acting-out behaviors, cannot be tolerated. The manner in which they are addressed, however, makes a difference in the patient's reaction to limit setting. For example, suppose that the patient with acting-out behaviors invades your personal space, sits too close, and cannot be deterred from asking personal questions. You might say to such a patient, "Why don't you sit over there. That way we can talk more comfortably." A therapeutic response to the request for personal information might be: "I'm sorry but I don't feel comfortable answering your questions about my personal life. We need to concentrate on your situation." By respecting the patient's behavior, valuing one's own rights in relationship, and suggesting alternatives that will allow the relationship to develop, you help make the relationship safe.

When the patient appears receptive but does not initiate conversation, there is a tendency for nurses to become overactive, especially with psychotic or depressed patients. This can frighten the patient. Frequent, short interactions work better, with small talk about such neutral topics as common interests, pastimes, places visited, and patient interests. Casual conversation about neutral topics, important in the beginning of most relationships, is particularly important with the psychiatric patient. It allows the patient to become more comfortable and to experience the nurse as a person without revealing too much initially. The needs of the patient direct the pacing of the relationship. With most patients, it is important to use an informal format that respects the shifting demands of the interpersonal situation and suggests inquiry rather than interrogation. Important material emerges only as the patient begins to trust in the relationship.

COLLECTING ASSESSMENT DATA

Once initial rapport is established, you can move into asking for basic information that will form the initial database. Collecting assessment data has both a content and a process aspect. The process dimension helps establish the relationship as a partnership (Kasch, 1986), in which the patient has the most accurate knowledge of his or her desires, hopes, strengths, and weaknesses, whereas you have the necessary knowledge base and objectivity to help the patient make maximum use of his or her personal characteristics.

It is important to start where the patient is, by carefully listening to the patient's personal story. This personal accounting usually builds on but is not entirely determined by either the psychiatric or the nursing diagnosis. A psychiatric diagnosis tells you something about the particular symptoms the patient presents. The nursing diagnosis specifies the particular dynamics and functional patterns in need of nursing intervention. Each patient also is special with a unique set of values, conflicts, wishes, and perceptions of reality that require consideration. Again *The Little Prince* suggests a personalized approach to assessment that recognizes the uniqueness of the person behind the symptoms:

> Grownups love figures. When you tell them that you have made a new friend, they never ask you any questions about essential matters. They never say to you, "what does his voice sound like? Does he collect butterflies?" Instead they demand: How old is he? How many brothers has he? . . . Only from these figures do they think they have learned anything about him. . . . But certainly, for us who understand life, figures are a matter of indifference. I should have liked to begin this story in the fashion of the fairytales. I should have liked to say: "Once upon a time there was a little prince who lived on a planet that was scarcely bigger than himself, and who had need of a sheep. . . . To those who understand life, that would have given a much greater air of truth to my story." (de Saint-Exupéry, 1943, pp. 16–17).

Personal data about one's life journey, developed from the story told by the patient, produce unique information that helps you individualize nursing interventions. Often, this information might not otherwise be available; it cannot be seen, and others in the patient's environment have no knowledge of its existence. These data can point to the areas in which the patient demonstrates the most flexibility, which, in turn, enhances the possibility of therapeutic movement (Busch, 1987).

In collecting data, try to obtain a comprehensive picture of the patient that includes an understanding of the reasons for seeking treatment, basic characteristics of the patient's personality development, personal resources, strengths, and limitations. *A history of the patient's normal functioning and personal strengths is as important to assess as the problem areas* (Havens, 1984). Too often the patient's many areas of normal functioning are overlooked in favor of considering the patient's dysfunctional behavior patterns.

Although data about the patient's mental disorder and functional ability may be developed quickly, personal assessment data often unfold only as the patient's trust level increases, and it may require an extended time to collect. It is important to give each patient the time and space he or she needs to reveal the self and to use language that has meaning to the patient. Schweitzer (Bugental, 1992) notes: "Only those who respect the personality of others can be of real use to them."

When collecting data, you need to *seek the truth with care.* For each patient, there are two realities: the external, which exists in objectivity, and an inner reality, which interprets objective reality through the filter of past experience (Casement, 1991). The role of the psychiatric nurse is to recognize the interplay between the two realities. This can be a challenge with mentally ill patients because they frequently combine reality elements with unconscious remnants of the past without conscious awareness. Although you may see the patient as capable of working through distressing events, the same events may appear overwhelming to the patient, producing intense anxiety. The anxiety may take on a life of its own, further interfering with effective problem solving. Respect for the person should be first and foremost in developing a clear understanding of the problem, from the patient's perspective.

The accuracy of your understanding of each unique patient rests in a fundamental way on the comprehensiveness of the assessment data. During the initial interview, observe behaviors, gestures, and body movements, particularly as they relate to the patient's verbal messages. How the patient answers provides valuable data about ways of thinking about things, ability to make choices, level of knowledge, interests, and personal strengths. For example, are there a lot of "I don't know" responses to routine questions? Is the patient able to identify personal strengths? Listening to the patient's account of his or her current situation, you should begin to notice connections and discrepancies between parts of the data. The process of telling the story to a person who cares to listen also enhances the sense of connectedness. In most cases, the initial interview does not elicit all of the information needed for the assessment. Try to address assessment questions of major importance, without creating undue anxiety or fatigue in the patient.

If there is reason to suspect the patient's reliability as a historian, significant others can supply information. Relying exclusively on patient information without soliciting the perceptions of significant others can distort and limit history taking, particularly with organically impaired or substance-abusing patients. Other times, information is sought from significant others to establish the family as part of a team approach to treatment. Moreover, contrasting patient and family data is another important source of information. The differences can be just as important as the similarities in developing the most appropriate nursing interventions. When others are to be involved in data collection, the patient needs to be aware that you will be talking with the family or significant others and what information will be sought or shared.

A comprehensive psychosocial assessment gives you an understanding of the basic issues and the immediate health care needs that the patient perceives are relevant. The objective problems and the patient's perception of them are not necessarily the same. Knowledge of the patient's expectations for help ideally support the reality of the situation in providing appropriate corrective experiences (Orlando, 1990). Understanding the underlying dynamics of patient behavior and negotiating differences are part of the interpersonal exchange between nurse and patient. Out of these understandings, you and the patient develop a joint working perspective about the nature of the patient's problems and the interventions most likely to resolve them. In Chapter 13, there is a thorough discussion related to psychosocial assessment data.

VALIDATING ASSESSMENT DATA

An important part of data collection is validation. To be certain that what you observe is indeed an accurate perception of the patient's reality, you should verify your perceptions with the patient and significant others. *Validation*, discussed in Chapter 10 as a form of communication, also cements the relationship because it involves the means by which one person confirms another and his or her experience. Effective validation of the patient's experience requires that nurses:

- *Describe* the observed patient *behavior(s)* (verbal and nonverbal)
- *Verbalize* their *own perceptions* about the behavior's intended meaning, especially if the inference is made about hidden feelings
- Remain *nonjudgmental*

FORMULATING APPROPRIATE DIAGNOSES

Once the database is complete, the next step is to analyze and synthesize the data into a unified whole from which you begin to formulate nursing diagnoses that relate to and support the psychiatric diagnosis. The problem/need statements embodied in the psychiatric and nursing diagnoses become the basis for deciding what type of nursing intervention is required and what referrals are necessary. Most psychiatric settings use the DSM-IV psychiatric diagnosis, including all five axes (see Chapter 9) as the basis for a biopsychosocial definition of the patient's problem. Additionally the treatment team develops nursing diagnoses or interdisciplinary critical pathways as the groundwork to guide clinical interventions.

Although the psychiatric diagnosis clusters characteristic symptoms of mental illness in ways that give direction to preferred treatment methods, it fails to provide the nurse with direction regarding the patient's functional abilities. The nursing diagnosis identifies the specific functional behaviors and their hypothesized causes that are in need of nursing intervention. Both perspectives are essential as central organizing ideas about the most effective treatment approaches for each patient. Ideally the nursing diagnosis is congruent with the DSM-IV psychiatric diagnosis, the patient's personal story, and the reasons the patient is seeking treatment.

DEVELOPING A THERAPEUTIC CONTRACT

Once nursing diagnoses are established to the mutual satisfaction of nurse and patient, introduce the idea of a therapeutic contract. Therapeutic contracts have much in common with expectations about behavior. As the fox explains to the Little Prince:

> ". . . One must observe the proper rites. . . ."
> "What is a rite?" asked the Little Prince. "Those also are actions too often neglected," said the fox. "They are what make one day different from other days, one hour from other hours. There is a rite, for example, among my hunters. Every Thursday they dance with the village girls. So Thursday is a wonderful day for me! I can walk as far as the vineyards. But if the hunters danced at just any time, every day would be like every other day, and I should never have any vacation at all"
> (de Saint-Exupéry, 1943, p. 84).

Because the fox has developed an understanding of the hunters' expected behaviors on Thursdays, the fox has more flexibility to carry out other activities. The same process occurs in the nurse-patient relationship. Spelling out goal-related behaviors frees you to concentrate on matters other than continually defining expectations. The use of a therapeutic contract places the responsibility for taking actions related to goal achievement directly on the patient.

A *therapeutic contract* is a verbal or written agreement between the patient and nurse that supports the aims of the relationship and concretely spells out role expectations and goals. It is a dynamic process statement, requiring negotiation and updating, as the original circumstances prompting the details of the agreement change. Each therapeutic contract is unique from a content perspective because it is tailored to meet the individualized needs of the patient. Simple therapeutic contracts consist of information about the nature of the relationship; the place, time, and frequency of sessions; and length of the relationship, if known. Rules that the patient is expected to follow, such as giving notice if the patient cannot attend sessions, no drugs or alcohol, and paying for missed appointments, are included, when appropriate.

Written therapeutic contracts are particularly appropriate with adolescent problem behaviors and with patients who are acting out or experiencing impulse control, and they serve as an integral part of the nursing care plan. They also are used to deter the patient from harming himself or herself when there is reason to believe that the patient is so inclined. Written therapeutic contracts encourage the patient to think before he or she acts, and they return the responsibility for symptom control to the patient by lengthening the time between thought and action. The contracts often serve as a needed reminder for what patients need to do or not do to achieve a successful outcome.

Writing a therapeutic contract also removes you from the position of dictating or controlling what the patient does. By formalizing exactly what the patient consents to do and under what circumstances, therapeutic contracts increase safety in the relationship through explicating expectations that everyone agrees are valid. In developing a workable contract, patients also gain important feedback about the feasibility of their plan before they carry it out.

Contracts should be written in clear, concrete language, leaving little room for differences in interpretation. The terms should be discussed thoroughly and modified if necessary. Figure 11–2 shows a sample therapeutic contract. Once trust is established and the therapeutic contract is in place, the working phase of the relationship is ready to begin. Contracts should be rewritten when the patient consistently demonstrates the behaviors identified in the initial contract. New contracts would follow a similar format.

▶ Check Your Reading

13. What are the tasks of the nurse during the preinteraction phase?
14. How would you describe the nurse's role during the orientation phase?
15. What is the function of a therapeutic contract, and how would you use it in the clinical area?

I, ______________________, agree that I will attend all group meetings on the unit. If I am going to miss a meeting, I will notify the charge nurse prior to the scheduled meeting. I understand that if I miss a meeting without prior notification, for one week I will lose my privileges to go off the unit. I will complete this contract by ______________________ .

____

(Nurse's signature)

____

(Patient's signature)

____

(Date)

FIGURE 11–2
A sample therapeutic contract.

Working Phase: Outcome Identification, Planning, and Implementation

The **working phase** is the action phase of the relationship. Peplau (1952) originally subdivided the working phase into two components: the identification phase, in which the patient explores the nature of the problem and its associated feelings, and the exploitation phase, in which the patient maximizes use of all appropriate resources to resolve the problem. The identification phase of the relationship most directly parallels the outcome identification and planning steps of the nursing process, and the exploitation phase relates to the implementation step. During the identification phase, the nurse helps the patient identify problems that interfere with successful progression of the journey. The patient's problem areas and personal strengths are embedded in each person's unique story. With each discussion, they emerge with greater clarity. *The Little Prince* explains how this might occur:

> As each day passed I would learn, in our talk, something about the little prince's planet, his departure from it, his journey. The information would come very slowly, as it might chance to fall from his thoughts (de Saint-Exupéry, 1943, p. 19).

You can help patients tell their story in several ways. First, the simple act of putting the feelings into words puts boundaries on difficult feelings and situations. The patient hears the emotional tone of voice and inflections at the same time as you. The metacommunication about the meaning of the communication provides important information about the emotional intensity of the experience for the patient. As you use active listening responses, important details that have been left out of the story begin to emerge as relevant parts of the person's journey. Finally, you can provide feedback to the patient and consequently can validate the legitimacy of the feelings. This allows a patient to acknowledge his or her own role in maintaining the status quo. Evaluating the antecedent behaviors and situations allows a person greater flexibility in effecting mastery and change (Egan, 1986).

Assessment data continue to be incorporated into an evolving plan of care, but the focus in the working phase is on goal setting and implementation of planned interventions. The goal of planned interventions is to help patients use their inner resources to effect desired behavioral change. As patients achieve greater mastery over life situations, they are able to assume greater responsibility for creating their own life experiences, and this, in turn, increases self-esteem. Thus, although the conceptual threads of trust, empathy, and genuineness continue to be important, empowerment emerges as particularly significant during both the identification and the exploitation segments of the working phase.

The working phase offers you an opportunity to engage fully in the process of "taming." You and the patient begin to understand each other fully and the nature of the relationship in achieving treatment goals, as acceptance moves to a deeper experiential level. It is a powerful and affirming experience for both participants. The Little Prince describes this process by characterizing the relationship with his rose as one of unique caring:

> But in herself alone she is more important than all the hundreds of your other roses: because it is she that I have watered; because it is she that I have put under the glass globe; because it is she that I have sheltered behind the screen; because it is for her that I have killed the caterpillars (except for the two or three that we saved to become butterflies); because it is she that I have listened to, when she grumbled, or boasted, or even sometimes when she said nothing (de Saint-Exupéry, 1943, p. 87).

The unique design of nursing interventions develops from a mutual analysis of relevant assessment data, which are individually tailored to the patient's needs. The purpose of the relationship provides direction for implementation of mutually identified treatment goals and then prescribes measures to evaluate these goals. Box 11–10 summarizes the tasks of the working phase.

IDENTIFYING EXPECTED OUTCOMES AND PLANNING ACHIEVABLE SHORT-TERM GOALS

Once the problems have been identified to everyone's satisfaction, you and the patient develop achievable working objectives to meet treatment goals. Treatment goals are written as patient outcomes. Long-term goals (desired outcomes at time of discharge) direct the development of short-term goals (objectives needed to achieve expected outcomes). Expected outcomes related to the development of social skills and those skills needed for independent living are most appropriate for chronically mentally ill patients. Short-term goals can relate to the reduction of symptoms associated with the mental illness and the sequential steps needed to achieve expected outcomes. For example:

Expected Outcome
Mr. Jones will not experience any anxiety attacks by time of discharge.

Short-Term Goals
Mr. Jones will keep a daily journal of his behavior and environmental factors noted before experiencing each anxiety attack.

Mr. Jones will verbalize his anxiety to the nurse.

Mr. Jones will do his breathing exercises when he observes signs of increasing anxiety: flushing, rapid heart rate, panic feelings.

Short-term objectives can change as the patient masters each behavior needed for goal achievement or finds that it is not effective. As the relationship develops, you help the patient to clarify and refine goals (Bulechek and McCloskey, 1992).

Expected outcomes should be clear, realistic, and achievable. Overambitious goals create frustration for the mentally ill patient. Signs that the goals are overwhelming for the patient include withdrawal, regression, return of symptoms, or bizarre behavior. The patient is telling you by behavior rather than through words that he or she cannot achieve the goal. It may be that the task goes beyond the patient's personal sense of mastery. When this occurs, it helps to redefine the goal as smaller sequential steps. For example, grooming can be sequenced in simple incremental steps, such as taking a daily shower, using deodorant, brushing the hair, wearing a tie, and so forth. Each small success makes the next step possible. When simplifying a task, it is best to ". . . try the simplest intervention first . . . 'When you hear the sound of hoof-

BOX 11–10 Tasks of the Working Phase

- Identifying expected outcomes
- Planning achievable short-term goals
- Developing realistic solutions using a problem-solving approach
- Working through resistances and transference
- Implementing the chosen interventions

beats, think first of horses and not zebras' " (Anderson and Stewart, 1983, p. 42).

Goal setting is a mutual, interactive process in which you bring information about resources and behavioral dynamics, and the patient brings critical personal data that affect goal achievement. Assessment of patient strengths becomes significant because the strengths are the building blocks for the actions needed to achieve identified goals. You need to involve the patient as much as possible in developing relevant treatment goals. As Gerhart (1990) suggests, "persons, despite their mental illness, are often capable of making meaningful decisions relating to their care and the way in which they conduct their lives" (pp. 55–56). Self-determination enhances self-esteem. Helping the nurse develop mutually acceptable treatment goals ensures that they fit both the patient and the situation. Moreover, active participation by the patient promotes greater self-awareness and personal ownership of treatment goals and the behaviors needed to achieve them.

DEVELOPING REALISTIC SOLUTIONS USING A PROBLEM-SOLVING APPROACH

During the working phase, an important opportunity for developing realistic relationship skills as well as sound analytic and problem-solving skills related to the problem or need under discussion takes form. Mentally ill persons often have great difficulty identifying the complex factors involved in a decision or considering *ongoing* verbal negotiations as essential to effective living. For many patients, analyzing a problem situation and reaching an effective solution are not behaviors they typically engage in with any ease. The working phase thus becomes a carefully guided experience, ordered around the patient's interests and capabilities. Interventions emphasize healthy personal growth through the development of a more effective personal frame of reference, authentic personal expression, and personal peace with internal values. Selected nursing actions reflect the combined talents of patient and nurse. Included in their development are the free expression of the fears, doubts, and lapses of self-confidence that accompany most effective solutions.

The working phase of the relationship is always congruent with the functional level of the patient. Mentally ill patients vary widely in their functional capabilities, ranging from seriously compromised to functioning well in some but not all areas of their lives. Nursing interventions should be based on the patient's diagnosis and should reflect the patient's level of ego strength. In the service of protecting the self, many patients have developed crippling defenses, which prevent meaningful interactions because their thoughts and emotions are no longer consciously linked to relationships, life situations, or sense of self. When these separations are of sufficient magnitude to preclude successful problem solving, you need to guide inquiry to help patients to understand the structure and process of their interactions. You need to help the patient clarify meanings and experience thoughts and feelings in a different, more therapeutic context. This strategy helps the patient to name uncomfortable feelings and attach their significance to specific life events.

BOX 11-11 A Five-Step Problem-Solving Process

- Define the problem or conflict
- Analyze the nature of the problem or conflict
- Consider alternatives and their consequences
- Weigh the advantages and disadvantages of each alternative
- Take action on the decision

> *Nurse:* You've just told me how angry you are that your mother expects you to follow her directions about how you should conduct your life. That would be quite difficult for any adult to do and feel good about it.
>
> *Patient:* Yes, it has gotten so bad that I really don't want to have anything to do with her and I feel guilty about that.
>
> *Nurse:* That's a normal reaction when you love someone but don't like their behavior. Do you see any ways in which you could have a relationship with your mother in which you could feel more in control?

You can help the patient to recognize anxious feelings, identify how the anxiety gets translated into symptoms, and describe the triggers for an increase in anxiety. This process provides patients with a structured opportunity to reduce personal anxiety without placing any demands for a particular response. Once anxiety is reduced to a level that allows the patient to work effectively, a five-step problem-solving process, summarized in Box 11–11, identifies the actions needed to achieve therapeutic patient outcomes.

Define the Problem or Conflict. The nursing diagnosis specifies the most probable origin of the problem as well as naming the actual problem. The patient should assume primary responsibility for developing a workable problem statement. By using listening responses, you can help the patient identify the central issues. Stating the problem in concrete behavioral terms puts boundaries around it and serves as the basis for developing the most appropriate strategies to solve it.

Analyze the Nature of the Problem or Conflict. A critical thinking approach considers the problem from all angles and places it in the context of the patient's current life situation. Questions you might use to help the patient analyze the problem or conflict include: *How* does the patient view his problem? *What* is the patient feeling right now? *What* resources does the patient feel he has to resolve the problem? *Who* else is or may need to be involved? *What* behaviors and feelings would indicate that the problem has been resolved? *What* would be different in the patient's life and feelings about himself if the problems were resolved? From this discussion ideally emerges the development of a collective purpose.

Consider Alternatives and Their Consequences. Looking at alternatives requires interpersonal involvement. When people share their ideas, a broader range of options emerges than would be the case from any one individual perspective. Ideally, generation of alternatives stimulates creative thinking abilities and encourages personal mastery. Included in the process of looking at the alternatives are the following questions:

- What changes in the patient's behavior are needed to achieve therapeutic goals?
- What are all of the possible ways that the problem might be resolved?
- What are the consequences of taking each action, pro and con?

In developing alternatives, the patient needs to defer judgment until there is sufficient information to warrant a particular solution.

During this part of the problem-solving process, you can use a technique referred to as brainstorming. *Brainstorming* is a problem-solving strategy in which participants verbalize any thoughts they have about a situation, to consider new information and all possibilities even when they conflict with currently held strong ideas and feelings. The goal becomes identification of as many solutions as possible for a particular problem. All value judgments are suspended. Encourage the patient to let all ideas flow freely without censure. At the same time, use summary statements to zero in on the essentials and focus on what is important. The patient's commitment to the project and ownership of his or her solutions facilitates progress, allowing the patient to act rather than react to life situations.

Weigh the Advantages and Disadvantages of Each Alternative. Once all possible alternatives have been exhausted, the next step is to evaluate the advantages and disadvantages of each option and decide on one. This capacity to broaden and then narrow the scope of possibilities provides an efficient way first to consider all potential solutions and then to select the one with the best fit. This decision forms the basis for the strategies the patient will use to meet his or her goals. The practicality of choosing one option over another can include such consequences as the perceived reactions of others, personal feelings, changes in self-esteem, and the possibility of unexpected actions from choosing one alternative rather than another.

Specific questions to help a patient choose the most appropriate strategy, adapted from Egan (1986), include:

1. Is the strategy specific, concrete, and measurable?
2. Is the course of action realistic (within the patient's span of ability and resources)?
3. Is the strategy adequate to achieve the desired goal?
4. Is the patient willing to take the actions needed?
5. Are the contemplated actions consistent with the patient's belief and value system?
6. Can the strategy be completed within a reasonable amount of time?

Ideally, positive consequences outweigh the negative ones. Your role during this part of the problem-solving process is to provide valid information based on expertise and experience, to help the patient clarify underlying values, and to help the patient pull relevant themes together related to each option. Every effort should be made to let the patient explore all of the possible consequences of each idea. You guide the process, but the patient determines the content. The most important gift that you can give to a patient is to help him or her solve problems with the least amount of assistance. Otherwise, the patient never learns the process of problem solving as an independent agent.

Self-awareness is particularly important during this part of the process because so often there is a temptation to tell the patient what you think he or she should do. It is difficult to refrain from giving advice. It is difficult to avoid verbally anticipating areas that are problematic for the patient, for which he or she has not yet found words. The reason for doing so lies in the subtle shift in responsibility for the actions away from the patient to the nurse. Even correct, well-intended advice can have unwanted outcomes because the patient does not learn to use personal inner resources. Or the patient may take your advice but put a twist on it that then sabotages the intent of the advice. It is not unusual for a patient to ask for advice and then not follow it, leaving you feeling foolish or discounted. In each of these situations, an awareness of each person's role responsibility coupled with the self-discipline needed to allow patients to experience the effects of their own decision making can make a difference in the outcome. Once the patient chooses the most promising alternative, he or she is ready to take action on his or her decision.

Take Action on the Decision. Talk without action is of limited value. The ultimate goal of this problem-solving step is to develop a shared vision as to what needs to be done. This information forms the basis for focused dialogue about the actions needed to achieve the goals. Once the patient has decided on a particular alternative, the next step is formulating a plan to direct the patient's course of action. Actions that follow a logical, incremental sequence are easier to implement and provide the most satisfaction.

In deciding on the most appropriate actions, it is important to build in the possibility of early success. A lot of energy is required to take actions that create change. Success builds morale and reinforces motivation. When there are small successes, the work itself becomes a source of satisfaction and motivator for further efforts. Sequentially ordering the actions in a step-by-step manner provides the patient with a patterned logical way to meet identified objectives.

Actively incorporate patient strengths and resources into the planned interventions (Box 11–12). Including personal strengths as an important part of any treatment plan helps patients feel more in charge of their situation. They are more aware of the power already present in their living situations, and their behavior is more likely to have personal meaning. Chosen actions generally meet the needs of the situation more realistically because they draw on the skills, expertise, resources, and interests of the patient.

Frequent feedback is important during the action segment. Change involves a continuous learning process. Through consistent dialogue, improvements can be made, new facts revealed, and original plans enhanced or revised based on the new information. Many of the actions the patient needs to take may involve practicing new skills. Step-by-step rehearsal promotes mastery, and feedback given by you encourages the patient and suggests alternative strategies.

Taking new actions involves risk, and always there are feelings attached. You can help the patient reduce the impact of painful feelings and self-doubt by talking about them as they emerge. This strategy encourages the patient to explore problems or feelings that can sabotage the patient's efforts and may point to the need to revise goals. It also helps when you are able to recognize and reinforce progress.

WORKING THROUGH RESISTANCES AND TRANSFERENCE

The next segment of the working phase involves working through potential and actual problems that threaten the work of the relationship. Through functional interaction with you in the relationship, the patient begins to take charge of his or her life. It a scary process as well as a dynamic one to embrace the idea of change actively. Not all patients are eager to learn new behaviors and to establish and work toward goals. Not all patients are able to survive emotionally the inevitable setbacks and self-questioning that accompany any real change. Even with your help, some patients cannot or will not engage in the behaviors that would bring about a different, more satisfying outcome to their life journey. This patient right to self-determination must be accepted.

Altering one's lifestyle is difficult for anyone but particularly so when anxiety compromises adaptation and learning as it does for the mentally ill. Anxiety is a normal constituent of the human condition. Mild and even moderate anxiety can actually enhance learning. This is not the case with severe anxiety, which can present in the form of withdrawal, resistance, or transference behaviors. Peplau (1987) notes that, "Nurses can neither demand nor otherwise control the responses patients will make to nurse behavior" (p. 201). They can try, however, to understand and respond therapeutically to patient needs that are unique and unfamiliar. This is an important dimension of the work because otherwise the patient does not have the necessary trust and security in the relationship to use the relationship constructively. Working through resistances to treatment is an important aspect of the working phase.

Resistances

Rapid, steady progress in achieving treatment goals is not as common in mentally ill patients as it is with physically ill patients. The course of treatment is likely to be slower and less dramatic. Mental illnesses are chronic disorders characterized, as most are, by periods of exacerbation and intervals of remission. Consequently, temporary setbacks are a relatively common occurrence. In fact, even without being mentally ill, there is an ebb and flow to human activity that occurs simply because the patient is human. Deeply rooted in every human being are old insecurities

BOX 11-12 Questions You Might Ask to Elicit Information About a Patient's Personal Strengths and Resources

Personal Strengths

Does the patient have:
- Good physical health?
- Good grooming?
- A sense of humor?
- Special abilities such as artistic or vocal abilities?
- Persuasive verbal expression?
- Ethnic, religious, or cultural beliefs and resources?
- A good memory?
- Motivation and or a good attitude of responsibility for himself or others?
- The ability to live within her income?
- A good relationship with a mental health professional?
- Common sense in some areas, if not all?
- Good work habits?
- Good problem-solving abilities?
- A risk-taking nature?
- Persistence?

Resources

Does the patient have friends? To what extent is the patient involved in relationships in the family? Outside the family?
How well is the patient able to carry out the social tasks associated with his role within the family? At work?
Does the patient engage in any club or leisure activities?
What does the patient do to have fun?
What are the characteristics of the patient's living situation?
What are the availability and accessibility of social and environmental supports?
Does the patient have an adequate income?
Does the patient live in a safe neighborhood?
Is there easy access to shopping, churches, and medical and psychological care?
Do family norms support movement toward mental health and use of psychiatric services?
Does the patient have a car, and is the patient willing to drive?

and ways of being that continue to emerge in stressful situations.

Identifying and supporting areas of positive health give the patient hope. For example, you might say to the patient experiencing a temporary setback, "I can see you are disappointed that you weren't able to stay off the liquor, but the facts that you have been sober for a year now and you came back for treatment show motivation. You were able to do it before, and that should give you some evidence that you will be able to do it again."

Some resistances are harder to deal with than others, and nurses lose their personal bearings in knowing how to respond effectively. A nurse can experience the same helplessness de Saint-Exupéry (1943) felt in experiencing the pain of the Little Prince and not knowing how to respond:

> I did not know what to say to him. I felt awkward and blundering. I did not know how I could reach him where I could overtake him and go on hand in hand with him once more. It is such a secret place, the land of tears (de Saint-Exupéry, 1943, p. 31).

When such feelings occur, and they will occur, you need to linger awhile with the puzzlement until the next part of the patient's story gradually reveals itself and makes sense of what has come before. You must patiently go with the patient's flow and support any of his or her efforts to remain centered and forward moving. Recognizing slips and symptom return as temporary setbacks and stating this to the patient as such can be helpful. Feedback, supplying information about different options and helping the patient make choices about courses of action, enhances the patient's sense of autonomy and self-esteem. Also, you can identify small improvements as evidence of the patient's effort and remind the patient that the journey is a process, not an event. Making eye contact, combing hair, using makeup, making a comment, going to church, attending the ward movie, and saying hello are important signals of increased engagement that should be acknowledged. Patients with less regressive behaviors often demonstrate increased self-discipline, a willingness to examine their behaviors, and increased patience and courage in taking risks or in making small decisions. By noticing these behavioral changes, you can reinforce the patient's motivation for constructive change.

Withdrawal is a common form of resistance in the nurse-patient relationship. Patients frequently move away from taking conscious actions in anxiety-producing situations. This behavior is adaptive in that it temporarily helps the patient reduce his or her anxiety. It undermines the possibility of success in achieving goals, however. Many times a patient is unaware that this is the consequence of withdrawal and anticipates being successful without actually making the changes needed to ensure a desired outcome. Peplau (1987) suggests that the work cannot continue until the patient becomes aware of his or her behavior and how it is sabotaging the progress of the relationship.

Your task with withdrawal behaviors is to make the patient aware of his or her anxiety-reducing behaviors that are used automatically and without conscious awareness. Focusing on content or criticizing the behavior as not being productive is not particularly useful. The patient needs to control the situation at this moment in time because of its threat to survival of the self-system. The goal, therefore, is to help the patient reduce anxiety to a more moderate level. Recognizing and naming the anxiety are critical interventions. Instead of forcing the patient to reveal content, you can simply say, "Can you tell me what you are feeling now," and remain psychologically present. Short phrases rather than long commentaries should be used when you observe withdrawal in a patient. Acknowledging that the content is anxiety producing—"This must be very difficult for you to accept"—makes the patient aware that there is a reason for the withdrawal. Your use of clues in the patient's behavior in understanding the nature of the patient's difficulties provides evidence of your psychological presence, and this object constancy sometimes can allow the patient enough ego strength to return to the work of the relationship.

Transference

The emergence of strong feelings and behavioral attitudes during the course of the relationship are referred to as *transference* when they occur in the patient and *countertransference* when they occur in the nurse. At times transference can be helpful, but it also can threaten the relationship. Ulman and Stolorow (1985) note that "both the transference and the countertransference continually shape one another in a specific pattern of reciprocal mutual influence" (p. 50). Transference reflects emotions transposed from the past onto the present situation. In mental health settings, it is not unusual for the patient to construct images of the nurse that fit his or her inner models of reality. The patient frequently develops strong beliefs about the nurse that have little to do with reality. These images, affects, and thoughts are called transference because the person experiencing them usually cannot connect them consciously with his or her own history or with his or her personalized sense of self (Allen, 1993). In extreme cases, transference becomes known as *projective identification*, a process whereby unconscious and disowned characteristics of previous relationships are projected onto the present relationship and reacted to or relived as if the two relationships were the same. Transference sabotages the goals of relationship to the extent that the nurse and patient interact with them and, in the process, ignore the issues for which the patient sought treatment.

Transference is easy to see when it is blatant; for example, the patient thinks the nursing staff are policemen out to harm the patient physically. Transference also occurs in subtle behaviors, recognizable only with frequent self-reflection, collegial consultation, and comparison with data known about the patient. Examples of transference include either overvaluing or undervaluing the nurse's expertise, hostility, flattery, or obsequiousness. Transference should be suspected in arguments with the nurse or sexual overtures.

Transferences are informative because they reveal how the patient has experienced other relationships. They provide direct access to emotions that otherwise might not emerge. Whenever transferences appear, you will need to address them before proceeding with problem solving. There are several ways of doing this. If the patient is giving you a hard time or seems stuck in a certain pattern of nonfunctional relating, you can briefly describe your reaction to the patient's behavior. For example, you might say, "It seems like you say you will take your medication, but then you tell me you have forgotten it, or you just don't feel like taking it. It makes me feel as though what we talk about goes in one ear and out the other, without much benefit to you." The second part of this intervention includes asking the patient about the feelings you stir up or whether the behaviors directed toward you are similar to those directed to significant others. With an initial denial for example, you can say that, "Well, often your relationship with me is similar to the way you act with others, so it is important to consider all of your feelings about me at this time." This comment distances you from personalizing the transference. Although it is inappropriate to focus on the meaning of the transference without advanced education, emotions noted in the here and now can promote greater awareness of transference feelings and their impact on relationships.

Another strategy is the use of simple questions about the nature of an observation, as for example, noting sadness or belligerence. You might say, "I notice that you looked a little apprehensive when you came into the room. What were you thinking about when you came in?" The patient may respond, "Well I thought you might have forgotten our appointment," or "I was afraid you might reject me," and you can follow up with an exploration of how past relationships may be influencing the patient's perception of the present one. If the transference seems to occur in relation to material discussed during the interaction, evidenced by a change in expression, you might note the change: "I notice your facial expression changed just then. Can you tell me what was going on in your mind just now?" Appropriate observations and responses to transference establish and sustain trust.

Transference from the patient to you is not completely unidirectional. As the relationship develops, both you and the patient become sensitive to each other's feelings. The patient is able to sense anger or anxiety experienced by you just as you can with the patient. It is the awareness of the flow of feeling exchange between the two that enables you to use your own feelings about the patient with the patient for therapeutic purposes.

Countertransference refers to the psychiatric nurse's personal feelings about the patient. It develops "as a combination of the patient's transference acted out projections and the human vulnerability of a therapist" (Masterson, 1992, p. 181). Countertransference can be positive or negative. It can be useful when it serves to resonate the patient's feelings and alert you to the patient's underlying needs. It can be dangerous when you identify so strongly with the patient that there is an unconscious collusion with the patient's pathology. Although most people know the ethical responsibilities involved in treating patients, it is sometimes difficult to detach from feelings that represent extensions of compassion and empathy. For example, if you believe that only you have an intuitive understanding and calming effect on the patient, there is an emotional overinvolvement that is not good for the patient or you. Subtle, sexually tinged attachments can occur with attractive patients. From the patient's perspective, sexual feelings may unconsciously represent simply a desire for a close relationship; it is up to you to make the necessary distinction between having feelings and acting on them. The boundaries of the therapeutic relationship are so critical to the trust needed for healing that they should never be violated.

Nurses can become aware of countertransference by attending to exaggerated feelings about the patient or an uneasiness about the relationship. Behaviors suggestive of countertransference include thinking about the patient frequently outside of the clinical situation, feeling anger or pride in relation to the patient's behaviors, allowing patients to act out without comment on it, and recognizing any feelings that do not legitimately belong in a therapeutic relationship. When countertransference emerges, you should explore the following questions:

What is similar about this situation (feeling) and others I have experienced?
Does this person remind me of someone else or of myself?
How have I responded to such feelings in the past?
What is my part in the development of these uncomfortable feelings?
What is needed to resolve these feelings?

Talking with a knowledgeable colleague usually puts the situation in perspective. With strong countertransference, it may be necessary to develop a consistent treatment approach with limits on your involvement with the patient, until such time as the feelings are less intense. Occasionally, it is better for you to transfer care of a particular patient to another primary caregiver.

IMPLEMENTING THE CHOSEN INTERVENTIONS

Once you have identified expected outcomes, planned achievable short-term goals, developed realistic solutions using a problem-solving approach, and worked through resistances and transference, you are ready to implement the interventions that you have chosen.

Termination Phase: Evaluation

The termination phase of the relationship parallels the evaluation phase of the nursing process. Peplau (1952) refers to the ending of a relationship as the resolution phase of the nurse-patient relationship. Responsibilities in this phase of the relationship can be compared to the tasks of evening when people tend to put away the things of the day, reflect on important moments, and leave new

BOX 11-13 Tasks of the Termination Phase

Evaluating patient performance

Evaluating achievement of the expected outcomes

Evaluating future needs

Making appropriate referrals

Dealing with common behaviors associated with termination

initiatives for the next day. In this phase of the relationship, nurse and patient review all that the patient was able to accomplish during the course of the relationship. Box 11–13 summarizes the tasks of the **termination phase.**

Ideally the seeds of termination are sown in the first encounter, when you first inform the patient that the relationship is time limited. A simple statement such as, "Mr. Jones, we will be meeting four times, and our last session will be next Friday," is sufficient. References to termination should be made enough in advance to allow for thorough discussion of feelings related to ending the relationship. Statements such as, "Mr. Jones, we only have two more sessions; I would like you to think about what we have done together, and what plans you might have after you are discharged," set the stage for discussion of ending the relationship. For relationships that have extended over a significant period of time, it is helpful to space the interviews before termination at gradually lengthened intervals. This helps to diminish the involvement gradually rather than having an abrupt finish. Long-term relationships with mentally ill patients are somewhat different in that a longer time may be needed to work through feelings about termination. Unfortunately, terminations with psychiatric patients often are contingent on transfer of personnel or patient to a different unit. When this occurs, it is equally important to terminate with the patient and to explain the reasons for the sudden ending.

EVALUATING PATIENT PERFORMANCE

During termination, you and the patient review what the patient was able to accomplish during the relationship. The discussion can start with the behaviors that first attracted the patient's attention and proceed through discussion of changes in the patient's motivation, attention to task, and changes in behavior. Discussion of both positive and negative behaviors has a meaningful role in helping the patient understand his or her participation as the architect of his or her personal destiny. For example, you might note, "I think your experience of being put down at home might partially explain your panic whenever you thought I wasn't approving your actions in dealing with your wife. Acknowledging to yourself that approval is important to you, and to take the steps we talked about when you notice that you seem to be on edge will help you cope."

EVALUATING ACHIEVEMENT OF THE EXPECTED OUTCOMES

Ideally, nurses prepare themselves as well as the patient for termination by reviewing what has already been accomplished in the relationship. In the last few sessions, you should ask the patient to identify high and low points for him or her and to provide a summary of his or her progress toward goals. Inviting the patient to describe his or her experience of the relationship first and then providing a response allows you an opportunity to soften or expand on the patient's narrative.

Achievement of therapeutic goals requires examination of all outcomes, logically and step by step. This summary analysis reinforces the concept of process in attaining goals and the learning that took place in accomplishing the goal, and it helps the patient generalize the process to other life situations. If the goals were partially achieved, you can help the patient identify what still needs to be done. Hypotheses as to why goals were not met can be identified for those goals that were not met during the terms of the relationship.

EVALUATING FUTURE NEEDS

The termination phase blends the traditions of the past with the realities of the present and with the potential for future personal growth. In assessing future patient needs, you help the patient consider what it will be like for him or her after discharge. This information is used to help the patient anticipate potential problems and possible solutions for handling them successfully. For example, it might be important for a patient to develop a written prevention plan he or she could carry on a 3 × 5 card to handle angry feelings. Or by linking the past with the current reality of staying sober through attendance at Alcoholics Anonymous, a chemically dependent patient is able to anticipate its role in his or her life after discharge.

MAKING APPROPRIATE REFERRALS

In a societal age in which insurance reimbursement increasingly determines length and type of treatment, most patients require referral for follow-up treatment. You can play an important role in helping patients determine their needs for service and in assisting them to access them appropriately. Referrals may include legal as well as medical and psychological services. Having a comprehensive knowledge of available community resources is essential to providing quality care for psychiatric patients.

DEALING WITH COMMON BEHAVIORS ASSOCIATED WITH TERMINATION

In the termination phase of the relationship, it is normal for the patient to demonstrate a number of regressive behaviors that can be disturbing to you if they are not understood. Typical behaviors include return of symptoms, anger, withdrawal, and minimizing the relationship. Some patients complain of a new and terrible symptom in hopes of convincing you to remain involved with them. Usually maladaptive termination behaviors subside gradually. Recognizing that these symptoms are normal reactions to loss with mentally ill patients and usually temporary decreases the nurse's anxiety.

Ending a significant relationship can create sadness in both the nurse and the patient. In *The Little Prince*, the fox explains why this is so:

> So the little prince tamed the fox. And when the hour of his departure drew near—"Ah," said the fox, "I shall cry." "It is your fault," said the little prince. "I never wished you any sort of harm; but you wanted me to tame you. . . ." "Yes, that is so," said the fox. "Then it has done you no good at all!" "It has done me good," said the fox, "because of the color of the wheat fields." And then he added: "Go back and look again at the roses. You will understand now that yours is unique in all the world. Then come back to say goodbye to me, and I will make you a present of a secret.". . . And he went back to meet the fox. "Goodbye," he said. "Goodbye," said the fox. "And now here is my secret: It is only with the heart that one sees rightly; what is essential is invisible to the eye" (de Saint-Exupéry, 1943, pp. 86–87).

Therapeutic relationships, because they confirm the essential nature of another human being, are carried in the heart, even after they end. Although ending any meaningful relationship is painful and sad, the experience of being valued, often a first-time experience for the mentally ill patient, makes the sadness bearable for the patient. Seeing the patients progress to a higher level of functioning and knowing that he or she played a role in their evolving maturity makes the sadness bearable for the nurse.

During the relationship, you may assume several roles that begin when you and the patient first encounter each other, meeting as strangers (Figure 11–3). These roles overlap and reinforce the efficacy of one another in the service of the patient's welfare.

Gift giving is not an uncommon patient desire in the final stages of a meaningful relationship. Often, too, you may want to give the patient a gift. The patient may request to continue the relationship through the exchange of phone numbers or ask you to keep in touch through Christmas or birthday cards. These attempts to hold on to the meaning of the relationship need to be recognized as normal. In social relationships, gift giving and phone number exchange are appropriate and commonplace. Gift giving in a professional relationship, however, needs to be approached with deep caution. Extending the boundaries of the relationship to include gifts, phone number exchange, or additional visits to "see how the patient is doing" are inappropriate because they can confuse the patient, and the potential to learn about positive endings in relationships does not occur.

There are several strategies for dealing with gift giving in the nurse-patient relationship. One strategy is to reflect on all the intangible gifts that the patient has given you. The relationship itself, in which the patient shares

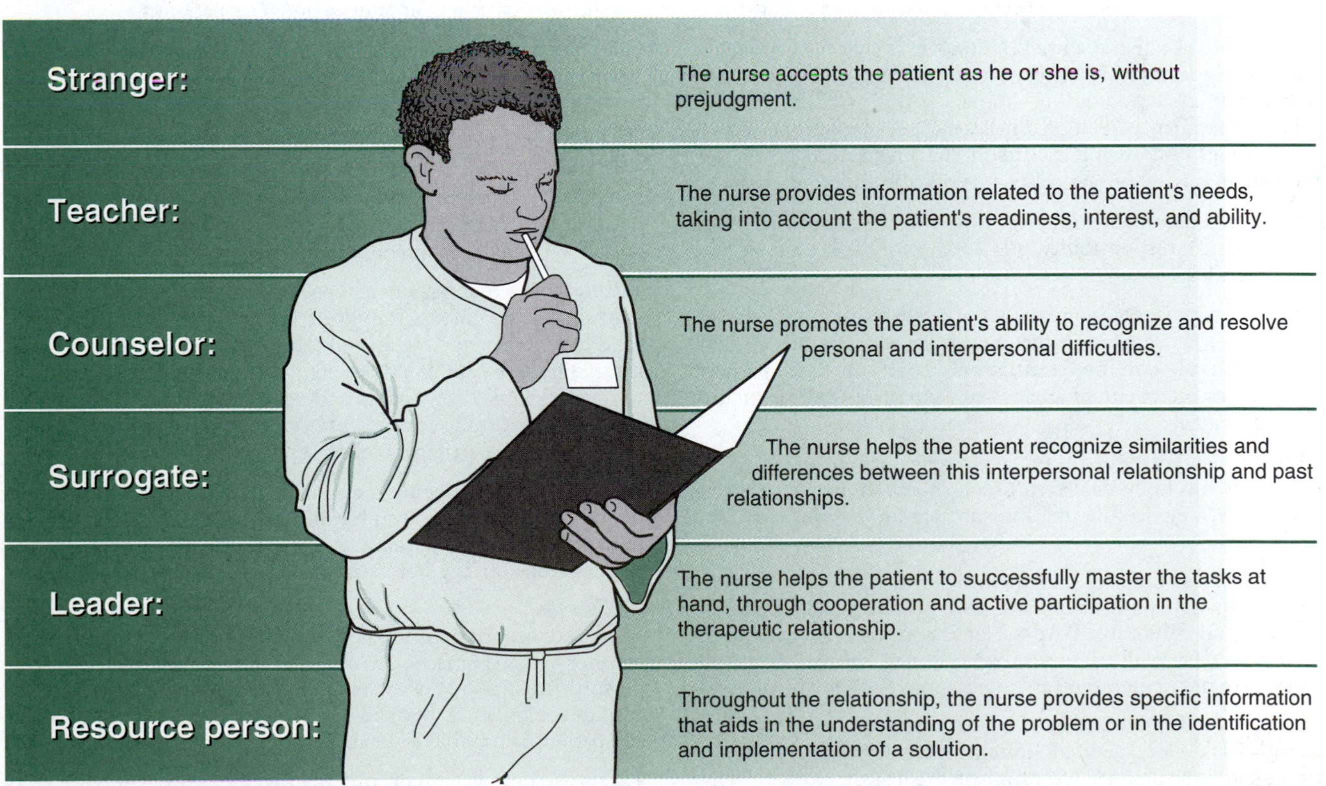

FIGURE 11–3
Roles that you may assume over the course of a therapeutic relationship.

deep feelings and revelations of self, is indeed a beautiful, lasting gift. In turning down a material gift, you need to acknowledge the value of all that you have received from a patient, thus reinforcing the worth of the patient and of the relationship that you have shared. There is no one answer about whether gifts should or should not be exchanged. In fact, if you handled every situation in the same fashion, you would be denying the uniqueness of each nurse-patient relationship. Each relationship has its own character and its own strengths and limitations, so that what might be appropriate in one situation would be totally inappropriate in another. Although the answer is not simple, it does involve being true to what you know and feel about the patient, assessing the meaning of the gesture, and using your best professional judgment in every situation. Most importantly, give freely of yourself.

▶ Check Your Reading

16. How would you distinguish between the identification and exploitation segments of the working phase, and how are they related to each other?
17. How would you describe the problem-solving process the nurse would use in the exploitation phase?
18. What are some of the behaviors the nurse would see during the termination phase?
19. What would be the best approach to handling the issue of gift giving in the termination phase?
20. In what ways do the phases of the nurse-patient relationship parallel those of the nursing process?
21. How would you characterize the differences between transference and countertransference feelings?
22. In what ways are they related to each other?

CONCLUSIONS

Each nurse-patient relationship represents a human encounter with the potential to heal, to support, and to provide guidance in negotiating the human journey. This chapter presents a framework for understanding the structure and conceptual components of the nurse-patient relationship. Psychological and nursing frameworks relevant to the study of therapeutic relationships identify and define boundaries, caring, respect, empathy, genuineness, authenticity, and trust as key conceptual elements threaded throughout the relationship. Nurses are in an excellent position to develop qualitative research studies exploring the nature of each of these key elements and how they contribute to the healing process in psychiatric nursing. In an era where health care is increasingly dehumanized with bureaucracy, human encounters in psychiatric nursing become extremely significant.

KEY POINTS TO REMEMBER

- A therapeutic relationship represents a time-bound alliance between nurse and patient, consciously entered into and characterized by respect, acceptance, empathy, and genuineness.
- The value of a therapeutic relationship is that it provides the mentally ill patient with an "experience of being understood and of being related to another human being" (O'Toole, 1989, p. 11). A therapeutic relationship offers the patient hope and the possibility of discovering that he or she has meaning, even if at the time it is to only one other person, the therapist.
- Social and therapeutic relationships differ in their (1) purpose, (2) focus, (3) responsibility, (4) level of self-disclosure, and (5) personal involvement.
- The conceptual components of the relationship—boundaries, caring, advocacy, unconditional acceptance, mutuality, authenticity, and trust—are the essential foundation on which patients begin to restructure their images of themselves and the nature of their journey.
- Boundaries are defined as "a dynamic line of demarcation separating an individual's internal (body, mind, and spirit) and external environments and varying in permeability and flexibility."
- Advocates are defined "as persons who stand along side of and empower patients and their families to have a voice when they are weak and vulnerable." Advocacy is a moral responsibility of the nurse designed to maximize patients' self-integrity and personal dignity when they are unable to do this for themselves.
- Caring is an intangible interactive process with physical, psychosocial, and spiritual dimensions that finds expression through actions designed to promote the health and well-being of patients. Caring is "to know that you would understand and care for me and dare to prove it."
- Mutuality in its most complete dimension involves inclusion. A connected relationship is one in which "the nurse views the patient first as a person and second as a patient."
- Unconditional acceptance is the capacity of the nurse to affirm the patient's humanity and to validate his or her life experience without questioning its validity or judging it in any way.
- Empowerment represents "the interpersonal process of providing the proper tools, resources and environment to build, develop, and increase the ability and effectiveness of others to set and reach goals for individual and social ends."
- Empathy is an interpersonal process in which the nurse is able to capture the inner struggle of the patient, is able to bring together different aspects of the patient's situation in a meaningful way, and is able to communicate that understanding to the patient in a way that is understood as truth by the patient. It is both an attitude and a communication strategy in which the nurse's role as participant observer is particularly relevant.
- Authenticity or genuineness refers to being "real" in therapeutic relationships. Although intimate aspects of the helping person's life are not shared with the patient, what is brought into the relationship are the natural feelings and attitudes of the nurse.
- The concept of trust involves a person's inner confidence that another person respects, understands, and responds fairly to that person. Trust is a mutual process. It begins with the nurse's confidence in his or her skills and includes the firm belief that the patient is capable of changing his or her behavior.
- Consistency is important to the development of trust. Structural consistency means that the nurse organizes the relationship around the health-related needs of the patient and

does not deviate from helping the patient achieve identified goals. Attitudinal consistency relates to the nurse's understanding of the professional role and equity in patient care.

• The structure of the therapeutic relationship consists of a preinteraction phase, which does not include the patient, and three sequential stages: the orientation, working, and termination phases.

• The goal of the preinteraction phase is to develop a safe environment for the development of the relationship. Specific tasks include identifying professional goals, establishing the physical setting, and working through arrangements with other members of the interdisciplinary health care team.

• The primary goal of the orientation phase is to establish a working alliance with the patient and to gain enough relevant assessment data to begin the development of a care plan. Specific tasks include defining the purpose of the relationship, establishing the role responsibilities of both participants, developing a rapport needed to accomplish the work, collecting relevant assessment data, identifying appropriate psychiatric and nursing diagnoses, and establishing a therapeutic contract.

• The working phase is the action phase of the relationship. Peplau originally subdivided the working phase into two components: the identification phase, in which the patient explores the nature of the problem and its associated feelings, and the exploitation phase, in which the patient maximizes use of all appropriate resources to resolve the problem.

• The termination phase of the relationship parallels the evaluation phase of the nursing process. Evaluation of the effectiveness of the problem-solving approach to the patient's problems can include evaluating the patient's performance, determining if the problem has been satisfactorily resolved, reviewing what has been learned in this situation that could prove useful in future situations, and analyzing the positive and negative behaviors that occurred during the problem-solving process.

• The emergence of strong feelings and behavioral attitudes during the course of the relationship are referred to as transference feelings when they occur in a patient and countertransference feelings when they occur in the helping person.

LEARNING ACTIVITIES

1. Think about a caring incident in which you were involved or one that you have observed. In one or two paragraphs, describe the incident using as much detail as possible. Bring the description of the caring incident to class. In small groups, share your caring incident. The group can then identify the characteristics of caring present in each student's description. Finally, small group attributes can be shared, compared, and contrasted with those of other class members.

2. John Antione is a 28-year-old schizophrenic single man, newly admitted to the hospital. He appears unshaven, with unkempt hair and loose clothing. He has a distinct body odor. Your instructor thinks working with this patient would be a good challenge for you. Have one student role-play the patient and another the nurse.

3. Before you enter the psychiatric unit, think through in your mind all of the images and ideas you have about mentally ill patients. What are your concerns? How do you think you will respond to the patients? What do you expect to find on the unit? How do you think the patients will respond to you? Be as honest as possible. There are no right or wrong answers. Write your answers to these questions and share them with your classmates. After the first 2 weeks on the unit, identify your current feelings. Compare them with your initial and preconceived ideas of what it would be like to work on a psychiatric unit. In what ways have your perceptions changed? If there are changes, to what do you attribute the change? Again, there are no right or wrong answers.

4. In small groups of three or four students, apply the five-step problem-solving format (see Box 11–11) to one of the following patient problems.

Carol Black was recently admitted to the inpatient unit with suicidal ideation and a severe depression following her husband's decision to leave her. Her husband wants to have joint custody of the children so he does not have to pay child support and wants to sell the house. Carol suspects but does not know that there is another woman. She has not worked in 10 years and feels betrayed because she always did what her husband wanted and has never had a life of her own.

Jeri Slovak has adult attention deficit disorder and learning disabilities that compromise her ability to complete written assignments on time. All her life she has felt vulnerable about her inability to organize her life and has defended herself by not telling anyone of her disability. Her college teachers are annoyed with her because obviously she is bright. They think she is either lazy or seriously mentally disturbed. She has been advised that unless she "cleans up her act," she will be dismissed from the program.

Pat Calhoun has a severe borderline personality disorder. When she becomes very anxious, she develops psychotic delusional thinking patterns. She believes that the world is coming to an end and that she must prepare ammunition and guns to protect herself. She has involved her 8-year-old son in helping her make the ammunition and regularly takes all of her children to a shooting range. Recently, Pat's husband lost his job and her oldest daughter was involved in an auto accident. Pat's anxiety is at a very high level.

CRITICAL THINKING EXERCISES

Mr. Kain, student nurse, begins to write a contract with Mr. Herman concerning his plan of care. The contract reads: Mr. Herman will meet with his nurse at least one time each day to discuss his plans for the day. He will notify his nurse if he has any feelings that frighten him. He will participate in one activity each afternoon.

1. Is the contract clear and precise?

2. What other information (evidence) do you need to determine whether the contract is therapeutic?

3. What assumptions is Mr. Kain making about contracts?

Mr. Kain sits down with Mr. Herman and reviews the content of the contract. His purpose is to give more structure to Mr. Herman's daily routine. He tells Mr. Herman that it is important for him to participate with others. Mr. Herman signs the contract and keeps a copy for himself. When Mr. Kain leaves the room, Mr. Herman crumples the contract and throws it in the garbage can.

1. What assumption did Mr. Kain make?
2. What point of view is Mr. Herman taking?
3. Consider alternate assumptions about this interaction.

REFERENCES

Allen, J. (1993). Dissociative processes: Theoretical underpinnings of a working model for clinician and patient. *Bulletin of the Menninger Clinic, 57*(3), 2811–308.

Anderson, C., and Stewart, S. (1983). *Mastering resistance: A practical guide to family therapy.* New York: Guilford Press.

Arnold, E., and Boggs, K. (1995). *Interpersonal relations: Communication skills for nurses* (2nd ed.). Philadelphia: W. B. Saunders.

Barnard, D. (1985). Psychosomatic medicine and the problem of meaning. *Bulletin of the Menninger Clinic, 49*(1), 10–28.

Benfer, B., and Schroder, P. (1985). Nursing in the therapeutic milieu. *Bulletin of the Menninger Clinic, 49*(5), 451–465.

Benner, P., and Wrubel, J. (1989). *The primacy of caring: Stress and coping in health and illness.* Menlo Park, CA: Addison-Wesley.

Berry, D. L. (1985). *Mutuality: A vision of Martin Buber.* Albany: State University of New York.

Brandon, D. (1983). Nowness in the helping relationship. In *Awakening the heart.* Boulder, CO: Shambala.

Brown, A. (1993). A conceptual clarification of respect. *Journal of Advanced Nursing, 16*(3), 354–361.

Buber, M. (1970). *I-thou.* (W. Kaufmann, Trans.). New York: Charles Scribner's Sons.

Bugental, J. (1992). The betrayal of the human: Psychotherapy's mission to reclaim our lost identity. In J. Zeig (Ed.), *The evolution of psychotherapy: The second conference.* New York: Brunner/Mazel.

Bulechek, G., and McCloskey, J. (1992). *Nursing interventions.* Philadelphia: W. B. Saunders.

Busch, P. (1987). Therapy with the uninvolved client. *Journal of Psychosocial Nursing, 25*(11), 21–25.

Casement, P. (1991). *Learning from the patient.* New York: Guilford Press.

Cashden, S. (1982). Interactional psychotherapy: Using the relationship. In J. Anchin and D. Kiesler (Eds.), *Handbook of interpersonal psychotherapy.* Elmsford, NY: Pergamon.

Connelly, L., Keele, B., Kleinbeck, S., Schneider, J., and Cobb, A. (1993). A place to be yourself: Empowerment from the client's perspective. *Image, 25*(4), 291–303.

Corcoran, S. (1988). Toward operationalizing a role. *Journal of Professional Nursing, 4*(4), 242–248.

Covey, S. (1991). *Principle-centered leadership.* New York: Simon & Schuster.

Curtin, L. (1979). The nurse as advocate: A philosophical foundation for nursing. *Advances in Nursing Science, 1*(3), 1–10.

de Saint-Exupéry, A. (1943). *The little prince* (K. Woods, Trans.). New York: Harcourt Brace.

Egan, G. (1986). *The skilled helper.* Monterey, CA: Brooks/Cole.

Forchuk, C. (1992). The orientation phase of the nurse-client relationship: How long does it take?" *Perspectives in Psychiatric Care, 28*(4), 1–10.

Forchuk, C., and Brown, B. (1989). Establishing a nurse-client relationship. *Journal of Psychosocial Nursing and Mental Health Services, 27*(2), 30–34.

Fox, R. (1993). *Elements of the helping process: A guide for clinicians.* New York: Haworth Press.

Friedman, M. (1985). Healing through meeting and the problematic of mutuality. *Journal of Humanistic Psychology, 25*(1), 11–40.

Gadow, S. (1989). Clinical subjectivity: Advocacy with silent patients. *Nursing Clinics of North America, 24*(2), 535–541.

Gardner, D. (1992). Presence. In G. Bulchek and J. McCloskey (Eds.), *Nursing interventions: Treatment for nursing diagnoses.* Philadelphia: W. B. Saunders.

Gebbard, G. (1992). Psychodynamic psychiatry in the decade of the brain. *American Journal of Psychiatry, 149*(8), 991–998.

Gerhart, U. (1990). *Caring for the chronic mentally ill.* Itasca, IL: F. E. Peacock Publishers.

Hagerty, B., Lynch-Sauer, J., Patusky, K., and Bouwsema, M. (1993). An emerging theory of human relatedness. *Image, 25*(4), 291–296.

Havens, L. (1984). The need for tests of normal functioning in the psychiatric interview. *American Journal of Psychiatry, 141*, 1208–1211.

Havens, L. (1986). *Making contact: Uses of language in psychotherapy,* Cambridge: Harvard University Press.

Havens, L. (1989). *A safe place: Laying the groundwork of psychotherapy.* Cambridge: Harvard University Press.

Hawks, J. H. (1992). Empowerment in nursing education: Concept analysis and application to philosophy, learning and instruction. *Journal of Advanced Nursing, 17*(5), 609–618.

Jacobs, L. (1978). *I-thou relation in Gestalt therapy.* Unpublished doctoral dissertation. Los Angeles: California School of Professional Psychology.

Kalisch, B. J. (1973). What is empathy? *American Journal of Nursing, 73*, 1548–1553.

Kasch, C. (1986). Establishing a collaborative nurse-patient relationship: A distinct focus of nursing action in primary care. *Image: Journal of Nursing Scholarship, 18*(2), 44–47.

Lego, S. (1980). The one to one nurse-patient relationship. *Perspectives in Psychiatric Care, 18*, 611–689.

Masterson, J. F. (1992). The vital therapeutic alliance with borderline and narcissistic patients: A developmental, self, and object-relations approach. In J. Zeig (Ed.), *The evolution of psychotherapy: The second conference.* New York: Brunner/Mazel.

Morse, J. M., Anderson, G., Bottorff, J. L., Yonge, O., O'Brien, B., Solberg, S. M., and McIlveen, K. (1992). Exploring empathy: A conceptual fit for nursing practice? *Image, 24*(4), 273–280.

Morse, J. M., Bottorff, J., Anderson, G., O'Brien, B., and Solberg, S. (1992). Beyond empathy: Expanding consciousness of caring. *Journal of Advanced Nursing, 17*(7), 809–821.

Morse, J. M., Bottorff, J. L., Neander, W., and Solberg, S. (1991). Comparative analysis of conceptualizations and theories of caring. *Image: Journal of Nursing Scholarship, 23*(2), 119–126.

Orlando, I. J. (1990). *The dynamic nurse-patient relationship: Function, process and principle.* New York: National League for Nursing.

O'Toole, A., and Welt, S. (Eds.) (1989). *Interpersonal theory in nursing practice: Selected works of Hildegard E. Peplau.* New York: Springer Publishing.

Peplau, H. (1952). *Interpersonal relations in nursing.* New York: G. P. Putnam Sons.

Peplau, H. (1962). Interpersonal techniques: The crux of psychiatric nursing. *American Journal of Nursing, 62*, 50–54.

Peplau, H. (1987). Interpersonal constructs for nursing practice. *Nurse Education Today, 7*(5), 201–208.

Peplau, H. (1992). Interpersonal relations: A theoretical framework for application in nursing practice. *Nursing Science Quarterly, 5*, 13–18.

Polster, E. (1987). *Every person's life is worth a novel.* New York: W. W. Norton.

Rieman, D. (1986). The essential structure of a caring interaction: Doing phenomenology. In P. L. Munhall & C. J. Oiler (Eds.), *Nursing research: A qualitative perspective* (pp. 86–108). Norwalk, CT: Appleton-Century-Crofts.

Roberts, K., and Fitzgerald, L. (1991). Serenity: Caring with perspective. *Scholarly Inquiry for Nursing Practice, 5*(2), 1211–1246.

Rogers, C. R. (1951). *Patient centered therapy: Its current practice, implications and theory.* Boston: Houghton-Mifflin.

Rogers, C. R. (1958). The characteristics of the helping relationship. *Personnel and Guidance Journal, 37*(1).

Safran, J., and Segal, Z. (1990). *Interpersonal processes in cognitive therapy.* New York: Guilford Press.

Satir, V. (1985). Going beyond the obvious: The psychotherapeutic journey. In J. Zeig (Ed.), *The evolution of psychotherapy.* New York: Brunner/Mazel.

Schmieding, N. (1993). Nurse empowerment through context, structure, and process. *Journal of Advanced Nursing, 9*(4), 239–245.

Schultz, J., and Videbeck, S. (1994). *Manual of psychiatric nursing care plans.* Philadelphia: J. B. Lippincott.
Scott, A. (1988). Human interaction and personal boundaries. *Journal of Psychosocial Nursing and Mental Health Services, 26*(8), 23–27.
Sullivan, H. S. (1954). *The psychiatric interview.* New York: W. W. Norton.
Tanner, C., Benner, P., Chesla, C., and Gordon, D. (1993). The phenomenology of knowing the patient. *Image, 25*(4), 273–283.
Thorne, S. E., and Robinson, C. A. (1988). Reciprocal trust in health care relationships. *Journal of Advanced Nursing, 13,* 782–789.
Tobias, M. (1990). Validator: A key role in empowering the chronically mentally ill. *Social Work, 35,* 351–359.
Ulman, R., and Stolorow, R. (1985). The "transference-countertransference neurosis" in psychoanalysis. *Bulletin of the Menninger Clinic, 49*(1), 311–351.
Uys, L. (1980). Towards the development of an operational definition of the concept "Therapeutic use of self." *International Journal of Nursing Studies, 17,* 175–180.
Zderad, L. (1969). Empathetic nursing: Realization of a human capacity. *Nursing Clinics of North America,* 655–662.

SUGGESTED READINGS

Benner, P., and Wrubel, J. (1989). *The primacy of caring: Stress and coping in health and illness.* Menlo Park, CA: Addison-Wesley.
Connelly, L., Keele, B., Kleinbeck, S., Schneider, J., and Cobb, A. (1993). A place to be yourself: Empowerment from the client's perspective. *Image, 25*(4), 291–303.
Hagerty, B., Lynch-Sauer, J., Patusky, K., and Bouwsema, M. (1993). An emerging theory of human relatedness. *Image, 25*(4), 291–296.
Kalisch, B. J. (1973). What is empathy? *American Journal of Nursing, 73,* 1548–1553.
Lego, S. (1980). The one to one nurse-patient relationship. *Perspectives in Psychiatric Care, 18,* 611–689.
Peplau, H. (1987). Interpersonal constructs for nursing practice. *Nurse Education Today,* 7(5), 201–208.
Peplau, H. (1992). Interpersonal relations: A theoretical framework for application in nursing practice. *Nursing Science Quarterly, 5,* 13–18.
Zderad, L. (1969). Empathetic nursing: Realization of a human capacity. *Nursing Clinics of North America,* 655–662.

CHAPTER 12

A MAP FOR THE JOURNEY
THE NURSING PROCESS

Science is simply common sense at its best that is rigidly accurate in observation, and merciless to fallacy in logic.

—Thomas Huxley

LEARNING OBJECTIVES

After studying this chapter, you should be able to:

1. Discuss the importance of the nursing process to the practice of psychiatric nursing.
2. Describe the steps of the nursing process.
3. Discuss the essentials of a comprehensive assessment.
4. Describe the diagnostic process from the nursing and medical perspectives, using both approved NANDA diagnoses and *DSM-IV* diagnoses.
5. List nursing diagnoses grouped under functional health patterns.
6. Identify the criteria of a well-formed expected outcome.
7. Identify expected outcomes for a given patient.
8. Describe the rationale for establishing priorities.
9. Discuss the relationship between the *Standards of Psychiatric-Mental Health Clinical Nursing Practice* and the implementation of the nursing process.
10. Discuss the importance of a theoretical underpinning to guide and direct nursing actions.
11. Discuss the most commonly used psychiatric nursing interventions.
12. Compare and contrast formative and summative evaluations.
13. Discuss the essentials of documentation.
14. Apply the entire nursing process to a given patient situation.

KEY TERMINOLOGY

Assessment
Diagnosis
Diagnostic and Statistical Manual of Mental Disorders (DSM-IV)
Documentation
Evaluation
Expected outcomes
Formative evaluation
Implementation
Interventions
North American Nursing Diagnosis Association (NANDA)
Nursing process
Planning
Prioritization
Standards of Psychiatric-Mental Health Clinical Nursing Practice
Summative evaluation

The **nursing process,** the basic "map" for nursing, is composed of five or six steps, depending on whether outcome identification and planning are viewed as one step or two. In this text, we use a six-step approach. The six steps of the nursing process are

1. Assessment
2. Diagnosis
3. Outcome identification
4. Planning
5. Implementation
6. Evaluation

Each of these steps is not a discrete entity. Rather, the steps flow in an interactive and continuous manner for the entire time during which care is provided (Ryan-Wenger, 1990; Sheehan, 1991). Figure 12–1 illustrates the interaction of the six steps. Keeping this interactive nature of the six steps in mind while studying each step separately will help you to better understand the entire process.

The nursing process provides a framework for the delivery of nursing care. It is a map for the journey of providing quality nursing care through the nurse-patient relationship. Without such a map, you and your patients would wander in diffuse directions through your interactions.

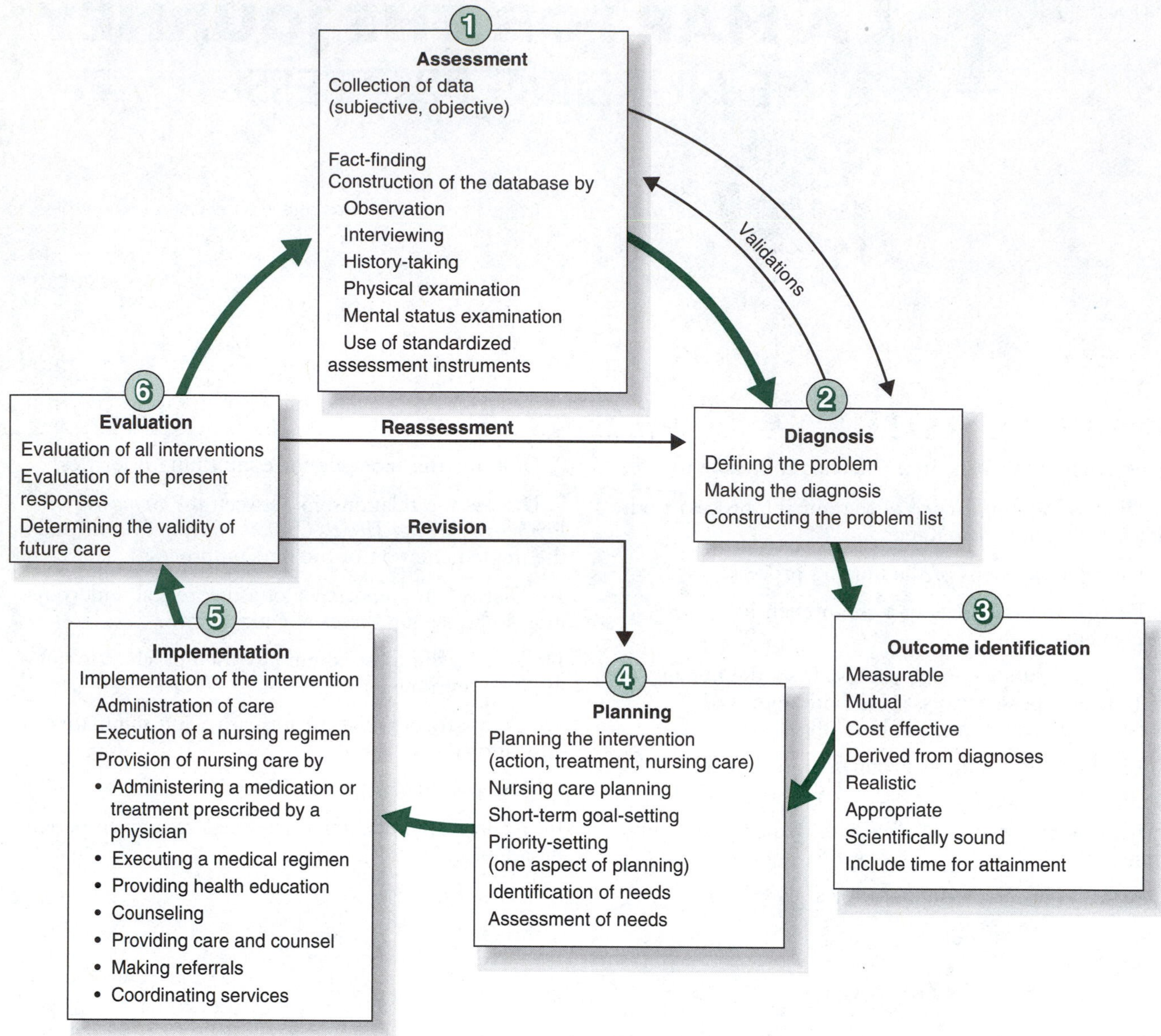

FIGURE 12–1

The six steps of the nursing process. (Modified from McCaffery, M., and Beebe, A. [1989]. *Pain: Clinical manual for nursing practice.* St Louis: C. V. Mosby. Reprinted with the permission of C. V. Mosby Company and J. B. Lippincott Company.)

The nursing process has been acknowledged as nursing's scientific method (Townsend, 1991). As with any scientific method of inquiry, it has its basis in the problem-solving approach (Table 12–1; Hurst et al, 1991).

The purpose of the nursing process is to provide a systematic and individualized method of fulfilling the goals of nursing: to help the patient to promote and maximize her or his level of health, to maintain the highest level of functioning, and to prevent illness and the sequelae of illness (Atkinson and Murray, 1990; Sheehan, 1991). The professional practice of psychiatric-mental health nursing is characterized by the use of the nursing process, with the application of theories of human behavior to provide the basis of nursing intervention, to facilitate patient-oriented health outcomes.

The nursing process is grounded in the nurse-patient relationship and is an interactive process. Using the nursing process in the delivery of care acknowledges the autonomy and integrity of the individual and facilitates his or her involvement in decisions about care. It is a deliberate approach, requiring thought, knowledge, and experience (Wilkinson, 1992; Sundeen et al, 1994; Arnold and Boggs, 1995).

To carry out the nursing process, to be technically efficient and provide quality professional care, you must have a sound knowledge base and think critically. All nursing actions are guided and reflected in the American Nurses' Association (ANA) *Standards of Clinical Nursing*

Practice (ANA, 1991)), which are generic standards for all nurses. As you learned in your introductory nursing courses, standards are authoritative statements that describe the responsibilities for which the nurse is accountable. They provide direction for professional nursing practice and a framework for evaluation of practice. In keeping with the metaphor of the journey, the 1991 generic *Standards* are the "atlas," providing the larger perspective for the journey on which you will use the nursing process "map." The 1994 ***Standards of Psychiatric-Mental Health Clinical Nursing Practice*** (ANA) provide the "regional" perspective for the journey; these standards are specific to psychiatric nursing. The standards clearly specify the role of the psychiatric nurse in carrying out the six-step nursing process; the standards delineate both basic and advanced nursing practice. These *Standards* appear in Chapter 4; a quick review of them will illustrate how the nursing process is integrated into their standards of care.

This chapter provides you with an overview of the entire nursing process and reviews each step. Because of the importance of the assessment step, we introduce it here and cover it in more detail in Chapter 13. This chapter also includes information on several documentation systems used in psychiatric nursing.

▶ Check Your Reading

1. What is the purpose of the nursing process?
2. How is nursing process related to problem-solving?
3. What are the phases of the nursing process?
4. What are the authoritative statements on nursing practice called?
5. What do the *Standards of Psychiatric-Mental Health Clinical Nursing Practice* describe?
6. How are the 1994 standards of care for psychiatric nurses related to the nursing process?

TABLE 12–1 Principles of Problem-Solving Used in the Steps of the Nursing Process

Step of the Nursing Process	Principle of Problem-Solving
Assessment: data collection	Observation
Diagnosis: formulation of nursing diagnoses	Definition of the problem
Outcome identification	Formulation of hypotheses
Planning: deciding what will be done, who will do it, and where and how it will be done	Planning of an approach
Implementation: carrying out the nursing actions	Testing of hypotheses and solutions
Evaluation: determining the success of the process and the outcomes	Formulation of conclusions

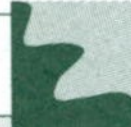

DENNIS'S STORY

Dennis was referred to psychiatric home care by the psychiatrist at a local community mental health center. Dennis had missed his last two appointments and had not received his intramuscular injection of fluphenazine (Prolixin), the antipsychotic medication that helped him deal with his suspicious thoughts. The doctor had received a telephone call from Dennis's mother, Mrs. S., because she and her husband were very concerned. She reported that Dennis was not sleeping at night, that he was barely eating, and that he had begun to treat his parents with hostility. Mrs. S. was terrified that Dennis would get violent, as he had many times in the past. She pleaded, "Please, can't you do something for Dennis?...for us?"

Initial Contact With a Home Care Nurse

On her initial visit, the psychiatric home care nurse, Susan, found Dennis to be anxious and guarded, as if he were being threatened. He looked exhausted and disheveled. Susan proceeded gently with Dennis, respecting his right to remain distant. On the first visit she asked him if it would be OK for her to sit in the room with him and ask him some questions. She assured him that he did not have to answer, but that the more information he shared with her, the better she would be able to help him. She observed that when she said this, the tension in his jaw noticeably slackened.

Dennis Responds to Susan's Approach

Dennis relaxed a bit with Susan's gentle approach, and she was able to complete most of her nursing assessment. Of particular importance was her finding that Dennis said he was hearing voices (auditory hallucinations) that frightened him, and that they were telling him to hurt himself and his parents. He stated, "I'm afraid.... Right now I can control the voices, but later I won't be able to, and I don't want to hurt anyone." Susan told Dennis that the doctor had given her an order to administer his fluphenazine if Dennis would allow her to do so. She explained to Dennis that the medicine would control the voices and allow him to get some rest so he could be strong enough to remain in control. With her assurances, Dennis allowed Susan to administer the injection. After administering the medication, Susan asked Dennis if she could speak with his parents to get information about what his life and theirs is like. He agreed, and Susan spoke with Mr. and Mrs. S. while Dennis remained in the room.

An Interview With Dennis's Parents

Mr. and Mrs. S. were eager to talk about their life with Dennis. His mother began. Looking straight ahead, she said, "He was such a wonderful boy, so smart. We really thought that he would be a doctor some day; that was what he always wanted to be. Then this happened." Her eyes filled with tears. His father then spoke. "He got sick when he was 20 years old, when he was at college. He was doing well, until one semester he just started acting peculiar. He never went back to school. It wasn't until almost six months later that we found out what was wrong."

Mrs. S. continued. "One day he came after his father and me. Thank God we weren't hurt. We got out of the house and ran next door to call the police. They came and took him away. That nearly broke our hearts. He's our only child, you know. Well, they took him to the emergency room, and then they admitted him to a mental hospital. He stayed there for three months, and while he was there, the doctors told us that he had something called 'paranoid schizophrenia.' We didn't even know what that was back then.... That was 15 years ago. My husband read all he could at the library about it. I wish we had never heard of it! Our lives have never been the same since."

After a pause, Mrs. S. continued. "We worry about what will happen to Dennis. We're getting older. Who'll take care of him when we die? We worry about our own safety. When he gets into these spells, you can't tell what he'll do.... We're afraid he'll hurt us. It has been so very hard. I don't know how we managed all these years, except for our faith and the prayers of the others at church. We are both praying people, and, believe it or not, so is Dennis when he's not in one of his spells. When his medicine is working, he reads the Bible every day. But we worry about him.... Things just don't seem to be working out. Isn't there something else?"

From her initial assessment information, Susan began to develop a map for the care of Dennis. With her skills in nursing, using the nursing process to chart the way, she knew where to start and where she hoped to go.

ASSESSMENT

As soon as the nurse-patient interaction is initiated, the **assessment** step of the nursing process begins. The focus of this step is on data collection. The information gathered provides the database for determining the direction of care for the patient. In the assessment step, you will gather information about the patient's past history, present situation, and health care expectations from a variety of sources. The patient is your first and primary source for data collection. However, you can often obtain additional information from family members, friends, significiant others, health team members, records, and the results of various tests and laboratory procedures. In some situations when the patient cannot provide the needed information, these additional sources become the primary sources.

On the initial visit of the psychiatric home nurse, Dennis's agitation and paranoia made it necessary for Susan to gather information about Dennis's past history from his parents. In addition, this provided Susan with information about the parental support system that was currently operating on Dennis's behalf.

Your focus is to gather complete biological, psychological, cognitive, sociological, and spiritual information about the patient. This includes physical assessment data, information about growth and development, descriptions of behaviors, and information about the patient's coping and emotions. Important cultural and ethnic variables; relationships with family, friends, groups, clubs, and other support systems; and involvement in work and school constitute the sociological information. The patient's religious affiliation and spiritual beliefs are important spiritual data to collect. These all contribute to the person's "basic make-up" and greatly influence perceptions and beliefs that underlie behaviors.

Once the data are sorted, the nurse is ready to move on to the next phase of the nursing process when the data are analyzed and nursing diagnoses are formed (Johnson et al, 1992).

▶ Check Your Reading

7. During the assessment phase, what is the focus of the nurse?
8. What or who is the primary source for data collection?
9. How can the quality of assessment be enhanced?
10. What is included in the psychological assessment?

DIAGNOSIS

The purpose of the **diagnosis** is to "name" the patient's problems. Once a problem is accurately defined and named, the possible solutions become more obvious. Naming focuses our thinking and problem-solving skills.

The advanced-practice certified specialist in psychiatric nursing "names" the patient's problems as both medical problems and nursing problems. To name medical problems, she or he uses the criteria in the ***Diagnostic and Statistical Manual of Mental Disorders–IV (DSM-IV)***. To name nursing problems, he or she uses the nomenclature specified by the **North American Nursing Diagnosis Association (NANDA)** for nursing diagnoses. Although the basic-level psychiatric nurse must understand the *DSM-IV*, only nursing diagnosis, using the NANDA diagnostic labels (Box 12–1), is within the scope of practice of the basic-level psychiatric nurse.

The basis for providing sound nursing care in the psychiatric setting is "the recognition and identification of patterns of response to actual or potential psychiatric illnesses and mental health problems" (ANA, 1994, p. 26). As a psychiatric nurse, you will compare information collected during the assessment against documented norms of health and wellness. Taking into account the

BOX 12-1 North American Nursing Diagnosis Association-Approved Nursing Diagnoses

This list represents the NANDA-approved nursing diagnoses for clinical use and testing for 1994.

Activity Intolerance
*Activity Intolerance, Risk for
†Adaptive Capacity: Intracranial, Decreased
Adjustment, Impaired
Airway Clearance, Ineffective
Anxiety
*Aspiration, Risk for
Body Image Disturbance
*Body Temperature, Risk for Altered
Breastfeeding, Effective
Breastfeeding, Ineffective
Breastfeeding, Interrupted
Breathing Pattern, Ineffective
Caregiver Role Strain
*Caregiver Role Strain, Risk for
Communication, Impaired Verbal
†Community Coping, Ineffective
†Community Coping, Potential for Enhanced
†Confusion, Acute
†Confusion, Chronic
Constipation
Constipation, Colonic
Constipation, Perceived
Decisional Conflict (Specify)
Decreased Cardiac Output
Defensive Coping
Denial, Ineffective
Diarrhea
†Disorganized Infant Behavior
†Disorganized Infant Behavior, Risk for
Disuse Syndrome, Risk for
Diversional Activity Deficit
Dysfunctional Ventilatory Weaning Response (DVWR)
Dysreflexia
†Energy Field Disturbance
†Environmental Interpretation Syndrome, Impaired
Family Coping: Compromised, Ineffective
Family Coping: Disabling, Ineffective
Family Coping: Potential for Growth
†Family Process: Alcoholism, Altered
Family Processes, Altered
Fatigue
Fear
Fluid Volume Deficit
*Fluid Volume Deficit, Risk for
Fluid Volume Excess
Gas Exchange, Impaired
Grieving, Anticipatory
Grieving, Dysfunctional
Growth and Development, Altered
Health Maintenance, Altered
Health Seeking Behaviors (Specify)
Home Maintenance Management, Impaired
Hopelessness
Hyperthermia
Hypothermia
Incontinence, Bowel
Incontinence, Functional
Incontinence, Reflex
Incontinence, Stress
Incontinence, Total
Incontinence, Urge
Individual Coping, Ineffective
Infant Feeding Pattern, Ineffective
*Infection, Risk for
*Injury, Risk for
Knowledge Deficit (Specify)
†Loneliness, Risk for
†Management of Therapeutic Regimen: Community, Ineffective
†Management of Therapeutic Regimen: Families, Ineffective
†Management of Therapeutic Regimen: Individual, Effective
Management of Therapeutic Regimen (Individual) Ineffective
†Memory, Impaired

BOX 12-1 North American Nursing Diagnosis Association-Approved Nursing Diagnoses *Continued*

Noncompliance (Specify)
Nutrition: Less than Body Requirements, Altered
Nutrition: More than Body Requirements, Altered
Nutrition: Potential for More than Body Requirements, Altered
Oral Mucous Membrane, Altered
†Organized Infant Behavior, Potential for Enhanced
Pain
Pain, Chronic
Parental Role Conflict
†Parent/Infant/Child Attachment, Risk for Altered
Parenting, Altered
*Parenting, Risk for Altered
†Perioperative Positioning Injury, Risk for
*Peripheral Neurovascular Dysfunction, Risk for
Personal Identity Disturbance
Physical Mobility, Impaired
*Poisoning, Risk for
Post-Trauma Response
Powerlessness
Protection, Altered
Rape-Trauma Syndrome
Rape-Trauma Syndrome: Compound Reaction
Rape-Trauma Syndrome: Silent Reaction
Relocation Stress Syndrome
Role Performance, Altered
Self Care Deficit
  Bathing/Hygiene
  Dressing/Grooming
  Feeding
  Toileting
Self Esteem, Chronic Low
Self Esteem Disturbance
Self Esteem, Situational Low
*Self-Mutilation, Risk for
Sensory/Perceptual Alterations (Specify)(Visual, Auditory, Kinesthetic, Gustatory, Tactile, Olfactory)
Sexual Dysfunction
Sexuality Patterns, Altered
Skin Integrity, Impaired
*Skin Integrity, Risk for Impaired
Sleep Pattern Disturbance
Social Interaction, Impaired
Social Isolation
Spiritual Distress (Distress of the Human Spirit)
†Spiritual Well-Being, Potential for Enhanced
*Suffocation, Risk for
Sustain Spontaneous Ventilation, Inability to
Swallowing, Impaired
Thermoregulation, Ineffective
Thought Processes, Altered
Tissue Integrity, Impaired
Tissue Perfusion, Altered (Specify Type) (Renal, Cerebral, Cardiopulmonary, Gastrointestinal, Peripheral)
*Trauma, Risk for
Unilateral Neglect
Urinary Elimination, Altered
Urinary Retention
*Violence: Risk for, Self-Directed or Directed at Others

*Diagnoses with modified label terminology in 1994. (This change was recommended by the NANDA Taxonomy Committee and adopted to remain consistent with the ICD.)
†New diagnoses added in 1994 classified at level 1.4 using new Criteria for Staging.

patient's individual variations (related to demographics, background, experiences, and situation), you can then make inferences about the patient's problems and needs. Using logical decision-making to apply knowledge and critical thinking, you will then analyze the data. This analysis logically progresses from the data to the identification of the nursing diagnoses (Wilkinson, 1992). Box 12–2 shows the steps in this process of logical decision-making for arriving at nursing diagnoses.

Nursing diagnoses are defined as clinical judgments about individual, family, or community responses to actual and potential health problems. Nursing diagnoses are used to describe a patient's condition, to prescribe nursing **interventions,** and to delineate the parameters for the establishment of outcome criteria. Nursing diagnoses focus on *responses* to an actual or potential unmet health need. These responses may be in the form of a response to a disease process, to a complementary concern along the health-illness continuum, or to some need unrelated to any identified medical diagnosis.

A nursing diagnosis states the existing or high-risk problems identified by the nurse. The statement consists of three parts:

- The health problem
- The etiological or contributing factors
- The defining characteristics

The health problem consists of the behavioral disruption, or potential disruption, that you have identified and that can be improved through nursing intervention: It is the patient's unmet need. The etiological factors include the stressors that contributed to the problem; these can be thought of as the probable causes of the problem. The defining characteristics describe signs and symptoms; these reflect the objective and subjective data that provide the supporting data for the nursing interventions (Alfaro, 1990; Doenges and Moorehouse, 1992; Gordon, 1994; Carpenito, 1995).

Often, nursing diagnoses flow from medical diagnoses. This is frequently the case in psychiatric nursing. Although the *DSM-IV* assists us in identifying symptom patterns and categorizing them into specific disorders, the *DSM-IV* fails to specify the suffering that the diagnostic label carries with it. A listing of symptoms does not provide the nurse with information about how the illness has affected the patient's life or how the illness has affected the patient's family. From the specific *DSM-IV* diagnosis, the nurse can identify a number of likely nursing diagnoses because the *DSM-IV* diagnostic criteria identify many patterns of behavior that provide clues to specific and appropriate nursing diagnoses. Let's look at Dennis.

The medical diagnosis for Dennis's condition is paranoid schizophrenia. Susan, Dennis's home care nurse, knew that certain behaviors often are evident with this diagnosis and that the patient has a basic problem with trusting others. In addition, she knew, based on the diagnosis, that Dennis might have hallucinations and delusions, aggression and guardedness, physical symptoms, and difficulty in communicating in a meaningful way with others. Given the diagnosis of paranoid schizophrenia, Susan knew that the nursing diagnoses would likely include the following:

Risk for Violence: Self-Directed or Directed at Others
Ineffective Individual Coping
Sensory/Perceptual Alterations: Auditory/Visual
Altered Thought Processes
Impaired Verbal Communication
Self Care Deficit
Social Isolation
Sleep Pattern Disturbance
Noncompliance
Ineffective Individual Coping

Susan then had to determine whether any of these diagnoses was appropriate for Dennis. Once she identified appropriate diagnoses, she tailored them to Dennis's unique situation by identifying the associated etiologies and defining characteristics. Her specific nursing diagnoses for Dennis were as follows:

Noncompliance with medication regimen related to anxiety as evidenced by missed appointments for injections of fluphenazine
Sensory/Perceptual Alterations: Auditory Hallucinations related to paranoia as evidenced by diverted attention, responses to an unseen being, and patient's report of hearing voices
Sleep Pattern Disturbance related to hallucinations and anxiety as evidenced by pacing, hypervigilance, and difficulty falling asleep
Risk for Violence: Directed at Others related to auditory hallucinations as evidenced by aggression toward parents

BOX 12-2 Steps in Logical Decision-Making for Arriving at Nursing Diagnoses

1. Identify the patient's behavioral, biological, psychosocial, and spiritual responses to stress.
2. Categorize the data into functional groups.
3. Identify missing data and any incongruencies.
4. Identify any patterns.
5. Compare the data to theoretical information, norms, and standards.
6. Identify basic needs and concerns, taking into account the patient's strengths and limitations.
7. Identify any causal relationships.
8. Identify the applicable nursing diagnoses.

After identifying the list of nursing diagnoses, the nurse uses **prioritization** to organize the identified diagnoses in order of importance. Highest priority is given to those problems that are life threatening. Next in priority are those problems that are likely to cause destructive changes. Lowest in priority are those diagnoses related to normative or developmental experiences (Sundeen et al, 1994). Psychiatric nurses often use Maslow's Hierarchy of Needs to help them prioritize nursing diagnoses (see Chapter 8).

At this point, the nurse validates the identified problems with the patient and discusses the next steps on the journey (Freund, 1993), which include establishing the desired outcomes and planning the interventions to accomplish these outcomes.

▶ Check Your Reading

11. What is the definition of a nursing diagnosis?
12. From what are nursing diagnoses derived?
13. What are the steps in logical decision-making?
14. What is the name of the group that develops the approved list of nursing diagnoses?

15. What are the three parts to a nursing diagnosis statement?
16. How are nursing diagnoses and the psychiatric diagnoses in *DSM-IV* related?

OUTCOME IDENTIFICATION

Nursing care is goal directed and outcome oriented. It is through the use of specific **expected outcomes**, with criteria for measurement, that you will formulate a plan of care. These expected outcomes are frequently referred to as long-term goals; in this text, however, we refer to long-term goals as expected outcomes.

Expected outcomes are the patient behaviors that the nurse anticipates will occur as a result of nursing interventions, indicating the resolution of—or progress toward the resolution of—the patient's unmet need or problem. The expected outcomes must be therapeutically sound and must reflect a scientific basis. The outcomes must be reasonable, attainable, cost effective, and realistic in relation to the patient's present and potential capabilities.

There are seven criteria for writing an expected outcome (Hickey, 1990, Redman, 1993). Expected outcomes must be

Patient centered
Singular
Observable
Measurable
Time limited
Mutual
Realistic

By incorporating all of these elements, the statement of expected outcomes provides information that can be readily evaluated; it designates information about *who* (the patient) will *do what* (the single behavior to be observed) *how, how much, how often, and to what degree* (criteria for measurement) and *when and where* (situational parameters).

Some expected outcomes are easily achieved, while others take longer for the patient to accomplish. To maintain a realistic focus, it is therefore advisable to organize the expected outcomes into a series of short-term goals that lead to the fulfillment of the longer-term expected outcome (Box 12–3).

Because most patients have a number of problems that you will want to address, you may need to identify several expected outcomes for each identified nursing diagnosis. When you plan care in this manner, you and your patients can experience increments of success while working toward the achievement of your shared vision. It is like stopping along the road at a variety of points before continuing the journey.

BOX 12–3 Example of an Expected Outcome and a Short-Term Goal for Dennis

Assessment

Patient statements:

- "I can control the voices now,
- but . . . ."
- "The voices keep telling me things."
- "I wish they would go away . . . like before."

Diagnosis

DSM-IV diagnosis—Paranoid schizophrenia

Nursing diagnosis—Sensory/Perceptual Alterations: auditory related to paranoia as evidenced by patient reports of hearing voices, averted gaze, and verbal responses to unseen beings

Outcome Identification, Planning, and Implementation

Expected outcome—By ______ the patient will report hearing no voices for a period of 2 weeks.

Short-Term Goals

During the one-to-one interaction with the home care nurse, the patient will

Identify each time he hears a "voice"

Identify, at least once during the second visit, what was happening when hearing "voices"

During the third visit, state one alternative response to control the "voices"

PLANNING

The particular routes that you and your patients take along the journey are represented in the plan of care. Once you have established expected outcomes, the **planning** step of the nursing process begins. In this step you will choose suitable strategies for intervention.

The selection of nursing interventions is a deliberate process of decision-making. It incorporates the priorities that you have already established to provide organized, efficient, and effective nursing care. In a plan of nursing care, it is helpful to categorize your interventions according to the types of interventions allowed by your level of practice. The psychiatric nurse with a *basic* level of practice focuses on the following categories of interventions:

- Counseling
- Milieu therapy
- Self-care activities
- Psychobiological interventions
- Health teaching
- Case management
- Health promotion and health maintenance

The psychiatric nurse with an *advanced* level of practice also uses the following categories of interventions:

- Psychotherapy
- Prescription of pharmacological agents
- Consultation

Selection of the best intervention to help the patient to resolve her or his problems depends on the complexity of the problems. The interventions can address *actual* problems, which require active management. Or, they can address *risk* problems—those that are likely to occur and for which preventive nursing strategies are necessary.

Once you have identified appropriate interventions, you will generate a plan of care, drawing upon your knowledge and experience, critical thinking skills, and research of the literature. You will develop the plan of care in collaboration with other members of the health care team and with the patient (Schultz and Videbeck, 1994).

Many references are available to help you plan psychiatric nursing care. For instance, care plan books provide standardized approaches to care that you can tailor to your particular patient situation. You can also base your interventions on a nursing intervention classification (NIC) system to ensure that the interventions that you choose are those supported by nursing research and accepted standards of practice (McCloskey and Bulechek, 1992).

Whatever resources you use, it is important that you consider the needs of the "whole patient," that you have a scientific rationale for all interventions, and that you communicate the plan to everyone involved in the patient's care. It is also important to include discharge planning in the plan of care to ensure continuity of care.

▶ **Check Your Reading**

17. What is the purpose of nursing outcomes?
18. What are the criteria for writing an expected outcome?
19. How are short-term goals related to expected outcomes?
20. How might nursing interventions be categorized in a plan of nursing care?

IMPLEMENTATION

According to the Standards of Care in the *Standards of Psychiatric-Mental Health Clinical Nursing Practice*, psychiatric nurses employ "a wide range of interventions designed to prevent mental and physical illness, and promote, maintain and restore mental and physical health" (ANA, 1994, pp. 28, 29; see also Chapter 4). As you learned in the preceding section, the interventions that you will use in psychiatric nursing depend on your level of practice. **Implementation** refers to all of the nursing actions that the nurse takes to facilitate the patient's achievement of identified patient outcomes.

Interventions Available to Psychiatric Nurses with a Basic or Advanced Level of Practice

Counseling. Counseling interventions include the use of communication and interviewing techniques (see Chapters 10 and 11), teaching problem-solving skills, intervening to resolve crises (see Chapter 15), helping patients manage stress (see Chapter 28), teaching relaxation techniques, training patients in healthy assertiveness, teaching patients how to resolve conflicts, and helping patients to modify behavior (see Chapter 18). Counseling is used to help patients modify or stop using unhealthy behaviors, to reinforce positive, healthy behaviors, and to facilitate the movement of patients toward personal and social integration. The exact focus of counseling depends on the unique needs of each patient. Chapter 16 covers individual therapy and provides additional information on counseling.

Milieu Therapy. Milieu therapy is the therapeutic use of the environment. It is important for the psychiatric nurse to be aware of the effects of the patient's environment and how the environment can help to provide boundaries for the patient's daily activities. It is vital to maintain a safe environment and to provide humane limits to protect the patient and others. For an in-depth discussion of milieu therapy, see Chapter 19.

Self-Care Activities. Self-care interventions are those that help patients to assume responsibility for the activities of daily living. The aim of these interventions is to maintain and improve the patient's functional status. Be sure to implement self-care interventions in such a way that you preserve the patient's dignity. Also ensure that the interventions are appropriate to the patient's age, developmental level, gender, sexual orientation, ethnic and social background, and educational level. Paying attention to the patient's functional level is of particular importance, because it often varies over the course of treatment (Johnson et al, 1992).

Psychobiological Interventions. Psychobiological interventions include psychobiological therapies and administration of psychopharmacological agents. All interventions that affect the patient's biological and physiological processes—be they electroconvulsive therapy, guided imagery, or administration of lithium carbonate—are considered psychobiological.

The basic-level psychiatric nurse is involved in the administration of these interventions, and the advanced-level psychiatric nurse may be involved in their prescription. Whatever your level of practice, it is important that you explore both the biological and the psychological impact of these interventions—that you consider *all* of the patient's responses to these treatments. Once these interventions have been administered, monitoring their actions and untoward effects is critical. For more information on psychobiological interventions, see Chapters 21, 23, and 30.

Health Teaching. Interventions that help patients to gain information are appropriate whenever you have identified the presence of the nursing diagnosis *Knowledge Deficit* (Redman, 1993). In psychiatric nursing practice, you will use health teaching to provide new information, to reinforce information and behaviors, and to teach alternative strategies and approaches to dealing with problems. For more information on health teaching, see Chapter 22.

Case Management. Case management includes all the interventions that are used to coordinate comprehensive health services and ensure continuity of care. These interventions include negotiating for services on behalf of patients, maintaining relationships with agencies and health care providers, and providing services that meet patient needs. The availability, accessibility, quality, and cost of care are among the factors that you will take into account when performing case management services (Girgenti and Mathis, 1994). Chapter 44 provides additional information about case management.

Health Promotion and Health Maintenance. As a psychiatric nurse, part of your role will be to employ strategies and interventions aimed at promoting and maintaining mental health and preventing mental illness. These interventions call for you to broaden your perspective to include the community.

Psychiatric nurses design interventions to promote mental health and prevent mental illness in clients identified as "at risk" for mental health problems. They also encourage consumer participation in identifying problems in the community and in planning, implementing, and evaluating programs to address those problems. They identify community resources to help consumers to use mental health services appropriately. Psychiatric nurses base all of these interventions on a knowledge of the health beliefs and practices of the population, a knowledge of the epidemiology of mental illness, and an awareness of the social, cultural, and political issues that affect mental health in the community.

Interventions Available Only to Psychiatric Nurses With an Advanced Level of Practice

Advanced psychiatric nursing interventions can be performed *only* by the psychiatric nurse who is certified as a specialist in psychiatric-mental health nursing. Also, the availability of these interventions depends on the Nurse Practice Act, statutes, and regulations covering the particular area where the nurse practices.

In addition to the interventions available to the basic-level psychiatric nurse, certified specialists may provide psychotherapy, prescribe pharmacologic agents, and perform consultation, in accordance with state regulations. The regulations vary among the states in the United States, and it is imperative that the advanced practice psychiatric-mental health nurse act within the limits of licensure.

▶ Check Your Reading

21. What are the interventions available to the psychiatric nurse at the basic level of practice?
22. What intervention includes communication and interviewing?
23. What is the focus of milieu therapy?
24. Maintaining and improving the person's functional status is the aim of which category of intervention?
25. Monitoring the effects of psychotropic medications is which type of nursing intervention?
26. What type of nursing interventions are directed to meeting the nursing diagnosis of knowledge deficit?
27. What is included in case management interventions?
28. Which type of intervention includes a broader community perspective?

EVALUATION

The last step of the nursing process, **evaluation**, is actually ongoing throughout the duration of the nurse-patient relationship. Changes in the patient's health status over time give rise to the need for modifications in the plan. Therefore, continuous monitoring of the effectiveness of nursing interventions and of the patient's attainment of expected outcomes is necessary.

Two types of evaluation—formative and summative—can be used. **Formative evaluation** includes reassessment of all aspects of the nursing process as you are implementing care to analyze the patient's responses. The success or failure of a nursing intervention may be due to any number of factors that occur throughout the nursing process (Harris and Gillien, 1992). In performing a formative evaluation, ask yourself these questions:

Is the assessment adequate and accurate?
Are the nursing diagnoses correctly stated to deal with the patient's needs?
Are the expected outcomes properly focused and written in a manner that facilitates evaluation of the achievement of expected outcome?
Are the planned interventions adequately thorough, based on sound principles, and efficiently implemented?
Can anything else be done if the interventions have not helped the patient to achieve the expected outcome?
Can the expected outcomes and short-term goals be modified to be more applicable to this patient at this time?
Can other, more relevant nursing diagnoses be considered?
Should any elements of the plan of care be discontinued? Why?

Evaluate each aspect of the nursing process continually, and make any necessary modifications. Even the best of plans can benefit from ongoing evaluation!

A **summative evaluation** is one in which you make a concluding statement about the entire nurse-patient journey. The summative evaluation includes information from the formative evaluation, as well as recommendations for future nursing care, as appropriate. The summative evaluation is most helpful when you are planning for the patient's discharge from care. It encompasses the status of all identified nursing diagnoses, the patient's current functional status, and recommended actions and referrals. A summative evaluation greatly assists in providing continuity of care. Box 12–4 shows a portion of a completed nursing care plan.

BOX 12-4 A Portion of a Completed Nursing Care Plan for Dennis

Assessment

Patient statements:

- "I can control the voices now, but . . . ."
- "The voices keep telling me things."
- "I wish they would go away . . . like before."

Diagnosis

DSM-IV Diagnosis: Paranoid schizophrenia

Nursing diagnosis: Sensory/Perceptual Alterations: auditory related to paranoia as evidenced by patient reports of hearing voices, averted gaze, and verbal responses to unseen beings.

Outcome Identification, Planning, and Implementation

Expected outcome: By ——— the patient will report hearing no voices for a period of 2 weeks.

Short-Term Goals	Nursing Interventions	Rationales
During the one-to-one interaction with the home care nurse, the patient will	1. Be aware of surrounding stimuli.	1. Provides information regarding potential triggers for hallucinations.
Identify each time he hears a "voice"	2. Decrease external stimuli.	2. Altered perceptions related to external stimuli in the environment are frightening to the patient and stimulate defensive coping behaviors.
Identify, at least once during the second visit, what was happening when hearing "voices"	3. Communicate verbally in direct, concrete, specific terms.	3. Schizophrenic patients have difficulty understanding and responding to abstract ideas.
During the third visit, state one alternative response to control the "voices"	4. Respond verbally to anything real that the patient talks about.	4. Reality orientation helps the patient to correctly interpret external stimuli.
	5. If the patient hallucinates, engage his attention. 6. Provide simple activities to help the patient distract himself from the voices.	5. and 6. External support from the nurse helps to provide the external controls needed to decrease the influence of internal voices.
	7. Encourage the expression of feelings related to the patient's awareness of the hallucinations.	7. Recognition of patient feelings enables the nurse to emotionally connect with the patient.
	8. Discuss alternatives to control the voices.	8. Providing concrete suggestions and anticipatory guidance helps the patient to take control of his symptoms.

Evaluation

Formative Evaluation:

1. The patient's communication is more reality based.
2. The patient has developed a list of three alternative activities and states he feels much better now that the voices are getting under control. Modification: Provide health teaching related to medications for controlling hallucinations.

Summative Evaluation:

1. The patient has been taking his medications, and he reports fewer episodes of hearing voices.

▶ Check Your Reading

29. What is a formative evaluation?
30. What is a summative evalution?
31. Why are both essential to excellent nursing care?

DOCUMENTATION

Communication among the members of the health care team through **documentation** is essential to the successful planning and implementation of nursing care. The nursing care plan is only one form of documentation that facilitates the process. Other methods of documentation can be used to reflect the use of the nursing process and to provide a legal record of the care that you have provided (Townsend, 1991; Town, 1993).

One method of documenting is to record, in a systematic manner, information from each step of the nursing process. The exact format for this method of documentation varies, depending on the forms and procedures preferred by each particular agency. However, the basic structure is to

- Document assessed information (A)
- Note the problems addressed (P)
- Describe briefly the nursing actions implemented as interventions (I)
- Document the outcomes in the evaluation section (E)

The acronym for this method is APIE.

Similar to this method is the problem-oriented record (POR) method of documentation. POR has as its basis a list of problems. For a given problem, you would record information about the nursing process using a "SOAPIE" format. The record begins with a notation, with date and time, of the problem. Next you would note the assessed information as subjective data (S) and objective data (O). Following that notation, you would indicate your interpretation of the assessed information (A), your plan (P) or activities to be carried out, what you actually implemented as the interventions (I), and your evaluation of the problem following the interventions (E).

Focused charting is another method of documentation, which uses a "specified" focus (as opposed to a "problem" focus). The focus may be a nursing diagnosis, a patient concern or behavior, a significant change in the patient's status, or a significant event that has some impact on the patient. For the specified "focus," you would describe data to support the focus, identify actions to address the focus, and note the patient's response to these interventions. This method of documentation is referred to as the DAR format, signifying *data*, *action*, and *response* (Townsend, 1991).

Carson (1994) has developed a documentation system for psychiatric home care that is applicable to other psychiatric health care systems. She designed the system to respond to Medicare criteria for reimbursement, which require that the psychiatric nurse deliver a skilled intervention that is documented in concrete terms with very specific and concrete outcome indicators. Carson describes the system, which uses a flowsheet format and coding, as "talking med-surg but doing psych" documentation. Carson's Psychiatric Care Plan is based on a psychoeducational approach and identifies standardized teaching interventions that psychiatric nurses perform. A sample portion of Carson's Psychiatric Care Plan form is shown in Figure 12–2.

The Care Plan, which contains 13 pages of psychiatric goals, the orders to support these goals, and the nursing interventions used to meet the goals, is used with a companion Clinical Nursing Note form. The Note form is brief and calls for little narrative. On it the nurse codes the identified goals and interventions, the patient's response to the interventions, and the degree of goal achievement. The Care Plan flowsheet allows the nurse to focus the care that he or she gives and to clearly document when the patient has met her or his goals or when the goals have been modified. Figure 12–3 shows a completed Psychiatric Nursing Clinical Note.

Evaluation of care and monitoring of quality are integral parts of your professional accountability. Health care agencies conduct surveys of nursing care as part of Quality Improvement (QI) functions. The emphasis of QI is on continuous improvement of care. Important aspects of QI include the monitoring and evaluation of patient care for the agency (Town, 1993; Girgenti and Mathis, 1994). This monitoring and evaluation may take the form of an audit of the outcomes of patient care ("outcome audit"), or it may take the form of an audit of the delivery of nursing care ("process audit"). Agency administrators then compare the documented data against established standards. If necessary, the agency will then take steps to improve the care (Sundeen et al, 1994).

At this time, most documentation relies on written notes in patient charts. However, as the health care system continues to develop in the area of technology and informatics, more and more documentation will rely on computerization. Eventually, computer data analysis may help to identify critical pathways for providing care and documenting activities and outcomes (Town, 1993). Yet all of these advances will still rely on the nursing process or a similar "map" to guide professional nursing practice.

▶ Check Your Reading

32. Why is documentation important?
33. What are the components of the APIE method of documentation?
34. What is the basis of the problem-oriented record?
35. What does SOAPIE stand for?
36. What is the method of documentation used in focused charting?
37. Agencies review nursing documentation as part of what functions?

BAY AREA HEALTH CARE
PSYCHIATRIC CARE PLAN

Patient's Name: ______________________ Date: ___/___/9___
Nurse's Signature: ______________________

Patient Outcomes/Orders/Interventions — Dates of Interventions and Resolution

PG = Patient Outcomes — PO = Orders — Letters = Interventions

___ PG.0 Patient Will Have Thorough Assessment
___ PO1 Skilled Nursing Visit Frequency = ______
___ PO2 Assess Vital Signs
___ PO3 Assess Medications
- ___ A. Assess Medication Effectiveness
- ___ B. Assess Medication Side Effects
- ___ C. Assess Medication Supply
- ___ D. Assess Medication Compliance

___ PO4 Assess Mental Status
- ___ A. Complete Mini Mental Exam
- ___ B. Complete Global Assessment Form
- ___ C. Complete Affective Scale
- ___ D. Complete Anxiety Scale
- ___ E. Other

___ PO5 Assess Social Support System
- ___ A. Complete Social Support Tool
- ___ B. Assess Who Is a Support
- ___ C. Assess What Kind of Support Is Given

___ PO6 Assess Nutrition/Hydration
- ___ A. Have Patient Do 24-Hour Diet Recall
- ___ B. Assess Food Likes/Dislikes
- ___ C. Assess Budgetary Restraints on Food Purchasing
- ___ D. Assess Nutrition Knowledge
- ___ E. Assess Cultural and/or Religious Impacts on Diet
- ___ F. Assess Physiological Impacts on Intake/Elimination
- ___ G Assess Adequacy of Diet

___ PO7 Assess Sleep Pattern
- ___ A. Assess Quantity of Sleep
- ___ B. Assess Quality of Sleep
- ___ C. Assess for Presence of Sleep Routines
- ___ D. Assess for Problems That Interfere with Restful Sleep

___ PG.1 Patient/Caregiver and Nurse Will Develop a Therapeutic Relationship

___ PO8 Develop a Therapeutic Nurse-Patient Relationship
- ___ A. Demonstrate Trustworthiness Every Visit
- ___ B. Develop Rapport With Patient/Caregiver by Listening Attentively to Concerns
- ___ C. Demonstrate Empathy by Reflecting Patient's Feelings and Reactions to Situations

Dr. Verna Benner Carson
Psychiatric Home Care Manual

FIGURE 12–2
A sample portion of Carson's Psychiatric Care Plan form. (From Carson, V. B. [1994]. *Bay Area psychiatric home care manual.* Baltimore: Bay Area Health Care.)

Illustration continued on following page

___ D. Demonstrate Therapeutic Communication Skills to Assist the Patient to Self-Disclose

___ E. Teach the Patient Regarding the Boundaries of the Relationship

___ F. Teach the Patient About the Importance of Discussing Thoughts and Feelings Honestly and Openly

___ G. Demonstrate Acceptance of Patient with Affirmation and Consistency

___ H. Teach the Patient the Impact of Patient's Behaviors on Others

___ I. Teach the Patient the Need for Limits on Inappropriate Behavior

___ J. Confront the Patient with Discrepancies in Behavior

___ K. Summarize the Accomplishments of the Relationship

___ L. Teach the Patient the Value of Terminating the Relationship in a Planned Way That Allows Open Discussion of Feelings and Thoughts

___ M. Other

___ N. Other

___ PG.2 Patient/Caregiver Will Demonstrate Criteria for MD Alert and Access to BAHC Personnel and On-Call Nurse

___ PO9 Teach Patient How to Use 911 and How to Access BAHC Personnel and On-Call Nurse

___ A. Teach How to Use 911

___ B. Teach What Situations Warrant Use of 911

___ C. Teach How to Contact On-Call Nurse

___ D. Teach What Situations Warrant Contacting On-Call Nurse

Patient's Name: ______________________

Dr. Verna Benner-Carson
Psychiatric Home Care Manual

FIGURE 12–2 *(Continued)*
A sample portion of Carson's Psychiatric Care Plan form. (From Carson, V. B. [1994]. *Bay Area psychiatric home care manual.* Baltimore: Bay Area Health Care.)

PSYCHIATRIC NURSING CLINICAL NOTE

PATIENT NAME: *Carl DeBeers* DATE: *3/5/96*

GOALS THIS VISIT (MUST BE TAKEN FROM CARE PLAN) *Assess the level of activity the pt. is capable of assuming. Ascertain the duties the HHA will need to assume.*

REASON HOMEBOUND (CHECK ALL THAT APPLY)

- ____ DISORIENTED
- ____ BEHAVIOR POSES RISK TO SELF/OTHERS
- ____ USES ASSISTIVE DEVICE TO AID MOBILITY (CANE, WALKER, WHEELCHAIR, BRACES)
- ✔ LIMITED ENDURANCE RELATED TO MEDICAL DX (BECOMES SOB WITH MILD EXERTION)
- ____ JUDGMENT IMPAIRED — REQUIRES 24-HOUR SUPERVISION
- ✔ LEAVING HOME IS NOT POSSIBLE WITHOUT TAXING EFFORT
- ✔ LEAVING HOME IS DEPENDENT ON ASSISTANCE FROM OTHERS
- ____ AGORAPHOBIC

VITAL SIGNS (IF APPLICABLE) BP *156/100 sitting 146/100 standing* P *88* TEMP ____ RESP *24* WT ____

ASSESSMENT: CHECK IF ASSESSED; RECORD ONLY SIGNIFICANT CHANGES

MENTAL STATUS:

- ORIENTATION ✔
- MEMORY ✔
- THOUGHT PROCESS *Focused on multiple symptoms*
- THOUGHT CONTENT ____
- EMOTIONAL TONE *"Hyper"*
- SUICIDAL/HOMICIDAL
  - IDEATION ____
  - INTENT *Denies*
  - PLAN ____
  - JUDGMENT/SAFETY ✔

MEDICATION ____

- EFFECTIVE ✔
- SIDE EFFECTS ✔
- COMPLIANT ✔ *Compliant*

ACTIVITIES OF DAILY LIVING

- ACTIVITY AND REST ✔ *Limited by dyspnea on exertion*
- NUTRITION/ELIMINATION ✔
- HYGIENE/APPEARANCE ✔
- DIVERSIONAL ACTIVITIES ✔
- SOCIALIZATION ✔

PATIENT BEHAVIOR/INTERACTION *Expending energies in various directions*

CAREGIVER BEHAVIOR/INTERACTION ____

EMERGENCY/CRISIS INTERVENTION SINCE LAST VISIT:

YES ____ (DESCRIBE) ____

NO ✔

COMPLIANCE WITH FOLLOW-UP APPOINTMENTS:

YES ____ DATE *3/2/96* FREQUENCY *Seen in clinic for complaints of left rib pain 3/4/96 To have chest film and angiogram. To see psychiatrist — Dr. Pearl*

NO ____ (ELABORATE) ____

ANY ADDITIONAL ASSESSMENT:

INTERVENTIONS: (IDENTIFY WITH CAREPLAN CODE AND INTERVENTION NUMBER: NEW INTERVENTIONS SHOULD BE ADDED TO CAREPLAN AND DESCRIBED HERE)

INTERVENTIONS	PATIENT/CAREGIVER OUTCOMES	EVALUATION
#3A-D	*Medication teaching on Desyrel. Compliant with meds*	*U.T., G.C.*
#10A, B, C #5B, C	*Using neighbors for hospital rides, shopping. Detests the dependence*	*U.T., G.C.*
#6B, F, G	*Puts little energy into meal preparation–using dietary supplements*	*U.T., G.C.*
#7A-D	*Sleeping can be a problem–discussed relaxation techniques*	*P.T., G.C.*
#12A, E, F	*Activities have ↑ anxiety–poor understanding of relaxation*	*P.T., G.C.*
#15I, K, H	*Bedtime routine lacking*	*U.T., G.C.*

HHA SUPERVISION (EVERY 14 DAYS):

VERBAL ORDERS NEEDED (IF SO, COMPLETE ORDER SHEET AND MODIFY CAREPLAN)

SIGNATURE: *Miriam Jacik, R.N.* REVISIT: *3/5/96*

GOALS FOR NEXT VISIT: *Teaching on addictive behaviors, decreasing cigarettes in light of ↑ COPD*

CODE FOR PATIENT/CAREGIVER OUTCOMES:	
UNDERSTOOD TEACHING	= UT
UNDERSTOOD PART OF TEACHING	= PT
DO NOT UNDERSTAND TEACHING	= NOT
LESS DEPRESSED	= LD
MORE DEPRESSED	= MD
LESS ANXIOUS	= LA
MORE ANXIOUS	= MA
FOLLOWED THROUGH WITH NURSE'S SUGGESTIONS	= FLU

CODE FOR EVALUATION OF GOALS:	
GOALS BEGUN	= GB
GOALS CONTINUING	= GC
GOALS MET	= GM
GOALS REVISED	= GR

Developed by Verna Benner Carson, R.N. (V.B. CARSON, 91)

FIGURE 12–3

A completed example of one of Carson's Psychiatric Nursing Clinical Notes. (Modified from Carson, V. B. [1994]. *Bay Area psychiatric home care manual.* Baltimore: Bay Area Health Care.)

CONCLUSIONS

The nursing process is a systematic, dynamic, interpersonal, interactive framework for problem-solving in the delivery of nursing care. The skilled and knowledgeable use of this "map" can help you provide quality psychiatric nursing care throughout your journey with patients who are facing mental illness.

KEY POINTS TO REMEMBER

- The nursing process is nursing's problem-solving approach.
- The nursing process includes six steps: assessment, diagnosis, outcome identification, planning, implementation, and evaluation.
- The ANA *Standards of Clinical Practice* and the *Standards of Psychiatric-Mental Health Clinical Nursing Practice* are authoritative statements that describe the responsibilities for which all nurses are accountable.
- The *Standards of Psychiatric-Mental Health Clinical Nursing Practice* identify specific interventions appropriate to the basic level practitioner and the certified specialist.
- The focus of assessment is comprehensive and holistic data collection.
- The patient is the primary source of data.
- The psychiatric nurse sorts collected data by functional health patterns.
- Nursing diagnoses represent clinical judgments about individual, family, or community responses to actual and potential health problems.
- The nursing diagnosis includes the health problem, the etiological or contributing factors, and the defining characteristics.
- Nursing diagnoses are often related to medical diagnoses, but rather than listing symptoms, nursing diagnoses focus on the human response patterns and suffering of the patient.
- Through prioritization, the psychiatric nurse ranks nursing diagnoses in order of their importance.
- Expected outcomes should be patient centered, focused on one behavior, observable and measurable, time-limited, mutual, and realistic.
- Interventions for the basic-level psychiatric-mental health nurse include counseling, milieu therapy, self-care activities, psychobiological interventions, health teaching, case management, and health promotion and health maintenance activities.
- Interventions for the certified specialist in psychiatric-mental health nursing include psychotherapy, prescription of pharmacological agents, and consultation.
- Evaluation continues throughout the entire nursing process.
- Formative evaluation covers all aspects of the nursing process *as the nurse is providing care.*
- Summative evaluation draws conclusions about the effectiveness of the entire nurse-patient interaction.
- Documentation can follow the APIE (assessment, plan, interventions, and evaluation) method, the problem-oriented record (POR) approach, or the focused charting approach using the DAR (data, action, and response) format.

LEARNING ACTIVITIES

1. Pair up with a classmate and practice collecting data from each other, using the assessment form provided in Chapter 13 or another tool that your instructor selects. Make your assessment complete enough that you can develop a list of nursing diagnoses.

2. Form a small work group with two to three other students. Using Dennis's story, develop a comprehensive list of nursing diagnoses for Dennis.

3. Using the list of nursing diagnoses that your team developed in activity 2, prioritize the list and provide the rationale for your decisions.

4. Using Dennis's story and the psychiatric diagnosis in Box 12–3, develop nursing actions that are appropriate to the nursing diagnosis Defensive Coping, Communication, Impaired, or Self-Care Deficit. Organize the activities with respect to the interventions described in the standards of care specified in the *Standards of Psychiatric-Mental Health Clinical Nursing Practice.*

CRITICAL THINKING EXERCISES

Ms. Rainner, a student nurse in the last week of her psychiatric clinical experience has just completed her initial assessment of Mr. Tabber, a newly admitted patient. She paints the following picture. Mr. John Tabber is a 20-year-old man who speaks softly, tilts his head to the left when spoken to, laughs when asked his name, and whistles "Oh Suzanna" when asked about his relationships with other people. His clothes consist of a white shirt that appears unironed, socks that do not match in color, and blue jeans with a tear at the knee. When asked if he ever thought about hurting himself, he replied, "Of course, hasn't everyone?"

1. What assumption can you make about Mr. Tabber's presenting picture?

2. What other information do you need?

3. What nursing diagnosis would you consider?

Later in the day Ms. Rainner observed Mr. Tabber talking on the telephone. He put his hand over one ear while he pressed the receiver into his ear so hard that another patient was prompted to say to him, "John, stop that or you're going to hurt yourself." After Mr. Tabber completed his phone call, Ms. Rainner saw him walk with a staggered gait down the hall.

1. What alternative reasons might explain these behaviors?

2. What conclusions can you make about Mr. Tabber's behavior?

3. How can you test your assumptions (and nursing diagnosis) to know if they are accurate?

REFERENCES

Alfaro, R. (1990). *Applying nursing diagnosis and nursing process* (2nd ed.). Philadelphia: J. B. Lippincott.

American Nurses' Association. (1991). *Standards of clinical nursing practice.* Washington, D.C.: American Nurses Publishing.

American Nurses' Association. (1994). *A statement on psychiatric-mental health clinical practice and standards of psychiatric-mental health clinical nursing practice.* Washington, D.C.: American Nurses Publishing.

American Psychiatric Association. (1994). *Diagnostic and statistical manual of mental disorders* (4th ed.). Washington, D.C.: American Psychiatric Association.

Arnold, E., and Boggs, K. (1995). *Interpersonal relationships: Communication skills for nurses.* Philadelphia: W. B. Saunders.

Atkinson, L. D., and Murray, M. E. (1990). *Understanding the nursing process* (4th ed.). New York: Macmillan.

Carpenito, J. (Ed.). (1995). *Nursing diagnosis: Application to clinical practice* (6th ed.). Philadelphia: J. B. Lippincott.

Carson, V. B. (1994). Doing psych, but talking med-surg language. *Caring,* June, 32–41.

Doenges, M. E., and Moorehouse, M. F. (1992). *Application of nursing process and nursing diagnosis: An interactive text.* Philadelphia: F. A. Davis.

Freund, B. (1993). Validating nursing diagnoses: An approach to reinforce nursing process with BSN-completion students. *Journal of Nursing Education, 32*(3), 140–141.

Girgenti, J., and Mathis, A. (1994). Putting psychiatric nursing standards into clinical practice. *Journal of Psychosocial Nursing and Mental Health Services, 32*(6), 39–42.

Harris, J., and Gillien, E. (1992). Psychiatric mental health nursing specialist process evaluation criteria. *Nursing Management, 23*(2), 54, 55, 58.

Hickey, P. (1990). *Nursing process handbook.* St. Louis: C. V. Mosby.

Hurst, K., Dean, A., and Trickey, S. (1991). The recognition and non-recognition of problem-solving stages in nursing practice. *Journal of Advanced Nursing, 16*(12), 1444–1455.

Johnson, P. A., Stone, M. A., Larson, A. M., and Hromek, C. A. (1992). Applying nursing diagnosis and nursing process to activities of daily living and mobility. *Geriatric Nursing, 13*(1), 25–27.

McCloskey, J. C., and Bulechek, E. M. (1992). *Nursing intervention classification (NIC).* St. Louis: C. V. Mosby.

NANDA nursing diagnoses: Definitions and classification 1995-1996. (1995). Philadelphia: North American Nursing Diagnosis Association.

Redman, B. (1993). *The process of patient education.* (7th ed.). St. Louis: C. V. Mosby.

Ryan-Wenger, N. M. (1990). A nursing process methodology. *Nursing Outlook, 38*(4), 190–193.

Schultz, J., and Videbeck, S. (1994). *Manual of psychiatric nursing care plans.* Philadelphia: J. B. Lippincott.

Sheehan, J. (1991). Conceptions of the nursing process among nurse teachers and clinical nurses. *Journal of Advanced Nursing, 16*(3), 333–342.

Sundeen, S. J., Stuart, G. W., Rankin, E. A., and Cohen, S.A. (1994). *Nurse-patient interaction: Implementing the nursing process* (5th ed.). St. Louis: C. V. Mosby.

Town, J. (1993). Changing to computerized documentation-plus! *Nursing Management, 24*(7), 44–46, 48.

Townsend, M. (1991). *Nursing diagnoses in psychiatric nursing* (2nd ed.). Philadelphia: F. A. Davis.

Wilkinson, J. (1992). *Nursing process in action: A critical thinking approach.* Menlo Park, CA: Addison-Wesley.

SUGGESTED READINGS

Carson, V. B. (1994). Doing psych, but talking med-surg language. *Caring,* June, 32–41.

Hurst, K., Dean, A., and Trickey, S. (1991). The recognition and non-recognition of problem-solving stages in nursing practice. *Journal of Advanced Nursing, 16*(12), 1444–1455.

Johnson, P. A., Stone, M. A., Larson, A. M., and Hromek, C. A. (1992). Applying nursing diagnosis and nursing process to activities of daily living and mobility. *Geriatric Nursing, 13*(1), 25–27.

Town, J. (1993). Changing to computerized documentation-plus! *Nursing Management, 24* (7),44–46, 48.

CHAPTER 13

GETTING TO KNOW THE TRAVELER

MENTAL HEALTH ASSESSMENT

Nursing assessment is not about facts; it is about our interpretation or translation of the facts.... In assessment, we compose a picture of the person, building up layers of information, adding more detail about his emotions, his thoughts, his behavior, his beliefs and so on. The picture is a composition because we construct it. It is only our representation of the reality that is the patient.

—*Phil Barker*

LEARNING OBJECTIVES

After studying this chapter, you should be able to:

1. Identify at least two theoretical frameworks for developing a nursing assessment tool.
2. Explain how the nurse uses the initial nursing interview to establish a therapeutic relationship.
3. State at least three reasons why a structured data collection tool is necessary for assessment.
4. Discuss the four therapeutic factors introduced by the nurse during the initial interview.
5. Give two reasons for incorporating standardized rating scales into the nursing assessment process.
6. List five significant dimensions in a holistic data collection tool, based upon the American Nurses' Association standard for assessment.
7. Describe how discharge planning begins in the assessment phase of nursing care.
8. Name at least three functions of the nursing database.

KEY TERMINOLOGY

Assessment
Cognitive assessment
Data collection tool
Discharge planning
Emotional assessment
Physical assessment
Self-awareness
Sociocultural assessment
Spiritual and philosophical assessment
Standardized rating scales

Whenever you meet a patient for the first time, it is like starting a new journey for you and the patient. The journey holds not only the promise of discovery as you and the patient learn about each other, but also for you, the promise of continued self-discovery.

The process whereby you learn about a patient is called **assessment.** It differs from getting to know someone in social situations, when the interaction is more spontaneous, less planned, and with a shared focus on you and your partner. In the relationships that you develop with patients, you become acquainted through thoughtful, deliberate, and frequently structured approaches, in which the patient is the focus of the interaction.

Getting to know psychiatric patients is often complicated because the symptoms of their illnesses are manifested in their thought processes or in their ability to relate to others. In the following story, you will observe how psychiatric nurses were challenged to get to know and understand a person whose thought processes and means of communication were severely impaired.

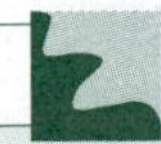

MRS. RYAN'S STORY

Mrs. Ryan is a 46-year-old, white, married, Roman Catholic woman who has been admitted to a university-affiliated psychiatric hospital. She has two school-age children and is a full-time homemaker. Her husband reports that, prior to admission, Mrs. Ryan had stopped eating and taking her medication and had begun to stay up all night pacing and talking to herself.

A Rough Beginning

On admission, Mrs. Ryan was disheveled and restless, and she alternated between refusing to answer questions and answering them incoherently. She had been hospitalized previously with a diagnosis of paranoid schizophrenia.

Because of Mrs. Ryan's intense physical activity and her inability to communicate verbally, the psychiatric nurses were unable to complete most of the nursing assessment. An assessment by the social work department, usually coordinated with the patient and family, was deferred because of Mrs. Ryan's disorganization.

The First Week of Hospitalization

During the first week of hospitalization, Mrs. Ryan took her medication and followed simple directions related to the activities of daily living. She dressed herself, but with uneven buttons and unmatched clothing, pushing away nursing staff who tried to assist. She needed supervision during meals and showers because she would not stay long enough to complete the tasks. She was able to toilet independently, and she began to sleep up to six hours at night. Mrs. Ryan often threw water on her face and hair and mumbled while looking at herself in the mirror.

The Second Week of Hospitalization

There was no change in Mrs. Ryan's behavior during the second week of hospitalization. Her physicians therefore increased her medication, and she began to nap during the day. When she wasn't napping, Mrs. Ryan paced alone in the hallway, talking softly to herself, or she isolated herself in her private room and did not interact with other patients on the ward. When her husband visited and brought her clothes or other items, she avoided him. He spent the visit times quietly sitting by himself in the dining area.

The nurses concluded that Mrs. Ryan was still too psychotic to try to complete the nursing assessment. They considered her too agitated to participate in group meetings and activity therapy.

The Third Week of Hospitalization

By the third week of hospitalization, Mrs. Ryan was pacing less. The night nurse reported that Mrs. Ryan cried at night and often said something that sounded like, "Who will feed the children?" Mrs. Ryan's psychiatric team discussed this observation, and they asked her if she was concerned about her children, but she refused to answer. Superficial conversations with Mr. Ryan gave the impression that he was managing the household adequately.

The Fourth Week of Hospitalization

At the end of the fourth week of hospitalization, there was no significant improvement in Mrs. Ryan's verbalization or hallucinations. She appeared to listen to staff members, but her answers to questions were incomprehensible. Every night she continued to cry. The staff began to give up hope for a quick recovery, calling her case "chronic." She participated minimally in the activities of the unit, and since she was not threatening to herself or others, she received a decreasing amount of attention from the nursing staff.

A consulting psychiatrist who visited weekly commented on Mrs. Ryan's lack of progress and encouraged the team to reevaluate her treatment plan. The treatment team then reviewed its assessment and noted how incomplete it was in the dimension of social/family issues. They agreed to hold a family meeting with Mr. Ryan to gather more history.

Mr. Ryan was cooperative, and his wife sat through most of the session and seemed to listen. As the team discussed family patterns and issues, Mr. Ryan admitted that he had a history of alcoholism and had had arguments with his wife over money prior to her hospitalization. One week, he said, he had spent his whole paycheck before buying groceries or paying any bills. Ever since his wife's hospitalization, he was staying sober, and the Ryan children were being cared for by a neighbor. Mr. Ryan reassured his wife that the children were safe, and the social worker arranged for them to visit briefly on the following evening.

Breakthrough

Within days of that family meeting, the staff noticed a decrease in Mrs. Ryan's pacing. She started to respond with a few words to questions about daily activities. Over the next few weeks, she made steady progress in her ability to communicate her needs and wishes. She requested a decrease in medication because she felt sedated. She asked to go to the beauty parlor on her first leave of absence because she looked "so horrible."

Mrs. Ryan was discharged after a 2-month stay. When she left, she was a quiet, soft-spoken woman who thanked the staff for helping her return to her family and home.

In the case of Mrs. Ryan and all psychiatric patients, the initial nursing assessment requires multiple skills in verbal and nonverbal communication, observation, self-awareness and relationship-building. As Mrs. Ryan's case illustrates, the psychiatric patient's ability to give an accurate history during admission may be quite limited. You must call on a creativity as well as sensitivity to gather the necessary information. The initial interview is the first step of the assessment stage of the nursing process. This stage establishes the framework for nursing diagnosis and development of the nursing care plan, including beginning phases of **discharge planning.** At the same time, the assessment interview sets the tone for your relationship with the patient as well as the shared journey on which you and the patient are about to embark. In this chapter you focus on your first contact with the psychiatric patient and the process for collecting objective data and establishing a therapeutic relationship. You are introduced to the use of standardized rating scales as part of a comprehensive assessment, as well as a holistic nursing assessment tool based on the American Nurses' Association (ANA) *Standards of Psychiatric-Mental Health Clinical Nursing Practice.*

THE NEED FOR STRUCTURED DATA COLLECTION

Although great variety exists among nurse theorists with regard to defining the proper dimensions of assessment, all agree on the need for a structured interview using a systematic **data collection tool.**

Data Collection Using Orem's Rehabilitation Model

One theory used to define a structure for data collection is Orem's rehabilitation model, which specifies seven areas of self-care for evaluation (Davidhizar and Cosgray, 1990):

- Intake of air, food, and fluid
- Elimination
- Maintenance of temperature and hygiene
- Balance between solitude and social activity
- Balance between rest and activity
- Prevention of hazards to life and functions
- Promotion of normalcy

Data Collection Using Roy's Adaptation Model

An alternative conceptual framework is the adaptation model, which defines five areas to explore (Johnson, 1984):

- Physiological
- Psychological
- Social
- Cultural
- Developmental

Data Collection Using Principles of Behavior Modification

Green (1987) suggests that behavior modification principles are applicable to the assessment process, with the following similarities in approach:

- The patient's behaviors are described in terms of frequency of occurrence and the context in which the behavior occurs.
- The description of behaviors includes a focus on preceding events and the consequences of particular behavior.
- The patient's skills and ability to learn are identified to plan appropriate interventions.

Data Collection Using Gordon's Functional Health Patterns

Gordon's functional health patterns provide still another structure for data collection. The functional health patterns are as follows (Hickey, 1990; Gordon, 1994):

- Health perception/health management
- Activity/exercise
- Nutrition/metabolic
- Elimination
- Sleep/rest
- Cognitive/perceptual
- Self-perception/self-concept
- Role/relationships
- Sexuality/reproductive
- Coping/stress tolerance
- Value/belief

The Focus of Assessment

Regardless of the theoretical approach to assessment, the focus of data collection is dependent on the patient's immediate condition or need. Accurate data collection reflects what the patient actually says, the behaviors observed, and specific information reported by others. It is imperative to distinguish accurate information from inferences, assumptions, interpretations, generalizations and judgments about the meaning of the information collected.

The database forms the baseline against which behavioral changes in the patient can be measured, indicating the effects of treatment. The database also contains the information necessary to formulate specific nursing diagnoses, identifying patient problems and responses; by the very nature of the questions, the patient is engaged as an active participant in planning care.

THE NEED FOR ATTENTION TO THE ART OF NURSING

Not only is it important for you to focus on collecting comprehensive data, but it also is equally important that you attend to the art of nursing through use of relationship-building skills during the assessment stage. The unique perspective of nursing, as compared with other health care professions, is its focus on the whole individual with his or her particular potential health problems, along with his or her particular responses. This approach is based on a number of factors:

- Respect for and acceptance of the individual
- The belief that mutually agreeable goals are essential for the patient's healing journey
- The belief in the importance of the patient's active participation in every phase of treatment

The ANA defines psychiatric mental health nursing as the "diagnosis and treatment of human responses to actual or potential mental health problems . . . a specialized area of nursing practice, employing theories of human behavior as its science and purposeful use of self as its art" (ANA, 1994). You must avoid following the medical model of seeking patterns of behavior and symptoms merely to establish a diagnosis and treatment plan (Salisbury, 1985).

Henderson (1987) warns nurses, as they collect assessment data, to avoid the specialized jargon so characteristic of medical assessment tools. Such jargon poses an unnecessary roadblock to the nurse-patient relationship, communication, and the nurse-patient journey. She encourages nurses to translate all of their observations and plans into simple terms that can be understood by patients and by other staff.

THE NEED FOR SELF-AWARENESS

The nursing assessment yields a database that provides objective details about patient problems and strengths, as well as the subjective nurse-patient reactions during the interview. To understand the subjective components of nursing assessment, you must possess **self-awareness;** you must be clearly aware of personal biases and have the ability to reflect on your own behavior throughout the interview. As one writer notes, "assessment packages are only as good as the expertise of the data collecting agent" (Farrell, 1991).

The quote at the beginning of the chapter implies that assessment data are more than facts; rather, they are the product of the interviewer, and they are not necessarily equal to the patient's perception of himself or herself or to the perceptions of others observing the same patient. This statement may have surprised you. However, we are not neutral in our responses to patients, and that lack of neutrality must be considered—not denied or ignored. In all communication situations both participants experience subjective responses. Relating to a patient who may be resistant or unable to verbalize clearly brings out various reactions in the nurse. These reactions must be recognized to differentiate your own responses from those of the patient. At the same time, an experienced nurse learns to use her or his feelings as a barometer to what is happening in the nurse-patient relationship. If the nurse feels anxiety only in the presence of a particular patient, it is probably indicative of some source of stress in the relationship that needs to be addressed.

Research comparing nurses' and patients' perceptions of needs has not shown consistent agreement. In one study comparing medical and psychiatric patients' self-report of needs with the nurses' perceptions of their needs, disagreement occurred in both specialties, with nurses tending to overestimate their patients' needs (Farrell, 1991).

The scientific approach to control this subjectivity includes the use of structured questions, observation, and standardized rating scales. Yet, even the use of measurement criteria may evoke a stereotype because the criteria automatically evaluate the patient against some standard of "normal" (Savage, 1991). It is important to prevent opinion from coloring both primary information, collected directly from the patient, and secondary information, obtained from other sources, including family, records, and other staff (Whyte and Youhill, 1984). With regard to secondary sources, you must be especially careful to seek current details rather than interpretations based on the past or based simply on appearances. Let's reflect on the journey of Mrs. Ryan.

> The staff assumed that the patient's family life was stable because the husband seemed "ok" during visits. Neither the nurses nor the other team members explored the social history as early as possible in the course of treatment, thereby delaying an effective intervention for the patient's tremendous anxiety level, namely, reassuring her that her children were safe. Mrs. Ryan's healing journey was delayed because of an incomplete database, which led to ineffective treatment.

Figure 13–1 illustrates the relationship between the nurse-patient relationship and the nursing process.

▶ Check Your Reading

1. Describe the three primary goals of the nursing assessment interview.
2. What are the seven aspects to evaluate in the rehabilitation model for nursing?
3. Name two main functions of the nursing database.
4. Why must the nurse be explicit about subjective impressions when interviewing the psychiatric patient?
5. Identify three ways to reduce the nurse's subjectivity in the assessment interview.

THE NEED FOR CONSIDERATION OF PATIENT PERCEPTIONS

Barker (1987) proposes that the interviewer proceed through five stages in the assessment interview in an

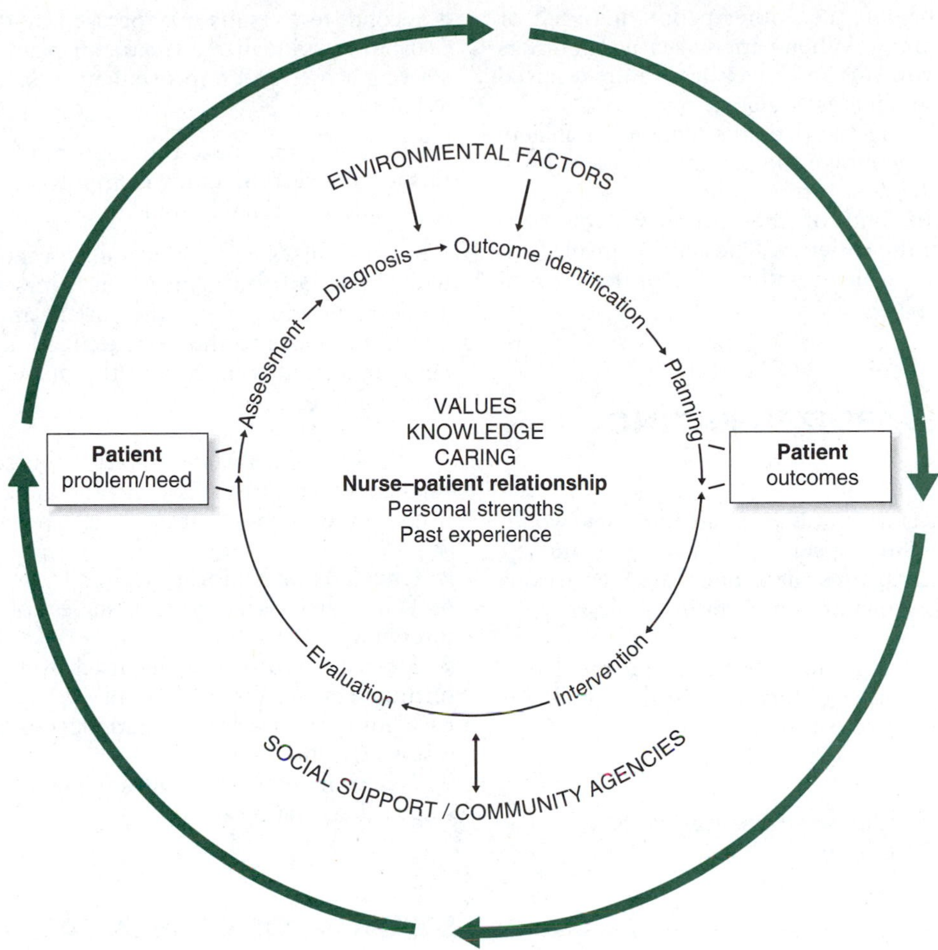

FIGURE 13–1

Significance of the nurse-patient relationship in the nursing process. (From Arnold, E., and Boggs, K. [1995]. *Interpersonal relationships: Professional communication skills for nurses* (2nd ed.). Philadelphia: W. B. Saunders.)

attempt to really learn about the patient's view of himself or herself and his or her problems. The first stage is identification of the problem from the patient's perspective, including how he or she feels about the problem, how it affects his or her relations with others, and whether it is inside of his or her head or his or her body. The second stage is measurement, a focus on the frequency of the problem behavior and the intensity of the patient's feeling about it. Third is clarification, asking about the effect of various situations or people on the problem behavior. Fourth is seeking the patient's explanation, a theory or belief about why this problem happened to him or her and what other people think and feel about him or her. The fifth stage is variation, looking for the patient's view of any patterns for his or her feelings and thoughts about the problem.

By placing a central focus on the patient's point of view, you are using the assessment interview to establish a relationship based on respect for the individual. Throughout the conversation, you listen attentively and accept the patient's report in a nonjudgmental way. The message given to the patient both verbally and nonverbally is that he or she is a partner in solving the problem. In addition to asking the required content of the data collection tool and conveying an attitude of respectful listening, you can give information that is immediately beneficial and therapeutic to the patient.

BEGINNING THE ASSESSMENT

Research into the factors that are most effective in psychiatric treatment has shown at least four elements that begin to operate in the initial interview, regardless of the discipline of the caregiver (Yalom, 1983; Hutton and Parkinson, 1993). First, merely providing information about the setting and admission procedures reduces the patient's anxiety about the unknown. A simple introduction and explanation about the purpose of the interview orients the patient to the current situation and establishes realistic expectations. Patients may not even remember how they got to a hospital, and they often may have misconceptions about the nature of psychiatric treatment.

Second, letting the patient know that he or she is not the only person with that particular problem brings out the factor of universality, i.e., other people have felt or believed the same thing. When patients learn that others have had similar problems and have successfully received treatment, they may feel less isolated.

Third, by reducing the patient's feelings of anxiety and isolation, you encourage the patient's sense of hope and positive expectations of treatment.

Fourth, by the end of the interview, you have communicated that the patient will be actively involved in decisions about care, which reinforces his or her sense of responsibility for self.

USING STANDARDIZED RATING SCALES

An overview of the nursing assessment interview would not be complete without special reference to the nurse's use of **standardized rating scales.** There are four reasons for you to become acquainted with rating scales:

- First, results of a standardized test enhance the data collection, adding another observation to the baseline that lends itself to future comparisons.
- Second, test results may be used by the treatment team to individualize a treatment plan, incorporating starting scores and improvement in scores as measurable goals.
- Third, you may have the opportunity to participate in formal research, and it is important to be familiar with valid and reliable tools.
- Finally, nurses and patients alike report satisfaction with the use of test instruments: Nurses feel that they are learning more about the patient and are able to contribute more to the team evaluation, and patients enjoy increased contact with the nurse, even if it is in a formal interview.

Table 13–1 lists standardized rating scales that are useful in mental health assessment and indicates how they are used. Some of these rating scales appear in Appendix I.

TABLE 13–1 Standardized Rating Scales and Their Use

Use	Scale(s)
Depression	Beck Inventory Hamilton's Depression Scale Montgomery-Asburg Depression Inventory Zung Self-Report Inventory
Anxiety	Modified Spielberger State Anxiety Scale Sheehan Patient-Related Anxiety Scale
Obsessive-compulsive behavior	Yale-Brown Obsessive-Compulsive Scale (Y-BOCS)
Mania	Mania Rating Scale
Schizophrenia	Scale for the Assessment of Negative Symptoms
Abnormal movements	Abnormal Involuntary Movement Scale (AIMS) Simpson Neurological Rating Scale CLAMPS Abnormal Movement Scale
General psychiatric assessment	Brief Psychiatric Rating Scale (BPRS) Global Assessment of Functioning Scale
Cognitive function	Mini-Mental State Examination
Assessment of children	Conners Parent Questionnaire Conners Teacher Questionnaire Children's Behavior Inventory Children's Psychiatric Rating Scale

▶ Check Your Reading

6. What are Barker's five stages of the assessment interview?
7. Describe two techniques used by the nurse to demonstrate respect for the patient.
8. Identify the four therapeutic factors that begin in the assessment interview.
9. Name at least three advantages of the nurse using standardized rating scales.

STANDARDS OF MENTAL HEALTH ASSESSMENT

The *Standards of Psychiatric-Mental Health Clinical Nursing Practice* published by the American Nurses' Association (ANA) provide a theoretical framework for a comprehensive assessment tool. In conjunction with the American Psychiatric Nurses Association, the Association of Child and Adolescent Psychiatric Nurses, and the Society for Education and Research in Mental Health Nursing, the ANA Council on Psychiatric and Mental Health Nursing revised its standards in 1994. The standards describe the nursing process in the six steps that we introduced in Chapter 12:

- Assessment
- Diagnosis
- Outcome identification
- Planning
- Implementation
- Evaluation

Standard I of the portion of those standards called the "Standards of Care" defines the rationale and measurement criteria for the assessment step as follows: "The psychiatric-mental health nurse collects client health data."

CONDUCTING THE ASSESSMENT

Now that we have outlined the nursing assessment process, identifying the need for objective data as well as for the therapeutic use of self in the interview, one sample of a holistic data collection tool using the ANA Standards as the framework can be examined.

Before explaining the tool itself, three overriding principles must be emphasized. First, upon admission to psychiatric care, the highest priority is placed on evaluation of the patient's safety. In fact, the defining criterion for hospital admission in many cases is literally dangerousness to self or others. You must be vigilant for any verbal or nonverbal signs of impending self-harm or destructive behavior.

Second, you must tailor the interview to the patient's immediate condition, prioritizing the questions to gain the most information possible at that time. The most elaborate tool is of little value when the patient is sedated or when he or she cannot sit still and verbalize clearly, as in the case of Mrs. Ryan. Using past experience and current cues from the patient, you select the most pertinent questions, realizing that an incomplete database becomes one of the first problems for the nursing care plan.

Third, data collection must be ongoing to complete the original database as soon as it is feasible. In the background story, the failure of the nurse to continue trying to complete the assessment contributed to the delay in helping Mrs. Ryan to face her major fear. Even when the patient cooperates with the full questionnaire, reassessment continues throughout the relationship to validate with the patient changes in priorities, plans, and effects of treatment. The following 11 sections explain the sample Psychiatric Nursing Assessment Tool that is found in Figure 13–2.

Patient Identification

After you introduce yourself and explain the purpose of the interview, it is important to ask the patient all of the basic questions listed in section I and to obtain a full set of vital signs. This initial information exchange provides a brief neutral zone in which the patient and nurse can observe each other and begin their journey. While the nurse may be analyzing the patient's orientation and general appearance, the patient is deciding if the nurse is trustworthy based on verbal and nonverbal signs of respect. The setting should be as quiet and private as possible. One small but important detail is to ask a patient his or her preference for the name that the staff will call them, i.e., Mr. X, the first name, or nickname. Without a preference, the patient is always addressed by his or her formal title. Last in this section, the vital signs are included—these data cannot be overlooked because the vital signs may be the first clue about a concurrent physical problem that the patient may not verbalize clearly (Dreyfus, 1987; Holmberg 1988).

► Check Your Reading

10. Identify the six stages of the nursing process as defined by the ANA.
11. What are the three significant principles guiding the nursing assessment, regardless of format?
12. What risk factor can be detected with routine vital signs?

Chief Complaint

This portion of the database requires much patience and encouragement on the part of the nurse as the patient begins to discuss potentially painful material. It is necessary to determine why the patient is seeking help at this point in time to allow the nurse to identify the precipitating event.

Questioning about suicidal and aggressive risks must be done in a matter-of-fact tone of voice. As the patient responds, the nurse has the opportunity to give information about hospital or agency procedures, e.g., precautions, privilege levels, and so forth. The nurse can also indicate that this problem is not totally unique and that other patients with similar concerns have been helped by treatment. It is imperative that the nurse record exactly what the patient says about his or her perception of the problem, regardless of what she or he may know from secondary sources. The patient's perceptions are the key to planning appropriate early interventions, and acceptance of his or her viewpoint engages the patient in planning for his or her own care (Whyte and Youhill, 1984; Wheeler, 1989). See Box 13–1 for sample interview questions to assess for suicidal or homicidal thoughts.

Medication History

The patient's use of medications is another crucial topic for you to explore because nursing staff members are involved in medication administration, and early treatment with an unknown patient poses certain risks. Ask the patient to recall as clearly as possible the names, dosage, and effects of all psychotropic medications. If a side effect or allergy is reported, a full description of the reaction is written because patients frequently use the term "allergy" when they mean minor side effect.

Studies have shown a high incidence of medication complications in patients receiving neuroleptics. It is estimated that 75% of all patients receiving antipsychotic medication suffer from extrapyramidal symptoms (EPS) (see Chapter 23 for a complete discussion of medication issues). For elderly patients, 17% of readmissions to hospitals may be due to adverse drug reactions (Blair, 1990). Because neuroleptic medication side effects range from minor (e.g., a tremor) to life-threatening (e.g., neuroleptic malignant syndrome), it is a serious nursing responsibility to try to prevent a recurrence in a susceptible patient. Prevention or prompt treatment of side effects not only minimizes patient distress during current treatment but also has an impact on the patient's future medication compliance. It is believed that one third of

Text continued on page 293

I. PATIENT IDENTIFICATION

Date and time of admission ______________________ By ______________________, R.N.

Name ______________________ Age __________ Sex __________ Race __________

Address ______________________ Phone __________

Significant other ______________________ Relation __________

Legal status ______________________ Referred by __________

Prefers to be called ______________________

Vital signs: BP __________ T__________ P__________ R__________ Ht __________ Wt __________

II. CHIEF COMPLAINT

Reason for seeking treatment ______________________

____

Recent history re: concerns ______________________

____

Any suicidal or aggressive ideation ______________________

____

Any history of suicidal or aggressive behavior ______________________

____

Any family history of suicide or violence ______________________

____

II. MEDICATION HISTORY (complete Medication Profile)

V. HISTORY OF PRIOR PSYCHIATRIC TREATMENT

Date(s), by whom, type ______________________

____

Compliance with treatment (any elopement or AMA D/C) ______________________

____

Effect of treatment ______________________

____

Goals for current treatment ______________________

____

V. EMOTIONAL ASSESSMENT

Mood: Anxious ☐ Depressed ☐ Euphoric ☐

Hostile ☐ Labile ☐ Other ☐

Describe (verbal and nonverbal signs): ______________________

____

Affect: Sad ☐ Elated ☐ Labile ☐

Flat ☐ Inappropriate ☐ Other ☐

Describe (verbal and nonverbal signs): ______________________

____

Coping patterns—describe usual behavior when feeling:

Anxious ______________________

Sad ______________________

Angry ______________________

FIGURE 13–2

A psychiatric nursing assessment tool.

VI. COGNITIVE ASSESSMENT

Orientation: Person ☐ Place ☐ Time ☐

Describe alteration ______________________________

Memory: Immediate ☐ Recent ☐ Remote ☐

Describe deficit(s) ______________________________

Attention: Alert ☐ Lethargic ☐ Distracted ☐

Other ☐ Describe other ______________________________

Fund of information: Last three presidents: ______________________________

Concentration: Serial 7s: ______________________________

Judgment: What would you do in a crowded movie theater if you smelled smoke?: ______________________________

Abstract thinking: Similarities (apple/orange): ______________________________

Proverb (glass houses): ______________________________

Perception: Hallucination ☐ Illusion ☐

Describe ______________________________

Communication: Verbal ______________________________

Nonverbal ______________________________

Any physical impairment No ☐ Yes ☐ Describe ______________________________

Thinking:

Logical ☐	Coherent ☐	Blocking ☐
Loose associations ☐	Disorganized ☐	Circumstantial ☐
Grandiose ☐	Paranoid ☐	Delusional ☐

Describe ______________________________

Self-concept: Strengths ______________________________

Weaknesses ______________________________

Insight: Recognizes need for help? Yes ☐ No ☐

Accepts responsibility for self? Yes ☐ No ☐

Describe ______________________________

FIGURE 13–2 *Continued*

Illustration continued on following page

VII. PHYSICAL ASSESSMENT

General appearance (include injuries, bruises, scars) ______________________________

Current physical complaints ______________________________

Current medications (add to profile on last page)
Previous illness/surgery/accident ______________________________

Any problem with:

Cardiac ☐	Respiratory ☐	Liver ☐
Urinary ☐	Brain ☐	Thyroid ☐
Reproductive/sexual ☐	Immune ☐	Bone/joint ☐
Blood sugar ☐	Other ______	

Describe onset, sx, tx ______________________________

Growth and development (family of origin, entering and leaving school, first job, first intimate relationship) ______________________________

TRIADS (Type, Role of offender, Intensity, Autonomic, Duration, Style) ______________________________

Activities of daily living (describe usual routine):

Sleep ______________________________

Eating (wt change) ______________________________

Elimination ______________________________

Exercise ______________________________

Work ______________________________

Leisure ______________________________

Use of caffeine, tobacco, alcohol, drugs ______________________________

Use of birth control/"safe sex" practices ______________________________

VIII. SOCIOCULTURAL ASSESSMENT

Living situation (spouse or significant other, children, home, responsibility) ______________________________

Support system (family, friends, agencies) ______________________________

Occupation/income ______________________________

Education ______________________________

Community involvement ______________________________

Current economic/legal/environmental stressors ______________________________

FIGURE 13–2 *Continued*

Ethnic background ______

Cultural beliefs related to current problem/treatment ______

IX. SPIRITUAL AND PHILOSOPHICAL ASSESSMENT

Spiritual beliefs ______

Participation in religious practices ______

Beliefs related to current problem ______

Beliefs related to current treatment ______

Most important life values ______

X. ADDITIONAL ASSESSMENT

Input from significant other/secondary source ______

Patient reaction to interviewer ______

Interviewer reaction to patient ______

XI. PROBLEM IDENTIFICATION AND NURSING DIAGNOSIS

(refer also to Medication Profile)

Prioritize the three most immediate needs by placing a number beside the appropriate description.

Emotional ______

Cognitive ______

Physical ______

Sociocultural ______

Spiritual ______

Discharge planning ______

Risk factors present (check all that apply or write N/A in each box):

Danger to self ☐ Danger to others ☐

Elopement ☐ History of noncompliance ☐

History of adverse medication reaction ☐ ______

Concurrent medical problem ☐ ______

Other ☐ Explain ______

If unable to complete full database, explain ______

(Follow up as necessary and write date and initials in each section when completed.)

FIGURE 13–2 *Continued*

Illustration continued on following page

III. MEDICATION PROFILE

Name ______ Age ______ Sex ______ Date of admission ______

Admission vital signs: BP ______ T ______ P ______ R ______ Ht ______ Wt ______

Allergies ______

Medication	Reason	Date Started	Dose	Effect	Side Effects/Adverse Reactions
I. Current prescriptions					
1.					
2.					
3.					
4.					
5.					
6.					
7.					
8.					
9.					
10.					
II. Current over-the-counter > weekly					
1.					
2.					
3.					
4.					
5.					
III. History of prescriptions					
1.					
2.					
3.					
4.					
5.					

FIGURE 13–2 *Continued*

BOX 13-1 Sample Interview Questions to Assess for Suicidal or Homicidal Thoughts

Suicidal Thoughts

- You say you are feeling very sad. Many times, when people feel sad they think about hurting themselves. Have you thought of hurting yourself?
- Are you thinking of hurting yourself now?
- If you would harm yourself, have you thought about how you would do it?
- Do you have a plan for hurting yourself?
- I would like to know what you are thinking and planning. I want to be able to protect you from hurting yourself, and I know that sometimes just talking about your ideas might make you feel less like hurting yourself.
- Have you thought of what life would be like if you were dead? What thoughts have you had?
- What has kept you from acting on these thoughts in the past?

Homicidal Thoughts

- You describe feeling uptight and angry. Have you thought of hurting someone else when you are feeling this way?
- Could you describe your hostile feelings to me?
- What have you done to control these feelings in the past?

schizophrenic patients on neuroleptics experience akinesia (patient complaint of stiffness in moving muscles, decreased motor activity) or akathesia (patient complaint of restlessness, inability to sit still), and they also have a relapse rate of 50% during the first year after hospitalization, largely because of noncompliance with medications (Michaels and Mumford, 1989; Blair, 1990). Not to be forgotten in this section is the patient's use of over-the-counter drugs or prescriptions for medical problems. In a state of emotional distress, patients may not produce a complete medical history, but they may tell you the names of prescription drugs they have been taking for medical problems.

History of Prior Psychiatric Treatment

It is important to get specific dates and effects of previous treatment to plan for the most effective current approach. As the patient describes his or her past care, you assess for patterns of compliance and begin to set realistic goals for treatment. Specifically, if the patient reports leaving treatment prematurely, either by elopement (running away) or by signing out against medical advice, this signals a potential risk for this admission. At the same time, it allows the patient to detail his or her dissatisfaction or disappointment with past treatment and encourages the setting of goals for this episode. Incorporating the patient's goals into the multidisciplinary treatment plan is one of the most important contributions made by the nurse.

▶ Check Your Reading

13. Why does the nurse record the patient's perceptions of the problem?
14. What questions must be answered in a medication history?
15. What is the primary reason for relapse in psychiatric patients?

Emotional Assessment

Even if the patient is unwilling or unable to discuss his or her coping patterns, much of the **emotional assessment** can be completed from previous observations. Again, record the exact words and actions that lead you to select a particular descriptive term. (For definitions and examples of terms commonly used to describe assessment findings, see Table 13–2.)

These behavioral snapshots compose the baseline picture against which comparisons are made to assess progress and to determine discharge criteria. If the patient can describe coping patterns, this information allows the nurse to support strengths and to identify areas of weakness in need of teaching.

Cognitive Assessment

Similar to the preceding part, **cognitive assessment** has already begun prior to these questions, and certain parts can be completed without further inquiry. But it is vital that you use precise questions to assess the patient's level of cognition because deficits are not always self-evident. The questions related to orientation, memory, attention, fund of information, judgment, and abstract thinking are derived from the Mini-Mental State Examination (MMSE). Studies have shown the MMSE to be an effective screening tool in identifying cognitive impairments, especially in the elderly (Rovner and Folstein, 1987). As before, whenever a descriptive term is checked, it must be accompanied by the specific words and actions of the patient.

The interview of the hallucinating patient requires additional attention to detail. Hallucinations may be present in a variety of conditions, including schizophrenia, mood disorders, and alcoholism. Not all hallucinations are considered unpleasant to the patient, and sometimes he or she hears multiple voices in dialogue that represent the positive and negative sides of an issue.

TABLE 13–2 Terms Commonly Used to Describe Assessment Findings

Term	Definition	Example
Affect		
Flat	Affect without any expression of feelings; unresponsive to varied topics or surroundings over time	Patient discusses the weather and her mother's death without any change in facial expression or tone of voice
Inappropriate	Affect does not match the feeling or topic being discussed	Person laughs when speaking of being afraid
Labile	Affect rapidly changes from one mood to another	During the course of a conversation, person cries and then laughs
Blocking	Involuntarily interrupting speech or train of thought	Patient begins to answer question but pauses at odd points while speaking
Circumstantiality	Pattern of speech in which irrelevant details are included with relevant details in describing an event, but follows through on one topic	Person describes his dinner but also describes what he was wearing and a phone call
Compulsion	An irresistible urge to repeatedly perform an act which may be contrary to one's usual standards due to extreme anxiety if the act is not completed	Person washes her hands five times each hour
Confabulation	Fabrication of events or situations to fill in gaps in memory, usually in a plausible way	Patient explains his black eye with elaborate story about a fight but his wife reports that he was home all evening
Delusion	A fixed belief that is defended intensely despite it's being illogical or unrealistic; paranoid with excessive suspiciousness; or grandiose with exaggerated view of self-worth	Patient believes the hospital food is poisoned and only eats food in sealed containers, or patient believes that she is an alien with supernatural powers
Echolalia	Automatic but meaningless repetition of another person's words	In response to question "Are you afraid?" patient answers "Afraid, afraid, afraid."
Echopraxia	Imitation of another person's body movements	Patient sits opposite the interviewer and copies the hand position and leg movements of the interviewer
Flight of ideas	Rapid stream of talk describing multiple topics unrelated to each other	Patient states, "I feel fine, the trees are green, the chairs are broken."
Hallucination	Sensory perception that does not result from real, external stimulus, most commonly auditory or visual but may be tactile, olfactory or gustatory	Patient hears voice of a relative talking about him or sees bugs on hands
Ideas of reference	Believing that statements or behavior of others are related to oneself even when no realistic connection exists	Patient believes talk show host is talking about him
Illusion	Misinterpretation of an external sensory stimulus, usually visual or auditory	Person sees clothing on a chair and thinks it is a cat
Loose associations	Pattern of speech in which the connections between ideas are so vague that, to the listener, they do not seem to follow any logical sequence	Patient talks about medication, then switches to describe a cat, and then changes the subject again
Neologism	Word invented by a person with a meaning specific to that person	A crying patient says, "My bermin hurts" but does not explain what that is
Obsession	Involuntary preoccupation with a particular thought or idea that seems irrational	A thin patient is preoccupied with fear of getting fat
Perseveration	Involuntary persistent or repetition of an idea or response	Patient keeps repeating one phrase over and over
Tangentiality	In conversation, the tendency for a response to digress from the original topic	When asked about sleep, the patient replies, "I sleep fine but my mother used to say that I sleep too much, she always criticizes me."

With prolonged hallucinations, many patients develop coping mechanisms to control them, e.g., wearing headphones, pacing, singing, humming, listening to loud music, and wearing ear plugs. If a patient is distracted and seems to be paying attention to internal rather than external stimuli, it may mean that the patient is hallucinating. Hallucinations can be auditory (hearing voices), visual (seeing things that others do not see), or olfactory (smelling things that others do not smell). If you think that your patient is hallucinating, inquire about (Williams, 1989)

- The type of perception
- How long it has been present and when it started
- How much the patient believes it is real
- The major emotional theme, i.e., is it harmful or helpful to the patient?
- The presence of any commands and the patient's response
- What coping strategies the patient uses to control the hallucinations

This knowledge is helpful in planning interventions that will support the patient's constructive coping patterns. It is important to recognize that it is not always possible to eliminate hallucinations in some patients; rather, the goal may be to help the patient to adapt to the impairment.

Physical Assessment

The abbreviated format used here for **physical assessment** is based on the assumption that the patient is receiving a physical examination and appropriate diagnostic tests as part of the admission procedure. If not, then the nurse needs to communicate with the patient's physician to compare her or his findings with the results of the most recent physical examination. Early identification of medical problems is essential to clarify the psychiatric diagnosis, to identify coexisting medical conditions, and to provide appropriate medical treatment.

Psychiatric patients are at increased risk for inadequate treatment of physical problems. Psychiatric illnesses frequently impair cognitive processes, which in turn results in impaired communication and social skills. These deficits pose a barrier to seeking help, verbalizing symptoms, and following through on treatment recommendations. Some studies point to a high incidence of cardiovascular and endocrine disorders in psychiatric patients that may go untreated without careful assessment (Holmberg, 1988).

Many times, a patient who has been reluctant to talk about emotions and thoughts will freely tell the nurse about physical complaints or difficulties in performing daily activities. In such cases, the nurse may decide that it is more productive to shift the conversation to physical issues for a period of time. Likewise, discussion of milestones in growth and development might also be less stressful for the patient. Once the patient is feeling more at ease, the nurse shifts back to a focus on emotions and feelings.

Two specific risk factors that may be uncovered by a thorough assessment of physical issues are risk for HIV infection and history of or current substance abuse. It is important to question knowledge of safer sex practice for all sexually active patients. Despite potential controversy related to staff or patient beliefs about contraception, precautions for safer sex are now frequently included as part of general health teaching for patients in hospital settings and nearly always involve the nurse (Davidhizar et al, 1990).

Signs of physical or sexual abuse may become apparent during evaluation of physical or social factors. The presence of physical injuries or a history of frequent accidents may signal an abusive relationship. Descriptions of conflict in the family of origin can hint at past abuse. If child abuse from the past is reported, it is important to gather information to assist in treatment. One strategy for collecting this information is the TRIADS system (Burgess et al, 1993):

- *T*ype of abuse
- *R*ole of relationship of the offender
- *I*ntensity of abuse
- *A*utonomic response
- *D*uration
- *S*tyle of abuse (access and pattern)

▶ **Check Your Reading**

16. Why must the nurse carefully explain each descriptive term?
17. What problems may be found through use of the Mini-Mental State Examination?
18. What specific information is gathered about hallucinations?
19. Name at least two risk factors that may be identified during the physical assessment.

Sociocultural Assessment

As illustrated in the case of Mrs. Ryan, performing a full **sociocultural assessment** with both the patient and significant others can have an impact on the course of treatment. Observations of the individual in a treatment setting, out of context of his or her usual social system, always present an incomplete picture. Data related to the patient's living situation and usual level of interpersonal activity are necessary to

- Understand the whole person
- Develop realistic treatment goals
- Clarify the presence or absence of the support system, which is relevant for successful discharge planning

Pressing financial or legal problems may need immediate attention to allow the patient to attend to even more abstract therapeutic goals. Appropriate referrals to other members of the treatment team or community resources need to be initiated as soon as the need is identified.

The patient's particular cultural or ethnic background contains further keys to treatment. It is essential for you to ask explicitly about the patient's values and beliefs related to

- What caused the present problem
- What will make it better

If the patient's or family's beliefs are at odds with the proposed treatment plan, increased risk for premature withdrawal from care or treatment failure exists.

Specific cultures have their own customs or traditional methods for healing, and increased awareness of these beliefs can facilitate selection of congruent treatment approaches. For example, Native Americans traditionally believe in the use of the "talking circle" to resolve problems; i.e., a group sits together in a circle, and everyone offers a prayer without interrupting each other. Thus, a Native American may benefit more from group therapeutic approaches than from a primary one-to-one relationship. At the same time, cultural belief systems may affect the patient's performance on testing instruments that were standardized with mainstream cultural values. For instance, it is culturally natural for an Inuit female to feel that she needs help with decision-making. Concluding that she is dependent and needs to increase assertiveness skills would be culturally inappropriate treatment (Manson et al, 1987; Campinha-Bacote, 1988).

Your awareness of your own cultural biases is essential to objectively evaluate and accept the patient's belief system. Studies evaluating the treatment effect of matching the patient and therapist according to race and ethnic background have had mixed results. Although similarity between the patient and therapist may make the therapist more of a role model to the patient, it does not necessarily improve the patient's general level of functioning. It seems that patient-therapist congruence in defining the problems and setting treatment goals is more important than matching their sociocultural backgrounds (Flaskerud, 1990). Chapter 14 offers suggestions for other cultural assessment inquiry.

Spiritual and Philosophical Assessment

Just as knowledge of sociocultural factors plays an important role in understanding the individual and formulating realistic treatment goals, so also a **spiritual and philosophical assessment** is important to complete. The presence and intensity of faith in God, degree of religious commitment, a sense of purpose and meaning, along with basic life values, strongly affect the patient's potential for recovery. Specific religious beliefs may be directly linked to the patient's view of the cause of illness and the direction for treatment. For example, it is common for people suffering from mental illness to seek assistance from a clergy person or spiritual leader before or concurrently to seeking professional help. It is important for the mental health team to recognize the importance of this spiritual support and to avoid minimizing it in any way. Box 13–2 offers specific questions to use in a spiritual and philosophical assessment.

The patient with a Judeo-Christian background may view his or her illness as a form of suffering for past sins. The patient may seek forgiveness as well as insight as a means of recovery and may respond well to insight-oriented one-to-one discussions. Prayer may be as much

BOX 13–2 Questions to Use in a Spiritual and Philosophical Assessment

Concept of God

Is religion or God important to you? If so, can you describe how?

Do you use prayer in your life? If so, does prayer benefit you in any way?

Do you believe God or a deity is involved in your personal life? If so, how?

What is your God or deity like?

Sources of Strength and Hope

Who are your support people?

Who is the most important person in your life?

Are people available to you when you are in need?

Who or what provides you with strength and hope?

Religious Practices

Is your religious faith helpful to you?

Are any religious practices meaningful to you?

Has your illness affected your religious practices?

Are any religious books or symbols helpful to you?

Meaning and Purpose

What gives your life meaning and purpose?

What makes you get up out of bed every morning and do what you have to do?

Do you feel that your life makes a difference? If so, in what ways?

In what ways has your illness had an impact on your meaning and purpose?

Modified from Carson, V.B. (1989). *Spiritual dimensions of nursing practice.* Philadelphia: W. B. Saunders.

a part of his or her healing as therapy (Hutton and Parkinson, 1993).

If the patient is unable to discuss spiritual issues during the initial assessment, it is valuable to follow up with these questions at a later time. This material allows the nurse to support positive beliefs and personal religious practices, but it also identifies an increased risk for the patient who feels hopeless and disengaged from any relationship to God.

Additional Assessment

This separate section is provided primarily for pertinent information from the family or other secondary sources regarding the patient's present behavior and past history. As noted earlier, these data supplement but do not substitute for the knowledge gained directly from the patient. Whenever a significant difference exists between the patient's and others' perceptions, you must respond first to the emotional needs of the patient to maintain the therapeutic relationship. For example, a patient arrives on the unit highly anxious, stating that he is being chased by enemy agents; but the police report that he was arrested for stealing food from a convenience store. Your initial intervention addresses the patient's feelings of fear and suspiciousness rather than focusing on socially appropriate behavior.

You also consider data collected by other health team members. For instance, if the patient has had psychological testing, the results of these tests are important pieces of data. Psychological tests provide information on personality styles, thought processes, and intellectual abilities. Tests might include the Minnesota Multi-Phasic Personality Inventory, the 16 P-F personality test, or the Rorschach Ink-Blot test.

Also included in this section is an explicit opportunity for the nurse to record subjective reactions during the interview. These observations acknowledge the importance of the nurse's continuous self-evaluation during the assessment interview and may be useful in interpreting the data.

▶ Check Your Reading

20. Identify three reasons to complete the sociocultural assessment.
21. What is the biggest risk if the patient's culture clashes with the treatment plan?
22. Must a match in ethnic background exist between the patient and therapist to allow a therapeutic effect to occur?
23. Name the significant risk factor that can be identified during the spiritual assessment.

Problem Identification and Nursing Diagnoses

The final section of the questionnaire documents your professional judgment about all of the data collected and deserves thoughtful attention. All problems and potential problems are identified using each major dimension, i.e., emotional, cognitive, physical, sociocultural, and spiritual. In addition, any needs related to discharge planning are summarized, including self-care deficits, support system, or referrals to other disciplines. The needs are prioritized to indicate at least the top three concerns that require immediate nursing attention. Risk factors are deliberately repeated to ensure that they are addressed in the initial treatment plan. Lack of completion of the full database calls for explanation and continued attempts until all information is obtained. (See Chapter 12 for a complete discussion of nursing diagnosis, outcome identification, planning, implementation, and evaluation.)

CONCLUSIONS

A thorough nursing database, concluding with appropriate nursing diagnoses, serves four vital functions: It defines the focus of nursing care for one particular patient, allowing for a comprehensive nursing care plan. It serves as a means of communication with nurses and other colleagues who read the database (or conclusions) as they collect and compare their own data. It interjects the input of nurses into the multidisciplinary treatment plan, advocating for recognition of the patient's own goals. And, finally, it facilitates continued learning on the part of the nurse interviewer as she or he uses nursing diagnoses to describe the problems faced by a unique individual. In some nursing systems, assessment data have even proven valuable as the foundation of a patient acuity system, which ultimately determines nursing staffing patterns (Hay and Nelson, 1988; Karshmer, 1991).

As you meet each new patient, another journey begins. Initially, you try to gather as much subjective and objective information as possible from a stranger who presents with impaired communication skills. At the same time, you begin to develop a therapeutic relationship with the patient to provide a basis for trust and hope in treatment. Ongoing assessment leads you to a fuller appreciation of the patient as a unique person with unique strengths, fears, hopes, and goals. And along the way, you discover more about yourself, enhancing both your professional growth and your personal growth.

KEY POINTS TO REMEMBER

- Psychiatric patients may be limited in their abilities to give an accurate history.
- The initial interview is the first step in the assessment process.
- The assessment phase of the nursing process establishes the foundation for nursing diagnoses, the development of the nursing care plan, and the beginning phases of discharge planning.
- Orem's Rehabilitation Model specifies seven areas for assess-

ment: intake of air, food, and fluid; elimination; maintenance of temperature and hygiene; balance between solitude and social activity; balance between rest and activity; prevention of hazard to life and functions; and promotion of normalcy.

- The adaptation model defines five areas for assessment: physiological, psychological, social, cultural, and developmental.
- The behavior modification model suggests describing the patient's behaviors in terms of frequency and the context in which the behavior occurs. The description of events includes a focus on those events immediately preceding and following a particular behavior, and the patient's skills and abilities to learn are identified; these elements allow you to plan appropriate interventions.
- Gordon's functional health patterns suggest another structure for assessing data. These include health perception/health management; activity/exercise; nutrition/metabolic; elimination; sleep/rest; cognitive/perceptual; self-perception/self-concept; role/relationships; sexuality/reproduction; coping/stress tolerance; and value/belief.
- The focus of attention in assessment is the patient's immediate condition or need.
- Assessment reflects what the patient says, the behaviors observed, and specific information reported by others.
- Assessment involves the art of nursing, as relationship and communication skills facilitate data collection.
- Assessment necessitates that the nurse continually evaluate his or her own reactions, values, and beliefs.
- Subjectivity can be controlled through the use of structured questions, observations, and the use of standardized assessment tools.
- Baker states that the assessment interview has five stages, including identification of the problem from the patient's perspective; measurement of the behaviors; clarification of problem; seeking of the patient's explanation; and variation.
- Beginning the assessment involves providing information to the patient; letting the patient know that she or he is not alone with the problem; reducing the patient's feelings of anxiety; and communicating that the patient is part of the decision-making process.
- Standardized assessment tools enhance data collection; the results are used in planning, the data are used in research, and nurses and patients experience satisfaction with using standardized instruments.
- The 1994 standards of psychiatric-mental health nursing published by the American Nurses' Association provide a framework for comprehensive assessment.
- The assessment collects data about patient identification, patient's chief complaint, medication history, history of prior psychiatric history, emotional and cognitive assessment, physical assessment, sociocultural assessment, spiritual and philosophical assessment, additional assessment, and problem identification and nursing diagnoses.

LEARNING ACTIVITIES

1. Practice the database with a friend and find out how much you do or do not know about the person.
2. Question yourself and identify which sections are the most personal and difficult to discuss.
3. Observe two people talking and look for the nonverbal signs of listening behavior that encourage the conversation.
4. Explore the standardized rating scales and score yourself on one of them.

CRITICAL THINKING EXERCISE

Mrs. James was admitted to the psychiatric diagnostic unit with difficulty concentrating, headaches, and sleeplessness. Past history shows two depressive episodes following surgery for cervical cancer two years earlier. Although her admitting diagnosis is depression, an MRI scan of her head was ordered because of her medical history. The patient fears that her cancer has returned. She tells her nurse that if they find another tumor she will kill herself.

1. What is the patient's point of view?
2. What assumption(s) is the patient making?
3. What inference(s) can the nurse draw from the patient's statement?

The head nurse believes in the Kantian imperative of always telling the truth and informs the patient that her cancer has spread without preparing her for the bad news.

1. What assumption is the nurse making about the truth?
2. What conclusions has she drawn about the patient's belief system?
3. What evidence suggests that the nurse's conclusion to inform the patient may be faulty?

REFERENCES

American Nurses' Association Council on Psychiatry & Mental Health Nursing, (1994). *A statement on psychiatric and mental health clinical nursing practice and standards of psychiatric-mental health clinical nursing practice* (p. 25). Washington, D. C.: American Nurses Publishing.

Barker, P. (1987). Assembling the pieces. *Nursing Times, 83* (47), 67.

Beeber, L. S. (1989). Enacting corrective interpersonal experiences with the depressed client: An intervention model. *Archives of Psychiatric Nursing, 3* (4), 211.

Berry, K. N. (1987). Let's create diagnoses psych nurses can use. *American Journal of Nursing*, May, 707.

Berthot, B. D., and Lapierre, E. D. (1989). What does it mean? A new scale for rating patients' behavior. *Journal of Psychosocial Nursing*, 27 (10), 25.

Blair, D. T. (1990). Risk management for extrapyramidal symptoms. *Quality Review Bulletin*, March, 116.

Burgess, A. W., Hartman, C. R., and Kelley, S. J. (1990). Assessing child abuse: The TRIADS checklist. *Journal of Psychosocial Nursing, 28* (4), 7.

Campinha-Bacote, J. (1988). Culturological assessment: An important factor in psychiatric consultation-liaison nursing. *Archives of Psychiatric Nursing, II* (4), 244.

Carson, V. B. (1989). *Spiritual dimensions of nursing practice.* Philadelphia: W. B. Saunders.

Catherman, A. (1990). Biopsychosocial nursing assessment: A way to enhance care plans. *Journal of Psychosocial Nursing, 28* (6), 31.

Crook, S., and Beail, N. (1987). Standing up to assessment. *Nursing Times*, March 25, 34.

Davidhizar, R., Boonstra, C., Lutz, K., and Poston, P. (1991). Teaching safer sex in a long-term psychiatric setting. *Perspectives in Psychiatric Care*, 27 (1), 25.

Davidhizar, R., and Cosgray, R. (1990). The use of Orem's model in psychiatric rehabilitation assessment. *Rehabilitation Nursing, 15* (1), 39.

Downing, A. R., and Brockington, I. F. (1978). Nurse-rating of psychotic behavior. *Journal of Advanced Nursing, 3*, 551.

Dreyfus, J. K. (1987). Nursing assessment of the E D patient with psychiatric symptoms: A quick reference. *Journal of Emergency Nursing, 13* (5), 278.

Farrell, G. A. (1991). How accurately do nurses perceive patients' needs? A comparison of general and psychiatric settings. *Journal of Advanced Nursing, 16*, 1062.

Flaskerud, J. H.: Matching client and therapist ethnicity, language and gender: A review of research. *Issues in Mental Health Nursing, 11*, 321.

Gordon, M. (1994). *Nursing diagnosis: process and application* (3rd Ed.). New York: McGraw-Hill.

Green, C. (1987). The importance of behavior modification for the nursing process in mental handicap. *Nurse Education Today*, 7, 59.

Hay, M. A., and Nelson, L. M. (1988). Client classification a "needs" approach. *Journal of Psychosocial Nursing, 26* (12), 23.

Henderson, V. (1987). Nursing process—a critique. *Holistic Nursing Practice, 1* (3), 7.

Hickey, P. (1990). *Nursing process handbook.* St. Louis: C. V. Mosby.

Holmberg, S. (1988). Physical health problems of the psychiatric client. *Journal of Psychosocial Nursing, 26* (5), 35.

Hutton, A. P., and Parkinson, A. R. (1993). Theoretical bases for nursing diagnosis in mental health nursing. In R. P. Rawlins, S. R. Williams, and M. N. Johnson (Eds.), *Nursing process in psychiatric nursing.* St. Louis: C. V. Mosby.

Kuhlman, T. L., Sincaban, V. A., and Bernstein, M. J.: Team use of the Global Assessment Scale for inpatient planning and evaluation. *Hospital and Community Psychiatry, 41* (4), 416.

Johnson, M. N. (1984). Theoretical bases for nursing diagnosis in mental health nursing. *Issues in Mental Health Nursing, 6*, 53.

Lesage, A. D., Cyr, M., and Toupin, J. (1991). Reliable use of the Present State Examination by psychiatric nurses for clinical studies of psychotic and nonpsychotic patients. *Acta Psychiatrica Scandinavica, 83*, 121.

Malone, J. A. (1991). The DSM-III-R versus nursing diagnosis: A dilemma in interdisciplinary practice. *Issues in Mental Health Nursing, 12*, 219.

Manson, S. M., Walker, R. D., and Kivlahan, D. R. (1987). Psychiatric assessment and treatment of American Indians and Alaska natives. *Hospital and Community Psychiatry, 38* (2), 165.

McDougall, G. J. (1990). A review of screening instruments for assessing cognition and mental status in older adults. *Nurse Practitioner, 15* (11), 18.

McGorry, P. D., Goodwin, R. J., and Stuart, G. W. (1988). The development, use and reliability of the Brief Psychiatric Rating Scale (Nursing Modification)—an assessment procedure for the nursing team in clinical and research settings. *Comprehensive Psychiatry, 29* (6), 575.

Michaels, R. A., and Mumford, K. (1989). Identifying akinesia and akathisia: The relationship between patient's self-report and nurse's assessment. *Archives of Psychiatric Nursing, III* (2), 97.

Morrison, E. F. (1990). Nursing adaptation evaluation: A method for evaluating nursing care. *Perspectives in Psychiatric Care 26* (4), 11.

Mulhearn, S. (1989). The nursing process: Improving psychiatric admission assessment? *Journal of Advanced Nursing*, 14, 808.

Reed, R. C. (1989). Chaining nursing diagnosis: The use of etiological sequencing in the development of a plan of care. *Archives of Psychiatric Nursing, III* (6), 344.

Reimer, T. T., Brink, P. J., and Saunders, J. M. (1984). Cultural assessment: Content and process. *Nursing Outlook, 32* (2), 78.

Richards, D. A., and Lambert, P. (1987). The nursing process: The effect on patients' satisfaction with nursing care. *Journal of Advanced Nursing, 12*, 559.

Robitaille-Tremblay, M. (1984). A data collection tool for the psychiatric nurse. *Canadian Nurse*, August, 36.

Rovner, B. W., and Folstein, M. F. (1987). Mini-Mental State Exam in clinical practice. *Hospital Practice*, January 30, 99.

Salisbury, D. (1985). Don't waste the process. *Nursing Times*, March 6, 42.

Sanger, E., Thomas, M. D., and Whitney, J. D. (1988). A guide for nursing assessment of the psychiatric inpatient. *Archives of Psychiatric Nursing, II* (6), 334.

Savage, P. (1991). Patient assessment in psychiatric nursing. *Journal of Advanced Nursing, 16*, 311.

Seymour, J., Saunders, P., Wattis, J. P., and Daly, L. (1994). Evaluation of early dementia by a trained nurse. *International Journal of Geriatric Psychiatry 9* (1), 37–42.

VanCott, M. L. (1993). Communicative competence during nursing admission interviews of elderly patients in acute care settings. *Qualitative Health Research 3* (2), 184–208.

Wheeler, S. Q. (1989). ED telephone triage: Lessons learned from unusual calls. *Journal of Emergency Nursing, 15* (6), 481.

Whyte, L., and Youhill, G. (1984). The nursing process in the care of the mentally ill. *Nursing Times*, February 1, 49.

Williams, C. A. (1989). Perspectives on the hallucinatory process. *Issues in Mental Health Nursing*, 10, 99.

Yalom, I. (1983). Inpatient group psychotherapy. New York: Basic Books.

Zimmerman, M. (1993). A five-minute psychiatric screening interview. *Journal of Family Practice* 37 (5), 479–482.

SUGGESTED READINGS

Burgess, A. W., Hartman, C. R., and Kelley, S. J. (1990). Assessing child abuse: The TRIADS checklist. *Journal of Psychosocial Nursing, 28* (4), 7.

Savage, P. (1991). Patient assessment in psychiatric nursing. *Journal of Advanced Nursing, 16*, 311.

Seymour, J., Saunders, P., Wattis, J. P., and Daly, L. (1994). Evaluation of early dementia by a trained nurse. *International Journal of Geriatric Psychiatry, 9* (1), 37–42.

VanCott, M. L. (1993). Communicative competence during nursing admission interviews of elderly patients in acute care settings. *Qualitative Health Research, 3* (2), 184–208.

Zimmerman, M. (1993). A five-minute psychiatric screening interview. *Journal of Family Practice*, 37 (5), 479–482.

CHAPTER 14

TRAVELERS FROM MANY LANDS

THE IMPACT OF CULTURE

The flow of cultural generations is a continuum to which each individual born contributes and from which each individual passing subtracts

—Theodore Schwartz

LEARNING OBJECTIVES

After studying this chapter, you should be able to:

1. Define the components of culture.
2. Discuss the differences between stereotypes and levels of prejudice.
3. Assess the importance of ethnic identity in patients and their extended families.
4. Recognize the significance of beliefs, perceptions, and values as facilitating or impeding help-seeking behavior.
5. Develop a frame of reference when interpreting cultural support systems.
6. Acquire the knowledge and skills needed to intervene appropriately for the patient's culture and difficulties.
7. Assess your journey to various cultures.

KEY TERMINOLOGY

Culture
Culture-bound syndrome
Ethnic competence
Ethnic identity
Ethnocentrism
Prejudice
Race
Racism
Stereotype
Transcultural identification

Nursing is a journey to many cultures, for every patient is a mosaic of cultural conditioning. Culture represents the interplay between individuals and their society. Patterns of behavior are learned, shared, organized, and transmitted by groups and individuals (Linton, 1945). Inherent in every culture are beliefs and values; behavior that is esteemed; and taboo, roles, and relationships that give meaning to human encounters.

Every culture has norms or standards of behavior that it considers reasonable and normal rather than disabling and abnormal. The diversity of patients seeking mental health care requires that caregivers have an understanding of cultural relativity. Brent and Callwood (1993, p. 293) suggest "viewing behaviors of other groups as different from those of one's own without value judgements. Not 'better' or 'worse' than, just 'different' from."

Nurses bring their own hierarchy of values and subjective view of the world to the art of healing. Every human being embraces a system of values, private or public, admitted or tacit (Harris, 1972). Understanding terms such as ethnic identity, culture, and stereotyping is therefore basic to the delivery of helpful and healing services. As professionals, the greatest challenge is to provide care that is culturally relevant to various ethnic groups.

This chapter provides you with an understanding of terms that will help you describe and understand culture: stereotyping, prejudice, ethnic identity, racism, race, culture-bound syndromes, ethnic competence, ethnocentrism, and transcultural identification. Each term identifies a concept that equips you to become a culturally sensitive nurse—one who can meet patients wherever they are on their journeys.

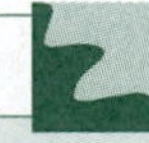

THAO'S STORY

Try to imagine a country scarred and broken by war. Intellectuals and professionals must hide their identity to survive. A new generation of citizens is forced to embrace an ideology foreign to their ancient traditions.

Imagine a young wife with three small children. She pondered her fate and the fate of her children as her husband was sent to a reeducation camp. His "crime" was that he had been a military officer in South Vietnam. Now he was doomed to years of torment, forced manual labor, and tedious hours of indoctrination. His sentence was indeterminate because he had to learn to be a good Communist. No one knew how long he would be held. Imagine the restless nights, the myriad questions, the "what ifs" endured by his young wife and family. Would he resist reeducation? Could he endure the indefinite years of isolation from family and friends? Would he survive the harsh prison environment? What would be the consequences for the family?

Thao's Decision to Leave

In the late 1970s, Saigon was still an important hub for making connections to the political taskmasters and for mastering the intricacies of escape. Thao, the young wife and mother, valued family, tradition, dignity, and education, but none of these could be realized without freedom. If she remained in Saigon, her three children—Leong, age 6; Fong, age 5; and Pguong, age 4—would never have an opportunity to live freely and follow the ancient traditions. Soon Thao realized her close-knit family and neighbors had come to the same conclusion. Because the Communists wanted to rid Vietnam of ethnic Chinese, Thao and some of her family and friends, more than 150 people, plotted their escape by obtaining false papers.

Imagine the grief in bidding goodbye to elderly parents, sisters, brothers, nieces, and nephews who elected to stay behind to care for the elderly and be a living presence in their ancient land. Imagine this young wife unable to have a final embrace with her spouse or even risk telling him of the escape plan. Imagine three wide-eyed youngsters who could not be told of the proposed journey and could not take any childhood mementos with them. The journey must be planned with no hint of deception to the new regime, who had eyes and ears everywhere!

The Family's Escape

The secret escape meant that 150 people had to travel in little groups, partially by bus and foot to reach a coastal town where a boat was waiting to take them to an unknown destination. Imagine sitting in a crowded bus and peering out windows to etch in one's memory the last scenes of home. How many times their hearts pounded with fear, anxiety, and sadness! Would their fake papers be uncovered? Would someone in the group become too ill to continue the journey? Imagine arriving in the coastal town where the sea of humanity surged relentlessly toward unstable boats. The exit price was exact—12 ounces of gold for each person stepping onto the boat.

Imagine the boat finally chugging toward open sea—would they encounter pirates or endure brutal rapes, starvation, and death? Imagine seeing the shoreline of one's beloved country fade in the mist and mingle with tears for what might have been and those who were left behind. Imagine being well educated, a professional, who must now endure a refugee camp in Indonesia. During her months in the refugee camp, Thao desperately tried to contact relatives in California—to no avail. They had moved, and their current whereabouts were unknown. Engulfed in hopelessness, Thao wondered, "Was I stupid? Did I make a mistake? Is this going to be the rest of my life?" Finally a sensitive immigration officer and a staff member with the Refugee High Commission learned that Thao's husband was a political prisoner in a reeducation camp, with no hope of release.

Thao sighed with relief and pent-up grief when informed in late 1979 that she and her children would be admitted to the United States as refugees. Imagine stepping off the plane in Norfolk, Virginia in December 1979. There was a chill in the air; there were no familiar faces, sights, sounds, or scents. Everything was different.

Life in a New Land

Imagine exchanging upper-middle-class status for a working-class life in a foreign country. Imagine having to search for stores where one could buy traditional foods. Imagine having no temple in which to worship and no extended community to celebrate religious festivals. Imagine trying to make children practice their native language when no neighbor or classmate could speak Vietnamese. Imagine working full time and striving to hold part-time and seasonal jobs to support not only the family in the United States, but also the loved ones left behind. Imagine getting word that your husband lay very ill and medication needed was costly and would not be provided because he had not yet demonstrated that he was reeducated.

Imagine the physical exhaustion of working untold hours, the constant anguish about loved ones left behind, and the strain of balancing raising one's children to be both American and Vietnamese. Imagine being robbed of years of marital companionship and children who could no longer recall what their father looked like.

Imagine the daily journey to be a good person, neighbor, citizen, and success by American standards. Throughout these years, Thao maintained her modest decorum, inspired her children to excel in their studies, and offered prayers to bless those left behind. Today, Thao jokes about retiring as she works as a cultural "broker" for the latest wave of refugees. Her three children attend Virginia universities on scholarships. Leong's goal is to be a medical doctor. Fong wants to be a psychologist. Pguong hopes for a career in international journalism. Their lives are now full of hope. For Thao and her children, the longing for loved ones in Vietnam has been answered: A local television station that documented the family odyssey is providing them a journey home.

UNDERSTANDING CULTURE-RELATED TERMS

Culture

Culture refers to the pattern of beliefs, behaviors, foods, dress, music, and traditions that gives a group its distinctiveness. Members of a cultural group share a consensus of beliefs, social norms, and ways of responding to life. Group members view the world through a distinctness engendered by religious tenets, philosophy of life, history, and lived experiences.

Cultures are made vibrant by both continuity and change. In Asia, for example, the elderly have traditionally been respected, with ancestors celebrated and remembered in ceremonial rituals and shrines. Social transformation, however, has diminished family support, even among the family-oriented Chinese (Heok, 1994). Cultures are not fixed in concrete but are subject to growth. Economic conditions, media influences, war, famine, and political upheavals can change even those cultures that have protected themselves from outside influences, as the Chinese have. Perception and interpretation of other cultures are ongoing processes.

Who has the knowledge to interpret or judge another's culture? Serving others as a nurse means developing universal love and acceptance of all people. Universal love is not only psychologically possible, but also essential, the only complete and final way to love (de Chardin, 1967). Understanding another's culture may be a lifelong task. Patience, persistence, effort, and real caring are necessary elements if you are to begin the journey of understanding a fellow traveler's culture.

▶ **Check Your Reading**

1. What is culture?
2. What external influences change cultures?

Stereotyping

A **stereotype** is an exaggerated belief or fixed idea about a person or group and is sustained by selective perception and selective forgetting. Stereotyping leads to tunnel vision, myths, and "isms" about an individual or a group of people. For instance, the term *old age* has different cultural interpretations. Chronological peers are not always psychological peers. A 65-year-old living in the United States, active and in good health, may contemplate taking on a second or even third career; a person of the same age, in poor health and with a diminished hope that life will improve, may act like a person decades older. Yet age 65 is commonly seen as the retirement age for those in their sixties. Beyond age 65, people are labeled senior citizens. Such a label hides individual identity, values, aspirations, and achievements.

Stereotypes relating to age, race, sex, and religion abound, resulting in rigid preconceptions used to label people. As a helping professional you need to engage individuals in the wholeness of their humanity. You must look beyond the surface, the label, and the diagnosis. Tap into the essence of the patient. What keeps the patient hoping? What brings comfort and joy? What causes anxiety, depression, or isolation? What experiences have significantly shaped the patient's personality? How does a particular culture define mental health and mental illness?

Concern about stereotyping also raises the concern about the role of ethnicity, social class, gender, help-seeking patterns, bias in psychiatric diagnosis, and involuntary commitment in minority populations (Good, 1993). Diagnosis involves complex relations, beliefs, language, and differential interpretations of illness. Good (1993, p. 431) cites the work of Snowden and Cheung (1990), who concluded:

> *Blacks and Native Americans are considerably more likely than Whites to be hospitalized; Blacks are more likely than Whites to be admitted as schizophrenic and less likely to be diagnosed as having an affective disorder. Asian-Americans/Pacific Islanders are less likely than Whites to be admitted, but remain for a lengthier stay, at least in state and county mental hospitals.*

Specific patterns of misdiagnosis, lack of culturally valid diagnostic instruments, and culturally competent mental health practitioners may, in fact, put minorities at greater risk for diagnosis of serious mental illness, hospitalization, and social stigma. These factors are intertwined with stereotyping and practitioner bias.

As early as 1968, Robert Butler, a physician, suggested that *ageism*, a stereotypical way of dealing with the elderly, was a prejudice toward a segment of society. Ageism is based on half-truths, apathy, and ignorance (McKenzie, 1980). Labels in mental health imply that precise distinctions can be made between "normal" and "abnormal" behavior. The process, however, raises serious questions of cultural relevancy and ethics in nursing care. Clinical assessment is a complex task. Interviewing techniques and other assessment tools may not be culture fair, compounding the problems of transcultural nursing.

Brink (1990, pp. 3–4) defines *transcultural nursing* as "the fusion of nursing and anthropology in both theory and practice." Brink offers an antidote to labeling:

> *If nurses, whatever their specialty, would view every patient care situation as a study sample of one, collect data on that case, and compare all cases at the end of a year's period, then generalizations could be made on the basis of that comparative data, and each nurse would have added to the body of nursing literature in that field.*

The issue of labeling and labeling theory is also central to Cohen's reevaluation of cross-cultural research. Cohen (1992, p. 60) cites Waxler's work, which found that specific social and cultural variables influenced the "molding" of mental illness in Sri Lanka:

> *The first factor was the Sinhalese family, described as being large, tolerant, and relatively strong; mentally ill members were neither alienated nor rejected, but rather cared for and given positive social support. The second factor was the treatment system in which there were many choices and all*

care was short-term. The family retains control not only over treatments themselves but also over the messages about illness given by treatment people. The Sinhalese explain mental illness in terms of external causation: gods, demons or sorcery are responsible for the aberrant behavior in the mentally ill. For these reasons, the mentally ill person's self and social past are not under suspicion, stigmatization can be avoided, and treatment follows a "standard and ritualistic" course.

Sinhalese culture mediates on behalf of the patient, thus eliminating the negative effects of labeling and stereotyping. The complications of labels such as *insane* or *schizophrenic* are long term: "Once a person is designated abnormal, all of his other behaviors and characteristics are colored by that label" (Rosenhau, 1990, p. 181).

As travelers trying to understand other cultures, we might recall the words of St. Paul: "I don't understand myself at all. The good that I would do, I do not, and that which I would not, that I do" (Rm 7:15). The desire to avoid stereotypes and labeling must commence with a desire to transform the dark corners of your being into areas of light (Catoir, 1990).

▶ Check Your Reading

3. How do stereotypes perpetuate "isms"?
4. Besides age, what other characteristics are subject to stereotyping?

Prejudice

Prejudice is a preconceived idea or attitude, which can be negative, formed before the facts are known, and sustained by overgeneralizations. Prejudice represents a bias without reason, resisting all evidence. Two essential ingredients of prejudice are (1) an attitude of favor or disfavor and (2) an erroneous belief.

Allport's (1979) classic book, *The Nature of Prejudice*, offers insight into levels of prejudice.

- *Antilocution* is talking about a targeted group of people with like-minded people or joking to demean members of a group that is ethnically or culturally different.
- *Avoidance* is an intentional way of behaving designed to forestall, inhibit, or diminish contact with others who are viewed as different.
- *Discrimination* is active exclusion of people who are different by contrived rules or regulations.
- *Physical attack* is violent touching that results from heightened emotions, inadequate facts, and closed minds, in which hatred and division are nurtured.
- *Extermination* is aimed at the deliberate and systematic destruction of a racial, political or cultural group as demonstrated by lynchings, pogroms, massacres, and genocide.

As the levels of prejudice intensify from antilocution to extermination, the targeted persons "develop social formation which appears to the surrounding oppressive culture to be excessive or pathological" (Lerner, 1972, p. 465). The coping mechanisms of the targeted group may result in extreme withdrawal or behavior marked by intense fear.

Those who are targets of prejudice are depersonalized and dehumanized, both of which mitigate against good mental health. Prejudice against those with mental health problems also exists worldwide and is operative at all levels beginning with antilocution. The misconceptions persist that persons with mental illness are "incurable and dangerous" and "to blame for their conditions." Former friends avoid the patient. Discrimination, sometimes subtle, sometimes overt, occurs in employment, particularly in promotion, professional, or political careers. In societies with low tolerance for persons with mental illness, cases of physical attack and extermination have been documented, especially during great upheavals, such as war and famine.

▶ Check Your Reading

5. How do levels of prejudice differ in intensity?
6. What prejudices are held toward the mentally ill?

Race and Racism

Race broadly distinguishes individuals or groups on the basis of appearance. Judging others simply on appearance leads to erroneous decision making, false assumptions, and denial of the uniqueness of each person. **Racism** is a belief that one racial or ethnic group is inferior to another and that unequal treatment is therefore justified. Understanding a specific individual and group in relation to other groups for Burke (1986) implies an investigation of five aspects of race:

- *Prejudice* on an individual level is evidenced by an attitude of derogation, avoidance, discrimination, or attack on another person.
- *Institutional racism* is supported by a belief in racial superiority of one group over another. Constraints are initiated and power controlled by one group.
- *Individual orientations to racism* can lead to specific behaviors: (1) a superiority position based on fear; (2) a "do-good" position with token gestures to eliminate the racism; (3) a nonreactor position owing to overwhelming anxiety; (4) the catastrophic reaction, in which an individual is prepared to justify a position by angry and irrational means; (5) the apathetic position, in which an individual goes along with the status quo.
- *Reactions of those affected by racism* include the ways fears, frustrations, and antagonisms affect mental health and adjustment.
- *Symbolic racism* emerges in labels of desirable and undesirable and perpetuates rigid patterns of relating between individuals and groups.

Racial characteristics are observable. Racism, however, involves prejudicial attitudes, and discrimination influences the self-image of those who endure racism. Rack (1982) contends that racism may be used as a metaphor for illness. A health professional who makes interpretations may be responding to ill-conceived racial stereotypes. Cultural differences in the manifestations of distress and the way such manifestations are interpreted represent diagnostic pitfalls for the psychiatric nurse and may be linked to racism.

▶ Check Your Reading

7. Define and discuss the various levels of racism.
8. Identify two ways in which racism might interfere in psychiatric nursing.

Ethnocentrism

Ethnocentrism is the making of one's own view the center or focal point for decisions. It implies an acceptance of one's culture as superior and relegates other individuals and groups to a position of inferiority. Individuals or groups are judged or rated against the standards of the ethnocentrist's world view. Although all individuals have a vested interest in their own cultural perspective, rendering nursing care to patients from other cultures means eliminating or diminishing the inherent bias of an ethnocentric viewpoint.

▶ Check Your Reading

9. Define ethnocentrism.
10. What are the implications of ethnocentrism when providing nursing care to those whose culture is different from your own?

Ethnic Identity

Ethnic identity encompasses the perception and inner sense of affiliation with a group that shares a racial, national, linguistic, or cultural background. Ethnic identity provides the security of knowing that one belongs, a sense of roots. How often have you heard the comment "he is so Americanized," meaning an immigrant has outwardly conformed to the dominant culture? How often have we attributed education to an implied acceptance of American standards: "She is a professional and still uses herbs"? In this instance, we assume that merely being a professional would cause one to shed the value that the ethnic group places on the use of herbs.

Understanding another person's deep sense of ethnic identity is not easy in a world in which labeling is based on cursory introductions. Consider the following poem by Paul Laurence Dunbar (1872–1906) entitled "We Wear the Mask":

We wear the mask that grins and lies,
It hides our cheeks and shades our eyes,—
This debt we pay to human guile;
With torn and bleeding hearts we smile,
And mouth with myriad subtleties.

Why should the world be overwise,
In counting all our tears and sighs?
Nay, let them only see us, while
We wear the mask.

We smile, but, O great Christ, our cries
To Thee from tortured souls arise.
We sing, but oh, the clay is vile
Beneath our feet, and long the mile;
But let the world dream otherwise,
We wear the mask.

Ethnicity is linked with an individual's social identity and includes history, language, and religion. Terms such as *ethnic group* or *ethnicity* describe a self-awareness possessed by the person(s) to whom the terms are ascribed. Members of an ethnic group think and behave similarly.

▶ Check Your Reading

11. What is the significance of ethnic identity?
12. What is included in the understanding of the term ethnicity?

Transcultural Identification

Transcultural identification is the degree to which the particular group modifies its customs and activities to blend with the dominant culture. Modification of a group's customs, however, can lead to blurring or even rejection of a group's original cultural values.

Considerable ethnic variation exists within many ethnic groups—differences attributed to level of ethnic identity, acculturation, family influences, sex-role socialization, religious and spiritual influences, immigration experience, and linguistic skills (Lee and Richardson, 1991). New immigrants are often faced with conflicting choices—to acculturate their children and grandchildren into the dominant culture, thereby fostering acceptance, or to nurture ethnic pride in their descendants. Regardless of how close-knit a family or ethnic group appears to be, you must be able to evaluate how fluently different generations can speak to each other in their native language. Not only do third-generation monolingual members clash with peers, who claim they are not really "ethnic" unless they can speak their native tongue, but also, increasingly, grandchildren cannot communicate with their grandparents. The mediator and translator may be the bilingual parent (Quintanilla, 1991).

You need to be tuned into the multiple losses and compromises engendered by immigration—one's country, culture, human attachments, family traditions, and ability to communicate are all threatened. Loss occurs not only by death, but also from leaving, separating, being left, changing, letting go, and challenging the status quo. Loss is viewed differently by different cultures. Often, collateral information about a patient must come from a family member who has shared the journey and understands the complexity of losses and the uniqueness of the patient.

The following American phrases illustrate transcultural conflicts: "The early bird gets the worm." "He who hesitates is lost." "Strike a bargain." "God helps those who help themselves." "The squeaky wheel gets the grease." "Tell it like it is." "Do it." "Just say no." These American expressions focus on decisiveness, independence, and a take-charge way of approaching life (Hanson et al, 1990). Many other cultures operate from a different set of beliefs: "Find your enjoyment in renunciation." "What God wills." "The nail that stands up gets pounded down." "Emptying the heart of desires." "It can't be helped." These beliefs underscore a nonattachment to fame, worldly success, and control and an acceptance of contemplation and fate as the appropriate means of dealing with life's challenges. Our story of Thao aptly illustrates that in Asian cultures, obligation to one's kin takes precedence over human fulfillment.

Patterns of kinship, education, religion, economics, and politics are interrelated with the lifeways of a particular group. When the geographical boundaries, social institutions, lines of authority, and family life patterns are significantly altered or completely eradicated, as they are for refugees, change has a profound impact on individual and group behavior. The trauma of being a refugee requires adaptation to meet a four-phase adjustment process:

1. *Culture shock* is the severe anxiety generated by being in a new culture with unfamiliar language and social norms.
2. *Social isolation* occurs when new refugees are housed where rent is affordable, not necessarily where their counterparts live.
3. *Status inconsistency* is a common experience. Many refugees who held professional credentials have to update or even requalify for licensing in a new country, without the benefit of fluency in the language of the credentialing examinations.
4. *Cultural conflicts* invariably occur when the woman is employed and the male head of the household is unemployed or working in a marginal job. The cultural conflicts can last a generation, creating both interpersonal and intrapsychic turmoil. This is an area in which the culturally competent nurse can be an educator, interpreter, mediator, and advocate and a link to support networks such as mutual assistance associations.

▶ Check Your Reading

13. Discuss how variations in transcultural identification can lead to conflicts, for both individuals and families.

14. Identify three losses that occur with transcultural identification.

Ethnic Competence

Ethnic competence means acting in a manner congruent with the behavior and expectations of a particular culture. According to Pittman and colleagues (1989), competence is linked with cultural acquisition through structures and processes that shape individuals. Yet competence does not imply complete mastery of the nuances of all other cultures. Rather, it commences with respect; sensitivity; and a willingness to observe, listen, and learn from others whose cultural backgrounds differ from one's own.

A wide range of conceptual frameworks and models is available for use in intercultural situations. Some models focus on the individual (Griffith-Kenney and Christensen, 1986); others adopt a group orientation (Hofstede, 1980). Dobson (1991) developed a detailed transcultural health visiting schema emphasizing similarity and reciprocity in using cultural frames of reference. Davis's (1980, p. 221) schematic representation offers four approaches to evaluating the complex relationships in caring for patients from a variety of cultures.

Davis's scheme examines caregiving of a British nurse to a British patient but with many geographical and ethnic nuances to be considered and raises the possibility that the nurse is not British but interacts with British patients. How does the nurse's training help or hinder the British patient's helping-seeking behavior? Davis's scheme also demonstrates the variability in transcultural nursing (i.e., the British-trained nurse must learn competency in other cultures). For example, in a pluralistic society such as the United Kingdom, an Ethiopian nurse may have a patient from Peru. Competent assessment thus depends on understanding dimensions of culture and the transactions that constantly occur between nurse and patient.

As early as 1967, Leininger argued that the Western criteria used in separating "normal" from "abnormal" may not be used by other cultures. Synthesizing and applying the findings of anthropological studies, Leininger (1978) formulated a culturological assessment paradigm based on

- Cultural life patterns
- Cultural values, norms, and expressions
- Cultural taboos and myths
- World view and ethnocentric tendencies
- Cultural diversities
- Life-caring rituals and rites of passage
- Folk and professional health-illness systems
- Specific caring behaviors and nursing care, values, beliefs, and practices
- Cultural changes and acculturation

Leininger's theory of cultural care incorporates decades of transcultural research and requires that "care knowledge and skills should always be repatterned for the best interests of the clients" (1991, p. 44). She believes cultural care goes beyond values, beliefs, and practices. Care is embedded in language; religion; kinship and social patterns; and political, legal, educational, economic, technological, ethnohistorical, and environmental components or institutions of a culture. (See Leininger [1991] for new insights about transcultural nursing care incorporating Leininger's theory of culture care.)

Although this form of assessment can be applied to individuals, groups, or societies, the question of diagnosis has generated a wealth of interest (Carnevali, 1983; Asuni, 1986; Rao, 1986; Tseng, 1986). Diagnosis creates labels and can mitigate against delivering nursing care that embraces a cultural care perspective.

Ethnic competence is an ongoing task, a perpetual learning process. Cultures are not stagnant. A culture continues to condition and shape coping styles and concepts of health and illness. Ethnic competence requires extensive knowledge of different assessment approaches as well as face-to-face interactions with individuals from different cultures. One of your roles is observer and learner.

▶ Check Your Reading

15. Why are assessment and diagnosis important considerations in a discussion of ethnic competence?
16. What is ethnic competence?

Culture-Bound Syndromes

A **culture-bound syndrome** is intrinsically ethnocentric and restricted to a specific people and locale. Such syndromes usually are evident by bizarre displays of behavior that are not congruent with traditional Western psychiatry classifications. Simons and Hughes (1985) believe that culture-bound syndromes raise issues about the differential contribution of biological and cultural factors in the cause and shaping of mental disorders. They consider the relativity of meaning across cultural contexts and the potential generalizability of psychiatric classifications developed in one culture. Culture-bound syndromes may be the result of factors operating in a particular culture. Therefore, when interpreting behavior, you must also consider the particular culture's defined ways of expressing normality.

For example, *amok* is characterized by a sudden frenzy and is a fully elaborated cultural complex found in Malaysia, Indonesia, and the southern Philippines. Rack (1982) notes that *amok* has been variously attributed to drug intoxication, psychogenic psychosis, and schizophrenia. *Latah*, found primarily in Malaysia, is considered a culture-bound form of hysteria.

Old hag is a culture-bound syndrome found in Newfoundland. The victim of old hag awakens terrified, unable to move, with a sensation of weight on the chest. Because the interpretation of this syndrome occurs in a society in which members share a belief in old hag, the syndrome involves neurophysiological factors and cultural shaping.

Koro and *jiryan* are psychosexual disorders. Koro patients have the delusional fear that the penis will retract into the abdomen and cause death. Cases of koro have been found among the Chinese community in Britain (Rack, 1982). Jiryan, a common complaint in Pakistan, is known as *dhat* syndrome in India. Complaints of jiryan/dhat evolve around a fixed belief that sperm is leaking from the body in the urine. The patient may not complain of anxiety about potency but of generalized weakness, malaise, and depression.

Windigo psychosis, reported among Native Americans, appears to be a form of severe depression in which culturally determined fears of cannibalism color the depressive delusions. Finally, *piblokto*, reported among Inuit women, has features of agitated depression and fuguelike withdrawal. Other culture-bound syndromes are identified in Chapter 10.

Although many researchers have recorded and attempted to explain culture-bound syndromes, Lefley (1990) concluded that culture-bound syndromes do not seem to fit a universal behavior pattern. The meaning of illness is therefore defined from a particular cultural perspective. Al-Issa (1982, p. 4) makes a point that must be considered when dealing with a patient whose presenting behavior is not congruent with good mental health: "[P]sychopathology is a universal phenomenon . . . and some cultural contexts may influence only the threshold of its manifestations." Al-Issa (1982, pp. 6–7) contends that "cultural variables may resist measurement and comparison across cultures because it is difficult to isolate them from the context and meaning in which they are embedded."

▶ Check Your Reading

17. What issues are raised by the term culture-bound syndrome?
18. Identify three culture-bound syndromes.

MAJOR CULTURAL VARIABLES AFFECTING MENTAL HEALTH CARE

Health care delivery is culture bound, laden with beliefs, values, practices, and ramifications. Eliason (1993) and West (1993) go so far as to contend that nursing practice and theory cannot be ethical unless nurses consider cultural factors and incorporate them into the plan of care. Understanding the relevance of all of these elements helps make one culturally competent.

Culture affects all aspects of communication, including concepts of time, space, touch, and tone of voice. These concepts are clues to accepted norms for daily functioning and important in rendering nursing care.

Time

Time is endowed with different meanings in various cultures. Hall and Whyte (1990, p. 51) have identified five aspects of time:

- Appointment time
- Discussion time
- Acquaintance time
- Visiting time
- Time Schedules

Each of these concepts of time has relevance in providing nursing care.

Throughout much of Asia, for example, because of traffic congestion, it is not unusual for individuals to be several hours late for an engagement but still believe they are on time. Also in Latin America, a 45-minute delay or a 45-minute wait is not unusual. You need to be aware that if you want a patient from those geographical areas to keep an appointment by American time standards, you may need to ask the patient to come earlier; that is, if the actual appointment is meant for 2:00 P.M., ask the patient to come at 1:00 P.M.

Discussion time in American culture actually means making your point quickly and efficiently. This concept in Asian and Latino cultures, however, implies that details are important. Therefore, the patient may try to explain the context and symptoms associated with the illness and the role the family is playing in the healing process. Listening to the patient conveys respect and patience and signals the family and extended family that your goal is to provide nursing care while cognizant of the patient's culture.

Acquaintance time is the period needed by the patient and family to "size up" the professional providing health care service. Hall and Whyte (1990, p. 53) write: "[I]n Central America, local custom does not permit a salesman to land in town, call on the customer and walk away with an order, no matter how badly your prospect wants and needs your product. It is traditional there that you must see your man at least three times before you can discuss the nature of your business." Applying this insight to psychiatric nursing, you might question how often has a patient been labeled resistive when the patient was looking for clues to established rapport. Rapport is conveyed by demonstrating awareness of some aspects of the patient's culture and by your own body language and sense of caring. Caring is almost universally recognized in a warm, polite, attending caregiver. Cultures around the world emphasize the importance of acquaintance time. Box 14–1 provides examples.

Treatment of a loved one, particularly in a foreign country, brings significant concern. The psychiatric nurse should use acquaintance time not only for dialogue, but also for validating cultural concepts about mental health, mental illness, and traditional treatment. You can then inform the patient about accepted psychiatric modalities currently used in the United States and Canada. We cannot assume that individuals from other cultures, even those from the highest socioeconomic levels, are familiar with American standards of mental health care or that these standards are amenable to their own values and beliefs.

"Visiting time involves the question of who sets the time for a visit" (Hall and Whyte, 1990, p. 53). In India, a person who says "come over and see me . . . see me anytime" means just that. You have crossed a boundary and are now friends. For the psychiatric nurse, this acceptance may facilitate follow-up with a patient.

Americans live by schedules, yet Hall and Whyte (1990, p. 54) write "not only is our idea of time schedules no part of Arab life but the mere mention of a deadline to an Arab is like waving a red flag in front of a bull." The implication for the psychiatric nurse is not to make a specific request for a decision but to work on building the relationship between the patient and mental health professional.

Time has a significance in all cultures. For each ritual surrounding births, weddings, funerals, and mourning, there is protocol. For instance, in remembrance of a deceased loved one, Filipinos are expected for family prayers for nine consecutive evenings following the person's death. For many refugees, particularly those with strong traditions of ancestor worship, the inability to comply with expected cultural norms honoring the deceased may lead to mental health problems.

▶ Check Your Reading

19. What is appointment time and its potential impact on a nurse-patient relationship?

BOX 14-1 Acquaintance Time Across Cultures

In Arab culture, the time required to get something accomplished depends on relationships. Trusting a loved one to the care of a psychiatric nurse, particularly a non-Arab, may require extensive application of acquaintance time to build trust and rapport

In Japanese culture, time is used to test patience. If you cannot demonstrate patience, you have lost the opportunity to build cultural bridges

In African-American and West Indian cultures, relationships are valued and built over time. Individuals from these cultures are not driven by the actual clock time; the quality of the relationship propels trust and confidence in the health care provider

Hispanics see time in terms of *mañana* (tomorrow), the exception being a family member's or friend's crisis. In this case, it is important to respond immediately

In Ethiopia, the time required for a decision is directly proportional to its importance

20. What significance does acquaintance time have for the development of a nurse-patient relationship?

Space

Space is an integral component in communication. Space connotes personal boundaries and conveys culture-specific meanings. Americans and Canadians, for the most part, consider 2 feet to be a proper or respectable distance when talking to another adult. Typically, Hispanic Americans and people of Arab culture converse at a more intimate distance, less than a foot. To them, this seems comfortable and implies a real personal conversation.

Asians are generally sensitive to each other's personal space and have definite rules concerning physical contact. They feel comfortable conversing with others who stand 5 to 6 feet away. An "outsider" earns acceptance by politeness and dress that conveys an attitude of respect for others.

For African-Americans, those who are close may engage in close contact; "outsiders" are expected to maintain at least an arm's length of distance. West Indians maintain little space between friends when communicating. The "outsider" needs to look for a signal that invites closeness.

Touch

Americans generally are uncomfortable with physical touch. In Arab and Hispanic American cultures, however, communication typically includes an embrace, particularly between men. Contact between men and women in Arab culture is prohibited; in Latin America, physical contact may extend to a kiss on the hand of the woman.

Hall and Whyte (1990, pp. 50–51) note that a handshake in Latin America, particularly between two men, is seen as cold and impersonal. The *doble abrazo* in which two men embrace by placing their arms around each other's shoulders is the accepted norm of greeting. Touching the shoulders of a Javanese, however, is seen as a humiliation and an unpardonable breach of traditional etiquette. Thai culture regards the head as sacred; patting a small child on the head is considered offensive. If the head needs to be touched for a medical purpose, always explain the reason and ask permission of the adults.

▶ Check Your Reading

21. Give two examples of different cultural views of space.
22. Give two examples of different cultural views of touch.

Voice Tone

The human voice also carries cultural connotations. In American culture, speaking distinctly in a well-moderated and self-controlled tone is the desirable norm. Hall and Whyte (1990) note, however, that a cool, logical approach to conversation may be regarded by Middle Easterners with suspicion. In the Middle East, "from childhood, the Arab is permitted, even encouraged, to express his feelings without inhibition. Grown men can weep, shout, gesture expressively and violently, jump up and down—and be admired as sincere" (Hall and Whyte, 1990, p. 49).

Throughout much of Asia, respect and communication are enhanced by speaking in polite but soft tones. Being gregarious or making self-referent statements is not well accepted in traditional Asian societies. One demonstrates manners and humility by listening more than speaking.

Color and Dress

In some Asian countries, white is associated with a funeral. In many African countries, red symbolizes witchcraft and death. Good mental health in the United States has often been associated with the ability to coordinate the color of one's wardrobe; in Africa, the Caribbean, and South Pacific, bright, multiple colors are the accepted norm of dress.

Much of the world still adheres to distinct uniforms for nurses. A patient from such a geographical region may have difficulty relating to an American nurse in an institution that no longer requires uniforms. You may want to explain to the patient how to recognize "the nurse" (i.e., a certain badge).

Gestures

Many gestures are subtle and easy to overlook. Although Americans use hand gestures for emphasis, people of Italian and Hispanic background feel comfortable with extensive hand movement to make a point. To an Arab, however, a quick wave of the hand or showing the sole of one's shoe is considered a violation of basic courtesy.

Words and Terms of Address

Words do not easily translate across cultures but must be understood from a group's frame of reference. You may therefore need to work not merely with an interpreter but with a culture broker, someone who has an insider's view of the patient's culture. For example, "old" in Iraq means 40 and above; for unmarried women, over 30 is old. In India, people over age 60 are considered old. In Japan, a man age 65 retires from his lifetime job, but survival depends on getting another job, at a lower salary (Maryknoll, 1994). Hatton (1992) distinguishes between translators and interpreters who appraise tasks, patients, providers, or information and have considerable power. The cultural broker is more than a translator. This person has ascribed or achieved acceptance in two distinct cultures.

Terms of address for an elderly patient vary across cultures. European Americans and African-Americans generally use the term grandmother or grandfather or some variation. Filipinos have specific cultural terms: *Lolo* is equivalent to grandfather; *lola* is the equivalent to grandmother. *Na ang bultok* means all white hair already. In Chinese culture, the middle-aged generation use *old Mr./old Mrs.* as a sign of respect, whereas the term *old big* is used by younger generations. Understanding how words can be interpreted and knowing the accepted form of address for a patient can enhance communication.

▶ Check Your Reading

23. Give an example of how voice tone and gestures differ across cultural groups.
24. How might the American practice of nurses wearing street clothes rather than uniforms affect someone from another cultural group?
25. Why is it important to know different terms of address in different cultures?

Perceptions of Mental Illness

The stigma attached to seeking mental health treatment appears to be universal. Throughout much of Asia, mental health problems are viewed as imbalances in the body. In Africa and much of the Caribbean, mental illness is viewed as suffering from a spell. Even in the United States, researchers have found that perceptions of elder abuse and help-seeking patterns differ among African-American, White, and Korean-American elderly women (Moon and Williams, 1993). These differences underscore cultural distinctions in communication, education, diagnosis, and intervention.

Decision Makers

When the patient is elderly, you need to consult cultural-specific informants and decision makers. For the African-American patient, the key decision maker is often the oldest daughter. In Filipino culture, the eldest child, whether son or daughter, makes the decisions. Among the Vietnamese, the eldest son is traditionally vested with decision-making power, although disruption of family patterns because of war may warrant that the child closest to the parent make decisions. Traditionally, in Chinese culture the eldest son and his wife were expected to be caregivers and decision makers; likewise among Hispanic-Americans, the eldest son is expected to care for elderly parents.

In many cultures, the mental health or subsequent mental illness of a member of that culture demands a communal response. Although Native Americans have sought services from Western practitioners and the Indian Health Service, the power of the group and use of ancient rituals in the healing process are well documented. Islanders of the South Pacific conform to communal decision making and a prescribed course of action for dealing with mental illness.

Religion

The role of religion varies across cultures and significantly affects the meaning ascribed to good and evil, suffering and salvation. Fervent Catholics rely on God's greatness and prayers to see them through a crisis, whereas Buddhists accept suffering as a reality of life. In Orthodox Judaism, all events of daily life are greeted with an appropriate blessing. Judaism is steeped in ritual for all occasions, with the most solemn blessing uttered at the synagogue service by the officiating rabbi (Catoir, 1992).

Substantial cultural and social differences are attached to significant events and the stresses of everyday life. Patients want relief from their symptoms and evaluate how well their needs are being met. You must realize that patients from other cultures may feel threatened, misunderstood, and mistrustful. In addition, the patient and family may have culturally conditioned beliefs regarding remedies for healing.

Newbold (1991, p. 98) asserts that nursing is a ministry: "[P]eople need people, not only to meet their own needs but to be needed by others. The relationship of patient and nurse is unlike any other, and part of its uniqueness is the intimacy with which one relates to a person."

▶ Check Your Reading

26. Give an example of how a culture understands mental illness.
27. Give two examples of how religion affects people across cultures.

SPECIFIC CULTURAL GROUPS

European Americans

European Americans comprise a heterogeneous group. Among their differences are beliefs, emigration patterns to the United States, and presenting forms of mental illness. The 1980 U.S. Census provided data about ethnic background. Respondents represented more than 100 groups. One hundred million Americans claimed their ancestors came from the British Isles; 49 million were of German background; 13 million were French; 12 million were Polish; still many others came from other European nationalities. Similar to all groups, European Americans share certain communication patterns, as summarized in Box 14–2.

Irish Americans

More than 40 million Americans claim Irish heritage. Some have experienced problems associated with alcoholism and concomitant depression. Relentless stereotyping, discrimination, and poverty have led the Irish to develop a strong sense of identity and cohesion, especially in the first and second generations. This ethnic group

BOX 14-2 Communication Patterns Among European Americans

Preference is for direct eye contact during speaking as signs of attention and respect

Getting to the point quickly is valued more by Northern Europeans. Southern Europeans are more gregarious and engage in unhurried small talk

Relative distance between two speakers in conversation is farther apart than with peoples from Latin or Arab cultures

Public behavior is expected to be modest and emotionally restrained, especially among Northern or Eastern Europeans. Emotional displays are seen as irresponsible or in bad taste

Southern Europeans (Spaniards, Italians) are more prone to show their emotions, and hand gestures are often used to make a point in a conversation

Hand-holding, hugging, and kissing between men and women in public is acceptable

A slap on the back denotes friendliness

It is customary to shake hands with persons of the opposite sex

traditionally has emphasized a strong oral tradition, the development of mythology, and a complex style of communication in which a question may be answered by asking another question.

Cultural characteristics and other mediating factors, such as role expectations and support networks, however, may hinder or facilitate recovery. Traditionally, Irish women have been expected to be strong and nurturing. There is a high tolerance for Irish men to gather in the pub. Mothers cater to sons, thus reinforcing a dependency role. Research (Al-Issa, 1982) suggests a high incidence of schizophrenia among Irish people.

Mental illness creates a sense of shame for the Irish-American patient and family. Although psychiatric facilities have existed for more than a century both in the United States and Ireland, a family might hide a mental problem in a loved one by keeping the person confined to one part of the house and seeking divine intervention for a cure through prayer.

Irish Americans, particularly first and second generation, are overwhelmingly Catholic. Catholicism postulates that God is Love. Religion offers hope but demands commitment. Catholicism also speaks to sin, repentance, and redemption. The psychiatric nurse working with a patient of Irish ancestry needs to address religious beliefs and practices. A pervasive sense of guilt and intrapunitiveness is often experienced by an Irish patient when mental illness occurs. The hopeful message of Catholicism, which focuses on love and forgiveness, is helpful to the patient trying to overcome mental illness: "[The Church] . . . is a refuge for sinners, a comforter of the afflicted and a source of spiritual nourishment on the journey of life" (Catoir, 1992, p. 57). The 12 steps of Alcoholics Anonymous are congruent therapeutic tools for this ethnic group.

▶ Check Your Reading

28. Give two characteristics of Irish Americans that affect their risks for mental illness.
29. What is the role of religion in the life of many Irish Americans?

Italian Americans

Most Italian Americans are descendants of people who immigrated to the United States from the southern part of Italy. Italians maintain strong family ties. Regionalism is also important, and Italians often want the listener to know they are Neapolitans, Calabrians, or Venetians. For the psychiatric nurse, this is important information for recognizing pronounced regional differences among Italians.

Although Catholicism is a factor in the life of most Italians, according to Sowell (1981), religious institutions are viewed distantly, sometimes cynically, by southern Italians. Italians believe that the well-being and honor of the nuclear family is to be preserved at all costs. Although strong family ties can reinforce good mental health, family bonds that are tenuous, critical, or hostile can lead to depression. So too, when religion is seen as external control, a sense of helplessness may propel the Italian American toward depression. For Sicilians, their spirituality or religion is not concerned with conformity to rules for personal salvation but in placating the capricious power of Satan, "the evil eye," or overcoming magic (Sowell, 1981). For the psychiatric nurse working with an Italian-American patient, assessment of family relationships, religious beliefs, and degree of emotional expression is important.

Jewish Americans

Jewish people came to the United States and Canada from many European countries, among them Spain, Portugal, Germany, Austria, Russia, and Poland. As a result, they adhere not only to Judaism, but also to the cultures from which they emigrated.

In Western Europe, those who practiced their religion could still be identified as French or German; in Eastern Europe, being a Jew was a separate identity isolated from the dominant culture.

Three branches of Judaism exist today. Orthodox believers follow the Talmudic teachings concerning Kosher (dietary) rules, Sabbath observance, and strict adherence to ancient rituals. Reform Judaism has discontinued some Talmudic practices and stresses adaptability, morality, and belief in God. Conservative Judaism follows prescribed holy days yet reinterprets Talmudic teachings for contemporary practice.

Judaism stresses that God has endowed every person with physical, intellectual, and emotional gifts. Individuals are expected to develop and use these gifts in harmony with all people. All branches of Judaism believe that one's actions become a living memorial in death. Harmonious relationships, good deeds, and praying for forgiveness for wrong deeds are the challenges Judaism presents to its adherents. Individuals are not passive but continuously shape attitudes, memories, and outcomes by the good they do or fail to do.

Over the centuries, the Jewish community has developed a strong ethnic self-consciousness as well as elaborate support systems to address the needs of its members, including those with mental illness. This network is important for the psychiatric nurse meeting a Jewish patient's needs. Adherents of Orthodox and Conservative Judaism tend to prefer treatment by a professional who espouses their religious beliefs. The psychiatric nurse needs to understand the significance of specific practices such as ritual baths, head coverings for women, and prescribed prayers.

▶ Check Your Reading

30. What is the role of the family in the mental health of Italian Americans?
31. What supports exist in the Jewish community to assist persons with mental illnesses?

African-Americans

African-Americans believe acceptance must be earned by being sincere and trustworthy. Brusque questioning can cause a patient to be resistive. A commonly held African-American cultural belief is that a person should not share personal information with outsiders. Therefore, professional help is more likely to be accepted if the nurse has earned the respect and trust of the pastor and extended family. Communication patterns among African-Americans are summarized in Box 14–3.

African-Americans gain strength from their nuclear and extended families, next-door neighbors, close friends, lodge brothers, sorority sisters, and church. Each family has a power source, a person who has control and who sets the rules. You need to identify this significant power source because this individual may influence the patient's acceptance or rejection of treatment interventions.

Some African-Americans harbor a distrust of "the system." Even the African-American nurse who works in the system may often be viewed as part of it. Therefore, you cannot presume an automatic bond between an African-American patient and an African-American nurse. If the nurse promotes a sense of empowerment in the African-American patient, advocacy and cultural brokering become part of the expanded professional's role (Jezewski, 1993). When access to health care is limited, biased, or fails to validate the African-American's feelings and experiences, you must function as both an advocate and cultural broker. The cultural broker's status facilitates a bond with the minority patient and enhances the patient's ability to operate in the dominant culture.

▶ Check Your Reading

32. Why might a cultural broker be useful for an African-American patient?
33. Why is trust so important in the African-American community?

BOX 14–3 Communication Patterns Among African-Americans

Touching of one's hair by another person is often considered offensive

Preference is for indirect eye contact during listening and direct eye contact during speaking as signs of attentiveness and respect

Public behavior may be emotionally intense, dynamic, and demonstrative

A clear distinction is made between "arguing" and "fighting." Verbal abuse is not necessarily a precursor to violence

Asking "personal questions" of someone one has met for the first time is seen as improper and intrusive

Interruption during conversation is usually tolerated. Competition for the floor is granted to the person who is most assertive

Conversations are regarded as private between the recognized participants. "Butting in" is seen as eavesdropping and is not tolerated

Use of the expression "you people" is seen as pejorative and racist

Hispanic Americans

Hispanic is a government designation that groups all people who speak Spanish and identify themselves as belonging to the Latin culture as a homogeneous group. Some Hispanic people prefer to be called Latino: "People from Central and South America and Mexico, although preferring to identify according to their national origin, such as Dominican or Colombian, are more responsive to the term Latino" (Arredondo, 1991, p. 143).

In actuality, Hispanic Americans vary widely in expressing their culture. In addition, their health care expectations and help-seeking behavior may differ widely depending on country of origin and social class. Mufford (1992) found that 50% were born in the United States, with the remaining coming from about two dozen other countries. Well-educated, upper-class immigrants may experience situational anxiety, whereas refugees from strife-torn Central America may suffer significant depression. Although only about 5% to 10% of Hispanics use folk medicine, including herbs and spiritual healers (Mufford, 1992), you need to elicit this information with culture sensitive interviewing skills.

Because Hispanics represent nearly 10% of the U.S. population, with Mexican Americans constituting the largest subgroup of Hispanics, an understanding of basic Hispanic cultural beliefs is paramount. Loyalty to the family takes precedence over social institutions or indi-

BOX 14-4 Communication Patterns Among Hispanic Americans

Hissing to gain attention may be acceptable

Touching is often observed between people in conversation

Avoidance of direct eye contact is sometimes a sign of attentiveness and respect; sustained direct eye contact may be interpreted as a challenge to authority

Relative distance between two speakers in conversation is closer than with European Americans

Official or business conversations are preceded by lengthy greetings, pleasantries, and other talk unrelated to the point of business

vidual preferences. Children learn early about unquestionable parental authority and loyalty. Respect and cooperation define social relationships and obligations. Typical communication patterns are summarized in Box 14–4.

Comas-Diaz (1989) believes that mental illness among Hispanics is a family affair because of the cultural emphasis on kinship, relationships, and identification of each patient with a namesake. Comas-Diaz recommends that nurses explore the myths and stories attributed to the ancestor for whom the patient was named.

Gender roles are clearly defined in Hispanic culture. This clear role definition is a source of conflict for those who question fixed roles, and as in all group-centered cultures, the individual who embraces different values, thinking, or emotional or communication styles may end up estranged. "The victim of mismatch feels alienation from individuals, groups and cultures, and institutions that play an important part in his or her life" (Ramirez, 1991, p. 3). Individuals who do not fit in their own culture may exhibit symptoms of depression and an inability to cope. Understanding the dynamics of "victim mismatch" is important in acknowledging the continuum of cultural differentiation or simply the broad range of behaviors within a culture that can merit approval or disapproval.

Folk healing, more commonly known as *espiritualismo* or *espiritismo*, is practiced among some Hispanic Americans. Its core belief is the soul voyaging, altered states of consciousness, and the presence of spirit-beings, who can enter into a person's body. According to Kearney (1978, p. 21), "in *espiritualismo*, trance states include *videncia*, the ability to 'see' spirit phenomena with the eyes shut and at a distance; *clarividencia*, the ability to 'see' spirit phenomena with opened eyes; and *oido*, the ability to 'hear' spirit-beings."

Religion remains a key factor in the life of most Hispanics. Help-seeking behavior may include prayers, novenas, pilgrimages, and directly seeking a priest's or pastor's advice. These religious leaders are usually significant supports.

The work of Rivera (1988) is particularly helpful for the psychiatric nurse working with the Hispanic patient. Rivera found that explaining mental illness as a physiological imbalance that can be corrected by medication is amenable to the Hispanic family's belief system. An educational problem-solving approach then helps mobilize all the family in a concerted effort to assist the ill member. Such an approach is consistent with the Hispanic system of extended interpersonal relationships and the cultural help-seeking behavior pattern. Mental health literature consistently indicates that Hispanic Americans desire treatment from a health professional who shows *personalismo*, or formal friendliness; *simpatía*, or warmth and concern; and *respeto*, or respect for the person and culture (Erzinger, 1991). Good communication demonstrating these qualities can be the beginning of a helping relationship.

▶ Check Your Reading

34. What are the three qualities that Hispanic Americans look for in a mental health professional?
35. What is the core belief of *espiritismo?*

Asian Americans and Pacific Islanders

Asia is a continent teeming with millions of peoples. Its geography includes towering mountains and majestic rivers. Asian class and caste systems define relationships, and religious movements, such as Buddhism, Islam, Hinduism, and Confucianism, have a profound impact on every aspect of life. Communication patterns common among Asian Americans are summarized in Box 14–5.

Indian Peoples

India is a heterogeneous country with 31 states and 630 million people speaking 15 major languages and hundreds of dialects. India's religion is predominantly Hindu. Hinduism asserts that people consist of an *atman*, which is an extension of the cosmic *brahman*, or universal energy, atmosphere, life, or soul. Accordingly, individuals continue to experience rebirth until they recognize the all-important truth: Present unhappiness is caused by ignorance, selfish attachments, and the seeking of earthly happiness. The individual seeking *nirvana* (oneness with the universal energy) and the end of the cycle of rebirths must lead a good life, have spiritual discipline, and eliminate any earthly attachments.

The Hindu religion exerts great influence on how individuals interpret suffering and human existence. The laws of *karma* ("action") and *samsara* ("reincarnation") were first articulated in the *Upanishads* (Hindu Scriptures). "Every individual deed or action was viewed as Karmic input that would inevitably lead to an output in kind, good deeds ripening as good fruit, evil deeds as evil" (Wolpert, 1991, p. 83). Therefore, according to the law of *karma*, depression is viewed as an atonement for some misdeeds in life. Depression results in fewer suicides in India than in other Western countries. Rao (1986) reports that both religious injunctions and social stigma may mitigate against completion of a suicide attempt.

Rao (1986) writes that disorders of the mind are mentioned in the *Upanishads*, and mental illness is estimated to affect some 2 to 7 persons per 1000 in India. Although many mentally ill people consult indigenous healers, who include shamans, depression is more often diagnosed through somatic complaints.

Rao (1986) found schizophrenia to be distributed across all socioeconomic groups and castes, with the catatonic form (characterized by psychomotor retardation or excitability) the more common expression of this illness. Rao (1986) notes that catatonic schizophrenia could be attributed to low linguistic competence, whereas those patients with highly developed linguistic skills might develop more delusional symptoms. For the nurse caring for patients from India, a precise understanding of their educational level, religious beliefs, and the family and communal support systems is important. If an Indian person becomes mentally ill while residing in another culture, the illness may not correlate with Rao's findings because the patient will have experienced a new set of environmental and social factors.

In India, culture-bound syndromes have been found to be common. Sexual neurosis and koro are two of these. Another is *possession syndrome*, in which a patient exhibits dissociation. Supernatural or religious frenzy is often the climax of possession.

Southeast Asians

The term *Southeast Asian refugee* masks differences among Vietnamese, Cambodians, and Laotians. Although hunger, exhaustion, and death were common experiences, Vietnamese are generally better educated than the other groups. Many have had years of exposure to French culture. Before the fall of Saigon in 1975, "several thousand military officers, governmental officials, the well-to-do, and the educated escaped to Thailand, from whence some made their way as refugees to the United States" (Chan, 1991, p. 155). "The more heterogeneous 'second wave' of refugees who started arriving in 1978 can be divided into the 'boat people' from Vietnam and the 'land people' from Kampuchea and Laos" (Chan, 1991, p. 157). These refugees were poorer and less educated than the 1975 group.

Cambodian and Laotian refugees came from rural areas. Some were Catholic, but more were Buddhist and animists. The term *refugee* masks the diversity and the different stresses experienced by waves of refugees. For the psychiatric nurse, understanding the different circumstances endured by refugees and the functional support systems they have created is important. If the patient is a refugee, focus on the circumstances of their journey to the United States or Canada. Many have endured great trauma and never received mental health treatment after their arrival. For some, experience has caused late-life flashbacks of earlier trauma and depression.

Among the boat people of Asia who arrived in the United States in the last two decades, mutual assistance associations (MAAs) have become their network for kinship, survival, and adjustment. The acknowledged leaders within the MAA are generally refugees who are bilingual and accepted for their leadership skills.

As a result of the 1987 Amerasian Homecoming Act, an influx of new Asian immigrants and refugees have entered the United States. Amerasians, the offspring of American fathers and Asian mothers, have endured years of hostility in Southeast Asia, being stereotyped as the "dust of the earth." They arrive with dreams of being reunited with an American parent, a dream that is seldom fulfilled. They also come to the United States with little formal education, few job skills, and significant identity confusion. Many, however, have mastered street survival skills.

In many cases, Amerasians enter the mental health system soon after arrival because of anxiety, severe depression, and suicidal ideation. Because of the patient's

BOX 14-5 Communication Patterns Among Asian Americans

In Vietnamese culture, the following is observed: (1) Touching or hand-holding between men may be acceptable; and (2) hand-holding, hugging, and kissing between men and women are unacceptable; (3) a slap on the back is insulting; (4) it is not customary to shake hands with persons of the opposite sex; (5) a verbal outburst is unacceptable

In Chinese culture, (1) respect is always accorded to an older person; (2) patience should be demonstrated; (3) speaking in a quiet, thoughtful manner helps promote communication

In Indian culture, (1) the older person takes the lead in conversation; (2) public displays of affection are taboo; (3) eyes are generally cast down when listening

Do not point your feet at a Cambodian; feet are the lowest point of the body spiritually. Similarly, do not step over a Cambodian's feet or legs

Do greet a husband before his wife, his wife before their children, and older children before the younger

Do appreciate that a Cambodian may agree to what you say or may indicate that he or she understands so as not to embarrass you by saying you made little sense at all. Not being embarrassed in front of others is one aspect of "saving face"

Cambodians do not shake hands. They place their hands, palms together, near their faces in greeting. They may shake hands as they try to learn American ways; but what awkwardness you may detect is less their feeling "shy" or "primitive" than their simply feeling awkward, much like you would if you tried to greet with your palms. Do not try this either. This can seem patronizing and is difficult to do because the height of the hands indicates esteem

Do not touch a Cambodian or his or her children on the head. This is the most important part of the body, where the spirit resides

Do not call a Cambodian solely by his or her first name. We think "Sam" or "Linda" is friendly; to a Cambodian, it may indicate an intrusion or lack of respect, perhaps like calling Sam "Sammy-boy" or Linda "Little Lady." Use Mr. or Mrs. or Miss and then the given name, which is usually noted last (as in Smith, Sam)

years of emotional pain, social dissonance, culture conflicts, poor sense of self-worth, and inability to trust or appreciate emotional intimacy, the psychiatric nurse confronts many challenges in helping the Amerasian patient. You can help Amerasian patients tell their stories, accept themselves, let go of the past, and move on with focused, achievable goals.

Buddhism, the religion of many Southeast Asian refugees, postulates that suffering is integral to human existence. Suffering is caused by desire, self-indulgence, or craving and leads to an unending cycle of birth, growth, decay, death, and rebirth. The Noble Eightfold Path to eliminate desire and suffering is achieved by

- Right views
- Right aims or intent
- Right speech
- Right conduct or action
- Right means of livelihood
- Right effort
- Right mindfulness
- Right meditation or contemplation

"This path leads to the cessation of craving and, finally, to nirvana, the cessation of rebirth" (Bradley, 1963, p. 112). Because Buddhism talks about abandoning the self, this religious tenet contradicts the Western psychiatric emphasis on self-worth and self-acceptance. How to reconcile these opposing views with a patient who professes Buddhism is a challenge. *Hakims*, traditional Asian healers, are successful because they are concerned with the whole patient and family—an important approach for psychiatric nurses to emulate.

Chinese Americans

China is an ancient civilization. Its people have emigrated to all corners of the globe, often suffering discrimination and resentment in their new homelands. As a result, tight-knit communities of Chinese people have stressed loyalty to one's family, one's clan, and support of mutual aid organizations as survival mechanisms.

When meeting a Chinese patient, determine whether that patient was born on the Chinese mainland or is a second-generation or third-generation Chinese living in the United States or Canada. Tseng (1986), in tracing the development of Chinese psychiatry, notes that Chinese medicine has been in existence for more than 3000 years, with herbal medicine frequently prescribed. In mainland China, however, the development of modern Chinese psychiatry and the treatment of mental illness has evolved only since the late 1950s. Traditional Chinese medicine considered weakness, exhaustion, emptiness, deficiency, and disharmony to be the reasons for illness. After the Cultural Revolution, Chinese psychiatry was revised, with psychological factors emphasized as the exclusive causes of mental illness. This orientation still persists on the Chinese mainland.

The "overseas Chinese" subject to discrimination lived their own separate cultural and social existence, in ethnic enclaves. The Chinese reaction to discrimination was withdrawal, timidity, and anxiety. "Overseas Chinese" developed Chinatowns complete with community organizations to meet the needs of citizens, including the needs of patients with mental illness. Second- and third-generation Chinese living in the United States still retain strong loyalty to family values and ethnic identity. This group has a high percentage of college-educated individuals who are increasingly more integrated into the dominant culture, both occupationally and residentially.

The religious traditions of Taoism and Confucianism have long been practiced by the Chinese. "Taoism holds that everything should be done according to Tao, the natural way; all else is madness and leads to disaster" (Bradley, 1963, p. 135). Although the Taoist reveres nature worship, over the centuries, Taoism became a religion of superstition; magical control; and a powerful Taoist priest clan consulted for amulets, potions, and incantations. Confucian belief stresses the tradition of ancestor worship, filial piety, benevolent love, duty, wisdom, integrity, and propriety.

Understanding the inherent hierarchy of all relationships is important in helping a Chinese American patient. "The son is inferior to his father and owes *Hsiao*, respect and obedience, to him. So, too, the wife is inferior to her husband and owes him corresponding *Hsiao;* the younger brother, servant, and citizen owe *Hsiao* to elder brothers, master and emperor" (Bradley, 1963, p. 144).

Japanese Americans

Individuals of Japanese origin suffered prejudice and discrimination, especially in the form of mass internment during World War II. This last experience shapes the attitudes of many Japanese Americans today. Among the Japanese Americans, the Issei were first generation; the Nisei are second generation; and the Sansei are third generation. "As of 1942, the average age of Issei males was fifty-five, while that of Nisei was only seventeen" (Sowell, 1981, p. 170). The third generation was born early in wartime internment camps or in postwar America, and many are militant about correcting past injustices against their ethnic group. The elder Issei Japanese consider the Sansei generation "too American"; hence there are some intergenerational strains.

Strong family and communal values with emphasis on education, self-control, and pressure to conform have resulted in little social pathology. Fear of failure, however, is an inherent motivator among Japanese. The Japanese American is expected to conform to family expectations and community norms. The psychiatric nurse needs to understand that individualism is frowned on, even today.

Shintoism is the indigenous religion of Japan. It is estimated that 70 million of Japan's 95 million people are adherents of Shinto. Shintoism has been influenced by Buddhist and Confucian practices as well as the religious thought of India. The basic concept of deity in Shinto is the concept of *Kami,* meaning something holy or connected with the spirit world. Two main causes of evil and misfortune for individuals, according to Shinto myths, are polluting actions, such as hanging a man's clothes on a hook intended for a woman's clothes, and displeasure of the ancestors (Bradley, 1963). When working with Japanese American patients, you need to explore religious beliefs, the Kami as lived daily, and the degree of stress imposed by the need to conform.

Filipino Americans

Although the Philippines have been strongly influenced by the cultures of Spain and the United States, the inherent values of Filipinos remain strongly oriented toward group and church. About 90% of Filipinos are Catholic; the remainder are Muslim or Protestant. More than 800 dialects are spoken in the Philippines. Different provinces, both urban and rural, create divergent forms of stress. Some Filipinos are proud of their Spanish origins; others adhere to the influences of Chinese culture; and those who identify themselves as Muslim are strongly influenced by the tenets of Islam.

For decades, the Philippines have had mental health practitioners, psychiatrists, and psychiatric nurses, yet they seek professional help only after a crisis. A widely inculcated belief is that the extended family can provide the listening ear and the guidance needed to resolve a psychological conflict. Belief in the preservation of the good name of the family and the power of prayer are strong behavioral determinants. As a nurse journeying with a Filipino patient, be aware of other behavioral modifiers influenced by cultural beliefs.

Despite differences, Filipinos as a group are sensitive and may be reluctant to ask questions for fear of appearing aggressive or embarrassing the health care provider. They respond better if you speak softly and unhurriedly and demonstrate an interest in the concerns of the family. A cardinal rule is not to say or do anything to embarrass the patient or the family. *Pakikisama* is a Tagalog word devised from the root *sama,* meaning to accompany, go along with. Avoid outward signs of conflict by focusing on smooth interpersonal relationships or use a go-between. Avoid shame *(hiya)* at all costs (Lynch, 1968, pp. 1–21).

Pacific Island Peoples

The Pacific Islands have seen European, Asian, and American influences, yet the significance of the social group remains a strong force for approval or disapproval. The Admiralty Island, situated about 150 miles north of New Guinea, came under German and Australian influence. Romanucci-Ross (1978, p. 129) provides insights into anger, shame, and suicide in these islands:

A person can be shamed to illness in several ways. A woman, for example, was seen by her husband's brother as she was in a treetop and her genitals were exposed to his glance. In another instance, a man was not paid by his wife's temporary consort for a sexual encounter. Both were undisputed reasons for shame suicide.

BOX 14-6 Communication Patterns Among Pacific Islanders

Pacific Islanders observe facial expressions for signs of trust and openness

Roles are ascribed, with elders permitted to take the lead in conversation

To refuse to accept hospitality offered through food or beverage is to insult the host

Friendship is based on reciprocity

Communication patterns among Pacific Island peoples are summarized in Box 14-6.

In most of the Pacific Islands, strong group mores also involve belief in spirits, ritual, and the equivalent of the Native American medicine man or woman. "A long illness constitutes a journey of self-discovery for the sick person and allows for the communication of formerly unspeakable subjects and decisions" (Romanucci-Ross, 1978, p. 133). The social definition of insanity in the Admiralty Islands is similar to that of India. If a woman goes against her husband's wishes or is too gregarious, she may be labeled mentally ill. Citing a case in which a young mother of three feared that her husband and his lover would take her children away by declaring her mentally ill, Romanucci-Ross (1978, p. 134) notes that assessments of this woman's sanity "varied with the degree of kinship and the quantity and quality of gain from her freedom or eventual confinement."

Dobson (1991) contends that in many cultures, the individual is seen as an integral part of the social group to which he or she belongs, especially in Samoa and the Fiji Islands, where health needs are an inherent aspect of group and community functioning. Al-Issa (1982, p. 9) indicates that the low rates of schizophrenia in the South Pacific "seem to be consistent with a cultural framework that provides communal decisions and clear-cut paths of action for individuals who are predisposed to schizophrenia." The competent transcultural nurse must recognize that attitudes are socially learned and often result in marked cultural differences for what is considered acceptable behavior.

▶ Check Your Reading

36. How might depression be understood in Hinduism?
37. What is the inherent conflict in the beliefs of American psychiatry and Buddhism?
38. Contrast the American and Japanese views on individualism.
39. What is the role of the Filipino extended family in responding to mental illness?

Native Americans

Native Americans come from at least 10 different cultural areas (e.g., California, Northeast, Plains, Southeast, Southwest, Arctic, Subarctic), more than two dozen language families (e.g., Algonquian, Siouan, Hokan,

Iroquoian, Eskimaleut), and numerous tribes (e.g., Chumash, Shawnee, Seminole, Crow, Blackfoot, Apache, Navajo). The greater diversity in Indian languages, sociopolitical organization, contact with Westerners, and contacts with other tribes has shaped intertribal relations. Communication patterns among Native Americans are summarized in Box 14–7.

Native Americans are not one people; between 1.5 and 1.8 milliion Native Americans live in the United States, with nearly 600 federally recognized native entities and more than 365 state-recognized Native American tribes. Each of these entities has unique customs, traditions, histories, and social organizations. There are still many Native American tribes, such as the Meherrin and Eno-Occaneechi, working to be federally recognized.

Native American societies were generally egalitarian. Custom and tradition prevailed. Leaders' influence sprang from personal qualities. Status and authority were derived from knowledge of tribal tradition and lore. To understand the mental health issues of Native Americans, you must know that the historical relationship between Native American tribes and the U.S. government has created dependency and identity confusion. Services offered by the government have sought to adapt and acculturate the Native Americans into the dominant society (Trimble, 1988).

The decision to leave or stay on an Indian reservation generates many issues and sharp distinctions between urban and rural reservation Native Americans. Urban Native Americans are more likely to be migratory, to become invisible in the dominant culture, and to have less contact with traditional support systems—all factors leading to greater stress, anxiety, and depression (Sage, 1991). Native American children raised in urban areas often lack traditional role models to develop self-esteem and assert their sense of identity. Such children often have more strained intergenerational ties, especially with grandparents still residing on reservations. On an Indian reservation, all members of a tribe know their genealogy, and even a person of mixed blood participates in traditional tribal ceremonies or seeks the service of a medicine man or woman.

BOX 14-7 Communication Patterns Among Native Americans

- Native Americans are generally reserved in conversation
- They do not engage in small talk, touching, hugging, or demonstrative displays of emotion
- They are comfortable with periods of silence
- To develop rapport, the nonindigenous communicator should know something of the group's real history and not succumb to the stereotypes presented in the media
- Sharing food and drink is a common form of hospitality
- Roles are formalized, with chiefs, elders, and shaman having a special place of respect
- When a significant decision needs to be made, the above-named persons need to be included
- There is a formal hierarchy surrounding roles and status that should be observed

Native Americans experience high rates of poverty and have less access to preventive medical care. Studies (Cheadle et al, 1994; Grossman et al, 1994) continue to document the prevalence of risk-taking behavior, especially a high incidence of alcohol and drug abuse and suicide, even among Native Americans who have achieved a higher socioeconomic status. Cheadle and colleagues (1994) suggest investigating other social and environmental influences to understand the factors that precipitate mental illness.

Although alcoholism has long been linked with depression and suicide, O'Nell (1993), in working with Flathead Indians residing on a reservation, discovered that heart and spirit are symbols central to an understanding of Flathead life and that for the tribe, depression and consequent drinking may have positive connotations: "Life within the Flathead community is characterized, ideally, by close affective ties of kinship and friendship as well as by expectations of generous sharing among one's group of family and friends" (O'Nell, 1993, p. 461).

Life is also characterized, however, by feelings of loneliness, of not being cared for, of having nothing, or, worst of all, by fears of being abandoned. It is a mark of maturity to feel profound loneliness when separated from loved ones, to feel sorrow for the pain one has caused others, and to feel pity for those who have nothing. "Depression, therefore, can be a positive expression of belonging in this milieu. To be sad is to be aware of human interdependence and the gravity of historical, tribal, familial, and personal loss. To be depressed, and that includes tearfulness and sleep and appetite disturbances, is to demonstrate maturity and connectedness to the Indian world. A carefree attitude is often thought of as indicative of immaturity" (O'Nell, 1993, p. 461).

Drinking is seen as a positive expression of sociability, a reaffirmation of the bonds of friendship and kinship. Not drinking may be interpreted as a slight against family and friends. Drinking is normally a group activity, yet alcoholism may interfere with the intended outcomes of this social custom. O'Nell also notes that it is inappropriate and culturally insensitive in the Flathead Indian community to ask direct questions about painful or shameful experiences.

In journeying to the world of the Native Americans, the precise meaning of customs, rituals, and taboos remains specific to each group. Native Americans are inherently reverent and exercise religion and ritual before undertaking all activities. They experience an intimate relationship with the natural world and see themselves as extensions of animate and inanimate nature. Yet they attribute human properties to plants, animals, inanimate objects, and natural phenomena. Native American religion generally involves the belief that the universe is suffused with preternatural forces and powerful spirits. Tribes generally have a shaman or medicine man or woman, who is thought to control the spirits through ritual, magic, incantations, sacred objects, or herbal remedies. All tribes emphasize wholeness and balance, each with its own understanding of equilibrium within its oral history and religion.

Ritual purification, through the use of sweat lodges, is practiced and more widely accepted on reservations and in urban areas. The sweat lodge combines ancient ritual and incantations to promote healing. The sweat lodge is a symbol of Native American religion and identity and is used by all Native American Indian groups. Its "common purpose is to bring the individual closer to the elemental forces of life, and to express unity between all humans, animals, the earth, and the physical forces in the universe" (Walker et al, 1993, p. 565). Because the medicine man or woman conducts the sweat lodge ceremonies, you should view this person as a collaborator in the healing process.

An interview with a Native American patient may take a different response pattern. For instance, the communication style of the Native American is often a sharp contrast to the dominant culture. Native American culture emphasizes symbols and periods of silence. Therefore, making small chit-chat with a Native American patient may only increase anxiety. Demonstrating reverence for the environment and knowledge of sacred symbols such as sacred pipes, medicine wheels, and eagle feathers promotes rapport.

When working with a Native American, recognize that many Native Americans believe that poverty means being without family and friends (Primeaux, 1977). Even when one opts to leave the reservation, there is considerable pressure from the family and the tribe to remain in contact and to return for visits.

Manson and colleagues (1987) advocate group therapy for Native Americans to clarify issues surrounding identity and the conflicts associated with feelings of being an "outsider." Family therapy, too, has been beneficial because elders can be role models, reinforce positive values, and reduce the patient's sense of stigma and isolation (Attneave, 1969).

Inuit and Aleut Peoples

Within the Arctic area, the Eskimaleut language family is used by two groups with ancestral links: the Inuit (Eskimo) and Aleut peoples. The name *Eskimo* means "eaters of raw meat" in the Algonquian language. This name was used by whites; people to whom it is applied prefer the name *Inuit*, which means "people" in their own language. In Canada, the Eskimos are officially called Inuit by the Canadian government. Lefever and Davidhizar (1991) wrote of the diversity of Inuit, some living in Canada and others in Alaska, Greenland, and Russia. Birket-Smith (1971, p. 56) carefully examined the interface between coastal Inuit and Europeans and concluded that "many superficial judgements have been passed on the character of the Eskimos . . ." contact between the Inuit and north Pacific cultures have resulted in greater assimilation with the European culture.

The most important support for the Inuit and Aleut peoples continues to be the extended family. Marriage is highly regarded. Children are welcomed and viewed as an assurance of care and support in old age. Among the Inuit, a person of importance is called *tsumatag*, "he who thinks" (Waldman, 1985). In the difficult Arctic environment, Inuit traditionally have created special partnerships with nonfamily members. "Sharing partners" participate in the preparation of food gathered through hunting and fishing; "song partners" perform religious rituals together.

Similar to other Native Americans, Inuit carve beautiful objects out of wood, bone, and ivory for their religious rituals. Many customs prevail for giving birth, cutting the umbilical cord, naming a child, celebrating a good fishing catch, and burying the dead. Some customs require the use of stone knives, mussel shells, and amulets. Ceremonial dances and masks representing the spirits of animals and the forces of nature are used under the direction of an Inuit shaman. Birket-Smith (1971, p. 178) found that an Inuit who becomes ill first consults the shaman, because disease is ascribed to witchcraft or the loss of the soul. As in some Asian cultures, Inuit stress respect for the dead and the burning of lamps to honor the dead. Inuit draw strength from nature, as the poem "Words to a Sick Child" (Bierhorst, 1983, p. 41) suggests:

Go up to the mountain
From the summit of the
mountain you shall seek health,
You shall draw life.

Despite their collaboration and dependence on nature, hysteria occurs with high incidence among Inuit (Davis, 1986). In reviewing the work of earlier researchers with this population, Abel and coworkers (1987, p. 55) note that "antic hysteria is an acute dissociative reaction," probably precipitated by the harsh environment and the anxiety that an individual may feel alone in a difficult situation. The climate, the struggle for food, and preservation of a traditional way of life are made particularly difficult because Inuit possess little capital, and large corporations remain eager to explore for minerals, oil, and gas in their natural habitat.

Similar to other native peoples, the Inuit are comfortable with periods of silence, with formal handshakes, with less need for personal space, and with reliance on nonverbal communication. Lefever and Davidhizar (1991) emphasize that "the nurse who understands Eskimo culture will look for nonverbal clues, such as watching the face for raised eyebrows (indicating 'yes') or a wrinkled nose (indicating 'no'). Although Inuit seldom disagree publicly with others, their nonverbal communication may mean not agreement but a simple acknowledgment of the speaker's words.

For the psychiatric nurse, examining the patient's support system and degree of felt interdependency may be a helpful starting point. Also, learn if the patient has used herbs or consulted a shaman. Determine the patient's relationship to the extended community. In turn, the community's endorsement of you does much to encourage the patient to seek and accept help.

▶ **Check Your Reading**

40. What effect might "chit chat" have on a Native American?
41. How is depression viewed in the Flathead Indian culture?
42. How is drinking viewed within the Flathead Indian culture?
43. What is a sweat lodge?
44. What is the role of the shaman in Native American cultures?

West Indian Peoples

West Indians are strongly influenced by African traditions and remnants of British, Spanish, Dutch, or French culture, depending on the island of origin and family traditions. Communication patterns among West Indians are summarized in Box 14–8. West Indians frequently speak their thoughts aloud. Brent and Callwood (1993) observed that such individuals are not hallucinating; rather, their speech is a manifestation of a cultural pattern. Children at play quickly dash to cover their heads when it rains, not because they fear getting wet but because they want to keep neatly groomed hair. Leff and Isaacs (1981) noted that a scarf tied around the forehead may not "indicate royalty" or schizophrenia but may be a cultural behavioral response to a headache. Superstitions—including belief in jumbies (spirits) and voodoo—abound in the Caribbean and modify behavior in countless ways. Yet you cannot assume that every patient from the Caribbean holds these beliefs. If serious mental illness is present, however, patients may report that the spirits have taken control or that God has destined them for great power.

Unusual behavior may be attributed to weather, nutrition, or a physical illness. Some West Indians seek healers experienced in herbs. The great array of herbs for sale at the open-air market in St. Thomas, U.S. Virgin Islands, attests to the extensive use of herbs by people from every socioeconomic class.

The family remains the key element to helping the patient explore emotional problems and engage in treatment. Sharing the degree or depth of distress may be especially difficult for a nurse from a different ethnic or cultural group. Valls (1983) noted that West Indian proverbs set the tone for understanding the West Indians' frame of reference: "[I]n times of adversity, it is best to be home; settle family matters in private; too much talk can get one in trouble."

McCartney (1971), a native Bahamian, writes in *Neuroses in the Sun* about the remnants of social, racial, and color prejudice. "Racial prejudice is an aspect of our culture that is as universally decried as it is deeply ingrained in our minds" (McCartney, 1971, p. 53). The effects of conquest and colonialism often create a long-term sense of inferiority, rejection of authority, and identity struggle, especially for those of mixed racial ancestry trying to accept all of their racial inheritance. You need to recognize that racism is an issue for some patients. McCartney (1971, pp. 64–65) notes that some individuals from the Caribbean who had "never given much thought to their social value in terms of colour experience some very painful shocks when confronted with the racial value system of an alien society. The psychic damage resulting from this kind of experience . . . is hard to assess." Although mental illness hospitals exist throughout the Caribbean, the stigma of mental illness is sometimes expressed in antagonism toward the mentally ill person and the search for a cure through the services of a spiritualist or an *obeah* practitioner.

BOX 14–8 Communication Patterns Among West Indians

- The communication style is "laid back" and indirect
- Conversation may ramble before one gets to the heart of the matter
- A non–West Indian should not touch the West Indian because this is considered impolite
- Making direct inquiries without first engaging the person in conversation may give the appearance of impatience
- Smiling and joking are acceptable ways of communicating

Religion is both a social and a spiritual resource in much of the Caribbean. Belief in the supernatural is found in Puerto Rico *espiritismo*, Afro-Cuban *santería*, and Haitian *voodoo*. Each of these religions has prescribed rituals for cleansing persons who believe their condition is due to failure to propitiate malevolent spirits or to perform obligatory rituals (Lefley, 1990). In cultures in which folk traditions abound and mental illness and healing are ascribed to outside forces or evil spirits, you may need to involve not only the family, but also a traditional healer, exorcist, or priest as educator, consultant, and cotherapist. Weiss (1992, p. 241) suggests that "strong disapproval of folk healing by Christian clergy and by Protestant fundamentalist mental health works caused patients and family members (of immigrants from Santo Domingo in the Caribbean) to deny such involvement."

Espiritismo is sought as a healing intervention during times of crisis. The cause of the individual's affliction is identified and resolved through a medium, an individual who can communicate with the spirits of the dead. *Espiritismo* and the Afro-Cuban religions share the view that supernatural entities may possess a living person and that the patient may present with symptoms of paranoia. In her research, Weiss (1992, p. 248) found that when patient's kin consulted healers, it was usually at the point "when patient's illness was especially difficult to manage at home." Both the family and the patient worried about being "branded as 'crazy' or 'loca'," either by action or by treatment rendered, and might refer to the patient's present state "as being on the brink of spiritual growth and, at worst, as succumbing to spiritual vulnerabilities or to the evil intent of persons or forces beyond the circle of intimates" (Weiss, 1992, p. 249).

When journeying to the culture of a person from the West Indies or one of the many islands of the Caribbean, you should recognize that European, American, Indian, and African beliefs are interlaced with religious rituals and folklore. Before attempting to diagnose a patient, you need to know if the patient attributes the distress to being hexed or possessed by evil spirits. For patients who think they have a hex put on them, ask by whom and why. Try to ascertain if family members are encouraging the patient to seek treatment only through a mental health setting or if healers or herbalists have been sought. The answers to these questions may reveal the respondent's perception of your role and intention. Trust must be earned.

▶ Check Your Reading

45. How might someone from the Caribbean explain mental illness?
46. What role does the family play in the treatment of a West Indian patient with a mental illness?

COMMUNICATION FOR CULTURAL UNDERSTANDING

Learning about a patient's culture is more than filling out forms and asking questions. It must be a journey to acquire perspective; to promote understanding; and to facilitate respect, trust, and the building of a relationship. This does not happen without time and effort. It implies that you have first taken the time to study the patient's culture and then to engage the patient and family without making significant cultural mistakes.

Among the immediate variables that may affect communication are (Hofling et al, 1976):

- The patient's behavioral symptoms and presentation or the degree to which in the patient's culture he or she may be considered mentally ill
- The psychiatric nurse's personality, sensitivity, and ability to be a transcultural communicator
- The degree to which the psychiatric nurse deemphasizes the use of medical jargon and speaks to the patient in a tone and manner that creates rapport. Use of culture-specific idioms or phrases may be helpful
- The environment for treatment and the emotional climate created by verbal tone and nonverbal signals
- Time as a factor in contributing to the patient's readiness to relate to the psychiatric nurse

Evaluate the following before beginning an intervention with a patient from another culture:

- Do I hold a theoretical orientation about the cause of a patient's mental illness that is in opposition to this patient's religious or cultural beliefs?
- What nonverbal signals do I send that may provoke anxiety, fear, or resistance?
- Does the mental health environment, beginning with the manner in which I receive the patient, signal that the patient's culture is important? Does the decor include pictures artifacts, and bilingual signs to reassure the patient?
- Do I assume that someone who speaks with an accent is uneducated?
- How much time do I take to learn how my patients are socialized?
- Do I pay attention to the impact of my personal style on particular patients?

Learn cross-cultural communication—the do's and don'ts that can provide you with communication tools (Taylor, 1989). See Box 14–9 for communicating strategies across cultural groups.

BOX 14–9 Suggestions for Effective Communication

Speak slowly, audibly, and distinctly and use terminology that patients from other cultures can understand

Use simple words and avoid jargon

Listen as much as you speak and do not interrupt because this can be seen as rude

Allow extra time to communicate with someone whose first language may not be your own. Trying to understand one another may require extra effort and time

Respect silence and do not fill every gap in the communication process

When you experience frustration or sense conflict or misunderstanding in a cross-cultural situation, stop and ask yourself if the conflict is due to a cultural difference. Try to see a common basis of understanding

Adapt your style to the demands of a situation. Speak the "language" of the patient

Do not make assumptions or judgments about people based on their accents or language fluency

Be open and sensitive as to how you give feedback

Know who in the family is the appointed "head" or decision maker

Understand the "hot bottoms" that can lead to conflict

Hot bottoms include the use of slang racial and ethnic stereotypes; it includes verbal and nonverbal behavior that does not meet accepted cultural norms. This includes making definite pronouncements about a culture that is not your own

Identify and network with the traditional cultural brokers and healers

Ask the patient if he or she uses herbs, and if so, what is the health benefit expected

Learn to identify culturally relevant rituals

Stress the patient's strengths; demonstrate respect and caring

CONCLUSIONS

Culture permeates every aspect of human behavior. It shapes perceptions and specific response patterns. No two cultures are exactly alike, and even within ethnic and cultural groups, differentiation and specificity mean that the competent nurse needs to consider specific patient needs before intervening. Not all researchers agree on the role culture plays in creating psychopathology, but psychopathology is a universal phenomenon. Cultural beliefs and expectations, however, shape levels of tolerance and support networks and either facilitate or hinder help seeking.

Spirituality or religion exists worldwide. Every religion postulates a set of beliefs, rituals, and practices that can empower or diminish the individual. Clergy representing many religious traditions as well as native healers and medicine men and women have roles in the healing of spiritual and emotional wounds.

Although the competent psychiatric nurse may not know every culture in detail, an understanding of cultural diversity leads to nursing care that is sensitive to the patient while promoting the patient's well-being within the norms of the ethnic group.

KEY POINTS TO REMEMBER

- Every culture has norms or standards of behavior.
- Cultural relevancy means seeing differences without value judgments.
- In the journey to another's culture, nurses need to be aware of their own values and subjective world view.
- Cultures undergo both continuity and change.
- Stereotypes perpetuate "isms" and fixed patterns of labeling others.
- Prejudice operates on different levels of severity. Patients who have suffered prejudice may appear more guarded or restrictive because of their experiences.
- Ethnic identity encompasses the deepest core of being. It encapsules the individual and provides a sense of affiliation and roots.
- Transcultural identification is the modification of customs and activities so that a particular group can more easily blend with the dominant culture. Language, dress, and sex-role socialization frequently change; such changes may ignite intergenerational conflict.
- Ethnic competence means acting in a manner that is accepted, expected, and congruent with the members of a particular culture.
- Space, time, and color are imbued with different cultural meanings.
- Within ethnic and cultural groups, beware of viewing all members of the group as the same.
- Assessing not only where the patient was raised, but also the parents' background promotes cultural relevancy.
- American cultural emphasis on independence, self-help, and individual rights can clash with both cultural beliefs and religious tenets that stress interdependence, passivity, group norms, punishment, fatalism, and destiny.
- Distinguish between an immigrant and a refugee. Immigrants usually plan their departure from their homeland. They do not always leave their country because of poverty. They simply may want to live abroad for a period and often return home to retire. Refugees flee from political, economic, and social upheavals.
- African-Americans believe trust must be earned. The extended family and the church are significant support systems.
- Hispanics value family loyalty; respect and cooperation is expected and accorded.
- Filipinos are strongly family and group oriented. They are sensitive to any appearance of aggressive behavior and go along with others to avoid conflict.
- West Indians, although strongly influenced by superstitions, do not equally use herbal medicine.
- Talking to oneself in West Indian culture is an accepted behavior.
- West Indians value the family, and in times of distress, it remains a critical element in the healing process.
- Amulets, feathers, and shells are used by various cultures to ward off evil spirits.
- Verbal and nonverbal communication is a significant part of the journey to another's culture. Persistent study, patience, and listening can facilitate admission to another culture.
- You are on a journey that requires you to change and grow.

LEARNING ACTIVITIES

1. Read an ethnic journal and determine what values are being conveyed. How do the values differ from your own? Ethnic journals and magazines include but are not limited to *Ebony*, *Irish-American*, *Chinese Studies for Pupils*, and *Hispanic-American*.
2. Visit a refugee resettlement office. Who works there? What messages does the environment suggest? How would you feel if you were a refugee seeking services in a new country? What would be your first priorities?
3. Ask a friend from another ethnic or cultural group if you may come to a religious service or cultural celebration.
4. Think about the world of cultural diversity. Which groups of people do you know least about? What do you need to do to be a competent psychiatric nurse as you journey toward understanding the cultures of others?

CRITICAL THINKING EXERCISES

Miss Sandra Banes, a community mental health nurse, visited Mrs. Jardee, a Filipino woman who had just lost her husband of 25 years. Miss Banes was told by Mrs. Jardee's youngest daughter that the mother had not eaten since the funeral 3 days before. When Miss Banes talked to Mrs. Jardee, who was lying in bed reading her Bible, she complained of back pain while crying incessantly. With her assessment of Mrs. Jardee, Miss Banes decided to talk to Mrs. Jardee's daughter about possible hospitalization. When she attempted to approach the daughter about this decision, the daughter said that she could not help her. Miss Banes was unsure what to make of this response.

1. What assumption(s) can be made about Miss Banes's understanding about cultural influences in decisions of health care?

2. What evidence do you have to support your assumptions?

3. Consider any bias.

Miss Banes was concerned and decided to talk to the daughter about the other children in the family. The daughter told the nurse that her older sister had gone to help the younger brother and his wife choose a new school for their children.

1. What other information does Miss Banes need to know to help Mrs. Jardee?

2. What are your reasons for saying this?

3. What conclusions (if any) can you draw about the outcome of this situation?

REFERENCES

Abel, T. M., Metraux, R., and Roll, S. (1987). *Psychotherapy and culture.* Albuquerque: University of New Mexico.

Aguilar, R. J. (1989). Hispanics Part II: Special treatment needs. *Professional Counselor,* 49–50.

Al-Issa, I. (1982). Does culture make a difference in psychopathology? In I. Al-Issa (Ed.), *Culture and psychopathology.* Baltimore: University Park Press.

Allport, G. W. (1979). *The nature of prejudice.* Reading, Massachusetts: Addison-Wesley Publishers.

Arredondo, P. (1991). Counseling Latinos. In C. C. Lee and B. L. Richardson (Eds.), *Multicultural issues in counseling: New approaches to diversity.* Alexandria, Virginia: American Association for Counseling and Development.

Asuni, T. (1986). African and Western psychiatry: A comparison. In J. L. Cox (Ed.), *Transcultural psychiatry.* London: Croom Helm.

Attneave, C. L. (1969). Therapy in tribal settings and urban network intervention. *Family Process 8,* 192–210.

Bierhorst, J. (Ed.) (1983). *The sacred path: Spells, prayers and power songs of the American Indians.* New York: Quill.

Birket-Smith, K. (1971). *Eskimos.* New York: Crown Publishers.

Bradley, D. G. (1963). *A guide to the world's religions.* Englewood Cliffs, New Jersey: Prentice Hall.

Brink, P. J. (1990). *Transcultural nursing: A book of readings.* Prospect Heights, Illinois: Waveland Press.

Burke, A. W. (1986). Racism, prejudice and mental illness. In J. L. Cox (Ed). *Transcultural psychiatry.* London: Croom Helm.

Caplan, N., et al (1989). *The Boat People and achievement in America (a study of family life, hard work and cultural values).* Ann Arbor: University of Michigan Press.

Carnevali, D. L. (1983). *Nursing care planning: Diagnosis and management* (3rd ed.). Philadelphia: J. B. Lippincott.

Catoir, J. T. (1990). *God delights in you.* New York: The Christophers.

Catoir, J. T. (1992). *World religions.* New York: Alba House.

Chan, S. (1991). *Asian Americans.* Boston: Twayne Publishers.

Cheadle, A., et al (1994). Relationship between socioeconomic status, health status and lifestyle practices of American Indians: Evidence from a Plains reservation population. *Public Health Reports, 109*(3), 405–413.

Cohen, A. (1992). Prognosis for schizophrenia in the Third World: A reevaluation of cross-cultural research. *Culture, Medicine and Psychiatry, 16*(2), 53–75.

Comas-Diaz, L. (1989). Culturally relevant issues and treatment implications for Hispanics. In D. R. Koslow and E. P. Salett (Eds.). *Crossing cultures in mental health.* Washington, D.C.: Sietar International.

Davis, B. D. (1980). *Nursing training and transcultural psychiatry.* Transcultural Psychiatry Society Conference, Bradford, England.

Davis, B. D. (1986). Culture and psychiatric nursing: Implications for training. In J. L. Cox (Ed.), *Transcultural psychiatry.* London: Croom Helm.

de Chardin, P. T. (1967). *On love.* New York: Harper & Row.

Dobson, S. M. (1991). *Transcultural nursing.* London: Scutari Press.

Eliason, M. J. (1993). Ethics and transcultural nursing care. *Nursing Outlook, 41,* 225–228.

Erzinger, S. (1991). Communication between Spanish-speaking patients and their doctors in medical encounters. *Culture, Medicine and Psychiatry, 15*(1), 91–110.

Fiske, A. P. (1993). Social errors in four cultures: Evidence about universal forms of social relations. *Journal of Cross-Cultural Psychology, 24* (4), 463–494.

Good, B. J. (1993). Culture, diagnosis and comorbidity. *Culture, Medicine and Psychiatry, 16*(4), 427–446.

Griffith-Kenney, J. W., and Christensen, P. J. (Eds.) (1986). *Application of theories, frameworks and models* (2nd ed.). St. Louis: C. V. Mosby.

Grossman, D. C., et al (1994). Health status of urban American Indians and Alaska Natives. *JAMA, 271*(11), 845–850.

Hall, E. T., and Whyte, W. F. (1990). Intercultural communication: A guide to men of action. In P. J. Brink (Ed.), *Transcultural nursing: A book of readings.* Prospect Heights, Illinois: Waveland Press.

Hanson, M. J., et al (1990). Honoring the cultural diversity of families when gathering data. *Topics in Early Childhood Special Education, 24*(1), 112–131.

Harris, S. J. (1972). *The authentic person.* Niles, Illinois: Argus Communications.

Hatton, D. C. (1992). Information transmission in bilingual, bicultural contexts. *Journal of Community Health Nursing, 9*(1), 53–59.

Heok, K. E. (1994). *Ageing and old age.* Singapore: Singapore University Press.

Hofling, C. K., Leininger, M. M., and Bregg, E. (1976). *Basic psychiatric concepts in nursing* (2nd ed.). Philadelphia: J. B. Lippincott.

Hofstede, G. (1980). *Culture's consequences. International differences in work-related values.* Beverly Hills, California: Sage.

Jezewski, M. A. (1993). Culture brokering as a model for advocacy. *Nursing and Health Care, 14*(2), 78–85.

Kearney, M. (1978). Spiritualist healing in Mexico. In P. Morley and R. Wallis (Eds.), *Culture and curing (Anthropological perspectives on traditional medical beliefs and practices).* London: Peter Owen.

Keefe, S. E. (1992). Ethnic identity: The domain of perceptions of and attachment to ethnic groups and cultures. *Human Organization, 51*(1), 35–43.

Lee, C. C., and Richardson, B. L. (1991). Promise and pitfalls of multicultural counseling. In C. C. Lee and B. L. Richardson (Eds.), *Multicultural issues in counseling: New approaches to diversity.* Alexandria, Virginia: American Association for Counseling and Development.

Lefever, D., and Davidhizar, R. E. (1991). American Eskimos. In J. N. Geiger and R. E. Davidhizar (Eds.), *Transcultural nursing assessment and intervention.* St. Louis: Mosby-Year Book.

Leff, J., and Isaacs, A. (1981). *Psychiatric examination in clinical practice.* St. Louis: C. V. Mosby.

Lefley, H. P. (1990). Culture and chronic mental illness. *Hospital and Community Psychiatry, 41*(3), 277–286.

Leininger, M. (1978). Culturological assessment domains for nursing practices. In M. Leininger (Ed.), *Transcultural nursing: Theories, concepts, practices.* New York: Wiley.

Leininger, M. (1991). The theory of culture care diversity and universality. In M. Leininger (Ed.), *Culture care diversity and universality: A theory of nursing.* New York: National League for Nursing Press.

Lerner, G. (Ed.) (1972). *Black women in white America.* New York: Random House.

Linton, R. (1945). *The cultural background of personality.* Westport, Connecticut: Greenwood Press Publishers.

Manson, S. M., et al (1987). Psychiatric assessment and treatment of American Indians and Alaska natives. *Hospital and Community Psychiatry, 38*, 165–173.

Maryknoll, March 1994, 8–9.

McCartney, T. O. (1971). *Neuroses in the sun.* Nassau, Bahamas: Executive Printers.

McKenzie, S. C. (1980). *Aging and old age.* Glenview, Illinois: Scott, Foresman & Co.

Moon, A., and Williams, O. (1993). Perceptions of elder abuse and help-seeking patterns among African-American, Caucasian-American and Korean-American elderly women. *The Gerontologist, 33* (3), 386–395.

Mphande, L., and James-Myers, L. (1993). Traditional African medicine and the optimal theory: Universal insights for health and healing. *Journal of Black Psychology, 19* (1), 25–47.

Mufford, C. (1992). A cure of many colors. *New Physician, Oct.*, 14–19.

Newbold, C. (1991). To walk with each other. In G. F. A. Pierce (Ed.), *Of human hands.* Minneapolis: Augsburg.

O'Nell, T. D. (1993). Feeling worthless: An ethnographic investigation of depression and problem drinking at the Flathead reservation. *Culture, Medicine, and Psychiatry, 16*(4), 447–469.

Pittman, M. A. Eisikovits, R. A., and Dobbert, M. L. (1989). *Culture acquisition: A holistic approach to human learning.* New York: Praeger.

Primeaux, M. (1977). Caring for the American Indian patient. *American Journal of Nursing,* 77, 91–94.

Quintanilla, M. (1991). The language gap. *Los Angeles Times,* pp. E1+.

Rack, P. (1982). *Race, culture and mental disorder.* New York: Tavistock Publishers.

Ramirez, M. (1991). *Psychotherapy and counseling with minorities.* New York: Pergamon Press.

Rao, A. V. (1986). Indian and Western psychiatry: A comparison. In J. L. Cox (Ed.), *Transcultural Psychiatry.* London: Croom Helm.

Rivera, C. (1988). Culturally sensitive aftercare services for chronically mentally ill Hispanics: The case of the psycho educational/treatment model. *Fordham University Hispanic Research Center Research Bulletin, 11.*

Rosenhan, D. L. (1990). On being sane in insane places. In P. J. Brink (Ed.), *Transcultural nursing: A book of readings.* Prospect Heights, Illinois: Waveland Press.

Sage, G. P. (1991). Counseling American Indian adults. In C. C. Lee and B. L. Richardson (Eds.), *Multicultural issues in counseling: New approaches to diversity.* Alexandria, Virginia: American Association for Counseling and Development.

Schwartz, T. (1976). Relations among generations in time-limited cultures. In T. Schwartz (Ed.), *Socialization as cultural communication.* Los Angeles, University of California Press.

Shuman, R. B. (Ed.) (1970). *A galaxy of black writing.* Durham, North Carolina: Moore Publishing Co.

Simons, R. C., and Hughes, C. C. (Eds.) (1985). *The culture-bound syndromes (folk illnesses of psychiatric and anthropological interest).* Boston: D. Reidel Publishing Co.

Sowell, T. (1981). *Ethnic American: A history.* New York: Basic Books.

Takaki, R. (1993). *A different mirror: A history of multicultural America.* Boston: Little, Brown & Company.

Taylor O. L. (1989). The effects of cultural assumptions on cross-cultural communication. In D. R. Koslow, and E. P. Salett (Eds.), *Crossing cultures in mental health.* Washington, D.C.: Sietar International.

The cultures of illness. *U.S. News and World Report,* Feb. 15, 1993, pp.73–76.

Trimble, J. E. (1988). Stereotypical images, American Indians and prejudice. In P. Katz and D. Tylor (Eds.), *Eliminating racism: Profiles in controversy.* New York: Plenum Press.

Tseng, W. S. (1986). Chinese psychiatry: Development and characteristics. In J. L. Cox (Ed.), *Transcultural psychiatry.* London: Croom Helm.

Valls, L. (1983). *Ole time sayings.* U. S. Virgin Islands: St. John.

Waldman, C. (1985). *Atlas of the North American Indian.* New York: Facts on File.

Walker, R. D., et al (1993). Treatment implications of comorbid psychopathology in American Indians and Alaska natives. *Culture, Medicine, and Psychiatry, 16*(4), 555–572.

Weiss, C. I. (1992). Controlling domestic life and mental illness: Spiritual and aftercare resource used by Dominican New Yorkers. *Culture, Medicine, and Psychiatry, 16*(2), 237–271.

West, E. A. (1993). The cultural bridge model. *Nursing Outlook, 41,* 229–234.

Williams, D. R. (1994). The concept of race and health status in America. *Public Health Reports, 109* (1), 26–41.

Wolpert, S. (1991). *India.* Berkeley: University of California Press.

SUGGESTED READINGS

Brink, P. J. (Ed.). (1990). *Transcultural nursing: A book of readings.* Prospect Heights, IL: Waveland Press.

Eliason, M. J. (1993). Ethics and transcultural nursing care. *Nursing Outlook, 41,* 225–228.

Geiger, J., and Davidhizar, D. (1991). *Transcultural nursing assessment and intervention.* St. Louis: CV Mosby-Year Book.

Leininger, M. (1991). *Culture care diversity and universality: A theory of nursing.* New York: National League for Nursing Press.

West, E. A. (1993). The cultural bridge model. *Nursing Outlook, 41,* 229–234.

UNIT III
FACILITATING THE JOURNEY

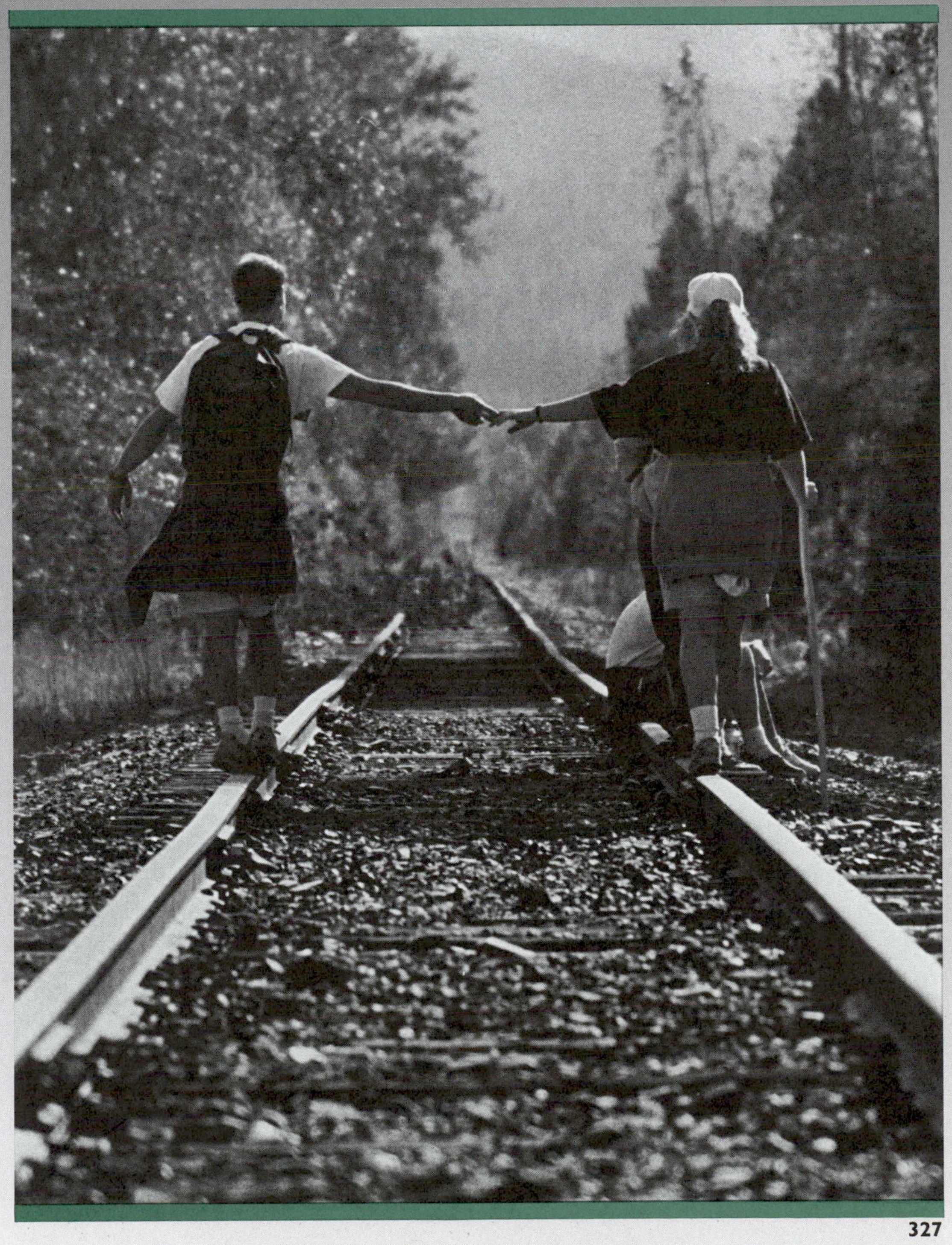

CHAPTER 15

CRISIS INTERVENTION

It is important to the healing process that you be with the pain, experience the desolation, feel the hurt. Don't deny it or cover it or run away from it. Be with it. Hurt for awhile.

—M. Colgrove, H. Bloomfield, and P. McWilliams

LEARNING OBJECTIVES

After studying this chapter, you should be able to:

1. Define "crisis" and "crisis state."
2. Specify relevant theoretical models of crisis and crisis intervention.
3. Describe the characteristics of the crisis state.
4. Identify risk factors associated with the development of the crisis state.
5. Distinguish between situational and developmental crises.
6. Use the nursing process to develop appropriate crisis intervention strategies.
7. Identify the legal implications of crisis situations.

KEY TERMINOLOGY

Balancing factors
Crisis
Crisis sequence
Crisis intervention
Critical incident debriefing
Critical stressor
Developmental (maturational) crisis
Situational crisis
Social support

Crisis is a term used to describe a serious life circumstance whose presence in one's life temporarily stuns the traveler and decisively interrupts the normal forward progression of the journey. Characterized by emotional disequilibrium, cognitive disorientation, and a perceived inability to use previous problem-solving skills, people in crisis experience the confusion and emotional pain of a crisis as an overpowering life experience.

Typically the appearance of a crisis offers a new, unsettling, and more complex point of view about life. Its impact on the patient's journey can include a tragic account of the struggle between life and death, between being and nonbeing, and between affirmation and perceived stigma. In a crisis, life seems out of focus. For the person in crisis, it is difficult to believe that life will ever be the same. In one sense, life *cannot* ever be quite the same again after a crisis. How a person handles a crisis determines whether it leads the traveler on a trail toward greater personal growth or whether it leads to psychopathology.

The immediate goal of **crisis intervention** is to stabilize the individual, family, or community—to restore those involved to precrisis function. To achieve resolution, however, the person or people experiencing a crisis ultimately need to integrate the meaning of the crisis into their unique personality structures and experiential backgrounds. Full reconciliation of the meaning of a crisis takes time.

This chapter describes the characteristics of and the immediate sequence of events that make up a crisis. It also provides general guidelines for intervention. Beginning with what constitutes a crisis, the chapter identifies what you can do to help people in crisis. It then describes how to help patients and families find opportunities for personal growth in these circumstances. Recognizing that crisis is an inevitable part of each person's personal journey, this chapter seeks to provide you with theory-based guidance in helping your patients understand and resolve their crises.

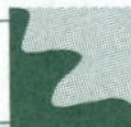

UPTON REHNBERG'S STORY

Upton Rehnberg sat in seat No. 8 in Row 9, reading a story about the Boeing Company in *Fortune* magazine. Feeling pleased with himself that he had been lucky enough to get this last seat on the plane, he settled in for a smooth flight to Chicago. A slight smile flickered across his face as thoughts of his son Lars's ninth birthday celebration punctuated Mr. Rehnberg's reading.

About an hour into the flight, Mr. Rehnberg's reading was interrupted again, but this time by the sound of a loud explosion. He immediately put on his seatbelt and noticed that the plane had begun to spiral slowly downward, turning to the right in a lazy descent. The pilot announced that they had lost engine number 2, but that they could still make it to Chicago with a little delay in the original schedule.

Mr. Rehnberg, a private pilot himself with a keen interest in the aerospace industry, commented to the flight attendant that the pilot was using engine power to steer. He suggested that that was indicative of serious trouble. The flight attendant gave some vague response, but the fear in her eyes indicated that Rehnberg's assessment was correct.

Half an hour later, the pilot again addressed the passengers and announced that the plane would make an emergency landing in Sioux City. The flight attendants prepared the passengers to brace themselves, look for exits, and keep their heads down until the plane came to a full stop.

Within minutes, the plane hit the runway, bouncing around and skidding hundreds of yards to an adjacent cornfield before coming to a stop resting on its top. Mr. Rehnberg found himself upside down with nothing in front of him. The galley was gone, and the whole first class section had disappeared. As he tried to dislodge himself, a small fireball moved through the left side of the plane. It hit Mr. Rehnberg, melting his nylon shirt and burning his face, arms, and right leg.

Ignoring his pain, Mr. Rehnberg struggled loose from his seat and lowered himself down. He pushed rubble out of the way and realized he could see directly outside into the cornfield. As passengers tried to move past Mr. Rehnberg, a maze of cables blocked their way and prevented their passage. Maintaining his composure, Mr. Rehnberg moved the cables away and directed the stunned, injured, and disoriented passengers to the cornfield. "Just move toward the corn," Mr. Rehnberg encouraged them. Several elderly people fell as they tried to climb out of the plane. Mr. Rehnberg dropped the cables to assist them and then returned to his self-appointed task of clearing the exit. After about 25 passengers had deplaned, Mr. Rehnberg himself left, still seemingly unaware of his own injuries. He then began to assist others who were on the ground.

The crash of United Flight 232 left at least 110 people dead, but more than 180 survived—thanks in part to people like Upton Rehnberg. Riding to St. Luke's Regional Medical Center, feeling the pain of second-degree burns over 6% of his body, Mr. Rehnberg felt relieved that he was going to the hospital. He then began to realize the impact of what had just happened.

The next day, reunited with his wife, Mr. Rehnberg commented that his life would never be the same. "I survived a major fatal airline crash." Recognizing the need to integrate this experience, Mr. Rehnberg stated, "I'm not particularly a spiritual individual, and it's frustrating to my wife because she is. You hear the old adage—try and live your life so that at any moment if you die you can be satisfied with your life. Well, I've had some minor illnesses and very little physical injury in my life. I've never felt close to death before this, and it's made me think. My five-year-old is just starting to learn to play chess, and I think sometimes the best possible use of time is sitting down to play chess with him. Just being aware of using time and not just letting it happen, those are the things I have to decide."

Story adapted from Alvarez, R. (1989, July 23). "One Seat Left: Luck Put Man on Flight 232." *Baltimore Sunday Sun, 89* (30), pp. 1A, 16A.

Upton Rehnberg's crisis was dramatic enough to receive news coverage. The life crises that most people face would not receive the same type of media attention. Yet every day, people experience life crises that, for them, can be equally dramatic and personally unsettling. Mr. Rehnberg faced a life-threatening crisis, and he emerged psychologically unharmed. The plane crash did not immobilize him, and he could be justifiably proud of his swift and heroic response to the crisis. But Mr. Rehnberg also notes the lingering personal effect of the crisis and describes it as a pivotal life event, bringing into sharper focus the people and life events that are of most value to him.

As it is with all crises, a sudden chance life event forced a reassessment of Mr. Rehnberg's priorities. His journey was interrupted in a dynamic way by a single unexpected event, which instantly and spontaneously became an integral part of a more complex life story. Once the immediate shock subsided, surprising feelings flooded Mr. Rehnberg, some in the form of questions, others in the form of decisions about the future directions of his journey. The feelings were about the meaning of his life. In his mind, he might have pondered: How can anyone really attribute meaning to this unfortunate event? Why did it occur? Why was he spared when 110 others died? These are all common questions that people in crisis ask themselves. Reflections about the past flashed through his mind and were interwoven into the present.

An invitation to change and broaden Mr. Rehnberg's perspectives about the journey appeared in the form of critical questions about the relationship of the crisis to the remainder of his journey. What can Mr. Rehnberg learn from this experience? Will he allow this event to mar his journey or to enrich it? How can he integrate the meaning of this event into his overall journey in ways that will transcend the tragedy of the particular circumstances? Each of the personalized answers to these difficult questions presents an opportunity for personal growth.

Failure to explore the meaning of a stressful life event can lead to the development of psychopathology. Unexamined the experience of crisis can forever limit the options of the traveler in many other portions of the human journey. The intensity of the immediate feelings subsides, but the feelings continue to resurface periodically, as unwelcome, intrusive, and unexpected intruders. The sharpness of potentially overwhelming feelings accompanying flashbacks of the original event continue to materialize with the trigger of a situational cue or when a person is alone in a wavelike form (Horowitz, 1986). Until the crisis is integrated as a necessary contributor to the journey and a potentially creative part of the life story, it continues to have a strong ripple effect—often years later.

THEORETICAL PERSPECTIVES

Eric Lindemann

In 1944, Lindemann developed a classic paper on bereavement that later evolved as a model for considering the nature and resolution of crisis in broader terms. He studied 101 patients who were in crisis as a result of personal loss. Included in this group were bereaved disaster victims and their relatives who had lost someone in the famous Coconut Grove fire and those of patients who had lost a relative during therapy. Other participants in the study were the relatives of armed service men either killed or lost in World War II and relatives of patients who had died in the hospital. His study of their behavior provided Lindemann with the observations of normal and morbid grief, which he later formulated into a stage theory concerning grief resolution. He noted that individuals experiencing a normal grief reaction suffered from physical complaints, preoccupation with memories of the deceased, anger, guilt, changes in patterns of activity, and imitating characteristics of the deceased. Some people had more difficulty accepting the reality of the loss, and others appeared to have a *delayed reaction* to the loss of a loved one. Distorted reactions included development of a physical illness or clinical depression. Unable to integrate the experience, the individual failed to ascribe a meaning to the loss that allowed life to continue. Prolonged intense grief represented the unresolved part of the relationship (Lindemann, 1944).

Lindemann became convinced that appropriate therapeutic intervention could help the patient disengage from disconcerting ties to the deceased and develop new patterns of interaction. He believed that the same interventions that were helpful in bereavement would prove just as helpful in other types of stressful events and proposed a crisis intervention model as a major element of preventive psychiatry in the community. Because Lindemann believed that crisis intervention should have a community focus, he worked with Caplan to establish the first mental health clinic devoted to preventive psychiatry (Baldwin, 1979).

Gerald Caplan

Caplan (1964; 1974), a colleague of Lindemann, receives credit for describing the sequence of the crisis state and for defining crisis intervention as a distinct form of preventive psychiatric therapy. The crisis intervention techniques developed through his research studies with the Harvard Family Health Clinic serve as a model for modern community mental health systems. Caplan believed that crisis represents a transitional period in a person's life characterized by emotional and cognitive disequilibrium forcing a reappraisal of previously held values and beliefs. It occurs when a person is faced with a potentially insoluble problem that has meaning for the person. The crisis situation does not occur in a vacuum, and the antecedents are usually identifiable. The crisis state is self-limiting, usually lasting four to six weeks. It is most accessible for treatment during the peak of the crisis, and it can be resolved successfully or incline the person to the development of a mental disorder. An inability to resolve a crisis successfully makes a person more vulnerable to difficulties in resolving other life crises.

Disruption in emotional homeostasis forms the cornerstone for Caplan's theoretical approach to crisis intervention. He describes four phases of escalating tension that leads to the crisis state. In the first stage, the person experiences increased tension related to the impact of an identifiable stressor. Failure of normal problem-solving strategies in the second stage results in a further increase of tension. When normal problem solving fails to counterbalance the increased tension, the individual mobilizes more vigorous and aggressive strategies characteristic of the third stage. It is possible to avert the crisis at this stage if the new coping strategies are effective, the person redefines the problem so it is resolvable, or the goals are abandoned as being unattainable. If the new strategies do not work, tension escalates to the breaking point. Readily observable emotional disorganization marks the fourth stage in the form of a crisis state.

According to Caplan, a crisis state does not develop spontaneously, nor does it unfold apart from the immediate environment of the person in crisis. To understand fully the nature of the crisis, it is necessary to assess the *context* in which the crisis arises. This assessment includes information about the nature of family bonds, work affiliation, and other significant relationships. The patient can avoid more serious dysfunction by altering the unhealthy environmental conditions that create a stress quickly. Caplan's work is particularly relevant for understanding interpersonal and developmental crisis states.

Caplan's ideas revolutionized previously held concepts of therapeutic intervention by suggesting the need for community-based intervention for basically healthy people in active crisis. His approach stresses the focus of intervention as being *problem-centered* rather than self-centered. This change in focus reframes the crisis state as a problematic issue in need of a solution rather than the consequence of a fatal flaw or personality defect in need of correction. Implicit in his construct is the need to reexamine what is useful in our lives and what is useless in light of the crisis and to restructure outmoded beliefs and actions.

Caplan (1974) recognized the important role nurses play in crisis intervention. He states, "I felt that among health professionals nurses were particularly well suited to stimulate such support and to act as bridges of communication and as mediators between their patients and other professional and non-professional agencies" (p. 215).

Erik Erikson

Erikson (1963; 1968) is important for his description of crisis as a natural part of personal maturation. He viewed developmental (maturational) crisis points as critical to normal healthy personality development. Erikson used an eight-stage model of human ego development (see Chapter 6) and proposed that personality growth could be divided into distinctive psychosocial developmental periods, or life stages. Each psychosocial crisis marks the transition to the next life stage. Although the critical demands of life differ from stage to stage, they are relatively similar for all members of a given society. The precise timing, however, and behavioral expression of a stage reflect an individual's culture, physical development, and life circumstances, such as illness or family norms. That culture plays a role is seen in the fact that societal expectations in Eastern cultures are quite different than they are in the West. For example, a woman's identity in many Eastern cultures is clearly tied to family and spouse, whereas in the West, women have more freedom to express their identity with ever-expanding career and life choices. The behavior of women in each culture reflects societal expectations.

Although developmental crises are directly related to social expectations, they also are age related. Psychosocial development emerges from a ground plan that uniquely defines each person's personality. In the beginning, the ground plan is not within the individual's conscious awareness but develops with greater clarity as the result of interactions with others and significant life experiences. A *crisis point* occurs when the self-understandings previously used by an individual to negotiate life no longer are sufficient to meet its social demands.

Each developmental crisis is systematically related to all others, and each has its own time of special focus or *ascendancy*. The task necessary for maturation exists in its purest form during the assigned stage but may also reappear during a later phase in a modified form. To move to the next stage of development, a person must successfully resolve each maturational crisis, the threads of which are incorporated into the higher level of psychosocial development.

Solutions to the tasks contained within each phase of development are established as a formative seed in previous phases, worked on in the present phase, and refined in subsequent ones. For example, the adolescent's focus on identity actually begins much earlier as the child engaged in social role behaviors during play and later developed fundamental skills in peer relationships with schoolmates. Following adolescence, identity becomes more complex and distinctive, as the individual increasingly incorporates social roles and life experience into his or her personal identity. In old age, mature adults reflect back on the meaning of their lives and share their insights with the younger generations.

The environment plays an important role in the development of a psychosocial crisis because it presents an individual with new defining characteristics about expected modes of behavior for each time period that are qualitatively different from the social expectations that preceded it. Rather than describing a psychosocial crisis as a purely situational response, however, Erikson (1963) viewed its development as an interactive process with personal factors. He describes an internal psychological process, "a necessary turning point, a crucial moment, when development must move one way or another, marshaling resources of growth, recovery, and further differentiation" (p. 16).

The central thread in Erikson's (1968) conceptualization of psychosocial crisis is the process of *identity consciousness*, ". . . which is always changing and developing; at its best it is a process of increasing differentiation, and it becomes ever more inclusive as the individual grows aware of a widening circle of others significant to him, from the maternal person to 'mankind' " (p. 23). Although Erikson specifies solutions to developmental crises in the extreme, for example, identity versus identity diffusion, he intended successful resolution to be framed as a balance between the two polarities. Table 15–1 identifies situational stressors that commonly occur during different stages of life. By understanding common situations occurring during transitional stages, such as marriage, first pregnancy, and retirement, you can help people anticipate developmental passages and provide special help to these individuals and their families with the psychosocial needs that characteristically emerge at this time.

Donna Aguilera

Aguilera (1994) and Aguilera and Messick (1974) provide a nursing framework for understanding the nature of balancing factors related to crisis and crisis intervention. They identify **balancing factors** as related to

- The patient's realistic perception of the problem
- The number and quality of social supports
- The caliber of coping mechanisms relevant to the resolution of the problem

Your assessment should focus on the presence or absence of these balancing supports in developing a relevant treatment plan. If a person has several balancing factors, it is much easier to resolve a crisis than if the person demonstrates lack of insight, has deficient coping skills, and has limited social supports. Overwhelming stressful situations are mediated through positive balancing supports, and without them, a crisis situation can become self-destructive in its intensity and in the amount of personal energy it requires.

People may lack an accurate perception of a crisis situation for a number of reasons. They can feel lost in the mire of confusion because of the suddenness of the threat, previous unresolved conflicts, mental illness, drug abuse, or lack of education and life experience. Some individuals are more prone to the development of a crisis state and may not recognize it as such because their lifestyle continuously exposes them to more personal threats, losses, or role changes. Because crisis is such an integral part of their lives, they may interpret it as just one more inevitable overwhelming circumstance in a life filled with chaos. Failure to achieve developmental tasks at the appropriate time also leaves a person poorly prepared to cope successfully with unexpected life circumstances, for example, the teenage mother with a special needs child.

TABLE 15–1 **Situational Stressors That Commonly Occur During Different Stages of Life**

Developmental Stage	Stressor
Trust vs. mistrust	Rejection by primary caregiver Physical illness or trauma Hospitalization, separation from parent
Autonomy vs. shame and doubt	Illness or trauma requiring restraint Rigid toilet training Loss of a parent
Initiative vs. guilt	Physical injury Entering school Loss of parent
Industry vs. inferiority	Peer or teacher conflicts Dyslexia Moving or changing schools
Identity vs. role confusion	Teenage pregnancy Graduation from high school Entering college First job Loss of parent
Intimacy vs. isolation	Unwanted pregnancy Separation, divorce, death of partner Birth of a child
Generativity vs. stagnation/self-absorption	Illness of self or family member Care of compromised parents Children leaving home Layoffs from employment Changes in job responsibilities
Ego integrity vs. despair	Death of spouse, family members, friends Failing senses, disability Retirement, financial difficulties Neglect or abuse by adult children

Aguilera (1994) identifies supportive relationships, defined as **social support,** as being important balancing factors. Social supports can include family, neighbors, friends, clergy, and health professionals from any of the health disciplines; they can occur with informal and chance encounters as well as from longer-term relationships with professionals and significant others. A taxi cab driver, sympathetic teacher, or even a stranger can provide a casual remark or brief opportunity to share human pain. Individuals without the support of an extended family or friends are more prone to the development of crisis. Social support is a critical mitigating factor in whether or how quickly a crisis state is resolved. In the clinical setting, you may become a significant social support for the patient in crisis.

The presence or absence of coping skills is classified as an important balancing factor. Deficient coping skills can occur as a result of unresolved personal issues or excessive anxiety, which leads to the development of defensive coping strategies and postponement of constructive efforts. The presence or lack of personal resources in terms of attitudes, creativity, intelligence, money, health, and interpersonal relationship skills can significantly influence the threat, development, and treatment of a patient in crisis. Successful past coping with difficult situations provides the foundation for developing new initiatives with the current crisis. The patient has more options to draw from in designing corrective mechanisms and a history of success that increases self-efficacy in the present.

The Aguilera/Messick model is useful as an assessment framework for evaluating the impact of a crisis event in functional terms (Figure 15–1). It also serves as a nursing theory–based guidepost for identifying where the intervention needs to focus. For example, one patient may have an accurate perception of the hazardous event and full awareness of being in a crisis state but may lack knowledge about potential resources or have a meager support system. Another patient may lack all of the above and require more specialized nursing intervention. Each patient needs an individualized treatment plan that supports careful attention to the specific needs presented by the individual. Specific knowledge of the personal attributes and social supports available to the individual as balancing factors in mastering difficult stress situations should guide the treatment process.

▶ Check Your Reading

1. In what ways does crisis represent an interruption in the human journey?

2. What do you see as the value (if any) of using theoretical frameworks in crisis situations?
3. What implications does Caplan's model have for preventive psychiatry?
4. How would you use Erikson's model to help a patient in crisis?
5. In what ways is the Aguilera/Messick model useful in crisis intervention?

NATURE OF CRISIS

A crisis is both an occurrence and a psychological state precipitated by a hazardous event. The hazardous event, labeled a **critical stressor,** creates great emotional upheaval and temporary personality disorganization.

Definitions

Crisis

A crisis is a "serious or decisive state," a "turning point." The word *crisis* is a derivative of the Greek word meaning "decision," but the Chinese provide two alternative definitions for it: "danger" and "opportunity."

Caplan (1964) suggests that "[a] crisis occurs when a person faces an obstacle to important life goals that is, for a time, insurmountable through the utilization of his

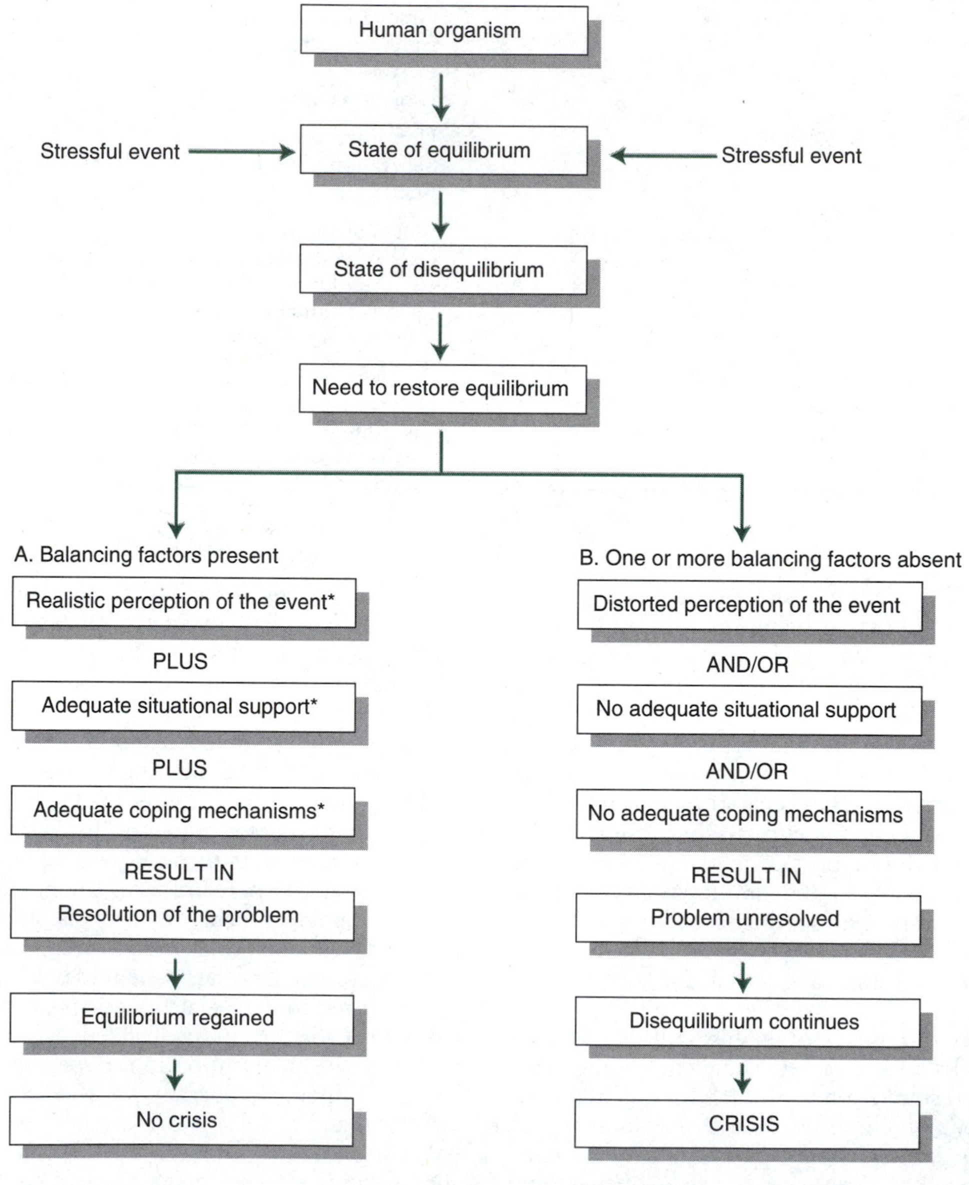

FIGURE 15–1
The Aguilera/Messick model, which is useful for assessment of the functional impact of a crisis. (Redrawn from Aguilera, D. [1994]. *Crisis intervention: Theory and methodology* [7th ed.]. St. Louis: Mosby-Year Book.)

customary methods of problem solving" (p. 18). What is clear in all of these definitions is that one event, a single moment in time, can forever change the course of one's life. It is, as Caplan postulates, "an upset in a steady state" (quoted in Rapoport, 1965, p. 24).

Characteristic of all definitions of crisis is the notion that something extraordinary has happened that requires a person to make a decisive paradigm shift in responding to abnormal circumstances. By definition, if a person knew how to cope with the crisis easily, it would not be classified as a true crisis. Crisis is experienced as unexpected, uncontrollable, and a personal threat to self-concept, and it usually involves a loss of something important to the individual. When a person experiences a crisis, he or she typically knows little about how to do the things that he or she has to do to meet the needs of the situation and function appropriately. Moreover, what the person does need to know about coping with the crisis situation must be learned in a relatively short period of time. Each particular crisis situation presents the person with uncharted territory, and this fact alone can be potentially overwhelming. Its precise meaning and subsequent effect on personal functioning depend on many factors.

Case Example 15–1 Christine's Story

Christine Belmont is 23 and has been married for 18 months. She has just given birth prematurely to identical twin daughters. At the time of the birth of the twins, it was apparent that one of the infants had meconium staining (an indicator of fetal distress). The infant was rushed to the neonatal intensive care unit, where neonatologists determined that the infant had aspirated meconium. Despite intensive medical and nursing intervention, the infant died six days later.

The other infant weighed 4 pounds at birth. Despite her size, she appeared to be healthy and was released to her parents. Nevertheless, the young parents were instructed that their surviving infant should not be taken out of the house until she weighed five pounds.

Instead of enjoying the birth of their babies, this couple now has to plan a funeral to which they cannot even bring their surviving infant. It is a confused, painful, and emotionally charged situation that most couples having their first baby do not encounter. The couple is experiencing a roller coaster of conflicting emotions—joy over the birth of their infants, interlaced with profound sadness and grief over the loss of one of them.

In Case Example 15–1, there are many factors to consider. First, the hazardous event meets all of the criteria for a crisis in that it is unexpected, it is uncontrollable, and there is a profound loss. The crisis this young woman and her husband face, however, is not simply the loss of an infant. It instantly reorders the mental map the couple have carried about themselves as human beings, and it momentarily undermines their understanding of reality. Christine and her husband have to come to terms not only with the physical reality of their baby's death, but also with their self-image as parents, the meaning of their youth, and the uncompromising nature of the events that have taken place over the past week. All of the plans and shared goals that involved two babies have to be modified. The joy of giving birth is tempered by the decisive unexpected death issue accompanying it. Moreover, having twins is physically more demanding than having a single birth, which means that Christine is less physically able to cope with this unforeseen set of circumstances than she might be otherwise. Theirs is not an ordinary experience, so although their peers may be highly supportive, they may be of little practical assistance in working through the roller coaster emotions and reality functions required to resolve this crisis.

Crisis intervention in this case would consist of providing guidance and support to the couple in coping with their grief about the loss of one infant and reducing their anxiety about caring appropriately for the surviving infant. The professional help given to Christine and her husband would be designed to complement their own personal resources. To direct the couple effectively, you need to have a general understanding of the nature of the crisis state and the progressive steps involved in crisis intervention.

Crisis State

The term *crisis state* is used to describe a personal response—physical, emotional, spiritual, and behavioral—to a crisis situation. Some crises, for example, loss of an important relationship, characteristically induce "a state of crisis of lesser or greater intensity, or of lesser or greater duration, in nearly all individuals" (Rapoport, 1965, p. 23). The response to a hazardous event or critical stressor can be highly specific to each person's interpretation of the threat that a particular stressor poses for him or her. Although each crisis response can be described in similar terms as far as presenting symptoms are concerned, what constitutes a crisis for one person may not be a crisis for another person because each is a unique individual. Understanding the individualized response to crisis is essential to successful implementation of the nursing process in crisis situations.

The precise causes of the crisis state defy any real attempt to categorize them. For the person experiencing it, the crisis state represents a cosmic freezing of time. Being in the crisis state does not mean that the individual is suffering from an emotional or mental illness. Although the behaviors observed in crisis may be severely dysfunctional and may mimic definable psychiatric symptoms, they are not necessarily evidence of pathology. The mother who has just a buried a child may "hear" the child's voice coming from the back seat as she drives. Yet she is not schizophrenic or comparably psychotic. Her response is quite "normal" for the acute phase of the grieving process. Tyhurst (1957) notes that an individual may already have chronic psychiatric symptoms when he or she experiences the crisis state, and this comorbidity needs to be assessed as part of the overall treatment protocol.

A crisis situation typically sets the stage for the development of a crisis state, but understanding the "facts" of a crisis situation is not enough to help someone through a crisis. Rather, it is knowing the crisis "from the inside," that is, the personal way in which each person experiences a particular situation, that is most important. For instance, in the Case Example 15–1, you would want to let Christine and her husband talk a lot about the births—and the death of one daughter—what it meant to them to have their babies, and how they would like to proceed. Inquiries about the mother's physical well-being, the couple's perception of their living infant, and their concerns about her care also would be important. This personal knowledge helps you guide the parents in selecting from the different paths leading to a constructive resolution of the crisis.

Thus, your assessment embraces validation of feelings as well as data collection. In Case Example 15–1, you would acknowledge how incomprehensible the event must be for the couple and their extended families. In the course of developing an accurate assessment, you should confirm the human suffering attached to losing an infant and all that it stirs up in terms of self-perceptions, death of a dream, and the meaning to each partner.

Attention should be paid to the meaning of the event to other significant people involved in this case. The input of others usually colors the meaning of a crisis. Family members and nursing staff select different elements to observe and comment on, partially because they each have a different experiential background. They also have different purposes in considering the circumstances. One set of grandparents might focus on the sadness of their daughter, whereas another might think more about the loss of the infant. You might gather data about the grandparents' involvement or response. Availability and connectivity to a church and the cultural implications of the crisis situation for the family are also important. These perspectives provide an integrated understanding of its meaning to guide your future work and thinking. There also is another benefit to this intervention. A simple, empathetic understanding of the position of each family member holds, as you inquire about the nature of the crisis event, helps to organize the family into a self-supporting network, which can help restore the balance in a temporary state of emotional disequilibrium.

Elements Contributing to the Onset of a Crisis State

Caplan (1964) identifies five elements that typically contribute to the development of a crisis state (Box 15–1). These elements are interactive.

BOX 15–1 Five Elements That Typically Contribute to the Development of a Crisis State

A critical stressor
Vulnerability
Failure of previous coping strategies
Intolerable tension
Lack of social support

Hazardous Events

A hazardous event usually ushers in the development of the crisis state. Referred to as a critical stressor, the personal disequilibrium associated with a crisis state starts with self-awareness of an external event or internal critical stressor. Perceived as acutely dangerous to the well-being of an individual, family, or community, the precipitating factor in a crisis state can occur as a single incident, or it can be the result of a combination of factors that exceed a person's coping capacity. Common hazardous events include loss through death, divorce, accidents, disasters, serious illness, loss of a job, injury to self, or injury to another. Internal critical stressors can encompass loss of expected promotion, change in role or relationship, or a perceived alteration in either status or responsibilities. In defining a problem stressor, it is important to note that not all hazardous events or critical stressors are negative or undesired turning points in a personal journey. The birth of a baby, a new job or desired promotion, or getting better after a long, debilitating illness can stimulate the development of a crisis state.

To qualify as a precipitant of a crisis state, a critical stressor may or may not be objectively catastrophic. Being bypassed for promotion is a single critical stressor, enough to create a crisis, but a person with a strong marriage and social support in the community might weather it satisfactorily with little intervention. Coupled with a problem marriage, financial difficulties, or loss of a friend at the same time, the combination of factors could promote a full-blown crisis state requiring crisis intervention and perhaps follow-up treatment. Thus, it is as crucial to assess the personalized meaning of the critical stressor as it is to gather facts about the crisis. How an individual interprets its intrusion in the journey affects every segment of planning and intervention.

A critical stressor can be perceived as a threat, a loss, a challenge, or an opportunity to change how one conducts life. For example, a forced change in territory can be devastating for a fledgling salesman, but the same circumstance may be simply an unwelcome irritant to a more experienced salesman who has been through the scenario before and has learned how to respond successfully. Or the new assignment may be viewed as a challenge and new opportunity for professional growth. The intervention in each case would start with the individual's interpretation of the event and support the strengths while minimizing the potential maladaptive responses.

Vulnerability

An individual's response to the stressor often depends on his or her personal vulnerability at the time a critical stressor occurs. Vulnerability is a highly individual phenomenon, which, in part, depends on how a person characteristically handles problems or learns to negotiate the environment effectively and, in part, on the meaning and timing of the crisis. Thus, personal and environmental factors play a role in vulnerability. To begin with, people demonstrate markedly different attitudes, codes of conduct, life goals, and ways of responding to a crisis that reflect their past history and unique perceptions of the current situation. When two people are confronted with the same set of circumstances, each selectively chooses different aspects as being most important. The patient's perspective on his or her vulnerability is important assessment data because interventions have the greatest chance of success when they emphasize issues of importance to the patient. Physical illness, lack of social support, and the presence of concurrent stressors create additional vulnerability and increase the intensity of a critical stressor.

Failure of Previous Coping Strategies

Crisis lies always in the "I" of the beholder. In some cases, the intensity of a critical stressor for a given individual has its roots in the past, and a person is more at risk for the development of a crisis because of previous experiences. For example, loss of a parent in childhood can make responses to any threat of loss in adulthood much more acute. Lack of experience with previous failure or the expectations of significant others can predispose a person to experiencing a single event as an earth-shattering life experience, an insurmountable crisis resolvable only through extreme measures. A single failed test or a disappointment in a hoped-for relationship has caused some people to commit suicide.

Handling a crisis situation typically is less difficult for the person who is accustomed to meeting his or her own needs and has the knowledge, resources, and skills needed to seek out the appropriate solution. It is most difficult for the person for whom working out ways of meeting personal needs and dealing with people and institutions has never been a strength and less so for people who simply lack experience.

Self-efficacy plays a role in determining vulnerability (Bandura, 1977). Some people perceive an objectively crisis-producing life situation as being within their ability to cope. They turn a potential crisis into an opportunity for growth with a little imagination, or they have strong social support as a balancing factor. Such people respond with resiliency (see Chapter 9) rather than vulnerability, and the potential crisis resolves of its own accord or with minimal professional intervention. They draw immediately on personal strengths, such as faith or a sense of humor to regain perspective.

Intolerable Tension

The third factor in the development of a crisis state is intolerable tension that brings the person to a breaking point. Tension can build in relation to the situation itself or with the personal immobilization created by a protracted attempt at resolution without needed respite.

Case Example 15–2 Mrs. Dittman's Story

Margaret Dittman is a hospitalized four-year-old newly diagnosed with leukemia. Her parents insist on being involved with all aspects of her care. They make frequent trips to the hospital, attend support group meetings, and interact frequently with hospital staff. The staff views the family as a model of successful coping. One day, however, the mother's emotional reserve seems to "snap." Her coping structure, which up until this point was strong enough to prevent a crisis state, becomes ineffective. Both she and others around her are aware of a significant change in her behavior that resembles symptoms of a psychiatric problem. This mother, however, is simply experiencing a crisis state stemming from exhaustion—a nonpathological emotional response to overwhelming stress.

Consider Case Example 15–2. The initial strategies used with this mother would be to support her obvious investment in her child's well-being, to validate her current feelings as a nonpathological response to an overwhelming turn of life events, and to assist her in ventilating her concerns and negative feelings. You should also help both parents understand what is happening to their child and use the Aguilera/Messick model to help them shift the weighting of balancing factors in a more positive direction.

Prolonged, unrelieved excessive tension leaves the person in a dangerous condition. In its early stages, excessive tension can be brought under control with the standard crisis intervention strategies described later in the chapter. Unfortunately, without help, a crisis can result in a lower level of functioning, for example, alcohol or drug abuse, chronic psychological symptoms, or social isolation. In its most extreme form, an active crisis state can precipitate a brief reactive psychosis that warrants a specific psychiatric diagnosis. The symptoms produced by a brief reactive psychosis are florid, out of character for the patient, and quite frightening for both patient and staff. Stabilizing the patient with medication and ensuring a secure, protected environment are essential before using more traditional crisis intervention strategies. One way of distinguishing between a brief psychotic state and other forms of pathology is through past history and current drug use.

Lack of Social Support

Social support given by someone in the external environment strengthens a person's resolve and promotes resiliency. It can be delivered through words, actions, or simply the committed presence of another human being during a difficult time. Identified earlier as being an important balancing factor in assessing the intensity of a crisis and in directing the focus of treatment (Aguilera, 1994), social support is perhaps the most essential balancing factor. In almost every instance, lack of such external support plays a decisive role in the creation of a crisis state. Figley (1985), for example, found that the family members suffering the most psychological damage in a crisis situation were those who were denied social support within the family. Unfortunately, family members closest to the member actually experiencing the crisis can become "infected" with similar anxiety and also require crisis intervention, particularly if they enter the situation in a vulnerable state (Figley, 1988).

Although lack of social support is a critical dimension of crisis risk in outpatients, it also plays a role in inpatient settings. Psychiatric hospitalization in and of itself can represent a critical stressor, and how it is handled is extremely important. Patients admitted to a psychiatric unit are cut off from their normal social supports, and consequently their perception of the attitudes of their caregivers assume greater importance. If they are in touch with reality, the experience of hospitalization coincides with feelings of shame, lack of self-confidence, and powerlessness in being able to manage their own affairs. Consider the reaction of a nurse consumer of inpatient services in Case Example 15–3. Social support provided by the nurse in the form of explanations and interventions designed to promote mutuality and inclusion of the patient as a partner rather than object of the admission process could have significantly decreased this patient's sense of crisis.

Case Example 15–3 Gretchen's Story

Admission to a psychiatric hospital is not easy. I did not want to be there, but I felt I had no choice. Walking into the hospital made me feel ill at ease and embarrassed. I was very grateful to have a friend with me to ease the emotional pain. The unit was supposed to be open, but it was locked at the time of my admission. Realizing I was to be held behind locked doors made me feel very humiliated. I also felt like a prisoner, an outcast of society. This was the beginning of the stripping of my personhood—my body and soul.

I was taken to a small, bare room that looked like a jail cell. It had three chairs and a desk. There were no pictures on the walls, flower arrangements, or anything to make me feel welcome. The room seemed very small and needed a coat of paint. It was here that I was "interrogated." Form after form was presented to me to sign. It was difficult at best to keep the forms straight. I signed eight forms, one of which was called "Patient's Rights," which I was told would be good to read some time. After signing all of the forms, the psychiatric technician left and the primary nurse entered to get my history. While she was obtaining my history, my suitcase was taken out of the room.

At the completion of the history-taking, I was shown to my room. On the way, I had to stop at the desk to have my purse gone through. It made me sick. I wanted to cry. I felt like a very bad person who couldn't be trusted. At the time, I also noticed that many things had been removed from my suitcase. I felt like I had been punched in the stomach or assaulted. Things taken away from me included all aerosols, glass bottles, and electrical appliances such as blow dryer; my embroidery, because it was in a plastic bag; mirrors, tweezers, needles, keys, and even my pillow. Taking my pillow seemed to be the last straw. Everything had been taken from me. I felt angry at these people for taking my things. I felt very alone because I knew none of the patients or staff. I was upset because no one seemed to know that I was a person—a nurse with a doctoral degree. I was on the wrong side of the desk. Then I felt embarrassed. I shouldn't be here. I was a respectable person, but no one seemed to know or care.

When I got to my room, I was shocked not to have a bathroom or telephone in my room. Again, I felt like I had been hit in the stomach. Tears, tears, tears—they just wouldn't stop. My roommate came and introduced herself. She was nice. Another patient on the "welcome committee" oriented me to the unit and told me about community life. She also seemed nice and was helpful to me. A physician came and wrote an order so that I could have my pillow. As I lay awake that first night, crying, I wondered how I had ever gotten here. What had I done to deserve this punishment? Why couldn't anyone see *me* and know how scared I felt?

Maintaining continued casual contacts that are caring and respectful of the patient as a unique person also can reduce the incidence of inpatient crisis states. Cardell and Horton-Deutsch (1994) note that selected research studies support the hypothesis that "patients who felt uncared for and/or misunderstood by the staff reported continued or increased suicidal ideation" (p. 369).

Risk Factors for the Development of a Crisis State

No one is immune to developing a crisis state. Given the right set of circumstances, everyone is capable of experiencing the startling and profound disequilibrium associated with crisis (Gulliland and James, 1993). Unexpected life events fail to respect race, creed, or socioeconomic status. Crisis events happen to good people who put a lot of effort into making their lives successful as well as to those who do not plan their lives effectively. Nevertheless, there are risk factors that enhance the probability of life events or personal circumstances resulting in a crisis state. The nature of the crisis and number of sequential or concurrent stressors make the possibility of crisis more likely because they affect the perception of a potential crisis event. Previous life experience with similar stressors, physical and emotional state, age, and developmental stage contribute to the individual's coping responses, and level of social support interacts with all of the aforementioned as balancing factors.

"Unacceptable" Stressors

The nature of a crisis affects its perception and its acceptability. Disasters caused by "acts of God," such as cyclones or flooding, are more acceptable than crises precipitated by humans. Events caused by people that actually produce less objective damage frequently create higher levels of perceived crisis (Melick et al, 1982) because people believe that their actions could have prevented them. Following an accident, it is common for those closest to the victim to blame themselves or others for "causing" the accident by not being home or by choosing a different plan for the evening, even when this was not a determining factor. The role of chance needs to be emphasized in such circumstances.

Concurrent Stressors

Coinciding life events influence the perception of a crisis and its manageability. For example, the family with many small children and circumscribed social support may have more limited options for regrouping and replacing what is lost than a family in which these circumstances were not an issue. An elderly person with limited financial and social resources may suffer a greater sense of depression and demoralization following a disastrous flood. For this person, the tragic event parallels a time period in which there characteristically are many losses and fewer options. Compounding the sense of loss may be a lack of resiliency; the adaptive process and physical stamina needed to respond effectively to the crisis are lacking.

Insufficient Exposure or Poor Response to Prior Stressors

A lack of experience with normal stresses can magnify the meaning of a commonly occurring stressor. For example, a popular teenage athlete who experiences the loss of a significant relationship or failed expectations in the first semester of college may be at high risk for a crisis state. His less noticed friend, for whom disappointment is a more natural part of the journey, may weather a similar loss with greater equanimity. Previous experience with similar stressors can either make a situation more manageable or increase its impact. Knowing that one has survived a crisis makes the next one a little easier, whereas unsuccessful resolution can heighten its intensity.

Holmes and Rahe (1967) believed that individuals have a limited tolerance for repeated crisis and developed a research tool to prove their hypothesis. Their *Schedule of Recent Experiences* (Figure 15–2) is used to describe common life change events that qualify as crisis; each was given a quantitative weighting. Their tool is based on the premise that the number and nature of significant life

Forty-three common life events are listed in the order of their importance. Total score predicts likelihood of developing a serious illness within the next two years. Scores of more than 300 indicate a high probability (80%) of developing a serious illness within the next few years. Scores between 150 and 300 have a 51% probability, and scores of less than 150 within a year have a 37% probability of developing a major physical or psychological illness.

Life Event	Your Value Score	Life Event	Your Value Score
1. Death of spouse	100 ____	23. Son or daughter leaving home	29 ____
2. Divorce	73 ____	24. Trouble with in-laws	29 ____
3. Marital separation	65 ____	25. Outstanding personal achievement	28 ____
4. Jail term	63 ____	26. Spouse begins or stops work	26 ____
5. Death of a close family member	63 ____	27. Starting or finishing school	26 ____
6. Personal injury or illness	53 ____	28. Change in living conditions	25 ____
7. Marriage	50 ____	29. Revision of personal habits	24 ____
8. Fired at work	47 ____	30. Trouble with boss	23 ____
9. Marital reconciliation	45 ____	31. Change in work hours, conditions	20 ____
10. Retirement	45 ____	32. Change in residence	20 ____
11. Change in family member's health	44 ____	33. Change in schools	20 ____
12. Pregnancy	40 ____	34. Change in recreation	19 ____
13. Sex difficulties	39 ____	35. Change in church activities	19 ____
14. Addition to family	39 ____	36. Change in social activities	18 ____
15. Business readjustment	39 ____	37. Mortgage or loan under $10,000	17 ____
16. Change in financial state	38 ____	38. Change in sleeping habits	16 ____
17. Death of close friend	37 ____	39. Change in number of family get-togethers	15 ____
18. Change to different line of work	36 ____	40. Change in eating habits	15 ____
19. Change in number of arguments with spouse	35 ____	41. Vacation	13 ____
20. Mortgage over $10,000	31 ____	42. Christmas	12 ____
21. Foreclosure of mortgage or loan	30 ____	43. Minor violation of law	11 ____
22. Change in work responsibilities	29 ____		Total ____

FIGURE 15–2

The Holmes-Rahe "Schedule of Recent Experiences." (Reprinted with permission from *Journal of Psychosomatic Research, 11,* 213–218. Holmes, T. H., and Rahe, R. H. The social readjustment rating scale. 1967. [The scale gives complete wording of the items.] Elsevier Science, Ltd., Pergamon Imprint, Oxford, England.)

crises over a short period of time directly correlate with the development of physical illness. The larger the number of serious life events, the more likely the development of a stress-related physical illness within a three-year period.

Prolonged Stress

In addition to the number of stressors a person experiences, the length and unremitting nature of a single chronic stressor can intensify the current experience. A lifetime of chronic illness or a dysfunctional family background makes a current crisis more difficult. Crisis always involves a threatened loss of control and a diminished sense of coping ability. With prolonged stress, each new situation takes a toll that is qualitatively different than suffering from an isolated crisis incident. Intense feelings from previous encounters with stressful situations typically are pushed out of memory or minimized as people struggle for survival in dealing with the chaos of the current crisis. Although their beat is faint, memory keeps intruding, creating and magnifying the rhythms of the current crisis situation.

Physical and Emotional Depletion

Depletion in a patient's physical and emotional state blurs or distorts the meaning of a crisis. Physical factors contribute to a person's vulnerability because needed energy is tied to responding to bodily tension rather than to a focus on the tension of the crisis. It is more difficult for anyone to maintain a balanced perspective when one is tired, in pain, or distracted by physical symptoms. Drugs or alcohol cloud and distort the meaning of a situation, causing some to be overlooked as potential crisis and creating bizarre or numbed responses to others.

The presence of concurrent psychiatric symptoms makes realistic assessments of a crisis situation less probable. Most patients with a premorbid depressive disorder experience a potential crisis situation with greater intensity and deepening of symptoms, whereas those with behavioral disorders tend to act out rather than try to resolve the anxiety associated with the crisis state. Particularly problematic are those patients who impulsively and characteristically take self-destructive actions in response to a crisis because they can hurt themselves unintentionally in the heat of a crisis state.

Ironically, certain patients seem to be at their best coping with crisis situations with high drama, yet they are unable to contend with similar resolution of more deeply rooted psychiatric symptoms and unresolved responses to life. Crisis superimposed on an underlying behavioral disorder obviously is a more complex condition, which usually warrants careful observation and referrals once the immediate crisis is resolved.

Crisis as an Opportunity

In the throes of a crisis state, it is difficult to think of it as having a positive value, and yet it can be a significant turning point in an individual's life journey. A crisis state has the capacity to propel a person into an entirely different mode of thinking. It is a summons to action, in which old habits are called into question and new responses become imperative. Because a crisis situation is so disruptive to the journey, it sets off an inner revolution of meaning into motion, capable of inspiring a person to consider new and different directions. Rapoport (1965) suggests that "the challenge it provokes may bring forth new coping mechanisms which serve to strengthen the individual's adaptive capacity, and thereby in general, to raise his level of mental health" (p. 23).

The presence of a crisis state can act as a brief and unexpected window in time during which individuals are more open to change and therefore more likely to reorganize their priorities in light of the changed circumstances. For this reason, you can work more intensively with the person involved, and the possibility for personal growth in a shortened period of time is much higher. Second, a crisis often brings to light earlier unresolved and related problems that suddenly become available and amenable to treatment. Without the crisis to magnify the problem areas, many people live with problems that chronically exist in a lesser intensity. Thus, crisis intervention has important implications for preventive psychiatry (Case Example 15–4).

Case Example 15–4 Norma's Story

Norma Byron's youngest daughter was recently diagnosed with anorexia nervosa. The girl was hospitalized in her first semester of college. This illness served as an impetus for Norma to scrutinize more closely her own seriously dysfunctional marriage. Contributing to the marriage problems were Norma's chronic depression and her husband's need to control. Neither partner was good at expressing feelings that could be heard by the other. Norma and her husband now have the opportunity, in coping with the crisis of their daughter's illness, and with appropriate help, to resolve a longstanding dysfunctional communication pattern that otherwise might not have surfaced with such clarity.

From Williamson, J. (1990). Reaching children at greatest risk. *Child World, summer/fall,* 3–5.

You can be a valuable resource in joining the patient as a professional ally, in a therapeutic process designed to help a patient explore, learn from, and resolve serious life events. Ideally, *successful resolution of a crisis leads to greater self-awareness of what is truly important about the journey.* A crisis can invite a person to experience a new or broader sense of self. Successful coping with a crisis situation can enhance a person's competency in coping with other difficult life issues, and it has the potential to deepen the meaning of existentially important life circumstances.

Types of Crises

Crises typically are classified as situational or maturational (developmental) types for description purposes. Situational crisis occurs unpredictably, whereas maturational crises are identifiable in relation to predictable stages of human development.

Situational Crises

Characteristically, a **situational crisis** is a random event, coming without warning and entirely nondiscriminatory in its choice of victim. The critical stressor can occur as an unbalancing community, personal, or family circumstance. Situational crises can develop simultaneously for many people at the same time and extend over a period of time, as in a war situation, or they can transpire as a singular event affecting a particular person or family.

DISASTERS

Disasters are communal crises. They occur as natural or human-caused large-scale disasters, affecting large numbers of people simultaneously. Melick and colleagues (1982) suggest that "[a] disaster is not a single event occurring in the life of an individual; rather it is a series of events preceding and following impact whose sequelae are likely to be experienced over time by exposed individuals, and by the community in which the disaster occurred" (p. 624).

Although disasters always present personal dilemmas for individual members of a community, the initial focus of crisis intervention is on restabilizing the whole community. Most disasters are reported extensively in the press and immediately generate an outpouring of sympathy and social and practical support from strangers as well as those involved with the victims. Examples of disasters include airplane crashes, earthquakes, war casualties, nuclear plant accidents, forest fires, hurricanes, droughts, and floods. Governments classify disasters as federal major disasters or federal emergency disasters, depending on their magnitude and severity, for federal relief purposes.

In 1957, Tyhurst studied individual responses to community disaster and was one of the first psychiatrists to propose that a state of crisis does not represent a psychiatric illness. According to Tyhurst, a crisis offers a unique opportunity for personal growth, no matter how severe the symptoms might appear. He described three identifiable phases of adjustment in the **crisis sequence.** Initially, people in crisis experience a *period of impact,* which activates a psychological state of shock. The feeling of wholeness is irrevocably shaken, and individuals in crisis experience a sense of unreality. This phase is followed by a *period of recoil,* which represents an emotional retreat from the event in the form of denial, feelings of hopelessness, and limited attention to working through the problem. Usually the period of recoil yields to more productive reality testing and reframing of the original incident. Tyhurst refers to a third phase of adjustment as the *posttraumatic period,* during which a person begins to integrate the crisis experience into the larger tapestry of life in a more productive way. Tyhurst's work is particularly useful in understanding the sequence of feelings following a catastrophic crisis and helping therapists deal with their own feelings in relation to it.

People experiencing disaster tend to act informally and spontaneously to help each other weather the impact of the crisis. The level of mutual helpfulness is distinctive, people share scarce resources impartially, and individual needs are subsumed into meeting the needs of the larger aggregate (Tidmarsh, 1969). Mr. Rehnberg's response in the air crash is a good example of a person acting altruistically and spontaneously to help others with little regard for his own well-being in a disaster situation.

During a disaster, crisis intervention strategies that directly support and empower the efforts of the local citizenry are most productive for two reasons. First, they take advantage of the personal resources available in the group, and second, they serve to help the community reestablish a sense of personal control at a time when typically there is a general feeling of helplessness. Attempts by the professional helper to provide direct assistance often are viewed as an intrusion during the period of *altruistic community* characteristic of disaster crisis situations.

COMMUNITY CRISES

A community crisis may or may not reach disaster proportions. It represents a more personalized situational crisis affecting one person or a small segment of the community. An individual's crisis can capture the attention of an entire community if it symbolizes behaviors that potentially can alter the journey for other members. The abduction of a child, a brutal murder, or discovery of a public official's misconduct all provide examples of individual crises instantly affecting an entire community almost as if it is a personal experience. For example, in 1994, a mother's murder of her two children in North Carolina shocked an intact community, creating a crisis not only for the family, but also for others symbolically touched by it. Families confronting relocation and urban renewal typically describe their situation as a major community crisis. Faced by a common difficulty, the community tends to draw more closely together. Crisis intervention, both generic and individual, helps families and communities adjust to new roles and shifts in position or status.

PERSONAL CRISES

Other situational crisis states emerge from unexpected externally created circumstances or personal illness that affects a single person or a smaller nucleus of family and friends. For example, an auto accident, divorce, rape, terminal medical diagnosis, and severe illness in a previously healthy individual can create instantly a state of psychological shock that is potentially overwhelming for the individual or family. So out of the ordinary is the circumstance that the individual literally does not know how to think about the problem, much less how to

BOX 15-2 Examples of Personal Crises

Mrs. Jackson's husband died suddenly of a heart attack 6 weeks ago. They had been married for 24 years.

Maria Porter got engaged at Christmas. Her fiance was involved in an auto accident over New Year's and it looks as though he will be a paraplegic.

Mr. Francis went to the doctor with double vision last week, and learned that he has Graves' disease and that there is a strong possibility that he will be completely blind in 2 years.

Mr. Maxwell has been surplused from his job as middle manager after 18 years of employment with the same company.

Mrs. Braxton has become increasingly frail and can no longer live by herself. She must move in with her daughter and her family.

Mrs. DiNola's husband has been diagnosed with Alzheimer's disease. She is 51 and has just started a new job.

formulate strategies to resolve it. Symptoms of shock emerge quickly. Initially an individual may use defensive coping patterns to reduce the tension. This is the mind's way of cushioning the shock of the new information. It also is quite normal in the early stages of a crisis to feel disoriented and dazed. A common thought is "This can't be happening to me" or "I must not have all the facts, I can't believe that this is happening." Previous adaptive patterns may be called on to correct the tension. In addition to the psychological shock of the crisis, an individual may experience somatic symptoms and physical responses in the form of insomnia and changes in eating patterns. A personal crisis can stimulate a roller coaster of emotions normally associated with any loss: shock, anger, anxiety, shame, and despair. Your primary goal is to provide the type of help that restores at least a previous level of functioning.

Personal crisis inevitably precipitates an identity turning point, typically requiring a *major shift* in thinking about oneself. In each case, the patient's crisis of identity does not represent a simple cause-effect relationship to the event but rather needs to take into account each individual's interpretation of the events and the social supports available to them in resolving it. Examples of personal crises are found in Box 15–2. Consider the meaning that each of these personal crisis situations might have on lifestyle, sense of identity, and role relationships.

FAMILY CRISES

Individuals are members of families and communities. An individual family member in crisis can precipitate a family unit crisis that is separate from but related to the individual's crisis. For example, jailing of an individual family member, death, or hospitalization creates financial and emotional consequences for all family members. Hoff (1989) outlines three potential sources of family crisis: (1) loss of a family member, (2) addition of a family member, and (3) loss of morale occasioned by the deviant or abnormal behavior of one or more of the family members. Examples include divorce, death, birth of an infant, addition of a frail elder to the family unit, alcoholism, and mental illness.

Other critical stressors that can directly affect normal family functioning include moving to a different geographical area; bankruptcy; marriage; caring for elderly parents; delinquency; illegitimacy; adult children moving home; spousal, child, or elder abuse; and serious illness regardless of the family member it directly affects.

Just as individuals focus on different parts of a crisis, so do individual parts of the family unit. For example, the birth or illness of a child needing special care obviously creates a crisis situation for the parents, but what about the impact on the other children? The crisis affects their ability to complete their own developmental tasks and their interaction with the child, with the parents, and with their friends. Yet often the needs of the other children are forgotten in the heat of a crisis situation. It is not until much later that the child even has either the awareness or the words to describe what happened. For children, who cannot give voice to their concerns, a crisis in the family can be a hidden turning point with long-term psychological fallout.

The relationship between individual and family crisis is a reciprocal one. Admitting a loved one to a nursing home, having to initiate commitment proceedings for a mentally ill relative, and enduring the criminal trial of a family member present critical stressors to all family members as well as to the individual involved. Sometimes a family crisis erupts to reveal an underlying psychodynamic problem within the family. For example, as one drug-abusing child is admitted to a treatment center, a second child assumes the delinquent or drug-abusing role in the family. In many instances, the identified patient in crisis actually is either acting out or reacting to the larger context of a crisis in the family (Benglesdorf and Alden, 1990). Thus, a crisis provides not only the family's initial entry into the health care system, but also a unique opportunity for individual personal growth within the family context. Many of the same strategies used to treat individuals in crisis are extended to the treatment of family members as a collective unit.

In assessing and responding to family crisis, it is important to explore with the family their beliefs about the crisis and its impact on the family. This information can be obtained through conversations about how the family handles problems, their expectations of each other, and the meanings of such a crisis in their family. Interventions in a family crisis need to consider the family instead of the individual as the decision-making unit, and it is important to regard all family members' viewpoints as important pieces of data. Knowledge of the family strengths, previous coping strategies, their perception of the problem, and the resources available to them in the crisis period provides a baseline of data from which to select the most appropriate interventions (Case Example 15–5).

Case Example 15–5 Martha's Story

Martha Miller is a 75-year-old widow living on the East coast of the United States. She has osteoporosis and was successfully treated for colon cancer about two years ago. She describes herself as a loner who likes to read and prefers to live by herself. She does not have a good relationship with her daughter, who lives in the area, and is pained with their estrangement. Recently, Martha fell and broke her ankle. Her son, who has suggested that she move near him in California, is now insisting on it. She has to decide whether to move near her son or to continue to live in a house in which she finds it increasingly difficult to care for herself. Although she has a good relationship with her son, she has a strained relationship with her daughter-in-law, and she fears that living near the couple would not be a good situation.

In Mrs. Miller's case, it is obvious to everyone that she needs a different level of care. She realizes she is unable to cope effectively by herself, but she is disturbed and unclear as to whether leaving her home and moving across the country is the answer. Although she may not appear to her neighbors as particularly anxious because her style is to internalize her anxiety, and although the solution seems perfect because her son wants to take care of her, Mrs. Miller is experiencing a crisis state. It is hard for her to sort out what is best in the situation, and she feels an emotional paralysis that prevents her from deciding on an appropriate behavioral solution. As a first step, you would need to help Mrs. Miller organize her dilemma into verbal terms. Moreover, her daughter, son, and daughter-in-law may not have thought through what would be in their own interest as well as their concern for their mother. A significant part of the intervention process would be to explore Mrs. Miller's relationship with her daughter, son, and daughter-in-law in more detail. Other possible supports in her community would be of interest. You should not assume that Mrs. Miller's problems will be helped by direct problem-solving. Rather, your role is to help Mrs. Miller regain a sense of control by converting experiences and vague perceptions into words and subsequently validating them with the individuals involved. By helping the patient reflect on what has happened and what needs to be done, you can assist Mrs. Miller in asking the right questions and in building bridges with her adult children that ultimately will prove more beneficial for her and her family.

Families typically resolve crisis states by making important changes in the way they function or approach a crisis situation. But they often need help from you in fully understanding the nature of the problem and what it entails for the family. Good intentions are not enough, and you play an important role in helping families organize their immediate situation into workable terms and in assisting them to generate creative alternatives in difficult situations. Table 15–2 identifies relevant family interventions for different behavioral symptoms.

Developmental (Maturational) Crises

The other major categorization of crisis is a **developmental (maturational) crisis**. These crisis states relate to normal periods of maturational transition, as described by Erikson (1963; 1968) and typically are associated with age-related life events. They tend to arise more gradually than situational crisis and usually can be resolved without professional intervention (see Table 15–1 for examples).

Typical markers associated with the emergence of developmental crisis (e.g. marriage, first job, first home, first baby, children entering school, leaving home, caring for aging parents, retirement, divorce, death of a child) create potentially overwhelming feelings. Anticipatory guidance, recognition, and educational support are early interventions that help an individual recognize and pass through a transitional crisis state successfully. Ironically, many people do not recognize age-stage developmental crises as they go through them, and, consequently, they experience them as strange and unnatural. Explaining that many parents have difficulty with the teenage years or that teenagers often appear rebellious and immature because they are trying to establish their own sense of identity helps parents understand difficult behaviors from a different perspective. A simple discussion of normal adolescent rapid swings of mood and behavior is a highly effective strategy in many cases.

When a situational crisis is superimposed on a normal developmental psychosocial crisis point, professional assistance may be necessary. Examples include mastectomy during perimenopause, birth of a special-needs child to an adolescent mother, cancer diagnosis in a teenager or young adult, or early loss of a parent or spouse. Sometimes the only understanding comes from the spiritual aspect of oneself (Case Example 15–6). Symptoms of a maturational crisis are typically categorized in DSM-IV as one or more "additional conditions that may be a focus of clinical attention," as follows:

V62.3 Academic Problem
V62.2 Occupational Problem
313.82 Identity Problem
V62.89 Phase of Life Problem

Case Example 15–6 Edward's Story

Edward, once a vigorous athlete and an active man who swore he would never work behind a desk, was injured in an accident that left him completely paralyzed from the neck down. His fast-paced, perfectionistic lifestyle was suddenly changed. He recalls the following thoughts as he was being taken into the emergency room 15 years ago: "I felt as if God were speaking to me: 'You take control of the physical circumstances. I'll cover everything else.' I had a special feeling of warmth and security in my body." One week after the accident, Edward had an experience "that was like starting my life all over, being born again. I had to throw out everything I knew before starting all

TABLE 15–2 **Relevant Family Interventions for Different Behavioral Symptoms**

Symptom	Interventions
Anxiety, shock, fright	Giving information that is brief, concise, explicit, and concrete Repetition of information and frequent reinforcement—encourage families to record important facts in writing Ascertain comprehension by asking family to repeat back to you what information they have been given Provide for and encourage or allow ventilation of feelings, even if they are extreme Maintain constant, nonanxious presence in the face of a highly anxious family Inform family as to the potential range of behaviors and feelings that are within the "norm" for crisis Maximize control within hospital environment, as possible
Denial	Identify what purpose denial is serving for family (e.g., is it buying them "psychological time" for future coping and mobilization of resources?) Evaluate appropriateness of use of denial in terms of time; denial becomes inappropriate when it inhibits the family from taking necessary actions or when it is impinging on the course of treatment Do not actively support denial but do not dash hopes for the future (e.g., "It must be very difficult for you to believe your son is nonresponsive and in a trauma unit") If denial is prolonged and dysfunctional, more direct and specific factual representation may be essential
Anger, hostility, distrust	Allow for ventilation of angry feelings, clarifying what thoughts, fears, and beliefs are behind the anger; let them know it's "OK" to be angry Don't personalize family's expressions of these strong emotions Institute family control within the hospital environment when possible (e.g., arrange for set time(s) and set person(s) to give them information in reference to the patient and answer their questions) Remain available to families during their venting of these emotions Ask families how they can take the energy in their anger and put it to positive use for themselves, for the patient, for the situation
Remorse and guilt	Do not try to "rationalize away" guilt for families Listen, support their expression of feeling and verbalizations (e.g., "I can understand how or why you might feel that way; however . . .") Follow the "howevers" with careful, reality-oriented statements or questions (e.g., "None of us can truly control another's behavior"; "Kids make their own choices despite what parents think and want"; "How successful were you when you tried to control ____________'s behavior with that before?"; "So many things have happened for which there are no absolute answers")
Grief and depression	Acknowledge family's grief and depression Encourage them to be precise about what it is they are grieving and depressed about; give grief and depression a context Allow the family appropriate time for grief Recognize that this is an essential step for future adaptation—do not try to rush the grief process Remain sensitive to your own unfinished business and hence comfort or discomfort with family's grieving and depression
Hope	Clarify with families what their hopes are, individually, and with one another Clarify with families what their worst fears are in reference to the situation—are the hopes or fears congruent? Realistic? Unrealistic? Support realistic hope Offer gentle factual information to reframe unrealistic hope (e.g., "With the information you have or the observations you have made, do you think that is still possible?") Assist families in reframing unrealistic hope in some other fashion (e.g., "What do you think others will have learned from ____________ if he doesn't make it?" "How do you think ____________ would like for you to remember him/her?")

From Kleeman, K. (1989). Families in crisis due to multiple trauma. *Critical Care Nursing Clinics of North America, 1*(1), 25.

over again from scratch." Among the major changes that Edward says he made were developing a more compassionate and trusting sense of others, an appreciation of beauty in the world, and "a deeper, more enhanced dependence on God in controlling things we don't understand."

From Miller, W., & C'deBaca, J. (1994). Quantum change: Toward a psychology of transformation. In Heatherton, T., & Weingerger, J. (Eds.), *Can personality change?* (p. 269). Washington, D.C.: American Psychological Association. ©1994 by the American Psychological Association. Reprinted with permission.

▶ Check Your Reading

6. How do the characteristic elements of a crisis interact with one another to create a crisis state?
7. In what ways is knowledge of risk factors helpful in assessing patient needs and planning appropriate nursing interventions?
8. What are the fundamental differences between a situational and a maturational crisis?

CRISIS INTERVENTION

Caplan (1964) identifies crisis intervention as a form of preventive psychiatry that he developed as a result of his work with people in crisis. It is a specialized construct of short-term, goal-directed therapy designed to help patients and families mobilize resources quickly in unstable, emotionally charged situations. By definition, a person in a crisis state requires immediate action to resolve the problem. It cannot be tolerated indefinitely. The time frame generally associated with crisis intervention is four to six weeks.

The American Nurses' Association (1994) specifies crisis intervention as a "basic level psychiatric-mental health nursing clinical practice function":

Psychiatric-mental health nurses provide direct crisis intervention services to persons in crisis and serve as members of crisis teams. Crisis intervention is a short-term therapeutic process that focuses on the resolution of an immediate crisis or emergency through the use of available professional personnel, family, and/or environmental resources (p. 15).

Knowledge of crisis intervention strategies becomes increasingly important as psychiatry moves into the community. Outpatient management of emotional disturbances has expanded dramatically in preference to hospitalization as the treatment of choice in acute situations. Patients in psychiatric crisis, previously stabilized with short-term hospitalization, are being treated in the emergency room or crisis centers. For many chronically mentally ill patients, psychiatric emergency services are their only source of therapeutic intervention (Slaby, 1994).

Orientation Phase

Assessment

Effective crisis intervention depends on an accurate, comprehensive assessment. The focus of the assessment is slightly different from other forms of treatment in that it is more immediately and closely associated with crisis resolution (Hoff, 1989). Thus, assessment and intervention are joined together from the beginning. The crisis, perception of hazardous events leading to the state of crisis, and accompanying feelings are the primary concern. Knowledge of previous coping strategies with other stressful life circumstances is important because of its relationship to the current crisis, but most other information is left for follow-up treatment. Exploration of underlying personality dynamics is useful only as it relates to the immediate crisis. Excessive focus on emotional deficits undermines the crisis intervention process, and the therapy is likely to be less than optimal in resolving the crisis.

A full inquiry into the nature of the crisis and its meaning to the patient, including evaluation of risk related to self-harm or harm of others, is absolutely essential. If the assessment is too narrow in scope, the intervention will probably be ineffective. Looking only at the immediate facts of a situation and not considering the patient's perceptions, risk of lethality or violence, sources of social support, or previous coping mechanisms suggests a failure to recognize the many levels of observation required in crisis situations.

As with other forms of interpersonal relationships in psychiatric nursing, the orientation phase in crisis intervention parallels the assessment phase of the nursing process. Initially, you are concerned with three tasks: (1) triage assessment for medical and psychiatric emergency, (2) engagement of the patient in the treatment process, and (3) development of a comprehensive database to serve as the foundation for planning and intervention.

Triage Assessment

Crisis interventions in the emergency room and initial stages of treatment typically require a first-level assessment of the level of acuity and emergency medical management of critical physical and psychiatric symptoms before proceeding to a second-level therapeutic response. The crisis state is one of urgency and racing emotions. A sense of intolerable tension invades the entire person, physically, psychologically, and spiritually. Profound anxiety takes over and narrows perceptions. There is an inability to focus on much other than the object of the crisis and its immediate impact on self. For some people, the only solution they see is taking their own life or that of another. Before proceeding with a standard psychiatric interview, you need to evaluate the physical condition of the patient, potential for self-harm, and potential for harm to others.

MEDICAL CONDITION

Obviously the first consideration in a triage assessment is to identify or rule out physical causes of toxicity and to treat the patient's symptoms appropriately. Failure to recognize the physical symptoms of overdose or drug toxicity can result in permanent damage or death. Patients with a cognitive disorder precipitated by alcohol-induced or drug-induced intoxication present a frightening appearance in the emergency room. Typically the patient with a cognitive disorder presents with symptoms of delirium (see Chapter 38). Confused and disoriented to time and place, these patients may appear drowsy or stuporous or agitated and belligerent depending on the cause of the delirium. Symptoms of tachycardia, elevated blood pressure, sweating, and dilated pupils should alert you to the presence of respiratory or cardiac decompensation and *must always be treated as a first-order medical emergency.* Questions about drug use, dosage, and last intake are important. Because of the patient's confusional state, relatives or significant others may have information about the patient's past history and events leading up to arrival in the emergency room that make for a more informed and accurate diagnosis.

Following assessment of cardiac and respiratory status and physical stabilization of the patient, proceed with a mental status examination. This begins with an appraisal of the patient's appearance, gait, movements, and speech. Making the patient comfortable while asking the person accompanying the patient questions may prove more fruitful than asking the patient directly. It also is possible to help the organically impaired patient feel more relaxed by offering a glass of water or a visit to the rest room. A calm, understanding, and sympathetic attitude is much more productive than approaching the patient with an initial show of strength. It is important to set realistic limits, particularly with belligerent patients, who can be highly provocative and attention grabbing. These patients are more easily handled in a smaller room, apart from the mainstream of activity, where distracting stimuli that can further disorganize or anger the patient can be limited.

POTENTIAL FOR SELF-HARM

A key factor in first-level assessment, particularly if the person appears disorganized or impulsive, is lethality potential. In a crisis state, perceptions are limited, and a patient may view suicide as his or her only option. Patients are at higher risk for suicide if they have a history of dual diagnosis of mental illness and substance abuse (Brown et al, 1989) or personal or family history of suicide attempts, depression, alcoholism, or psychotic episodes. Individuals with borderline or antisocial personality disorders have a higher incidence of suicide. Suicide increases with age, and having a serious illness escalates suicide potential. Rates are higher for Protestants and lower for those of the Jewish and Catholic religions, which have strict sanctions against taking one's life. Unemployment and loss of a spouse are correlates of increased suicide potential. Although women attempt suicide more often, men complete the act more frequently. Suicide rates are higher during spring and fall (Slaby, 1994) and occur more often among the widowed, divorced, and separated. Margo and Finkel (1990) report a higher than normal risk among early dementia victims. Copycat suicides are risk factors, particularly among adolescents (Rosen and Walsh, 1989), and the likelihood of suicide increases among young people with a history of criminal behavior (Keitner et al, 1990). White men over the age of 50 are at higher risk, and "severe insomnia, even in the absence of depression, is associated with higher risk" (Slaby, 1994, p. 420).

Schneidman (1987) contends that most people who commit suicide have thought about it beforehand and that there is a predictable pattern related to their choosing suicide as a viable option to difficult life issues. Because most individuals provide clues to suicidal intent, it is important for nurses to be aware of risk factors and to ask appropriate questions. Many verbalize their feelings more readily than one would expect and are relieved when asked directly about their suicidal ideation.

Having a plan, particularly if the method is immediate and available, makes the individual a very high risk. It can be likened to an individual who is searching for a new job or home. If the search is just a passing thought, it is far less likely to be vigorously pursued than if the same individual reads the Sunday paper each week and knows exactly where to look and all of the details when the moment for decision presents itself. Asking direct questions about suicidal ideation and as to whether there is a plan can save a patient's life. Assessment questions should focus on the following elements:

- Acuity
- Suicidal ideation
- Plan
- Means availability
- Social support

Case Example 15–7 John's Story

John Lambert is a 51-year-old engineer who has trouble expressing his feelings. He came to the emergency room because he was experiencing heart palpitations and was afraid he was going to have a heart attack. Mr. Lambert's physical findings are normal. In general, Mr. Lambert is emotionally distant, but when he drinks, he has episodic uncontrolled rages that frighten his wife and children. The combination—the emotional abuse that occurs when he drinks and the controlling, distant behavior he portrays in the marriage—have caused his wife to seek a legal separation. His children are teenagers and are occupied with their friends, partially as a way of staying out of the marital troubles of their parents.

Once Mr. Lambert's physical condition has been assessed, he tells the nurse about the impending separation. The assessment of suicide potential includes exploration of whether the patient has entertained thoughts of suicide. The conversation proceeds in the following manner:

Mr. Lambert: I just can't see any way out of this situation. My life is a nightmare, but it's the only life I know.

Nurse: Mr. Lambert, I can see that you are very distraught. Can you tell me how bad you feel, say on a scale of 1-10? *(Assessment of acuity)*

Mr. Lambert: At least a 9.

Nurse: That sounds really bad. I'm wondering if you have felt bad enough to hurt yourself? *(Assessment of suicidal ideation)*

Mr. Lambert: I have thought about suicide, but I don't think I would ever do it.

Nurse: When you have thought about it, have you thought about how you might do it, and when or where? *(Assessment of a plan)*

Mr. Lambert: Well, I would probably shoot myself because it's quick, and I'd do it when everyone was out of the house.

Nurse: Do you own a gun or have one readily available?

Mr. Lambert: Yes, I have a gun collection, but I have them locked up so we don't have accidents. I keep the only key.

Nurse: What about ammunition? *(Assessment of means availability)*

Mr. Lambert: Yes, I have ammunition, but I keep it in the same cabinet, locked up.

Nurse: It sounds pretty serious. The fact that you have thought about suicide, and you have given some thought to how you would do it, makes you a suicide risk. How do you think your wife and children would respond if you were to end your life? *(Assessment of social support)*

Mr. Lambert: Well, obviously my wife would be relieved, and I don't think my children would care at all because they're busy with their own lives.

Consider Case Example 15–7. Note that the nurse does not directly challenge the patient's statement that "he would never do it" but asks for more information. This is because the patient sees limited options, lacks a social support system, and does not appear to have successful coping mechanisms. The fact that he does not perceive that those in his immediate environment care increases his risk. In asking questions about level of social support, it is important to assess not only the patient's perception of accessibility and nature of the support, but also to verify the patient's perceptions with the actual people named. Sometimes a patient tells you that social support is either available or not available, when in fact just the opposite is the case.

You should consider the patient in this case example to be a strong suicidal risk until proved otherwise. He has suicidal ideation and a definite plan that could be implemented rather easily. He also expresses feelings of worthlessness and hopelessness and, by history, demonstrates a lack of control over his anger. His drinking patterns further predispose him to suicide in that they loosen his inhibitions, and he is more likely to act impulsively. In gathering relevant data, you should inquire about a family history of suicide. If present, the patient's risk further increases. Giving away possessions, feeling excessive guilt, or making amends for bad behaviors would make the suicide risk greater. Factors that might mitigate the suicide risk would be religious codes of conduct against suicide, presence of a support system, and successful coping with other difficult situations. The availability of meaningful social support is particularly important in deciding whether to admit a suicidal patient to the unit or to treat the patient in an outpatient setting.

Not all patients would be as forthcoming as Mr. Lambert in Case Example 15–7. Frequently, individuals tell their significant others, family, or friends of their suicidal ideation but not the professional caregiver, particularly if there is no previously established relationship. Hence, it is important to interview those involved with the patient on a daily basis. If the patient has a regular therapist, this person should be notified, and additional information may be obtained from this source. Usually the patient has to give written permission for any exchange of information unless the patient is a minor or unable to give consent. In such cases, you would seek permission from a responsible party and document carefully all aspects of the information exchange. The patient has the right to know who will be involved in having knowledge of his or her condition and what information is being sought. Chiles and Strosahl (1993) suggest the use of a crisis card, which is completed in the first session and consists of specific written instructions agreed to by the patient in the event of a suicidal crisis. A sequential listing of steps provides additional think time that can prevent impulsive acting out of death wishes, for example, contacting social support or local crisis agencies. The important element in the crisis card is contact between the potential suicidal patient and others that might be able to help the patient in the immediate situation. For a more complete understanding of potential suicide victims and their treatment, see Chapter 36.

POTENTIAL FOR HARM TO OTHERS

The second factor to consider in a triage assessment is potential for harm to others. Symptoms cover a wide variety of behaviors ranging from abuse (verbal, sexual, physical) to homicide and physical maiming. Table 15–3 summarizes indicators of potential violence. Sometimes

TABLE 15–3 Indicators of Potential Violence

Category	Indicators
Mental status	Confused Paranoid ideation Evidence of drug involvement Organic impairment
Motor behavior	Agitated Pacing Aggressive gestures
Speech patterns	Rapid Incoherent Menacing tones Verbal threats
Affect	Belligerent Labile

From Arnold, E., and Boggs, K. (1995). *Interpersonal Relationships: Professional skills for nurses* (2nd ed.) (p. 507). Philadelphia: W. B. Saunders.

the violence is focused on the actual caregiver, but many times it is randomly exercised against whomever is unfortunate enough to be in the patient's path.

Violence in crisis situations typically represents a serious stress response, usually covering feelings of anxiety, powerlessness, and loss of control. Before any other assessment is made, you need to distinguish organic violence from other forms of potential violence and abuse. *Violence should be considered organic, until proved otherwise.* Organic causes include retardation (the person does not have as many options), use of psychedelic drugs, and paranoid psychotic disorders.

Safety of the patient, other patients, and staff is of prime concern. For this reason, you must present a professional demeanor with a calm authoritative tone and be fully aware of the impact of the patient's behavior on other patients as well as on the actual interaction between the particular patient and yourself. Moreover, it is important to recognize that the organically impaired individual, regardless of appearance, has the strength many times his or her weight. Trying to talk about it may be out of the question. Medication usually is warranted, and it may be necessary to restrain or seclude a patient temporarily until he or she is no longer a danger to others. Table 15–4 presents guidelines for intervening for the potentially violent behaviors of nonorganically impaired patients.

Asking the patient about the presence of violent feelings is appropriate. For example, you might inquire, "Have you thought of hurting your (wife, son) when you are this angry?" Any time you feel really uncomfortable, it is better to verify your intuitions with the patient rather than watch the behavior escalate before intervening.

The treatment obviously is different for each case and dependent on symptoms or cause. If the person is not too out of control, it is useful to encourage ventilation, avoid challenge, and speak calmly. Offering alternatives and expressing confidence reinforces the patient's sense of control. "I know this is difficult for you, but I think you can control yourself," or "Mr. Sims, what has happened is terrible, but I think you can be more help to your wife if we can talk about your anger in a private area." Taking the patient out of an overly stimulating environment usually helps diffuse anger and anxiety. If this is not possible, remove other patients and visitors from the area. When the patient is very upset, it is critical to allow enough space between you and the patient. A cramped examining room in an emergency suite is not appropriate. There should be no sharp instruments or medications in the room selected as a quieter area. In addition to providing enough space between the patient and you, movement should be slow and deliberate. Moving in quickly often is misinterpreted as an attack. You should always maintain a safe distance, with the exit clearly available to the patient. At the same time, you need to have full access to a graceful exit. Under no circumstances should you be in a position where you can be backed into a corner. Having sufficient trained staff is important. Often a simple show of force is sufficient to quiet out-of-control behaviors. If medication is given, and usually it is, you should briefly state what the purpose of the medication is, for example, "Joe, we're going to give you some medication that will help relieve your anxiety and make you more comfortable." The patient has the right to refuse antipsychotic medication, and there are legal restraints on giving medication to voluntarily hospitalized patients who refuse medication except in emergency situations, in which there is immediate danger of serious and irreversible harm (Slaby, 1994; Beck and Staffin, 1986). Table 15–5 provides guidelines for handling different levels of aggressive behavior.

Sometimes patients are so out of control they need to be secluded or temporarily restrained. Although nurses can legally implement these procedures without an immediate physician's order in emergency situations, most hospitals specify a limited time period, ranging from 1 hour to 24 hours, to obtain the order. *The only reason to seclude or restrain a patient is to provide safety for the patient and other patients on the unit* if the patient is out of control. Careful written documentation of the date, time, name of the physician notified, and reason for the procedure is essential.

Whenever a patient is to be secluded or restrained, there should be a plan and one person in charge of the operation. There should be a clear delineation of tasks, *before implementation.* Anything that potentially could be used as a weapon needs to be removed, and a body search for weapons (e.g., concealed knife taped to back) may need to be initiated.

Staff training is essential to prevent injury to patients or staff. During the procedure, one staff member should talk to the patient in reassuring, calm, nonretaliatory tones and in simple words about what is happening. The patient needs to be reassured that the restraint or seclusion is temporary and necessary only until his or her behavior is under better control. Vital signs should be taken and recorded once the patient is in the seclusion room or in restraints. The patient requires focused intensive care during the entire process. Typically, there is a stated protocol for observation every 15 minutes or every hour. The patient should be toileted at regular intervals, and food is served on disposable paper products. It is important to address the patient by name and to treat the patient with dignity. Feelings of anger toward the patient for his or her behavior need to be addressed outside of the therapeutic situation. Box 15–3 provides guidelines for the use of seclusion and restraints in emergency psychiatry.

Later, it is important to discuss the restraining process and to encourage discussion of the behavior that resulted in the confinement, with the development of a prevention plan. Moreover, the staff needs to process the incident—all areas of it. Once the incident is over, it is also helpful to develop a standardized care plan to cope with future incidents because patient violence of all types is increasing.

Whenever a patient is considered to be a danger to self or others or is unable to care for himself or herself (and the latter is defined quite narrowly), the decision of whether to admit the patient to inpatient treatment becomes an issue. Patient rights require that the patient be cared for in the least restrictive environment. At the same time, acutely psychotic patients and those with a potential to harm self or others must be detained until their condition stabilizes. Some hospitals use a small number of "holding beds" to allow for emergency treatment and medication stabilization for patients requiring a longer time for evaluation and symptom reduction. Gillig and colleagues (1989) reported a study in which the rate of hospitalization for acute psychiatric symptoms was 36% for emergency services with holding beds compared with 52% for those without holding beds. A more complete discussion of violent behavior and strategies other than those required in emergency situations is presented in Chapter 40.

TABLE 15–4 **Guidelines for Intervening for the Potentially Violent Behaviors of Nonorganically Impaired Patients**

Don'ts	Dos
Don't overlook your feeling that your patient is growing hostile and showing inappropriate anger	Document your observations (even though your patient has not behaved in an overtly dangerous way), and share your feelings and suspicions with the staff and the nursing administration Request medication as needed (medication prescribed early enough and in adequate doses can help prevent violence) Review your patient's history, searching purposefully for signs of alcoholism, drug addiction, reaction to a change of medication, or a metabolic or emotional disturbance
Don't undervalue what others (family or staff) tell you about your patient's behavior in the belief that he'll be different with you or that you can handle it	Use what the family and other staff members already know about the patient. This information is significant—especially information about previous violence, about what's apt to provoke the patient, and how the patient behaves when provoked
Don't continue with a treatment or interview if a patient is obviously growing more and more agitated. Do not touch him or move toward him. He may misinterpret your gesture and react with physical aggression	Ask the patient why he's angry or agitated—and what's making him act this way. Also, ask him how he handles such feelings ordinarily and what others can do to help him. You want him to know that his feelings and point of view are being respected so he'll feel less powerless, less victimized. Be sure he understands that violence on his part will not be tolerated
Don't isolate yourself with a patient who has a record of or potential for violence. Don't corner yourself in a setting without a clear exit. (Elevators may prove particularly troublesome since you have no instant exit)	Put the patient in a room near the nurses' station—not at the end of a long, relatively unprotected corridor. Keep the door open when working with the patient—and face him (or align yourself literally and figuratively beside him), rather than turning your back on him Have a security officer or male aide within immediate call if you suspect violence is imminent Study the contents of the patient's room carefully, with an eye to what he could use to harm himself or one of the staff
Don't disturb the patient (with treatments or taking vital signs) any more than is necessary. He may need his own territory	Arrange opportunities for physical activities if these seem to help the patient siphon off his excess energies. Arrange for time out of his room, if this seems appropriate—and he agrees to it
Don't assign a timid, inexperienced nurse to a potentially violent patient	Assign a mature, easy-going, experienced nurse to care for the patient. (In this kind of powderkeg situation, it is axiomatic that there should be only one anxious person in the room: the patient)
Don't overlook the significance of gender in the assignment of a nurse to the patient	Therefore, you might want to consider assigning a male staff nurse to a female patient who's potentially violent and a female nurse to a male patient. Observers have learned that a female patient may be inclined to react negatively to another woman, but positively to a male staff member. This gender crossing also works for the male patient, who might hesitate to strike or injure a female nurse

Developed by Joyce Wallskog, Ph.D., R.N., Marquette University, Milwaukee, Wisconsin. From Arnold, E., and Boggs, K. (1995). *Interpersonal relationships: Professional communication skills for nurses* (2nd ed.) (p. 508). Philadelphia: W. B. Saunders.

TABLE 15–5 **Guidelines for Handling Different Levels of Aggressive Behavior**

Level	Patient Behavior	Nurse Actions
Environmental trigger	Stress response	Encourage ventilation: avoid challenge, speak calmly, clearly, offer alternative
Escalation period	Movement toward loss of control	Take control: maintain safe distance, acknowledge behavior, medicate if appropriate, remove to quiet area, "show force" if necessary
Crisis period	Emotional/physical discharge	Apply external control: implement emergency protocol, initiate confinement, give focused intensive care
Recovery	Cool down	Reassure: support, no retaliation; encourage to discuss behavior and alternatives; release when in control; assess reaction to release; assist in reentry toward environment; conduct sessions for staff to process all areas of incident
Postcrisis and letdown	Reconciliatory	Demonstrate acceptance while continuing clarification of unit standards and expectations

From Steele R. L. (1993). Staff attitudes toward seclusion and restraint: Anything new? *Perspectives in Psychiatric Care, 29*(3), 28. Reprinted with the permission of Nursecom, Inc.

Clinical judgments about the need for immediate hospitalization related to potential harm to self or others revolve around the answers to the following questions:

- Is the patient able to maintain self-care without a structured, monitored setting?
- How significant is the risk of self-destructive behavior?
- What is the level of the patient's reality testing capacity?
- What is the level of the patient's anxiety, rage, or fear that might precipitate a lethal response?
- Is the patient able to engage with the nurse and willing and able to provide meaningful information?
- Does the patient have an immediate support person who is willing to monitor and respond appropriately to decompensation and changes in the patient's behavior?

If hospitalization is indicated, the patient should be encouraged to seek this form of treatment voluntarily. Although treatment considerations ultimately lie within the physician's realm of decision making, you play an important role in obtaining appropriate information, making cogent observations, and acting as advocate of the patient. Record keeping of all pertinent observations and data collection is essential. Any gaps in information and the reasons why they occurred also are recorded (Kaplan and Sadock, 1993).

Engaging the Patient

The first contact between you and the patient in a crisis situation sets the stage for all that follows. In acute crisis situations, you may forget to introduce yourself by name, to specify your role, or to acknowledge the patient by name, as a unique individual. There is a tendency to respond to the acuteness of the situation rather than to the patient as a person. Yet this simple intervention of taking

BOX 15-3 Guidelines for the Use of Seclusion and Restraints in Emergency Psychiatry

1. Initiate seclusion or restraint only after:
2. (a) It is determined that the patient is a danger to self or to others
3. (b) Other, less restrictive measures have been implemented without success
4. Physicians' orders for and nursing documentation of seclusion or restraint must indicate clinical justification, specifics of the type of seclusion or restraint to be used, time limitations, and specific behavioral criteria for discontinuation.
5. In the absence of a physician's order during an acute emergency, document all of the information in #2, along with the date, time, name, and response of the physician who was contacted to write the order.
6. There must be an automatic review of patients restrained more than 12 hours or discharged within 48 hours of use of seclusion or restraint.
7. Review patient and staff injuries during seclusion and restraint.
8. Ensure that the chart contains documentation of patient behavior following release from seclusion or restraints.

Adapted from Slaby, A. (1994). *Handbook of psychiatric emergencies* (p. 15). Norwalk, CT: Appleton-Lange.

the time to introduce yourself, calling the patient by name, and describing your role directs the patient to the type of information you need and the kind of help the patient can expect from you. You can begin the first session by introducing yourself and identifying your role with a simple statement such as:

"Mrs. Tisedale, I'm Marcia Cohen, the crisis intake nurse tonight. My job is to help people sort out the events, thoughts, and feelings in crisis situations, in order to help them come to terms with what has happened. Won't you have a seat over here?"

As can be seen in this statement, your first priority is to put the patient at ease and to establish the direction of assessment and intervention. Every effort should be made to reduce the patient's anxiety. Simple informal and inviting gestures, such as extending a handshake, offering to take the patient's coat, providing a comfortable chair, and suggesting a glass of water, enhance comfort. Next the focus is on establishing the interview as a collaborative process, which is not always easy when people are acutely anxious.

Crisis intervention is an art as well as a skilled nursing function. Although the concept of patient uniqueness is paramount in considering any treatment approach, it sometimes loses its significance in serious crisis situations because of acuity. Yet patients in severe crisis particularly need to know that their unique needs are of concern to their caregivers. This in itself has a calming effect because the patient feels that there is a possibility of joining with an expert to solve a problem that is mutually understood. The interview should begin where the patient is and with the patient's description of what brought him or her to seek treatment. No two people are exactly alike, and although their presentation of symptoms in crisis may appear similar, it is important to look beyond the superficial facts in the situation to each person's interpretation of its unique meaning.

Typically, patients in crisis are scared, confused, and anxious. How you respond, what is said, and the manner and tone of its delivery serve to increase or decrease the patient's anxiety. A calm, even voice can secure the patient's attention much better than a more excited tone. Language and content need to be suited to the maturity and readiness of the patient. In fact, anything that adds to the human qualities of crisis intervention enhances its effectiveness.

Ideally the interpersonal climate in a crisis situation is one that is free flowing, changing, but, at the same time, highly focused on here-and-now problem resolution. Every effort should be made to ask only those questions that are relevant and directly related to the situation under discussion. It is important to encourage the patient to speak personally about what he or she is experiencing and the particular issues the patient feels are critical to resolving the crisis.

The therapeutic approach in a crisis situation is much more structured than in other forms of nurse-patient relationships, with much closer time linkage between assessment and intervention. A delicate balance exists between helping the person in crisis to express his or her feelings and structuring the encounter in ways that bring about quick resolution of the crisis state. Obviously, it is important to convey empathetic understanding for the patient's predicament and to encourage the patient to talk about perceptions of the experience. Simple sharing of the events and associated feelings can reduce tension significantly. Time is of the essence, however, and consequently, intervention to stabilize the patient begins as a necessary part of the assessment phase.

RECOGNIZING POWERLESSNESS

It is not always easy to engage the patient in meaningful dialogue before trust is established. Extreme patience, understanding, and empathy for the patient or family's sense of lost control, helplessness, and powerlessness are necessary elements. During a crisis, patients typically demonstrate a cognitive rigidity resulting in unreasonable demands, constricted problem solving, tunnel vision, and overreaction. It is not uncommon for patients and their families to display confusion and project anger onto the health care system and specific health care providers as defensive maneuvers to reestablish personal strength. If you can realize that this behavior may be the only way a person can feel control in a situation experienced as potentially overwhelming and ego shattering, it is possible to react with acceptance rather than anger or frustration.

Another characteristic of the crisis state is decreased perceptual attention. People simply do not hear much of the information given to them. Although they may appear attentive and respond appropriately, their anxiety typically gets in the way of full comprehension. Consequently, frequently repeating information, asking the patient to invite a trusted family member or friend to listen with him or her to instructions and explanations, and providing written instructions can prove quite helpful. These interventions also have ramifications for increasing the potential of fully informed consent in crisis situations. In general, the more involved the patient is in the interview process, the better the quality of the assessment data. Initial efforts to reduce or compensate for excessive anxiety make this possible. Although the specific interviewing strategies and formats depend on the needs of the individual patient, the patient is more likely to be compliant with treatment suggestions and to experience the mutuality in the relationship.

Follow-up between sessions helps reduce the sense of helplessness. A flexible policy whereby the patient can contact the crisis center or receive support by phone if the tension becomes intolerable is useful. Few patients abuse this type of consultation.

Finally, in the early stages of a crisis state, many people want to make binding but impulsive and unwise decisions that they would never make in ordinary circumstances. This is to be discouraged because often other facts come to light, feelings change, and possibilities may emerge that were not apparent in the initial stages of a crisis situation. You can be quite helpful in directly making a statement, such as, "I know you are upset right now, but it usually works better to postpone any decisions about major changes until we can get your situation stabilized and the air clears a little bit. Lets look at your situation and see if we can understand what is going on that we can do something about."

INSTILLING HOPE

An important element of the orientation phase is the instillation of hope. Although it is most important to recognize the profound impact of a crisis, you can portray the crisis as an opportunity for reclaiming the essential parts of the human journey. For example:

At times, it is appropriate to identify specifically to patients after an overdose that there must have been a part of them that wanted to die (e.g., the part that led them to take the pills), or else they wouldn't be talking to you, but there also must be a part that wanted to live (e.g., the part that warned a relative to look for them) or else they wouldn't be talking to you. It may be useful to tell patients explicitly that "I want to work with the part of you that wants to live. I'm glad that part of you will have another chance" (Hillard, 1990, p. 119).

Recognizing the "Repeater"

As many as one third of the patients presenting in psychiatric crisis in the emergency department are repeaters who use the emergency department as their first-line intervention in crisis situations (Fisher, 1989). Drawn from the poorest socioeconomic groups, these patients are frequently alcoholic, schizophrenic, homeless, or without significant social supports. Usually, they lack insight despite the greater majority of them being in psychiatric treatment. This population requires a special set of skills because resistance to treatment and an unwillingness to engage in a treatment process that requires suspension of immediate gratification or resolution of their problem preclude easy engagement of the patient. They need to be taken seriously because they can inadvertently commit suicide. The patient may present with vague medical symptoms or attribute their origin to an accident or medical disorder. For example, a severely ill borderline patient presented in the emergency department, having "fallen down the stairs in her house." She suffered a concussion and had broken her nose. What she neglected to tell the staff was that she had been drinking heavily and that this incident was one of many in which she entered the health care system with physical symptoms reflective of self-mutilation and passive self-destructive acts. Frequently, chronic psychiatric patients, presenting with medical emergencies, forget to tell the staff that they are in ongoing active treatment. Or they may tell the crisis intervention team information they feel uncomfortable sharing the level of their stress with their primary therapist. For this reason, all information gathered in the emergency department should be shared with the patient's primary therapist. Consistency and follow-through with frequent and thorough sharing of information is crucial to the successful management of frequent emergency department users. The goals of treatment should focus on resolving the immediate crisis and strengthening the treatment already in progress.

Developing a Comprehensive Database

ELICITING THE PRECIPITATING EVENT

Before any action can be taken, you must understand the nature of the crisis and its personal meaning to the patient. Most crisis situations have a factual component and a critical emotional impact. The experience of a crisis has a shattering effect on all previous assumptions, and often an individual may be genuinely baffled in attempting to understand what has happened and why it happened. Because of the large role perception and experience play in development of a crisis state, the individual's unique account of the crisis is extremely important as a starting point. In addition to providing the nurse with necessary baseline data, the development of an explanation of how the crisis came to be helps the patient make sense out of the change in his or her reality. A good place to begin is with *identification of the precipitating factors.* You can structure your comments in a simple way, such as:

Jean, I know this is a very difficult situation for you. I wonder if you could start at the beginning, and tell me a little of what led up to your coming to the emergency department (crisis center, hospital unit).

Verbally ordering the information sought in a logical, sequential manner and starting with the triggering circumstances helps the patient stay focused on important relationships between the event and corresponding feelings. Guidelines for general assessment questions are presented in Box 15–4.

Validation by you, acceptance of the patient's accounting, and neutralizing of upsetting emotions through discussion help confirm the patient at a time when confidence in one's personal abilities is at a low point.

DEFINING THE PROBLEM

In the course of telling the story of a crisis, you can help patients develop a realistic perception of their crisis. A concrete problem definition provides an inner contact with the personalized meaning of a crisis, which is essential to its resolution. Frequently a patient's understanding is aware only of diffuse outlines of the problem. The patient's perceptions are so clouded by anxiety that it is almost impossible to sort out the actual events in ways that permit realistic solutions. Actively listening for verbal and nonverbal cues regarding important points and feelings helps communicate interest and compassion. A comprehensive patient assessment in an emergency situation focuses on the patient's stated complaints, observations by you regarding level of functioning, and reports of others for the purpose of developing a succinct and realistic problem statement. Assessment of the risk factors described earlier in the chapter provides insight into the contributing factors in the development of the crisis state. The problem statement is validated with the patient and forms the basis for developing relevant nursing diagnoses.

PACING THE NARRATIVE

In a crisis situation, thoughts become jumbled, and you can get caught up in the patient's anxiety. There is a tendency in emergency situations to make assumptions or to become overactive. Although it is important to ask for clarification in obtaining an accurate and complete understanding of the patient's situation, it is critical to not anticipate the story. Because, in the final analysis, only the patient can resolve his or her crisis and the patient must do it in his or her own way, it is important that the patient relive the story of the crisis in his or her own way. Moreover, how the patient relates the story and what the patient feels is important gives you useful information that would not be available with a more programmed approach to getting information.

Active listening strategies previously identified in Chapter 10 form the basis for gathering data, defining the problem, and identifying personal strengths. When you lack information about a key part of the problem, it is critical to seek clarification by asking for concrete details.

The conversation should not be allowed to move ahead of either party's understanding. Using the patient's verbal and nonverbal cues to paraphrase and reflect back key ideas and themes helps the patient stay focused and expand on the story. Whenever possible, you should use the patient's own words in listening responses because this feedback reinforces the reality of the person describing his or her experience.

Pacing also involves monitoring the patient's statements so that therapeutic suggestions parallel the patient's level of understanding and acknowledgment. For example, the parents of a newly admitted trauma victim may not be ready to hear the full extent of their son's injuries in the initial sessions. *It is critical to stay with the patient or family's level of readiness and understanding, rather than to impose a suggestion that may be objectively correct but may not be a good "fit" with the patient's perception of the problem or potential solution.*

Therapeutic suggestions and verbal interventions should be concise, empathetic, and related only to the crisis, the patient's perceptions, and his or her feelings surrounding the events. This can be done in one or two sentences. Longer explanations often are not heard because of the patient's anxiety. Periodically summarizing what you understand and what you tell the patient reinforces or corrects key points.

ASSESSING FOR PERSONAL STRENGTHS

Personal strengths form the backbone for deciding on individualized nursing interventions. When a person feels out of control, typically there is limited awareness of personal strengths. Building from a person's strengths reinforces the positive elements that are already present as personality characteristics in working with difficult life issues. Strengths might include the ability to communicate thoughts and express feelings, the ability to perform more than one family role, and the willingness to look at the crisis as an opportunity for change.

BOX 15-4 Guidelines for Asking General Assessment Questions

Begin with the History of Presenting Symptoms

When did the symptoms begin?
How are they described by the patient?
What else is going on simultaneously in the patient's life?
Is there any evidence of a psychiatric emergency (suicidal ideation, hallucinations)? (if suicidal, does the patient identify a plan?)
What medication is the patient on at this time? (dosage, time of last intake)?
Is the patient currently using recreational drugs (marijuana, hallucinogens, cocaine, alcohol, amphetamines)?
Is the patient currently in treatment with a therapist?
Is this the first emergency room visit?

Inquire About Past Relevant History and Coping Mechanisms

Has the patient had other similar crisis events?
Is there a patient or family history of mental illness or drug abuse?
Has the patient or anyone in the family ever attempted suicide?
Has a family member or significant person in the patient's life ever experienced a similar crisis?
How has the patient coped with difficult life situations in the past? (past medical/psychiatric evaluations, hospitalizations, or treatment?)
Is there a history of any previous neurological disease or dysfunction?

Assess the Patient's Level of Social Support

To whom does the patient turn in times of stress?
Who are the people important and accessible in the patient's life at the present time?
What is the patient's perception of their willingness to be involved with the current crisis?
If the patient is in treatment, what is the patient's perception of the contract, availability, and therapist involvement?
What is the nature of the home environment?
What is the nature of the patient's work and social environment?

BOX 15-5 Diagnostic Stems for Problems Commonly Experienced by Patients in Crisis

Anxiety
Community Coping, Ineffective
Confusion, Acute
Decisional Conflict (Specify)
Defensive Coping
Denial, Ineffective
Energy Field Disturbance
Environmental Interpretation Syndrome, Impaired
Family Coping: Disabling, Ineffective
Grieving, Dysfunctional
Home Maintenance Management, Impaired
Hopelessness
Individual Coping, Ineffective
Management of Therapeutic Regimen: Community, Ineffective
Management of Therapeutic Regimen: Families, Ineffective
Management of Therapeutic Regimen: Individuals, Ineffective
Nutrition: Less than Body Requirements, Altered
Parenting, Altered
Powerlessness
Rape-Trauma Syndrome
Rape-Trauma Syndrome: Compound Reaction
Rape-Trauma Syndrome: Silent Reaction
Relocation Stress Syndrome
Risk for Injury
Risk for Self Mutilation
Role Performance, Altered
Self Esteem Disturbance
Sensory/Perceptual Alterations (specify) (visual, auditory, kinesthetic, gustatory, tactile, olfactory)
Sleep Pattern Disturbance
Social Interaction, Impaired
Spiritual Distress (distress of the human spirit)
Thought Processes, Altered
Violence: Risk for, Self-Directed or Directed at Others

Working Phase

Diagnosis, Outcome Identification, and Planning

Nursing diagnoses identify the functional deficits found in crisis situations that are amenable to nursing intervention. Box 15–5 presents the NANDA-approved diagnostic stems for problems commonly experienced by patients in crisis. Once you have enough information to formulate relevant nursing diagnoses, you can direct the conversation toward the concrete difficulties that need resolution first. Doing something about the problem reduces the sense of helplessness. Emphasis on immediate concerns and "thinking aloud" about issues in need of more immediate resolution, versus issues to address later, is helpful in focusing the client and fostering self-monitoring of tasks needed to resolve the crisis (Case Example 15–8).

Case Example 15–8 Ann's Story

Ann Bartholomew is a 19-year-old single white woman who has been living with her boyfriend for the past year. She has a part-time job as a stripper in a local bar. Her parents have "disowned" her because they don't approve of her lifestyle, and the money she brings in from her job is insufficient to support her needs. Moreover, Ann is addicted to marijuana and uses cocaine and alcohol on a fairly regular basis.

Ann just found out that her boyfriend has been cheating on her, and she feels that she can't live without him. Her boyfriend accompanied her to the emergency room after finding that she had just ingested large amounts of alcohol and marijuana. Her parents are concerned about her current condition and have agreed to participate in her treatment.

Ann is initially triaged as a medical/psychiatric emergency. She is evaluated as a moderately low suicidal risk that can be handled outpatient once her condition is stabilized. Her risk is increased because of drug use, but her lack of a plan, her gender, and the willingness of the family to be involved in treatment lower it. The plans for Ann's care were as follows:

Nursing Interventions	Rationales
1. As a means of reducing lethality without hospitalization, obtain from Ann a commitment to treatment and a contract that she will not do anything self-destructive.	1. Even though the nurse evaluates Ann as a moderately low suicidal risk, her methods for coping do not give much evidence of prethought, range of options, or constructive problem solving. The contract will help her think before acting.
2. Prioritize problem areas as a way of helping Ann to distinguish between major and minor life events needing immediate solutions.	2. In crisis situations, most people have trouble prioritizing their problems or taking charge. A sharp focus on the circumstances needing prompt attention reduces the sense of disorganization and makes the problem areas more manageable.
3. Provide direct intervention with the drug abuse problem.	3. Drug abuse enhances the chances of an unintentional suicide and clouds the clarity of thinking needed to resolve the crisis.
4. Set short-term goals directly related to the resolution of specific parts of the identified problem areas.	4. Successful coping with the manageable parts of the crisis helps patients feel more capable, and the learned coping skills enable them to respond more effectively.

5. Refer for case management and mobilization of community resources.	5. Ann's current crisis situation is more intense because of underlying personal and family dynamics that increased her vulnerability. Providing ongoing support to work through these issues will reduce the likelihood of similar crisis episodes.

Planning care for patients takes into careful consideration the three elements that Aguilera (1994) considers as balancing factors: (1) realistic assessment of the crisis event, (2) coping resources, and (3) sources of personal support. For many patients, a realistic perception of the crisis event eludes them. Your role is to help establish some sense of order in the current chaos and to begin to identify appropriate resources. Simple interventions to contact family or to involve community agencies early in the patient's care can greatly reduce anxiety for both patient and family. You can help patients clarify who could be important to them at this time and how to access them appropriately.

The goal of crisis intervention is to restore the patient to precrisis functioning. Goals that are *acceptable to the client, affordable, accessible, and appropriate to the resolution of the crisis* are most likely to be successful (Beckingham and Baumann, 1990). You play an important role in structuring interventions that emphasize patient mastery. Crisis intervention depends on developing a mutual understanding of the problem and the strategies most likely to resolve it. Consequently, you need to be aware of the patient's response and should use frequent validation (see Chapter 10) as a listening response strategy. Planning to include the family and other support systems in the resolution of a crisis offers one of the greatest modifiers of unfortunate circumstances. Selection of behavioral tasks should focus first on areas of change needed in the immediate present because these most often also affect the final resolution of the crisis situation. Another consideration is choosing tasks that are easiest for the patient to implement. This strategy provides patients with ready-to-use successful coping strategies and empowers them to risk trying harder tasks. When it is obvious that the patient is not familiar with or able to grasp the entire sequence of events needed to achieve a goal, a useful strategy is to break goals down into small achievable segments. Steps involved in reaching the proposed solution should fit both the problem and the resources available to the patient.

► Check Your Reading

9. How does the assessment phase in crisis intervention differ from that in other types of therapeutic relationships?
10. What are the factors the nurse should consider in planning care for patients in crisis?

Implementation

Intervention in crisis specifically calls for a different perspective of the hazardous event or critical stressor that allows for the possibility of an acceptable solution. In crisis situations, the steps in problem solving and the decision-making process parallel those described in Chapter 11. The time frame for intervention is accelerated, however, and scope of intervention is restricted. Time is of the essence, so only those problems in need of prompt attention to lessen the impact of the stressor are addressed. All interventions are deliberately structured to stabilize the patient immediately, with more extensive intervention planned for a later time.

Once the problem is defined, you and the patient mutually review possible alternatives. When looking at alternative solutions, it is critical to explore and anticipate potential consequences. The patient needs to list and prioritize all possible decisions that could be undertaken, using the criteria (acceptable, affordable, and accessible). Just as in other relationships with patients, avoid the temptation to "tell the patient what to do." Instead, prompt the patient to consider alternatives, pose questions to stimulate broader thinking about a topic, provide information the patient does not have, and simply be emotionally present as the patient struggles with difficult life issues. Unless the patient presents a danger to self or others, the locus of control should remain with the patient. The objective in providing advice is to help the patient postpone impulsive decision making when he or she is not in full charge of his or her faculties. Your role in the working phase is to take the least directive posture possible and to encourage the patient to identify each "best next step" (Slaikeu, 1990, p. 225). This means looking at what must be done this day or in the next week, rather than focusing on the ultimate outcome. For the patient to have cognitive mastery over the current situation is the overriding goal of successful crisis intervention.

STRUCTURING THE ENVIRONMENT

By contrast with purely insight and behavioral interventions, the emphasis in crisis intervention is on the development of concrete strategies to reduce the impact of the stressor. Structuring the environment to maximize patient control and to minimize conflict often reduces tension immediately. The object of this intervention is to provide prompt external support to prevent further chaos or to reduce the patient's stress by removing a tangible stressor in the environment. For example, you might take the patient to a quiet, low-stimuli environment. In the community, the simple intervention of encouraging a young mother to engage the babysitting services of a teenager for several hours a day, thereby providing some respite from child care, can make a potential crisis more manageable. Or arranging for Meals on Wheels for an isolated elder can reduce the anxiety of meal preparation. To a college student experiencing conflict with a roommate, you might suggest a temporary return to home while other living arrangements can be explored. Sometimes just a brief respite from stress allows the patient to move to a more adaptive mode of problem solving and prevent a crisis from erupting.

REINFORCING STRENGTHS

As you become aware of the patient's strengths, it is important to point them out. Simple statements such as, "This is difficult, but I think you are capable of coping with it," or encouraging the patient who is berating his or her current coping skills to wait until he or she is in a better position to make realistic judgments about self-worth reframes the current crisis as a temporary setback rather than a permanent condition. Asking questions about how the patient dealt with previous stresses helps the patient recall past mastery of difficult times, and recognizing previous achievements helps sustain motivation when current outcomes are uncertain. Credit for managing small tasks in the immediate situation and taking initial steps toward problem solving encourages the patient to take the "next best step."

ENCOURAGING VENTILATION

Encouraging the patient to verbalize about emotionally charged events generally promotes emotional relief and a reduction in distress. In crisis, some patients need permission to express their feelings because they feel shameful, whereas others simply are unaware of the feelings being experienced. You can directly state that unusual and disturbing feelings are a normal part of the crisis state and use active listening to help patients define the issues as the patient perceives them. Anger and confusion are emotions frequently experienced in crisis situations. It is important not to discourage crying or anger, unless the expression of feelings is out of control or threatening. If the patient's expression of feelings is out of control, however, or if the patient is talking about harming someone else, feelings may need to be harnessed and redirected toward a more productive outcome.

NORMALIZING FEELINGS

Closely related to encouraging expression of feeling is the concept of normalizing. Frequently, people in crisis feel they are "losing it" or "falling apart" because the distress is so great and the feelings are so strange. Your assurance that crisis precipitates a wide range of reactions can be consoling to the person experiencing these feelings. Another strategy to help the patient normalize the situation is to focus fully on the *immediate* problem and help the patient develop concrete mini-solutions for the immediate concerns. For example:

Jane Corbett is experiencing a crisis state related to her husband's sudden request for a divorce. Whether or not she should leave the home without legal advice, what to say to her husband when she returns home, and how to respond to the children who will realize that she is not herself are issues that need to be dealt with immediately. By breaking the hazardous event down into smaller units with the patient, the situation appears more manageable, and the patient begins to feel more in control. This intervention allows Jane to choose and prioritize the specific actions needed to make an "abnormal" situation more normal and workable.

CLARIFYING DISTORTIONS

Earlier in the chapter, a realistic perception of the crisis event was identified as a critical balancing factor for resolving a crisis. You can play an important role in gently guiding patients to consider alternative explanations and in reducing the sense of blaming that so frequently accompanies a crisis situation. Distortion of the crisis events creates an unnecessary self-inflicted stress on the person experiencing the crisis state, whereas correcting distorted perceptions of the crisis situation greatly facilitates development of a workable plan. Sometimes the crisis is intensified by distorted perceptions, fears, and beliefs about its origin and who is responsible for its development. For instance, a patient may take full personal blame for a situation in which he or she may have played a minor part and one that actually was caused by many factors. Hoff (1989) notes, "The tendency to blame and scapegoat is especially strong in family and marital crises."

Another common feeling is that of helplessness and perceptions of being a victim destined to be battered by life circumstances. Statements such as, "If I had done it differently, this wouldn't have happened," or "My life is not worth anything unless I have this job, this girl friend, etc," indicate this feeling. For example, a young man who had done well with a bank as a computer programmer was laid off suddenly. Intellectually, he recognized that he was one of many laid off by the bank in a period of recession. Emotionally, he struggled with the perception that even if you did a wonderful job and gave everything to the organization, you could be eliminated with the stroke of a pen. Although partially correct in his assumption, he narrowed his perception of this critical life event to reflect his sense that it was him as an individual that was at fault rather than simply being in the wrong place at the wrong time. Your listening responses help the patient define central concerns and provide the patient with a unique opportunity to challenge the correctness of such assumptions. In implementing this intervention, you need to be aware of psychosocial differences in how people perceive and respond to crisis. Special consideration of difficulties in language, information processing, or cultural norms that interfere with a mutual understanding of the crisis acknowledges human diversity, which is always present in crisis situations. For example, a young Mexican patient told her physician that she slept in the same bed with her father. This "fact" was recorded as an incestuous relationship when, in reality, it was quite common for children to sleep in the same bed as their parents, and the fact was culturally but not pathologically significant.

SUPPORTING DEFENSES

When a patient exercises defenses in an adaptive manner, it is important to provide an immediate reinforcement that links the behavior with a particular result. For example, you might tell a patient who has decided to call the police instead of beating his disorderly son up, as he normally does, "Making that phone call was a really good thing to do. You dealt with the problem without getting yourself in trouble." In this situation, you explicitly link the patient's reframing of a defensive posture as an adaptive response to an outcome that benefits the patient. This may seem rather obvious, but often patients do not consciously link behavior to outcome, and maladaptive defenses to difficult situations persist, whereas they might not if the new behavior is reinforced so that it becomes a more automatic response.

Maladaptive defenses tend to reinforce the intensity of the crisis. Examples include ego mechanisms that deny, falsify, or distort reality. Although a patient may need to do this initially to buffer the full effect of the crisis, maladaptive defenses in general provide a roadblock to resolving the crisis (see Case Example 15–9).

Case Example 15–9 Kevin's Story

Kevin Waller, age 16, has been arrested for selling cocaine in school. His mother is a single parent who works long hours and was unaware that Kevin had been taking drugs, let alone selling them. She comes to the emergency room in crisis and distraught but convinced that there must be some mistake. Her son is a good boy who would never be involved with something like this. She tells the nurse that she knows he has recently gotten mixed up with some bad friends, and they must have set Kevin up for this to avoid their own involvement. The nurse knows that there is considerable legal evidence to indicate that Kevin has been dealing drugs for some time.

The nurse's approach needs to be sensitive to the mother's need for denial at this time but not supportive of it or encouraging toward it. It is also important for the nurse to make the assessment, as well as the interventions, immediately therapeutic and relevant to the needs of the situation.

At this time, the nurse recognizes that Kevin's mother has limited ability to absorb the shock of her son's arrest. The nurse also recognizes that the mother has limited ability to imagine alternative explanations for either her son's involvement or the resolution of the crisis.

Because a realistic appraisal of the problem is essential to the development of appropriate interventions, the nurse knows that she must address the problem directly and quickly. As a first level of response, the nurse attempts to widen the mother's constricted view of the situation. To rebut the mother's denial, the nurse begins by acknowledging the mother's pain and reframing her current dilemma as a life problem in need of a solution:

> *Nurse:* Mrs. Waller, I know this must be a terrible shock for you. It's not uncommon for parents to find out about their children's drug use in just this way. Our job will be to help you make some sense out of what has happened and to look at some ways that we might use this situation as a positive turning point in your family. You say that you know that Kevin has gotten involved recently with bad companions. What has this been like for you?

Note that in the nurse's response, she does not refute Mrs. Waller's description. Instead, she implicitly broadens the implications of Mrs. Waller's findings by suggesting that her experience is not uncommon. Immediately following this suggestion, the nurse moves the discussion toward the idea of intervention and toward the idea of finding meaning in the event for purposes of assessment and intervention.

REINFORCING BEHAVIOR

The desired outcome in crisis intervention is behavioral change that allows the client to assume some sense of control over his or her life comparable to or exceeding precrisis functioning (Slaikeu, 1990). Reinforcement of behavior plays an important role in empowering patients to take charge of their lives. It takes many avenues. For example, it may include behavioral modeling or role playing. You can take the role of an employer or significant family member in helping patients make crucial requests or respond to difficult dialogue. This strategy is particularly helpful in situations in which the predicted responses are likely to be accusatory or rejecting. Direct interventions, such as anticipatory guidance, specific assertiveness training, or behavioral rehearsal, also support desired behaviors.

Basic exploration of the consequences to various choices proves helpful for many patients for two reasons: First, it provides a forum for discovering and resolving cognitive distortions, and second, it helps patients problem solve possible objections and consider ways to resolve them. Strategic questions might include:

- "What would happen if you decided to do this instead of . . . ?"
- "What is the worst possible scenario if you decide to do . . . ?"
- "How do you think your husband (parent, friend, boss) will react if you do . . . ?"

Depending on the situation, it may be advantageous to point out that change in one person always makes those around them a little uncomfortable, and even a desired change initially can breed objections. This strategy is particularly relevant for use with maturational crisis. Developing alternative strategies in case the first initiative does not work should be the norm rather than the exception in crisis intervention.

ACKNOWLEDGING EFFORTS

Acknowledgment of the patient's efforts can be as effective as noting successful achievement. It is a particularly important strategy when the expected outcome does not occur, as it frequently does not, the first time around. Efforts can be reworked into the necessary modifications more easily if the patient can see the relationship between the previous efforts and the next step. The nurse's statement in the following example acknowledges the patient's efforts and reframes her concern within the broader context of developing alternative options to resolving her problem.

> *Nora:* I did as you told me, I asked my husband to come into the crisis center for this appointment, but he refused to come. It's really pretty hopeless. There's no one that can help me at home.
>
> *Nurse:* Nora, I know that you would like to get his cooperation, and it took courage to ask him. But I wouldn't look at it as a failure. You may have "seeded" the idea of help with him, and more important, you were able to say what you needed. That's a new behavior for you that you will need to resolve this situation. Now, let's look at some other options for getting you the help you need.

Termination Phase

Evaluation

Termination dates and goals to be accomplished are established within the first or second contact. Because crisis intervention is of limited time duration, time frames should be honored. Crisis intervention strategies always entail a review process that is both self-reflective and planned. It is important for patients to see the significance of their efforts, to articulate sources of social support, and to identify in closing not only strategies to reduce stress, but also those competencies needed to promote personal well-being. During the final session, you and the patient mutually assess goal accomplishment or lack of attainment. Reasons why certain outcomes occurred during the intervention process are discussed in detail. Particularly relevant are the mention of changes the patient has made in attitude and mastery of coping skills. This discussion fosters further consolidation and internalization of more effective coping strategies. Anticipatory guidance helps the patient foresee future situations that may become problematic.

As you review goal achievement with the patient, it is important to focus on what this event means to the patient and what has been learned from living through the stress. This learning may prove helpful to the patient in the future as other stressful situations are encountered. Included in the formative evaluation is the degree to which the patient seemed to be handling feelings associated with the crisis as well as the concrete action steps taken to resolve the crisis. For example, has the patient achieved a reality-based perception and cognitive mastery over the crisis event and surrounding circumstances? Were there earlier unresolved issues that contributed to the development of the current crisis, and, if so, have they been addressed?

The summative evaluation criteria relate to the questions: "Is the patient's basic level of functioning at or above the precrisis state? Should this case be closed, or are there other agencies or referrals that should be contacted?" An evaluation of progress assists the patient in placing the whole sequence of events in a positive perspective and brings closure to an important period in the patient's life. Without attention to the evaluation phase of the nursing process, an excellent assessment and comprehensive, appropriate nursing interventions are rendered ineffective.

Identifying the Need for Further Treatment

Not every crisis situation is resolved satisfactorily within the given time frame. Although the goal of crisis intervention is to enhance the coping skills, effectiveness, and competence of the patient in the short term, individuals may need assessment of potential in the long term for stabilities of these adjustment skills. Three identifiable coping patterns usually suggest the need for further treatment. First, some people seem to cope successfully with a difficult crisis-producing situation for some time and then fall apart. Emotional exhaustion ensues because the person runs out of energy. Or a person in the midst of a crisis develops a physical illness. Patients or family members who appear to be the rock of Gibraltar, able to weather and coordinate all aspects of a crisis situation, are particularly vulnerable to fallout once the crisis is under control. A second pattern you might observe involves a person's attempts to cope with stress by becoming more and more involved with extraneous activities. These activities can become a trap with no exit because the reflective time needed for transformation and growth is missing. A third pattern emerges when a person becomes so involved in a crisis situation that everything else in the person's life becomes connected with the crisis. Earlier conflicts resurface and are interwoven with the current circumstances without the person being able to distinguish between past and current history.

Crisis intervention, by definition, is short term, and it is not designed to deal with larger life issues. At the same time, it often pokes at the edges of a personal journey and permits access to a more detailed portrait of self with unbelievable vividness. In the face of crisis, emotional barriers are lifted, and feelings previously denied emerge spontaneously into view. Travel to emotional health and well-being, although still not easy, at least becomes more understandable. Because crisis often offers an opportunity to delve into previously unavailable personal accounts of a journey, you can use it as the springboard for engaging the patient traveler in a deeper search for personal truth. You need to "seize the moment" to provide information that otherwise might fall on deaf ears or to suggest further referral for a more careful review of underlying personality dynamics. Because a relationship between you and the patient now exists, it is easier to propose further intervention within the context of the crisis intervention. An example of a useful way to propose follow-up treatment is as follows:

John, you know we have done some really good work together in getting you stabilized about your wife's decision to get a divorce. But this is a very hard situation for you to deal with, and you probably will continue to have feelings that will come in potentially overwhelming waves at times when you least expect it. I would like to suggest that you consider making an appointment with ______, for follow-up continuation of your care related to these issues and what to expect as you work through this difficult time in your life.

Establishing the link between the good work accomplished to date and future opportunities for personal growth helps facilitate compliance. If the patient is not interested in follow-up care at this time, you still can furnish written information about resources should the need for further treatment arise.

Making Appropriate Referrals

In most communities, there are social service and legal agencies or services specifically designed to aid the traveler in crisis—and beyond. Community agencies and professionals frequently used as referral resources include private and public social services, the police, lawyers, physicians, clergy, school personnel, self-help groups (e.g., Shanti for the AIDS victims, Alzheimer's and related disorders support groups for family members, Candlelighters), and financial resource agencies such as Social Security. Giving patients information about resources empowers them and gives them more leverage in difficult interpersonal situations.

Making referrals is an art. It begins with your knowledge of relevant referral sources and the best ways to access them. By calling different service agencies in one's community, you can learn important information about fees, accessibility, means of contact, and services offered. Giving a phone number to a patient usually is not sufficient. It is not always as easy as it looks to access important referral resources even when your coping skills are intact. For the patient emerging from a crisis, trying to access social services through the general information number and either being put on hold or directed through a maze of different departments is frustrating. A quick call from you can ensure contact when the patient's coping skills are deficient. When more than one agency or professional is involved in the care of the patient, coordination of efforts and frequent contact become essential. Otherwise the interventions may work at cross purposes or represent duplicative efforts that are confusing to the patient and ultimately frustrating for the professionals or agencies involved. Table 15–6 summarizes the do's and don't's of psychological first aid.

Record-Keeping

Although record-keeping is always important, it is critical that it be accurate and complete as it relates to crisis intervention treatment. The patient record should contain the date and time of admission, interview notes containing a precise description of the patient, an initial treatment plan, behavioral notes, treatment, and behavioral responses. Notations regarding physician and family notifications should be made with name, date, time, and response included. Rationale for exceptions to regular protocols should be entered in the documentation. For example, if the patient is not allowed to see his or her family because of impending violence, the reason for postponing the visitation should be written in the nursing notes.

When individuals or families are in crisis, they frequently act irrationally. It is not uncommon for a patient who clearly needs crisis intervention to refuse treatment or to decide he or she wants to leave the treatment center, emergency room, or psychiatric unit before being fully evaluated or against medical advice. Unless the patient is a danger to self or others, he or she must be allowed to leave. It is important, however, not only to have a dialogue with the patient about the risks of taking this action, but also to record the nature of the discussion, the patient's response, behaviors noted, and the time and date of departure in the patient's chart. Matter of record information also should include the names of the physician, social worker, family members who were notified, the time, date, and their response. It should be clearly stated that the patient left against medical advice, what instructions were given if any, and further treatment or referrals suggested.

▶ Check Your Reading

11. How might the nurse use a patient's strengths in crisis intervention?
12. What is meant by normalizing feelings?
13. What should be included in a nursing note for a patient in crisis?

GENERIC CRISIS INTERVENTION IN DISASTERS

Crisis intervention in disaster situations requires a generic rather than individual approach. Generic support as a crisis intervention strategy is based on a public health model and is designed to reach large numbers of individuals in as short a time as possible. Obviously, it is most effective in large-scale disasters and community crisis situations. *Generic support* interventions focus on facilitating needed connections with appropriate agen-

TABLE 15–6 **Dos and Don'ts of Psychological First Aid**

Dos	Don'ts
Contact	
Listen carefully	Ignore either facts or feelings
Reflect feelings and facts	Judge or take sides
Communicate acceptance	
Dimensions of the problem	
Ask open-ended questions	Rely on yes/no questions
Ask person to be concrete	Allow continued abstractions
Assess lethality	Ignore "danger" signs of lethality, violence, or physical emergency
Possible solutions	
Encourage brainstorming	Allow tunnel vision
Deal directly with blocks	Leave obstacles unexplored
Set priorities	Tolerate a jumble of needs
Concrete action	
Take one step at a time	Attempt to solve it all now
Set specific short-term goals	Make binding long-term decisions
Confront when necessary	Be timid
Be directive, if and only if you must	Retreat from taking responsibility when necessary
Follow-up	
Make a contact for recontact	Leave details up in the air, or assume that client will follow through on plan on his or her own
Evaluate actions steps	Leave evaluation to someone else

From Slaikeu, K. (1984). *Crisis intervention: A handbook for practice and research.* ©1984 by Allyn and Bacon. Reprinted by permission.

cies, provisions, and basic supplies such as food, water, and shelter to sustain the individual temporarily until more permanent arrangements can be made. Treatment goals emphasize relief for groups rather than individuals. Providing immediate, tangible relief and mobilizing large groups of people to understand the meaning of the crisis and the tasks needed for return to equilibrium are central goals. By contrast with the directive role you assume in individual crisis situations, crisis intervention in large-scale disasters supports the sense of participation by the local citizens rather than assuming the primary role for decision making. Research studies (Farbarow, 1978) document quicker recovery rates and less negative long-term effects when local citizens participate actively in the recovery process. Generic crisis intervention strategies generally are used in disasters in which large numbers of people have experienced loss and disruption (Baldwin, 1979). Case Example 15–10 illustrates this approach.

Case Example 15–10 The Story of a Virginia Flood

On November 4, 1985, the city of Roanoke, Virginia experienced a flood that resulted in the deaths of 10 people, left hundreds homeless, and caused an estimated $750 million worth of damage. Following this disaster, Mental Health Services of the Roanoke Valley launched a plan to facilitate recovery. The agency immediately distributed educational materials to explain the normal emotional reactions to such a catastrophe. They encouraged people to come and seek help at the Mental Health Center. A program for flood victims and for rescue and medical personnel was organized by a team of specially trained counselors.

Following the immediate impact, your role shifts to strengthening the individual coping strategies of the person or persons involved. Research (Farbarow, 1978) suggests that young children, the elderly, and ethnic subcultures within the community are particularly vulnerable populations to long-standing emotional strain as a result of a disaster. Parents may need particular attention to resume their parental responsibilities as soon as possible. Encouraging children to express their feelings through words, images, or the use of play therapy helps mitigate the anxiety and stimulates a sense of mastery over an incomprehensible situation. Children are particularly susceptible to misinterpretation of events (Cochrane and Myers, 1980). They may not appear upset, but they are absorbing all of the data surrounding the hazardous event without necessarily being able to understand or integrate it. For example, a girl of nine witnessing the sudden and precipitous death of a favorite grandmother went with her in the ambulance to the emergency room. Everyone assumed she was old enough to understand what had happened and undervalued the meaning of the experience for her. Twenty years later, this young woman is unable to enter an emergency room or hospital.

PSYCHIATRIC EMERGENCY SERVICES

Psychiatric emergency services have taken a proactive community-based approach in the form of mobile crisis teams. These teams are composed of interdisciplinary specially trained crisis intervention workers. The mobile crisis service functions as an outreach mechanism for people who might not seek treatment on their own initiative. The evaluative emergency psychiatric service provides the initial point of entry into the larger mental health system for patients in psychiatric crisis. Operating around the clock, the mobile crisis team responds to calls in the community and does a preliminary assessment and first-order intervention of persons in crisis with concurrent probable mental illness or situational crisis in the field. Patients served might include a frail elderly patient who refuses to eat, an agoraphobic patient, or a confused schizophrenic patient living in the community. Usually, it is the family rather than the patient who initiates the request for treatment because either they are unable to provide the required care or the patient is unwilling to consider hospital-based services. Frequently the person or family requesting the service as well as the patient is in a state of acute crisis. By providing immediate support, reinforcing family strategies and referral to the appropriate support services, an acute crisis can be reduced and it is possible to avert the need for rehospitalization of a chronically ill mental patient. Acutely suicidal, homicidal, or intoxicated patients are not treated by the team. This form of alternative mental health services for the patient in crisis is particularly effective for treating transitory psychiatric crisis in the deinstitutionalized mentally ill (Gurian, 1978; Benglesdorf and Alden, 1987).

CARING FOR YOURSELF

Working with acute crisis situations is emotionally draining. For many crisis situations, there are no authoritative or definitive answers to serious life questions. The human carnage and destruction of all that is important to a person's sense of self and well-being, often occurring in a matter of moments, affects the caregiver as well as the victim. There remain existential questions that continue to haunt the crisis worker, about their own contributions, the meaning of life, and their place in it. Careful retrospective analysis of a crisis situation and one's role in helping patients resolve it can reveal its truth and transform its meaning, thereby putting it in perspective.

Nurses actively engaged in crisis work need a formalized mechanism for understanding their reactions to catastrophic events beyond their control. Providing consistent, caring support to persons in acute states of emotional equilibrium demands a steadiness and balance that simultaneously requires understanding and backing of the caregiver. If the crisis affects the individual worker, personally as well as professionally, the problem is more complex. For example, a disaster, such as a hurricane or earthquake, can create a role conflict for nurses who are torn between attending to their personal family needs and their professional responsibility to those of the larger community (Stanley, 1990).

With every crisis situation, professional caregivers have certain fears and discomforts that cannot be addressed in the critical moments of crisis intervention. These feelings need to find their voice once the immediate crisis subsides. Usually, this is best accomplished with a group format. It is important for nurses working with crisis situations to understand that they are not alone with their reactions. What nurses find in postcrisis group recall is that other workers' experiences parallel and echo their own, and this can be reassuring to the individual nurse. There is common recognition that one's own sense of discomfort is embedded in the context of an unfamiliar world in which previously learned coping strategies did not hold up. Although talking about it may not fully resolve a personal ache, the level of discomfort generally is less following a **critical incident debriefing.** Talking, expressing feelings, and exploring ways to deal with the feelings are all positive ways to cope with stress and to put it in perspective. The balancing factor of having a designated time and place to talk about the fears and discomforts of working with people in terrible circumstances helps to mitigate the tension and resolve a personal sense of feeling out of control. Moreover, shared experiences and actions broaden nurses' professional framework for understanding and coping with potentially awkward, confusing, and untenable feelings.

Rubin (1990) describes a "critical incident stress debriefing" approach to stress reduction of personnel in high stress settings. This technique was first used informally to reduce the impact of psychological stress casualties among emergency service personnel dealing with war casualties (Mitchell, 1988) and has been broadly applied across a wide variety of clinical settings. Debriefing after major or cumulative crisis circumstances, such as an unusual number of deaths on a critical care unit, mass casualties, or environmental devastation, obviously is an effective and essential way of reducing collective stress among nursing personnel. The concept can also be used with any group of nurses routinely working with patients to resolve crisis situations in psychiatric and medical settings, for example, with case management in which crisis situations are compounded by limited resources.

The goals of the debriefing process relate to helping the individual understand what happened from a "big picture" perspective, providing a safe place to ventilate feelings, assisting the nurse with differentiating between the things that can and cannot be controlled related to resource allocation and ultimately to reduce the tension to a workable level and restore the nurse to precrisis functioning.

The critical incident stress debriefing includes a five-phase format: (1) fact, (2) thought, (3) reaction, (4) teaching, and (5) reentry. In the *fact phase*, each participant is invited to share his or her perception of the incident. As the group members describe the incident, new information and pieces of information are integrated into a more understandable whole. The *thought phase* builds on this information by asking participants to reflect on the incident and to share what they were feeling personally during different parts of the crisis. In the *reaction phase*, participants are asked to evaluate the impact of the emotional aspects of the incident, e.g., "what was the worst part of the incident for you." Previously undiscussed and less acceptable feelings are allowed to emerge in a safe environment. Knowing that other people experience the same feelings as you do and that those feelings are normal behavioral responses to abnormal circumstances often is a relief to people who work with intense stress and have no place to share their feelings and concerns. Participants discuss stress-related symptoms they had during the incident or are experiencing currently. The *teaching phase* focuses on specific stress management strategies to reduce stress and ways to enhance group support of each other. In the final *reentry phase*, the facilitator encourages questions designed to put closure on the incident and provides a summary of the process. Individual referrals for further counseling, if needed, are provided at this time (Rubin, 1990).

▶ Check Your Reading

14. In what ways are mobile crisis units forms of preventive psychiatry?
15. What factors should be considered in a patient referral?
16. Why is it important for nurses to engage in a critical stress debriefing following a crisis incident?

CONCLUSIONS

The psychiatric-mental health nurse plays a key role in crisis intervention, whether the crisis be a psychiatric emergency involving a drug overdose, a community crisis such as a flood, or a disaster such as a plane crash. In the initial stages of crisis, the psychiatric nurse's role is to stabilize the person, family, or community whose journey is in crisis. Later, after stabilization, the psychiatric nurse helps the victims of crisis integrate the meaning of the crisis into the story of their life's journey.

KEY POINTS TO REMEMBER

- Crisis is a time of decision.
- Elements of a crisis include a critical stressor, a vulnerable state, failure of normal problem-solving methods, lack of social supports, and intolerable tension.
- Balancing factors, such as social support, redefining the goals, and a realistic appraisal of the crisis situation, can avert a crisis state.
- A crisis state is not a pathological state.
- A crisis is categorized as situational or maturational.
- Evaluation of lethality is a first-order consideration in assessment in crisis intervention.
- Assessment and intervention strategies are linked closely together in crisis intervention.
- Interventions are based on the problem-solving mode, with attention focused on the immediate situation.
- Referral is an important part of crisis intervention.
- A critical incident stress debriefing format provides a formalized opportunity for nurses to gain new understanding and personal awareness of reactions to difficult crisis situations.

LEARNING ACTIVITIES

1. Think back to a time when you confronted a potential crisis. Perhaps it involved the death or illness of a family member, friend, or pet; the suicide of a classmate; the loss of a first love; or moving to a new area. Or perhaps it was an experience that was personally significant to you because it was a first experience. Perhaps it was your first day of clinical as a nursing student or maybe your first semester away from home. Next, identify the factors that made the crisis potentially overwhelming and those that helped reduce the sense of crisis. What were the balancing factors that helped to reduce the effects of your stress or added to them? How did you cope? Were you able to talk with sympathetic friends, student support services, or family who could console and support you? Next, share your experience with your classmates and develop a list of the defining characteristics of the crisis and the most successful coping strategies that you discovered. Discuss how these experiences can be used to shape your responses to patients in crisis.

2. Consider the following scenario: Mr. Terrera has brought his wife to the emergency department because he is worried about her. Their son committed suicide about three weeks ago. According to Mr. Terrera, Mrs. Terrera has not been able to sleep and refuses to eat. She says, over and over again, "Why did it have to happen this way?" She cries all the time since her son's death. The couple is Spanish, and Mrs. Terrera does not speak English fluently.

Using the strategies presented in this chapter, role play the initial interview in groups of four students. One student should act as observer and feedback to the "nurse interviewer."

3. Consider the following scenarios:

a. Joan Ferrenz is 24. Her mother drove her to the emergency department after Joan told her she had swallowed a significant number of Co-Tylenol pills and consumed a fifth of whiskey.

b. John Taylor was brought by the police to the emergency room. He seems easily distracted and very angry.

c. Carol Moore is a borderline schizophrenic patient who is well-known to the emergency room staff. She has just cut her wrists with a knife and appears quite distressed.

d. Tim Jackson's girlfriend told him she didn't want to see him anymore. He doesn't know how he will live without her and has come to the emergency room complaining of shortness of breath, profuse sweating, and heart palpitations.

Analyze these scenarios and identify the following for each:

1. Central or immediate problem
2. Contributing factors
3. Obstacles to problem solving
4. Desired outcomes

First, on your own, develop a nursing strategy, including prioritized nursing actions, for each case. Then discuss your results in small groups. Come to a consensus as to how you would approach each of the patients, what considerations would be most important, and who should be involved in the treatment process.

CRITICAL THINKING EXERCISES

The community health nurse, Mrs. Peabody, was making a 10-day follow-up visit to Mrs. Alverez after her abdominal surgery. As Mrs. Peabody entered the house, Mrs. Alverez's daughter, Maria, met her at the door stating, "My brother has been shot by a gang member and my mother is dying. Please help us."

1. What assumption(s) is Maria making about Mrs. Peabody?
2. What assumptions can Mrs. Peabody make about what has happened?
3. What other information is needed to assess the crisis level accurately?

Recognizing a crisis situation, Mrs. Peabody makes an assessment of everyone's coping behaviors. She notes that Maria is crying hysterically, that Mrs. Alverez is lying in bed in a fetal position, and that the son is sitting in his room watching MTV. He does not appear to be upset.

1. What conclusion(s) can be drawn about this scene?
2. How would Mrs. Peabody check out her assumptions about this crisis situation?
3. What alternative interpretation could explain the characters' behavior?

REFERENCES

Abbott, K. (1990). Therapeutic use of play in the psychological preparation of preschool children undergoing cardiac surgery. *Issues in Comprehensive Pediatric Nursing, 13* (4), 265–277.

Aguilera, D. (1994). *Crisis intervention: Theory and methodology* (7th ed.). St. Louis: Mosby-Year Book.

Aguilera, D. C., and Messick, J. M. (1974). *Crisis intervention: Theory and methodology.* St. Louis: C. V. Mosby.

Alvarez, R. (1989, July 23). One seat left: "Luck put man on flight 232." *Baltimore Sunday Sun, 89* (30), pp. 1A, 16A.

American Nurses' Association (1994). *Standards of psychiatric mental health clinical nursing practice.* Washington, D.C.: American Nurses' Association Press.

Anonymous (1992). Open learning programme. M#: Managing stress. The stress question (continuing education credit). *Nursing Times, 88* (20), 13–19.

Arnold, E., and Boggs, K. (1995). *Interpersonal relationships: Professional communication skills for nurses.* Philadelphia: W. B. Saunders.

Back, K. (1992). Critical incident stress management for care providers in the pediatric emergency department. *Critical Care Nurse, 12* (1), 78.

Baldwin, B. A. (1979). Crisis intervention: An overview of theory and practice. *The Counseling Psychologist, 8,* 43–52.

Bauduea, A. (1977). Cognitive processes mediating behavioral change. *Journal of Personality and Social Psychology, 35* (3), 125.

Beck, J., and Staffin, R. (1986). Patients' competency to give informed consent to medication. *Hospital and Community Psychiatry, 37,* 400–402.

Beckingham, A., and Baumann, A. (1990). The ageing family in crisis: Assessment and decision making models. *Journal of Advanced Nursing, 15,* 782–787.

Benglesdorf, H., and Alden, D. C. (1987). A mobile crisis unit in the psychiatric emergency room. *Hospital and Community Psychiatry, 38,* 662–665.

Berman, A., and Jobes, D. (1991). *Adolescent suicide: Assessment and intervention.* Washington, D.C.: American Psychological Association.

Brandon, J. E., Loftin, J., and Curry, J. (1991). Role of fitness in mediating stress: A correlational exploration of stress reactivity. *Journal of Perceptual and Motor Skills, 73,* 1171–1180.

Brown, V., Ridgely, M., Pepper, B., Levine, I., and Ryglewicz, H. (1989). The dual crisis: Mental illness and substance abuse. *American Psychologist, 44,* 565–569.

Caplan, G. (1964). *Principles of preventive psychiatry.* New York: Basic Books.

Caplan, G. (1974). *Support systems and community mental health: Lectures on concept development* (p. 215). New York: Behavioral Publications.

Cardell, R., and Horton-Deutsch, S. (1994). A model for assessment of inpatient suicide potential. *Archives of Psychiatric Nursing, 8* (6), 366–372.

Chiles, J., and Strosahl, K. (1993). The suicidal patient: Assessment, crisis management, and treatment. In J. Dunner (Ed.), *Current Psychiatric Therapy.* Philadelphia: W. B. Saunders.

Cochrane, C. T., and Myers, D. V. (1980). *Children in crisis: A time for caring, a time for change.* Beverly Hills, California: Sage Publications.

Cohen, R. (1978). Tarasoff vs. Regents of the University of California. The duty to warn: Common law and statutory problems for California psychotherapists. *California Western Law Review, 15,* 153–182.

Colgrove, M., Bloomfield, H., and McWilliams, P. (1976). *How to survive the loss of a love.* (p. 42). New York: Leo Press.

David, J. (1991). How well do nurses care for their own? *Journal of Advanced Nursing, 16* (8), 887–888.

Davidzer, R. (1991). How to stay sane as a student of nursing. *Imprint, 38* (4), 96–98.

Davis, J. M., Hoshiko, B. R., Jones, S., and Gosnell, D. (1992). The effect of a support group on grieving individuals' level of perceived support and stress. *Archives of Psychiatric Nursing, 6* (1), 35–39.

Dooley, D., and Catalano, R. (1991). Unemployment as a stressor: Findings and implications of a recent study. *WHO Region Publications European Series, 37*, 313–339.

Dunne, E., McIntosh, J., and Dunne-Maxim, K. (Eds.) (1987). *Suicide and its aftermath: Understanding and counseling the survivors.* New York: W. W. Norton.

Edens, J. L., Larkin, K. T., and Abel, J. (1992). The effect of social support and physical touch on cardiovascular reactions to mental stress. *Journal of Psychosomatic Research, 36* (4), 371–381.

Emmons, R. (1991). Personal strivings, daily life events and psychological and physical well-being. *Journal of Personality, 59* (3), 453–472.

Epstein, S., and Katz, L. (1992). Coping ability, stress, productive load and symptoms. *Journal of Personality and Social Psychology, 62* (5), 813–825.

Erikson, E. H. (1963). *Childhood and society.* New York: W. W. Norton and Co.

Erikson, E. H. (1968). *Identity, youth, and crisis.* New York: W. W. Norton and Co.

Farbarow, N. (Ed.) (1978). *Training manual for human service workers in major disasters*, DHEW Publication No. (ADM) 77-538. Washington, D.C.: Superintendent of Documents, U.S. Government Printing Office.

Felsten, G. (1991). Influences of situation-specific mastery beliefs and satisfaction with social support on appraisal of stress. *Psychological Reports, 69* (2), 483–495.

Figley, C. R. (1985). From victim to survivor: Social responsibility in the wake of catastrophe. In C. R. Figley (Ed.), *Trauma and its wake: The study of post-trauma stress disorder.* New York: Brunner/Mazel.

Figley, C. R. (1988). Post-traumatic family therapy. In F. M. Ochberg (Ed.), *Post traumatic therapy and victims of violence* (pp. 83–113). New York: Brunner/Mazel.

Fisher, H. (1989). Psychiatric crises: Making the most of an emergency room visit. *Journal of Psychosocial Nursing and Mental Health Services, 27* (11), 4–8.

Folks, D. G., and Kinney, F. C. (1992). The role of psychological factors in dermatologic conditions. *Psychosomatics, 33* (1), 45–54.

Fujimura, L., Weis, D., and Cocran, J. (1985). Suicide: Dynamics and implications for counseling. *Journal of Counseling and Development, 63*, 612–615.

Gadzella, B., Ginther, D., Tomcala, M., and Bryant, G. (1991). Differences between men and women on stress producers and coping strategies. *Psychological Reports, 69* (2), 561–562.

Gillig, P., Hillard, J., Bell, J., et al (1989). The psychiatric emergency service holding area: Effect on utilization of inpatient resources. *American Journal of Psychiatry, 146*, 369–372.

Gray, S., and Diers, D. (1992). The effect of staff stress on patient behavior. *Archives of Psychiatric Nursing, 6* (1), 26–34.

Gropper, E. (1992). Promoting health by promoting comfort. *Nursing Forum, 27* (2), 5–8.

Gulliland, B., and James, R. (1993). *Crisis intervention strategies.* Pacific Grove, California: Brooks/Cole Publishing.

Gurian, B. E. (1978). The psychiatric house call. *American Journal of Psychiatry, 135*, 592–593.

Hersh, J. B. (1985). Interviewing college students in crisis. *Journal of Counseling and Development, 63*, 286–289.

Hillard, J. (1990). *Manual of clinical emergency psychiatry.* Washington, D.C.: American Psychiatric Press.

Hoff, L.A. (1989). *People in crisis.* Redwood City, California: Addison-Wesley.

Holmes, T. H., and Rahe, R. H. (1967). The social readjustment rating scale. *Journal of Psychosomatic Research, 11*, 213–218.

Horowitz, M. J. (1986). *Stress response syndromes.* New York: Jason Aronson.

Hughes, R. (1988). Grief counseling: Facilitating the healing process. *Journal of Counseling and Development, 67*, 77.

Janosik, E. (1984). *Crisis counseling: A contemporary approach.* Belmont, California, Wadsworth.

Jin, P. (1992). Efficacy of Tai Chi, brisk walking, meditation and reading in reducing mental and emotional stress. *Journal of Psychosomatic Research, 36* (4), 361–370.

Kaplan, H., and Sadock, B. (1993). *Pocket handbook of emergency psychiatric medicine.* Baltimore: Williams & Wilkins.

Keitner, G., Ryan, C., Miller, et al (1990). Family functioning, social adjustment, and recurrence of suicidality. *Psychiatry, 53* (1), 17–30.

Kleeman, K. (1989). Families in crisis due to multiple trauma. *Nursing Clinics of North America, 1* (1), 25.

Langley, R., and Levy R. (1977). *Wife beating: The silent crisis.* New York: Dutton.

Lepore, S., Evans, G., and Schneider, M. (1991). Dynamic role of social support in the link between chronic stress and psychological distress. *Journal of Personality and Social Psychology, 61* (6), 899–909.

Lindemann, E. (1944). Symptomatology and management of acute grief. *American Journal of Psychiatry, 101*, 151–158.

Margo, G., and Finkel, J. (1990). Early dementia a risk factor for suicide. *Hospital and Community Psychiatry, 41*, 676–678.

McFarland, P. H., and Stanton, A. L. (1991). Preparation of children for emergency medical care: A primary prevention approach. *Journal of Pediatric Psychology, 16* (4), 489–504.

Melick, M., Logue, J., and Frederick, C. (1982). Stress and disaster. In L. Goldberger and S. Breznitz (Eds.), *Handbook of stress: Theoretical and clinical aspects.* New York: The Free Press.

Miller, W., and C'deBaca, J. (1994). Quantum change: Toward a psychology of transformation. In T. Heatherton and J. Weinberger (Eds.), *Can personality change?* Washington, D.C.: American Psychological Association.

Mitchell, J. T. (1988). Stress: The history, status and future of critical incident stress debriefings. *Journal of Emergency Medical Services, 13*, 43–46.

Niaura, R., and Goldstein , M. G. (1992). Psychological factors affecting physical condition: Cardiovascular disease literature review. *Psychosomatics, 33* (2), 150–155.

November, M. T., Morris, M., Litton, J., and Stabler, B. (1992). Stress buffering effect of psychological support in a diabetic camp. *Diabetes Care, 15* (2), 310–311.

Nurius, P. (1984). Stress: A pervasive dilemma in psychiatric emergency care. *Comprehensive Psychiatry, 25*, 345–354.

Nyamathi, A., Jacoby, A., Constancia, P., and Ruvich, S. (1992). Coping and adjustment of spouses of critically ill patients with cardiac disease. *Heart and Lung, 21* (2), 160–166.

Ostell, A. (1991). Coping, problem solving and stress: A framework for intervention strategies. *British Journal of Medical Psychology, 64*, 11–24.

Parachin, V. M. (1991). Pressure-proof your life: Creative ways to reduce stress. *Today's OR Nurse, 13* (12), 9–11.

Pelletier, M. (1992). The organ donor family members' perception of stressful situations during the organ donation experience. *Journal of Advanced Nursing, 17* (1), 90–97.

Perry, S., Fishman, B., and Jacobsberg, L. (1992). Stress and HIV infection. *American Journal of Psychiatry, 159* (3), 416–417.

Rapoport, L. (1965). The state of crisis: Some theoretical considerations. In *Crisis intervention.* New York: Family Service Association of America.

Rice, M., Helzel, M., Varney, G., and Quinsey, V. (1985). Crisis prevention and intervention training for psychiatric hospital staff. *American Journal of Community Psychiatry, 13*, 289–304.

Roberts, A. R. (Ed.) (1991). *Contemporary perspectives on crisis intervention.* Englewood Cliffs, New Jersey: Prentice Hall.

Rosen, P., and Walsh, B. (1989). Patterns of contagion in self-mutilation epidemics. *American Journal of Psychiatry, 146*, 656–658.

Rubin, J. (1990). Critical incident stress debriefing: Helping the helpers. *16* (4), 255–258.

Russler, M. (1991). Multidimensional stress management in nursing education. *Journal of Nursing Education, 30* (8), 341–346.

Ryan-Wenger, N. M. (1992). A taxonomy of children's coping strategies: A step toward theory development. *American Journal of Orthopsychiatry, 62* (2), 256–263.

Schaefer, K., and Peterson, K. (1992). Effectiveness of coping strategies among critical care nurses. *Dimensions of Critical Care Nursing, 11* (1), 28–34.

Schafer, J., and Fals-Stewart, W. (1991). Issues of methodology, design and analytic procedure in psychological research on stress. *British Journal of Medical Psychology, 64*, 375–383.

Schneidman, E. (1987). At the point of no return: Suicidal thinking follows a predictable path. *Psychology Today, March*, 54–58.

Schonfeld, D. (1989). Crisis intervention for bereavement support: A model of intervention in the children's school. *Clinical Pediatrics, 28*, 27–33.

Schutte, N., Bouleige, L., Fix, J., and Malouff, J. (1986). Returning to partner after leaving a crisis shelter: A decision faced by battered women. *Journal of Social Behavior and Personality, 1*, 295–298.

Scrignar, C. B. (1988). *Post-traumatic stress disorder.* New York: Praeger Publishing.

Shaw, M., and Halliday, P. (1992). The family, crisis, and chronic illness: An evolutionary mode. *Journal of Advanced Nursing, 17*, 537–543.

Shore, B. J., Tatum, E., and Vollmer, W. (1986). Psychiatric reactions to disaster: The Mount St. Helens experience. *153*, 590–595.

Slaby, A. (1994). *Handbook of psychiatric emergencies* (4th ed.). Norwalk, Connecticut: Appleton-Lange.

Slaikeu, K. (1990). *Crisis intervention: A handbook for practice and research* (2nd ed.). Boston: Allyn and Bacon.

Stanley, S. (1990). When the disaster is over: Helping the healers to mend. *Journal of Psychosocial Nursing and Mental Health Services, 28* (5), 12–16.

Steptoe, A. (1991). Invited review: The links between stress and illness. *Journal of Psychosomatic Research, 35* (6), 633–644.

Terry, D. J. (1992). Stress, coping and coping resources as correlates of adaptation in myocardial infarction patients. *British Journal of Clinical Psychology, 31*, 215–225.

Thompson, B. T., Brantley, P. J., Jones, G. N., Dyer, H. R., and Morris, J. L. (1992). The relation between stress and disease activity in rheumatoid arthritis. *Journal of Behavioral Medicine, 15* (2), 215–220.

Thompson, S. W. (1991). Communication techniques for allaying anxiety and providing support for hospitalized children. *Journal of Child and Adolescent Psychiatric and Mental Health Nursing, 4* (3), 119–122.

Tidmarsh, S. (1969). *Disaster* (pp. 20–21). Middlesex: Penguin.

Turner, S., and Shapiro, C. (1986). Battered women: Mourning the death of a relationship. *Social Work, 31*, 372–376.

Tyhurst, J. (1957). The role of transition states—including disasters—in mental illness. In *Symposium on Preventive and Social Psychiatry.* Washington, D.C.: Walter Reed Army Institute of Research.

Wakefield, M. (1992). Stress control for nurses. *Canadian Nurse, 88* (4), 24–25.

Weinberger, R. (1991). Teaching the elderly stress reduction. *Journal of Gerontological Nursing, 17* (10), 23–27.

Weincourt, R. (1985). Never to be alone: Existential therapy for battered women. *Journal of Psychosocial Nursing, 23*, 24–29.

Williams, R., and Stafford, W. (1991). Silent casualties: Partners, families, and spouses of persons with AIDS. *Journal of Counseling and Development, 69*, 423–427.

Wilson, L. (1981). Thoughts on Tarasoff. *Clinical Psychologist, 34*, 37.

Wright, B. (1993). *Caring in crisis: A handbook of intervention skills.* London: Churchill Livingstone.

Wurzbach, M. E. (1992). Assessment and intervention for certainty and uncertainty. *Nursing Forum, 27* (2), 29–35.

Zinner, E. (1987). Responding to suicide in schools: A case study in loss intervention and group survivorship. *Journal of Counseling and Development, 65*, 499–501.

SUGGESTED READINGS

Aguilera, D. (1994). *Crisis intervention: Theory and methodology* (7th ed.). St. Louis: C. V. Mosby.

Back, K. (1992). Critical incident stress management for care providers in the pediatric emergency department. *Critical Care Nurse, 12* (1), 78.

Davidzer, R. (1991). How to stay sane as a student of nursing. *Imprint, 38* (4), 96–98.

Dunne, E., McIntosh, J., and Dunne-Maxim, K. (Eds.) (1987). *Suicide and its aftermath: Understanding and counseling the survivors.* New York: W. W. Norton.

Hersh, J. B. (1985). Interviewing college students in crisis. *Journal of Counseling and Development, 63*, 286–289.

Janosik, E. (1984). *Crisis counseling: A contemporary approach.* Belmont, California: Wadsworth.

McFarland, P. H., and Stanton, A. L. (1991). Preparation of children for emergency medical care: A primary prevention approach. *Journal of Pediatric Psychology, 16* (4), 489–504.

Ostell, A. (1991). Coping, problem solving and stress: A framework for intervention strategies. *British Journal of Medical Psychology, 64*,11–24.

Perry, S., Fishman, B., and Jacobsberg, L. (1992). Stress and HIV infection. *American Journal of Psychiatry, 159* (3), 416–417.

Russler, M. (1991). Multidimensional stress management in nursing education, *Journal of Nursing Education, 30* (8), 341–346.

Ryan-Wenger, N. M. (1992). A taxonomy of children's coping strategies: A step toward theory development, *American Journal of Orthopsychiatry, 62* (2), 256–263.

Schaefer, K., and Peterson, K. (1992). Effectiveness of coping strategies among critical care nurses. *Dimensions of Critical Care Nursing, 11* (1), 28–34.

Schafer, J., and Fals-Stewart, W. (1991). Issues of methodology, design and analytic procedure in psychological research on stress. *British Journal of Medical Psychology, 64*, 375–383.

Schonfeld, D. (1989). Crisis intervention for bereavement support: A model of intervention in the children's school. *Clinical Pediatrics, 28*, 27–33.

Schutte, N., Bouleige, L., Fix, J., and Malouff, J. (1986). Returning to partner after leaving a crisis shelter: A decision faced by battered women. *Journal of Social Behavior and Personality, 1*, 295–298.

Scrignar, C. B. (1988). *Post-traumatic stress disorder.* New York: Praeger Publishing.

Steptoe, A. (1991). Invited review: The links between stress and illness. *Journal of Psychosomatic Research, 35* (6), 633–644.

Terry, D. J. (1992). Stress, coping and coping resources as correlates of adaptation in myocardial infarction patients. *British Journal of Clinical Psychology, 31*, 215–225.

Thompson, B. T., Brantley, P. J., Jones, G. N., Dyer, H. R., and Morris, J. L. (1992). The relation between stress and disease activity in rheumatoid arthritis. *Journal of Behavioral Medicine, 15* (2), 215–220.

Thompson, S. W. (1991). Communication techniques for allaying anxiety and providing support for hospitalized children. *Journal of Child and Adolescent Psychiatric and Mental Health Nursing, 4* (3), 119–122.

Turner, S., and Shapiro, C. (1986). Battered women: Mourning the death of a relationship. *Social Work, 31*, 372–376.

Wakefield, M. (1992). Stress control for nurses. *Canadian Nurse, 88* (4), 24–25.

Weinberger, R. (1991). Teaching the elderly stress reduction. *Journal of Gerontological Nursing, 17* (10), 23–27.

Weincourt, R. (1985). Never to be alone: Existential therapy for battered women. *Journal of Psychosocial Nursing, 23*, 24–29.

Williams, R., and Stafford, W. (1991). Silent casualties: Partners, families, and spouses of persons with AIDS. *Journal of Counseling and Development, 69*, 423–427.

Wilson, L. (1981). Thoughts on Tarasoff. *Clinical Psychologist, 34*, 37.

Wurzbach, M. E. (1992). Assessment and intervention for certainty and uncertainty. *Nursing Forum, 27* (2), 29–35.

Zinner, E. (1987). Responding to suicide in schools: A case study in loss intervention and group survivorship. *Journal of Counseling and Development, 65*, 499–501.

CHAPTER 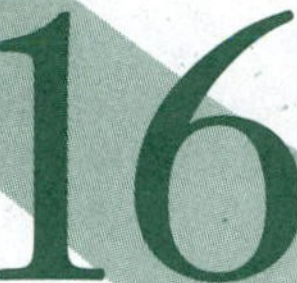

16 INDIVIDUAL THERAPY

And, therefore if the head and the body are to be well, you must begin by curing the soul; that is the first thing. And the cure, my dear youth, has to be effected by the use of certain charms, and these charms are fair words; and by them temperance is implanted in the soul, and where temperance is, there is health speedily imparted, not only to the head, but to the whole body.

—*Plato*

LEARNING OBJECTIVES

After studying this chapter, you should be able to:

1. Describe several different approaches to individual therapy.
2. Discuss the differences between long-term therapy and short-term therapy.
3. Identify the influence of rising health care costs on the techniques of individual therapy.
4. Appreciate the unique journey of the nurse therapist.
5. Describe the attitude and skills necessary for beginning the patient journey in individual therapy.
6. Describe the attitude and skills needed to continue the patient journey in individual therapy.
7. Appreciate the role of self in empowering the patient journey in individual therapy.

KEY TERMINOLOGY

Automatic thinking schema
Behavior therapy
Cognitive distortions
Cognitive psychotherapy
Countertransference
Insight
Long-term therapy
Psychoanalysis
Psychoanalytical psychotherapy
Psychodynamic short-term therapy
Psychotherapy
Short-term therapy
Supportive psychotherapy
Transference

Psychotherapy is often referred to as the talking cure. Today's form of psychotherapy is an outgrowth of the work of Freud and his colleagues in the late 19th century. The goal of psychotherapy is to help the patient overcome or modify feelings, behaviors, and thoughts that are getting in the way of the patient meeting goals for self. Since Freud's time, countless volumes and papers have been written on the theory of psychotherapy as well as how to practice psychotherapy. Nursing is part of this tradition. The following story is about Peggy, who came to a clinical nurse specialist hoping for relief from her pain and suffering.

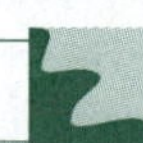

PEGGY'S STORY

Peggy finally had an appointment in mental health with a clinical nurse specialist. The people at the clinic told her that a clinical nurse specialist has a master's degree in psychiatric nursing. For months, Peggy had been struggling with a kind of drowning feeling mixed with anxiety that made her irritable and feel mean. During these months, there were times when she couldn't get out of bed in the morning to attend her college classes. The odd thing was, there were many nights that she couldn't sleep at all. She was the first in her family to go to college, and she really wanted to succeed. Oh, she could just hear her mother yelling at her, "Who do you think you are anyway? Good enough to go to college—huh." And she was really scared that she was like her mother. There were days at a time that her mother never got out of bed. And those scenes where her mother would blame her and her brother for how horrible she felt. The anxiety was something her mother had too. Peggy supposed that was why her mom drank so much. But that was another thing. Peggy couldn't handle alcohol. She knew that after three or four drinks she sort of "lost it." Often she could not remember anything at all after that point. She felt that the rape two summers ago would not have occurred if she had not had those drinks. In fact, she didn't remember ever having a sexual experience without alcohol. And her brother had well-known substance abuse problems.

Peggy wasn't sure what this appointment could do for

her except make her more anxious and irritable. She had to wait two weeks between the phone call and the appointment. Her roommates made her call because they said she was unbearable; they were tired of it and were considering asking her to move somewhere else. She had punched a wall once, and she stayed in her room a lot lately, often drinking beer, smoking cigarettes, and not wanting anything to do with her roommates. Their threat to call her family had done it—she was so ashamed of her family and she didn't want anyone to know how awful it really was. Her mom never was able to keep the house clean, and her dad seemed to spend all his time on his boat. She remembered when she was about seven that her family spent a lot of time near the water and how she used to dive in the ocean and spend as long as possible under the water. No one ever seemed to worry about her. Soon she found that under the water was the only safe place to let herself cry or yell. Being upset in front of her parents only led to name-calling, usually "fat little cry-baby." Her feelings were not important. The other safe thing she could do was eat, so she was fat and ugly most of her life. But eating felt so good! Even now she was 50 pounds overweight after countless diets. The last time she had lost weight, about four years ago, she was still at home and suddenly her father stopped yelling at her and began to be nice to her and call her his little princess. Was this really true or a dream? Did he come into her room at night after he had been out with his buddies and kiss her over and over again telling her how lovely she was? Phew, the smell of him is there with her now.

Peggy wondered what talking to someone would help—she couldn't possibly tell this nurse everything! If she did, the nurse wouldn't want anything to do with her anyway. Besides, she herself didn't even know what everything was. What if the nurse laughed at her?

HISTORY OF PSYCHOTHERAPY

As the quote that opens this chapter indicates, ancient scholars recognized that talking can often bring healing. Aristophanes, a great ancient Greek writer, wrote *The Clouds*, a dialogue between Socrates and Strepsiades. Strepsiades has come for counsel over his worry about his debts.

> *Socrates:* Come, lie down here.
>
> *Strepsiades:* What for?
>
> *Socrates:* Ponder a while over matters that interest you.
>
> *Strepsiades:* Oh, I pray not there.
>
> *Socrates:* Come, on the couch!
>
> *Strepsiades:* What a cruel fate.
>
> *Socrates:* Ponder and examine closely, gather your thoughts together, let your mind turn to every side of things. If you meet with difficulty, spring quickly to some other idea; keep away from sleep.

Although Socrates may have had the right treatment, his wisdom went largely unheeded because ancient people attributed emotional disorders to outside forces. Strepsiades, engaging in an early analysis in the previous dialogue, eventually decides to try controlling the cycles of the moon as a way to solve his problems (Alexander and Selesnick, 1968). Indeed, early peoples thought that emotions were controlled by the lunar cycles (thus, the term *lunacy* to describe mental illness). Individuals were reluctant to recognize and take responsibility for personal feelings. As civilization progressed, blame for mental illness went from celestial bodies to magical fluids such as black bile, to spirits, and to the devil. Mental illness was often considered a permanent affliction, and those who suffered were often condemned to die or were imprisoned, chained in dungeons, for life. Some were hanged for practicing witchcraft or burned for sorcery or committing acts directed by the devil (Brigham, 1994).

The greatest change in thinking about the origins of emotions came from St. Augustine, an early leader of the Christian church. Although his teachings were the pathway to faith in God, he believed in the necessity for psychological self-understanding as a pathway to changing behaviors by first changing inner values. St. Augustine undertook and wrote the first self-analysis, exposing a truthfulness about inner motivations on behavior and feelings that Sigmund Freud, 1400 years later, would validate. St. Augustine's psychology tells about the feelings, conflicts, and anguish of an individual of greatest sincerity and introspective power, and it can be justly considered as the earliest forerunner of psychoanalysis. (Alexander and Selesnick, 1968, p. 87).

PSYCHOANALYTICAL PSYCHOTHERAPY

Psychoanalytical psychotherapy is an outgrowth of the work done by Freud. Freud lived in an era when science was flourishing, great advances were being made in medicine, and there was beginning recognition that human behavior came from self rather than outside forces. Freud postulated that all mental illnesses are due to the influences of early interpersonal experiences and that to understand a person's illness, these early experiences must be explored and systematically observed. He developed the technique of **psychoanalysis**, which often involves daily visits to the physician to help the patient with memory recall of childhood. The role of the physician is to observe these memories and help guide the patient on the journey toward understanding their influence on present behavior. This technique may take years because some memories, lodged in the unconscious (see Chapter 6), are not part of the patient's everyday awareness. Therefore, memory recall can be slow and difficult. Although psychoanalysis is still practiced, few patients can afford the cost of daily visits for years, and so, a century after Freud's teachings, **psychoanalytical psychotherapy**, using Freud's theories, is the more common treatment.

Psychoanalytical psychotherapy usually is done once or twice a week until the patient is better. The psychotherapist assesses the patient using Freudian theory that early experiences are pleasurable instincts, such as bodily pleasures experienced from early infancy, and aggressive instincts are the impulses to get what one wants. These instincts are largely unconscious and are labeled the id. Freud postulated that as a person grows, the id is often in conflict with reality and the need to behave and get along in family and society. Freud labeled this reality and the need to behave appropriately the ego. Depending on the quality of early childhood relationships, the pleasure and the aggressive instincts give into healthy life forces (a healthy ego) or become maladaptive, manifesting as anxiety, depression, and countless frustrating interpersonal relationships at work and home (an unhealthy ego) (Strachey, 1958). Freud believed that the primitive impulses of the id were kept in check by both the ego and a third concept, the superego. He considered the superego as the place where values and morals were located and often helped the ego or conscious self perform in a healthy manner (see Chapter 6).

If a person's ego is not healthy, the goal of psychoanalytical psychotherapy is to explore the development of the id, ego, and superego through memory recall of childhood experiences and exploration of dream content. Dreams are important in psychoanalytical psychotherapy in that they often reveal hidden messages about a patient's struggle with life. The patient describes memories and dreams in the therapy session, recreating them and using the therapist as a neutral sounding board. The patient is reacting to the therapist as if reexperiencing these early conflicts. This process is called **transference**. It is important for the therapist to remain neutral as the patient reveals memories so that the patient can experience any conflicts, through the transference, in a different and more healthy way than in the childhood experience. Because the therapist does not react the way a caretaker did, the patient is free to respond in a different manner. As the transference continues, the therapist guides the patient, through careful observations and questions, to an understanding, called **insight**, into how their early childhood experiences are influencing their present difficulties. As the patient's insight becomes more sophisticated, the patient begins to understand how he or she developed certain ways of responding to events and people based on these early childhood experiences. These responses are known as defense mechanisms. With these new insights, the patient is able to "unhook" himself or herself from these past defense mechanisms and begin to explore more satisfying ways of relating to others. This exploration also occurs through the relationship with the therapist.

To receive help from psychodynamic psychotherapy, a person must be able to tolerate intense scrutiny into the inner self. The patient should have a relatively stable lifestyle so that constant change and crisis are not distracting from the transference process. Because psychodynamic psychotherapy requires deep exploration, the patient may be going to therapy once or twice a week so that time is required to commit to therapy. The duration of therapy is relatively long-term, lasting anywhere from six months to three years. The patient needs the financial resources to tackle such long-term work because insurance companies have become unwilling to reimburse for long-term therapy. Table 16–1 summarizes the essential features of psychoanalytical psychotherapy.

TABLE 16–1 Essential Features of Psychoanalytical Psychotherapy

Duration	Long-term 1–4 times a week
Therapist's role	Neutral
Main techniques	Exploration of childhood memories Transference (understanding patient's feelings toward therapist) Insight (understanding childhood influences) Interpretation (linking past memories with present difficulties)
Patient's role	Tolerance of scrutiny of the inner life Remembering childhood experiences Free-association Remembering dreams Developing a stable lifestyle Developing transference

When Peggy left the nurse therapist's office, she was unsure of herself. The office was nice enough but didn't have any personal touches in it like photographs or flowers or notes all over the place like her internist's office. That office was cluttered and comfortable. The nurse had hardly said anything at all during the 50 minutes, and she did not seem to react at all as Peggy was telling her story. Of course, Peggy did not tell her all the family stuff.

Neutral

Neutral

The nurse seemed quite calm and only asked her a few questions about how this or that situation made her feel. She did not even care when Peggy was silent. Once she did ask Peggy to "free associate," which meant that she wanted Peggy to just say whatever came into her head. That was weird—she actually had just finished talking about an assignment at school that she was having trouble with and the first thing that popped into her head was her father yelling at her mother for being too stupid to get a job. The nurse said "uh, huh, and what do you remember about that?" Peggy did not say anything right away, and the nurse didn't either. It seemed like a long time, and Peggy remembered that being silent was one way to hope that her parents would not notice her and yell. She had a special spot that she went to behind a big old dirty chair where no one could see her. At just the right angle she could watch TV and no one would know. — *Childhood memories* / *Childhood memories*

But there was some of that familiar anxiety again. She supposed that keeping quiet was the best way to make sure that the nurse did not hate her. She heard the nurse wonder if her father's anger had anything to do with her difficulties at school? That's funny—the anxiety is sort of the same when she thought about the teacher. Peggy did not know how she felt about the nurse. She was relieved that the nurse did not seem upset by her feelings and that she had not commented on her weight. Peggy had agreed to return two times a week—for how long she didn't know. — *Interpretation* / *Transference* / *Insight*

▶ Check Your Reading

1. What did ancient people attribute emotions to?
2. How did St. Augustine change thinking about emotions?
3. What is the id?
4. What is the ego?
5. What is the superego?
6. Why is it important for the therapist to remain neutral in the transference process?
7. What are the reasons that psychoanalysis and psychoanalytic psychotherapy are long-term?

LONG-TERM THERAPY TO SHORT-TERM THERAPY

Long-term therapy flows from the psychoanalytical model as developed by Freud and his medical doctor colleagues. The reason for the long-term approach was not only that the journey through a patient's childhood memories took a long time to pursue, but also that psychoanalysis and psychodynamic psychotherapy sought to change the personality characteristics of the patient. Psychotherapy was viewed as the most important part of a patient's life. Being in psychotherapy defined the patient as ill. As such, the patient was expected to bring mental processes to the medical doctor for care and was not expected to help in the journey toward wellness outside the psychotherapy room. In fact, major life events, such as weddings or birth of a child, were considered distracting to the therapeutic process because they disrupted the patient's ability to have thoughts (free associate) about the childhood memories and were discouraged. The medical doctor was considered all wise in his or her listening, reflecting, and questioning and in knowing when the therapeutic journey would be over and the patient cured.

When long-term therapy first began to flourish, in the early 1900s, there were no insurance companies, so the economics of mental health care were not of particular importance. It was comfortable and easy to have the same patient returning over and over again, and patients invariably benefited from psychoanalysis or psychodynamic psychotherapy. Some people were in therapy for years, and therapy became part of who they were. Early insurance policies gave unlimited coverage for long-term therapy. In the 1970s and 1980s, however, health care costs rose. Mental health care was targeted for its perceived excesses, and insurance companies began to put limits on the amount of therapy a person could have. This was the beginning of managed care, in which a third party (the insurance company) outside the therapist-patient relationship became an overseer and tied payment for therapy to third-party approval.

The insurance company also controlled who could provide therapy by stipulating that only therapists who were credentialed by the company were eligible for reimbursement. Therapists were forced to apply to the insurance company to become providers for them. In addition, the insurance company hired utilization managers to review the therapy and progress of patients. Therapists had to present a written treatment plan to the utilization manager and justify how therapy would help the patient get better. Filling out those insurance company forms began to force mental health therapists to think more clearly about therapy goals. The insurance companies' unwillingness to pay for open-ended therapy forced therapists to think about how to help patients in shorter periods. Thus, the philosophy around long-term therapy shifted, and shorter-term treatment models were explored, written about, and practiced by mental health professionals.

The effect of health care economics was also felt on inpatient psychiatric care. Patients used to spend many months to years in hospitals. With the increased cost of health care, the expense of hospitalizations went up. Between 1986 and 1991, the cost for inpatient psychiatric services went from \$2.9 billion to \$5.3 billion (Talbott, 1994). Patients who had long-term hospitalizations were no longer welcome to stay. Other treatment modalities such as day treatment and evening treatment were developed as alternatives. Further hospitalizations, if indicated, became short-term because managed care capped the number of allowed hospital days. For a patient to be admitted to a hospital, permission had to be obtained from the insurance company through the utilization manager.

Today, patients must be in crisis to gain admission. This means that the acuity level in the hospital is quite high, and rapid progression through assessment, stabilization, and discharge planning is a must. Hospitalization is three to four times more expensive than day treatment or outpatient treatment so that managed care encourages short hospital stays. Stabilization of acute symptoms becomes the focus of the hospital stay rather than long-term issues underlying the acute episode. Symptoms that indicate the patient is harmful to self or others are aggressively treated, and intense issues likely to regress the patient are handled by teaching patients coping skills and careful planning for follow-up. Hospitalization should be seen as only the beginning stage of recovery—more in-depth work can take place in outpatient therapy (McGihon, 1994). Again the utilization manager is often in the inpatient setting evaluating treatment and limiting the number of days reimbursed for that particular admission.

Thus, psychiatric nurses who work in inpatient settings only have a short period to help patients stabilize. The work that the psychiatric nurse performs in the hospital is indeed short-term, perhaps only five or six hours because the patient is often stabilized and discharged within one week. Discharge planning takes on a high priority with the focus on four areas: medication compliance, symptom recognition and management, relapse prevention, and planning for follow-up treatment (McGihon, 1994). Learning short-term therapy techniques is helpful in maximizing the nursing care plan, and in giving optimal care. Knowledge of how to move a patient to other alternatives in the psychiatric care continuum is also important.

Along with the above-mentioned economic incentives, schools of nursing and social work, having developed graduate programs in the 1950s and 1960s with specialties in mental health, were graduate students trained at the master-degree level or above in psychotherapy. Students were now being trained to do psychotherapy in four disciplines: medicine, psychology, nursing, and social work. As more of the nonmedical students graduated, the traditional medical approaches to psychotherapy were questioned and other views tried, such as family therapy and behavioral therapy and biofeedback. As the nonmedical disciplines became recognized, with reimbursement, and as the public became more informed and less willing to accept traditional medical treatment, long-term therapy has become a privilege for only a few people who can afford it.

SHORT-TERM PSYCHOTHERAPY

For the purposes of this chapter, **short-term therapy** (also called brief therapy) refers to models of therapy that use techniques to help patients return to health in a short period. The models described in this chapter include psychodynamic short-term therapy, cognitive therapy, behavior therapy, and supportive psychotherapy. Initially, some short-term therapy models were developed to treat specific patient problems or diagnostic categories (for instance, cognitive therapy initially was developed for patients with depression). Today the short-term therapy model that is used is not defined by the patient's diagnoses but by the training of the therapist and the patient's biological, psychological, social, and cultural presentation. Although the techniques used for each of these models may be different, the framework for assessing and planning for short-term therapy remains the same.

Psychodynamic Model

Psychodynamic short-term therapy flows from psychoanalytical theory as developed by Freud as well as early writings by Malan (1976), Mann (1973), and Sifneos (1972), which describe short-term therapy using an analytic perspective. The term *psychodynamic* means that the unconscious plays a role in the emotions and that past events as well as genetics and present reality influence current behavior. The psychodynamic short-term therapist assesses patient problems using Freud's theories but does not have the goal of childhood memory exploration for the purpose of personality change. Rather the goal is to help the patient with here-and-now issues based on the patient's biological, psychological, social, cultural, and spiritual presence.

This psychotherapist uses a variety of techniques including making psychodynamic interpretations for patients to help them gain insight more quickly. These techniques include joint sessions with significant others, and use of time outside the therapy session through homework assignments, role playing, recognizing and promoting patient strengths, and expectations that the patient will take care of the self through proper exercise, nutrition, and soul-fulfilling or life-giving activity. Patients are often asked to learn more about their problems through reading assignments. Additionally, groups and classes on such themes as stress management and assertiveness are encouraged as an adjunct to the therapy. Psychodynamic short-term therapy techniques place increased responsibility for cure on the patient and less on the patient-therapist relationship as in the analytic model. Table 16–2 summarizes the essential features of psychodynamic short-term therapy.

All short-term therapy uses the patient's strengths and existing resources to facilitate change and alleviate the presenting problems. The short-term therapist views the patient as basically well but at a point in life at which new behaviors need to be learned. The therapeutic approach underscores the positive attributes a person brings to therapy; facilitates the development of a working partnership between the nurse and the patient; helps the patient develop future-oriented, positively worded goals; and identifies actions necessary for reaching those goals (Mason, 1994). The therapist functions as the patient's mental health consultant and brings to the therapy a unique knowledge of psychology (for instance, the effect of early childhood loss on adult relationships). With this knowledge, the therapist often teaches the patient about what the patient is experiencing. With knowledge of the patient's history and the current problem, the short-term therapist defines, along with the patient, goals for treatment and the approximate length of time to reach these goals. The therapist actively presents ideas for change with the expectation that the patient is motivated and will use these ideas outside the therapy session.

Flexibility to try different ideas and therapeutic techniques as well as to plan therapy sessions for times when the sessions will most benefit the patient is important. Termination in short-term therapy occurs when the mutually defined goals are reached. Often, work on the presenting problem has a positive effect on other areas of the patient's life. Termination is an opportunity to review new behaviors and plan with the patient how these behaviors can be used in the future to enhance the patient's overall health. There is understanding between the therapist and the patient that there may be other points in the patient's life, such as periods of high stress or times of developmental transitions, when the patient may need a mental health consultant to maximize health potential. The patient is welcome to return. Because the door is left open for the patient to return and because the relationship with the therapist is one of mutuality, termination often does not bring up strong feelings of loss and abandonment as it may in long-term therapy (Tables 16–3 and 16–4).

TABLE 16–2 Essential Features of Psychodynamic Short-Term Therapy

Duration	Short-term—up to 20 sessions Frequently flexible
Therapist's role	Active
Main techniques	Psychodynamic interpretation Patient education about psychodynamics "Homework" Using supports outside therapy (e.g., self-help groups, family) Mutual definition of goals Assessment and use of patient strengths Teaching importance of self-care skills
Patient's role	Willingness to work outside therapy sessions Tolerance of interpretations Mutual definition of goals

▶ Check Your Reading

8. What role did insurance companies play in the evolution of short-term therapy?
9. What beliefs does a psychoanalytical psychotherapist hold about a patient?
10. In contrast, how does a psychodynamic short-term therapist view a patient?
11. What is a utilization manager?
12. What is the focus of an inpatient hospitalization?
13. Name the four areas important for discharge planning.
14. Name several techniques that the psychodynamic short-term therapist might use.
15. From what theory base does the psychodynamic short-term therapist operate?

First Interview

The initial contact with the patient is a most important part of the journey in short-term therapy. As a nurse therapist, one's knowledge about health care from a biological, psychological, social, cultural, and spiritual domain allows one to consider the patient from a unique holistic perspective. The wholeness of that view empowers both the patient and the nurse to reach for higher levels of wellness. The nurse brings to the initial interview a high degree of respect for human potential. The nurse recognizes that each encounter with a patient is an opportunity for growth for the patient as well as for the

TABLE 16–3 Comparison of Short-Term and Long-Term Therapy

Short-Term Therapy	Long-Term Therapy
Seeks change in the presenting problem	Seeks major personality change
Sees the patient as healthy	Sees the patient as ill
Therapy reinforces strengths and teaches new behaviors	Therapy is the most important part of the person's life
Therapy is helpful during certain times of life	Therapy is ongoing over a long period
The patient works toward goals outside therapy sessions	The patient brings memories to the session to work through during sessions
The therapist is active, and presents ideas like a consultant	The therapist is a listener, reflector, questioner
The goals of therapy are mutually defined	The goal of therapy is known only to the therapist
The termination time is known	The termination time is unknown

Adapted from Budman, S., and Gurman, A. (1988). *Theory and practice of brief therapy.* New York: Guilford Press.

TABLE 16–4 Models of Long-Term and Short-Term Psychotherapy

Long-Term Therapy	Short-Term Therapy
Psychoanalysis Psychoanalytic psychotherapy Supportive psychotherapy	Psychodynamic short-term therapy Cognitive therapy Behavioral therapy Supportive therapy Alternative therapy

Adapted from Budman, S., and Gurman, A. (1988). *Theory and practice of brief therapy.* New York: Guilford Press.

nurse. As such, journeying into the therapeutic relationship is a privilege.

During the initial interview, you convey respect for the relationship and set the tone and the boundaries for how the therapy will proceed. After initially listening to the patient's presenting problem and gathering beginning information on the patient's history, explain your role and the patient's role in the therapy. Explain that you are like a mental health consultant who will help the patient understand problems and come up with ideas to alleviate them. Make it clear that you need the patient's help to do that. After the initial interview, you have enough information about the patient to begin analysis and treatment planning and can share with the patient some ideas to assess further the patient's willingness to journey with you to solve the problem. The more mundane side of the therapy needs to be discussed, such as telephone calls, length of sessions, being late for sessions, billing procedures, missed appointments, vacations, and what the patient should do if he or she cannot reach you in an urgent or emergency situation.

Last, the initial interview includes a discussion of informed consent and confidentiality. Informed consent implies that you and the patient are aware that you are entering into a therapeutic relationship. The outcome of this relationship should be a positive change in the patient's life. The patient needs to be aware that effecting such a change may require work outside as well as during the therapy session. Inform the patient that such work may be hard and emotionally painful. Explain that the patient is expected to take care of himself or herself through exercise, proper nutrition, rest, and life-fulfilling activities that enrich the soul.

Confidentiality is also discussed with the patient. Assure the patient that everything told to you stays with you unless these conditions exist:

- You think that the patient is a danger to self or others.
- You are under court order to discuss the patient's mental health records.
- The treatment is part of an overall treatment plan where the shared information would be needed for planning purposes.

Assessment

A good deal of the first interview is devoted to assessment of the patient, but more in-depth assessment may need to be gathered over the next several interviews. The assessment process is covered in Chapter 13. Highlighted here is the knowledge particularly necessary for short-term therapy.

PRESENTING PROBLEM

Listen to the presenting problem with utmost care and concern. You can elicit much information about the patient by carefully asking questions such as

- Has this problem ever occurred before?
- Does this problem feel familiar to you?
- What have you tried to do to make this better?
- What has worked for you in the past?
- Has it been more severe some times than others?

Finally, ask the patient what he or she wishes would happen to solve the problem. The answer to this question gives you an idea of how powerless the patient feels about the problem and what strengths the patient can bring toward alleviating the problem. This information gives you an idea of how the patient views a therapeutic partnership as well as how severe or chronic the patient's problem is.

PSYCHIATRIC HISTORY

In addition to data about past treatment for psychiatric illness, membership in self-help groups is important information for you to know, as is knowledge about psychiatric issues, such as any books read or courses taken in school. Such knowledge assists you in assessing the patient's understanding of his or her illness as well as capacity to seek help.

MEDICAL HISTORY

Of particular note would be any chronic conditions, such as asthma, gastrointestinal problems, headaches, and joint pains. Many visits to the physician for these problems can give you a clue as to how much the patient expresses feelings through physical ailments. Additionally, asking a female patient about her periods, whether they are normal, and how she feels premenstrually may provide vital information about her moods. If her periods have stopped, asking about her journey through menopause adds assessment data on how she feels about aging. A woman's decision about estrogen replacement helps assess not only the level of knowledge about self, but also how she approaches decision making. Did she decide not to take estrogen because her mother didn't? Did she make her decision based on consultations with her gynecology practitioner? Did she base her decision on knowledge from readings? Did she evaluate her risk based on her family history of cancer? Assessing when her last pelvic examination was done and whether she does a self-breast examination is important for the patient's overall health. All of this information, although important for a complete medical history, also provides you with clues as to the patient's attitude about self and ability to care for self. These are strengths important to short-term work.

DEVELOPMENTAL HISTORY

Educating the patient about psychological issues early in the relationship in important so that the patient has a knowledge base from which to work. As you move through the interview, there are many opportunities to educate. Explaining to the patient that often childhood transitions or milestones have an influence on how we continue to grow helps the patient begin to connect past events to the present.

Ask the patient what he or she remembers about going off to school, a sibling being brought home from the hospital, moving into grade school, and being an adolescent. As the patient answers each of these questions, you should be particularly interested in how the patient made friends, how the patient related to teachers, and what the patient did when there was a problem to solve. Who did the patient go to for support and advice? Again, this information allows you to assess the patient's strengths in making relationships, which is important in establishing mutuality in the short-term therapy process.

FAMILY HISTORY

Family history is of major importance in understanding the patient because early family life offers our first opportunities to form relationships and learn how to be behave in a civil and social manner. Additionally the family history clarifies what the patient has learned about formal religion and the concept of spirituality as well as problem solving. Helpful questions include

- What do you remember about discipline in your family?
- What happened if your parents disagreed about something?
- How did your parents show love?
- How did you know the rules in your family?

A patient's sense of belonging and connectedness is often tied to family.

Last, the family history includes any history of mental illness, substance use, or trauma. Reviewing this history provides an opportunity to educate the patient about familial tendencies of many mental health disorders. A genogram is often helpful, not only to remember the patient, but also to educate the patient about family dynamics and relevant family history (see Chapter 20). Learning about the patient's current familial environment helps you assess how much support the patient has.

TRAUMA OR ABUSE

You are responsible for as complete an assessment as possible. Often, patients do not speak of painful events because they were not asked about these events. For purposes of short-term therapy, it is necessary to assess the amount of traumatic events in a patient's life and the patient's perceptions of those events. If the patient's response indicates that trauma and abuse are issues, assess acuity level and the kind of resources outside therapy that might be helpful.

SLEEP, NUTRITION, AND EXERCISE

Asking the patient about the basic requirements of life is particularly important in assessing the level of distress the patient is experiencing. Additionally, you can further assess knowledge of self-care and attitude about wellness.

STRENGTHS AND UPLIFTS AND FRIENDSHIPS

Patient strengths are an important tool to the short-term therapist. These strengths help guide you and the patient in treatment planning and goal formulation. Using what patients bring with them to help meet their needs so that they can live a satisfactory life is key to short-term therapy (deShazer et al, 1986).

Analysis and Planning

The analysis phase of individual therapy is a challenging and fun part of the nurse therapist's work. From the history, you have a good knowledge of the patient from a biological, psychological, social, cultural, and spiritual perspective. Consider how your knowledge and skills in psychiatry and nursing can best promote wellness in the patient. Ask yourself:

- What can I offer this patient based on my knowledge of the patient and what I know about psychiatry, nursing, and my skills as a therapist?
- What strengths does the patient bring into this therapeutic journey?
- What short-term therapy techniques seem particularly helpful for this patient and would build on the patient's strengths?

Together, you and the patient plan goals for therapy. In establishing goals, you may need to help the patient think of ways that he or she will know if the goal is met. For instance, if the patient says, "I want to be rid of this anxiety," you can help the patient decide what behavior will exist when the anxiety is gone. This may include

- Being able to stay focused on and finish one report at work before starting another rather than having six uncompleted reports
- Being able to sleep at night without grinding teeth
- Being able to go through an entire day without shortness of breath.

As you and the patient work together, these goals can be evaluated as to whether they are being met. You may supplement the therapy sessions with readings on anxiety. You may teach the patient relaxation techniques or perhaps encourage the patient to take a class on stress management. Written exercises designed to help the patient observe himself or herself and the environment in which the patient becomes most anxious are helpful. As you are thinking of ways you can help the patient in the journey toward the goals, you can also decide how many therapy sessions you need to work with the patient. Included in the planning stage, too, is how frequently you think the patient needs to be seen. Because managed care pays for a certain number of sessions, it is up to you and the patient to decide on frequency. Often the initial two or three visits are weekly. Once you and the patient have devised a mental health plan with goals for the patient to work toward, the visits may become biweekly and then monthly.

The longer frequency between sessions coincides with the patient's learning what must be done outside the sessions to promote mental health. You become a consultant whose role is to provide information and support while the patient journeys toward wellness. Often an analogy about a commonly understood medical problem, such as diabetes, is helpful in guiding the patient to understanding his or her role. Explain that after a patient is diagnosed with diabetes, the patient is taught about diabetes and then taught how to monitor some aspects of life, to understand how the diabetes works in the body. Most notably, the patient may need to check blood sugar throughout the day and respond to an abnormal blood sugar level with dietary changes. The dietary changes are individualized and necessary for normal blood sugar levels. If blood sugar levels do not return to normal, medication may be indicated. The homework the patient will be doing in the therapeutic journey is analogous to monitoring blood sugar levels but instead involves monitoring mood and modifying behavior to promote the return of the patient's mental health to normal. If the patient's mental health problems are severe enough or do not respond to the patient's attempt to change, psychopharmacology may be indicated. Again the analogy with the diabetic patient can be helpful, explaining that sometimes the only way for blood sugar levels to remain within normal limits is through chemical intervention. The patient's mood disorder may be severe enough that there is a chemical imbalance that can be helped with medication to bring the imbalance within normal limits.

Psychopharmacology is often included in the analysis stage, particularly if the patient has neurovegetative symptoms (problems such as lack of appetite, sleep disturbance, constipation, and general physical slowing) and lack of interest in activities (see Chapter 30). Many states now have legislation that allows for an advanced-practice nurse or clinical nurse specialist to prescribe psychotropic medications. Prescription writing has allowed the nurse therapist to provide holistic rather than fragmented care by sending the patient to a psychiatrist. Helping the patient decide on psychopharmacology, helping with decisions on the right dosage, and helping monitor side effects, if any, all become part of the helping relationship. Often, your ability to prescribe is helpful for the patient on a short-term basis and necessary to understand the patient better. For instance, if a patient comes in complaining of sleep deprivation as a presenting problem, it is difficult to obtain an adequate history and mental status because sleep deprivation itself causes lack of focus, irritability, decreased concentration, hypervigilance, and sometimes confusion. If you can help the patient sleep with two or three nights of psychopharmacology, a much more accurate assessment can be done.

Implementation

The implementation phase of the relationship is also called the working phase of the journey and usually begins with the first interview (see Chapter 11). During the implementation phase, emphasize your role as the mental health consultant, guiding the patient to do the work. During this phase of working with the patient, transference and countertransference are important. Transference refers to the patient's responses to or feelings toward the therapist. In long-term therapy, transference behavior and feelings are important for the patient to work through childhood experiences and influences. In short-term therapy, transference is important to consider if the patient is resisting doing any work outside the therapy session. If the patient does not bring into the session the agreed-on homework, you need to consider whether this lack is due to the patient's disorganization or to the patient's feeling toward the therapist as an authority figure. You must consider the following:

- How does the patient explain not doing the homework?
- Is the patient angry about it despite having agreed with the therapist in the previous session that it was a good idea?
- Did the patient lose the homework sheet and therefore not follow through?
- Why didn't the patient call and get another sheet?
- Does the patient think he or she will not meet the nurse therapist expectations?
- Does the patient want to avoid exploring the particular topic under discussion?
- If the answer to question 6 is yes, why is the topic an uncomfortable one?

You need to explore these questions actively with the patient and try to help the patient figure out how to do the homework so that the goals can be met in the timeframe allotted. It is helpful to remember that not making progress in the journey toward goals only gives the patient negative feedback about self. Explain your concern for the patient by emphasizing the capacity to use help. The goals may need to be changed if both you and the patient agree no progress is being made.

Another aspect of the implementation phase that becomes important is **countertransference**, which refers to your responses to or feelings toward the patient. Because entering into a therapeutic relationship is a privileged journey, respect for that privilege carries with it not only a belief in the potential in human life for healthy attachment, love, and community, but also a great respect for the diversity of others and what can be learned from that diversity. To be open to that learning, however, you must have a high degree of respect for yourself. Sullivan often taught that one could respect another only if he respected himself (Sullivan, 1954). You must be on a journey of your own so that you have an awareness of the areas in your life that influence your behavior (see Chapter 8). When those areas intersect with a patient's experience, you must be able to respond in a way that is helpful to the patient's therapeutic journey. Human potential implies movement forward. You should be open to learning from your patient but in a way that is silent and reflective. Much of this awareness and learning can be accomplished through supervision with another mental health clinician. You may notice that at times during your sessions with patients you day dream or feel indifferent, bored, irritable, or sad toward the patient. These behaviors and feelings are often signals of countertransference and need to be discussed with another clinician so that they do not get in the way of patient care. Additionally, in your efforts to help, you need to be aware that the relationship is one-sided in that the patient has come for help. You need to be clear about the boundaries involved in providing that care (Gutheil and Gabbard, 1993). The following quote speaks to the nurse's need to know the self:

> Then the wise or temperate man, and he only, will know himself, and be able to examine what he knows or does not know, and to see what others know and think that they know and do really know; and what they do not know and fancy that they know, when they do not (The Charmides in the Dialogues of Plato, 375 B.C.).

▶ Check Your Reading

16. What is the focus during a first interview?
17. What areas should assessment cover?
18. Why are written exercises useful during analysis and planning?
19. Explain the importance of transference and countertransference during therapy.

Cognitive Psychotherapy

Cognitive psychotherapy is descended from the work done by Beck (1976) and colleagues at the University of Pennsylvania. Beck postulated that the patient's way of perceiving events in life prevents the patient from reaching goals. Thus, in cognitive psychotherapy, the patient's subjective experience is explored. This exploration includes studying the patient's current thoughts and feelings about events and investigating how these thoughts and feelings contribute to and perpetuate the patient's difficulties and mood. Thoughts that flow from the patient in a negative manner are called distorted thinking or **cognitive distortions**. For example, a man, recently separated from his wife, might want to see a movie and can find no one to go with him, so he decides to go alone. He may interpret his not finding a companion to accompany him as proof of his being unacceptable to others, and as a result he might feel sad and depressed (cognitive distortion), or he may think that the next time he will plan further ahead and feel proud of himself for going to the movie anyway.

Cognitive psychotherapy is based on the belief that people express their illness through thoughts and attitudes (Burns, 1985). For instance, patients who are depressed interpret events around them as negative, dangerous, and burdensome. They interpret their relationship to these events as hopeless, undesirable, and worthless. Looking ahead into the future only brings more of the unpleasant present. These cognitive distortions become the patient's way of interpreting the world and thus become the first thoughts that come to mind as the patient perceives events of the day. Thus, these thoughts are automatic and continual. There are several components of distorted thinking:

- *Arbitrary inference* is the drawing of a conclusion about an event without any evidence. For example, a patient sees his therapist in the grocery store, but the therapist has not seen the patient. The patient believes that the therapist finds him too unlikable to acknowledge him.

- *Selective abstraction* is the drawing of a conclusion on the basis of one fact rather than considering all facts. For example, a therapist is able only to get through to a patient's answering machine to cancel an appointment because a snowstorm has already accumulated five inches, the highways are dangerous, and many phone lines are down. The patient considers the therapist uncaring because he did not call the patient's car phone.

- *Overgeneralization* is the drawing of a conclusion about oneself on the basis of a single fact or event. For example, after five years of successfully teaching special education to inner-city high school students, a current student who is continually truant does not pass. The parents sue the teacher. The teacher tells her therapist that she is a failure as a teacher.

- *Magnification and minimization* is the drawing of a conclusion through exaggeration or underestimation. Looking at the mess in her house, the patient thought she couldn't clean it in less than a week and began to panic. In reality, she and a friend took four hours to bring it to order.

- *Inexact labeling* is the drawing of a conclusion on the basis of emotional response rather than facts. The patient's teenage child came home, slamming the door and going to his room saying "Don't speak to me." The patient tells her therapist how much her son hates her.

The goal of cognitive psychotherapy is to train patients to recognize their automatic thoughts and cognitive distortions. During the initial interview, the therapist assesses for cognitive distortions in the patient's responses. The therapist then explains the theory of cognitive distortions and educates the patient about how problems are perpetuated by these distortions. This is further explored by having the patient review his or her thoughts each day. Or the patient might be asked to write thoughts about a specific ongoing negative situation, such as the patient's relationship with his or her boss. The patient is asked to keep a journal, or log, of this work, which is then brought to therapy and explored. Figure 16–1 shows a blank cognitive distortions log, and Figure 16–2 shows a completed one. The therapist helps the patient identify the distorted thinking and explore whether there might be other objective and logical ways to think about his or her response to the event.

After several instances of distorted thinking have been explored, a theme, or **automatic thinking schema**, may begin to emerge. These schema are different from cognitive distortions in that they are usually well hidden from the patient's consciousness. They are basic attitudes about self, such as being stupid or unworthy, that have been learned in childhood and have been fueled and supported by the cognitive distortions. These schema can also be explored in helping the patient formulate more healthy perceptions and thoughts.

To benefit from cognitive psychotherapy, the patient must be willing to do the homework (for example, the journal) and be able to tolerate exploring his or her thoughts. The patient must also be from a social, family, and community environment that supports change. Cognitive psychotherapy is usually short-term, anywhere from 8 to 20 sessions. It is goal oriented in that the patient and the therapist have agreed that they will work toward alleviating specific problems. The patient may begin treatment with several sessions a week but rapidly distribute the sessions weekly and biweekly as the patient becomes familiar with recognizing his or her cognitive distortions and able to think about upsetting events differently. Insurance companies generally pay for cognitive psychotherapy because a well-defined goal can be accomplished within the sessions authorized by the insurance company. (Table 16–5 summarizes the essential features of cognitive psychotherapy. Case Example 16–1 shows how cognitive psychotherapy helped one patient, Janet.)

NEGATIVE SITUATION	AUTOMATIC THOUGHTS AND ASSOCIATED FEELINGS OR EMOTIONS	REVISED THOUGHTS

FIGURE 16–1
A cognitive distortions log used for keeping a journal of thoughts about a negative situation.

NEGATIVE SITUATION	AUTOMATIC THOUGHTS AND ASSOCIATED FEELINGS OR EMOTIONS	REVISED THOUGHTS
My 3-year-old daughter was crying because I would not let her watch TV after one hour. She banged her fists on the floor and said she hated me! She said her Dad would let her watch as much as she wanted.	I'm a bad mother. He's better than I am. She will love him and not me.	All the early childhood experts, including my nurse practitioner, say that watching more than an hour of TV per day is harmful to intelligence. It is much better that I help my daughter set up play with her toys. Perhaps she can have a friend over this afternoon. I think I will set some TV rules with her so that this will not happen again.

FIGURE 16–2
A completed cognitive distortions log.

TABLE 16–5 **Essential Features of Cognitive Psychotherapy**

Duration	Short-term—up to 20 sessions Frequency flexible, usually weekly
Therapist's role	Active
Main techniques	Training patients to recognize automatic thoughts Exploration of the patient's current thoughts (cognitive distortions) Educating patients about cognitive distortions Assigning homework Exploring alternative ways to think Exploring attitudes beneath cognitive distortions
Patient's role	Learning about cognitive distortions Tolerance of exploration of thought contents Doing homework

Case Example 16–1 Janet's Story

Boy was I a wreck when I went into that therapy session today! I sure dumped a lot of stuff on that nurse. As I was telling her my history, I realized how I haven't really dealt with my father's never being around and my always disappointing him. And my mother! Always traveling to one fancy place or another and always worried that everything looked OK—including me. Oh, I tried so hard to be good enough for Dad and it just never seemed to work. I went to an Ivy League school for pete's sake. I'll never forget his joking at that Christmas party about the finishing college I was going to, and then with a chuckle saying that the college was going to have to work hard. I went to therapy back then because I was so unhappy I tried to kill myself. I thought I had learned a lot about my family and how come I felt so unsuccessful and so unloved. I could never find a boyfriend who seemed just right and respected me for who I was. But then again, who I was was pretty bad.

For a few years after therapy and college I did some art and developed a nice portfolio. Even entered some shows and did OK. That's where I met my husband—one of those outdoor craft fairs—he was admiring my art work. I really studied him hard. Was this a man who would stay with me, be honest with me, and share with me? I thought so and we married. Now it's five years later and I know he's having an affair. I feel like I'm going crazy. How could I have been so wrong? How can I be such a failure? And now nothing is going right . . . he's so mean and says that I am not the woman he married, that I'm no fun and that all I care for is our daughter. I'm not even doing that right. I made her come in for supper the other night and both of them said I was wrong to do that, that we should eat when we want instead of as a family. He says I am too rigid about the TV. The painter disappeared, too, and he took our ladder. I know it's my fault because I only got a reference from one person. The one woman in the neighborhood I felt close to is moving away—she probably didn't like me much anyway because she always seems to be with her sister now.

The nurse said that it certainly seemed like there were a lot of negative happenings in my life and asked me how they were all my fault. Boy, did I tell her how I screwed up! She said she would like to learn more about that and began telling me about how automatic thoughts sometimes get in the way of being able to evaluate situations appropriately. She said that sometimes these negative thoughts come so easily because they are based on deeply and long-held thoughts about ourselves. She asked me what my first thought was in the morning and I told her that it was wondering what would go wrong today. She asked what it would be like if I woke up pondering what I would handle well today? While it seemed like a relief to think that, I quickly knew better.

She then said it would be worthwhile to explore these negative thoughts and gave me some interesting homework. I am supposed to keep a chart and describe a situation, my automatic thoughts about it, and then rewrite the situation in a way that comes out better for me. If I was having trouble with rewriting, she suggested I call some friends and get their ideas. She said there are usually different ways to respond to situations and the charting would help me see that. She said with practice, the goal of all this charting is to interrupt automatic negative responses and replace them with responses that are more positive. We did a sample one during the session.

▶ Check Your Reading

20. Describe two techniques often used in cognitive therapy.
21. What are cognitive distortions?
22. Describe two components of cognitive distortions.
23. What is an automatic thinking schema?

Behavior Therapy

Behavior therapy involves identifying events in the patient's environment that have caused the patient to behave in a maladaptive way (for instance, becoming nauseous from anxiety) and either changing the environment or changing the patient's response to the environment so that the patient's behavior changes. There is little, if any, focus on psychodynamics. Behavior theory evolved in the 1940s as a new way to understand human behavior. Behavior theorists believed that human behavior was a learned phenomenon, so that if behavior was maladaptive, it could be unlearned through therapy. (See Chapter 18 for complete discussion of behavior therapy.)

The behavior therapist works with the patient to choose the behavior that needs changing. Because behavior therapy addresses one behavior at a time, it is often short-term. Additionally, many of the techniques that the behavior therapist uses the patient can use outside the therapy session.

Supportive Psychotherapy

Supportive psychotherapy evolved because other psychotherapies were not helpful to some patients. **Supportive psychotherapy** involves the therapist becoming a sort of role model or parent figure for the patient in a supportive and understanding manner. As such, the therapist helps the patient maintain the best level of functioning. Often, patients with long histories of mental health problems benefit from supportive psychotherapy. In general, patients who are particularly suited for supportive psychotherapy have poor interpersonal skills and consequently are somewhat isolated. Often, this isolation leads to poor reality-testing ability and thus poor problem-solving ability. Frequently the patient also has poor affect regulation so that he or she experiences either inappropriate emotional responses to events or little response when one is warranted. Additionally the patient may have poor impulse control. To help the patient, the therapist must be well trained in psychodynamic theory and know the patient's history. The therapist uses that knowledge to help the patient understand current problems and handle those problems rather than waiting for the patient to gain insight or to complete homework assignments (Werman, 1984).

The therapist doing supportive psychotherapy is an active part of the relationship and may use many therapeutic techniques to be helpful to the patient. Of primary importance is that you establish a good working relationship with the patient by demonstrating concern and involvement. Strive to support the patient's strengths while providing guidance to build on those strengths. You need to be available to the patient outside the scheduled hour for phone consultations and for referrals to other helpful resources. You must be able to help the patient express intense feelings in a contained manner. This effort supports the patient's expression of feelings rather than acting out feelings through aggression. Your careful reflection about what the patient is saying helps the patient feel understood. You may use some cognitive psychotherapy to help the patient see certain situations differently, or you may use some behavior therapy techniques to help the patient deal more effectively with a certain situation. Helping the patient problem solve and explore options slowly to improve the patient's predicament may be learned by the patient and become part of how the patient operates outside the therapy room.

To benefit from supportive psychotherapy, the patient needs to have had other successful relationships in life. The length of supportive psychotherapy is almost completely determined by the patient's situation. Relatively healthy patients who have experienced extremely stressful events in their lives may need only a few sessions for stabilization. They may find that talking through the confusion engendered by the event is sufficient to restore their coping abilities. Other patients with more chronic life situations and mental health problems may need more frequent therapy sessions and for longer periods of time. In general, to convince insurance companies to cover extended mental health visits, the therapist may have to show that the supportive psychotherapy is diverting the patient from more costly services, such as hospitalization. (Table 16–6 summarizes the essential features of supportive psychotherapy. Case Example 16–2 shows how supportive psychotherapy helped Bob.)

Case Example 16–2 Bob's Story

The physician who had been seeing me for the last two years left today and instead I now have a nurse. I wondered what the physician had told her about me. Did she tell her about all the children I have populated the world with and how guilty I feel about not taking care of these kids? I guess it doesn't matter anyway since this is something he wouldn't let me talk about—always waving his hand as if my concerns about this were a pesky fly. I wonder why I'm not doing so well in art school? I used to love art and now I'm always in trouble with my teacher. Pretty soon I'm going to explode about it. I probably should get some coffee before I meet my new therapist. Ha! If she says something I don't like, I'll just spill it in her office.

Well, I met this nurse and you would not believe what happened. She listened to what I had to say and then repeated it back to me. She said I could talk about my kids, especially if my feelings about them were causing me to act in certain ways I didn't like. Then she said that most people have things that they carry in their hearts that make them feel sad, and that it's OK—that you have to accept those things, not try to deny them, and move on. She said she would like to help me do that! Then she asked if I had any ideas how she could help me. I was so surprised that I said no. She asked me to think about this and bring a list in next time of what would be helpful to me. The other thing that happened was she asked about drinking coffee and when I told her that I was drinking 10 to 12 cups from noon to midnight, she seemed very concerned and started telling me about the effects of caffeine on mood. I'll have to ask about it again, but I wonder if it may have anything to do with my trouble at school? Finally she wondered why I had missed appointments with the doctor. I had to admit to being disorganized and all. She asked what would be the best time for me and now I can go at that time—every other week. I think I can remember that.

TABLE 16–6 Essential Features of Supportive Psychotherapy

Duration	Long-term or short-term Frequency flexible
Therapist's role	Active Concerned Involved
Main techniques	Use of many therapeutic techniques Establishment of a good working relationship Supporting and building on patient strengths Availability Teaching problem solving Being a role model
Patient's role	Mutually define goals Work on goals outside session Openness to therapist's feedback

Let's look now at how a short-term therapy model might be applied to Peggy's case.

Peggy's health insurance company was bought by a managed care company. They informed her that her mental health benefit was now 20 visits a year with a co-pay. The co-pay for the first six visits or so was $2.00, but then it got higher the more visits she used. She was lucky that her nurse could refer her to a colleague whom the insurance company had listed as a provider. After a year in psychoanalytic therapy, Peggy felt like she could understand a lot of how her childhood influenced the way that she was now. She knew, for instance, that in new situations in which she did not know what to expect, she was often silent and her posture almost shrinking. She knew this was related to trying to stay out of her father's way for she never knew what mood he would be in. She understood that her doing this got in the way of completing her school projects, particularly if the teacher was a man. She also knew that she ate to try to fill herself up with good things—almost as if she were trying to fill up with love that she didn't have as a child. She knew that she had trouble expressing emotions because she was never allowed to as a child, and often she did not recognize what emotions she was feeling. It was exhausting work remembering all those things and then trying to figure out how they affected her now. She still had not talked about her father kissing her, though. And she still had days where she had trouble getting out of bed and felt mean toward her roommates. She still hated her family!

When Peggy left her first session with the new nurse therapist, she was amazed at how different the new nurse was. The new nurse said that therapy would involve a lot of planning between them and she asked Peggy to prioritize her problems. Peggy decided that not being able to get out of bed several times a month was highest on the list. Then she said that she wanted to work on her relationship with men because there was one guy at her part-time job that she thought she might like. She also said that she would like to feel more friendly toward her family. With these problems outlined, she and the nurse established goals to work toward. Together they decided that staying in bed one weekend day per month when Peggy chose to would be a goal. To reach that goal, there were several things that Peggy needed to do. First, she needed to establish consistent bedtime rituals and not have any caffeine after 12 noon. Then she needed to start getting some exercise every other day. The nurse gave her some articles on exercise, caffeine, and sleep. The nurse also told her how sleep deprivation affects mental health. The nurse said that if these ideas did not help, she might be able temporarily to prescribe some medication to help with sleep. All of that happened in the first session! The nurse invited her to call if anything should come up and said that they would work on making goals for her other high-priority problems in future sessions. She suggested they meet every other week so that Peggy had time to work on her goals before the next session.

As Peggy continued to define her goals and find ways with the nurse's help to meet them, she became more confident in herself and more able to see how she could have control over many things in her life. With her new boyfriend, for instance, her goal was to move slowly in the relationship and not have any alcohol. With the nurse, she was able to role play telling her boyfriend about herself without alcohol to calm her anxiety. When the time came, although she was nervous, she did it! She found herself hanging out less and less with her old buddies who drank. She discovered that what she really wanted to do was help disadvantaged kids like herself who don't have love while growing up. She switched her major at school to emphasize child health. As a part-time job, she worked in a home for emotionally disturbed children. There was a period of time during her therapy when her family became especially difficult, calling on her to come home and to help them with cleaning and driving places. Her goal with the family was to invite them over for her Christmas party, then three months away. No way she was having them over! Peggy got an answering machine, and told her family that their calling all the time was getting in the way of her studying. She asked them not to call. Peggy and the nurse devised a way that she could keep in touch with them but also set limits on what she could do for them. What Peggy did was write a note to them weekly letting them know what she was doing and that she was fine. As she studied her family genogram with the nurse, she learned more about how hard their lives were and that the choices they made they needed to be responsible for. She also made a list of awful childhood memories, including the one of her father kissing her, and buried them in the park. When the nurse first suggested this, Peggy thought it was pretty strange, but as she was preparing to do this ritual, the nurse was helping her recognize some positive aspects of herself that she had because of her family. Believe it or not, Peggy realized that her work ethic was from her Dad. He went to work every day no matter what and she thought her willingness to struggle with school work and part-time work and difficult finances must be influenced by him. She realized from her mother's situation that she early in life had decided to educate herself so that she could support herself. As she recognized these positive aspects, she began to feel a lot softer about her family. Also, they didn't call her now unless something really needed to be communicated. She found that she soon dropped the note writing and called them once a week. They came to the Christmas party. Peggy planned it so that they came from 5 o'clock to 7 o'clock. That way her apartment wasn't so crowded, and her mother would not have time to drink too much. They were fine!

Peggy was now only meeting with the nurse once a month. They had a total of 12 sessions (plus a few phone calls). The nurse felt that Peggy had good solutions to her problems if she would give herself time to problem solve and continue to take care of herself. At the last session, the nurse suggested that perhaps a break in therapy would be appropriate—that Peggy needed to take her new life skills and practice them so they became a part of her. At the last session, the nurse and Peggy summarized everything that Peggy had learned and then made a list of the important things for Peggy to remember when taking care of herself. The nurse suggested she tape that list where she could see it daily. Finally, the nurse said that Peggy might find there are other times in her life that she may need to return for therapy and that was just fine.

▶ Check Your Reading

24. What role(s) does the therapist have in supportive psychotherapy?
25. What techniques does the therapist use in supportive psychotherapy?
26. What kind of patient benefits from supportive psychotherapy?

CONCLUSIONS

As the psychiatric nurse journeys with the patient toward optimum mental health, the nurse demonstrates respect for human potential that includes all spheres—biological, psychological, social, cultural, and spiritual. The nurse strives to understand how each of the spheres affects the patient's life and uses the patient's strengths in each sphere in planning treatment. The nurse joins with the patient and offers knowledge in psychiatry and nursing as well as skills in listening, supporting, and understanding, as she journeys with the patient. The nurse conveys to the patient that the patient is the most important part of the treatment, particularly in the implementation phase. As the patient's mental health consultant, the journey toward health is guided by the nurse, and the work is done by the patient.

Aristotle said, "*A thing may be accompanied by another in three ways, either simultaneously, subsequently, or potentially. Life accompanies health simultaneously (but not health life).*" *(Book One, The Rhetoric of Aristotle, 334 B.C.).* Psychiatric nursing is for helping patients return to optimal mental health. In the ongoing effort to reduce health care costs, psychiatric nurses need to insist on appropriate mental health care. Insurance companies and health care planning groups are asking for outcome data to support the importance of individual psychotherapy. They are asking how we know the problem (depression, for instance) won't go away on its own with some time? How do we know that psychotherapy is really helpful? Studies, mostly done by physician groups, have been unable to show one type of psychotherapy is better than another for relieving symptoms (Crits-Christoph, 1992). A few studies of cognitive therapy have shown cognitive therapy to be more effective than no psychotherapy in treating both depressed volunteers and psychiatric patients with diagnosis of depression (Stoudemire, 1994, p. 490). There is also a growing body of research showing that supportive psychotherapy is helpful in treating various psychiatric illnesses as well as mental health problems that may arise because of medical illness (Stoudemire, 1994). The general agreement is that, with major mental illness, treatment that combines psychotherapy and pharmacology is more effective than either one alone. Nurse therapists need to devise outcome studies for various psychotherapies practiced by nurses and define that practice as unique to nursing. With such studies, nurses could advocate for patients with data showing that mental health care is an important aspect of patient's overall health.

KEY POINTS TO REMEMBER

- Psychotherapy is frequently referred to as the "talking cure."
- Psychoanalytic psychotherapy grew out of the work of Freud.
- Freud developed the technique of psychoanalysis, which involves memory recall of unconscious childhood memories.
- Transference occurs when the patient reacts to the therapist as if the therapist were the significant other in the patient's early conflicts.
- Long-term therapy flows from the psychoanalytic model developed by Freud.
- Insurance companies seldom reimburse for long-term therapy that is open-ended in its projected length of time.
- The development of short-term psychotherapy was driven by economics as much as by clinical issues.
- Psychodynamic short-term therapy places responsibility for cure on the patient. It uses techniques such as homework assignments, role playing, recognizing and promoting patient strengths, and placing expectations on the patient regarding taking care of self through proper exercise, nutrition, and soul-giving activity.
- During the first interview of short-term therapy, the nurse therapist conveys respect for the nurse-patient relationship and sets the tone and the boundaries for how the therapy will proceed. The nurse also discusses confidentiality and informed consent.
- Assessment begins in the first interview and may continue into subsequent therapy sessions. The nurse therapist gathers information regarding the presenting problem; the patient's psychiatric, medical, developmental, family, and abuse or trauma history; the patient's sleep, nutrition, and exercise habits; and the patient's strengths, uplifts, and friendships.
- During the analysis phase of therapy, the nurse considers what skills can best assist the patient. Together the nurse and patient establish goals for the relationship and frequency of the visits. The nurse also analyzes whether or not the patient needs psychopharmacology.
- The implementation phase of therapy begins during the first interview and involves working through transference as well as countertransference. The nurse and patient actively work to achieve goals previously established.
- Cognitive psychotherapy focuses on correcting the cognitive distortions that influence the patient's behavior and feelings.
- Cognitive psychotherapy works to identify automatic thinking schema and change them.
- Behavior therapy views all behavior as learned, so that if the behavior is maladaptive, new behaviors can be learned.
- Supportive psychotherapy involves the therapist becoming a sort of role model or parent figure for the patient. This type of therapy works well with patients with long histories of mental health problems, who have poor interpersonal skills, and who have poor affect regulation.
- The therapist doing supportive psychotherapy draws on skills from other types of therapy, including cognitive and behavioral therapy.
- There is a need for studies that evaluate the effectiveness of therapy.

LEARNING ACTIVITIES

1. Do you know what mental health benefits your insurance covers? If you do not know, review your health care benefits.

2. Interview a nurse psychotherapist to discover the types of patients that are coming for psychotherapy. What are the nurse's greatest challenges as a therapist? What are the nurse's greatest frustrations as a therapist?

3. In your clinical experience, use several of the techniques identified as part of short-term therapy. Homework assignments or role playing can be effectively used with patients. After you have used these techniques, evaluate their effectiveness.

4. There are many movies that depict the therapy process. Try to watch one of them and identify the techniques. Some suggestions include "Coming Out of the Darkness," a made-for-television movie with Diana Ross depicting a patient diagnosed with paranoid schizophrenia. Another is "Dream Team," a movie that focuses on the adventures of a group of

patients who leave the hospital for a community outing and become separated from their psychiatrist. "Ordinary People" tells the struggle of a family that has lost a son through suicide and how each family member copes with this loss.

CRITICAL THINKING EXERCISE

Nurse Sweeney recently attended a course on cognitive psychotherapy. She plans to incorporate the concepts into her practice as a nurse psychotherapist. To formulate her nursing interventions using Beck's concepts, she presented the following patient to the course instructor. Mrs. Kennal, a 60-year-old school teacher, recently had surgery for breast cancer. She was unable to return to teaching because she did not want to touch anyone or anything. She believed that she would contaminate others and give them cancer. Because of a fear of being alone and helpless, Mrs. Kennal refused to drive to her doctor's appointments.

1. What assumptions can Nurse Sweeney make about Mrs. Kennal's behaviors?

2. What evidence supports these assumptions?

3. What cognitive distortions might Mrs. Kennal be making about her physical health?

Nurse Sweeney determined that Mrs. Kennal had used distorted thinking when she believed the cancer had contaminated her and in turn she would contaminate others. She also used it in her belief that the stress of teaching and controlling children in the classroom caused her to get cancer.

1. How would Nurse Sweeney test her conclusions?

2. Suggest other alternatives to those stated.

REFERENCES

Adler, E. (1982). Supportive psychotherapy revisited. *Clinical Psychiatry, 4;* 3–13.

Alexander, F., and Selesnick, S. (1968). *The history of psychiatry.* New York: New American Library.

Aristotle (1954). *The rhetoric and poetics of Aristotle.* New York: Random House, Modern Library Series.

Barth, K., et al. (1988). Comprehensive assessment of change in patients treated with short-term dynamic psychotherapy: An overview. *Psychotherapy Psychosomatics, 50,* 141–150.

Beck, A. (1976). *Cognitive theory and emotional disorders.* New York: International University Press.

Bennett, M. (1984). Brief psychotherapy in adult development. *Psychotherapy: Theory, Research and Practice, 21,* 171–177.

Brigham, A. (1994). The moral treatment of insanity (July, 1847). *American Journal of Psychiatry, 151*(6), 11–16.

Brodady, J. (1983). Techniques in brief psychotherapy. *Australia New Zealand Journal of Psychiatry, 17,* 109–115.

Buckley, P. (1986). Supportive psychotherapy, a neglected treatment. *Psychiatric Annals, 16,* 515–521.

Budman, S., and Gurman, A. (1988). *Theory and practice of brief therapy.* New York: Guilford Press.

Burns, D. (1980). *Feeling good: The new mood therapy.* New York: Plume.

Burns, D. (1985). *The feeling good handbook.* New York: Plume.

Colby, K. (1951). *A primer for psychotherapists.* New York: Ronald Press.

Crits-Christoph, P. (1991). *Handbook of short-term dynamic therapies.* New York: Basic Books.

Crits-Christoph, P. (1992). The efficacy of brief dynamic psychotherapy: A meta-analysis. *American Journal of Psychiatry, 149*(2), 151–158.

Davanloo, H. (1980). *Short-term psychotherapy.* New York: Jason Aronson.

deShazer, et al (1986). Brief therapy: Focused solution development. *Family Process, 25,* 207–221.

Dimascio, A. et al (1979). Differential symptom reduction by drugs and psychotherapy in acute depression. *Archives of General Psychiatry, 36,* 1450–1456.

Gutheil, T., and Gubbard, G. (1993). The concept of boundaries in clinical practice: Theoretical and risk management dimensions. *American Journal of Psychiatry, 150*(2), 188–196.

Harden, S., and Durham, J. (1985). First rate: Exploring the structure, process, and effectiveness of nurse psychotherapy. *Journal of Psychosocial Nursing and Mental Health Services, 23,* 19–15.

Heber, S., et al (1984). The nurse as short-term psychotherapist. *Canadian Nurse, 80*(6), 32–35.

Hollander, M. (1965). *The practice of psychoanalytic psychotherapy.* New York: Grune & Stratton.

Leibenluft, E., and Goldberg, R. Guidelines for short-term inpatient psychotherapies. *American Journal of Psychiatry, 143*(12), 1507–1517.

Luborsky, L., and Crits-Christoph, P. (1990). *Understanding transference: The Core Conflictual Relationship Theme Method.* New York: Basic Books.

Malan, D. (1976). *The frontier of brief psychotherapy.* New York: Plenum.

Malan, D. (1979). *Individual psychotherapy and the science of psychodynamics.* Oxford: Butterworth-Heinemann.

Mann, J. (1973). *Time-limited psychotherapy.* Cambridge: Harvard University Press.

Mason, W. (1994). Solution-focused therapy and inpatient psychiatric nursing. *Journal of Psychosocial Nursing, 32*(10), 46–49.

McGihon, N. (1994). Health care reform: Clinical implications for inpatient psychiatric nursing. *Journal of Psychosocial Nursing, 32*(11), 31–33.

Moore, T. (1992). *Care of the soul.* New York: Harper Collins Publishers.

Plato (1952). *The dialogues of Plato.* Chicago: William Benton.

Sifneos, P. (1972). *Short-term psychotherapy and emotional crises.* Cambridge: Harvard University Press.

Sifneos, P. (1987). *Short-term dynamic psychotherapy: Evaluation and technique (2nd ed.). New York: Plenum.*

Stouchmere, A. (Ed.) (1994). *Clinical psychiatry for medical student.* In R. Ursano, et al. (Ed.), *The psychotherapies: Basic theoretical principles and techniques* (2nd ed.). Philadelphia: J. B. Lippincott.

Strachey, J. (Ed.) (1958). *Standard edition of the complete psychological works of Sigmund Freud.* Vol. 12. London: Hogarth Press.

Sullivan, H. (1954). *The psychiatric interview.* New York: W. W. Norton.

Talbott, J., et al (1988). *Textbook of psychiatry.* Washington, D.C.: American Psychiatric Association Press.

Talbott, J. (1994). Tighter controls urged in federal payments for psychiatric patients. *Hospital Community Psychiatry, 45* (1), 86–87.

Ursano, R., and Hales, R. (1986). A review of brief individual psychotherapies. *American Journal of Psychiatry, 143* (12), 1507–1517.

Ursano, R., et al (1991). *Concise guide to psychodynamic psychotherapy,* Washington, D.C.: American Psychiatric Association Press.

Werman, P. (1984). *The practice of supportive psychotherapy.* New York: Brunner-Mazel.

Wolberg, L. (1988). *The technique of psychotherapy,* Vols. 1 and 2. New York: Grune & Stratton.

Wolpe, J. (1973). *The practice of behavior therapy,* (2nd ed.) (p. 17). New York: Pergamon Press.

SUGGESTED READINGS

Crits-Christoph, P. (1992). The efficacy of brief dynamic psychotherapy: A meta-analysis. *American Journal of Psychiatry, 149*(2), 151–158.

Harden, S., and Durham, J. (1985). First rate: Exploring the structure, process, and effectiveness of nurse psychotherapy. *Journal of Psychosocial Nursing and Mental Health Services, 23*, 19–15.

Heber, S., et al (1984). The nurse as short-term psychotherapist. *Canadian Nurse, 80*(6), 32–35.

Mason, W. (1994). Solution-focused therapy and inpatient psychiatric nursing. *Journal of Psychosocial Nursing, 32*(10), 46–49.

CHAPTER 17

GROUP PSYCHOTHERAPY

A human being is part of the whole, called by us "Universe"—a part limited in time and space. He experiences himself, his thoughts and feelings as something separated from the rest—a kind of optical delusion of consciousness.

—Einstein

LEARNING OBJECTIVES

After studying this chapter, you should be able to:

1. Identify the historical context for the development of group psychotherapy.
2. Describe the structural elements of group psychotherapy.
3. Specify the stages of group development and relevant tasks related to each stage.
4. Analyze the conceptual components of group psychotherapy.
5. Characterize group leader tasks and functions.
6. Apply therapeutic strategies with group members having special problems.
7. Describe appropriate therapeutic group formats for special populations.
8. Identify legal and ethical issues related to professional leadership in conducting therapeutic groups.

KEY TERMINOLOGY

Adjourning phase
Altruism
Catharsis
Cohesion
Coleadership
Curative factors
Forming phase
Functional similarity
Group as a whole
Group contract
Group dynamics
Group think
Interpersonal learning
Maintenance role functions
Norming phase
Norms
Performing phase
Psychodrama
Psychoeducational groups
Reminiscence groups
Resocialization groups
Scapegoating
Self-roles
Storming phase
Task role functions
Therapeutic community
Universality

Psychological health is inextricably interwoven with community. Simple but enduring statements such as "No man is an island" and "Man cannot live by bread alone" metaphorically convey the idea that human beings basically need others as companions in successfully negotiating a safe, successful passage through life. Rarely can individual people perform all major life tasks entirely on their own. Moreover, one's life journey can be more complex and less clearly understood than it needs to be when the traveler takes to the road unaccompanied. Without the counsel of others, without regularly receiving strength and emotional nourishment from fellow travelers, the journey can be barren and devoid of meaning. In the absence of meaningful relationships with others, much emotional and spiritual suffering takes place. Such suffering is not at all necessary. Personal wholeness and psychological well-being depend on having dynamic interactions with other people who affirm, challenge, and validate an individual's sense of self and reality.

Psychotherapy groups build on a natural learning-based format associated with informal groups. Human beings experience similar milestones on their personal journeys. These include birth, death, and physical and emotional growth. These events occur with regularity, regardless of socio-economic status, race, creed, or color. All people share parallel human experiences of joy, pain, laughter, and tears. Much can be learned about the many possible choices for reaching personally meaningful solutions and ways to handle difficult situations from others who have successfully "met the challenge." In all walks of life, the paths people choose to travel are influenced by those they meet along the way and by their interactions. Even a brief encounter can be important. Many of these rich human-to-human interactions occur in small-group formats.

Group psychotherapy uses basic principles of communication and relationship within a formal therapeutic context. In a therapy group, people can experience a deeper level of communication than is possible in informal groups, a level that helps people change maladaptive patterns of socially relating to each other. Clinicians also use group therapy as a powerful tool to correct personal behaviors that get in the way of meeting life's challenges. Therapy supports individual travelers in sorting out the most appropriate ways to meet their personal goals.

Group psychotherapy enhances a person's ability to function as a contributing member of the community. The experience of being in a group does not deny the uniqueness of each person. The group's organizing principles bring people in touch with their collective humanity and responsibility. Having a role to play in helping others achieve their personal goals and experiencing the give and take of community interaction enables people to recognize themselves as a part of the whole. In a group, members experience themselves playing a role in writing the full story of their own lives and in contributing to the narrative of the community. Although group psychotherapy does not guarantee mental health, it can be a powerful contributing factor when human circumstances threaten the natural and satisfying progression of the journey.

Group psychotherapy is a *process*, not an event. The essence of the encounter in each person's experience is an intensely personal process. Its benefits are measured and explained in different unique ways. Galway Kinnel's (1980) poem "Saint Francis and the Sow" captures the essence of effective group psychotherapy as reframing each participant's experience of self into a composite human likeness of beauty and worth. This is the goal of all successful group approaches. Group psychotherapy is designed to touch the soul of the traveler as well as to offer practical problem-solving help in negotiating the journey.

When most people first engage in group psychotherapy, regardless of their stated reasons or problems, they enter convinced of their unloveliness. Like the sow mired in mud, these individuals have forgotten or have never been told they are creatures of beauty or worthy of attention. And so they deplore who they are or what has happened to them, without fully realizing that they have untouched beauty and can rewrite the story of their journey in a different way.

In a manner similar to the gentle minstering of Saint Francis, group members use the human touch of words and caring actions to affirm each other's humanness. They tell each other that their despised or disowned qualities are capable of transformation into wholeness, as in "the long, perfect loveliness of sow." Within the group, members help each other understand what it means to be fully human. They learn to reclaim a more vibrant sense of self. The group invites its members to integrate the parts of self that are shameful and despised with the inner lovable parts hidden in the shadow, unseen and unheard. The group may further suggest that because of, and not in spite of, the shadow side, human beings, like the sow, can begin to appreciate their own innate, unique loveliness. As members learn to recognize these characteristics as an essential part of their wholeness, they begin to experience their humanness as composed of beauty and value. The experience of being accepted and affirmed by their peers as a person of worth and the sheer number of affirmations delivered simultaneously by group members is extremely powerful and very difficult to turn aside as being irrelevant.

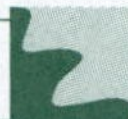

SAINT FRANCIS'S STORY

The bud
stands for all things,
even for those things that don't flower,
for everything flowers, from within, of self-blessing;
though sometimes it is necessary
to reteach a thing its loveliness,
to put a hand on its brow
of the flower
and retell it in words and in touch
it is lovely
until it flowers again, from within, of self-blessing;
as Saint Francis
put his hand on the creased forehead
of the sow, and told her in words and in touch
blessings of earth on the sow, and the sow
began remembering all down her thick length,
from the earthen snout all the way
through the fodder and slops to the spiritual curl
of the tail,
from the hard spininess spiked out from the spine
down through the great broken heart
to the blue milken dreaminess spurting and shuddering
from the fourteen teats into the fourteen mouths
sucking and blowing beneath them:
the long, perfect loveliness of sow.

"Saint Francis and the Sow" from MORTAL ACTS, MORTAL WORDS.

HISTORICAL DEVELOPMENT OF GROUP PSYCHOTHERAPY

Since the beginning of time, group discussion has been an important part of effective problem-solving and creative thinking about life. The value of group formats in promoting healing and fostering behavioral change was acknowledged in early tribal rituals and medieval morality plays. Ceremonial rituals specifically identified people as valid members of their community or religious group, thereby symbolizing their "belonging" to something larger.

Medieval morality plays used human dilemmas and direct audience participation for encouraging the audience to share vicariously with the actors. The plays often required successful solutions to difficult life problems. Group psychotherapy as a recognized form of psychological treatment, however, is a relatively recent phenomena. It began in the 20th century, sparked by observations about personal change occurring as the result of group participation. These analyses of group influences were conducted by those outside the field of psychology, as well as by those within it.

The historical experiences with group psychotherapy are rich and varied. With limited third-party reimbursement for individual treatment of mental disorders, group therapy probably will become even more important in the next decade. As Scheidlinger (1994, p. 223) observes,

The pressure of the market place may compel a much needed interdisciplinary elaboration of group psychotherapy's scientific base as well as a more precise delineation of its therapeutic elements and its applicability to specific maladaptive conditions. In a broader sense, group treatment modalities are uniquely suited to play a vital role in the alleviation of the serious problems of our day, a time characterized by alienation and a general anxiety created at least in part by the unprecedented nature and rate of societal change.

Joseph Pratt

In 1907, Joseph Pratt, an internist in Boston, developed a psychoeducational method for teaching patients with tuberculosis about their disease and improving their morale. He used informal group meetings. He described the weekly meetings held in conjunction with his more formal presentations (Pratt, in MacKenzie, 1992, p. 29) as

the most important feature of the class system. It is held every Friday in a large, cheerful room at Massachusetts General Hospital. The class meeting is a pleasant social hour for the members. One confided to the friendly visitor that the meeting was her weekly picnic. Made up as our membership is of widely different races and different sects, they have a common bond in a common disease.

Many of Pratt's patients continued with the informal groups because of the camaraderie they offered, even after their disease had resolved. The success of his group-treatment approach inspired Pratt and others to use a group format in the treatment of other chronic diseases such as diabetes. Later, Pratt expanded its use to the treatment of neurotic disorders. The idea of sharing a "common bond in a common disease," which Pratt advocated at the turn of the century, serves as the basis for many contemporary mutual help groups. For example, support group methods for addressing the needs of AIDS patients use a combination of psychoeducational and inspirational techniques to help patients cope with the limited treatment options and high mortality of their disease.

Samuel R. Slavson

Samuel R. Slavson (1890–1981) is recognized as a pioneer in the development of group formats for children and adolescents. Considered the father of group psychotherapy in America (MacKenzie, 1992), Slavson founded the American Group Psychotherapy Association in 1942 and served as its first president. Born in Russia, Slavson immigrated to New York at the age of 13 and became interested in group work as a result of community service work with adolescents in "self-culture" groups. Slavson's observations that withdrawn inner-city youth engaged spontaneously with their peers when presented with games and a structured group experience led him to use this format for a therapeutic purpose. He described his group therapy approach as therapy *by* the group rather than therapy *in* the group, meaning that the relationships individual members developed with each other constituted the primary healing force. Slavson used a combination of games, tools, and food to engage groups of children in actively communicating with each other. This work laid the groundwork for activity therapy, in which arts and crafts help children experience and direct their energies in productive ways.

Slavson used an activity group composed of eight same-sex children of approximately the same age. The accepting group climate allowed the children to share their experiences and to work out emotional tensions in a productive way. Today, Slavson's principles of group treatment are found in elementary school short-term psychoeducation and in focus groups related to parental divorce, drug abuse, and social skills training (Scheidlinger, 1994).

Jacob L. Moreno

In 1925, Jacob Moreno, known as the "father of psychodrama," introduced action-oriented group therapy in the United States. This theory of group psychotherapy originated from Moreno's earlier work in Vienna with the "theatre of spontaneity," in which role-playing techniques were employed as an extension of life actions. Moreno later founded the American Society for Group Psychotherapy and Psychodrama in 1942. He viewed psychodrama as an unique way of helping patients overcome maladaptive behavior patterns and develop new perspectives through the reenactment of emotionally difficult interpersonal situations. As patients assumed different roles in the scenario, they were able to experientially perceive both parts of a situation and personal reactions not within their awareness.

Moreno is credited with introducing the phrase "here and now" to psychotherapy (Kaplan and Sadock, 1993). Psychodrama bridges reality and fantasy by creating a stage that provides the patient with a "space for living." The patient or subject is referred to as the protagonist and is requested by the director (psychotherapist) to act as himself or herself, not to perform but to respond spontaneously as ideas and feelings come to mind. Other people (staff, patients) serve as auxiliary egos and aid the patient's enactment by representing the person's opposing thoughts, feelings, and delusions, or absent people. The audience is all the other people watching the psychodrama. They provide spontaneous feedback and act as a sounding board for the patient.

While Moreno was a charismatic leader, he was also quite abrasive. His strong personality and insistence on acknowledgment by others as the founder of group psychotherapy alienated many of his colleagues. Moreno never really earned the respect and recognition he felt he deserved (Kaplan and Sadock, 1993). His theoretical feud with Slavson had a divisive effect on group psychotherapy, as their individual group psychotherapy associations seriously splintered the group therapy movement. Nevertheless, psychodramatic approaches are the basis of many group workshop formats in industrial settings, and the techniques Moreno pioneered are the basis for other forms of psychiatric treatment, such as role-playing, role reversals, mirroring, and the empty chair technique used in gestalt therapy.

World War II

Public awareness of group psychotherapy as a form of treatment for people with emotional problems developed during World War II. Concurrently, a significant number of war-related psychiatric casualties and a limited number of psychiatrists to treat military personnel caused group psychotherapy to become the primary treatment for mental illness in the military. Although born of necessity, the efficacy of the treatment method was indisputable. Other clinicians outside the military began to consider group therapy. Its success became its strongest marketing tool.

Today, group therapy is considered a legitimate form of psychiatric treatment in a wide range of practice settings: inpatient hospitals, outpatient clinics, correctional institutions, and rehabilitative or supportive centers (Kaplan and Sadock, 1993). Patients of all ages with varied medical and psychiatric diagnoses appear to benefit from group therapy. In fact, contemporary estimates are that over half of "all psychiatric inpatient settings in the U.S. currently employ group treatment modalities" (Scheidlinger, 1994, p. 223).

Kurt Lewin

Kurt Lewin (1890–1947), a German social psychologist, is credited with using "here and now" experiential techniques to expand human consciousness and enhance human potential. Lewin founded the National Training Laboratories (NTL) in Bethel, Maine, in which experiential training groups enable group therapists the unique experience of studying their own reactions and responses in group formats. Lewin proposed a way to study group interactions as integrated components of a larger social field. Within this social field, he believed that people could explore their self-definition unfolding in the group, but only if they were willing to integrate their personal needs with the overall requirements of group membership. Lewin (1951) described the group as a dynamic whole, in which "the whole and parts are equally real, and the whole has definite properties of its own."

Lewin is best known for his work in developing a social field theory to facilitate the change process in a group format. He envisioned the group as a social field in which change could be orchestrated by examining the *driving* and *restraining* forces operating in individual and group perceptions about a selected issue. Lewin identified driving forces as those that moved the group toward its goal and restraining forces as those that inhibited the group's ability to reach its goal. Lewin believed that change could occur on both an individual and a group level through understanding the nature of restraining forces and working through them while simultaneously strengthening the driving forces. Still in use, the fundamental principles of Lewin's theory are presented in his text *Field Theory in Social Science*, published in 1951.

Lewin's work has had far-reaching consequences for group psychotherapy. He first introduced the concept of **group dynamics,** a term he used to describe group actions regularly occurring throughout the life of the group. Carl Rogers was greatly influenced by Lewin's work in developing the encounter group movement in the 1960s. Experiential group principles and techniques are currently found in many sensitivity and human potential groups. Robert Bales's (1950; Bales and Cohen, 1979) *System of Interaction Process Analysis*, a research tool widely used to study group dynamics empirically and William Schultz's (1966) FIRO (Fundamental Interpersonal Relations Orientations), a research instrument developed to measure group cohesion and outcome, are based on Lewin's social field theory of group dynamics.

S. H. Foulkes

S. H. Foulkes (1898–1976) was a German psychoanalyst who migrated to England and established the British Group-Analytic Society. Despite his training, Foulkes is recognized as a forerunner of here and now group interactions. He viewed the group experience as a "hall of mirrors" in which people can see themselves reflected in others. According to Foulkes (1975), the interactions that occur among group members offer an understanding of individual patients that is not available in a reflective discussion of past life events. By understanding each person's picture of other members in the group, including the leader, the therapist has a glimpse of that person's matrix of earlier personal relationships.

The group experience offers immediate and ongoing opportunities to observe self in relation to others and to receive feedback about their observations as a revealing mirror of the patient's personality. Personal mental health and wholeness develop from acceptance of both desired and undesired aspects of self-image. Foulkes viewed the group leader as the "conductor" of the group, charged with orchestrating emerging material in a helpful way, while considering the performance of all members simultaneously and maintaining a neutral, accepting stance toward each player. His model of group therapy is presented in his text *Group Analytic Psychotherapy: Method and Principles*, published in 1975.

Wilfred Bion

Wilfred Bion also introduced group methods into human relations training, and his work led to the development of the Tavistock Institute of Human Relations (1959; 1961). The training model used at the institute blended Bion's concept of "group assumptions" with Lewin's ideas about field theory. The Tavistock group has had an important influence on the development of human relations training programs in industry and on the education of mental health professionals (Trist and Murray, 1990).

Bion is credited with developing an intervention design referred to as a **group as a whole** model. He proposed that human beings cannot be completely understood apart from the interactions and membership in the groups to which they belong. Bion held that the basis of pathology was to be found in primitive anxieties associated with that membership. According to Bion, groups develop "basic assumptions" that direct their behavior in defending against primitive anxieties. As described in MacKenzie (1990), these primitive assumptions fall into three distinct categories:

- Dependency, in which the group acts as though it can function effectively only if a superior and wise person is leading. Group members in this state behave as if they were helpless to direct their activities and instead address their problems passively.
- Fight or flight, in which the group clusters together as if threatened by a dangerous force. The language of the group centers on themes of threat and the need to defend itself or escape. Such groups may experience rapid alterations between fear and revenge. The group may turn on the group leader for failure to resolve issues and provide answers.
- Pairing, in which the group is preoccupied with issues concerning two of its members and acts as if a resolution of the problems presented by this pair would be therapeutic to the entire group. Pairing may have a voyeuristic quality with sexual overtones. As in the other two assumption states, responsibility for direction is displaced from the individual to another source.

The shared anxieties of the group as a whole become the focus of treatment. This is accomplished by a leadership style referred to as the Tavistock method. The group leader assumes a passive role, sitting silently and refusing to be drawn into the group except for infrequent group interpretations of resistance to the group task (MacKenzie, 1990). The leader comments only on the collective responses (basic assumptions) of the group as a whole and does not directly address individual or content concerns of members.

When this technique is applied, everything that happens in the group is up to the discretion of its members. Typically a Bion group begins in silence until one of the members breaks it and introduces a topic for discussion. When resistance occurs or group discussion breaks down, the leader might make a single process comment, such as "the group is acting as if members are unable to continue the discussion without the leader's approval." The comment is followed by silence from the leader. No further explanation is given, even though individual members may press for it. If the group chooses not to terminate with closing statements, the group ends abruptly, and group members are faced with drawing their own conclusions about the group's meaning.

The Bion group as a whole method produces much anxiety in members, particularly those who find it more difficult to enter group discussions without the support of the group leader. On the other hand, it is a powerful way to learn about group phenomena. It remains a useful method for use in training groups with mentally healthy participants. Because of its potential to activate primitive affects without providing the corrective mechanisms to understand and discharge them constructively, it should be used with extreme caution in psychotherapy groups. This leadership style is likely to be harmful for some participants, particularly those who do not have a clear idea of its purposes and progression (MacKenzie, 1990).

Maxwell Jones

Maxwell Jones carried the group concept to a broader level by applying group principles to the unit in psychiatric hospitals. His interest began in response to a dissatisfaction with the status differentiation between staff and patients. Jones felt that differences accentuated the patient's mental deficits. Consequently, he developed the concept of a **therapeutic community** in the 1950s as a way of establishing greater equality and communication among professionals and their patients. Jones believed that eradicating what he viewed as the artificial partitioning of professionals and patients into a caste system would allow patients to emphasize their strengths for the good of the community rather than focus on their pathology. Jones developed the concept of a community milieu that simulates social situations and highlights difficulties of social adaptation. He proposed a combined methodology of catharsis, reeducation, and experiential learning from others as primary means of encouraging mental patients to rely more on their own personal resources.

The therapeutic community is a large group experience specifically designed to help patients acquire needed skills to cope with the stressors outside the hospital. Patients can practice these skills in a protected therapeutic setting. The therapeutic community represents a microcosm of society in which maladaptive behaviors can be reframed in a more positive manner. The method uses a democratic format with established parliamentary procedures. An elected patient leader and secretary preside. Matters of concern to the unit involving other patients and issues with staff are addressed in the full community. Patients and staff have an equal voice, although staff retains administrative control over individual and unit decisions. The equal voice of staff and patient members allows staff to relate to individual behaviors in a less formal manner than is possible in psychotherapy groups. In addition to their use in inpatient and partial hospitalizations units, therapeutic communities are found in half-way houses, substance abuse units, and group homes. They are a major organizing structure for group communication and governance. Chapter 19 addresses the use of therapeutic community group principles in milieu therapy.

BOX 17–1 Characteristics of Effective and Ineffective Groups

Effective Groups	Ineffective Groups
Goals are clearly identified and collaboratively developed.	Goals are vague or imposed on the group without discussion.
Open, goal-directed communication of feelings and ideas is encouraged.	Communication is guarded: Feelings are not always given attention.
Power is equally shared and rotates among members, depending on ability and group needs.	Power resides in the leader or is delegated with little regard to member needs. It is not shared.
Decision-making is flexible and adapted to group needs.	Decision-making occurs with little or no consultation. Consensus is expected rather than negotiated based on data.
Controversy is viewed as healthy because it builds member involvement and creates stronger solutions.	Controversy and open conflict are not tolerated.
A healthy balance exists between task and maintenance role functioning.	One-sided focus on task or maintenance role functions to the exclusion of the complementary function.
Individual contributions are acknowledged and respected. Diversity is encouraged.	Individual resources are not utilized. Conformity, the "company man," is rewarded. Diversity is not respected.
Interpersonal effectiveness, innovation, and problem-solving adequacy are evident.	Problem-solving abilities, morale, and interpersonal effectiveness are low and undervalued.

From Arnold, E., and Boggs, K. (1995). *Interpersonal relationships: Communication skills for nurses.* Philadelphia: W. B. Saunders, p. 273.

Irving Yalom

In 1975, Irving Yalom published the first edition of his classic text, *Group Psychotherapy.* Yalom developed an interpersonal model of group psychotherapy based on Harry Stack Sullivan's individual model of psychotherapy (see Chapter 6). Like Sullivan, Yalom believes that the relationship developed within the context of treatment should be the focus of the therapeutic process. Today, it is almost impossible to consider serious study of group psychotherapy without referring to Yalom's classic works in the area of group psychotherapy. Yalom's videotapes (1990) on the subject provide a vivid picture of group therapy in action.

▶ Check Your Reading

1. In what ways are the early models of group psychotherapy similar and different from one another?
2. What role did World War II play in the development of group psychotherapy?
3. What role does group therapy play in helping people bring about behavioral change?

CHARACTERISTICS OF GROUP PSYCHOTHERAPY

Group psychotherapy is defined as a structured meeting between two or more people who meet on a regular, predetermined basis for the purpose of achieving identified health-related goals. Group therapy is a form of psychological treatment that uses peer as well as professional relationships in a collaborative, structured, time-limited format. The expected outcomes of group psychotherapy include both symptom relief and resolution of interpersonal problems. The characteristics of effective and ineffective groups are presented in Box 17–1. The key to the development of effective therapy groups is a sound knowledge of basic group principles, a flexible leadership style, and careful selection of patients.

Within a safe, healing interpersonal environment, a person reexperiences emotional pain and can learn to respond to it differently. As Alonso and Swiller (1992, p. xxii) note:

> *Group psychotherapy offers individuals an unprecedented opportunity to explore personal responses in relationships. In the group, every member is bound to have his or her problems, not just to talk about them. Interpersonal problems and distress are actually experienced as part of the group process. Members can feel their own authenticity, their powerful affects, the tolerable exposure of their injured selves, and the support of others. They can learn how they are experienced by others and how their own perceptions may be distorted. Group members have the opportunity to observe the interpersonal skills and deficiencies of others and to experiment with methods of interaction that are new to them. They can learn both the universality of human anguish and the uniqueness of the potential value of every individual.*

Each psychotherapy group develops a unique collective personality. When human beings come together, the group immediately becomes more than the sum of its parts. Each group is made up of individual people, each bringing to a specific group his or her personal interpretation of reality, set of values, communication, and experiences that combine to form the group's character. Within the psychotherapy group, each member influences group dynamics and in turn is affected by the group as a whole. A healthy group personality has a direct effect on task accomplishment and satisfaction with outcomes.

Purpose

The purpose of therapeutic groups is to provide a consistent forum for human contact and community around selected issues of mental health and well-being. This human contact is described as the "life-blood of growth, the means of changing one's self and one's experience of the world" (Leepson, 1980, p. 122). Human contact does not take place randomly but is part of a clearly prescribed, sequential format directed toward identified group goals (Table 17–1).

Realistic group goals form the infrastructure of the group's existence. They give meaning and direction to the group's struggle. Group goals represent the identified outcomes that each group seeks to achieve through its common effort. Group goals differ from personal goals in that they are broader. They represent a composite rather than an individual aim. Each member is expected to contribute to the achievement of stated group goals.

Group goals should support the overall aims of the patient's treatment plan. Effective goals are at least indirectly related to the personal and cooperative resources of group members. Thus, goals for a group of low-functioning patients would be quite different than those for a highly functional outpatient group. For a low-functioning group, the goal might be simple communication with one another; a higher-functioning group might center on personality change. Goals also need to be appropriate to the setting and reinforced through collective support and encouragement. To whatever extent possible, members should have an opportunity to develop their own goals for personal development. This involvement ensures ownership. It encourages group members to work toward goals that are achievable and personally meaningful.

TABLE 17–1 Identifying Group Purpose

Type of Group	Opportunities Provided by Group Category
Therapy groups	Reality-testing Encouraging personal growth Inspiring hope Strengthening personal resources Developing interpersonal skills
Support groups	Giving and receiving practical information and advice Supporting coping skills Promoting self-esteem Enhancing problem-solving skills Encouraging client autonomy Strengthening hope and resiliency
Activity groups	Getting people in touch with their bodies Releasing energy Enhancing self-esteem Encouraging cooperation Stimulating spontaneous interaction Supporting creativity
Education groups	Learning new knowledge Promoting skill development Providing support and feedback Supporting development of competency Promoting discussion of important health-related issues

From Arnold, E., and Boggs, K. (1995). *Interpersonal relationships: Communication skills for nurses* (p. 264). Philadelphia: W. B. Saunders.

Types of Groups

Current group models favor a psychodynamic, action-oriented, or interpersonal focus. Psychodynamic models are concerned with identifying underlying group dynamics, linking past with present. Members are expected to talk about transference, countertransference, and resistance issues. Interpretation of group themes takes place throughout the group's existence, with a stronger focus on process rather than content. Action-oriented models make use of the member's past and use goal-setting, cognitive reframing, and role-playing to help individuals develop different coping strategies. These groups emphasize behavioral practice. They provide immediate feedback regarding group achievement. Interpersonal models focus on the immediate group interactions between members. Like psychodynamic formats, they have a stronger focus on process versus content. The difference lies in the focus on the here and now, in the group sharing of their personal reactions. Valued aspects are member openness and the integration of underlying dynamics with manifest content and cohesiveness.

Tasks

Psychotherapy groups have individual and group tasks that become integrated in the process of helping people achieve increased self-awareness and improved psychosocial functioning. The group format provides a safe place and a structured blueprint for practicing interpersonal behaviors and responses. Ideally, these new skills generalize to other parts of the individual's life. The primary task of group therapy, however, is not change. This is up to members to accomplish at their own speed, and in their own way. Goal achievement for each person differs, if for no other reason than that individual needs are different.

Beyond individual goal achievement, however, a collective task is common to all group therapy formats. The prescribed group format specifically offers an "opportunity for group members to participate in an evolving social microcosm that is the object of continual review and self-examination, and the relatively unique opportunity to function in an open social system that values authenticity, candor, and the open expression of feelings" (Bednar and Kaul, 1994, p. 642). The group process sets forth supportive, interpersonal conditions to which all group members adhere in their conversations with each other. This cooperation allows individual group members to engage in a process of communicating their feelings, concerns, and life issues, thereby stimulating further personal growth.

Communication

Communication is the primary means of healing in most psychotherapy groups. The communication process in group therapy is similar to that of individual therapy. Active listening and empathy are equally critical elements. Many of the same listening responses and verbal communication strategies described in Chapter 10 are applicable. The difference is that in group therapy, more interactions are possible. Therefore, you should listen for common themes expressed among members and observe their interactive behaviors with each other rather than simply those that patients address to the leader.

The role of the therapist differs from that in individual therapy. In a group setting, the leader encourages interaction between members. Instead of answering the member directly, the question is redirected back to the group for discussion. The therapeutic alliance thus develops among members of the group rather than solely between therapist and patient and is referred to as **cohesion.** Cohesion contains the same dimensions as one-to-one relationships: unconditional acceptance, genuineness, empathy, and valuing of the individual as a unique person (MacKenzie, 1990).

Ideally, the mode of communication in psychotherapy groups is one of inquiry. How the group member sees the problem is the critical issue. Group therapy works best when members can put aside preconceived notions and stereotypes, striving to comprehend what can be understood both about each group member and about the group as a whole. At times, communication is supportive; at other times it becomes confrontive. Both forms are directly linked to the achievement of identifiable group goals. The purpose of the group and the nature of its membership dictate the most effective approach in each group situation. As a source of support, group members act as a social and informational link for many people, particularly for those who feel socially isolated or who have lost faith in themselves or others. Loss of hope can temporarily paralyze people, rendering them vulnerable to feeling helpless and hopeless about a situation. Group support includes not only affirming a person's efforts but also providing each group member with the interpersonal tools needed to understand and negotiate the journey successfully.

Most groups use some form of confrontation to correct faulty thinking. When done with care and respect for the receiver's position and feelings, confronting misperceptions and reality testing about inappropriate attitudes can be extremely helpful. Although the change for each individual traveler must come from within, change usually requires a new way of thinking. If heard, the story of the journey challenged by a caring confrontation becomes one of renewal. The traveler returns to the world a wiser, more fully developed, and sensitive human being.

STRUCTURAL COMPONENTS OF PSYCHOTHERAPY GROUPS

Group structure plays an indirect yet highly significant role in a group's dynamics. Lack of attention to member selection, group size, time frame, and setting can sabotage effectiveness in meeting desired outcomes. Consistency in group structure is just as important to group psychotherapy as it is to individual relationships. Many of the same considerations apply (see Chapter 11).

Patient Selection

Patient selection refers to the choice of appropriate individuals for the group experience. Typically, group members do not know each other before entering the group, and it is best not to include people who socialize with each other in the same group. Patient selection is based on treatment need and capacity to contribute to group goals. These become strong therapeutic and ethical responsibilities because the structure of the therapeutic process requires each group member to function as a primary source of therapeutic value for other members. In a sense, each shares the therapist role for the group. Yalom (1985) believes that patients should be diagnostically heterogeneous and functionally homogeneous in a mixed therapy group. Matching the patient, the nature of his or her problems, the degree of disturbance, and current circumstances with the group goals, member composition, and stage of development leads to the formation and maintenance of a cohesive group culture. Yalom suggests that group members should have enough in common with each other to feel interpersonally comfortable in the group. **Functional similarity** describes comparable levels of functional ability and social recognizability, which members need to engage in meaningful conversation. Significant differences in educational level, life experiences, or developmental level are barriers to full participation. When group members feel uncomfortable, they are not as likely to talk with each other.

MacKenzie (1992) refers to the "Noah's Ark" phenomenon as important in member selection, so that the group has at least two members with similar characteristics. Pairing members in this way precludes the creation of a group social isolate. "One of a kind" characteristics in a group, such as gender or race, and significant differences in age or experience can present the single member with an unnecessary handicap and isolation in the group. For example, it would not be appropriate to place a single adolescent girl in a group of adolescent boys. When one therapist made this error and the girl's mother told the psychiatrist her daughter was uncomfortable, the psychiatrist's response was that they were all adolescents and had similar issues. Not so! The adolescent girl continued for a few more sessions and then dropped out, feeling like a failure. Had one other female been in the group or had this young girl been placed in a different adolescent group of a mixed membership or only females, the outcome might have been different. Being one of a kind is a common experience of women and minorities in Alcoholics Anonymous, which often is predominantly white and male. In making a referral to a self-help group, encourage the person to try several and find the one that best fits her or his needs.

Psychiatric symptoms also can pose issues for ensuring functional similarity. For example, creating an interpersonal climate responsive to the needs of both actively psychotic and nonpsychotic patients in the same group would be almost impossible. Including a psychotic patient who cannot tolerate the anxiety of deep emotional exploration in a group of nonpsychotic patients would not be appropriate. Placing a psychotic patient instead in a group focused on concrete problem-solving, reality-testing, and socialization skills would be highly beneficial. Yet this group might prove boring to the nonpsychotic patient. In a similar way, elderly patients feel out of place in a group emphasizing the here and now but would profit from placement in a group emphasizing reminiscence (Lappe, 1987).

Another component of member selection is the capacity to contribute to group goals. Persons with significant cognitive disorders, for example, are not good candidates for psychodynamic groups. Their deficit precludes processing here-and-now communication. These patients derive benefit from **reminiscence groups** in the early stages, which capitalize on remote memory retention, and from **resocialization groups,** which require little cognitive processing. Patients with active manic symptoms, antisocial personality disorder, and significant paranoid features typically are not good candidates for group therapy. First, their symptoms disrupt the group functioning. Second, their pathologies interfere with their own ability to derive benefit as their symptoms preclude the necessary cooperation with other members. They should be included only after their symptoms are under sufficient control to gain some benefit from group membership and to be able to contribute in a meaningful way.

As mentioned earlier, another factor to consider in group composition is the issue of a homogeneous or heterogeneous group membership. Homogeneity is achieved by grouping patients of similar diagnosis or age in a particular group. An adolescent group might exclude young adults from membership because adolescents' issues are different from those in adulthood. Homogeneous grouping of patients with eating disorders is more effective than heterogeneous grouping because everyone is in touch with the denial and evasive nature of symptoms (Harper-Giuffre & MacKenzie, 1993). The same would be true for a substance use group.

Group Size

The size of the group is another structural consideration. Large-group formats are the most cost-effective way to deliver didactic educational material, but they also limit the amount of interaction that can take place. Typically, psychoeducational groups consist of 10 to 15 members, and the group process centers on discussion of a particular topic.

Psychodynamic and interpersonal therapy groups try to limit membership to six to eight members. This size allows for a variety of interpretations but also permits sufficient interpersonal space for intimate sharing. Groups containing more than 10 members allow less potential for intimacy and self-disclosure needed for effective problem-solving and goal accomplishment. Groups that are too small, however, create an emotional intensity or the formation of subgroups that is difficult to regulate. When groups contain fewer than five members, the dialogue suffers greatly when more than one member is absent. The group may never get beyond the engagement stage because any turnover suggests a need to replace the members who have resigned from the group. Moreover, groups of three members often form a subgroup coalition of two, excluding the third person and thereby affecting morale and effective decision-making. Such small groups also increase the anxiety of the therapist because of the need for a leader to fill in the gap.

Group Environment

Frequency of Meetings

The nature and goals of the group determine the frequency of meetings. Educational groups provide participants with concentrated information and limited dialogue. Depending on the nature of the information, psychoeducation groups can consist of one to four sessions and are held in blocks of up to four hours each at designated times. The group disbands when it has achieved its educational purpose.

Human potential encounter groups count on extensive time exposure to break down defenses quickly. Marathon encounter groups represent a one-time extended group in which group members are continuously together for large time spans, ranging from 8 to 48 hours. Mutual-help support group meetings vary from once a week to one a month. They can last up to two hours, with a break in the middle for refreshments and networking.

Psychotherapy groups need considerable time before members can feel comfortable sharing intimate details about themselves. Traditional psychotherapy groups are held once a week in outpatient settings and more often in the inpatient environment. Outpatient groups meet for 45 to 90 minutes. Inpatient groups are scheduled in 45- to 60-minute blocks. Attention to time boundaries respects the need of individuals to have lives outside the group and firmly integrates the group as a set pattern in the patient's life. The group space becomes a special agreed-upon time for self-exploration. Nothing interferes with it, and members can then plan activities in their lives to include their commitment to the group. Most begin to depend on it and block out the time as "their" group time. Rescheduling meetings without having a definite rationale communicates to group members that the leader does not consider the group space to be very important.

Equally important is the need to begin and end groups on time. Otherwise, members may become fidgety, making explorations in the last few minutes of the group impossible because selected individuals already have left the group, at least psychologically. Beginning before the group is scheduled means that some patients will not have the same opportunity to benefit from opening statements. Waiting until all members are present before beginning unfairly penalizes those who have made the effort to be on time. Moreover, it can lead to overlooking behaviors that need to be strengthened for effective social interaction. Leader sensitivity in allowing a few minutes between group sessions in inpatient or day hospital settings for members to arrive at their next destination makes patients and staff less frantic.

The total period for the group to achieve its goals also bears some discussion. Some groups are open-ended, but many have built-in time frames. If group members accept a defined period, say 8 to 12 weeks as the life of the group, stick to the initial contract. A new contract may be renegotiated with members if they achieve the original goals or the period elapses. Assuming that the group should continue without further negotiation, however, is a mistake. Members can construe this assumption as a "bait and switch" that will affect further group participation. A more straightforward approach is to review members' progress and to solicit input as to how each group member would like to proceed. Individual decisions to leave the group at this point should be honored without any undue pressure to continue.

Setting for Meetings

Group psychotherapy settings reflect their purpose. The room for group meetings should be well ventilated and large enough to accommodate all participants. It should be set apart from the general flow of traffic. During the meeting, it should be inaccessible to intrusion. A simple sign of the door, stating "Meeting in Session" usually is sufficient to deter unintentional intruders. Always using the same room under the same conditions fosters a feeling of safety that cannot be achieved otherwise.

Seating should allow for meaningful interaction. Because interaction is verbal, group members should see each other's nonverbal facial expressions and body posture in an open, face-to-face position. Most psychotherapy groups are seated in comfortable chairs arranged in a circle, equidistant from each other. This arrangement allows the fullest exposure of each member to other member communications. If cushions rather than chairs are used, they are organized in a similar manner. If a member is absent, the empty chair or cushion remains in its designated position.

The seating arrangement should be set up before the meeting. Nothing is more disconcerting than to arrive at the designated time only to find that the chairs must be set up or the room cleaned before it can be used for the group. Enough chairs for each member, no more and no less, should be provided. Most therapy groups require only simple room arrangements, but if supplies such as a flip chart, handouts, or paper and markers are going to be used, they should be prepared beforehand.

Group Contract

Once the leader establishes the physical environment as safe and consistent, the next step is to define the psychological structures needed to support group aims. These are identified in the form of a group contract. The preliminary **group contract** spells out the boundaries of the relationship, confidentiality, the behaviors expected of the patients and what behaviors the group members can anticipate from the group therapist. The contract represents the working agreement among individual members and the group leader. It forms the interpersonal structural guidelines and expectations under which the group will operate. The contract defines how the group will proceed and identifies rules to govern behavior. Space, time, and behavioral expectations for absences are established from the outset.

A group therapy contract should reflect the specific goals and purposes for which the group was formed and the rationale for the group's existence. The contract can be simple and direct. Without a contract to guide the course of the group life, however, detours regarding important issues may prevent the group from achieving stated therapeutic goals. While it is important to incorporate current trauma into the group discussion, the group contract keeps the leader and members focused on the reasons for the group's existence and its established therapeutic goals. Other possibilities for treatment exist. When significant individual issues cannot be addressed fully within the group, the leader may need to refer the individual in crisis for individual consultation. Such intervention is a legal and ethical responsibility.

Group Norms

Norms are behavioral standards of conduct and basic operating procedures that provide structural boundaries and guidelines for expected behaviors. Norms are part of the collective forces that operate within a psychotherapy group and pressure members to conform to expected behavioral standards. Conceptual norms provide structural interpersonal boundaries. They help determine how individual members should relate with each other. Once established, they are difficult to overturn or modify.

Universal Norms

Some norms are essential to the life of any group. These are *universal* norms because they are absolutely critical to effective group functioning. For example, regular attendance, member verbal interaction, confidentiality, and respect for other group members are all universal norms. Regular attendance is important not only for individual learning purposes but also for the entire group. Often group members have comments or reactions to another member's contribution that would go unheard without a follow-up in the next session. The value of many different reactions is lost with irregular attendance. Moreover, individual absences are of concern to other members, who typically develop all sorts of fantasies as to why the person is missing. If the issue of attendance is not addressed, the irregular attender tends to be scapegoated or ignored after returning to the group.

Confidentiality means that nothing personal and nothing that would identify an individual group member can be shared outside the group without the group's permission. Confidentiality is a universal norm in all groups. One exception to this rule is that the data presented in group meetings are recorded in each individual patient's chart as it relates to each patient's treatment plan. Patients need to be forewarned that an overall description of their participation will be entered into their patient record for treatment purposes. They should be informed about this disclosure from the outset of treatment.

Confidentiality is such a fundamental norm of group life that typically the leader specifies it as a behavioral standard during preinterview selection. The leader also should reinforce its importance during the group orientation. Each time the group adds a new member, this norm gets restated. Although it may sound redundant to the leader, the group generally appreciates the marking of its importance.

Another reason for emphasizing confidentiality in group life is that patients have no professional standards for monitoring their behavior. Although confidentiality is ethically dictated, patients are not legally bound to protect the communication of other group members (Applebaum and Greer, 1993). Thus, if the patient chooses to share a confidence outside the group, the therapist has no recourse other than to strengthen the norm of confidentiality as a standard of common decency in the group and to make it a criterion for continued membership. By stressing the role of group members as therapists for each other and the ethical principles involved with confidential material, most group members will recognize the importance of confidentiality. (See Chapter 11 for a fuller explanation of confidentiality in therapeutic relationships.)

Group-Specific Norms

Other group norms are referred to as group-specific norms. These differ from group to group. Typically, these are defined as behavioral standards developed by the group to facilitate goal achievement. Simple examples of group specific norms are asking members for updates on their accomplishments in the past week or determining how people are to be addressed. Other group-specific norms represent standards unique to the needs of the membership and specifically related to stated group outcomes. For example, the group treatment of alcoholic patients might contain group behavioral standards related to not drinking and strategies to maintain sobriety. Group-specific norms for low-functioning groups may need to include very explicit behavioral standards, such as talking one at a time, not leaving the room during the session, and refraining from violent behavior toward other group members and from obscene language. Case 17–1 illustrates the importance of group-specific norms in member behavior.

Case Example 17–1 One Participant's Story

A voluble young man revealed a torrent of private details about himself in the first few sessions of a new group. This pronounced level of self-disclosure remained unmatched by his peers and unchecked by the therapist. Before long, the patient became identified as deviant in respect to a prevailing norm in the group, a norm that pointed to a gradual entry into personal exchanges. The group, intimidated by the pace of the deviant member's self-disclosures, steered a self-protective course around him. His subsequent sense of isolation was the prelude to bitter disillusionment that culminated in his premature dropping out.

From Bloch, S., and Crouch, E. (1985). *Therapeutic factors in group psychotherapy.* Oxford: Oxford University Press, p. 4, by permission of Oxford University Press.

Differences in Structuring Inpatient and Outpatient Groups

Inpatient groups differ from outpatient groups in several ways. Group membership in inpatient groups tends to be more diverse. It reflects the current population rather than a deliberate attempt to match treatment with patient needs. Although the focus of inpatient and many outpatient groups is on the here and now, a qualitative difference exists in the level of interpersonal analysis. Outpatient groups typically last over a greater span of time (minimum 8 to 12 weeks). Inpatient groups, because of short-term stays, do not deal in the same depth with long-standing interpersonal communication styles. Instead, Yalom (1985) suggests that the inpatient group helps to "spot" maladaptive behavioral patterns, which are later worked through in outpatient therapy. Noting this difference is highly relevant in helping patients select appropriate treatment agendas in inpatient groups.

During inpatient treatment, you need to support the patient's ego growth. The task is to help the patient learn to cope with the inner chaos and overwhelming emotions that precipitated admission to the hospital. The goal is to return the patient to the community with the ability to interact successfully. The group task is to provide the corrective emotional experiences that will make return possible. With inpatient therapy, the therapist takes a much more active role, clarifies more often, and directs the process of establishing appropriate norms.

Because most inpatient treatment groups tend to be part of an integral part of a larger therapeutic protocol, always establish in the initial session that the leader will be sharing information from group sessions with other health team members. This disclosure is an explicit group norm. Closely correlated with this universal norm on inpatient units is that the leader and other group members must have the freedom to share information of relevant unit events that could affect group treatment (Kibel, 1993). For example, members are bound to report any clandestine activities, such as outside intimate relationships between group members or members smoking pot or having access to alcohol. To withhold this kind of information constitutes secrecy that can be damaging to the trust needed in group sharing.

Socialization among members of both inpatient and outpatient groups is an issue. In the inpatient setting, activities that promote socialization receive support. The leader encourages members to continue the dialogue begun in the therapy group. The work of the outpatient group, however, depends on limited social contact outside the group. Members need to experience the full impact of the group dynamics within the group, where all of the data are equally available for the group members to explore with each other.

Intimate relationships are not acceptable outcomes of the socialization process in either inpatient or outpatient groups. Closeness develops among group members, but relationships that extend beyond the social group format into serious personal relationships usually are problematic for the two people involved, as well as for the group at large. They should be discouraged. The group leader may need to explain that, "in my experience, the group relationship is so special that having personal relationships tends to dilute its effectiveness."

▶ **Check Your Reading**

4. How does the size of the group affect interaction?
5. In what ways are time boundaries important to the structural framework of the group?
6. What are the significant differences between inpatient and outpatient group psychotherapy?

DEVELOPMENT OF PSYCHOTHERAPY GROUPS

Defined stages of development occur in group psychotherapy relationships, just as they do in one-to-one therapeutic relationships. MacKenzie (1992) observes that "In the stage model, group development is conceptualized as an epigenetic process, in which adequate resolution of any one stage is in part dependent on the satisfactory mastery of the preceding stage or stages" (p. 49). The stages of group development are categorized as preinteraction, engagement (forming, storming), working phase (norming, performing), and termination (adjourning). As the group develops, the tasks associated with each phase become increasingly more complex and fully integrated. As with individual therapy, time spent in the termination phase of group life is important.

Preinteraction

Group psychotherapy actually begins before the first meeting, as the leader carefully establishes a suitable foundation for the group to begin. During the preinteraction phase, the group leader carefully aligns professional goals with desirable group goals. Other decisions include whether the group should have an open or closed group membership. Open groups are those in which group membership changes frequently. This type of group is found in inpatient settings that depend on member residency and in many mutual help/support groups. Closed group membership means that the group membership will not change for the life of the group or only for a clearly understood reason. Members often must meet certain diagnostic criteria for acceptance. Some groups, such as Alcoholics Anonymous, offer both open and closed groups to its members and potential members. Anyone can attend some meetings, whereas others are closed to all but the designated member population. Psychotherapy groups also can share characteristics of both open and closed membership. They are open in that as one member leaves the group, another fills the empty slot, but they have a closed membership in that members cannot arbitrarily enter the group simply because they have similar interests or problems.

Many pregroup considerations required for successful group relationships parallel those for all therapeutic relationships (see Chapter 11). As with individual relationships, group therapy requires the leader to cultivate a working alliance with other members of the health care team. You need to develop a mutual understanding of the goals, time frames, and other logistical considerations with other health team members. Otherwise, conflicts in treatment goals and time commitments may prevent the patient from fully engaging in the group. Moreover, these negotiations permit you to educate the interdisciplinary team about the purposes and design of the group.

The initial assessment interview takes place as an individual session before the first group session. The interview should achieve several goals simultaneously. First is the need to determine the patient's suitability for the group, with attention to matching functional similarity and degree of emotional disturbance with the current composition of the group. Too many active or passive patients in the same group affect group interaction.

Assessment interviews also provide you with an important opportunity to evaluate motivation and personal commitment. A potential member can be quite suitable for the group but for a variety of reasons lack the necessary commitment for group membership. Unless the person can be encouraged to find a reason for joining the group or is able to see the possible benefit, postponing membership or selecting a different treatment format would be better. For example, a schizoid patient with little chance of participating because of extreme discomfort in group situations probably would not be a good candidate. Potential group members who cannot make the time commitments necessary for regular attendance may need to postpone their entry. For example, some individuals travel as part of their job and cannot attend on a regular basis. Their "in and out" attendance pattern can be very disruptive and usually is not tolerated well by other group members.

The final goal of a pregroup interview is to make entry into the group easier. Validating important issues with each patient and assessing for potential interpersonal strengths such as humor or honesty can be useful (MacKenzie, 1992). By demonstrating the connection between serious life issues and the purpose of the group, you introduce the work of the group in a personable, nonthreatening manner. During initial discussion, the patient begins to experience the "person" of the leader and to view the leader as an ally. Experiencing the group leader as a human being and consistent member of the group beforehand often reduces patient anxiety about joining the group (Piper and Perrault, 1989).

In the pregroup interview, you can provide necessary information about the group purpose, format, and expectations and address common misperceptions about group therapy. Time with the therapist concurrently offers a patient an opportunity to ask the questions that may make a difference between accepting or rejecting group membership. In fact, MacKenzie (1990) specifically suggests that pretherapy preparation is a crucial element in reducing the number of group dropouts.

Engagement (Forming) Phase

The engagement phase, or **forming phase** of group therapy is similar to the orientation phase in individual therapy; the purpose and tasks of both modalities are parallel. The first meeting is introductory and sets the stage for the development of the group. Having an overall plan of action developed for the first meeting increases the comfort of the leader. Some leaders prepare an outline as a guide. Others simply prepare their thoughts.

Usually you begin the group with a self-introduction and ask members to say their names and tell the group something about themselves. The precise format is left open to encourage the participants to present in ways that are comfortable. The manner in which individuals express themselves and the type of information they choose to share give you important data that can be used later, in the working phase. At the same time, make sure that individual members do not prematurely disclose lengthy intimate details about themselves. Otherwise, the sharing may lead to intense discomfort when the patient reflects on it. The result could be premature termination from the group—sometimes psychologically, but more often altogether. Should a "show stopper" occur, thank the member for the contribution but say that the individual might want to bring the issue up later when the group members knew each other better (Case Example 17–1). Try to discourage a patient's vulnerable frankness in initial group sessions, without turning the patient off to the idea of presenting an important personal situation later.

Leadership Tasks

In the beginning of the group, the members need structure, so you are more active than is necessary later. Keep the conversation supportive and flowing in the first meeting. Lack of initial structure leaves the group floundering and uncertain (Corey and Corey, 1990). A standard first-meeting format is to identify the group's purpose and goal, specify technical details, and name fundamental structural norms such as expected attendance, confidentiality, what to do in case of absence, and how the group will function.

A general statement about the nature of the work (i.e., that the group is a place where members can discuss serious personal issues and get feedback from each other) establishes the task of the group as serious. Reality testing begins with the first meeting. Sometimes, individuals enter groups with unrealistic perceptions of what the group experience can offer. They have little or no experience with interacting in groups (Yalom, 1985). If members have never had group therapy before, briefly educate them as to their role as members. Provide a simple statement about group goals and assist members to clarify their meaning. Letting members ask questions consistent with their personally held values tends to encourage greater commitment. Sufficient time to review and respond to individual concerns helps members feel heard and saves later frustration from unclear expectations.

Common Communication Patterns

Acceptance, inclusion, and trust are primary values in beginning group meetings. Initially, group communication tends to be tentative, polite, and guarded, as members explore their values and ideas with each other. They need to know that other group members, including the leader, will respect their contributions and will not make them look foolish to their peers. Finding commonalities in experiences and related feelings helps strengthen initial emotional bonding among group members. Statements that link member contributions point out similarities and indirectly stress the importance of group members as therapists for each other.

Resistance may be an issue in the early stages of group, particularly if the membership is involuntary, as it frequently is on inpatient units. During the initial stages of group development, more so than at later stages, members may show opposition to the idea of group therapy. Sometimes, it is helpful to ask patients about their previous experiences with groups and to inquire about similarities and contrasts with the current group therapy format. You also can note the resistance and address it as being a normal reaction, while requesting members to withhold judgment about the group's efficacy. For example, noting some reluctance to be in the group, you might say "I know that some of you have reservations about group psychotherapy; this is a very normal reaction, but I am hoping that you will give it a chance because it is a treatment method that works for many people. If you have any questions or if you know of any ways I can help you feel more comfortable in the group, I'd like to hear about them."

You can reinforce the norm of group psychotherapy as a reflective process with comments such as, "What about asking the group how they think you might proceed" or "I think it would be important for you to get the group's feedback on . . ." Unless you are fairly insistent about this format from the beginning, it becomes increasingly difficult to shed the mantle of the expert and director of the action.

Toward the end of each meeting, even the first one, ask members to summarize their reactions to the discussion. This process helps put closure on issues. A strong summary statement also allows a concentrated glimpse at possible misperceptions or important feelings that have not emerged into full view and otherwise might go unaddressed. In such a situation, do not extend group time, because ignoring time constraints is a boundary violation. Instead you might say, "This would be a good topic for us to start with next time."

Transition (Storming) Phase

The initial stage of group development brings a strong emphasis on finding commonalities. Once group members feel more comfortable with each other, the focus of group interaction changes from a focus on similarities to a period in which differences become critically important.

The **storming phase** of group development is uncomfortable for the leader and many group members. Issues of control and power replace those of inclusion and acceptance. Strong feelings and open conflict are typical. Just how stormy this phase will be depends on the members and their typical ways of interacting. For example, a women's group may approach this phase in a much less aggressive manner than an all-male group. Although uncomfortable, this stage of group development is absolutely essential because it sets the stage for the development of the group-specific norms that will guide the group in the working phase. Fortunately, this stage is short lived. This fact can help you tolerate the discomfort.

During the storming phase, your role is to act as the gatekeeper in helping individual group members identify but move beyond their personal agendas and engage in collective and collegial dialogue. Usually essential at this stage is to provide an interpersonal climate in which it is legitimate to express strong feelings and have them heard, even if one cannot agree with their substance.

Most significant for the group's development is your ability to act as a nonanxious presence to help members maintain a positive attitude and commitment during the storming stage. This task is not easy, particularly when you come under attack. Staying the course, however, often helps the group to rebalance itself. Identifying personal reactions to challenging behaviors helps you maintain perspective so you will not respond inappropriately and escalate conflict. Here is an opportunity in which a coleader can help deflect intense emotion directed toward you. During the transition stage, you become an "affirmer of standards"; through words and actions you reflect a basic respect for each person's contribution. This attitude encourages patients to take risks in communicating by making the interpersonal environment safe for each group member.

Norming Phase

During the **norming phase,** the group develops behavioral standards needed to meet stated goals. These goals help ensure interpersonal safety and facilitate goal accomplishment. Establishing norms to direct the work of the group naturally follows from the members' blended experience of identifying their commonalities and differences. The more ownership individual members take of standards, the more effective the group is likely to become. Group pressure on members who do not conform to expected norms helps reinforce bonding. Compassion and respect, however, are important. Confrontation tends to reinforce the group's seriousness in belonging to all members. Inevitably, norm violations by one member affect the entire group.

Performing (Working) Phase

Once the ground rules for operating the group are in place, members actively engage in working on group identified problems. The **performing phase** is characterized by cohesion and productivity (Corey, 1990). Most of the in-depth work of the group takes place during this phase. Without the preliminary stages of forming, storming, and norming, however, the work could not be accomplished because the necessary trust and cooperation would not be present. In the performing stage, group communication reflects cooperation rather than competition, and within the group, self-disclosure is spontaneous and honest. Members know what to expect from each other. In the process of working through differences, a genuine respect for other members develops. The sense of belonging is at its highest peak. It is in this phase of group development that individual members are most likely to experience fully validation of their worth from other group members.

Throughout the group's life, your primary function is to facilitate interactions among group members and to provide an accepting interpersonal environment in which group members can feel supported in exploring difficult issues. The degree to which active interventions by you is necessary, however, changes as other group members take responsibility for leadership activities, and in essence, become therapists for each other. Although you still retain overall accountability for the group structure and progression toward group goals, leadership is shared with other group members, who assume both task and maintenance functions. Keeping the group focused on therapeutic goals is an important leadership task, as Case Example 17–2 illustrates.

Case Example 17–2 A Leader's Story

A chemical substance abusers' group has maintaining sobriety as an immediate goal. During the group's history, several crises have occurred—a member's father died, another person lost his job, and a third was raped. The leader may be tempted to deal with these issues at length, but the group's purpose could well be lost. These concerns need to be tied into the goal of maintaining sobriety. If they are not, intervention in all these crises could direct the group from the overriding goal of focusing on sobriety. Current crises could all be resolved, but in the process, many of the group members could have returned to patterns of chemical abuse.

Data developed from Buchanan, D. (1980). The central concern model, a framework for structuring psychodynamic production. *Group Psychotherapy, Psychodrama, and Sociometry 33*, 25–32.

Orchestrate the direction of the group when it gets lost in detail or stuck in superficial discussion by asking relevant open-ended and focused questions. These help the group explore problem areas in depth. Using a variety of strategies to broaden the expressiveness of members helps deepen their connections. Neutral probes that encourage further details provide another helpful strategy.

Themes that typically emerge in groups are dependency versus independence, power versus powerlessness, and enmeshment versus abandonment. Individual themes of loneliness, isolation, alienation, loss, or self-protection can trigger group themes surrounding similar issues. Homogeneous groups engaged in treatment around their diagnosis may develop group themes related to their lived experience of their disorder. When helping members discover the themes presented by individual group members, you need to be aware that "confusion is not a theme, but rather a smokescreen that prevents either an individual or the group from uncovering feelings" (Buchanan, 1980, p. 52). You will want to help the group sort out its confusion as a group dynamic, rather than consider it an underlying content theme.

Effective therapy group in the working phase provides a democratic atmosphere in which each person can experience different social models of relating and varied ethical lines of reasoning. You can foster bonding among group members by linking their comments, making observations about helpful statements, and drawing attention to common concerns and similar responses. Structure the experience so that it brings out the "best" in a patient.

While supporting patient contributions is important, also try to bring the group as a whole into the problem-solving mode, so that all can learn from the shared experience. For example, you might invite other group members to share their observations of the patient in the here and now or to relate their sense of how the problem might be addressed.

Seeking solutions consistent with treatment goals is an important function of group process. The format of identifying problem statements or themes, generating ideas, choosing between alternatives and implementing chosen actions is quite similar to the problem-solving process described in Chapter 11. The difference is that other group members and you participate as equals in identifying the problem and developing solutions. Often group involvement with one member's dilemma mirrors other group members' difficulties with similar issues.

Adjourning (Termination) Phase

Termination, the **adjourning phase** of group relationships, occurs in a variety of ways: members leave; the group disbands; a member is terminated. Most often, individual group members leave a psychotherapy group because their work is finished or they are discharged from the hospital or treatment program. Any of these actions initates an **adjourning phase.** Sometimes you add new members to offset the loss.

Preparation for voluntary endings in an outpatient group can begin with a norm established in the first meeting: Ask members to tell the group of impending departure one week and to return the next to say good-bye. If the group member enters after the group is well established, this norm can be addressed in the pregroup interview. Prolonging the departure provides sufficient time to allow both the patient and other group members to say a proper good-bye.

Terminations are important for the group as well as for the patient. Arrangements to provide sufficient time for a fitting good-bye should be factored into the last session. Ask the patient to tell the group what has been helpful and what he or she would like to say to each group member. Another strategy is to ask each group member to share perceptions of the exiting patient with him or her. Generally, you will save your remarks for last, to emphasize or neutralize other patient comments, if necessary. Sometimes, when a group member has been very important to the group, the group is angry about the departure, and the words are not particularly supportive. You may have to suggest gently that the group is having trouble giving up a valued member. If done with tact, this intervention can help members get in touch with their feelings. When eliciting feeling from other group members, Buchanan (1980) advises "keep it simple. Ask the group members how they feel and they will usually respond with short and direct statements" (p. 52).

When the allotted time for group is almost up, you can say to the group and the exiting member, "Our time is almost up. Is there anything any of you would like to add to what has already been said?" While not a part of normal group protocol, members often hug or shake the hand of the parting member. Recommendations for further referral usually are done individually and are not a legitimate part of the group's termination process.

If the group as a whole is ending, help the group summarize goal achievement and gain closure on any unresolved issues. End on a relaxed note, with good feelings. By contrast with the performing (working) phase, the task of the adjourning phase is not to open new business. Rather, the intent is to gain closure on the experience. Avoid the introduction of emotionally charged material during the patient's last session. Good endings are as important as good beginnings. For many, the ending in one group frequently serves as an important element in considering membership in another therapy group.

CONCEPTUAL COMPONENTS OF PSYCHOTHERAPY GROUPS

Curative Factors

In 1975, Yalom identified 11 **curative factors,** or therapeutic factors, in successful small group treatment. Curative factors are an element of group therapy that contributes to improving a patient's condition. Curative factors are a function of the actions of the group therapist, the other group members, and the patient himself or herself (Bloch and Crouch, 1985, p. 4).

Catharsis

Catharsis refers to the expression of emotion. In group therapy, patients are taught to identify and differentiate their feelings, to express them honestly and openly in a socially acceptable manner, and to become the master rather than the victim of their emotions. Honest communication of feelings with respect for the rights of self and others is essential for satisfying interpersonal relationships. Mentally ill patients typically have trouble recognizing and sharing deep personal feelings. To the extent that emotions are suppressed or unconsciously repressed, a person feels emotionally constricted, lonely, and alienated from society. At the other end of the spectrum are intense feelings expressed without considering the impact on the other person. While this catharsis momentarily discharges the anxious feelings of the sender, it can be quite damaging to a relationship. Both positive and negative feelings can be problematic. For example, constantly proclaiming love for another can be just as harmful to a relationship, as burning it up with anger.

Although catharsis of any emotion is useful if the feeling has been repressed, anger and guilt bear special mention. Chronic reactive anger tends to push people away. Indiscriminate expression at inappropriate times can be highly destructive to interpersonal relationships. When pent-up angry feelings build and are suddenly released, the receiver literally may not know how to respond. The anger may be out of proportion to the incident and often may be intense and extreme.

While violence in the group cannot be permitted, group psychotherapy offers patients a structured format where expression of anger and effective responses are heard without either party suffering in the process. Here group members can learn to express anger and to respond effectively to strong anger presentations without fear of retaliation. This experiential knowledge, learned in a safe interpersonal environment, helps patients take charge of their feelings instead of being bound by the negative energy of anger and unexpressed feelings of resentment. In the group, members are encouraged to take responsibility for their own anger and anxiety, to recognize when they feel threatened, and to channel their emotional feelings into appropriate expressions of needs and fears. It is thus easier to look at negative emotions more objectively. Most important, acceptance of powerful feelings by the group can lead to greater self-acceptance, as shown by a group member quoted in Bloch and Crouch (1985, p. 102):

> *I had been silent and tense and was suddenly asked by the group to disclose what I was feeling. I exclaimed vehemently that I was feeling angry, particularly at my mother; I burst into tears and bolted from the room. When I returned, I felt embarrassed and upset, but the group showed much concern and assured me that I was welcome back and supported me about feeling angry in the first place.*

Another emotional catharsis treated in group psychotherapy is guilt. Rollo May (1969) states that "when a person denies his potentialities, fails to fulfill them, his condition is guilt" (p. 35). Guilt typically relates to a situation in which a person wishes he or she had acted in a different way. Unfortunately, accompanying feelings of inadequacy and an inability to accept oneself rather than who one might have been only intensify the guilt feelings. As the person relives the trigger events stimulating the guilty feelings, they assume new dimensions that often are not totally based in reality. Statements of self-blame and sentences beginning with "if only I had . . . " suggest guilt feelings.

Group interventions can help a patient recognize guilt as a wasted emotion. Members can respond to catharsis of painful guilt feelings by reminding the person that most people have 20/20 hindsight about what they might have done but not before or while they did it. Moreover, it is impossible to do a precise retake of the situation, except in one's mind.

Through careful questioning, the group members act as witness in observing with the patient an unacceptable self-image in the original guilt-producing situation. By separating the observer from what is observed, group members can help a patient burdened by guilt to reframe an experience. Subjective descriptions of reality in which the patient was the villain can be called into question. Understanding the arbitrary nature of perception can lead to increasing self-acceptance. Members can draw attention to factors that might otherwise be ignored and so provide new insight. Members also provide valuable counsel about guilt as shaped by beliefs, values, and attitudes that may not be truly valid.

Group interventions for guilt feelings also include helping the person maximize his or her potential in the present. With the support of the group, individual members can learn to intensify feelings for clarification and to release or change their meaning when needed. This process requires deliberate actions and full responsibility for self, but the group supplies the support and encouragement needed to let go of negative emotions. Group members can help people develop ways to make amends for past transgressions, thereby releasing the emotional energy associated with guilt. Through dialogue, the individual can move to accepting oneself as an imperfect human being, living in an imperfect world, always with the possibility of learning from mistakes and letting go of irrational feelings.

Cohesion

Yalom (1985) describes group **cohesion** as the "we-ness" of the group, the sense that the group is important to the group members. Cohesion is composed of all the factors that make the group attractive for a member. In a cohesive group, the members like and respect one another, strongly desire to achieve identified group goals, and are willing to lend their efforts to making it happen. Task performance in cohesive groups tends to be higher because higher levels of cooperation stimulate greater involvement. Group members take pride in their group, and the group boasts a record of low absenteeism and membership turnover. Cohesive groups foster a sense of belonging. Typically, members are glad they are part of their group, rather than any other. In fact, Yalom argues that cohesion is the most powerful source of motivation for group participation (Case Example 17–3). Outsiders also perceive cohesive groups as friendly and committed to group goals.

Case Example 17–3 Paul's Story

Paul, absent from the group for two weeks, seemed tense and eventually brought up the possibility that he might drop out. Others commented that they would feel very unhappy to see him go. One member even got angry, calling Paul selfish to consider leaving, as he was needed by the group. Paul relaxed and said that hearing the group's responses convinced him that he should stay.

From Bloch, S., and Crouch, E. (1985). *Therapeutic factors in group psychotherapy.* Oxford: Oxford University Press, p. 102, by permission of Oxford University Press.

Variables such as a good match between individual needs and group goals, recognition of functional similarity with other members, and an esprit de corps stemming from having a shared common experience facilitate the development of cohesiveness. You can help promote cohesiveness by guiding the group to establish realistic norms, seeing that they are applied in a consistent manner, and role-modeling respect and acceptance of members' ideas and feelings. Allowing certain members special consideration, however, or not confronting dominating or blocking members who threaten group goals makes the development of cohesion more difficult.

Group Think

Cohesion as a curative factor does have limits. Some groups become too cohesive, and the need to be accepted by the group supersedes critical thinking and realistic objections. In its most extreme form, cohesiveness can exert pressure on members to accept ideas and decisions that are truly incongruent with their personal beliefs and values. Janis (1971) coined the term **group think** to describe a mindless group decision-making process in which the value of group membership becomes so important that opposing opinions or conflicting values and ideas are suppressed in favor of group harmony and consensus. Group members abandon creative problem-solving as a legitimate part of the process. They fail to consider the rights of others to hold different opinions. The costs of disagreeing with the predominant view can be exclusion from the group and the questioning of one's integrity. Those who oppose the majority view are treated as troublemakers, excluded from full participation in decision-making, or ridiculed for their ideas. In either case, the dissenting member feels diminished and becomes silent, leaves the group voluntarily, or is asked to leave. Alternative solutions are simply ignored or dismissed as being unworkable. The group acts on decisions that appear to be consensus but actually do not represent the critical thinking of the group.

Group think is particularly dangerous when a group bands together in rationalizing decisions that are morally wrong or that would adversely affect a given population without their input. The phenomenon is at the base of sorority cliques, and at its extreme, in the group beliefs of the Nazis about their right to persecute the Jews. Characteristics of group think are presented in Table 17–2. Although more prevalent in work and political groups, group think can cause scapegoating in a therapy group.

Frequent reality checks and a leadership style that encourages critical thinking help prevent group think. So does the emergence of constructive conflict as a necessary part of group process. Guiding group members to consider the consequences and implications of their decisions also helps reduce the possibility of group think solutions.

Self-Understanding

Self-understanding, insight and the acceptance of personal responsibility for behavior are important dimensions of the healing process in group psychotherapy. Yalom (1985) emphasizes insight as it relates to interpersonal functioning rather than the etiology of symptoms. While Yalom believes the patient should perceive the link between current behavior and memories of past relationships and experiences, more important is self-understanding of the role one now plays in interpersonal relationships. To remain mentally healthy, each person must strive to face reality without self-deception or loss of self-respect. When thoughts, feelings, words, and actions are consistent with a person's values and with the norms of society, internal consistency leads to well-being. By contrast, mental illness typically involves self-concept distortion. Group psychotherapy helps patients develop insight into their actions, to notice behaviors that otherwise might be overlooked while providing the interpersonal support for individuals to speak the truth about themselves to self and others (Case Example 17–4).

Case Example 17–4 Charles's Story

Charles, a quiet shy group member, told the group that it was up to others to help a person through depression. The group disagreed, pointing out that this placed an unfair burden on others; also that it was not adultlike for the depressed person to abdicate all responsibility. It was then mentioned by the group that Charles's reticence in the meetings was similarly unfair to them. Although Charles seemed to resist the other members' arguments at the

TABLE 17–2 **Characteristics of Group Think**

Attitude	Explanation
Invulnerability	Strong feeling that nothing can interfere with proposal or decisions; minimizing or ignoring danger signals
Rationalization	Developing a unified justification about success; gathering only positive evidence without looking seriously at limitations
Morality	Unquestioned sense of morality without considering the ethical consequences of decisions or impact on people affected by them
Stereotypes	Nonmembers are viewed as weak, nonessential stake holders, stupid or evil; no effort is made to include or consider their position
Pressure	Individual members who disagree with decision are eliminated, ignored, ridiculed, or silenced through social pressures from real opposition
Self-censorship	Individual members do not express their misgivings during the crucial discussion phase
Unanimity	An assumed consensus exists with little basis in reality
Mindguards	Members who have opposing information protect the leader and other group members from hearing information in conflict with the group think decision

From Arnold, E., and Boggs, K. (1995). *Interpersonal relationships: Communication skills for nurses* (p. 266). Philadelphia: W. B. Saunders. Adapted with permission from Janis, I. (1971). Groupthink. *Psychology Today Magazine* 44–46, 74 (November). Copyright © 1971 (Sussex Publishers, Inc).

time, these did appear to have given him insight into how he affected others. His group participation increased greatly following this event.

From Bloch, S., and Crouch, E. (1985). *Therapeutic factors in group psychotherapy*. Oxford: Oxford University Press, p. 29, by permission of Oxford University Press.

Telling the truth about oneself in a group format is easier than it would be otherwise because truth-telling is integrated into the group process. It is an essential characteristic, reinforced as an implicit norm. Group members, by their presence and feedback, remind each other that they are all part of the human condition and that their actions are important. This process often represents a new way of looking at life and one's place in it as an active contributor to its design.

Universality

Universality is the mutual human recognition of common life experiences, conflicts, and emotional reactions. When individuals feel badly about themselves, they automatically assume that no one else could possibly understand or feel as they do. Yet most life circumstances occur with regularity to many people. It is very reassuring to most patients to find that they are not alone and to discover that others have experienced similar problems and feelings. Learning that others feel the same way that they do enables patients to view their own situation with greater objectivity and lessens the sense of shame, aloneness, and isolation. The leader can help foster feelings of universality by linking together different members' reactions to the same issue and by making explicit comparisons around common themes, such as, "John, I'm wondering if what Jane just said about her relationship with her mother strikes any similar cords with you." As one participant, quoted in Bloch and Crouch (1985, p. 189), explained,

I told the group how I sometimes feel unbearably insecure in large groups. I find that I am thinking that anything I say will be stupid so I clam up and say nothing at all. This makes me feel even more inadequate. Both Martin and Anne told me that precisely the same thing happens to them. It was a relief for me to know that others suffer from the same problem.

Altruism

Altruism is different from, but related to, universality. The term refers to the self-recognition of emotional support, reassurance, practical advice, affirmation, of effort that group members offer one another. It is rewarding to understand the plight of another human being and, through that understanding, be a tremendous help and support. Most people experience an increase in self-esteem simply from the act of being helpful. Altruism allows a group member to step outside a personal circle and become involved in the life of another. The process of touching the other through an extension of self usually benefits the giver as well as the receiver (Case Example 17–5).

Case Example 17–5 Yvonne's Story

Yvonne was feeling very depressed and upset. I desperately wanted to help her. After she had said that nobody seemed to find her or what she said interesting, I was able to say to her quite genuinely "You're interesting *to me.*" It was very difficult for me to do this. Since then Yvonne has spent more time on her appearance and seems to be in high spirits. This pleases me very much.

From Bloch, S., and Crouch, E. (1985). *Therapeutic factors in group psychotherapy.* Oxford: Oxford University Press, p. 192, by permission of Oxford University Press.

Altruism is a particularly important curative factor with patients who suffer from low self-esteem and feel they have little to offer others. Usually the help given to another is visible and/or is acknowledged as valuable by the receiver. This reciprocity reinforces the giver's actions. Mutual altruism is a primary factor in mutual help groups and an important element found in 'sponsor' system in Alcoholics Anonymous. This is a mechanism by which those who have achieved sobriety are expected to act as "on call resource support persons," to those who have difficulty maintaining abstinence. The altruistic act of helping the other resist the impulse to drink simultaneously reinforces the helper's resolve to remain sober.

You can facilitate the development of altruism by encouraging members to help other members be more involved with the group. Assign group tasks. In some situations, you might identify altruism if members fail to pick up on it. For example, after a patient makes a supportive remark or demonstrates interest nonverbally, the group leader might comment, "Bob, it sounds to me as if Mary is really trying to 'be there' for you. What does this feel like to you?"

Interpersonal Learning

Interpersonal learning describes people's developing interpersonal skills from one another through observation, feedback, and practice. The small psychodynamic or interpersonal therapy group represents a social microcosm in which patients actually live their experiences in the here and now and receive immediate feedback. When individuals see that other members can express themselves without reprisals or can influence others through their words, the experience can become the impetus to try new communication behaviors, first within the group and then with significant others in their lives. Self-disclosure promotes corrective and supportive feedback. Patients can revisit painful emotional traumas in a safe interpersonal environment and develop more constructive ways of dealing with current interpersonal situations. Patient efforts can be reinforced by strategies such as affirmations and values clarification (Case Example 17–6).

Case Example 17–6 Corinne's Story

Corinne revealed more about herself than she had in the past. I made an effort to understand her since we seem to be on the same wavelength. I came away with more knowledge than ever before. I realized that her talking at cross-purposes with her husband was very similar to my own marital problems. I learned quite a bit from her revelations about the basis for my own troubles with Bob.

From Bloch, S., and Crouch, E. (1985). *Therapeutic factors in group psychotherapy.* Oxford: Oxford University Press, p. 192, by permission of Oxford University Press.

Instillation of Hope

Hope takes many forms but is for members the explicit or implicit belief that participation in a therapeutic group will be beneficial. Most people join therapy and support groups in the hope that they will feel better and be able to conduct their interpersonal lives more effectively. MacKenzie (1990) argues that the sense of hope is what motivates people to continue treatment. Hope is the foundational element in "providing exposure to other therapeutic factors" (p. 40).

Groups awaken hope among members in a number of ways. Within the group context, people see their peers struggle with difficult issues, then see them emerge from the struggle with a new set of coping skills. As members find they can be accepted "just as they are" and that others really care to help them become "all that they can be," they begin to trust the prospect of relationships. Trust and hope, as Erikson points out, are interrelated concepts.

The leader can make hope explicit as a curative factor by commenting on improvements at different stages. For example, you might make a simple statement such as, "Jane, I know that it is hard for you to feel comfortable sharing your experience with the group. I think it is a breakthrough that you were able to share enough so that we can help you with resolving the pain and betrayal you have been feeling for such a long time." You can also prompt member acknowledgement of changes, by stating, "I wonder what others notice about Jane's sharing today."

Identification

Identification occurs when members see implications for themselves in hearing others' stories and watching others struggle and resolve difficult life issues. Individuals see parallels in their own situations and note relevant features of their own circumstances in the dilemmas other group members face. Simultaneously, patients begin to identify with others' efforts to risk new behaviors. Alternative solutions become visible. This curative factor helps patients to relate with one another in ways that are mutually understood and highly satisfying (Case Example 17–7).

Case Example 17–7 Albert's Story

Albert complained that he had not yet learned how to be properly assertive. Sometimes he is too assertive, sometimes too passive. Others reminded him of occasions in the group when he had been both appropriately and inappropriately assertive. Joan identified with Albert's problems and felt the group's work with him was also helping her to understand her own difficulties in "speaking her mind."

From Bloch, S. and Crouch, E. (1985). *Therapeutic factors in group psychotherapy.* Oxford: Oxford University Press, p. 195, by permission of Oxford University Press.

You can encourage identification with comments such as, "Albert, what is it like to hear that Joan can really identify with your situation and appreciates your sharing your experience with the group?" The dialogue used to facilitate identification focuses on here-and-now data that all group members are privy to, thus sharpening the identification. Words are not the only source of identification. Group members view the group leader as a role model; therefore, your therapeutic attitudes of acceptance, unconditional positive regard, empathy, respect, and genuineness are important resources. Even if you are not verbally active, the presence or absence of these therapeutic attitudes will be duly noted by the patient group members. The same is true for the behaviors of other group members. People in groups learn as much from what is caught nonverbally as from what is verbally taught.

Recapitulation of the Primary Family

Group therapy often stimulates a secondary examination of a member's primary family. This curative factor develops because the unconscious paradigm of family dynamics represented by the group offers unique opportunities to work through habitual defenses and maladaptive coping mechanisms. These once may have been needed for survival but now are self-destructive. According to Yalom, the group format prompts memories of the original family constellation, with group members assuming the role of parent and taking sibling positions in the patient's mind.

In a supportive environment, patients begin to recognize their maladaptive patterns of interacting with other people. Other group members help the patient to see a tendency to relive the dynamics of past traumatic relationships in present relationships. Member comments provide significant reality testing, because group members do not know the earlier script and can pose thoughtful questions about intense emotional experiences. Moreover, group members are not bound by the same neutrality as the group leader. Feedback can be very personal. It is more believable when delivered by a peer rather than the leader because it comes from direct experiencing of a similar situation. Consequently, the group can make significant inroads into the patient's defensive structure without incurring the intense rage an individual approach sometimes engenders. Such intimate sharing of experiences and feelings without negative repercussions is a new and healing experience for many patients.

Potential transferences are diluted in group formats. For example, the leader often is thrust into the role of parent by group members. Seeing how others respond positively to the leader can encourage a person to reconsider the possibility that all men (or women) authority figures do not typically respond as his or her father or mother did at an earlier time. Members are able to say to the leader what they were unable to say to their parents and to learn different responses. For certain members, when the leader acknowledges their contribution or constructive effort, it is as if they finally received the sought-after positive comment from their own parent. For example, Bloch and Crouch (1985, p. 30) describe a patient who saw the group leader as a mother figure:

I became very antagonistic to the female therapist, saying that she had not been at all helpful to me. I did not see any point in coming to the group any more. The therapist pointed out that, since my mother died when I was very young, I seemed to be searching for a substitute mother, and I seemed to want her to become my "super mother." I felt this struck a chord in me, and it helped me to explain much about my difficult relationship with women.

Here, as with all of the curative factors, the leader reinforces the presence of the curative factor in helping individual members develop a different attitude about past relationships.

Guidance

One of the primary benefits of a therapy group is the rich opportunity for gaining practical advice and guidance borne of member experiences with similar problems and issues. MacKenzie (1990) notes patient reports of situations in which, "simple instructions to stop destructive behavior or to follow through on socially appropriate action have been quite helpful in moving them through a phase of resistance" (p. 45). Appropriately given, guidance can provide the individual with ideas he or she might not have thought of on his or her own. However, the balance between giving constructive advice or guidance and coercive recommendations that compromise the patient's autonomy is a thin one. Giving guidance needs to be based on the patient's need and readiness to hear the suggestion. Otherwise it will fall on deaf ears. From time to time, you may need to step in when members are telling another patient, "you *should* do . . . ," instead of providing a suggestion that the patient is equally able to reject or accept. A tactful approach is to suggest a number of alternative tactics and to solicit other suggestions or to ask the patient directly how the strategy might need modification. If other group members deliver a "should" message, you might intervene with a simple statement to the patient that several options have been proposed, but "only you can decide what will work for you."

Existential Factors

Yalom (1985) identified existential factors as an important curative consideration. In today's uncertain world, therapy groups often take a broader perspective than simply focusing on personal needs. Human beings are seeking ways to understand and respond to unprecedented threats to human survival. One of the realities of human existence is that what happens to a person is not always fair. Bad things happen to very good people, and good things happen to people who do not seem to deserve them. Here, spiritual support can help a patient work through the meaning. In some cases, the patient may need to work through his or her anger at a God who let this happen. An inescapable existential anxiety about the meaning of life, aloneness, and death accompanies every human being. Mental health involves accepting the finite nature of our human existence and becoming "meaning makers" within the confines of whatever limitations life presents. Journeying with fellow travelers grappling with similar existential issues provides a camaraderie that facilitates inner development and peace in the search for deeper meaning. The interpersonal exchange with other group members about existential issues, not typically discussed in social circles, helps surmount the boundaries of an isolated human existence.

Salience of Individual Curative Factors

Yalom (1985) argues that the value of each curative factor shifts in relation to group development. For example, universality is more important in early group sessions. Later, as members develop confidence and trust each other, interpersonal learning may emerge as more important. A study conducted by Kivlighan and Mullison (1988) using critical incident reports confirmed these findings. In other studies of outpatient groups, cohesion and catharsis emerged as more important than insight (Fuhriman et al, 1986).

Specific diagnoses also influence the importance of one curative factor over another. For example, in group treatments for incest victims (Bonney et al, 1986) and bulimia patients (Hobbs et al, 1989), the highest therapeutic value was placed on self-understanding. Ultimately, a particular group personality and the specific needs of members determine the therapeutic factors that become most important. Very clear, however, is the consistency with which most of these curative factors are present in effective groups.

Role Functions

Leader Functions

The role of the leader in group treatment is not one simply of neutral observer or facilitator of the action. Part of the healing process involves members' getting to know you as a real person. Group members need to be able to experience you as compassionate, trustworthy, and competent. Effective leaders are sensitive to their own feelings and concerns as they emerge within the context of the group. Self-awareness allows you to keep the necessary rein on personal feelings and to act as an objective participant observer. You need not completely suppress personal feelings. In fact, it often is important to bring them forward in ways that help group members clarify concerns and feelings in the group. Expression of feeling can counteract group projections, but only if it relates to the concerns and feelings of the group members, not solely your own. For example, you might say to a highly resistant group, "I know this is frustrating for you to feel so stuck, and I share your frustration. Any ideas what we might do about it?"

The role of leader in a psychotherapy group is one of *conductor* and *artist.* As conductor, you are constantly aware of the structure that the group needs, and you provide it. For example, psychotic patients need structured leadership. Those with intact interpersonal skills require a less directive leadership style. You are responsible for ensuring that the boundaries of the group are intact and that the group is moving toward achievement of group goals.

The artistry of leadership is reflected in how you promote a spontaneous, interpersonal flow of communication among group members. It involves knowing when to confront and when to use a more laid-back approach, when to comfort and when to take a stern stand about an issue. As with individual formats, therapeutic use of self becomes the primary tool (see Chapter 11). You, together with group members, act as a cheerleading section, applauding member efforts, and offer corrections in direction when the travelers stray off course. Group members can share leadership responsibilities with you as the group progresses. The continued presence of a caring, competent leader who reinforces member feedback equips patients to become primary therapists for each other.

Coleadership

Coleadership refers to an equal peer relationship in which two professional leaders assume shared responsibility for the conduct of the group. There are many advantages to coleadership, but one of the most important is having someone available to process the group after each session. An equally informed and competent member who has shared in the same experience can be extremely valuable. The opportunity to share insights about the group process is an important source of clarification and support. Coleadership is particularly relevant in large groups. An old "rule of thumb" is to insist on a coleader for groups having 10 or more members.

Within the group itself, coleadership is useful in picking up on issues and feelings that the other leader may have missed. The coleader can bring an issue forward directly or can cue the leader to its presence nonverbally. If one leader makes a mistake in processing, the other can correct it and model for group members that differences in opinion and personal reactions need not be destructive. Patients sometimes split the coleaders into polarities—nurturing versus harsh, bumbling versus competent. Whereas the leader under attack cannot always respond directly without appearing defensive, the coleader can redirect the transference focus without incurring the rage of the patient. This can be done with a statement such as, "It seems as though you are having a great deal of conflict with your feelings about Joan [group leader]. Any ideas what that is about?"

Cotherapy potentially is a growth experience for the therapists involved, as well as for the group. The two leaders can learn from each other, and in a sense, the coleadership experience becomes one of peer supervision. However, it also is hard work because it demands a high level of trust between the leaders. Philosophically, leaders who choose to work together should be in agreement, although their basic communication style may differ. Ideally, their individual communication styles will complement rather than mirror or conflict with each other. As equal partners in developing and responding to group process issues, the coleaders need to establish norms of openness, honesty, and respect for each other's opinions even when they disagree about how something should be handled. This format works best when the leaders involved have basically the same value orientations and operate from different strengths and sensitivities but genuinely respect their differences. Sufficient time for pre- and postgroup sessions allows the necessary dialogue to occur. New strategies or a different course of action should be discussed between the coleaders before being implemented in the group. When properly implemented, cotherapy offers the group a rich and diverse interpersonal experience.

Establishing the Group Culture

Initially, the primary task of the leader is to establish a safe, supportive, working environment in which patients can feel comfortable addressing personal issues. Yalom (1985) suggests that the leader is responsible for establishing a group "culture" in which norms support members taking responsibility for their actions and using the group to experiment with different ways of behaving with others. As they begin to take interpersonal risks with one another, members are better able to generalize their actions to interpersonal situations in their outside lives.

Once the group is underway, you can employ many of the same strategies of active listening presented in Chapter 10. Above all, you should maintain the same sensitive, reflective, and respectful attitude. Group culture also describes the therapeutic relationships with the group. It is important to discuss content in the context of the group as a whole and in relation to specific group members. Group issues include anxiety that initial meetings arouse, the effect of premature termination, leader or member absence, and the shut-down of emotion that often occurs in a meeting following one of deep personal disclosure.

Giving Feedback

You need to be simultaneously aware of shifts in the group's attention, multiple patterns of interaction (i.e., who withdraws or interrupts and around what situations, how members respond to confrontation or praise, which patients are supported, and which are challenged). The artistry of group therapy will determine which of the multiple ways to respond you can use effectively. You need to determine whether to intervene on an individual level, e.g., "Jack, I notice that you clammed up when Bob got angry with Jill," or to make a group-focused comment, e.g., "Bob and Jill seem to be hopelessly deadlocked around this issue; how do group members perceive they might handle this in a better way?" Comments about group participation as a whole provide another way of responding, e.g., "People seem hesitant to express their opinion about what is going on in group today; it might be important to explore what is going on here." One-sentence statements usually are more effective than more lengthy discourse.

Providing effective feedback for group members becomes the shared responsibility of you and the members. In general, feedback that is clear, immediate, and relevant to the issue under discussion is most effective (Rothke, 1989). It becomes more difficult to discount if the sender delivers the message as an "I" message. For example, you might say to a defensive member, "I am feeling left out of your conversation about your son's drug habit because there isn't any room for me to tell you what I think might be helpful."

Activating the Here and Now

Reflection related to what is happening interpersonally in the group, as it is actually occurring, provides significant information that deserves careful attention. A here-and-now approach helps members reflect on the meaning of their communication patterns. This experiential movement simultaneously allows members to learn constructive ways to handle affectively laden material in a supervised therapeutic environment. Noting changes in response to content and nonverbal reactions to other patients involved with the discussion can facilitate here-and-now interaction about the theme. You can assist members to assess their own, and other patient's vulnerability or readiness to hear an interpretation. Modeling respectful confrontation marked by appropriate choice of words, and proper assessment of timing keeps the dialogue within a supportive framework and helps move the group to a deep level of engagement (Case Example 17–8).

Case Example 17–8 Martha's Story

Martha Brownell is a 58-year-old patient who has just finished a long discourse on how lonely and depressed she has been since her husband died a year ago. The group is silent, and Martha does not seem to have benefited from her catharsis. At this point the leader might suggest to Martha, "Martha, I wonder if it might be helpful for you to explore how you are experiencing a sense of loneliness and social isolation right here in the group, Is this something you think you might be able to do?" By bringing the theme of loneliness and social isolation into the present situation, the group leader makes it a concrete issue that the group members can work with directly. Otherwise group members have knowledge of the patient's experience only as an abstract circumstance in which they can play a limited role.

Member Role Functions

Group member role functions are those behaviors a person demonstrates in the group related to achieving group goals and morale that facilitate group achievement and satisfaction. Role functions ideally advance the goals of the group. Successful group functioning depends on members striking a balance between task and maintenance role functions. **Task role functions** refer to those directly associated with task completion. Members assuming task roles are concerned with helping the group stay on course with the group task. They generate new ideas, stimulate discussion about issues, and identify strategies needed for goal achievement. By contrast, **maintenance role functions** help sustain member interest and personal involvement in achieving group goals. Members assuming maintenance functions are concerned with the morale of the group. They are sensitive to individual needs for inclusion and emotional support. Consequently, their contributions to group interaction focus on areas of agreement and resolution of conflict. Issues of respect and group cohesiveness depend on members willing to assume maintenance role functions (Box 17–2).

A balance between task and maintenance role functions produces an intellectually stimulating and emotionally satisfying capacity to achieve desired outcomes, while providing information mechanisms that allow members to remain committed and satisfied with the process. Without a focus on task (goal) achievement, group life suffers because the rationale for its existence is unclear. Yet without attention to the relations between members, the task becomes sterile and burdensome. Although group members do assume different roles in a group, usually some members are more attuned to task role functions and others to maintenance roles.

Benne and Sheats (1948) identify a maladaptive set of group roles, **self-roles,** which are nonfunctional and destructive to group life (Table 17–3). Self-roles gratify individual concerns but fail to account for the needs of the group as a whole. In doing so, they tend to splinter group interaction. Self-roles emerge when members get caught up with their own needs and are unable to contribute fully to overall goals. Moreover, their contributions tend to distract the rest of the group from its task (Case Example 17–9). Other group members typically experience these members as annoying and tend to discount their contributions as irrelevant.

BOX 17–2 Task and Maintenance Role Functions in Group Relations

Task Role Functions: Behaviors Relevant to the Attainment of Group Goals

Initiating: Identifies tasks or goals; defines group problem; suggests relevant strategies for solving problem.

Seeking information or opinion: Requests facts from other members; asks other members for opinions; seeks suggestions or ideas for task accomplishment.

Giving information or opinion: Offers facts to other members; provides useful information about group concerns.

Clarifying elaborating: Interprets ideas or suggestions placed before group; paraphrases key ideas; defines terms; adds information.

Summarizing: Pulls related ideas together; restates key ideas; offers a group solution or suggestion for other members to accept or reject.

Consensus-Taking: Checks to see if group has reached a conclusion; asks group to test a possible decision.

Group Role Maintenance Tasks: Behaviors That Help the Group Maintain Harmonious Working Relationships

Harmonizing: Attempts to reconcile disagreements; helps members reduce conflict and explore differences in a constructive manner.

Gatekeeping: Helps keep communication channels open; points out commonalities in remarks; suggests approaches that permit greater sharing.

Encouraging: Indicates by words and body language unconditional acceptance of others; agrees with contributions of other group members; is warm, friendly, and responsive to other group members.

Compromising: Admits mistakes; offers a concession when appropriate; modifies position in the interest of group cohesion.

Standard-setting: Calls for the group to reassess or confirm implicit and explicit group norms when appropriate.

Every group needs both types of functions and needs to work out a satisfactory balance of task and maintenance activity.

From Rogers, C. (1972). The process of the basic encounter group. In R. Diedrich and H. A. Dye (Eds.), *Group procedures: Purposes, processes and outcomes.* Boston: Houghton Mifflin.

TABLE 17–3 Nonfunctional Self-Roles

Role	Behavior
Aggressor	Criticizes or blames others. Personally attacks other members. Uses sarcasm and hostility in interations.
Blocker	Instantly rejects ideas or argues an idea to death. Cites tangential ideas and opinions. Obstructs decision-making.
Joker	Disrupts work of the group by constantly joking and refusing to take group task seriously.
Avoider	Whispers to others, daydreams, doodles, acts indifferent and passive.
Self-confessor	Uses the group to express personal views and feelings unrelated to group task.
Recognition seeker	Seeks attention by excessive talking, trying to gain leader's favor, expressing extreme ideas, or demonstrating peculiar behavior.

From Arnold, E., and Boggs, K. (1995). *Interpersonal relationships: Communication skills for nurses* (2nd ed) (p. 269); developed from Benne, K. D., and Sheats, P. (1948). Functional roles of group members. *Journal of Social Issues*, 4 (2), 41–49.

Case Example 17–9 Jean's Story

Jean Murphy is a 36-year-old woman who entered group therapy because of a troubled marriage and her son's arrest for marijuana possession. She monopolized the group sessions with her dissatisfaction about most things in her life. Although other group members tried to engage her in working on these issues, Jean refused to consider their suggestions while maintaining that her own desires and interests were consistently ignored. Finally, the group leader asked other group members directly for their feedback about Jean's behavior, saying "What has your experience of Jean's dilemma been like today?" The leader also asked Jean to consider how she was ignoring the group's input as a corollary to the way she perceived others acting towards her. Jean was angry at first, but she began to realize that she perpetuated her own problems in some ways by not listening to suggestions or considering others' needs when they were different from her own. As she became better able to align her personal goals with group goals, she was able to check herself when her anxiety tempted her to monopolize the group's attention. Laughingly she would say, "There I go again."

Behaviors associated with maladaptive self-roles include monopolization, withdrawal from group dialogue, constant joking, and verbal attacks on the leader or other group members. If the group member displaying self-role behavior can be persuaded to drop the personal agenda in favor of the group's work, the behavior can sometimes benefit the group. In all other cases, self-roles prove destructive both for the individual and for the group as a whole. In Case Example 17–9, the leader was able to help Jean become a participant observer of her own behavior. Her willingness to reexamine her behavior earned her the respect and support of her peers, which reinforced her desire to learn different, more productive behaviors.

▶ Check Your Reading

7. What is the significance of curative factors in group psychotherapy?
8. How do task and maintenance role functions work together to support group goals?
9. What are the necessary elements of successful coleadership?
10. What is group think? Why is it potentially so dangerous?

COMMON COMMUNICATION PROBLEMS IN GROUP PSYCHOTHERAPY

Certain communication problems occur more commonly in group situations than in other treatment modalities.

Scapegoating

Scapegoating represents group projection of an undesired characteristic onto a single member or social condition. Those who scapegoat act as if the offending member is the sole possessor of the characteristic. Projection can relate to sexual or power issues, noncompliance, or undesired personal characteristics. Scapegoating is always a group issue, despite its focus on a single object. Behaviors that indicate scapegoating include disregarding the presence of a member, making snide remarks, or discounting the member's contributions. Often the person being scapegoated is a little different from other group members in behavior, physical appearance, level of assertiveness, or verbal abilities. The human scapegoat implicitly colludes with the other group members to maintain the projection (Case Example 17–10).

Case Example 17–10 Betty's Story

Betty is a 16-year-old in an adolescent psychotherapy group. She is a little overweight but not dramatically so. Other group members dress in ways that are becoming, but Betty chooses to wear no makeup and to dress like a tomboy in drab, ill-fitting clothing. When Betty enters the room, the other girls either do not pay any attention to her or snicker when she sits down. They tell her she should lose weight and have little sympathy for her big-boned physique. Betty does not speak often. When she does, the other group members either disagree with her or discount what she is saying.

After several weeks of this interactive behavior, the group leader asked Betty if she could tell the group what the group was like for her. As Betty described how uncomfortable she felt, the leader asked other group members if they could share what it was like for them when they did not quite fit in with a particular group. Broadening Betty's feelings into a group theme helped all the group members own the undesired emotion and took the pressure off Betty as its sole repository.

MacKenzie (1990) suggests that "a variant on this process is for the group to agree on an external source of the problem. This may be a collective agreement that men are the problem in a group of women or that the school system is the problem in a group of parents" (p. 153). Unless the problem can become a group issue and is owned by the group, the group projection will continue to be a source of conflict without the possibility of resolution.

Scapegoating can be handled in several ways. You may choose to ask the group, "Why is this an issue? Is it possible that the group's annoyance with Jack relates to something deeper that the group needs to address?" Another strategy is for the leader to pair for a short time with the scapegoat with a statement such as, "Jack may be a little too strong on this issue, but he may be raising an important point that the group needs to address." Still another way to handle scapegoating is to ask the individual directly about the experience of group censure, e.g., "Jack, the group seems pretty disturbed by. . . . I wonder how you are experiencing their comments?" The scapegoat, while appearing aggressive or comfortable with his or her position, often can state how he or she really feels. A follow-up exploration of the member responses to the scapegoat's revelations results in greater group ownership of the problem. Without any intervention, the scapegoated member is most likely to drop out of the group.

Monopolizing

Sometimes, a member will monopolize the group's attention with personal data that grabs attention but forces the group to digress from its purpose. When monopolizing occurs and the group has tried but seems unable to confront the issue, you may have to take a more proactive stance. Tactful confrontation not only can help the member take a different position but also can serve as an important role-modeling technique.

You can make a transitional statement such as, "What you are saying clearly is very important to you, but I'm wondering how others are feeling right now in listening to you. I think it might be helpful to hear their feedback." Or "You are making an interesting point, but I think we need to move on so that everyone will have a chance tonight. Is that ok with you?" Another way to deflect the monopolizer is to throw a comment into the group such as "I wonder if others in the group share Bob's perception that . . . ?" If none of these comments works, you may need to set limits directly: "Bob, what you are saying here obviously is important to you, but it doesn't really fit with the purpose of our group, so I'm going to have to ask you to stop and let the group move on in a different direction."

Member Conflicts

Expression of negative feelings is grist for the group mill, but expression of anger without reflection from which all can learn can be damaging to the group and the self-esteem of members. You can help diffuse anger and personal attacks on group members—and yourself—by remaining calm and treating the feelings as important pieces of information. Negativity indicates feelings rather than specific commentary about individuals. Treating explosive or defensive feelings as neither right nor wrong but as an expression of differences that may be important for group life can be an important source of learning. Members learn that agreement is not always necessary, that people can have entirely different perspectives and can draw radically distinct conclusions about the same phenomena. This recognition is important for successful negotiation of conflict, in the group and in life.

SPECIAL TYPES OF GROUPS

Cognitive Behavioral Groups

Cognitive behavioral therapy groups build on behavioral principles (presented in Chapter 18). At the high end of the functional spectrum, these groups assist patients with distorted thinking patterns that threaten successful functioning. Patients help one another recognize crooked thinking patterns and begin to replace them with more productive ways of relating. Cognitive behavioral strategies use task assignments, modeling, role-playing, and assertiveness training to help individuals take charge of their lives. At the lower end of the functional spectrum are social skills training for patients with serious deficits. Steps in the group process are presented in Box 17–3.

Groups for the Chronically Mentally Ill

Chronically mentally ill patients usually need more flexible group boundaries regarding attendance. Many need more reminders to attend. Group participation with lower-functioning patients can appear erratic, but a smaller core of patients often attends on a regular basis, with a peripheral subgroup attending irregularly (DeBosset, 1982; McIntosh et al, 1991). More peripheral members may appear not to be as involved but if asked, these members would state that they considered themselves a regular part of the group, despite the irregularity of their attendance. Regular members would agree.

Psychotic patients, even after they have been stabilized with medication, frequently talk in metaphor about their experience. Their limited emotional responsiveness and peculiar language make it difficult for the therapist and other members to decode their conversation. Their speech may seem to have no meaningful connection with the situation at hand, or the patients may use repetitive phrases. Remember that verbalized thoughts, while out of context in ordinary conversation, have meaning and connection with the patients' experience of the current situation. Their meaning lies in the concrete, specific, personal experiential life of the patient rather than on those meanings more routinely encountered in poetry or analogy. Typically, the psychotic patient's seemingly unconnected remarks are deemed irrelevant. The person uttering them tends also to be dismissed psychologically, thereby adding to social isolation.

The personal metaphors of the mentally ill can take on common meaning for the whole group if you recognize symbolic expressions and translate metaphors into here-and-now language the group can respond to effectively. Inevitably, you will find clues to private meanings and relation to the patient's experience. Other members can sometimes decode a patient's meaning, but more often, you need to consider all the possible (and tangential) meanings of a word in trying to make sense of a metaphor. Once patients' symbols are understood, their communication makes sense and typically contributes to understanding important themes.

In Case Example 17–11, the therapist took the patient's metaphor and brought it into the group for discussion. The group used the metaphor, stimulated by the therapist's absence, to explore the meaning of anger to these patients and how they handled it. Opportunities to consider alternative meanings of the underlying theme suggested in the patient's metaphor, rather than its explicit content, promoted fascinating group solutions.

BOX 17–3 Applications of Cognitive-Behavioral Group Psychotherapy in Social Skills Training

1. Discuss the rationale for the procedures, provide examples, and ask for feedback before implementing.
2. Ask participants to help set goals and discuss ways they can be achieved.
3. Ask members to provide each participant suggestions to finalize the agreed-upon strategy for goal achievement.
4. If needed, you or a group member demonstrates the desired behavior.
5. Each patient practices or rehearses the agreed-upon behaviors. Should a patient experience difficulty in implementation, coach this patient until he or she is able to do the action independently. Coaching is then discontinued.
6. The patient receives "homework" assignments to reinforce the new learning outside the group situation.

Case Example 17–11 One Patient's Story

In one group after the therapist's absence, one of the schizophrenic members reported a dream in which her father adopted a younger sister "who was just like me until she became violent and blew up a building" (similar to the one in which the group met) because she had become angry with her father. The patient had no thoughts about the dream. The therapist asked what the others thought, and the response was a series of associations to mistreatment by parents or authority figures. The therapist wondered how they could let parents know that they had been hurt. This led to a lively discussion of their helplessness as children and several members' animated illustrations of their successes in standing up to mistreatment. The angry feelings directed at the therapist were not explored. The dream was used to explore adaptive solutions.

From Alonso, A., and Swiller, H. (1992). *Group therapy in clinical practice* (pp. 86, 87). Washington, D.C.: American Psychiatric Press.

With the chronically mentally ill, you will need to be much more proactive, eliciting comments from patients and making the linkages. To accomplish group goals, you may have to employ a variety of activities and provide direct instructions on how to respond. Appreciation of the difficulty that psychotic and low-functioning patients have with abstract data and processing abilities helps you use concrete language and frequent interpretations of member dialogue. The role-modeling such patients see in you helps them become clearer in their own communication. Small tangible rewards, such as coffee served at the end of the session, may be necessary to increase motivation.

Support/Mutual Help Groups

Lock (1986) defines a self-help support group as "a voluntary organization, usually of peers, who have come together for mutual help and support in satisfying a common need, overcoming a common handicap or life-disrupting problem, and bringing about desired or personal change, or both" (p. 1596). Support groups are problem specific and situation or symptom focused. They are organized to provide emotional support and practical advice to others with the same problem or a similar life issue. Originally developed in response to shrinking resources for health care, particularly for supportive care for patients and families coping with a chronic illness, support/mutual help groups are likely to become increasingly important. Capitated care and privatizing of publicly funded mental health care mean that these groups

TABLE 17–4 Essential Characteristics of Self-Help/Mutual Support Groups

Characteristic	Typical Pattern
Criteria for membership	Common problem, predicament, or illness
Purpose	To provide emotional and other support through sharing of personal lived experience as well as exchanging other resources
Structure	Nonhierarchal, voluntary association: • Members give and receive from each other as facilitators of each other's healing • Reciprocal, no-fee relationship, rather than a contractual relationship based on fees for services rendered
Role functions	Members take responsibility and actions to resolve their problem issues (self-help) Group members help each other with practical advice and support (mutual aid)

Developed from Borkman, T. (1991). Introduction to the special issue: Self-help groups. *American Journal of Community Psychology*, 19 (5), 643–649.

may be some people's only link with such support. Some support groups are short term, but most are designed as long-term, open-ended groups with loose boundaries. Because group members, including the leader, typically have personal experience with the problem, they bring an authenticity that is difficult to match in most group formats. Joining with others who have experienced similar difficulties is a source of unparalled support. Mutual help groups are organized around universality as a healing factor in coping with chronic disease and shameful feelings. The group becomes a reference point to which individuals can return time after time, drawing support, understanding, and practical advice about how to handle difficult situations. (Table 17–4).

Meetings can be held in any regularly established site, in a variety of settings, from hospitals to public libraries and churches. At the beginning of each meeting, briefly introduce the purpose of the group and ask members to introduce themselves. Each describes a bit about his or her situation. A sample format is presented in Table 17–5.

Some meetings may be designated as topic meetings and feature special themes such as legal issues. Meetings may be followed by a question-and-answer period. Light refreshments are sometimes served, and the meetings are open to all individuals with similar concerns. Unlike formal psychotherapy groups, no fee is required for service, and the leadership responsibility falls on volunteers, who may or may not have formal training. Hepworth and Larsen (1986) note that a particularly effective and unique aspect of such groups is that "self-help groups generally have effective communication networks among members that, in addition to regular

TABLE 17–5 Sample Format for Leaders of Support Groups

Procedure	Sample Statements
1. Introduce self	"I am Christy Atkins, a staff nurse on the unit, and I am going to be your group facilitator tonight."
2. Explain purpose of the group	"Our goal in having the group is to provide a place for family members to get support from each other and to provide practical information to families caring for Alzheimer victims."
3. Identify norms	"We have three basic rules in this group: we respect each other's feelings; we don't preach or tell you how to do something; and the meetings are confidential; everything of a personal nature stays in this room."
4. Ask each member to identify self and something about his or her situation	"I'd like to go around the room and ask each of you to tell us your name and something about your situation."
5. Link common themes	"It seems as if feeling powerless and out of control is a common theme tonight. What strategies have you found help you to feel more in control?"
6. Allow time for informal networking (optional)	Providing a 10-minute break with or without refreshments allows members to talk informally with each other.
7. Provide closure	"Now I'd like to go around the room and ask each of you to identify one thing you will do in the next week for yourself to help you feel more in control."

From Arnold, E., and Boggs, K. (1995). *Interpersonal relationships: Professional communication skills for nurses* (p. 288). Philadelphia: W. B. Saunders.

group meetings, provide opportunities for both telephone and face-to-face contacts" (p. 549). Examples of mutual help/support groups are identified in Table 17–6.

Psychodrama

Psychodrama is a kind of action-oriented therapy. It is a therapeutic tool through which the individual acts out problems and concerns in life. The therapeutic goal "is not to analyze the patient, but to help him dream again" (Moreno, 1964). Moreno felt that traditional methods of group psychotherapy did not allow patients to really get in touch with their feelings, which they described but did not reexperience. The focus on description of feelings, he believed, limited the patient to the illness rather than to the healing possibilities in a situation. Through active participation in psychodrama, patients could get in touch with the more imaginative sides of themselves and develop strategies that they might not otherwise think of (Table 17–7).

With psychodrama, the patient (protagonist) is brought directly into the situation as an active participant. The director coordinates the process so that the group and the protagonist (the person portraying the problem) receive maximum benefit. Other group members act as auxiliary egos or play the roles of significant others with whom relationships are being explored. The action takes place as if it is unfolding in the present, even if the incident took place many years ago (Moreno, 1978). The primary advantages of psychodrama are its direct access to reenacting painful situations and the potential for learning new responses in a safe therapeutic environment. Its purpose is to promote a therapeutic environment where the individual's spontaneity may be rekindled and guided toward insightful, responsible, creative living (Vander-May and Peake, 1980, p. 27). Psychodrama is action oriented and uses a format more symbolic than in other forms of therapy. With psychodrama, participants can become emotionally involved observers in their own and others' scenarios.

Warm-Up

The here-and-now quality of psychodrama can produce initial anxiety. Careful preparation of the patient and enough time for warming up the group are essential. Describe the purposes of psychodrama and let patients know that they have control over the setting of the scene. Patients should be reassured that most people initially experience anxiety but that anxiety typically abates as the enactment progresses.

Setting the scene is part of the warm-up, which allows the protagonist time to get acquainted with the format and others who will take part in the psychodrama. The same rules about confidentiality that apply to other therapeutic relationships and explanations of what will be placed in the patient's chart apply to psychodrama.

A double is used when the protagonist has difficulty expressing feelings about all or part of the situation. Doubles can be used for the duration of the session or to add emphasis and clarity to certain ideas. The double might return to his or her original seat once the issue is fully developed. The double mimics the protagonist's body posture and gestures and puts into words the feelings suggested in the protagonist's description. The individual playing the role double can be a group member, a staff member, or the director. By reinforcing appropriate feelings or strengthening the focus on an issue, the

TABLE 17–6 **Examples of Mutual Help/Support Groups**

Name of Group	Population Served
Candlelighters	Families of children with cancer
Make Today Count	People with cancer and their families
Compassionate Friends	People who have lost a significant person through death
Alcoholics Anonymous	Adult alcoholics
Al-anon	Spouses and significant others involved with the alcoholic
Alateen	Adolescent children of alcoholics
ACOA (Adult Children of Alcoholics)	Adult children of alcoholics
Narcotics Anonymous	Adults with a drug problem
Fly without Fear	People with phobias about flying
Overeaters Anonymous	People with a significant weight problem
Gam-Anon	Families of gamblers
Parents Anonymous	Parents who abuse their children
NAMI (National Alliance for Mental Illness)	Family members of the mentally ill
Resolve	Infertile people and couples
National Conference of Stutterers	People who stutter

TABLE 17–7 **Psychodrama Techniques**

Task	Procedure
Setting the scene	The protagonist chooses and sets the scene by describing what is happening. Strategic questions include "Where did this situation occur?" "Who was with you at the time?" "What did they say to you?" "Where were the other people who were with you?"
Role reversals	Role reversals are conducted by the director. Moreno (1964) believed that the protagonist should take the role of all significant persons so that distortions may be explored and reintegrated.
Soliloquy and aside	The actor or actress speaks aloud the thoughts and feelings that usually go unspoken.
Doubling	The double becomes an auxiliary ego that represents a part or parts of the protagonist.
Concretization	Concretization makes visible through deliberate action and visual stimuli what otherwise exists only as symbol or feeling. For example, an authority figure might be placed on a higher level than the protagonist, or physically hanging onto someone can represent clinging behaviors (VanderMay and Peake, 1980).
Mirroring	Mirroring is similar to the role of double, except that the auxiliary ego actually replaces the protagonist in the scene and mirrors observed behavior. By observing an auxiliary ego acting out his or her own situation, the protagonist frequently is able to develop alternative solutions that were unavailable when he or she was enmeshed in his or her own situation.
Self-counseling	Self-counseling requires the protagonist to take the role of counselor to the individual playing his or her auxiliary ego. The protagonist gains enough distance to reality-test resistances, and offers practical solutions to his or her auxiliary ego. The result is greater insight about what might work in his or her own situation.

protagonist can deepen the meaning or develop new understandings of a situation.

For example, Sacks (1993) suggests the following sequencing of a scenario. The *protagonist* might say, "My mother went to the A&P and bought those stupid kiwis for a dollar each. Then she came back and paid the mortgage three weeks before it was even due. Then she bought this big stupid thing that. . . ." The double might respond, "She *always* throws her money away, and it drives me crazy" (p. 217). Psychodrama is a very intense form of group psychotherapy for the protagonist. Periodically asking the protagonist how he or she is doing is essential. This brief questioning allows the patient to reflect on what is happening and to make necessary corrections if the process is too intense.

Achieving Closure

Another critical dimension of the psychodrama process is achieving closure. Because of the often powerful feelings that emerge from a psychodrama session, you have an ethical and therapeutic responsibility to allow enough time for closure and to provide for follow-up support with unit personnel, if warranted. Otherwise, an individual can have a powerful experience but little opportunity to integrate it into other parts of life or to consider the meaning of uncomfortable feelings associated with the psychodrama encounter.

GROUPS FOR THE ELDERLY

Group psychotherapy for the elderly has become an increasingly important treatment modality in recent years, particularly for depressed patients. Burnside and Schmidt (1995) have authored an excellent text on group work with the elderly for those that might be interested in working as group therapists with this segment of the population. Special modifications of group strategies for the elderly include a slower pacing of interventions, taking into consideration the longer reaction or processing time typically associated with aging. Allowing extra time for members to assemble and holding groups during daylight hours when sensory attributes are highest and patients typically have more energy are significant to patient enjoyment and participation.

Burnside and Haight (1994) note that the total population in the year 2030 will include 60 million people over the age of 65, roughly 20% of the population, with those over 85 compromising the fastest-growing segment of the population. Validation, life review, and reminiscence groups are beneficial formats for the elderly. They provide a scheduled social environment at a time when the elderly traveler's social connections typically are shrinking. They offer an opportunity for people to reframe earlier life experiences in a more positive light (White and Ingersoll-Dayton, 1989).

Reminiscence groups allow members to revisit past times and see that while some of those times were unfortunate, they responded to them in the only way possible at the time. Developed as an experience rather than as the human failing of an individual member, life review can rework past traumas. Burnside and Haight (1994) submit that "reminiscence provokes shared feelings and boosts self-esteem while the group process produces validation for each member. . . . Often members not only affirm their own lives, but in an interesting parallel process, they affirm others in the group" (p. 56). As individual members share their feelings, a sense of universality emerges. It becomes clear that most experiences are not completely unique and can be enjoyed by all members.

The elderly typically respond better to a reminiscence group than to one focused on current events. This trend matches Erikson's characterizing this stage as integrity versus despair over the conduct of one's life. Fielden (1990) describes two types of group intervention with elderly patients, one using slides and current discussion of health issues from a here-and-now perspective, and the other employing a reminiscence format. Slides, pictures, and audio helped participants discuss their reminiscences. Members were encouraged to bring personal mementos to the meetings. Results of the study indicated significant improvement in communication among the reminiscence group but no significant change in members of the here-and-now group. Similar findings about reminiscence groups were reported by Lappe (1987), who found that patients involved in a reminiscence group demonstrated higher self-esteem than those in here-and-now groups.

Leading a reminiscence group does not require special training other than a knowledge of basic group dynamics. The group focuses on patients' perceptions of life events, not on intrapsychic dynamics. Patience, understanding of aging, and a healthy respect for the elderly traveler are relevant skills. Box 17–4 provides guidelines for leading a reminiscence group.

Reality Orientation Groups

Reality orientation groups are used with cognitively impaired patients. The therapist meets with a group of four to six patients for 20 to 30 minutes daily, depending on the patient's attention span. The leader assumes a directive role and addresses each patient by name before introducing simple information about the date, season of the year, time, weather, menu for the day, and common object recognition. Each patient is expected to respond. Correct responses are rewarded with praise and sometimes by checks on a board. Although the questions may seem tedious, they are quite effective with seriously regressed patients in keeping them from total passivity and withdrawal from unit life.

Remotivation Groups

Remotivation groups were initiated in the 1960s by Dorothy Hoskins Smith in a Pennsylvania State Hospital. She used a five-step process centered around the introduction of nonthreatening material such as poetry or pictures of trees and plants to reach the still-intact portions of a person's experiences (Table 17–8).

After an introduction and asking each patient's name, the therapist introduces the object for discussion; for example, an apple and a picture of an apple tree. Each

BOX 17–4 Guidelines for Leading Reminiscence Groups

Before the Group Begins

1. Identify possible group outcomes to share with group members.
2. Obtain administrative permission to conduct the group.
3. Assess member capacity to contribute and derive benefit from group.
4. Identify primary themes, and alternate ones for use if the first theme is unsuccessful.
5. Select appropriate props to trigger memories. Props should be situation and gender appropriate. Introduce props one at a time to prevent sensory overload.
6. Set up the room beforehand, making accommodations for special limitations.
7. Make name tags for each group member.

Beginning the Group

1. Introduce yourself and explain the purpose of the group.
2. State the norms, i.e., confidentiality, sharing what they feel comfortable with disclosing, dates and time of the group. (Should be held at the same time on the same day each week.)

Conducting the Reminiscence Group

1. Select a theme; for example, first job, most satisfying experience, birth of first child. If a prop is used, this can be passed around the group. Sometimes, you can share a memory that triggers discussion if the group seems reluctant to develop one.
2. Use reflective open-ended questions such as, "Does what Martha says about her experience with . . . remind you of anything?" and linking statements such as, "It sounds as if Martha's experience of . . . is similar to what others in this group have experienced," to facilitate discussion.
3. Refreshments can enhance the social aspects of the reminiscence group. If used, they should be nutritious, simple to eat, and provided at the beginning or end of the meeting to ensure full concentration during the session.
4. Acknowledge each person's contribution, and encourage each member to provide at least one memory. If an individual is unable to do this, the leader can make a simple comment such as, "It's OK not to share right now, but we would like to hear your ideas if you would feel comfortable sharing later." This strategy reinforces the expectation of sharing without placing undue pressure on the member.

Ending the Meeting

1. Shake hands with each member and thank him or her individually for coming.
2. Record salient issues and patient responses in the patient record.
3. Share observations with other members of the interdisciplinary health care team.

Data developed from Burnside, I., and Haight, B. (1994). Reminiscence and life review: Therapeutic interventions for older people. *Nurse Practitioner, 19* (4), 55–61.

TABLE 17–8 **Guidelines for Leading Remotivation Groups**

Strategy	Introductory Comment
1. Welcome and greet each group member by name	"Welcome, Mary, I'm so glad you could join us today."
2. Provide a bridge with the introduction of a simple, universal topic	"Today, we are going to talk about the spring season. This is a time when the weather begins to be warm, and plants begin to bloom."
3. Develop the topic through use of props, pictures, and simple questions	"I have some pictures of things that happen in the spring on this felt board." (Discussion, followed by another introductory comment.) "Can you think of anything else that happens in the spring?"
4. Encourage personal reflections about the topic	"I wonder if any of you would be willing to share with us your favorite memory of spring?"
5. Thank each member personally for coming to the group, and specifically mention his or her contribution	"Mary, I want to thank you for coming to the group, and for telling us about your lilac bush. It helped me remember how beautiful the lilac really is."

patient is asked to talk about the object. The therapist acknowledges each person's contribution and ends the group by thanking each member for attending.

ACTIVITY GROUPS

Activity groups are an outgrowth of Slavson's (see Chapter 6) earlier work in which he used situational actions to help patients develop more constructive social skills. Still one of the best treatment modalities for use with behaviorally disordered children and adolescents, activity groups have also proven quite successful in teaching basic social skills, such as table manners and meal planning, to severely regressed mental patients and to those with brain trauma.

Most activity groups are composed of six to eight members. The group meets for one and a half hours once or several times a week. In a structured format, the leader directs a specific activity such as a sport, arts and crafts, planning a meal, or eating together. As with other group formats, patient selection is important. Criteria are the ability to contribute to group goals and the group's potential benefit to the patient. Balanced membership is important, with membership drawn from a wide variety of personality types. Too many aggressive or withdrawn patients can sabotage the goals of the group. Through play materials and selected social activities, patients work together in a planned but permissive and supportive social environment. Being accepted by their peers and the group leader helps patients be themselves and enhances personal growth and living situations with here-and-now issues. Specific strategies include a combination of education, guidance, and social support about effective ways of behaving in social situations.

As a leader, you will need to provide ground rules and assume the surrogate role of the good parent. Observe the interaction among the patients to obtain a more comprehensive portrait of each individual's interpersonal conflicts and personal insecurities.

PSYCHOEDUCATION GROUPS

Health teaching is identified as a standard of care in psychiatric mental health nursing. Mohr (1993) notes that "psychoeducation provides patients with the tools necessary for social reintegration through education; the practice of skills has the potential to empower mentally ill clients" (p. 38). **Psychoeducation groups** are becoming increasingly popular in inpatient and outpatient settings where patients are in direct treatment for relatively short periods. Typically, the format consists of an informal class or a scheduled educationally oriented activity led by nurses or allied health personnel. Each session addresses a topic such as medication management, coping strategies, or social skills training.

The process of a psychoeducation group is different from that of a psychodynamic group. Psychoeducation involves significant didactic material about a selected topic, medication, or the symptoms or treatment of a specified mental disorder determined through a needs assessment. Group discussion is focused on the designated topic. The leader is responsible for directing the patients attention back to the subject if discussion takes a different focus. Evaluation is an important component of psychoeducation. A simple pre- and posttest for important elements helps stimulate patient interest and gives you important feedback about the efficacy of the psychoeducation.

Psychoeducation groups are particularly well formulated for nurses to lead. Major prerequisites are a thorough knowledge of the topic and a working knowledge of group dynamics. Psychoeducation groups can be a lot of fun to lead. Preparation helps reduce anxiety. An outline and handouts related to the topic are useful. Begin by asking members to state their names and perhaps something they would like to learn about their disorder (or other issue). Then present didactic information and follow it with questions and answers. Learn to "read" the audience, so that if interest seems to flag, you can comment appropriately, or if a puzzled look appears on faces, you can use a different way of presenting the material. At the end of the session, summarize the information and ask members to comment on what they have learned in the session.

HUMAN RELATIONS GROUPS

Human relations training groups were initiated in the 1960s to educate group leaders in the experience of group dynamics. Experiential learning involves an actual exercise in which group members participate. The exercise is followed by spontaneous sharing about participants' experience of the exercise. Not until participants have cognitively and affectively processed the meaning of the exercise for the individual or for the group as a whole is learning completed. This processing leads to the development or the sharpening of knowledge that would not otherwise be available. The new learning is experienced as "insight or an 'aha' experience," in which the learner gets in touch with a new or previously unacknowledged part of self. In turn, experiential learning helps individuals generalize or transfer experience to the larger world. New responses become automatic parts of a person's behavioral repertoire. Self-confidence in initiating new actions outside the group becomes possible.

Sensitivity and encounter groups are also used to increase human awareness and to enhance human potential. In 1962, Michael Murphy founded Esalan, which became the prototype for this innovative method. The format used action-oriented group dynamics, mediation, and movement to facilitate self-awareness. A time-limited but authentic experience became a primary value. Participants were encouraged to be themselves as much as possible and to express their feelings openly. Together for long periods with time out only for toileting, participants were to break down personal defenses and share more of themselves.

The popularity of sensitivity/encounter groups decreased after the 1960s for a number of reasons. First was the variation in training for leaders; some were professionally trained, but others developed their skills simply by having joined a previous group. Designed to challenge habitual ways of thinking, encounter groups had no follow-up mechanisms to handle primitive emotions brought to the surface. Consequently, results were controversial. For some, the format increased personal awareness and social functioning. For others, it was a destructive psychological experience (Lieberman et al, 1973).

▶ Check Your Reading

11. Compare and contrast the roles participants take in psychodrama.
12. In what ways will the group leader have to modify group formats for the chronically mentally ill?
13. What are some of the distinguishing characteristics of a reminiscence group for the elderly?

ETHICAL AND LEGAL ISSUES

Boundary Violations

Problems with boundary violations are always a possibility in group psychotherapy, as intimate relationships invariably set up the possibility of strong feelings emerging among participants. Business arrangements, social encounters, and sexual intimacy between therapist and patient are gross violations of ethical standards. In one-to-one therapeutic relationships, the patient is protected from mistreatment by professional ethical standards and legal practice requirements related to intimacy, conduct, and engaging with patients in friendships outside therapy.

As mentioned earlier, group members do not have the same formal bounds on their actions with each other. Although an ethical violation of the group psychotherapy relationship that alters the effectiveness of the treatment, no legal sanctions prevent consenting adults from sometimes engaging in intimate relationships originating from therapy. Boundary violations between group members represent an abuse of the therapy process, but no formal legal sanctions exist against member-to-member abuse. Lymberis (1993) notes that the "competence of the group leader is the best defense against member-to-member exploitation" (p. 352). Initially establishing clear boundaries and expectations for group member behavior as explicit group norms reduces the possibility of abuse. For example, you might say to the group, "Even though you may think that it is harmless, having relationships with group members outside of the group diminishes its effectiveness, because feelings are handled outside the group rather than within it so that we can all learn from them. Therefore, I am asking that you do not have contact with each other outside of the group session." Some outpatient group contacts allow patients to have conversations outside the group session but you should make it a group norm that anything discussed outside a session is brought back to the group.

Record-Keeping

You need to take responsibility for ensuring that completed records for each patient reflect the following data:

- Initial evaluation summary
- Patient diagnosis (*Diagnostic and Statistical Manual-IV* and related nursing diagnosis)
- Specific recommendation for group therapy based on diagnosis
- Delineation of treatment goals for the specified patient
- Summary of each group session and patient response

• Periodic clinical summary of the patient's progress related to the group experience

• Documentation of consultations with colleagues and/or referrals based on the patient's lack of progress in the group

CONCLUSIONS

In a time of cost containment, group psychotherapy is likely to become the treatment of choice for many people. As people live longer and assume greater responsibility for their health care, psychoeducation and mutual support groups will become increasingly important. Designing short-term group interventions for different subpopulations is the next step in the development of group psychotherapy. Research is needed to evaluate the efficacy of group psychotherapy and to provide information that will help clinicians tailor specific interventions to meet the selected treatment needs of different populations.

KEY POINTS TO REMEMBER

• Group psychotherapy is a growth-producing treatment strategy that stresses peer relationships as a supportive structure designed to enhance the healthy parts of an individual rather than the illness aspects.

• The goal of group psychotherapy is to assist patients to resolve behavioral symptoms and to develop higher levels of functioning in interpersonal relationships.

• Yalom identifies 11 curative factors found in effective psychotherapy groups. These are catharsis, cohesion, universality, altruism, self-understanding, interpersonal learning, recapitulation of the primary family, instillation of hope, identification, guidance, and existential factors.

• Most psychotherapy groups are made of 7 to 10 patients. This group size permits greater emotional sharing.

• Psychotherapy groups typically meet once a week in outpatient settings and more often on a regularly scheduled basis on inpatient units.

• The interaction in a therapy group is verbal. Recreational and movement groups focus on nonverbal actions.

• Group members usually do not know each other before entering the group. It is best not to include people who socialize with each other in the same group.

• Some group norms such as confidentiality, attendance, the way absences will be handled are universal behavioral standards.

• The content of most psychotherapy groups relates to emotional sharing in a here-and-now context.

• Group members generally have some say in setting goals and establishing group-specific norms that are comfortable for all group members.

• Group members are encouraged to discuss all problems within the group and should be discouraged from seeking individual consultation with either the leader or other group members outside the group.

• The socialization and supportive interaction that typically occurs in a group reinforces a feeling of belonging that is difficult to experience as powerfully in a one-to-one relationship.

• Psychodrama is action-oriented group psychotherapy in which participants reenact past experiences in the present.

• In group formats with the chronically mentally ill, boundaries need to be looser and leadership needs to be more structured.

• Elderly patients profit more from reminiscence groups rather than those dealing with current events.

LEARNING ACTIVITIES

1. Pick a topic of interest to psychiatric nursing such as caring, empowerment, or belonging. Develop an incident related to the topic and write a description of nurses employing the concept. Include participants, the scene, and an explanation of the incident's meaning for you. Share your story with a small group of students. As each student shares a story, identify underlying themes. Have one student act as scribe and record the results. Define the concept by identifying themes discussed in small groups. Develop a common definition.

2. Identify a support group in your community and arrange to talk with the contact person or attend the group. (Usually community support groups are identified with time, place, and contact person in the community newspaper.) Ask about purpose, format, session times, fees, and any other information you can get about the group. Share this information with the larger clinical or student group.

CRITICAL THINKING EXERCISE

Susan and Ron are senior nursing students during their psychiatric nursing experience. Their assignment was to organize a medication teaching group for the patients on the general psychiatric unit. They recruited five patients: Mrs. G, a 45-year-old school bus driver admitted because of a recent accidental medication overdose; Mr. Z, a 22-year-old college student recently admitted with a delusion that the devil was stealing his mind and soul; Mr. S, a 40-year-old depressed secretary ready for discharge; Mr. J, a 42-year-old paranoid computer operator; and Miss B, a 33-year-old phobic telephone operator. Everyone met in the conference room sitting in chairs around a long table.

1. What assumptions can you make about Ron and Susan's knowledge of groups?

2. What evidence do you have to support your assumptions?

3. Give an alternate explanation of why this group might have been chosen.

At the beginning of group, Ron and Susan asked each patient to introduce themselves and identify which medications they were taking. When Mrs. G began to talk about the sadness she felt and how the Paxil that she was taking helped her, Mr. Z stood up and announced that she should read the Bible more and then she would not be sad. At this time, Miss B covered her ears and started to cry. She stated, "I want to leave."

1. Put yourself in each patient's place and identify their point of view.

2. Make sense out of what might be happening.

3. What conclusions, if any, can be drawn from the information given?

REFERENCES

Agazarian, Y. M., and Janoff, S. (1993). Systems theory and small groups. In H. Kaplan and B. Sadock (Eds.), *Comprehensive group psychotherapy.* Baltimore: Williams & Wilkins.

Alonso, A., and Swiller, H. (1992). *Group therapy in clinical practice.* Washington, D.C.: American Psychiatric Press.

American Group Psychotherapy Association. (1991). *Guidelines for ethics.* New York: American Group Psychotherapy Association.

Applebaum, P., and Greer, A. (1993). Confidentiality in group therapy. *Hospital and Community Psychiatry, 44* (4), 311, 312.

Bales, R. F. (1950). *Interaction process analysis.* Cambridge: Addison-Wesley.

Bales, R. F., and Cohen, S.P. (1979). *SYMLOG—A system for multiple level observation of groups.* New York: Free Press.

Bednar, R., and Kaul, T. (1994). Experiential group research: Can the cannon fire? In A. Bergin and S. Garfield (Eds.), *Handbook of psychotherapy and behavior change* (4th ed.). New York: John Wiley & Sons.

Benne, K. D., and Sheats, P. (1948). Functional roles of group members. *Journal of Social Issues, 4* (2), 41–49.

Bion, W. R. (1959). *Experiences in groups.* New York: Basic Books.

Bion, W. R. (1961). *Experience in group and other papers.* London: Tavistock.

Bloch, S., and Crouch, E. (1985). *Therapeutic factors in group psychotherapy.* Oxford: Oxford University Press.

Bonney, W., Randall, D., and Cleveland, J. (1986). An analysis of client-perceived curative factors in a therapy group of former incest victims. *Small Group Behavior, 17,* 303–321.

Buchanan, D. (1980). The central concern model, a framework for structuring psychodramatic production. *Group Psychotherapy, Psychodrama, and Sociometry, 33,* 25–32.

Burnside, I., and Schmidt, M. (1995). *Working with the elderly: Group process and techniques.* Boston: Jones and Bartlett Publishers.

Burnside, I., and Haight, B. (1994). Reminiscence and life review: Therapeutic interventions for older people. *Nurse Practitioner, 19* (4), 55–61.

Corey, G., and Corey, M. (1990). *Groups: Process and practice* (3rd ed.). Monterey, CA: Brooks/Cole.

DeBosset F. (1982). Core group: A psychotherapeutic model in an outpatient clinic. *Canadian Journal of Psychiatry, 27,* 123–126.

Fielden, M. A. (1990). Reminiscence as a therapeutic intervention with sheltered housing residents: A comparative study. *British Journal of Social Work, 20,* 21–44.

Foulkes, S. H. (1975). *Group analytic psychotherapy: Method and principles.* London: Gordon & Breach.

Fuhriman, A., Drescher, S., Hanson, E., Henrie, R., and Rybicki, W. (1986). Refining the measurement of curativeness: An empirical approach. *Small Group Behavior, 17,* 186–201.

Harper-Giuffre, H., and MacKenzie, R. (1993). Group psychotherapy with eating disorders. In H. Kaplan, and B. Sadock (Eds.), *Comprehensive group psychotherapy* (p. 449). Baltimore: Williams & Wilkins.

Hepworth, D., and Larsen, J. (1986). *Direct social work practice: Theory and skills.* Chicago: Dorsey Press.

Hobbs, M., Birtchnell, S., Harte, A., and Lacey, H. (1989). Therapeutic factors in short-term group therapy for women with bulimia. *International Journal of Eating Disorders, 8,* 623–633.

Janis, I. (1971). Groupthink. *Psychology Today Magazine, 74* (November), 44–46.

Kaplan, H., and Sadock, B. (1993). *Comprehensive group psychotherapy.* Baltimore: Williams & Wilkins.

Kibel, H. (1993). In A. Alonso, and H. Swiller (Eds.), *Group therapy in clinical practice* (pp. 93–111). Washington, D.C.: American Psychiatric Press.

Kinnel, G. (1980). St. Francis and the sow. In *Mortal acts, mortal words.* Boston: Houghton Mifflin.

Kivlighan, D., and Mullison, D. (1988). Participants' perceptions of therapeutic factors in group counseling: The role of interpersonal style and stage of group development. *Small Group Behavior, 19,* 452–468.

Lappe, J. (1987). Reminiscing: The life review therapy. *Journal of Gerontological Nursing, 13* (4), 12–16.

Leepson, E. (1980). Psychodramatic treatment of the schizoid personality. *Group Psychotherapy, Psychodrama, and Sociometry, 33,* 25–32.

Lewin, K. (1992). Frontiers in group dynamics: Concept, method and reality in social science. Social equilibria and social change. In K. R. MacKenzie (Ed.), *Classics in group psychotherapy.* [Originally published in *Human Relations, 1*(5–41), 72–87, 1947.]

Lewin, K. (1951). *Field theory in social science.* New York: Harper.

Lieberman, M., Yalom, I., Miles, M. (1973). *Encounter groups: First facts.* New York: Basic Books.

Lock, S. (1986). Self-help groups: The fourth estate in medicine? *British Medical Journal, 293,* 1596–1600.

Lymberis, M. (1993). Ethical and legal issues in group psychotherapy. In A. Alonso, and H. Swiller (Eds.), *Group therapy in clinical practice.* Washington, D.C.: American Psychiatric Press.

McIntosh, D., Stone, W., and Grace, M. (1991). The loosely bound group: Format, technique, and patient perceptions. *International Journal of Group Psychotherapy, 41,* 49–64.

MacKenzie, K. R. (1990). *Introduction to brief group psychotherapy.* New York: Harper & Row.

MacKenzie, K. R. (1992). *Classics in group psychotherapy.* New York: Guilford Press.

Mohr, W. (1993). Nurse-led educational program in psychiatric settings. *Journal of Psychosocial Nursing, 31* (3), 34–46.

Moreno, J. L. (1964). *Psychodrama.* Vol. I. New York: Beacon House.

Piper, W. E., and Perrault, E. (1989). Pretherapy preparation for group members. *International Journal of Group Psychotherapy, 38,* 17–34.

Polster, E. (1973). *Gestalt therapy integrated.* New York: Brunner/Mazel.

Pratt, J. (1992). The class method of treating consumption in the homes of the poor. In K. R. MacKenzie (Ed.), *Classics in group psychotherapy.* New York: Guilford Press. [Originally published in 1907.]

Rothke, S. (1989). The role of interpersonal feedback in group psychotherapy. *International Journal of Group Psychotherapy, 36,* 225–240.

Sacks, J. (1993). Psychodrama. In H. Kaplan, and B. Sadock (Eds.), *Comprehensive group psychotherapy* (3rd ed.). Baltimore: Williams & Wilkins.

Scheidlinger, S. (1994). An overview of nine decades of group psychotherapy. *Hospital and Community Psychiatry, 45* (3), 217–224.

Schultz, W. (1960). *FIRO: A three-dimensional theory of interpersonal behavior.* New York: Holt, Rinehart and Winston.

Slavson, S. R. (1979). In M. Schiffer (Ed.). *Dynamics of group psychotherapy.* New York: Aronson.

Stone, W. (1993). Group psychotherapy for the chronically mentally ill. In A. Alonso, and H. Swiller (Eds.), *Group therapy in clinical practice.* Washington, D.C.: American Psychiatric Press.

Trist, E., and Murray, H. (Eds.). (1990). *The social engagement of social science: The Tavistock anthology.* Philadelphia: University of Pennsylvania Press.

Tuckman, B. (1965). Developmental sequence in small groups. *Psychological Bulletin, 63,* 384–399.

VanderMay, J., and Peake, T. (1980). Psychodrama as a psychotherapy supervision technique. *Group Psychotherapy, Psychodrama, and Sociometry, 33,* 25–32.

White, D., and Ingersoll-Dayton, B. (1989). Life review groups: Helping the member with an unhappy life. *Clinical Gerontology, 8* (4), 47–50.

Yalom, I. D. (1975). *The theory and practice of group psychotherapy* (1st ed.). New York: Basic Books.

Yalom, I. D. (1985). *The theory and practice of group psychotherapy* (3rd ed.). New York: Basic Books.

Yalom, I. D. (1990). [Videotape.]

SUGGESTED READINGS

Burnside, I., and Schmidt, M. (1994). *Working with the elderly: Group process and techniques.* Boston: Jones and Bartlett.

Kaplan, H., and Sadock, B. (Eds.) (1993). *Comprehensive group psychotherapy* (3rd ed.). Baltimore: Williams & Wilkins

MacKenzie, K. R. (1992). *Classics in group psychotherapy.* New York: Guilford Press.

Yalom, I. D. (1985). *The theory and practice of group psychotherapy* (3rd ed.). New York: Basic Books.

CHAPTER 18

BEHAVIORAL THERAPY

Take my hand my child
and I will show you the morning sun.

I will teach you all that I know,
and you will share with me the secrets of the heart.
It may not be an even exchange,
but it is all that I have to offer.

—*Author unknown*

LEARNING OBJECTIVES

After studying this chapter, you should be able to:

1. Specify three theory-based approaches to behavioral therapy.
2. Identify terms relevant to the practice of behavioral therapy.
3. Differentiate between observational learning and self-management.
4. Discuss social skills training.
5. Apply behavioral techniques, using the nursing process in the care of the mentally ill patient.

KEY TERMINOLOGY

Antecedent
Behavioral therapy
Chaining
Classical conditioning
Consequence
Contiguity
Cueing
Discrimination
Distraction
Extinction
Fading
Flooding
Generalization
Modeling
Negative reinforcement
Observational learning
Operant conditioning
Positive reinforcement
Premack principle
Punishment
Reinforcement
Reinforcement schedule
Response
Satiation
Self-management
Simple association
Social-cognitive theory
Social reinforcement
Social skills training
Stimulus

Behavior therapy provides a systematic way of examining and changing human behavior by manipulating its **antecedents** (things that precede it) and **consequences** (the payoffs a person receives for performing it). According to behavior therapists, most human behavior can be understood in this way. Behavior therapy can be used as a primary unit of intervention, or it can be packaged as one of several integrated therapeutic interventions for a patient. Conscious use of behavioral principles occurs in a wide variety of applications, including business, education, clinical settings, and parenting.

Behavior therapy is one of the major forces in psychotherapeutic thinking (see Chapter 6). Many clinical psychologists identify their therapeutic orientation as behavioral or cognitive-behavioral. (**Behavioral therapy** addresses *observable* behavior; thoughts and emotions are not addressed because they cannot be directly observed). Cognitive-behavioral therapy recognizes learning as an internal process that cannot be observed directly, so that change occurs in a person's ability to respond in a particular situation. Behavioral therapy associations now exist in many countries. Behavioral approaches are used in the treatment of a wide range of psychiatric disorders, ranging from obsessive-compulsive disorder, attention deficit disorder, sexual dysfunction, drug abuse, socially learned violent behavior, depression, adolescent conduct disorders, anxiety and panic disorders, phobias, and mental retardation. Token economies can help severely regressed patients learn basic activities of daily living (ADLs) and social skills. The therapist or treatment team aims to increase the patient's level of comfort, satisfaction with life, or ability to function in a social setting. These concerns, in turn, help the patient continue with life's journey.

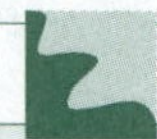

ANDY'S STORY

Along with three classmates and our instructor, I entered the children's psychiatric unit. I was eager for my first child assignment yet highly anxious. What if, after all the time and energy I'd invested so far, I would fail? My mind was full of all the new reading I had been doing, and I began grabbing snatches of it as a way to deal with my anxiety. I remembered "To the extent that he can find gratifying channels of expression for his impulses, the child will be psychologically healthier" (Josselyn, 1955). So this would be my goal: goals for my patient would, of course, depend on his needs.

When I received my assignment, my instructor said, "And, Susan, I'm assigning you to *Andy*." She pointed him out and gave me a brief history. "He is eight years old (he looked three or four). His IQ is estimated to be between 33 and 50, but he is really not "testable" because of his behavior. He is wantonly destructive, withdrawn, obstreperous, and negativistic. He frequently strikes out. In addition, he is regressed to very infantile levels. For example, he toilets indiscriminately, which includes smearing feces, and often clings to the adults near him. He uses only single words, approximately 75, and most of them are negative. You'll soon learn what those are! He is the scapegoat of the other children and seems only tolerated by the adults."

I looked at Andy with a sinking feeling! My first impulse was to turn and run! What could I do to help this very disturbed and disturbing little boy? As I watched him, he obviously was not comfortable, satisfied, or able to function smoothly. He walked with a semistooped, stiff-legged gait, had a blank or frowning countenance, often pushed others or threw things at them, yelling "Shup!" (shut up). He periodically pulled up the skirts of women staff members shouting, "Boo!" He occasionally spit on the floor. There was *nothing* positive to say about him. He apparently had no concept of self. He did not play, seem to be interested in play, or seem to understand what play was all about. Later I often reminded myself of my goal: to help him find "gratifying channels of expression for his impulses." I posted a card with Alfred Adler's words on the dashboard of my car: "The life of the human being is not a 'being' but a 'becoming.'"

Setting Goals for Andy

After my assessment of Andy's needs, I identified three for initial intervention:

1. To stop feces-smearing
2. To improve language skills
3. To improve social skills

To stop the feces-smearing, I decided to use the techniques of substitution and positive reinforcement. I introduced home-made finger paint as a means for receiving attention rather than using feces-smearing for attention getting.

The finger paint was taken into the bathroom at the time of his bath. I demonstrated the way to smear the bright colors over the tiles above and in the tub. At first he said, "Not nice" and put his hands behind his back. After several demonstrations, he eventually, hesitantly put a minuscule bit of red paint on one finger and made a very short smear. He immediately looked at me to see my reaction. Of course, I was smiling and shaking my head, "Yes." By the third session he would meet me when I arrived, take my hand, and lead me to the closet where he knew the paint was stored. Later, we began to include other children in the unit with us. The activity greatly helped improve his image with the other kids, who would vie for a chance to "paint" with him.

To address his lack of language, I used the techniques of modeling and positive reinforcement in the context of play. Using concise sentences, and incorporating these into a game format, I would name everyday items such as food, clothing, or toys. Sometimes, I would say what I thought he was feeling. Andy would repeat my words and actions and began to demonstrate affect. In addition to learning new words, he also began to distinguish himself from others. I decided not to reinforce (to extinguish) undesirable language but to state acceptable alternative language with the expectation that he would learn it. He did.

His lack of social skills was one of Andy's most obvious difficulties. To help him gain positive social reinforcement for improved social skills, I used modeling and cueing. Also using a game format, I would demonstrate the desired behavior, state what was expected, and provide praise for his achievement. Undesirable behavior was ignored, or limits were set by stopping him, either physically or verbally, if it appeared he would hurt himself or another person or seemed likely to destroy property. His interest and participation in the "games" was a delight.

Andy After Intervention

When summarizing the experience at termination time, I was pleased with our work together. Andy now had a vocabulary of about 300 words, very few of them negative. He differentiated himself from things and from others. He had transferred his smearing urges to using a sponge to wipe the tables after meals (after helping with the clearing). He had playmates among the other children. He no longer pulled up skirts, spit, or yelled. We both had experienced a gratifying journey together. He had discovered useful and satisfying channels for expressing his impulses and had become more psychologically healthy. He was accepted as a resident of a prestigious school for the retarded, and I went on to begin my career as a child psychiatric nurse.

THEORETICAL PERSPECTIVES

Behavioral methodologies are based on three theoretical approaches to learning. These focus on the ways learning occurs. All three approaches can help facilitate the patient's journey.

Learning Through Simple Association

Also known as contiguity, the theory of learning through **simple association** grew out of the work of Thorndike (1913) who, using cats as his subjects, described the law of effect: Whenever two sensations occur together over and over again, each will become associated with the other. Later, when only one of these sensations (a stimulus) occurs, the other (a response) will also be remembered. **Contiguity** is the association of two events in the mind, which occurs because of their repeated pairing. Thorndike defined **stimulus** as an event that activates behavior, and **response** as an observable reaction to a stimulus. Much of our learning in school is done through deliberate and repeated pairing of a stimulus and a correct response. Not all learning, however, is deliberate on the part of the learner. Learning depends on what is "caught" from the behavior of others as well as what is actually taught to them. As the result of things they see and hear from the media or from their parents and friends, children and adults develop stereotypes about the way things should be. For example, we may believe that all mothers work only in the home when, in fact, that is the exception. Or we may perceive that all men are "macho" when, in fact, many men are quiet and sensitive. All patients, but mentally ill ones in particular, learn compassionate ways of being indirectly from the modeling of the nurse. This principle of contiguity is the one upon which all other behavioral approaches are based.

Classical Behavioral Conditioning

Classical conditioning is credited to Pavlov, a Russian scientist in the 1920s (see Chapter 6), who used cues to stimulate desired behavioral change. Using dogs as his subjects, Pavlov demonstrated that they could learn to respond automatically to a stimulus that once had no effect on them. He noted that whenever the dogs were given food, they salivated. He then started playing a tuning fork along with the presentation of the food. After he paired the tone with the food repeatedly and then only played the tone, the dogs salivated without the presentation of the food.

One needs only to look at personal experiences to recall situations in which desirable results came from conditioning. If you have been successful in school, you are likely to anticipate new learning experiences eagerly. You might also remember undesirable results from conditioning.

For example, Andy received disapproving attention from others when he aggressively grabbed them or pulled up their skirts. What he wanted and needed was to be held and cuddled, but lacking that, *any* attention would do.

The hitting, spitting, and negative language all gradually diminished when Andy was given numerous cues about more appropriate behavior from those in his environment. Pavlov used a process called **cueing,** in which a stimulus "sets up" a desired behavior. During the conditioning process, **generalization,** or responding to similar stimuli in the same way, also took place. Finally, Andy demonstrated **discrimination,** or the ability to respond differently to similar stimuli, after behavioral treatment. When playing with his toys, for example, Andy frequently hit and yelled at them, although he learned not to behave this way with people. Thus, he had learned to express his negative feelings in a socially acceptable manner, and he was able to discriminate between toys and people.

Discrimination occurs in part because of another process, **extinction,** a gradual disappearance of a learned response. If a conditioned stimulus is presented repeatedly but is not followed by the unconditioned stimulus (e.g., Pavlov's tone but no food), the conditioned response (e.g., salivating after the tone) will finally go away, or extinguish. Another technique for stopping an undesirable behavior is through the use of **satiation,** repeating a problem behavior beyond the point of interest or motivation. For example, one of the most successful programs to help smokers quit involves satiation at the beginning of the program. Smokers are directed to smoke to the point that they become physically ill or repulsed, and they are later reminded of their feelings during the period of satiation. Box 18–1 provides general guidelines for using classical conditioning strategies.

Operant Conditioning

Operant conditioning largely focuses on controlling behavior by controlling consequences. Several types of operant conditioning are relevant: reinforcement, extinction, and punishment. **Reinforcement** is any behavioral consequence that strengthens behavior. The strengthening can occur as a reward (positive reinforcement), or as the removal of a negative contingency (negative reinforcement). Box 18–2 lists guidelines related to operant conditioning.

Operant conditioning was introduced as a treatment modality for people in the late 1960s but was viewed with considerable distaste by those in the mental health fields, who deemed it mechanistic and inhumane. (As Chapter 6 explains, the early work on behavioral learning was done with animals.) The contention was that animal work was conducted in controlled laboratory settings not possible when working with humans. Cognitive psychologists were more interested in explaining how human learning actually takes place, but researchers studying conditioning felt that their intent was simply to identify a few general principles of learning that could also apply to all higher organisms. Skinner (1953) is generally credited with developing operant conditioning (built upon the principles of classical conditioning) as it is currently used

BOX 18-1 Guidelines for the Use of Classical Conditioning Techniques in Psychiatric Settings

- Associate positive, pleasant events with desired behaviors.
- Create a comfortable, nonthreatening environment.
- Avoid competitive and other undesirable situations.
- Choose situations in which limited negative effects will occur.
- Encourage the patient to volunteer to go into the situation.
- If fears are too strong for immediate participation, devise small steps toward the goal (use shaping).
- Help the patient recognize differences and similarities among situations.
- Demonstrate how to discriminate, to respond differently to similar stimuli.
- When appropriate, teach how to generalize, to respond to similar stimuli in the same way.
- Tell the patient that no positive reinforcement will be given unless the desired behavior occurs and that aversive stimuli will occur following undesired behavior (e.g., tell the patient that pushing the button on the patient-controlled-analgesia apparatus will stop pain—providing positive *and negative* reinforcement—and that forgetting to press it will allow pain to recur [aversive stimulus]).

BOX 18-2 Guidelines for Operant Conditioning Strategies

- Make sure that only positive behavior is reinforced.
- Make sure reinforcement is truly reinforcing (Premack principle).
- Give sufficient reinforcement for attempts at tackling new material or trying new skills.
- Use teaching, demonstrating, or modeling to help establish new behaviors.
- When necessary, use shaping to establish a new behavior.
- Gradually decrease reinforcement on an unpredictable schedule to encourage persistence after new behaviors are established.

in education and treatment. The term *operant* refers to any voluntary behavior. Skinner's work, originally using pigeons, demonstrated that many behaviors are not simple responses to stimuli but represent deliberate actions, or operants. According to Skinner, these operants are affected by what happens after them, whether they are rewarded (reinforced):

$$\text{ANTECEDENT} \rightarrow \text{BEHAVIOR} \rightarrow \text{CONSEQUENCES, or } A \rightarrow B \rightarrow C$$

▶ Check Your Reading

1. In what ways are classical and operant conditioning strategies similar to and different from one another?
2. What role does behavioral learning play in everyday life?

PRINCIPLES OF APPLICATION

Defining the Problem: Assessment

Assessment is a critical element of behavioral methodologies before, during, and after intervention. Before any intervention is applied, assessment provides a baseline for evaluating the nature and extent of the problem behavior that is affecting the patient's journey. Also included in the baseline assessment is an examination of the antecedent conditions that support the targeted behavior. During treatment, behaviors continue to be analyzed for the purpose of determining needed modifications. Failure to meet behavioral expectations can occur for a variety of reasons related to the problem description, the nature of the intervention, or the relevancy of the reinforcer.

For example, a behavioral expectation may have been set too high. Careful analysis reveals that it needs to be broken down into smaller steps for successful achievement. Or the converse may happen, and the patient achieves the desired behavior with less effort than originally anticipated. Then the behavioral expectation might be expanded to include a more complex behavioral repertoire. Evaluation after treatment serves as the basis for judging the treatment's effectiveness, so that data are used continuously as an essential component of behavior therapy to inform, plan, implement, and evaluate future treatment efforts.

Defining the Problem Behavior

For purposes of assessment, behavior is simply what a person does in a particular situation. You can think of behavior as being sandwiched between two sets of environmental influences: those that precede it (its antecedents) and those that follow it (its consequences). When behavioral therapy is used, each patient may be viewed as an experimental subject in which specific behavior can be directly observed and described. Just as with any research study, the appropriateness and adequacy of the problem definition has direct implications for the interventions and discussion of results.

Effective behavioral methodologies are based on a blending of behavioristic and humanistic learning principles. It is important to assess whether the problem represents a skill deficit or a performance deficit because the interventions for each will be different. Skill deficits require learning the steps involved in successful performance. Performance deficits require a different motivation to make successful performance more rewarding.

Children and adults with behavior problems can exhibit symptoms from a variety of diagnostic categories, including phobias, obsessive-compulsive traits, attention deficit disorders, eating disorders, cluster A personality disorders, and conduct disorders. The behaviors that become the target of behavioral interventions typically contribute to the development of maladaptive interpersonal relationships that interfere with personal productivity and growth and thus are considered problematic.

Targeting Behaviors

When targeting behaviors, you need to approach the process from a purely scientific perspective. Consider only behavioral activities that interfere with the patient's functioning and are amenable to change. Behavioral therapies are not concerned with insight or motivation. Problem behaviors are identified as discrete actions; for example, in a 24-hour period, Andy uses 25 words, 15 of which have a negative connotation. The behavioral actions are counted precisely over an identified period, usually three days to one week. The data form the baseline. Data can be recorded as a number or can be graphed. Continuous plotting of data provides a living record of change. A written record is particularly useful when the behavior changes are small and might go unnoticed without such precision.

Also record behaviors occurring spontaneously in the environment that appear to evoke or maintain the behavior. For example, the nurse working with Andy would note whether certain situations seemed to stimulate negative language or make him silent. Similarly, if Andy received reinforcement in the form of attention from staff when he used negative language, this attention would be fully described. Boehm (1992, p. 425) identifies three components of a behavioral assessment:

- Antecedent events that precede the behavior
- Small steps that make up the behavior
- Consequences that follow the behavior

By noting the actual baseline behaviors in a logical and sequential format, you can easily see how you might rearrange either the antecedent conditions or the consequences of the behavior to support behavioral change. Interrupting any part of the sequence by altering the meaning provides a new direction for behavioral change. Furthermore, as Lazarus (1978) suggests, "Not only do *counting*, *charting*, and *graphing* establish a base rate (often essential for estimating the severity of any problem), but the very act of keeping records often lends some control to the behaviors one wishes to modify" (p. 32). Box 18–3 presents the steps involved in identifying target behaviors.

As you use behavioral analysis with a patient, look for action descriptors of the behavior. Target behaviors must be described in specific, clear, observable, and measurable terms, as behavioral units. Behavioral descriptions such as, "the patient is noncompliant with medication" or "Johnny is hostile toward peers and staff," provide little information to either nurse or patient about the exact nature of the patient's undesirable behavior. It would be almost impossible to measure progression toward goal achievement with such baseline data. Instead, use a behavioral problem statement such as, "when medication is offered, the patient responds by stating that he will not take his medicine and does not come to receive his medication, except for his bedtime meds, resulting in inadequate symptom control." This statement describes the patient's response in behavioral terms that can be measured easily and also identifies the specific situations in which the behavior occurs. Other health team members reading this behavioral statement would know immediately what behavior to expect from this patient. The problem statement might then read, "Johnny makes threatening remarks to staff and does not interact spontaneously with staff."

Once the behavioral unit is properly identified, the next step is to specify the *measurement unit*, which identifies the exact count or frequency occurrence of the problem. For a behavioral intervention to work, everyone involved in the treatment must agree that the behavior and the behavioral change are counted similarly by those in charge or by one person for all occurrences. The measurement unit is judged to be reliable when those involved with the implementation are viewing the occurrence of the same behavior in the same way. Establishing a unit of measurement that is both reliable and consistent is essential; otherwise, the feedback to the patient is limited, and the intervention may or may not be replicated as intended by other staff members. The best method for specifying the frequency of a target behavior is observation or patient recording of data. The latter helps the patient (if able) to take responsibility for identification of the problem. Patient responsibility also reinforces the notion that behavioral change ultimately is in the hands of the patient. Lazarus (1976) describes a patient-therapist dialogue related to targeting a client's

BOX 18–3 Guidelines for Targeting Behaviors

- Distinguish between behavioral and nonbehavioral causes of the problem. Is the behavior contributing to the problem, or is the problem due to some factor outside the client's control?
- List behaviors the client must exhibit to follow the recommendations.
- Rank each behavior listed in order of importance (e.g., smearing of feces is more important to address than negative social behaviors).
- Rank each behavior according to the extent to which it is changeable (e.g., lack of language is changeable but only to the extent of the patient's capability to learn).

headache behaviors. Such a dialogue might proceed in the following manner (Case Example 18–1).

Case Example 18–1 Jim's Story

Therapist: Does anything in particular bring on these headaches? For instance, do you notice them more at certain times or in certain places?

Jim: (Pause) I can't say I do. No, not really.

Therapist: Well, will you keep tabs on these headaches? What I want you to do is to make a note each and every time you have a headache. Will you record the time of day, where you are, and more or less what you were doing just before the headache came on. Jot down exactly what you were doing, feeling, and thinking. I'd like you to do this very thoroughly. Will you do it?

Jim: Sure, You want to see if there is some pattern?

Therapist: Right. Also, let's get a baseline. Let's see exactly how many times you have a headache over a period of two weeks. Could you also make a notation as to the severity of each attack?

Jim: Like "mild," "moderate," or "severe?"

Therapist: Right. And would you keep track of how many aspirins you take? By the way, can you tell me what the consequences are when you do have a headache?

Jim: How do you mean?

Therapist: I mean, does it spoil your fun? For instance, do you cancel appointments or not go out?

Jim: Well, my wife was mad at me only last night because we had tickets for a show and my head was splitting and I opted out.

Therapist: Do you like shows? Especially the one you missed last night. Were you honestly looking forward to it?

Jim: (Laughs) Well, I'll have to put it to you this way. If it had been a poker game, I just might have made it.

In this sample dialogue, the therapist accomplishes several tasks essential to targeting the behavior in need of change. First, he engages Jim's interest and actively involves him in the process of looking at his behavior in an analytical manner. He proceeds sequentially to establish baseline data by asking Jim to note what is occurring just before the behavior (antecedent conditions), to record the frequency of the behavior, and to specify its severity. The therapist also engages Jim in observing the consequences, both positive and negative, of the baseline targeted behavior. In one encapsulated conversation, the therapist has covered all the essential elements necessary for targeting a behavior in need of change and developing the basis for intervention.

Frequently, occurrences of problem behaviors can serve as rationales for intervention and can be useful in evaluating progress toward goal achievement. Occurrences of problem behaviors can be charted or graphed. Children frequently enjoy recording the number of times they engage in a task or perform a desired behavior by marking a chart with stars or check marks. Many patients like to self-monitor their behavior and work with their charts. The action of participating in the assessment and problem definition increase the patient's participation and responsibility for problem resolution. The actual numbers of behavioral occurrences can be transferred to standardized observation sheets that are initially shared with the patient and interdisciplinary staff.

Using Multiple Sources of Data

The general assessment process is thoroughly described in Chapter 13. When considering behavioral techniques, you will need to collect assessment information from

- *Patient self-report.* The patient may state, "I become so anxious at a party that I stammer, blush, and sweat." The difference in self-report for behavioral intervention is that it must be focused on specific behavioral actions and observable data.
- *Administration of appropriate tests.* Examples include the Subjective Units of Distress Ratings (SUDS) and the Beck Depression Scale.
- *Ratings of others.* Consider family, friends, and other professionals.
- *Direct observation* of patient behaviors. Note explicit definitions of behavior and the number of times it is observed during a 24-hour period.

Obviously, the needs of the patient and the patient's capabilities will dictate which sources of assessment data are most relevant. If a patient is cognitively able to provide self-report information, incorporating the patient's perceptions and definitions of behavior has several benefits. It promotes mutuality, and it stimulates more interest in the project. Most important, it helps the patient become a more critical observer of his or her own behavior and the antecedents and consequences of certain behaviors. From the patient's perspective, knowledge is power. An accurate assessment of specific behaviors gathered with the patient's cooperation makes him or her responsible for the behavioral change and serves as the foundation for recording progress toward desired behaviors that makes sense and is easily understood.

Direct observation is useful particularly when the patient is either cognitively or emotionally unable or disinclined to identify target behaviors. The patient should be carefully observed around the clock for at least two weeks, if possible, to see

- What he or she does that he or she shouldn't do

- What he or she *prefers* doing (potential positive reinforcers)
- What he or she does not do that he or she should do
- What he or she doesn't like (potential aversive stimuli and basis for reinforcement)

Videotapes are very useful direct observation tools. The assessment of Andy involved only reports of others and personal observations. Assumptions were made that it was in his best interest and that of those in his social setting to eliminate feces smearing, indiscriminate toileting, negative language, and other antisocial behavior. Adult patients can be engaged in the actual tabulation of troublesome behaviors.

Detailed interviews and observations provide information about environmental factors that may be subtly reinforcing undesirable behavior. For example, the father of an adolescent with an eating disorder would carefully watch what his daughter ate and was very concerned and tender with his daughter around this issue but spent very little time with her otherwise. The implicit message his daughter received was that her eating disorder got her the attention she so badly needed and that this attention was unavailable without her behavioral symptoms. Neither the father nor the daughter was consciously aware of how her father's behavior actually reinforced her symptoms.

Specific behaviors targeted for change must be considered within the context of the whole person and that person's environment. People are different, and different behaviors require different interventions. Some people learn faster than others, and reinforcers in the patient's social environment may influence treatment outcomes. For optimal success, consider only those behaviors that are amenable to change and for which the person has the necessary resources and support to modify within a reasonable amount of time. This limitation is important because treatment planning is based upon the integration of all findings from the diagnostic process, the internal and external factors affecting the patient (i.e., behavioral, biological, psychological, genetic, religious, sociocultural, familial, as well as community values and availability of support resources).

Developing Nursing Diagnoses

Behavioral strategies are based on nursing diagnoses and focus on behavioral actions needed to move the patient toward his or her goals. In describing a nursing diagnosis amenable to behavioral intervention, always specify the precise behaviors. For example, a patient with mental retardation may present with a nursing diagnosis of Ineffective Individual Coping, but the precise behaviors associated with the diagnoses may be quite different. Nursing diagnoses might be

- Ineffective Individual Coping related to mental retardation, as evidenced by episodic verbal outbursts, physical aggression towards peers when stressed, and property destruction
- Ineffective Individual Coping related to mental retardation, as evidenced by inability to dress self, use toilet, or practice personal hygiene

Goal-Setting: Outcome Identification

Once the target behaviors have been identified, linked to an appropriate nursing diagnosis, and operationally defined, the next step is to define behavioral goals. Behavioral outcomes must be described with a set of criteria establishing that the treatment outcome has been achieved. For example, if the terminal outcome for Andy is that he will not use negative language, the nurse needs to specify what level of performance is required. Should he use no such language, or will the acceptable criterion initially be that he will reduce his negative language by 10%? Moreover, is the expectation that Andy will not express *any* negative language, even when it is appropriate for him to express displeasure or anger?

Although the treatment outcomes (goals) focus on the problem presented in the nursing diagnosis, the particular objectives to achieve those outcomes will focus on the symptoms (evidence). The behavioral goals for the first diagnosis would center on helping this patient assume better control of his or her anger and its associated behavior. Interventions would concentrate not only on providing rewards for behavior control but also on manipulating the environment so that trigger events (antecedents) would occur less often. Negative reinforcement might be necessary in the form of time outs. With the second nursing diagnosis, the goals would shift to consideration of the tasks needed for activities of daily living associated with personal hygiene. Then the behavioral nursing interventions and reinforcement would concentrate on assisting the patient to take individual responsibility for his or her personal needs. The content of the behavioral intervention would be quite different, although the basic principles would remain the same.

▶ Check Your Reading

3. Why is it important to precisely define target behaviors?
4. What sources of data might you use in targeting behaviors, and how would you decide which was the most appropriate?

Choosing Reinforcement: Planning

The planning phase of behavioral management focuses on identifying behavioral reinforcers that have meaning to the patient, communicating with other health team members about the elements of the treatment plan to ensure continuity, and developing an appropriate reinforcement schedule. This plan will become part of the patient's journey during the course of treatment.

Identifying Behavioral Reinforcers

Designing behavioral strategies can be a highly creative and enjoyable component of nursing care for the mentally ill patient. One of the most rewarding and challenging techniques for the therapist is to be able to anticipate what a patient will do in a given situation and introduce an alternative activity that will be just as satisfying to the patient, if not *more* satisfying, in time to prevent the inappropriate behavior. For example, the nurse working with Andy found that by introducing a game before transitional times in his schedule, Andy's undesirable behavior was eventually prevented, and he and the staff found it more rewarding than the previous undesirable behavior.

Types of Reinforcers

Reinforcers can be tangible items or social activities. Tangible reinforcers need little explanation. They take the form of tokens to be exchanged for actual goods, privileges, or opportunities (such as candy) when the patient does a desired activity. Social reinforcers are equally effective for many patients. Andy's increased use of socially acceptable behavior was facilitated by the use of **social reinforcement,** expressions of praise, approval, and affection given for performing the desired behavior. With social reinforcement, always provide feedback about the behavior or the child's mastery of a task rather than praising the child as "being good." The emphasis in behavioral therapy is on the actual behavior rather than on the personal characteristics of the patient. Behavioral principles associated with social reinforcement are presented in Box 18–4.

Premack Principle

When choosing reinforcers, select those that have meaning to the patient and are strong enough to motivate him or her to perform the designated behaviors (Premack, 1965). Choice of the most appropriate reinforcer depends both on the patient's preferences and on the situation. If possible, choose reinforcers that are present naturally in the real world because they allow the patient to experience positive and negative reinforcement in a real situation. For this reason, the use of a token economy in a unit setting is particularly appealing.

In some situations, a more preferred activity can serve as a reinforcer for a less preferred activity. This phenomenon was first described in 1965 by David Premack, who asserted that a high-frequency behavior (preferred activity) can be especially effective as a reinforcer for a low-frequency behavior (a less preferred activity). The **Premack principle** is sometimes referred to as "Grandma's rule": First do what I want you to do; then you may do what you want to do. For example, patients can earn tokens for appropriate behavior (low-frequency behavior), which entitle them to purchase time, objects or treats, or special privileges (high-frequency behavior).

BOX 18-4 Basic Principles of Social Reinforcement

- Be sure the patient understands and is able to do the target behavior (consider the patient's limitations)
- Be clear and systematic when giving praise following each occurrence of the target behavior
- Reward specific, genuine achievement
- Give recognition to the patient's effort and ability, which will raise self-confidence
- Do not give undeserved praise

When using this principle, remember that the low-frequency behavior must happen first (Case Example 18–2). For example, telling children that they must eat everything on their plate before they will get dessert and that they must complete their homework assignments before they can watch television are examples in everyday life.

Case Example 18–2 Larry's Story

Larry is a strapping adolescent who enjoys active sports. On the unit, he has high energy, which he uses to disrupt the activities. He enjoys being the center of attention but chooses to do it in a negative way that lands him in seclusion for much of his time. Larry is not getting the treatment he needs, and the unit is in an uproar.

Using the Premack principle, the nurse targets certain negative behaviors for problem management. She makes participation in basketball (high-frequency behavior) contingent on Larry's not engaging in negative behaviors on the unit (low-frequency behavior). Simultaneously, time would be spent teaching Larry more productive ways of interacting. This is important; it is not enough to help this patient eliminate an undesirable behavior without helping him develop a different behavior to fill the void.

Another advantage in using the Premack principle as the basis for choosing reinforcers is that careful observation usually reveals potential reinforcers already in the environment. These can be reframed without additional cost. For example, noting that Andy liked to smear feces, the nurse substituted finger painting, which has a similar movement, and paired it with praise to help Andy modify his smearing behavior.

Positive Reinforcement

One of the most useful and successful techniques is positive reinforcement, which is simple to use and rewarding for the therapist as well as the patient. **Positive reinforcement** is any consequence that strengthens behavior by presenting a desired consequence after the behavior. With Andy, the attention, acceptance, and approval positively reinforced his more acceptable behavior. In real life, positive reinforcement is used to modify the behavior of local citizens in a number of ways. For example, some freeways now have special lanes for high-occupancy vehicles, reinforcing (strengthening) the behavior of car-pooling. Drivers who wish to get to work faster can engage other people in car-pooling and therefore take advantage of the special lane to enjoy the consequence of arriving at work more quickly. The bonuses and merit raises that employees earn for high productivity and the high grades earned by students for superior work are other examples of positive reinforcement.

Negative Reinforcement

Another form of reinforcement is **negative reinforcement,** a consequence that strengthens desired behavior by removing an aversive stimulus. Understanding negative reinforcement is important because many professionals tend to view negative reinforcement as something bad, a strategy to be avoided. Yet negative reinforcement is an important behavioral strategy that is very effective in removing habitual reinforcers for an undesired behavior. In fact, recent studies demonstrate that negative contingencies, for example, loss of recess time for children with attention deficit hyperactive disorder, are actually more effective as reinforcement of appropriate behavior and maintain the behavior for longer periods than rewards do (Sullivan and O'Leary, 1989).

If you have been reinforced negatively—that is, avoided the aversive stimulus—you are likely to repeat a desired action when again faced with a similar situation. Negative reinforcement is an important component of behavioral choice in everyday situations. For example, if you have a toothache, any response—for example, taking aspirin, which alleviates the pain (negative reinforcer)—will be more likely to recur when a toothache recurs. Thus, you "escape" from the unpleasant situation. Penalties and late charges are used as negative reinforcers to encourage payment of bills on time, and people are conscious of car and mortgage payments in part because of the danger of repossession should their financial obligations be neglected.

Punishment

Unfortunately, the line between negative reinforcement, which strengthens desired behavior, and punishment sometimes gets crossed, and one danger in using behavioral strategies is that this distinction is not made. **Punishment,** which reinforces behavior in a disapproving and nonconfirming manner, actually weakens the potential for desired behavior change. For example, it is common in the grocery store to observe a parent criticizing a child for whining or running around. Usually, the child does not respond well to this intervention. The behavior continues because what the child really wants is to leave the store. The child's behavior is being reinforced, but the desired outcome (from the parent's perspective) frequently is not achieved. We seldom hear a parent say to a child, "Gee, you were really good in the store today. You sat quietly in the cart and were very pleasant!" Of course, in that situation, the parent could use some preventive techniques like taking toys or books or using the grocery store experience as a mental stimulation exercise, pointing out the various colors and shapes and talking about the items on the shelves.

Using positive reinforcement rather than punishment not only is preventive but also helps to improve the self-image of the other person. Although primary reinforcement strategies eliminate punishment or aversive stimuli because they are not of value for most patients, punishment and adversive stimuli are useful in eliminating certain types of symptomatology, as is described later in the chapter.

A special type of aversive reinforcement is the use of "time outs," which essentially remove the patient from the milieu and from participation in earning points or tokens for behavior. If time outs must be applied, the procedure is more caring when coupled with opportunities for the patient to have appropriate behaviors strengthened with other forms of reinforcement.

Extinction

Extinction is a behavioral strategy to decrease the frequency of an undesirable behavior by *ignoring* it. Dollard and Miller (1976) state that, "When a learned response is repeated without reinforcement, the strength of tendency to perform that response undergoes a progressive decrease" (p. 173). However, when a targeted behavior is first ignored, it may actually increase in frequency as the patient attempts to obtain the previous reinforcement. Furthermore, Bandura et al (1969) suggest that the rapidity of behavioral change with extinction depends somewhat on the degree to which the behavior was reinforced on an irregular basis, the distinction between previous reinforcement and withholding of the reinforcement, perception of deprivation during extinction, and the degree to which alternative behaviors are available. Behavior that has been reinforced irregularly and behaviors in which the difference between the external reinforcer of behavior and the absence of that reinforcer is minimal are harder to extinguish. Also, if few alternatives to the target behavior are available, it is more likely to be resistant to extinction procedures. If the therapist continuously ignores it, however, the behavior will decrease over time and eventually be eliminated.

Identifying and Controlling Antecedents

Antecedents are those behaviors or circumstances that contribute to the problem or make it more likely to occur.

Environmental manipulation is a simple intervention often used to change the direction of behavior. In many situations, a simple reorganization of the environment will change inappropriate behavior. A child who is easily distracted can be helped to concentrate by being placed in a quiet corner with a partial screen. "Baby-proofing" a house will prevent accidents. Children traveling in a car will learn to occupy themselves if provided with interesting activities. The same is true for mentally ill patients. It is possible to use distraction to reduce stimuli for a patient threatening property destruction or harm to others before the behavior actually occurs.

By observing a patient closely, you can modify the environment to support the functional well-being of a patient. For example, colors used and the arrangement of the furniture contribute toward the comfort of those sitting in a room, thus modifying their behavior. Furthermore, research documents that music playing in waiting rooms and elevators increases the comfort of persons using them, and it is well known that a change of environment is usually a benefit of a vacation. Environmental manipulation is a preventive technique that psychologically healthy persons use often, and it can be taught to others. Engaging patients in painting a room, rearranging the furniture, or even thinking about such activities can encourage them to use their creative abilities, become more self-reliant, and raise their levels of self-esteem. Simply changing the behavior of one person in an environment can change behavior in the others there.

In the clinical setting, the environment can be manipulated to support patients in regaining control over their behavior. Seclusion or time out periods may be effective when their behavior threatens appropriate functioning on the unit. Later, patients usually are grateful that you took control of the situation when they were unable to do so. A behavior-oriented treatment plan and a written contract in which patients and staff know contingencies for certain behaviors before they occur provide a sense of safety without constant vigilance and, in many cases, without avoidance of the patient.

Determining Schedules of Reinforcement

Too much positive reinforcement tends to *stop* desired behaviors. A **reinforcement schedule** determines the frequency with which reinforcement occurs. Although continuous reinforcement is an advantage initially, the patient needs to develop internal motivation and satisfaction for performing. This development cannot occur if the reinforcement remains solely external. Reinforcement schedules are described as continuous, intermittent, and variable ratio or variable interval, as summarized in Table 18–1.

The critical principle in determining schedules of reinforcement is *that they must be applied in a systematic manner and that the reinforcers are clearly linked to behavior performance.* An intermittent schedule of reinforcement tends to have the strongest and longest-lasting effect on behavior because of the anticipation of a reward, even when it is not immediately forthcoming. But when evaluating behavioral change, be sure that scheduling is conducted in a systematic rather than a random manner.

TABLE 18–1 **Types of Reinforcement**

Schedule	Definition
Continuous	Reinforcement given after each behavioral response
Intermittent	Reinforcement given randomly after some, but not all, behavioral responses
Variable ratio	Reinforcement given after a certain percentage of responses
Variable interval	Reinforcement given after a certain time interval of response

Continuous reinforcement is most useful when behavior therapy begins, as reinforcement changes behavior fastest if applied immediately after every desirable response. Once a patient has mastered the required response, reinforcement is better on an intermittent schedule. If not, the patient often will stop the new behavior when reinforcement stops. Reinforcing on an intermittent schedule is best if done systematically. Once a desired behavior is established and a reward is expected, the reinforcement should be withdrawn using a variable ratio schedule or a variable interval schedule. Desired behavioral responses are reinforced frequently but not with each occurrence. Ultimately, the desired behavior should occur consistently because the person never knows when reinforcement might occur.

Two methods are used in applying reinforcement on a variable basis. The first, a variable ratio schedule, involves systematically reinforcing a behavior based on a varying number of responses. Usually, the response ratio is known to the nurse but not to the patient and is lengthened gradually—for example, every three times, then every fifth. The other method, a variable interval schedule is similar but is based on time rather than response ratio. It refers to the reinforcement of behavior based on selected, varying intervals. Using a variable ratio schedule, the therapist may decide to give positive reinforcement after every 5th, then 10th, then 7th, then 12th desired response. The patient who cannot predict the time of reward for desirable behavior will be more likely to continue at a high level. Using a variable interval schedule, the therapist will reinforce the desirable behavior at unpredictable (to the patient) intervals.

Behavioral Contracting

Contracting was first introduced in Chapter 11 as the transition point into the working phase of the nurse-patient relationship. In behavior therapy, the contract is an essential component that spells out exactly what the patient must do to bring about the desired behavioral change. A contract represents a negotiated agreement between the nurse and patient, in which the reinforcement contingencies for demonstrating appropriate behavior are clearly identified in advance. The consequences may be either tangible or social rewards or primary or secondary reinforcers, but both parties must agree on what they are and how they will be allocated.

Patient expectations should be stated objectively and clearly in positive terms, with the level of behavior expected—for example, "Jane will brush her teeth after every meal." If the behavioral expectation simply read, "Jane will brush her teeth," then she could brush them once a day and receive the reinforcement. Specificity also allows for more flexibility in modifying the behavioral expectation, should it become necessary. If the nurse finds that a patient is unable to complete the full task, the behavior can be broken down into the smaller steps required to complete the task. If the contract calls for a minimum level of performance that the patient exceeds, the contract is more easily renegotiated to provide for more complex behavioral achievement.

The contract should specify the monitoring system to be used. If penalties for failure to engage in the desired behaviors are employed, they should be stated specifically. Strive for achievable goals that will promote patient success and mastery and work on having the reward system match the level of effort required. Some behavioral contracts also include a bonus system for sustained excellent performance. Figure 18–1 shows a sample behavioral contract.

▶ Check Your Reading

5. What is the Premack principle, and how would you apply it?
6. How do different types of reinforcers affect behavior?
7. In what ways are negative reinforcement and extinction different?

Treatment Applications: Implementation

Basic Tools

The basic tools used in the implementation phase vary in direct application but require learning principles involved with shaping, flooding, fading, reinforcing, modeling, and cueing. Distraction and substitute gratification help to shape behavior of lower-functioning patients. The choice of tool depends on the targeted behavior and on the plan for facilitating the patient's journey.

SHAPING

Shaping is a technique used by the therapist to reward behaviors that are approximations of the desired behavior and gradually to increase expectations as the patient masters smaller approximations until the goal is met. The reinforcers are used to encourage behavioral responses in the desired direction. Additionally, the therapist chooses to comment on any action that represents the patient's effort to achieve the goal. Simultaneously, the therapist ignores or extinguishes behaviors that move the patient in the opposite direction. With this strategy, the patient's behavior begins to take shape in the way negotiated and identified in the nurse-patient contact. For example, in Andy's case, he had never used finger paints. The nurse acted as a **model** by finger-painting, and she showed Andy

This is a contract between *Jack McLaughlin* and *Jennifer Jones, RN*, which begins on *January 19, 1996* and terminates on *discharge from Unit 3B* and consists of the following terms:

Jack McLaughlin will: (1) attend all scheduled activities on the unit; (2) approach the nurse and ask for help when feeling out of control; (3) not display any physical or verbal aggression to others on the unit.

If *Jack McLaughlin* fulfills his contract from Monday through Friday each week, he will be granted a weekend pass. However, if he fails to complete the contract, this privilege will be withheld.

Date *January 18, 1996*

Patient's signature *Jack McLaughlin*

Nurse's signature *Jennifer Jones, RN*

FIGURE 18–1
A sample behavioral contract.

where the paints were kept. Each time he showed an interest in wanting to finger-paint by taking the nurse to the closet where the paints were kept, the nurse rewarded him with a smile and encouragement, and she showed him how to use the finger paint.

There are times when the goal behavior is too complicated or impossible, for the patient to accomplish as a one-step process. Shaping is particularly effective when the patient needs to learn a complex behavior that either is too difficult or is currently not within his or her behavioral repertoire. If the patient has never performed a behavior before, it may be necessary to start from scratch in teaching the patterned steps to reaching a desired outcome; this need may become apparent after the protocol is in place. Shaping allows the therapist the flexibility of breaking down the terminal outcome into smaller segments without losing the overall intent. It is a teaching tool in which subsets of a behavioral outcome are presented to the patient in a series of smaller, sequential steps, with reinforcement of each step toward the goal. As the patient masters each step, another is added to the protocol, and the patient must perform the additional step to earn the reward. In this way, the patient learns the desired behavior through a series of small steps that can be reinforced and strengthened. Guidelines for shaping behaviors are presented in Box 18–5.

BOX 18–5 Guidelines for Implementing Shaping Procedures

- Break the target behavior down into a series of smaller increments
- Reinforce each of these smaller behaviors as they occur
- Gradually link two or more desired steps together before reinforcement
- Gradually require *all* of the smaller behaviors to occur so that the target behavior occurs before reinforcement
- Gradually require longer periods of attending to the task before reinforcement

Chaining and Fading

Chaining and fading are two operant techniques designed to facilitate the shaping of behaviors. Most complex behaviors are composed of sequences or chains of behavior that, when linked together, form the complex behavior. For example, the process of eating a meal in the cafeteria involves picking up a tray, silverware, and plate and placing food on the tray; getting condiments and a drink; walking to the table; sitting down; placing the napkin on your lap; picking up the silverware; and eating. **Chaining** is a behavioral technique that involves unifying or "chaining" together individual behaviors in a progressively more complex skill or task expectation. The seriously mentally ill patient may have significant difficulty eating in a socially acceptable manner, but with chaining, each subset of behavior can be taught and reinforced sequentially. The logical sequencing and immediate reinforcement will aid the internal processing required to learn the behavior.

Fading involves the gradual phasing out of stimulus prompts related to achievement of a desired behavior as the patient is able to accomplish it without the prompts. For example, once the patient spontaneously puts toys away without prompting, discontinue the reminders. The principle behind fading is that it is important for the individual to internalize the behavior steps and essentially to become his or her own behavioral therapist.

FLOODING AND RESPONSE PREVENTION

Flooding (gradually increasing exposure to anxiety-provoking situations within the context of a therapeutic relationship) and response prevention are used to treat obsessive-compulsive disorder (OCD) (for example, compulsive hand-washing and neck-posturing). Repeated incremental exposure to anxiety involves actual contact with the feared stressor. Instead of facing it alone and without reflection, however, the patient is encouraged to talk about his or her fears, face them with support, and through exposure with no untoward consequences, to reduce their power.

Response prevention serves to stop the ritualistic responses typically used by the patient to reduce anxiety, for example, excessive hand-washing. The combination of strategies, rather than the use of either flooding or response prevention, results in success. In a study of patients with OCD, Steketee et al (1982) used flooding or response prevention alone and a combined treatment for excessive hand-washing. Patients treated with the combined treatment protocol demonstrated the most improvement.

Harris and Wiebbe (1992) had a patient self-monitor his hand-washing for two weeks to establish a baseline. A nurse then monitored the patient for one day. Direct observation of neck posturing was conducted by two independent raters. The patient also completed the Subjective Units of Distress Scale (SUDS). Flooding and response prevention were spread over a period of 58 days of hospitalization, during which time graded exposure followed by response prevention in increasing time increments was applied. The patient went from 14 to 16 hand-washings a day to 2 to 3 per day.

CUEING

Cues are used as prompts that "set up" the desired behavior. For example, the therapist may wish to set a timer as a cue or to rise from sitting, while at the same time reminding the patient that their time together is almost over. Alternatively, as a prompt, the therapist may say, "Our time together is almost over." Such techniques not only help the patient prepare for the transition but prevent negative reactions. Thus, cueing, providing an antecedent stimulus just before a particular behavior is to take place, can be used deliberately to encourage the behavioral occurrence. Cues can be used to build trust in the relationship or as self-management prompts for individual patients. Identifying and purposefully employing behavioral cues in treatment also proves useful, particularly in the early stages of treatment. As treatment progresses, the reinforcers themselves will act as cues, and statements by the therapist are not needed for behavioral performance.

Cueing can be taught to patients and can be generalized to other situations. For example, patients can be instructed to recognize trigger events for panic attacks and to employ deep breathing or thought replacement to counter their effect. Cues such as alarms or visual prompts are useful for prompting appropriate responses in dementia victims. Thus, the therapist by "holding the patient's hand along the journey" can teach the patient to provide his or her own cues and prompts, thereby controlling some of his or her emotional responses. The use of mental images, listening to music, or self-talk (e.g., "I am not afraid," "I can breathe deeply") may prove effective.

DISTRACTION

Distraction is a behavioral strategy whereby you can prevent or change inappropriate behavior by simply distracting the patient's attention. Distraction is a particularly useful strategy for use with the dementia victim. For example, Bill was very concerned about his bank statements. He was sure that his banking matters were not being taken care of, and neither his wife nor the nurse could convince him otherwise. A student nurse developed the idea of taking laboratory forms and letting Bill fill them out as bank slips. This simple act of distraction completely calmed his fears, much to the relief of his wife and the nursing staff. For another example, when Andy appeared to be contemplating some negative action, starting a game or pointing out something interesting to him was usually easy.

Mentally healthy individuals often use distraction deliberately as a way of restoring emotional balance. For example, a person might think "I feel really down in the dumps today. I think I'll go for a walk, read, garden, or call a friend." Using distraction can significantly change a person's mood. Again, the therapist can serve as a teacher of coping skills. The emotionally deprived patient has a very limited coping repertoire.

SUBSTITUTE GRATIFICATION

Emotionally deprived patients are unable to see that they have alternatives. The grossly obese person who uses eating as a way to alleviate feelings of emptiness is one example. The need for oral gratification is very strong and goes back to infancy. One often hears obese persons say, "Eating is my only joy." Such a situation illustrates the classic vicious circle in which the more one eats the more one feels negative about oneself. Many other scenarios cause similar feelings and processes. Similar substitute gratification can be used as a deliberate strategy to positively affect behavior.

With Andy, substitute gratification was the introduction of finger painting as a substitute for smearing feces.

The psychologically handicapped person who needs to make major lifestyle or mind-set changes, however, often feels trapped with no choices. You will be most effective by assuming a nonjudgmental manner and stating some alternatives. Again, select alternatives that are more acceptable than those behaviors currently employed by the patient (Kendall, 1985).

The following sample care plan, developed for Andy, is based on behavior strategies.

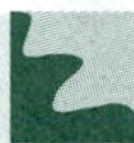

Assessment

Baseline data were collected on Andy over a one-week period. The nurse noted the number of times he smeared feces and did not use the toilet. She noted his used vocabulary, which consisted of approximately 70 words.

In assessing Andy's behavior, the nurse observed that no child proactively approached Andy. He received more attention from staff for his negative behaviors such as lifting the dress of female staff and feces-smearing than he did for any other behavior. When he was not acting out, Andy was likely to be avoided, or "erased," as a person worthy of notice on the unit.

Planning

The overall goal in behavioral treatment is always to provide intervention enabling the patient to lead a more satisfying and comfortable life. In Andy's case, the treatment plan consisted of the following areas of focus:

- To eliminate feces smearing and indiscriminate toileting, substitution with social reinforcement was selected as the intervention of choice. Finger painting was used as a substitute activity because it allowed Andy similar movement and a more positive creative and socially acceptable outlet. Social reinforcement took the form of appreciating his product and praising his efforts.
- To improve language skills, positive reinforcement, modeling, cueing, and social reinforcement were chosen. It was decided that undesirable language would be ignored (fading) and acceptable alternate language would be verbalized (cueing), with the expectation that Andy would learn it (modeling). Each time Andy would use appropriate language, the nurse would acknowledge it (positive reinforcement).
- To increase Andy's repertoire of social skills, modeling, cueing, prompting, and positive reinforcement were selected. Appropriate social behavior would be demonstrated within play activities and the routine activities of daily living of the milieu. Andy was helped by the nurse to rehearse specific social skills. Praise was given for successful performance. Undesirable behavior would be ignored, or limits would be set by stopping him, either physically or verbally, if it appeared that he would hurt himself or another person or destroy property. Andy was told specifically of the limits set on his behavior (a form of negative reinforcement).

Implementation

First, the protocol was introduced to Andy. Then, to begin treatment to stop feces-smearing, finger paint was taken into the bathroom at the time of his bath. The method for smearing it over the tiles above and in the tub was demonstrated. At first he did not want to enter into the activity, but after several demonstrations, along with positive affect and verbal encouragement, he hesitantly began to experiment. After each session he helped to clean up with a sponge. Once the routine was established, other children from the unit were invited to participate in the sessions. Soon they were vying for chances to paint. Andy received frequent social reinforcers, and his status within the unit was elevated.

To increase language skills the nurse named everyday items, such as food, clothing or toys, or would say what she thought he was feeling. He would repeat the words and actions and began to demonstrate positive affect. All these activities were carried out within the context of games or in a playful manner. When he used undesirable language, the nurse would either ignore it or state acceptable alternate language with the expectation that he would learn it.

To improve social skills, also using a game format, the nurse would demonstrate the desired behavior, state what was expected, and provide praise for Andy's achievement. As with helping him increase his language skills, undesirable behavior was ignored or limits were set by stopping him, either physically or verbally, if it appeared he would hurt himself or another person or destroy property. Statements such as, "Hitting hurts. You can hit your bed or pillow, but not Billy," when he hit another child or "Beds are for sitting or sleeping; floors are for standing" (along with lifting him down and placing him on the floor) when he jumped on the beds. He was praised when he complied. His interest and participation in the "games" was enthusiastic.

Evaluation

After three finger painting sessions, Andy no longer smeared feces or eliminated indiscriminately. He had transferred (generalized) his smearing of finger paint and cleaning it up with a sponge to helping clean off tables after meals. He obviously showed pleasure in his accomplishments and their side effects. By the end of the seven months of twice-weekly interventions, his vocabulary had increased to about 300 words, and he was using minimal negative language. He was accepted by his peers and the staff as a result of his greatly improved social skills and obvious positive self-image. He also was accepted for admission to a private school for the retarded that had previously rejected him.

▶ Check Your Reading

8. What are three of the basic tools of behavioral therapy?

9. Which basic tool of behaviorism might be more appropriate for patients with lower levels of functioning?

TREATMENT APPLICATIONS BASED ON BEHAVIORAL APPROACHES

Token Economy

Token economies grew in popularity in the 1960s and 70s, especially in the treatment of children and adolescents with behavior problems (Kazdin and Bootzin, 1972). They still are used as the organizing structure for the unit in many inpatient settings for children and adults. Tokens are awarded for demonstrating appropriate behavior. With a total milieu approach, the patient earns tokens for demonstrating designated behaviors (see Chapter 19 for a description of the concept of milieu therapy). When a patient enters the unit, he or she is given an explanation of the token system and what he or she must do to earn tokens. The tokens have no value in and of themselves but can be used to obtain specified rewards such as tangible goods, activities, or privileges. For desired behavior, the patient receives tokens for a better bed, dessert, books, time in activity areas, better clothes, field trips, and so on.

The use of a token system is based on the principle of generalized reinforcers. The token serves as a primary reinforcer with more than one secondary reinforcer available for patient selection. Having more than one reinforcer as a backup allows much more flexibility in using the Premack principle to change reinforcers in line with the patient's desires and encourages personal decision-making. Tokens also lessen the danger of *reinforcer satiation*, which occurs when a primary reinforcer no longer has meaning for a patient. For example, a patient may tire of a certain candy, and going out for recess may not be as important during the winter months. Moreover, tokens can be assigned different values. As behavior improves, more complex behaviors can be required to earn a token, or the value of an individual token can be reduced. The use of a token system also has the advantage of directly teaching the patient the value of delayed gratification because the token is given at the time of behavior performance, but the exchange of the token for a tangible item or privilege generally occurs later. Box 18–6 outlines the steps in implementing a token economy.

In selecting tokens, choose those that cannot be duplicated easily and are easy to carry or store. Poker chips, play money, paper punches, and squares from colored construction paper are common tokens. Who will assess behavior performance—therapist, other patients, patient, parents—should be established clearly. During the initial stages, set strict guidelines for monitoring procedures and have them in writing. Written evidence of behavioral change is much more compelling than spoken descriptions.

The range of secondary (backup) reinforcers should reflect those of interest and importance to the patient. They can be tangible objects or food items, activities, or privileges. When the system is first initiated, make the earning of tokens relatively easy to accomplish (more behaviors worth a small number of tokens, and fewer behaviors requiring many tokens). Once the system is in place and accepted as valid, the value ratio of token to behavior performance can be increased. *The secondary*

BOX 18-6 Steps in Implementing a Token Economy

- Decide on the token, and the value of each token. Specify the behaviors that will earn tokens and their token value (a written list is helpful).
- Decide on the backup reinforcers. Backup reinforcers are most effective when they reflect use of the Premack principle in their selection.
- Determine the cash value for each backup reinforcer, with the most highly valued by the patient assigned the greatest cash value.
- Establish exchange times.
- Explain the token system to the patient and allow for questions.
- Careful monitoring of the relevance of the system, the patient's response, and possible complications such as other patients stealing tokens, and the consistent application across patients are elements sometimes overlooked, but these factors are very important to the success of the technique.

reinforcers, number of tokens for behaviors, behavior definitions, and progress toward identified outcomes need to be evaluated frequently.

Exchange times need to be carefully established and adhered to consistently. When patients are doing well, it is tempting to sometimes bend the rules and reward them at different times. Unfortunately, this practice tends to undermine the strategy. Initially, exchange times occur closer to the time the behavior is actually performed, but once the system is in place, these times need to be gradually lengthened.

Token economies have been used to establish social, self-care, and functional behaviors in children, adolescents, and the seriously mentally ill. The adaptability of token economies to the patient and the unit situation makes them a very useful tool in behavior management.

Social Skills Training

Social skills training is a learning process in which people learn functional ways of interacting. In discussing social skills training, first ask the question, "What distinguishes people who are socially skillful (competent) from those who are not?" Yahraes (1978) states that the socially competent person can

- Get and maintain the attention of others and use others as resources in socially acceptable ways
- Express both affection and hostility to others
- Lead and follow peers
- Compete with others
- Express pride in something he or she has done or is doing or in something he or she possesses

The socially competent individual also possesses a number of nonsocial abilities that directly affect his or her social capacity:

- Linguistic competence
- Intellectual competence (i.e., ability to sense dissonance or discrepancies in the environment; to anticipate the consequences of whatever is occupying the person's attention; to deal with abstractions, such as numbers, letters, and rules; to take another person's perspective; and to make interesting associations between something he or she sees or hears and something from his or her experience, whether real or imaginary)
- Executive abilities, as indicated by the planning and execution of activities requiring several steps and by the effective use of resources
- Ability to attend to two things at once—for instance, to concentrate on the task at hand yet to be aware of what is going on

The person who is socially incompetent because of mental illness, retardation, or poor role modeling lacks most of these characteristics and is unable to function smoothly in society because of feelings of low self-esteem, isolation, and anger. Such persons often resort to violent behavior as a way to express feelings. Increasing concern about violent behavior is evidenced by preventive measures included in the August 1994 Anti-Crime Bill passed by Congress. Violence prevention programs include social skills and anger management training. Most schools have introduced anger management and conflict resolution training for staff, students, and parents. Typical problems addressed in a behavioral context can include disruptiveness, poor self-management, social withdrawal, emotional control, and low achievement.

One model for the training is a cognitive/problem-solving approach in which interpersonal and problem-solving skills are taught. The goal is to look at alternative solutions, means-ends situations, consequential/causal thinking, and sensitivity to interpersonal problems. The person learns to ask "What is my problem?" "What am I supposed to do?" "What is my plan?" and "How do I do it?" (Kazdin, 1985).

Another model for social skills training uses a combination of behavioral techniques, verbal cues, self-talk, and inclusion of the family in environmental manipulations for patients who have difficulty in social settings (Uomoto and Brockway, 1992). Modeling, role-playing, rehearsal, and positive reinforcement, used alone or in combination with pharmacotherapy, have been found effective in increasing positive social behavior and in reducing displays of depressive affect (Kazdin, 1992).

Behavior management through social skills training is used as both a primary and secondary prevention strategy. Parents of children lacking appropriate social skills are taught behavioral management and communication skills (e.g., to listen and communicate, praise and support acceptable behavior, set appropriate limits, encourage mutual respect, interact consistently, and respond effectively when limits are exceeded) (Green, 1992; Wender and Solanto, 1992).

Cognitive Behavioral Models

Compared with a strict behavioral theorist, cognitive psychologists Piaget (1970), Bruner (1973), Ausbel (1977), and Lazarus (1976) believe that learning is an internal process and cannot be observed directly. Change, they contend, occurs in a person's ability to respond in a particular situation. According to the cognitive view, the change in behavior that behaviorists call learning is a reflection of internal change. Thus, in contrast to the behaviorists, cognitive psychologists studying learning are interested in such intangible factors as knowledge, meaning, intention, feeling, creativity, expectations, and thought, not just observable behavior (see Chapter 30 for a more complete discussion of the use of cognitive behavioral models in the treatment of depression).

Bandura (1971), a leader in developing **social-cognitive theory** (which equates learning with more than observable behavior), suggests that people "know" more than their behavior indicates (see Chapter 6). He wrote

> *Man is a thinking organism possessing capabilities that provide him with some power of self-direction. To the extent that traditional behavioral theories could be faulted, it was for providing an incomplete rather than an inaccurate account of human behavior. The social learning theory places special emphasis on the important roles played by vicarious, symbolic and self-regulatory processes.*

The major difference between traditional operant models of behavior therapy and social learning theory is the thesis in the social learning model that the subject is able to perform a response without its actually being reinforced. Reinforcement, however, can affect the level of response rate and its intensity.

Bandura (1986) is responsible for much of what we know about **observational learning,** which takes place when one sees others rewarded or punished for their actions. Observational learning also occurs when an observer simply copies behavior of a model whom he or she admires. Models, in fact, do not need to be real people but may be characters from a favorite television program or story. If models other than those from "real life" are used, the therapist frequently uses cueing statements to help shape the patient's behavior by focusing on the salient issues in discussing the model's behavior.

Bandura postulated that an individual's learning a new behavior is contingent on four variables: attention, retention, motor reproduction, and incentive. To learn a behavior through modeling, the individual's attention must be directed toward the target behavior of the model. Second, the individual must have the intellectual capacity to retain image of the modeled behavior. It is not possible to learn complex behavior or to make sense of the steps involved in it without having a certain level of mental ability. The patient also must have the physical capacity to reproduce the behavior. Finally, the individual must see some value in learning the behavior. Without motivation, the individual is unlikely to direct attention to the model. Box 18–7 presents basic principles of observational learning.

When using observational learning as a behavioral strategy, consistently model those behaviors you want to teach. Encourage patients to observe behavioral models whom they admire (e.g., peers, favorite sports figures, characters in books or on TV). Positive reinforcement is another strategy to ensure repetition of modeled behavior (Woolfolk, 1987).

Aversive Behavioral Reinforcers in Treatment

Punishment is anything that weakens or suppresses behavior. To be used successfully, punishment should be viewed as negative by the person receiving it. For example, in 1994 Attorney General Reno noted the high recidivism rates of expensive "model" programs for juveniles and emphasized the need for aftercare. This should be no surprise. Incarcerated juveniles do not experience incarceration as punishing. When asked why, many say, "If they made it rough here—like beating us, or putting us in isolation, or giving us bread and water to eat, then we might try harder to stay out."

The use of aversive therapy, since its inception, has been controversial (Murphy, 1993). When using punishment, examine the issues thoroughly beforehand. In addition, do not expect a patient to change current coping behavior unless you can offer an alternative that is more acceptable (rewarding) to the patient.

Today, aversive procedures are used widely to treat such behaviors as alcoholism, sexual deviation, shoplifting, hallucinations, violent and aggressive behavior, and self-mutilation. Punishment is sometimes the treatment of choice when other less drastic measures have failed to produce the desired effects. Three paradigms for using aversive techniques are

- Pairing of a maladaptive behavior with a noxious stimulus (e.g., pair the sight and smell of alcohol with

BOX 18-7 Basic Principles of Observational Learning

Attention: to learn through observation one must *pay attention.*

Retention: to imitate the behavior of a model, one must *remember* it.

Production: once one knows how a behavior should look and remembers the steps, one needs to *practice* and *get feedback and coaching* about subtle points.

Motivation or *reinforcement:* one may acquire the new behavior but not perform it until *adequate incentive* is present.

electric shock), so that anxiety or fear becomes associated with the once-pleasurable stimulus

- Punishment (e.g., applied after the patient has had an alcoholic drink)
- Avoidance training (e.g., the patient avoids punishment by pushing a glass of alcohol away within a certain time limit)

Some other examples of aversive procedures are electric shock, nausea and vomiting chemicals, noxious odors, verbal aversion such as descriptions of disturbing scenes, costs or fines in a token economy, and denial of positive reinforcement (isolation).

Before initiating any aversive protocol, the therapist/treatment team/society *must* answer the following questions: "Is this in the best interest of the patient?" "Does its use violate the patient's rights?" "Is it in the best interests of society?" And ongoing supervision, support, and evaluation of those administering the aversive therapy *must* occur.

For example, mild electric shock and shock in combination with positive reinforcement have been demonstrated to eliminate self-injurious behavior (Williams et al, 1993), and a bitter-tasting substance on the fingers of nail-biters, a mild aversive treatment, has been found effective (Silber and Haynes, 1992). (For those interested in further information, Silber and Haynes have done a broad and comprehensive review of the literature.) Behaviors such as thumb-sucking, hair-pulling, and nose-picking have responded to mild aversive therapy, which was found most effective when the cooperation of the patients played an integral part of the treatment program.

Holmstrom (1988), a nurse, describes how, in her experience, behavior modification was used in Canadian institutions for the mentally handicapped in the 1960s and 1970s. At that time, emphasis usually was on the use of aversive therapy without positive reinforcement to stop undesirable behavior. Institutions also tended to rely upon regimented protocols, which created rather intense environments. The author's description of Canadian practices of that time reflects similar practices in the United States.

▶ Check Your Reading

10. How does a token economy work?
11. What criteria might you use to distinguish between a socially competent and a socially incompetent person?
12. How has cognitive theory been integrated with behaviorism?
13. In what situations are aversive reinforcers likely to be used?

BEHAVIORAL STRATEGIES IN SELF-MANAGEMENT

Self-management, involving the patient in developing the treatment plan, is probably the umbrella under which behavior therapy is currently most used. Self-management provides the patient with the tools for guiding the therapeutic journey. Those in the health care fields are increasingly aware that to increase the possibility of success they need to help patients express their own expectations. Patients need consciously to make lifestyle or mindset changes as they work toward reaching their personal goals. Thus, although behavior therapy still is often used in its simple forms, many current protocols use complicated, multifaceted models. The literature includes numerous examples: a combination of pharmacological interventions, a series of pretreatment interviews and a dual-component stress management program including home practice of antistress imagery, and cue-controlled relaxation procedures for patients with tics and Tourette's syndrome (Azrin and Peterson, 1988; Michultka et al, 1989).

Biofeedback

Biofeedback and related techniques help patients learn to control hypertension, headaches, dysmenorrhea, and chronic orofacial pain (Beaton et al, 1984; Nakagawa-Kogan and Betrus, 1984). At the Management of Stress Response Clinic at the University of Washington, for example, patients are taught to take their own blood pressure, and they participate in 14 biofeedback sessions (three EMG sessions, three autonomic nervous system–focused sessions, and seven pulse wave velocity sessions). Throughout each session, blood pressure is monitored. Quieting responses and muscle relaxation are taught, along with coping and cognitive skills. Lifestyle factors such as diet and exercise are monitored. Finally, each patient is discharged on the same protocol and followed for six months, at which time three group sessions present information about hypertension.

Desensitization

Desensitization is part of a standard behavioral approach in which patients develop behavioral tasks customized to their specific fears. First, the fear is broken down into its component parts through the exploration of the particular stimulus cues the patient presents. For example, certain situations may precipitate a phobic reaction, whereas others will not. Crowds at parties may be problematic, whereas similar numbers of people will not cause the same distress in other settings. Or a person may have an avoidance reaction with dogs or with certain types of dogs but not with other animals. Desensitization procedures owe their origins to Wolpe's method of increasing comfort with an anxiety-provoking stimulus through graduated exposure. Fear of flying has been significantly reduced by exposing a person incrementally to visual presentations of the feared stimuli. A number of research studies report that repeated exposure to models involving feared or phobic behaviors tends to reduce the anxiety of the observer (Bandura et al, 1969).

Fears of flying and actual flight experiences are common areas for cognitive restructuring. For fears of flying, an eight-week educational program held in a busy airport follows these procedures. The process involves a combination of techniques, including relaxation and systematic desensitization (patients are instructed on designing their own hierarchies of fear, developing a set of statements representing the stages of the flight, ordering the statements from most fearful to least fearful, using relaxation techniques to reach a level of relaxation, and then progressing through the list). Patients practice these techniques every day. With cognitive restructuring, patients are encouraged to think about the effects their belief systems have on their feelings and actions and how these can be changed as a result of the desensitization. They draw up a chart containing their old belief system and their new belief system. Group support is provided through the course of treatment (Roberts, 1989).

Desensitization and modeling in dentistry help to decrease the anxiety of child patients. Before treatment, child patients are shown a tape-slide series demonstrating all aspects of the examination. Music and sounds are included, along with a female voice. Evaluation of the children includes heart rate monitoring, dentist's subjective observations, parents, comments, and a behavioral rating scale (Boj and Davila, 1989).

Guided Mastery

Guided mastery has been used in conjunction with desensitization to help people with cardiopulmonary disease manage dyspnea. Guided mastery focuses upon guiding the patient to relax and follow step-by-step instructions. Patients also learn coping skills, which provide an increased sense of self-mastery. While patients exercise on a treadmill at increasing levels of speed and grade, they experience greater-than-usual levels of potentially fearful stimulus (dyspnea) in a monitored, safe environment. They are then instructed to take long steps and to relax their shoulders, arms, and hands. Being able to determine the treadmill speed and grade gives patients a feeling of control over the level of dyspnea.

Desensitization, used with guided mastery, includes supervision, which provides the patient with constant monitoring. Patients learn that they can tolerate greater intensity of dyspnea at higher levels of exercise than they previously thought they could (Carrieri-Kohlman et al, 1993). Eye-movement desensitization is reported to be a rapid, effective treatment for posttraumatic stress disorder (Spector and Huthwaite, 1993). Patients are instructed to focus on the traumatic memory or image. They are asked to list their negative perceptions about themselves or the image of the event. They are then asked to assess (on a 0 to 10 scale) the intensity of their anxiety by completing the Subjective Units of Distress Scale (SUDS), identifying the physical location of the anxiety, and giving a statement about the validity of their cognitions. The therapist then has the patient visually track a finger, which is moved rapidly and rhythmically back and forth across the line of vision from left to right 30 to 35 cm from the patient's face, two back and forth movements per second (a saccade). The back and forth movements are repeated 12 to 14 times (a "set"). After each set, patients are instructed to "blank out the picture and take a deep breath." Then, they bring back the picture and feelings and assign a rating to their intensity. (This procedure requires previous practice by the therapist to ensure fluent performance.) When the intensity level reaches 0 or 1, the patient's belief in the desired cognition is tested by asking the patient "How do you feel about the change?" If the treatment is successful, patients will report increased positive perceptions about themselves and the image of the event (see Chapter 28 for integration of behavioral strategies in the treatment of anxiety disorders).

Applied Relaxation

Relaxation training was originally developed by Jacobson in 1938. His progressive relaxation techniques involve systematic muscle relaxation with instructions given by the therapist in a calm, even tone. Once these techniques are learned, the patient can use them whenever he or she feels anxious and tense. They have been used as part of a protocol to decrease fear of blushing and trembling (Scholing and Emmelkamp, 1993).

Applied relaxation and cognitive methods are used in the treatment of panic disorders (Ost et al, 1993). The authors describe a study in which patients attended 12 one-hour sessions over a three-month period. The treatment program was followed by a maintenance program that ran for six months after the end of the therapy. During that time, the therapist had a total of 90 to 120 minutes of telephone contact with the patient. During the first two sessions, the treatment was described and followed by a specific analysis concerning both anxiety-arousing aspects of the phobic situations and the patient's physiological reactions. Relaxation therapy consisted of practicing progressive relaxation and tension release of muscles, learning to recognize early signs of anxiety, learning some rapid relaxation skills, applying training in phobic situations, and reviewing treatment and maintenance instructions.

The cognitive therapy protocol also was applied over a 12-day period (Ost et al, 1993). During that time, the treatment and its rationale were described. The patients, in a specific diary, recorded cognitive reactions and negative thoughts while confronting phobic situations. Patients were instructed to identify self-instructions that they found useful in natural phobic situations and summarize them on index cards, which they carried at all times. Patients also were taught to recognize alternative explanations, besides anxiety, to various negative emotions. Cognitive restructuring and guided imagery focused on attitudes to phobic problems. The last two sessions summarized and described the maintenance program. After each session, homework assignments required patients to record time frames for exposure to the anxiety-producing situation. Patients also practiced respective treatment conditions. Treatment protocols resulted in significant improvement that lasted at least for the year of follow-up.

In some situations, amazing results are achieved with very short-term interventions. Significantly beneficial effects with only one rehearsal and recording session help chronic nightmare sufferers (Neidhardt et al, 1992). Patients keep a one-month record of their nightmares. Half of the patients do only the recording, while the other half also receive a lesson on imagery to reduce the nightmare frequency. At the inception and at the three-month follow-up, both groups experienced a significant decrease in nightmare frequency.

Failure to comply with prescribed regimens and educational interventions is a primary reason for lack of satisfactory results. Gilpatrick (1989) uses behavioral techniques in conjunction with an educational program to improve compliance. She lists steps for identifying specific behaviors that are linked to the health problem: reminding, tailoring, contracting, shaping, self-monitoring, and reinforcing. Gilpatrick uses self-reinforcement, self-monitoring, and spouse participation as maintenance reinforcers, which help sustain improvements.

Patients are most likely to continue compliance if they have a satisfactory social support system. Components of a social support system are communication of positive affect with others, a sense of belonging or social integration, and elements of reciprocity (Dimond and Jones, 1983). Increasingly popular supports for those attempting to make major lifestyle changes, and a valuable resource for nurses, are the innumerable "mutual help" groups, in which persons experiencing problems such as obesity, alcoholism, gambling, and other ongoing problems gather to share, give, and receive support from others. When used in conjunction with behavioral strategies, each tends to reinforce the other. The behavioral strategies foster mastery, and the social support obtained through the mutual help group helps reinforce motivation.

BEHAVIORAL STRATEGIES IN PREVENTIVE PSYCHIATRY

Behavioral techniques can facilitate our collective journey by preventing major health problems for large numbers of people. Because "vascular diseases and cancer are currently the major contributors to morbidity and mortality" (Elder and Neef, 1986), chronic health problems are considered lifestyle diseases warranting nationwide intervention. For example, excessive smoking and drinking are considered "volitional" acts and present a major challenge to public health and behavioral medicine professionals. For the last 15 to 20 years, population-based behavior modification programs using cognitive educational techniques (frequent offerings of printed materials and TV public service presentations) for addictive conditions and chronic disease control have been attempted. Conditions such as high blood pressure, cholesterol, and obesity have also been targeted, but results of such campaigns are hard to document. Attitudes toward smoking, however, have changed remarkably. Many restrictions have been placed upon smoking. Still, current information indicates that young people are increasingly taking up smoking. More recently, attempts at cancer prevention involve encouragement to obtain early screening (e.g., mammograms, fecal smears). At present, a nationwide educational campaign to decrease exposure to HIV has been launched.

High birth rates among unmarried adolescent mothers plague the United States, with increasing awareness of babies adversely affected by their mothers' high-risk lifestyles. In an attempt to design programs to change such behavior, the U.S. Department of Health and Human Resources, the Public Health Service, and the Alcohol, Drug Abuse, and Mental Health Administration are focusing on raising awareness and developing community resources.

Of course, conditions requiring major lifestyle changes are more complicated than those in which one behavior is targeted for addition or extinction. To treat obesity, programs combining diet, structured physical activity, behavioral techniques, and group therapy are the most effective (Wilson, 1992). Anorexia nervosa and bulimia typically require inpatient treatment and sophisticated cognitive-behavioral techniques. Programs to treat drug addiction also require a combination of several types of intervention, often including a period of residential treatment.

To address some of the most pressing nationwide problems affecting children (e.g., child abuse, sexually transmitted diseases, alcoholism, fetal alcohol syndrome, drug and tobacco addiction, teenage pregnancy, and violence), emphasis is on the need for community-wide awareness and prevention or early intervention. Community Mobilization Against Substance Abuse (CMASA) is one program in which government monies are awarded to counties, which decide how to use the funds. The federal government also is providing intensive team-building conferences to further develop local capabilities.

Basic to effective preventive programs for at-risk children are education and ongoing support for their parents. Such parents, many of whom have had inadequate or inappropriate parenting themselves, need help to feel competent and satisfied in their roles. The federal government has many free publications readily available to help professionals plan intervention strategies. One of these, *What Every Parent Should Know* (Gordon, 1987) includes many concrete suggestions for dealing with real-life situations. Advice is based on behavioral principles, one of which is environmental manipulation. Those entering the field of psychiatry and mental health will wish to become familiar with a variety of available materials.

▶ Check Your Reading

14. How are behavioral strategies applied to techniques of self-management?
15. Give some examples of how behaviorism has been applied to preventive psychiatry.

CONCLUSIONS

Because behavior therapy is based on learning principles, behavioral management techniques are used widely in education, psychiatry/mental health, business, public relations, and politics. Psychiatric nurses have had a role in teaching behaviorist principles to educators, parents, and managers in a great range of fields. For those working within the constraints of today's health care settings, behaviorism can offer short-term interventions for those unable to undergo long-term therapy. For patients who seek techniques for self-management, behaviorist strategies can improve the quality of their lives. By focusing on observable actions, health care professionals—and their patients—can achieve measurable results.

KEY POINTS TO REMEMBER

- Behavioral therapy provides a systematic way of examining and changing human behavior through manipulation of its antecedents and consequences.
- Target behaviors need to be defined operationally as discrete behavioral actions.
- The Premack principle postulates that a high-frequency behavior (preferred activity) can be especially effective as a reinforcer for a low-frequency behavior (a less preferred activity).
- Reinforcers can be positive or negative, tangible or social. Secondary reinforcers are most effective because they are attached to a number of reinforcers from which the patient can choose.
- Shaping is a technique used by the therapist to reward behaviors that are approximations of the desired behavior and gradually to increase expectations as the patient masters smaller approximations until the goal is met.
- People learn from observation of others as well as from direct behavioral strategies.
- Relaxation strategies, biofeedback, and flooding are important self-management strategies that can be used whenever needed and at relatively low cost.

LEARNING ACTIVITIES

1. Identify a behavior that you would like to change. Develop an operational definition of the behavior, and count the number of times you do it in a week. For example, snacking may be a problem. Keep a journal for two weeks and count the number of times a day you snack. Note the times and what you are doing just prior to having the urge to snack. Identify what happens after you snack and the consequences of your snacking.

2. Select a complex behavioral outcome, for example, conducting an election for class office, planning a party, cleaning the house, planning Thanksgiving dinner, or completing an assignment. Specify all of the behavioral components incorporated in the final outcome and order them sequentially as subsets to achieving the goal.

3. Plan a behavioral program to change the specific behavior of a friend, colleague, relative, or yourself. Specify your observational method and justify its selection. Collect the baseline data over a period. Identify the desired outcome. Describe the reinforcers and reasons for selection. Consider any negative implications or unexpected consequences. Pick a child and use behavioral strategies to teach the child a skill.

CRITICAL THINKING EXERCISE

Ms. Trudy Henry, a student nurse, has just learned about behavioral conditioning therapy in her psychiatric nursing class. Two days earlier, Trudy found a young kitten in the parking lot of her apartment building that was very thin and looked as though it had not eaten for days. When she offered it food, the cat attempted to bite her. She managed to feed the animal and gave it shelter in her home without getting bitten. She noticed that any time that she attempted to touch the cat (which she named Nipper) for any reason, it used a biting movement with its jaw but did not inflict harm. She wondered if biting was Nipper's means of relating. Armed with her new knowledge about behavioral conditioning, Trudy set out to test her hypothesis and to make a plan to decrease the biting.

1. What assumption(s) is Trudy making about Nipper's behavior?

2. What assumption(s) is Trudy making about behavioral conditioning?

3. What are possible ways that she could test her assumptions?

Trudy's plan was this: "Each time Nipper attempts to bite, I will hold and stroke his back, gently touch his nose, and say to him in a soft quiet tone, 'you're such a beautiful kitty cat.'" Trudy decided against spanking him on the tail with a newspaper each time he attempted to bite.

1. What evidence does the reader have to determine Trudy's understanding of behavioral conditioning?

2. What alternative approaches, using behavioral conditioning concepts, could be considered?

3. What conclusion(s) can the reader draw from the above data?

REFERENCES

Ausbel, D. P. (1977). *The psychology of meaningful verbal learning.* New York: Grune & Stratton.

Azrin, N. H., and Peterson, A. L. (1988). A simple skill using behavioral strategies. Incorporate shaping, use of rewards in your teaching. Behavior therapy for Tourette's syndrome and tic disorders. In Cohen et al (Eds.), *Tourette's syndrome: Clinical understanding and treatment.* New York: John Wiley & Sons.

Bandura, A. (1971). *Social learning theory.* New York: General Learning Press.

Bandura, A. (1986). *Social foundations of thought and action.* Englewood Cliffs, NJ: Prentice-Hall.

Bandura, A., Blanchard, E., and Ritter, R. (1969). The relative efficacy of desensitization and modeling approaches for inducing behavioral, affective, and attitudinal changes. *Journal of Personality and Social Psychology, 13,* 173–199.

Beaton, R., Egan, K., and Mitchell, P. (1984). Frontalis and trapezius electromyographic activity in healthy nonpatients and in clinical headache samples. *American Journal of Clinical Biofeedback,* (7), 3–11.

Boehm, S. (1992). Patient contracting. In G. Bulechek and J. McCloskey (Eds.), *Nursing interventions.* Philadelphia: W. B. Saunders.

Boj, J. R., and Davila, J. M. (1989). A study of behavior modification for developmentally disabled children. *Journal of Dentistry for Children,* November-December, 452–457.

Bruner, J. S. (1973). *Beyond the information given: Studies in the psychology of knowing.* New York: Norton.

Carrieri-Kohlman, V., Douglas, M. K. Gormley, J. M., and Stulbarg, M. S. (1993). Desensitization and guided mastery: Treatment approaches for the management of dyspnea. *Heart & Lung, 22,* 226–234.

Dimond, M., and Jones, S. L. (1983). Social support: A review and theoretical integration. In P. L. Chinn (Ed.), *Advances in nursing theory development.* Rockville, MD: Aspen.

Dollard, J., and Miller, N. (1976). Learning theory psychotherapy. In W. S. Sahakian (Ed.), *Psychotherapy and counseling.* Chicago: Rand McNally.

Elder, J. P., and Neef, N. A. (1986). Behavior modification and the primary and secondary prevention of cancer. *Family Community Health, 9* (3), 14–24.

Gilpatrick, D. M. (1989). Moving clients toward wellness: Behavioral change. *Clinical Nurse Specialist, 3*(1), 25–28.

Gordon, T. (1987). *What every parent should know.* National Committee for Prevention of Child Abuse.

Green, J. L. (1992). Parenting skills and discipline. Hoekelman et al (Eds.), *Primary pediatric care.* St. Louis: Mosby-Year Book.

Harris, C. V., and Wiebe, D. J. (1992). An analysis of response prevention and flooding procedures in the treatment of adolescent obsessive compulsive disorder. *Journal of Behavioral Therapy and Experimental Psychiatry, 23*(2), 107–115.

Holmstrom, C. (1988). Behavior modification for the mentally handicapped. *Psychiatric Nursing,* July–August, 6, 7.

Jacobson, E. (1938). *Progressive relaxation.* Chicago: University of Chicago Press.

Jankowski, J. J. (1985). Treatment planning. In A. J. Solnit et al (Eds.), *Child psychiatry.* New York: Basic Books.

Josselyn, I. (1955). *The happy child.* New York: Random House.

Kazdin, A. E., and Bootzin, R. R. (1972). The token economy: An evaluative review. *Journal of Applied Behavioral Analysis, 5,* 343–372.

Kazdin, A. E. (1985). Behavior therapy. In A. J. Solnit et al (Eds.), *Child psychiatry.* New York: Basic Books.

Kazdin, A. E. (1992). Depression. In Hoekelman et al (Eds.), *Primary pediatric care.* St. Louis: Mosby-Year Book.

Kendall, P. C. (1985). *Cognitive-behavior therapy for impulsive children.* New York: Guilford Press.

Lazarus, A. (1966). *Psychological stress and the coping process.* New York: McGraw Hill.

Lazarus, A. (1978). *In the mind's eye.* New York: Rawson.

Michultka, D. M., Blanchard, E. B., and Rosenblum, E. L. (1989). Stress management and Gilles de la Tourette's syndrome. *Feedback and Self Regulation, 14*(2), 115–123.

Murphy, G. (1993). The use of aversive stimuli in treatment: The issue of consent. *Journal of Intellectual Disability Research, 37,* 211–219.

Nakagawa-Kogan, H. N., and Betrus, P. A. (1984). Self-management: A nursing mode of therapeutic influence. *Advances in Nursing Science,* July, 55–73.

Neidhardt, E. J., Krakow, B., Kellner, R., and Pathak, D. (1992). The beneficial effects of one treatment session and recording of nightmares on chronic nightmare sufferers. *Sleep 15*(50), 470–473.

Ost, L. G., Westling, B. E., and Hellstrom, K. (1993). Applied relaxation, exposure in vivo and cognitive methods in the treatment of panic disorder with agoraphobia. *Behavioral Research Therapy, 31*(4), 383–394.

Piaget, J. (1970). *The science of education and the psychology of the child.* New York: Orion Press.

Premack, D. (1965). Reinforcement theory (pp. 123–180). In D. Levine (Ed.), *Nebraska symposium on motivation.* Lincoln, NE: University of Nebraska Press.

Nebraska symposium on motivation. Vol. 13. Lincoln, NE: University of Nebraska.

Roberts, R. J. (1989). Passenger fear of flying: Behavioural treatment with extensive in-vivo exposure and group support. *Aviation, Space, and Environmental Medicine,* April, 342–348.

Ross, A. O. (1981). *Child behavior therapy: Principles, procedures, and empirical basis.* New York: John Wiley & Sons.

Scholing, A., and Emmelkamp, P. M. G. (1993). Cognitive and behavioural treatments of fear of blushing, sweating or trembling. *Behavioral Research Therapy, 31*(2), 155–170.

Silber, K. P., and Haynes, C. E. (1992). Treating nailbiting: A comparative analysis of mild aversion and competing response therapies. *Behavioral Research Therapy, 30*(1), 15–22.

Skinner, B. F. (1953). *Science and human behavior.* New York: Macmillan.

Spector, J., and Huthwaite, M. (1993). Eye-movement desensitisation to overcome post-traumatic stress disorder. *British Journal of Psychiatry, 163,* 106–108.

Steketee, G., Foa, E., and Grayson, J. (1982). Recent advances in the treatment of obsessive-compulsives. *Archives of General Psychiatry, 39,* 1365–1371.

Sullivan, M., and O'Leary, S. (1989). Differential maintenance following reward and cost token programs with children. *Behavior Therapy, 21,* 139–151.

Thorndike, E. L. (1913). Educational psychology. In *The Psychology of Learning.* Vol. 2. New York: Teachers College, Columbia University.

Uomoto, J. M., and Brockway, J. A. (1992). Anger management training for brain injured patients and their family members. *Archives of Physical Medicine and Rehabilitation, 73,* 674–679.

U.S. Department of Health and Human Services. (1991). *Prevention plus III: A four-step guide to useful program assessment,* Washington, D.C.: U.S. Department of Health and Human Services.

Wender, E. H., and Solanto, M. V. (1992). Attention-deficit hyperactivity disorder. In Hoekelman et al (Eds.), *Primary pediatric care.* St. Louis: Mosby-Year Book.

Williams, D. E., Kirkpatrick-Sanchez, S., and Iwata, B. A. (1993). A comparison of shock intensity in the treatment of longstanding and severe self-injurious behavior. *Research in Developmental Disabilities, 14,* 207–219.

Wilson, F. R., Omeltschenko, L., and Yager, G. G. (1991). Coping with test stress: Microcomputer software for treatment of test anxiety. *Journal of Behavioral Therapy and Experimental Psychiatry, 22*(2), 131–139.

Wilson, M. H. (1992). Obesity. In Hoekelman et al (Eds.), *Primary pediatric care.* St. Louis: Mosby-Year Book.

Woolfolk, A. E. (1987). *Educational psychology.* Englewood Cliffs, NJ: Prentice-Hall.

Yahraes, H. (1978). *Developing a sense of competence in young children.* DHEW Publication No. (ADM) 78-643.

SUGGESTED READINGS

Bandura, A. (1971). *Social learning theory.* New York: General Learning Press.

Holstrom, C. (1988). Behavior modification for the mentally handicapped. *Psychiatric Nursing,* July–August, 6, 7.

Lazarus, A. (1978). *In the mind's eye.* New York: Rawson.

Premack, D. (1965). Reinforcement theory. In D. Levine (Ed.), *Nebraska symposium on motivation.* Lincoln, NE: University of Nebraska Press.

CHAPTER 19

MILIEU THERAPY

Every moment instructs, and every object: for wisdom is infused into every form.

—Ralph Waldo Emerson

LEARNING OBJECTIVES

After studying this chapter, you should be able to:

1. List three historical precursors to milieu therapy.
2. Define milieu therapy.
3. List the components of milieu therapy.
4. List contemporary settings for milieu therapy.
5. Identify nursing roles in milieu therapy consistent with the process criteria of American Nurses' Association (ANA) Standard Vb.
6. Refer to Joint Commission on Accreditation of Healthcare Organizations (JCAHO) criteria for therapeutic environment.
7. List three ways to support spirituality within the therapeutic milieu.

KEY TERMINOLOGY

Holding environment
Milieu
Milieu environment
Milieu therapy continuum
Residential/therapeutic community
Therapeutic milieu community

We all have experienced environments that make us feel good—where we can be ourselves and know that we are accepted, where we can enjoy the people around us, and where we feel comfortable and at ease. Yet we have all been in surroundings that make us feel tense—where we are uneasy and anxious, where we feel self-conscious or inadequate, and where we know that we are not at our best. The significance of the environment is also recognized in psychiatry as a factor with the potential to help in the recovery of people with mental illness. When we talk about the environment in psychiatry, we usually are referring to the **milieu**, which is defined as the "surroundings, especially of a social or cultural nature" (Flexner, 1993, p. 1220). When we talk about **milieu therapy**, we are referring to the management of the environment to create and/or facilitate a healing context for the patient (Mosher et al, 1986).

Milieu therapy takes naturally occurring events from the environment and uses them as rich learning opportunities for patients. These naturally occurring events include interactions and the daily ebb and flow of routine activities. These events are referred to as the **therapeutic milieu** (Rubin, 1991).

Abroms (1969, p. 557) offers a more detailed definition of milieu therapy as

> *the means of organizing a treatment environment so that every treatment technique (including somatic therapies, individual and group psychotherapies, occupational therapies, etc.) can be systematically utilized to further the patient's aim of controlling symptomatic behaviors and of learning appropriate psychosocial skills.*

This chapter provides the historical perspective of milieu therapy, as well as its components and setting. You will also learn its current uses and possible future developments. Peter's story illustrates several therapeutic milieu settings for treatment. Peter is a young chronically mentally ill patient who has used several psychiatric care milieus over a brief period. Because his stays within psychiatric facilities were short, Peter will need assistance to use different levels of care safely along the milieu therapy and therapeutic community continuums.

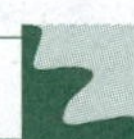

PETER'S STORY

Peter is in the outpatient clinic this morning for an emergency visit. He is met by Marianne, a psychiatric nurse. Peter is accompanied by Kim, his case manager, who is concerned about Peter's behavior over the last 24 hours. Kim reports, "I got a call early today from the residential program director who said that Peter has been more irritable and argumentative. He has been verbalizing threatening statements that have something to do with someone's trying to get him kicked out of town. Peter has not been sleeping well lately—in fact, the last two nights he slept only one to two hours. I'm worried about him.

Until today I have never been afraid of him, but today he threatened to hurt me if I didn't get him out of town."

Peter's History

Marianne reviewed Peter's history and found that he had been out of a state hospital for only one month. There he had received treatment for six months, but before entering the state hospital, Peter had been in another hospital close to his parents' home, which had closed units and relocated Peter. Peter's history included three psychiatric admissions as well as placements in several residential settings in his home county from which he ran away many times, often back to the state hospital. Peter has been threatening to the staff in the past, but has never harmed himself or others while hospitalized. He assaulted his father and a police officer several years ago. Peter has demonstrated impaired judgment by running away without money or resources in cold weather, and he has been consistently unable to manage his resources when in the community. In addition to the residential placements, Peter has lived at the YMCA and a group home, but he always ran out of money and ran away from these settings.

Peter's Current Condition

In the waiting room, Peter sits several seats away from Kim. He appears restless. He scans his environment, mumbles, smiles, and giggles to himself. Abruptly Peter stands up and yells, "I have to see the doctor now... or somebody's gonna be sorry!"

Marianne observes Peter's distress and sees him promptly. Peter appears a little more comfortable in Marianne's office, away from the busy waiting room. Marianne asks Peter to tell her what is happening with him. Peter states, "There are forces that want me out of this town; if I can't get help, I might have to hurt somebody. I have been hearing voices... they say they will kill me. Can you help me?" Marianne responds, "You are in a safe place, Peter. We will help you. You will not be alone, and we will not let anything harm you." Marianne documents evidence of auditory hallucinations, delusional thoughts, high anxiety, and feelings of being unsafe. Peter appears calmer and agrees to remain in Marianne's office with Kim while he waits to see the psychiatrist. Marianne uses another office to make calls to determine the available resources that may be needed to help Peter remain safe. She finds that a bed is available in the local hospital's acute psychiatric unit, and a direct admission is possible with the treatment team's referral.

Peter is seen by the psychiatrist, and the treatment team refers Peter to the acute care setting for stabilization of his schizophrenia. Marianne meets with Peter to tell him of the recommendation for inpatient care. Peter seems relieved and agrees to enter the hospital as a voluntary patient.

HISTORICAL PERSPECTIVE

Milieu therapy is based on the concept that, in a supportive environment, people are able to change. Milieu therapy has foundations in the moral treatment of the late 18th and early 19th centuries (Tuck and Keels, 1992) and includes a systematic, responsible, patriarchal approach to the care of the mentally ill (Almond, 1974). For example, Dr. Philippe Pinel of Paris used the Quaker moral approach for the treatment of prisoners in the 1700s (LeCuyer, 1992). Moral treatment also was the norm at the York Retreat in England and at the Friends Asylum in Philadelphia.

Dorthea Dix, a nurse, reported to the Massachusetts legislature in 1843 regarding the poor conditions of the incarcerated insane. (Chapter 2 provides a complete discussion of Dorthea Dix's work.) As a result of Ms. Dix's national efforts, 15 states established special hospitals for psychiatric patients. Large state hospitals, however, never became the centers for the moral treatment that Dix had envisioned. Rather, overcrowding and lack of funding plagued these institutions.

Henry Burdett, a British reformer, wrote in 1891 of the conditions under which American psychiatric patients were detained. These included overcrowding, deteriorating facilities, and extensive physical restraint (Almond, 1974). During this time, Hermann Simon, a German, developed a more active therapy with rehabilitative work in a supportive atmosphere and called it "milieutherapie" (Almond, 1974). Simon's work was curtailed by the rise of Hitler in the 1920s.

The years between the 1940s and late 1960s were marked by expanding interest in the treatment possibilities inherent in milieu therapy. This interest began after World War II, when Maxwell Jones integrated social context as an important aspect in the treatment of returning soldiers. Jones' concept of the therapeutic community, which he began in London, spread to the United States (Watson, 1992). By the 1950s, the concept of milieu therapy had expanded to include social and cultural values as important factors.

The Community Mental Health Act of 1963 also contributed to a rising interest in milieu therapy as effective treatment of the mentally ill (Krauss, 1987). The new focus was reflected in an explosion of articles dealing with the treatment environment and with stigmatization experienced by the mentally ill (Mosher et al, 1986).

Milieu therapy is based on psychoanalytical theory with careful diagnosis and a prescriptive environment. Harry Stack Sullivan, at Chestnut Lodge, and Austin Riggs, at Menninger Clinic, began to prescribe staff attitudes and responses based on psychodynamic theories (LeCuyer, 1992). As milieu therapy evolved, the concept changed from the milieu as the setting for treatment to the milieu as an aspect of treatment to the milieu as a free-standing therapeutic factor capable of changing behavior and personality (Cumming and Cumming, 1962). Figure 19–1 illustrates the evolution of milieu therapy.

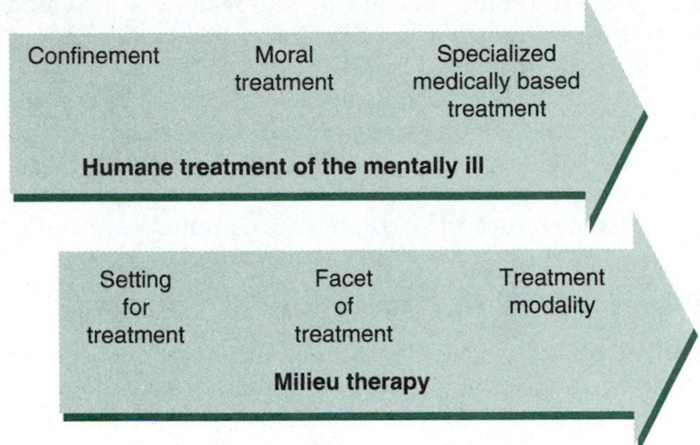

FIGURE 19–1
The evolution of milieu therapy.

▶ **Check Your Reading**

1. Who was the nurse of the 1800s who advocated for improved conditions for the incarcerated insane?
2. What legislative act renewed interest in milieu therapy after WWII?

COMPONENTS OF MILIEU THERAPY

According to Warner (1984, p. 19), "A milieu which promotes reintegration (psychological, social and physical) is therapeutic." LeCuyer (1992, p. 108) states, "Milieu therapy is an interdisciplinary theoretical and clinical approach to inpatient psychiatric treatment in which the total environment is thought to have therapeutic potential." The responsibility for maintaining this environment as a therapeutic entity lies with you, the nurse. The American Nurses' Association (ANA) (1994) states that "the psychiatric-mental health nurse provides, structures, and maintains a therapeutic environment in collaboration with the client and other health care providers." Specifically, the ANA standard Vb states that the nurse is responsible for the therapeutic milieu.

Traditionally, milieu therapy was considered an inpatient modality. Now, however, as treatment settings increase and patients move more quickly between settings, you need to view the milieu as part of a treatment continuum rather than a specific setting.

Milieu Therapy Versus Therapeutic Community: Two Different Journeys

It is important to distinguish between milieu therapy and therapeutic community. Although the terms are often used interchangeably, they represent real differences in approach. Milieu therapy has a medical framework and includes a psychiatrist, a diagnosis, and a prescribed staff approach (Almond, 1974). **Therapeutic community** uses the environment as therapy but moves away from the medical model (Almond, 1974). Group decision-making, use of democratic procedures, and more emphasis on group process characterizes the therapeutic community (Gerson et al, 1983).

Thomas Main coined the term therapeutic community (Tuck and Keels, 1992), but it was Maxwell Jones who developed the concept. Jones, an Englishman, wrote *Therapeutic Community* in 1953 (Yurkovich, 1989) after addressing the need to treat the large number of World War II veterans who required psychiatric care (Almond, 1974). Within the therapeutic community, patients, nurses, and attendants made most of the decisions about daily life rather than having them prescribed by a physician (Almond, 1974). Within the therapeutic community, the social context was considered the most curative factor (Yurkovich, 1989). Rapoport (1960) identified the themes of this modality as democratization, permissiveness, reality confrontation, and communalism.

The therapeutic community concept proliferated during the 1960s (Almond, 1974) and paralleled the antipsychiatry sentiment (Kennard, 1983) of that time. Also during the 1960s, addiction treatment expanded and integrated the therapeutic community model. Synanon, Dayton Village, and Phoenix House were examples of therapeutic communities for the treatment of addictions (Kennard, 1983).

Assumptions of Milieu Therapy

The curative nature of the therapeutic environment is based on four assumptions.

The Therapeutic Relationship Is Worthy of Respect

A therapeutic relationship characterized by respect, support, and genuine interest is healing and may be a prototype for other relationships. Hildegard Peplau was instrumental in defining the psychiatric nurse's relationship with a patient as having curative potential (Peplau, 1952; Peplau, 1964; Peplau, 1969). A leader in nursing education who taught interpersonal skills, Peplau explicated this interpersonal theory of nursing (Peplau, 1964). She espoused the importance of a nursing assessment to determine the patient's ability to relate, so that on the basis of this assessment, nurses make themselves available to relationships with patients.

Defense mechanisms operate within staff members and patient alike. Each has a need to recognize, process, and adjust the therapy to avoid potential negative effects of therapy (Gutheil, 1985). The nurse working in mental health-psychiatric settings needs supervision to assist him or her in recognizing these patterns and to work effectively with them.

Personalities in the Therapeutic Milieu Are Heterogeneous

An important aspect of milieu therapy is that the patient has opportunities to interact and relate to multiple personalities in different roles (LeCuyer, 1992). An interactive approach to care can provide for meaningful exchange between staff and patients. The patient may work on different relationship issues with different staff members. For example, the patient may work on relating to authority figures with one staff member while working on gender issues with another. In addition, by relating to several staff members in one-to-one relationships, patients give a clearer picture of their personalities (Mulvihill, 1989).

Patient Ego Strengths Can Be Built Upon

The strengths of the patient can be utilized within the milieu as each patient participates in treatment, helps others, and participates in the running of the setting. By encouraging each patient to participate in acceptable ways within the protective setting, all staff members have the potential for therapeutic influence.

Group and Community Processes Provide Learning Opportunities

The social behavior of the patient provides a wealth of information about the patient's motives, defenses, and strengths (Mulvihill, 1989). This information is useful to you because you often have the responsibility of making decisions about components of individual and group involvement in different treatment modalities (Tuck and Keels, 1992). In addition, you need knowledge of group process and self-awareness about transference and countertransference (Tuck and Keels, 1992).

Goals of Milieu Therapy

The overriding goal of milieu therapy is to provide a patient with a safe environment in which he or she can try new, more adaptive behaviors. This safety is accomplished through four subgoals:

- Providing for basic needs, including structure
- Supporting the patient's ego
- Promoting coping
- Supporting the patient's spirituality

In expectation of patient change, you must promote coping skills and support patient spirituality for each setting of the milieu therapy continuum.

Maintaining a Safe Environment

Frequently, patients need protection from themselves and others and require assistance with environmental safety, both in the hospital and in the community. Inpatient safety is provided by one-to-one staffing for suicidal, homicidal, or self-mutilating patients. Voluntary "time out" and one-to-one observation are the first line of helping patients feel safe. Psychopharmacology is used to decrease symptoms. Seclusion and restraints are used when these impulses cannot be controlled by the patient and staff through less restrictive interventions.

In the community, patients need places to live that are safe from crime and street violence. They need secured buildings and advocates for safe housing. Rehabilitation housing, group homes, adult foster homes, and secure private housing are all alternatives in community housing.

Providing for Basic Needs, Including Structure

Patients must have basic needs met, including the need for structure, before they can work on behavioral or personality changes. Food, clothing, safety, and medical care must be assured. Often, mentally ill patients neglect medical problems, which can result in their requiring medical treatment concurrently with psychiatric treatment.

Structure is provided on the inpatient unit with schedules, routines, and a rhythm of daily life. Structure and routine frequently break down in the patient's life as symptoms increase. Providing structure is often overlooked in establishing community care. Programs and activities may be available, but factors like transportation or expenses may make participation difficult.

To prevent the regressive effects of hospitalization or supported living, the patient is encouraged to participate as much as possible in obtaining basic needs (LeCuyer, 1992). If others provide services that the patient is able to do alone, the skill may be forgotten, so that over time the patient becomes apathetic and more dependent. To prevent unnecessary dependence, it is critical in each setting to continue to assess patient strengths and abilities and to incorporate this knowledge into the care plan. However, dependence in areas where the patient has deficits is actually a strength; i.e., the patient who can identify when and where assistance is needed is far more functional than the patient who is unable to recognize the need for assistance. Supporting the patient to gain this awareness is important for the patient's coping and adaptation. This strategy is especially critical for the patient with serious and persistent mental illness.

Patient Change via Support of Ego Strengths

The expectation of change provides hope that is essential to healing and growth. Such hopeful expectation is based on realistic expectations of the staff that come from working with patients with similar difficulties. Ego strengths are identified, stimulated, and built upon (Tuck and Keels, 1992).

Promoting Coping Skills in a Teaching and Learning Environment

Coping is emphasized in a teaching and learning environment (Benfer and Schroder, 1985). Teaching the patient that growth is a process and that coping skills will be needed to make lasting changes is essential. Achieving mental health and coping with psychiatric illness are life-long ventures for many patients.

Resocialization is important for many patients who may have severely restricted their interactions as a way of coping with symptoms (LeCuyer, 1992). When symptoms decrease, the patient needs to reaffiliate with others but may feel ill at ease in doing so. The role-modeling of social skills by staff is essential in teaching the patient how to reach out to others.

Supporting Patients' Spirituality

Mental health workers have resisted attending to the spiritual needs of patients (Carson, 1994; Lannet, 1991). Pollner (1989) points out that patients' need for social support is well documented, but the relationship with the divine or spiritual is often overlooked when considering healing because it is sometimes difficult to separate psychotic symptoms from spiritual issues or because practitioners have difficulty with their own spiritual issues. Nursing strives to provide holistic care, and part of that care involves alleviating spiritual distress. Therefore, you need to support patients' spirituality.

A broad definition of spirituality makes this aspect of care more applicable to a wide variety of patient situations and psychiatric nursing care. Shafranski and Gorsuch (1984, p. 233) provide an existential definition of spirituality as ". . . . the courage to look within and to trust. What is seen and what is trusted appears to be a deep sense of belonging, of wholeness, of connectedness, and of openness to the infinite." Carson (1994) specifically identifies the need for connection with God as essential to the well-being of the psychiatric patient.

Supporting spirituality in the therapeutic milieu may range from having an environment that fosters reflection to having religious advisers available. You can facilitate and honor religious practices by understanding a broad spectrum of cultural and religious practices.

American Nurses' Association Standards for Milieu Therapy

The psychiatric nurses' responsibilities in the therapeutic environment are defined in the *Statement on Psychiatric-Mental Health Clinical Nursing Practice* (American Nurses' Association [ANA], 1994, pp. 29, 30).

Gunderson's Components of Milieu Therapy

Gunderson (1983) identified five components of milieu therapy. The interaction of the components promotes change by providing a safe environment that allows for intrapsychic growth (Gunderson, 1983; Walker, 1994). Illustrated in Figure 19–2, these components are solid for the inpatient milieu and permeable for the community setting. The illustration demonstrates that the components of milieu therapy can constrict or expand like a lens, depending on the patient's needs.

Structure

The goal of having a structured environment is to provide opportunities for interactions at both individual and group levels (Gunderson, 1983). These interactions may be both formal and informal. A structured and orderly environment assists the patient to feel secure and allows the patient to choose from available activities as much as possible.

The environment is designed to have daily patterns and predictable rhythms. The mentally ill sometimes demonstrate changes in circadian patterns and are often awake when opportunities for interaction are limited.

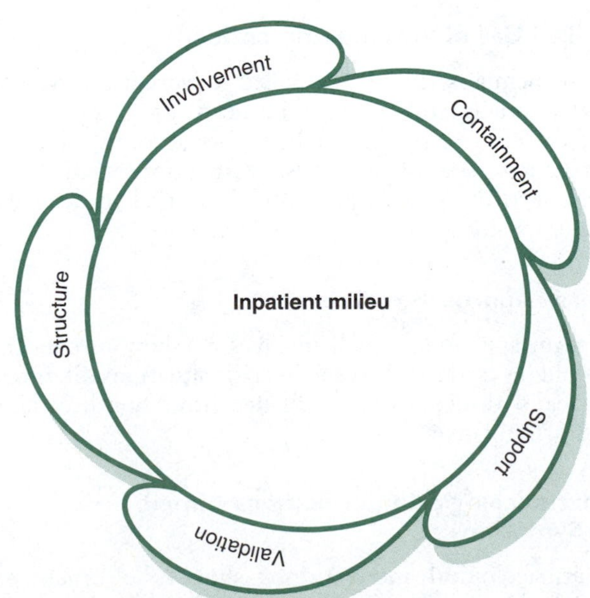

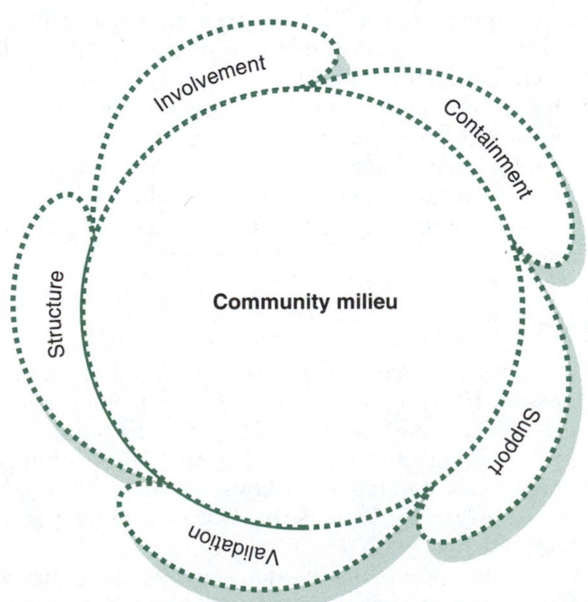

FIGURE 19–2
Gunderson's components of milieu therapy.

Assisting them to reestablish normal circadian patterns may help make more social opportunities available.

Level systems (patient privilege systems) may be used as a form of structure in the inpatient setting (Walker, 1994). Such systems allow patients to earn privileges by meeting behavioral expectations. For example, on admission, all patients begin at the lowest level with the fewest privileges. As patients demonstrate behavioral control, compliance with treatment, and symptom control, the privileges increase. Changes in the level usually require a written physician's order. The privileges may include permission to leave the unit, permission to leave the hospital, special activities, and use of certain facilities.

Involvement

Interacting with others provides an opportunity to increase ego strength and modify one's personality (Gunderson, 1983; Walker, 1994). The milieu promotes interpersonal and interactional skills. The level of involvement is matched with the abilities of the individual. For example, persons with symptomatic thought disorders tolerate interaction less well than other patients and may require low stress involvement.

The settings for interactions vary greatly. In inpatient settings, one-to-one relating groups, community meetings, and free social time provide opportunities for involvement. In the community, partial hospitalization programs, psychosocial programs, outpatient therapy groups, individual therapy, volunteer work, support groups, and employment are but a few of the settings for involvement.

Containment

Containment involves assisting the patient to be safe and to learn to discharge unaccepted burdens in an acceptable manner (Gunderson, 1983). Teaching appropriate expression is done in one-to-one interactions as well as through group activities. Patients are given the opportunity to learn that if they cannot contain themselves, then society has mechanisms to assist. The inpatient setting provides one-to-one verbal interventions, time out, seclusion, as-needed medication, and restraints, whereas police, courts, and emergency mental health workers are used in the community.

Support

Safety, support, and control are important milieu factors (Gunderson, 1983). Patients need protection from themselves if they are suicidal, homicidal, or self-mutilating. This protection takes the form of periodic observation at needed intervals ranging from constant one-to-one supervision to every 15 minutes to monthly monitoring in the community.

The milieu provides a holding environment that is supportive without excessive demands. Such an environment is often required for patients with chronic or serious mental illness. Winnicott (1960) describes a **holding environment** as one that provides consistency, caring, and object constancy, thereby facilitating growth, intimacy, and possibly use of higher defenses.

Validation

Validation is affirmation of individual worth. It involves reassuring patients that what they are experiencing is within the realm of human experience (Gunderson, 1983; Walker, 1994). The staff's demonstration of care and concern serves to substantiate a patient's self-worth. The milieu provides an opportunity to have symptoms validated and taken seriously. This information can teach patients how to cope with symptoms and life experiences.

Validation and human connectedness belong to the dimension of caring for the spiritual being. In connecting with others in a safe relationship, both patient and nurse have an opportunity to experience the spirituality of reflective relating.

Maintaining a Safe Milieu for the Therapeutic Journey

Psychiatric nursing includes the maintenance of a safe environment for the patients and staff. Sclafani (1986) identifies five factors for a safe milieu.

High-Quality Environment

Both the therapeutic environment and programing must be of a high quality. The setting should be attractive and comfortable and should provide privacy. The social climate should be positive and the staff attitude affirming. Routines should be reasonable and flexible, with staffing at an appropriate level to meet the needs determined by the functional levels of the patients.

Skilled Use of Verbal Intervention

Staff members should be skilled in verbal intervention that is timely and caring. The need for personal space should be assessed and taken into account when approaching patients in crisis. Verbal interventions are helpful to the patient and should be used to deescalate rising tensions.

Team Approach to Crises

A team approach, which involves a "show of concern" should be used to intervene in crisis situations. Staff need to deal with behavioral problems with a nonthreatening "security blanket."

Pharmacological Interventions Aimed at Symptoms

Pharmacological interventions should be timely and matched to patients' symptoms. The effective use of medications is highly dependent on your ability to recognize worsening symptoms and to obtain appropriate orders.

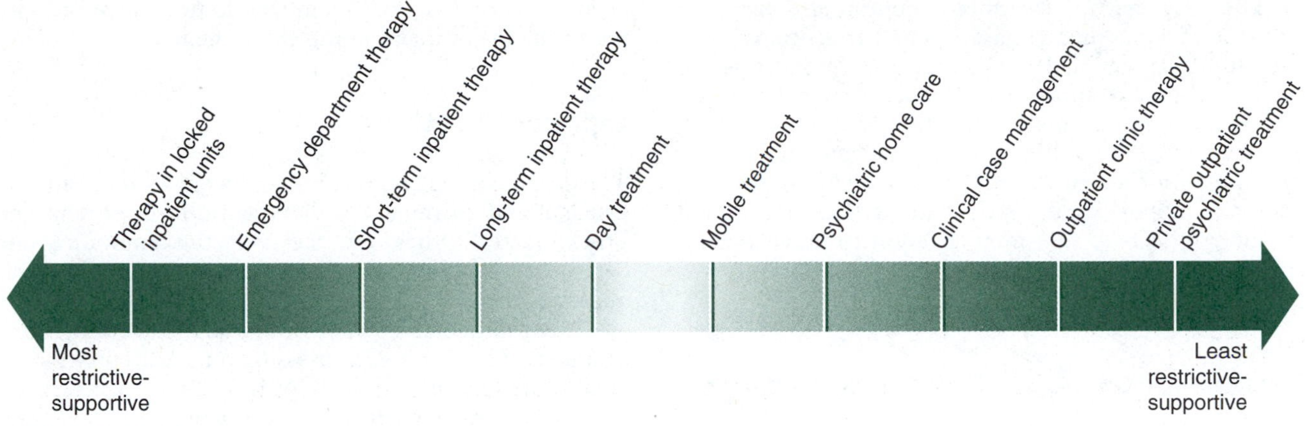

FIGURE 19–3
The continuum of milieu therapy.

Safe Use of Restraints

Physical restraints require a sufficient number of staff members. To protect the patient and themselves, staff members must be trained and practiced in physical restraint. Mechanical restraints are used only in conjunction with one-to-one staffing, verbal intervention, and pharmacological intervention, if ordered, to minimize the time a patient is restrained (Sclafani, 1986).

▶ **Check Your Reading**

3. Describe two assumptions of milieu therapy.
4. Discuss the issue of dependence as it applies to ensuring that the basic needs of patients are met.
5. Describe a holding environment.
6. Describe considerations for the safe use of restraints.

SETTINGS FOR MILIEU THERAPY

The Continuum of Milieu Therapy

Psychiatric treatment settings may be viewed on a continuum, from most restrictive-supportive to least restrictive-supportive. The placement of treatment settings on the continuum depends on the individual setting (Figure 19–3). The **milieu therapy continuum** includes

- Inpatient settings
- Community treatment settings
- Community residential settings
- Psychosocial settings

"Viewing the environment as a continuum between community and hospital settings gives direction for planning change" (Forchuk, 1991, p. 166). In contemporary psychiatric care systems, patients have very short inpatient experiences. Therefore, patients proceed rapidly between inpatient and community settings. To assist the patient in making a transition, you must know about the settings across the milieu therapy continuum.

Locked inpatient psychiatric treatment, in which the patient is involuntarily committed, is the most restrictive treatment setting. The psychiatric emergency department is a restrictive-supportive setting with intensive treatment and support provided to the patient. Short-term inpatient care with continuing assessment and intensive acute treatment may also be restrictive-supportive. Long-term inpatient care with more community outings and privileges often is less restrictive. Day treatment, also called partial hospitalization, provides intensive support and treatment during the day time, with the patient returning to a community residential setting at night. Mobile treatment is a less restrictive community treatment in which the treatment team delivers intensive support, often on the patient's own turf. Psychiatric home care may be toward the center of the continuum, with treatment provided in the patient's environment because of the patient's psychiatric homebound status. Clinical case management provides intense support in a less restrictive environment. The case manager is part of the treatment team and assists in making sure that all patient needs are met and coordinated. The outpatient clinic generally provides for a full range of outpatient treatment that can be supportive but unrestrictive. Private outpatient psychiatric treatment may be the least restrictive-supportive. The private setting often offers a narrow range of services but may be very supportive within a single modality of treatment. Private community treatment is often the least restrictive; its success or effectiveness depends on the patient's motivation for treatment.

The concept of a treatment continuum is especially important for the seriously and persistently mentally ill. These people often require treatment for extended periods in several settings along the continuum. While mobility across the treatment continuum is common for the patient who is seriously and persistently mentally ill, it is uncommon for the staff (Forchuk, 1991). Staff members may have a limited view of the patient's experience. Yet for comprehensive planning, staff members need to be well acquainted with the other treatment settings so they may assist patients in making the transition from one setting to another.

The psychiatric treatment continuum may be viewed as having three phases: acute, transitional, and follow-up (Segal et al, 1990) (Figure 19–4). Patients use transitional care to move out of acute care or follow-up care. When patients make transitions from acute care, they may move to follow-up care or remain in transitional care for an extended period, depending on their needs for support. Sometimes patients use transitional care after follow-up care in an attempt to prevent acute care.

Contemporary Issues Related to Settings

Current factors affecting mental health care such as decreased length of stay in inpatient settings, maintenance of more seriously mentally ill patients in less restrictive settings (LeCuyer, 1992), advances in biomedical treatment of psychiatric illnesses, cost-containment efforts, and the aging population (Watson, 1992) have significantly changed the settings for psychiatric treatment. Therefore, milieu therapy, originally conceived of as a long-term inpatient treatment modality, must evolve. (For an extensive discussion of these trends in health care see Chapter 3.) These contemporary issues are external factors affecting the journey across the socioenvironmental treatment continuum.

The contemporary environment, characterized by rapid patient turnover, decreased length of stay, and heterogeneity of patient population, presents many challenges to the establishment and maintenance of a therapeutic environment. Strong treatment team concept, creativity, commitment, and excellent staff communication (Watson, 1992) are important for milieu therapy in the current health care delivery system.

Staff must have the opportunity for timely communication about individual treatment and the maintenance of milieu therapy. Expertise, guidance, and support must be available so that staff members do not feel alone with the problems of maintaining the milieu.

Inpatient Settings

The hospital milieu is powerful and requires attention and management to remain a therapeutic force (Frank and Frank, 1991). Otherwise, the collective emotional and behavioral problems of patients lead by default to a negative milieu.

Environmental considerations are basic and often assumed. The Joint Commission on Accreditation of Healthcare Organizations (JCAHO) mandates criteria for the therapeutic inpatient environment. Many of these considerations apply to community settings as well (see Box 19–1).

Two tools measure aspects of the milieu in the inpatient setting. These are the Moos Ward Atmosphere Scale (Moos, 1974; Moos and Houts, 1968) and the Patient Perception of Ward Scale (Graham et al, 1971). Both tools are over 20 years old and reflect the assumption of long-term stays. Now, because long-term stays are no longer the norm, nurses need new tools to assess contemporary milieu settings.

Locked Inpatient Units

Locked units are designed to provide containment and structure to involuntary patients who are at risk of harming themselves or others. The laws that define involuntary psychiatric containment vary between states; for all, however, eminent harm to self or others is the major criterion. Although locked units are designed to provide treatment to involuntary patients, voluntary patients may also be treated for an acute crisis in such settings. Also, admission units in larger psychiatric hospitals are usually locked to provide containment while a comprehensive patient assessment is conducted.

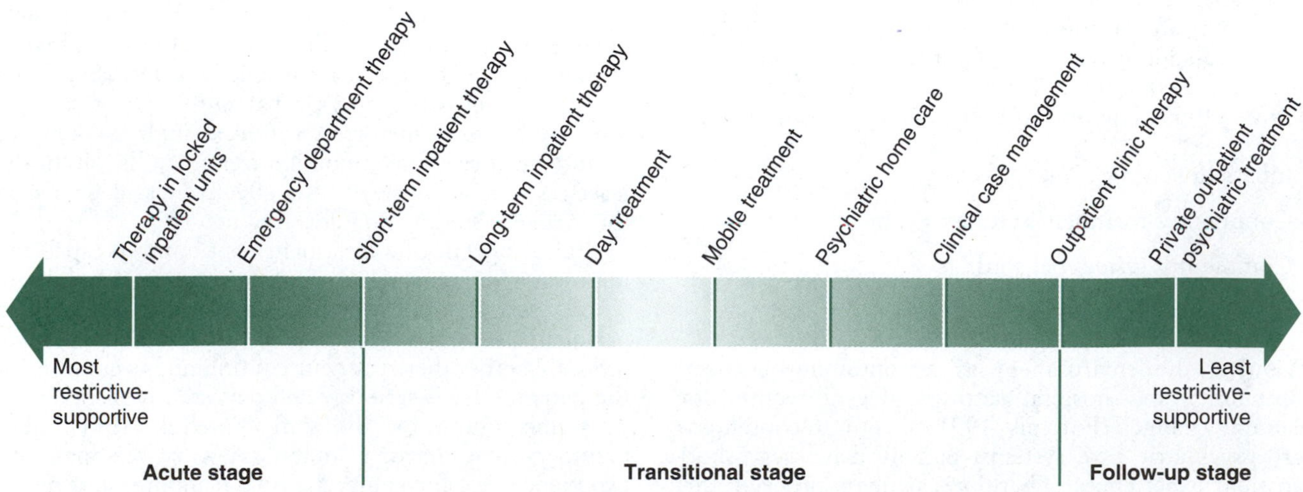

FIGURE 19–4
The stages of milieu therapy.

BOX 19-1 Joint Commission on Accreditation of Healthcare Organizations (JCAHO) Criteria for the Therapeutic Milieu

EC.4 The organization establishes an environment of care that enhances the positive self-image of individuals served and preserves their human dignity.

EC.4.1 Waiting or reception areas are comfortable; their design, location, and furnishings accommodate the characteristics of visitors and individuals served, the anticipated waiting time, the need for privacy and/or support from staff, and the organization's goals.

EC.4.2 Restrooms are available for individuals served.

EC.4.3 The design, structure, furnishing, and lighting of the individual environment promote clear visual perceptions of people and functions.

- EC.4.3.1 Lighting is controlled by individuals served, when appropriate.
- EC.4.3.2 The environment provides views of the outdoors, where possible.
- EC.4.3.3 Appropriate mirrors that distort as little as possible are placed at reasonable heights in appropriate places to aid in grooming and to enhance the self-awareness of individuals served.
- EC.4.3.4 The environment minimizes distractions that interfere with therapeutic activities.
- EC.4.3.5 The environment maximizes the involvement of the individual in leisure activities.

EC.4.4 The organization promotes awareness of time and season.

EC.4.5 A telephone is available for private conversations.

EC.4.6 Ventilation contributes to the habitability of the environment.

- EC.4.6.1 All areas and surfaces are free of undesirable odors.

EC.4.7 Door locks and other structural restraints are used in accordance with the organization's mission and program goals.

EC.4.8 Furnishings and equipment suitable to the population served are available.

- EC.4.8.1 Furnishings are clean and in good repair.
- EC.4.8.2 Broken furnishings and equipment are repaired promptly.

EC.4.9 Dining areas are comfortable, attractive, and conducive to pleasant living.

- EC.4.9.1 Meal and snack times are appropriate to the ages served and facilitate commonly recognized conventions concerning the times when meals and snacks are served.
- EC.4.9.2 Depending on the program goals, facilities are available for serving snacks, preparing meals for special occasions, and for recreational activities.
- EC.4.9.3 The facilities for serving snacks, preparing meals, and for recreational activities permit participation by the individuals served.

EC.4.10 The dining rooms are adequately supervised.

- EC.4.10.1 Staff is provided to assist individuals when needed.
- EC.4.10.2 Staff is provided to ensure that each individual served receives an adequate amount and variety of food.

EC.4.11 Sleeping rooms have doors for privacy unless clinically contraindicated.

- EC.4.11.1 In rooms containing more than one individual, privacy is provided by partitioning or furniture placement.

EC.4.12 The number of individuals in a room is appropriate to the organization's goals and to the ages, developmental levels, and clinical needs of individuals served.

- EC.4.12.1 Except when clinically justified in writing, based on program requirements, no more than eight individuals sleep in a room.
- EC.4.12.2 Sleeping areas are assigned based on individual need for group support, privacy, or independence.

EC.4.13 In accordance with the needs of the individuals served, good standards of personal hygiene and grooming are taught and maintained, particularly in regard to bathing, brushing teeth, caring for hair and nails, and using the toilet, with due regard for privacy.

- EC.4.13.1 Individuals served have the personal help needed to perform these activities and, when indicated, assume responsibility for self-care.
- EC.4.13.2 Incontinent individuals are cleaned and/or bathed immediately following voiding or soiling, with due regard for privacy.
- EC.4.13.3 The services of a barber and/or beautician are available to individuals served, either in the organization or in the community.
- EC.4.13.4 Articles for grooming and personal hygiene that are appropriate to the individual's age, developmental level, and clinical status are readily available in a space reserved near his or her sleeping area.

EC.4.14 Closet and drawer space are provided for storing personal property and property provided for use by individuals served.

- EC.4.14.1 If clinically indicated, an individual's personal articles may be kept under lock and key by staff.

EC.4.15 Individuals served are allowed to keep and display appropriate personal belongings and add suitable personal touches to their surroundings.

EC.4.16 Individuals served are encouraged to take responsibility for maintaining their own living quarters and day-to-day housekeeping activities of the program, as appropriate to their clinical status.

EC.4.17 Individuals served wear suitable clothing.

EC.4.18 The organization formulates a policy regarding the availability and care of pets and other animals, consistent with the organization's goals and good health and sanitation requirements.

EC.4.19 Unless contraindicated for therapeutic reasons, the organization accommodates the needs of individuals to be outdoors through the use of nearby parks and playgrounds, adjacent countryside, and organization grounds.

Peter's story continues in a locked inpatient unit as a treatment setting. The acute care setting admits Peter, and he remains an inpatient for five days. Medication is adjusted, Peter benefits from a low-stress environment, and an attempt to identify stressors is made.

Peter is accompanied to the hospital by Kim. Because Marianne has arranged for a direct admission to the psychiatric unit, Peter did not go to the emergency department before admission to the psychiatric unit. Peter was pacing and talking about people who want to run him out of this town. Now, however, Peter seems to be familiar with hospital routines and appears less agitated.

Miguel, a psychiatric nurse, is Peter's primary nurse. His completed initial assessment of Peter includes psychiatric and medical history, presenting problem, medications, psychosocial history, and mental status. Miguel reviews and provides a copy of patient rights to Peter. When Peter is calm, Miguel gives Peter a tour of the unit and introduces him to other patients and to staff members. The unit routine is discussed.

Peter's medication is adjusted, and Miguel documents Peter's response and assesses for side effects. Miguel remains in contact with Kim (Peter's case manager) and Marianne (Peter's outpatient clinic nurse) regarding discharge plans. Peter's symptoms stabilize within four days. He no longer refers to being run out of town. He reports a decrease in auditory hallucinations and is less frequently mumbling to himself. No stressor that contributed to the increased symptoms was identified during hospitalization. Peter does admit that he does not have any friends and is away from his family. For support, Peter is discharged to the crisis unit, with a plan to return to residential housing in about a week.

Consistent with JCAHO criteria (Box 19–1), it is your responsibility as a nurse to provide an appropriate environment for patients. You coordinate treatment provided directly by nurses and by other professionals. Usually, you are responsible for the development of an interdisciplinary treatment plan. Nurses provide 24-hour care and have an opportunity to both observe and influence the patient's ability to cope with daily life.

Familiarization. You should orient patients initially and at appropriate intervals. Because patients may be acutely ill with thought disorders and high levels of anxiety, orientation may need to be frequent and ongoing. Schedules, routines, and rules are explained and posted.

Assessment of Environmental Effects. Complete nursing notes at least once a shift and more frequently for significant events that reflect patient response to milieu factors.

Consideration of Physical, Social, and Cultural Environment. The therapeutic potential of the milieu is assessed and developed as an ongoing process that requires continuing adjustment in response to the rapidly changing needs of patients on the locked unit. Physical safety and physical needs of patients and staff are important considerations on locked units.

The American Nurses' Association (ANA) Standard Vb does not specifically address spirituality. A humane environment, however, is mandated. The locked unit is the setting in which persons with spiritual distress are more likely to be found. The nursing role for supporting spirituality on the locked unit includes

- Assessing the patient's spiritual or religious practices and needs
- Advocating and facilitating for the patient to see a spiritual or religious leader if desired
- Supporting spiritual or religious practices within the milieu
- Providing humane treatment with an opportunity for connecting with others

Communication. You should teach and model effective communication patterns with patients and staff. Clear communication is essential within the rapidly changing locked unit. You will often provide other professionals with a daily report of each patient's ability to participate, and activities are adjusted accordingly.

Activities. The locked unit often contains psychotic and violent patients. Therefore, safety is a prime consideration when you select activities for patients. Simple, concrete, quiet activities often work best in this setting. The use of objects that can harm self or others is avoided.

Limits. Limit-setting, time outs, restraint, and seclusion are used on locked units when patients are unable to control their behavior. Staffing must be adequate to meet the special needs of patients on the locked unit and to avoid the excessive use of restraints. You must be sure patients and staff understand the rationale and the behavioral expectations for release from limitations.

Opportunity for Questions. You will provide the patient and significant others opportunities to ask questions. The locked unit admission often represents a crisis for the patient and family. Education and communication with the patient and significant others assist them in coping and in adaptation to the situation. You will use discharge planning to assist patients to resume life outside of the hospital. Linkage with needed community services before discharge is an essential part of this planning.

Emergency Departments

Emergency departments have become the "new asylum for the poor" (Weissberg, 1991). The impoverished mentally ill often have no resources for emergency or follow-up care (Weissberg, 1991); therefore, the emergency department may provide the primary care for the seriously mentally ill and for mentally ill chemical abusers (Oldham et al, 1990). This population often presents an increased potential for violence, and referrals for aftercare planning may be difficult.

As a psychiatric nurse in the emergency department, you will be responsible for

- Providing an environment with a lower level of stimulation
- Patient assessment (including suicide potential)
- Crisis intervention with patient and care providers
- Treatment with neuroleptics, as ordered
- Teaching patient and family about mental illness and treatment resources
- Referral to inpatient or community treatment

Familiarization. You will provide orientation to the purpose and process of the emergency evaluation both to the patient and to care providers.

Assessment of Environmental Effects. To protect the patient and others in waiting and treatment areas, you will provide a less stimulating environment. The emergency department milieu is one of high activity, and the sights and sounds of medical crises are often apparent to the emergency psychiatric patient. Examine and treat the patient in a quiet, or counseling, room to provide protection and decreased stimulation for the psychiatric patient in the emergency department. You will record responses to treatment in the nursing notes.

Consideration of Physical, Social, and Cultural Environment. Patients presenting to the psychiatric emergency department often have both mental and physical problems. Medical problems in the psychiatric patient may be identified in this setting because some of these patients lack consistent medical care. Physical care may include assessment for psychoactive drug use. Social and cultural sensitivity and awareness are especially important in providing emergency mental health services. Spiritual caring in the emergency department includes respect for religious and spiritual practices, providing privacy during the psychiatric emergency, and avoiding disruption of practicing beliefs where possible.

Communication. The therapeutic potential of the psychiatric emergency department milieu is best used when it is connected to the larger mental health system of the community. However, the emergency department is often the least well connected link on the treatment continuum (Figure 19–3). The emergency department provides emergency evaluation, treatment, and referral. You will coordinate with professionals across the treatment continuum by teaching patients about the appropriate use of the emergency department, including having them seek referral when necessary. You should work toward congruence between policy and procedure of the hospital, nurse practice standards, and the milieu needs of the patient to promote the therapeutic potential of the emergency setting.

The emergency department may be staffed by an emergency psychiatric service (EPS) worker, usually a social worker or a psychiatric nurse. This person assesses, treats, coordinates with emergency department physicians, and plans inpatient or community care. You may be the only mental health professional in the emergency department, with a psychiatrist on call and the emergency department physicians available for medical care. Therefore, you should communicate the psychiatric needs of the patient clearly and understandably to other professionals. As applicable, you will communicate with the referring professional and with professionals where the patient is to be referred.

Support. The primary milieu activity of the psychiatric emergency department is the provision of patient and staff safety while emergency assessment and treatment occur. To protect the patient and others, you may identify the need for one-to-one staff support for the psychiatric patient.

Limits. Limit-setting, restraint, seclusion, and one-to-one staffing are used in the emergency department when patients are unable to control behavior. The least restrictive method is used, in accordance with humane treatment. You must be sure that patients and staff members understand the rationale and the behavioral expectations for release from the restraint or seclusion.

Opportunity for Questions. Teaching is essential for patients and significant others during crises, treatment, and appropriate referrals. You should give patients and families an adequate opportunity to ask you any questions.

> Peter did not have to go to the emergency department before admission to the acute psychiatric unit because the psychiatric assessment was completed in the outpatient clinic, and direct admission was arranged by Marianne and Peter's treatment team. If he had had medical problems that needed to be assessed before admission to the psychiatric unit, Peter might have had to go to the emergency department from the outpatient clinic. Peter also might have been seen in the emergency department if his treatment team did not have an arrangement for direct admission with the hospital.

Short-Term Psychiatric Units

The creation of the therapeutic milieu is more difficult in short-term inpatient units because of the rapid patient turnover (Long et al, 1992). Patient needs are highly varied in the short-term setting. They include crisis intervention, symptom stabilization, help in restoring previous level of functioning, and assistance in strategies to lengthen community tenure (LeCuyer, 1992).

Hospitalization of the psychiatric patient at the time of admission usually requires that he or she assume the patient role, in which he or she is generally passively accepting of the ministrations of clinicians. The patient may be upset, confused, psychotic, and experiencing other symptoms of psychiatric illness. Because the level of distress is elevated, the patient may be more willing to accept treatment. Patients who are acutely ill often require assistance in managing the expectations of the milieu. They need to be told the purposes of procedures and reminded of the routine. They also need frequent supportive interactions so they may participate.

The journey toward psychiatric recovery includes decreases in symptoms and in patient distress. The psychiatric patient is then expected to relinquish the sick role and to demonstrate more adaptive behavior. You should explain to the patient the purpose of changing expectations.

Short-term inpatient units require a milieu approach that is individualized and consistent with the group and environment. The staff needs to maintain close attention to the environmental stimuli to which acutely ill patients are exposed. Low stress interactions must be made available to offset the effect of having many patients in crisis in the environment.

As in the locked inpatient environment, you will coordinate and manage the short-term inpatient milieu. The focus is on crisis intervention, structure, and support (Kahn and White, 1989). Yet "Treatment outcome research shows little measurable benefit for patient and sometimes harm, when classic milieu techniques are applied in short term, acute treatment settings" (Kahn and White, 1989, p. 609). Kahn and White (1989) propose a short-term inpatient milieu approach that takes into account both biological and psychosocial research:

- A focus on the crisis that led to hospitalization
- Provision for a holding environment
- Integration of the social and emotional context
- Provision for an aftercare plan that is consistent with patient needs and resources
- Graduated therapy

Focus on Issues. When you focus on issues that have lead to the patient's hospitalization, make sure to identify what happened to disrupt coping (Kahn and White, 1989) and to initiate problem-solving around these issues. This focus may include interfacing with the patient's community support network. Questions include

- Did the patient experience difficulty with roommates in a group setting?
- Did financial problems lead to isolation or eviction from an apartment?
- Have symptoms of the illness kept the patient from outpatient treatment?
- What led to decompensation or disruption of coping—consider both symptoms and everyday stressors

Providing a Holding Environment. A holding environment is therapeutic in that it positively influences cognition, behavior, and emotion. Here and now interactions within the holding environment are positive healing factors that staff members can provide for the patient (Kahn and White, 1989).

Integrating the Emotional and Social Context of the Patient's Illness. The integration of emotional and social context requires an assessment of the patient's illness experience in a familial and social context. Are the patient's symptoms or behavior within the norms of the family or social or ethnic group? What is the meaning of these emotions or behaviors to the family or group? Help the patient integrate cultural values with personal goals.

Aftercare Planning. Aftercare plans begin on admission. Primary considerations are what the patient perceives as needs and what is available. The referring agency, if there is one, provides a beginning. What has the patient previously done in outpatient treatment? If the patient is dependent on public transportation, sending the patient to a clinic where no public transportation connection exists will be of no value. Aftercare must be practical, perceived as relevant, affordable, and located where the patient can get to it regularly. Kahn and White's (1989) view is that responsibility for the patient does not end with discharge but ends when the patient is engaged in outpatient treatment. Here transitional treatment settings focused on helping patients reintegrate with the community can be invaluable.

Graduated Therapy. The graduated therapy is represented by a spiral moving from the center focus outward, in an unfolding way, as it moves toward outpatient treatment (Figure 19–5).

The phases of graduated therapy are orientation, engagement, education, and understanding. Orientation includes familiarization with the unit and treatment program, expectations, and goal setting. Engagement is actively giving and receiving feedback to other patients and staff. Education includes learning about the illness, treatment, and coping strategies. Understanding is the ability to integrate the crisis episode and translate that into applications for real life (Kahn and White, 1989). When the patient has reached the point of understanding, discharge to community treatment is the next step.

Long-Term Psychiatric Units

The patients served in long-term facilities include those who

- Have not stabilized in short-term settings
- Have been involuntarily committed
- Are chronically ill and unable to safely maintain self in the community

The patients in longer-term treatment settings are younger, sicker, and more violent than ever before. Treatment should be provided in the least restrictive setting; however, it is difficult to predict violence in this population (Sclafani, 1986). Staff members are challenged to provide least restrictive care while providing for the safety of the patient, other patients, and staff.

Long-term facilities often have a shortage of staff, especially RNs, and maintaining order and safety in long-term psychiatric settings is generally a higher

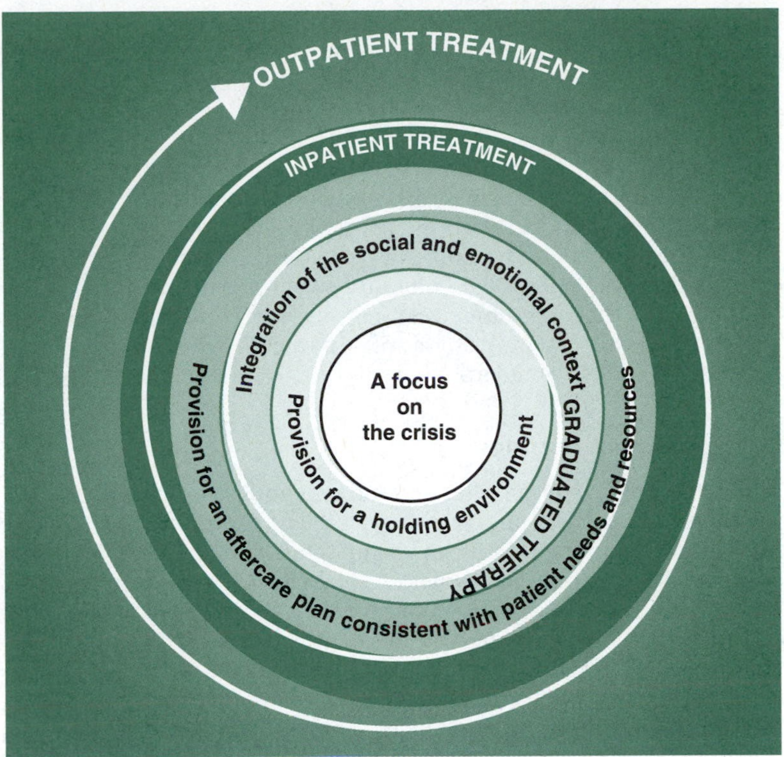

FIGURE 19–5
Kahn and White's factors to incorporate into short-term milieu therapy.

priority than maintaining a therapeutic milieu. However, in these settings, you must continue your efforts toward the development and maintenance of a therapeutic milieu as outlined in the criteria of Standard Vb.

Familiarization. Reality orientation is maintained by having clocks, calendars, and schedules posted. Many long-term settings have personalized patient schedules initialed by the staff when a patient attends a prescribed activity. You will often prompt and remind patients of daily routines.

Assessment of Environmental Effects. Psychiatric technicians and nursing assistants may provide much daily care, including writing notes of patient response to the milieu. You will supervise technicians and nursing assistants, write treatment plans, and periodically document patient response to the milieu. You will consult with other staff regarding behavior management and milieu adjustment.

Coping With Limited Resources. Nurses in long-term settings often have been creative in developing a therapeutic milieu with limited resources. In such settings, you will advocate for needed facilities and work toward congruence between policy and procedure of the institution, nurse practice standards, and the milieu needs of the patient to promote the therapeutic potential of the setting.

Nursing care to meet the patients' spiritual needs in the long-term setting is aimed at assessment of religious needs and practices of patients, providing privacy for spiritual or religious practice, assisting with dietary restrictions as needed, assisting with access to spiritual or religious leaders, and providing an opportunity for connectedness with others.

Communication. You are a role model for the appropriate and effective use of communication for patients and staff. Much effort in the long-term setting, including the appropriate use of communication, is aimed at resocializing patients.

Activities. You will work with activity, art, and occupational therapists to develop activities that meet the needs of patients.

Limits. Limit-setting, restraint, seclusion, and behavioral codes (code team response to dangerous behaviors) are used in long-term psychiatric settings when patients are unable to control their behavior. You must be sure that patients and staff understand the rationale and the behavioral expectations for release.

Opportunity for Questions. Many questions may arise at the time of admission and discharge planning from long-term care. Patients and significant others are encouraged to question and confirm their understanding of recommended treatment.

▶ Check Your Reading

7. Why is the concept of a treatment continuum important in caring for the serious and persistently mentally ill?
8. Name the three phases of the treatment continuum.
9. List at least four factors to be considered for milieu therapy in short-term inpatient units.
10. List and describe the phases of graduated therapy.

Community Treatment Settings

Tuck and Keels (1992, p. 54) state "The essential difference between inpatient and outpatient care is the controlled milieu in which it occurs." Although this assertion is true, the therapeutic setting continuum has increasingly blurred the clarity between inpatient and community settings. The advent of crisis units, residential settings, and intensive outpatient services has led to milieu considerations in community settings. The psychiatric mental health nurse—with a biopsychosocial and spiritual orientation and skills in facilitating the patient's journey—is the uniquely qualified professional to deliver care to those in need of community-based treatment. Nursing roles for community treatment settings correlate with the measurement criteria of American Nurses' Association (ANA) Standard Vb.

Day Treatment Settings

Individual therapy, group therapy, and psychopharmacological treatment are the mainstays of day treatment. Modalities are similar to those in hospitals but without the evening and nighttime components. Dealing with behavioral crises in a free-standing nonacute setting is a milieu consideration. Free-standing settings may have fewer staff members and resources available. Therefore, the staff needs strategies for handling potential crises. Because stays in the day program are longer, ranging from weeks to months, patients have more time for cohesion and group process to develop. It is important that staff members be skilled in group process.

Mobile Treatment Settings

Mobile treatment is a community treatment modality that provides clinical services to seriously and persistently mentally ill patients residing in homes, neutral settings, or anywhere the patient can be engaged. The seriously and persistently mentally ill are those with major symptoms of schizophrenia, bipolar disorder, schizoaffective disorder, severe personality disorders, and severe major depression. Many highly symptomatic patients with these disorders have great difficulty coming into traditional outpatient settings. Either they are unable to coordinate the steps to get to the clinic, or their symptoms are so severe they fear the clinic or are unable to see the need for treatment. These patients are met anywhere they will agree to meet; e.g., at a fast-food restaurant, at home, at the coffee shop, or in a store-front clinic. Patients in mobile treatment often develop long-term relationships with staff.

The clinical staff members attempt to provide holistic care. Intensive case management with supportive therapy is provided in a one-to-one relationship, which grows as the patient is able to tolerate the interaction. Note, however, that meeting patients on their own turf is very different from meeting them in inpatient settings. These patients need to be accepted despite the choices that they make. Staff members need to be tolerant and to be satisfied with slow gains. Constant respect for the patient's personal choices and own home are necessary. Only when the patient's choices present a danger to self or others may the staff intervene against the patient's wishes.

The mobile treatment environment provides a milieu that is under greater patient control. It is the staff's responsibility to provide for safety when meeting the patient in the community. That the patient controls the milieu allows staff members to engage with patients who would otherwise not seek out treatment where the milieu is controlled by staff.

Psychiatric Home Care

Psychiatric home care is an emerging modality that is important for the home-bound patient with psychiatric illness (see Chapter 44). The condition that renders the patient home bound may be either somatic or psychiatric. The goals of psychiatric home care and psychiatric home health care populations are listed in Chapter 43.

The staff evaluates the home milieu, makes recommendations to family and care providers, and sometimes refers to community agencies. Again, the milieu is controlled more by the patient than by the staff, and staff members must plan for their own safety.

Outpatient Clinics

Outpatient psychiatric clinics provide individual therapy, psychiatric evaluation, psychopharmacology and medication monitoring, group therapy, case management, and crisis intervention. The milieu in these settings is not well recognized. They contain waiting rooms, group therapy rooms, and the environment of individual therapy. Recognizing the milieu factors means considering

- Access to services
- Safety of the environment
- Barriers to care
- Managing the interactions within the clinic setting

Facilitating Access to Care. The referral and intake processes determines accessibility of care. Referrals may come from other agencies, practitioners, and self-referrals. An outpatient clinic must be approachable to persons in the community who have mental health issues. The clinic must have an admission process that considers that the patients may be highly symptomatic when he or she initiates the contact. Waiting lists, directives to call another person or to call at another time, and other requirements are often inappropriate. Intake needs to be timely, friendly, and free of barriers. Barriers to care include the size of fees, lack of accessibility to public transportation, and poor staff attitudes. Each must be monitored so that patients can afford care, can get to the clinic, and will feel welcome in the treatment setting. Otherwise, the patient will not follow through with treatment.

Providing a Safe Environment. A safe, physically accessible environment is essential. Safety includes protecting support staff, patients, and clinicians from violence. Support staff members—including secretaries, receptionists, and medical records personnel—all have patient contact. Support staff members need to know when to alert clinical staff. They need to be able to observe waiting areas and initiate a plan to deal with a patient presenting with an acute problem.

Support staff generally see patients before they are seen by clinical staff, so these staff members provide a first impression. Patients in crisis may be initiating services for the first time and may benefit from being greeted by friendly, calm, and prompt staff. Support staff therefore need training about mental illness.

The outpatient clinic, especially if it is a government-funded community mental health center (CMHC), often has the responsibility to influence the community milieu. This responsibility includes being a resource to the community regarding mental health issues and providing service in a community disaster.

Patients, families, and care providers need to be told that treatment may be delivered in several settings during the course of illness. Patients and families need to know about the resources available and how and when to access these resources. Most important, patients need to know that using resources of both inpatient and outpatient settings is not a sign of failure.

Peter receives treatment in the outpatient clinic, and over the course of his lifetime, most of his treatment will be provided in this setting. The outpatient clinic, or CMHC, provides evaluation, medication, emergency evaluation, and case management. The clinic is the hub of Peter's treatment.

Before Peter leaves the hospital, Miguel, his nurse, arranges with Marianne, the clinic nurse, for an appointment at the clinic to monitor Peter's medication. Individual therapy is arranged with Marianne, who is an advanced practice clinician (i.e., clinical specialist).

Marianne provides monitoring of medication, mental status, and community adjustment. She provides psychoeducation to Peter, his family, and his care providers at the residential program. Within the nurse-patient therapeutic relationship, Peter expresses to Marianne his distress with his diagnosis, loss of potential, and his questioning of religious beliefs related to having a chronic illness. Peter and his family have a strong religious faith, and Peter's illness has been perceived as a loss of faith. Additionally, he is in another community, no longer near his church. He expresses guilt that he has not attended religious services, as was his practice in his home community.

Kim, Peter's case manager, works to link Peter with needed medical services. For example, Kim arranges for Peter to have some dental work done by a dentist who donates services to disabled persons. She helps Peter contact his pastor and arranges for a visit.

Familiarization. As a nurse in a day treatment or outpatient clinic setting, you will teach patients about expectations, routines, and schedules of activities. When providing treatment in mobile treatment and psychiatric home care, you will work with patients in finding treatment times that are mutually agreeable. Assure safety of both patient and staff.

Assessment of Environmental Effects. In each community setting you have the opportunity to observe, analyze, interpret, and record the effects of the environment and patient response. The day treatment setting provides the most potential to manipulate the treatment environment. You may use a consultation approach to advise the patient about milieu in the home setting.

Consideration of Physical, Social, and Cultural Environment. In the day treatment and outpatient settings, you must consider milieu factors, including barriers to care and safety. Identify and monitor potential barriers and work toward solutions. Monitor the setting for physical, social, and cultural barriers. Educate support staff about mental illness and develop plans handling behavioral incidents. You can maintain awareness and teach support staff about cultural diversity.

Assess the physical environment of mobile treatment and home care patients for any potential environmental hazards that require correction. The setting should be free of hazards for the patient and care providers. Is the home setting secure and free of danger from the community? In home care and community psychiatric nursing, you will promote the therapeutic potential of these milieus by teaching self-care, supporting family and care providers, and consulting with other community health care providers. You need to work toward congruence between the policy and procedure of the employing agency, nurse practice standards, and the milieu needs of the patient to promote the therapeutic potential of community treatment settings.

Often, when practicing in community settings, you will have larger caseloads and a more complex organization within which to work. You must be careful to retain a holistic view of the patient, who has a full range of basic needs, including the need for spiritual meaning. Providing and promoting spiritual care in the community involves respecting spiritual and religious practices, providing the opportunity for meaningful one-to-one interaction, and promoting settings conducive to respect and human dignity.

Communication. In community settings, you will model appropriate communication patterns for patients, support staff, and other clinicians. Communication patterns are aimed at conveying respect of others and self.

Activities. In day treatment and outpatient clinics, you will collaborate, formulate, and provide direct milieu activities. In mobile treatment and psychiatric home care, you will provide direct one-to-one milieu activities. In each setting, you may refer to other milieu activity providers, as the patient is able. Such referrals might include psychosocial programs, community support and activity programs, self-help groups, and referrals for additional home care modalities, if indicated.

Limits. You may use limit-setting in each of the community settings. Clearly articulate the rationale for limits. Restraints and seclusion are not used in community settings. Instead, staff members use verbal deescalation techniques, remove themselves from harm, and use law enforcement, if necessary. If the patient is demonstrating potential harm to self or others and is unwilling to follow treatment recommendations, emergency petition for psychiatric evaluation may be used within the laws of the state. You must know the laws regarding emergency petition and be able to complete a petition or assist staff members or care providers in completing a petition.

Opportunity for Questions. A major goal of community psychiatric treatment modalities is the maintenance of patients in their homes and promotion of optimum health. This process includes referral and advocacy for services and facilities in the community that support the maintenance of home life while receiving needed psychiatric treatment. Patients and significant others may have questions and may require explanation, rationale, and education, especially for referrals.

▶ Check Your Reading

11. Describe mobile treatment including the target population.
12. List at least three considerations for the outpatient clinic milieu.
13. Describe limit-setting, including the emergency petition, in community settings.

Community Residential and Psychosocial Settings

Sommers (1987, p. 170) states "the character of a psychiatric patient's residential surroundings and social milieu can influence the success she/he experiences in attempting to adjust to life in the community." These settings are generally organized by psychosocial community nonprofit agencies. The focus of psychosocial rehabilitation services is the development and maintenance of social networks and social supports (Stroul, 1989). Often these programs do not include a treatment component but coordinate services with the community treatment programs. Therefore, diagnosis and treatment may come from the outpatient psychiatric clinic, and housing and support may come from the residential program. Figure 19–6 shows the continuum for milieu therapy and the continuum of the **residential/therapeutic community.**

The residential continuum, like the treatment continuum and the therapeutic community continuum, extends from the most restrictive-supportive to the least restrictive-supportive. A patient, however, may receive one level treatment service and another level of residential service. Generally, if the patient is in a highly supportive residential arrangement he or she may use a lower level of treatment over the long term. For example, a paranoid schizophrenic patient living in a 24-hour supervised residential setting would probably use less crisis intervention or psychiatric home care than the same patient living independently. The converse may also be true—the more clinical treatment that is provided, the lower the level of residential support that is needed. Because treatment is generally more costly than residential services, however, a relatively higher level of treatment would generally be used only on a short-term basis.

Notable exceptions to the separation of treatment and residential services exist. For example, Way Station in

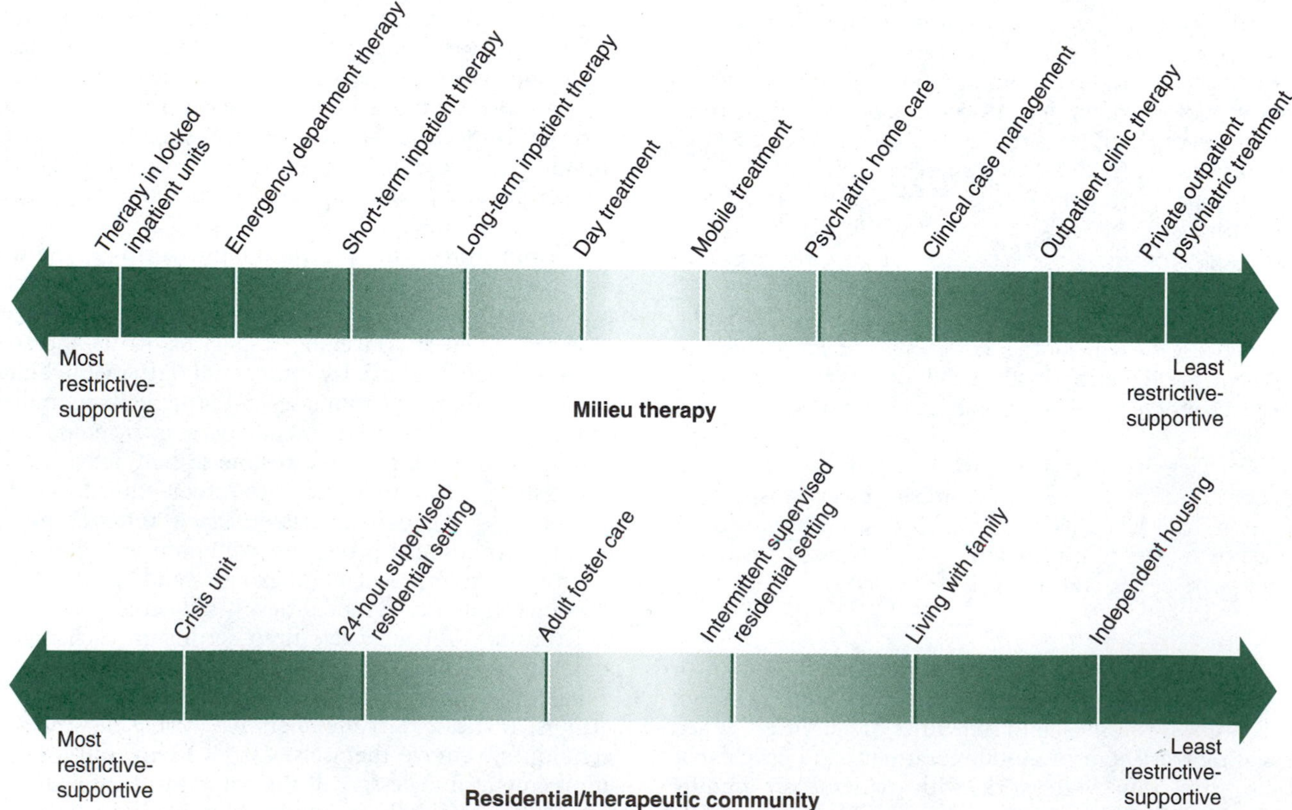

FIGURE 19–6
The continuum for milieu therapy and the continuum of the residential/therapeutic community.

Frederick, Maryland, a national model for psychosocial rehabilitation programs, and a few other programs throughout the country offer treatment and residential and psychosocial programs within one agency. The advantage is coordination among treatment, residential, and psychosocial components.

Crisis Units

The crisis unit is generally an extension of a residential program where 24-hour staff coverage is provided by paraprofessionals who provide a supportive, low-stress environment. Generally, no clinicians work at the site. The patient must be voluntary, able to physically care for himself or herself, and willing to follow treatment recommendations of clinicians. The order for the crisis unit services comes from the emergency department or the clinical component of the patient's treatment team. The service is usually limited to two weeks or less. The goal is to prevent hospitalization and stabilize the patient. The crisis unit may provide all factors of short-term inpatient therapy except graduated therapy (see Figure 19–5) and biological interventions. The holding environment is often the most important factor in crisis unit services.

The story of Beatrice in Case Example 19–1 is an example of a journey that includes the use of the crisis unit.

Case Example 19–1 Beatrice's Story

Beatrice, age 29, has worked at the travel agency for the past four years. She has a diagnosis of bipolar disorder, which was made after a manic episode that led to month-long hospitalization when she was 25 years old. She has been stable on lithium carbonate and outpatient therapy and had one other manic episode that was treated without hospitalization.

Beatrice sees her therapist on an emergency basis. She is upset and crying. Her mother, with whom she lives, had a heart attack and was hospitalized. Her father died 15 years ago of a myocardial infarction. Beatrice is afraid that she will get sick again and require hospitalization. Then who would visit her mother and help her come home? She is also afraid that her mother will die. She fears losing her job. Beatrice is frightened and confused but is not experiencing an exacerbation of her mental illness. Rather she is having a life crisis.

With Beatrice's permission, the therapist makes the referral to the crisis unit. Beatrice is able to stay in the crisis unit until her mother improves and plans are made for her to come home. Beatrice is able to maintain her employment and take only one day off from work. The crisis unit staff assisted Beatrice by providing staff support, assistance in making arrangements for her mother to come home, and encouragement to continue working. The support and holding environment helped Beatrice avoid decompensation and hospitalization.

The inpatient unit refers Peter to the crisis unit for a one-week stay. The purpose is to have Peter return to his day program and have staff available at night. When Peter returns to his day program, it is discovered that there were irreconcilable differences between Peter and the two other men that lived in his residential apartment. The other men had played a couple of jokes on Peter and have been doing pranks to get a rise out of him. Peter had difficulty coping with being the brunt of the jokes because he was new and without supports and because his illness makes environmental stress difficult to handle. A team meeting is called, including Peter, Marianne, Kim, and residential and crisis unit staff. Now less symptomatic, Peter is able to ask for a different residential arrangement. Another apartment is found with one other male patient. Peter agrees to a two-week trial of living in the new apartment. Until he demonstrates that he is comfortable, Peter will have increased staff support in his residential setting.

Residential Settings

Residential programs are often offered as part of psychosocial spiritual rehabilitation programs. Levels of residential supervision range from having 24-hour on-site staff to having staff work only a few hours a week. These programs offer patients a place to live and assistance with and teaching of activities of daily living. A therapeutic community may involve house meetings and democratic house rules. Because treatment is often provided from the clinical component of another agency, communication between residential staff and the clinical team is essential.

Adult Psychiatric Foster Care Settings

In adult foster care arrangements, psychiatric patients live in family homes for support and assistance with activities of daily living. This service may be provided by the Department of Social Services (DSS). The DSS case manager, working in cooperation with the foster family and treatment team, is responsible for maintaining an appropriate milieu for the patient. Adult foster care provides care for psychiatric patients who have been released from state hospitals after long stays (deinstitutionalized) and often works well for the elderly psychiatric patient. Patients with a potential for violence should not be placed in families with vulnerable members such as children or the elderly. Canada uses regulated private lodging homes for provision of therapeutic residential services for the chronically mentally ill (Chambers et al, 1988).

Nursing Roles in Community Treatment Settings. Your role within these settings may be more consultive because you generally would be employed by the agencies providing treatment. You do provide direct services within these programs, however, and you have the knowledge and experience with milieu therapy that may be useful to these programs. Your current and potential nursing roles are correlated with the measurement criteria of American Nurses' Association (ANA) Standard Vb.

Familiarization. When referring patients or residential or psychosocial programs, you will orient patients to the purpose of the organization and the reason for referral and provide an overview of the milieu that they will encounter. The programs are responsible for specific orientations to rules and activities.

Assessment of Environmental Effects. You will monitor and support patient participation in residential and psychosocial programs, and you may include such participation in treatment plans. Knowledge of these programs allows you to advise patients about the components of these programs that may be most beneficial as milieu therapy or therapeutic community for the individual patient.

Consideration of Physical, Social, and Cultural Environment. You will work to develop the therapeutic potential of these settings by providing direct care (such as psychiatric home care or mobile treatment) and by consulting to these agencies. When providing direct care, you must know who is responsible for the milieu and advocate for patients if necessary. This requires careful coordination of the policy and procedure of the employing or consulting agency, nurse practice standards, and the milieu needs of the patient to promote the therapeutic potential residential and psychosocial settings.

Spiritual caring for the mentally ill within community programs includes assessing the spiritual and religious needs and preferences of patients, supporting the opportunity for religious practice, and supporting access to spiritual and religious leaders and services. Do patients in these programs have access to transportation to see spiritual and religious leaders or services of their choice? Are patients able to carry out dietary or prayer practices within program settings? Is the atmosphere conducive to reflection, human contact, and dignity? These are issues related to supporting spirituality.

Communication. Use communication with patients and staff that is clear and consistent with maintaining a therapeutic milieu. Protect patient confidentiality between agencies by obtaining release of information, reviewing what information will be exchanged, and identifying circumstances information will be exchanged.

Activities. You may serve in many capacities that foster the development and institution of milieu activities designed to meet patient needs. These include serving as board member or consultant to program agencies, serving on community coordinating committees, and serving as a member of community placement teams (determines appropriateness of residential placement as patients leave hospital settings).

Limits. You may use limit-setting when providing direct care within these settings or may consult with care providers within these settings about limit-setting. The purpose of limits must always be clearly communicated to patient and staff. Restraints and seclusion are not used in the community. Emergency petition for psychiatric evaluation may be necessary.

You will assist the mentally ill to live at home by providing direct care within crisis units, residential programs, and adult foster care programs. Appropriate referral to these programs supports the patient in maintaining community life. You also may advocate for needed community facilities and services supporting healthy community life for the mentally ill.

▶ Check Your Reading

14. Describe the relationship between level of treatment and level of residential services.
15. What is a crisis unit? What is the goal of treatment in this setting?
16. Describe adult psychiatric foster care.

CONCLUSIONS

The therapeutic milieu exists on a continuum of treatment settings. Milieu therapy includes a treatment component, and nurses often provide that treatment component. Because nurses provide treatment in many therapeutic community settings, the nurse needs to make sure that the result is a therapeutic milieu. If you are providing the treatment plan and the referral to a setting, you are responsible for ensuring that the resulting milieu is therapeutic.

Individual treatment planning and service delivery in the form of case management have been the focus of much attention in recent literature. The result has been less attention to milieu and group process. Case management is essential, especially for the seriously and persistently mentally ill, to assure coordination of care across the treatment continuum. This concern does not, however, preclude the need to attend to the milieu process. The milieu will exist with or without explicit attention. To assure that the milieu is positive, psychiatric and mental health providers are responsible for managing socioenvironmental factors. Mentally ill individuals need nurses to develop, monitor, provide consultation, and maintain the therapeutic milieu in both inpatient and community treatment settings. Chapter 44 discusses case management as a modality of psychiatric care.

The future of nursing in the development of therapeutic milieus that meet the needs of mentally ill patients in contemporary health care is shifting from traditional inpatient settings to community settings. The inpatient milieu will remain important as a treatment setting for containment of sicker and potentially violent mentally ill individuals. The inpatient milieu must help patients regain behavioral control and become oriented to the therapeutic work that they will do in community treatment after discharge. Nurses need to be prepared to deliver direct care in communities, provide consultation to community settings, and advocate for safe and appropriate environments for the mentally ill. These are important elements in a patient's therapeutic journey.

If milieu therapy is a nursing domain and responsibility, nursing professionals must find methods to measure milieu therapy efficacy. Nurses need tools to measure inpatient and community therapeutic milieu efficacy. Perhaps a tool that measures patient satisfaction, psychiatric symptom levels, and hospital days used annually would reflect the effectiveness of the therapeutic milieu.

KEY POINTS TO REMEMBER

- Historical precursors to milieu therapy include moral treatment, therapeutic community, and psychoanalytical theory.
- Milieu therapy is the scientific management of the environment that is aimed at assisting the patient to change (Mosher et al, 1986).
- Gunderson's (1983) components of milieu therapy include structure, involvement, containment, support, and validation.
- Contemporary settings for milieu therapy include the following inpatient settings: locked inpatient units, emergency departments, short-term psychiatric units, and longer-term psychiatric units. Community milieu settings include day treatment, mobile treatment, psychiatric home care, and outpatient clinics. Nurses may provide direct care and consultation in residential and psychosocial program settings.
- Nursing roles are consistent with the eight process criteria of the American Nurses' Association (ANA) Standard Vb for nurses in the milieu.
- The Joint Commission of Accreditation of Healthcare Organizations (JCAHO) provides criteria for the therapeutic environment for the inpatient milieu. These criteria may also apply, in part or in total, to community settings.
- Spirituality is supported and promoted within milieu settings in many ways, some of which include
  - Assessing patients' spiritual or religious beliefs and practices
  - Providing privacy for spiritual or religious practice
  - Assisting patients with access to spiritual leaders and services
  - Providing an environment conducive to reflection and human dignity
  - Assisting patients in following dietary or prayer practices
  - Providing an opportunity for human connectedness

LEARNING ACTIVITIES

1. Read current journal articles on milieu therapy. What milieu settings and factors are described?
2. What milieu therapy settings have you seen in clinical environments or while visiting or working in health care settings? What settings do you want to know more about? Visit at least one new setting.
3. Which of Gunderson's components have you observed in a setting? Try to observe each next time you are in a setting.
4. Think about the milieu in community settings. What are some milieu factors that may have a negative impact on patients? Do psychiatric nurses have a role in the development and maintenance of the milieu in community settings?
5. Think about your own environment. What are the positive and negative factors of your milieu? Could you adjust anything to make your own environment more conducive to working toward your personal goals?

CRITICAL THINKING EXERCISE

Mrs. Rosa was admitted with back pain and depression to the acute care psychiatric unit. During the first four days of her stay, she rarely left her bed to attend community meetings. John Bailey, a new student nurse, was assigned to assess Mrs. Rosa's needs and develop a plan using milieu therapy as his focus of intervention.

1. What assumption(s) can be made about Mrs. Rosa?
2. How would Mr. Bailey test these assumptions?
3. Suggest some possible plans that Mr. Bailey could use.

After reading about milieu therapy, John decided to meet with Mrs. Rosa to develop a map of planned activities, discuss the reasons why she was able or unable to attend them, and develop alternate activities that could be attended. After three days, John reported his plans and interventions to his instructor. He reported, "Mrs. Rosa is now getting out to attend meetings, but I don't think I've been very therapeutic." When his instructor asked why, John said, "Because she hasn't talked to me about anything very 'deep.' " To John's amazement, Mrs. Rosa was discharged from the unit the following week feeling much better and capable of functioning as the secretary of the community meeting.

1. What assumption(s) might Mr. Bailey have about milieu therapy?
2. What evidence suggests that his assumptions were clear? Unclear?
3. What do you wish to tell Mr. Bailey about milieu therapy?

REFERENCES

American Nurses' Association. (1994). *Standards of psychiatric and mental health nursing practice and standards of psychiatric-mental health clinical nursing practice.* Washington, D.C.: ANA.

Abroms, G. M. (1969). Defining milieu therapy. *Archives of General Psychiatry, 21,* 553–560.

Almond, R. (1974). *The healing community: Dynamics of the therapeutic milieu.* New York: Jason Aronson.

Benfer, B. A., and Schroder, P. J. (1985). Nursing in the therapeutic milieu. *Bulletin of the Menninger Clinic, 40,* 451–465.

Carson, V. B. (1994). Spirituality and depression: An important relationship. *Smooth Sailing: DRADA Newsletter,* January.

Chambers, L., Forchuk, C., Munroe-Blum, H., Woodcox, V., Moore, G., and Wigmore, D. (1988). The development of guidelines to promote a therapeutic environment in lodging homes. *Canada's Mental Health,* December, 14–18.

Cumming, J., and Cumming, E. (1962). *Ego and milieu.* Chicago: Atherton.

Flexner, S. B. (Ed). (1993). *Random house unabridged dictionary* (2nd ed.). New York: Random House.

Forchuk, C. (1991). Reconceptualizing the environment of the individual with a chronic mental illness. *Issues in Mental Health Nursing, 12,* 159–170.

Frank, J. D., and Frank, J. B. (1991). Psychotherapy in a controlled environment. In J. D. Frank and J. B. Frank (Eds.), *Persuasion and healing* (pp. 274–294). Baltimore: Johns Hopkins University.

Gerson, S., Leingraber, J., Painter, M., and Ross, D. (1983). From custodial treatment to therapeutic community. Part I: Management of resistance to change process. *International Journal of Therapeutic Communities, 4,* 38–46.

Graham, J., Friedman, I., Lilly, R. S., and Allon, R. (1971). Factor analysis of the patient perception of the ward scale. *Journal of Clinical Psychology, 267,* 278–284.

Gunderson, J. G. (1983). An overview of modern milieu therapy. In J. G. Gunderson, O. A. Wills, Jr., and L. R. Mosher (Eds.), *Principles and practice of milieu therapy* (pp. 1–13). New York: Jason Aronson.

Gutheil, T. G. (1985). The therapeutic milieu: Changing themes and theories. *Hospital and Community Psychiatry, 36,* 1279–1285.

Joint Commission on Accreditation of Hospitals. (1987). Therapeutic environment. In *Consolidated standards manual for children, adolescent, and adult psychiatric, alcoholism and drug abuse facilities and facilities serving the mentally retarded/developmentally disabled* (pp. 177–182). Washington, D.C.: Author.

Kahn, E. M., and Fredrick, N. (1988). Milieu-oriented management strategies on acute care units of the chronically mentally ill. *Archives of Psychiatric Nursing, 2,* 184–140.

Kahn, E. M., and White, E. M. (1989). Adapting milieu approaches to acute inpatient care for schizophrenic patients. *Hospital and Community Psychiatry, 40,* 609–614.

Kennard, D. (1983). *An introduction to therapeutic communities.* Boston: Routledge & Kegan Paul.

Krauss, J. B. (1987). Nursing, madness, and mental health. *Archives of Psychiatric Nursing, 1,* 3–15.

Lannet, J. L. (1991). Resistance and countertransference issues with spiritual and religious patients. *Journal of Humanistic Psychology, 31,* (4) 68–76.

LeCuyer, E. A. (1992). Milieu therapy for short stay units: A transformed practice theory. *Archives of Psychiatric Nursing, 6,* 108–116.

Long, C. G., Blackwell, C. C., and Midgley, M. (1992). An evaluation of two systems of inpatient care in a general hospital psychiatric unit. I: Staff and patient perceptions and attitudes. *Journal of Advanced Nursing, 17,* 64–71.

Moos, R. (1974). *Evaluating treatment environments.* New York: Wiley Interscience.

Moos, R., and Houts, P. (1968). Assessment of the social atmosphere of psychiatric wards. *Journal of Abnormal Psychology, 73,* 595–604.

Mosher, L. R., Kresky-Wolff, M., Matthews, S., and Menn, A. (1986). Milieu therapy in the 1980's: A comparison of two residential alternatives to hospitals. *Bulletin of the Menninger Clinic, 50,* 257–268.

Mulvihill, D. (1989). Therapeutic relationship in milieu therapy. *Canadian Journal of Psychiatric Nursing, 30,* 20–22.

Oldham, J. M., Lin, A., and Breslin, L. (1990). Comprehensive psychiatric emergency services. *Psychiatric Quarterly, 61,* 57–67.

Peplau, H. E. (1952). *Interpersonal relationships in nursing.* New York: Putnam.

Peplau, H. E. (1964). *Basic principles of patient counseling.* Philadelphia: Smith, Kline, & French.

Peplau, H. E. (1969). Professional closeness . . . as a special kind of involvement with a patient, patient, or family. *Nursing Forum, 8,* 342–360.

Pollner, M. (1989). Divine relations, social relations & well being. *Journal of Health and Social Behavior, 30,* 92–104.

Rapoport, R. N. (1960). *Community as a doctor.* London: Travistock.

Rubin, R. L. (1991). Child psychiatric nursing. In G. W. Stuart and S. J. Sundeen (Eds.), *Principles and practice of psychiatric nursing* (pp. 852–877). Washington, D.C.: Mosby.

Sclafani, M. (1986). Violence and behavior control. *Journal of Psychosocial Nursing, 24,* 9–13.

Segal, S. P., Hazan, A. P., and Kotler, P. L. (1990). Characteristics of sheltered care facility operators in California in 1973 and 1985. *Hospital and Community Psychiatry, 41,* 1245–1248.

Shafranski, E., and Gorsuch, R. (1984). Factors associated with the perception of spirituality in psychotherapy. *Journal of Transpersonal Psychology, 16,* 231–241.

Sommers, I. (1987). Tolerance of deviance and community adjustment of the mentally ill. *Community Mental Health Journal, 23,* 159–171.

Stroul, B. A. (1989). Community support systems for persons with long-term mental illness: A conceptual framework. *Psychosocial Rehabilitation Journal, 12,* 9–26.

Tuck, I., and Keels, M. C. (1992). Milieu therapy: A review of this concept and its implications for psychiatric nursing. *Issues in Mental Health Nursing, 13,* 51–58.

Walker, M. (1994). Principles of a therapeutic milieu: An overview. *Perspectives in Psychiatric Care, 30* (3), 5–8.

Warner, S. L. (1984). Humor & self disclosure within the milieu. *Journal of Psychiatric Nursing, 22,* 17–21.

Warner, S. (1993). The cost-effectiveness of a nursing demonstration project, Part II. *Archives of Psychiatric Nursing, 7,* 61–67.

Watson, J. (1992). Maintenance of therapeutic community principles in an age of biopharmacology and economic restraints. *Archives of Psychiatric Nursing, 6,* 183–188.

Weissberg, M. (1991). Chained in the emergency department: The new asylum for the poor. *Hospital and Community Psychiatry, 42,* 317, 318.

Winnicott, D. W. (1960). The theory of the patient-infant interaction. *International Journal of Psycho-analysis,* 41, 585–595.

Yurkovich, E. (1989). Patient and nurse roles in the therapeutic community. *Perspectives in Psychiatric Care, 25,* 18–22.

SUGGESTED READINGS

Forchuk, C. (1991). Reconceptualizing the environment of the individual with a chronic mental illness. *Issues in Mental Health Nursing, 12,* 159–170.

LeCuyer, E. A. (1992). Milieu therapy for short stay units: A transformed practice theory. *Archives of Psychiatric Nursing, 6,* 108–116.

Tuck, I., and Keels, M. C. (1992). Milieu therapy: A review of the concept and its implications for psychiatric nursing. *Issues in Mental Health Nursing, 13,* 51–58.

Walker, M. (1994). Principles of a therapeutic milieu: An overview. *Perspectives in Psychiatric Care, 30* (3), 5–8.

Watson, J. (1992). Maintenance of therapeutic community principles in an age of biopharmacology and economic restraints. *Archives of Psychiatric Nursing, 6,* 183–188.

Yurkovich, E. (1989). Patient and nurse roles in the therapeutic community. *Perspectives in Psychiatric Care, 25,* 18–22.

CHAPTER 20

FAMILY THERAPY

The beauty of loving someone is the feeling of "wholeness" that I experience. The need for that individual in my life, the "I'm part of you and you're part of me" feeling that connects two people and makes them necessary to each other.

—Kathleen Andrus

LEARNING OBJECTIVES

After studying this chapter, you should be able to:

1. Identify trends in today's families.
2. Identify central concepts that organize families.
3. Discuss the history of family therapy.
4. Describe some recent directions in family therapy.
5. Explain the concepts of family systems theory.
6. Explain essential components of a family assessment.
7. Identify family diagnoses.
8. List principles related to family interventions.
9. Identify techniques used in family therapy approaches.
10. Explain the evaluation stage related to family intervention.
11. Apply the nursing process to the family as a patient in the mental health setting.

KEY TERMINOLOGY

Anxiety
Boundaries
Conflict
Developmental tasks
Differentiation of self
Distance/pursuit
Emotional cutoff
Family
Family myths
Family secrets
Genogram
Hierarchy
Level of differentiation
Multigenerational transmission
Nonnormative events
Normative events
Overresponsibility/underresponsibility
Pileup
Projection
Roles
Rules
Sibling position
Societal regression
Spirituality
System
Subsystems
Triangle

Closeness and distance, togetherness and separateness, wanting to merge with another and wanting to remain an individual . . . these opposite concepts are the keys to understanding families and family therapy. Life would be flat without the fulfillment of being close to other human beings. Yet few among us do not sometimes wish for more separateness, more identity, and more sense of self.

This dance, moving between closeness to another and space for self, is part of the journey that describes families and perhaps all human relationships. The family is a special case, however, because it is within the family unit that one grows, develops, establishes self-worth, and forms beliefs about life. The family, in some form, has been in existence since the beginning of human history. No other unit is quite like the family, which continues over our lifespan. Some say that the family is dying in today's society. Others are convinced that by strengthening the family we can strengthen our future.

Families are part of the context in which everyone lives. Families influence our life's journey as individuals. Families are the arena in which most of our important relationships with others are maintained. Families are resources to help people maintain their health and to provide support when illness strikes. In the past, families were sometimes blamed or identified as the cause of mental illness. Current thinking emphasizes family strengths as well as weaknesses. Today we recognize that families are valuable and resilient resources.

You will encounter families at various points along their journey and in multiple ways in the mental health setting. Family theory can be used by nurse generalists as well as by nurse specialists. At the simplest level, family theory requires changing your perspective to include the whole family rather than only the individual. Certainly a depressed woman can be understood in terms of psychiatric medical theory. The picture becomes broader and clearer, however, if she is understood as an overburdened member of a family struggling against poverty and the drug addictions of several family members.

Families are important to nurses as both the context in which individuals live and as units to be analyzed as "patients." Sometimes gathering data on the family situation is necessary to support the individual patient fully. At other times, however, the family needs treatment, and the entire family becomes the "patient."

Family-centered practice occurs in all phases of the nursing process. A comprehensive family assessment identifies strengths that can be useful in the plan of care. During the analysis stage, you might identify family-related problems such as family violence or altered parenting skills. Family-centered interventions might suggest alternative family coping skills or teaching healthier communication patterns. A family-centered evaluation appraises individuals as well as the family as a whole.

Family therapy is a specialized modality in psychiatric treatment, preferably practiced by a nurse with a master's degree and specific training in family therapy. The psychiatric nurse who intends to use family therapy as a treatment should have formal instruction and clinical supervision in family therapy. Many training programs are available in family therapy throughout the United States. At the present time, advanced practice nurses recognized by the American Nurses' Association (ANA) must present evidence of sufficient theoretical and clinical content in an accredited master's program, satisfactorily complete an examination that tests knowledge, and participate in supervised postgraduate clinical practice. Common to both general and specialized practice is a broader understanding of the individual as a member of family system.

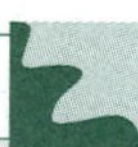

THE BLOUNTS' STORY

Ken and Diane Blount have just decided to enter family therapy. Ken, age 39, and Diane, age 37, have been married for 16 years. They have an 8-year-old son, Billy, and a 10-year-old son, Jason. Neither had been married before. They are choosing family therapy now because things have come to a crisis within their family. Not only is their marriage "on the rocks," but Jason has been diagnosed with depression and has recently attempted suicide. Jason is in therapy with a child psychiatrist, and the "whole family" is now entering family treatment.

This recent turn of events is not the first time troubles have appeared for this family. Diane had great difficulty getting pregnant. The Blount's first child, a girl, was stillborn. Things looked fine for a while after Jason was born. Ken had a good job with an accounting firm, and Diane worked out of the home doing word processing.

Shortly after Billy was born, though, it became apparent that something was wrong. Billy was eventually diagnosed as autistic. Management of him at home was incredibly time consuming and energy draining. Ken started working longer and longer hours. Most of the care was left to Diane. She threw her whole self into learning to care for Billy. She hoped for a miracle that would cure the autism and make Billy normal. Meanwhile, Jason was getting along as best he could. Actually, he became a model child who tried to do anything he could to take the burden off his mother and not be a bother.

Ken's parents lived in another city. They saw the kids only on holidays but sent money to help with Billy's care. Diane began to use a network of neighbors and friends to help her with Billy. Her mother and Dad frequently came to give her some relief, but this assistance was still not enough for a child who required constant attention.

At one point, Ken became extremely critical of Diane. Diane had gained a lot of weight and was totally involved with Billy's care. They separated for a short time about two years ago and eventually got back together. After a time, Diane began to deal with the situation by ignoring Ken most of the time.

Within the last year, the care of Billy has become more problematic because of his increasingly unpredictable aggressive outbursts. The doctor suggested that the family consider institutionalization for Billy. Ken would not agree. He believed Billy should be handled at home, even though he gave little of the care. Diane eventually made the decision that she would institutionalize Billy and return to school to complete her teaching certificate. At this point, she and Ken separated. About three weeks later, Jason swallowed a bottle of aspirin.

UNDERSTANDING FAMILIES

Family Forms

In defining family many questions arise. Does a family contain just parents and children, or are grandparents included? Is it a "real" family if a married couple chooses not to have children? Is a gay couple with children a family? Can a family consist of people living together who are not related? Family forms in today's society have become increasingly diverse (Table 20–1). The traditional view of a typical family consisting of two parents and several children, a nuclear family, is not the dominant family form (Box 20–1). Single-parent families, individuals living alone or together without being married, divorced and remarried individuals, and widows and widowers account for more of our nation's families than do nuclear families. Each family form has strengths and weaknesses—no one form is healthiest. Our definition of **family** is a group of people related by blood, marriage, or emotional ties, who define themselves as a unit and cooperate to accomplish the normal tasks of daily life.

▶ Check Your Reading:

1. Discuss at least two different roles for nurses using a

TABLE 20–1 **Family Forms**

Term	Definition
Nuclear	A father, mother, and at least one child living together but apart from both sets of their parents
Extended	Three or more generations including married brothers and sisters and their families
Three generational	Any combination of first-, second-, and third-generation members living within a household
Dyad	Any two members, typically husband and wife, living alone without children
Single parent	Divorced, never-married, separated, or widowed male or female and at least one child; most single-parent families are headed by women
Step-parent	One or both spouses are divorced or widowed and remarry into a family with at least one child
Blended or reconstituted	A combination of two families with children from one or both families and sometimes children of the newly married couple
Single adult living alone	An increasingly common occurrence for the never-married, divorced, or widowed
Cohabiting	An unmarried couple living together
No-kin	A group of at least two people sharing a relationship and exchanging support who have no legalized or blood ties
Compound	One man (or woman) with several spouses
Gay	A homosexual couple living together with or without children
Commune	More than one monogamous couple sharing resources
Group marriage	All individuals are married to each other and are considered parents of all the children

BOX 20–1 Demographic Trends in Family Forms

Smaller families—decreased family size results in stronger emotional bonds and more investment in each child.

Increase in empty nest time—longer life spans result in a longer empty nest stage and possibly relate to increased divorce rates.

Increase in number of dependent elderly—longer life spans increase the number of elderly who may be dependent on others.

Increase in number of older women living alone—the increased chance of survival for women has lengthened the period of widowhood. This group is bimodal economically.

Increase in number of never-married adults— more and more couples postpone marriage or decide not to get married at all.

Older first-time mothers—postponement of marriage and dual-career families result in older first-time mothers and children spaced farther apart.

Separation of children from biological parents— increased divorce rates result in greater numbers of children living with a single-parent or blended families.

Increase in number of children born outside legal marriage—new technologies, changes in societal values, and increasing teenage pregnancy result in more children being born into alternate family forms.

Unavailability of family to care for dependent members—the increase of females in the work force removes family members to care for young, elderly, and ill members.

Adapted from Glick, P. C. (1988). Fifty years of family demography: A record of social change. *Journal of Marriage and the Family, 50,* 861–873.

family focus in their care. How does a nurse prepare to be a family therapist?

2. Name at least three family forms common in the United States today other than the traditional nuclear family.

3. What are some of the implications of recent demographic trends for nurses as they offer health care to families?

4. How would you define *family*, and what would you say about emerging family trends?

Families as Systems

Families have many different characteristics. Any family can be thought of as a **system**, a whole in which the sum of the parts is greater and different than the separate pieces. We can look at individual members of a family, such as Mary, John, Jimmy, and Marie. But when they are together as the Smith family, something more than the sum of their individual personalities exists. Systems have **boundaries** or imaginary walls, both around them and between their subsystems. **Subsystems** are subgroups of people within the family. Subsystems include siblings, parents, or coalitions of like-minded family members. Boundaries that are permeable and clear, allowing information to flow in and out, lead to open, healthier systems. Boundaries that are impermeable shut the system off from information, resources, and sources of support. Closing a system tends to increase the anxiety and intensify the patterns of interaction within the system. Boundaries between subsystems should be clear and appropriate to each family member's age. For example, a 13-year-old boy does not belong in a parental subsystem. He should be acting like an adolescent in the family power structure, or **hierarchy**. **Roles**, defining who does what and under what circumstances, should be clearly spelled out.

It is easy to see that the Blount family as a whole was more than its separate parts. It helped that the family opened its boundaries to allow others to offer support and physical help when it was desperately needed. The subsystems in this family included an altered parental subsystem with Jason in the parental role rather than the role of a child most of the time. The sibling system for him was unique because his brother was not able to function as a brother, and his father was not acting like a father. Roles in this family were very clearly spelled out, but they left an inequitable distribution of tasks. Who had the power in the family? Surprisingly, it may have been Billy. Everyone else needed to adjust to him.

Family Communication

Families have **rules**, or norms that govern their behavior. Right or wrong, conscious or unconscious, family rules structure life's journey in the way that individual family members relate to each other and operate towards the outside world. Often these rules define the patterns that families use in their communication with each other. These rules help the family create meaning for themselves about their behaviors and the events that occur in their lives. For example, a healthy family rule might be to respect the privacy and decisions of each of the members. The meaning this creates when a family member is given the autonomy to make personal choices validates the self-worth of the family member. A dysfunctional rule that hinders healthy family operation might be an injunction that the family is never to talk about an angry encounter. Shutting off communication about feelings and events interferes with understanding and problem-solving.

Sometimes family rules evolve over the years or even over generations into rules that carry anxiety and shame. These rules turn into **family secrets**, private information that shuts down communication and intensifies anxious behavior around similar incidents. Family secrets might include hiding an illegitimate pregnancy, a divorce, or a "black sheep" family member. **Family myths** are long-time beliefs that shape a family's interactions with each other and the outside world. Myths are distorted family perceptions that have evolved, like family secrets, over time and become more intense. A family myth might be a belief that "no matter what you do, you are doomed to be poor" or "men are not strong enough to deal with emotions."

Communication in families is healthier when it is open, honest, clear, direct, and congruent. Communication facilitates problem-solving. Satir (1972), a family therapist, believes that healthy communication promotes self-esteem by validating each person's worth and purpose within the group. The goals of healthy communication are openness (members discuss events with each other rather than engage in circuitous ways of transmitting the information), honesty (members feel free to say what they think and feel), clarity (communication is simple and understandable), directness (members go directly to the person involved rather than communicate through another), and congruence (verbal messages match internal feelings). The family may not be able to communicate in these ways.

Unhealthy ways of communicating, such as adopting the roles of placater, computer, distracter, or blamer, detract from exchange of information and also erode individual members' self-esteem. For example, the blamer is really adopting a life stance that he or she is not capable of accepting responsibility for his or her own actions. The placater is communicating that others' wishes are more important than his or her own. The computer is very analytical and denies the emotional content of family issues. The distracter fears conflict and attempts to distract the family's attention away from the conflict. Some families have difficulty with problem-solving. They will either bury problems because they hesitate to discuss tense material, detour or shift responsibility to other family members, or engage in conflict that does not negotiate an acceptable solution. Families that transcend these patterns and problem-solve effectively cope better with life problems (Case Example 20–1).

Case Example 20–1 The Walker Family's Story

The Walker family needs to learn healthier patterns of communication. Tom and Beth Walker are a middle-age couple with two college-age children, Kathy and Dave. Tom has an alcohol problem that is getting more severe. He has begun to miss work and is having problems with high blood pressure and esophageal varices. Beth is a placater. She tries to smooth everything over so no one is upset or unhappy. Dave is a distracter. When the family gets close to talking about an anxiety-provoking issue, he jokes or diverts the attention to himself. The family also has a secret. Beth's father was a drinker who abandoned her and her younger brothers when she was only 10 years old. Few people in the family know that he left after he lost his job because of his drinking.

This family has always operated with three major rules to guide their communications:

- Do not speak about unpleasant or upsetting things to each other.
- Do not let outsiders know the family business.
- If bad news needs to be communicated to Dad, Mom is the one to do it.

There is nothing inherently bad about these rules or styles of communication. They have a function, such as protecting people from upsetting information or interpersonal conflict. A family that uses these patterns, however, has difficulty discussing problems openly and honestly. Problems are often swept under the table and not addressed, or one family member or a small subsystem will attempt to solve the problem for the whole family. When family members attempt to keep things calm no matter what or to keep the lid on a family secret, they pay a price. It takes great energy to hide the truth. Everyone in the family system usually ends up feeling the anxiety in some way.

It has become popular in lay thinking to believe that in any situation people will do better if feelings are expressed. The Walker family is an example of a family that needs to work on expressing feelings. In some families, however, expressed emotion is very high. Family members exhibit a pattern opposite from the Walkers. They express anything that they feel at inappropriate times. Such a family could benefit from learning the principle of recognizing the difference between thinking and feeling. When a person can become clear about thoughts and feelings and is able to express them to another in a nonreactive way, information can be received and acted upon appropriately.

The nurse who worked with the Walker family was contacted by Kathy through the college counseling center. Kathy was the family member most open to outside help. The nurse believed the family needed to learn more open communication patterns. She was also aware of the denial that takes place with alcoholism and knew that the denial would be difficult to work against. She provided Kathy with information about Al-Anon and encouraged her to attend meetings while she was coming to therapy sessions. Eventually, Beth also attended the counseling, but Tom and Dave did not.

Initial sessions dealt with defining the extent of the problem and its effects on all family members. Education about alcoholism as a disease and family communication behaviors that enabled the alcoholic behavior was provided. The nurse was careful to model healthy communication herself. For example, when Kathy called to tell her that her father had recently been reprimanded at work and asked her not to tell her mother, the nurse refused to keep this secret and calmly brought it up in the next session, modeling the way to communicate distressing information. Beth responded by saying she knew it already and had been afraid to talk about it with the children. A discussion followed where Kathy and Beth agreed to stop keeping information from other family members.

Beth and Kathy began to identify and change the ways they were enabling Tom's behavior at home. A change in their behavior, however, was not enough to get Tom to stop drinking. Eventually, a family intervention was organized with the help of a professional rehabilitation program. Tom entered treatment and now has two years of sobriety. The whole family continues "one day at a time."

Let's return to the Blount family and examine the rules that shaped their journey. The Blount family had a rule that no one should complain about the troubles the family was having. The sacrifices that were required were expected to be borne without comment. When Ken began treating Diane poorly, a family secret developed. Actually, there was more to the secret than Ken's behavior. Before they were married, Diane had become pregnant. She had not wanted to have the baby and had an abortion even though it was contrary to both her personal spiritual values and those of her family. Keeping this secret was related to a family myth because Ken and Diane both believed that their children's afflictions were somehow related to this earlier mistake. Another operating myth was that "Billy would get better if Diane would just do the things required of a good mother." The Blounts were not using open, honest, and direct communication. Diane blamed Ken for his nonparticipation in Billy's care. Ken responded by becoming superreasonable and explaining why he needed to focus all his energy on the financial concerns of the family.

Families and Time

Families are different from other social groups in that they share a unique journey together (Skolnik and Skolnik, 1986). Few social groups span the time frame that family does . . . from womb to tomb . . . and beyond. Families create patterns, identities, and expectations across generations. The influence of the extended family helps to explain current events because present lives are so intertwined with the lives that came before. Genetic and physical influences are increasingly important as we learn to understand the interconnections of illness and genetic predisposition. For example, schizophrenia, bipolar illness, and even substance abuse may be influenced by special susceptibilities to these illness (Scheflin, 1981). Others suggest that much more than physical characteristics are transmitted through generations. The **multigenerational transmission** process, a concept proposed by family systems theory suggests that a level of emotional health is transmitted or passed down to the next generation. The level of emotional health is influenced by the degree of fusion (need for togetherness) one has with one's parents (Kerr and Bower, 1988).

Families have another time-related characteristic. The function of many families is to reproduce and protect the development of their members. Families are organized to care for their dependent members who cannot care for themselves—infants, children, people who are ill or disabled, and the elderly. Family development theory suggests that families have identifiable stages with tasks that need to be accomplished around specific times. For example, a childbearing family needs to reorganize itself to accept the introduction of the baby and to provide safe care for its newest member. A launching family prepares to release functional members into the community (Duvall, 1957). Duvall outlined eight stages of the family life cycle:

1. Married couple
2. Childbearing family
3. Family with preschooler
4. Family with school-age children
5. Family with teenagers
6. Family as a launching center
7. Middle-aged parents
8. Aging family

Duvall further specified **developmental tasks**, specific kinds of goals to be accomplished at each stage of a family's journey. Others (Carter and McGoldrick, 1988) have expanded this work to more closely match today's families. In their scheme, they recognize that families may not have children and may include several generations alive at the same time.

Family Functioning

Some families are healthier or more functional than others. Families differ in their ability to cope with extraordinary life stress (**nonnormative events**) and to deal with everyday life tasks (**normative events.**) Many theories attempt to describe differences among families in their functional abilities. Bowen (1978) suggests the family **level of differentiation** (how comfortable the family is in accepting individual differences among its members) is an important predictor of function and is related to physical, social, and emotional function. Structural therapists suggest that organization and structure of the family determine its health (Minuchin, 1974). Communication therapists look at communication patterns (Satir, 1967). Developmental theorists look for transitions that are early, late, or atypical to the societal norm. Clusters of transitions and insufficient accomplishment of task from preceding transitions detract from a family's ability to deal with a current transition. Nonnormative or unusual events, such as a fire or a sudden death, also weaken a family's response.

Family coping theory (Hill, 1949) suggests the ABC-X (Crisis) Model of Family Coping. A (the event) interacts with B (resources) interacts with C (family's definition of the event) to produce X (the crisis). The roller-coaster course of adjustment represents a process involving disorganization, recovery, and a subsequent level of reorganization as a family proceeds through a crisis. McCubbin's model (McCubbin et al, 1982) adds the concept of **pileup** of demands. Families differ in their ability to adapt to a stressor and manage it. If, over time, the family has been exposed to a series of stressors that deplete the family's resources, then the family will experience greater difficulty adjusting to a present crisis. Families that are exposed to stress over long periods of time end up in a situation of maladaptation, in other words, being worn out and functioning less well over time (Case Example 20–2). Characteristics of functional families are outlined in Box 20–2.

Case Example 20–2 The Miller Family's Story

The Miller family was seen at a community mental health center. Carl, age 62, is a retired steelworker who recently suffered a cerebral vascular accident that left him partially paralyzed and unable to speak. He lives with his wife, Emma, age 59. Also living in the home are their daughter Elise, age 35, and her daughter Lisa, age 7. Elise is a divorced single parent. Recently, the family was joined by Emma's brother, Michael, age 43, who is HIV positive and becoming fairly ill.

Emma and Carl are upper middle class. Carl owned his own printing business. Since the stroke, Emma has returned to work as a secretary at an investment house. Elise also works at a furniture showroom. The family income has been greatly reduced but is being supplemented by Carl's disability. Michael is currently without financial resources.

On a typical day, Emma and Elise get up and care for Carl and Lisa before they go to work. Michael drops Lisa at school and then returns home to sit with Carl. Most of their day is spent watching television until Lisa returns home from school. Then Michael helps Lisa with her homework and starts dinner. Carl watches the activity from his bed. Elise and Emma return home about 6:00 p.m. Sometimes in the evening, Michael and Emma go to church or to choir practice. The family socializes in the church, and the church frequently sends visitors to help out where they can.

The family is coping well, but Michael has suffered his second bout of pneumocystic pneumonia this month and is beginning to feel weaker. Emma and Elise are beginning to feel exhausted as they try to care for the other members of the family and also work. At this point, the family has no plans for handling the demands posed by the progression of Michael's illness.

The nurse working with this family recognized the areas of family competence or strength that have served the family well in the past. The nurse also recognized that the family is at a transition point when life events such as Carl's illness and retirement, the financial adjustments, and the demands of a school-age child are adding increased stress and may tax the family's resources to the point the family no longer is able to cope without help.

The nurse focused his strategies on helping the family recognize its resources and coping styles, analyzing which are functional at this point, and mobilizing additional resources. The nurse discovered that this family's boundaries are pretty closed. They are willing to accept help from their church and people they know, but it is difficult for them to accept help from others.

Eventually, the nurse working with this family gained their trust. As Michael's illness progressed, the nurse worked to keep family members calm and thoughtful about choices. He acknowledged their desire to handle the problem themselves but helped them explore other choices. At a family session, Emma, Michael, and Elise reviewed what was happening and decided that the family needed more help. The church was contacted, and more help was provided. Lisa was put in an after-school program. The nurse helped the family arrange for homecare for both Carl and Michael. Meals on Wheels made

BOX 20-2 Characteristics of Functional Families

Developmental Stages and Tasks

A family goes through predictable stages according to the age and development of its members. Tasks need to be achieved at the stage-appropriate time or they may never be achieved. Maturational crises are predictable. Some crises are unpredictable and interfere with achievement of tasks.

Roles

Roles define certain patterns of expected behavior and are often gender linked. Roles need to be appropriate for age and sex, flexible rather than rigid, and able to support family functioning.

Boundaries

Boundaries exist around the system to handle exchange between the system and the environment. Boundaries exist between subsystems to differentiate members belonging to each subsystem. They need to be permeable to allow information and resources in and out of the system. Boundaries between subsystems should have clear generational lines and support a strong parental coalition. Boundaries should be neither too rigid nor too diffuse.

Subsystems

Each member of the family belongs to several subsystems simultaneously: spousal, parental/child, sibling, grandparents. Subsystems should include all age-appropriate members.

Patterns of Interaction

Patterns repeat themselves and are healthier when one member is not blamed, left out, or put down in the interaction.

Power

Power results from clear role definition and appropriate rules. Power should be somewhat shared, appropriate to age, and located within the parental subsystem until the children are independent.

External Stressors

External stressors usually are present at some point. If they are not intense, of long duration, or occurring simultaneously, the family may be able to adapt. Illness brings its own set of demands to the family.

Open/Closed System

As the system closes, all variables and patterns become fixed and less able to adapt. Energy is used in dysfunctional ways. Open systems can adapt and change as feedback is received from inside as well as outside the system.

Communication

Healthy communication is clear, honest, direct, congruent, and specific. Healthy communication becomes a mechanism for the family to resolve conflict.

Encouragement of Autonomy/Acceptance of Difference

A balance needs to exist between the autonomy of family members and the need to be a cohesive group.

Level of Anxiety

When the family is calmer, people in the family can think and problem-solve better. Families tend to do better when things are calm than when they are in times of stress. Anxiety can be due to a transition or it can be long term. Long-term anxiety tends to wear down the ability of the family to function well.

Resources/Social Support

Resources are available to most families from within and outside the family, but the family needs to be able to use them. Extended family is often used. All families have some strengths.

Perception

Perception refers to the way a family sees a situation, the meaning it attaches to the events influence family reactions.

Adaptability

Flexibility, adaptability, and resilience are necessary for a family to be able to cope with changing demands. A family needs to maintain a degree of flexibility and also a degree of cohesiveness and predictability.

deliveries during the day. Emma and Elise were both encouraged to learn to rest and take some time for themselves to maintain their own functioning as the situation became more difficult. The family's spiritual resources were assessed, providing a source of comfort and strength.

Carl and Michael both lived about another year and died at home—three days apart from each other. Emma and Elise were constantly supported by members of the church and the health care resources that were drawn upon to help them.

Let's turn our attention again to the Blount family. This family has been exposed to multiple stressors—nonnormative events over time. They dealt with initial crises well, but as the events piled up, their emotional and physical resources became depleted. Eventually, they moved into a state of maladaptation and were not as functional as they had been. The family's ability to achieve its expected developmental tasks, like getting Jason to sports and Boy Scouts, going to church to maintain their spiritual support, or creating a meaningful family life, was dissipated. In many ways the Blounts were no longer fulfilling the functions required of a healthy family.

▶ Check Your Reading

5. Discuss the difference between an individual and a systems way of looking at an emotional problem.
6. What happens inside a family when boundaries are more closed and impermeable? What happens inside a family when boundaries are open or permeable?
7. What does it mean when one says "boundaries around and between subsystems should be age-appropriate?" Can you give an example of inappropriate behavior within a subsystem?
8. Name four dimensions of healthy communication.
9. Describe some family roles that detract from open communication.
10. How do family myths and family secrets affect communication in families?
11. What is the result of the multigenerational transmission process?
12. According to Duvall, in what developmental stage was the Blount family? What tasks would you expect them to accomplish at this stage of their family life?
13. Of what importance is a transition or pileup of events to a family? How does one predict if a family would do better or worse when certain events occur?
14. List five characteristics of functional families. Explain how these characteristics vary in dysfunctional families.

FAMILY INTERVENTIONS

History of Family Therapy

The evolution of family therapy is itself a journey. Until the 1950s when family therapy first began to appear, most psychiatric professionals were treating individuals. Some clinicians believed that relationships with other people might be important to the understanding of an individual's illness. For example, in his interpersonal theory of psychiatry, Harry Stack Sullivan (1953) related the functioning of the individual to the messages about self received from interactions with others. Most psychiatrists however, were wedded to the idea that the patient was sick and had to be treated on an individual basis. Some psychiatric clinicians who were treating individuals—such as Bowen, Ackerman, and Jackson—began to orient their thinking to the family group. These schools of therapy later emerged as theoretical approaches in their own right. In 1961, the journal *Family Process* was first published (American Association for Marriage and Family Therapy [AAMFT], 1981). In 1966, the Group for Advancement of Psychiatry (GAP) distributed a questionnaire that documented the wide interest in family psychiatry (Committee on the Family, 1970). The family movement was on its way!

In 1963, California became the first state to pass a licensing law for marriage and family counselors. At that time, people were being trained in family therapy in two ways: in accredited training centers specifically for family therapists and within graduate schools in their own profession (e.g., medicine, nursing, social work, ministry). The GAP became the AAMFT in 1978. In 1980, the AAMFT was accepted as the official accrediting agency for marriage and family therapy by the U.S. Department of Health, Education, and Welfare (AAMFT, 1981). At this time, the AAMFT's position is that family therapy is a profession in its own right. The AAMFT specifies curricula and training requirements for clinical members and approved supervisors, credentials members, and accredits approved training centers. It helps its membership define the extent of their practice, deals with ethical issues, and supports its credentialed members who are dealing with legal and ethical concerns. Professionals can currently become credentialed by attending an accredited training program and participating in 200 hours of supervision with an approved AAMFT supervisor. While this position has furthered the professionalism of marriage and family therapy, the practical considerations of participating in the training have limited the numbers of credentialed family therapists.

Emerging Family Treatments

Both psychoeducation and marital/divorce therapy are emerging as useful family treatments.

Psychoeducation

Psychoeducation is becoming increasingly popular and is used in several ways to provide

- Information and training about a specific area of family life, such as communication skills training or parent effectiveness training
- Information and support to families dealing with a

specific stress or crisis, such as a family support group for Alzheimer's

- Prevention and enrichment, such as premarital counseling, for families not in crisis

Research supports the effectiveness of psychoeducation in a variety of ways. For example, the improvement of communication skills enhances the marital relationship and parent-child relations (Hawkins and Roberts, 1992; Meyers, 1993). Parent Effectiveness Training (Gordon, 1980) improves parent-child openness and empathy (Grando & Ginsberg, 1976). Roosa and others developed a program directed at preventive intervention for children in alcoholic families, which resulted in less depression and acting out and more positive coping for children who participated in this eight-week program (Roosa et al, 1989). Psychoeducational programs are relatively inexpensive and often effective in influencing family life.

The National Alliance for the Mentally Ill (NAMI) has become very active in providing psychoeducation for families of the mentally ill. This group advocates for improved treatment and services for the chronically mentally ill. They also share information and challenge stereotypes about the mentally ill and their families. When concepts about family systems were first published, some clinicians thought dysfunctional families were the "cause" of emotional symptoms. NAMI counters this assumption and helps families learn to cope with the effects of the illness on the individual as well as the family (Hatfield and Lefley, 1988) (Case Example 20–3).

Case Example 20–3 The Thomas Family's Story

The Thomas family was having a difficult time as the teenage children grew up. Josh, the 15-year-old child, was skipping school and getting bad grades. Josh frequently stayed out beyond his 11:00 p.m. curfew and refused to do his chores. He was constantly argumentative, and family members found themselves frequently involved in fights that ended in Josh's storming out of the house. Sometimes Luann, a single parent, became so frustrated she would slap Josh across the face. When this happened, her mother, Dorothy, and Julie, the 13-year-old daughter, retreated to their rooms.

Josh complained that he did not have the freedom he deserved as a 15-year-old. He believed his life and his school performance were his own business and that his mother should stay out of the picture. Luann was very worried about Josh's educational success. Luann interpreted Josh's current behavior to mean that he was likely to have trouble in adapting to a difficult world. Her behavior was fueled by worry. Luann believed that she was struggling to help him learn to be a functional adult. This family was able to tolerate individual differences but was struggling to allow Josh some autonomy.

Luann happened to run across an advertisement for parent effectiveness training for parents of adolescents. The series of classes ran for 12 weeks and was open to anyone in the community as a service of the community mental health clinic. The series was run by a nurse in the clinic and was attended by a group of 17 parents, who met weekly for the 12 weeks. The class consisted of a 30-minute educational session followed by a group discussion. Luann learned some effective techniques to help her set limits on Josh's behavior. She also learned information about adolescence and the importance of providing freedom when possible. By listening to other families' experiences, she began to see how her problems with Josh were universal and to get ideas about how to deal with them.

At every session, reading and homework was assigned. In the third session, every parent mapped out a plan for dealing with the behavior of the adolescent and providing realistic consequences. Luann sat down with Josh and explained carefully what his limits were and took an "I position" that stated what she was going to do. Support from the group helped her maintain her objective plan and decrease her tendency to react to Josh automatically. At first Josh acted out even more, but when he realized that she was not going to back down, he began to obey the family rules. Luann, however, had to work to keep her mother from interfering with her discipline. Dorothy thought the punishments were too harsh and felt sorry for Josh. A triangle had developed in which Josh would run to Grandma for protection when he was in conflict with Mom.

Luann began to realize the techniques she learned would also be helpful with Julie, even though Julie reacted to her in different ways. Eventually, Luann became a peer counselor who helped run the classes. Josh stayed in school and graduated. He is now attending a community college.

Marital and Divorce Therapy

Marital therapy today can take many forms including maintenance of a marriage in crisis, treatment of sexual problems, movement towards a successful divorce, or helping a stepfamily or blended family adjust. Marital enrichment is also a goal of this treatment.

The American Association of Marriage Counselors was formed in 1942. Before that time, most marital problems were treated by having each spouse work separately with an individual counselor. In the 1960s, therapists began leading weekend retreats or enrichment programs for people who wanted to avoid the problems they had seen in other marriages. Emphasis in these workshops was on open communication, encouragement of trust, sharing experiences, and building positive feedback patterns. The retreats usually took place in a group setting with a "facilitator" rather than a therapist. The facilitator set the stage for the couples to rediscover the vitality in their marital relationships. In 1973, the Association of Couples of Marital Enrichment (ACME) was established. The facilitators in marital enrichment programs work towards three goals:

- Dispelling the myth that marriage is living happily ever after. Marital enrichment emphasizes the series of

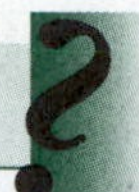

WHAT PATIENTS NEED TO KNOW Common Questions When Beginning Therapy

How do I decide if our problems could be helped with family therapy?

Family therapy can be useful for problems, such as marital conflict, that are clearly identified as family problems. It is also often useful when the issue involves disturbances in family relationships such as occur between parent and child, caregiver and care receiver, or siblings. Waiting until the problem is out of hand is like waiting until one's blood pressure is too high. Often therapy can be useful in a preventive way to help people work on their relationships before they are in serious trouble. Many therapists use family systems concepts with individuals who are interested in working on their own functioning. Some therapists see only one person in the family.

How do I know the theoretical orientation of the therapist, and does it matter?

When the call is made to set up the first appointment, you can ask the therapist to explain his or her theoretical orientation. The style in which a therapist works will become clearer after you are actually in therapy. Although some would disagree, the theory used may not be as important as the fit between the particular therapist and the patients. Gender should also be considered. Will someone in the family be uncomfortable or feel as if sides are being taken if the therapist is a male or a female? Once therapy begins, if the style of the therapist is not helpful, you can always ask for a referral to someone else.

Is therapy covered under my insurance, and how much will it cost?

Emotional problems that are clearly identified as psychiatric illnesses in the *Diagnostic and Statistical Manual-IV (DSM-IV)* are often more likely to be reimbursed than family therapy. However, health care plans differ as to what is covered. The best advice is to call your representative and ask if the therapy is covered. Sometimes there is a deductible or copayment. Therapists also differ in the ways they manage their billing. At times, one family member may be the identified patient and other family members will join in the treatment sessions under that billing.

What can I expect to happen during the first session?

For some therapists, the therapeutic process begins with the first telephone call. The therapist may want to discuss the problem on the telephone or develop some sense of what the family is like before the family comes to the office. The therapist may set some rules; for example, a therapist might insist that all family members come to the appointment. Sometimes homework is given for the family to complete before the first appointment. The first session is usually an information-gathering session. The therapist attempts to gain some understanding of the problem and help the family reframe the problem. Although patients may experience some relief, it often takes several sessions before anything is "resolved."

How long will therapy take?

Time varies according to the problem and many other factors. The therapist sets mutual goals and discusses the expected time with the family early in the encounter.

tasks and adjustments to new situations that make up married life.

- Building an effective communication system. An enrichment program stresses creation of daily sharing times, use of complete rather than inferred communication cycles, and frequent mutual affirmation.

- Learning to use conflict constructively. Conflict can become an effective means to an end if it is used to solve problems and address troubling situations. Couples learn to accept anger as a signal that other feelings, such as fear or hurt, also are present and move towards effective ways of negotiation or compromise.

Sometimes, however, marriages do move toward divorce. Today's marital therapist will not necessarily view divorce as a failure but as one outcome of the process. If a couple divorces, helping the family move toward the divorce while maintaining other functions is a goal of some therapists (Haber, 1993). For example, the therapist assists the partners to negotiate child custody without encouraging the children to align with one or the other partner; to assist each parent to deal with the issues of loss and grief and still provide some support for the child; to assist the partners to leave the emotional marriage with an understanding of the reciprocity in the breakdown of the relationship without blaming the other. At some stages in the process, the divorce therapist helps the partners make decisions; protect legal, financial, and social arrangements; and prepare for life as autonomous individuals.

Family members often remarry, and many bring children from previous marriages. Treating blended families involves helping families establish an identity as a new family without invalidating ties or values held by the original family. The discipline of children, financial arrangements, chores and household tasks, values, holiday rituals, inlaws, and religion become frequent issues. Strengthening and empowering the marital bond of the new couple is necessary and often difficult if the couple is trying to establish bonds with children. Frequently the couple has little time alone in the face of competing family responsibilities. "What Patients Need to Know: Common Questions When Beginning Therapy" suggests responses to typical patient concerns.

▶ Check Your Reading

15. Briefly describe the emergence of family therapy.
16. What is the name of the national professional association of family therapists? What functions does it perform?
17. How does psychoeducation differ from family

therapy? Describe a potential nursing role in a psychoeducational program.
18. Name three goals of marital therapy.

THE PROCESS OF FAMILY THERAPY

Family therapy refers to a wide variety of interventions, skills, and techniques that are drawn from a variety of theoretical approaches (Box 20–3).

The theory or framework that directs the family work is inside the therapist's head and is used as a map to guide the therapist's actions with the family. These theoretical maps have emerged from many different schools of thought. An overview of some theoretical approaches is presented in Table 20–2.

Murray Bowen is the founder of a school of family therapy that developed the family systems approach in more specific ways. Bowen's thinking about families was stimulated during his work at the National Institute of Mental Health where he began observing the interactions of families of schizophrenics on a psychiatric inpatient research unit (Bowen, 1978). His observations of first the mother, then the nuclear family, and eventually generations of the family, has been articulated in Bowen's family systems theory.

Bowen family systems theory views the family as a system. The goals of the therapy are to

- Improve the ability of each family member to be able to differentiate their thinking and feeling
- Differentiate self or become less emotionally reactive to others with a more solid sense of self

Bowen family therapists view themselves as *coaches* to the family. The role of the therapist is to help the family decrease its anxiety, gain a broader perspective on problems, and become aware of the ways emotional reactivity influences individual and family functioning. Coaching people to define self, that is, to develop a more solid self in the face of forces to fuse with others, is one of the main strategies.

Starting with a **genogram** (family diagram), a Bowen family therapist will gather information that helps the family look at relationships between family processes and events, track multigenerational patterns, and connect with important relationships. Education, questioning, analogies, and observations are techniques used as the coach attempts to maintain a neutral position, manage anxiety, and define self to the family. In this school of thought, the therapist considers it essential that each patient continues to work on his or her own level of differentiation concurrently to participating in family therapy. In recent years the theory has turned towards natural systems. Observing patterns over time in other types of organisms adds breadth to understanding the family system.

BOX 20–3 Types of Family Therapy

Individual Family Therapy

Individual family therapy occurs when each family member has a therapist. The family may meet together from time to time to work on issues of family conflict and interaction. The family is not the focus of treatment, but understanding the family context is believed to be important to the growth of the individual member.

Couples Therapy

Couples therapy is for married or unmarried individuals who are seeking help for a troubled relationship or attempting to prevent problems in an impending marriage. The couples may be heterosexual or gay, intending to live together or to live separately, recently together or about to separate.

Conjoint Family Therapy

Conjoint family therapy is for a single nuclear family. Typically, the family presents with a problem, then both the family and the therapist work together to define the goals that will be addressed during the contacts. The family is typically viewed as a system in which all members have a part to play in the issue. Individual concerns are addressed within an effort to support the family unit.

Multiple-Family Group Therapy

Multiple-family group therapy is for several families meeting together at one time. The families often have issues and concerns in common. Learning occurs from observing and listening to the other families present their concerns and work on their issues.

Multiple-Impact Therapy

Multiple-impact therapy is intense therapy similar to multiple group family therapy but is focused during a short encounter like a weekend or week. Typically, several therapists conduct intense and focused therapy while living in a community setting with the families. The therapy is usually directed toward a specific problem or issue like child discipline, marital enrichment, or sexual concerns.

Network Therapy

Network therapy moves into the community where people actually live. All persons who are interested or connected with the crisis are invited to participate. The network group may include professionals, neighbors, community members, friends, and family. A team enters the home to address the immediate crisis. During this process, energy is often mobilized to create a longer-lasting network of support for the family.

TABLE 20–2 **Models of Family Therapy**

	Significant Therapists	View of Treatment	Interventions
Psychoanalytic	Ackerman	A corrective relationship between therapist and family will heal the family	1. Tackling the defenses—confronting the discrepancies between thoughts and feelings 2. Re-creating a family environment that can act as a parent
Strategic and structural	Bateson Haley Minuchin	Needs to focus on the "here and now" by changing the structure and operations of the family	1. Reframing 2. Suggesting paradoxes (opposites) 3. Changing the hierarchy by joining, enacting, marking boundaries
Experiential	Whitaker	A humanistic experience directed by spontaneity and focus on feelings Encounter groups Psychodrama	1. Using the therapist's own "craziness" 2. The therapist taking charge of the "battle" for the structure of sessions 3. The family taking charge of the "battle" for initiative or ultimate outcome
Communication	Jackson Satir	Helping the family modify dysfunctional communication to reduce symptoms and increase self-esteem	1. Role-modeling 2. Education 3. Confrontation of double-binds 4. Use of the "meta" (observer) position

The two most important concepts, anxiety and differentiation of self, target the difference between thinking and feeling. **Anxiety** is viewed as the arousal of the organism upon perceiving a real or imagined threat (Papero, 1990). The higher the level of chronic anxiety in the family, the more each individual life course becomes determined by reactive mechanisms rather than thought. **Differentiation of self** refers to the degree to which an individual can separate thought from feeling. An individual with a high degree of differentiation of self will react with a high degree of thought and less emotional reactivity. Emotional reactivity is a tendency to react automatically to a situation without being able to separate thoughts from feelings. This tendency tends to produce more difficult life courses. Gavazzi (1993) tested the assumption that level of differentiation is related to increased life problems in an adolescent sample. He found level of differentiation, or the family's tolerance for individuality and intimacy, to be significantly correlated with presenting problems of adolescents in a clinical setting. Problems such as depression, use of substances, running away, lack of friends, and academic difficulties were associated with lower levels of differentiation.

Differentiation of self is related to the forces of togetherness and separateness. Individuals with less differentiation are more fused with other people and more relationship oriented. Individuals with more differentiation are more able to maintain autonomous or separate selves and tend to act on beliefs and principles rather than on an urge to be fused with another person.

In any two individuals, most noted in a marriage, tension lies in the struggle between togetherness and separateness. It is difficult to sustain a close twosome for too long. Typically, the twosome will attempt to manage this tension by triangling in a third person. The **triangle** then becomes the basic building block of interpersonal relationships. In any triangle, there is a close side, a distant side, and a side where tension or conflict occurs between the two people (Figure 20–1).

Any mother who has invited children to visit knows what a triangle is. Two children who usually play well together will suddenly explode into trouble when a third is added. "Mommy, he won't play with me!" is a familiar refrain as one child sides with another and the third is left out in the cold. In times of calm, being in the most distant position is uncomfortable. People struggle to regain closeness. When the situation is tense, however, the most distant position is usually the most comfortable. People in the triangle will maneuver to get to that outside position.

Triangles are present in all areas of life. The psychiatric nurse, patient, and psychiatrist become a triangle. The nurse manager and his or her two best staff nurses become a triangle. The spouse of a patient, the patient, and the therapist are a triangle. The three people in the car pool form a triangle. When tension increases, people in a triangle find it difficult to manage tension and will triangle in a third or fourth person, forming more triangles. In times of anxiety, these interlocking triangles can escalate tension so that people are caught reacting automatically to each other rather than dealing thoughtfully with the issue at hand. The key to managing triangles is not to avoid them—an impossibility—but to learn to manage and retain a self within them. This detriangling requires remaining connected with all the people while defining a self or stating an "I position." The natural tendency is to desire approval or to seek distance to escape the tension. Detriangling requires thinking one's way out of the reactivity.

Marriages typically use one of four patterns within the primary family triangle of mother, father, and child. These emotional processes are distance/pursuit, overresponsibility/underresponsibility, conflict, and projection to a child.

Distance/pursuit is like a dance in which one partner wants more emotional closeness than the other. Typically, although not always, the female is the pursuer and chases the other until he or she becomes uncomfortable and distances. The plea "Let's talk more. Let's spend more time together" results in the distancer spending more time at work, reading the newspaper, or working in the garage on the car. When the pursuer gives up and retreats, however, the distancer has more comfort in the relationship and will often return or even become the pursuer. "Why don't we go out tonight?" is the next step in the dance.

The pattern of **overresponsibility/underresponsibility** is also called under- and overadaptation or dysfunction in a spouse. We are most familiar with this pattern in alcoholic families in which one partner enables or takes care of the other. The person in the "one-up" position looks like a hero. His or her overdoing—assuming tasks, decisions, and emotional responsibility for the other—looks helpful. The consequences, though, tend to hold the spouse in the "down-one" position in check. It is very difficult for someone who is already having trouble functioning to pull up out of this position. It is much easier for the spouse who is overfunctioning to pull back and do less.

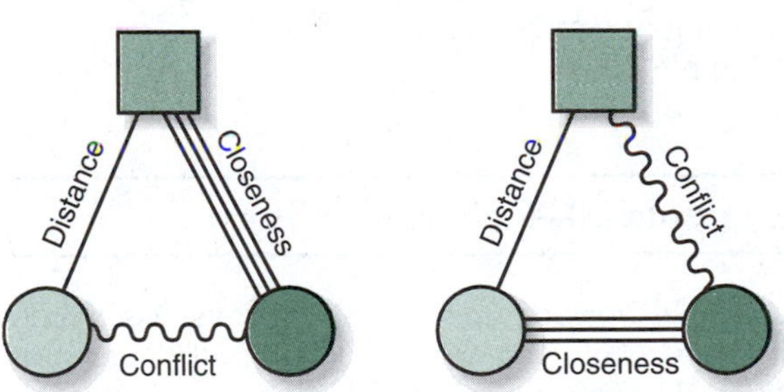

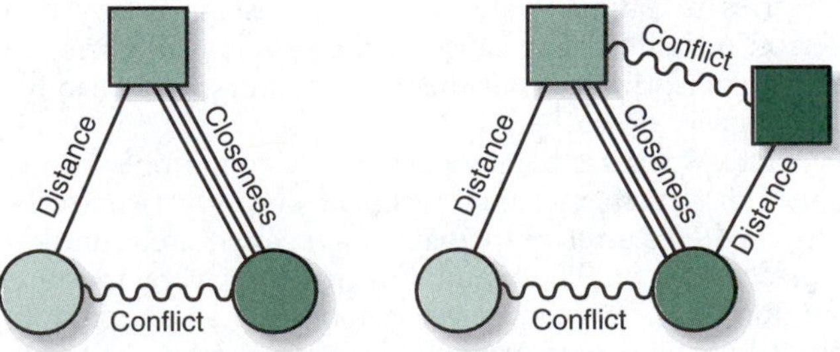

FIGURE 20–1
Solutions to tension or conflict in relationships: **A,** Switching roles. **B,** Triangling-in a fourth person.

Nurses and others entering the helping professions are sometimes overresponsible. Our positions within our families of origin often have placed us in this role. An overresponsible person is most comfortable when doing for or taking care of another. The cost for this pattern of behavior, however, is that the spouse, child, or patient who is being taken care of does not learn to function for herself or himself. Another cost for the overfunctioner is spending so much time responding or caring for others that he or she neglects himself or herself—his or her health, personal development, and need for relaxation.

Conflict is the third mechanism within the patterns of the nuclear family emotional process. Conflict is a repeated pattern used to manage anxiety within the family where the situation that triggers the conflict is never actually resolved. Typically, tension builds up between two people with neither able to state an "I position" and stick to it. Finally, the conflict escalates into a crisis. In some families, the conflict is loud and may even involve physical violence. In other families, the conflict may not be observable to an outsider. The twosome tend to settle the conflict by making up, reestablishing a harmonious twosome, and enjoying a short honeymoon from the conflict. Shortly, though, the tension and conflict begin to build again. In some families, these situations are forms of tension management—the family literally blows off some steam and then settles down. Police and law enforcement professionals know this pattern well. They are frequently called to the house of conflictual families to settle a dispute, only to have the situation dropped and start again days later.

The fourth mechanism is **projection**, a pattern so important that Bowen named it one of the nine concepts of this theory. When a couple cannot manage tension between them, they may project by turning to another, often a child. Unresolved issues or need for emotional closeness are then removed from the marriage and focused instead on the child. The projection may take a negative form—such as scapegoating or focusing on a child's behavior. It may be expressed in what looks like a more positive form such as excessive attention and concern about a child's school performance, development, or potential. Often, the mother will begin to live through the child—that is to focus her own desires and worries on the other person. Bowen (1978) suggests that this child focus leads to the next concept, the multigenerational transmission process.

The multigenerational transmission process suggests that some children will receive more emotional fusion than others. Circumstances surrounding the child's birth, gender, appearance, or birth order may predispose the child to this process. Therefore, some children in a family will have less differentiation of self than their parents, some about the same, and some more (those with the most freedom from projection). If one traced these levels of differentiation over generations, one would be able to see the level of differentiation of different family lines increase and decrease in health.

Emotional cutoff is a way of handling tension in a family by separating self from the process. Cutoff may vary from intrapsychic separation to physical distancing

(Papero, 1990). On a simple level, people speak of "needing space." On more intense levels, cutoff may take the form of psychosis or moving to a distant locale to avoid uncomfortable contact. The problem of cutoff is that it makes people more vulnerable to other intense relationships and toward repeating patterns that are unresolved within their family of origin. People who cut off from families are more vulnerable to life problems.

Sibling position, a concept Bowen borrowed from Walter Toman (1969), suggests that people develop certain personality characteristics related to their birth order and gender within their family of origin. Oldest children tend to be responsible, even overachieving, and they tend to look for positions of leadership and authority. Middle children tend to get along well with others and to know how to negotiate. Younger children focus less on responsibility and more on social and recreational pursuits. They are comfortable letting others assume the more dominant roles and taking a follower position. Whether people are born into a constellation of brother or sisters also affects personality. For example, an older sister of brothers is most comfortable taking care of men. She would do well as a secretary with a male boss or as a Cub Scout den mother. A younger brother of an older sister will often not object to the female taking a leadership role. He might be comfortable with a female boss. He might marry a woman used to being "in charge."

Some factors skew these tendencies. Losses, such as divorce or the death of a parent, alter the usual picture. If siblings are separated by more than four years, the younger sibling will tend to develop more like an older or an only child. Toman suggests that successful marriages may be related to complementary sibling positions between spouses. An older brother of a sister should do well married to a younger sister of a brother, for example.

Societal regression suggests that crowding and environmental pressures are more likely to push levels of differentiation down rather than up. As society becomes increasingly more populated, with more people responding automatically, evidence suggests individual dysfunction—with physical, emotional, and social symptoms—and increasing societal irresponsibility. For example, as violence in America continues to increase, we seem unable to set limits that will send clear messages to offenders. American society may not have enough individuals with high levels of differentiation who are able to take "I stands" on the problem. A society with more people having higher levels of differentiation would take a position and effectively enforce the consequences. Adequate differentiation may be important in responding effectively to societal as well as personal challenges.

Spirituality is the final concept of Bowen's theory. Bowen was reluctant to talk much about spirituality, suggesting that it is something that each person needs to define personally. Yet at the end of Bowen's life, it became such an important concept to him that he augmented his theory, believing it to be incomplete without a spiritual component.

▶ Check Your Reading

19. Describe a triangle. What purpose does a triangle serve?
20. Define emotional cutoff.
21. What does "differentiation of self" mean?
22. What does Bowen mean when he talks about societal regression?
23. What effect does taking an "I stand" have on a triangle?
24. What does Toman say about the effect of sibling position?
25. What is meant by multigenerational transmission process?

NURSING PROCESS

Whether you practice as a generalist or a specialist, the nursing process continues to be a useful guide for thinking about families and intervening along their journey. *Assessment* means gathering information about the family "problem" and making a contract for the nursing contact. Goals are mutually identified and established with the family. Goals should specify time limits and expectations. Interventions are based on family theories and knowledge about families. Evaluation is included at every step of the process and must consider the individuals within the family as well as the family unit.

ASSESSMENT

Every professional encounter begins with assessment. This is the first step to participating in the family's journey. Gathering comprehensive information is essential for understanding the family's problems. Assessment of families in the psychiatric setting includes an understanding of the presenting problem as well as an understanding of family functioning and family dynamics (Case Example 20–4).

Case Example 20–4 Patrick's Story

Patrick, an RN working on an inpatient psychiatric unit, attempts to use family systems theory in all his professional work. He tries to use the ideas to help him think more clearly about work and personal issues, with the goal of keeping his own functioning at a reasonably high level. He tries to "think systems," not focusing on any one person or issue as the cause of the problem. He tries to collect facts, think about the broad picture, and keep his own anxiety down.

This week has been a particularly rough one for the unit. The nurse manager resigned abruptly two weeks ago, and an interim manager was appointed until a replacement could be found. For the past several months, the unit has been fairly anxious about a change in billing procedures and patient admission. Rumors suggest that layoffs may occur. The patients have been acting out. Several were restricted to the dayroom after being caught smoking in the bathroom. During the community meeting, many complaints were made about the heavy-handed style of the nursing staff.

At noon, the chief psychiatrist approached Patrick and questioned his care of one of the young male patients on the unit. At first, Patrick responded angrily and automatically. He defended himself and suggested the psychiatrist was not on the unit enough to see what was going on. Quickly he realized that he was in the middle of a triangle with himself, the patient, and the psychiatrist. He realized his typical automatic response was to get angry and blame the other person. He recovered by clearly stating what he had said to the patient and allowing the psychiatrist to draw his own conclusions.

Later in the staff lounge Patrick gave some thought to what had occurred. He realized the entire unit not only was more anxious today, but also had been anxious since the administrative changes had begun to occur. Most staff members had responded by choosing sides or clumping into little groups. The togetherness seemed to help people feel better. He realized that he too had been pretty anxious, even though he usually worked on monitoring his own anxiety.

Another of Patrick's typical reactions during times of stress is overfunctioning. As an oldest child in a family of five, he learned early in life to take over to get things done. This functioning for others sometimes left him tired, with little time for himself. Pat realized not only that he was overfunctioning with the patient who had complained about him but also that he was doing it at home in his personal life. He was tired and feeling stressed even before he came into work.

Patrick resolved to be more aware of the current emotional intensity of the unit and try to work to keep himself calm in the midst of the emotional field. He would attempt to detriangle himself by keeping in contact with both the psychiatrist and the patient without complaining or talking about either person to the other. Most important, he needed to start to take care of himself and decrease his efforts at taking over others' problems. His attempt to become clearer about his thinking and feeling states is an example of using Bowen family systems theory in a work setting.

As with all assessment, you will use all available sources of data to help fill in a complete picture of the family and each member. Of course whenever discussing a family with another member of the health team or reviewing records, the family's permission must be secured first. Sources of data can include but should not be limited to

- Charts and written health records
- Biological data such as blood pressures or specimens
- Phone calls and conversations with other health team members
- Information from social service agencies involved with the family
- Environmental and community information

However, the most accurate and complete information must be obtained from observing and interviewing the family itself.

Interviewing families can be more difficult than interviewing an individual patient, and when you are not familiar with this situation, it can be a little frightening. After all, the family has been together for a long time and has a history that gives even the most dysfunctional family strength and collective power. Interviewing families can also be a rich source of information and a path to establishing relationships that are fulfilling and meaningful for you and for family members. The first contact with a family might occur in the hospital, clinic, community setting, or family home. Seeing families in their own environment is, of course, preferable because you can observe first hand the physical and environmental conditions, as well as the way family members respond to each other on their own turf.

The First Interview

Family assessment within a family therapy setting is more controlled. Some therapists believe the therapeutic process begins the moment a family member picks up the telephone to call for an appointment. An experienced therapist learns a great deal about the family's perception of the problem and how family members are managing tension by assessing how the family presents the problem on the telephone, whom they single out as the sick or problem individual, and whom they expect will attend the therapy. Most professionals are careful to structure even beginning contacts with families to maximize information. The first interview also can set the stage for the family to begin to see a family problem rather than an individual concern. Neutrality, honesty, and careful statement of boundaries or the limits both of the therapy and the helper are important in the first encounters.

The initial interview has many purposes. Information about family dynamics and family history must be obtained. Practical concerns such as phone numbers, health insurance information, and other health care sources are addressed. The family may come to the session wanting to talk about the problem and expecting that one session will even determine a solution. Most often the nurse must help family members broaden perception to include the whole family. At times the family is very anxious or angry, and this first session is used to help the family become calmer. Your challenge is to remain neutral and yet connect with each family member. Ask each member for a perception of the problem and indicate that all family members are important.

Gather information about the presenting problem. Why has the family come for help now? How do family members describe the problem? One of the family members may be the symptom bearer—the one who is acting out or holding the tension for the family by becoming identified as sick. Sometimes one or more family members have an emotional illness or carry a *Diagnostic and Statistical Manual-IV* (*DSM-IV*) diagnosis, such as a phobia or major depressive disorder. Sometimes the family defines the issue as a family one—marital conflict or problems with discipline. Discuss the history

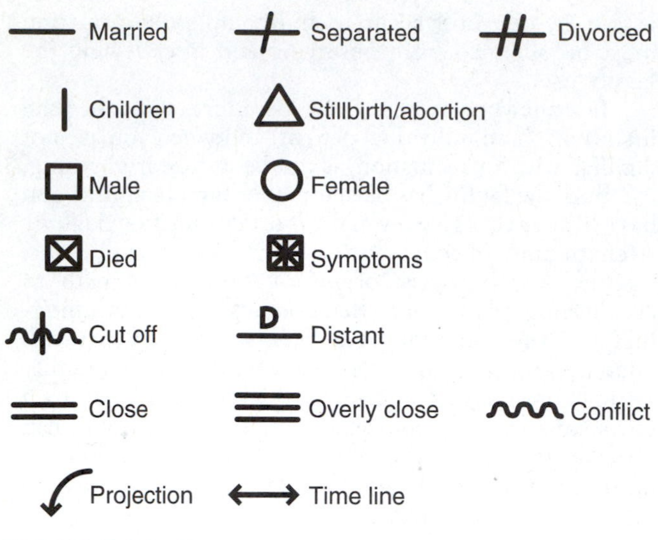

FIGURE 20–2
Symbols used in genograms.

of the problem, events surrounding its onset, and previous attempts to correct it.

During the first encounter, begin forming hypotheses or informed guesses about the family issues. Evaluate family functioning. How much anxiety is the family experiencing now? How much have family members experienced in the past? What are the current indicators of social, emotional, and physical health or dysfunction? Historically, what has the level of functioning been for each member and the family? Is this a family that typically functions well but is now under stress? Or is this a family that functions with a high level of anxiety all the time and has chronic problems?

During the first session, attempt to engage the family in therapy. The goal of this engagement is to convince family members that counseling is valuable and that they should come back. Although some people would use charisma or an interpersonal approach to engage the family, most family therapists attempt to summarize the family's perceptions of the problem, present their own view of the problem, and discuss what sorts of interventions might be attempted. Before the family leaves the session, an initial contract is formulated that describes the expected encounters, the time and frequency, and the responsibilities of nurse and patients. The family should emerge from the session with a calmer and clearer view of the problem and some hope that family life can be strengthened by the contact.

Assessment Tools

Depending on the therapist's theoretical approach, different assessment tools may be used. Box 20–4 presents some specific family assessment tools.

A **genogram** is a format for drawing a family tree that records information about family members and their relationships for at least three generations (McGoldrick and Gerson, 1985). An assessment tool useful throughout the contact with the family, a genogram makes it easier for a clinician to think about the family members, patterns, and significant events that are important in the family's care. A genogram also may be used as a therapeutic tool to help individuals see family processes more clearly. Although the therapist may think he or she knows what the family should do, interpretations that come from family members themselves are usually more accurate and useful for change. The picture of the family that is presented on the genogram helps the observer think about the family systemically and over time. Sometimes when a larger picture is presented, connections between events and relationships become clearer and are viewed in a more objective way.

Genograms serve several other functions. The process of collecting and recording information for the genogram is a way for the interviewer and family to connect in a personal but emotionally safe way. It also provides the interviewer with information about how the members of the family think about the family problems and interact with other members. Beginning to record information on a genogram can detoxify issues or reduce anxiety about the family problem. During the process, people are required to think, organize, and present facts. The therapist joins the family and helps to normalize and reframe problems so that they are viewed in a larger context. This type of interaction helps individual family members to step back and think about an issue in a calmer way.

Typically the genogram is constructed in the beginning of therapy and revised as new information becomes available. Three parts to genogram construction must be considered:

1. Mapping the family structure
2. Recording family information
3. Delineating family relationships

First, the person and family completing the assessment fill in the facts about the family and later return to describe the process of family interaction. A diagram of family members placed in each generation is drawn using horizontal and vertical lines. Symbols are used to represent pregnancies, miscarriages, marriages, and deaths (Figure 20–2). Males are placed on the left of the horizontal line; females on the right. Birth order is represented by placing the oldest sibling on the far left and progressing toward the right. In the case of multiple marriages, the earliest is placed on the left, with the most recent on the right.

Family information that is helpful includes ages, dates of births and deaths, geographical location, occupation, and educational levels. Critical family events such as moves, marriages, divorces, losses, and successes are recorded. Family members' physical, emotional, or social problems or illnesses are identified. A chronology or time line of family events is often very useful to help people see relationships between events and behavior changes. Observing and describing family relationships is the most crucial stage and often the most helpful to the family but is often ignored. Relationship patterns that are quite complex can be inferred from observations and from family members' comments and analyses. Triangles are present in every family. Attempting to map the primary or most influential triangles in the family is a part of describing the family relationships. Figure 20–3 shows the genogram of the Blount family.

DIAGNOSIS

The various assessment instruments mentioned in Box 20–4 provide a comprehensive assessment but also a massive amount of data. Family assessments can be complex and confusing if data are not sorted and analyzed in some way. What does this information all mean? In what way can it be used to help the nurse and family plan their work together? The information must be integrated and analyzed before decisions about the plan of care can be made. Several steps in organizing include

- Determination of needs or areas of concern
- Assessment of family functioning
- Determination of patterns of family interaction
- Identification of components or targets of care
- Determination of the therapist's contribution
- Priority-setting of identified needs

The North American Nursing Diagnosis Association (NANDA) has been identifying and listing diagnostic nomenclature since the early 1970s (NANDA, 1995). These diagnoses are formulated to help nurses choose and direct nursing interventions by focusing on patient responses to existing or high-risk problems rather than on the disease process. Each diagnosis consists of three parts:

- Health problem
- Etiological or contributing factors
- Defining characteristics

The health problem consists of the identified behavioral disruption, or potential disruption, that can be improved through nursing intervention; it is the unmet need of the patient. The etiological factors include the stressors that contribute to the problem; these can be considered the probable causes of the problem. The defining characteristics describe the concomitant signs and symptoms, which reflect the objective and subjective behaviors that provide the supporting data for the nursing interventions.

The North American Nursing Diagnosis Association suggests several diagnoses that relate to interpersonal relationships and family, such as Altered Parenting. Some examples of these diagnoses are presented in Box 20–5. NANDA includes four nursing diagnoses specific to family functioning:

- Altered Family Processes
- Ineffective Family Coping: Compromised

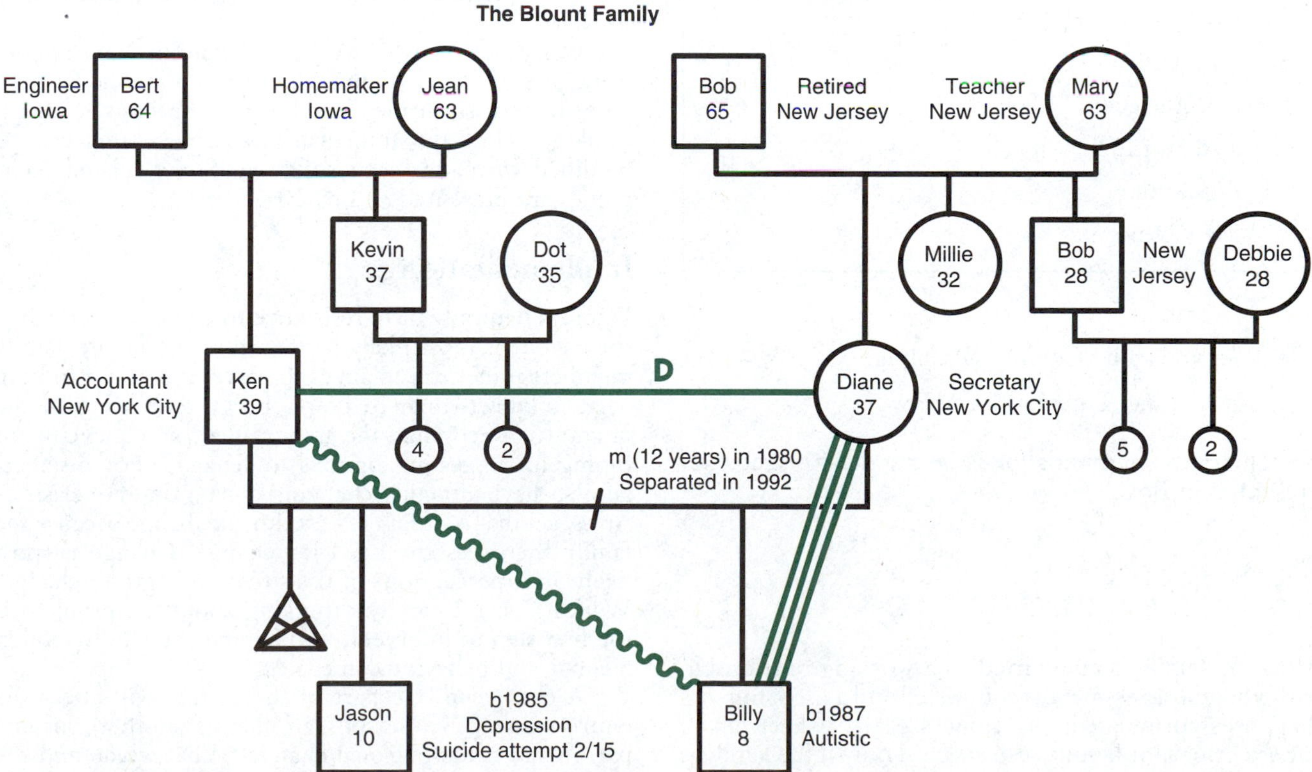

FIGURE 20–3
A sample genogram.

BOX 20–4 Examples of Family Assessment Instruments

Family APGAR of Family Functioning (Smilkstein, 1978)

Family Coping Index (Freeman and Heinrich, 1981)

Family Inventory of Life Events and Changes (FILE) (McCubbin and Thompson, 1987)

Family Map (Minuchin, 1974)

Family Nutritional Assessment Tool (James, 1989)

Family Self-Care Patterns (Pender, 1987)

Genogram (McGoldrick and Gerson, 1985)

Family Strengths (Otto, 1973)

BOX 20–5 Interpersonal Nursing Diagnoses

Impaired Adjustment

Ineffective Breastfeeding

Impaired Verbal Communication

Impaired Home Maintenance Management

Ineffective Individual Coping

Altered Parenting

Altered Role Performance

Self-Care Deficit

Sexual Dysfunction

Impaired Social Interaction

Social Isolation

Risk for Violence

- Ineffective Family Coping: Disabling
- Family Coping: Potential for Growth

An elaboration of criteria for assigning these diagnoses is presented in Box 20–6.

OUTCOME IDENTIFICATION

After the family is committed to a working relationship with you, the assessment is completed and a list of nursing diagnoses formulated; priorities are then determined. Interventions for families can succeed only if the family is sincere in wanting to change and agrees with the goals set for the contacts. Choosing priorities is a mutual process in which you as therapist provide information to the family that summarizes what has been said and observed. Use theory, training, and experience to communicate informed knowledge to the family. You need not insist on being the expert who controls every decision, but you should communicate what you know about families in a clear way. Even so, what the family sees as a problem or need will ultimately determine where they will focus their energies.

Goals must be specific, communicated to all, and include long- and short-term outcomes. For example, long-term goals for a family with a child who is wetting the bed might be to reduce the frequency of bed-wetting to an occasional accident and to defuse the family process so that no anger is expressed when it occurs. In the first week, the short-term goal for the family might be that the mother awakens the child at 3:00 a.m. to go to the bathroom. In the second week, the short-term goal might be that father checks on the bed in the morning instead of the mother. Short-term goals progress toward long-term goals with expected modifications as the family and you learn what works and make adjustments to new information.

PLANNING

Interventions are directed by principle rather than by rote. Basically, the therapist helps the family see its own patterns of operation in a different way. Once the family can become thoughtful about its own operation, family members will begin to think themselves out of the problem. The family will create solutions that are likely to work.

Every person who works with families and applies principles of family therapy does so in a unique fashion. The framework inside your head is the basis to direct thinking. How the framework is implemented can be modified to match each situation. Some related techniques are presented in Box 20–7.

Implementation

Families naturally have resistance to change. Even when the change is most likely beneficial to the family, family members prefer to remain as they are. It is easier to keep what is known than to exert energy to move into the unknown. Recognize the importance of sequencing or timing in suggesting options for change. For instance, families have difficulty changing during times of crisis or stress, yet that is often the best time to change because the family then sees the need for change. Change is most likely after perceptions of the situation begin to change. Working on the family's thinking about the problem is the first step to intervention. Helping the family modify feelings and behavior comes next.

A change in one part of the system will affect the entire system. No person can change another, but any person can make personal change. What we do and the way we react has an impact on others. When any one person in a system changes, the system will automatically change. When priorities are determined, an awareness of the systemic nature of the family may show that a positive change in one member may actually end up being a negative change for another or for the whole family. For example, suppose a family coping with a chronic illness depends mostly on the caregiving of a 40-year-old sister. If the sister changes her behavior and starts claiming some time for herself, the care for the ill member might deteriorate; other family members pulled in to assist may experience more stress; and the family dynamics will change. The sister's choice was not necessarily an incorrect one. It simply points out how interconnected individual family members' behaviors are with the functioning of the entire family system.

The more important a family member is to the family functioning, the more impact a change in that member will have on the family. Not all family members will

BOX 20-6 Major Defining Characteristics of Family Diagnoses

Altered Family Processes

Definition

The state in which a family that normally functions effectively experiences a dysfunction.

Defining Characteristics

Family system unable to meet physical needs of its members; family system unable to meet emotional needs of its members; family system unable to meet spiritual needs of its members; parents do not demonstrate respect for each other's views on child-rearing practices; inability to express/accept wide range of feelings; inability to express/accept feelings of members; family unable to meet security needs of its members; inability of the family members to relate to each other for mutual growth and maturation; family uninvolved in community activities; inability to accept/receive help appropriately; rigidity in function and roles; family not demonstrating respect for individuality and autonomy of its members; family unable to adapt to change/deal with traumatic experience constructively; family failing to accomplish current/past developmental task; unhealthy family decision-making process; failure to send and receive clear messages; inappropriate boundary maintenance; inappropriate/poorly communicated family rules, rituals, symbols; unexamined family myths; inappropriate level and direction of energy.

Ineffective Family Coping: Disabling

Definition

Behavior of significant person (family member or other primary person) that disables his or her own capacities and the capacity to effectively address tasks essential to either person's adaptation to the health challenge.

Defining Characteristics

Neglectful care of the client in regard to basic human needs and/or illness treatment; distortion of reality regarding the health problem, including extreme denial about its existence or severity; intolerance; rejection; abandonment; desertion; carrying on usual routines, disregarding needs; psychosomaticism; taking on illness signs of client; decisions and actions by family, which are detrimental to economic or social well-being; agitation, depression, aggression, hostility; impaired restructuring of a meaningful life for self, impaired individualization, prolonged overconcern for client; neglectful relationships with other family members; client's development of helpless, inactive dependence.

Ineffective Family Coping: Compromised

Definition

A usually supportive primary person (family member or close friend) is providing insufficient, ineffective, or compromised support, comfort, assistance, or encouragement which may be needed by the client to manage or master adaptive tasks related to his or her health challenge.

Defining Characteristics

Subjective: Client expresses or confirms a concern or complaint about significant other's response to his or her health problem; significant person describes preoccupation with personal reaction (e.g., fear, anticipatory grief, guilt, anxiety to illness, disability, or to other situational or developmental crises); significant person describes or confirms an inadequate understanding or knowledge base, which interferes with effective assistive or supportive behaviors.

Objective: Significant person attempts assistive or supportive behaviors with less than satisfactory results; significant person withdraws or enters into limited or temporary personal communication with the client at the time of need; significant person displays protective behavior disproportionate (too little or too much) to the abilities or need for autonomy.

Family Coping: Potential for Growth

Definition

Effective managing of adaptive tasks by family member involved with the health challenge, who now is exhibiting desire and readiness for enhanced health and growth in regard to self and in relation to the client.

Defining Characteristics

Family member attempting to describe growth impact of crisis on his or her own values, priorities, goals, or relationships; family member moving in direction of health-promoting and enriching lifestyle which supports and monitors maturational processes, audits and negotiates treatment programs, and generally chooses experiences that optimize wellness; individual expressing interest in making contact on a one-to-one basis or on a mutual-aid group basis with another person who has experienced a similar situation.

From North American Nursing Diagnosis Association (1994): *Nursing diagnoses: Definitions and classification.* Philadelphia: NANDA.

BOX 20-7 Family Systems Interventions

- Decrease anxiety by focusing on thinking rather than feeling.
- Broaden the perspective by mapping the multi-generational family system, gathering facts, and reframing individual interpretations.
- Manage your own self by monitoring anxiety.
- Identify the primary triangles and teach family to manage self within them.
- Track the family emotional process.
- Explore connecting to others and healing cutoffs.
- Coach the family toward identifying possible solutions that come from family members.
- Help family members monitor and become more aware of individual reactions to emotional triggers.
- Increase awareness by teaching the family aspects of the theory.
- Coach family members towards defining a self.
- Maintain neutrality.
- Define an "I position" for yourself as therapist.

change equally or have equal capacity to change. Identifying the family member most likely to be able to change is a good strategy when you are helping the family to modify its functioning. The member who is healthy is more likely to be able to change than the member who is dysfunctional.

Family strengths are as important as family problems. The perception of the family problem is often unhealthier than the problem. When one family member is blamed, scapegoated, or held responsible for others, the shared family problem cannot be recognized. For example, at times Harry is lazy and irresponsible. Is it also possible that Harry adds humor and genuineness to a restricted family environment? Can the problem be reframed and seen as an asset?

A family's capacity to change will be related to the level of functioning. The family has probably operated at a certain level of health for a long time before you appear on the scene. Having realistic ideas about what can be accomplished for each family is necessary. If you can help the family think about their issues in ways that lead to a small improvement or maintenance, you will leave the family in better shape than if it had no intervention at all.

Boundaries around a system regulate information to and around a system. Families that are closed (i.e., families with boundaries that are not very permeable) often like to try to deal with problems themselves. These families may have strong beliefs that they should manage troubles themselves. Helping them accept help from extended family, the community, or professionals may involve exploring their beliefs and offering help while acknowledging the family's preferred style. Other families may have had past experiences with resources that turned out to be ineffectual or inadequate. Making sure that resources are reliable and that family members have realistic expectations of what the resource can provide is a way to circumvent a repeat of earlier experiences.

Two-person systems are unstable. Triangles, coalitions, and alliances are facts of family life. A relationship with only one part of a family will activate triangles and decrease the effectiveness of intervention. You need to relate to the entire system in a neutral way. Work to detriangle self and maintain connections with everyone.

High levels of anxiety decrease a person's ability to think and increase automatic behaviors. You temper the amount of anxiety by being a calm person in touch with the system. Adding a more anxious person hinders the process. Constantly be aware of your own anxiety and its influences on behavior.

Evaluation

Evaluation is the final step of the nursing process, but it is also a step that begins with the first contact and occurs continuously as the contact progresses. The word *evaluate* means to determine the worth of something. Many methods can be used to evaluate family nursing care. The key to evaluation is to determine the correct criteria that demonstrate the value of the nursing contact. Criteria for evaluating patient outcomes are derived from the objectives developed with the family. Because the outcomes of nursing interventions occurring during one session may not be apparent until later, both formative and summative evaluative criteria should be developed.

WHAT TO EVALUATE

In looking at the specific areas to evaluate, recognize that the process of evaluation takes place with each interaction between you and the family. The evaluative process is formative at the beginning. The end result of therapy is summarized as part of the summative evaluative process.

Examination of Goals. At the beginning of the planning process, you and the family have stated criteria for goal achievement. If the criteria were clearly stated and data are available, evaluation is simply a matter of determining goal achievement. Goals should be written in the form of outcomes so that the true impact of the nursing intervention can be determined. For example, knowing that a family member wants to be a more effective parent is not the same as observing how many visits the family member kept with the child.

Remember that families may have both short-term and long-term goals. During the evaluation process, examination of short-term goals (formative evaluation process) may make it evident that the long-term goal (summative evaluation process) is not going to be achieved. Revision of the long-term goal or revision of the actions performed to accomplish the care may be necessary.

Examination of Effect on the "Sick Member." Many encounters are initiated because someone in the family has been identified as sick. The person who is the focus of care, especially one who has been identified by an agency or reimbursement mechanism, is the primary person to be evaluated. What effect have nursing actions had on the "sick member?" Has this person's health status improved? Has this person's position and role within the family changed in any way? To what extent is this person satisfied with the nursing contact?

Examination of Effect on Individuals. Many times other individuals within the family have needs of their own. Other members will be involved in offering care to the ill person or in coping with necessary changes. Family nursing interventions often upset the balance within a family. What is the impact on each member of the family? To what extent have individual health needs been met? To what extent is each person satisfied with the nursing contact?

Examination of Effect on Subsystems. A subsystem of the family may have been the target of care or may be particularly affected by the activities of the family. For example, the nurse may have been working with a single mother and her parenting of a toddler. The sibling subsystem, two older children of the family, may feel left out or may have benefited by the mother's new skills. As families learn new behaviors, other groups within the family may be affected. Have the changes been beneficial and satisfying for all the members of the system? Do interventions need to be planned for another portion to balance recent activity?

Examination of Effect on the Whole Family. Families are more than collections of individuals; the family is a unit that can stand on its own. How has the family as a whole benefited or responded to the nursing interventions? Is the family able to function more effectively? Does the family operate more smoothly as a unit? What is the affective response to the interactions? Is the family better able to master situations and solve problems for itself?

How to Terminate the Nurse-Family Relationship

Ending a meaningful relationship always elicits feelings for both family and you. In any relationship that is defined as potentially therapeutic, attention must be paid to the termination process. Terminating is a time when everyone involved must deal with personal feelings about separation. Many people have a preferred way in which they separate; people may distance, attempt to prolong the contact, become angry or sad, act out, or deny that the relationship has been important. The type of reaction depends to some extent on the way separations were handled in the past.

In the health setting, you will frequently experience termination. Patients also experience terminations when you are transferred or when cases are discharged without much notice. Effective handling of termination involves careful planning, advance notice, and talking about the emotions and issues that arise. Often you bring up the issue of termination before the patient is ready. Allowing patients to express reactions and helping families perceive themselves as able to master upcoming situations independently will help the family make the transition to independence and termination.

During the final contacts, you begin to prepare the family by reminding members that their time together is limited. A date or goal is set as the marking point for termination. Discuss goal accomplishment, satisfaction with the process, and plans for continuation of health maintenance. If referrals or transfers are needed, arrange these during the termination process. Establish criteria for the family to know when to seek health care again. For example, the reappearance of the signs and symptoms of a chronic mental illness would be a signal for the family to contact the clinic. Try to find a way to frame the outcomes of the visits to indicate success for the family, even if the original goals were not met. In almost every contact, you and the family learned something or grew in some way that could be presented as success. The Blount family's story illustrates varying success.

The first interview with the Blount family was conducted with Ken, Jason, and Diane together. Later, Jason spent some time in the waiting room while the nurse talked to the couple. The Blounts were asked to describe their view of the problem. Ken said that it was Diane's selfishness that was driving the couple apart and affecting Jason. Diane felt pretty guilty about her recent choices and was willing to accept the blame but did not see much hope for the marriage. After completing a genogram with the family, the nurse made some statements of how he viewed the problem and what he thought could be done in therapy. Meeting times, payment, and other issues related to establishing a clear contract for the sessions were settled.

The nurse communicated that he saw the problem differently from the way either Ken or Diane described it. He was struck by the prior events within their life as a couple—the abortion, the stillbirth, and the recognition of Billy's autism. He also thought he recognized a pattern within the family relationships. Information about the extended family showed that Ken's mother had devoted herself tirelessly to the care of a retarded sister. This effort was expected of her as the oldest daughter, yet the stress of that responsibility drove a wedge between her and Ken's father that was always present. In many ways, Diane's mother followed a similar path. She did not care for an ill relative, but she did compromise most of what she wanted out of life—to live in the city and be close to people—for the sake of her relationship with Diane's dad. Both mothers accepted the belief that responsibility to another, even if it compromises self, is the most important thing in a woman's life. The nurse described his role as trying to help the family accurately describe the patterns of relationships within their families. He communicated hope for this family with the belief that being able to make some choices for self to improve one's own functioning would result in improved health for the whole family. The concepts from family theory, such as the dance between separateness and closeness, are evident here.

Ken and Diane each struggled to maintain a balance between closeness and responsibility to others and some sense of separateness for self. Over the next several sessions, the Blounts continued to investigate these patterns. Ken became more aware of his reactivity to Diane when she did what he expected—took care of Billy—and his anxiety about having to relate to Billy or Diane as this difficult task was occurring. He began to recognize his distancing and criticism as ways of getting himself out of the "hot seat" that occurred in the tense relationship between himself and Diane.

In turn, Diane began to look at her pattern of responsibility to Billy as having some irresponsible parts. Her intense focus on him had left little time for herself, her other child, or her husband. Diane experienced intense anxiety about Billy's care, a reaction that might have been related to her dismay about the abortion. When she finally decided to claim some space for herself, she did it as a reaction to what was happening. It was not clear how much of her decision was based on what she really believed she should do and how much was based on her need to cut off completely from the situation.

When the nurse assessed the family, he concluded that the family level of differentiation was actually moderate to high but that the level of anxiety the family was experiencing was also high. Principles he used to direct his thinking included the idea that the whole family must be seen as a system. Notice that little attention has been paid to Jason, the one identified as having the problem. The nurse worked first to decrease anxiety by asking thoughtful questions and trying to get family members to see present circumstances within the broader context of their whole history together. He identified primary triangles and tracked family process. He began teaching aspects of the theory. Through all the contacts, he worked on maintaining neutrality and objectivity.

It would be easiest to see Ken as the offending party in this situation. Diane was working hard, and Ken was critical of her efforts. But this interpretation does not take into account Diane's part in this situation. Her intense focus on Billy turned her away from other people important to her, yet what else was she to do when someone needed to care for the child? A family perspective tries to avoid focusing blame on any member. It suggests that families react as best they can to given life circumstances.

Family members began to see some of their patterns and to understand the part that each played in family patterns. The nurse coached them to define self, to allow principles rather than automatic reactions to direct behavior. When this happened, they each began to make plans for changing the way they operated. Ken began working on his relationship with Jason. He spent less time at work and more time with Jason several afternoons a week. He also began to visit Billy in the institution. At first he was angry with Diane, but eventually he began to see the whole picture and began to wonder how he could develop a different kind of relationship with her. Diane also began to work on herself. She began to practice taking small stands whenever she was confronted with a situation in which her wishes would be compromised. She got a part-time job in a jewelry store and was soon promoted to evening manager. She worked on balancing her life with Jason, Billy, and herself. But the distance she felt with Ken had gone too far, and she was not interested in pursuing a relationship with him. Ken moved out but continued to see the children.

Jason began acting like the 10-year-old that he was. He began to have friends at school, joined the swimming team, and learned to rollerblade with the neighborhood kids. As he was parented more appropriately, his depression decreased, and his suicidal thoughts went away. The nurse helped Jason work out a way to relate to Billy; Jason began to take his old cars and trucks with him when they went to visit. Billy would not play with Jason, but he would play with the cars and trucks while Jason was there. Jason had a relationship with his mom, his dad, and his brother. He now thought of himself not as the problem but as one player in the family drama.

How did the nurse evaluate his interaction with the family? The family's initial goal was to help Jason recover from his depression and to understand the role the family dynamics played in that situation. This goal was achieved with positive outcomes for the identified member (Jason), for each individual, and for the family as a whole. Jason was returned to an appropriate child subsystem, and the parents were returned to the parental subsystem. Another goal of the family—to get the marriage back together—was not achieved, and the marital subsystem was disturbed. When the family revised their goals—to deal successfully with the separation—they were able to achieve more success.

▶ Check Your Reading

26. What is a genogram?
27. How is a genogram used?
28. What are the functions of a genogram?
29. How are goals determined for family therapy?
30. What is evaluated in family therapy?
31. Identify at least three of the principles of family intervention.

CONCLUSIONS

A family approach is different from individual therapy. Family therapy offers a broader view of the problem and helps people avoid the natural tendency to look for "quick fixes" to complex human phenomena. Families differ widely in structure and function. There is no one right way to be a healthy family. Families develop behavior that helps them adapt to life circumstances and cope with stress as best they can.

As a nurse, you can work with families as a trained therapist or in more informal encounters. You will use the nursing process to assess, diagnose, identify outcomes, plan, implement, and evaluate care with families. When a family can be helped to observe itself and think its way through its own problems and find solutions, therapy has been successful. Family health is the basis for our society's future. Strengthening family functioning is a worthy goal for anyone in nursing practice.

KEY POINTS TO REMEMBER

- Current family forms include many more types than the traditional nuclear family.
- No best family form exists.
- Families are systems in which the whole becomes greater than and different from the individual parts.
- Opening the boundaries of a system permits freer exchange of information and resources.
- Healthy communication is open, honest, direct, clear, and congruent with feelings.
- Families exist over a lifespan and have a history that influences current and future actions.
- Healthy families can vary along a range of characteristics.
- Family therapy sprang from individual therapy in the 1950s but has become a modality with many different approaches.
- The American Association of Marriage and Family Therapy (AAMFT) is the current family therapy professional organization.
- Bowen's family systems theory stresses identifying thoughts versus feelings.
- According to Bowen, the two important variables in human functioning are level of differentiation and anxiety.
- The triangle is a three-person emotional system that shapes most human interaction.
- The use of the nursing process is the basis for family-focused as well as individual nursing.
- A useful family assessment tool is the genogram.
- Genograms are used to describe facts and family interactions.
- Planning care for families must be a mutual process between you and the family.
- Family interventions are based on understanding the family as a system.
- Evaluating the effectiveness of family therapy includes an examination of the effects on different members and subsystems as well as on the entire family unit.

LEARNING ACTIVITIES

1. Take an informal survey of the different types of family forms in your nursing class. What percentage of the students currently live in a traditional family? What other family forms are represented? Are some of these family forms not defined in the text?

2. During one weekday evening, browse through all the sitcoms on TV. What family forms are represented in the sitcoms? Are the forms presented as a problem, a resource, or simply as a fact of modern everyday life? Rate the level of health of the families in the sitcoms. What factors do you notice that contribute to the function or dysfunction of these families?

3. During a meeting with one of your psychiatric patients, construct a time line that indicates all the important or nodal events or family stressors that have occurred for the patient during the past 10 years. Include both normative and nonnormative events. Does the patient describe any relationship between these events and personal health?

4. Make a list of all the possible behaviors a family can use to help them cope with a serious illness. See if your classmates can add to it. Which of these behaviors does your own family use? How difficult would it be for your family to try some new ones?

5. Spend one evening observing family communication in a family other than your own. Can you identify rules and roles within this family? How do you rate the communication for openness, clarity, directness, honesty, and congruency?

6. Spend some time constructing a genogram with one of your patients. Try to collect data on at least three generations. Be sure to include both facts and emotional relationships. Does the genogram help the patient see anything not seen before? Do you think the patient is fairly objective or fairly blaming in describing the family?

7. Family systems theory suggests that families resist change. Known patterns of relating to each other are more comfortable than new ones. Without announcing your intentions, try making a minor change in your family like changing your seat at the dinner table, doing something unusual at breakfast, or behaving differently during a family holiday. Watch to see if the family exerts any pressure on you to revert to your typical behavior. How much pressure would be exerted if this change held more importance for the family?

8. Family theory can be used by nurse generalists or nurse specialists. Make a list of family situations or problems that you have encountered during your clinical experience. Which do you think are appropriate for a nurse generalist? Which for a nurse specialist? What criteria did you use to decide?

9. Using the local telephone book or other referral sources available to you, construct a list of potential places of treatment for families within your community. Can you locate sources that use a sliding-scale reimbursement schedule to treat families with few economic resources? In your community, how would you get information about the quality of each of these treatment sources?

CRITICAL THINKING EXERCISE

Keeping in mind the family system concepts as defined by Bowen, consider the following family interactions. Mary and Mike Adamm live in a quiet suburban community. They have two children, John, age 11, and Susie, age 17. Mary works part time as a telephone operator, and Mike has his own construction company. Mike's mother recently had a stroke and was hospitalized. Because he builds homes, Mike decided to build a house specially designed for the disabled for his mother so that she would be able to care for herself more easily when she recovered. Since Mike was working so hard on his mother's house, Mary decided to cut back on her work hours so that she could be more available to John, who has lost his "fishing buddy."

1. What assumption(s) can be made about the degree of differentiation for each member of the Adamm family?

2. What further evidence is needed to support your assumptions?

3. Consider alternative reasons why Mary cut back her work hours?

Susie had planned to attend junior college 10 miles away from the family home after graduation, but about a month later, she announced to her parents at dinner one evening that she was going away to a private college. She stated that her basketball coach could get her help and she could get a 50% scholarship. She failed to tell her mother that her boyfriend was also going to this school.

1. What would Bowen say about triangles in this family?

2. What assumption(s) might Susie be making and/or reacting to?

3. Consider possible reactions that Mary and Mike might have to Susie's announcement.

REFERENCES

American Association for Marriage and Family Therapy. (1981). AAMFT Commission on Accreditation receives Department of Education approval. *AAMFT Newsletter, 12*(1).

Artinian, N. (1994). Selecting a model to guide family assessment. *Dimensions of Critical Care Nursing, 14*(1), 4–13.

Berkey, K. M., and Hanson, S. (1991). *Pocket guide to family assessment and intervention.* St. Louis: Mosby–Year Book.

Bowen, M. (1978). *Family therapy in clinical practice.* New York: Jason Aronson.

Combrinck-Graham, L. (1985). A developmental model for family systems. *Family Process, 24*(2), 139–150.

Committee on the Family. (1970). *The field of family therapy.* Vol. VII. Report No. 78. New York: Group for the Advancement of Psychiatry.

Duvall, E. M. (1957). *Marriage and family development.* New York: J. B. Lippincott.

Freeman, R., and Heinrich, J. (1981). Family coping index. *Community health nursing practice.* Philadelphia: W. B. Saunders.

Gavazzi, S. (1993). The relation between family differentiation levels in families with adolescents and the severity of presenting problems. *Family Relations, 42*(4), 463–468.

Glick, P. C. (1988). Fifty years of family demography: A record of social change. *Journal of Marriage and the Family, 50,* 861–873.

Gordon, T. (1980). Parent effectiveness training: A preventative program and its effect on families. In M. J. Fine (Ed.), *Handbook on parent education.* New York, Academic Press.

Grando, R., and Ginsberg, B. G. (1976). Communication in the father-son relationship: The parent-adolescent relationship development program. *The Family Coordinator, 25,* 465–473.

Hartman, S. A. (1978). Diagrammatic assessment of family relationships. *Social Casework,* 59.

Hatfield, A., and Lefley, H. (Eds.). (1988). *Families of the mentally ill.* New York: Guilford Press.

Hawkins, A. J., and Roberts, T. A. (1992). Designing a primary intervention to help dual-earner couples share housework and child care. *Family Relations, 41,* 169–171.

Hill, R. (1949). *Families under stress.* New York: Harper & Row.

Jacob, S. (1991). Support for family caregivers in the community. *Family & Community Health, 14*(1), 16–21.

James, K. (1989). Family nutrition and weight control. In P. Bomar (Ed.), *Nurses and family health promotion: Concepts, assessments, and interventions.* Baltimore: Williams & Wilkins.

Kerr, M., and Bowen, M. (1988). *Family evaluation.* New York: Norton.

McCubbin, H. I., Cauble, A. E., and Patterson, J. M. (1982). *Family stress, coping, and social support.* Springfield, IL, Charles C. Thomas.

McCubbin, H., and Thompson, A. (1987). Family inventory of life events and changes. *Family assessment inventories for research and practice.* Madison, WI: University of Wisconsin at Madison.

McGoldrick, M., and Gerson, R. (1985). *Genograms in family assessment.* New York: Norton.

Minuchin, S. (1974). *Families and family therapy.* Cambridge, MA: Harvard University Press.

North American Nursing Diagnosis Association. (1995). *Nursing Diagnosis: Definitions and Classification 1994–1995.* Proceedings of the Eleventh National Conference, April, 1994. Nashville, TN: North American Nursing Diagnosis Association.

Otto, H. (1973). A framework for assessing family strengths. In A. Reinhardt and M. Quinn (Eds.). *Family-centered community nursing.* (pp. 87–93). St. Louis: Mosby.

Papero, D. (1990). *Bowen family systems therapy.* Boston: Allyn & Bacon.

Pender, N. J. (1987). *Health promotion in nursing practice.* Norwalk, CT: Appleton & Lange.

Roosa, M., Gensheimer, L., Short, J., Ayers, T., and Shell, R. (1989). A preventive intervention for children in alcoholic families: Results of a pilot study. *Family Relations, 38,* 295–300.

Satariano, H. H., and Briggs, N. J. (1989). The good family syndrome. *Pediatric Nursing, 15*(3), 285–286.

Satir, V. (1972). *Peoplemaking.* Palo Alto, CA: Science and Behavior Books.

Scheflen, A. E. (1981). *Levels of schizophrenia.* New York: Bruner/Mazel, Inc.

Skolnik, A. S., and Skolnik, J. H. (1986). *Family in transition.* Boston: Little, Brown, & Co.

Smilkenstein, G. (1978). A proposal for family function test and its use by physicians. *Journal of Family Practice, 6*(6).

Toman, W. (1969). *Family constellation.* New York: Springer Publishing.

SUGGESTED READINGS

Bowen, M. (1978). *Family therapy in clinical practice.* New York: Jason Aronson.

Carter, E. A., and McGoldrick, M. (1988). *The changing family life cycle.* New York: Gardner Press.

Hatfield, A., and Lefley, H. (Eds.). (1988). *Families of the mentally ill.* New York: Guilford Press.

Satir, V. (1972). *Peoplemaking.* Palo Alto, CA: Science & Behavior Books.

CHAPTER 21

MIND-BODY-SPIRIT THERAPIES

We shall not cease from exploration and the end of all our exploring will be to arrive where we started and know the place for the first time.

—*T.S. Eliot*

LEARNING OBJECTIVES

After studying this chapter, you should be able to:

1. Describe traditional Chinese medicine.
2. Define "life force."
3. Define acupuncture and discuss its use.
4. Discuss two conditions for which herbal therapy is used.
5. Define imagery and discuss its use.
6. Define therapeutic touch and discuss its use.
7. Define therapeutic massage and discuss its use.
8. Discuss the concept of energy transformation.
9. Define bioenergetics and discuss its use.
10. Define biofeedback and discuss its use.
11. Identify Western mind-body-spirit therapies including electroconvulsive therapy (ECT), hydrotherapy, psychotropic pharmacology, nutritional and exercise interventions, prayer, meditation, religious practices, and "doing good works."

KEY TERMINOLOGY

Acupuncture
Bioenergetics
Biofeedback
Ch'i
Electroconvulsive therapy
Exercise
Hydrotherapy
Imagery
Life force
Meditation
Nutrition
Orthomolecular therapy
Prayer
Psychotropic pharmacology
Relaxation
Religious practices
Traditional Chinese medicine
Transcendental meditation
Therapeutic massage
Therapeutic touch
Traditional acupuncture
Yin and yang

In Chapter 1, we introduced the idea of a world view and said that this textbook is based on a theistic world view, which holds that God exists, and that He is all powerful, personal, and intimately involved in our everyday lives. Yet even those who share a theistic world view—and certainly those who hold other world views—hold different beliefs about the role of alternative therapies in mental illness.

Each nurse and each patient must make an informed choice about these therapies. To make such a choice, you and your patients need to understand the basis for these therapies. You need to be able to compare and contrast your own world views with the beliefs upon which these therapies are based. And you need to decide whether these therapies are consistent with your world views.

Two principal types of alternative therapies for mental illness exist: those stemming from an Eastern tradition and those stemming from a Western tradition. In this chapter we present a brief overview of the alternative therapies stemming from both traditions. As you read and study this material, we encourage you to think critically about the alternative therapies. Consider how they fit with your own world view. Consider how they fit with a theistic world view. Consider the degree to which these therapies find support in objective research.

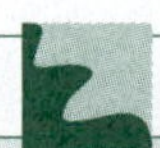

MILLIE'S STORY

Millie is 52 years old, very much overweight, depressed, and about ready to give up. Let's hear her tell her story to an acupuncturist: "I've seen them all—doctors, therapists, even nutritionists—not one of them has been able to provide me with any relief. I'm broke and still sick. Life is so difficult. I decided you were my last shot. I'm always in the dumps; I feel nauseated most of the time. I am so sensitive to foods and lots of other things around me. I have a spastic colon, chest problems, abdominal gas, and dizziness, and I'm fat. I'm so tired I can barely get started each day. I know my thyroid is slow. I suffer from migraine headaches; I also have sugar problems, but I crave chocolates.

"I wish I could have made something of myself. I had the ability . . . just didn't have any motivation. The closest I ever came to success was when I owned my own flower shop. I had to sell it about four years ago—the allergies became too much for me. Sure I had allergy tests . . . but I didn't believe the results. The tests showed that I had no allergies. Why would I want to cut myself off from something that I was good at? I used to treat projects in the flower shop as people. I could make flowers blend from being nothing to being beautiful in an arrangement. This is something I have never been able to do with myself.

"I have always been weird, and I have never belonged anywhere. When I was a little girl I hated school. That's when I started to have stomach pains and would throw up. I just wanted to stay home with my mother.

"No, my mom was not affectionate, but somehow I felt safe with her. She didn't talk much either. It's funny—I remember her telling me that I was an accident and that I wasn't wanted, but I still felt good being with her. I didn't have any friends. In fact I tried to stay away from other kids. I even quit high school because I didn't like to be around other kids. I worked for a while and then decided that I ought to go back to night school and get my high school diploma. After that I went to college. I did well and graduated with a degree in early childhood education. And you know what? I do not like children or understand them. I don't have a clue why I did that.

"I got married for the first time in 1965. I knew almost immediately that I had made a mistake. My life went downhill fast; I developed more physical problems, and I started to see a psychiatrist. Finally, in 1971, my husband came home, packed his bags, and just left.

"In 1974 I married again. The marriage is okay. Am I happy? No, but it's better than being alone. Sometimes my husband gets on my case for being fat. He never says anything positive about me. We don't talk much either.

"I think I believe in God or at least in a higher power. I pray to Him to take care of me, but He doesn't seem to listen. I guess there are others with more important problems than mine. I think maybe some of my problems are related to my karma—you know, I need to work out my bad deeds from a former life.

"I take Nardil every day, Synthroid, Phenergan, and lots of herbs and megavitamins."

Millie's journey is clearly a complicated tapestry. Millie has many problems, and she has found no lasting solutions in traditional medical, psychiatric, and spiritual care. She has now turned to an alternative therapist.

EASTERN MIND-BODY-SPIRIT THERAPIES

Historical Development

Taoism

Taoism came into being as a guiding philosophy around 2500 B.C.—perhaps even earlier. Taoism teaches that the reality of existence is us—that if we live within the natural rhythms of the universe, we will be whole. Taoism teaches that we are one with all that is around us. If we pay attention to nature and all her changes (endless birth, growth, death, and renewal), we will sense that we are no different from what we see around us. Taoism teaches a respect for the **life force** of nature and emphasizes that we should recognize a oneness of ourselves with the universe.

According to the Taoist view, we are essentially divine. We ourselves therefore possess the creative energy or life force to change. This energy is called the **Ch'i**, or **yin and yang**.

According to Taoists, this life force is a two-part force, with each part complementary to the other and neither part more important than the other. Good and evil, birth and death, action and inaction, flexibility and inflexibility, and love and fear are but a few facets of this two-part force. Health, according to Taoism, is the balance between these parts.

Taoism therefore focuses on understanding imbalances. According to Taoism, health involves being balanced in our natural rhythms, and illness emanates from imbalances. For example, humans are by nature diurnal beings, awake and active during the day and asleep and inactive during the night. If we adopt a nocturnal pattern, we are out of balance with our nature. Taoism teaches that this imbalance may harm our well-being, because fighting our natural rhythms consumes a great deal of energy (Chia, 1983; Cleary, 1992).

Taoists believe that staying in tune with the natural rhythms is what we are to do to complete our life journey. In Taoism, the goal of life is transformation, or movement toward one's completion (returning to and being reabsorbed into the life force). Taoists also believe that nature gives us guidance in our quest for balance.

A practitioner operating from a Taoist perspective therefore teaches patients to remain balanced between the two parts. The premise is that it is better to maintain order than to spend time correcting disorder (Dreher, 1990; Chopra, 1991a, 1991b).

▶ Check Your Reading

1. What is Taoism?
2. What is the Ch'i, or life force?
3. What does Taoism say about the role of balance in achieving healing of mind, body, and spirit?

Traditional Chinese Medicine

Traditional Chinese medicine is based on Taoist natural philosophy. The goal of traditional Chinese medicine is therefore to promote harmony (health), or order, out of chaos (illness) (Larre et al, 1986).

Traditional Chinese medicine is a vast system of medicine based on a constellation of concepts, theories, laws, and principles of energy movement within the body. Specific modes of therapy in traditional Chinese medicine include acupuncture, diet therapy, exercises, herbal therapy, and manipulation of the musculoskeletal system. These modes of therapy are aimed at addressing the patient's illness in relation to the complex interaction of mind, body, and spirit. Adherents of traditional Chinese medicine say that not only does it address symptoms, it addresses what they call "cosmologic" events—events that relate to the dynamics of the universe.

According to traditional Chinese medicine, the Ch'i, or life force, circulates throughout the universe, as well as in our bodies, in precise channels called meridians. (These meridians become significant in the practice of acupuncture.)

Traditional Chinese medicine incorporates a five-element theory that is a concrete expression of the Taoist concept of Ch'i, yin and yang, or life force. In this five-element theory, every substance, including the elements of the body, is classified as one of five primordial elements: wood, fire, earth, metal, and water (Figure 21–1). For instance, a practitioner of traditional Chinese medicine would say that the spleen and stomach "are of the realm of earth." The lungs and large intestines, on the other hand, "belong to metal."

These elements are said to act on one another as part of a dynamic system. For example, a practitioner of traditional Chinese medicine would say that fire "animates" earth, that earth produces metal, that metal enriches water, that water produces wood, and that wood gives rise in turn to fire. In this system, the *transition* of the five elements reflects the human condition of transformation, and transformation, in this system, is the essence of healing (Feng and English, 1973; Kaptchuk, 1981).

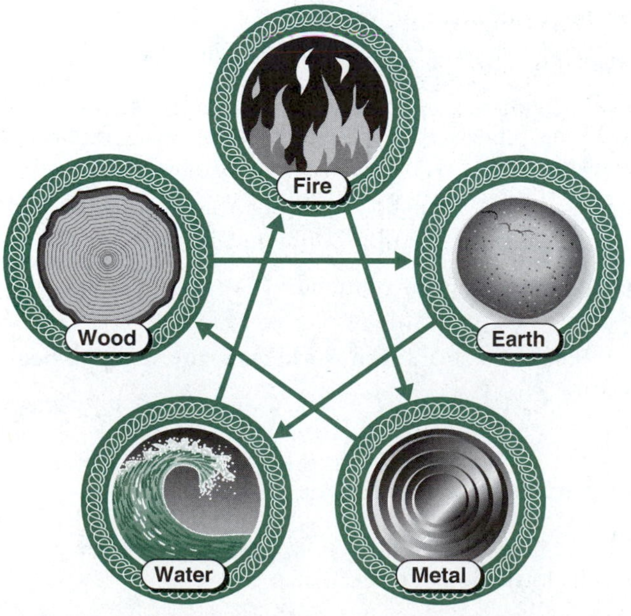

FIGURE 21–1
The ancient Chinese five-element model of energy transformation.

According to traditional Chinese medicine, the relationships among the elements can be both nurturing or destructive. Thus, they illustrate the delicate interaction between yin and yang and the need to maintain balance.

According to traditional Chinese medicine, health depends not only on the web of relationships within the five-element energy system, it also depends on the relationships within the patient's environment, including

- Relationships with individuals, families, and communities
- Relationships with seasons, climates, and other physical phenomena
- Relationships with emotional, mental, and spiritual influences

Just as any other health care practitioner would, a practitioner of traditional Chinese medicine assesses the patient through a thorough history and physical examination. However, the practitioner of traditional Chinese medicine uses the history and physical examination to gain an understanding of the imbalances of mind, body, and spirit that have caused the patient's illness.

Diagnosis, in traditional Chinese medicine, involves not only questioning but also observing body structure, skin color, breath, body odors, nail condition, voice, gestures, mood, and pulse.

Practitioners of traditional Chinese medicine say that *pulse diagnosis* is an art requiring years of practice. The practitioner identifies six pulses in each wrist, using both a light and a firm touch. She or he then describes the qualities of the pulses, using terms such as "fast," "slow," "weak," "slippery," "astringent," "stretched," and "tardy." Practitioners of traditional Chinese medicine believe that they are able to identify not only the patient's current health status but also past health history as well as a prognosis for future health (Connelly, 1987).

The acupuncturist, a practitioner of traditional Chinese medicine, describes Millie's problems as follows: "Millie, based on my assessment, I believe that you are stuck in transformation from early in life. You are unfulfilled in what we call your *earth nature.*

"First of all, I believe that you have what we call a *disturbance in earth as your center.* You see, earth is our center, our soul, where our sense of self resides. Earth flourishes in our late summer, when the spring's birth comes to fruition. It is our ripening stage. It is the element within us that has to do with bonding and nourishment. The digestive organs (where we 'rot and ripen' our foods) are the targets of illness in our earth nature.

"From birth, you did not seem to bond spiritually with your mother, and perhaps not even physically. Your mother fed you from a bottle rather than from her breasts. Not surprisingly, you developed a milk allergy early on. From earliest infancy, you could not digest and assimilate all that was around you—not only foods but also, metaphorically, your family and others.

"Also, Millie, your ripening, or maturity, is yet to come. Transformations are difficult for you. Your organs of birth (your ovaries and uterus) have been targets of disease. You have never been able to conceive and bear children. Indeed, your reproductive abilities floundered before they began.

"Earth is our 'mother,' from whom we derive all nourishment. Your history of disease in your uterus (including irregular and troublesome periods, fibroids, endometriosis, and early menopause), reflect this unfulfillment in your earth nature. Your organs of fruition failed. Your sense of career never germinated. You were not able to give birth, so to speak, to your life's ambitions. Consequently, you have had no ambitions. You have not been able to nourish yourself, let alone others. All of these problems deal with nourishment or lack of nourishment in mind, body, and spirit.

"Second, I believe that you have a *disturbance in earth as your protector.* Earth is not only our center but also our protector, where we live and thrive. If our earth within is imbalanced, we develop problems with nourishment and our immune systems. Conceiving anything, including children and ideas, and bringing projects to fulfillment, become difficult, if not impossible. Life is stuck in incompleteness, with no forward movement.

"Third, I believe that you have a *disturbance in earth as your rootedness.* You see, our earth is our rootedness. If we are not properly rooted, we cease to be grounded and balanced. Our self-esteem then becomes vulnerable to forces outside ourselves, as does our sense of purpose. Because earth normally provides our stability, instability is a sign of imbalance in our earth nature. Thus, your life has been characterized by wandering—nothing that you have ventured has come to fruition. Your only identity is manifested in symptoms to be addressed and cured. Your symptoms give you substance. Weight or body fat is protective. With excessive body fat, your earth nature is expressing imbalance by establishing a protective wall of insulation from life.

"In addition to disturbances in your earth nature, I believe that you also have some disturbance in what we call your *fire nature.* Fire nourishes earth. Warmth and caring (the fire of life) allow the fruits of the earth to grow. Millie, you never experienced this vital essence. How could you thrive? You never experienced a sense of belonging, a sense of being held in the bosom of the earth mother or in the bosom of your family. You never experienced touch, which is essential for grounding the human spirit and connects us all to one another. Without the ultimate communicator—touch—in your life, you have never felt connected with anyone.

"What I would like to do now is to work with you on a treatment plan that will address these disturbances in your earth nature and fire nature."

▶ Check Your Reading

4. What is traditional Chinese medicine?
5. What are the five elements in traditional Chinese medicine?
6. What are yin and yang?
7. How is healing defined in traditional Chinese medicine?

An Eastern View of Healing

To understanding healing from an Eastern world view, we must examine the goals, principles, and stages involved in healing. From an Eastern world view, the goals of healing are

- To be in harmony with one's environment and all of creation in mind, body, and spirit.
- To reawaken the spirit to its possibilities.
- To reconnect with life's meaning.

According to this world view, the principles of healing are

- All nature (i.e., all living systems) tends toward order and harmony.
- All living systems are interdependent.
- Illness, or "dis-ease," is a pattern or patterns in the healing continuum of life.
- Healing is transformational and evolutional.
- All healing is manifested as a simultaneous, yin and yang reflection of the whole being in a state of transition.
- All healing is engendered through love and compassion. Love is the "author" of all healing.
- All healing is spirit centered.

Finally, in an Eastern world view, the stages of healing are

- Awakening
- Intentionality and focus
- Commitment
- Transformation
- Attainment
- Empowerment

In an Eastern view of healing, the stage of *awakening* represents a time—often triggered by crisis or illness—in which the person is said to sense a need for change, a feeling of diminution in the quality of life. The stage of *intentionality and focus* is when the person desires to change his or her consciousness from patterns of "disharmony" to patterns of healthy behaviors. He or she seeks to ease the pain of spiritual discomfort and to obtain help. The stage of *commitment* is when the person forges healing relationships and establishes goals for change. The stage of *transformation* is when mutual, creative, active participation occurs between practitioner and patient toward ongoing change in mind, body, and spirit. The stage of *attainment* is when the patient incorporates new, healthy behaviors, has a sense of well-being, and accepts new challenges for growth. He or she has a willingness to evaluate and change toward greater levels of wholeness. The final stage, the stage of *empowerment*, is when the person feels a sense of stability and harmony.

▶ Check Your Reading

8. List two of the goals of healing from an Eastern world view.
9. Identify two of the principles of healing from an Eastern world view.
10. Identify the stages of healing from an Eastern world view.

Specific Therapies

Some specific body-mind-spirit therapies stemming from an Eastern world view are

- Acupuncture
- Imagery
- Therapeutic touch
- Therapeutic massage
- Relaxation
- Bioenergetics
- Biofeedback

This list of therapies, each of which we discuss in more detail in the following sections, is not all inclusive. However, it is representative of the more common approaches used by practitioners of the therapies stemming from the world view of Eastern pantheistic monism.

Acupuncture

Traditional **acupuncture** is a system of health care and treatment based on the concept of *energetics*. According to Seem (1987), in his book *Body Mind Energetics*, "this view of functional energetic systems and their interrelation portrays the body as a microcosm of the forces of the universe, with man situated between heaven (the sun and moon and the cosmos) and Earth. A dynamic series of energetic fluctuations, working on the human organism from above and below, constitutes the body of a living system."

As we saw earlier when we discussed traditional Chinese medicine, practitioners of acupuncture believe that energy courses through human beings in precise meridians. They believe that this energy is flowing, dynamic, observable, and measurable, and that its transition affects the balance of health.

A practitioner of acupuncture identifies this balance by examining the ways in which people respond to problems. The practitioner then uses the technique of acupuncture to address the promotion of health and the prevention of illness (Requena, 1986).

The practitioner first performs an in-depth assessment of the patient's history. She or he then performs a thorough Eastern physical examination, in which she or he assesses the patient's energy balance by several means. For example, she or he might employ pulse diagnosis, temperature-taking, examination of the facial features (called *physiognomy*), examination of the dynamics of the patient's structure and functioning, and observation of the patient's skin color, voice, and emotions.

Based on the collected data, the practitioner identifies the pattern of disruption of the patient's energy. She or he states the diagnosis in terms of the five-element system of traditional Chinese medicine and the networks of the acupuncture meridians (see Figure 21–1). The practitioner identifies these disruptions as energy blockages manifested in mind, body, and spirit.

The practitioner then develops a comprehensive treatment plan unique to the particular patient. Where the practitioner has identified energy blockages, she or he inserts long needles, which look rather like small knitting needles, into specific points along the imbalanced meridians. Acupuncturists have identified at least 722 such acupuncture points, though only about 40 to 50 are in common use. By inserting these needles, practitioners believe that they can manipulate, disperse, or reactivate energy.

Acupuncturists also practice the less well known but related procedure known as *moxibustion*. In this procedure, the practitioner burns a substance called *moxi*, which is derived from the plant *Artemesia vulgaris*, a member of the chrysanthemum family. This burning produces heat over the patient's energy points. This heat penetrates the skin and, practitioners believe, alters the flow of Ch'i, or energy (Chow, 1984).

Acupuncturists evaluate the impact of their interventions both by how the patient feels in mind, body, and spirit and by what the practitioner observes. Interestingly, an acupuncturist considers all change positive. An acupuncturist considers the absence of change "energy stagnation."

A unique aspect of acupuncture is that the practitioner provides hands-on patient care 100% of the time during acupuncture therapy. Another benefit, according to practitioners, is that because the acupuncture needles

TABLE 21–1 **Herbal Remedies**

Detoxifying Herbs	Red clover Alfalfa Passion flower Dandelion Elderberry Catnip
Nerve Tonics	Valeriun Skullcap Hops Passion flower
Antifungal Herbs	Pau d'arco Aloe vera Tea tree oil
Antibiotics	Goldenseal Echinacea Myrrh Garlic
Digestive Herbs	Licorice Peppermint Ginger Slippery elm Chamomile

actually penetrate the patient's energy field, the energy of the practitioner is always joined with that of the patient.

Focus and intent of both the patient and the practitioner are said to be essential to the process of acupuncture. The practitioner focuses entirely on the patient and teaches the patient to focus inward to try to feel the energy flowing or not flowing. When the patient experiences a sensation that might indicate energy blockage, the practitioner asks him or her to focus on the meaning of that blockage. Practitioners view this process of focusing as essential for achieving balance. For example, if the patient experiences a "knot" in the stomach, the acupuncturist might ask him or her to focus on what he or she is not able to digest in life.

Acupuncturists also utilize herbs, nutrition, and exercise to promote health. According to acupuncturists, herbs promote healing by influencing the energy field internally by altering ingestion and assimilation, much as the needles would act externally. Likewise, they say that diet and exercise keep energy flowing through nourishment and movement. Table 21–1 lists some herbal remedies commonly used in acupuncture.

Let's return now to Millie, to see how her acupuncturist addressed her problems.

Millie's acupuncturist determined that Millie's healing required that she enter into what he called "a journey of transcendence—a rising above your symptoms and an opening of the window to your truth." Her practitioner therefore chose counseling, teaching, and traditional acupuncture as primary interventions. She also interspersed other therapies to complement and enhance these primary modes of treatment. These secondary interventions included imagery, therapeutic massage, and simple exercise. She also focused on proper nutrition.

The practitioner stated her goal for Millie's acupuncture as follows: "By the end of the first acupuncture treatment, Millie will experience changes in the sound of her voice, her emotions, and her general well-being." The practitioner tried to meet this goal by administering three acupuncture treatments to help Millie "open her energy fields," thereby allowing Millie to unblock behavioral patterns and create change.

▶ **Check Your Reading**

11. To what does the term *energetics* refer?
12. Describe the process of acupuncture.
13. What is unique about the process of acupuncture?

Imagery

Imagery, simply put, is "the mind thinking in pictures" (Epstein, 1989). The idea of using imagery as an intervention is to visualize not only what is real but also what one wants to *become* real. The idea is that our mental pictures actually change reality. In some situations, imagery does indeed seem to change reality; why that happens, however, is the subject of controversy.

From an Eastern perspective, the spiritual basis of using imagery as an intervention is the belief that the only reality is Brahman, the universal energy. By creating an image, we can thus change reality and move toward healing.

The science of psychoneuroimmunology offers an alternative explanation for the success of imagery. Psychoneuroimmunology does not suggest that cancer, pain, or any disease process is unreal. Instead, it suggests that as human beings we are created in such a way that when we think positive thoughts (the process of thinking being in itself biochemical), we generate a health-enhancing effect in our immune systems (Olness, 1981). Conversely, when we are besieged by stress and we perceive our situation to be hopeless, we produce a different type of biochemical process, resulting in a depletion of our immune systems (Carson, 1993). For more information on this perspective, see Chapter 7.

As used in health care, imagery is the imagination of health. As Thomas Moore says in his popular book *Care of the Soul* (Moore, 1992, p. 159), "a poetic reading of the body as it expresses itself in an illness calls for a new appreciation for the laws of imagination. . . ." Imagery is often used in patients with medical disorders resistant to traditional approaches: patients with AIDS, patients in hospice care, patients with chronic pain, and adults and children with cancer. Case Example 21–1 illustrates the use of imagery in a patient with cancer.

Case Example 21–1 C.R.'s Story

The following abstract from a medical journal illustrates the successful use of imagery as an adjuctive treatment in a 13-year-old with advanced cancer:

C.R., aged 13, was admitted to our center with the diagnosis of Ewing's sarcoma Stage IV with bilateral lung metastasis. Cyclic chemotherapy was initiated during the four-day hospitalization. We were asked to see the patient on the last day because of pain. In the initial conversation with the parents they expressed great interest in having their son learn imagery exercises for pain control and sleeping and also asked if the patient could use this "to fight cancer."

Patient was in bed on the initial visit. He was irritable, tense, and complaining of pain in his back at the intravenous site. When asked if he wanted to move via wheel chair to our office, he declined. The initial practice was conducted in a four-bed room where we made a tape of the initial exercise. Patient indicated that he could not visualize switches and preferred to focus on the perception of numbness in the areas of discomfort. He relaxed very well using favorite place imagery, which included imagining that he was playing with his cat. The patient was given the option of deciding when to practice although we recommended B.I.D. practice. It was suggested that he induce numbness for gradually increasing periods of time. It was suggested that, although he could use the tape when he wished, at least half the practice should be without assistance of the tape. The patient quickly demonstrated improvement in pain control and decrease in requirements for pain medications. After discharge he was followed on an ambulatory basis with three individual practice sessions and group practice sessions. He spoke frequently about his imagery to combat cancer. The Acterberg-Lawlis interview concerning cancer imagery was filled out by him as follows:

He said that his cancer cells looked like black knights lined up for attack. He perceives them being "not strong enough to beat the white knights" who are the white blood cells. He sees the white blood cells charging all over the place and sees more of them than the black knights. The cancer cells are smaller than a white cell. The white knights fight the black knights by "piercing them, chopping them up with their daggers, they always do their job." The drugs are vicious beasts that go along with the white knights and eat up what's left. To the question, "How well does your treatment work to kill off disease," he answers, "The white knights and vicious beasts always win—they don't have much to do now." He stated that he thinks about his imagery treatment on and off every day.

Thirty months after diagnosis he continues to do well in remission. Recently, given the option of practicing peripheral temperature control, he quickly demonstrated the ability to change fingertip temperature ±5°F over a 5-minute period and, on several occasions, raised his fingertip temperature 17°F.

Abstract from Olness, K. (1981). Imagery (self hypnosis) as adjunct care in childhood cancer: Clinical experience with 25 patients. *American Journal of Pediatric Hematology/Oncology, 3,* 313.

Millie's practitioner initiated the use of therapeutic imagery after three acupuncture treatments so that Millie could begin to visualize a more balanced body, functioning as it should without allergies and illness. According to her practitioner, "Body image was an ongoing issue of malfunction and helplessness for Millie."

The practitioner stated the goal of imagery for Millie as follows: "Millie will state that she can imagine living her life allergy free and with a healthy body."

The practitioner helped Millie meet this goal by teaching Millie how to practice imagery and encouraging her to do so on a regular basis. The rationale for this intervention was that the use of imagery could help Millie to change her image of her self and her health, and, subsequently, to lead to change in the reality of her health as well.

▶ Check Your Reading

14. Define the term *imagery.*
15. What is the purpose of imagery?

Therapeutic Touch

Dolores Krieger (1981), a pioneer in **therapeutic touch,** describes the technique as "a conscious intentional therapy." It is a spiritual intervention without a basis in established religion. On the surface, it appears to be similar to the Christian practice of "laying on of hands," but in reality it is worlds—and world views—apart.

According to Macrae (1991, p. 18), "The practice of therapeutic touch involves the use of oneself (that is, one's own localized energy field) as an instrument to help whatever areas within the patient's field that have become obstructed and disordered by disease."

Essential to the practice of therapeutic touch are the beliefs that we are all healers and that a life force that we can manipulate is present in all of us. This universal energy is said to seek balance on all levels of mind, body, and spirit.

According to practitioners of therapeutic touch, the practitioner places his hands over a person, intentionally intervening in that person's energy field. The practitioner moves the person's life force to areas of depletion and clears blockages in the energy field to allow a free and ordered flow of energy and to promote healing (Hamilton, 1991; Heidt, 1991).

The practice of therapeutic touch involves five steps (Kreiger, 1979):

1. The practitioner *centers* himself or herself.
2. The practitioner assesses the patient's energy field.
3. The practitioner *unruffles* the patient's energy field.
4. The practitioner directs and modulates the energy field.
5. The practitioner stops the therapy when he or she can no longer recognize bilateral differences in the patient's energy field.

To assess the patient's energy field, the practitioner sweeps his or her hands over the patient's body. During this sweep, he or she is said to feel a number of sensations, which are described as follows (Macrae, 1991, pp. 31–34):

- Healthy energy flow—evenly distributed and unbroken

- Loose congestion—a cloud or wave of heat or heaviness
- Light congestion—coldness, or no response to the vibrations
- Deficit—a hollowness, or depletion of vibration
- Imbalance—an area's vibrations not flowing in harmony with the whole

Practitioners of therapeutic touch say that their assessment involves total interaction with the patient's energy field; they listen, observe, and *feel* in such a way as to gain an in-depth understanding of the patient's energy balance. The practitioner intuits the patient's vibrations, so to speak.

The aspect of therapeutic touch aimed at healing involves a second sweep across the patient's body. This time, the practitioner focuses on trying to manipulate energy imbalances and on transferring energy from himself or herself to the patient in an effort to create balance (Hanley, 1991; Hover-Kramer, 1991).

A good deal of research on therapeutic touch has been conducted, some of it funded by the Office of Alternative Medicine of the National Institutes of Health. Grad's 1963 and 1969 studies of therapeutic touch are particularly noteworthy, and Dolores Krieger cites them as foundational to her own work. Interestingly, Clark and Clark (1984) recently reviewed Grad's work, as well as the work of other nurse researchers on therapeutic touch, and concluded that research on therapeutic touch showed transient benefits, no significant benefits, or a need for replication of the research.

Janet Quinn (1989), a nurse researcher whose work was funded by the National Institutes of Health, tested the theories of intentionality and energy exchange—both of which are central to the practice of therapeutic touch. Quinn hypothesized that patients who were treated with therapeutic touch would experience a decrease in anxiety, as measured by decreased blood pressure, decreased heart rate, and reduced anxiety scores compared with patients who were treated with a technique that mimicked therapeutic touch. In her studies, Quinn found that the benefits of therapeutic touch were not significantly different from the effects of the technique that mimicked therapeutic touch.

Nevertheless, many nurses who use therapeutic touch cite anecdotal evidence of the technique's effectiveness in calming patients and instilling a sense of peace. It seems reasonable to ask, therefore, whether the effects of therapeutic touch observed by nurses are related to the technique of therapeutic touch, or whether they are related to the bestowing of kindness, a gentle touch, and focused attention.

▶ Check Your Reading

16. Define the term *therapeutic touch*.
17. What is the purpose of therapeutic touch?
18. What is the spiritual basis of therapeutic touch?

Therapeutic Massage

Therapeutic massage is an alternative approach to healing that employs a "systematic manipulation of soft body tissue by such movements as rubbing, kneading, pressing, rolling, slapping and tapping" (Beck, 1988, p. 12). Therapeutic massage, which includes such variations as shiatsu, acupressure, tui na, Swedish massage, rolfing, and polarity therapy, derives from Japanese, Chinese, European, and North American traditions.

Therapeutic massage has been reported as effective in calming infants and has been used to improve immune function in people infected with HIV, the agent responsible for AIDS.

Depending on the provider's point of view, the purposes of therapeutic massage may include opening *energy channels*, releasing a *blocked life force*, and promoting relaxation. Therapeutic massage is said to have a systemic effect, in that it promotes better circulation in the blood vessels and lymphatics, leading to metabolic balance. Additionally, practitioners say that it enhances detoxification and excretion of built-up waste products from both muscles and organs.

The practitioner assesses the patient through a brief history and physical examination. Depending on her or his perspective, the practitioner may look for areas of blocked energy by examining the patient's musculoskeletal structures and soft tissues, as well as by observing the patient's gait, posture, and expressions. The practitioner may attempt to reestablish the patient's energy flow by manipulation and what is called *healing intent*. The practitioner may also try to help the patient to release pain or blocked emotions in the process of relaxation.

According to experienced practitioners with an Eastern world view, the massage practitioner becomes attuned to the life force as he or she reads the symptoms of imbalance (e.g., muscle spasms, fatigue, and depression) and validates with the patient the changes resulting from therapy.

From a secular as well as a theistic perspective, therapeutic massage works because a patient who receives the massage interprets the actions of the practitioner as loving and caring. Biochemical changes result, leading to feelings of calm and peacefulness.

Millie's acupuncturist determined that it would be appropriate to use therapeutic massage to alleviate Millie's "stuckness" in circulation and her issues of "bound-up muscular tension" and "holding onto" emotional tension. The practitioner selected therapeutic massage in particular to address these problems because she felt that Millie needed a "hands-on" therapy to "ground" her through human contact.

The practitioner stated the goal of therapeutic massage with Millie in this way: "Millie will verbalize greater connectedness with others after one month of therapeutic massage sessions."

▶ **Check Your Reading**

19. Define the term *therapeutic massage.*
20. What is the purpose of therapeutic massage?
21. What is the Eastern spiritual explanation of the effectiveness of therapeutic massage?
22. What is a Western spiritual/biochemical explanation of the effectiveness of therapeutic massage?

Relaxation

Relaxation is a technique that combines imagery with progressive tensing and relaxing of muscle groups throughout the body. It is an intervention that can be interpreted through either an Eastern pantheistic or a Western theistic perspective. From an Eastern pantheistic perspective, relaxation is therapeutic because it enables a person to achieve harmony with the universal energy force. From a theistic perspective, relaxation is therapeutic because it activates God-given biochemical mechanisms for healing. The therapeutic use of relaxation is discussed in more detail in Chapters 28 and 37.

Bioenergetics

According to practitioners of **bioenergetics**, *bioenergy* (another name for the life force, or Ch'i) is a force that can be manifested in physical or emotional *planes.* If a person experiences distress in the physical plane, say these practitioners, it will also be manifest in the emotional plane. Healthy people are said to experience a free flow of bioenergy; they are emotionally responsive and physically relaxed. Unhealthy people, they say, often block the expression of feelings. According to practitioners of bioenergetics, this blockage is transformed into rigid musculature. Healing is said to come about through the release of physical tensions, which allows the expression of repressed feelings and eventual resolution of conflict.

The practitioner of bioenergetics is in direct contact with the patient. The practitioner helps the patient to complete exercises that result in the stretching of muscles and the highlighting of areas of tension. The practitioner then participates with the patient in the acting out of emotional responses; he or she encourages the open expression of feelings, which in turn is said to result in freer flow of bioenergy, and healing.

Transcendental Meditation

Transcendental meditation is a process whereby a person strives to experience pure consciousness, or oneness with the universal energy force. Transcendental meditation was introduced into the United States by the Maharishi-Mahesh Yogi in the late 1950s and 1960s. The Maharishi-Mahesh Yogi said that his purpose in spreading the technique of transcendental meditation was to encourage people to focus less on the material (which he viewed as unreal) and more on the immaterial energy force (which he viewed as real). He said that as we focused less on the material world and more on the spiritual world, social problems would be eliminated. The Maharishi-Mahesh Yogi did not propose that meditation led to good works or social action, but that meditation itself changes reality.

Transcendental meditation is a technique that must be taught and requires a number of steps:

1. A teacher initiates the person into transcendental meditation with an initial instructional presentation covering the benefits of the practice.
2. In a second presentation, the teacher presents the steps of transcendental meditation.
3. The teacher interviews the person.
4. The teacher provides individual instruction.
5. The teacher gives the student a unique *mantra*, frequently a word with spiritual significance, which the student is to focus on and repeat hypnotically.
6. The individual practices transcendental meditation independently but returns at least three times for monitoring by a mentor who ascertains the student's progress and answers questions.

▶ **Check Your Reading**

23. What is bioenergy?
24. Define the term *transcendental meditation.*
25. What is the purpose of transcendental meditation?
26. What is the purpose of bioenergetics?
27. What did the Maharishi say that he hoped that transcendental meditation would accomplish?

Biofeedback

Like relaxation, **biofeedback** is an effective technique that we can explain through both an Eastern pantheistic perspective and a Western theistic perspective. From an Eastern pantheistic perspective, biofeedback is therapeutic because the body is basically an energy field that needs to be rebalanced and brought into harmony with the universe. From a Western perspective, biofeedback is therapeutic because it taps into a God-given biochemical healing mechanism.

Biofeedback teaches the patient to bring under conscious control such functions as respiratory rate, heart rate, blood pressure, and skin temperature. The goal of bringing these functions under voluntary control is to relieve such physiological problems as migraine headaches, stuttering, insomnia, chronic pain, and anxiety.

Biofeedback training involves several steps:

1. Becoming aware of the functioning associated with the targeted symptom (e.g., noting the changes that occur preceding and during a migraine headache)
2. Learning to recognize internal changes associated with the targeted symptom
3. Learning to voluntarily alter those internal changes
4. Becoming motivated to learn this control

Practitioners of biofeedback facilitate the process of acquiring sensitivity to internal changes through the use of electronic equipment. This equipment measures biochemical changes in the body and signals the patient of these changes. The equipment includes:

• An EEG to monitor changes in brain waves (alpha, delta, and theta). This device is used for patients with anxiety and general tension, stuttering, insomnia, and chronic pain.

• A thermistor, to measure skin temperature. This device is used in patients with migraines to help them learn to shift blood volume from central to peripheral sites, such as the hands.

• An EMG to measure muscle relaxation. This device is used in patients with bruxism (grinding of the teeth) and spasticity.

• A galvanometer, to measure galvanic skin response (GSR). This device is used to help patients recognize unconscious emotional states.

▶ **Check Your Reading**

28. What is biofeedback?
29. Identify at least four conditions in which biofeedback could be used.
30. Identify at least two of the electronic instruments used in biofeedback.
31. What are the four steps used in the process of biofeedback?

WESTERN MIND-BODY-SPIRIT THERAPIES

In addition to the Eastern mind-body-spirit therapies explored in this chapter, several Western mind-body-spirit therapies can be used in the treatment of psychiatric patients. These include **electroconvulsive therapy,** the use of **psychotropic medications** (covered in depth in Chapter 23), hydrotherapy, nutrition, exercise, prayer, meditation, performing religious practices, and doing "good works."

Hydrotherapy

Hydrotherapy involves the use of water in the treatment of mental illness. Traditionally, it called for the patient to be wrapped in wet packs or cold sheets. This technique resulted in subduing and quieting the patient. Historically, the practice was often associated with the early insane asylums, where the treatment was punitive. However, this technique, which may sound punitive and primitive, is less restrictive than medication and is very effective in calming patients who are out of control.

Nutrition

Nutrition is an essential consideration when working with a patient who has a mental illness. Because psychiatric illnesses affect the whole person, it is not surprising that patients with mental illnesses frequently have inadequate diets. Often, either their diets are deficient in the proper nutrients, or they eat too much or too little. As you conduct patient assessments, be sure to assess the patient's nutrition, and be prepared to address this area in health teaching.

Medications and Food

One important area of nutrition to consider is the interaction of foods and medications. For instance, some medications, such as antidepressants classified as monoamine oxidase inhibitors, involve dietary restrictions. Patients taking monoamine oxidase inhibitors are instructed to avoid eating foods that contain a substance called tyramine. These foods, taken with monoamine oxidase inhibitors, could cause a hypertensive crisis, in which the patient's blood pressure soars to dangerous levels.

Millie takes Nardil, a monamine oxidase inhibitor, and yet she continues to eat chocolate, which contains tyramine. Consequently, she becomes very ill.

Caffeine and Other Stimulants

Another important area of nutrition to consider is the ingestion of foods or substances that produce or exacerbate psychiatric symptoms. For instance, patients with an anxiety disorder should avoid stimulants, such as those found in over-the-counter diet and cold preparations, as well as caffeine. These substances can intensify anxiety in patients already struggling with an anxiety disorder.

For instance, caffeine triggers increased activity of the sympathetic nervous system, which causes the "fight or flight" physiological response typical of an anxiety attack. It is helpful to advise patients to cut down on caffeine slowly over a period of months, for example, first substituting decaffeinated coffee and then herbal teas for regular coffee. In fact, many herbal teas, such as chamomile, hops, and peppermint, actually have a relaxing effect on the body (Hunt, 1989; Communication Channels, 1994; Danton et al, 1994).

Foods High in Sugar

Another important area of nutrition to consider is the ingestion of large quantities of refined simple sugars. Refined simple sugars can affect mental health by causing a "roller coaster" effect in energy levels, leading to anxiety and depression. Foods such as cookies, candies, cakes, pies, soft drinks, ice cream, and other sweet foods quickly break down into glucose in the digestive tract. Glucose then moves rapidly into the bloodstream and is taken up by the cells of the body to satisfy their energy needs.

To handle this overload of glucose, the pancreas releases large amounts of insulin, an important protein that helps transport glucose from the blood into the cells of the body. Frequently, however, the pancreas "overshoots" and releases too much insulin. This results in a rapid fall in blood glucose, producing the roller coaster effect typically felt by a person with hypoglycemia or premenstrual syndrome.

To correct this situation, the adrenal glands release cortisol and other hormones. These substances cause the liver to release stored sugar to return blood sugar levels to normal. Unfortunately, as the adrenal glands are at work boosting blood sugar levels, they are simultaneously heightening alertness and producing symptoms of anxiety.

Eating complex carbohydrates is better for our physical and emotional well-being than eating refined sugars. Our bodies must work harder to break down complex carbohydrates into glucose than they need to work in order to process simple sugars. The sugars in complex carbohydrates therefore enter our bloodstream at a more even rate than do simple sugars. Fruit-based desserts and fruit salads can be satisfactory substitutes for foods high in simple sugars. Fruits also contain fiber, which delays the rate at which sugars are absorbed into the bloodstream (Lark, 1994).

Alcohol. People with moderate to severe anxiety and mood swings should avoid alcohol entirely or limit its use to occasional small amounts. Alcohol is a simple sugar, which is rapidly absorbed by the body. Like other simple sugars, alcohol worsens the symptoms of hypoglycemia, causing an increase in anxiety and mood swings. Additionally, the use of alcohol is contraindicated with most psychotropic medications (Lark, 1994; Seligman, 1994).

Food Additives

Some people are sensitive to food additives, which can produce anxietylike symptoms including rapid heartbeat, shallow breathing, headaches, "spaciness," or dizziness. Aspartame (Nutrasweet) and monosodium glutamate (MSG) are two of the most popular additives that have been repeatedly implicated in the production of unpleasant physical and psychological reactions.

Dairy Products

For some people, eating dairy products worsens symptoms of depression and fatigue. To ensure adequate intake of calcium and protein, counsel such patients to substitute beans, peas, soybeans, sesame seeds, and green leafy vegetables for dairy products. Soy milk, potato milk, and nut milk, which are available at natural food stores, are excellent substitutes for cow's milk (Lark, 1994).

Wheat and Other Gluten-Containing Grains

In anxious and depressed people who are sensitive to some foods, the ingestion of wheat may worsen the anxiety and depression. The causative component of wheat appears to be gluten, a protein derivative that gives dough its tough, elastic character. People suffering from severe anxiety should therefore eliminate wheat from their diet for at least one to three months during the early stages of recovery. Oats, barley, and rye, which also contain gluten, should be eliminated initially. For some people, even corn and rice can increase symptoms of anxiety, fatigue, and depression.

Buckwheat, on the other hand, is easily digested by most people who are sensitive to gluten. It comes from a different plant family than wheat and other gluten-rich grains. Quinoa and amaranth are other good choices; all are available at natural food stores. Buckwheat, quinoa, and amaranth are also excellent sources of the B vitamins, vitamin E, many essential minerals, complex carbohydrates, essential fatty acids, and fiber. For people sensitive to wheat and other gluten-containing foods, a good meal might consist of beans and buckwheat bread with vegetables, or corn bread and split pea soup (Lark, 1994).

Vegetables and Fruits

Swiss cheese, chard, broccoli, beet greens, mustard greens, kale, raisins, blackberries, and bananas are rich in calcium, magnesium, and potassium—important minerals that help improve endurance, stamina, and vitality.

Brussels sprouts, parsley, peas, tomatoes, potatoes, berries, and melons supply a good dose of vitamin C, which is essential for the production of adrenal hormones (Lark, 1994).

Seeds and Nuts

Raw flax seeds and pumpkin seeds are excellent sources of two essential fatty acids: linoleic acid and linolenic acid. Adequate levels of essential fatty acids are important in preventing both the emotional and physical symptoms of premenstrual syndrome, menopause, emotional upsets, and allergies. Sesame and sunflower seeds are excellent sources of linoleic acid (Hunt, 1989; Communication Channels, 1994; Danton et al, 1994).

Vitamins, Minerals, and Amino Acids

The use of specific vitamins, minerals, and amino acids in tablet, capsule, or powder form to balance a person's nutritional needs is called **orthomolecular therapy**. Orthomolecular therapy is not synonymous with megavitamin therapy. In megavitamin therapy, a person consumes massive quantities of vitamins, far exceeding recommended daily allowances, in an attempt to achieve overall health; in orthomolecular therapy, the person consumes specific vitamins, minerals, and amino acids (*sometimes* in large quantities, when a deficiency is severe) to correct a specific imbalance thought to underlie a specific problem.

A number of conditions appear to respond to orthomolecular therapy. For instance, brewer's yeast (500 mg three times daily with meals) along with B-complex vitamins with niacin (50 mg three times daily with meals), has been effective in treating anxiety and exhaustion. Rheumatoid arthritis, a severe, crippling form of arthritis, sometimes responds to treatment with pantothenic acid (500 mg four times a day). Likewise, phenylalanine seems to increase the body's pain tolerance, and senility and senile dementia may respond to L-glutamine (1 g daily, progressing to 2 g by the end of a month). Similarly, antioxidants (vitamin C, vitamin E, selenium, zinc, and beta carotene) may bind with pesticide residues on fruits and vegetables and protect us from the harmful effects of these chemicals (Salaman, 1989). Niacin and foods high in fiber also seem to act as detoxifiers.

Exercise

Exercise is as important for the psychiatric patient as it is for any other patient and should be a part of your care of people with mental health problems. Some psychiatric illnesses and some psychotropic medications produce lethargy and listlessness. Patients may become sedentary and may therefore benefit from health teaching, encouragement, and concrete suggestions about ways to increase physical activity in their lives.

Additionally, physical exercise, particularly aerobic exercise, discharges the "fight or flight" energy associated with anxiety. Exercising results in increased oxygenation and blood circulation and revitalizes organ systems. The removal of waste products such as carbon dioxide, lactic acid, and other products of metabolism is more efficient with increased exercise.

Exercise results in the release of hormones called beta endorphins, substances thought to be responsible for the "runner's high" experienced by marathon runners. Exercises such as running, bicycling, walking, and swimming can increase beta endorphin levels significantly and should be included in the treatment plan of all patients with mental illness (Hunt, 1988; Communication Channels, 1994; Danton et al, 1994).

Prayer

Prayer, simply stated, is "talking to God." In a theistic world view, prayer is one of the main spiritual tools for seeking God's help. People with a theistic world view pour out their hearts to God, believing that He understands their struggles, accepts them as they are, sustains them in their sorrows, celebrates with them in their joys, and strengthens them in their journeys. Prayer is a powerful form of communication. It allows a person to feel connected to someone who not only is greater and more powerful but also loves unconditionally (Poloma, 1993). People have few other (if any) resources to which to turn for such *communion.* However, prayer recognizes that God is the creator, and that the person praying is the *created.* Although many people view prayer as a means of manipulating God, the authors of this book believe that the person who is praying *cannot* manipulate God, because we see God as sovereign—as exercising absolute authority over the universe (Carson, 1989; Carson and Green, 1992; Carson, 1993). Nevertheless, we believe that through prayer we sometimes receive authentic healing from our pain.

Studies have shown that Americans are a "praying" people (Paloma, 1993; Gallup and Jones, 1989). In fact, four decades of Gallup polls have consistently demonstrated that 9 of 10 Americans pray on occasion (Gallup and Jones, 1989).

In a study by Poloma (1993), prayer was associated with mental health. A positive relationship existed between prayer and three out of four indicators of quality of life: life satisfaction, general happiness, and existential well-being. Poloma also found that prayer contributes as much as a comfortable income and contributes more than gender, education, or age to one's sense of being satisfied with life. What is it about prayer that makes this difference? It is not the frequency or type of prayer that contributes to well-being; it is the extent and depth of intimacy with God that most contributes to such well-being.

In two other studies by Carson and Green (1992) and by Carson (1993), participants who tested positive for HIV who were spiritually well and who were hardy indicated that the most important behavior in which they engaged was prayer.

Meditation

Meditation, when viewed from a theistic perspective, is quite different from transcendental meditation and other Eastern forms of meditation. From a theistic world view, the purpose of meditation is "to be still and know that God is God" (Poloma, 1993, p. 49). The focus is not on overcoming self-identity so as to be one with an impersonal, universal energy force, but rather on communing in deep relationship with the Almighty. The 1989 Gallup poll (Gallup and Jones, 1989) found that people who engaged in meditative prayer stated that they spent time "quietly thinking about God," "feeling the presence of God," "trying to listen to God speaking," and "worshipping and adoring God." The focus of meditation or meditative prayer is on God—not on one's own needs or problems; this focus on God, with its interior stillness, allows for an inner response. People who engage in this type of prayer experience a positive effect on measures of mental health and well-being.

Religious Practices

Religious practices, such as attending services at a synagogue or church; reading the Bible, Torah, Koran, or other religious writings; and participation in activities sponsored by religious organizations generally correlate positively with measures of mental health. Religious commitment, measured in part by participation in religious activities, is associated with lower rates of suicide, drug and alcohol abuse, divorce, depression, and anxiety.

Doing "Good Works"

In his book *Man's Search for Meaning*, concentration camp survivor Viktor Frankl (1965) says that two factors determined whether a prisoner of a World War II concentration camp survived. The first factor was the good fortune of not being selected for extermination in the gas chambers. *The second factor was the prisoner's level of spiritual well-being—his ability to find meaning in the most bestial of conditions.* Frankl notes that many of the prisoners who survived were the first to share a piece of bread with another who seemed more in need, who managed to keep a sense of humor, who focused on others at their own expense, who encouraged others when circumstances seemed bleak, and who led others in prayer or song to raise hope.

Doing such "good works"—helping others even when our own circumstances would have us act selfishly and shun others—somehow exerts a transforming power on ourselves. In reaching beyond ourselves and our own difficulties, we somehow ultimately bring good upon ourselves. Doing "good works" is love in action, and love in action is a strong tool for promoting physical, mental, and spiritual health—in others, and, ultimately, in ourselves.

CONCLUSIONS

Sometimes patients do not find relief from their mental illnesses through traditional methods of Western medicine. Consequently, they may turn to alternative mind-body-spirit therapies.

Many of these therapies, such as acupuncture, imagery, therapeutic touch, therapeutic massage, relaxation, bioenergetics, transcendental meditation, and biofeedback, are rooted in the spiritual world view of Eastern pantheistic monism. Other alternative therapies are rooted in Western medicine or in a Western, theistic world view. These therapies include electroconvulsive therapy, psychotropic medications, hydrotherapy, nutrition, exercise, prayer, meditation, religious practices, and doing "good works."

We encourage you to think critically about these alternative mind-body-spirit therapies. Keep abreast of the research being conducted on these therapies. Think about the degree to which they are consistent with your own world view. Think about the implications of these therapies when dealing with patients and other health care professionals who hold different world views.

KEY POINTS TO REMEMBER

- Taoism teaches that reality is energy and that our goal is to live in unity with all that surrounds us.
- According to pantheistic monism, the Ch'i (life force, or yin and yang) is the divine energy within and outside of us.
- Traditional Chinese medicine is the foundation of the current mind-body-spirit therapies rooted in pantheistic monism. Traditional Chinese medicine focuses on our unity with nature and on maintaining balance in our energy systems and relies on a five-element energy system.
- Acupuncture deals with moving energy through the *meridians* of the body to restore energy balance.
- Imagery is a technique that focuses on changing reality by creating a different mental image. From a pantheistic view, the basis for this practice is the belief that the only reality is the divine energy—all else is illusion.
- Therapeutic touch attempts to manipulate energy through the practitioner's use of her or his hands to move energy from one area of the patient's body to another and to direct energy from the practitioner to the patient for the purpose of enhanced healing.
- From the viewpoint of pantheistic monism, therapeutic massage unblocks energy flow and connects patient and practitioner through human touch.
- Relaxation is a technique that combines imagery with progressive tensing and relaxing of muscle groups throughout the body.
- Bioenergetics is concerned with removing blockages to promote the flow of *bioenergy*, or Ch'i.
- Transcendental meditation focuses on getting beyond the self and becoming one with the universal energy force.
- Hydrotherapy, which has traditionally involved wrapping patients with wet packs, is a Western mind-body-spirit therapy used to calm agitated patients.
- Nutrition is an important consideration in mental health.
- Exercise is beneficial to mental health as it decreases anxiety and increases a sense of well-being.
- Prayer, especially meditative prayer, is associated with mental health and well-being.
- Religious practices, including attendance of religious services, reading religious works, and participating in activities sponsored by religious groups are all positively related to measures of mental health and well-being.
- Doing "good works" contributes to a sense of spiritual well-being and is a powerful tool for promoting physical, mental, and spiritual health.

LEARNING ACTIVITIES

1. Examine your own world view. Does your world view allow for the use of any of the alternative therapies discussed in this chapter? If so, which ones? On what basis do you draw your conclusions?

2. Imagine that a patient for whom you are caring for tells you that she is also seeing an acupuncturist. What would your reaction be? What would you say to your patient?

3. Interview two other health professionals. Ask them to define the concept of world view. Ask them if they understand the world views undergirding the alternative therapies rooted in Eastern medicine. What is your reaction to their responses?

4. Investigate what types of alternative therapies are practiced in your area. Call two of these practitioners and ask what types of patients seek help from them. Ask them to explain their world view or the belief system undergirding their practice.

CRITICAL THINKING EXERCISE

Mrs. Robinson, a 36-year-old woman, had been admitted to the inpatient psychiatric unit with a diagnosis of depression. During her seven-day inpatient treatment, Mrs. Robinson complained about frequent low back pain. When Nurse Chelo approached her room to discuss discharge plans, Mrs. Robinson asked Nurse Chelo what she thought about her getting acupuncture for her low back pain. When Nurse Chelo asked the patient if she had discussed it with her doctor, Mrs. Robinson stated, "I asked him about it once and he just laughed. He told me that as soon as my depression disappeared, my back pain would also disappear."

1. What is Mrs. Robinson's doctor's point of view regarding acupuncture?

2. What assumptions can you draw about Mrs. Robinson's point of view?

3. What other evidence would you need to support your assumptions about Mrs. Robinson's doctor and her points of view?

Nurse Chelo had just read about acupuncture in her new psychiatry textbook and decided to give Mrs. Robinson some information about the treatment.

1. What else could happen as a result of Nurse Chelo giving information?

2. If Nurse Chelo's response had been different, what else might have happened?

3. What conclusions (if any) can you make about the decision that Mrs. Robinson will make about acupuncture?

REFERENCES

Alexander, K. (1989). Orthomolecular survey demonstrates effectiveness: Patients recount benefits of nutrients. *Health News and Review,* 7(4), 5, 6.

Beck, M. (1988). *The theory and practice of therapeutic massage.* New York: Milady Publishing.

Carson, V. B. (1989). *Spiritual dimensions of nursing practice.* Philadelphia: W. B. Saunders.

Carson, V. B. (1993). Prayer, meditation, exercise, and vitamin use: Behaviors of the hardy individual who is HIV+, diagnosed with ARC or AIDS. *Journal of the Association of Nurses in AIDS Care, 4*(3), 18–28.

Carson, V. B., and Green, H. (1992). Spiritual well-being: A predictor of hardiness in the AIDS patient. *Journal of Professional Nursing, 8*(4), 209–220.

Chia, M. (1983). *Awaken healing energy through the Tao.* New York: Aurora Press.

Chopra, D. (1991a). *Creating health.* Boston; Houghton Mifflin.

Chopra, D. (1991b). *Perfect health—The complete mind/body guide.* New York: Harmony Books.

Chow, E. P. Y. (1984). *Traditional Chinese medicine: A holistic approach.* Diamond Bar, CA: Quest.

Clark, P., and Clark, M. J. (1984). Therapeutic touch: Is there a scientific basis for practice? *Nursing Research, 33*(1), 37–40.

Cleary, T. (1992). *I Ching—The book of change.* Boston and London: Shambala.

Communication Channels, Inc. (1994). Supplements can help some anxiety disorders. *Better Nutrition for Today's Living, 56*(6), 20, 21.

Connelly, D. M. (1987). *Traditional acupuncture: The law of the five elements.* Columbia, MD: The Centre for Traditional Acupuncture.

Danton, W. G., Altrocchi, J., Antonuccio, D., and Basta, R. (1994). Nondrug treatment of anxiety. *American Family Physician. 49*(1), 161–177.

Dreher, D. (1990). *The Tao of inner peace.* New York: HarperCollins.

Epstein, G. (1989). *Healing visualizations: Creating health through imagery.* New York: Bantam Books.

Feng, G., and English, J. (1973). *Tao Te Ching. A new translation of Lao Tsu.* London: Wildwood House.

Frankl, V. E. (1965). *Man's search for meaning.* New York: Washington Square Press.

Gallup, G., and Jones, S. (1989). *100 questions and answers: Religion in America.* Princeton, NJ: Princeton Religion Research.

Goble, F. (1971). *The third force—The psychology of Abraham Maslow.* New York: Pocket Books.

Grad, B. (1963). A telekinetic effect on plant growth. *International Journal of Parapsychology, 5,* 117–133.

Grad, B. (1969). Some biological effects of the laying-on-of-hands: A review of experiments with animals and plants. *Journal of the American Society for Psychical Research, 59,* 96–127.

Hamilton, D. (1991). Vital energy: The antebellum health movement. *Journal of Holistic Nursing, 9*(3; Winter), 10–18.

Hanley, M. A. (1991). Therapeutic touch—The art of improvisation. *Journal of Holistic Nursing, 9*(3; Winter), 26–31.

Heidt, P. R. (1991). Therapeutic touch—The caring environment. *Journal of Holistic Nursing, 9*(3; Winter), 19–25.

Hover-Kramer, D. (1991). Energy fields: Implications for the science of human caring. *Journal of Holistic Nursing, 9*(3; Winter), 5–9.

Hunt, D. (1989). *No more fears.* New York: Warner Books.

Kaptchuk, T. (1983). *The web that has no weaver: Understanding Chinese medicine.* New York: Congdon and Weed.

Kreiger, D. (1979). *The therapeutic touch* (pp. 62, 63). Englewood Cliffs, NJ: Prentice-Hall.

Kreiger, D. (1981). *Foundations for holistic health nursing practices—The renaissance nurse.* Philadelphia: J. B. Lippincott.

Lark, S. M. (1994). Strike back at high anxiety: Natural ways to stay calm in stressful times. *Vegetarian Times,* #198, 90–93.

Larre, J., and Rochat, de la Vallee, E. (1986). *Survey of traditional Chinese medicine.* Columbia, MD: Traditional Acupuncture Foundation; Paris: Institut Ricci.

Macrae, J. (1991). *Therapeutic touch.* New York: Alfred A. Knopf.

Moore, T. (1992). *Care of the soul.* New York: HarperCollins.

Olness, K. (1981). Imagery (self hypnosis) as adjunct care in childhood cancer: Clinical experience with 25 patients. *American Journal of Pediatric Hematology/Oncology, 3,* 313.

Poloma, M. (1993). The effects of prayer on mental well-being. *Second Opinion, 18*(3), 37–51.

Quinn, J. (1989). Therapeutic touch as energy exchange: Replication and extension. *Nursing Science Quarterly,* 2(2), 79–87.

Requena, Y. (1986). *Terrains and pathology in acupuncture.* Brookline, MA: Paradigm Publications.

Salaman, M. (1989). Super nutrition for super health. *Bestways, 17*(4), 38–42.

Seem, M. (1987). *Body Mind Energetics.* Rochester, VT: Thorsons Publishers.

Seligman, M. E. P. (1994). What you can change & what you cannot change. *Psychology Today, 27*(3), 34–47.

SUGGESTED READINGS

Carson, V. B. (1993). Prayer, meditation, exercise, and vitamin use: Behaviors of the hardy individual who is HIV+, diagnosed with ARC or AIDS. *Journal of the Association of Nurses in AIDS Care, 4*(3), 18–28.

Clark, P., and Clark, M. J. (1984). Therapeutic touch: Is there a scientific basis for practice? *Nursing Research, 33*(1), 37–40.
Hanley, M. A. Therapeutic touch—The art of improvisation. *Journal of Holistic Nursing; 9*(3; Winter) 26–31.
Hunt, D. (1989). *No more fears.* New York: Warner Books.
Lark, S. M. (1994). Strike back at high anxiety: Natural ways to stay calm in stressful times. *Vegetarian Times,* #198, 90–93.
Oliveira, A., and Crowe, R. (1995). Complementary therapies. In P. Kelly, S. Holman, R. Rothenberg, and S. P. Holzemer (Eds.). *Primary care of women and children with HIV infection.* Boston: Jones & Bartlett Publishers.
Poloma, M. (1993). The effects of prayer on mental well-being. *Second Opinion, 18*(3), 37–51.
Quinn, J. (1989). Therapeutic touch as energy exchange: Replication and extension. *Nursing Science Quarterly, 2*(2), 79–87.

CHAPTER 22

PATIENT AND FAMILY EDUCATION

The journey begins with the first step.

—Confucius

LEARNING OBJECTIVES

After studying this chapter, you should be able to:

1. Differentiate among the basics of education and learning.
2. Identify different types of education and learning.
3. Compare and contrast theoretical perspectives of learning.
4. Identify the major principles of learning.
5. Describe the elements involved in the process of education.
6. Identify different styles of learning.
7. Identify educational considerations for the adult learner.
8. Describe the components of the biopsychosocial-spiritual model.
9. Describe the basic elements of a learning plan.
10. Compare and contrast individual and group learning approaches.
11. Identify a variety of teaching techniques for patient education.
12. Identify the role of the family and significant others in patient education.

KEY TERMINOLOGY

Accommodation
Active learning
Affective domain
Assimilation
Behavioral learning theory
Cognitive domain
Cognitive learning theory
Convergent learning style
Demonstration
Divergent learning style
Health education
Learning
Learning style
Lecture
Motivation
Objective
Passive learning
Patient education
Psychomotor domain
Psychosocial learning theory
Readiness
Return demonstration
Self-efficacy
Social cognitive learning theory

One of the most important actions that you will perform as a nurse is assisting the patient to prepare for self-care. The activities of patient education provide the foundation for this assistance. Patient education has long been recognized as an important part of the general care for almost any medical diagnosis and more recently as an essential component of nursing care. Health teaching has gained prominence in the past decade largely because of the increased focus on health rather than on mere treatment of disease states, shortened hospital stays requiring patients to assume greater responsibility for convalescence, and the increased incidence of long-term illness and disabilities. In addition, the consumer has more questions and is better informed than in past decades, in part because of the numerous health-oriented messages that have appeared in the media. These messages tend to be directed toward promoting healthier lifestyles.

Still, effective patient education for the mentally ill has been lacking. Patient education in this area must expand to include all aspects of psychological functioning, from promoting wellness to maximizing functioning of the seriously mentally ill. It is possible to promote, maintain, and modify a number of behaviors by teaching patients to care for themselves more effectively.

Patient education makes a difference in the patient's journey. These differences include decreased length of hospital stay, fewer complications, and enhanced compliance with a medical regimen (Haggard, 1989). These benefits are cost saving for both patients and the health care delivery systems. In addition, intrapersonal and emotional benefits from consumer/patient education lead to enhanced patient satisfaction.

The teaching role of the nurse has long been recognized as an integral part of nursing practice. The important role of educating patients is included in the American Nurses' Association *Standards of Clinical Nursing Practice* (1991) as well as in the standards of the Joint Commission on Accreditation of Health Care Organizations (Redman, 1993). Yet teaching invariably receives the lowest priority and least attention in planning for staffing needs.

All too often teaching activities are identified as "extra" rather than "integral" aspects of the journey of care. Given the pressures, time constraints, and multiple demands that each nurse must face; taking time for effective patient education is often difficult. Constraints are especially problematic when hospitals hire insufficient staff or apply insufficient financial resources to provide for effective patient education services. Although many hospitals for the mentally ill have been conducting different types of didactic therapeutic programs since the 1970s, the individualized learning needs of patients are often overlooked, and collaborative education for families is lacking (Bisbee, 1991).

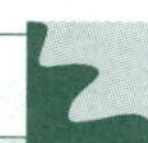

DEEDRA'S JOURNEY

Deedra first sought help because she was "really sad all of the time," she "couldn't cope," she suffered from "insomnia," and she was having recurring thoughts of "just quitting...ending it all." She had many of the classic symptoms of depression. She said she wished that she could control her feelings. She was frightened that she was "really losing her mind and couldn't stop what was happening to her."

Deedra's History

Deedra reported that when she was growing up, her mother had been very moody and withdrawn; she felt that she could never really please her mother. Her father worked two jobs and, when he was home, spent most of his time with her brothers. Although things were "strict at home," she reported that she had a "normal" upbringing. She had three brothers, two older and one younger. After leaving home, the members of her family of origin seldom communicated, except for holiday greetings.

Deedra was an "above-average student" in school. She said she liked to learn but that it put a lot of pressure on her. She said that if she brought home a grade that was not an A, she felt she was a disappointment to her parents. She won a scholarship to a local business school after graduation from high school.

As she was growing up, she had very few friends. She "didn't date much" and after graduation lost all contact with her high school acquaintances. Deedra reported that she had had one good friend, but the friend's husband was transferred and they had moved about six months previously. During the initial interview, Deedra stated that she did not have anyone she considered a "real friend."

Deedra's Condition

At the time she sought treatment, Deedra was 31 years old and had a job as a legal secretary for a prestigious law firm. She looked very young for her age; she was underweight and pale, stating that she "did not eat properly;" and she suffered from chronic headaches and pains due to work-related wrist problems. She reported that she often felt "so down and out" that she had trouble functioning and had been missing many days from work. For hours, she would sit in the family room, staring out the window.

Like many working women, Deedra felt the pressures of multiple role demands. She had been married at the age of 21 to a man who she described as "very stern and rigid." Although she and her husband shared a "loving relationship," they "seldom did anything together any more;" she experienced no pleasure from their intimate relations. She knew she was having trouble keeping up with the things she needed to do around home and work, but the more she thought about it, the more guilt ridden and immobilized she became. She spent hours thinking about her problems and how she had disappointed her family. She said that she was neither a good wife nor a good mother to her 10-year-old daughter. Deedra said that she just couldn't deal with her daughter, her husband, work, or life. She was "so tired of being so tired."

Deedra's Treatment Plan

The treatment plan for Deedra included individual psychotherapy with the certified nurse specialist, antidepressant medication, and patient education to start as soon as she was off suicide precautions. Deedra began treatment with her nurse psychotherapist, meeting three times a week. To facilitate her treatment progress, the nurse psychotherapist incorporated education about depression and coping skills into their sessions. To better provide this educational information, the nurse psychotherapist and the staff collaborated in their treatment efforts, reviewing patient education information and learning theories.

FOUNDATION FOR THE JOURNEY INTO PATIENT EDUCATION

Education and Learning

Mental health professionals generally agree that patients need assistance with understanding the full scope of their individual health/illness situations. Education is an integral part of providing quality, cost-effective patient care. Today more than ever before, complex treatment modalities require more education with active participation by patients and their families. Educational needs are intensified because less care is provided by the traditional "family" physician and more specialized care requires interaction with a greater number of caregivers. Shortened hospital stays and economic factors related to health insurance further complicate the situation.

Patient education is a process of deliberately creating cognitive, affective, behavioral and psychomotor changes (Redman, 1993). The function of education is to develop organized bodies of knowledge and generic problem-solving skills (Hatfield, 1990). **Health education** involves the dissemination of information to foster a state of well-being of mind and body so the individual can strive toward achieving the highest level of functioning. Mutual responsibility and collaboration between patient and caregiver mark this process.

Learning is a dynamic process that results in the acquisition of new knowledge and behaviors on the part of the learner. Learning takes place in a variety of ways and in numerous situations. **Active learning** involves the investment of time and energy in activities that lead to the acquisition of the desired knowledge and skills. **Passive learning** occurs when the learner is expected to absorb or internalize information that is conveyed by others without active participation.

Learning takes place through formal and informal modes of education. Education involves teaching, defined as "activities that allow the teacher [facilitator] to help students learn" (Redman, 1993, p. 8). Teaching communicates specific knowledge about a given subject in a manner to facilitate learning. The multidimensional process of learning is influenced by the social and cultural context of the learning. The individual's past experiences, perception of the current situation, and appraisal of a "need to know" interact to create the sense of readiness to learn.

▶ **Check Your Reading**

1. What is patient education?
2. What is health education?
3. What is learning?

Theoretical Perspectives on Learning

Learning involves a change in the journey, either through the knowledge base or through the development of new motor skills. Different theoretical approaches and principles provide insight into the dynamics of learning (Table 22–1).

Learning Theories

Behavioral learning theory has as its basis the stimulus-response patterns of conditioning and reinforcement. Most behaviorists classify conditioning as either classical or operant. These are important concepts that form the basis for the behavior modification approaches to treatment. (This theory is fully discussed in Chapter 18.)

Psychosocial learning theory was proposed by Lewin in the late 1940s. Defining an outgrowth of "field theory," Lewin (1947) proposed three phases that precede learning. First, the person must recognize the need to learn and be willing to work toward the goal of learning. This phase is termed "unfreezing." Second, the person must actively engage in learning new behaviors and testing them. This phase is called the "moving" phase. Third, the behaviors are solidified; new patterns adopted; and the behavior is learned and integrated. This phase is the "refreezing" phase (Lewin, 1947).

In learning a new procedure, for example, the patient must first come to terms with the need to learn a new procedure and the consequences of not learning it (unfreezing). Once motivated, he or she will learn the steps and skills involved in the procedure and practice the new behaviors (moving). Once the behavioral change of doing the procedure has become integrated, behavior becomes a part of the person's repertoire (refreezing). Lewin's psychodynamic perspective suggests a greater investment on the part of the patient than does behavioral theory.

Cognitive learning theory builds upon one aspect of the psychodynamic theory of learning. Cognitive learning involves the development of insights or understanding of the meaning of situations that provide impetus to behavior change. New insights foster a reorganization of the person's internal cognitive structure of storing, appraising, and retrieving information. Motivation to take action results from a decision that the patient needs to make changes, to adapt to the world, and to solve problems. Thus, when the patient realizes what effects new procedure will have for his or her life, he or she will readily learn the procedure because it is recognized as something desirable.

Social cognitive learning theory, largely developed by Bandura (Rankin and Stallings, 1990), incorporates principles of behaviorism with cognitive theory. This perspective is based on the proposition that a person responds to the world with information, values, attitudes, and standards of behavior that are learned from observing others. The observations are encoded and the information stored mentally so that it then serves as a guide for

TABLE 22–1 Educational Theories

Theory	Major Concepts and Features
Behavioral	Classical conditioning Operant conditioning Reinforcement
Psychosocial	Unfreezing Moving Refreezing
Cognitive	Meaning/appraisal Storing Retrieving
Social cognitive	Significant others Modeling Expectations

all future learning. Behavior becomes regulated by the perceived effects, the expectation that the behavior will have a certain outcome. Much of the behavior is motivated and regulated by internal standards and evaluations that have developed over time from the observations of life and significant others' responses.

In addition, believing that one can carry out certain behaviors, **self-efficacy,** is based on cognitive perspectives that have been integrated. When learning, the patient's decision to learn new behaviors will include attitudes about the situation, past experiences, the social context, expectations that are held for oneself, and the perceived expectations of significant others in relation to learning the new procedure. If the person is capable, if his or her belief system supports the successful accomplishment of newly learned behaviors, and if the person values the expected outcomes from learning the procedure, the procedure will be learned because all the reinforcers are operating in the context of that learning.

▶ Check Your Reading

4. What is the basis for behavioral learning theory?
5. What are the phases of psychosocial learning theory?
6. What does the cognitive learning theory espouse?
7. What does the social cognitive learning theory espouse?
8. What is self-efficacy?

Principles of Learning

Although learning is an individualized experience, 16 general principles are important in planning any educational endeavor. Each principle influences how the learning progresses and how the educational endeavor is organized. These principles are summarized in Box 22–1.

The first five principles are related to the individual's perception and past experiences. The first is that life experiences contribute to a person's resources for further learning. In any learning situation, the person brings all of the experiences of his or her life to date. These life experiences influence the way problems are perceived and appraised; similar experiences from which the person can draw facilitate the learning process in a new situation. Past experiences may also negatively influence the learning process.

Perception plays an influential role in all life experiences, including the process of learning. The second principle is that the person's beliefs, values, and attitudes affect the perception of a need to learn (i.e., that a problem exists that must be solved). Third, taking into account the individual's social and cultural background is important because each strongly influences that person's perception of learning needs. Sociocultural context includes primary relationships, secondary social influences, ethnic practices, and societal norms and values.

Fourth, the learning process is stimulated by the person's perception of a problem, usually arising out of some unmet need. Resolving the situation and meeting the need provides the main goal of the learning endeavors. The fifth principle is therefore that the priority given to any perceived problem is influenced by the person's beliefs, values, attitudes, and past experiences. The problem with the highest priority will be the one that the person has the strongest commitment to resolving. Priority is strongly related to motivation to learn.

These five principles are applied while working with Deedra. Her past experiences were reviewed, especially those related to learning situations. According to the initial history, she had been successful in learning situations, yet she felt pressure to please others. Exploring the positive aspects associated with her learning experiences should identify what she can gain from them. In addition, exploring her past experiences can serve as a helpful resource. For example, she had certain ways of studying and learning that had been successful.

BOX 22–1 Principles of Learning

1. Life experiences contribute to the resources for further learning.
2. Individual beliefs, values, and attitudes affect the perception of the need to learn.
3. Social and cultural context strongly influence perception.
4. The learning process is stimulated by the person's perception of the problem/need to learn.
5. Priority given to learning is influenced by perception, beliefs, values, attitudes, and experiences.
6. Motivation to act depends on the person's perceived susceptibility to and severity of the problem.
7. A person will engage in learning activities if that person believes a solution exists.
8. Belief in one's ability to carry out activities toward a solution is influential in motivation to take action.
9. Stages of cognitive development influence the organization of learning processes and activities.
10. Learning progresses from simple to complex.
11. Cognitive, affective, and psychomotor learning activities have different levels.
12. Individuals have a preferred method to access information (visual, auditory, kinesthetic, olfactory/gustatory).
13. Individuals use different strategies to learn (modeling, trial and error, problem-solving).
14. In any single situation, different people will be at different points in the learning process.
15. In different situations, the same person will be at different points in the learning process.
16. Learning involves change, and change can be stressful to a person (ranging from motivational to overwhelming levels).

Also apparent is that Deedra believes she has a problem. She sought help and treatment and stated that she wished she could control her situation. She also reported that her work was being influenced by her problem. These statements support the identification of a perceived need and provide information about the social/relationship context that influences her need to learn. Her perception of the problem will influence how to proceed with instruction.

The next three principles bridge the concepts of perception and health behaviors. For a person to be motivated to learn new behaviors that influence health status, the person must perceive a risk for developing a problem or situation that will be of sufficient severity to warrant engaging in the learning process. Thus, the beliefs of existence of or susceptibility to a problem, as well as the perceived severity of the situation (if left unattended), influence motivation. Often, some event acts as a trigger stimulus to motivate the person to proceed.

Motivation is a person's willingness to take action (to learn something) because of the perceived existence and severity of the problem and his or her susceptibility to it. The person then engages in the search for some effective way to resolve the situation and to take action. In addition, one must recognize that he or she has the ability to carry out the tasks to learn what is necessary and to overcome any perceived barriers to resolving the situation. Thus, the sixth principle is that the person must perceive a problem or unmet need that is of sufficient severity to warrant action. This perception leads to motivation to learn. Seventh, a person will learn if that person believes that some solution to the problem is possible. Eighth, the person must perceive that he or she is capable of overcoming any barriers to learn and resolve the perceived problem.

Deedra's level of motivation was high, even though she was depressed. She felt that she had a problem, that it was getting worse; and that it needed to be controlled. The therapist's job was to help Deedra identify her options and potential solutions so that she herself would be able to do something. When she entered treatment, Deedra felt powerless and desperate for change. Her level of depression made it initially difficult to focus beyond the immediate despair. After she began taking the antidepressant medication, however, she began to focus, to learn to control her sense of depression, and to "be happier." The therapist assisted Deedra by providing information about the depressive process and treatment options. Focusing on past successes helped Deedra learn that she was a capable and competent person. Eventually, this process led to Deedra's ability to identify former "hurdles" in her life that she had overcome and recognize the potential to conquer her current situation.

BOX 22-2 Learning Levels From Simple to Complex

Cognitive	Affective	Psychomotor
Remember	Recognize	Perceive
Understand	Respond	Manipulate
Apply	Verbalize	Combine
Analyze	Utilize	Perform
Evaluate	Conceptualize	Adapt

The next three principles emerge from the educational field. The ninth principle is that stages of cognitive development must be taken into account when organizing learning. According to Piaget, human beings proceed through five cognitive stages, depending on their growth and development: sensorimotor (0 to 2 years), preoperational perceptual (2 to 4 years), preoperational intuitive (4 to 7 years), concrete operations (7 to 11 years), and formal operations (11 to 15 years) (Sundeen et al, 1994). Most adult learners can reason and be critically reflective, but not all adult mentally ill patients have these capabilities.

Principle number 10 is that learning progresses from simple to complex. Organizing the educational situation to progress from simple to complex enhances the efficiency and effectiveness of the learning process. This principle is closely related to the 11th principle—that levels of learning apply to cognitive, affective, and psychomotor learning. These levels progress from simple to complex and are summarized in Box 22–2.

Deedra was identified as an adult learner who was able to reason and be critically reflective. At the onset of therapy, she was hypercritically reflective, leading to negative evaluations of most situations, an attribute that contributed to her depression. The educational approach taken provided basic descriptive information about depression and then moved into more complex explanations, including the influence of brain chemistry and thought processes. After each piece of information was presented (cognitive), the therapist and Deedra discussed how it applied to Deedra's case. This discussion allowed Deedra to express her concerns, her feelings about her situation, and the meaning of the experience on a personal level (affective). In addition, Deedra kept a journal of her experiences, insights, and feelings. To reinforce learning, the therapist had Deedra role play situations to act out her feelings and practice different postures to use when dealing with different individuals (psychomotor).

The next four principles reflect individual differences in any learning situation. The 12th principle is that individuals have preferred methods to access information.

The different ways a person may access information depend on major sensory functions—visual, auditory, kinesthetic, and olfactory/gustatory modes. Educational endeavors that include aspects of each of the primary accessing modes are more successful than those that rely on one mode to convey information.

Principle 13 is that individuals use different strategies to learn. In some situations, modeling may work best; in others, trial and error may be used; and in still others, problem-solving is the strategy of choice. Principles 14 and 15 are closely related. Principle 14 is that in any situation, different people will be at different points in the learning process. Number 15 reflects the same notion for one person; in different situations, any one person will be at different points in the learning process. Each learning situation requires an assessment of "where" each of the participants needs to begin the process of learning.

For Deedra, these four principles are evident in the following ways. Early in her interactions, the therapist realized that Deedra expressed herself using sensory-based kinesthetic words like "feel," "can't stand it," "feeling lost," and "not able to do anything about it." To make the learning experiences more familiar to Deedra, the therapist made certain that kinesthetic verbs and activities were incorporated into the treatment. Because Deedra had reported earlier that she had been successful when learning things, time was spent exploring the learning strategies that she used to "be successful." Her method was taking notes and writing things down, so an assignment to keep a journal of experiences was well suited for Deedra's learning style.

Deedra was at a different point in learning about depression than she was in learning how to cope better at work and to deal with her husband. In these situations, role play was more helpful for Deedra to learn new ways to act. In keeping with the 14th principle, Deedra handled the relationship problems with her husband in one way; he handled them in another. Deedra's husband felt that their problems originated from Deedra's depression and had nothing to do with how they related to each other. Deedra's husband was at a different learning point.

The 16th principle is that learning involves change at some level and change can be stressful. The stress of learning may be challenging, motivational, or overwhelming, depending on the individual's attributes and the multifaceted context of the situation. The challenge of solving a significant problem presents an ideal opportunity for effective learning.

Deedra recognized a strong need for her to change how she processed her life experiences. She was motivated now to learn to move out of her painful state. In some ways it was a difficult process, because it affected how she related to those around her. Her relationship with her daughter markedly improved when she was able to share and attend more to her daughter's needs. Changes in her relationship with her husband eventually led them to seek marital counseling.

► Check Your Reading

9. How does perception influence learning?
10. What is motivation?
11. What are the different methods of accessing information?
12. Why is it advisable to progress from simple to complex?
13. What are Piaget's stages of cognitive development?

Adult Learning

In addition to the general principles that guide educational endeavors, specific attributes of adult learners are also important. Adult learners use reasoning and reflectively critique situations. In addition, because most adult learners have many other responsibilities, time constraints impinge on the learning process.

Adult learners want pragmatic information to solve real-life problems. What is taught must be relevant and applicable to the patient's concerns. The patient must be kept at the center of all learning activities and must perceive the value of spending time in learning new information. Otherwise, the patient will be a passive participant in the learning process.

The adult learner has many experiences from which to draw to enhance the relevance of new skills and information. Providing examples that demonstrate the usefulness of the new information in real-life situations will facilitate the learning process. In addition, providing opportunities for practice and feedback will enhance the learning process and improve competence related to any new skill or integration of information.

Adult learners are accountable for their own learning. Your role as an educator is to be a motivator and facilitator for the patient, so that the patient can discover the new insights and skills that accompany learning.

► Check Your Reading

14. Identify two characteristics of adult learners.
15. Who is accountable in adult learning?

Motivation

Motivation describes the combination of factors that stimulate, drive, direct, and maintain any behavior. Motivation may originate from within the person or from external factors. It is at the root of the learner's willingness to engage in the educational endeavors and to internalize learning. Evidence of motivation at any point is called **readiness** (Redman, 1993).

Early in the learning process, the learner's values, attitudes, beliefs, perceptions, and needs are motivational factors to address. During learning, ongoing stimulation of the learner's interest and emotional (affective) experience stimulate motivation. Once the learner has developed a sense of competence, motivation becomes more internal. Success breeds more success!

Motivation and readiness to learn are factors that you must consider. Internal motivation, self-directed by the patient, lasts longer than external motivation. Reaffirming the learner's internal motivations strengthens the learning process and the interaction between learner and instructor. Incentives also assist in motivating the person.

▶ Check Your Reading

16. What is readiness?
17. How do readiness and motivation affect learning?

NURSING PROCESS

Patient education does not mean handing out instruction sheets. Rather, it involves a process similar to the nursing process. You are engaged with multiple assessments, nursing diagnoses, identifying outcomes, developing a specific plan, implementing activities, and completing evaluations at every phase of the educational process. Keep in mind that this dynamic, interactive process flows back and forth with some overlap depending upon the events that occur within any given phase.

Assessment

To clarify the exact learning needs of the individual, a thorough assessment is necessary. It is important *not* to assume that you know what the patient needs. Always assess. Careful assessment prevents needless repetition of already known information, saves time, enhances learning, and increases the rapport between learner and teacher. The result will be more satisfactory for all persons involved.

Learning Needs

Identification of the learning needs provides the "what" of the educational endeavor. You will use many methods to discover the learning needs of patients. Information may be garnered from patients themselves, from family members, from representatives of any social support networks, from records and charts, and from input from other staff. Direct conversations, interviews, and questionnaires can be used to gather information. In addition, observation and ongoing patient interactions provide salient information about possible learning needs.

Learning Style

Assessing the learning style of the patient tells you "how" this patient learns. **Learning style** refers to the manner in which a person perceives and processes information in a learning situation. Among the styles of learning are those identified by Kolb (DeCoux, 1990): convergent, divergent, assimilation, and accommodation.

The **convergent learning style** is when a person likes a single solution to a problem. The convergent learner enjoys dealing with things rather than people. For such a learner, reading information, handouts, diagrams, and specific demonstrations are preferred learning activities.

The individual who has a **divergent learning style** prefers learning situations that call for the generation of ideas and has a sincere interest in people and working with groups. Group discussions, brainstorming, and individual problem-solving activities stimulate the divergent learner.

A person who likes to create theoretical models is likely to rely on the **assimilation** style of learning. Such an individual is more concerned with abstract concepts than with people, while paying close attention to details. The assimilation learning style lends itself to studying theories, detailed interactional models, and diagrams as well as diaries or experiential recordings, which can then be used to create a model. Planned activities that are detailed and complex are preferred.

With the **accommodation** learning style, the learner relies heavily on information from other people rather than on personal analytical abilities. The person with this learning style enjoys preplanned experiments or carrying out the steps of a planned activity. Written directions and procedures, lectures with some directed question and answer sessions, or a specific demonstration that requires a return demonstration suit this learner.

Learning Readiness

Assessing readiness shows you "when" the best learning moment may occur. In addition, you need to identify potential obstacles to the educational endeavor. Obstacles to the learning process must be assessed to proceed properly with the educational endeavors. One of the foremost potential obstacles to education is the health care system itself. The structure of health care organizations, the current methods of payment and insurance coverage, and the procedures followed for any patient may negate opportunities for patient-centered education.

The individual may also present obstacles. Psychosocial factors and past experiences may become formidable barriers to learning. Sensory deficits and severity of illness must be considered. In addition, the amount of information that the person must assimilate and the amount of change necessary can halt the learning process if these are perceived and appraised as being too much of a burden.

Environmental factors may impede the learning process. If the educational endeavor takes place in an area filled with distraction, the learning process can be thwarted. Also, if learning a psychomotor skill is the focus of the instruction, setting up the environment to practice the procedure and skill is essential. Then accommodating the new learning in the actual environment in which the patient functions daily becomes the challenge. Often, new information is not easily transferred to other settings, and the individual may require specific assistance to do so.

▶ **Check Your Reading**

18. What is a learning style?
19. What are the four learning styles identified by Kolb?
20. What are the areas that we assess in regard to a potential learner?

Diagnosis

The specific nursing diagnosis provides the basis and direction for the health teaching that follows. Arnold (1995) proposes that the nursing diagnosis should specify "whether the knowledge deficit is related to lack of exposure or experience, cultural values, misinformation, lack of interest or motivation, unfamiliarity with support resources in the community, or a lack of confidence in the health care system" (p. 385). These data will direct the nurse in selecting the most appropriate information and learning format for each patient. Nursing diagnoses most amenable to educational information include knowledge deficit and ineffective coping, individual and family, although almost every nursing intervention ideally contains an educational component.

Outcome Identification

The development of an education plan begins with determining the long-term outcome, or goal, for the educational endeavor. Frequently, the goal has to do with expanding the knowledge base of an individual patient and family members. The goal may focus on developmental issues, legal aspects, coping, rehabilitation, self-care, or compliance with treatment regimens. The major goal helps in developing objectives.

An **objective** is a behavioral statement that guides the learning process and establishes the parameters for evaluating the success of the learning. Two major factors to consider in constructing an objective are content and form. The learning objective should be precisely stated. A well-formed objective includes the specific behaviors to be demonstrated, the situation or conditions surrounding the performance, and the criteria for measuring acceptable performance. To minimize alternative interpretations of a word and thus avoid misinterpretations; specificity of behavioral terms is important. Examples of precise behavioral terms are found in Box 22–3.

An objective states the expected behaviors of the patient, not the teaching activity. In addition, each objective is stated singly. When behaviors are clumped together with compound verbs, the learner may experience confusion about what is expected, and evaluation of the outcome becomes inconsistent. Brevity and clarity are the keys to writing useful learning objectives. Avoid excess words and make each objective a simple behavioral statement. The objective should identify "who" is required to do "what behavior," in "what situation," and "when, how often, or how much."

An additional organizing principle in writing any learning objective is specifying the level of behavior. Behaviors can be divided into three large groupings called domains. The **cognitive domain** deals with intellectual abilities. The **affective domain** deals with psychological aspects such as values, attitudes, feelings, interests, and general appreciation. The **psychomotor domain** encompasses motor skills. Each domain is arranged in a hierarchical array called a taxonomy, which reflects less complex behaviors and then progresses to more complex behaviors within the domain. An example of the levels of the cognitive domain, based on the classic work of Bloom and Krawnthol (1984), appears in Box 22–4.

BOX 22–3 Commonly Used Behavioral Terms for Identifying Learning Objectives

Administer	Design	Organize
Analyze	Develop	Perform
Apply	Differentiate	Predict
Assess	Discuss	Prepare
Calculate	Evaluate	Recall
Categorize	Explain	Recognize
Choose	Formulate	Record
Classify	Identify	Report
Compare	Initiate	Select
Compare and contrast	Institute	State
Compile	Instruct	Synthesize
Conduct	Interpret	Tabulate
Construct	Label	Tally
Contrast	List	Translate
Demonstrate	Measure	Volunteer
Describe	Order	Write

Planning

Once you have confirmed the major area of concern, you can initiate the planning phase of the educational process. When the patient has several specified needs, the most immediate concerns are addressed first. Prioritizing salient needs makes it easier strategically to plan for educational endeavors. At this point, identify alternative concerns and any potential restraining factors so that you can reach a clear agreement with the learner as to the focus of the educational endeavors. Your communication skills are especially important to establishing rapport between you and the patient. The context of the discussions, the language used, and the nonverbal cues are all part of the strategic communications that facilitate the learning process.

Planning then means selecting initial approaches and alternatives used to teach the information and assist the patient to meet the objectives. A succinct, step-by-step

BOX 22-4 Taxonomy of Cognitive Behavioral Domain Summarized

1.00 Knowledge—recall/remembering information
- 1.10 Knowledge of specifics
  - 1.11 Knowledge of terminology
  - 1.12 Knowledge of specific terms
- 1.20 Knowledge of ways and means of dealing with specifics
  - 1.21 Knowledge of conventions
  - 1.22 Knowledge of trends and sequences
  - 1.23 Knowledge of classification and categories
  - 1.24 Knowledge of criteria
  - 1.25 Knowledge of methodology
- 1.30 Knowledge of universals and abstractions
  - 1.31 Knowledge of principles and generalizations
  - 1.32 Knowledge of theories and structures

2.00 Comprehension—lowest level of understanding
- 2.10 Translation
- 2.20 Interpretation
- 2.30 Extrapolation

3.00 Application—use of abstractions in particular and concrete situations

4.00 Analysis—breakdown into constituent elements; the relative hierarchy of ideas or relationships are expressed
- 4.10 Analysis of elements
- 4.20 Analysis of relationships
- 4.30 Analysis of organizational principles

5.00 Synthesis—putting together elements to produce a whole
- 5.10 Synthesis of a unique communication
- 5.20 Synthesis of a plan or set of operations
- 5.30 Synthesis/derivation of a set of abstract relations

6.00 Evaluation—judgment about the value of material/methods for a given purpose
- 6.10 Judgment of internal evidence
- 6.20 Judgment of external criteria

Adapted from the *TAXONOMY OF EDUCATIONAL OBJECTIVES. HANDBOOK I: COGNITIVE DOMAIN*, edited by Benjamon S. Bloom. Copyright © 1956, renewed 1984 by Longman Publishers.

approach allows the patient to process the information provided. Moving from basic, foundational material to more complex topics facilitates information processing.

At this point you also need to clarify the role of the patient, the family/support network, and other health care personnel in the educational endeavor. In many cases, the primary participants are you and the patient. In other situations, you may need to focus aspects of the teaching plan on the family/support network representatives to best meet the needs of the patient. To identify the role of each potential participant, be sure to appraise each situation.

The plan also identifies the parameters of implementation. Establishing specific learning sessions generally provides the mechanism for the largest part of the educational endeavors. These learning sessions must include time for feedback and reinforcement of information and skills. In addition to the planned sessions, a "teaching moment" sometimes will arise during the day. To capitalize on such opportunities and further the learning, all the people who have significant interactions with the patient should know the educational plan. Opportunities to continue reinforcement of progress toward the objectives occur throughout the day. Such reinforcement may fall on the family or on other staff/personnel. When these people are well informed concerning the learning goals, they can better assist in the learning process. One method of communicating the specifics of an educational endeavor is through the use of an educational lesson plan form that contains the essential information (Figure 22–1).

▶ Check Your Reading

21. What is an objective?
22. What is included in an objective?
23. How do we arrive at goals for teaching?

Implementation

To select the particular strategies for implementing the plan, you first need to decide on the approach to follow. Should the strategies be carried out with an individual approach, as one-on-one instruction, or as independent study? Should the approach be focused on a group of learners, either in a small- or a large-group arrangement? Selecting the approach depends on many variables, including the needs of the patient, the content to be learned, the environment, time constraints, and economic limitations. A group approach is cost effective when instructor time is at a premium. Yet some learners are intimidated in group settings and therefore would probably do better in directed one-to-one instruction. Internally motivated individuals do well with independent self-study modules to learn information that can be reinforced during associated feedback periods.

After you decide about the approach, select strategies and techniques to implement the educational plan (Box 22–5). No single technique is best in all situations, and incorporating several techniques tends to enhance the learning experience. Studies have shown that only a small percentage, up to 30%, of information transmitted verbally is remembered unless information is specifically targeted (Haggard, 1989). Communication is the main determinant of effective teaching; how the information is transmitted makes a decided difference. One of the most important qualities of effective patient education is to stimulate and engage the interest of each learner. As such, your enthusiasm is very important. Unless you convey a true interest in the learning process, the learner becomes cynical and disillusioned. In addition, your philosophy about education, learning, and people influences the learning process.

EDUCATIONAL LESSON PLAN

PATIENT ______________________ DATE ____________

TOPIC ______________________

SHORT-TERM GOAL	CONTENT OUTLINE	METHODS/STRATEGIES	TIME FACTORS

FIGURE 22–1
A sample educational lesson plan form.

One instructional technique is individual **lecture,** a didactic explanation. Lectures provide the opportunity to transmit information, as well as a chance to explore for understanding. Any information must be presented in a way that allows for assimilation by the particular patient. Reinforcement and praise are important. The addition of a discussion session following the presentation of information reinforces the learning process.

Group lecture format also can be used for instruction. When you present information to a group, however, be prepared for a variety of different responses from the participants. It is useful to anticipate the questions that may be asked. Also useful are audiovisual tools, such as transparencies and slides, which highlight important points and synthesize information. Teaching the actual class is likely to take longer than interacting with a single individual. Advance preparation and practice of the content presentation are advisable.

Similar to group lecture, group discussion techniques are used for patient teaching. The purpose of group discussion is to allow learners to exchange ideas, opinions, and feelings about content areas. Active learning is encouraged as more of the group participants are drawn into the discussion. Encourage full participation by asking quiet group members direct nonthreatening questions such as "What do you think about that . . . ." Reinforce their contributions with positive remarks and also keep the discussion on target and summarize salient points as the session ends.

BOX 22-5 Teaching Techniques

Individual lecture/explanations

Individual discussion

Demonstration/return demonstration

Self-study programs

Workbooks

Journal writing and review

Group lecture

Discussion groups

Role play

Games/simulation

Computer-based instruction

Another technique is the question and answer format of interacting with the learner. Open-ended questions stimulate discussion and problem solving. Independent thought and reinforcement of the learner's abilities to think through situations are enhanced using this technique.

Often it is important for the patient to learn a new procedure. Two invaluable educational techniques used for such situations are **demonstration,** in which the learner is shown a procedure, and **return demonstration,** in which the learner performs the procedure as demonstrated. The patient must first understand the purpose of the demonstration, what is to be learned, and the sequence to be used. All equipment must be prepared in advance. Actual use of objects that the patient needs to learn about makes teaching more realistic and pragmatic. Encourage the learner to handle all equipment and become comfortable with manipulation of the objects to be used in the teaching session. Then the demonstration can proceed with sequenced segments that are eventually put together to provide the whole. Reinforce these increments of learning as the learner practices each one. Then ask the learner to perform a return demonstration of the whole procedure. When a patient is learning procedures, frequent practice of each step is encouraged, especially because overlearning procedures encourages compliance. The key component in using demonstration and return demonstration as teaching techniques is that practice is supported without threat of failure. The learner is able to explore, experience mistakes, and rectify them in learning the correct procedures.

Independent learners may profit from self-directed teaching techniques. Information can efficiently and effectively be presented for individuals who have good reading skills and enjoy written materials. A self-study educational piece should be focused on a few succinct learning objectives. The information should be divided into small segments with frequent checkpoints where the learner can examine his or her understanding of the material and review, if necessary. Limit the information to what is essential. Generally, at the completion of the self-study, a posttest validates that learning has been achieved.

Workbooks are used as teaching tools in much the same way as self-study instruction, or they may be used to reinforce information presented in other ways. A workbook allows the learner systematically to use, review, or apply information. Journal writing provides learners with a chance to express their thoughts and feelings on a variety of topics. Clarify the purpose of keeping a journal. Generally, journals provide a way to explore how their life is being affected and to enhance personal understanding of a situation. Give the learner directions for keeping a journal. Reviewing the journal entries with the patient is the most important part of journal learning. Through this discussion, the learner gleans the meaning of what he or she has written.

A technique that allows groups to actually participate in and learn from structured situations is role-playing. This experience is purposeful simulation of a life event. Each participant is assigned a role. The instructor spends a few minutes with each learner to ensure that everyone understands their part. Observers are also specifically alerted as to what behaviors to notice during the role play. After the role play, always debrief participants, allowing them to discuss the exercise and share their perceptions.

Another learning technique is the use of games. Games allow the learner to review material and work through a simulated situation. The game is designed to accomplish a particular objective. Each participant is provided with rules and information about that objective. When the game is over, participants discuss what they learned from the experience.

Special techniques that use advanced technology can also be used to enhance the learning experience. Computer-based instruction can range from specific learning modules to interactive video disk presentations that require the participants to respond at certain points. The potential applications of technology to learning techniques is endless. The cost of equipment and necessary hardware and software, however, can be restrictive.

The choice of teaching technique that best suits the learning objectives for the individual participant(s) is of utmost importance in successful educational endeavors. Likewise, you must enter into each teaching situation prepared and committed to facilitate the learning process.

▶ Check Your Reading

24. List at least five different teaching strategies.
25. What is the purpose of journal-writing?
26. How is role-playing used in patient education?
27. What is the benefit of individual lecture?
28. Identify one constraint of group lecture.

Evaluation

The last part of the educational process is evaluation. Evaluation is necessary to determine whether the learning objectives have been met (Walsh, 1992). The most simple evaluation method is to review each objective for the criteria for measurement. This is most readily accomplished on an individual basis.

To check the learner's retention and understanding of information that has been presented, a test can be constructed. A well-constructed test can measure the learner's progress, diagnose difficulties, and determine the effectiveness of teaching. Using a pretest and post-test is a variation of testing for knowledge acquired. The pretest can provide you with information about what the learner already knows, thus allowing for the most efficient use of the instruction time. In some situations, an oral test may be preferable, especially for those individuals who have reading problems or test anxiety that severely compromises their ability to perform on a written test.

Evaluation of the learner's performance of procedures using psychomotor skills requires a different form of testing. Usually, simulations and demonstration of the skill are used to evaluate the learner's ability to perform. This method requires that you be as objective as possible when checking for precise behaviors. The mere presence of the observer may cause the learner to have difficulty in demonstrating proficiency in a specified skill.

In addition to evaluation, the accomplishment of the learning objectives, the learning process, and educational endeavor effectiveness can also be evaluated. Each participant is asked for feedback related to the organization of content, the learning environment, instructor effectiveness, and suggestions for change. In this way, you can examine the effectiveness of the educational endeavor itself. This overall evaluation is often accomplished with a participant feedback form. Questions may be open

ASSESSMENT

Assessment data are as follows:

- *Readiness: The patient expresses a desire to learn how to control and to deal with her diagnosis of depression*
- *Learning Style: Assimilation — concepts and details*
- *Resources: Post–high school education; likes to learn; successful legal secretary; motivated at this time*
- *Obstacles: Minimal emotional support from spouse; prefers totally quiet environment — needs to learn how to work with others in the area*

DIAGNOSIS

DSM-IV Diagnosis: *Depression*

Nursing Diagnosis: *Knowledge Deficit related to depressive disorder, treatment, and medications*

OUTCOME IDENTIFICATION, PLANNING, AND IMPLEMENTATION

Expected Outcome 1: *By discharge, the patient will understand depression as a disease process and will understand the coping skills necessary to avoid relapse, cope better, and gain a sense of control.*

Short-Term Goal	Nursing Interventions	Rationales
(See Educational Lesson Plan.)	*(See Educational Lesson Plan.)*	

EVALUATION

Formative Evaluation: *Deedra enjoys the educational approach. She is a quick learner who scored 100% in a quiz related to depression. Deedra is able to state the reasons for taking her medications and to explain the dosage schedule and side effects.*

Summative Evaluation: *Deedra has achieved greater insight into her responses to stress. She has begun to try new coping skills but continues to need support in the area of relationships. I am recommending that she attend a social support group.*

FIGURE 22–2

A sample care plan for Deedra with an educational lesson plan.

ended or worded in a manner to allow the learner to rate each area from poor to excellent. Regardless of the method chosen, a section can be added for further comments and suggestions. These evaluations provide data that can be useful in modifying or strengthening educational efforts (Figure 22–2).

▶ Check Your Reading

29. Identify two methods of evaluating the effectiveness of patient education.
30. When would demonstration and return demonstration be used?
31. How would a workbook be used in patient education?

EDUCATIONAL LESSON PLAN*

PATIENT: *Deedra* DATE: *3/5/96*

TOPIC: *Depression*

SHORT-TERM GOAL	CONTENT OUTLINE	METHODS/STRATEGIES	TIME FACTORS
After the 1:1 session, the patient will: *1. Identify behaviors associated with depression*	*Define depression.* *List behaviors.* *Describe the cycle of negative thoughts and feelings.*	*Didactic*	*10 minutes*
2. Identify one positive feeling *3. Identify a thought that she can "stop"*	*Explore the desired positive feelings.* *Explore the feelings with the patient.* *Identify trigger events.* *Explore potential resources.*	*Discussion*	*15 minutes*
4. List a "replacement" thought that is neutral	*Describe negative thought ruminations.*	*Discussion*	*15 minutes*
	Demonstrate the thought-stopping technique.	*Role play*	*10 minutes*
	Indentify replacement thoughts.	*Discussion*	*5 minutes*
	List alternatives.	*Journal (homework)*	*15 minutes qod*

This is a partial lesson plan.

FIGURE 22–2 *Continued*
A sample care plan for Deedra with an educational lesson plan.

EDUCATING PATIENTS ABOUT MENTAL ILLNESS

Serious mental illness is debilitating to both patient and the family and disruptive in almost every aspect of their lives. To deal with these life situations and solve problems, all involved need a sound foundation of relevant information. The seriously mentally ill person may be incapable of making relevant decisions or solving problems, so the responsibility often falls on a family member, especially with increasing numbers of the mentally ill cared for outside hospital settings (Hatfield, 1988).

Providing a solid knowledge base to the family, as well as the patient, within the limits of each patient's capabilities, assists in developing reasonable and realistic expectations. This knowledge becomes important for planning and carrying out the strategies of care for the patient. Such knowledge should guide the journey. Teaching programs for the psychiatric patient and family are applicable in acute treatment situations and in management of chronic mental illness. Such programs support the treatment and rehabilitative efforts of care.

THE BIOPSYCHOSOCIAL-SPIRITUAL MODEL

A number of different models for understanding mental illness are found in the literature. Each model offers a method of examining information and organizing one's thoughts. If the model is restrictive, then the approaches that flow from it will be limited. If a combination of models is used, then the process is expanded. One model frequently used by nurses for organizing the educational endeavors is the biopsychosocial model. This model encompasses biological, psychological, and sociological theories. The spiritual component makes the model more holistic, thus forming the biopsychosocial-spiritual model.

The basic tenet of biological theory is that psychiatric disorders are diseases caused by biological or neurochemical imbalances within the brain. Psychological theory holds that psychiatric illness is due to psychodynamic interactional factors, and sociological theory suggests that behavioral disorders result from social learning experiences. The spiritual component focuses attention on the essential being of the individual, the role of the transcendent in the person's life, and the spiritual qualities and belief systems that the person holds.

Using a combined biopsychosocial-spiritual model allows you to account for a variety of factors that contribute to the development, manifestation, and outcomes of any one mental disorder. In addition, this model suggests a multifaceted treatment approach.

VARIABLES THAT LIMIT LEARNING

Psychiatric patient education is tailored to the specific needs of patients. A comprehensive, structured, time-limited program helps each participant assimilate the information regardless of the form of the teaching. The teaching may be formal or informal and may use any approach. Often, the group-learning approach is chosen to facilitate patient interactions and support, especially when the education is for the family members or for groups of both patients and family members.

The characteristics of the person suffering from the mental illness have an impact on the educational endeavor and its content. Symptoms such as hallucinations make it difficult for the person experiencing schizophrenia to deal with educational stimuli. An individual in the manic phase of a bipolar disorder cannot focus on the information. Consider each person's illness experience, readiness to learn, temperament, style of learning, and academic ability, especially when providing patient education to someone diagnosed with a mental illness. Generally, education is delayed until the psychotic symptoms are no longer a problem.

CHOICES IN EDUCATIONAL CONTENT

In developing the learning plan for the person with a mental illness or for the family, you need to do a thorough assessment of the patient's learning needs and decide on the approach and methods of teaching. A learning plan, with specific lesson plans for each segment, must then be developed. Implementation requires the artful use of nursing, interpersonal, and communication skills. Evaluation allows for modification and revisions of the educational plan as well as evaluating the responses of the participant(s).

Broad Content Areas and Themes

When you develop the learning plan for the mentally ill person and/or the family, content can be organized around the major concerns expressed. The teaching sessions reflect answers to the questions most frequently raised by patients and family members. They want to know what is "wrong," What caused it? Will the patient get better? What treatment(s) are available? What else can be done? Who can or will do it?

On the basis of these concerns, relevant content includes information about different diagnoses, associated symptoms, probable causes, treatment options including specifics about medications, prognosis, and problems involved in living with serious mental illness. Much time is spent discussing each patient's experiences with respect to learning to live effectively (Ascher-Suanum and Krauss, 1991). Box 22–6 summarizes broad educational content areas for persons diagnosed with mental illness. These areas can be subdivided to allow for better instructional pacing and assimilation of content.

Including certain themes throughout the sessions further enhances the learning experience of both patient and family. These themes include

- Control of illness versus cure
- Balance between rights and responsibilities
- Illness-monitoring techniques

When these themes are woven throughout the classes, they reinforce the content presented in previous sessions.

BOX 22–6 Core Content Areas for Education of Mentally Ill Patients and Family Members

Definition of mental illness

Aspects of different diagnoses

Explanation of symptoms

Causes of mental illness

Treatment options

Medication management

Coping and stress management

Communication and relationship skills

Support systems

BOX 22-7 Content Outline: Educational Learning Plan for Educating Patients About Mental Illness

I. Patient education overview
   A. Purpose
   B. Introduction of instructor and participant(s)
   C. Role of the participant(s)
   D. Rights and responsibilities
   E. Expectations regarding participation, assignments, acceptable behavior
   F. Role of the instructor
   G. Topics for the different sessions
   H. Any materials (as necessary)
   I. Participant questions
II. Definition of mental illness
   A. Definition
   B. Overview of types of mental disorders
      1. Schizophrenia
      2. Other psychotic disorders
      3. Depressive disorder
      4. Anxiety disorder
      5. Bipolar disorder
      6. Cognitive disorders
      7. Personality disorder
      8. Substance-use disorder
   C. Major symptoms experienced
      1. Behavioral symptoms
      2. Thought disturbances
      3. Perceptual disturbances
      4. Mood and emotional disturbances
   D. Variability of experiences
      1. Range of responses
      2. Participant responses
   E. Diagnostic procedures
      1. Physical examination
      2. Psychiatric examination
      3. Psychological tests
      4. Psychosocial assessment
   F. Treatment approaches
      1. Medical
      2. Medication
      3. Psychotherapies
      4. Educational
   G. Participant questions
III. Medications
   A. What each participant should know
      1. Name and type of medication
      2. Dosage and administration schedule
      3. Actions and side effects
      4. Special instructions
   B. Categories of major psychotropic medications
      1. Antipsychotic drugs
      2. Antidepressant drugs
      3. Antianxiety agents
      4. Mood stabilizers
      5. Medications to treat side effects
   C. General principles of taking medications
      1. Rules
      2. Proper storage
      3. Cautions
   D. Importance of adhering to medication regimens
   E. Hazards of substance abuse
   F. Participant discussion of different experiences with medications
   G. Participant questions
IV. Monitoring mental illness
   A. The concept of illness
      1. Acute versus chronic nature
      2. Cyclic dynamics
      3. Relapse
   B. Symptoms
      1. Meaning of symptom
      2. Recognizing symptoms
      3. Self-monitoring
      4. Individual symptom list
      5. Signs of relapse
   C. Response needed
      1. Communication of concern
      2. Communication with family/support personnel
      3. Communication with health care provider
      4. Decrease environmental stress
      5. Active positive response to seek assistance
   D. Participant exchange on the meaning of mental illness as a chronic disorder
   E. Participant discussion of experiences related to different symptoms
   F. Participant questions
V. Coping and management of stress
   A. Definition of stress and coping
   B. Stress response
      1. Physiological effects
      2. Psychological effects
      3. Behavioral effects
      4. Sociological effects
   C. Stress and mental illness
   D. Reducing stress
      1. Lifestyle factors
      2. Environmental factors
      3. Relaxation techniques
      4. Cognitive coping techniques
   E. Developing individualized techniques to manage stress
   F. Participant discussion of stress management experiences
   G. Participant questions
VI. Communication and relationship skills
   A. Definition of communication and relationship
   B. Types of communication
      1. Verbal
      2. Nonverbal
   C. Styles of communicating
      1. Direct
      2. Indirect
      3. Active
      4. Passive
      5. Assertive
      6. Aggressive
   D. Relating communication style to situation
   E. Conversations
      1. Initiation interactions
      2. Topics
      3. Roles
   F. Effective communication
      1. Principles
      2. Communication techniques
   G. Role of communication in relating to others

BOX 22-7 Content Outline: Educational Learning Plan for Educating Patients About Mental Illness *Continued*

- H. Interpersonal interactions
  1. Social versus therapeutic relationship
  2. Phases of a relationship
- I. Participant practice in effective communications and relating to others
- J. Participant questions

VII. Interactions with family and support network representatives
- A. Roles of family members/support network representative
- B. Effect of patient's mental illness on others
- C. Effect of temperament on coping with patient's mental illness
- D. Rights and responsibilities of family members/ support network representatives
- E. Role of members in assisting management, treatment, and rehabilitation of the patient
  1. Gaining access to services
  2. Monitoring
  3. Medication management
  4. Partnership for care
- F. Communication with family members and others
- G. Participant practice and role play of interactions with family members/support network representative

VIII. Community resources
- A. Identifying available resources
- B. Access to resources
  1. Procedures
  2. Strategies
- C. Categories of resources
  1. Housing/shelter
  2. Food
  3. Income
  4. Health care
  5. Rehabilitation
  6. Leisure activities
- D. List potential resources
  1. Social Security income
  2. Social Security disability income
  3. Public housing
  4. Private groups (e.g., Salvation Army, National Alliance for the Mentally Ill)
  5. Department of mental health (local and state)
  6. Subsidized living residences
  7. Medicare/Medicaid
  8. Hospitals/clinics
  9. Hotlines
  10. Vocational rehabilitation services
- E. Participant discussion about experiences with community resources
  1. Positive
  2. Negative and how resolved
- F. Participant questions

IX. Detailed investigation of specific diagnoses of mental illness (as appropriate for participant[s] or group)

Detailed Content

The organization of content varies greatly among learning programs. To assist in planning an educational endeavor for psychiatric patients, Figure 22–2 outlines the various core content areas. To implement any aspect of this outline, a learning plan will need to be developed (see Figure 22–1). A very useful resource for the development of a detailed lesson plan for most of these content areas can be found in *Educating Patients and Families About Mental Illness: A Practical Guide* (Bisbee, 1991). Always remember that the specific needs of the participant(s) may necessitate presenting in small pieces of information over a longer period than you first planned. At other times, the participant(s) may be ready for more information than you initially considered. Having each lesson plan fall within specific time constraints facilitates the accomplishment of the entire learning plan. The balance between desired content and the actual flow of the learning session is a skill that develops with experience (Box 22–7).

Family Education

In addition to the content taught to the patient, several other areas need to be addressed when planning sessions for teaching family members of the mentally ill patient. Family members need to review not only the rights and responsibilities of the patient but also the rights and responsibilities of family members in various relationships to the patient. Acknowledging these rights and responsibilities facilitates a partnership in treatment between the patient and the health care providers.

Another area of focus is the many roles a patient may assume within the family. These include the sick role, disabled role, recovering role, and well role. The role of the family in treatment, management of illness, and rehabilitation are other areas for discussion and teaching. Several areas relate to the family role in management of the patient's illness. Monitoring the progress of treatment includes learning about relapse and its prevention (Daley et al, 1992). Encourage the learning of skills in maintaining a therapeutic living environment. In most cases, these skills include medication management, promoting a healthful lifestyle, and coping and stress management techniques for the caregiver.

Another focus of family education is managing behaviors, including concrete plans for coping with the behaviors manifested by the mentally ill patient and the family members' response. In addition, learning to respond in potential emergencies is useful. Having the opportunity to practice the plan and contingency plans using role play or "drills" assists in learning skills needed to manage behavioral aspects of the illness.

Often the family is called upon to assist the patient in learning general activities of daily living. Personal skills such as hygiene, grooming, and household care are included. Other aspects of training include social skills and vocational skills. Also teach the role of the family in facilitating skills development and strategies for skill building.

▶ Check Your Reading

32. Give one reason for educating family members about the patient's illness.
33. What is unique about the biopsychosocial-spiritual model?
34. How does the patient's illness act as a constraining variable in teaching?
35. Identify three common questions posed by family members.
36. Identify three broad content areas that would most likely be included in patient/family education.
37. What are the three themes that are woven throughout the teaching sessions?
38. What are some of the specific content areas presented in patient education?
39. In addition to teaching families about mental illness, what else is reviewed with them?
40. What is the family's role in illness management?

CONCLUSIONS

Education about psychiatric illness and how to manage it is one of the most helpful strategies that we can offer patients and families. By increasing their knowledge, we make a direct and lasting impact on their journey; we provide them with the tools and information to make informed decisions, to handle symptoms, to understand their rights and responsibilities, and to journey with a bit more control and choice. By sharing knowledge, we affirm the collaborative and partnership roles we have with patients and families. We are not in charge of the patient's journey. We are more like coaches. We run alongside. We encourage. We challenge, and we support. We affirm, and we stimulate hope.

KEY POINTS TO REMEMBER

- The mentally ill person and the family have a need to understand fully the scope of the individual illness.
- Activities of patient education provide the means to understanding.
- Patient education is an integral part of quality and cost-effective care, and it is the process of deliberately creating cognitive, affective, behavioral, and psychomotor changes.
- The function of education is the development of organized bodies of knowledge and generic problem-solving skills.
- Learning is a dynamic process that incorporates readiness to learn, motivation, acquisition of new knowledge, attitudes and skills, and the resulting ability to change behavior.
- Learning takes place in both formal and informal contexts.
- The learning process is influenced by a person's cognitive and sensorimotor abilities, past experiences, perception, and sociocultural factors.
- The theoretical basis used—be it a behavioral, psychodynamic, cognitive, or social cognitive learning theory—provides the framework for understanding the ongoing dynamics of learning.
- Principles of learning guide you in carrying out the phases of the educational endeavor.
- The principles of adult learning guide you in developing learning programs that take into account the attributes of the adult learner.
- The process of education involves the phases of assessment, diagnosis, outcome identification, planning, implementation, and evaluation.
- The process begins with a thorough assessment of the learner's needs, learning style, and any obstacles to learning.
- On the basis of assessed information, planning proceeds with the identification of the overall goal and long-term outcomes.
- Next, behavioral objectives, which are specific, measurable, and patient centered, are delineated to guide the learning process and set the parameters for the implementation and evaluation phases of the process.
- Succinct activities are set forth to meet the learning behavioral objectives.
- Implementation of the plan involves either an individual or a group approach to the learning endeavors.
- Different learning activities may include lectures, discussions, question and answer sessions, demonstrations and return demonstrations, self-study programs, workbook assignments, role play, and games. The teaching activity chosen must be best suited for each patient's learning needs, style of learning, and behavioral objectives.
- The last phase of the process is evaluation of how well criteria were met, both for each learning objective and for the overall educational endeavor.
- Retention of information and understanding can be evaluated through direct discussion, observation, or testing.
- Often, a combination of methods of evaluation are employed.
- Educating patients about mental illness incorporates all of the information about general patient education, taking into account that serious mental illness is debilitating to the patient and the family.
- The mentally ill person may not be capable of making relevant, competent decisions or carrying out problem-solving activities as other patients can.
- Often the responsibility for decision-making falls to a family member or a representative of the support network—an important factor in planning and carrying out educational endeavors for the mentally ill.
- The necessary information incorporated into teaching patients about mental illness flows from expressed major concerns.
- A method for presenting information depends on the choice of a theoretical framework to assist in educating the learners about mental illness.

• The biopsychosocial-spiritual model provides one of the broadest frameworks from which to teach about the many facets of living with mental illness.

• The most relevant content includes information about the nature of mental illness, information about different diagnoses, associated symptoms, probable causes, treatment options, medications, prognosis, coping, and managing stress.

• The content can be tailored by pacing to meet the patient's specific learning needs.

• Education of those responsible for patient care—the family or representative from a support network includes other supportive information.

• For patients unable to care for themselves, content related to monitoring the patient, managing various situations, maintaining a therapeutic living environment, and coordinating all aspects of care needs to be developed.

• A group approach provides learning opportunities to family/support representatives and allows participants to share experiences and express concerns in a supportive and understanding situation.

• Your collaborative role in patient education assists in providing quality care, fostering self-care whenever possible, and supporting all the participants.

• Because the bulk of care for the mentally ill population occurs outside the traditional hospital, opportunities for linking the health care system and the community continue to grow.

LEARNING ACTIVITIES

1. Review the detailed content outline. Develop a sample teaching plan for one topic that you would like to present to a patient with whom you are working.

2. What teaching strategies are most effective in facilitating your learning? Why is this so?

3. What is your learning style? On what do you base your conclusion? How would you determine the learning style of a patient with whom you were working?

4. What is your preferred method of accessing information? How do you know that about yourself? How would you assess this issue in a patient?

CRITICAL THINKING EXERCISE

Sabrina, a student in her first week of the psychiatric clinical, was assigned to Miss Kim Kenny, a depressed 28-year-old woman. Sabrina noticed in the patient's chart that she had a history of asthma, had smoked for 15 years, and was a waitress in a gambling casino. She decided to do some health teaching with Miss Kenny. Because this was her third meeting with her, Sabrina felt comfortable approaching her, stating, "Kim, I think you need to stop smoking. I have a lot of good pamphlets that tell you why smoking is bad for you. You, of all people, should know that smoking will only make your asthma worse." Miss Kenny sat listening as she was told about how bad smoking was. At the end of the talk Miss Kenny said, "I know I should stop, but where I work everybody smokes."

1. Under what assumption(s) is the student operating in this interaction?

2. What could she have assumed instead?

3. Why do you think she made these assumptions?

The next day, Sabrina had a meeting scheduled with Miss Kenny at 11:00 a.m. At 11:30, Miss Kenny ran up to Sabrina, apologizing for being late. It seems that one of the other patients was showing her how to make an ashtray in ceramics class.

1. Make sense out of the data.

2. What conclusions can you draw about Miss Kenny's readiness to stop smoking?

3. Suggest other approaches. Might they have had a different result?

REFERENCES

Arnold, E. (1995). Health teaching in the nurse-client relationship. In E. Arnold and K. Boggs (Eds.), *Interpersonal relationships: Communication skills for nurses.* (pp. 374–413). Philadelphia: W. B. Saunders.

Ascher-Suanum, H., and Krause, A. (1991). *Psychosocial educational groups for patients with schizophrenia: A guide for practitioners.* Gaithersburg, MD: Aspen Publications.

American Nurses' Association. (1991). *Standards of clinical nursing practice.* Kansas City, MO: American Nurses' Association.

Bisbee, C. (1991). *Educating patients and families about mental illness: A practical guide.* Rockville, MD: Aspen Publications.

Bloom, B., and Krawnthol, D. (1984). *Taxonomy of educational objectives: The classification of educational goals. Handbook I: Cognitive domain.* New York: Longman Publication Group.

Daley, D., Bowler, K., and Cahalane, H. (1992). Approaches to patient and family education with affective disorders. *Patient Education and Counseling, 19*(2), 163–174.

DeCoux, V. (1990). Kolb's Learning Style Inventory: A review of its applications in nursing research. *Journal of Nursing Education, 29*(5), 202–207.

Haggard, A. (1989). *Handbook of patient education.* Rockville, MD: Aspen Publications.

Hatfield, A. (1988). Issues for psychoeducation for families of the mentally ill. *International Journal of Mental Health, 17,* 48–64.

Hatfield, A. (1990). *Family education in mental illness.* New York: Guilford Press.

Lewin, K. (1947). Frontiers in group dynamics. *Human Relations, 1,* 5–41.

Lipkin, G., and Cohen, R. (1992). *Effective approaches to patient behavior* (5th ed.). New York: Springer-Verlag.

Opdycke, R., Ascione, F., Shimp, L., and Rosen, R. (1992). A systematic approach to educating elderly patients about their medications. *Patient Education and Counseling, 19*(1), 43–60.

Rankin, S., and Stallings, K. (1990). *Patient education issues: Principles and practice* (2nd ed.). Philadelphia: J. B. Lippincott.

Redman, B. (1993). *The process of patient education* (7th ed.). St. Louis, MO: C. V. Mosby.

Sundeen, S., Stuart, G. Rankin, E., and Cohen, S. (1994). Nurse-client interaction: Implementing the nursing process (5th ed.). St. Louis, MO: C. V. Mosby.

Walsh, J. (1992). Methods of psychoeducational program evaluation in mental health settings. *Patient Education and Counseling, 19*(2), 205–218.

SUGGESTED READINGS

Daley, D., Bowler, K., and Cahalane, H. (1992). Approaches to patient and family education with affective disorders. *Patient Education and Counseling, 19*(2), 163–174.

Dickey, L. (1993). Promoting preventive care with patient-held minirecords: A review. *Patient Education and Counseling, 20*(1), 37–47.

Opdycke, R., Ascione, F., Shimp, L., and Rosen, R. (1992). A systematic approach to educating elderly patients about their medications. *Patient Education and Counseling, 19*(1), 43–60.

Walsh, J. (1992). Methods of psychoeducational program evaluation in mental health settings. *Patient Education and Counseling, 19*(2), 205–218.

CHAPTER 23

PSYCHOPHARMACOLOGY

At this point in my life, I cannot imagine leading a normal life without both taking lithium and being in psychotherapy. Lithium prevents my seductive but disastrous highs, diminishes my depression . . . but ineffably psychotherapy heals.

—A patient with manic depressive illness

LEARNING OBJECTIVES

After studying this chapter, you should be able to:

1. State the mechanism of action of each family of psychotherapeutic drugs.
2. State the principal uses of each family of psychotherapeutic drugs.
3. State the major adverse effects, and related nursing interventions, of each family of psychotherapeutic drugs.
4. State the major drug interactions of each family of psychotherapeutic drugs.
5. Apply the nursing process to a patient requiring psychotherapeutic drugs.
6. Identify the spiritual implications of taking psychotherapeutic drugs.

KEY TERMINOLOGY

Acute dystonia
Agranulocytosis (clozapine induced)
Akathisia
Antianxiety agent (anxiolytic drug)
Antidepressants
Antipsychotic agents
  Atypical
  High potency
  Low potency
Benzodiazepines
Butyrophenones
Carbamazepine
Chlorpromazine
Clozapine
Extrapyramidal reactions
Haloperidol
Lithium
Monoamine oxidase inhibitors (MAOIs)
Monoamine hypothesis of depression
Negative symptoms (of schizophrenia)
Neuroleptic malignant syndrome
Parkinsonism (antipsychotic induced)
Phenothiazines
Positive symptoms (of schizophrenia)
Psychotherapeutic drug
Receptor
Reuptake (of transmitter)
Selective serotonin reuptake inhibitors (SSRIs)
Synaptic transmission
Tardive dyskinesia
Transmitter (neurotransmitter)
Tricyclic antidepressants
Valproic acid

Our topic for this chapter is **psychotherapeutic drugs**—drugs used to treat psychiatric disorders. This group of drugs has four major divisions: (1) antipsychotic agents (used primarily for schizophrenia), (2) antidepressants, (3) lithium and other drugs for bipolar disorder (manic-depressive illness), and (4) anxiolytics (used to relieve anxiety). None of the psychotherapeutic agents is curative: These drugs only offer symptomatic relief. Furthermore, none represents ideal therapy by itself; rather, all of these agents are best used in conjunction with some form of psychotherapy. Unfortunately, not all patients receive ideal treatment: Many are left to rely on drug therapy alone. Conversely, patients who could benefit from drug therapy (along with their psychotherapy) may fail to receive the medication that they need—thus needlessly prolonging discomfort. The journey of Dr. Royce Opara, which follows, illustrates the consequences of failing to prescribe psychotherapeutic drugs for the patients who need them.

This chapter including Figs. 23–1 and 23–2 and Tables 23–1 to 23–12, is adapted from Chapters 11 and 24 through 27 of Lehne, R. A., et al. (1994). *Pharmacology for nursing care*. (2nd ed.). Philadelphia: W. B. Saunders.

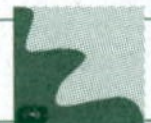

DR. ROYCE OPARA'S STORY

Dr. Royce Opara, a 37-year-old physician, was admitted to a private psychiatric hospital in early January of 1979. He was board certified as an internist and was also a subspecialist in nephrology. He had been married three times and had three children, one with his current wife and two with his second wife.

Dr. Opara had a past history of brief periods of anxiety and depression that had been treated on an outpatient basis. Before this admission he had been suffering from anxious and depressive symptoms for approximately two years, although he had received treatment during periods of difficulty during his prior marriages. From 1977, he had been treated as an outpatient with a combination of individual psychotherapy and tricyclic antidepressant medication. He did not maintain the recommended dose of antidepressant medication, and his condition deteriorated as problems with his wife increased over conflict about her desire for another child. Because of strong cultural biases, he resisted the suggestion of family therapy. Hospitalization was recommended when he became suicidal and had increased his consumption of cocaine from occasional to daily use.

On admission to the facility, the admitting psychiatrist found him verbally abusive, obstinate, and agitated. He was diagnosed as suffering from major injuries to an underlying narcissistic personality disorder and secondarily from a manic-depressive illness, depressed type. He was hospitalized for several months. He was often unpleasant; he would make aggressive gestures; and he was often not compliant. During this time he continued to be treated with individual psychotherapy four times a week but with no psychotherapeutic medications. He lost a considerable amount of weight, experienced severe insomnia, and had marked psychomotor agitation. His agitation, manifested by incessant pacing, was so extreme that his feet became swollen and blistered, requiring medical attention. His progress was minimal, forcing the family to become increasingly concerned. Finally, a brother, who was a cardiologist, convinced the family to seek a second opinion from a psychiatrist who lived in a nearby metropolitan area. In response to his inquiry, the clinical staff at the hospital held a clinical case conference to review the patient's treatment. They decided to make no major changes and specifically decided not to institute any medication regimen. Dr. Opara's condition did not improve. Later, in an unpublished diary, he described his hospitalization in terms that were reminiscent of an experience in Hades.

After several months, his relatives convinced him to leave the hospital. He was subsequently transferred to a private psychiatric facility in another state. His discharge diagnosis was manic-depressive illness, depressed type. At the new facility, he was diagnosed as having a psychotic depression, agitated type, and treatment with a combination of phenothiazines and tricyclic antidepressants was initiated. Within three weeks his condition had improved, and within three months he was discharged (with a final diagnosis of manic-depressive illness, depressed type with psychotic features). He resumed his professional work, and as of 1990 he continued to function well without rehospitalization.

He subsequently initiated a lawsuit against the first facility claiming that as a result of negligence in not administering drug treatment—to which he had responded favorably in the past—he lost his standing in the professional community and custody of his children. He was awarded financial damages by an arbitration panel in an amount agreed upon by both parties, thus averting the need for a jury trial.

Although Dr. Opara may have received some benefit from treatment with antidepressant medications in past episodes of illness, for the first seven months of hospitalization on this admission, pharmacological agents were withheld in favor of a treatment approach based on psychodynamic formulations of the etiology of anxiety and depression. Thus, the influence of possible endogenous genetical and biological dysfunction was ignored.

MECHANISMS BY WHICH CENTRAL NERVOUS SYSTEM DRUGS ACT

All of the psychopharmacological drugs produce their therapeutic effects by altering communication between neurons within the CNS. In all cases, this is accomplished by influencing synaptic transmission (rather than by axonal conduction). Accordingly, in order to understand how these drugs act, we need to know the ways in which they can alter communication between neurons at synapses. To establish this understanding, we will first review the steps in **synaptic transmission,** after which we will discuss the ways in which drugs can affect each step.

Steps in Synaptic Transmission

Synaptic transmission takes place in five basic steps. These are depicted in Figure 23–1 and discussed below.

Step 1: Synthesis

For synaptic transmission to take place, molecules of **transmitter** must be present within the nerve terminal. Hence, we can look upon synthesis of transmitter as being the first step in transmission. In Figure 23–1, the letters Q, R, and S represent the precursor molecules from which the transmitter (T) is made.

Step 2: Storage

Once transmitter is synthesized, it must be stored until the time of its release. Storage of transmitter molecules takes place within *vesicles,* which are tiny packets present in the axon terminal. Each nerve terminal contains a large number of transmitter-filled vesicles.

Step 3: Release

Release of transmitter is triggered by the arrival of an action potential at the axon terminal. The action potential initiates a process in which vesicles undergo fusion with the terminal membrane, causing release of vesicular contents into the synaptic gap. With each action potential, only a small fraction of all vesicles present in the nerve terminal are caused to discharge their contents.

Step 4: Receptor Binding

Following their release, transmitter molecules diffuse across the synaptic gap and then undergo *reversible* binding to *receptors* on the postsynaptic neuron. This binding initiates a series of events that result either in excitation or inhibition of the postsynaptic neuron; thus, binding of transmitter can either increase or decrease the chances that the postsynaptic neuron will fire an action potential of its own.

Step 5: Termination

Transmission is terminated by dissociation of transmitter from its receptors, followed by removal of free transmitter from the synaptic gap. Transmitter can be cleared from the synaptic gap by three processes: (1) **reuptake** into the presynaptic neuron, (2) enzymatic degradation, and (3) diffusion. In those synapses where transmission is terminated by reuptake, axon terminals contain "pumps" for the active transport of transmitter molecules back into the neuron (see step 5a in Figure 23–1). Following reuptake, molecules of transmitter may be degraded, or they may be repackaged in vesicles for reuse. In synapses where transmitter is cleared by enzymatic degradation (see step 5b in Figure 23–1), the synapse contains large quantities of transmitter-inactivating enzymes. Although simple diffusion away from the synaptic gap (see step 5c in Figure 23–1) is a potential means of terminating transmitter action, this process is very slow and generally of little significance.

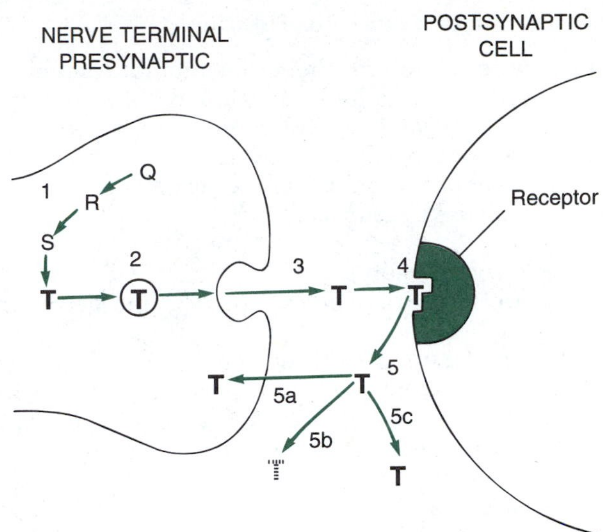

FIGURE 23–1
Steps in synaptic transmission. **Step 1,** Synthesis of transmitter (T) from precursor molecules (Q, R, S). **Step 2,** Storage of transmitter in vesicles. **Step 3,** Release of transmitter. In response to an action potential, vesicles fuse with the terminal membrane and discharge their contents into the synaptic gap. **Step 4,** Action at receptor. Transmitter binds (reversibly) to its receptor on the postsynaptic neuron, causing a response in that cell. **Step 5,** Termination of transmission. Transmitter dissociates from its receptor and is then removed from the synaptic gap by (a) reuptake into the nerve terminal, (b) enzymatic degradation, or (c) diffusion away from the gap.

Effects of Drugs on Synaptic Transmission

In this section, we will look at the specific ways in which drugs can alter the steps of synaptic transmission. By way of encouragement, although this information may appear complex, it isn't. In fact, most of it is self-evident.

Transmitter Synthesis

Drugs can either increase or decrease transmitter synthesis—the impact of which should be obvious. A drug that increases synthesis will increase the amount of transmitter stored in presynaptic vesicles. As a result, when an action potential reaches the axon terminal, more transmitter will be released, and therefore more transmitter will be available to **receptors** on the postsynaptic cell, thus intensifying transmission at that site. Conversely, a drug that decreases transmitter synthesis will cause the transmitter content of vesicles to decline, resulting in reduced transmitter release and suppression of synaptic transmission.

Transmitter Storage

Drugs that interfere with transmitter storage will reduce synaptic transmission. This is because disruption of storage depletes vesicles of their transmitter content, thus decreasing the amount of transmitter available for release.

Transmitter Release

Drugs can have one of two effects on transmitter release: They can *promote* release or they can *inhibit* release. Drugs that promote release will intensify transmission; conversely, drugs that inhibit release will suppress transmission.

Receptor Binding

Many neuropharmacological drugs act directly at receptors. Drugs in this category are known to act one of three ways: (1) they can bind to receptors and cause receptor activation; (2) they can bind to receptors and therefore prevent receptor activation by the natural transmitter at that site (or by other drugs that bind to that receptor); and (3) they can bind to the receptor complex and thus enhance the actions of the natural transmitter at that site. Drugs that directly activate receptors are called *agonists*. Conversely, drugs that prevent receptor activation are called *antagonists*. The receptor agonists and antagonists constitute the largest and most important groups of neuropharmacological drugs.

Termination of Transmitter Action

Drugs can interfere with the termination of transmitter action by two mechanisms: (1) blockade of transmitter reuptake or (2) inhibition of transmitter degradation. Drugs that act by either mechanism will cause the concentration of transmitter in the synaptic gap to rise, thus intensifying transmission.

▶ Check Your Reading

1. How are neurotransmitters stored in the nerve terminal?
2. What are the two possible outcomes when a transmitter binds to its receptor on a postsynaptic neuron?
3. What is the general term for a drug that causes receptor activation when it binds to a receptor? What about a drug that prevents receptor activation as a result of receptor binding?
4. What is the effect of a drug that blocks transmitter reuptake?

ANTIPSYCHOTIC AGENTS

The **antipsychotic agents** are a chemically diverse group of compounds that are used to treat a broad spectrum of psychotic disorders. Specific indications include schizophrenia, delusional disorders, acute mania, depressive psychoses, and drug-induced psychoses.

Since their introduction in the early 1950s, the antipsychotic agents have catalyzed revolutionary change in the management of psychotic illnesses. Before these drugs became available, psychoses were largely untreatable and patients were fated to a life of institutionalization. With the advent of antipsychotic medications, many patients with schizophrenia and other severe psychiatric disorders have been able to leave psychiatric hospitals and return to the community. Others have been spared hospitalization entirely. For those who must remain institutionalized, antipsychotic drugs have at least been able to reduce suffering.

The antipsychotic drugs fall into two major groups: *traditional antipsychotics* and *atypical antipsychotics*. All of the *traditional* agents block receptors for dopamine in the CNS, and they all can cause serious *movement disorders*, referred to as *extrapyramidal reactions*. Although the atypical agents also block dopamine receptors, the pattern of blockade differs from that of the traditional agents. As a result, the risk of extrapyramidal reactions with the atypical agents is low.

Traditional Antipsychotic Agents

In this section we will discuss pharmacological properties shared by all of the traditional agents. Much of our attention will focus on adverse effects. Of these, the extrapyramidal reactions are of particular concern. Because of these neurological side effects, the traditional antipsychotics are known alternatively as **neuroleptics.**

Classification

The traditional antipsychotics can be classified according to potency or chemical structure. From a clinical viewpoint, classification by potency is more informative.

CLASSIFICATION BY POTENCY

Traditional antipsychotic agents can be classified as **low potency,** medium potency, or **high potency** (Table 23–1). The low-potency drugs, represented by *chlorpromazine (Thorazine)*, and the high-potency drugs, represented by *haloperidol (Haldol)*, are of particular interest.

It is important to note that although the neuroleptics differ from one another in potency, all of these drugs are essentially equal in their ability to relieve symptoms of psychoses. (In pharmacology, the term potency refers only to the size of the dose needed to elicit a given response; potency implies nothing about the *maximal effect* that a drug can produce. Hence, when we say that haloperidol has a higher potency than chlorpromazine, we mean only that the dose of haloperidol required to relieve psychotic symptoms is smaller than the required dose of chlorpromazine; we do not mean that haloperidol can produce greater effects. If administered in therapeutically equivalent doses, both drugs will elicit an equivalent antipsychotic response.)

If the low-potency and high-potency neuroleptics possess the same therapeutic ability, why should we distinguish between them? The answer is that although these agents produce identical *antipsychotic effects*, they differ significantly in their *side effects*. Hence, by knowing the potency category to which a particular neuroleptic belongs, we can better predict that drug's undesired responses. This knowledge is useful in drug selection and providing patient care and education.

CLASSIFICATION BY CHEMICAL STRUCTURE

The traditional antipsychotic agents can be placed into five major groups based on their chemical structures (Table 23–2). One of these groups, the phenothiazines, has three subdivisions. Drugs in all groups are equivalent with respect to antipsychotic actions.

Two chemical categories—the **phenothiazines** and the **butyrophenones**—deserve special attention. The phenothiazines were the first of the modern antipsychotic agents. Chlorpromazine, the prototype of the low-potency neuroleptics, is a member of the phenothiazine family. The butyrophenones stand out because they are the family to which haloperidol belongs. Haloperidol is the prototype of the high-potency antipsychotics.

Mechanism of Action

The traditional antipsychotic drugs block a variety of receptors within the outside the CNS. To varying degrees, these drugs produce blockade at receptors for dopamine, acetylcholine, histamine, and norepinephrine. There is little question that blockade at these receptors is responsible for the major adverse effects of the antipsy-

TABLE 23–1 Traditional Antipsychotic Drugs: Relative Potency and Major Side Effects

			Incidence of Major Side Effects			
Potency Class	**Drug**	**Equivalent Oral Dose (mg)***	***Sedation***	***Orthostatic Hypotension***	***Anticholinergic Effects***	***Extrapyramidal Effects†***
	Chlorpromazine	100	High	High	Medium	Low
Low	Thioridazine	100	High	High	High	Low
	Chlorprothixene	100	High	High	High	Low
	Mesoridazine	50	High	Medium	Medium	Low
	Triflupromazine	25	High	High	Medium	Medium
	Acetophenazine	20	Medium	Low	Low	Medium
Medium	Loxapine	10	Medium	Medium	Medium	High
	Molindone	10	Medium	Low	Medium	Medium
	Perphenazine	8	Low	Low	Low	High
	Trifluoperazine	5	Low	Low	Low	High
	Thiothixene	4	Low	Low	Low	High
High	Fluphenazine	2	Low	Low	Low	High
	Haloperidol	2	Low	Low	Low	High
	Pimozide	1	Low	Low	Low	High

*Doses listed are the therapeutic equivalent of 100 mg of oral chlorpromazine.
†Incidence refers to *early* extrapyramidal reactions (acute dystonia, parkinsonism, akathisia). Incidence of *late* reactions (tardive dyskinesia) is the same for all of these drugs.

TABLE 23–2 Traditional Antipsychotic Drugs: Chemical Classification, Routes, and Dosages

Chemical Class and Generic Name	Trade Name	Routes	Dosage Range (mg/d)
Phenothiazine: aliphatic			
Chlorpromazine	Thorazine, Ormazine	PO, IM, R	30–800
Triflupromazine	Vesprin	IM	60–150
Phenothiazine: piperidine			
Mesoridazine	Serentil	PO, IM	30–400
Thioridazine	Mellaril	PO	150–800
Phenothiazine: piperazine			
Acetophenazine	Tindal	PO	60–120
Fluphenazine	Prolixin, Permitil	PO, IM	2–40
Perphenazine	Trilafon	PO, IM	12–64
Trifluoperazine	Stelazine	PO, IM	2–40
Thioxanthene			
Chlorprothixene	Taractan	PO, IM	75–600
Thiothixene	Navane	PO, IM	8–30
Butyrophenone			
Haloperidol	Haldol	PO, IM	1–15
Dihydroindolone			
Molindone	Moban	PO	15–225
Dibenzoxazepine			
Loxapine	Loxitane	PO, IM	20–250

PO = oral; IM = intramuscular; R = rectal (suppository)

chotics. However, since the etiology of psychotic illness is entirely unknown, the relationship of receptor blockade to therapeutic effects can only be guessed. One theory suggests that neuroleptics suppress symptoms of psychosis by blocking specific subtypes of *dopamine receptors* in the mesolimbic and mesocortical areas of the brain, regions thought to be involved in the expression of psychotic symptoms. In support of this theory is the observation that all of the traditional antipsychotics produce dopamine receptor blockade.

Therapeutic Uses

SCHIZOPHRENIA

Schizophrenia is the most common indication for antipsychotic drugs. These agents effectively suppress symptoms during acute psychotic episodes, and, when taken chronically, can greatly decrease the risk of relapse. *Initial* effects are seen in one to two days, but *full* effects develop gradually—over six to eight weeks. So-called **positive symptoms** (e.g., agitation, tension, delusions, hallucinations) generally respond better than do the **negative symptoms** (e.g., social withdrawal, blunted affect, motor retardation). All of the traditional antipsychotic agents are equally effective, although individual patients may respond better to one drug than to another. Consequently, selection among these drugs is based primarily on their side-effect profiles, rather than on their therapeutic effects. Because the high-potency agents generally cause fewer side effects than do the low-potency agents, many clinicians select a high-potency agent for initial treatment.

Please note that antipsychotic drugs do not alter the underlying pathology of schizophrenia. Treatment, therefore, is not curative—it offers only symptomatic relief.

BIPOLAR DISORDER (MANIC-DEPRESSIVE ILLNESS)

Most patients with bipolar disorder are managed with lithium, the drug of choice for this disease. Neuroleptics may be used in acute cases (in combination with lithium) to help manage patients who are going through a severe manic phase. Drugs for bipolar disorder are discussed later in the chapter.

TOURETTE'S SYNDROME

This rare, inherited disorder is characterized by severe motor tics, barking cries, grunts, and outbursts of obscene language, all of which are spontaneous and beyond the control of the patient. At least two antipsychotic drugs—haloperidol and pimozide—can help to suppress symptoms.

OTHER USES

Neuroleptics can be used for dementia and other organic mental syndromes (psychiatric syndromes resulting from organic causes, such as infection, metabolic disorders, poisoning, and structural injury to the brain), delusional disorders, and schizoaffective disorder. In addition, these agents can relieve symptoms of Huntington's chorea.

Adverse Effects

Although antipsychotic agents produce a variety of undesired effects, these drugs are generally very safe; death by overdose is almost unheard of. Of the many side effects that these drugs can produce, the most troubling are the **extrapyramidal reactions**—especially **tardive dyskinesia.** It is important to note that the adverse effect profile of the low potency agents differs from that of the high-potency agents. Specifically, the low-potency agents are associated with a higher incidence of sedation, hypotension, and anticholinergic effects, whereas the high-potency agents are associated with a higher incidence of early extrapyramidal reactions (see Table 23–1).

EXTRAPYRAMIDAL REACTIONS

Extrapyramidal reactions are movement disorders resulting from effects of antipsychotic drugs on the extrapyramidal motor system. The extrapyramidal system is the same neuronal network whose malfunction is responsible for the movement disorders of Parkinson's disease.

Four types of extrapyramidal reactions occur. These differ from one another with respect to time of onset and management. Three of these reactions—**acute dystonia, parkinsonism,** and **akathisia**—occur early in therapy and can be managed with a variety of drugs. The fourth reaction—tardive dyskinesia—occurs *late* in therapy and has no satisfactory treatment. Characteristics and management of the four extrapyramidal reactions are summarized in Table 23–3.

The *early* reactions occur less frequently with low-potency agents (e.g., chlorpromazine) than with high-potency agents (e.g., haloperidol). In contrast, the risk of tardive dyskinesia is equal with *all* antipsychotics.

Acute Dystonia. Acute dystonia develops within the first few days of therapy—frequently only hours after the first dose. The reaction can be both disturbing and dangerous. Typically, the patient develops severe spasm of the muscles of the tongue, face, neck, or back. Oculogyric crisis (involuntary upward deviation of the eyes) and opisthotonus (tetanic spasm of the back muscles causing the trunk to arch forward, while the head and lower limbs are thrust backward) may also occur. Severe cramping can cause joint dislocation. Laryngeal dystonia can impair respiration. The cause of acute dystonia is unknown.

Intense dystonia constitutes a crisis that requires rapid intervention. Initial treatment consists of anticholinergic medication (e.g., benztropine, diphenhydramine) administered IM or IV. As a rule, symptoms resolve within five minutes of IV administration and within 15 to 20 minutes of IM administration.

It is important to differentiate between acute dystonia and psychotic hysteria. Misdiagnosis of acute dystonia as hysteria could result in escalation of antipsychotic dosage, thus causing the acute dystonia to become even worse.

TABLE 23–3 **Extrapyramidal Reactions to Antipsychotic Drugs**

Type of Reaction	Time of Onset	Features	Management
Early Reactions			
Acute dystonia	1 to 5 days	Spasm of muscles of tongue, face, neck, and back; opisthotonus	Anticholinergic drugs (e.g., benztropine) IM or IV
Parkinsonism	5 to 30 days	Bradykinesia, masklike facies, tremor, rigidity, shuffling gait, drooling, cogwheeling, stooped posture	Anticholinergics (e.g., benztropine, diphenhydramine), amantadine, or both
Akathisia	5 to 60 days	Compulsive, restless movement; symptoms of anxiety, agitation	Reduce dosage or switch to a low-potency antipsychotic. Anticholinergic drugs, beta blockers, and benzodiazepines may help
Late Reaction			
Tardive dyskinesia	Months to years	Oral-facial dyskinesias, choreoathetoid movements	Best approach is prevention; no reliable treatment. High-dose diazepam may help.

Parkinsonism. Antipsychotic-induced parkinsonism is characterized by bradykinesia, masklike facies, drooling, tremor, rigidity, shuffling gait, cogwheeling, and stooped posture. Symptoms develop within the first month of therapy and are indistinguishable from those of idiopathic Parkinson's disease.

Neuroleptics cause parkinsonism by blocking dopamine receptors in the striatum. Since idiopathic Parkinson's disease is also due to reduced activation of striatal dopamine receptors, it is no wonder that Parkinson's disease and neuroleptic-induced parkinsonism share the same symptoms.

Neuroleptic-induced parkinsonism is treated with some (but not all) of the drugs used to treat Parkinson's disease. Specifically, centrally acting anticholinergic drugs (e.g., benztropine [Cogentin], diphenhydramine [Benadryl], and amantadine [Symmetrel]) may be employed. Levodopa, however, should be avoided, because this drug promotes activation of dopamine receptors and might therefore counteract the beneficial effects of antipsychotic treatment.

Use of antiparkinsonian drugs should not continue indefinitely. Antipsychotic-induced parkinsonism tends to resolve spontaneously, usually within a few months after its onset. Hence, antiparkinsonian drugs should be withdrawn after a few months to determine if they are still required.

Akathisia. Akathisia is characterized by pacing and squirming brought on by an uncontrollable need to be in motion. This profound sense of restlessness can be very disturbing. The syndrome usually develops within the first two months of treatment. The cause is unknown. Like other early extrapyramidal reactions, akathisia occurs most frequently with high-potency antipsychotics.

Three types of drugs have been used to suppress symptoms: (1) anticholinergic agents, (2) beta-adrenergic blockers, and (3) **benzodiazepines.** Although drugs can be helpful, a reduction in antipsychotic dosage or switching to a low-potency agent may be more effective.

It is important to differentiate akathisia from worsening of psychosis. If akathisia were to be confused with anxiety or psychotic agitation, it is likely that antipsychotic dosage would be increased, thus making akathisia more intense.

Tardive Dyskinesia. Tardive dyskinesia develops in 20% to 40% of patients during long-term therapy and is the most troubling of the extrapyramidal reactions. The risk increases with duration of treatment and dosage. For many patients, symptoms are irreversible.

Tardive dyskinesia is characterized by involuntary choreoathetoid (twisting, writhing, wormlike) movements of the tongue and face. Patients may also present with lip-smacking movements, and their tongues may flick out in a "fly-catching" motion. One of the earliest manifestations is the appearance of slow, wormlike movements of the tongue. Involuntary movements that involve the tongue and mouth can interfere with chewing, swallowing, and speaking. Eating difficulties can result in malnutrition and weight loss. Over time, tardive dyskinesia produces involuntary movements of the limbs, toes, fingers, and trunk. For some patients, symptoms decline following a dosage reduction or drug withdrawal; for others, tardive dyskinesia is irreversible.

The cause of tardive dyskinesia is complex and incompletely understood. One theory suggests that symptoms result from excessive activation of dopamine receptors. It is postulated that, in response to chronic receptor blockade, dopamine receptors of the extrapyramidal system undergo a functional change such that their sensitivity to activation is increased. Stimulation of these "supersensitive" receptors produces an imbalance in favor of dopamine and thus produces abnormal movement. In support of this theory is the observation that symptoms of tardive dyskinesia can be reduced (temporarily) by *increasing* antipsychotic drug dosage, which will cause greater receptor blockade. (Since symptoms eventually return even though antipsychotic dosage is kept at an elevated level, dosage elevation cannot be used to manage tardive dyskinesia.)

Tardive dyskinesia has no reliable means of treatment; hence, prevention is the best approach. Antipsychotic drugs should be used in the lowest effective dosage for the shortest time required. After 12 months, the need for continued therapy should be assessed. If drug use must continue, a neurological evaluation should be done at least every three months to detect early signs of tardive dyskinesia. For patients with chronic schizophrenia, dosage should be tapered periodically (at least annually) to determine the need for continued treatment.

If signs of tardive dyskinesia appear but the patient requires continued antipsychotic therapy, what should be done? Unfortunately, this question has no easy answer. If drug use continues, tardive dyskinesia may become progressively worse; thus discontinuation would seem desirable. If treatment ceases, however, relapse of psychosis may occur; hence, discontinuation may well be harmful. In the face of this dilemma, the clinician should discuss the options with the patient and a family member so that the patient can make an informed decision regarding continued treatment. It has been noted that symptoms of tardive dyskinesia have abated in some patients following substitution of an atypical antipsychotic agent (e.g., clozapine) for a traditional antipsychotic agent. Accordingly, a trial with an atypical agent may be a reasonable choice for the patient who cannot simply discontinue antipsychotic treatment.

OTHER ADVERSE EFFECTS

Neuroleptic Malignant Syndrome. Neuroleptic malignant syndrome (NMS) is a rare but serious reaction that carries a 4% risk of mortality (decreased from 20% just a decade ago because of early recognition and treatment). Primary symptoms are "lead-pipe" rigidity, fever (temperature may exceed 41°C), sweating, and autonomic instability, manifested as dysrhythmias and fluctuations in blood pressure. Level of consciousness may rise and fall; the patient may appear confused or mute; and seizures or coma may develop. Death can result from respiratory failure, cardiovascular collapse, dysrhythmias, and other causes. NMS is more likely with high-potency agents than with low-potency agents.

Treatment consists of supportive measures, drug therapy, and immediate withdrawal of antipsychotic medication. Hyperthermia should be controlled with antipyretics and cooling blankets. Hydration should be maintained with fluids. Two drugs—*dantrolene* and *bromocriptine*—are helpful. Dantrolene, which is a direct-acting muscle relaxant, reduces rigidity and hyperthermia. Bromocriptine, which is a dopamine receptor agonist, helps to relieve CNS toxicity.

Resumption of antipsychotic therapy following an episode of NMS carries a significant risk that NMS will recur. Since NMS has a high rate of morbidity and mortality, the decision to resume treatment must be made with great care. If continued treatment with an antipsychotic is clearly required, the lowest effective dosage should be employed, and high-potency agents should be avoided.

Anticholinergic Effects. Antipsychotic drugs produce varying degrees of muscarinic cholinergic blockade (see Table 23–1). By blocking muscarinic receptors, these drugs can elicit a full spectrum of anticholinergic responses (e.g., dry mouth, blurred vision, photophobia, urinary hesitancy, constipation, tachycardia). Patients should be informed about these responses and taught how to minimize danger and discomfort. As indicated in Table 23–1, anticholinergic effects are more likely with low-potency agents than with high-potency agents.

Orthostatic Hypotension. Antipsychotic drugs promote orthostatic hypotension by blocking alpha$_1$-adrenergic receptors on blood vessels. Alpha-adrenergic blockade prevents compensatory vasoconstriction when the patient stands; thus, blood pressure falls. Patients should be informed about signs of hypotension (e.g., lightheadedness, dizziness) and advised to sit or lie down if these signs occur. In addition, patients should be informed that hypotension can be minimized by moving slowly when assuming an erect posture. With hospitalized patients, blood pressure and pulses should be checked before drug administration and one hour after. Measurements should be made while the patient is lying down and again after he or she has been sitting or standing for one to two minutes. If blood pressure is low and pulse rate is high, the drug should be withheld and the physician consulted. Hypotension is more likely with low-potency antipsychotics than with the high-potency drugs (see Table 23–1). Tolerance to hypotension develops in two to three months.

Sedation. Sedation is common during the early days of treatment but subsides within a week or so. Neuroleptic-induced sedation is thought to result from blockade of histamine receptors in the CNS. Daytime sedation can be minimized by administering the entire daily dose at bedtime. Patients should be warned against participation in hazardous activities (e.g., driving) until sedative effects diminish.

Seizures. Antipsychotic drugs can reduce seizure threshold, thus increasing the risk of seizure activity. The risk of seizures is greatest in patients with epilepsy and other seizure disorders. These patients should be monitored, and, if loss of seizure control occurs, the dosage of their antiseizure medication must be increased.

Sexual Dysfunction. Antipsychotics can cause sexual dysfunction in women and men. In women, these drugs can suppress libido and impair the ability to achieve orgasm. In men, neuroleptics can suppress libido and cause erectile and ejaculatory dysfunction; the incidence of these effects is 25% to 60%. Drug-induced sexual dysfunction can make treatment unacceptable to sexually active patients, thus leading to poor compliance. A reduction in dosage or switching to a high-potency antipsychotic may reduce effects on sexual function. Patients should be counseled about possible sexual dysfunction and encouraged to report problems.

Dermatologic Effects. Drugs in the phenothiazine class can sensitize the skin to ultraviolet light, thus increasing the risk of severe sunburn. Patients should be warned against excessive exposure to sunlight and advised to apply a sunscreen or wear protective clothing. Phenothiazines can also produce pigmentary deposits in the skin, cornea, and lens of the eye.

Handling antipsychotics can cause contact dermatitis in patients and health care personnel. Dermatitis can be prevented by avoiding direct contact with these drugs.

Neuroendocrine Effects. Antipsychotics increase levels of circulating prolactin by blocking the inhibitory action of dopamine on prolactin release. Elevation of prolactin levels promotes *gynecomastia* (breast growth) and *galactorrhea* in up to 57% of women. Up to 97% experience menstrual irregularities. Gynecomastia and galactorrhea can also occur in males. Since prolactin can promote growth of prolactin-dependent carcinoma of the breast, neuroleptics should be avoided in patients with this form of cancer. (It should be noted that although antipsychotic drugs can promote the growth of cancers that already exist, there is no evidence that antipsychotic drugs actually cause cancer.)

Agranulocytosis. Agranulocytosis is a rare but serious reaction. Among the traditional antipsychotics, the risk is highest with chlorpromazine and certain other phenothiazines. Since agranulocytosis severely compromises the ability to fight infection, white blood cell counts should be made whenever signs of infection (e.g., fever, sore throat) appear. If agranulocytosis is diagnosed, the neuroleptic should be withdrawn. Agranulocytosis reverses upon discontinuation of treatment.

Physical and Psychological Dependence

Development of physical and psychological dependence is rare. Patients should be reassured that addiction and dependence are not likely to occur.

Although physical dependence is minimal, abrupt withdrawal of antipsychotics can precipitate a mild abstinence syndrome. Symptoms result from chronic cholinergic blockade and include restlessness, insomnia, headache, gastric distress, and sweating. This syndrome can be avoided by withdrawing antipsychotic medication gradually.

Drug Interactions

ANTICHOLINERGIC DRUGS

Drugs with anticholinergic properties will intensify anticholinergic responses to *neuroleptics*. Patients should be advised to avoid all drugs with anticholinergic actions, including antihistamines and certain over-the-counter sleeping aids.

CNS DEPRESSANTS

Neuroleptics can intensify CNS depression caused by other drugs. Patients should be warned against using alcohol and all other drugs with CNS-depressant actions (e.g., antihistamines, opioids, barbiturates).

LEVODOPA

Levodopa (a drug used to treat Parkinson's disease) may counteract the antipsychotic effects of neuroleptics. Conversely, neuroleptics may counteract the therapeutic effects of levodopa. These interactions occur because levodopa and neuroleptics have opposing effects on receptors for dopamine: Levodopa activates these receptors, whereas neuroleptics cause blockade.

Toxicity

The traditional antipsychotic drugs are very safe; death by overdose is extremely rare. With chlorpromazine, for example, the therapeutic index is about 200; that is, the lethal dose of this drug is 200 times greater than the therapeutic dose.

Overdosage produces hypotension, CNS depression, and extrapyramidal reactions. Extrapyramidal reactions can be treated with antiparkinsonian drugs. Hypotension can be treated with IV fluids plus an alpha-adrenergic agonist (e.g., phenylephrine). There is no specific antidote to CNS depression. Excess drug should be removed from the stomach by gastric lavage. (Emetics cannot be used because their effects would be blocked by the antiemetic action of the neuroleptic.)

Depot Preparations

The depot antipsychotics are long-acting, injectable preparations used to treat patients with chronic schizophrenia. The objective is to prevent relapse and maintain the highest possible level of functioning. The rate of relapse is lower with depot therapy than with oral therapy. Depot preparations are valuable for all patients who need long-term treatment—not just for those who have difficulty with compliance. There is no evidence that depot preparations pose an increased risk of side effects, including neuroleptic malignant syndrome.

Three depot preparations are available: haloperidol decanoate (Haldol Decanoate), fluphenazine decanoate (Prolixin Decanoate), and fluphenazine enanthate (Prolixin Enanthate). Following IM or SC injection, active drug (fluphenazine or haloperidol) is slowly absorbed into the blood. Because of this slow, steady absorption, plasma drug levels remain relatively constant between injections. The dosing interval is two to four weeks. Typical maintenance dosages are presented in Table 23–4.

Atypical Antipsychotic Agents

Atypical antipsychotic agents differ from traditional agents in that they cause few or no extrapyramidal symptoms, including tardive dyskinesia. In fact, tardive dyskinesia may actually remit when patients are switched from a traditional antipsychotic drug to an atypical one. Several others are being tested in clinical trials.

TABLE 23–4 **Depot Antipsychotic Preparations**

Generic Name (Trade Name)	Route	Typical Maintenance Dosage
Haloperidol decanoate (Haldol decanoate)	IM	50 to 200 mg every 4 weeks
Fluphenazine decanoate (Prolixin decanoate)	IM, SC	2.5 to 25 mg every 2 weeks
Fluphenazine enanthate (Prolixin enanthate)	IM, SC	2.5 to 25 mg every 2 weeks

Clozapine

Clozapine (Clozaril) is a relatively new antipsychotic drug that is indicated for patients with schizophrenia who have not responded to traditional agents or who cannot tolerate their extrapyramidal effects. The drug's major adverse effect is agranulocytosis, and a few deaths have occurred despite weekly hematologic monitoring.

MECHANISM OF ACTION

Like traditional antipsychotic agents, clozapine blocks receptors for dopamine. However, the pattern of blockade is unique: compared with traditional agents, clozapine produces relatively strong blockade of $dopamine_1$ receptors and relatively weak blockade of $dopamine_2$ receptors. This pattern of receptor blockade may explain the drug's relative lack of extrapyramidal effects and may also underlie its therapeutic effects. In addition to blocking receptors for dopamine, clozapine blocks receptors for serotonin, norepinephrine, histamine, and acetylcholine.

THERAPEUTIC USES

Because of the risk of fatal **agranulocytosis,** clozapine is generally reserved for patients with severe schizophrenia who have not responded to traditional antipsychotic drugs. In this treatment-resistant group, clozapine has had a 40% to 60% success rate. Not only have patients responded, but the quality of the response is often superior to that seen with traditional drugs. Patients are more animated, behavior is more socially acceptable, and rates of rehospitalization are lower. Because the incidence of extrapyramidal effects with clozapine is low, the drug is well suited for patients who have experienced severe extrapyramidal symptoms with a traditional antipsychotic drug.

ADVERSE EFFECTS

In contrast to traditional antipsychotics, clozapine carries a low risk of extrapyramidal effects. Tardive dyskinesia has not been reported. In fact, tardive dyskinesia may improve when patients switch to clozapine from a traditional agent. Neuroendocrine effects (e.g., galactorrhea, gynecomastia, amenorrhea) and interference with sexual function are minimal.

Agranulocytosis

Clozapine produces agranulocytosis in 1% to 2% of patients. The overall risk of death is about 1 in 5000, the usual cause being gram-negative septicemia. Agranulocytosis typically occurs during the first six months of treatment, and the onset is usually gradual. It is not known why agranulocytosis occurs.

Because of the risk of fatal agranulocytosis, *weekly* hematologic monitoring is mandatory. If the total white blood cell (WBC) count falls below $3000/mm^3$ or if the granulocyte count falls below $1500/mm^3$, treatment should be interrupted. When subsequent *daily* monitoring indicates that counts have risen above these values, clozapine can be resumed. If the total WBC count falls below $2000/mm^3$ or if the granulocyte count falls below $1000/mm^3$, clozapine should be permanently discontinued. Blood counts should be monitored for four weeks after drug withdrawal.

Patients should be informed about the risk of agranulocytosis and told that clozapine will not be dispensed if the weekly blood test has not been made. Also, patients should be informed about early signs of infection (e.g., fever, sore throat, fatigue, mucous membrane ulceration) and instructed to report these signs immediately.

Seizures

Generalized tonic-clonic convulsions occur in 3% of patients. The risk of seizures is dose related. Patients who have experienced a seizure should be warned not to drive or to participate in other potentially hazardous activities.

Other Adverse Effects

The most common side effects are drowsiness and sedation (40%), dizziness (20%), hypersalivation (30%), tachycardia (25%), and constipation (14%). Additional effects include postural hypotension (9%) and elevation of body temperature (5%).

DRUG INTERACTIONS

Because of its ability to cause agranulocytosis, clozapine is contraindicated for patients taking other drugs that can suppress bone marrow function (e.g., many anticancer drugs).

DOSAGE AND ADMINISTRATION

To minimize side effects, treatment should begin with a 12.5-mg dose, followed by 25 mg once or twice daily. Dosage is then increased by 25 mg/day until it reaches 300 to 450 mg/day. Further increases can be made once or twice weekly, in increments no larger than 100 mg. The usual maintenance dosage is 300 to 600 mg/day in three divided doses.

Risperidone

Risperidone (Risperdal) produces strong blockade at $serotonin_2$ receptors and weaker blockade at $dopamine_2$ receptors. Antipsychotic effects are equivalent to those of haloperidol and may have a more rapid onset. Both positive and negative symptoms are improved. Interestingly, lower doses of risperidone (less than 10 mg/day) are more effective than high doses. Like clozapine, risperidone causes fewer extrapyramidal symptoms than do the traditional agents. In comparison with clozapine, risperidone does not cause agranulocytosis.

Using Antipsychotic Drugs to Treat Schizophrenia

Characteristics of Schizophrenia

Before discussing drug therapy of schizophrenia, we need to review the characteristics of schizophrenia itself. For a more complete discussion of the illness, refer to Chapter 29.

Schizophrenia is a chronic psychotic illness characterized by thought disorders and a reduced ability to comprehend reality. Symptoms usually emerge during adolescence or early adulthood.

ACUTE EPISODES

During an acute psychotic episode, delusions and hallucinations are frequently prominent. Delusions are typically religious, grandiose, or persecutory. Auditory hallucinations, which are more common than visual hallucinations, may consist of voices arguing or commenting on one's behavior. The patient may feel that he or she is under the control of external influences. Disordered thinking and loose association may render rational conversation impossible. Affect may be blunted or labile. Misperception of reality may result in hostility and uncooperativeness. Impaired self-care skills may leave the patient disheveled and dirty. Patterns of sleeping and eating are usually disrupted.

RESIDUAL SYMPTOMS

After florid symptoms (e.g., hallucinations, delusions) of an acute episode remit, less vivid symptoms may remain. These include suspiciousness; poor anxiety management; and diminished judgment, insight, motivation, and capacity for self-care. As a result, patients frequently find it difficult to establish close relationships, maintain employment, and function independently in society. Suspiciousness and poor management of anxiety contribute to social withdrawal. An inability to appreciate the need for continued drug therapy may cause noncompliance, resulting in relapse and possibly hospital readmission.

LONG-TERM COURSE

The long-term course of schizophrenia is characterized by episodic acute exacerbations separated by intervals of partial remission. As the years pass, some patients experience progressive decline in mental status and social functioning, whereas others may stabilize. Maintenance therapy with antipsychotic drugs reduces the risk of acute relapse but may not prevent long-term deterioration.

POSITIVE VERSUS NEGATIVE SYMPTOMS

The symptoms of schizophrenia can be divided into two major groups: positive symptoms and negative symptoms. Positive symptoms can be viewed as an exaggeration or distortion of normal function, whereas negative symptoms can be viewed as a loss or diminution of normal function. Positive symptoms include hallucinations, delusions, agitation, tension, and paranoia. Negative symptoms include lack of motivation, poverty of speech, blunted affect, poor self-care, and social withdrawal. In general, antipsychotic drugs have a greater impact on positive symptoms than on negative symptoms.

Drug Therapy for Symptoms of Schizophrenia

Drug therapy of schizophrenia has three major objectives: (1) suppression of acute episodes, (2) prevention of acute exacerbations, and (3) maintenance of the highest possible level of functioning. A discussion on measures to achieve these objectives follows.

PREADMINISTRATION ASSESSMENT

Prior to treatment, patients should undergo a thorough mental status examination and a physical examination. They should be observed for overt behavior (e.g., gait, pacing, restlessness, volatile outbursts), emotional state (e.g., depression, agitation, mania), intellectual function (e.g., stream of thought, coherence, hallucinations, delusions), and responsiveness to the environment.

Patients who must avoid certain antipsychotics or use them with caution must be identified. Traditional antipsychotic agents are *contraindicated* for patients who are comatose or severely depressed and for patients with Parkinson's disease, prolactin-dependent carcinoma of the breast, bone marrow depression, and severe hypotension or hypertension. These drugs should be used cautiously in patients with glaucoma, adynamic ileus, prostatic hypertrophy, cardiovascular disease, hepatic or renal dysfunction, or seizure disorders. *Clozapine* is *contraindicated* for patients with a history of clozapine-induced agranulocytosis and for those with bone marrow suppression and those taking myelosuppressive drugs (e.g., many anticancer drugs).

DRUG SELECTION

Treatment is usually initiated with one of the traditional antipsychotic agents. Although all of the traditional agents produce equivalent therapeutic effects, some patients may respond better to one agent than to another. Accordingly, if treatment with one traditional agent is unsuccessful, a trial with a drug from a different chemical class should be made.

Selection among the traditional antipsychotic drugs is based largely on side effects: The patient should not be given a drug that, because of its side-effect profile, is especially likely to cause discomfort, inconvenience, or harm. For example, certain patients (e.g., those with prostatism or glaucoma) are especially sensitive to anticholinergic drugs. Accordingly, these patients should not be treated with low-potency neuroleptics. By similar logic, if the patient has a history of extrapyramidal reactions, high-potency agents should be avoided. By properly matching patients and drugs, side effects can be minimized, comfort can be maximized, and compliance can be promoted. Table 23–5 indicates the neuroleptics that should be avoided in the presence of certain predisposing factors.

In the United States, *clozapine* and *risperidone* are currently the only alternatives to the traditional antipsychotic agents. Because these drugs are associated with a low incidence of extrapyramidal reactions, they are especially well suited for patients who have experienced severe extrapyramidal reactions to traditional agents. Also, because of their superior ability to relieve negative symptoms, both drugs may be beneficial for patients whose negative symptoms have not responded to traditional agents. Because clozapine can produce fatal agranulocytosis, it is not considered a drug of first choice; rather, clozapine should be reserved for patients who have not responded to trials with at least two of the traditional agents.

TABLE 23–5 **Antipsychotics That Should Be Avoided in the Presence of Certain Predisposing Factors**

Predisposing Factor	Antipsychotic Agents to Avoid
Glaucoma, prostatism, adynamic ileus, urinary hesitance	Low potency agents (anticholinergic actions can exacerbate these disorders)
Use of anticholinergic drugs (e.g., tricyclic antidepressants)	Low-potency agents (anticholinergic effects will intensify muscarinic blockade)
Old age	Low-potency agents (the elderly are especially sensitive to the anticholinergic and sedative effects of these drugs)
Active life-style	Low-potency agents (sedative effects can interfere with function)
Delirium	Low-potency agents (anticholinergic action can exacerbate delirium)
Cardiovascular disorders	Low-potency agents (anticholinergic and hypotensive actions can exacerbate these disorders)
History of extrapyramidal reactions	High-potency agents (disruption of extrapyramidal function is greatest with these drugs)
Active sex life in males	Thioridazine (this agent inhibits ejaculation)

DOSING

Dosing with neuroleptics is highly individualized. Unresponsive patients may need doses that are 10 to 20 times greater than those used for highly responsive patients. Elderly patients require relatively small doses—typically 30% to 50% of those taken by younger patients.

Dosage size and timing are likely to change over the course of therapy. During the early phase of treatment, antipsychotics should be administered in divided daily doses. Once an effective dosage has been determined, the entire daily dose may be given at bedtime. Since antipsychotics cause sedation, this practice can promote sleep and decrease drowsiness during the day. During long-term therapy, the dosage should be gradually reduced to the lowest effective amount.

Routes of Administration

Antipsychotic drugs are administered orally, IM, SC, IV, and by rectal suppository. Routes for individual agents are summarized in Tables 23–2 and 23–4.

Oral

Oral administration is preferred for most patients. Antipsychotics are available in tablets, capsules, and liquids for oral use.

The liquid formulations require special handling. These preparations are concentrated and must be diluted prior to use. Dilution may be performed with a variety of fluids, including fruit juices, milk, and carbonated beverages. The oral liquids are sensitive to light and must be stored in amber or opaque containers. Liquid formulations of *phenothiazines* can cause contact dermatitis; nurses and patients should take care to avoid skin contact with these preparations. If a spill occurs, the affected area should be flushed.

Intramuscular

Intramuscular injection is generally reserved for patients with severe, acute schizophrenia and for long-term maintenance therapy. Injections should be made into the deltoid or gluteal muscle, and the site should be rotated. Depot preparations are given every two to four weeks (see Table 23–4).

INITIAL THERAPY

With adequate dosing, symptoms begin to resolve within one to two days. However, the full therapeutic response develops gradually over six to eight weeks.

Some symptoms resolve sooner than others. During the first week, the goal is to reduce agitation, hostility, anxiety, and tension, and to normalize sleeping and eating patterns. During the next six to eight weeks, symptoms should continue to steadily improve. The goals over this interval are increased socialization, improved self-care and mood, and improved formal thought processes. Of the patients who have not responded within six weeks, 50% are likely to respond by the end of 12 weeks.

It is important to note that not all symptoms respond equally. As discussed earlier, positive symptoms generally respond better than do negative symptoms.

MAINTENANCE THERAPY

Schizophrenia is usually chronic and requires prolonged treatment. The purpose of long-term therapy is to reduce the recurrence of acute florid episodes and to maintain the highest possible level of functioning. Unfortunately, although long-term treatment can be very effective, it also carries a risk of adverse effects, especially tardive dyskinesia.

Following control of an acute episode, antipsychotic therapy should continue for at least 12 months. Withdrawal of medication prior to this time is associated with a 55% incidence of relapse, compared with only 20% in patients who continue drug use. Accordingly, patients must be convinced to continue therapy for the entire 12-month course, even though they may be symptom free and consider themselves "cured."

After 12 months, an attempt should be made to discontinue drug use, provided that symptoms are absent. About 25% of patients will not need drugs beyond this time. To avoid adverse reactions to drug withdrawal, dosage should be reduced gradually. It is important that medication not be withdrawn at a time of stress (e.g., when the patient is being discharged following hospitalization). If a relapse occurs in response to withdrawal, treatment should be reinstituted. For many patients, resumption of treatment controls symptoms and prevents further relapse.

When long-term therapy is conducted, dosage should be adjusted with care. To reduce the risk of tardive dyskinesia and other adverse effects, a minimum effective dosage should be established. Annual attempts should be made to lower the dosage or to discontinue treatment entirely.

Long-acting (depot) antipsychotics are especially well suited for long-term therapy. Depot therapy has three major advantages over oral therapy: (1) the relapse rate is lower with depot therapy, (2) depot therapy maintains steady drug levels between doses, and (3) the total dose per unit time is lower, thus reducing the risk of side effects. There is no evidence that depot preparations carry a higher risk of tardive dyskinesia or NMS. In the United States, only 10% of patients receive depot therapy. This low rate of use is based in large part on the widely held (but incorrect) perception that depot therapy is for "losers"—patients who suffer recurrent relapse because of persistent noncompliance with oral therapy.

PROMOTING COMPLIANCE

Poor compliance is a common cause of therapeutic failure, and is responsible for a substantial number of hospital re-admissions. Compliance can be difficult to achieve because treatment is prolonged and because patients may fail to appreciate the need for therapy, or they may be unwilling or unable to take medicine as prescribed. In addition, side effects can discourage compliance.

Compliance can be enhanced by:

- Ensuring that medication given to hospitalized patients is actually swallowed and not "cheeked."
- Encouraging family members to oversee medication by outpatients.
- Providing patients with written and verbal instructions on dosage size and timing, and encouraging them to take their medicine exactly as prescribed.
- Informing patients and their families that antipsychotics must be taken regularly to be effective and thus cannot be used on a PRN basis.
- Informing patients about side effects of treatment and teaching them how to minimize undesired responses.
- Assuring patients that antipsychotic drugs do not cause addiction.
- Establishing a good therapeutic relationship with the patient and his or her family.
- Using a depot preparation (e.g., fluphenazine decanoate, haloperidol decanoate) for long-term therapy.

▶ Check Your Reading

5. What is the major indication for antipsychotic drugs?
6. How are antipsychotic drugs thought to act?
7. What are the early extrapyramidal reactions, and how are they treated?
8. What is tardive dyskinesia, and how is it treated?
9. What is the neuroleptic malignant syndrome?
10. What is the significance of clozapine-induced agranulocytosis?

ANTIDEPRESSANTS

As their name suggests, **antidepressants** are drugs used to treat depression. These agents fall into four groups: (1) tricyclic antidepressants, (2) monoamine oxidase inhibitors (MAOIs), (3) selective serotonin reuptake inhibitors (SSRIs), and (4) miscellaneous antidepressants. The principal indication for these drugs is major depression. As a rule, antidepressants are not indicated for uncomplicated bereavement. It should be noted that antidepressants are not merely general psychic stimulants; rather, these drugs act selectively to alleviate symptoms of depression.

Major Depression: Characteristics, Pathogenesis, and Overview of Treatment

Characteristics

Before discussing the antidepressant drugs, it will be helpful to briefly review characteristics of depression itself. For a more complete discussion of depression, refer to Chapter 30.

The principal symptoms of depression are (1) depressed mood and (2) loss of pleasure or interest in all or nearly all of one's usual activities and pastimes. Associated symptoms include insomnia (or sometimes hypersomnia); anorexia and weight loss (or sometimes hyperphagia and weight gain); mental slowing and loss of concentration; feelings of guilt, worthlessness, and helplessness; thoughts of death and suicide; and overt suicidal behavior. For a diagnosis to be made, symptoms must be present most of the day, nearly every day, for at least two weeks.

Major depression is a frustrating illness because symptoms may not correspond with external events. That is, rather than occurring in response to life's tragedies, symptoms of major depression may descend "out of the blue"; otherwise healthy individuals—unexpectedly and without apparent cause—find themselves feeling profoundly depressed.

It is important to distinguish between major depression and normal grief or sadness. Whereas major depression is an illness, grief or sadness is not. Rather, grief and sadness are appropriate reactions to a major life stressor (e.g., death of a loved one, loss of a job). In most cases, grief and sadness resolve spontaneously over several weeks and do not require medical intervention. If, however, symptoms are unusually intense, and if they fail to abate within an appropriate time, a major depressive episode may have been superimposed. In these cases, treatment is indicated.

Pathogenesis

The etiology of major depression is undoubtedly complex and not yet known. Since depressive episodes can be triggered by stressful life events in some people but not in others, it would appear that, for some people, a predisposition to depression exists. Social, developmental, and biological factors, including genetic heritage, may all contribute to that predisposition.

Clinical observations made in the 1960s led to formulation of the **monoamine hypothesis of depression,** which asserts that depression is caused by a functional insufficiency of monoamine neurotransmitters (norepinephrine, serotonin, or both) in the brain. This hypothesis is based mainly on two observations: (1) depression can be induced with reserpine, a drug that depletes monoamines from the brain, and (2) the drugs used to treat depression intensify monoamine-mediated neurotransmission. Although these observations do indeed support the monoamine hypothesis, it is likely that this somewhat simplistic theory will need refinement as our understanding of the brain deepens. However, despite its shortcomings, the monoamine hypothesis does provide a useful conceptual framework for understanding the antidepressant drugs.

Treatment

Depression can be treated with three modalities: (1) drugs, (2) electroconvulsive therapy (ECT), and (3) psychotherapy. Each modality has a legitimate role.

Drugs are the primary therapy for major depression. Currently available antidepressants are listed in Table 23–6. For many patients, the **tricyclic antidepressants** are drugs of first choice. These agents are effective and relatively safe and can be administered easily. The SSRIs are as effective as the tricyclics and are better tolerated. As a result, fluoxetine (Prozac), the prototype of the family, has achieved widespread popularity. MAOIs are generally reserved for patients who have not responded to tricyclics or to one of the SSRIs. However, for patients with atypical depression, MAOIs are the drugs of choice. *Antianxiety agents* (e.g., diazepam) can be employed in depression, but their use is not routine. As a rule, CNS stimulants (e.g., amphetamines, methylphenidate) are without benefit in depression. As discussed later, patients with *bipolar depression* can be treated prophylactically with lithium.

ECT is a valuable tool for treating depression. This procedure is effective, and beneficial responses develop more rapidly than with drugs. Accordingly, ECT is indicated when speed is critical (i.e., in severely depressed, suicidal patients) or when a patient has failed to respond to antidepressants.

The role of psychotherapy in major depression is largely supportive; symptoms do not respond nearly as well to psychotherapy as they do to medication. However, although of less direct benefit than drugs, psychotherapy can help to relieve suffering by providing insight, reassurance, and caring.

Tricyclic Antidepressants

The tricyclic antidepressants are drugs of first choice for many patients with major depression. The first tricyclic agent—imipramine—was introduced to psychiatry in the late 1950s. Since then, the ability of the tricyclics to relieve depressive symptoms has been firmly established. The most common adverse effects of the tricyclics are sedation, orthostatic hypotension, and anticholinergic effects. The most hazardous adverse effect is cardiac toxicity.

TABLE 23–6 **Antidepressants: Adverse Effects and Effects on Neurotransmitters**

	Transmitter Reuptake Antagonism							
	NE	***5-HT***	**Anti-cholinergic Activity**	**Sedation**	**Hypo-tension**	**Seizure Risk**	**Cardiac Toxicity**	**Other Side Effects**
Tricyclic Antidepressants								
Amitriptyline	++	++++	++++	++++	+++	+++	++++	
Desipramine	++++	+	++	++	++	++	+++	
Doxepin	++	++	+++	++++	++	+++	++	
Imipramine	+++	+++	+++	+++	+++	+++	++++	
Nortriptyline	+++	++	++	+++	+	++	+++	
Protriptyline	++++	++	+++	+	++	++	++++	
Trimipramine	+	+	+++	++++	+++	+++	++++	
Monoamine Oxidase Inhibitors								
Isocarboxazid	[a]	[a]	0	+	++	0	0	Hypertensive
Phenelzine	[a]	[a]	0	+	++	0	0	crisis from
Tranylcypromine	[a]	[a]	0	[b]	++	0	0	tyramine in food
Selective Serotonin Reuptake Blockers								
Fluoxetine	0	++++	0	[b]	0	+	0	Skin rash
Fluvoxamine	0	++++						
Paroxetine	0	++++	0	0	0		0	
Sertraline	0	++++	0	[b]	0	+	0	
Miscellaneous Antidepressants								
Amoxapine	+++[c]	++[c]	+++	++	+	+++	+	Parkinsonism
Bupropion	[d]	[d]	++	[b]	+	+++++	+	Seizures
Maprotiline	+++	+	+++	+++	++	++++	+++	Seizures
Trazodone	0	++	0	+++	+++	++	+	Priapism

NE = norepinephrine; 5-HT = serotonin; DA = dopamine.
[a]MAOIs do not block transmitter reuptake. Rather, they increase intraneuronal stores at NE, 5-HT, and DA.
[b]Produces moderate *stimulation*, not sedation.
[c]In addition to blocking NE and 5-HT *reuptake*, amoxapine blocks *receptors* for DA.
[d]Bupropion primarily inhibits reuptake of DA rather than NE or 5-HT.

MECHANISM OF ACTION

The tricyclic drugs are blockers of monoamine (norepinephrine and serotonin) reuptake. By blocking reuptake, the tricyclics can increase the amount of these transmitters available for receptor binding, thereby intensifying their effects. Such a mechanism would be consistent with the monoamine hypothesis of depression. The monoamine hypothesis, which asserts that depression stems from a *deficiency* in monoamine-mediated neurotransmission, predicts that drugs capable of *increasing* the effects of monoamines reduce symptoms of depression. This prediction is fulfilled by the tricyclic drugs. The relative abilities of individual tricyclics to block reuptake of norepinephrine and serotonin are summarized in Table 23–6.

We should note that blockade of reuptake, by itself, cannot fully account for the therapeutic effects of the tricyclics. This statement is based on the observation that clinical responses to the tricyclics (relief of depressive symptoms) and the biochemical effects of the tricyclics (blockade of transmitter uptake) do not occur in the same time frame. That is, whereas the tricyclic drugs block transmitter uptake within hours of administration, relief of depression takes several weeks to develop. Hence, it would appear that in the interval between the onset of uptake blockade and the onset of a therapeutic response, intermediary neurochemical events must be taking place. Just what these events might be is unknown.

PHARMACOKINETICS

Tricyclic antidepressants have half-lives that are long and variable. Since their half-lives are long, the tricyclic antidepressants can usually be administered in a single daily dose. However, because their half-lives are variable, the tricyclic drugs require individualization of dosage.

THERAPEUTIC USES

Depression

Tricyclic antidepressants are preferred drugs for treatment of major depression. These medicines can elevate mood, increase activity and alertness, decrease morbid preoccupation, improve appetite, and normalize sleep patterns.

It is important to note that the tricyclic agents, and all other antidepressants, do not relieve symptoms immediately. *Initial* responses take from one to three weeks to develop. One or two months may be needed before a *maximal* response is achieved. Because therapeutic effects are delayed, tricyclic antidepressants cannot be used on a PRN basis. Furthermore, because responses are delayed, a therapeutic trial should not be considered a failure until medication has been administered for at least one month without success.

Suicide is always a concern during the treatment of depression, since the patient may be so despondent as to perceive suicide as the only means of relieving his or her suffering. To reduce the chances of suicide, several precautions can be taken. First, since antidepressants take several weeks to alleviate symptoms, the patient presenting with suicidal tendencies should be hospitalized until treatment has had time to substantially reduce suicidality. In addition, since the antidepressants themselves can be vehicles for suicide, the patient should not be given access to a large supply of these drugs. Accordingly, you should ensure that each dose is actually swallowed and not "cheeked." This precaution prevents the patient from accumulating multiple doses that might be taken with suicidal intent.

Bipolar Disorder

Bipolar disorder (manic-depressive illness) is characterized by alternating episodes of mania and depression (see Chapter 30). Tricyclic antidepressants can be helpful during the depressive phase of this illness.

Panic Disorder

Panic disorder is characterized by spontaneous panic attacks. Primary associated symptoms are anticipatory anxiety and phobic avoidance (agoraphobia). Tricyclic antidepressants can eliminate panic attacks in approximately 75% of those treated. The associated symptoms (anticipatory anxiety and phobic avoidance) are not affected.

ADVERSE EFFECTS

The most common undesired responses to tricyclics are orthostatic hypotension, sedation, and anticholinergic effects. The most serious adverse effect is cardiac toxicity. Adverse effects of individual tricyclics are summarized in Table 23–6.

Orthostatic Hypotension

Orthostatic hypotension is the most serious of the common adverse responses to treatment. Hypotension is caused mainly by blockade of alpha-adrenergic receptors on blood vessels. The patient should be informed that orthostatic hypotension can be minimized by moving slowly when assuming an upright posture. Also, the patient should be instructed to sit or lie down if symptoms of hypotension (dizziness, lightheadedness) occur. For the hospitalized patient, blood pressure and pulse rate should be monitored on a regular schedule (e.g., four times daily). These measurements should be taken while the patient is lying down and again after the patient has been sitting or standing for one to two minutes. If blood pressure is low and pulse rate is high, medication should be withheld and the physician should be notified.

Anticholinergic Effects

The tricyclic antidepressants can block muscarinic-cholinergic receptors, thus causing an array of anticholinergic effects (e.g., dry mouth, blurred vision, photophobia, constipation, urinary hesitancy, and tachycardia). The patient should be informed about possible anticholinergic responses and instructed in ways to minimize discomfort.

Diaphoresis

Despite their anticholinergic properties, tricyclic antidepressants often cause diaphoresis (sweating). The mechanism of this paradoxical effect is unknown.

Sedation

Sedation is a common response to the tricyclic drugs. This response is probably due to blockade of histamine receptors in the CNS. The patient should be advised to avoid hazardous activity if prominent sedation occurs.

Cardiac Toxicity

Tricyclics can adversely affect cardiac function; however, in the absence of overdosage or pre-existing cardiac impairment, serious cardiotoxicity is rare. These drugs affect the heart by decreasing vagal influence on the heart (secondary to muscarinic blockade) and by acting directly on the bundle of His to slow conduction. Both effects increase the risk of dysrhythmias. To minimize adverse cardiac effects, patients older than 40 years of age and those with heart disease should undergo an electrocardiographic evaluation prior to treatment and periodically thereafter.

Seizures

Tricyclic antidepressants lower seizure threshold. Caution must be exercised in patients with epilepsy and other seizure disorders.

Hypomania

Occasionally, the tricyclics produce too much of a good thing, elevating mood from depression all the way to hypomania (mild mania). If hypomania develops, the patient should be evaluated to determine whether elation is drug-induced or symptomatic of manic-depressive illness.

DRUG INTERACTIONS

Monoamine Oxidase Inhibitors

The combination of a tricyclic antidepressant and an MAOI can lead to *severe hypertension* from excessive adrenergic stimulation of the heart and blood vessels. Excessive adrenergic stimulation occurs because (1) inhibition of MAO causes accumulation of norepinephrine in adrenergic neurons and (2) blockade of norepinephrine reuptake by the tricyclics decreases norepinephrine inactivation. Because of the potential for hypertensive crisis, combined therapy with tricyclic antidepressants and MAOIs is generally avoided.

Direct-Acting Sympathomimetic Drugs

Tricyclic antidepressants potentiate responses to direct-acting sympathomimetics (i.e., drugs such as epinephrine and norepinephrine that produce their effects by direct interaction with adrenergic receptors). Stimulation by these drugs is increased because tricyclics block their uptake into adrenergic terminals, thus prolonging their presence in the synaptic space.

Indirect-Acting Sympathomimetic Drugs

Tricyclic antidepressants decrease responses to indirect-acting sympathomimetics (i.e., drugs such as ephedrine and amphetamine that produce their effects by promoting release of transmitter from adrenergic nerves). Effects of indirect-acting sympathomimetics are reduced because tricyclics block uptake of these agents into adrenergic nerves, thereby preventing them from reaching their site of action within the nerve terminal.

Anticholinergic Agents

Since the tricyclic antidepressants exert anticholinergic actions of their own, these drugs will intensify the effects of other medications that exert anticholinergic actions. Consequently, patients receiving tricyclic agents should be advised to avoid all other drugs with anticholinergic properties, including antihistamines and certain over-the-counter sleeping aids.

CNS Depressants

Depression of the CNS caused by the tricyclics will increase with that caused by other drugs that have CNS-depressant properties. Accordingly, the patient should be warned against taking all other CNS depressants, such as alcohol, antihistamines, opioids, and barbiturates.

TOXICITY

Overdosage with tricyclic antidepressants is often life threatening. (The lethal dose is only eight times the average daily dose.) To minimize the risk of death by suicide, the acutely depressed patient should be given no more than a one-week supply of medication at one time.

Clinical Manifestations

Symptoms result primarily from *anticholinergic* and *cardiotoxic* actions. The combination of cholinergic blockade and direct cardiotoxicity can produce *dysrhythmias*, including tachycardia, intraventricular blocks, complete atrioventricular block, ventricular tachycardia, and ventricular fibrillation. Responses to peripheral muscarinic blockade include hyperthermia, flushing, dry mouth, and dilation of the pupils.

CNS symptoms are prominent. Early responses are confusion, agitation, and hallucinations. Seizures and coma may follow.

Treatment

Absorption of ingested drug can be reduced with gastric lavage followed by administration of activated charcoal. Physostigmine (a cholinesterase inhibitor) is given to counteract anticholinergic actions. Propranolol, lidocaine, or phenytoin can be given to control dysrhythmias. Dysrhythmias should not be treated with procainamide or quinidine, because these drugs aggravate cardiac depression.

DOSAGE AND ADMINISTRATION

Dosage

Dosages for individual tricyclics are summarized in Table 23–7. General guidelines on dosing follow.

Initial doses of tricyclic antidepressants should be kept *low* (e.g., 50 mg of imipramine/day for the adult outpatient). Low initial doses minimize adverse reactions and, as a result, help to promote compliance. High initial doses are both undesirable and unnecessary. They are undesirable because they pose an increased risk of adverse reactions. They are unnecessary in that onset of therapeutic effects is delayed regardless of dosage, and therefore aggressive initial dosing offers no benefit.

Because of interpatient variability in metabolism of tricyclics, dosing is highly individualized. As a rule, dosage is adjusted on the basis of *clinical response*. However, in the absence of a therapeutic response, *plasma drug levels* can be used as a guide for dosage determination. Levels of imipramine, for example, must be above 225 ng/ml for antidepressant effects to occur. If a patient has not responded to imipramine, measurements should be made to ensure that plasma drug levels are greater than 225 ng/ml. If drug levels are below this value, the dosage should be increased.

Once an effective dosage has been established, most patients can take their entire daily dose at bedtime, since

TABLE 23–7 **Adult Dosages for Antidepressants**

Generic Name	Trade Name	Initial Dose*† (mg/d)	Dose After 4–8 weeks* (mg/d)	Maximum Dose‡ (mg/d)
Tricyclic Antidepressants				
Amitriptyline	Elavil, Endep	50–150	100–200	300
Desipramine	Norpramin, Pertofrane	50–150	75–200	300
Doxepin	Adapin, Sinequan	50–150	100–200	300
Imipramine	Tofranil	50–150	100–200	300
Nortriptyline	Aventyl, Pamelor	25–100	75–150	150
Protriptyline	Vivactil	10–40	15–40	60
Trimipramine	Surmontil	50–150	75–250	250
Monoamine Oxidase Inhibitors				
Isocarboxazid	Marplan	20–30	20–30	30
Phenezine	Nardil	45–75	45–75	75
Tranylcypromine	Parnate	20–30	20–30	30
Selective Serotonin Reuptake Inhibitors				
Fluoxetine	Prozac	20	20–40	80
Fluvoxamine	Luvox	50–100	50–300	300
Paroxetine	Paxil	20	20–50	50
Sertraline	Zoloft	50	50–200	200
Miscellaneous Antidepressants				
Amoxapine	Asendin	50–150	200–300	400
Bupropioin	Wellbutrin	200	300	450
Maprotiline	Ludiomil	50–100	100–150	225
Trazodone	Desyrel	150	150–200	400

*Doses listed are *total daily doses*. Depending on the drug and the patient, the total dose may be given in a single dose or in divided doses.
†Initial doses are employed for 4–8 weeks, the time required for most symptoms to respond. The smaller dose within the range listed is used initially. Dosage is gradually increased as required.
‡Doses higher than these may be needed for some patients with severe depression.

the long half-lives of the tricyclic antidepressants make divided daily doses unnecessary. Once-daily dosing at bedtime has several advantages: (1) it is simple to perform, and thus facilitates compliance; (2) it promotes sleep by causing maximal sedation at night; and (3) it reduces the intensity of side effects during the day. Although once-a-day dosing is generally desirable, not all patients can use this schedule. The elderly, for example, can be especially sensitive to the cardiotoxic actions of the tricyclics. As a result, if the entire daily dose were taken at one time, effects on the heart might be intolerable.

Once remission has been produced, therapy should continue for at least six months. Failure to take medication for this period is likely to result in relapse. Patients should be encouraged to continue drug therapy even if they are symptom free and feel that further medication is not needed.

Routes of Administration

All of the tricyclic agents can be administered by mouth, the usual route for these drugs. Two agents—*amitriptyline* and *imipramine*—may also be given by IM injection. Intravenous administration is not used. Since effects take weeks to develop, there would be no advantage to this route.

DRUG SELECTION

In the United States, seven tricyclic antidepressants are available (see Tables 23–6 and 23–7). When administered in adequate doses, all seven agents are equally effective at reducing symptoms of depression and panic disorder. Principal differences among these agents concern side effects (see Table 23–6).

Selection among tricyclic agents is made on the basis of side effects. For example, if the patient has been experiencing insomnia, a drug with prominent sedative properties (e.g., doxepin) might be selected. Conversely, if daytime sedation is undesirable, a weakly sedative agent (e.g., desipramine) might be preferred. Elderly patients with glaucoma or constipation and males with prostatic hypertrophy can be especially sensitive to anticholinergic effects; for these patients, a drug with weak anticholinergic properties (e.g., desipramine) would be appropriate.

Monoamine Oxidase Inhibitors

The MAOIs are second- or third-choice antidepressants for most patients. Although these drugs are as effective as the tricyclics, they are more dangerous. Of particular concern is the risk of hypertensive crisis in response to ingestion of certain foods and drugs. With the advent of newer alternatives to the tricyclic antidepressants, indications for the MAOIs continue to decline.

Only three MAOIs are approved for use in the United States (see Tables 23–6 and 23–7). One of these drugs—isocarboxazid—is essentially obsolete. Hence, only two MAOIs—phenelzine and tranylcypromine—are employed to any significant degree.

MECHANISM OF ACTION

Before discussing the MAOIs, we need to discuss MAO itself. MAO is an enzyme present in the liver, the intestinal wall, and the terminals of adrenergic nerves. The function of MAO in nerve terminals is to convert monoamine transmitters (norepinephrine, epinephrine, serotonin) into inactive products. In the liver and intestine, MAO serves to inactivate biogenic amines present in food; in addition, these enzymes can inactivate biogenic amines administered as drugs.

Antidepressant effects of the MAOIs appear to result from inhibition of MAO within nerve terminals (Figure 23–2). By inhibiting intraneuronal MAO, these drugs increase the amount of norepinephrine and serotonin available for release from neurons of the CNS. The intensified transmission that occurs when these transmitters are released in supranormal amounts is thought to be responsible for relief of depression.

The MAOIs can act on MAO in two ways: reversibly and irreversibly. Phenelzine and isocarboxazid produce *irreversible* inhibition. Tranylcypromine produces *reversible* inhibition. Recovery from irreversible inhibition requires synthesis of new enzyme, a somewhat slow process. Hence, the effects of the irreversible inhibitors persist for about two weeks after drug withdrawal. Recovery from reversible inhibition is more rapid, occurring in three to five days.

It should be noted that antidepressant effects of the MAOIs cannot be fully accounted for by MAO inhibition alone. This statement is based on the fact that the biochemical action of these drugs (inhibition of MAO) takes place rapidly, whereas the clinical response (relief of depression) takes weeks to develop. Hence, it would appear that in the interval between initial inhibition of MAO and alleviation of depression, additional neurochemical events must be taking place. It is these as yet unknown events that are ultimately responsible for the beneficial response to treatment.

THERAPEUTIC USES

Depression

The MAOIs are as effective as the tricyclic agents for relieving depression. However, because their use can be hazardous, MAOIs are generally reserved for patients who have not responded to tricyclics or the newer antidepressants. For one group of patients—those with atypical depression—MAOIs are drugs of first choice. As with the tricyclic agents, beneficial effects take a week or more to develop.

Other Uses

MAOIs have been used with some success in the treatment of bulimia and other obsessive-compulsive

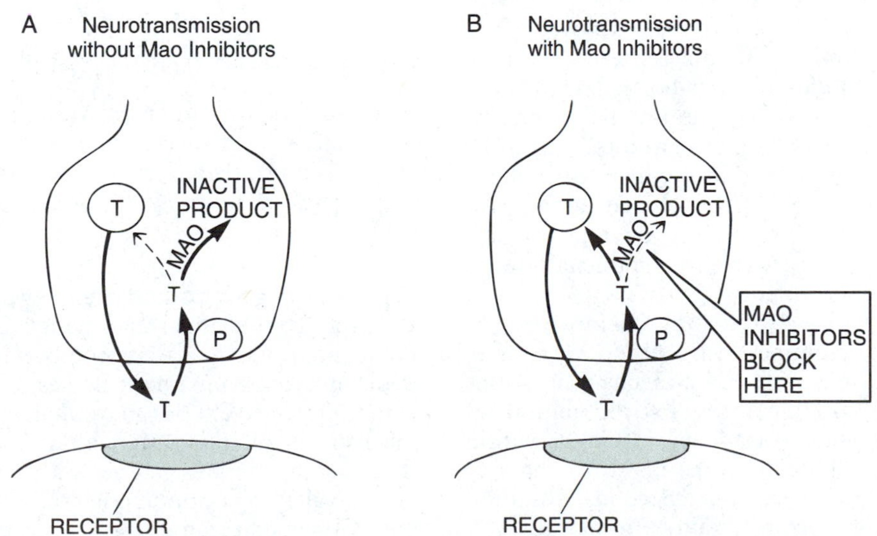

FIGURE 23–2
Mechanism of action of monoamine oxidase (MAO) inhibitors. **A,** Under drug-free conditions, much of the norepinephrine or serotonin that undergoes reuptake into nerve terminals becomes inactivated by MAO present within the terminal. This inactivation process helps maintain an appropriate concentration of transmitter within the terminal. **B,** MAO inhibitors prevent inactivation of norepinephrine and serotonin, thereby increasing the amount of transmitter available for release. Release of supranormal amounts of transmitter intensifies transmission. P—uptake pump; T—transmitter (norepinephrine or serotonin).

disorders. Like the tricyclics, MAOIs can eliminate spontaneous *panic attacks* in patients with panic disorder.

ADVERSE EFFECTS

CNS Stimulation

Unlike the tricyclic agents, MAOIs cause direct CNS stimulation (in addition to acting as antidepressants). Excessive stimulation can produce anxiety, agitation, hypomania, and even mania.

Orthostatic Hypotension

Despite their ability to increase the norepinephrine content of peripheral sympathetic nerves, the MAOIs reduce blood pressure when administered in usual therapeutic doses. The patient should be informed about signs of hypotension (dizziness, lightheadedness) and advised to sit or lie down if these occur. Also, the patient should be informed that hypotension can be minimized by moving slowly when assuming an erect posture. For the hospitalized patient, blood pressure and pulse rate should be monitored regularly (e.g., four times daily). These measurements should be taken while the patient is lying down and after the patient has been sitting or standing for one to two minutes.

Hypertensive Crisis From Dietary Tyramine

Although the MAOIs normally produce *hypotension,* these drugs can be the cause of severe *hypertension* if the patient should ingest foods that contain *tyramine,* a substance that promotes the release of norepinephrine from sympathetic nerves. Hypertensive crisis is characterized by headache, tachycardia, hypertension, nausea, and vomiting.

Before considering the mechanism by which hypertensive crisis is produced, let's consider the effect of tyramine under drug-free conditions. In the absence of MAO inhibition, dietary tyramine does not represent a threat. Much of the tyramine in food is metabolized by MAO in the intestinal wall. Furthermore, any dietary tyramine that does get absorbed passes directly to the liver via the hepatic portal circulation. Once in the liver, tyramine is immediately inactivated by MAO. Hence, as long as hepatic MAO is functioning, dietary tyramine is prevented from reaching the general circulation and, therefore, is devoid of adverse effects.

In the presence of MAOIs, the picture is very different: Dietary tyramine can produce a life-threatening hypertensive crisis. The mechanism of this reaction has three components. First, inhibition of neuronal MAO augments norepinephrine levels within the terminals of sympathetic neurons that regulate cardiac function and vascular tone. Second, inhibition of hepatic MAO allows dietary tyramine to pass directly through the liver and enter the systemic circulation intact. Third, upon reaching peripheral sympathetic nerves, tyramine stimulates the release of the accumulated norepinephrine, thus causing massive vasoconstriction and excessive stimulation of the heart; hypertensive crisis results.

To reduce the risk of tyramine-induced hypertensive crisis, the following precautions must be taken:

- MAOIs must not be dispensed to patients who are considered incapable of rigid adherence to dietary restrictions.
- Before an MAOI is dispensed, the patient must be fully informed about the hazard of ingesting tyramine-rich foods.
- The patient must be provided with a list of specific foods and beverages to avoid. These foods—which include most cheeses, yeast extracts, fermented sausages (e.g., salami, pepperoni, bologna), and aged fish or meat—are listed in Table 23–8.
- The patient should be instructed to avoid all drugs that are not specifically approved by the physician.

The patient should be informed about the symptoms of hypertensive crisis (headache, tachycardia, palpitations, nausea, vomiting) and instructed to notify the physician immediately if these develop. If the physician is unavailable, the patient should go directly to an emergency room. In the event of hypertensive crisis, blood pressure can be lowered with 10 mg of nifedipine (Procardia), a calcium channel blocker; blood pressure declines because of vasodilation secondary to blockade of calcium channels on blood vessels.

In addition to tyramine, several other dietary constituents (e.g., caffeine, phenylethylamine) can precipitate hypertension if ingested by patients taking MAOIs. Foods that contain these compounds are listed in Table 23–8. The patient should be instructed to avoid them.

DRUG INTERACTIONS

The MAOIs can interact with many drugs to cause potentially disastrous results. Accordingly, *the patient should be instructed to avoid all medications—prescription agents and over-the-counter drugs—that have not been specifically approved by the physician.*

Indirect-Acting Sympathomimetic Agents

Indirect-acting sympathomimetics (e.g., ephedrine, amphetamine) are drugs that promote the release of norepinephrine from sympathetic nerves. Use of these agents by patients taking MAOIs can result in *hypertensive crisis.* The mechanism of this interaction is the same as that described for tyramine. The patient should be instructed to avoid all sympathomimetic drugs, including ephedrine, methylphenidate, amphetamines, and cocaine. Sympathomimetic agents may be present in cold remedies, nasal decongestants, and asthma medications; all of these preparations should be avoided unless approved by the physician.

TABLE 23–8 **Foods That Can Interact with MAO Inhibitors**

Foods That Contain Tyramine

Category	*Unsafe Foods (High Tyramine Content)*	*Safe Foods (Little or No Tyramine)*
Vegetables	Avocados, especially if overripe; fermented bean curd; fermented soybean; soybean paste	Most vegetables
Fruits	Figs, especially if overripe; bananas, in large amounts	Most fruits
Meats	Meats that are fermented, smoked, or otherwise aged; spoiled meats; liver, unless *very* fresh	Meats that are known to be fresh (exercise caution in restaurants; meat may not be fresh)
Sausages	Fermented varieties: bologna, pepperoni, salami, others	Nonfermented varieties
Fish	Dried or cured fish; fish that is fermented, smoked, or otherwise aged; spoiled fish	Fish that is known to be fresh; vacuum-packed fish, if eaten promptly or refrigerated only briefly after opening
Milk, milk products	Practically all cheeses	Milk, yogurt, cottage cheese, cream cheese
Foods with yeast	Yeast extract (e.g., Marmite, Bovril)	Baked goods that contain yeast
Beer, wine	Some imported beers; Chianti wine	Major domestic brands of beer; most wines
Other foods	Protein dietary supplements; soups (may contain protein extract); shrimp paste; soy sauce	

Foods That Contain Other Vasopressors

Food	*Comments*
Chocolate	Contains phenylethylamine, a pressor agent; large amounts can cause a reaction.
Fava beans	Contain dopamine, a pressor agent; reactions are most likely with overripe beans.
Ginseng	Headache, tremulousness and manic-like reactions have occurred.
Caffeinated beverages	Caffeine is a weak pressor agent; large amounts may cause a reaction.

Interactions Secondary to Inhibition of Hepatic MAO

Inhibition of MAO in the liver can decrease the metabolism of several drugs, including epinephrine, norepinephrine, and dopamine. These drugs must be used with caution since their effects will be intensified and prolonged.

Tricyclic Antidepressants

The combination of tricyclic antidepressants with MAOIs may produce hypertensive episodes or hypertensive crisis. As a result, this combination is not employed routinely. However, although potentially dangerous, the combination can benefit certain patients. If this combination is employed, caution must be exercised.

Antihypertensive Drugs

Combined use of MAOIs and antihypertensive agents may result in excessive lowering of blood pressure. This response should be no surprise considering that MAOIs, by themselves, can cause hypotension.

Meperidine

Meperidine (Demerol) can cause hyperpyrexia (excessive elevation of temperature) in patients receiving MAOIs. Accordingly, if a strong analgesic is required, an agent other than meperidine should be chosen. Furthermore, the analgesic should be administered in its lowest effective dosage.

Selective Serotonin Reuptake Inhibitors

In recent years, drugs that produce selective blockade of serotonin reuptake have become available (see Tables 23–6 and 23–7). These new drugs are as effective as the tricyclic antidepressants and appear to be safer, although possible long-term effects are not yet known. Fluoxetine, the most popular of these drugs, can be considered the prototype for the group. Accordingly, we will focus our discussion on this agent.

Fluoxetine

Since its introduction a few years ago, fluoxetine (Prozac) has become the most widely prescribed antidepressant in the United States. The drug is as effective as the tricyclic agents, causes fewer side effects, and is less dangerous when taken in overdosage.

MECHANISM OF ACTION

Fluoxetine causes selective inhibition of serotonin reuptake. This action is thought to underlie its antidepressant effects. The drug has no effect on dopamine or norepinephrine. In contrast with the tricyclic agents, fluoxetine does not block cholinergic, histaminergic, or alpha-adrenergic receptors. Furthermore, fluoxetine produces CNS excitation rather than sedation.

PHARMACOKINETICS

Fluoxetine is well absorbed following oral administration, even in the presence of food. The drug is widely distributed throughout the body and is highly bound (94%) to plasma proteins. Fluoxetine undergoes extensive hepatic conversion to norfluoxetine, a metabolite with pharmacological actions like those of fluoxetine itself. Norfluoxetine is eventually converted to inactive metabolites that are excreted in the urine. The drug has a long half-life (approximately seven days). As a result, steady-state plasma drug levels are reached after about four weeks.

THERAPEUTIC USES

Fluoxetine is used primarily to treat *major depression.* Antidepressant effects begin in one to three weeks and are equivalent to those produced by the tricyclics. The drug is also approved for *obsessive-compulsive disorders* and has been used on an investigational basis to treat bulimia and to *suppress appetite in obese patients.*

ADVERSE EFFECTS

The most common reactions are nausea (21%), headache (20%), and manifestations of CNS stimulation, including nervousness (15%), insomnia (14%), and anxiety (10%). Anorgasmia and other sexual dysfunctions occur frequently. Fluoxetine can cause dizziness and fatigue; patients should be warned against participation in hazardous activities (e.g., driving). Skin rash, which can be severe, has occurred in 4% of patients; in most cases, rashes readily respond to drug therapy (e.g., antihistamines, glucocorticoids) or to withdrawal of fluoxetine. Other common reactions include diarrhea (12%), excessive sweating (8%), and anorexia with associated weight loss (11%).

In contrast with the tricyclic agents, fluoxetine produces little or no cardiotoxicity, hypotension, or muscarinic blockade.

Overdosage causes nausea, vomiting, and signs of CNS stimulation (e.g., agitation, restlessness, hypomania, seizures). Because fluoxetine is not cardiotoxic, overdosage is less dangerous than with the tricyclics.

DRUG INTERACTIONS

Fluoxetine should not be combined with MAOIs, since severe adverse effects have been reported. MAOIs should be withdrawn at least 14 days before starting fluoxetine. When fluoxetine is discontinued, at least five weeks should elapse before an MAOI is given.

Fluoxetine inhibits a liver enzyme system (the cytochrome P450 system) that is responsible for metabolizing many other drugs, including the tricyclic antidepressants. As a result, concentrations of these other drugs may increase, possibly to dangerous levels. Accordingly, caution should be exercised if these combinations are used.

DOSAGE AND ADMINISTRATION

Fluoxetine may be taken with or without food. The initial dosage recommended by the manufacturer is 20 mg/day. If needed, the dosage may be increased gradually to a maximum of 80 mg/day; however, doses greater than 20 mg/day may increase toxicity more than they increase beneficial effects. If daily doses above 20 mg are used, they should be divided. Elderly patients and patients with impaired liver function should take lower doses.

Other SSRIs

In addition to fluoxetine, three other SSRIs are available: *fluvoxamine* (Luvox), *sertraline* (Zoloft), and *paroxetine* (Paxil). All three drugs have properties similar to those of fluoxetine. They all produce selective blockade of serotonin reuptake, relieve symptoms of major depression, and cause CNS stimulation rather than sedation. Like fluoxetine, these drugs cause fewer anticholinergic effects than the tricyclics and less orthostatic hypotension. In addition, they are much safer than the tricyclics when taken in overdose. Common side effects include nausea, headache, nervousness, and insomnia. As with fluoxetine, the incidence of sexual dysfunction (especially anorgasmia) is high.

Miscellaneous Antidepressants

Trazodone

Trazodone (Desyrel) blocks serotonin reuptake and may also stimulate serotonin receptors directly. Antidepressant effects take several weeks to develop and are equivalent to those of the tricyclic agents.

Common side effects are sedation, orthostatic hypotension, nausea, and vomiting. In contrast with the tricyclic agents, trazodone lacks anticholinergic actions and is not cardiotoxic. Accordingly, trazodone may be preferred for elderly patients and other persons for whom the cardiac and anticholinergic effects of the tricyclics may be intolerable.

Trazodone can cause *priapism* (prolonged, painful erection of the penis). In some cases, surgical intervention has been required. Priapism itself or the procedures required for relief can result in permanent impotence. Patients should be instructed to notify the physician or to go to an emergency room if persistent erection occurs. (Prolonged clitoral erection has not been reported.)

Overdosage with trazodone is considered safer than with tricyclic agents or MAO inhibitors. Death from overdosage with trazodone alone has not been reported (although death has occurred following overdosage with trazodone plus other CNS depressants).

Amoxapine

Amoxapine (Asendin) has both antidepressant and neuroleptic properties. Antidepressant effects are equivalent to those of the tricyclics.

Amoxapine has relatively weak anticholinergic and sedative properties. Following overdosage, the risk of seizures with this drug is greater than with the tricyclics. Caution should be exercised in patients with epilepsy.

Like the antipsychotics, amoxapine can block receptors for dopamine. As a result, the drug can cause *extrapyramidal side effects* (e.g., parkinsonism, akathisia). Because of the risk of tardive dyskinesia (an extrapyramidal effect that develops with prolonged use of dopamine antagonists), long-term use of amoxapine should be avoided.

Bupropion

Bupropion (Wellbutrin) is a unique antidepressant similar in structure to the amphetamines. Like the amphetamines, this agent has stimulant properties and suppresses appetite. Bupropion is devoid of the anticholinergic, antiadrenergic, and cardiotoxic effects associated with the tricyclic agents. Antidepressant effects begin in one to three weeks and are equivalent to those of the tricyclics. The mechanism by which depression is relieved is unknown.

Bupropion is generally well tolerated. The most common adverse effects are weight loss, dry mouth, and dizziness. Other undesired responses include tremor, agitation, and insomnia.

At doses greater than 450 mg/day, bupropion produces seizures in about 0.4% of patients. The risk of seizures is greatly increased in patients with predisposing factors, such as head trauma, pre-existing seizure disorder, CNS tumor, and use of other drugs that lower seizure threshold.

Dosing must be done carefully to minimize the risk of seizures. Dosage escalation must be done slowly. The initial dosage is 100 mg twice a day. After four days, the dosage can be increased to 100 mg three times a day. If necessary, the dosage can be increased to a maximum of 150 mg three times a day.

Maprotiline

Although maprotiline (Ludiomil) is structurally different from the tricyclic antidepressants (maprotiline has four rings rather than three), this drug is very similar to the tricyclics with respect to therapeutic effects and side effects. The principal difference between these drugs is that maprotiline is more likely to cause seizures, even when used in moderate doses; following overdosage, about 30% of patients experience seizures. Because of the risk of seizures, maprotiline should not be taken by patients with a history of seizure disorders. The drug's side effect profile is summarized in Table 23–6. Usual dosages are shown in Table 23–7.

▶ Check Your Reading

11. What is the usual time course for developing a therapeutic response to antidepressant drugs?
12. What are the *most common* adverse effects of the tricyclic antidepressants?
13. What is the *most serious* adverse effect of the tricyclic antidepressants?
14. Why are tyramine-containing foods dangerous for patients taking MAOIs?
15. What is the principal advantage of SSRIs over tricyclic antidepressants?

LITHIUM AND OTHER DRUGS FOR BIPOLAR DISORDER

Our topic in this section is drug therapy of bipolar disorder, also known as manic-depressive illness. The mainstay of therapy is lithium and discussion focuses largely on this agent.

Bipolar Disorder (Manic-Depressive Illness): An Overview

Clinical Manifestations

Before considering drug therapy, it will be helpful to briefly review the characteristics of bipolar disorder. A more complete discussion of this illness can be found in Chapter 30.

Manic-depressive illness is a cyclic disorder characterized by recurrent fluctuations in mood. Typically, patients experience alternating episodes of mania and depression separated by periods in which mood is normal. The characteristics of depressive episodes are described in the preceding section and are not repeated here.

Manic episodes are characterized by heightened mood (euphoria), hyperactivity, excessive enthusiasm, and flight of ideas. Manic individuals display overactivity at work and at play and have a reduced need for sleep. Mania produces excessive sociability and talkativeness. Extreme self-confidence, grandiose ideas, and delusions of importance are common. Manic individuals frequently indulge in high-risk activities (e.g., questionable business deals, reckless driving, gambling, sexual indiscretions), giving no forethought to the consequences. Symptoms in the late stages of a manic episode may resemble those of paranoid schizophrenia (hallucinations, delusions, bizarre behavior).

As noted, most individuals with bipolar disorder go through alternating episodes of mania and depression. Untreated episodes of mania or depression generally last from 4 to 13 months. For the majority (approximately 70%) of patients, periods of normal mood separate the episodes of mania and depression. As time passes, manic and depressive episodes tend to occur more frequently.

Overview of Drug Therapy

DRUG SELECTION

Drug therapy of bipolar disorder is summarized in Table 23–9. As indicated, the mainstay of therapy is *lithium.* Lithium can provide symptomatic control during both the manic phase and the depressed phase. In addition, when taken *prophylactically,* lithium can reduce the frequency and severity of recurrent manic and depressive episodes. When used to control acute mania, lithium is often combined with a *benzodiazepine* (if symptoms are mild) or with an *antipsychotic agent plus a benzodiazepine* (if symptoms are severe). When used during the depressed phase, lithium is usually combined with an *antidepressant* (a tricyclic or bupropion [Wellbutrin]). However, there is a risk that the antidepressant will transport the patient from depression into mania.

In recent years, two antiseizure drugs—*carbamazepine* (Tegretol) and *valproic acid* (Depakene, Depakote)—have been used on an investigational basis to treat manic-depressive illness. Both drugs can control symptoms during manic episodes and depressive episodes, and both can provide prophylaxis against recurrent mania and depression. These agents represent an alternative to lithium for patients who fail to respond to lithium or who find its side effects intolerable.

TABLE 23–9 Drug Therapy of Bipolar Disorder

Illness Phase	Drugs
Manic phase	
Moderate symptoms	Lithium* + a benzodiazepine
Severe symptoms	Lithium* + an antipsychotic agent + a benzodiazepine
Depressive phase	Lithium + a tricyclic antidepressant or bupropion
Normalized mood	Lithium (for prophylaxis against recurrence of mania or depression)

*For lithium nonresponders, addition or substitution of carbamazepine or valproic acid may be helpful.

PROMOTING COMPLIANCE

Poor patient compliance can frustrate attempts to treat acute manic episodes. Patients may resist treatment because they fail to see anything wrong with their thinking or behavior. Furthermore, the experience is not necessarily unpleasant. In fact, individuals going through a manic episode may well enjoy it. As a result, in order to ensure adequate treatment, hospitalization is often needed. To achieve this, collaboration with the patient's family may be required. Since hospitalization per se won't guarantee compliance, lithium administration should be observed to ensure that each dose is actually taken.

After an acute manic episode has been controlled, long-term prophylactic therapy is indicated, making compliance an ongoing concern. To promote compliance, the patient and family should be educated about the nature of manic-depressive illness and the importance of taking medication as prescribed. Family members can help to ensure compliance by overseeing medication use and by urging the patient to visit a physician or psychiatric clinic if a pattern of noncompliance develops.

Lithium

Lithium can provide symptomatic control in patients with manic-depressive illness. Beneficial effects were first described by John Cade, an Australian, in 1949. However, because of concerns about toxicity, lithium was not approved for use in the United States until 1970. Since lithium has a low therapeutic index, toxicity is a concern. Because significant injury can occur when plasma drug levels are only slightly greater than the therapeutic level, monitoring of lithium levels is mandatory.

Lithium is a simple inorganic ion that carries a single positive charge. In the periodic table of elements, lithium falls within the same group as potassium and sodium. Accordingly, lithium has properties in common with these two elements. Lithium occurs naturally in animal tissues but has no known physiologic function.

PHARMACOKINETICS

Absorption and Distribution

Lithium is well absorbed following oral administration. The drug distributes evenly to all tissues and body fluids.

Excretion

Lithium has a short half-life, owing to rapid renal excretion. Because of its short half-life (and high toxicity), the drug must be administered in divided daily doses; large, single daily doses cannot be used. Because lithium is excreted by the kidneys, it must be used with great care in patients with renal impairment.

Sodium depletion will *decrease* renal excretion of lithium, causing the drug to accumulate. Toxicity may result. Accordingly, it is important that sodium levels remain normal. Patients should be instructed to maintain normal sodium intake; a sodium-free diet cannot be used. Since diuretics promote sodium loss, these agents must be employed with caution. Sodium loss secondary to diarrhea can be sufficient to cause lithium accumulation, and the patient should be forewarned of this possibility.

Plasma Lithium Levels

Measurement of plasma lithium levels is an essential feature of treatment. *Lithium levels must be kept below 1.5 mEq/L; levels greater than this can produce significant toxicity.* For initial therapy of a manic episode, lithium levels should range from 0.8 to 1.4 mEq/L. Once the desired therapeutic effect has been achieved, the dosage should be reduced to produce maintenance drug levels of 0.4 to 1.0 mEq/L. Blood for lithium determinations should be drawn in the morning, 12 hours after the evening dose.

THERAPEUTIC USES

Manic-Depressive Illness

Lithium is the drug of choice for controlling manic episodes in patients with manic-depressive illness and for long-term prophylaxis against recurrent mania and depression in these patients.

In manic patients, lithium reduces euphoria, hyperactivity, and other symptoms but does not cause sedation. Antimanic effects begin five to seven days after the onset of treatment. However, full effects may not be seen until two to three weeks. For many patients, adjunctive therapy with a benzodiazepine or an antipsychotic agent can be helpful. Benzodiazepines (e.g., diazepam [Valium]) are used to provide sedation in patients with relatively mild symptoms of mania. Antipsychotics (e.g., haloperidol [Haldol]) may be required to provide rapid control in patients with severe symptoms.

Prophylaxis with lithium may not prevent episodes of depression. If depression occurs, adjunctive therapy with an antidepressant is indicated.

Other Uses

Although approved only for treatment of manic-depressive illness, lithium has been used with varying degrees of success in other psychiatric disorders, including alcoholism, bulimia, schizophrenia, and glucocorticoid-induced psychosis. Nonpsychiatric uses include hyperthyroidism, cluster headache, migraine, and syndrome of inappropriate secretion of antidiuretic hormone. In addition, lithium can raise neutrophil counts in children with chronic neutropenia and in patients receiving anticancer drugs or zidovudine (AZT).

MECHANISM OF ACTION

We do not know the underlying cause of manic-depressive illness, nor do we know how lithium stabilizes mood. Lithium has multiple effects on the nervous system. The drug can alter the synthesis, storage, release, and reuptake of neurotransmitters (norepinephrine, serotonin, dopamine, acetylcholine, GABA). Also, lithium can alter the distribution of neuronally important ions (calcium, sodium, and magnesium). In addition, lithium can influence the function of second-messenger systems. Which, if any, of these actions underlies lithium's therapeutic effects is unknown.

ADVERSE EFFECTS

Adverse effects of lithium can be divided into two categories: (1) effects that occur at excessive drug levels, and (2) effects that occur at therapeutic drug levels. In the discussion that follows, adverse effects produced at excessive lithium levels are considered as a group. Effects produced at therapeutic levels are considered individually.

Adverse Effects When Lithium Levels Are Excessive

Certain toxicities are closely correlated with the concentration of lithium in plasma. As indicated in Table 23–10, mild responses (e.g., fine hand tremor, gastrointestinal upset, thirst, muscle weakness) can develop at lithium levels that are still within the therapeutic range (i.e., below 1.5 mEq/L). When plasma levels exceed 1.5 mEq/L, more serious toxicities begin to appear. At drug levels above 2.5 mEq/L, death has resulted. Patients should be informed about early signs of toxicity and instructed to interrupt lithium use if these appear. The most common cause of lithium accumulation in compliant patients is sodium depletion.

To keep lithium levels within the therapeutic range, plasma drug levels should be monitored routinely. Levels should be measured every two to three days at the beginning of treatment and every one to three months during maintenance therapy.

Treatment of acute overdosage is primarily supportive; there is no specific antidote to lithium toxicity. The

TABLE 23–10 Toxicities Associated with Excessive Plasma Levels of Lithium

Plasma Lithium Level	Signs of Toxicity
<1.5 mEq/L	Nausea, vomiting, diarrhea, thirst, polyuria, lethargy, slurred speech, muscle weakness, fine hand tremor
1.5 to 2.0 mEq/L	Persistent GI upset, coarse hand tremor, confusion, hyperirritability of muscles, EKG changes, sedation, incoordination
2.0 to 2.5 mEq/L	Ataxia, giddiness, high output of dilute urine, serious EKG changes, fasciculations, tinnitus, blurred vision, clonic movements, seizures, stupor, severe hypotension, coma, death (usually secondary to pulmonary complications)
>2.5 mEq/L	Symptoms may progress rapidly to generalized convulsions, oliguria, and death

severely intoxicated patient should be hospitalized. Hemodialysis is an effective means of lithium removal and should be considered whenever drug levels exceed 2.5 mEq/L.

Tremor

Patients may develop a fine hand tremor, especially in the fingers, that can interfere with writing and other motor skills. Lithium-induced tremor can be augmented by stress, fatigue, and certain drugs (e.g., antidepressants, antipsychotics, caffeine). Tremor can be reduced with a beta-adrenergic blocking agent (e.g., propranolol [Inderal]) and by measures that reduce peak levels of lithium (i.e., dosage reduction, use of divided doses, or use of a sustained-release formulation).

Renal Toxicity

Chronic administration of lithium has occasionally been associated with degenerative changes in the kidney. The risk of renal injury can be reduced by keeping the dosage low and, when possible, avoiding long-term lithium therapy. Kidney function should be assessed prior to treatment and once a year thereafter.

Goiter

Long-term use of lithium can cause goiter (enlargement of the thyroid gland). Although usually benign, lithium-induced goiter is sometimes associated with hypothyroidism. Treatment with thyroid hormone or withdrawal of lithium reverses thyroid hypertrophy. Measurement of thyroid hormones (T_3 and T_4) and thyroid-stimulating hormone (TSH) should be obtained prior to treatment and annually thereafter.

Teratogenesis

Use of lithium during the first trimester of pregnancy is associated with an 11% incidence of birth defects (usually malformations of the heart). Accordingly, *lithium is contraindicated during the first trimester of pregnancy.* Furthermore, unless the benefits of therapy clearly outweigh the potential risk to the fetus, lithium should be avoided during the remainder of pregnancy as well. Women of child-bearing age should be counseled about the importance of avoiding pregnancy while taking lithium.

Adverse Effects During Lactation

Lithium readily enters breast milk and can achieve concentrations that are potentially harmful to the nursing infant. Consequently, breast-feeding during lithium therapy should be discouraged.

Polyuria

Polyuria occurs in 50% to 70% of patients taking lithium chronically. In some patients, daily urine output may exceed 3 L. Lithium promotes polyuria by antagonizing the effects of antidiuretic hormone. To maintain adequate hydration, patients should be instructed to drink 8 to 12 glasses of fluids daily. Polyuria, nocturia, and excessive thirst can discourage patients from complying with the prescribed regimen.

Lithium-induced polyuria can be *reduced* with a *thiazide diuretic.* The mechanism of this paradoxical effect is not known. Unfortunately, thiazides can increase plasma levels of lithium (perhaps by promoting sodium excretion). Accordingly, a reduction in lithium dosage is required.

DRUG INTERACTIONS

Diuretics

Diuretics promote sodium loss and can thereby increase the risk of lithium toxicity. Toxicity can occur because, in the presence of low sodium, renal excretion of lithium is reduced, causing lithium levels to rise.

Anticholinergic Drugs

Anticholinergic drugs can cause urinary hesitancy. Combined with lithium-induced polyuria, this effect can result in considerable discomfort. Unfortunately, the combination of lithium plus an anticholinergic drug cannot always be avoided: Patients frequently require concurrent therapy with agents that have prominent anticholinergic properties (e.g., antipsychotics, tricyclic antidepressants).

PREPARATIONS AND DOSAGE

Lithium is available as two salts: *lithium carbonate* and *lithium citrate.* With either salt, administration is oral. Lithium formulations and trade names are summarized in Table 23–11.

Lithium can cause gastric upset. This can be reduced by administering lithium with meals or with milk.

Dosing with lithium is highly individualized. Dosage adjustments are based on plasma drug levels and clinical response.

Plasma drug levels should be kept within the therapeutic range. Levels between 0.8 and 1.4 mEq/L are generally appropriate for *acute therapy* of manic episodes. For *maintenance therapy,* lithium levels should range from 0.4 to 1.0 mEq/L. (Levels of 0.6 to 0.8 mEq/L are effective for most patients.) To avoid serious toxicity, *lithium levels should not exceed 1.5 mEq/L.*

Knowledge of plasma drug levels is not the only guide to lithium dosing; consideration of the clinical response is at least as important. When evaluating the appropriateness of a lithium dosage, we must not forget to look at the patient. Laboratory tests are all well and good, but they are not a substitute for clinical assessment. If, for example, blood levels of lithium appear proper, but clinical evaluation indicates toxicity, there is no question as to the action that should be taken: The dosage should be reduced—despite the apparent acceptability of the dosage as reflected by plasma drug levels.

Because of its short half-life and low therapeutic index, *lithium cannot be administered in a single daily dose;* with once-a-day dosing, peak drug levels would be excessive. Hence, a typical dosage is 300 mg (of lithium carbonate) taken three or four times a day. A dosage of 600 mg twice daily is acceptable, provided that an extended-release formulation is employed; however, even these preparations cannot be given on a once-daily basis.

TABLE 23–11 **Lithium Preparations**

Lithium Salt	Formulation	Lithium Content*	Trade Name
Lithium carbonate (Li_2CO_3)	Capsules	4.06 mEq lithium (150 mg Li_2CO_3) 8.12 mEq lithium (300 mg Li_2CO_3) 16.24 mEq lithium (600 mg Li_2CO_3)	Eskalith, Lithonate
	Tablets	8.12 mEq lithium (300 mg Li_2CO_3)	Eskalith, Lithane, Lithotabs
	Tablets: slow-release	8.12 mEq lithium (300 mg Li_2CO_3)	Lithobid
	Tablets: controlled release	12.18 mEq lithium (450 mg Li_2CO_3)	Eskalith CR
Lithium citrate	Syrup	8 mEq lithium/5 ml (equivalent to 300 mg Li_2CO_3)	Cibalith-S

*Lithium content is expressed in two ways: (1) mEq of lithium ion and (2) mg of the particular lithium salt of which the preparation is composed.

Carbamazepine and Valproic Acid

Carbamazepine (Tegretol) and valproic acid (Depakene, Depakote) were originally developed and marketed for treatment of seizure disorders. In recent years, these drugs have been used with success to treat patients with bipolar disorder. At this time, carbamazepine and valproic acid are reserved for patients who have failed to respond to lithium or who cannot tolerate the side effects of lithium.

Carbamazepine was the first drug to be widely studied as an alternative to lithium for patients with manic-depressive illness. Like lithium, carbamazepine reduces symptoms during manic episodes and depressed episodes. In addition, the drug appears to provide effective prophylaxis against recurrence of mania and depression. For patients with severe mania, and for those who cycle rapidly, carbamazepine may be superior to lithium. When given to manic patients who have failed to respond to lithium, carbamazepine has had a success rate of about 60%. For treatment of acute manic episodes, the dosage should be low initially (200 to 400 mg/day) and then gradually increased to as much as 1.6 to 2.2 g/day. Lower doses should be employed when carbamazepine is used together with lithium, valproic acid, or an antipsychotic drug. The mechanism by which carbamazepine stabilizes mood is unknown.

Valproic acid is another promising alternative to lithium for manic-depressive patients who have failed to respond to lithium or who cannot tolerate its side effects. Clinical studies indicate that valproic acid can control symptoms in acute manic episodes and can provide prophylaxis against recurrent episodes of mania and depression. Like carbamazepine, valproic acid appears especially useful for patients with rapid-cycling bipolar disorder. Dosing should be initiated at 300 to 500 mg/day and then gradually increased to between 750 and 3000 mg/day. Valproic acid alters GABA-mediated neurotransmission, and this action may underlie the drug's mood-stabilizing effects.

▶ Check Your Reading

16. What is the role of lithium in the treatment of bipolar disorder?
17. What is the reason for monitoring lithium blood levels?
18. What blood level of lithium should not be exceeded?
19. What is the relationship of sodium intake and sodium levels to lithium toxicity?
20. Which drugs are used as alternatives to lithium in treating bipolar disorder?

ANTIANXIETY AGENTS

Anxiety is a common complaint, and the drugs employed for treatment are prescribed widely. Drugs used to relieve anxiety are called **antianxiety agents** or **anxiolytics;** an older term for these drugs is *tranquilizer.*

Before the benzodiazepines became available, anxiety was treated with barbiturates and other general central nervous system (CNS) depressants—drugs with multiple undesirable qualities: First, these drugs are powerful respiratory depressants that can readily prove fatal in overdosage. As a result, they are "drugs of choice" for suicide. Second, because they produce subjective effects that many people find desirable, general CNS depressants often have a high potential for abuse. Third, with prolonged use, most general CNS depressants produce significant tolerance and physical dependence. Fourth, barbiturates and certain other CNS depressants stimulate synthesis of hepatic drug-metabolizing enzymes and can thereby decrease responses to other drugs. Since benzodiazepines are just as effective as the general CNS depressants, but do not share their undesirable properties, benzodiazepines have largely replaced the general CNS depressants for managing anxiety and insomnia.

Benzodiazepines

Benzodiazepines are drugs of first choice for treating anxiety. In addition, these agents are used to promote sleep, induce general anesthesia, and manage seizure disorders, muscle spasm, panic disorder, and withdrawal from alcohol.

Benzodiazepines were introduced in the early 1960s and are among the most widely prescribed drugs in the United States. Perhaps the most familiar member of the benzodiazepine family is diazepam (Valium). The most frequently prescribed members are lorazepam (Ativan) and alprazolam (Xanax).

The popularity of benzodiazepines stems from their clear superiority over the alternatives: barbiturates and other general CNS depressants. Benzodiazepines are safer than the general CNS depressants and have a lower potential for abuse. In addition, benzodiazepines produce less tolerance and physical dependence and are subject to fewer drug interactions.

Since all of the benzodiazepines produce nearly identical effects, we will consider the family as a group, rather than focusing on individual agents.

OVERVIEW OF PHARMACOLOGIC EFFECTS

Practically all responses to benzodiazepines result from actions in the CNS. Benzodiazepines have few direct actions outside the CNS. All of the benzodiazepines produce a similar spectrum of responses. However, because of pharmacokinetic differences, individual benzodiazepines may differ in their clinical applications.

CNS. All beneficial effects of benzodiazepines and most adverse effects result from depressant actions in the CNS. With increasing dosage, effects progress from sedation to hypnosis to stupor.

Benzodiazepines depress neuronal function at multiple sites throughout the CNS. These drugs *reduce anxiety* through effects on the limbic system, a neuronal network associated with emotionality. They *promote sleep* through effects on cortical areas and on the sleep-wakefulness clock. They *induce muscle relaxation* through effects on supraspinal motor areas, including the cerebellum. Two important side effects—*confusion* and *amnesia*—result from effects on the hippocampus and cerebral cortex.

Cardiovascular System. When taken orally, benzodiazepines have negligible effects on the heart and blood vessels. In contrast, when administered *intravenously*—even in therapeutic doses—benzodiazepines can produce profound hypotension and cardiac arrest.

Respiratory System. Compared with the barbiturates, the benzodiazepines are weak respiratory depressants. When taken alone in therapeutic doses, these drugs produce little or no depression of respiration; and with toxic doses, respiratory depression is moderate at most. With oral therapy, clinically significant respiratory depression occurs only when benzodiazepines are combined with other CNS depressants (e.g., opioids, barbiturates, alcohol).

MECHANISM OF ACTION

Benzodiazepines *potentiate the actions of gamma-aminobutyric acid* (GABA), an inhibitory neurotransmitter found throughout the CNS. These drugs enhance the actions of GABA by binding to specific receptors in a supramolecular structure known as the GABA receptor-chloride channel complex. Benzodiazepines do not act as direct GABA agonists.

Because benzodiazepines act by amplifying the actions of endogenous GABA, rather than by directly mimicking GABA, there is a limit to how much CNS depression that these drugs can produce. This explains why benzodiazepines are so much safer than the barbiturates—drugs that can directly mimic GABA. Since benzodiazepines simply potentiate the inhibitory effects of endogenous GABA, and since the amount of GABA in the CNS is finite, there is a built-in limit to the depth of CNS depression that the benzodiazepines can produce. In contrast, since the barbiturates are direct-acting CNS depressants, maximal effects are limited only by the amount of barbiturate administered.

PHARMACOKINETICS

Absorption and Distribution

Most benzodiazepines are well absorbed following oral administration. Because of their high lipid solubility, benzodiazepines readily cross the blood-brain barrier to reach sites within the CNS.

Metabolism

Most benzodiazepines undergo extensive metabolic alterations. With few exceptions, the *metabolites are pharmacologically active*. As a result, responses produced by administering a particular benzodiazepine often persist long after the parent drug has disappeared from the plasma. Hence, there may be a poor correlation between the plasma half-life of the parent drug and the duration of pharmacological effects. Flurazepam, for example, whose plasma half-life is only two to three hours, is converted into an active metabolite with a half-life of 50 hours. Hence, administration of flurazepam produces long-lasting effects, despite the fact that within 8 to 12 hours of its administration, flurazepam itself can no longer be detected in the blood.

In patients with liver disease, metabolism of benzodiazepines can decline, thereby prolonging and intensifying responses. Because certain benzodiazepines (oxazepam, temazepam, and lorazepam) undergo very little metabolic alteration, these agents may be preferred for patients with hepatic impairment.

Time Course of Action

Benzodiazepines differ significantly from one another with regard to time course of action. These agents differ in onset of action, duration of action, and tendency to accumulate with repeated dosing.

Because all of the benzodiazepines have essentially equivalent pharmacological actions, selection among these drugs is based in large part on differences in time course. For example, if a patient needs medication to accelerate falling asleep, a benzodiazepine with a rapid onset of action (e.g., triazolam) would be indicated. However, if medication is needed to prevent waking later in the night, a benzodiazepine with a slower onset (e.g., estazolam) would be preferred. For treatment of anxiety, a drug with an intermediate duration of action is desirable. For treatment of any benzodiazepine-responsive condition in the elderly, a drug such as lorazepam, which is not likely to accumulate with repeated dosing, is generally preferred.

THERAPEUTIC USES

The benzodiazepines have three principal indications: (1) anxiety, (2) insomnia, and (3) seizure disorders. In addition, these drugs are employed as preoperative medication and in the management of muscle spasm, panic disorder, and withdrawal from alcohol. Although all benzodiazepines share the same pharmacological properties, and therefore might be equally effective for all of these applications, not every benzodiazepine is actually employed for all potential uses. The principal factors that determine the actual applications of a particular benzodiazepine are the pharmacokinetic properties of the drug itself and the research and marketing decisions of pharmaceutical companies.

Anxiety

Benzodiazepines are drugs of first choice for treating anxiety. Although all benzodiazepines have anxiolytic properties, only eight are marketed for this indication (Table 23–12). Anxiolytic effects result from depressing neurotransmission in the limbic system and cortical areas. Guidelines for managing anxiety with benzodiazepines are presented later in the chapter.

Insomnia

Benzodiazepines are drugs of first choice for treating insomnia. These drugs decrease latency time to falling asleep; they reduce awakenings; and they increase total sleeping time. Although all benzodiazepines can relieve insomnia, only a few are actually marketed for this use.

Panic Attacks

Alprazolam (Xanax), in high doses, provides effective treatment of panic disorder. Although several other medications, including SSRIs (e.g., fluoxetine [Prozac]), imipramine (a tricyclic antidepressant), and phenelzine (an MAOI) are also effective, alprazolam is the only drug actually approved by the FDA for this indication.

ADVERSE EFFECTS

Benzodiazepines are generally well tolerated, and serious adverse reactions are rare. Compared with the barbiturates and other general CNS depressants, the benzodiazepines are remarkably safe drugs.

CNS Depression

When taken in sleep-inducing doses, benzodiazepines cause drowsiness, lightheadedness, incoordination, and difficulty in concentrating. When these effects occur at bedtime, they are generally inconsequential. However, if sedation and other manifestations of CNS depression persist beyond waking, interference with daytime activities can occur.

Paradoxical Psychological Effects

When employed to treat anxiety, benzodiazepines sometimes cause paradoxical responses, including insomnia, excitation, euphoria, heightened anxiety, and rage. If these reactions occur, benzodiazepines should be withdrawn.

Anterograde Amnesia

Benzodiazepines can cause anterograde amnesia (impaired recall of events that take place after commencement of treatment). Anterograde amnesia has been especially troublesome with *triazolam* (Halcion). If patients complain of forgetfulness, the possibility of drug-induced amnesia should be evaluated.

Respiratory Depression

Benzodiazepines are only weak respiratory depressants. Death from overdosage with oral benzodiazepines *alone* has never been documented. Hence, in contrast to the barbiturates, benzodiazepines present little risk as vehicles for suicide. It must be emphasized, however, that although respiratory depression with oral therapy is rare, benzodiazepines can cause severe respiratory depression when administered *intravenously*. In addition, substantial respiratory depression can result from combining oral benzodiazepines with other CNS depressants (e.g., alcohol, barbiturates, opioids).

Potential for Abuse

The abuse potential of the benzodiazepines is lower than that of the barbiturates and most other general CNS depressants. The behavior pattern that constitutes "addiction" is uncommon among patients who take benzodiazepines for therapeutic purposes. When asked about drug-use patterns, people who regularly abuse drugs rarely indicate a preference for benzodiazepines over barbiturates. Because their potential for abuse is low, benzodiazepines are classified under Schedule IV of the Controlled Substances Act. This contrasts with the barbiturates, most of which are classified under Schedule II or III.

Adverse Effects During Pregnancy and Lactation

Benzodiazepines are highly lipid soluble and can readily cross the placental barrier. Reports based on benzodiazepine use during the first trimester of pregnancy suggest an increased risk of congenital malformations, such as cleft lip, inguinal hernia, and cardiac anomalies. Use near term can cause CNS depression in the neonate. Because they present a risk to the fetus, most benzodiazepines are classified in FDA Pregnancy Category D (i.e., there is a proven risk of fetal harm, but, depending on the patient, the potential benefits of use during pregnancy may justify

TABLE 23–12 **Major Drugs for Anxiety**

		Adult Oral Dosage		
Generic Name	***Trade Name***	***CSA Schedule***	***mg/dose***	***doses/d***
Benzodiazepines				
Alprazolam	Xanax	0.25–0.5	3	IV
Chlordiazepoxide	Librium, others	5–25	3 or 4	IV
Clorazepate	Tranxene, Gen-Xene	7.5–15	2 to 4*	IV
Diazepam	Valium, others	2–10	2 to 4*	IV
Halazepam	Paxipam	20–40	3 or 4	IV
Lorazepam	Ativan	1–3	2 or 3	IV
Oxazepam	Serax	10–30	3 or 4	IV
Prazepam	Centrax	10	3†	IV
Nonbenzodiazepine				
Buspirone	BuSpar	5–10	3	—

CSA = Controlled Substances Act
*With the sustained-release formulation, the total daily dose is administered in a single dose.
†May also be administered in a single 20–40 mg dose at bedtime.

the risk). Four of these drugs—estazolam, quazepam, temazepam, and triazolam—are classified in Category X (i.e., the risks of use during pregnancy clearly outweigh any possible benefits). *Women of child-bearing age should be warned about the potential for fetal harm and instructed to discontinue benzodiazepines if pregnancy occurs.*

Benzodiazepines enter breast milk with ease and may accumulate to toxic levels in the breast-fed infant. Accordingly, these drugs should be avoided by nursing mothers.

TOLERANCE AND PHYSICAL DEPENDENCE

With prolonged use of benzodiazepines, tolerance develops to some effects—but not to others. No tolerance develops to anxiolytic effects, and tolerance to hypnotic effects is generally low. In contrast, significant tolerance develops to antiseizure effects. Patients who are tolerant to barbiturates, alcohol, and other general CNS depressants show some cross-tolerance to benzodiazepines.

Benzodiazepines can cause physical dependence, but the incidence of *substantial* dependence is low. When benzodiazepines are discontinued following short-term use at therapeutic doses, the resultant withdrawal syndrome is generally mild and often goes unrecognized. Symptoms include anxiety, insomnia, sweating, tremors, and dizziness. Withdrawal from long-term high-dose therapy can elicit more serious reactions, such as panic, paranoia, delirium, hypertension, muscle twitches, and outright convulsions. Symptoms of withdrawal are usually more intense with benzodiazepines that have a short duration of action. With one agent—*alprazolam* (Xanax)—dependence may be a greater problem than with other benzodiazepines. Because benzodiazepine withdrawal syndrome can resemble an anxiety disorder, care must be taken to differentiate withdrawal from the return of original symptoms.

The intensity of withdrawal symptoms can be minimized by discontinuing treatment gradually. Doses should be tapered over several weeks. Substituting a benzodiazepine with a long half-life for one with a short half-life is also helpful. Patients should be warned against abrupt cessation of treatment. Following discontinuation of treatment, patients should be monitored for three weeks for indications of withdrawal or recurrence of original symptoms.

DRUG INTERACTIONS

Benzodiazepines undergo very few important interactions with other drugs. Unlike barbiturates, benzodiazepines do not induce hepatic drug-metabolizing enzymes. Benzodiazepines, therefore, do not accelerate the metabolism of other drugs.

CNS Depressants. The CNS-depressant actions of benzodiazepines will combine with those of other CNS depressants (e.g., alcohol, barbiturates, opioids). Although benzodiazepines are very safe when used alone, these drugs can be extremely hazardous in combination with other depressants. *Combined overdosage with a benzodiazepine plus another CNS depressant can cause profound respiratory depression, coma, and death.* Patients should be warned against use of alcohol and all other CNS depressants.

DOSAGE AND ADMINISTRATION

All benzodiazepines can be administered orally. In addition, three agents—diazepam, chlordiazepoxide, and lorazepam—may be administered parenterally (IM and IV). When used for sedation or induction of sleep, benzodiazepines are almost always administered by mouth. Intramuscular and intravenous administration are reserved for acute management of alcohol withdrawal, severe anxiety, status epilepticus, and other emergencies. Dosages for anxiety are summarized in Table 23–12.

Oral

Patients should be advised to take oral benzodiazepines with food if gastric upset occurs. Also, they should be instructed to swallow sustained-release formulations intact, without crushing or chewing. Patients should be warned not to increase the dosage or discontinue therapy without consulting the physician.

For treatment of insomnia, benzodiazepines should be given on an intermittent schedule (e.g., three or four days a week) in the lowest effective dosage for the shortest duration required. This minimizes physical dependence and associated drug-dependency insomnia.

Intravenous

Intravenous administration is hazardous and must be performed with care. Life-threatening reactions (e.g., severe hypotension, respiratory arrest, cardiac arrest) have occurred. In addition, IV administration carries a risk of venous thrombosis, phlebitis, and vascular impairment.

To reduce complications from IV administration, the following precautions should be taken: (1) inject the drug slowly; (2) take care to avoid intra-arterial injection and extravasation; (3) if direct venous injection is impossible, make the injection into infusion tubing as close to the vein as possible; (4) follow the manufacturer's instructions regarding suitable diluents for preparing solutions; and (5) have facilities for resuscitation available.

ACUTE TOXICITY

Oral Overdosage

When administered in excessive dosage by mouth, benzodiazepines rarely cause serious toxicity. Symptoms include drowsiness, lethargy, and confusion. Significant cardiovascular and respiratory effects are uncommon. If an individual known to have taken an overdose of benzodiazepines does exhibit signs of serious toxicity, it is probable that another drug was taken as well.

Intravenous Toxicity

When injected intravenously, even in therapeutic doses, benzodiazepines can cause severe adverse effects. Life-threatening reactions (e.g., profound hypotension, respiratory arrest, cardiac arrest) occur in approximately 2% of patients.

Treatment

General Treatment Measures. Benzodiazepine-induced toxicity is managed in the same fashion as toxicity from barbiturates and other general CNS depressants. Oral benzodiazepines can be removed from the body with gastric lavage followed by ingestion of activated charcoal and a saline cathartic; dialysis may be helpful if symptoms are especially severe. Respiration should be monitored, and the airway should be kept patent. Support of blood pressure with IV fluids and norepinephrine may be required.

Treatment with Flumazenil. Flumazenil (Romazicon) is a competitive benzodiazepine-receptor antagonist. The drug can reverse the sedative effects of benzodiazepines but may not reverse benzodiazepine-induced respiratory depression. Flumazenil is approved for treatment of benzodiazepine overdosage and for reversing the effects of benzodiazepines following general anesthesia. The principal adverse effect is precipitation of convulsions. This effect is most likely in patients taking benzodiazepines to treat epilepsy and in patients who are physically dependent on benzodiazepines.

Buspirone

Buspirone (BuSpar) is a new and different antianxiety medication. The drug has minimal CNS-depressant actions and does not enhance the depressant effects of alcohol, barbiturates, and other general CNS depressants. Buspirone is said to reduce anxiety while producing even less sedation than benzodiazepines. The drug is devoid of hypnotic, muscle relaxant, and anticonvulsant actions.

MECHANISM OF ACTION

The mechanism by which buspirone acts has not been established. The drug binds with high affinity to receptors for serotonin and with lower affinity to receptors for dopamine. Buspirone does not bind to receptors for GABA or benzodiazepines.

THERAPEUTIC USES

Buspirone is labeled for *short-term* treatment of *anxiety;* however, when taken for as long as one year, the drug showed no reduction in antianxiety actions. For treatment of anxiety, the drug appears to be as effective as benzodiazepines. Buspirone lacks sedative effects and is not indicated for insomnia. Use of buspirone is discussed further under *Management of Anxiety* later in the chapter.

ADVERSE EFFECTS AND DRUG INTERACTIONS

Buspirone is generally well tolerated. The most common reactions are *dizziness, nausea, headache, nervousness, lightheadedness,* and *excitement.* The drug is nonsedative and does not interfere with daytime activities. Furthermore, the drug poses little or no risk of suicide; huge doses (375 mg/day) have been given to healthy volunteers with only moderate effects (e.g., nausea, vomiting, dizziness, drowsiness, miosis). Buspirone does not enhance the depressant effects of alcohol, barbiturates, and other general CNS depressants.

TOLERANCE, DEPENDENCE, AND ABUSE

Buspirone has been used for up to one year without evidence of tolerance, physical dependence, or psychological dependence. No withdrawal symptoms have been observed upon termination of treatment. There is no cross-tolerance between buspirone and benzodiazepines, barbiturates, or other sedative-hypnotics.

To date, there is no evidence that buspirone has a liability for abuse. Accordingly, the drug is not regulated under the Controlled Substances Act.

Management of Anxiety

Anxiety is a nearly universal experience that often serves an adaptive function. When anxiety is moderate and situationally appropriate, drug therapy may not be needed or even desirable. In contrast, for patients with generalized anxiety disorder, symptoms are prolonged and potentially disabling; hence, anxiolytic therapy is frequently required.

Situational Anxiety Versus Generalized Anxiety Disorder

SITUATIONAL ANXIETY

Situational anxiety is a normal response to a stressful situation (e.g., family problems, examinations, financial difficulties). Although symptoms may be intense, they are also temporary. If necessary, drugs can be used to provide relief, but treatment should be short-term. Situational anxiety is common among patients with medical illnesses and those anticipating surgery.

GENERALIZED ANXIETY DISORDER

The hallmark of generalized anxiety disorder (GAD) is unrealistic or excessive anxiety about two or more life circumstances that lasts for six months or longer. Other psychological manifestations include vigilance, tension, apprehension, poor concentration, and difficulty falling asleep or staying asleep. Somatic manifestations include trembling, muscle tension, restlessness, and signs of autonomic hyperactivity (e.g., palpitations, tachycardia, sweating, clammy hands).

Treatment of GAD consists of psychotherapy and anxiolytic drugs. Psychotherapy provides support and encouragement and can improve coping abilities in anxiety-provoking situations. For some patients, this therapy may be all that is needed. However, if symptoms are intensely uncomfortable or disabling, antianxiety drugs are indicated. In most cases, benzodiazepines are preferred. Along with psychotherapy and drugs, the treatment program can include relaxation therapy (e.g., meditation, relaxation exercises, biofeedback) to reduce tension.

Drug Therapy of Anxiety

BENZODIAZEPINES

Benzodiazepines are drugs of first choice for anxiety. These widely used agents have rendered older anxiolytics obsolete. Since all benzodiazepines have very similar CNS effects, selection among these drugs is largely a matter of prescriber's preference. Dosages for anxiety are summarized in Table 23–12.

Since the introduction of benzodiazepines in the 1960s, attitudes toward these drugs have changed. When they first became available, benzodiazepines were used somewhat indiscriminately. In all probability, many people who did not really need these drugs were receiving them. Because of the freedom with which benzodiazepines had been dispensed, physicians were sometimes accused of poor medical practice. Furthermore, the frequent use of benzodiazepines led to public concerns about "addiction." In response to these developments, two changes took place: (1) physicians restricted their prescribing of benzodiazepines, and (2) patients tended to self-administer less medication than had been prescribed. The unfortunate result is that overtreatment was to some extent replaced with undertreatment.

The current consensus is that benzodiazepines have a completely legitimate role in the therapy of severe anxiety and that these drugs, like all others, must simply be used with discretion. When they are clearly indicated, benzodiazepines should be prescribed in a sufficient dosage and for a sufficient duration to achieve their objective: relief of symptoms and improvement of overall function. To help ensure that benzodiazepines are taken as prescribed, patients should be made to feel that their use of an anxiolytic is appropriate and that they should not be ashamed of their legitimate medical need. Also, patients should be made aware that significant tolerance and physical dependence are unlikely.

It is difficult to predict how long anxiolytic drugs should be taken. To determine the need for continued therapy, patients should be re-evaluated on a regular basis. In some cases, use of an "on-off" dosing schedule may be helpful. In such a regimen, treatment is interrupted periodically (e.g., every six to eight weeks). If anxiety returns, treatment can resume.

BUSPIRONE

Buspirone (BuSpar) is an alternative to benzodiazepines for treating anxiety. This drug differs from benzodiazepines in four important ways: (1) it does not cause sedation, (2) it has no abuse potential, (3) it does not potentiate other CNS depressants, and (4) its antianxiety effects take one week to begin and several weeks to reach their peak. Because therapeutic effects are delayed, buspirone is not suitable for patients who need immediate relief, nor is it suitable for PRN use. Since buspirone has no abuse potential, the drug may be especially appropriate for patients known to abuse alcohol and other drugs. Because it lacks depressant properties, buspirone is an attractive alternative to benzodiazepines in patients who require long-term therapy but who cannot tolerate benzodiazepine-induced sedation and psychomotor slowing. Buspirone does not display cross-dependence with benzodiazepines. Hence, when patients are switched from benzodiazepines to buspirone, the benzodiazepine should be tapered off prior to initiating buspirone (in order to prevent a withdrawal syndrome). Patients who have taken benzodiazepines should be told that buspirone will not produce sedation and that its effects will take one week or more to develop; this information will allow expectations to be realistic.

BETA BLOCKERS

Beta-adrenergic blocking agents (e.g., propranolol) can relieve symptoms caused by autonomic hyperactivity (tachycardia). These drugs may be most valuable as an aid to coping with situational anxiety, such as that experienced by individuals who are overly apprehensive about public speaking.

▶ Check Your Reading

21. Why are benzodiazepines preferred to barbiturates and other general CNS depressants for treating anxiety?
22. Are physical dependence and withdrawal concerns with benzodiazepine therapy?
23. What are the principal differences between benzodiazepines and buspirone?
24. How long should antianxiety therapy last?

NURSING PROCESS

In the past, initiation of psychopharmacological intervention was the prerogative of the treating psychiatrist, but currently over 40 states have granted prescriptive authority to Certified Specialists in Psychiatric and Mental Health Nursing. Regardless of whether the prescriber is a psychiatrist or an advanced practice nurse, the decision about which medication to use is based on several factors, including the patient's preference and responsiveness to a particular drug(s) in the past; a family member's treatment response; the drug's side effect profile; and the clinician's own observations about efficacy. Often, however, the decision to change to another medication is based on the observations and documentation of nurses regarding the patient's responsiveness or lack of responsiveness to a medication. Therefore, it is imperative that you understand not only the goals of treatment but also the effects of medications. The application of the nursing process to the patient receiving psychopharmacologic therapy will of course depend on the specific patient and the specific disorder being treated. However, to give an example of the application of the nursing process to the patient receiving psychopharmacologic therapy, we will consider the psychopharmacologic treatment of schizophrenia. To begin, let's take a look at Loren's story to understand the importance of medication issues to the schizophrenic patient (Case Example 23–1).

Case Example 23–1 Loren's Story

Loren Evans was a 35-year-old white female who was separated from her husband. The couple had been married for 15 years and were parents of two boys, ages 8 and 11, who were in the custody of their father. Loren had a diagnosis of schizophrenia—chronic undifferentiated type (CUT). The onset of her illness occurred at age 18 when she was a sophomore in college majoring in nursing. She reported several inpatient admissions and was being treated on an outpatient basis at a research center. She attended weekly group therapy sessions. Over the past three years, Loren participated in several drug treatment protocols and was now on a study designed to determine the lowest possible dose of a neuroleptic required to control for psychotic symptoms. The protocol required that Loren go on a drug-free trial period from the medication regimen of Prolixin 10 mg t.i.d. To observe for signs and symptoms of recurring illness, she had been referred to a home health agency. A request was made for a psychiatric certified specialist to perform weekly assessments to monitor mental status as Loren was titrated off medication and to perform health teaching about the earliest prodromal symptoms signaling impending acute recurrence. Loren has been medication free for the past three months. During that time, she experienced three major stressors: (1) the break-up of a relationship with an older man; (2) an allergic reaction to penicillin, which was treated with prednisone; and (3) refusal by her estranged husband to allow Loren unsupervised visits with her children. Over the past two weeks, Loren has exhibited mild anxiety and difficulty sleeping. She also has expressed dissatisfaction with her outpatient treatment and has expressed an intent to withdraw from the program. The certified specialist was concerned that Loren was beginning to exhibit subtle signs and symptoms of impending illness and reported her observations to the treatment team at Loren's outpatient program. Two days following the last home visit, Loren presented at her therapy session in an acutely agitated state and was subsequently admitted to an inpatient unit with a diagnosis of acute exacerbation of schizophrenia—CUT. She was again started on an antipsychotic medication, and two weeks following the admission was discharged to an outpatient program. She exercised her right to refuse treatment at the research center and opted instead for a day treatment program, which combined pharmacological interventions with a psychosocial component.

INITIAL PHASE OF ILLNESS

Assessment

During the initial phase of the patient's illness, you assess the presence of psychotic behavior. Questions you might ask include:

Is the patient willing to take the medication? If so, by what route?
Is the patient likely to "cheek" or hide pills in his or her mouth?
Is he or she more likely to swallow a liquid preparation?

Will the patient require intramuscular administration of medication?

Is the patient aggressively acting out? If so, will you need help in administering medication?

Does the patient understand the need for medication?

Diagnosis

The nursing diagnosis during the initial phase of treatment might be Ineffective Individual Coping related to auditory hallucinations as evidenced by agitation, pacing, insomnia, and threatening gestures.

Outcome Identification

The expected outcome of the initial phase of treatment is normalization of behavior and is expressed as follows:

> The patient's behavior will return to normal as evidenced by cessation of agitation, pacing, and threatening gestures and by sleeping 7 to 8 hours per night at the end of one week of receiving antipsychotic medication.

Planning and Implementation

Because the patient is in a state of acute psychosis and may be uncooperative to the point of refusing medication (particularly with pills, which are easily cheeked), you need to plan "how" medication will be administered. For instance, in the case of a patient who is a threat to others, you might obtain an order to administer the medication intramuscularly. You must know which medications are available in intramuscular and in liquid forms and which are not. You can change the form of medication (pill to liquid) without the physician's order, but you cannot change the route of administration (oral to intramuscular) without a specific written order. Indeed, in an acutely ill patient a liquid preparation has a more rapid onset of action than the pill form. You are exercising clinical judgment in determining the form of medication to readily achieve the aim of bringing behavior under control.

Evaluation

In the first phase of treatment, successful medication management is demonstrated by a decrease in the level of agitation, hostility, combativeness, and aggressiveness displayed by the patient. Also, usual patterns of sleep and eating patterns begin to return.

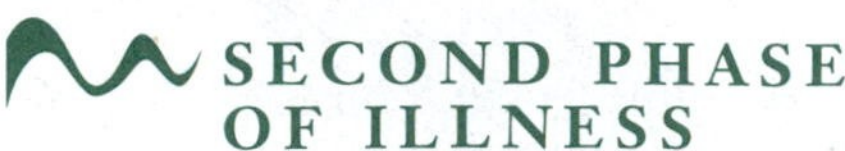

SECOND PHASE OF ILLNESS

Assessment

The second phase of the patient's illness is characterized by stabilization. This phase extends from one to three weeks and is characterized by the gradual reduction in the medication dosage. During the phase of stabilization, you monitor the patient's behavior for any signs and symptoms of recurring illness. It is during this phase that you assess for improvement in socialization, mood, and self-care activities. Because the patient may no longer be acutely psychotic and may be amenable to health teaching, you assess the patient's level of knowledge about the illness and the medications.

Diagnosis

The nursing diagnosis during the phase of stabilization might be: Knowledge Deficit about the effects and side effects of antipsychotic medications related to the unfamiliarity with the illness and treatment as evidenced by patient's verbalization of incomplete or inaccurate information.

Outcome Identification

The expected outcome of the stabilization phase is as follows:

> The patient/family will be able to state the effects and side effects of the prescribed antipsychotic medication and will verbalize willingness to adhere to medication schedule.

Planning and Implementation

Plan how to teach the patient and the patient's family about the illness as well as the medications that the patient is taking. Teaching focuses on identifying prodromal signs and symptoms and on encouraging the patient's active cooperation in self-reporting symptoms. The patient can be taught to be aware of even the slightest feelings of tension, anxiety, and unusual thoughts. Medication teaching focuses on knowing what the medication does, what side effects it produces, how to cope with side effects, and any adverse effects that the patient need to monitor.

Figures 23–3 through 23–5 show sample medication teaching tools that are appropriate to use in patient/family education for patients with schizophrenia. Figures 23–7 to 23–9 show similar teaching tools for use in patient/family education for patients with depression, mania, or anxiety.

Evaluation

Evaluation of the teaching plan can be done by verbal return demonstration to show that the patient understands the teaching, or a written test can be used to evaluate the level of learning that has taken place. Figure 23–6 shows a sample medication pre-post test used in evaluation.

Patient: ______________________________

Provider: ______________________________

Date: ______________________________

THORAZINE FACT SHEET

Trade Name: Thorazine

Generic Name: chlorpromazine

Purpose: To relieve the symptoms of your illness, including voices, visions, bothersome thoughts that you can't control, excessive fearfulness, believing people are saying bad things about you, thinking you have special powers, etc.

Warnings:

- Notify your doctor if pregnant or planning a pregnancy.
- Do not drive or operate machinery until you know how you will react to this medicine.
- Avoid drinking alcohol while taking this medicine.
- If your skin or the whites of your eyes get yellow or you get unexplainable sore throat, fever, and weakness, call your doctor *IMMEDIATELY.*
- Can cause tardive dyskinesia (TD). *IF* this occurs, it is slowly progressive, potentially irreversible involuntary movements of mouth, lips, and extremities. Your doctor will monitor and discuss continuing this medication with you.
- Always tell your doctor *all* medicines you are taking.
- Do not stop taking your medicine without your doctor's approval. The dosage should be slowly decreased. Stopping all at once may cause withdrawal symptoms.
- Do not give this medication to other people.
- If you need an antacid, take it two hours before or after this medication.
- During summer when it is hot and you are sweating more, increase fluids.
- If you have a seizure disorder, the frequency or severity of seizures may increase. Tell your doctor right away.

Common Side Effects	What To Do
Shakiness, restlessness, stiffness, thick tongue, neck twisting, eyes rolling up	Take your ________________ as prescribed. This medication is used to treat these symptoms. If you have no medication to treat these symptoms, call your doctor or go to Emergency Room.
Dizziness	Drink fluids, change position slowly.
Blurred vision	Should clear up in 2–3 weeks.
Sensitivity to the sun	Wear a sun block outside. Wear protective clothing.
Constipation	Eat bulk foods, drink fluids, drink prune juice, exercise.
Dry mouth	Suck on sugarless hard candy or chew gum. Practice meticulous dental care.

- You are taking _______ mg _______ times a day. Do not stop taking without your doctor's supervision as your symptoms may occur.
- If you miss a dose and remember within 2–3 hours, take it. Otherwise, skip it and take remaining doses as scheduled. DO NOT double up.

FIGURE 23–3

Medication teaching tool for Thorazine (chlorpromazine). (From Carson, V. B. [1994]. *Bay area psychiatric home care manual.* Baltimore: Bay Area Health Care. Copyright © 1994, Bay Area Health Care.)

Patient: ______________________________

Provider: ______________________________

Date: ______________________________

CLOZARIL FACT SHEET

Trade Name: Clozaril

Generic Name: clozapine

Purpose: To relieve the symptoms of your illness, including voices, visions, bothersome thoughts that you can't control, excessive fearfulness, believing people are saying bad things about you, thinking you have special powers, etc.

Warnings:

- This drug can cause your white blood cell count to fall very low (agranulocytosis) and reduce your ability to fight infection. Weekly blood tests are essential. Your prescription cannot be filled without proof of weekly blood tests.
- Do not drive or operate machinery until you know how you will react to this medicine.
- Avoid drinking alcohol while taking this medicine.
- Always tell your doctor *all* medicines you are taking.
- Do not stop taking your medicine without your doctor's approval. The dosage should be slowly decreased. Stopping all at once may cause withdrawal symptoms.
- Do not give this medication to other people.
- If you need an antacid, take it two hours before or after this medication.
- During summer when it is hot and you are sweating more, increase fluids.
- Keep all appointments with your doctor and the laboratory so that your response to this drug can be evaluated. Your dose may need to be adjusted, especially during the first few weeks.

Common Side Effects	What To Do
Flu-like symptoms, sore throat, weakness, fever, mouth sores, any sign of infection	Stop taking clozapine and contact your prescriber immediately.
Seizures, tremor	Stop taking clozapine and contact your prescriber immediately.
Fast or irregular heart beat, difficulty breathing	Stop taking clozapine and contact your prescriber immediately.

- You are taking _______ mg _______ times a day. Do not stop taking without your doctor's supervision as your symptoms may occur.
- If you miss a dose and remember within 2–3 hours, take it. Otherwise, skip it and take remaining doses as scheduled. DO NOT double up.

FIGURE 23–4

Medication teaching tool for Clozaril (clozapine). (Modified from Carson, V. B. [1994]. *Bay area psychiatric home care manual.* Baltimore: Bay Area Health Care. Copyright © 1994, Bay Area Health Care.)

Patient: ______________________________

Provider: ______________________________

Date: ______________________________

PROLIXIN FACT SHEET

Trade Name: Prolixin

Generic Name: fluphenazine

Purpose: To relieve the symptoms of your illness, including voices, visions, bothersome thoughts that you can't control, excessive fearfulness, believing people are saying bad things about you, thinking you have special powers, etc.

Warnings:

- Notify your doctor if pregnant or planning a pregnancy.
- Do not drive or operate machinery until you know how you will react to this medicine.
- Avoid drinking alcohol while taking this medicine.
- If your skin or the whites of your eyes get yellow or you get unexplainable sore throat, fever and weakness, call your doctor *IMMEDIATELY.*
- Can cause tardive dyskinesia (TD). *IF* this occurs, it is slowly progressive, irreversible involuntary movements of mouth, lips and extremities. Your doctor will monitor and discuss continuing this medication with you.
- Always tell your doctor *all* medicines you are taking.
- Do not stop taking your medicine without your doctor's approval. The dosage should be slowly decreased. Stopping all at once may cause withdrawal symptoms.
- Do not give this medication to other people.
- If you need an antacid, take it two hours before or after this medication.
- During summer when it is hot and you are sweating more, increase fluids.
- If you are allergic to aspirin or yellow dye (present in some foods and medications), tell your doctor.
- If you have ever had a bad reaction to insulin, shock therapy or any other tranquilizer, notify your doctor immediately.
- Before *any type* of surgery with a general anesthetic, tell the doctor you are taking prolixin.

Common Side Effects	What To Do
Shakiness, restlessness, stiffness, thick tongue, neck twisting, eyes rolling up	Take your ______________ as prescribed. This medication is used to treat these symptoms. If you have no medication to treat these symptoms, call your doctor or go to Emergency Room.
Dizziness	Drink fluids, change position slowly.
Blurred vision	Should clear up in 2–3 weeks.
Sensitivity to the sun	Wear a sun block outside. Wear protective clothing.
Constipation	Eat bulk foods, drink fluids, drink prune juice, exercise.
Dry mouth	Suck on sugarless hard candy or chew gum. Practice meticulous dental care.

- You are taking ________ mg ________ times a day. Do not stop taking without your doctor's supervision as your symptoms may occur.
- If you miss a dose and remember within 2–3 hours, take it. Otherwise, skip it and take remaining doses as scheduled. DO NOT double up.

FIGURE 23–5

Medication teaching tool for Prolixin (fluphenazine). (From Carson, V. B. [1994]. *Bay area psychiatric home care manual.* Baltimore: Bay Area Health Care. Copyright © 1994, Bay Area Health Care.)

MEDICATION PRE-POST TEST

PATIENT: ______________________________

NURSE: ______________________________

DATE: ______________________ **SCORE:** ______________

1. I am taking (name medication[s]).
2. I am taking ______________ mg ______________ times per day.
3. My schedule is ______________________________.
4. My medication helps me:
   a. Feel less sad.
   b. Feel less nervous.
   c. Feel less bothered by bad thoughts I can't control.
   d. Other (list any other benefits).
5. If I miss a dose of my medicine, I should:
   a. Double up on the next dose.
   b. If I remember to take it close to the regularly scheduled time, I should take it and stay with my normal schedule.
   c. If it is several hours from when I should have taken it, I will forget the missed dose and get right back on my normal schedule with the next dose.
6. My medication may make me feel drowsy and even clumsy. When I first begin taking the medicine it is a good idea to:
   a. Stay at home all the time until I feel more alert and sharper in my thinking.
   b. Avoid driving a car or operating machinery until I know how I will react to this medicine.
   c. Avoid taking the medicine right before I need to be alert in my actions and thinking.
   d. Tell my doctor I want another medication.
7. If I am going to have surgery, even dental surgery, I should:
   a. Stop taking medication the day before the surgery.
   b. Tell my surgeon all the medications I am taking.
   c. Take more of my medication right before surgery to put me in a better state of mind.
8. Before drinking any alcohol, whether in beer, wine, whiskey, wine coolers, or over-the-counter medications, I should:
   a. Stop taking my medication.
   b. Talk to my doctor about whether it is safe or not to mix alcohol with this medicine.
   c. Read the label on the bottle or package containing the alcohol to see what I should do.
9. If I am taking this medicine, there are certain things that I should tell my doctor. Please check off at least three things from the following list:
   ___ a. I have a history of an eating disorder.
   ___ b. I have a history of seizures.
   ___ c. I am pregnant or want to become pregnant.
   ___ d. I am breast-feeding.
   ___ e. I am taking other medications.
   ___ f. I have certain allergies.
   ___ g. I have a history of heart problems or high blood pressure or have had a recent heart attack.
   ___ h. I have a history of kidney disease.
   ___ i. I am a diabetic.
10. A friend asks me for a dose of my medicine to help him/her feel better. I should:
    a. Refuse and explain that the medicine may make him/her sick.
    b. Give one dose away just so the friend can see if it helps or not.
    c. Freely share my medicine with other people who have the same symptoms as I.

If you are taking a medication to make you feel less sad, please answer the next four questions.

11. My medication can produce some side effects that are bothersome but not serious. These include (please choose at least two from the following list):
    ___ a. Drowsiness, feeling tired, weak.
    ___ b. Excitement, insomnia, blurred vision.
    ___ c. Lightheadedness when I get up too quickly from lying down or sitting to a standing position.
    ___ d. Sensitive to sunlight.
    ___ e. Dry mouth.
    ___ f. Constipation, blurred vision, difficulty urinating.

FIGURE 23–6

Medication pre- post test. (From Carson, V. B. [1994]. *Bay area psychiatric home care manual.* Baltimore: Bay Area Health Care. Copyright © 1994, Bay Area Health Care.)

12. My medication does not make me feel better right away. It may take as long as:
    a. Two to three weeks.
    b. Three to four weeks.
    c. Five to six weeks.

13. Most of the side effects that my medication produces can be dealt with easily. Column A lists the side effects and Column B lists the common remedies. Please match the remedy with the side effect.

Column A	**Column B**
____ a. Drowsiness	____ 1. Take medicine with meals
____ b. Excitement, insomnia	____ 2. Wear sunblock and hat
____ c. Sensitive to sunlight	____ 3. Chew sugarless gum and suck on sugarless hard candy.
____ d. Dry mouth	____ 4. Eat more bulk foods, drink more water.
____ e. Constipation	____ 5. Take medicine at bedtime.
____ f. Nausea	____ 6. Take medicine in morning.

14. There are some side effects that I should immediately tell my doctor about. Which of the following fall into that category (check all that apply)?
    ____ a. High fever, chills, sore throat.
    ____ b. Change in skin color.
    ____ c. Any unusual bleeding.
    ____ d. Swelling of feet and lower legs.
    ____ e. Headache.
    ____ f. Diarrhea.

If you are taking medicine to make you feel less nervous, please answer the next three questions.

15. My medication can be habit forming. I should:
    a. Take the medication exactly as my doctor tells me to.
    b. Only take the medication when I feel desperate.
    c. Stop taking the medication as soon as I feel better.

16. When I feel better, I should:
    a. Stop taking the medication.
    b. Work with my doctor on a schedule to wean me off the medication.

17. Stopping the medication abruptly can cause me to:
    a. Have a heart attack and other coronary complications.
    b. Have seizures and experience withdrawal.
    c. Need more of the medication.

If you are taking a medicine to help you feel less bothered by troublesome thoughts you cannot control, please answer the following four questions.

18. My medicine can cause some unpleasant side effects that involve unusual movements. If I notice that I can't sit still (I have dancing feet) and I feel jittery inside, or I am experiencing spasms of my muscles in my face or other places in my body, I probably need to take some cogentin, benadryl, artane, or amantadine as ordered by my doctor. If I do not have any of these medicines available, I should:
    a. Stop taking my medicine.
    b. Call my doctor immediately or go to an emergency department.
    c. Take a double dose of my medication.

19. My medication can cause tardive dyskinesia, a more serious movement disorder with jerky movements of the face and extremities. If this happens to me, my doctor will probably:
    a. Increase the dose of my medicine.
    b. Decrease the dose of my medicine.
    c. Stop my medication immediately.

20. Because of the side effects of my medicine, my doctor may have also placed me on another medication, such as benadryl, cogentin, artance, kemedrin, akineton, or amantadine. These medications are used to control:
    a. The movement problems that come with my medicine.
    b. The dry mouth and constipation that come with my medicine.
    c. The blurred vision that comes with my medicine.

FIGURE 23–6 *Continued*

Illustration continued on following page

21. These additional drugs also have side effects. These include:
    a. Dry mouth, blurred vision, constipation.
    b. Fast heart beat.
    c. Seizures.
    d. Parkinson's disease.

If you are taking Tegretol or Dilantin please answer the following question.

22. Sometimes the dose of my medicine must be adjusted. Because of this it is important that I:
    a. Get my blood drawn so that my doctor can monitor how much of the medicine is in my system.
    b. Eat a balanced diet with 8 full glasses of water a day.
    c. Collect my urine for 24 hours to see that I am urinating the right amount.

FIGURE 23–6 *Continued*

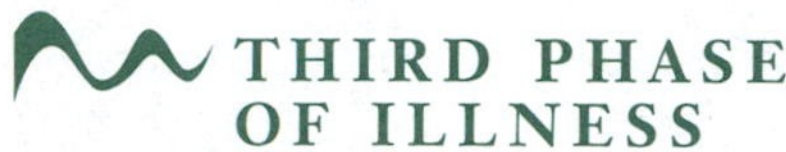

THIRD PHASE OF ILLNESS

Assessment

The third stage is the *maintenance* phase of treatment. The goal of maintenance is to maintain the patient on the lowest possible dose of medication. At this stage, the patient is probably being treated as an outpatient. Those who have experienced a first episode may not require prolonged treatment and may be gradually withdrawn from medications over a period of three to six months. During the third phase of the patient's illness assess for:

Stress in the patient's life (beginning employment, returning to school)
Level of knowledge and compliance with medication
Emotional issues such as powerlessness
Spiritual issues such as the belief that the individual is lacking in faith if he relies on medication; that he or she must not be good enough for God to heal him or her; that the illness is a punishment from God therefore he or she should not take medication.

Diagnosis

The nursing diagnoses during the maintenance stage focus on coping with stress, increasing knowledge, enhancing compliance, decreasing feelings of powerlessness, and relieving spiritual distress in the patient. Appropriate nursing diagnoses might include:

- Ineffective Individual Coping related to multiple stressors as evidenced by verbalizations of nervousness and decreased ability to concentrate
- Knowledge Deficit related to medication action as evidenced by patient's inability to state reason for taking medication
- Noncompliance related to discomfort of side effects of antipsychotic medication as evidenced by increasing disorganization in thoughts and verbalizations regarding the negative effects of medication
- Powerlessness related to inability to control illness as evidenced by verbalizations that medication is a crutch and that patient is weak
- Spiritual Distress related to patient's disappointment that God does not heal him or her as evidenced by verbalizations such as "I must not be good enough, or God would cure me without medications"

Outcome Identification

The expected outcome of the maintenance stage is reducing the medication to the lowest level that maintains stable behavior and could be expressed as:

- The patient's behavior will remain stable, oriented to reality, and nonaggressive while on a low dose of antipsychotic medication.
- The patient will exhibit effective coping strategies.
- The patient will verbalize an understanding of medication purpose, side effects, and schedule.
- The patient will verbalize that control over illness exists in decisions to understand and take medications.
- The patient will discuss feelings toward God and recognize that God uses multiple avenues for healing including medications.

Planning and Implementation

Your nursing interventions include the following:

Teach the patient coping abilities to deal with stress.

Reinforce medication and other health-related teaching with emphasis on acknowledging the role of stress in precipitating acute exacerbations of illness.

Negotiate with the patient ways to increase compliance, i.e., changing the time the medication is taken or the form or using medication boxes to assist patient in remembering when to take medication.

Acknowledge the patient's feelings of powerlessness over the illness and the inability to control symptoms without medications.

Emphasize the areas of life where the patient retains control.

Empathize with the spiritual distress that frequently accompanies chronic illnesses where medication useage is a fact of life.

Discuss spiritual beliefs that impact on medication use and offer alternative view on the use of medication as a healing tool of God

Patients whose illness is chronic (two or more episodes) may be maintained on a single dose of medication that can be administered at bedtime. Nighttime administration helps to minimize the sedative effect of many of the antipsychotics. This sedative effect during the daytime interferes with social participation as well as participation in nonpharmacological treatments, which are also of value in returning the patient to an optimal state of functioning. Chronically mentally ill patients may display persistent symptoms that are not responsive to traditional medication management, i.e., fixed systematized delusions, impaired insight, inappropriate effect. These patients may be excellent candidates for the use of clozapine or risperadone.

Evaluation

Evaluation includes reviewing whether the patient's symptom profile is improved, whether he or she is compliant with the medication regimen, and whether he or she is knowledgeable about the prescribed medication.

Patient: ______________________________

Provider: ______________________________

Date: ______________________________

PAMELOR FACT SHEET

Trade Name: Pamelor

Generic Name: nortriptyline

Purpose: This drug is used to treat depression.

Warnings:

- This drug can take 2–3 weeks to work.
- Do not drive or operate machinery until you know how you'll react to this medication.
- Always tell your doctor *all* medicines you are taking.
- See your doctor regularly for check-ups.
- Ask your doctor for advice about drinking alcoholic beverages.
- Women who are pregnant, plan to become pregnant, or are breast-feeding should inform their doctor.
- Do not allow anyone else to take this medication.
- Before surgery, inform your doctor you are taking this drug.
- This drug can cause an irregular heart beat.

FIGURE 23–7

Medication teaching tool for Pamelor (nortriptyline). (From Carson, V. B. [1994]. *Bay area psychiatric home care manual.* Baltimore: Bay Area Health Care. Copyright © 1994, Bay Area Health Care.)

Illustration continued on following page

Common Side Effects	What To Do
Drowsiness, weakness, tiredness, excitement, insomnia, blurred vision, difficulty urinating	Take this drug at bedtime if it causes drowsiness. Take this drug in the morning if it causes insomnia. If you take the drug more than once a day, ask your doctor if you can take it all at once. These symptoms should decrease over time. If they do not, contact your doctor.
Dizziness, lightheadedness, faintness when getting up from a sitting or lying position	Get up slowly.
Persistent fine tremor; shuffling walk; slow speech; difficulty swallowing; drooling; slow, jerky movements; jaw, neck, and back muscle spasms; inability to sit still; sore throat; fever; skin rash; yellowing of skin or eyes; irregular heart beat	Contact your doctor.
Sensitivity to the sun	Wear protective clothing and sunscreen when out in the sun.
Constipation, difficulty urinating, blurred vision	Contact your doctor if these symptoms are severe or persist.

- You are taking ______ mg ______ times a day. Your schedule is ______________________________ .
- If you miss a dose and remember within 2–3 hours, take it. Otherwise, skip it and take the remaining doses as scheduled. DO NOT double up.

FIGURE 23–7 *Continued*

Patient: ____________________

Provider: ____________________

Date: ____________________

NARDIL FACT SHEET

Trade Name: Nardil

Generic Name: phenelzine

Purpose: This drug is a monoamine oxidase inhibitor (MAOI) and is used to treat depression and anxiety.

Warnings:

- Avoid foods and beverages containing tyramine while taking medication and for two weeks after stopping medication. These foods and beverages include avocados (especially if overripe); fermented bean curd; fermented soybean; soybean paste; figs (especially if overripe); bananas (in large amounts); meats that are fermented, smoked, or otherwise aged; spoiled meats; liver (unless *very* fresh); fermented sausages such as bologna, pepperoni, and salami; dried or cured fish; fish that is fermented, smoked, or otherwise aged; spoiled fish; practically all cheeses; yeast extract (e.g., Marmite, Bovril); imported beers; Chianti wine; protein dietary supplements; soups (may contain protein extract); shrimp paste; and soy sauce. Also avoid chocolate, fava beans, ginseng, and caffeinated beverages.
- If you experience a severe headache, neck stiffness or soreness, nausea or vomiting, sweating (with fever or cold, clammy skin), dilated (large) pupils and increases sensitivity to light, and rapid or slow heart beat with chest pain, stop taking the medication and call your doctor immediately. These may be signs of an extreme rise in blood pressure.
- Do not drive or operate machinery until you know how you will react to this medication.
- Always tell your doctor *all* medicines you are taking and never take any medicines or drugs without asking your doctor first.
- See your doctor regularly for check-ups.
- Do not stop taking this medication without talking to your doctor.
- Ask your doctor for advice about drinking alcoholic beverages.
- Women who are pregnant, plan to become pregnant, or are breast-feeding should inform their doctor.

Common Side Effects	What To Do
Dizziness; lightheadedness; faintness when getting up from a sitting or lying position.	Get up slowly.
Dry mouth.	Suck sugarless hard candy or chew sugarless gum.
Restlessness; difficulty sleeping; constipation; difficulty urinating; loss of appetite; drowsiness; weakness; fatigue; rash; swelling of feet, ankles or lower legs; blurred vision; decreased sexual ability.	Contact your doctor if these symptoms persist or are severe.

- You are taking ______ mg nardil ______ times a day. Your schedule is ____________________
- If you miss a dose and remember within 2–3 hours, take it. Otherwise, skip it and take remaining doses as scheduled. DO NOT double up.

FIGURE 23–8

Medication teaching tool for Nardil (phenelzine). (Modified from Carson, V. B. [1994]. *Bay area psychiatric home care manual.* Baltimore: Bay Area Health Care. Copyright © 1994, Bay Area Health Care.)

Patient: ______________________________

Provider: ______________________________

Date: ______________________________

LITHIUM FACT SHEET

Trade Names: Cibalith-S, Eskalith, Eskalith CR, Lithane, Lithobid, Lithonate, Lithotabs

Generic Name: lithium

Purpose: This drug stabilizes the mood of people with manic-depressive illness (extreme mood changes from depression or anger to elation). It is also used investigatively to treat other mental conditions and illnesses.

Warnings:

- Lithium can decrease alertness and coordination. Do not drive a car or operate dangerous machinery until you know how this drug affects you.
- Keep all appointments with your doctor and the laboratory. You probably will have blood tests periodically to monitor the amount of lithium in your blood and also urine tests, especially if you experience side effects. Your dose may need to be adjusted occasionally.
- Drink 12 full glasses of water or other beverages each day (unless your doctor tells you otherwise) and use a moderate amount of salt on your food. However, if your doctor puts you on a low-salt or low-sodium diet, follow it.
- Avoid beverages with sugar because sugar causes cavities in your teeth and caffeine increases urination, which may alter the effect of lithium.
- If you are pregnant, may become pregnant, or are breast-feeding, tell your doctor before taking lithium. If you become pregnant, notify your doctor promptly.
- Many drugs can alter the effect of lithium. Before you take lithium, tell your doctor what prescription and nonprescription drugs you are taking. All of your doctors and dentists should know that you take lithium so that they can avoid prescribing drugs, especially ibuprofen (Advil, Motrin, or Nuprin) and sodium bicarbonate and other antacids containing sodium without consulting your doctor.
- If you are allergic to aspirin or tartrazine (yellow dye present in some processed foods and medications, including lithium) or have thyroid, kidney, heart or blood vessel disease, tell your doctor before taking lithium.
- Do not allow anyone else to take this medication.

Common Side Effects	What To Do
Nausea; loss of appetite; stomach bloating; abdominal pain.	Take lithium with meals. If these effects persist, contact your doctor.
Fine tremor of the hands.	Avoid beverages that contain caffeine (coffee, tea and cola). If the tremor worsens, spreads to other parts of the body, or is bothersome, call your doctor.
Headache; mild loss of memory; confusion; acne.	If these problems are bothersome, contact your doctor.
Dry, coarse skin; hair loss; mental dullness; sensitivity to cold; fatigue; sleepiness; slow reflexes; weight gain.	Contact your doctor.

FIGURE 23–9

Medication teaching tool for lithium. (From Carson, V.B. [1994]. *Bay area psychiatric home care manual.* Baltimore: Bay Area Health Care. Copyright © 1994, Bay Area Health Care.)

Common Side Effects	What To Do
Dry mouth; thirst; increased urination.	Drink plenty of water (or other beverages), especially if you have vomiting, diarrhea or a fever. Contact your doctor if you have increased urination or prolonged vomiting, diarrhea or a fever.
Lithium intoxication: shaking of the hands; muscle twitching; weakness or incoordination; vomiting; diarrhea; drowsiness.	Stop taking the medication and contact your doctor immediately.

- You are taking ______ mg nardil ______ times a day. Your schedule is ______________________________ ____.
- If you miss a dose and remember within 2–3 hours, take it. Otherwise, skip it and take remaining doses as scheduled. DO NOT double up.

LITHIUM TOXICITY

Symptoms: Feels like you are drunk (slurred speech, staggering walk, bad shakes, confused) and with the "flu" (nausea, vomiting, diarrhea).

If you have these symptoms, it may mean you have too much lithium in your blood. DO NOT TAKE THE NEXT DOSE OF LITHIUM. CALL YOUR DOCTOR OR GO TO EMERGENCY ROOM TO HAVE SOME BLOOD DRAWN FOR A LITHIUM LEVEL.

How to prevent this from happening:

1. Take lithium *exactly* as prescribed by your doctor.
2. Get lab work done as soon as doctor requests it.
3. DO NOT change the amount of salt or fluids you are taking in.
4. Tell your doctor if you are sick with the flu—vomiting or diarrhea—or if you have a kidney infection.
5. Tell your doctor if you get put on "water pills."
6. Drink a bit more fluid when it's hot and you are sweating.
7. Let your doctor know if you go on any special diet for weight, blood pressure, etc.

FIGURE 23–9 *Continued*

CONCLUSIONS

As with drug therapy of somatic disorders, drug therapy of mental illnesses has made a lot of progress but still has a long way to go. During the last four decades, we have developed powerful drugs that can provide symptomatic relief for many patients. Unfortunately, for many others, treatment remains largely ineffective. Much of the difficulty resides with our incomplete understanding of mental illness: if we don't really understand the disorders we are trying to treat (and we don't), we have no rational basis for developing new drugs to treat them. Fortunately, with the rapid advances being made in psychiatry and neuroscience, there is reason to hope that safer and more effective psychotherapeutic agents will soon be forthcoming.

Does the availability of psychotherapeutic drugs relieve you of your responsibility to provide good nursing care? Obviously not. In fact, with the advent of these drugs, nursing responsibilities have actually increased. If treatment is to be optimal, the nurse must evaluate the patient for a therapeutic response. Armed with this information, the prescriber will be in a better position to make dosage adjustments or the decision to switch to another drug (if your evaluation shows that the current selection is not working). In addition to helping optimize therapeutic effects, it is your responsibility to help minimize adverse effects. This is done by observing the patient for adverse effects and intervening as needed. Of equal importance, you must educate patients and their families about possible adverse effects along with measures to minimize discomfort or harm. Clearly, by providing informed and conscientious nursing care and patient education, you can greatly increase the chances of achieving the therapeutic goal: production of maximum benefit with minimal harm. Conversely, if the care and education that you offer are inadequate . . . well, we know that won't happen.

KEY POINTS TO REMEMBER

• When a neurotransmitter binds to its receptor on a postsynaptic neuron, it can either increase or decrease the chances that the postsynaptic neuron will initiate an action potential of its own.

• Two major mechanisms can terminate neurotransmission: enzymatic degradation of neurotransmitter and reuptake of transmitter back into the presynaptic nerve terminal.

• A drug that blocks reuptake of a neurotransmitter will intensify synaptic transmission by that transmitter.

• The major indication for antipsychotic drugs is schizophrenia.

• Antipsychotic drugs are thought to produce their therapeutic effects by blocking receptors for dopamine.

• Responses to antipsychotic drugs develop slowly, requiring a month or more to produce a full effect.

• Antipsychotic drugs cause three types of early extrapyramidal reactions: acute dystonia, parkinsonism, and akathisia. Acute dystonia and parkinsonism can be treated with anticholinergic drugs (e.g., benztropine). Akathisia, although more difficult to treat, may respond to anticholinergic drugs, benzodiazepines, and/or beta blockers.

• Tardive dyskinesia—a *late* extrapyramidal reaction—has no reliable treatment.

• Neuroleptic malignant syndrome, a life-threatening reaction to antipsychotic drugs, is characterized by muscular rigidity, high fever, and autonomic instability.

• Low-potency antipsychotics and high-potency antipsychotics produce equal therapeutic effects. These drugs differ, in that low-potency agents cause more anticholinergic effects, sedation, and orthostatic hypotension, whereas high-potency agents cause more *early* extrapyramidal reactions. Tardive dyskinesia is equal with both groups.

• Traditional antipsychotic drugs and atypical antipsychotic drugs differ in two principal ways: atypical antipsychotics are less likely to cause extrapyramidal reactions (including tardive dyskinesia), and atypical agents are more effective than traditional agents at relieving negative symptoms of schizophrenia.

• The major adverse effect of clozapine (Clozaril) is agranulocytosis. Because of this potentially fatal effect, weekly blood tests are mandatory.

• As with the antipsychotics, therapeutic responses to antidepressants develop slowly (over a month or more).

• The *most common* adverse effects of the tricyclic antidepressants are sedation, orthostatic hypotension, and anticholinergic effects.

• The *most serious* adverse effect of the tricyclic antidepressants is cardiotoxicity, which can be fatal.

• Patients taking MAOIs must be warned against eating foods that contain tyramine because tyramine can cause a fatal hypertensive crisis in these people.

• The principal advantages of SSRIs over tricyclic antidepressants are that SSRIs cause fewer side effects (hypotension, sedation, anticholinergic effects) and SSRIs are not cardiotoxic, which makes them much less dangerous when taken in overdose.

• Lithium is the principal treatment for bipolar disorder.

• To minimize the risk of toxicity, blood levels of lithium must be kept below 1.5 mEq/L. Monitoring of blood levels is essential.

• A reduction in sodium levels will reduce lithium excretion, causing lithium levels to rise—possibly to toxic concentrations. Patients must maintain normal sodium intake and sodium levels.

• Two anticonvulsants, carbamazepine (Tegretol) and valproic acid (Depakene, Depakote), are alternatives to lithium for treating bipolar disorder.

• Benzodiazepines are preferred to barbiturates and other general CNS depressants for treating anxiety because benzodiazepines are much safer and cause fewer side effects.

• Although benzodiazepines can cause physical dependence, the withdrawal syndrome associated with these drugs is usually mild (although it can be intense with some patients).

• Four principal differences exist between buspirone (BuSpar) and the benzodiazepines: buspirone lacks CNS-depressant actions; buspirone does not intensify the CNS-depressant effects of other drugs; antianxiety effects of benzodiazepines develop "immediately," whereas therapeutic effects of buspirone may take a week to begin and a month or more to reach their peak; and buspirone has even less potential for abuse than the benzodiazepines.

• When patients are taking any type of medication, you are responsible for assessing mental status, effectiveness of medications, presence of side effects, degree of compliance, and the patient's and family's level of knowledge about the medication(s) and the illness that the medication is being used to treat.

• One of the most common nursing diagnoses for patients taking psychotropic medication is Knowledge Deficit regarding medication use and side effects.

• The expected outcomes for patients taking any type of psychotropic medication focus on improvement in the patient's symptoms and functioning, increased knowledge regarding the illness and the medication, and appropriate levels of compliance with the medication regimen.

• Appropriate nursing interventions for patients taking any type of psychotropic medication include education of the patient and family regarding the illness and the medication(s) and exploration of ways to improve compliance.

• Evaluation of the nursing care focuses on whether the patient's psychiatric symptoms decrease, whether the patient experiences side effects and how effectively these side effects are controlled, whether the patient's level of functioning improves, and whether the patient is compliant with taking the medication.

LEARNING ACTIVITIES

1. Write in your journal your own reactions to the idea that you would have to take medication most of your life. Would it be difficult on you? What impact would this have on your self-concept? Your spirituality?

2. Interview two other people and ask the following questions:
What is your attitude about taking medications?
Do you have trouble remembering to take medications as they are prescribed?
Would/Does taking medications on a regular basis affect on your sense of well-being?

3. Begin to develop a medication file box. Write on three by five-inch index cards the name of every medication that your patients are taking. Describe the purpose of the medication, the side effects, the dosage range, what dose your patient is on, how the drug works, and any precautions that must be observed while taking the drug. Summarize what the ways in which the medication benefits your patient. What side effects does your patient experience? How are these side effects handled?

CRITICAL THINKING EXERCISE

Lillian, a 40-year-old schoolteacher was admitted to the inpatient unit for depression. She was overwhelmed with conflicts at work and with an impending divorce at home. Part of her treatment involved group counseling. Another part of her treatment involved the medication Prozac. Prior to discharge, the nurse provided Lillian with some educational information about her newly prescribed drug, Prozac.

1. What information would you give to Lillian about Prozac?

2. What assumptions can the nurse make about Lillian's use of the drug?

3. What evidence would convince the nurse that the patient understood her information about the drug?

Lillian was discharged to the outpatient clinic. Two weeks later, when she arrived for her first appointment, she had the New York Times best seller book *Listening to Prozac*. Lillian seemed very concerned about the stories that she heard from her friends about Prozac causing suicidal or homicidal tendencies.

1. What evidence does the nurse need to provide clear and precise information about what the patient is telling her?

2. What are alternative explanations why Lillian might have expressed such concerns to the nurse?

3. What conclusions (if any) can be drawn about Lillian's comments to the nurse?

REFERENCES

Abramowicz, M. (Ed.) (1994). Drugs for psychiatric disorders. *The Medical Letter on Drugs and Therapeutics, 36*, 89–96.

Byrd, C. (1993). Neuroleptic malignant syndrome: A dangerous complication of neuroleptic therapy. *Journal of Neuroscience Nursing, 215* (1), 62–65.

Brasfield, K. H. (1991). Practical psychopharmacologic considerations in depression. *Nursing Clinics of North America, 26* (3), 651–663.

Drug Facts and Comparisons. (1994–1995 monthly updates) *Facts and comparisons* (Loose-leaf ed.). St. Louis: C. V. Mosby.

Glod, C. A. (1991). Psychopharmacology and clinical practice. *Nursing Clinics of North America, 26* (12), 375–399.

Goodwin, K. R., and Jameson, K. R. (1990). *A patient with manic depressive illness*, (p. 725). Oxford: Oxford University Press.

Hamilton, D. (1990). Clozapine: A new antipsychotic drug. *Advanced Practice Nursing, 4* (4), 278–281.

Land, W., and Salzman, C. (1994). Risperidone: A model antipsychotic medication. *Hospital and Community Psychiatry, 45* (5), 434–435.

Lehne, R. A. (1994). Antidepressants. In R. A. Lehne, *Pharmacology for nursing care* (2nd ed.) (pp. 277–294). Philadelphia: W. B. Saunders.

Lehne, R. A. (1994). Antipsychotic agents and their use in schizophrenia. In R. A. Lehne, *Pharmacology for nursing care* (2nd ed.) (pp. 259–276). Philadelphia: W. B. Saunders.

Lehne, R. A. (1994). Basic principles of neuropharmacology. In R. A. Lehne, *Pharmacology for nursing care* (2nd ed.) (pp. 101–108). Philadelphia: W. B. Saunders.

Lehne, R. A. (1994). Benzodiazepines and other drugs for anxiety and insomnia. In R. A. Lehne, *Pharmacology for nursing care* (2nd ed.) (pp. 303–323). Philadelphia: W. B. Saunders.

Lehne, R. A. (1994). Drugs for bipolar disorder. In R. A. Lehne, *Pharmacology for nursing care* (2nd ed.) (pp. 295–302). Philadelphia: W. B. Saunders.

Marder, J. R., and Meibach, R. C. (1994). Risperidone in the treatment of schizophrenia. *American Journal of Psychiatry, 151* (6) 825–835.

SUGGESTED READINGS

Byrd, C. (1993). Neuroleptic malignant syndrome: A dangerous complication of neuroleptic therapy. *Journal of Neuroscience Nursing, 215* (1), 62–65.

Brasfield, K. H. (1991). Practical psychopharmacologic considerations in depression. *Nursing Clinics of North America, 26* (3), 651–663.

Glod, C. A. (1991). Psychopharmacology and clinical practice. *Nursing Clinics of North America, 26* (12), 375–399.

Hamilton, D. (1990). Clozapine: A new antipsychotic drug. *Advanced Practice Nursing, 4* (4), 278–281.

Land, W., and Salzman, C. (1994). Risperidone: A model antipsychotic medication. *Hospital and Community Psychiatry, 45* (5), 434–435.

Marder, J. R., and Meibach, R. C. (1994). Risperidone in the treatment of schizophrenia. *American Journal of Psychiatry, 151* (6) 825–835.

UNIT IV
TRAVELERS ACROSS THE LIFESPAN

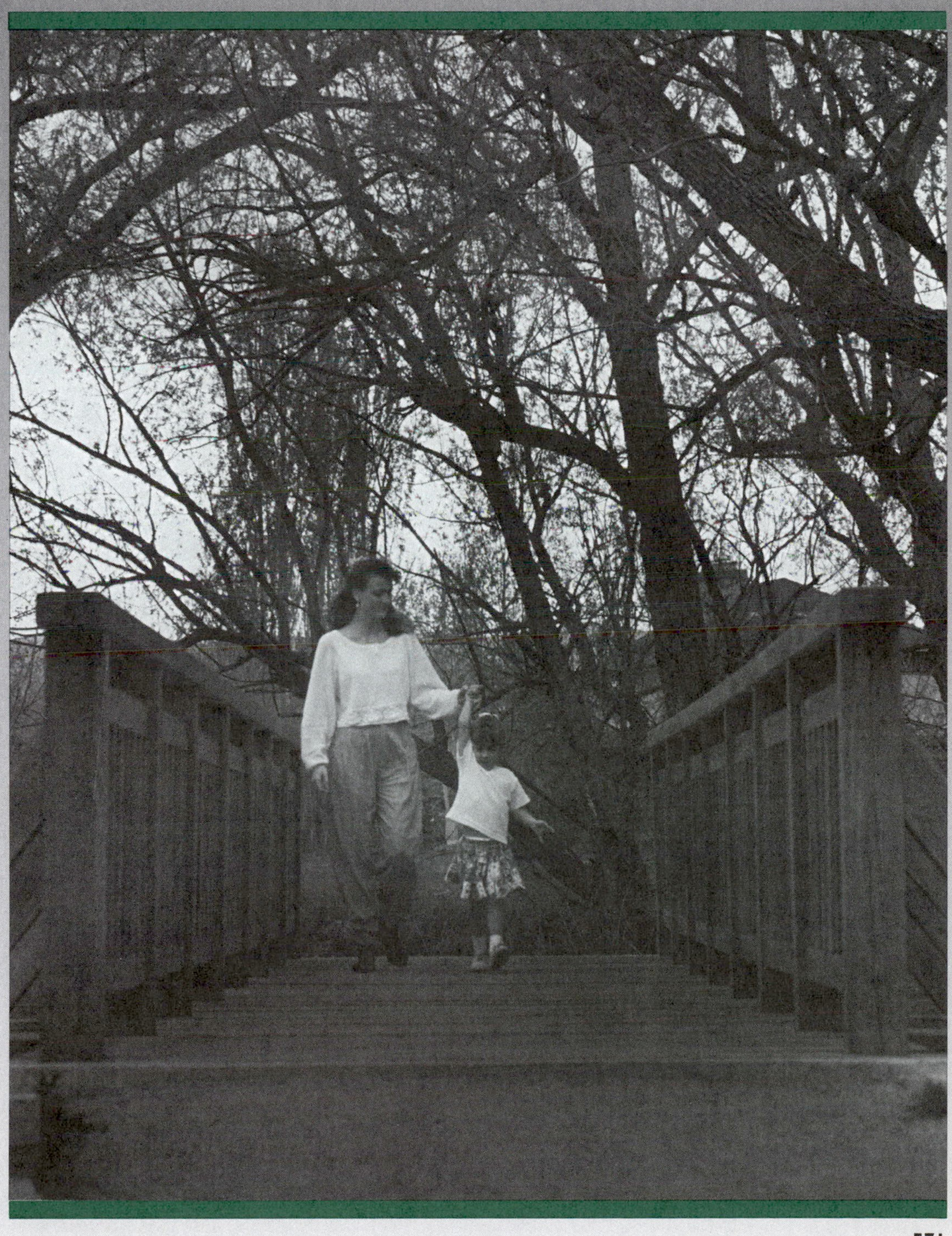

CHAPTER 24

THE PEDIATRIC TRAVELER

Today, as in times past, the most important and also the most difficult task in raising a child is helping him to find meaning in life.

As an educator and therapist of severely disturbed children, my main task was to restore meaning to their lives. This work made it obvious to me that if children were reared so that life was meaningful to them, they would not need special help.

—*Bruno Bettelheim*

LEARNING OBJECTIVES

After studying this chapter, you should be able to:

1. Outline the stages of normal child and adolescent development according to the major theorists.

2. Describe various coping strategies and their appropriateness to each developmental level.

3. Describe the risk factors associated with emotional disturbance in children and adolescents.

4. Outline the salient features of the physical and mental status examinations for this population.

5. List specific areas of assessment and features to be observed within each area.

6. Identify the broad categories of childhood and adolescent diagnoses according to the DSM-IV.

7. Suggest one nursing diagnosis appropriate to each disorder.

8. Apply the nursing process to a patient situation.

9. Describe the various treatment modalities and the settings in which these are used.

10. List the principles of medication use in children.

KEY TERMINOLOGY

Anal phase
Attachment
Early adolescence
Genital phase
Late adolescence
Latency phase
Middle adolescence
Oedipal phase
Oral phase

In getting to know a troubled child, whether a toddler, a school-age child, or an adolescent, you need to come to the encounter with your whole self—memories, knowledge, hope, earnestness, and also playfulness. Young people, whether eagerly or reluctantly, entrust themselves to a caring nurse. This trust can be seen as an act of courage and of hope.

To recognize this courage, to offer the help a child needs, and to participate in hoping with a child are acts of love for the nurse. In the words of Bettelheim (1950), however, "love is not enough." Neither is intuition, nor empathy—"a corrective experience is not enough" (Winnicott, 1965). These attributes are important, but you must also have a special kind of understanding guided by a basic knowledge of child and adolescent development—physical, social, and psychological—and by a capacity to enjoy the intellectual challenge of learning about psychopathology. Understanding is informed by a deep interest in the inner lives of others and a willingness to examine yourself honestly and continually. With this understanding comes a chance for both nurse and child to learn and to be changed.

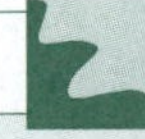

JORDI'S STORY

He woke up suddenly, looked around the room, and jumped out of bed. People were talking in the kitchen. The woman's voice was high-pitched, tremulous, and sounded angry. The man's voice said, "Yes—OK, already, OK," and then the door slammed and it was quiet again. He felt like eating but was afraid to go into the kitchen. The garbage pail under the sink, with its greasy, gaping, smelly hole, frightened him awfully.

Shaking miserably, he finally opened the door and walked into the room backward. The woman shook her head and said, "Why can't you walk like all of us, Jordi?" He couldn't answer—the pail might hear him. The big hole was like an ear, and it could hear everything—sometimes even his thoughts. If he kept quiet and thought nothing, maybe he could shut it out and make himself safe.

It rained that morning. He liked the lightning, and the thunder was rumbly and warm. It was the rain that scared him. Every time it came, the same thought was there—rain forest—and it would repeat over and over again—rain forest, rain forest—and the same picture popped into his head—only lately he was more and more in the picture.

The trees were raining down. They weren't the tall, nice ones. They were short, fat, heavy, and stubby. They had giant roots that spread all over. And they came down from the sky to look for him, and one day one would come—the one that hated him most. It would crush him into the dirt. The roots would strangle him. He would be buried deeper and deeper.

They led him out of the house into the bus. It was different from the trains and their routes that he knew so well. Then they went out of the familiar neighborhood.

He was afraid to sit, and nobody objected to his standing the whole way. He felt very small. It made him feel a little bit bigger to stand. He kept his fist clenched tightly on the seat, and his body became more rigid. As familiar surroundings disappeared, he clenched the seat even tighter, feeling that this would keep him from disappearing too.

He felt that if he held himself tightly and didn't budge, he would not come apart. It took immense concentration to hold himself together. Each bump and jolt threatened to make him scatter into little pieces. A private battle was taking place between him and the lurching of the bus.

The attendant talked to him. He didn't answer. He couldn't hear her. Keeping himself in one part absorbed him totally. All of his senses were concentrated on the terrible effort.

Dear God,

I didn't think orange went with purple until I saw the sunset you made on Tue. That was cool.

EUGENE

From Hample, S., and Marshall, E. (Eds.) (1991). *Children's letters to God: The new collection.* New York: Workman Publishing.

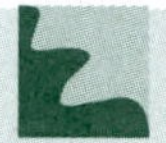

"What's wrong, Jordi? What? Tell me."

He hit himself with his closed fist again and again.

"Hold my hand, Sally. Help me—hold me."

She held his hands between hers as he moaned, "Oh, oh." Then she managed to get him on her lap. She bent over him, held her arms around him, and hugged him tightly.

He felt warm and safe (Rubin, 1960, p. 46).

THE BEGINNING OF THE JOURNEY: CONSIDERATIONS IN WORKING WITH CHILDREN AND ADOLESCENTS

The Child as Sojourner

One reason some people give for choosing to work with children is their pleasure in childhood spontaneity and creativity. Although there are certainly elements of these qualities in child psychiatric nursing, disturbed children often experience themselves as out of control and terrified or inhibited and joyless. Such children can be helped by adults who can tolerate terror and unhappiness and can imagine and hope for a renewal of their joyfulness.

Normal Development

Child and adolescent development has been described by different theorists over the last century. Psychoanalytic theorists have each proposed a number of discrete phases that correspond to the individual's mastery of physical, environmental, and—primarily—emotional tasks. Freud (1938) described these phases as follows:

1. The **oral phase,** from 0 to 18 months, so named because of the central role of the mouth in satisfying needs, experiencing intimacy, exploring the world, and expressing distress and satisfaction.
2. The **anal phase,** from 18 to 36 months, referring to the important role that control of the urethral and anal sphincters (*toilet training*) plays in the young child's life. Control involves both the regulation of pleasurable sensations and the assertion of autonomy.
3. The **Oedipal phase,** from 4 to 6 years, named, of course, for the Greek myth. This term describes the child's wish for exclusive possession of the parent of the opposite gender. In this phase children are believed

to develop a capacity for *triadic* relationships. The child can now appreciate the parents' relationship with one another as well as their joint relationship with the child.

4. The **latency phase,** roughly the period between the ages of 6 or 7 and 10 or 11. During this period, according to Freud, the urgent striving for a romantic attachment to the opposite-sex parent becomes *latent* (dormant).
5. The **genital phase,** from 12 to 20, the hallmark of which is a reworking of the original Oedipal conflict. Its successful completion results in the young adult's forming an emotional and sexual attachment to an appropriate person outside of the family.

Building on her father's work but focusing more on the child's adaptation, Anna Freud (1936) described several *lines of development* in different spheres of functioning, such as in care of the body and all of its needs and in relationships, both intimate and social. Erikson (1963) proposed that maturation involves the mastery of a series of basic developmental crises across the life span. In Erikson's view, successful resolution of each crisis allows the individual to move ahead in a satisfactory manner. Failure to negotiate the crisis at any of these phases, however, results in a diminished sense of self and a lack of readiness to face the next challenge. Piaget (1965) concentrated on the child's cognitive development, labeling styles of intellectual reasoning that move from simple to complex and from concrete to abstract. Kohlberg (1981) postulated distinct stages in the development of moral reasoning that follow a similar progression. Each of these theorists is represented in Table 24–1.

CHILDHOOD

Childhood is a time of growth, increasingly complex socialization, increasingly sophisticated learning about all aspects of a particular culture, and a gradual movement from the personal productivity of play to the societal productivity of work. Each stage of development is complete in itself, so that the child is not merely an incomplete adult. Each stage along the journey has its own unique appeal and infuses the world with its own unique energy. Play, which is often called both the language and the business of childhood, can serve as a window into the child's life.

ADOLESCENCE

Adolescence has also been broken down into three general phases: early, middle, and late. **Early adolescence** corresponds to the beginning of physical maturation and the development of primary and secondary sex characteristics. **Middle adolescence** is marked by the well-known struggle for independence, which often involves an uncomfortable degree of defiance and limit-testing. By **late adolescence,** some stability has generally been attained—in peer relationships, academic and leisure interests, and financial responsibility.

Adolescence in U.S. culture is known as a turbulent and stormy time, which many clinicians see as exciting

TABLE 24–1 **Models of Child Development**

Theorist and Orientation	Age and Developmental Phase (*0 1 2 3 4 5 6 7 8 9 10 11 12 13 14 15 16 17 18*)
Freud Psychosexual	Oral — Anal — Phallic-Oedipal — Latency — Genital
Erikson Social-emotional	Trust vs. Mistrust — Autonomy vs. Shame and Doubt — Initiative vs. Guilt — Industry vs. Inferiority — Identity vs. Role Confusion
Piaget Cognitive	Sensorimotor — Preoperational — Concrete operational — Formal operational
Kohlberg Moral	Preconventional: avoids punishment, satisfies own needs — Conventional: pleases others, obeys rules — Postconventional: personal values, universal principles
Anna Freud Lines of development	Dependency---Part-object---Family romance-------Ambivalence---Adult object relationships Dual unity Suckling--Self-feeding---Rational eating Weaning Food fads Wetting and soiling---Bladder and bowel control Egocentricity-------Companionship Body—Toy Play-------Work Irresponsibility in body management----Responsibility in body management

and filled with potential. Winnicott (1965) describes it as "defiance mixed with dependence." The vast majority of adolescents do weather the storm of changing bodies, changing feelings, and the search for identity. One study found that approximately 80% of all adolescents "enjoy life, are happy with themselves, and have positive feelings toward their parents" (Offer et al, 1991). Nevertheless, about 20% of teenagers are in a significant degree of distress.

Understanding the Individual Journey

A solid grounding in child and adolescent development is essential for *anyone* working with children and adolescents. Reading original works by the major theorists is useful. Reading fictional and autobiographical accounts—particularly accounts from different racial or cultural perspectives—and watching movies that explore the child's experience can be helpful too.

As always, however, going directly to the source still is more helpful. Children and adolescents can be the best teachers when the subject is themselves. You might begin by arranging to observe in a day care center or in an elementary, middle, or high school. Or you can simply drop by a playground or spend time in malls, restaurants, and clubs where teenagers "hang out." Ask the children and adolescents you meet straightforwardly about their lives. They are often glad to be taken seriously, listened to, and offered a chance to help an adult learn.

Any understanding of a child's own journey, no matter how deep or rich, is incomplete without a sense of the child's place in the family. Chess and Thomas (1986) propose the paradigm of "goodness of fit" as a way of approaching the parent-child relationship. This deceptively simple idea is important: It "is best if the children are valued for their unique and idiosyncratic traits, temperaments, skills, and weaknesses" (Pruett, 1991).

▶ Check Your Reading

1. Name Freud's developmental stages and the ages to which they refer.
2. Why is play important?
3. What did Erikson contribute regarding child development?
4. What does Kohlberg's theory contribute to our understanding of child development?
5. What are the three phases of adolescence, and what characterizes each phase?

The Journey as It Touches the Family

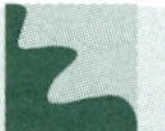

"I was with strangers the whole Saturday and Sunday—the whole weekend."

"But you were home, Jordi."

"Home, home with the public—with strangers."

"Your mother and father were home, Jordi."

"They were public also—they were all away from me..." (Rubin, 1960, p. 49).

The modern family is in peril. All too often, a family exists in isolation from any real sense of community. Within the family, individuals may feel isolated too. This sense of anomie appears to pervade all levels of American life. Kendall (1989, p. 145) writes of her work as a child psychiatric nurse consultant in a poor urban hospital setting:

> *Frequently, inner-city children from socially deprived environments are discharged home where the pressures of poverty, violence, overcrowding, separation (if placed in a foster home), apathy, and a myriad of additional problems again jeopardize the child's development, potentiating further crises and disturbances.*

Kendall proposes that nurses use critical theory—a theory of social conflict originating with Habermas (1971) and the Frankfurt School—as a means of gaining deeper understanding and challenging the traditional ideal of the "normal family." Kendall suggests that nursing as a profession remains mired in a conservative world view that does a disservice to the families it is trying to help. The application of critical theory may lead to "a rapprochement, or coming together . . . between nursing and the family in today's society." Describing the middle-class nuclear family as unrepresentative of the human species, Konner (1982) states that "subtly, deeply, persistently, it continues to serve as a yardstick for us, and this has to stop."

Regardless of social status or the constellation of family members, families of disturbed children often report that life at home holds little pleasure. So much time and energy are expended in efforts to manage the child's behavior, whether oppositional, withdrawing, or compulsive, that none is left for having fun. Siblings frequently feel cheated of a "regular life." A common cycle is that a relatively minor upset or transgression becomes an enormous to-do, as parents increase their demands and the child his resistance until both reach a crisis. The crisis may take the form of a verbal or physical outburst or the announcement of a consequence so dire that it momentarily makes everyone pause. Then, typically, remorse overwhelms the parents and often the child, and the temptation to draw close again, to repair and to indulge, is overwhelming. This sequence can become so habitual that the child is compelled to accelerate every request or refusal until the predicted outcome is attained. It has become the only relief available.

For the parents of an adolescent, the main task of this stormy period is to survive. Most parents know that this goal is serious: Psychoanalytically, adolescence is a time for reworking the family rivalries that characterize toddlerhood. Only now, as Winnicott (1971) puts it, "growing up means taking the parent's place. *It really does.*" Other cultures may have incorporated rituals that structure and contain this rite of passage more successfully than we have done in the United States. In the United States, even in the smoothest of transitions, normal adolescents appear to be compelled to ask parents both to leave them alone and to take care of them. As always, your treatment goal is to help family members increase their enjoyment of one another, not to impose change merely for the sake of order.

Nurses often work with young children and adolescents in an unusually close and intimate manner, acting at times as *parent surrogates.* It is a difficult challenge in these circumstances to resist the temptation to become a better mother or father than the child's own—or perhaps even a better mother or father than the *nurse's* own. Becoming a better parent can be quite gratifying (for both nurse and child) but only for a short while. Becoming a parent surrogate poses risks. One is that competition may result in the withdrawal of the child's real parents, who are likely to feel inadequate, rejected, or angry. Or the parents may rely on the nurse to go on providing a high level of involvement, beyond what is reasonable or possible. Both of these risks touch on the nature of therapeutic work with children and families, on the difference between gratifying immediate needs and offering the possibility of long-term change. This dilemma might be summed up here by quoting a proverb:

Give a man a fish and you feed him for a day. Show him how to fish and you feed him for a lifetime.

Nurses are in a position to teach parents the skills they need, both to care for their children and to anticipate developmental challenges and to use available resources for support.

Broadening the Path: The Outside World

School

You need only reflect on your own childhood memories to know that school is an extremely important part of a child's life. A good school not only educates a child, but also teaches a lifelong learning. A good school experience can enhance a child's social skills, self-esteem, and preparedness to meet many different kinds of challenges adaptively.

The school experience depends, in part, on the following characteristics (Comer, 1980; Linney and Seidman, 1989; Combrinck-Graham, 1991):

- Reasonable school size
- Collaborative relationships between school personnel and parents
- Strong administrative leadership
- A high degree of teacher autonomy
- Orderly structure that involves students rather than oppressing them
- Staff and parents maintaining high expectations for children

For disturbed and learning-disabled children, the school experience also depends heavily on the school's ability to recognize and provide for these special needs, regardless of the child's age.

Friends

Traditional models of personality development have given little attention to "the influence of children upon children" (McDermott, 1991). Yet from toddlerhood on, a child's interactions with other children are crucial in trying out empathy, reciprocity, self-assertion, self-regulation, and intimacy. The peer group takes on increasing importance until eventually—by adolescence—it overshadows the family in the child's involvement and allegiance."[S]elf-evaluation and evaluation of others, attachment and loyalty, and attribution of qualities evolve primarily through the peer culture" (Combrinck-Graham, 1991). Gang membership may be an expression of the need for teenagers to establish a sense of identity and efficacy by affiliation with a group (Rodriguez, 1994).

One of the most frequent complaints of disturbed children and their parents is that they have great difficulty making and sustaining friendships. Hyperactive children are frequently unpopular or may play only with children younger than themselves. Depressed or anxious children often withdraw from social contact. Impulsive and aggressive children tend to alienate peers by their actions. Developmentally delayed children may lack the skills needed to engage in reciprocal social exchanges. Psychotic children may appear bizarre or frightening to others. Such children need direct help negotiating more satisfactory relationships. Part of the plan of treatment should address the means by which this help is to be carried out.

Community

A fortunate child's community may include a neighborhood; a church, a synagogue, or mosque; a circle of family friends and acquaintances; and familiar people encountered day to day in local shops, libraries, YMCAs, or museums. An African saying captures this concept: "It takes a whole village to raise a child."

Yet many children do not grow up with a real sense of community. Their world may be narrowed by danger, homelessness, or isolation. Or they may attend a school far from home and have no friends nearby. The more you know about resources within the child's community, the more helpful you can be to parents who may themselves feel disconnected and alone. (Chapter 43 talks more about the place of the community in addressing the mental health needs of families.)

▶ Check Your Reading

6. What do you consider to be the most significant consideration in understanding each of the following: the child, the family, the outside world?
7. Why do nurses need to consider models other than the middle-class nuclear family when evaluating family functioning?
8. What tasks are facilitated through friendships?

9. Why do nurses need to be aware of community resources?

Racial, Ethnic, and Cultural Differences

Nurses who have an opportunity to work with children and families from backgrounds markedly different from their own have lives immeasurably enriched by what they learn. Both patient and nurse are part of a larger ecological system, and each comes to an encounter with a lifetime of cultural experiences (see Chapter 14). Nurses from majority racial or ethnic groups may be blind to their own assumptions because "cultural influences are woven into the personality like a tapestry" (McDermott, 1991).

The best way to understand what a child and family experience, value, and believe is to learn from the child and other family members themselves. Two general principles can guide your approach:

- Child-rearing practices do differ from culture to culture and between subgroups within the larger culture as well. These differences in practice have a strong effect on personality development in children (Caudill and Schooler, 1973; Whiting and Edwards, 1988; McDermott, 1991).
- Minority status is intrinsically neither a risk factor nor a protective factor but carries the potential to become one or the other. The influence of minority status depends on the pervasiveness of societal discrimination against the minority group; the fit between majority and minority beliefs, norms, and values; and the availability of strong adult role models and community support.

JOINING THE JOURNEY: THE THERAPEUTIC RELATIONSHIP

> Wherever he went, she was there. Whatever he did, she was there. For a long time they said nothing to each other and never even touched each other. But—no matter what—there she was, close to him.
>
> After a long time, a change took place. . . . He no longer felt that she was separate from him . . .
>
> And then they began to talk (Rubin, 1960, p. 24).

The therapeutic relationship is at the heart of child treatment, regardless of the modality or the setting. The phrase *continuity of care* is often stretched almost beyond recognition to include institutions and entire service systems, but true continuity is provided by an ongoing relationship with an individual person. You need not do all of the work alone. True collaborative involvement of other members of the "team" is essential. This team involves a partnership not only with other professionals, but also with the child and family. Take into account that a child, regardless of age, is a complete human being embedded in a family and community. In developing goals for treatment, incorporate these interlocking spheres of interest. In the words of Winnicott (1957), include "the child, the family and the outside world."

Frequently a disturbed child has become "stuck" in a cycle of maladaptive behaviors that draw forth unhelpful responses from those in the family and community who have also become "stuck" in responding a certain way. Thus, weaknesses and problems appear in both the child and others. Your challenge is to recognize and to draw on ways in which these three spheres can become sources of strength. As Rutter (1987) found in his studies of resilience in children, each of these areas has the potential to become *protective factors.*

Transference

The psychoanalytic concept of transference is complicated in child treatment. As Anna Freud (1946) pointed out, because children are generally still living with their parents and are still in the midst of a primary relationship with them, transference in the strictest sense of the word cannot occur. In addition, the more closely and intimately a nurse must interact with a child—for example on an inpatient ward for young children—the more their relationship is an immediate and *real* one for both nurse and child. Yet elements of this relationship are transferential. Chethik (1989) calls this displacement of ongoing issues from the family onto the nurse or therapist a "transference of current relationships." Thus, "dealing with the child's projected feelings is inevitable when working with children" (Critchley, 1985).

Teenagers also project feelings onto a caregiver. In their search for identity, adolescents are especially susceptible to idealizing or devaluing important adults. They may identify a primary nurse or therapist as being like a restrictive parent or attempt to persuade this person to ally with them in revolt against such a parent.

Countertransference

Feelings of countertransference are similarly inevitable when working with children and adolescents. Your goal is not to do away with or avoid such feelings but to make use of them for a deeper understanding. By examining these feelings, which involve unconscious communications, you can further the work of bringing hidden material to consciousness. This examination may be done with the assistance of a clinical supervisor.

Certain kinds of behavior in children are especially likely to evoke strong feelings in a caregiver (Lewis, 1991). Among these are expressions of hostility, destructiveness, aggression, extreme excitement, sexualized behavior, and seductiveness. Many nurses find working with adolescents to be especially challenging because of the potential for stirring up unresolved issues from their own adolescence. Also, in conflicts between a child and a parent, you may overidentify with one or the other. Some common signals of countertransference can alert you:

- Noticeable increase in anxiety
- Sudden rush of any strong emotion
- Persistent feeling of dislike for a child or parent
- Unusually compelling tenderness for a child or parent
- Boredom or sleepiness in the absence of real fatigue
- Urge to argue with a child or parent
- Wish to elicit gratitude from a child or parent

Equipment for the Journey: Coping Mechanisms

Anna Freud, in her 1936 monograph, *The Ego and the Mechanisms of Defense*, outlined a developmental progression of unconscious mental processes that people use to mediate their experiences of both the inner world and the disappointments and dangers of external reality. Table 24–2 lists common unconscious strategies and the age groups in which they are typically seen. Such strategies are inherently neither negative nor positive. They cause a person trouble only when they interfere with satisfactory living. The most primitive are most useful for young children; older children and adolescents who rely only on these early defenses have a hard time adapting successfully to the demands of their lives.

▶ Check Your Reading

10. Name one feature of transference unique to children.
11. What is countertransference?
12. Describe at least three manifestations of countertransference.
13. Give four examples of coping mechanisms and the developmental phase(s) to which each is appropriate.

Stumbling Blocks Along the Path: Epidemiology and Risk Factors

In a summary of 30 years of worldwide studies including more than 123,000 children, Verhulst and Koot (1992) reported that an average of 13% had a psychiatric disturbance of some kind. Five more recent studies cited by the same authors show an even higher range, between 17% and 26%. Overall, boys tend to have more problems with disruptive activity (also called *externalizing behaviors*).

In a national and world community increasingly beset by a host of social ills, children are especially vulnerable. Nurses must remain at the forefront of efforts to reverse this trend, as stated by Kendall (1989, p. 151):

TABLE 24–2 Common Coping Mechanisms Grouped by Developmental Appropriateness

Age in Years	Coping Mechanisms
0–5	"Delusional" projection Denial Distortion
3–15	Projection Fantasy Somatization Acting out Passive-aggressive behavior
3–Adulthood	Intellectualization Repression Displacement Reaction formation Dissociation
12–Adulthood	Altruism Humor Suppression Anticipation Sublimation

Adapted from Valliant, G. E. (1971). Theoretical hierarchy of adaptive ego mechanisms. *Archives of General Psychiatry, 24*, 107–118. Copyright 1971, American Medical Association.

> *The nurse in the clinical area is in an especially important position to challenge the prevailing ideological perspectives by focusing clinical interventions toward empowerment over oppressive family situations. Some of these interventions might include assessing for the political and social factors that influence familial relationships, helping to empower politically and socially disenfranchised groups by providing alternative and critical explanations for their situations, or aligning with families against the structures and systems that oppress them.*

At the very least, nurses must be alert to certain risk factors as they look for ways to prevent or ameliorate mental illness in children. In the words of Solnit (in Provence and Naylor, 1983 p. viii):

> *A high-risk environment is one which tends to complicate rather than facilitate a healthy development; it is one that uncovers and magnifies the [child's] and parents' vulnerabilities rather than providing the built-in support that will enable them to overcome weaknesses or deficits.*

Poverty

The single most prevalent risk factor among children with behavior problems is a low socieconomic status (Verhulst and Koot, 1992). Obviously, simply being poor does not cause difficulties. Children from extremely poor families can do extraordinarily well, and many do. As Winnicott (1971) puts it, there is even "the possibility that for a baby or a small child a slum family may be more secure and 'good' as a facilitating environment than a family in a lovely house."

Poverty makes it far more likely, however, that a child will be deprived of optimal nutrition and stimulation, exposed to environmental dangers, given inadequate health care, poorly educated, and in many ways cut off from a rich cultural heritage and from opportunities for creative expression. The effects of poverty on families—particularly on children—are at the root of an enormous social policy dilemma often portrayed as a burden on the middle classes. Instead, poverty represents a tragic loss of human potential in every generation. Children and families in the mainstream of society are also deprived, although in different ways, by this stratification of human activities.

Poor children, especially poor children of minority races and ethnic groups, are more likely to be channeled through the juvenile justice system than are middle-class and white children displaying the same behavioral symptoms (Children's Defense Fund, 1989). A study led by Kazdin (in Rierden, 1993) found that 80% of children with chronic conduct problems grow up to become adults with similar chronic problems, such as unemployment, criminal behavior, failed marriages, alcoholism, substance abuse, and other psychiatric disorders. "This is," Kazdin remarks, "probably the most costly mental health problem we face in the United States. Not only in terms of dollars but also in terms of human suffering." (Chapter 39 discusses some of the effects of poverty on individuals and families.)

Neglect and Abuse

In all states, nurses are among the professionals who are mandatory reporters of suspected child maltreatment. In practice, abuse or neglect rarely conforms to the prototype of a major physical injury caused by an obvious assault whose discovery leads to the removal of the child from the home. The reality is that defining neglect and abuse has been difficult and controversial (Korbin, 1987). The American Humane Association (1981) describes *neglect* as the "deprivation of necessities" such as food, clothes, shelter, health care, education and responsible supervision." Yet, as Helfer (1987) points out, there is no consensus on the point at which a relative deprivation of any of these becomes clearly definable as neglect.

Abuse, a widely used and easily misunderstood term, may be broadly intended to include severe emotional maltreatment or confined to a serious physical injury or (far more frequent) repeated episodes of minor injuries (Wolfe, 1987). Because of these ambiguities, you should try to be as specific as possible about the actual events and any physical evidence present rather than relying on vague terminology.

The short-term effects of parental violence include physical, developmental, and psychiatric symptoms (Kashani et al, 1992). Children who have suffered maltreatment are more likely to have difficulties in the security of attachment (Schneider-Rosen and Cicchetti, 1984; Crittenden, 1985), control of aggression (Hoffman-Plotkin and Twentyman, 1984; Lahey et al, 1984), mood (Kazdin et al, 1985), self-esteem and social competence (Wolfe and Moske, 1983; Kazdin et al, 1985), academic performance (Hoffman-Plotkin and Twentyman, 1984), and juvenile crime (Tarter et al, 1984). They are also more likely to become abusing parents, although the great majority of abused children do *not* grow up to commit abuses (Wolfe, 1987). Efforts to establish characteristic patterns among abusing parents have been largely inconclusive, although Wolfe (1987) lists a number of attributes that have been correlated with abuse. Among these are isolation, low frustration tolerance, and unrealistic expectations of the child.

The importance of specifying what actually happened rather than using a term such as *abuse* is equally true in sexual abuse, a phrase that also can refer to a broad range of inappropriate behaviors, from exposure of genitalia to rape. Estimates suggest that as many as 38% of all girls are exposed to some form of inappropriate sexual contact during childhood (Russell, 1986), and this figure is likely to be even higher for girls in impoverished circumstances (Wyatt et al, 1993). The sexual maltreatment of boys is less common but may be less likely to be reported than that of girls. Effects of sexual abuse include fearfulness, a sense of being "damaged goods," depression, impaired peer relations, and a drop in academic performance (Sgroi, 1982). Frequently, such children become preoccupied by sexual matters and may become highly stimulated by the intimacy of a therapeutic relationship.

The degree and nature of harm are certainly related in part to the age and temperament of the child. Harm is more directly related to the relationship with the person committing the offense, the manner and duration of the abuse, whether it involved affection and "specialness" or coercion and pain, and how the disclosure is handled by the caretaking adults. Research to date suggests that the degree of trauma experienced by a child depends significantly on whether sexual contact was initiated by an adult or by an older child (McLeer et al, 1988).

Take care not to approach a discussion of sexual abuse with any assumptions about its meaning for a child. Children tend to be acutely sensitive to what an adult wants to hear about such matters or wants *not* to hear. Sometimes a child is experiencing a great deal of conflict between negative and positive feelings related to the event, and often a child is overwhelmed with guilt on disclosure.

Exposure to Violence

The average American child watches about three hours of television a day and by age 12 "has witnessed eight thousand murders and more than a hundred thousand other acts of violence, according to the American Psychological Association" (Auletta, 1993). Fortunately the average American child normally appears to be able to maintain a sense of all of this as make-believe, although studies to date suggest that exposure to media violence can increase the likelihood of aggressive behavior (Lagerspetz, 1989; Centerwall, 1992). Anecdotal evidence leads one to conclude that under extreme stress or in the presence of a thought disorder, a child has far more difficulty separating fiction from reality. Instances of violent action have been apparently directly linked to the perpetrator's identification with a fictional aggressor. Incidents such as the killings of several youths in street fights immediately after showings of violent movies such as "The Warriors" in 1979 and "New Jack City" in 1991 are hard to ignore (Auletta, 1993).

Although some argue that violent television shows and movies provide a cathartic outlet (Derdeyn, 1992), it is still difficult to justify their sheer degree and volume. Because children of all ages can suffer from nightmares about such fictional characters, defending the aesthetic value of some movies seems impossible. In one, for example, an indestructible, grotesque, and terrifying child molester kills his victims by appearing to them *in their dreams*, even in the supposed safety of a locked adolescent psychiatric ward.

Another layer of exposure to violence is the relentless reporting of "news" about real-life beatings, murders, war, and other disturbing events in all the media. Still closer to home is the awareness of urban children of violence in their own neighborhoods. Many disadvantaged young people, especially poor, African-American teenage boys, express a sense of hopelessness about the future based on a belief that they are more likely to die in such neighborhood violence than to reach adulthood (Garbarino, 1992).

By far the most immediate ill effects of exposure to violence are in children from violent households. Children who are the targets of such violence may experience fear, anger, sadness, and depression (Brown & Finkelhor, 1986). Even when children are only witnesses, they grow up with role models of violence and victimization and are more likely to engage in violent behavior themselves (Farrington, 1978; Kashani et al, 1992) or to be repeatedly victimized in future relationships (Russell, 1986).

Parental Psychopathology

CONDUCT DISORDER IN EITHER PARENT

Conduct disorder or criminal behaviors in either parent or in both parents have been associated with psychiatric disturbance in children (Rutter and Quinton, 1984; Kazdin, 1992). Whether this effect is due to inadequate parenting, modeling, or the greater likelihood of parental maltreatment—or to some combination of factors—remains unclear.

DEPRESSION IN MOTHER

The other characteristic most strongly correlated with childhood psychopathology is maternal depression (Rutter, 1966, 1986). Although genetic factors are likely to be involved in this association, parental availability and the quality of caretaking are clearly important variables. Children of depressed mothers are more likely to have problems not only with mood disorders, but also with a range of other difficulties, including anxiety, poor self-esteem, and academic and conduct problems (Weissman et al, 1992; Weissman et al, 1987).

Medical Illness and Disability

A number of authors have studied the relationship between psychiatric disturbances and medical illness (Eason et al, 1985; Pless and Perrin, 1985; Lambert and Lambert, 1987; Pollock, 1987) or disability (Breslau, 1985; Rose and Thomas, 1987; Sacks, 1988). According to Mrazek (1991), "serious physical illness should be conceptualized as one of the most important early risk factors for emotional disturbance." In a nursing study of behavioral disturbances in medically hospitalized children, McClowry (1991) points out that, although the hospitalization may be in itself a stressor, other causes may underlie both the need for hospitalization *and* the emotional problems. Socioeconomic disadvantage is once again implicated as a contributing factor.

Nurses are often in a position to be especially helpful to children with medical illnesses or disabilities, whether they encounter such a child in a medical setting, an educational setting, or a psychiatric setting. It is especially important that you understand that illness and disability have a *meaning* to a child and family. As stated by Kleinman (1988), health care providers have an "existential commitment to be with the sick person and to facilitate his or her building of an illness narrative that will make sense of and give value to the experience." With the help of a committed nurse, an illness or disability can even provide a child and family with an opportunity for mastery and life-enhancing growth.

Medical illness or disability in the parent is also a risk factor for a child (Rutter, 1966). A number of hospitals in the United States are adopting the "Planetree" model, named after a National Institutes of Health (NIH)–funded study of factors that enhance healing in hospitals (Belkin, 1992). Two of the amenities included are the provision of a kitchen enabling families to prepare and eat meals together and unrestricted visiting by family members, including children. Experience and common sense suggest that such an approach, when handled well by parents and professionals, could be helpful for children, consistent with a commitment to support the integrity of the family as a whole. Nurses can also encourage family discussions about the child's inevitable questions and fears and about the realities of an illness or disability.

Divorce

The divorce rate in the United States has climbed sharply in the second half of the century, leveling off at approximately 50% (Hernandez, 1988). Children of divorce represent a significant and disproportionate percentage of child psychiatric patients. In inpatient settings, this figure approaches 100% (Wallerstein and Corbin, 1991).

Divorce has an immediate, often obvious impact on children's lives. It is related to family conflict, disruption, loss, diminished parenting, frequently diminished financial support, and at times increased dependence of the parent on the child (Hodges et al, 1983; Peterson et al, 1984; Emery, 1982; Wallerstein and Corbin, 1991).

Although the initial impact can be addressed immediately and may be mitigated by time, social support, and treatment, divorce has also been found to have profound long-term effects on development, especially as adolescents take on the tasks of young adulthood and face the prospect of repeating a pattern of failure in intimate relationships (Wallerstein, 1985; Kalter, 1987; Wallerstein and Blakeslee, 1989).

Longitudinal studies have indicated a complex blending of factors that contribute to postdivorce adjustment. These include individual resilience and the availability of encouragement either within or outside of the family. Wallerstein (1983) formulated six *psychological tasks* for the child of divorce:

- Acknowledging the reality of the marital rupture
- Disengaging from parental conflict and distress and resuming customary pursuits
- Resolving losses
- Resolving anger and self-blame
- Accepting the permanence of divorce
- Achieving realistic hope regarding relationships

▶ Check Your Reading

14. Up to what percentage of children are believed to have a psychiatric disturbance?
15. List six risk factors associated with mental illness in children and adolescents.
16. Which of these factors is most strongly correlated?
17. Identify three of the six psychological tasks facing a child after parental divorce.
18. What effect does living in a violent household have on a child?
19. Why is poverty a risk factor for children?
20. Define neglect.

NURSING PROCESS

ASSESSMENT

Jordi was observed for hours. There were rooms with one-way mirrors and interviews and tests of all kinds. He played with blocks, ink blots, and little statues of children and adults (Rubin, 1960, p. 12).

You can apply the same observational skills you learned in assessing a child's physical condition to assessing a child's psychiatric condition. The cornerstone of your assessment is a carefully gathered history that includes the child's motor, cognitive, and social development, past illnesses and injuries; daily living skills; school performance; and course of symptoms. One nursing approach to information gathering and organization is the functional health patterns proposed by Gordon (1987), which divide data into 11 categories:

- Role/relationship
- Health perception/health management
- Nutritional/metabolic
- Elimination
- Activity/exercise
- Sleep/rest
- Cognition/perception
- Self-perception/self-concept
- Sexuality/reproduction
- Coping/stress tolerance
- Value/belief patterns

Box 24–1 provides another way of organizing a psychiatric nursing assessment. Figure 24–1 is a sample child/adolescent/family assessment tool.

Physical Examination

A physical examination should be careful and thorough and performed with sensitivity to the child's feelings. Obvious findings, such as abnormal head circumference, bruises, or abdominal distention, should, of course, be noted. *Any* unusual observation should also be recorded, however, because some rare neurodegenerative and neuromuscular disorders may be mistaken for primarily psychiatric illnesses.

BOX 24–1 Important Aspects of a Psychiatric Nursing Assessment

History
- Developmental milestones
- Socialization
- School performance and behaviors
- Eating, sleeping, and elimination patterns
- Medical illnesses or injuries

Physical examination

Neurological examination
- Frank central nervous system anomalies
- Presence of *soft signs*

Mental status examination
- Appearance
- Anxiety level
- Attention span
- Relatedness
- Orientation
- Mood
- Thought processes
- Memory
- Presence of suicidal or homicidal ideation
- Coping mechanisms
- Quality and content of play

Child's Name: ______________________ Date: ____________

Nurse's Name: ______________________

Goals for Visit: ______________________

Vital Signs (If Appropriate): T________ P________ R________ B/P________

Allergies NKA:________ Drugs:________ Food:________ Other:________

Reason for Referral (Need for Control; Safety; Behavioral Interventions; Family Support): ______________________

____

____

Family History (Genogram; Any Recent Stress; Who Resided in Home; Child's Relationship with Family Members; Patterns of Communication; Disciplinary Practices): ______________________

____

____

____

____

____

Developmental History (Child's Growth; Developmental Milestones; Current Level of Functioning; Parental Expectations): ____________

____

____

____

History of Previous Treatment (When? With Whom? Where? Outcomes?): ______________________

____

____

____

History of Medical/Physical Problems: ______________________

____

____

Current Medical/Physical Problems: ______________________

____

____

Current Drug Therapy: Yes________ No________

If yes, what medications does child take?______________________

Dose______________________ Frequency______________________

Nutrition and Sleep:

Appetite Change Yes________ No________

Weight Gain: Yes________ No________

Weight Loss: Yes________ No________

Eating Problems: ______________________

Diet Restrictions: ______________________

Caffeinated Beverage Intake: ______________________

Food Allergies: ______________________

Overall Physical Appearance: Well Nourished ________ Obese ________ Poorly Nourished ________

Frail ________ Run Down ________ Other________

Regular Hours of Sleep: Yes______ No______

Difficulty Falling Asleep: Yes______ No______ Restlessness: Yes______ No______

Early A.M. Awakening: Yes______ No______ Nightmares: Yes______ No______

Dr. Verna Benner Carson
Psychiatric Home Care Manual

FIGURE 24–1

A sample child/adolescent/family assessment tool. (From Carson, V. B. [1994]. *Psychiatric home care manual.* Baltimore: Bay Area Health Care. Copyright © Bay Area Health Care, 1994.)

Pay special attention to the neurological examination. The presence of asymmetries, delays in coordination or speech, mixed or delayed "handedness," poor right-left discrimination, and visual difficulties may suggest organic dysfunction. When mild, these have been referred to as *soft signs*, a vague and imprecise term and one poorly correlated with *specific* psychiatric disorders. Nevertheless, evidence suggests that "soft signs on the neurological examination do reflect brain dysfunction in most cases and are influenced by heredity" (Pincus, 1991).

Mental Status Examination

Although numerous questionnaires and structured interviews have been developed to ascertain the presence of psychiatric symptoms in children, they are currently most useful for research. The mental status examination remains the primary tool of assessment for the child, as for the adult, but the interviewer conducting such an examination with a child must be more flexible and informal, providing both structured and unstructured opportunities for interaction.

You may be conducting the mental status examination alone or observing or assisting another clinician. The interview should take place in a private space with play items, such as paper and crayons, clay, dolls, animal figures (dinosaurs are particularly appealing to young children exploring their own feelings of power and powerlessness), toy telephones, and a toy medical kit. The inclusion of toy guns is a personal choice and a controversial question with no "right" answer. Be prepared for the child to express aggression regardless of the toys provided. For adolescents, have comfortable chairs; more sophisticated drawing materials; and a small selection of games, such as chess, checkers, or a deck of cards.

Pay special attention to the beginning of an encounter, even before entering the office or playroom. The manner in which the child greets (or refuses to greet) you is significant, as is the way the child parts from the accompanying adult. Equally valuable are any comments made while *approaching* the interview room, especially by adolescents. Such comments are often unguarded and can be extremely revealing. The ending of the interview is similarly rich in possibility.

During the interview, which unfolds in much the same way as a conversation, note the child's appearance, coordination, tolerance of separation from the accompanying parent, mood, range of emotion, relatedness, and understanding of the reason for the interview. Questions can determine the child's orientation, general comprehension, and memory (for example, making a game of listing three unrelated items and asking the child to recall them after five minutes). As the play or talking progresses, be attentive to the child's thinking—its content, speed, and order of flow. At some point, you must ask directly about hallucinations, suicidal thoughts and plans, sexual experience, and (depending on the age of the child) alcohol and substance use. Ask these questions in an empathic, straightforward, and low-key manner.

You should be developing working hypotheses about the *DSM-IV* differential diagnoses as well as tentative nursing diagnoses that will be solidified in planning treatment with the family. Throughout both the evaluation and the treatment, remember that much of a child's *and* an adolescent's communication happens indirectly, sometimes hidden in distracting chatter, sometimes in metaphors, and sometimes without any words at all. Pay careful attention both to what children say and to what they do. Watch how they relate to the people around them, how they show they are anxious, and what comforts them. Consider your own feelings and associations and ask yourself what these might mean. By watching and listening and keeping children company, try to understand what it is to *be* a particular child.

Specific Areas of Assessment

PLAY

The essential feature of my communication is this, that playing is an experience, always a creative experience, and it is an experience in the space-time continuum, a basic form of living (Winnicott, 1971).

For a child, play means many things. It has been called "the vehicle by which the child masters the environment and his own impulses and increases his adaptive behavior" (Critchley, 1985). Play is also a young child's main form of communication, and you need to observe and respond to it with this in mind. Box 24–2 outlines some important features of a child's play.

BOX 24–2 Important Aspects of Play

- Content: Themes such as aggression or nurturing may appear repeatedly, or play may involve a wide range of thematic material.
- Anxiety: Play may involve a manageable—even pleasurable—level of tension, or the child may be overwhelmed by anxiety and interrupt the play.
- Imagination: Imagination can range from simple manipulation of objects to richly elaborated fantasy play.
- Discrimination between make-believe and reality: Some children get lost in the play; others may assure the nurse "it's just pretend."
- Narrative line: Actions may be repeated endlessly, may jump from one to another, or may flow smoothly with a sense of a beginning and an ending.
- Persistence: One child may be easily frustrated and another may stick to a task such as building a tower until it is completed.
- Reciprocity: Some children ignore an onlooker completely; others invite the nurse to participate actively, seeking a shared experience.
- Adherence to rules: Blatant cheating is seen in young children and sometimes in older children with poor self-esteem; obsessional children may become so preoccupied by the rules that the point of the game is obscured.

"He took the doorknob attached to a long string and ran past her out of the house. He had his jiggler now and was truly safe.

He let his jiggler hang down in front of him and waited. Soon it would tell his feet where to go. . . . He walked and walked." (Rubin, 1960, p. 5)

Jordi's early play behavior was solitary, repetitive, and lacking in imagination and narrative line. Jordi could not use play to explore or master his fears because he was unable to distinguish between fantasy and reality.

"The monkey bars, crisscrossing up and down, forward and backward intrigued him. . . . He walked over cautiously and touched the closest bar. It was cold. A sinister chill ran through him. . . . It looked like a wonderful toy to climb over and swing from. And it looked like an awful monster that could tangle you up, crush you, and kill you. Her voice, soft and smooth, said, "Try it. It's fun, Jordi—fun—a toy. I'll show you." (Rubin, 1960, p. 39)

Over the course of his treatment, through teaching by example, through discussions, and mostly through the development of trust, Jordi gradually learned turn-taking in verbal play, the usefulness of rules, and the pleasure of mastery. Finally, he was able to take part in school-age games with other children.

For an adolescent, play may take the form of a structured game that becomes the underpinning of a conversation. It may involve creating something during a session. Or it may simply be talking itself, with its risk of intimacy, its humor, and the building of a shared vocabulary. In interviewing an adolescent, apply your observations to what is spoken rather than acted, for an adolescent can express a good deal verbally. If a game *is* the focus of a session, pay careful attention to both the adolescent's and your own response to a competitive situation. Even a structured game can become a vehicle for exploring dynamic issues in a displaced manner, as long as you keep sight of the goal of the session (Beiser, 1979). You should also be attentive to the authenticity or use of the adolescent's full self.

ATTACHMENT/SEPARATION

In the narrowest sense of the word, **attachment** refers to the reciprocal relationship between a mother and an infant during the first months of the child's life. Long regarded as a critical aspect of human development, attachment became the focus of much scientific concern and interest during the 1940s and 1950s (Spitz, 1945; Harlow and Harlow, 1962; Robertson, 1970).

Two decades later, researchers began to study the primary attachment relationship in a systematic way (Bowlby, 1969). The phrase *secure attachment* (Ainsworth et al, 1973) described an infant's sense of basic trust in the reliability of a supportive caretaker, or "good-enough mother" (Winnicott, 1971). Secure attachment contrasted with *insecure attachment*, which has since been further broken down into three categories based on infants' responses to a reunion with an absent caretaker: insecure-avoidant, insecure-resistant, and insecured/disorganized/disoriented (Main and Cassidy, 1988). These are believed to grow out of the infant's experiences of not being helped or comforted by a parent.

Studies to date have suggested that a secure attachment is strongly correlated with greater adaptive functioning in childhood (Thompson, 1991). Although the mother's role has been well defined by the theory, however, the *infant's* contribution is not as clearly understood. Researchers continue to look at the complex interaction between the two partners of this dyad (Stern, 1985).

In a broader sense, attachment also includes the capacity to form meaningful relationships with others throughout life. Studies have still not shown how, in the absence of a secure attachment in infancy, a child might with the proper support go on to develop better attachments. Numerous authors have cited this capacity to form attachments as an important *source of resistance* to risk (Garmezy, 1987) or a *protective factor* (Rutter, 1987). To assess this capacity in a child or adolescent, observe interactions with others and gauge the quality of the growing therapeutic relationship.

SEXUALITY

The bath felt very nice. It was warm, and he was alone. He pushed the piece of wood around the tub and watched it skim over his knees and then back again over his belly. Then he held it down on the bottom of the tub and let it go suddenly, watching it shoot to the surface. Then he thought of his penis. First he squeezed it; then he rubbed it up and down. It felt nice, and it was good to be alone. When his penis stood up, he stared at it a while and wondered how this magic took place (Rubin, 1960, pp. 51–52).

One of Freud's most revolutionary ideas was infantile sexuality. Yet, although it came as a disagreeable shock to turn-of-the-century Vienna, for most of recorded human history and prehistory, not only was infantile and childhood sexuality universally accepted, but also children were exposed to a full range of adult sexual expression, from birth onward, with no concern for their "corruption." Although we have scant record of their thoughts on the subject, Viennese *mothers* could hardly have been surprised to learn that infants are sensual creatures.

Children explore their bodies and find pleasure in exploration. Modern parents have become slightly more tolerant of this process, although tolerance often depends on the child's gender. For example, boys are now more frequently given the correct words for *penis*, *testicles*, and *scrotum*, whereas girls are often taught a substitute word or only the word *vagina*, not *vulva*, *labia*, or—particularly—*clitoris*. Boys are more likely than girls to be discouraged from affectionate physical contact with others.

Despite relatively minor changes, parents continue to be at a loss in providing for their children's sexual development and safety. For the most part, they avoid sexual topics and redirect children's interest in their own and others' sexuality. Some clinicians have expressed worry that, in a climate of pervasive concerns about sexual molestation, the trend toward fathers' greater involvement in all aspects of child care may be hindered by fears of accusation (Levenkron, 1993). This hindrance would be especially unfortunate because fathers who are closely involved in caring for their infants are *less* likely to engage in sexual behavior with children (Parker and Parker, 1984).

Worldwide studies of sexual mores place the United States among the most restrictive cultures in terms of childrearing practices. As Konner (1982) puts it, "the Western family, including that of the United States at mid-century as well as that of Freud's Vienna, afforded children much less experience and information regarding sex, playful or serious, than did the average nonindustrial society." Further, "everything we know about higher primates points to a crucial role for experience in the growth of normal behavior, and this is no less true of sexual than of other forms of behavior." Yates (1991) calls the constraints that cultural expectations place on children the "most pervasive influence on human sexual appetite and function."

One unfortunate outcome of these limitations is that while children and adolescents are strongly discouraged from learning about sexual pleasure and eroticism, the media bombard everyone with cultural messages that adults should know how to be sexy and to "perform" unfailingly well. This discrepancy appears to contribute to an extraordinarily high rate of sexual dysfunctions—approaching 50%—in both men and women (Yates, 1991). Another contributing factor to adult sexual dysfunction is a history of sexual molestation as a child (Groth, 1979). Although most children who have been molested do not repeat this pattern in adulthood, some sexual dysfunctions in men *are* associated with pedophilia, and sexual problems between married couples are positively correlated with father-daughter incest (Groth, 1982).

During an assessment, ask the parents about what the child has been taught and any other information that might be relevant. A good starting point is to invite the parents to speak about any concerns or questions they might have regarding their child's sexuality. Without an invitation, parents may hesitate to bring up this topic. In counseling parents, keep the following points in mind:

- You can model an approach to the subject that is direct, unembarrassed, and sensible, using language appropriate to the parents' background and educational level.

- Ask parents to clarify their attitudes and wishes about their child's sexuality by talking openly in a supportive environment.

- If frank discussion reveals major conflict or sexual difficulties between parents, they should be encouraged to take this up in separate couples' treatment.

- Your objective is to see that the child is protected as far as possible from *any* activity or event that is frightening, painful, overstimulating, or coercive.

Also observe the child for either overly inhibited or hypersexual behavior. Frank preoccupation with explicit sexual themes or knowledge of detail not explained by the parents' account of the child's experience should lead you to wonder about the possibility of sexual molestation or exposure to adult sexual activities. Ask the child a question such as "Have you ever been touched, or been asked to touch someone, in a way that made you feel excited, worried, or uncomfortable?"

Although Freud's term *latency* delineates the years (roughly between the ages of 6 or 7 and 10 or 11) when the child's hormone levels are stable and the Oedipal preoccupation with the parents goes temporarily "underground," experience tells us that latency-age children do continue to be interested in sex. They are, however, enlarging their repertoire of adaptive defense mechanisms and tend to become more private about all bodily functions (although not necessarily in their humor!). A striking increase in erotic preoccupation is a hallmark of adolescent development, along with physical maturation. The body is flooded with gonadal hormones. Most girls begin puberty approximately two years before most boys and reach maturity more quickly once puberty begins. Ask for information regarding Tanner staging, which tracks the emergence of secondary sex characteristics (Tanner, 1974), from an adolescent's most recent physical examination. Ask adolescents directly about sexual activity, keeping in mind that they may not yet trust you well enough to be candid.

Fisher (1992), a Darwinian anthropologist, suggests that teenagers in hunter-gatherer societies have traditionally enjoyed many years of learning about and trying out sexual relationships without fear of pregnancy because of the late menarche of slim, physically active girls. The average age of menarche in the developed world has dropped rapidly from age 17.5 in the early part of the century to 12.2 for white and 11.5 for African-American girls (Lauton and Freese, 1981). Now, of course, in addition to the risk of pregnancy, adolescents face the risk of contracting serious sexually transmitted diseases, including HIV. You can assess the need for appropriate guidance or health care. Do answer any questions in a direct and factual way.

MORAL DEVELOPMENT

The development of moral decision-making skills has been relatively little studied. Philosophers, early psychoanalytic theorists, and behaviorists have based speculations about moral development largely on self-reflection and extrapolation from studies of adults. Piaget (1965) observed children's behavior and reasoning in normative settings and plotted timelines of moral reasoning that correspond with cognitive phases.

Kohlberg (1981) took this stage theory a step further, proposing a sequence of six stages of moral development grouped in three levels: the premoral level, the level of

Dear God,
I do not think anybody
could be a better
God. Well I just
want you to know but
I am not just saying
that because you
are God. Charles

From Hample, S., and Marshall, E. (Eds.) (1991). *Children's letters to God: The new collection.* New York: Workman Publishing.

conventional role conformity, and the level of self-accepted moral principles. Gilligan (1982) criticized Kohlberg's conclusions, arguing that because the 25-year longitudinal study on which his work was based included only boys and men, it was not equally applicable to girls and women. Instead, she proposed a three-level theory of moral development for girls: concern for the self, caring for others in need, and concern and caring for all people (Gilligan, 1985). Gilligan hypothesized that, *for girls*, basing moral decisions on the primacy of caring relationships (for Kohlberg, a stage-three characteristic) is a higher value than basing moral decisions on universal ethical principles (for Kohlberg, stage six). A study designed to examine this question, however, suggests that this gender difference is not statistically significant (Walker, in Wolff, 1991). The study did show that both males and females tend to judge real-life situations on the basis of care and responsibility and hypothetical situations on the basis of justice and rights.

Another approach to the investigation of moral development is Hoffman's (1984) proposed four levels in the development of empathy: global empathy, egocentric empathy, empathy for another's feelings, and empathy for another's general condition. Coles (1986) conducted phenomenological research with children who have maintained a highly evolved moral stance despite adverse social circumstances. Kagan and Lamb (1987) collected essays from studies in anthropology, philosophy, and developmental psychology in an attempt to answer four long-standing questions:

- Is morality innate or learned?
- How do standards for moral judgment develop as children grow older?
- Are there universal standards that all children acquire?
- Do gender and cultural differences have any bearing on moral development?

All of these questions still need investigation and inquiry, so that you might ask how parents can best meet their children's needs in this regard. The answer is probably disarmingly simple: If parents who demonstrate a belief in their own values raise their children lovingly, the children are likely to grow up with similar values. "Moral education follows naturally on the arrival of morality in the child by the natural developmental processes that good care facilitates" (Winnicott, 1965). During assessment, try to get a preliminary sense of the child's social judgment and capacity for empathy, the level of excitement evoked by cruelty or identification with an aggressor, and any expression of regret or remorse for transgressions.

SPIRITUAL DEVELOPMENT

Perhaps even less well studied than moral development is the spiritual development of children and adolescents. Yet, as Coles (1990) reminds us, the "child's house 'has many mansions'—including a spiritual life that grows,

Dear God
It is great
the way
you always
get the
stars in
the right
places.

Jeff

From Hample, S., and Marshall, E. (Eds.) (1991). *Children's letters to God: The new collection.* New York: Workman Publishing.

TABLE 24–3 **Spiritual Development**

Developmental Stage	Erikson	Aden	Fowler	Westerhoff
Infancy	Hope	Faith as trust	Stage 0 Undifferentiated	
Early childhood	Will	Faith as courage		
			Stage I Intuitive-projective	Experienced faith
Preschool	Purpose	Faith as obedience		
School-age	Skill	Faith as assent	Stage II Mythical-literal	
Adolescence	Fidelity	Faith as identity	Stage III Synthetic-conventional	Affiliative faith
Young adulthood	Love	Faith as surrender	Stage IV Individuality reflexive	Searching faith
Adulthood	Care	Faith as unconditional surrender	Stage V Polar-dialectical	
Maturity	Wisdom	Faith as unconditional acceptance	Stage IV Universalizing	Owned faith

changes, responds constantly to the other lives that, in their sum, make up the individual we call by a name and know by a story that is all his, all hers" (p. 308).

Carson (1989) proposes that spiritual development takes place as a *two-directional process.* The horizontal dimension is concerned with the pervasive presence of spiritual values in day-to-day living, the vertical with the individual's relationship to a higher power. Carson further distinguishes between spirituality and religiosity because many people carefully abide by religious traditions without experiencing spiritual awakening, just as people without any religious affiliation may espouse an essential spirituality.

Building on these stages of the development of faith put forward by Fowler, Aden, and Westerhoff, Carson weaves in Erikson's (1961, 1963) belief in the importance of hope, as shown in Table 24–3. As Carson points out, these theories have been formulated in the context of Western cultures and Judeo-Christian values. One of the most striking differences between the industrialized nations and the rest of the peoples of the world is that in many indigenous cultures spiritual teaching is part of daily life and childhood education. Children's heritage is inseparable from their responsibility to safeguard the tenets and practices of their creed. For example, writing of the Australian Aborigines, Lawlor (1991) states that for them, "childhood emerges out of the depths of the spirit of the natural world and is inseparable from that world."

Hollander (1981) emphasizes the parents' role in assisting children to develop a spiritual awareness, particularly in families cut off from communal practices and rituals and a context to support spirituality in daily activities. Sometimes, catastrophic events can bring a child face to face with a spiritual crisis. Sometimes, with help, the child can make good use of such a crisis to develop a profound inner strength.

Not part of any model of spiritual development, however, is the view that the child is *innately* religious, inhabiting a world suffused with undifferentiated Godliness. This idea has run like a thread through Western mystical thought for thousands of years. From this perspective, promoting spiritual growth is less an obligation to teach and more an obligation to protect the child's inborn capacities from the negative influences of the material world. This belief can be traced as far back as Socrates, who expressed a conviction that each person is born endowed with complete knowledge and that this knowledge can be brought to consciousness by careful questioning. It appears in the words of Jesus to his disciples: "Except ye be converted, and become as little children, ye shall not enter the kingdom of heaven" (Matthew, XVIII, 3). And it appears nearly 2000 years later, in Wordsworth's "Intimations of Immortality":

> But trailing clouds of glory do we come
> from God, who is our home:
> Heaven lies about us in our infancy!

More recently, this idea can be found in Haun's *Celestial Interlude* (1993), in which a wind spirit recollects the spiritual wholeness of human childhood:

> *At six or seven . . . one summer afternoon, one may lie on its back on a cellar door, look up through the leaves of an ancient oak tree, and feel the movement of the earth. At this moment, it realizes that it is not just a six or seven year old kid; it is also the cellar door, and the house to which the door is attached, and the little green yard where the house was built, and the whole neighborhood it's in. It feels itself encompassing the town, the country, land and sea, and, closing its eyes, it is revolving in the air, slowly circling the sun, and knows that it is the earth onto which it was born.*

When considering a child's spiritual development, question both parents and child about spiritual faith, religious practices, and their importance to the family. Understanding another's values is an important part of empathy. As Carson (1989) reminds us, "spirituality is not something to be judged but rather to be assessed and accepted."

SUICIDALITY

No statistics are kept of suicides among children under 5, and records of death by suicide are extremely rare in children between the ages of 5 and 9. The most prevalent methods of suicide in young children involve impulsive actions such as jumping from a height or running in front of a car, so separating possible suicides from the high number of accidental deaths in this age group is difficult. In older children, even despite a likelihood of underreporting, the suicide rate is alarmingly high. As many as 60% of adolescents have considered suicide (Garrison et al, 1991). Girls have a higher rate of suicidal gestures, most often by means of overdose; boys have a slightly higher rate of completion, with hanging and firearm use the most common methods.

The management of suicidal behavior is "probably the most difficult issue in child psychiatric outpatient treatment and causes the most sleepless nights" (Lewandowski: Personal communication, 1990). Risk factors include

- History of suicide attempt
- Mood disorder, disruptive disorder, substance abuse disorder, anxiety disorder, or schizophrenia
- Recent significant loss
- Death of friend or family member by suicide, especially if recent
- Perception of isolation

The most immediate risk factor is *current suicidal ideation*, particularly in the presence of a lethal plan. Beware of making assumptions in evaluating the lethality of the plan. A young child may truly believe that squeezing his own throat will be fatal, and a bright teenager may lack a sophisticated knowledge of pharmacology. The best way to determine whether the child has such a plan is to ask. Approach the topic naturally in the context of the mental status examination, but even with a gentle approach, make your questions direct and unambiguous: "Have you ever thought of hurting yourself, or killing yourself? How would you do this? Are you feeling this way now?" A child at high risk for committing suicide must be kept safe and should be hospitalized if necessary.

▶ Check Your Reading

21. What do you assess as part of the physical examination?
22. Give one example to illustrate each of at least five important features of a play assessment.
23. Name at least four specific areas of assessment.
24. What is the most immediate risk factor for a potentially suicidal child?
25. Give one reason why a spiritual assessment is included in the overall assessment of children.

DIAGNOSIS

Naming a psychiatric "disorder" does not mean that it exists the way an object or physical disorder exists. This ambiguity may be especially true of many psychiatric diagnoses given to children, which, although they may be related to a neurological problem, are based on a cluster of attributes or behaviors and are not diseases. Also keep in mind that these attributes and behaviors are almost always just exaggerated versions of characteristics that all people share. The diagnosis is "not an end in itself, but a strategic doorway to treatment" (Nurcombe and Fitzhenry-Coor, 1987).

As Chapters 3 and 12 explain, you need to be familiar with the currently used psychiatric nosology, or classification system. The *DSM-IV* begins with a section addressing disorders "usually first diagnosed in infancy, childhood, or adolescence." These psychiatric diagnoses in turn suggest related nursing diagnoses.

For Jordi, the overriding nursing diagnosis is Social Isolation related to profound developmental delays, poor reality testing, and anxiety, as evidenced by lack of social skills and immature and bizarre behaviors.

Assessment data that support this finding might be stated as follows:

- Jordi's parents state "He has no friends."
- Jordi makes poor eye contact and rarely interacts with others.
- Jordi displays several unusual sensitivities and fears.
- Jordi appears to be responding to internal stimuli at times.

▶ Check Your Reading

26. Explain why most children's psychiatric disorders are different from a medical disease such as diabetes.

Attention Deficit and Disruptive Behavior Disorders

ATTENTION-DEFICIT HYPERACTIVITY DISORDER

A diagnosis of *attention-deficit hyperactivity disorder* (ADHD) is based on symptoms that occur before age 7 and have lasted at least six months. This diagnosis is further codified by the predominating symptoms—that is, whether the child is mainly inattentive, mainly hyperactive, or both.

In any classroom in the United States you may see a child like this: He is in constant motion, running when others walk, fidgeting as he waits in line, jumping up out of his seat, making mistake after mistake on his worksheets, not paying attention, or—when he *has* heard the question—blurting out the answer without waiting to be called.

A large epidemiological study found that ADHD is the most common psychiatric diagnosis given to children between the ages of 4 and 11 (Szatmari et al, 1989). In the representative sample of 1617 children studied, 9% of all boys and 3.3% of all girls were found to have ADHD. Other similarly broad population surveys suggest that a genetic contribution to this disorder is probable (Weiss, 1991).

The first line of treatment for ADHD is often a stimulant medication such as methylphenidate or dextroamphetamine. Because the vast majority of children with ADHD show situational differences in hyperactivity (Weiss, 1991), however, the child's environment clearly plays a key role and must be taken into account.

CONDUCT DISORDER

Conduct disorder is a label for disturbances of behavior contradictory to accepted social norms. These behaviors usually involve harming others or violating a trust. At least 3 of 15 criteria must have been present for six months or more; including stealing, running away, lying, fire-setting, truancy, and cruelty to animals.

A conduct disorder represents a description of a group of behaviors—such as impulsivity and violence—frequently clustered together. A number of investigators have begun studying the possible neurochemical contributions to such behaviors, most notably decreased noradrenergic and serotoninergic functioning (Eichelman, 1992; Quay, 1993). As always, however, you must also look beyond the behavior, or within it, to the communicative function it serves. The outside observer can easily recognize anger in a conduct-disordered child, but the child may be less clear about anger and less clear still about the other feelings underlying the actions. As Winnicott (1958) suggests, "there is a direct relationship between the antisocial tendency and deprivation," and, further, "*the antisocial tendency implies hope.*"

Your first response is to help provide what the child is missing: that is, not some material thing, but the safety of being contained and prevented from doing harm. With containment (which can be provided in a home or an institution), you can begin to link behaviors with feelings in a way that becomes comprehensible for a child.

OPPOSITIONAL DEFIANT DISORDER

Oppositional defiant disorder is another diagnosis given to children who are often more readily perceived as troubling than troubled. Similarly, this diagnosis requires a minimum of four out of eight designated behaviors present for at least six months, including: temper tantrums, arguing with adults, actively defying adult requests, provocative behavior, blaming others, and being easily angered. Again, because these behaviors are common, they must occur far more frequently than in others of the same mental age.

As Rey (1993, p. 1775) points out:

> *Symptoms of oppositional defiant disorder may be the final common pathway of many etiological factors, alone or in combination, including genetic, constitutional, social, and psychological mechanisms.*

Nevertheless, an oppositional, defiant child is relatively rare in a household in which parents agree on consistent, loving methods of providing structure and discipline. Oppositional children often have low self-esteem and may actually find their own behavior quite frightening. But they may also be frightened of giving up their defiance. It probably serves several functions, including distraction from fearfulness, sadness, and anxiety.

Although parents complain that they want their child to do as the child is told, the situation is likely to be quite a bit more complicated. It may be that both child *and* parents are wary of simple compliance yet have not found a way to manage aggression in a useful, life-affirming way. The object of socializing such children is not to break them in or even to domesticate them. As Cotton (1993, p. 2) writes:

> *Our patients are the discontented, sad and angry lions in the playing fields and classrooms of childhood. We want them to keep their lion strength, passion, and aggression, within the treatment settings and strategies we create for them. We don't want them to abandon the inner lion, but to befriend and tame it.*

A combination of externally imposed limits, cognitive teaching of problem-solving skills, and insight-oriented therapy can address both behaviors and feelings.

▶ Check Your Reading

27. Name at least two characteristics of a child with ADHD.
28. Suggest two nursing diagnoses for an adolescent with a disruptive behavior disorder.

Anxiety Disorders

The *anxiety disorders* of childhood and adolescence include both specific and general disturbances. Anxiety, fear, and impaired social interaction are potentially useful nursing diagnoses in these disorders. You need to distinguish, however, between children who experience realistic—if extreme—anxiety about actual threats and children whose anxiety is increasingly understood to have an important neurobiological component.

Of the anxiety disorders, only *separation anxiety disorder* is listed in *DSM-IV* as a childhood disorder. It is most commonly seen in early childhood and in preadolescence. It is characterized by at least a four-week duration of excessive and unrealistic worry about separation from the child's major attachment figures (usually but not always parents). Anxiety may be manifested by

***DSM-IV* Diagnosis:** Attention-Deficit Hyperactivity Disorder

DIAGNOSTIC CRITERIA

A. Either (1) or (2):

(1) Six (or more) of the following symptoms of *inattention* have persisted for at least six months to a degree that is maladaptive and inconsistent with developmental level:

Inattention

(a) Often fails to give close attention to details or makes careless mistakes in schoolwork, work, or other activities.
(b) Often has difficulty sustaining attention in tasks or play activities.
(c) Often does not seem to listen when spoken to directly.
(d) Often does not follow through on instructions and fails to finish schoolwork, chores, or duties in the workplace (not due to oppositional behavior or failure to understand instructions).
(e) Often has difficulty organizing tasks and activities.
(f) Often avoids, dislikes, or is reluctant to engage in tasks that require sustained mental effort (such as schoolwork or homework).
(g) Often loses things necessary for tasks or activities (e.g., toys, school assignments, pencils, books, or tools).
(h) Is often easily distracted by extraneous stimuli.
(i) Is often forgetful in daily activities.

(2) Six (or more) of the following symptoms of *hyperactivity-impulsivity* have persisted for at least six months to a degree that is maladaptive and inconsistent with developmental level:

Hyperactivity

(a) Often fidgets with hands or feet or squirms in seat.
(b) Often leaves seat in classroom or in other situations in which remaining seated is expected.
(c) Often runs about or climbs excessively in situations in which it is inappropriate (in adolescents or adults, may be limited to subjective feelings of restlessness).
(d) Often has difficulty playing or engaging in leisure activities quietly.
(e) Is often "on the go" or often acts as if "driven by a motor."
(f) Often talks excessively.

Impulsivity

(g) Often blurts out answers before questions have been completed.
(h) Often has difficulty awaiting turn.
(i) Often interrupts or intrudes on others (e.g., butts into conversations or games).

B. Some hyperactive-impulsive or inattentive symptoms that caused impairment were present before age 7 years.
C. Some impairment from the symptoms is present in two or more settings (e.g., at school [or work] and at home).
D. There must be clear evidence of clinically significant impairment in social, academic, or occupational functioning.
E. The symptoms do not occur exclusively during the course of a Pervasive Developmental Disorder, Schizophrenia, or other Psychotic Disorder and are not better accounted for by another mental disorder (e.g., Mood Disorder, Anxiety Disorder, Dissociative Disorder, or a Personality Disorder).

Code based on type:

314.01 Attention-Deficit/Hyperactivity Disorder, Combined Type: If both Criteria A1 and A2 are met for the past six months.
314.00 Attention-Deficit/Hyperactivity Disorder, Predominantly Inattentive Type: If Criterion A1 is met but Criterion A2 is not met for the past six months.
314.01 Attention-Deficit/Hyperactivity Disorder, Predominantly Hyperactive-Impulsive Type: If Criterion A2 is met but Criterion A1 is not met for the past six months.

Coding note: For individuals (especially adolescents and adults) who currently have symptoms that no longer meet full criteria, "In Partial Remission" should be specified.

***DSM-IV* Diagnosis:** Conduct Disorder

DIAGNOSTIC CRITERIA

A. A repetitive and persistent pattern of behavior in which the basic rights of others or major age-appropriate societal norms or rules are violated, as manifested by the presence of three (or more) of the following criteria in the past 12 months, with at least one criterion present in the past 6 months:

Aggression to people and animals

(1) Often bullies, threatens, or intimidates others.
(2) Often initiates physical fights.
(3) Has used a weapon that can cause serious physical harm to others (e.g., a bat, brick, broken bottle, knife, gun).
(4) Has been physically cruel to people.
(5) Has been physically cruel to animals.
(6) Has stolen while confronting a victim (e.g., mugging, purse snatching, extortion, armed robbery).
(7) Has forced someone into sexual activity.

Destruction of property

(8) Has deliberately engaged in fire setting with the intention of causing serious damage.
(9) Has deliberately destroyed others' property (other than by fire setting).

Box continued on following page

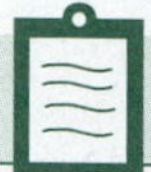

MEDICAL DIAGNOSES AND RELATED NURSING DIAGNOSES **Attention-Deficit and Disruptive Behavior Disorders** *Continued*

Deceitfulness or theft

(10) Has broken into someone else's house, building, or car.
(11) Often lies to obtain goods or favors or to avoid obligations (i.e., "cons" others).
(12) Has stolen items of nontrivial value without confronting a victim (e.g., shoplifting, but without breaking and entering; forgery).

Serious violations of rules

(13) Often stays out at night despite parental prohibitions, beginning before age 13 years.
(14) Has run away from home overnight at least twice while living in parental or parental surrogate home (or once without returning for a lengthy period).
(15) Is often truant from school, beginning before age 13 years.

B. The disturbance in behavior causes clinically significant impairment in social, academic, or occupational functioning.
C. If the individual is age 18 years or older, criteria are not met for Antisocial Personality Disorder.

Specify type based on age at onset:

Childhood-Onset Type: Onset of at least one criterion characteristic of Conduct Disorder before age 10 years.
Adolescent-Onset Type: Absence of any criteria characteristic of Conduct Disorder before age 10 years.

Specify severity:

Mild: Few if any conduct problems in excess of those required to make the diagnosis *and* conduct problems cause only minor harm to others.
Moderate: Number of conduct problems and effect on others intermediate between *mild* and *severe.*
Severe: Many conduct problems in excess of those required to make the diagnosis *or* conduct problems cause considerable harm to others.

***DSM-IV* Diagnosis:** Oppositional Defiant Disorder

DIAGNOSTIC CRITERIA

A. A pattern of negativistic, hostile, and defiant behavior lasting at least six months, during which four (or more) of the following are present:

(1) Often loses temper.
(2) Often argues with adults.
(3) Often actively defies or refuses to comply with adults' requests or rules.
(4) Often deliberately annoys people.
(5) Often blames others for his or her mistakes or misbehavior.
(6) Is often touchy or easily annoyed by others.
(7) Is often angry and resentful.
(8) Is often spiteful or vindictive.

Note: Consider a criterion met only if the behavior occurs more frequently than is typically observed in individuals of comparable age and developmental level.

B. The disturbance in behavior causes clinically significant impairment in social, academic, or occupational functioning.
C. The behaviors do not occur exclusively during the course of a Psychotic or Mood Disorder.
D. Criteria are not met for Conduct Disorder, and, if the individual is age 18 years or older, criteria are not met for Antisocial Personality Disorder.

RELATED NURSING DIAGNOSES	DEFINITION	EXAMPLE
Risk for Violence	A state in which an individual experiences behaviors that can be physically harmful either to the self or others.	Potential for Violence related to Conduct Disorder as evidenced by intermittent aggressive outbursts.
Ineffective Family Coping: Compromised	A usually supportive primary person (family member or close friend) is providing insufficient, ineffective, or compromised support, comfort, assistance, or encouragement that may be needed by the client to manage or master adaptive tasks related to his or her health challenge.	Ineffective Family Coping related to oppositional defiant disorder as evidenced by cycle of harsh punishment followed by overindulgent compensation.

Diagnostic criteria from American Psychiatric Association (1994). *Diagnostic and statistical manual of mental disorders, fourth edition.* Washington, D.C.: American Psychiatric Association.

such things as persistent worries about possible harm to the parents and reluctance or refusal to be separated from them—for example, to attend school or to go to bed. These children often complain of a wide variety of physical symptoms as well.

Separation anxiety in the child is often seen concurrently with a similar anxiety in the parent, lending support to the theory of a genetic contribution to the disorder. In this instance, both child and parent can be helped by the experience of surviving separations.

Overanxious disorder of childhood, included in the category of *generalized anxiety disorders*, is diagnosed based on symptoms present for six months or more. Symptoms include excessive or unrealistic worries about several events or activities, past or future; irritability; difficulty concentrating; and difficulty falling asleep. A problem in offering comprehensive treatment for any of these disorders is that antianxiety medications, such as the benzodiazepines, which are traditionally used to help anxious adults, have not been found to be particularly effective or helpful in children. Somewhat more helpful are antidepressants, such as bupropion or nortriptyline.

Obsessive-compulsive disorder, now generally believed to be a neurophysiologically based illness with a genetic component, has also been noted to occur at a higher rate in relatives of people with Tourette's disorder (Pauls, 1991). Although a single specific mechanism has yet to be

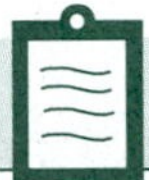

MEDICAL DIAGNOSES AND RELATED NURSING DIAGNOSES — **Anxiety Disorders**

***DSM-IV* Diagnosis:** Separation Anxiety Disorder

DIAGNOSTIC CRITERIA

A. Developmentally inappropriate and excessive anxiety concerning separation from home or from those to whom the individual is attached, as evidenced by three (or more) of the following:

(1) Recurrent excessive distress when separation from home or major attachment figures occurs or is anticipated.
(2) Persistent and excessive worry about losing, or about possible harm befalling, major attachment figures.
(3) Persistent and excessive worry that an untoward event will lead to separation from a major attachment figure (e.g., getting lost or being kidnapped).
(4) Persistent reluctance or refusal to go to school or elsewhere because of fear of separation.
(5) Persistently and excessively fearful or reluctant to be alone or without major attachment figures at home or without significant adults in other settings.
(6) Persistent reluctance or refusal to go to sleep without being near a major attachment figure or to sleep away from home.
(7) Repeated nightmares involving the theme of separation.
(8) Repeated complaints of physical symptoms (such as headaches, stomachaches, nausea, or vomiting) when separation from major attachment figures occurs or is anticipated.

B. The duration of the disturbance is at least four weeks.
C. The onset is before age 18 years.
D. The disturbance causes clinically significant distress or impairment in social, academic (occupational), or other important areas of functioning.
E. The disturbance does not occur exclusively during the course of a Pervasive Developmental Disorder, Schizophrenia, or other Psychotic Disorder and, in adolescents and adults, is not better accounted for by Panic Disorder With Agoraphobia.

Specify if:
Early Onset: If onset occurs before age 6 years.

***DSM-IV* Diagnosis:** Generalized Anxiety Disorder (includes Overanxious Disorder of Childhood)

***DSM-IV* Diagnosis:** Obsessive-Compulsive Disorder

***DSM-IV* Diagnosis:** Posttraumatic Stress Disorder

RELATED NURSING DIAGNOSES	DEFINITION	EXAMPLE
Anxiety	A vague, uneasy feeling whose source is often nonspecific or unknown to the individual.	Anxiety related to separations, as evidenced by rapid heartbeat, clinging, and inconsolable crying.
Spiritual Distress	Disruption in the life principle that pervades a person's entire being and that integrates and transcends one's biological and psychosocial nature.	Spiritual Distress related to witnessing mother's murder, as evidenced by preoccupation with death, expressions of hopelessness.

Diagnostic criteria from American Psychiatric Association (1994). *Diagnostic and statistical manual of mental disorders, fourth edition.* Washington, D.C.: American Psychiatric Association.

demonstrated, studies suggest the involvement of the serotoninergic system of the brain (Scahill et al, 1993).

The defining characteristics of obsessive-compulsive disorder are obsessions (recurring, distressing thoughts or images), compulsions (repetitive, driven behaviors performed in response to obsessions), or both. Treatment has focused on the use of medications (such as clorimipramine or fluoxetine) that block the reuptake of the neurotransmitter serotonin to support behavioral approaches. Typically, parents of a child with this disorder find themselves gradually accommodating to increasingly outlandish demands in a well-meaning but futile effort to help the child function. Learning to set limits supportively and to work with the child on such treatment interventions as *exposure* (intentionally confronting the child with provocative stimuli) and *response prevention* (not allowing the compulsion) are important for both parents and nurses (Scahill et al, 1993).

Posttraumatic stress disorder is now recognized in children as well as in adults. Either posttraumatic stress disorder or *acute stress disorder* may follow a child's experiencing or witnessing a terrifying event in which threat of harm or death or actual harm or death occurs. The difference between the two disorders is largely a matter of time of onset and duration of symptoms, both involving recurrent recollections of the event, disturbing dreams, increased anxiety, and avoidance of anything likely to remind the child of the event. Some symptoms may respond to antidepressant medication (see Table 24–4). Children who have had such experiences tend to recreate them repeatedly in play; it is possible for a helping adult to guide this repetition into a sense of mastery.

▶ Check Your Reading

29. Give an example of an unrealistic worry one might see in an overanxious child.
30. What is meant by *exposure* and *response prevention* in the treatment of obsessive-compulsive disorder?
31. Name two symptoms of posttraumatic stress disorder in children.

Feeding and Eating Disorders

Feeding and eating disorders, listed in DSM-IV in both the childhood section and a later, separate section, include a number of potentially serious problems in infants, children, and adolescents.

The diagnosis of *anorexia nervosa* is based on four major identifying features: (1) a refusal to maintain minimum weight normal for height and age; (2) an intense fear of becoming fat; (3) a distorted body image; and (4) in females, the absence of at least three consecutive, postmenarchal menstrual cycles. Extremely rare in boys and in prepubertal children, anorexia is primarily an illness of adolescent girls.

Recognized as a psychiatric disturbance more than 100 years ago, anorexia has been the subject of intensified interest since the 1960s. It is extremely difficult to treat and potentially fatal. With more public awareness and earlier recognition, however, more girls may receive treatment early, when they have the best chance for recovery. One reason for the difficulty of treatment is that girls and women affected by this illness generally do not wish to be "cured"—that is, to gain weight. The further the illness progresses, the more deeply entrenched is their resistance (Levenkron, 1993). Anorexia is frequently seen comorbidly with depression, anxiety disorders, and characterological disorders, such as borderline and dependent personality disorders (Hoffman and Halmi, 1993).

Wachsmuth and Garfinkel (1993) review the four basic goals of treatment:

- Establishing and maintaining an ongoing treatment alliance
- Weight restoration and reversal of the associated physical signs and symptoms of starvation
- Improvement in eating behavior
- Improvement in social functioning (p. 146)

They also note that a wide range of types of therapy has been recommended, including, either singly or combined, family therapy, individual psychotherapy, psychoanalysis, group therapy, and behavioral therapy. These recommendations have been based largely on clinical experience rather than on controlled outcome studies. One study by Russell and colleagues (in Wachsmuth and Garfinkel, 1993) compares the effectiveness of individual to family treatment on an outpatient basis. This study found that for adolescents under 18 and for patients with illness lasting less than three years, family therapy was significantly more effective. Although most anorectic adolescents do improve or recover, the illness is associated with a significant mortality rate of between 2% (Hall et al, 1984) and 18% (Theander, 1985). When the child's weight loss is extreme enough to warrant hospitalization, treatment may include tube feedings and strict behavioral contracts based on daily weights, with increasing privileges and autonomy in response to continued weight gain.

Bulimia nervosa, defined as episodes of binge eating alternating with extreme weight loss measures (such as self-induced vomiting or use of laxatives), is seen most frequently in high school–age and college-age young women. The subjective experience is typically reported to involve a feeling of being out of control and of being anxious about bodily appearances. Although this disorder is often associated with anorexia, bulimic individuals may range in weight from thin to obese and may keep their bulimia secret for many years before seeking help (Wozniak and Herzog, 1993). Bulimia can lead to significant medical problems ranging from erosion of tooth enamel to serious—even fatal—electrolyte imbalances. A promising treatment approach combines an exploration of interpersonal dynamics and behavioral interventions.

Pica is defined as the ingestion of nonnutritive substances over a period of one month or more. Pica appears to occur in three distinct groups: severely and profoundly mentally retarded children, young children in deprived environments, and chronically anxious children (Woolston, 1991). In each of these instances, the pica should be addressed by a behavior management plan, while the related condition must also be considered and included in a broader plan of care.

TABLE 24–4 **Commonly Used Medications in Child Psychiatry**

Medications	Common Uses	Recommended Dosages	Adverse Effects	Nursing Considerations
Stimulants				
Methylphenidate (Ritalin)	ADHD	0.9–2.1 mg/kg/d in divided doses Not approved for children under 6		Observe for a *rebound effect* in the late afternoon, with return or increase of the original behaviors Be aware that stimulants may increase or "unmask" tics in children. Similarly, stimulants can make compulsive behaviors more marked Monitor for lowering of the seizure threshold Note any changes in mental status. Stimulants may, in rare cases, precipitate psychotic episodes
Dextroamphetamine sulfate (Dexedrine)	ADHD	0.3–1.5 mg/kg/d in divided doses Not approved for children under 3	Decreased appetite Insomnia Growth delays Irritability Tachycardia	
Tricyclic antidepressants	Depression		Dry mouth Visual disturbances Sedation or insomnia Worsening psychoses Seizures Blood dyscrasias Cardiovascular changes, including rare fatal cardiac dysrhythmias	Insist on close monitoring for any ECG changes Educate patients about reporting and alleviating uncomfortable side effects Be aware that medication must be tapered to discontinue; abrupt withdrawal can cause extreme discomfort
Nortriptyline (Pamelor)	Depression	30–50 mg/d Not recommended for children under 12		
Norpramine (Desipramine)	Depression ADHD	25–100 mg/d, not to exceed 150 mg/d Not recommended for children under 12		
Amitriptyline (Elavil)	Depression	50–100 mg/d Not recommended for children under 12		
Imipramine (Tofranil)	Depression Enuresis	Up to 100 mg/d, not to exceed 2.5 mg/kg for treatment of enuresis Not recommended for children under 12 except for treatment of enuresis (in children age 6 and older)		

continued

Rumination disorder, a rare, poorly understood phenomenon, has been linked to serious difficulties in the parent-child relationship. It describes a pattern of regurgitating, rechewing, and swallowing food, although not due to a medical condition. At times, this disorder may occur in a biologically well-endowed infant because of maternal inadequacy, but it is more often seen in children with serious developmental delays.

Obesity, although not included in the *DSM-IV* as an eating disorder, is important to consider because it represents a serious, potentially life-threatening condition with psychological correlates. Essential to

TABLE 24–4 **Commonly Used Medications in Child Psychiatry** *Continued*

Medications	Common Uses	Recommended Dosages	Adverse Effects	Nursing Considerations
Clomipramine (Anafranil)	Depression Obsessions	Up to 3 mg/kg/d Not recommended for children under 10		
MAO inhibitors			Orthostatic hypotension Headache Sleep disturbances Gastrointestinal upset	Be aware that combining MAO inhibitors with tricyclics can cause severe seizures or hypertensive crises. A hypertensive crisis can also be induced by interaction with foods containing tyramine (cheese, beer, wine) as well as with amphetamines, cocaine, and caffeine. Because normal developmental issues make it unlikely that children can safely monitor their own use of such medications, the nurse should advocate an alternative
Phenelzine sulfate (Nardil)		Not approved for use in children under 16 (but may still be prescribed)		
Tranylcypromine sulfate (Parnate)		Not approved for use in children (but may still be prescribed)		
Other antidepressants				
Paroxetine hydrochloride (Paxil), fluoxetine hydrochloride (Prozac), sertraline hydrochloride (Zoloft)	Depression	Safety and efficacy not established, but these drugs are increasingly prescribed for children	Nausea Nervousness Sleep disturbances	Fluoxetine (Prozac) in particular may rarely be activating. Monitor children for increased agitation, aggression, or self-injurious behavior. None of these drugs should be given in conjunction with an MAO inhibitor (at least 5 weeks should intervene between medications). These drugs are presumed to work by inhibiting reuptake of the neurotransmitter serotonin. Because of a potential interaction, parents should be warned not to give the nutritional supplement tryptophan (sometimes used to promote sleep)

working with an obese child is the participation of a nutritionist, good medical management, and vigorous treatment of any underlying depression or anxiety. Without the sustained interest and motivation of the child and the active participation of the family, the child has little chance for successful weight reduction. If the child is still growing, attempting weight stabilization may be more realistic. (See Chapter 35 for more information on eating disorders.)

TABLE 24–4 **Commonly Used Medications in Child Psychiatry** *Continued*

Medications	Common Uses	Recommended Dosages	Adverse Effects	Nursing Considerations
Bupropion hydrochloride (Wellbutrin)	Depression ADHD	Not approved for use in children. If prescribed, likely dosage is 100–250 mg/d	Lowering of seizure threshold Dry mouth Sleep disturbances Gastrointestinal symptoms Tremor Rash or other allergic reactions	Never administer to children with seizure disorders, anorexia, or bulimia. Never give in conjunction with an MAO inhibitor (at least 2 weeks should intervene between medications)
Antihistamine: Diphenhydramine (Benadryl)	ADHD Anxiety Bedtime sedation	Not approved for behavior disorders but used in child psychiatry for decades	Dry mouth Sedation or dullness Overexcitement	Be aware that parents may be using diphenhydramine without any medical supervision (the drug is readily available) Warn parents that overdoses may be dangerous or fatal, as can use of this drug in infants (including ingestion through breast milk) Asthma may be aggravated by use of diphenhydramine
Anticonvulsants	Seizures			Administer regularly and accurately Decrease gastrointestinal upset by administering with food or liquid Observe and report any and all seizure activity
Carbamazepine (Tegretol)	Seizures Mood and behavioral disorders	15–30 mg/kg/d	Blurred vision Lethargy	
Sodium valproate (Depakene)	Seizures	15–50 mg/kg/d	Tremors Gastrointestinal symptoms	
Phenytoin (Dilantin)	Seizures	4–7 mg/kg/d	Rash Hyperplasia of the gums Hirsutism	Nurse, patient, and parents must pay special attention to oral hygiene
Phenobarbital	Seizures	3–6 mg/kg/d	Lethargy Hyperactivity	
Clonazepam (Klonopin)	Seizures	0.02–0.2 mg/kg/d	Lethargy Excessive salivation	
Diazepam (Valium)	Status epilepticus	IM: 2–5 mg in single dose IV: 5–10 mg at < 2 mg/min		

▶ **Check Your Reading**

32. Compare and contrast anorexia and bulimia.
33. What is pica?

Gender Identity Disorders

Gender identity disorders should be clearly distinguished from sexual orientation, which is *not* classified as a disorder. Homosexuality (a sexual orientation) *is* seen in latency-age children and adolescents but is separate from confusion or unhappiness about one's gender (an indication of an identity disorder). Homosexual children and adolescents often clearly recognize quite early that they are romantically interested in and sexually aroused by same-sex individuals. It is generally difficult for such children to find someone to talk to about their concerns,

TABLE 24–4 **Commonly Used Medications in Child Psychiatry** *Continued*

Medications	Common Uses	Recommended Dosages	Adverse Effects	Nursing Considerations
Antipsychotics (neuroleptics)	Schizophrenia and other psychotic disorders		Sedation Hypotension Extrapyramidal reactions	Because of their serious and wide-ranging adverse effects, neuroleptics should be used with extreme caution in children. Each drug has a unique combination of beneficial and adverse effects. Research each prescribed medication, and educate parents about expected responses and reportable reactions. A low-dose anticholinergic such as biperiden (Cogentin) may be used to mitigate extrapyramidal effects of some neuroleptics
Phenothiazines				
Chlorpromazine (Thorazine)	Psychotic disorders	1–3 mg/kg/d in divided doses		
Thioridazine (Mellaril)	Psychotic disorders	1–3 mg/kg/d in divided doses		
Perphenazine	Psychotic disorders	Pediatric doses not established Most often prescribed at 0.1–0.4 mg/kg/d in divided doses		
Butyrophenone: Haloperidol (Haldol)	Psychotic disorders	0.05–0.15 mg/kg/d (up to 6 mg)		
Thioxanthine: Thiothixene (Navane)	Psychotic disorders	6–10 mg/d in divided doses Not recommended for children under 12		

and clinicians should not respond to such a disclosure as if it were an indication of pathology.

Gender identity disorder in children is characterized by a persistent wish to be or a belief that one is of the opposite gender. *Gender identity disorder in adolescents* is characterized by a preoccupation with altering one's sexual characteristics. Nursing diagnoses to consider are Personal Identity Disturbance and Social Isolation.

Tic Disorders

Tic disorders include *transient tic disorder, chronic motor or vocal tic disorder,* and *Tourette's disorder.* Tics are defined as "sudden, repetitive, stereotyped motor movements or phonic productions." A significant percentage of all children; particularly school-age boys, are affected by tics at one time or another (Leckman and Cohen, 1988). Most of these tics, whether motor or (less commonly) vocal, disappear spontaneously within a few weeks or months, although they may recur from time to time. If the tics persist for more than a year, the disorder is classified as chronic. If both motor and vocal tics have occurred in the same chronically affected individual, the child is given the diagnosis of Tourette's. A genetic link has been suggested between Tourette's and obsessive-compulsive disorders.

"The first step in management of children with Tourette's syndrome is understanding them and their world" (Silver, 1988). An upsurge of public interest and knowledge about Tourette's has been helpful for these children. A child with Tourette's is now more likely to be recognized and offered treatment rather than punished and ostracized. Nevertheless, parents (and teachers) often

TABLE 24–4 **Commonly Used Medications in Child Psychiatry** *Continued*

Medications	Common Uses	Recommended Dosages	Adverse Effects	Nursing Considerations
Dibenzodiazepine: Clozapine (Clozaril)	Refractory schizophrenia in adults and some adolescents	Pediatric dosages not established		Because clozapine can cause life-threatening agranulocytosis, it must be used according to the guidelines of the Clozaril National Registry.
Benzisoxazole derivate: Risperidone (Risperdal)	Psychotic disorders	Pediatric dosages not established		
Antimanic agents: Lithium carbonate (Eskalith), lithium carbonate time release (Lithobid)	Bipolar disorders	900–1200 mg/kg/d in divided doses Not recommended for use in children under 12 but may still be prescribed	Gastrointestinal symptoms Weight gain Tremors Polyuria and polydipsia Fatigue	In both children and adolescents, dosage must be titrated carefully, according to serum lithium levels. Therapeutic levels range between 0.6–1.2 mEq/L. Levels even slightly above this range can be toxic, and sensitive individuals may experience toxicity at lower ranges. Nurse, patient, and family should be alert for signs of toxicity. These include worsening of expected adverse effects, dizziness, ataxia, slurring of speech, and blurred vision
Antihypertensive agents: Clonidine (Catapres)	Tourette's disorder ADHD Opiate withdrawal	0.2–0.6 mg/d Not recommended for children under 12 but may still be prescribed	Dry mouth Drowsiness Gastrointestinal symptoms Orthostatic hypotension	Check orthostatic blood pressures before administering each dose. Be aware that clonidine should not be stopped abruptly; dosage should be tapered over 3–4 d before discontinuing, to prevent rebound hypertension

are still at a loss as to how and when to set limits and to hold the child responsible for his or her behavior. Keep in mind that tics *can* be suppressed, so that one of the goals of treatment is to find ways of strengthening the child's ability to suppress tics. These methods can include social sanctions, behavioral reinforcers, and medication. The child can also be encouraged to take an interest in identifying the precipitating urge to tic and developing alternative strategies for handling this feeling.

▶ **Check Your Reading**

34. What is the difference between sexual orientation and a gender identity disorder?
35. Give a short definition of Tourette's disorder.

Elimination Disorders

Functional *enuresis* is involuntary wetting not caused by an identifiable physiological condition (such as urinary tract infections, which should be carefully ruled out). Enuresis can occur diurnally but is far more frequent at night. No single theory as to cause has been universally accepted, but most studies are now focusing on sleep and arousal patterns. Left untreated, it resolves spontaneously in most cases by age 13 or so. The condition is usually a source of considerable embarrassment and even shame for a child, however, and may interfere with such important social activities as sleepovers and camp attendance.

Although numerous approaches, such as fluid restrictions, awakening schedules, and aversive consequences, have historically been tried, the most effective methods have been shown to be medication and the *bell-and-pad* system (Mikkelsen, 1991). The bell-and-pad system uses an alarm triggered by the child voiding. It is most successful if the parents participate by waking the child at the first sound of the alarm, supervising any necessary clean-up, and rewarding progress. If the child and family are motivated and willing to work at it, the bell-and-pad method offers the decided advantages of a sense of pride and mastery as well as an absence of serious potential adverse reactions.

Functional *encopresis,* or fecal incontinence, is far rarer than enuresis. Three categories of encopretic children have been proposed by Hersov (1985):

- Children who volitionally soil
- Children who have inadequate bowel control
- Children who soil by leakage.

This last category includes children who have frequent diarrhea as well as those who experience retention with overflow. In all cases, medical causes must be ruled out. Then treatment should take the category into account, although aspects of the treatment may be similar. For example, children who retain feces probably need a bowel-cleaning regimen followed by daily laxatives, whereas children with loose stools may need a daily bulking agent. For all children, education about bodily signals is helpful, as is a plan for sitting on the toilet for 10 or 15 minutes following meals. The child who has been deliberately soiling as a means of communication can be helped toward self-expression through other means. If words are too difficult, art activities may be more satisfying.

▶ Check Your Reading

36. Suggest a treatment plan for nocturnal enuresis.
37. Define functional encopresis.

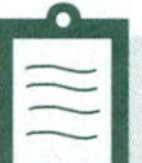

MEDICAL DIAGNOSES AND RELATED NURSING DIAGNOSES

Feeding and Eating Disorders

***DSM-IV* Diagnosis:** Anorexia Nervosa

***DSM-IV* Diagnosis:** Bulimia Nervosa

See Chapter 35 for details.

***DSM-IV* Diagnosis:** Pica

DIAGNOSTIC CRITERIA

A. Persistent eating of nonnutritive substances for a period of at least one month.
B. The eating of nonnutritive substances is inappropriate to the developmental level.
C. The eating behavior is not part of a culturally sanctioned practice.
D. If the eating behavior occurs exclusively during the course of another mental disorder (e.g., Mental Retardation, Pervasive Developmental Disorder, Schizophrenia), it is sufficiently severe to warrant independent clinical attention.

***DSM-IV* Diagnosis:** Rumination Disorder

DIAGNOSTIC CRITERIA

A. Repeated regurgitation and rechewing of food for a period of at least one month following a period of normal functioning.
B. The behavior is not due to an associated gastrointestinal or other general medical condition (e.g., esophageal reflux).
C. The behavior does not occur exclusively during the course of anorexia nervosa or bulimia nervosa. If the symptoms occur exclusively during the course of mental retardation or a pervasive developmental disorder, they are sufficiently severe to warrant independent clinical attention.

Medical Diagnosis: Obesity

Definition: The condition of weighing more than 120% of one's ideal body weight.

RELATED NURSING DIAGNOSES	DEFINITION	EXAMPLE
Body Image Disturbance	Disruption in the way one perceives one's body image.	Body Image Disturbance related to anorexia, as evidenced by weight at 70% of ideal body weight and patient's insistence that she looks "fat."
Altered Nutrition: More Than Body Requirements	The state in which an individual is experiencing an intake of nutrients that exceeds metabolic needs.	Alteration in Nutrition related to excessive caloric intake, as evidenced by weight of 325 lbs.
Risk for Injury	A state in which the individual is at risk for injury as a result of environmental conditions interacting with the individual's adaptive and defensive resources.	Risk for Injury related to ingestion of objects, as evidenced by history of swallowing toy parts or paint chips.

Diagnostic criteria from American Psychiatric Association (1994). *Diagnostic and statistical manual of mental disorders, fourth edition.* Washington, D.C.: American Psychiatric Association.

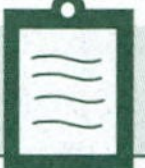

MEDICAL DIAGNOSES AND RELATED NURSING DIAGNOSES — Tic Disorders

***DSM-IV* Diagnosis:** Tourette's Disorder

DIAGNOSTIC CRITERIA

A. Both multiple motor and one or more vocal tics have been present at some time during the illness, although not necessarily concurrently. (A *tic* is a sudden, rapid, recurrent, nonrhythmic, stereotyped motor movement or vocalization.)
B. The tics occur many times a day (usually in bouts) nearly every day or intermittently throughout a period of more than one year, and during this period there was never a tic-free period of more than three consecutive months.
C. The disturbance causes marked distress or significant impairment in social, occupational, or other important areas of functioning.
D. The onset is before age 18 years.
E. The disturbance is not due to the direct physiological effects of a substance (e.g., stimulants) or a general medical condition (e.g., Huntington's disease or postviral encephalitis).

***DSM-IV* Diagnosis:** Chronic Motor or Vocal Tic Disorder

DIAGNOSTIC CRITERIA

A. Single or multiple motor or vocal tics (i.e., sudden, rapid, recurrent, nonrhythmic, stereotyped motor movements or vocalizations), but not both, have been present at some time during the illness.
B. The tics occur many times a day nearly every day or intermittently throughout a period of more than one year, and during this period there was never a tic-free period of more than three consecutive months.
C. The disturbance causes marked distress or significant impairment in social, occupational, or other important areas of functioning.
D. The onset is before age 18 years.
E. The disturbance is not due to the direct physiological effects of a substance (e.g., stimulants) or a general medical condition (e.g., Huntington's disease or postviral encephalitis).
F. Criteria have never been met for Tourette's Disorder.

***DSM-IV* Diagnosis:** Transient Tic Disorder

DIAGNOSTIC CRITERIA

A. Single or multiple motor or vocal tics (i.e., sudden, rapid, recurrent, nonrhythmic, stereotyped motor movements or vocalizations).
B. The tics occur many times a day, nearly every day for at least four weeks, but for no longer than 12 consecutive months.
C. The disturbance causes marked distress or significant impairment in social, occupational, or other important areas of functioning.
D. The onset is before age 18 years.
E. The disturbance is not due to the direct physiological effects of a substance (e.g., stimulants) or a general medical condition (e.g., Huntington's disease or postviral encephalitis).
F. Criteria have never been met for Tourette's Disorder or Chronic Motor or Vocal Tic Disorder.
Specify if:
Single Episode or *Recurrent*

***DSM-IV* Diagnosis:** Tic Disorder, Not Otherwise Specified

RELATED NURSING DIAGNOSIS	DEFINITION	EXAMPLE
Knowledge Deficit	Absence or deficiency of cognitive information related to specific topic.	Knowledge Deficit related to Tourette's Disorder, as evidenced by self-blame and uncontrolled rage.

Diagnostic criteria from American Psychiatric Association (1994). *Diagnostic and statistical manual of mental disorders, fourth edition.* Washington, D.C.: American Psychiatric Association.

Developmental Disorders

The *developmental disorders* are listed in the DSM-IV as *mental retardation, learning disorders, motor skills disorder, communication disorder,* and *pervasive developmental disorders.*

Mental retardation is defined by the American Association of Mental Deficiency as including both "significantly subaverage" intelligence and "deficits in adaptive behavior" (Grossman, 1973). Cognitive functioning is usually measured by a standardized test such as the Stanford-Binet or the Wechsler Intelligence Scales for Children, Revised (WISC-R). Adaptive functioning may also be assessed by a standardized formal interview such as the Vineland Adaptive Behavior Scales (Sparrow et al, 1984), or it may be described informally by the child's parents.

In practice, far more weight is given to a child's score on cognitive tests. These *intelligence quotient* or IQ tests measure a particular set of skills and "may not tell us much about *intelligence*" (Tanguay and Russell, 1991). What they do provide is a delineating boundary for the diagnosis of mental retardation, which the DSM-IV specifies as a score of 70 or below. Remember that the vast majority of retarded children have an IQ score of at least 55 (Tanguay and Russell, 1991) and the potential to enjoy a productive, loving, and fulfilling life. Psychiatric disorders do, however, occur at a disproportionately high rate among mentally retarded children (Rutter et al, 1970; Tanguay, 1990).

Clinicians sometimes hesitate to use the phrase *mental retardation* when talking to parents, but it is extremely important for parents to have as complete an understanding as possible of their child's cognitive limitations as well as strengths. When parents have an inaccurate idea of their child, their expectations may not match the child's capacities, and they may be unable to provide appropriate support to enable their child to reach full potential. Parents also need guidance in advocating for their child's special needs, both present and future.

Based on the teachings of Steiner, a number of model communities have been developed under the name "Camphill." There people with mental retardation, autism, and other developmental disorders live and work alongside people who do not have developmental disorders (Baron-Cohen and Bolton, 1993). This model should apply to every community, large or small, because segregation of people by any attribute or characteristic has historically led to extraordinary problems. Although the benefit to the "handicapped" of integrated living may

MEDICAL DIAGNOSES AND RELATED NURSING DIAGNOSES — Elimination Disorders

***DSM-IV* Diagnosis:** Enuresis

DIAGNOSTIC CRITERIA

A. Repeated voiding of urine into bed or clothes (whether involuntary or intentional).
B. The behavior is clinically significant as manifested by either a frequency of twice a week for at least three consecutive months or the presence of clinically significant distress or impairment in social, academic (occupational), or other important areas of functioning.
C. Chronological age is at least 5 years (or equivalent developmental level).
D. The behavior is not due exclusively to the direct physiological effect of a substance (e.g., a diuretic) or a general medical condition (e.g., diabetes, spina bifida, a seizure disorder).
Specify type:
Nocturnal Only
Diurnal Only
Nocturnal and Diurnal

***DSM-IV* Diagnosis:** Encopresis

DIAGNOSTIC CRITERIA

A. Repeated passage of feces into inappropriate places (e.g., clothing or floor) whether involuntary or intentional.
B. At least one such event a month for at least three months.
C. Chronological age is at least 4 years (or equivalent developmental level).
D. The behavior is not due exclusively to the direct physiological effects of a substance (e.g., laxatives) or a general medical condition except through a mechanism involving constipation.
Code as follows:
787.6 With Constipation and Overflow Incontinence
307.7 Without Constipation and Overflow Incontinence

RELATED NURSING DIAGNOSES	DEFINITION	EXAMPLE
Functional Incontinence	The state in which an individual experiences an involuntary, unpredictable passage of urine.	Functional Incontinence related to enuresis, as evidenced by daily soiling of bedding.
Self-Esteem Disturbance	Negative self-evaluation/feelings about self or self capabilities that may be directly or indirectly expressed.	Self-Esteem Disturbance related to encopresis, as evidenced by embarrassment, shame, and secretiveness.

Diagnostic criteria from American Psychiatric Association (1994). *Diagnostic and statistical manual of mental disorders, fourth edition.* Washington, D.C.: American Psychiatric Association.)

be more immediately obvious, it could also offer an incalculable benefit to the "normal" others.

The *pervasive developmental disorders* include *autistic disorder, Rett's disorder, childhood disintegrative disorder, Asperger's disorder,* and *pervasive developmental disorder, not otherwise specified.*

Autism may be viewed as the extreme end of a spectrum of deficits in the areas of relatedness, communication, and imaginative play. It is characterized by such features as a lack of awareness of other people or the use of people as if they were things, abnormal verbal and nonverbal communication, and a preoccupation with repetition and sameness. Autistic children frequently display a number of distinctive movements called *stereotypies,* such as hand flapping or rocking.

Autism is a poignant and thus far poorly understood disorder that has kindled a spark in popular interest over the last several decades, in part because of high functioning in some autistic children with such skills as advanced reading skills or savant qualities (for example, an ability to multiply large numbers or to memorize calendars or telephone listings). Autism has been the subject of a number of books and movies, some autobiographical, which have unfortunately contributed to the misperception of autistic individuals as normal or even quite brilliant children mysteriously kept "asleep" and awaiting a magic cure to "awaken" them (D'Ambrosio, 1970; Greenfeld, 1972, 1978, 1986; Kaufman, 1976).

Work with autistic children must rely heavily on concrete behavioral interventions, but "this is not to imply that psychodynamics are unimportant. On the contrary, all children are influenced by psychodynamics, and interactions with caretakers and environment have a deleterious, benign or beneficial effect on autistic children" (Campbell and Green, 1984).

Both *Rett's disorder* and *childhood disintegrative disorder* involve periods of normal development followed by the loss of previously acquired skills in several areas of development. *Asperger's disorder* was first described by Asperger (1944) as involving generally higher cognitive functioning than in most autistic children, along with difficulties with reciprocal relationships and characteristic preoccupations with such things as mechanical objects, telephone numbers, or bus schedules.

Pervasive developmental disorder, not otherwise specified (PDD-NOS), remains a sort of catch-all diagnosis whose broad application will probably be yet further categorized in the years to come. Globally, children considered to have PDD-NOS are those who have some autistic features but do not meet the criteria for autism or the other three pervasive disorders. It is unfortunate that, despite the fact that PDD-NOS children are statistically far more prevalent, little research has been done on this disorder.

Specific developmental disorders include the following:

- Learning disorders: reading disorder, mathematics disorder, disorder of written expression
- Motor skills disorder: developmental coordination disorder
- Communication disorders: expressive language disorder, mixed receptive/expressive language disorder, phonological disorder, stuttering

Although the prevalence of learning disabilities has not been firmly established, it is believed to be somewhere between 5% and 10% of the general population (Centers for Disease Control, 1987). Among psychiatrically disturbed children, however, the proportion is far higher because most learning-disabled children "have secondary emotional, social, and family problems" (Silver, 1991). Kazdin (1992) identifies learning disabilities as one of four major risk factors in developing serious behavior problems. A sad fact is that as many as one third of adolescent boys who end up in juvenile detention are learning-disabled (Lewis and Balla, 1980; Robbins et al, 1983).

Learning disbilities have also been correlated with diagnoses of conduct disorder and borderline personality disorder in adolescents (Hunt and Cohen, 1984). Regarding the communication disorders, Scahill proposed in a 1989 nursing research study that "children with speech and language delays are at risk for accruing additional problems—including emotional and behavioral disturbances."

Learning disorders can take many different forms and are not always easily recognized, involving as they do a "complex interweaving of neuropsychological and psychodynamic factors" (Rothstein et al, 1988). State educational systems generally specify diagnostic criteria for the provision of special education services. Nurses should be alert for any signs that a child has problems with perception, memory, understanding, verbal expression, abstraction, reading, writing, or problem-solving. A nurse may recommend that a battery of psychoeducational tests be ordered to identify specific developmental disorders. Testing can be critical, not only for the creation of a good educational plan, but also to guide nursing treatment. Parents, clinicians, and the child should be sensitively informed of learning strengths and weaknesses.

▶ Check Your Reading

38. List the five broad categories of developmental disorders.
39. Make a statement about the association of learning disorders to other childhood and adolescent adversities.

Disorders Not Specific to Children

Several other categories in the *DSM-IV* are not specific to children and adolescents but do occur in this population. Foremost among these are *mood disorders. Depressive disorders* do present in children with such classic signs as sadness, irritability, changes in appetite, and sleep disturbances. Another common symptom is a series of somatic complaints. At times, though, depression can be obscured by a child's inability to verbalize, by a high level of motor activity or impulsivity, and even by a veneer of cheerfulness.

Both *major depressive disorder* and the more chronic *dysthymic disorder* can be treated with a combination of psychotherapy and an antidepressant agent, such as one of the tricyclics or a newer medication such as fluoxetine. Nursing diagnoses include Impaired Adjustment, Sleep Pattern Disturbance, Social Isolation, Hopelessness, Spiritual Distress, and Potential for Self-Directed Violence. (See Chapter 30 for more complete discussion of mood disorders.)

Bipolar disorders have only relatively recently been diagnosed in children and adolescents and are often difficult to differentiate from other illnesses. They should be considered for such symptoms as lability of mood, pressured speech, sleeplessness, tangentiality, paranoia, and bizarre behavior, especially when the onset is sudden and in the presence of a positive family history. As in adult psychiatric assessments, it is essential to rule out alcohol-induced or drug-induced changes or other organic mental disorders, such as delirium or dementia.

Similarly rare, *schizophrenia* has been diagnosed in children as young as 5. Onset is usually gradual, with auditory hallucinations, delusions, and thought disorders the most common manifestations. Positive family history is a risk factor. As in adult schizophrenia, useful nursing diagnoses include Alteration in Thought Process, Potential for Injury, and Self-Care Deficit. Treatment includes the use of neuroleptics.

Substance-related disorders are often overlooked by child mental health clinicians, but they are commonly seen not only in adolescents, but also increasingly among younger children. Macdonald (in Bailey, 1992) calls substance abuse "the most commonly missed pediatric diagnosis." Symptoms of substance abuse may be missed, in part, because they can resemble some of the normal behavioral changes of adolescence. In addition, substance abuse frequently occurs in young people with other psychiatric disorders, such as depression, anxiety, and conduct problems, further obscuring the picture (Stowell and Estroff, 1992). Unrecognized and untreated, however, substance abuse undermines the most earnest therapeutic efforts. (See Chapter 31 for more details regarding adolescent substance use.)

Be alert to the ease of availability of alcohol and drugs in the child's community. Attendance at local Al-Anon, Nar-Anon, or Families Anonymous meetings may help to raise awareness. Substance abuse can impede normal development, impair judgment, exacerbate emotional problems, and cause irreversible physical harm. It may even be fatal.

▶ Check Your Reading

40. Name at least four possible signs of depression in children.
41. Suggest two nursing diagnoses for an adolescent with major depressive disorder.
42. What has been referred to as "the most commonly missed pediatric diagnosis"?

OUTCOME IDENTIFICATION

Identifying the outcome(s) of care for a child depends on the diagnoses, both DSM-IV as well as nursing. In Jordi's case, for example, expected outcomes might be

- The patient will demonstrate improved social skills.
- The patient will employ more adaptive coping skills when frightened, upset, or angry.
- The patient will begin to seek adult help and reassurance when confused by thoughts and perceptions.

PLANNING

Once you have, with the help of the child and parents, identified the central problems and the available resources and strengths, you need to develop a plan of care or treatment. A nursing care plan itself is one way to organize and plan care. Including a brief paragraph can enable others involved in carrying out the plan to have a better understanding of the child's strengths, weakness, and inner life.

> Jordi is a boy with fundamental deficits in relatedness whose isolation has been made worse by a thought disorder. These problems, along with a high degree of anxiety, have resulted in a profound delay in acquiring skills of social interaction. Strengths for Jordi are his tentative wish for interpersonal contact and his ability to use the structure of a well-known environment for support.

The plan specifies expected outcomes and the short-term goals likely to lead to these outcomes. Although objectives are written from the child's perspective, interventions are described from the nursing perspective.

Expected Outcome	Short-Term Goals
1. The patient will demonstrate improved social skills.	The patient will successfully interact in a play situation with a trusted adult. The patient will begin to develop greater comfort and facility as he increases his contacts with other children.
2. The patient will employ more adaptive coping skills when frightened, upset, or angry.	The patient will decrease unsafe outbursts from several times a week to fewer than once a month. The patient will use words to describe his thoughts and feelings.

3. The patient will begin to seek adult help and reassurance when confused by thoughts and perceptions.	The patient will remain in verbal or physical contact with a trusted adult during episodes of disorganization.

▶ **Check Your Reading**

43. Identify at least two expected outcomes for Jordi.
44. Why would the nurse not "humor" a patient by temporarily going along with a delusion?

IMPLEMENTATION

Individual Therapy

Psychotherapy takes place in the overlap between two areas of playing, that of the patient and that of the therapist. Psychotherapy has to do with two people playing together. The corollary of this is that where playing is not possible then the work done by the therapist is directed towards bringing the patient from a state of not being able to play into a state of being able to play (Winnicott, 1971).

The same basic principles that apply to individual therapy also apply to child therapy, although the means of communication, especially for younger children, are rather different. As Axline (1982) points out, there are some general "rules" that should apply to *all* adult interactions with children, both in therapy and in day-to-day life. These have to do with respecting and accepting children as they are, maintaining sufficient limits to provide a sense of reassurance and security, encouraging the expression of feelings, letting them take their time, providing opportunities for creativity and spontaneity, and recognizing that immaturity is a phase of development and not a *deficit*.

In most settings, a nurse is required to have a master's degree to provide individual psychotherapy. At times, the nurse-psychotherapist plays along with the child; at other times, the nurse maintains a reflective stance. In either case, a balance between permissiveness and structure must be sought. Letting children explore their fantasies—however messy and dangerous—is necessary, but, letting children actually destroy toys or hurt themselves *or* the therapist is likely to disrupt treatment seriously:

For a pretend or imaginary attack is one thing. It can ultimately be countered by the knowledge that the attack was not real. But as soon as an attack is made on a physical level, it acquires the possibility of actual hurt . . . of taking away the person who is struck. It can terrify the child (Baruch, 1952).

Generally, for young children especially, it is best to meet at a consistent time, in a consistent place, making the same toys and materials available each session and confining the therapeutic work to the playroom. Interpretations should be used sparingly and in the initial phase of treatment should be made in the language of the play itself. That is, if a child is playing out a parent-child scenario, the therapist can comment on the interaction in the third person rather than abruptly (and intrusively) shifting to a direct reference to the child and parent. Children do extremely well with metaphors. Children also do astonishingly well making their own interpretations when they are engaged in therapeutic work.

Facility in verbalizing what a child is unable to express is an invaluable gift. When the time is opportune for making an important observation, the nurse-therapist should not hold back. Gently the nurse can create a vocabulary that is incorporated both in the play and in the child's growing self-understanding. A skilled therapist can engage in this delicate balancing act intuitively, making it appear effortless, but this level of expertise requires years of training and experience to achieve. Some of the interventions presented as appropriate to Jordi's story can be applied to the individual treatment of many adolescent patients.

- Build Jordi's capacity for reciprocal interactions; for example, practice turn-taking and other elements of conjoint play with him. The nurse's relationship with the patient can function as a bridge to other relationships of trust.
- Introduce Jordi to other children in a safe, familiar setting, allowing him to watch them for extended periods without interaction. The nurse can minimize the patient's anxiety by maintaining sameness and allowing for gradual accommodation.
- Gradually encourage Jordi to play alongside another child. Support Jordi in brief, structured interactions such as familiar turn-taking activities with other children. The nurse can help the patient increase a sense of control through mastery of each successive step before going on to the next one.
- Maintain neutrality while keeping Jordi safe during outbursts. Avoid reinforcing behavior. High expressed emotion, either negative or positive, can become a reinforcer for maladaptive behavior.
- Initially, use a safe holding technique during outbursts; gradually increase expectation that Jordi will regain self-control without physical intervention. The nurse provides containment until the patient learns to take over that function for himself.
- Help Jordi practice alternative expressions of upset and anger, including words. Having satisfactory experiences with more adaptive forms of self-expression can be self-reinforcing.
- Assist Jordi to recognize cues to his own increasing agitation and positively reinforce adaptive coping techniques. The nurse's aim is to help the patient learn a skill that can be built over the life span. Self-awareness is an important therapeutic tool.
- During calm moments, help Jordi come up with words and phrases to represent his delusional ideas and his feelings. Use examples from stories or from other people if this is less threatening. The nurse appeals to the patient's strengths to help him understand his own illness in simple, concrete, benign terms.

- Verbalize your understanding of Jordi's feeling-states when he appears disorganized. The nurse helps the patient to shift focus from the unreality of his disordered thinking to the reality of his feelings.
- Reassure Jordi of his safety; describe the real context he is in. The nurse is careful not to collude with the patient's distorted perceptions.

Family Therapy

Family work has a special significance in child treatment because, as Critchley (1985) states, "Most child therapists agree that, to achieve any long-term therapeutic gains, the child's family must be involved in the treatment process." This work may be approached through various means, including family sessions, parent support groups, or direct modeling and education (see Chapter 20). You can offer invaluable help because it is difficult to proceed further until the home situation is stabilized.

A few essential principles of behavior management can be taught:

- The parents are responsible for making decisions, including decisions about what choices the children can make.
- The family should agree on a simple set of rules based on safety and respect for one another.
- The family should agree on a set of consequences for breaking the rules—these must firm enough that the parents will not feel compelled to exceed them in the heat of the moment but reasonable enough that they will be stuck to after the upset subsides.
- The family should agree on a set of rewards that will be available for following the rules—preferably these will rely heavily on family members doing enjoyable things together rather than on material objects.
- The parents must keep in mind that all behavior is a form of communication: The goal is to help the child recognize this and find acceptable ways of expressing feelings.

When difficulties arise, the parents should be encouraged to let the child's struggle be against the *rule*, not against the parents. In that way, they may even allow themselves to feel frustrated along with the child instead of feeling frustrated by the child. Behavior management works to change the behaviors of the child by first changing the behaviors of the "managers."

Group Therapy

The history of group therapy is a brief and dynamic one (see Chapter 17). Similarly the application of treatment theories to children's psychotherapy groups is still a fledgling discipline. The first children's therapeutic play groups were organized in 1934 by Slavson (Critchley, 1985). These were structured by the therapist, both in the selection of membership and in the nature of the play, to provide *corrective life experiences.* Most groups for children since then have focused on socialization, self-disclosure, or particular activities with the intention of preparing for similar situations in daily life. In the last two decades, clinicians have explored the usefulness of the British group-as-a-whole theory for these age groups (Moss and Moss, 1990). This theory holds that the group itself must be seen as the patient, as an entity greater than the sum of its individual parts. The same defensive *group* behaviors and responses to therapy seen in adult groups can also be recognized and brought to awareness in groups of children as young as 3.

▶ Check Your Reading

45. What level of educational preparation is generally required to do individual psychotherapy?
46. Give one reason why it is important not to allow a child to hurt the therapist.
47. Why is it important for a child's family to be involved in treatment?
48. List five basic principles of behavior management techniques.
49. Name the fundamental belief of the British group-as-a-whole school.

Treatment Settings

Because some children require more intensive treatment and greater containment than can be provided by outpatient services, individual, family, and group therapy can all be offered on an *outpatient* basis or as part of a comprehensive inpatient, day treatment, or residential program.

Inpatient hospitalization is the most restrictive modality and is generally reserved for comprehensive evaluation and treatment of the most seriously disturbed children. It is an extremely expensive intervention, not only in money, but also in the emotional investment and time commitment required of the entire family. When successful, however, hospitalization can act as a catalyst for permanent changes in the child, family, and community and can dramatically improve the trajectory of a child's life.

As in adult psychiatry, the therapeutic milieu is one of the most powerful components of inpatient treatment. A well-functioning milieu provides *containment, structure, support, involvement,* and *validation* (Delany, 1992). Figure 24-2 shows a schedule from a child and young adolescent inpatient unit. For both children and adolescents, the participation of the family in the milieu work can make the difference between temporary gains and permanent growth.

Residential treatment programs are neither as restrictive nor as intensive as inpatient wards. They provide structured living and education to children who have been unable, for whatever reason, to function adaptively at home. The availability of such programs varies drastically from region to region, as does the quality of the facilities themselves. At their best, they offer stability and ongoing treatment while a family continues to work toward

CHILDREN'S SCHEDULE							
	MONDAY	TUESDAY	WEDNESDAY	THURSDAY	FRIDAY	SATURDAY	SUNDAY
7:30–8:00	Wake-up/room inspection	Wake-up/room inspection	Wake-up/room inspection	Wake-up/room inspection	Wake-up/room inspection		
8:00–8:30	BREAKFAST	BREAKFAST	BREAKFAST	BREAKFAST	BREAKFAST	Wake-up	Wake-up
8:30–9:00	Community meeting	Community meeting	Community meeting	Community meeting	Community meeting	BREAKFAST	BREAKFAST
9:00–10:00	School	School	School	School	School	Community meeting	Community meeting
10:00–12:00	Testing Appointments	Testing Appointments	Testing Appointments	Testing Appointments	Testing Appointments	Super clean-up Fun time	Clean-up Room inspection Fun time
12:00–12:30	LUNCH	LUNCH	LUNCH	LUNCH	LUNCH	LUNCH	LUNCH
12:30–1:00	Quiet time	Quiet time	Quiet time	Quiet time	Quiet time	Personal time	Personal time
1:00–2:00	Group therapy	Life skills activity group	Video club/ fitness fun	Group therapy	Fitness fun/ success club	Family activity (1:00–2:30)	Family activity (1:00–2:30)
2:00–3:00	Physical education	Free play outside	Library Read-aloud	Creative expression	Physical education	Personal time (2:30–3:00)	Personal time (2:30–3:00)
3:00–3:30	Snack	Snack	Snack	Snack	Snack	Snack	Snack
3:30–5:00	Game time/ individual therapy	Game time/ individual therapy	Game time/ individual therapy	Game time/ individual therapy	Game time/ individual therapy	Game time/ individual therapy	
5:00–5:30	Community meeting	Community meeting	Community meeting	Community meeting	Community meeting	Visiting (3:30–5:00)	Visiting (3:30–5:00)
5:30–6:00	DINNER	DINNER	DINNER	DINNER	DINNER	Community meeting DINNER	Community meeting DINNER
6:00–6:30	Rewards	Rewards	Rewards	Family night		Special activity	Rewards
6:30–7:15	Physical therapy/baths	Personal time	Personal time	Support groups	Personal time	Personal time	Personal time
7:15–8:00	Snack Bedtimes begin	Snack	Snack	Snack	Movie night	Snack	Snack Goodbye party

FIGURE 24–2
A sample schedule from an inpatient psychiatric unit for children and adolescents.

returning the child permanently to the home. At worst, they may function as a sort of temporary orphanage, a way station between a terrible beginning and an uncertain future.

Partial hospitalization and—still less restrictive—*day treatment* programs generally follow a daily structure similar to the inpatient milieu, although usually with less stringent rules and with higher behavioral expectations for children or adolescents. These patients can maintain sufficient self-control to live at home. Whether a child is being seen in outpatient therapy or in a day program, there is frequently an unmet need for *home-based services.* More and more agencies are establishing programs to meet this need, sometimes with a parent aide working with the child and family for several hours a week, sometimes with a visiting nurse meeting with the family to continue therapeutic work begun earlier. The potential for useful change with a home-based model of care is enormous. Currently, however, the existing programs are diverse and frequently not coordinated with the other components of the child's care, so that it is difficult to evaluate their efficacy.

Fragmentation of treatment delivery is perhaps the single greatest weakness in the system of mental health care available to children in the United States. Many advanced-practice nurses looking toward children's future psychiatric needs advocate nursing case management as most effective in meeting those needs. A nursing case manager not only provides direct care and supervises an in-home aide, but also functions as coordinator of various mental health services a child might need throughout development.

► **Check Your Reading**

50. Briefly describe the characteristics of the different settings in which child psychiatric treatment is provided.
51. List the five descriptors of the well-functioning therapeutic milieu.

Psychopharmacology

Some experts decry the use of psychopharmacology under any circumstances; they point to the long-term adverse effects of neuroleptic medications and the common occurrence of stimulants prescribed by pediatricians without adequate monitoring (Breggin, 1994). Psychopharmacological agents do carry dangerous potential for unnecessary and even harmful use, and medication should *never* be a substitute for needed environmental changes. Clinical experience suggests, however, that some children benefit enormously from a carefully controlled, judicious use of medication and that to deny those children such a benefit is inhumane. Box 24–3 lists some basic principles of medication use in children.

BOX 24-3 Principles of Medication Use in Children

- Inclusion of parents and child in any decision regarding use of medication. *Any medication should be presented and used in the context of a comprehensive plan of treatment*
- Completion of a thorough assessment, including an accurate diagnosis, before considering a medication trial
- Weighing of risks and benefits associated with each agent, paying special attention to developmental concerns
- Completion of requisite baseline measures, such as blood counts, vital signs, weight, electrocardiogram
- Clear identification of target symptoms and selection of an objective means to evaluate the efficacy of the medication
- Awareness that children frequently show different responses from those of adults with similar symptoms
- Use of extreme caution. The least dangerous agent should be tried first, begun slowly and tapered if stopped unless immediate discontinuation is indicated by an adverse reaction
- Completion of an adequate trial and thorough documentation to prevent subjecting the child to unnecessary risk in the future
- Continued careful monitoring of both beneficial and adverse effects, with the active participation of parents and child
- Avoidance of polypharmacy

Be sensitive to the family members' feelings about medication and about any previous experiences with either prescription or nonprescription drugs. It takes time and patience to discuss this important matter thoroughly. Often, even in the presence of strong ambivalence, the family's "expectations of pharmacotherapy's effects may be unrealistically high and attended by anxious hopes" (Munir, 1989).

You also need to be familiar with the most commonly used psychiatric medications. Parents and children need education and support to make the best use of this intervention. Table 24–4 gives uses, dosages, adverse effects, and nursing considerations for these medications.

EVALUATION

"I can climb the bars now, Sally."

"What was that, Jordi? I didn't hear you."

"The bars, the monkey bars—now I can climb on them and play."

"Yes, you sure can."

"Sally, it's the bars and things, other things too."

"Yes, there's been much, Jordi—many things."

And there were things, many things. There was incident after incident. There were bars, many bars—bars to cross, bars to climb, bars to knock down—and they did it. And it was hard work. But they struggled, and the bars came down (Rubin, 1960, p. 62).

When the initial treatment goals and objectives are established, the nurse, the child, and the child's family should plan to review their progress periodically at reasonable intervals and to revise goals as may be appropriate. As with Jordi's care plan, it can be extremely helpful to include some measures of progress easily recognized by everyone. Losing sight of a child's gradual improvement causes family and child to become discouraged. Also, identify what should be accomplished to bring treatment to a successful conclusion.

The trend in child psychiatric treatment has been steadily away from long-term, exploratory work toward shorter-term, specific, identifiable behavioral achievements. Although short-term goals help focus treatment, limited time frames sometimes have the effect of replacing the forest with a succession of trees. As goals are attained, reviewed, and revised, keep a perspective on the longer view of this journey. Hold onto hope for the child so that goals achieved truly do become steps toward a richer, more fulfilling life. As feelingly expressed by Herskowitz (1989):

To be totally alive with one's senses, fully perceptive, emotionally unrestricted, to have a mind free to explore and make new connections, and a strong, agile body, is to live in a state of grace.

Termination

Then he ran out of the room and out of the building. . . . He rode all over New York and cried most of the time. Then he thought about Sally and the times gone by. Then he thought about their talks of the last six months.

When he got back, it was six o'clock, but everybody was still there. . . .

He looked at her and said, "I came back, I came back. Sally, I came back to leave."

(Rubin, 1960, p. 73).

Whether one works with a child for a brief time or for many years, the moment of ending the relationship is important and must be acknowledged as such. It is a time for reviewing the child's accomplishments, for expressing both the sadness of loss and the security in knowing that something within the child, something strengthening and life-giving, which the relationship created, will never be lost. Be cautious about responding to a child's anger or distress out of personal feelings or out of an identification with the child. Right up to the instant of departure, your focus is on the meaning of this event to the child and the child's need to master this separation.

Because the work of ending will have been done in the days, weeks, or months leading up to it, the actual moment of "goodbye" may seem surprisingly anticlimactic, for if all has gone well, the child is now ready to move ahead, despite a sense of loss and sadness. The child will be looking forward, toward the journey to come.

CASE STUDY: BETSY

Betsy is the 11-year-old daughter of Margaret, a 29-year-old single parent. Margaret brought Betsy to the clinic because she was "depressed" and not doing well in school. Two months ago, Margaret was hospitalized for two weeks because she was suicidal. When she was in the hospital, she began to resolve issues related to childhood sexual abuse by her father. She is currently being treated for depression with outpatient therapy and fluoxetine (Prozac). Margaret has full custody of both Betsy and her younger sister, Amy.

During the initial session, Betsy would not answer specific questions but did participate in drawing on the blackboard. Margaret stated that Betsy and Amy fight a lot and that they have no specific rules about bedtimes or mealtimes. Betsy cries frequently in the evening because she misses her father and grandparents. She is currently not doing well in school and spent the last two days in the nurse's office because she was too upset to be in class.

ASSESSMENT

Assessment data are as follows:

- Child and mother anxious and upset
- Mother describes feeling "overwhelmed"
- Poor grades
- Poor parenting skills
- Lack of structure in home
- Ambiguity regarding child and parent roles

DIAGNOSIS

***DSM-IV* Diagnoses:** Separation Anxiety Disorder
Generalized Anxiety Disorder

Nursing Diagnoses: Altered Parenting related to inadequate role identity evidenced by description of feeling overwhelmed by task of parenting two children and maintaining full-time employment while recovering from depression, inadequate support system, and lack of appropriate role models

Altered Growth and Development related to inadequate maternal and paternal caretaking evidenced by poor performance in school, inability to concentrate in class, absences from class, and verbalizations of hopelessness and depression

EXPECTED OUTCOME 1: By ____ the parent and child will interact in a positive manner.

SHORT-TERM GOALS	NURSING INTERVENTIONS	RATIONALES
The child will remain psychologically safe.	1. Assess the parent's awareness of the child's needs. 2. Determine the parent's ability to nurture both child and self.	1–2. Ability to provide safety and nurturing is a basic function of parenting. Child may need to be removed from the home if child cannot perceive minimal psychological security at home.
By ____ the mother will begin to verbalize the child's need for nurturing.	1. Encourage the mother to verbalize the differences between ideal and actual parenting behaviors. 2. Encourage the mother to verbalize the need for self-nurturing as well as nurturing the child. 3. Provide opportunity for mother to explore role identity through counseling (group or individual).	1–3. Parenting is a learned behavior. Often parents rely on how they were parented. The fact that the mother sought help for her child is one indication of her desire to learn different ways to parent.

EXPECTED OUTCOME 2: By ____ the parent and child will demonstrate decreased anxiety.

SHORT-TERM GOALS	NURSING INTERVENTIONS	RATIONALES
By ____ mother and child will describe at least two ways they have learned to cope with anxiety in a positive manner.	1. Assess previous coping behaviors for dealing with anxiety. 2. Focus on positive behaviors and individual and collective strengths. 3. Teach mother and child some positive ways of coping with anxious feelings, such as relaxation exercises, drawing, painting, and affirmations.	1–3. Assists the mother and child in cognitive awareness of ways to decrease anxiety and of the relationship between anxiety and behavior. Empowers the mother and child to manage their own care eventually.
By ____ the child will be able to spend at least two hours away from the mother without increasing signs of anxiety.	1. Arrange for gradually increasing times for the child to be away from the mother. 2. Monitor for evidence of increased anxiety, such as increased vital signs, restlessness, apprehension, or increase in somatic complaints. 3. Encourage the child either to verbalize feelings or to express feelings through play or drawing.	1–2. Behavioral methods assist in the desensitization process. Gradual time away helps the child to learn to trust. 3. Enables child to work through fearful situations without somatization.

EXPECTED OUTCOME 3: By ____ the parent and child will demonstrate clear role identities.

SHORT-TERM GOALS	NURSING INTERVENTIONS	RATIONALES
By ____ the mother will verbalize expectations for self and child.	1. Encourage mother to express her expectations freely. 2. Encourage mother to determine how expectations were derived.	1. Parents may have unrealistic expectations of their ability to parent. 2. Expectations may reflect cultural or family of origin values. Increasing mother's awareness may help her to be more realistic.
By ____ the mother will verbalize areas of failure to meet expectations.	1. Listen attentively. 2. Show empathy and understanding.	1–2. Failure to meet expectations leads to anger and frustration. The mother needs your unconditional acceptance.
By ____ the parent will develop parenting strategies that more clearly define the role of parent and child.	1. Help parent develop more realistic expectations of an 11-year-old child. 2. Teach mother appropriate growth and development for an 11-year-old child. 3. Assist mother with limit-setting strategies and age-appropriate disciplinary measures.	1–3. Based on her own parenting history, mother may be unaware of the norms for growth and development. Based on the history of abuse in her family, the mother may rely on ineffective ways of discipline and may be unaware of any other alternatives.

EXPECTED OUTCOME 4: By _____ the child will perform at age-appropriate level in school and home.

SHORT-TERM GOALS	NURSING INTERVENTIONS	RATIONALES
By _____ the child will express a willingness to attend school.	1. Explore with the child all possible reasons for not wanting to attend school. 2. Discuss the potential benefits of attending school. 3. Devise a behavioral chart that allows for rewards for days of school attended.	1–2. An 11-year-old child is old enough to reason. Exploring benefits of an education is beneficial. 3. The use of positive reinforcement is valuable when attempting to change behavior.
By _____ the family will be able to use appropriate support services.	1. Make appropriate referrals to parenting classes, social worker, and school counselor. 2. Monitor family progress. 3. Collaborate with involved health professionals.	1–3. This family has multiple needs and will require the use of various health care professionals. Collaborating is an essential part of planning, maintaining, and evaluating care.
By _____ the parent will be able to set appropriate guidelines for bedtime and meals within one week.	1. Assess current routines at home. 2. Assist mother in defining routines that are compatible with adequate time for daily routines for the family and allow for adequate amounts of sleep and recreation. 3. Develop a chart for the family to follow for the following week. 4. Monitor progress. 5. Offer praise where indicated.	1. It is important to begin where the family is in regard to routine. If you change routines too quickly or severely, noncompliance can be expected. 2–3. Behavior modification is useful when providing structure for a family. 4–5. Positive reinforcement of efforts on a regular basis strengthens desired behavior.

EXPECTED OUTCOME 5: By _____ the mother and child will verbalize hopefulness and meaning in life.

SHORT-TERM GOALS	NURSING INTERVENTIONS	RATIONALES
By _____ the mother will express hope for her own well-being as well as the well-being of her daughters.	1. Assess for suicidal ideation. 2. If present, determine the level of suicidality and initiate plan of care for suicidal patient. If not present at this time, encourage client to explore internal resources, such as significant others, a higher power, or God. 3. Encourage mother to talk about her hope for the future. 4. Emphasize strengths and positive statements. 5. Assist to develop short-term goals.	1–2. Assessing for suicidality is always a priority intervention from an ethical/legal standpoint and may require immediate intervention. 3–5. These interventions aid in restoring esteem and confidence in self.
By _____ the daughter will express feelings of hope for her future.	1. Assess for suicidal ideation. 2. If present, determine the level of suicidality and initiate plan of care for suicidal patient.	1–2. Assessing for suicidality is always a priority intervention from an ethical/legal standpoint and may require immediate intervention.
	3. Encourage the child to identify her losses. 4. Use a variety of modalities such as art, play, music, and drama to help the child work through the identified losses.	3–4. Unidentified, unresolved grief often leads to loss of hope.

EVALUATION

Formative Evaluation: The nurse observed that Betsy and her mother met each of the short-term goals in the time frames allotted. As her mother developed confidence in their ability to identify and respond to Betsy's needs, Betsy could tolerate longer periods away from her without increased signs of anxiety.

Summative Evaluation: Betsy was able to meet all of the expected outcomes with the help of the nurse and Margaret's referral to the local family mental health clinic for treatment of her depression. Over a six-month period, Betsy's grades improved dramatically. Betsy looked forward to going to school and being with her friends. Both mother and child expressed satisfaction with their relationship.

CONCLUSIONS

Even with many similarities between the adult journey and the pediatric journey, children also present important differences. Most childhood and adolescent psychiatric disorders refer to a number of attributes and behaviors that can be modified through a combination of treatment approaches. Mere recognition of these disorders does not tell us what the child's experience is or allow us into the child's inner world.

The story of Jordi is the tale of a child whose development is placed in jeopardy by his own constitutional vulnerability and by a poor fit with his family and community. But it is also the story of a child protected by his intelligence, by his parents' unselfish love for him, and most of all by the dedication and skill of a woman who learned to accompany Jordi on his journey, to share a vision of the world with him.

The practice of child psychiatric nursing is a rare experience, involving the nurse in work that is extraordinarily complex: It is at once beautiful and horrifying, intellectually challenging, emotionally demanding, and deeply fulfilling. It requires dedication to a kind of professionalism that does not distance the nurse from a patient but makes you even more immediately available. If you choose this journey in nursing, you must have a solid knowledge of physical, cognitive, social, spiritual, and psychological development. You must enjoy and respect children. You must be prepared for serious self-examination. In return, you will be welcomed into the lives and hearts of children and their parents in a unique way: as a fellow sojourner, as a guide who is at the same time being guided, as a fully alive human being connecting with others in that momentary state of grace.

KEY POINTS TO REMEMBER

- Child psychiatric nurses must have a basic knowledge of normal child and adolescent development.
- Psychiatrically disturbed children may experience themselves as out of control, terrified, inhibited, and without joy or hope.
- Each stage of child and adolescent development should be thought of as complete in itself, with characteristic challenges and tasks appropriate to the child in each stage.
- Adolescence can be described as a time of "defiance mixed with dependence" (Winnicott, 1965).
- Any understanding of a child's individual journey is incomplete without a sense of the child's place in the family.
- The nurse need not compete with the child's parents but rather should support and teach them.
- The nurse should have an understanding of and an appreciation for the community in which a child lives.
- Minority status is in itself neither a risk factor nor a protective factor but has the potential to become either one.
- The therapeutic relationship is at the heart of child treatment.
- Transference and countertransference are important concepts in child psychiatric nursing.
- Coping mechanisms are unconscious strategies for managing conflicts. They are not good or bad but can be either useful or troublesome depending on the person and the situation.
- A nurse should be alert to the presence of such risk factors as poverty, neglect and abuse, exposure to violence, parental psychopathology, divorce, and medical illness or disability.
- The nurse draws on the same observational skills used for physical assessments to assess a child's psychiatric status.
- The cornerstone of a thorough assessment is a carefully gathered history.
- Particular attention must be paid to the neurological examination.
- The nurse should attend to such areas of a child's life as play; attachments; sexual, moral, and spiritual development; and the presence of suicidal ideation.
- The nurse should be familiar with the DSM-IV nomenclature. The nurse should also be aware that most psychiatric diagnoses of childhood and adolescence describe a cluster of attributes or behaviors that are an exaggeration of normal characteristics.
- Nurses and other mental health professionals frequently miss substance abuse, not only in adolescents, but also in younger children.
- The child psychiatric nursing formulation provides an opportunity to convey a sense of who a child is.
- A nursing care plan should specify expected outcomes and short-term goals.
- Treatment modalities with children include individual therapy, group therapy, and family therapy. Treatment settings include outpatient clinics, inpatient and partial hospitalization programs, day treatment, and residential centers.
- Parents and children should be involved in making decisions about medication. Any medication should be used as part of a comprehensive plan of treatment.
- The nurse, the child, and the child's parents should plan to review their progress periodically.
- Regardless of how long a therapeutic relationship has lasted, the process of ending it is important and must be given attention.

LEARNING ACTIVITIES

1. Take an informal survey of your friends and family members. Ask them to tell you about what helped them through any difficult time as they were growing up.

2. Arrange to observe for an hour at a school or a day care center. Write a process recording of an interaction there.

3. Call your local reference librarian or Chamber of Commerce and ask for statistics on the number of children in your area living below the poverty level. Call the local court and ask for statistics on the number of children involved in the criminal justice system annually. Call the local child welfare department and find out what mental health services for children are in place in your area.

4. Find out if your place of worship offers any programs that would be helpful to troubled children and their families.

CRITICAL THINKING EXERCISE

Nurse Hadden was approached by the second grade teacher, Mrs. Lane, to discuss her concerns about one of her students, Timmy. Mrs. Lane reported that since Timmy started second grade, she noticed that he never stopped moving. He could not sit still to finish the reading assignment, he was always asking to go to the bathroom, he never seemed to listen when she told the children their directions, he blurted out words at unexpected times, and he recently started to push other children at recess.

1. What assumptions can you make about Timmy's behavior?

2. What evidence suggests that your assumptions are accurate or faulty?

3. If you are the nurse, what other evidence do you need to draw a conclusion about Timmy's behavior?

Two months later, Timmy's mother called the nurse to inform her that Timmy was taking Ritalin. She requested that the nurse help monitor Timmy's medication.

1. What conclusion(s), if any, can be drawn about the outcome of the nurse-teacher discussion?

2. Suggest possible alternate explanations about Timmy's condition.

3. Assuming an alternate explanation, would the results be the same?

REFERENCES

Ainsworth, M. D. S., Blehar, M. C., Waters, E., et al (1978). *Patterns of attachment.* Hillsdale, N.J.: Lawrence Erlbaum.

American Humane Association (1981). *National study on child abuse and neglect reporting.* Denver: American Humane Association.

American Psychiatric Association (1994). *Diagnostic and statistical manual of mental disorders* (4th ed., rev.). Washington, D.C.: American Psychiatric Association.

Asperger, H. (1944). Die "autischen psychopathen" im kindersalter. *Archive fur Psychiatrie und Nervenkrankheiten, 117,* 76–136.

Auletta, K. (1993). What won't they do? *The New Yorker,* May 17, 45–53.

Axline, V. (1982). Entering the child's world via play experiences. In G. L. Landreth (Ed.), *Play therapy: the dynamics of the process of counseling* (pp. 47–57). Springfield, Ill.: Charles C. Thomas.

Bailey, G. W. (1992). Children, adolescents and substance abuse: Special section. *Journal of the American Academy of Child Psychiatry, 31,* 6, 1015–1017.

Baron-Cohen, S., and Bolton, P. (1993). *Autism: The facts.* Oxford: Oxford University Press.

Baruch, D. (1952). *One little boy.* New York: Julian Press.

Beiser, H. R. (1979). Formal games in diagnosis and therapy. *Journal of the American Academy of Child Psychiatry,* 480–491.

Belkin, L. (1992). Hospital study testing the benefits of comfort. *New York Times,* Sept. 26, vol. 142, p. 16.

Bettelheim, B. (1950). *Love is not enough.* Glencoe, Ill.: Free Press.

Bettelheim, B. (1975). *The uses of enchantment.* New York: Random House.

Bowlby, J. (1969). *Attachment and loss. Vol. I: Attachment.* New York: Basic Books.

Breggin, P. R. (1994). Toxic psychiatry. Why therapy, empathy and love must replace the drugs, electroshock and biochemical theories of the "new psychiatry." New York: St. Martin.

Breslau, N. (1985). Psychiatric disorders in children with physical disabilities. *Journal of the American Academy of Child Psychiatry, 24,* 1, 87–94.

Brown, A., and Finkelhor, D. (1986). Impact of child sexual abuse: A review of the research. *Psychology Bulletin, 99,* 66–77.

Carson, V. B. (1989). *Spiritual dimensions of nursing practice.* Philadelphia: W. B. Saunders.

Caudill, W., and Schooler, C. (1973). Child behavior and child rearing in Japan and the United States: An interim report. *Journal of Nervous and Mental Disorders, 157,* 323–338.

Centers for Disease Control (1987). Assessment of the number and characteristics of persons affected by learning disabilities. In Interagency Committee on Learning Disabilities: *Learning disabilities. A report to the U.S. Congress.* Washington, D.C.: U.S. Department of Health and Human Services.

Centerwall, B. S. (1992). Television and violence: The scale of the problem and where to go from here. *Journal of the American Medical Association, 267,* 22, 3059–3063.

Chess, S., and Thomas, A. (1986). *Temperament in clinical practice.* New York: Guilford Press.

Chethik, M. (1989). *Techniques of child therapy: Psychodynamic strategies.* New York: Guilford Press.

Children's Defense Fund (1989). *A vision for America's future.* Washington, D.C.: Children's Defense Fund.

Cohen, D. J., Bruun, R. D., and Leckman, J. F. (1988). *Tourette's syndrome and tic disorders.* New York: Wiley & Sons.

Coles, R. (1986). *The moral life of children.* Boston: Atlantic Monthly Press.

Coles, R. (1990). *The spiritual life of children.* Boston: Houghton Mifflin.

Combrinck-Graham, L. (1991). Development of school-age children. In M. Lewis (Ed.), *Child and adolescent psychiatry.* Baltimore: Williams & Wilkins.

Comer, J. (1980). *School power.* New York: Free Press.

Cotton, N. (1993). *Lessons from the lion's den.* San Francisco: Jossey-Bass.

Critchley, D. L. (1985). Individual and play group therapy. In D. L. Critchley & J. T. Maurin (Eds.), *The clinical specialist in psychiatric mental health nursing.* New York: John Wiley & Sons, pp. 229–257.

Crittenden, P. M. (1985). Maltreated infants: Vulnerability and resistance. *Journal of Child Psychology and Psychiatry, 26,* 85–86.

D'Ambrosio, R. (1970). *No language but a cry.* New York: Doubleday.

Delaney, K. R. (1992). Nursing in child psychiatric milieus. Part I: What nurses do. *Journal of Child Psychiatric Nursing, 5,* 1, 10–14.

Derdeyn, A. (1992). Resolved: Horror films are good for children. *Journal of the American Academy of Child and Adolescent Psychiatry, 31,* 1, 165–166.

Eason, L. J., Finch, A. J., Brasted, W., and Saylor, C. F. (1985). The assessment of depression and anxiety in hospitalized pediatric patients. *Child Psychiatry and Human Development, 16,* 1, 57–64.

Eichelman, B. (1992). Aggressive behavior: From laboratory to clinic. *Archives of General Psychiatry, 49,* 488–492.

Emery, R. E. (1982). Interparental conflict and the children of discord and divorce. *Psychological Bulletin, 92,* 310–330.
Erikson, E. H. (1961). In J. Huxley (Ed.), *The humanist frame.* London: George Allen & Unwin.
Erikson, E. H. (1963). *Childhood and society.* New York: W. W. Norton.
Farrington, D. P. (1978). The family backgrounds of aggressive youths. In L. Hersov, et al (Eds.), *Aggression and antisocial behavior in childhood and adolescence.* Oxford: Pergamon Press.
Finch, S. M. (1952). Psychosomatic problems in children. *Nervous Child, 9,* 261–269.
Fisher, H. E. (1992). *The anatomy of love: the natural history of monogamy, adultery and divorce.* New York: W. W. Norton.
Freud, A. (1936). *The ego and the mechanisms of defense.* London: Hogarth.
Freud, A. (1946). *The psycho-analytic treatment of children.* London: Imago.
Freud, S. (1938). *The basic writings of Sigmund Freud* (A. A. Brill, Ed. & Trans.). New York: The Modern Library.
Garbarino, J. (1992). The meaning of poverty in the world of children—Special issue: The impact of poverty on children. *American Behavioral Scientist, 35,* 3, 220–237.
Garmezy, N. (1987). Stress, competence and development. *American Journal of Orthopsychiatry, 57,* 2, 159–173.
Garrison, C. Z., Addy, C. L., Jackson, K. L., McKeown, R. E., and Waller, J. L. (1991). A longitudinal study of suicidal ideation in young adolescents. *Journal of the American Academy of Child and Adolescent Psychiatry, 30,* 4, 597–603.
Gilligan, C. (1982). *In a different voice: Psychological theory and women's development.* Cambridge: Harvard University Press.
Gilligan, C. (1985). *Remapping development.* Paper presented at the biennial meeting of the Society for Research in Child Development, Toronto.
Gordon, M. (1987). *Nursing diagnosis: Process and application.* New York: McGraw-Hill.
Greenfeld, J. (1972). *A child called Noah: A family journey.* New York: Holt, Rinehart, Winston.
Greenfeld, J. (1978). *A place for Noah.* Washington, D.C.: Holt, Rinehart, Winston.
Greenfeld, J. (1986). *A client called Noah: A family journey continued.* Washington, D.C.: Henry Holt.
Grossman, H. J. (1973). *Manual on terminology and classification in mental retardation.* Washington, D.C.: American Association on Mental Deficiency.
Groth, A. N. (1979). Sexual trauma in the life histories of rapists and child molesters. *Victimology, 4,* 10–16.
Groth, A. N. (1982). The incest offender. In S. Sgroi (Ed.), *Handbook of clinical intervention in childhood sexual abuse.* Lexington Mass.: Lexington Books.
Habermas, J. (1971). *Knowledge and human interests.* Boston: Beacon Press.
Hall, A., Slim, E., and Hawker, F. (1984). Anorexia nervosa: Long term outcome in 50 female patients. *British Journal of Psychiatry, 145,* 407.
Harlow, H. F. and Harlow, M. K. (1962). Social deprivation in monkeys. *Scientific American, 207,* 136–146.
Haun, C. (1993). *Celestial interlude.* Unpublished manuscript.
Helfer, R. E. (1987). The litany of the smoldering neglect of children. In R. E. Helfer and R. S. Kempe (Eds.), *The battered child* (pp. 301–311) (4th ed.). Chicago: University of Chicago Press.
Hernandez, D. J. (1988). Demographic trends and the living arrangements of children. In E. M. Hetherington and J. D. Arsteh (Eds.), *Impact of divorce, single-parenting and stepparenting on children.* Hillsdale, N.J.: Lawrence Erlbaum.
Herskowitz, M. (1989). The nature of human nature. *Annals of the Institute for Orgonamic Science, 6,* 60–68.
Hersov, L. (1985). Faecal soiling. In: M. Rutter & L. Hersov (Eds.), *Child and adolescent psychiatry: Modern approaches.* London: Blackwill Scientific. 482–489.
Hodges, W., Buchsbaum, H. K., and Tierney, C. W. (1983). Parent-child relationships and adjustment in preschool children in divorced and intact families. *Journal of Divorce,* 7, 2, 43–58.
Hoffman, L., and Halmi, K. (1993). Comorbidity and course of anorexia nervosa. *Child and Adolescent Psychiatric Clinics of North America, 2,* 1, 129–144.
Hoffman, M. L. (1984). Moral development. In M. H. Bornstein and M. E. Lamb (Eds.), *Developmental psychology: An advanced textbook.* Hillsdale, N.J.: Lawrence Erlbaum.
Hoffman-Plotkin, D., and Twentyman, C. T. (1984). A multimodal assessment of behavioral and cognitive deficits in abused and neglected preschoolers. *Child Development, 55,* 794–802.
Hollander, A. (1981). *How to help your child have a spiritual life.* New York: Bantam.
Hunt, R. D., and Cohen, D. J. (1984). Psychiatric aspects of learning difficulties. *Pediatric Clinics of North America, 31,* 471–497.
Kagan, J., and Lamb, S. (1987). *The emergence of morality in young children.* Chicago: University of Chicago Press.
Kalter, N. (1987). The long term effects of divorce on children: A developmental vulnerability model. *American Journal of Orthopsychiatry, 57,* 4, 587–600.
Kashani, J. H., Daniel, A. E., Dandoy, A. C., and Holcomb, W. R. (1992). Family violence: Impact on children. *Journal of the American Academy of Child and Adolescent Psychiatry, 31,* 2, 181–189.
Kaufman, B. (1976). *Son-rise.* New York: Harper & Row.
Kazdin, A. E. (1992). Overt and covert antisocial behavior: Child and family characteristics among psychiatric inpatient children. *Journal of Child and Family Studies, 1,* 1, 3–20.
Kazdin, A. E., Moser, J., Colbus, D., and Bell, R. (1985). Depressive symptoms among physically abused and psychiatrically disturbed children. *Journal of Abnormal Psychology, 94,* 298–307.
Kendall, J. (1989). Child psychiatric nursing and the family: A critical theory perspective. *Journal of Child and Adolescent Psychiatric and Mental Health Nursing, 2,* 4, 145–153.
Kleinman, A. (1988). *The illness narratives.* New York: Basic Books.
Kohlberg, L. (1981). *The philosophy of moral development: Moral stages and the idea of justice. Essays on moral development* (vol. 1). San Francisco: Harper & Row.
Konner, M. (1982). *The tangled wing: Biological constraints on the human spirit.* New York: Henry Holt.
Korbin, J. E. (1987). Child abuse and neglect: The cultural context. In R. E. Helfer and R. S. Kempe (Eds.), *The battered child* (4th ed.). Chicago: University of Chicago Press.
Lagerspetz, K. (1989). Media and the social environment. In J. Groebel and R. A. Hinds (Eds.), *Aggression and war: Their biological and social bases.* New York: Cambridge University Press.
Lahey, B. B., Conger, R. D., Atkeson, B. M., and Treiber, F. A. (1984). Parenting behavior and emotional status of physically abusive mothers. *Journal of Consulting and Clinical Psychology, 52,* 1062–1071.
Lambert, Jr., C. E. and Lambert, V. A. (1987). Psychosocial impacts created by chronic illness. *Nursing Clinics of North America, 22,* 3, 527–533.
Lauton, B., and Freese, A. S. (1981). *The healthy adolescent: A parents' manual.* New York: Scribner & Sons.
Lawlor, R. (1991). *Voices of the first days: Awakening in the aboriginal dreamtime.* Rochester, Vt.: Inner Traditions.
Leckman, J. F., and Cohen, D. J. (1988). Descriptive and diagnostic classification of tic disorders. In D. J. Cohen, R. D. Bruun, and J. F. Leckman (Eds.), *Tourette's syndrome and tic disorders.* (pp. 3–19). New York: John Wiley & Sons.
Levenkron, S. (1993). *Addictions treatment with the eating disorders patient.* Presented at Greenwich Hospital, Greenwich, Conn.
Lewis, D., and Balla, D. (1980). Psychiatric correlates of severe reading disabilities in an incarcerated delinquent population. *Journal of the American Academy of Child Psychiatry, 19,* 611–622.
Lewis, M. (1991). Psychiatric assessment of infants, children, and adolescents. In M. Lewis (Ed.), *Child and adolescent psychiatry.* (pp. 447–463). Baltimore: Williams & Wilkins.
Linney, J. A., and Seidman, E. (1989). The future of schooling. *American Psychologist, 44,* 336–340.
Main, M., and Cassidy, J. (1988). Categories of response to reunion with the parent at age 6: Predictable from infant classifications and stable over a 1-month period. *Developmental Psychology, 24,* 415–426.

McClowry, S. (1991). Behavioral disturbances among medically hospitalized school-age children. *Journal of Child and Adolescent Psychiatric and Mental Health Nursing, 4*, 2, 62–67.

McDermott, Jr., J. F. (1991). The effects of ethnicity on child and adolescent development. In M. Lewis (Ed.) *Child and adolescent psychiatry.* Baltimore: Williams & Wilkins.

McLeer, S. V., Deblinger, E., Atkins, M. S., Foa, E. B., and Ralphe, D. L. (1988). Post traumatic stress disorder in sexually abused children. *Journal of the American Academy of Child and Adolescent Psychiatry, 27*, 650–654.

Mikkelson, E. J. (1991). Modern approaches to enuresis and encapresis. In M. Lewis (Ed.), *Child and adolescent psychiatry* (pp. 583–591). Baltimore: Williams & Wilkins.

Moss, N., and Moss, G. (1990). *The application of British group-as-a-whole theory to group therapy with young children.* Presented at the Interdepartmental Conference at the Yale Child Study Center, New Haven, Conn.

Mrazek, D. A. (1991). Chronic pediatric illness and multiple hospitalizations. In M. Lewis (Ed.), *Child and adolescent psychiatry*, (pp. 1041–1050). Baltimore: Williams & Wilkins.

Munir, K. (1989). Child and adolescent psychopharmacology comes of age. In J. Ellison (Ed.), *Psychotherapist's guide to pharmacotherapy.* Chicago: Year Book.

Nurcombe, B., and Fitzhenry-Coor, I. (1987). Diagnostic reasoning and treatment planning: I. Diagnosis. *The Robinson Memorial Lecture*, Perth, Australia.

Offer, D., Howard, K. I., Schonert, K. A., and Ostrov, E. (1991). To whom do adolescents turn for help? Differences between disturbed and nondisturbed adolescents. *Journal of the American Academy of Child and Adolescent Psychiatry, 30*, 4, 623–630.

Parker, H., and Parker, S. (1984). Cultural roles, ritual and behavior regulation. *American Anthropologist, 86*, 584–600.

Pauls, D. L. (1991). Genetic influences on child psychiatric conditions. In M. Lewis (Ed.), *Child and adolescent psychiatry.* Baltimore: Williams & Wilkins.

Peterson, G. W., Leigh, G. K., and Day, R. D. (1984). Family stress theory and the impact of divorce on children. *Journal of Divorce*, 7, 3, 1–20.

Pfeffer, C. R. (1991). Attempted suicide in children: Causes and management. In M. Lewis (Ed.), *Child and adolescent psychiatry.* Baltimore: Williams & Wilkins.

Piaget, J. [1932] (1965). *The moral judgment of the child.* New York: Free Press.

Pincus, J. H. (1991). The neurological meaning of soft signs. In M. Lewis (Ed.), *Child and adolescent psychiatry.* Baltimore: Williams & Wilkins.

Pless, I. B., and Perrin, J. M. (1985). Issues common to a variety of illnesses. In N. Hobbs & J. M. Perrin (Eds.), *Issues in the care of children with chronic illness.* San Francisco: Jossey-Bass.

Pollock, S. E. (1987). Adaptation to chronic illness: Analysis of nursing research. *Nursing Clinics of North America, 22*, 3, 631–643.

Provence, S., and Naylor, A. (1983). *Working with disadvantaged parents and their children.* New Haven: Yale University Press.

Pruett, K. D. (1991). Family development and the roles of mother and father in child rearing. In M. Lewis (Ed.), *Child and adolescent psychiatry* (pp. 215–221). Baltimore: Williams & Wilkins.

Quay, H. C. (1993). The psychobiology of undersocialized aggressive conduct disorder: A theoretical perspective. *Development and Psychopathology, 5*, 165–180.

Rey, J. M. (1993). Oppositional defiant disorder. *American Journal of Psychiatry, 150*, 12, 1769–1774.

Rierden, A. (1993). Ties that bind poverty's children. *The New York Times*, Sunday, March 21, p. 1.

Robbins, D. M., Beck, J. C., Preis, R., Jacobs, D., and Smith, C. (1983). Learning disability and neuropsychological impairment in adjudicated, unincarcerated male delinquents. *Journal of the American Academy of Child Psychiatry, 22*, 40–46.

Robertson, J. (1970). *Young children in hospital* (2nd ed.) London: Tavistock.

Rodriquez, L. J. (1994). Gangs are part of the solution. *The Utne Reader, 64*, 58–59.

Rose, M., and Thomas, R. (1987). *Children with chronic conditions: Nursing in a family and community context.* New York: Grune & Stratton.

Rothstein, A., Benjamin, L., Crosby, M., and Eisenstadt, K. (1988). *Learning disorders: An integration of neuropsychological and psychoanalytic considerations.* Madison, Conn.: International Universities Press.

Rubin, T. I. (1960). *Jordi.* New York: Macmillan.

Russell, D. E. H. (1986). *The secret trauma: Incest in the lives of girls and women.* New York: Basic Books.

Rutter, M. (1966). *Children of sick parents: An environmental and psychiatric study.* Institute of Psychiatry Maudsley Monographs, no. 16. London: Oxford University Press.

Rutter, M. (1986). The developmental psychopathology of depression: Issues and perspectives. In M. Rutter, C. E. Izard, and P. B. Read (Eds.), *Depression in young people: Developmental and clinical perspectives.* New York: Guilford Press.

Rutter, M. (1987). Psychosocial resilience and protective mechanisms. *American Journal of Orthopsychiatry, 57*, 3, 316–331.

Rutter, M., Graham, P., and Yule, W. (1970). *A neuropsychiatric study in childhood.* London: Heinemann.

Rutter, M., and Quinton, D. (1984). Parental psychiatric disorder: Effects on children. *Psychological Medicine, 14*, 853.

Sacks, O. (1987). *The man who mistook his wife for a hat.* New York: Harper & Row.

Sacks, O. (1988). *Seeing voices: A journey into the world of the deaf.* Berkeley: University of California Press.

Scahill, L. (1989). *Detecting communication disorders in child psychiatric inpatients.* Unpublished Master's thesis.

Scahill, L., Walker, R. D., Lechner, S. N., and Tynan, K. T. (1993). Inpatient treatment of obsessive compulsive disorder in childhood: A case study. *Journal of Child Psychiatric Nursing, 6*, 3, 5–14.

Schneider-Rosen, K., and Cicchetti, D. (1984). The relationship between affect and cognition in maltreated infants: Quality of attachments and the development of visual self-recognition. *Child Development, 55*, 648–658.

Sgroi, S. (1982). *Handbook of clinical intervention in childhood sexual abuse.* Lexington, MA: Lexington Books.

Shaywitz, S. E., and Shaywitz, B. A. (1992). *Attention deficit disorder comes of age.* Austin: Pro-ed.

Silver, A. A. (1988). Intrapsychic processes and adjustment in Tourette's syndrome. In D. J. Cohen, R. D. Bruun, and J. F. Leckman (Eds.), *Tourette's syndrome and tic disorders.* New York: John Wiley & Sons.

Silver, L. B. (1991). Developmental learning disorders. In M. Lewis (Ed.), *Child and adolescent psychiatry* (pp. 522–528). Baltimore: Williams & Wilkins.

Smith, L. (1949,1961). *Killers of the dream.* New York: W. W. Norton.

Sparrow, S., Balla, D., and Cicchetti, D. (1984). *The Vineland adaptive behavior scales* (interview edition, expanded form). Circle Pines, MN: American Guidance Service.

Spitz, R. A. (1945). Hospitalism: An inquiry into the genesis of psychiatric conditions in early childhood. *Psychoanalytic Study of the Child, 1*, 53–74.

Stanley, S. R. (1989) Disclosure of sexual abuse: The secret is out—what now? *Journal of Child and Adolescent Psychiatric and Mental Health Nursing, 2*, 4, 154–160.

Stern, D. (1977). *The first relationship: Mother and infant.* Cambridge: Harvard University Press.

Stern, D. (1985) *The interpersonal world of the infant.* New York: Basic Books.

Stowell, R. J. A., and Estroff, T. W. (1992). Psychiatric disorders in substance-abusing adolescent inpatients: A pilot study. *Journal of the American Academy of Child and Adolescent Psychiatry, 31*, 6.

Szatmari, P., Offord, D. R., and Boyle, M. H. (1989). Ontario Child Health Study: Prevalence of attention deficit disorder with hyperactivity. *Journal of Child Psychology and Psychiatry, 30*, 219–230.

Tanguay, P. E. (1990). Mental retardation. In B. D. Garfinkel, G. A. Carlson, and E. B. Weller (Eds.), *Psychiatric disorders in children and adolescents.* Philadelphia: Harcourt, Brace, Jovanovich.

Tanguay, P. E., and Russell, A. T. (1991). Mental retardation. In M. Lewis (Ed.), *Child and adolescent psychiatry* (pp. 508–516). Baltimore: Williams & Wilkins.

Tanner, J. M. (1974). Sequence and tempo in the somatic changes in puberty. In M. M. Grumbach, G. D. Grave, and F. E. Meyer (Eds.), *Control of the onset of puberty.* New York: John Wiley & Sons.

Tarter, R. E., Hegedus, A. E., Winsten, N. E., and Alterman, A. I. (1984). Neuropsychological, personality and family characteristics of physically abused delinquents. *Journal of the American Academy of Child Psychiatry, 23,* 668–674.

Theander, S. (1985). Outcome and prognosis in anorexia nervosa and bulimia: Some results of previous investigations, compared with those of a Swedish long-term study. *Journal of Psychiatric Research, 19,* 493–508.

Thompson, R. A. (1991). Attachment theory and research. In M. Lewis (Ed.), *Child and adolescent psychiatry* (pp. 100–108). Baltimore: Williams & Wilkins.

Vaillant, G. E. (1971). Theoretical hierarchy of adaptive ego mechanisms. *Archives of General Psychiatry, 24,* 2.

Verhulst, F. C., and Koot, H. M. (1992). *Child psychiatric epidemiology: Concepts and findings. Developmental clinical psychology and psychiatry* (vol. 23). Newbury Park, CA: Sage.

Volkmar, F. R. (1991). Autism and the pervasive developmental disorders. In M. Lewis (Ed.), *Child and adolescent psychiatry* (pp. 499–508). Baltimore: Williams & Wilkins.

Wachsmuth, J. R., and Garfinkel, P. E. (1993). The treatment of anorexia nervosa in young adolescents. *Child and Adolescent Psychiatric Clinics of North America, 2,* 1, 145–160.

Wallerstein, J. S. (1983). Children of divorce: The psychological tasks of the child. *American Journal of Orthopsychiatry, 53,* 220–243.

Wallerstein, J. S. (1985). Children of divorce: Preliminary report of a ten-year follow-up of older children and adolescents. *Journal of the American Academy of Child Psychiatry, 24,* 5, 545–553.

Wallerstein, J. S., and Blakeslee, S. (1989). *Second chances: Men, women and children a decade after divorce.* New York: Ticknor & Fields.

Wallerstein, J. S., and Corbin, S. B. (1991). The child and the vicissitudes of divorce. In M. Lewis (Ed.), *Child and adolescent psychiatry.* Baltimore: Williams & Wilkins.

Weiss, G. (1991). Attention deficit hyperactivity disorder. In M. Lewis (Ed.), *Child and adolescent psychiatry* (pp. 847–853). Baltimore: Williams & Wilkins.

Weissman, M. M., Fendrich, M., Warner, V., and Wickramarantne, P. (1992). Incidence of psychiatric disorder in offspring at high and low risk for depression. *Journal of the American Academy of Child and Adolescent Psychiatry, 31,* 4, 640–648.

Weissman, M. M., Gammon, D., John, K., and Merikangas, K. R. (1987). Children of depressed parents: Increased pathology and early onset of major depression. *Archives of General Psychiatry, 44,* 847.

Whiting, B., and Edwards, C. (1988). *Children of different worlds: The formation of social behavior.* Cambridge: Harvard University Press.

Winnicott, D. W. (1957). *The child, the family, and the outside world.* London: Tavistock.

Winnicott, D. W. (1958). *Collected papers.* London: Tavistock.

Winnicott, D. W. (1965). *The maturational processes and the facilitating environment: Studies in the theory of emotional development.* New York: International Universities Press.

Winnicott, D. W. (1971). *Playing and reality.* London: Tavistock.

Wolfe, D. A. (1987). *Child abuse: Implications for child development and psychopathology. Developmental clinical psychology and psychiatry* (vol. 10). Newbury Park, CA: Sage.

Wolfe, D. A., and Mosk, M. D. (1983). Behavioral comparisons of children from abusive and distressed families. *Journal of Consulting and Clinical Psychology, 51,* 702–708.

Wolff, S. (1991). Moral development. In M. Lewis (Ed.), *Child and adolescent psychiatry* (pp. 187–194). Baltimore: Williams & Wilkins.

Woolston, J. L. (1991). *Eating and growth disorders in infants and children. Developmental clinical psychology and psychiatry* (vol. 24). Newbury Park, CA: Sage.

Wyatt, G. E., Newcomb, M., and Rierderle, M. (1993). *Sexual abuse and consensual sex: Women's developmental patterns and outcomes.* Newbury Park, CA: Sage.

Wozniak, J., and Herzog, D. B. (1993). The course and outcome of bulimia nervosa. *Child and Adolescent Psychiatric Clinics of North America, 2,* 1, 109–128.

Yates, A. (1991). Childhood sexuality. In M. Lewis (Ed.), *Child and adolescent psychiatry* (pp. 195–215). Baltimore: Williams & Wilkins.

SUGGESTED READINGS

Kendall, J. (1989). Child psychiatric nursing and the family: A critical theory perspective. *Journal of Child and Adolescent Psychiatric and Mental Health Nursing, 2,* 4, 145–153.

Rubin, T. I. (1960). *Jordi.* New York: Macmillan.

Rutter, M. (1987). Psychosocial resilience and protective mechanisms. *American Journal of Orthopsychiatry, 57,* 3, 316–331.

Winnicott, D. W. (1971). *Playing and reality.* London: Tavistock.

CHAPTER 25

THE ADULT TRAVELER

Do what you can—and the task will rest lightly in your hand, so lightly that you will be able to look forward to the more difficult tasks that may be awaiting you.

—Hammarskjöld

LEARNING OBJECTIVES

After studying this chapter, you should be able to:

1. Identify theories of adult development.
2. Describe developmental tasks in early and middle adulthood.
3. Describe mental health issues commonly faced by the traveler in early and middle adulthood.
4. Identify nursing interventions to promote mental health in the adult traveler.

KEY TERMINOLOGY

Adult
Adult development
Developmental eras
Dual-career families
Horizontal stressors
Menopause
Midlife crisis
Novice adulthood
Organismic
Transitional periods
Vertical stressors

Adulthood is the segment of the life journey that typically begins to unfold in the 20s (early adulthood) and extends through middle adulthood (age 35 to 55) and into late middle adulthood (age 55 to 64). The word **adult** derives from the Latin *adultus* meaning to grow up. Adulthood is defined as being fully developed and mature. Another definition is a person after an age (as 21) specified by law. But what do we really mean by adulthood? Is adulthood best described as a dynamic process, a stage of human development, or is it better characterized as a state distinguished by responsibility, love, and commitment? Is the experience of adulthood different for men and women, and if so, in what ways? What are the critical mental health issues particular to adulthood? What do nurses need to know to facilitate the human development and psychological well-being of adults in the 1990s?

Normal early and middle adult development may be a seamless narrative from the individual traveler's perspective, but the prologue actually begins in childhood. Before adulthood, a person's perspectives and identity evolve in relation to the groups to which a person belongs, all of which influence ideas, emotions, and behavior in different ways. The foundation for understanding the journey first rests with the past as the individual experienced it: parenting, life experiences, role models, education, articles or books read, movies seen, and so on. These factors have an intimate bearing on how the present is perceived and interpreted. The way people interact is a little different, even if they have been exposed to the same set of circumstances because each person beholds reality differently. Reality is always shaped by the "I" of the beholder.

Adulthood offers each person a second chance to rewrite life's story. It provides an extended opportunity to shape a creative identity, this time with personal meanings reflective of personal choices. No matter how traumatic or disapproving childhood was, adulthood offers another possibility for personal fulfillment and satisfaction. Each human being comes face to face with an open invitation to shape values and develop a life story with characters and scenes truly of the individual's own making. Thus, the adult journey is distinctly and personally human, uniquely fitted to that person's travels, similar to but unlike any other.

In a sequential pattern experienced as a dynamic growth process, healthy adult travelers typically develop and refine their life stories, make necessary corrections, and embrace modes of behavior increasingly more consistent with their sense of self as a holistic being. Each day of adulthood offers its own opportunities for personal growth, but it is also important to "seize the moment" because it is impossible to fully predict when or how the story will end. For a significant number of adult travelers, the human meaning of the journey is compromised by serious physical or mental deficits or cut short by death in early or middle adulthood. Consequently, exploring the possibilities for each day in the life of the adult is as important as considering developmental potential over the life span.

The story of early and middle adulthood is also about

roles and relationships that can either support or contradict adult development, thereby enhancing or diminishing the skill of the traveler in negotiating the next step of the journey. Adulthood argues for responsibility, love, commitment, and balance as the defining characteristics of the journey to wholeness and maturity. In the final analysis, the quality of each adult traveler's journey is judged "by the content of their character" (King, 1963). Whether an individual is white or a person of color, rich or poor, handsome or ugly, too thin or too fat, educated or illiterate no longer matters. The manner in which each traveler has conducted the adult years is viewed as the only measure of success. The exemplar for the adult traveler is that of an extraordinary man whose adult life was relatively short but whose character and commitment to His destiny continue to shape the world in ways that are beyond our comprehension.

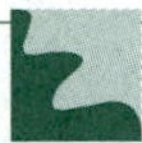

THE STORY OF A COMMITTED YOUNG MAN

A young man, adamant in His committed life. The one who was nearest Him relates how, on the last evening, He arose from supper, laid aside His garments, and washed the feet of His friends and disciples—an adamant young man, alone as He confronted His final destiny....

He had assented to a possibility in His being, of which He had had His first inkling when He returned from the desert. If God required anything of Him, He would not fail. Only recently, He thought, had He begun to see more clearly, and to realize that the road to possibility might lead to the cross. He knew, though, that He had to follow it, still uncertain as to whether He was indeed the "One who shall bring it to pass," but certain that the answer could only be learned by following the road to the end. The end might be a death without significance—as well as being the end of the road of possibility....

Is this hero of this immortal, brutally simple drama in truth "the Lamb of God that taketh away the sins of the world"? Absolutely faithful to a divined possibility—in that sense the Son of God, in that sense the sacrificial Lamb, in that sense the Redeemer. A young man, adamant in His commitment, who walks the road of possibility to the end without self-pity or demand for sympathy, fulfilling the destiny He has chosen—even sacrificing affection and fellowship when the others are unready to follow Him—into a new fellowship (Hammerskjöld, 1964, pp. 68–69).

BASIC ASSUMPTIONS ABOUT ADULTHOOD

The study of adult development begins with an assumption that *development in adulthood is much more complex than that of infant and child development* simply because for the adult, "the blending of past and present is a psychological reality" (Neugarten, 1969, p. 126). The past and present are interwoven to represent a deeper knowledge of life. Adulthood presents the opportunity for a much richer and longer experiential story, of which the individual is the primary author. As Costa and McCrae (1994) suggest, "personality cannot be grasped at a single cross section; it is necessary to see how it unfolds over a lifetime" (p. 64).

Related to the first assumption is a second: *Adulthood is a continuous, dynamic process of human development and adjustment, developed interactively through experience and education.* Kelly and Rasey (1952, pp. 34, 35) describe the role of experience as follows:

> *Experience, then, is the process of undergoing, the contact with the concrete, the working out of projected circumstances. It is built into structure, and man is made out of it. The organism is henceforth different, and if it were possible to repeat an experience, the outcomes would be different, since the repeated experience would really be encountered the second time by a different individual.*

The role of experience in shaping personal identity parallels the ideas of nursing theorists Rogers (1970) and Parse (1981). They assert that it is impossible to experience the same phenomena in exactly the same way because of intervening life experience. Thus, motherhood can be repeated several times, but the experience of pregnancy and birth is slightly different with each child. Moreover, no two individuals ever experience the same phenomena in exactly the same way because each person brings different life expectancies and tools of experience to each situation. For example, the experience of giving birth is different for the first-time mother who gives birth in her 30s and one who gives birth at age 21.

Education influences human development by bringing new experiences and different ways of thinking. Education links culture, theory, and practical applications together and encourages the student to enter into dialogue about its meaning. Atchley (1991) suggests that "the adult develops life principles—a philosophy of life—through an interaction between what is known, what is experienced, and his or her personality" (p. 120). Thus for each person, the journey is a little different because the philosophy of life that directs it is uniquely tailored to the individual traveler.

A third assumption is that *most people's experience of adulthood cannot be measured by a steady, orderly progression through life.* Adulthood can be described in general themes characterizing different developmental seasons. Although this information aids nurses in helping patients understand their journeys and anticipate the next steps, adulthood is a living process, and each person embraces it differently (Lerner and Hood, 1986). **Adult development** is not about linear progression to an ideal state but about *being* an adult person. Tournier (1957, p. 230) notes that maturity is more than simply, "an accumulation of knowledge and experience, as if it were stones placed one upon another to form a monument." Adulthood therefore needs to be conceptualized as a condition of "human *being*" directed by a person, who "imparts movement to our being, always refashioning our body and soul. The flowering of the person is not a state at which we arrive, it is the movement that results from our incompleteness. . . ." Accordingly "the concept of person belongs to the realm of quality, not quantity." The lived experience of adult development can be as passionate and varied as each person chooses to make it.

A fourth assumption is that *adult development is always contextually bound.* To understand each adult's journey, you need to consider the landscape that enables and maintains its progression. An informative data assessment always contains information about the interplay between the human organism and the environment in normal circumstances. An effective treatment plan respects and actively incorporates the integration between the patient and current circumstances in his or her environment. Understanding a person's context helps ensure interventions that are personally meaningful because they acknowledge the patient's world as a significant part of the story. As Hayes (1994) notes, "the client's history is not so much a record of one's life experience as it is a living representation of one's experience of life—of one *experiencing* life" (p. 72).

The fifth assumption is that *the experience of adulthood is different for women than it is for men.* There is growing recognition that men and women's psychological make-up may be as different as their physical differences and *as complementary to each other* in developing a holistic, realistic knowledge of a situation. We have moved in the professional and popular literature from narrowed thinking that "anatomy is destiny," as Freud suggests, to equally fallacious reasoning that there are no real gender differences other than those that can be explained by social learning factors, to a conclusion that there are recognizable complementary differences that complete adulthood as a portrait of wholeness. Popular nonfiction presents differences in communication and psychosocial approaches to situations that appear to be gender related. These books top the best-seller lists, finding avid readers trying to understand both themselves and their gender opposites. The two essential findings are that (1) there are real differences in the ways men and women seek and respond to their social world and (2) these need to be understood and appreciated as necessary to the larger purposes of our society. These realizations do not mean that only men have certain psychological characteristics or that women are the exclusive repository of others. The narrow attribution of characteristics as solely male or female is inaccurate. Also inappropriate is defining some traits as better or less effective and efficient in coping with life tasks. As both men and women recognize the value and uniqueness of each person, psychological differences begin to have the same potential for completion of wholeness as do physical differences.

THEORETICAL PERSPECTIVES ON ADULT DEVELOPMENT

In 1890, William James wrote that "[f]or most of us, by the age of thirty, the character has set like plaster, and will never soften again" (James, 1981, p. 126). Early psychologists, including Freud, asserted that personality characteristics were firmly established in early childhood and that modifying them in adult life was difficult, if not impossible. Few would disagree that an adult's response to life is deeply affected by innate temperament characteristics, position in family, and early childhood experiences. Each person establishes a continuity of self and personality, in which "changes can be incorporated into a whole that others still recognize as the same unique individual" (Atchley, 1991, p. 260).

In more recent times, such developmental theorists as Erikson (1978; 1980; 1982), Jung (1969b), and Maslow (1969) have argued that personality is *not* fixed in adulthood. They believe adulthood is a describable dynamic phase of human development in which men and women continue to develop psychologically into more complete human beings. Research of adult male development, for example, has characterized dynamic changes in middle-class men from young adulthood through middle age. Most significant changes are related to intimacy, career, and development of personal meaning (Vaillant, 1977; Levinson et al, 1978).

Current theories of adult development are drawn from the work of Jung (1969b), Erikson (1982), and Levinson and colleagues (1978). Their approach was **organismic** in that they believed that human development occurred as a natural qualitative maturation of personality. To a classic stage theorist:

> *Each stage is a more differentiated, comprehensive, and integrated structure than is the one before it. Each succeeding stage represents the capacity to make sense of a greater variety of experiences in a more adequate way (Hayes, 1994, p. 263).*

Each sequential stage brings the potential for greater adaptation and differentiation, as adults qualitatively reorganize their lives psychologically and socially to meet current demands (Commons et al, 1989).

Common to classic stage theories is the belief that young adults in their 20s are concerned with establishing themselves in a suitable occupation, selecting a life mate, and choosing a lifestyle with meaning. In their 30s, these same adults focus on stabilizing their career choices and maximizing family commitments. Adults in their 40s are occupied with making contributions to society. In the 50s and early 60s, they reassess life's meaning, and many redirect their energy. Finally, in old age, adults look back on their lives with either pride or regret—the final ending is determined by all the events leading up to it. Although modern thinking challenges the idea that adult development is stage related, stage theory continues to provide a relevant organizing framework that nurses can use with adult patients.

Carl Jung

In contrast to Freud, who believed that the early years of life experience could explain a person's adult life patterns, Jung (1969a, b) asserted that personality development is a lifelong process, with distinct changes occurring in midlife. According to Jung, the young adult strives for mastery over the external world, experienced in work and relationships. The dictates of society form the framework for development, with emphasis on competence in the work world and the development of ego-enhancing relationships. For both men and women, the approval of others is important. Jung was one of the first psychiatrists to recognize complementary differences and similarities between men and women. He advocated broadening of social roles and further suggested that adult development limited to traditional gender roles can lead to one-sidedness in personality development.

According to Jung, human beings begin to turn inward for sources of meaning in the second half of the life journey. He argued that adults cannot live the afternoon of life by the same rules that governed the morning. Around the age of 35 to 40, Jung noted, adults undergo a transitional stage of development, typically characterized by significant emotional turmoil. Although work and relationships remain important, most individuals begin to question what they are doing. In an unsettling inner stirring of emotions, people create an interior space for awareness of their previously ignored personality potentials. In describing Jung's midlife crisis, Staube (1981) suggested that the "essence and goal of individuation became clear to him at midlife through his personal experience and his artistic elaboration of images that came to him from the depths of the creative psyche" (p. 62). The period of self-questioning can last over a significant time span—sometimes years. With the crisis successfully negotiated, the integration of the inner self at midlife "can result in people who are wiser and more complete than they were during the energetic strivings of their youth" (Kastenbaum, 1993, p. 11).

Erik Erikson

Erikson's (1980, 1982) seminal work on personality development (see Chapter 6) is particularly important in considering adulthood. He argued convincingly that all people, whether famous or unknown, continue to develop during their adult years in similar ways. Erikson based his accounts on the study of adult development observed in the life stories of successful adults across diverse cultures. He researched major historical figures such Luther (1958) and Gandhi (1960).

The cornerstone of Erikson's theory is identity. The first four stages of human development begin the process by arranging the building blocks of childhood to form the edifice of personal identity. The psychosocial crisis of identity versus identity diffusion reaches its ascendancy in late adolescence. The adolescent then prepares to assume the mantle of adulthood. As an adult, identity is first chosen in work and love and later expanded to include generative efforts for the benefit of the larger society.

Erikson viewed adult maturity as an evolving developmental process occurring in sequential stages. During early adulthood, individuals begin to question the validity of cultural or family ideals. They no longer blindly follow standards of behavior as if these represent the only one-dimensional literal interpretation of life. Instead the developing person increasingly chooses attitudes, behaviors, and actions that become the foundation of an honorable woman or man.

Erikson's model of personality development is based on an epigenetic principle conceptualized in three adult stages: young adulthood, middle adulthood, and maturity. Erikson viewed the psychosocial tasks of young and middle adulthood as *intimacy versus isolation* and *generativity versus stagnation.* The final stage of adult development he labeled maturity *(ego integrity versus despair)* (see Chapter 26). For those who have successfully mastered psychosocial tasks during earlier phases of adult development, their identity is evidenced in their ego integrity. As mature adults reflect on the meaning of their lives, they achieve a wisdom that can only be acquired through fully lived experience. Although growing maturity brings with it an awareness of the finitude of life, fear of the unknown is significantly reduced when accompanied by feelings of a life well lived with few regrets. This understanding makes it easier for a person to face the inevitability of death. A sense of despair emerges for those who feel they have not led a meaningful life and are unsure of their place in the greater scheme of life. Attention to making the early and middle adult years meaningful helps prevent despair in old age.

Daniel Levinson

A theory of adult male development was described in the best-selling book, *The Seasons of a Man's Life*, published in 1978 by Levinson and colleagues. Their descriptions of milestones in adult development were based on a longitudinal series of interviews with 40 men who were between 35 and 45 years of age when first interviewed. The subjects represented a wide range in socioeconomic status, religious preference, and educational level. Five of the subjects were men of color. Adulthood, stated Levinson, is characterized by a series of negotiations between self and society. Figure 25–1 is a diagram of his theoretical model.

Levinson and associates emphasized developmental life structures considered to represent the underlying pattern of each man's life. Their findings suggest a distinctive sequence in a man's life patterns. The pattern consists of "a series of alternating stable [structure-building] periods" (1978, p. 49), with intervening transition periods. During the life cycle, therefore, each man goes through long periods (eras) of relative stability in which developmental tasks are pursued within an existing life structure.

Levinson and colleagues (1978) referred to the sequential structure-building periods as **developmental eras.** Accordingly, he staged his theory of human development as four developmental eras ranging from birth to death: childhood (0 through 22 years), early adulthood (17 through 45), middle adulthood (40 through 65), and late adulthood (60 through 85). Each era spans approximately 20 to 25 years. Levinson and colleagues mention the first era, childhood and adolescence (0 through 22), and the last era, late adulthood (60 through 85), as phases of human development, but they are not

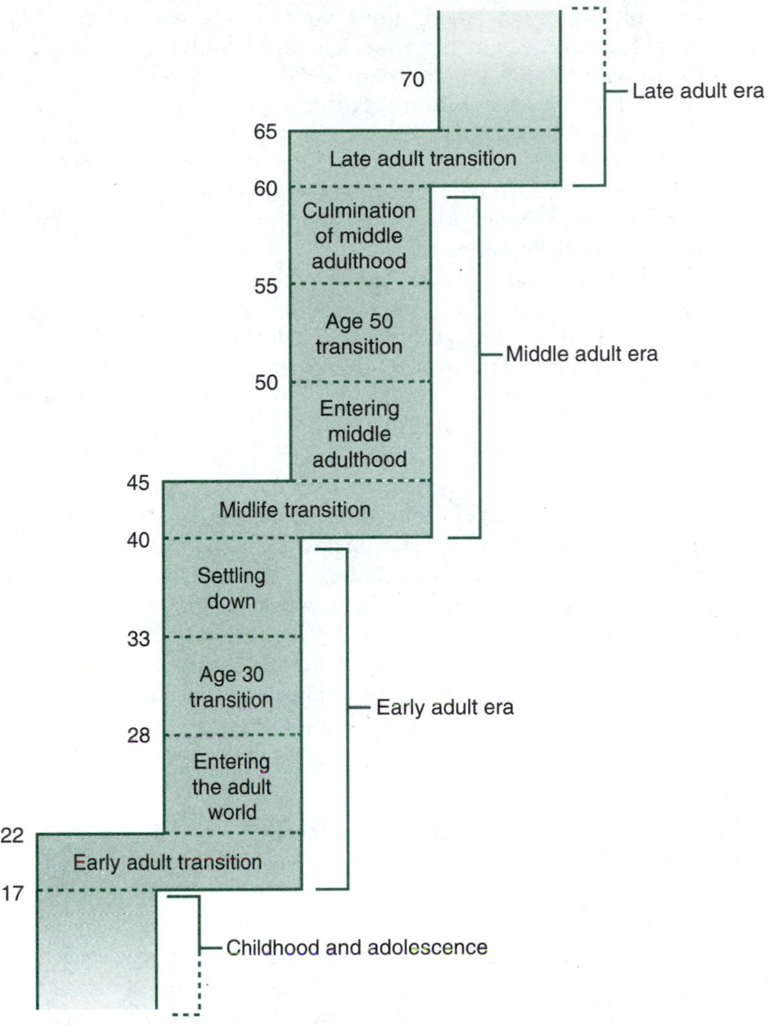

FIGURE 25–1
Levinson's theory of adult male development. (From THE SEASONS OF A MAN'S LIFE by Daniel J. Levinson, et al. Copyright © 1978 by Daniel J. Levinson. Reprinted by permission of Alfred A. Knopf Inc.)

explored in the depth he accords to early and middle adulthood.

Marking movement into each era of adult development is a **transitional period** in which people question previous life structures, consider new possibilities, and make crucial new choices. The transitional periods overlap the era left behind and the next era, extending over a five-year period. Transitions occur because the person no longer has confidence in the previous life structure and must consider new choices. Transitional periods typically are experienced as a personal crisis in which the past is integrated into the new future. Much of what has occurred before must be discarded or reworked in a new way. Each transition involves exit from past ideas about life; these are not lost but are necessary for a new beginning. Entitled "Graceful Exit," an anonymous passage describes transition to the next life stage:

There's a trick to a graceful exit. It begins with the vision to recognize when a job, a life stage, a relationship is over—and to let go. It means leaving what's over without denying its validity in our lives. It involves a sense of future, a belief that every exit line is an entry, that we are moving on, rather than out.

The trick of changing well may be the trick of living well. It's hard to recognize that life isn't a holding pattern but a process. It's hard to learn that we don't leave the best parts of ourselves behind. We own what we learned back there. The experiences and the growth are grafted into our lives. And when we exit, we can take ourselves along—quite gracefully.

Although individuals differ in the precise movement through transitional stages created by biological, psychological, spiritual, and social circumstances, Levinson contends that his theory is applicable transculturally. The concept of transition is particularly useful in thinking about adulthood because it emphasizes the dynamic nature of life experience. Nurses can help healthy adults understand transitions as being uncomfortable but necessary steps in their adult journey.

Carol Gilligan

Gilligan (1982) proposed a model of women's development based on the notion that there are distinctive differences in the ways women physically, emotionally, and spiritually approach their adult years. Her work suggests that differences in the experience of adulthood are both individual and gender related. Gilligan developed her theory in response to Kohlberg's research proposing that women display less moral maturity than men of the same age. Gilligan argued that the instrumentation used in the study put women at a disadvantage because it failed to account for values held by women in making their moral decisions.

Gilligan argued that women speak with a different voice—"a voice of 'care and connection' as opposed to the male voice of 'rights and justice,' and that this different moral voice arises out of a different sense of self" (Kitzinger, 1992, p. 241). Her model proposed that women's adult development occurs with the context of an *embedded self*. According to Gilligan, women strive to develop a sense of connectedness, whereas men struggle for autonomy. Self-realization for women comes from an involvement in meaningful relationships, "networks, sustained by activities of care-giving and response" (Gilligan, 1982, p. 40). Although her work has been criticized for lack of empirical support, it has raised serious questions about adult development in women and has firmly established the validity of equal but different gender-linked approaches to major life events.

THE ADULT TRAVELER IN EARLY AND MIDDLE ADULTHOOD

Physically, most people (except those with malnutrition or disease) have attained their full height by age 21 (Bogin, 1988). Legally a person becomes an adult at 18. Adulthood, as defined by age and physical maturity, generally occurs in a predictable and similar fashion whether the person is mentally healthy or mentally ill. People experience much variation, however, in their psychological maturity.

Normal adults of the same chronological age do not necessarily have comparable interests, nor are they working on similar developmental tasks. Life experience in adulthood is influenced by energy level, physical appearance, differences in health, self-management, and other social or organic factors that affect maturity. Unexpected twists to a life pattern and personal crises also affect the experience of adulthood. These factors help account for the wide range of interests, developmental tasks, and adjustment patterns found in adults. They are critical elements in the way individual adults perceive themselves, develop, and implement their life goals.

The call to assume the mantle of adulthood is one that people respond to differently for a variety of reasons. Some people never assume adult roles because of serious physical or emotional deficits, such as autism, active psychosis, head trauma, or profound mental retardation. Others discard adult roles as too confining and instead live their adult lives with the variations of personality disorders. Still others assume adulthood with a vengeance that stifles creativity and precludes giving time to the child that lives within. This narrowed, distorted adulthood takes the form of neurosis. Biological and social factors impede or facilitate a person's experience of the journey in adulthood.

Adult Travelers in Their 20s

A healthy transition from adolescence into adulthood is marked by excitement, confusion, and fear by most emerging young adults. They enter adulthood with a strong dose of idealistic thinking, filled with hope and dreams for the future, determined to make a difference. In early adulthood, life beckons with the promise of unlimited possibilities, and as Sheehey (1976) noted, "the tasks of this period are as enormous as they are exhilarating" (p. 85).

Levinson wrote of the early to mid 20s as **novice adulthood.** Seventeen to 22 is considered a transitional period. Extending from 22 to 33 years of age, the novice faces four developmental tasks: (1) constructing an occupation, (2) gaining a marriage and family, (3) procuring a mentor relationship, and (4) developing a dream. As they begin to form their first independent adult structures, novice adults need to develop a dream, "an imagined possibility that generates excitement and vitality" (Levinson et al, 1978, p. 91). This dream provides the energy needed to develop a career identity that is personally meaningful and satisfying.

Levinson believed that those who are most successful in their careers have benefited from a mentor relationship with a more experienced adult willing to share knowledge and be a guide through the difficult paths of career and life. The relationship itself offers support and encouragement of the young adult's efforts. The combination of expert advice and enthusiastic new ideas provides unparalleled opportunities for personal and professional growth for both novice and mentor. A number of studies have found that both men and women profit in their job advancement and satisfaction from mentor relationships (Noe, 1988; Burke & McKeen, 1990).

Society judges maturity by the individual's ability to assume adult roles. In the 20s, adult maturity is associated with the ability to establish financial and emotional independence from the family of origin. Typically, young adults choose to leave their family home, become self-supporting, choose a mate, and begin a meaningful career. Although each person's journey continues to reflect rituals, beliefs, and values that symbolize that individual's role within the family and community, young adults now have an element of choice. Adults in their 20s are intensely involved in and focused on their careers, or if they have not yet selected one, they are confused about which way to turn. As they progress through their 20s, the choice of a life work becomes clearer. By age 30, most young adults have established themselves. Delayed marriages and decisions to have no children or to delay having them then become critical issues. Comparing their lives to those of others in the same age bracket is significant to adults in their 20s. Consequently, social norms and expectations become measures of success for young adults.

Case Example 25–1 Ashley's Story

Ashley Bennett is 24 years old. She graduated from college two years ago, with a degree in interior design. Although her mother would have preferred that she stay in the area, Ashley was determined to start a life of her own. She selected Atlanta because it was a "young people's town," and the weather appealed to her. So she set out to seek her fortune.

Ashley found a job with a small interior design firm and began working as a design assistant. The pay was minimal, and like most young adults, Ashley found a gap between her current salary and what she would like to be earning. But she liked what she was doing, so she learned to budget her money and scaled her needs down to match her pocketbook. It was lonely away from home and school at first, with several crises of confidence. But Ashley was determined to make it on her own. Deciding to buy her first car was scary, but Ashley decided to go ahead anyway. She had to work at a second job to make her car payments and still feel comfortable financially, but it was worth it to her because she felt safe in her new car. She moved into a smaller apartment with two other roommates and took great pride in decorating it just as she wanted it. By the end of the first year, Ashley had successfully negotiated the transition from home and school to her own personally chosen living environment, from the security of family to an inner security based on her own accomplishments.

Case Example 25–1 illustrates the decision-making common to young adults. In making the transition from adolescence to adulthood, Ashley has learned many valuable lessons about money, friends, and negotiating her life circumstances. Has it been worth it? Yes. Can she expect to negotiate or relate to the future solely with what she has learned in her first year as an independent adult? No. But she is off to an excellent start in taking responsibility for her own actions and building a life that has meaning to her.

Adult Travelers in Their 30s

During their 30s, men and women further refine their life structures in ways that mature and stabilize their lives. Levinson and colleagues (1978) suggested that blending the lofty aspirations of the 20s with purposeful goals based in reality is the task of the 30s. Adults must become aware that a fruitful life requires a lot of care and effort. Consequently, developmental efforts in the 30s are characterized by finding career and role relationships that are life-affirming, morally worthwhile, and personally satisfying. People learn that they can influence the world in their own way by what they choose to do and how they do it. In contrast to those in their 20s, adults in their 30s are ready to expand their energies in ways that allow them to change and grow as responsible adults. They want to make a difference by extending their talents to others. As Case Example 25–2 shows, finding a congenial social group often becomes the means to achieving adult social and civic responsibility in the community.

Case Example 25–2 Marian and Dave's Story

Marian and Dave are in their early 30s. They have been married for six years and are expecting their first child. For the first few years of their marriage, they rented an apartment but recently moved into their first home. Both work full-time. They have recently joined a church and make genuine efforts to meet their neighbors because they want to become an active part of the community in which they hope to raise their child. Expenditures are now more carefully planned, more likely spent for the home or the birth of the baby rather than on spontaneous activities. While work commitments remain important, Marian is considering changing jobs, working for a company closer to home. Dave clearly has deepened his professional commitment to his firm and works long hours, not only for the paycheck but also for the satisfaction his work brings. Both Marian and Dave are aware that they have to make quality time for themselves a priority if they want their marriage commitment to continue to grow and develop.

A New Combination of Life Goals

Caring associated with generativity allows people to experience more humanized values and deeper interests in community with others. Although relationships remain significant, they become more reality-based. Important changes include a decreasing emphasis on appearances and developing comfort with imperfections, as this woman reveals:

The biggest difference for me is that I don't take myself so seriously. The other day I had some friends over for lunch. Just before they were set to arrive, I took a homemade quiche out of the oven, and it slipped out of my hands onto the floor. My beautiful quiche was completely destroyed. Had I been in my 20s, I would have thrown it out, gone quickly to the store to buy something else, or cried and taken my friends out to lunch. Instead I scooped the quiche back into the pan, served it with the explanation of what happened and we all had a good laugh. I realized they had come to see me, and that was the most important thing. I didn't have to be as perfect as I felt I needed to be in my 20s, and that is such a relief. (Arnold, 1994).

Toward the end of the 30s, Vaillant (1977) suggested, a phase of career consolidation between intimacy and generativity takes place. People seriously and methodically begin to examine life commitments and to evaluate their worth. Levinson's (1978) study reports similar findings. This transitional period sets the stage for a midlife crisis, which has typically affected men in their 40s. (Changes in work in the 21st century, however, may make the 30s a time of change rather than consolidation.)

Midlife Crisis

The pace and rhythm of adulthood change dramatically with the midlife crisis, a transitional period beginning anywhere from 35 to 50 (Kotre and Hall, 1990). A **midlife crisis** is an internal questioning of the meaning of one's life thus far. It represents an essential part of the life journey unique to each individual, yet commonly experienced in the fullness of a life well traveled as a turning point. Most people find that excessive reliance on the opinions of others gives way to a deeper understanding of what has true inner meaning for the person. The desired outcome of a midlife crisis is a realigning of attitudes and behaviors needed to complete the life cycle in a meaningful way.

Midlife crisis is forced on people by physical, social, and psychological factors needing attention in midlife. Initially the crisis can be experienced as loss (Kalish, 1989). In midlife, body contours change; facial appearance and hair color sometimes show marked differences; and energy levels shift. Physical changes occur graphically in midlife, signaling for many the passage of years in ways not easily avoided. Although a gradual decline in physical capacity occurs in midlife, most people can do many of the activities they performed in earlier life but at a slower pace. Most important for reframing the midlife experience is a strong correlation between physical well-being, full engagement with life, and mental health.

RELATIONSHIPS

Psychological concerns in midlife typically focus on professional or personal relationships (or both) and on self-definition. Critical reevaluations of professional and personal relationships and their relevance for future growth can be quite unsettling, as this traveler in midlife reveals:

I experienced a significant change in thinking about myself, signaled first by a period of intense disequilibrium about the meaning of my life. I noticed with some shock that things of importance and concern to me for many years, for example, meeting the expectations of others, status, and recognition, were no longer critical issues, but I had nothing to take its place (Arnold, 1994).

Divorce and remarriage are common outcomes of midlife evaluations. These changes may represent a creative life solution for those in long-term relationships that clearly have been destructive. For those whose personal needs transcend their long-term commitments, however, the outcome is clothed in irresponsibility and self-absorption. These people make choices for the wrong reason, as a way of retaining declining youth. The transitional midlife crisis, for some men and to a lesser extent for some women, can include turning to another person as the source of intimacy. Such a turning provides the middle-aged adult with feelings of renewed youthful vigor and freedom from thoughts of aging (Staube, 1981). The financial havoc and emotional carnage of such decisions, however, can be serious costs for families and adult children. For many middle-aged adults who choose divorce, any self-absorbed peace is marred by ongoing problems.

Nurses can help patients sort out the meanings of relationships and can coach patients in reworking relationships that have become stale or unworkable. Therapeutic strategies can enhance the ability to reflect on life with responsibility and compassion. Adults often need help in mastering the difficult ordering of relationships and their meaning for the second half of life.

OPPORTUNITY FOR SELF-DEFINITION

Many travelers speak of their midlife crisis as a rebirth—a freedom to be and to cherish—a turning point of great significance to the life journey. Painful choices and inevitable shifts in self-concept form the foundation in the midlife journey toward wholeness. As Jung suggests, the journey necessarily entails an integration of all parts of self—inner strivings and outer accomplishments. It also is a time, however, when care of the human spirit becomes an important, exhilarating task (Lane, 1987). In Case Example 25–3, a woman speaks of her personal midlife crisis as a pivotal point in her journey. The crisis allowed her to make choices that were painful but significant to the completion of her journey.

Case Example 25–3 Patricia's Story

Patricia grew up in a small town and became a nun in her late teens. For over 20 years, she lived the vowed religious life. Always a positive person, Patricia accepted that her life was unfolding as it should until her mother became gravely ill, and Patricia as her only child received permission to care for her at home. She viewed this time as a period of reflection in which she experienced a profound midlife crisis, brought to the forefront of her mind by her current crisis. The role reversal of parent care and an awareness that something was missing from her life led her to question what was truly important to her. Patricia made the decision to leave the religious life, the wisdom of which she felt was reaffirmed in many ways during the ensuing years. She described the changes she experienced during her midlife crisis as shifting from doing what others expected to a realization that she had choices in life, that she was in charge of her own destiny. In the process of developing a lifestyle based on choice rather than expectation, Patricia experienced a new peacefulness, a "freedom to be," which she characterized as being able to enjoy herself and her life in fresh ways that brought renewal and exhilaration to her human existence. Patricia's crisis of meaning in her forties contained many of the characteristics common to a midlife crisis:

- A life stressor (her mother's illness) requiring a different set of coping strategies
- Awareness of significant physical changes in herself and in her mother

• Realization of life's finiteness and that if changes are to occur, they must occur now

• A quest for meaning that arises as a powerful inner force in midlife.

Adult Travelers in Their 40s

Healthy adults in their 40s are much more complex human beings than they were in their 20s. They have gone forward and established careers and families, developed ideas about what is important to them, and contributed to their communities in meaningful ways. But life also changes for travelers in their 40s, and adults find it necessary to break with the past, to test and experiment with new lifestyles, to explore new modes of creativity and generativity, and to rediscover what is meaningful in life.

Generational Responsibilities

Because both men and women are living longer, adults in their 40s may be caregivers for elderly parents and simultaneously be parents of late adolescent or adult children. As their adult children extend their education, parents often provide financial assistance for a much longer period than previously was the case (Kingson et al, 1986). These demands create additional stress on adults already beginning to contemplate diminished income in their declining years. Adults in their 40s are more realistic and more sensitive to potential physical vulnerability in themselves (Buhler and Goldenberg, 1968; Gould, 1975). They pay more attention to their health.

In their 40s, healthy adults streamline their assets both figuratively and objectively (Thurnher, 1983). Although the process of consolidation takes place toward the end of the 30s, it reaches ascendancy in the early to mid 40s. Career reevaluation and significant career changes are common in the 40s, as individuals discover that their sense of self is in conflict with their chosen career. Even if the career has significant meaning, men and women at midlife generally are at the peak of their careers—and they know it. Moreover, current economic uncertainties have intensified the sense of midlife crisis for many, as midmanagement and senior-level workers in their 40s and 50s are often first cut in the "right sizing" of many companies and government jobs.

Typically the impetus to develop a meaningful path to fulfillment and to plan the direction of later life takes on greater energy. At the same time, the midlife adult senses the need to balance commitments, to go with the flow of life.

Menopause

Menopause typically occurs as a natural life process during the 40s or 50s, presenting the female traveler with significant hormonal symptoms and cessation of the menses. Menopause definitively marks the end of the reproductive years, and hormonal fluctuations associated with menopause frequently create mood changes that require psychiatric intervention (Mercer et al, 1989). Strategies that reframe menopause as a natural process, occurring as an unavoidable interval in the story of adult women, but one that need not become a defining characteristic, are important nursing interventions. Especially useful is psychoeducation regarding the benefits and risks of hormonal therapy, anticipatory guidance about what to expect, and creative ways to negotiate life in the postmenopausal years.

A deliberate reframing of a natural physical process is particularly important because many research studies of perimenopausal and postmenopausal women speak of this time in a woman's life as one of physical loss and depletion, to be corrected with estrogen therapy. Psychological issues raised in research include diminished sexual attractiveness and functioning. Absent are studies related to postmenopausal women as a time of positive transition, with potential for greater self-awareness, personal growth, and fulfillment, yet many women experience their postmenopausal years as positive. Once again, the popular literature takes the lead in addressing women's adult development (Sheehey, 1993), much as Levinson's work did for men in the 1970s.

Adult Travelers in Their 50s

The 50s offer a window in time, grasped by the healthy adult as a period of growth and renewed vitality. Referred to as late middle adulthood, the 50s typically are a time when much of what has gone before is integrated into a fuller life story, and many unimportant details are discarded as irrelevant. Sheehey (1981, p. 289) captures the essence of development in the second half of life with a quote from Shopenhauer:

The first 40 years of life furnish the text, while the remaining 30 supply the commentary; without the commentary we are unable to understand aright the true sense and coherence of the text, together with the moral it contains.

The renewed research interest in the period between 50 and 65 is partly a result of a dearth of information about this segment of adult development. Most studies of women in late midlife address this decade solely in relation to menopause or skip to the broader category of the *older woman,* as if this term equally described the psychological concerns of women in their 50s and women in their 70s. Studies of men in their 50s simply are not available. Part of the reason for fewer life scripts that cast men and women in their 50s in roles of renewal is that in the early part of this century, men and women reaching this age were considered old. Most could expect less than 20 more years of life, typically spent in retirement and ill health. Midlife men and women today can expect another 30 to 40 years in which the old rules about later adulthood no longer apply.

Many healthy adults describe the 50s as zestful, characterized by an appreciation of freedom from previous obligations and a chance to reprioritize role responsibilities. They describe the 50s as a *window of time* in which their physical and emotional energies can be focused in directions both meaningful and enriching.

Healthy adults in their 50s are able to "let go" of the need to control what is happening and are better able to go with the flow of life as it presents itself. Relationships with significant others have the potential for deepening, partially because people have more time and maturity to devote to their nurturance. Adults in their 50s have the health and energy to devote to the relationships that are important to them. At the same time, adults in their 50s are more aware of limitations in time to live a healthy and active lifestyle. They now recognize the need to use time well and that whatever they wish to do with the rest of their lives needs to be done now (Arnold, 1994). As health becomes more of an issue in the 50s, Fiske and Chiriboga (1990) note that "Health problems are not only major stressors in and of themselves, but they tend to precipitate a chain of secondary stressors. The onset of a serious health problem, especially during the later years, leaves a characteristic signature: the loss of a sense of personal security, a heightened sense of vulnerability, acceleration of the psychological processes of aging" (p. 284).

Nurses need to consider the 50s an important segment in the life journey. During this time, a person's life story can be enhanced by helping the older midlife adult get in touch with the creative aspects of later life. It is becoming more and more the norm that late middle life offers adults an opportunity to become reenergized, moved by a clear sense of direction, and empowered by their maturity to engage with life in a new and innovative manner.

▶ Check Your Reading

1. How would you describe the differences between adults in their 20s and those in their 50s?
2. What is meant by the midlife crisis, and what factors influence its development?

MENTAL HEALTH ISSUES IN NORMAL ADULTHOOD

In thinking about mental health issues facing the traveler in early and middle adulthood, first review the characteristics associated with emotional maturity (Box 25–1). No one is perfect and, consequently, people strive for but do not fully attain healthy maturity in all areas of their lives. Perhaps this is why people typically write their memoirs in their later years.

Self-Actualization

Maslow (1969) and other humanist psychologists point to self-actualization as a natural force in normal personality development (see Chapter 6). Mastery of developmental tasks required for self-actualization of adulthood is contingent on the sense of being needed, meaningful interaction with peers, and increasing skill in handling complex problems and decisions about difficult life issues. For the traveler, self-actualization brings an ever-present sense of freshness and excitement about possibilities. The adult develops an experiential awareness and delight that life makes a difference. Knowledge that one's efforts have meaning and are the best one can offer fosters serenity and satisfaction. Life remains full of possibility for the self-actualizing adult, but it is coupled with the realization that one must go with the flow and rhythms of the journey, accepting and working with all that life presents. Self-actualized travelers are able to make significant contributions to the community, simply through their presence. Reed (1994) refers to this self-transcendence as "a characteristic of developmental maturity whereby there is an expansion of self-boundaries and an orientation toward broadened life perspectives and purposes" (p. 64).

Vertical and Horizontal Stressors

Personal growth does not take place in a vacuum, and adult development closely interacts with a person's environmental context (Mercer et al, 1989). Vertical and horizontal stressors (Figure 25–2) are directly related to mental health issues in early and middle adulthood. They can prime the development of mental symptoms or lay the groundwork for personal growth. **Vertical stressors** are carried from generation to generation in the form of beliefs, values, and modes of conduct. Inherent in one's culture, social community, and family background, vertical stressors contribute to or raise questions about each

BOX 25–1 Suggested Measures of Maturity

- Openness to being personally challenged
- Dedication to the truth (reality principle)
- Having multiple perspectives (being able to see that it is possible to look at a situation from several different and equally valid viewpoints)
- Willingness to take responsibility for one's own actions
- Being able to let go of impossible expectations and situations
- Equal comfort in the company of others and in solitude
- Capacity to establish loving but not binding bonds with others
- Ability to make and keep commitments
- Capacity to delay gratification for a greater good
- Ability to admit when one is wrong and to make amends

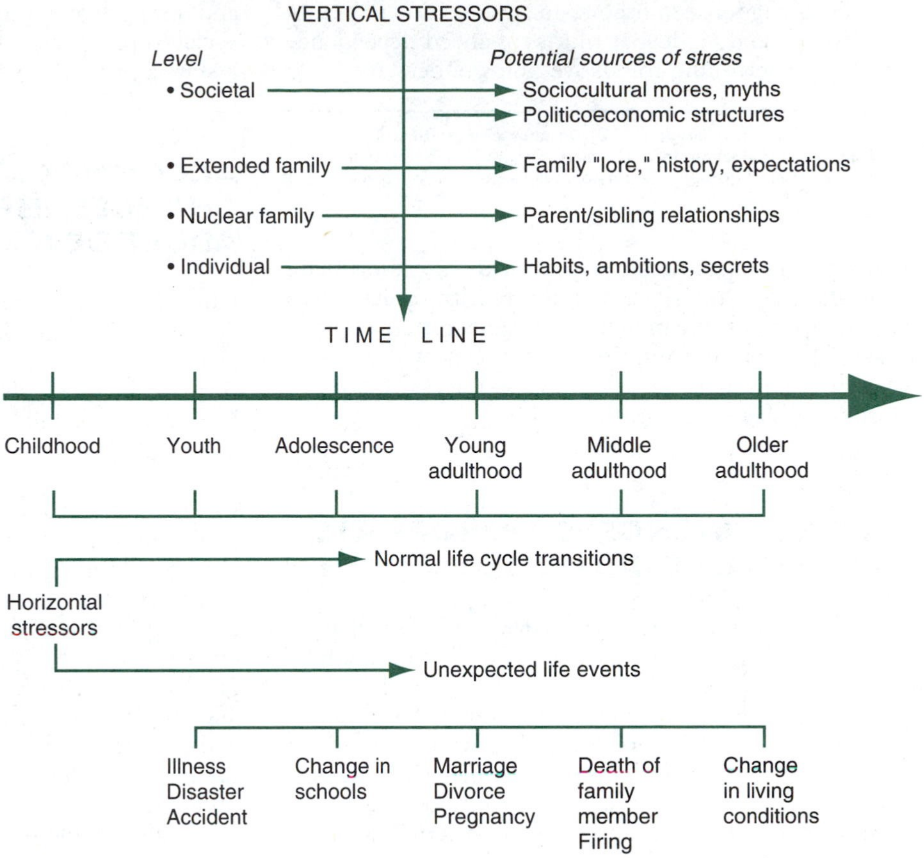

FIGURE 25–2
Vertical and horizontal stressors directly related to mental health in early and middle adulthood. (From Arnold, E., and Boggs, K. [1995]. *Interpersonal relationships: Communication skills for nurses* [2nd ed.]. Philadelphia: W. B. Saunders.)

individual's unique experience of adulthood. For example, the type of social support a person received as a child can later influence the adult's ability to use social support effectively in adult relationships. Bowlby (1977) describes three adult modes of maladaptive support-seeking behavior patterns stemming from inappropriate parenting:

- The compulsively self-reliant person who has difficulty forming attachments, resulting from parental rejections of the child's attempt to form attachments.
- The compulsive caregiver, often the result of having had a disabled or depressed mother who was unable to take care of the child and instead created a context in which the child takes care of the mother. This person develops many relationships but always is a caregiver. Being cared for is uncomfortable, so that this individual avoids being placed in such a position.
- The compulsive support seeker who develops many relationships but is constantly in need of support. This distortion of attachment arises when too much support has been given to a child, who then never develops self-efficacy, or when an individual so deprived consistently seeks in adulthood what was unavailable as a child.

Horizontal stressors occur as normative, expected or unexpected life events. Neugarten (1977) proposed that life events serve as symbols of transitions during the course of each person's life trajectory. Normative life events typically occur more gradually than situational stressors, which are abrupt changes in the conduct of a person's life. Typical horizontal stressors during early adulthood can include starting a job, getting married, and having a first child. Later in life, these stressors can include a last child leaving home, retirement, or birth of the first grandchild. The stressor can be pleasant or unpleasant, desired or undesired. Illness is an unexpected stressor that dramatically serves as a turning point in many adult journeys, as the following example illustrates:

Case Example 25–4 Edward's Story

Edward, a vigorous athlete and active man who swore he would never work behind a desk, was injured in an accident that left him completely paralyzed from the neck down. As he was being taken into the emergency room (15 years ago), he reported, "I felt as if God were speaking to me: 'You take control of the physical circumstances, I'll cover everything else.' I had a special feeling of warmth and security in my body." His fast-paced, perfectionistic life was suddenly changed. One week after the accident, he had an experience "that was like starting my life all over, being born again. I had to throw out everything I knew before starting all over again from scratch." Among the major changes he reported were a more compassionate and trusting sense of others, an appreciation of beauty in the world, and "a deeper more enhanced dependence on God in controlling things we don't understand."

From Miller, W. and C'deBaca, J. (1994). Quantum change: Toward a psychology of transformation. In T. Heatherton and J. Weinberger (Eds.), *Can personality change?* (p. 269). Washington, D.C.: American Psychological Association.

Here a young adult chose to cope with his unfortunate circumstances in a positive manner. Health professionals play an important role in helping patients reframe critical stressors that occur naturally or as unexpected crises in ways that continue to promote self-actualization in adulthood (Clayton & Birren, 1980).

NURSING DIAGNOSES APPROPRIATE TO NORMAL ADULTHOOD

Appropriate nursing diagnoses provide defining characteristics and name a cause for a vertical stressor in adulthood. Typically, nursing interventions for healthy adults correspond to one or more of the nursing diagnoses summarized in Box 25–2. There are many possible reasons for the development of symptoms warranting a general diagnosis. Therefore, carefully inquire about possible causes related to one or more of the following: lack of knowledge regarding developmental milestones, recent moves, unrealistic expectations related to parenting or a job, dysfunctional marital relationships, or role reversals.

A comparison of normal developmental patterns with the patient's presenting symptoms provides the data necessary to arrive at appropriate nursing judgments for each adult patient. Specific nursing interventions should relate to the particular phenomena of concern, the desired outcome, and underlying dynamics of the situation. Primary prevention strategies should reduce risk factors and strengthen protective factors. Psychoeducation and social support also help improve the self-esteem and restart a productive self-concept of adult travelers.

BOX 25–2 Nursing Diagnoses Related to Adult Mental Health

- Spiritual Distress
- Body Image Disturbance
- Compromised, Ineffective Family Coping
- Ineffective Individual Coping
- Altered Family Processes
- Sexual Dysfunction
- Parental Role Conflict
- Risk for Altered Parenting
- Powerlessness
- Knowledge Deficit
- Self-Esteem Disturbance

ACCOMMODATING TO SOCIAL CHANGES: IMPLICATIONS FOR ADULT DEVELOPMENT

Chronological adult development based on stage theories does not take into full account social changes affecting women who juggle career concerns with family obligations or the relatively recent phenomenon of competent, hard-working adults laid off because of corporate restructuring or downsizing (MacKinnon-Slaney, 1994). Dramatic social changes in the last 35 years have altered and will continue profoundly to affect our understanding of adult human development. The role of women has changed dramatically. Because these shifts affect family and work life, corresponding roles for men have undergone significant transformation (Carlsen, 1988). In most cultures, work roles for women for centuries have been gender linked, with a strong emphasis on homemaking and child-rearing. The euphemism "keep them barefoot and pregnant," described what most women could look forward to as their career. Should they work, the cultural milieu traditionally confined women to a narrow range of occupational roles—nurse, teacher, social worker, or secretary. Only in cases of extreme emergency were women permitted to assume work roles traditionally reserved for men. For example, during World War II, women were allowed to become military pilots and to assume traditional male jobs in private industry. Once the war ended, however, this window of opportunity evaporated as if it had never existed.

In the 1990s, greater flexibility of social roles allows both men and women a broader sense of identity and existential space to find their own truths. Men and women now can seek careers traditionally reserved for the opposite sex. For example, men become nurses; women become physicians and steam fitters; fire and police departments recruit women; traditionally male-exclusive military colleges are ordered to admit women to their ranks. These changes have also benefited men, who now feel freer to develop closer relationships with their children and to share some of the burden for maintaining the family's financial resources with a spouse. The term *househusband* is now a legitimate phrase to describe men who choose to be homemakers as their wives become primary breadwinners.

Only in the last few decades have women been able legitimately to expand their personal horizons beyond the home and to join men as equals in life and work (Baruch et al, 1983; Josselson, 1987). Salary discrepancies still exist, however, and men statistically hold an advantage. In many companies, a "glass ceiling" limits promotion of women to the highest ranks. Even so, the lot of women in the workplace has improved dramatically. Women now have consistent roles in most employment areas, and a great range of occupational choices is open to the imagination and talents of women. In providing culturally specific health care, however, you need to realize that in many cultures the role of women remains limited to subservient homemaker and childbearer.

Dual-Career Families

The past 30 years have seen a dramatic change in the structure of the family and a broadening of social role expectations. Parental units in which the father goes to work and the mother stays at home with the children are becoming increasingly uncommon. **Dual-career families,** those in which one partner works full-time and the other is employed at least 20 hours a week, are the rule rather than the exception. Yet women continue to consider home and work responsibilities in making career decisions (Paludi, 1991).

Research shows that greater flexibility of social roles for men and women are sources of satisfaction and benefit for children. Hoffman (1989) suggested that the cognitive, social, and emotional development of school-age children with working mothers parallels or is better than that of children with mothers at home. Employed mothers in Hoffman's study expressed satisfaction with their combined role and their relationship with their children. Moreover, their school-age children held less stereotyped views of male and female roles than the children of mothers who did not work. Gottfried and colleagues (1988) also found strong indications that paternal involvement enhanced their children's cognitive and psychosocial development. Still, many women experience deep personal satisfaction as full-time homemakers and mothers and select this option.

Changes in Family Structures

In addition to major changes in social roles occurring within the family unit, the definition of a family is much more diverse than it was 25 years ago. The traditional model of a married couple as mother and father and children who live with their biological parents still exists but is no longer the only acceptable option. The divorce rate has risen significantly, and more marriages terminate in divorce than in death. Households headed by a female single parent number more than one in five. For every three marriages that succeed, another two will be dissolved through separation and divorce (National Center for Health Statistics, 1987).

Joint custody and parental visiting rights are facts of life for many families, with more than 1 million marriages ending in divorce each year. Yet although many children grow up in single-parent or blended stepfamilies, Golombok and Fivush (1994) note that the diversity of family form does not necessarily have an adverse impact on children. Rather it is the quality of the parent-child relationships and alternative child care arrangements that accounts for differences in child development. (See Chapter 20 for issues and interventions related to families.)

In the 1990s, many men and women are choosing to remain single. No longer is single life a sign of failure when a woman makes a deliberate choice. Cohabitation between consenting adults, with or without children, has also become a common long-term alternative to marriage. Today, it is much more acceptable for homosexual couples to raise children and to live together openly as couples (Patterson, 1992). Divergent lifestyles for men and women are more acceptable, and having a homosexual orientation is viewed as a sexual preference rather than the consequence of faulty parenting or a symptom of mental illness.

Women's patterns of marriage, childbearing, and caregiving have also changed considerably. Just a few decades ago, the childbearing decades were culturally limited to the 20s and early 30s. Should a woman conceive a child in her late 30s or early 40s, the child was deemed a "change of life" baby, with the implication that conception was unplanned, an irregularity of nature associated with the beginning of menopause. Today, there is a "blurring of life periods" (Neugarten and Neugarten, 1986) as women postpone having children until they are older. Many adults approach marriage and childbirth as options rather than expectations of mature adulthood, and many more women have their first child in their late 30s and 40s. New reproductive technologies also allow women at older ages, women without partners, and homosexual couples to have children of their own.

The decision to postpone childbirth does not seem to carry adverse effects. In a comparative study of parents with first children born in the 20s, 30s, and 40s, Daniels and Weingarten (1982) reported that age variation did not significantly affect accomplishment of parenting tasks. Becoming a parent at a later age required more initial adjustment, but these parents also reported greater ultimate satisfaction with their parenting than they believed they would have experienced with a first child at an earlier age.

Infertility

Having children still establishes a sense of continued identity for women. Childbearing is a normal life process, a recognized symbol of adult status and feminine identity (Phoenix et al, 1991). Yet approximately 20% of women wishing to have children experience difficulty (Olschansky, 1994) or are unable to have biological children. **Infertility** is defined as the inability to have children for biological reasons. Causes of infertility are many and can occur in one or both partners. Infertility is not simply a biological crisis. It carries great potential for an identity crisis, particularly if the role of mother is central to a woman's identity or is viewed by the husband as important to the relationship. As one woman explained:

I think we've all grown up with the idea that pregnancy is what a woman does, it's the most natural thing, and we have a whole 2000 years of literature and culture that have always pointed in that direction. So there has been this tradition, and it's very hard at times to redefine oneself as a woman.

I figured I could sit in the backyard and make quilts and do handwork that I love to do, which in some ways I haven't done because now I see no purpose—it is more something to do if you're pregnant. There are some things I still haven't done, like fix up the patio with Astroturf, which would be nice for a child to play in. And some things I would do in the house that now really aren't needed since there are no kids. I had images and plans of things I would do (Phoenix et al, 1991, p. 177).

Although typically considered a woman's issue, infertility in men is quite common and of considerable concern to the men involved. The procedures for assessing fertility are invasive and time consuming. In vitro fertilization and adoption are possible solutions, but in vitro technology is expensive and not always successful. You can help patients work through the emotional aspects of infertility and can connect them with the appropriate medical services for explaining options or providing direct service. Note that people can be generative in many ways and that biological childbearing is only one of them. Helping men and women to see their reproductive capacity as something besides the defining characteristic of their masculinity or femininity is particularly important. (See Chapter 10 for communication and reframing strategies.)

Ending a Relationship

Achievement of intimacy is a significant psychosocial task of adulthood, so that the end of a relationship, whether in separation, divorce, or death, marks a turning point in the adult's journey. This process of loss applies to homosexual as well as heterosexual partners and can also apply to the end of a relationship with a dear friend, a meaningful job, or even a beloved pet.

Some of the factors affecting the intensity of the loss relate to the nature and length of the relationship, the level of conflict in or satisfaction with the relationship, and the amount of social support the person receives on an ongoing basis. Fiske and Chiriboga (1990) found that divorcing persons were more likely to experience both positive and negative changes in nearly all areas of their lives. One woman describes some of the complications induced by a lost relationship:

In my 40s I was very involved in education, family, and community. It was exciting and fulfilling. The change at age 54 to a single lifestyle was traumatic. I had always felt that being married had given me the freedom to explore and engage in new activities with home and husband as always an emotional and financial safety net. Now it seems tiresome to make all decisions—and do all thinking—alone. In the past six years, I've also had to come to terms with the basic fact that there are many things over which we have absolutely no control (Arnold, 1994).

In divorce, "burying" the partner is often harder than the separation when a partner dies. Frequently, the divorced parents face continued involvement. Opportunities for despair as well as for personal growth accompany the process of working through either the voluntary or the involuntary ending of a relationship.

Becoming widowed in early and middle stages of adulthood is particularly traumatic because these widowed women have few peers who understand or can respond to their pain. At a time when their contemporaries are walking through life with a partner, widows are at a distinct disadvantage. Atchley (1991) suggests that "the social disruption widowhood causes depends largely on the number of role relationships affected by the spouse's death (p. 250). Fiske and Chiriboga (1990) observed that loss of a spouse was more devastating for men than for women. They postulated that women are more likely to have close relationships with a number of people, whereas many men have close relationships only with their wives. But for many people, loss is poignant, as this woman describes:

At age 52, my husband of almost 33 years died. He was just 54 and had a brain tumor. This event so changed my life, my outlook, my future, my lifestyle that I have trouble thinking beyond it. His death is so all-consuming that age, stage, and outlook seem to be a result of that event (Arnold, 1994).

Although this woman had many friends, the loss was still devastating. When tragedy strikes, a person's developmental world stops—at least for a time. Some life issues are *not* particularly age related or more gracefully handled during one age period than another. Nor are the usual remedies useful, as another woman, an introvert by nature, states:

Social support is not a substitute for inner strength. Movies and dinner do not complete a sleepless night. I am a solitary person in most of life's crises and do not count on others to fill my needs or wipe my tears—a function of a miserable, bleak, and unsupported childhood. I have always worked at finding serenity and staying alive. I am no less in the world but embrace it more fully (Arnold, 1994).

We often equate maturity, mental health, and the ability to resolve grief with the level of social support a person receives or seeks. Yet, as this woman's testimony shows, social support is critical for some, but the route others must take is different. You therefore need to be aware and supportive of personal choices.

The Not-So-Empty Nest

In past decades, the *empty nest* was identified as the basis for depression in midlife women. Contrary to popular belief, a number of researchers (Neugarten, 1970; Cooper and Gutmann, 1987) report that the last child leaving home does not create depression for most women but that the empty nest actually liberates parents. Both working parents and home-oriented women experienced greater freedom, more free time, greater privacy, and more opportunities. This woman's statement captures her sense of personal growth:

My family has grown and gone, and the hectic pace of the 40s, which tore me between being a wife, mother, and caretaker for aging parents, has ended. Perhaps the very fact that the 40s were so full of obligations makes the 50s appear idyllic early on. I now have the time and means to work and play as I like. I am able to fulfill obligations because I want to, and not because I have to. I have passed the "have to" years and entered the "want to" years (Arnold, 1994).

Lowenthal and Chiriboga (1972) report exceptions to these findings in women with long-standing emotional problems whose lives have revolved around their children. For these women, therapy can help them reestablish a stronger sense of self.

The empty nest is not an abrupt change for many adults today. Changing social and economic realities have created different mental health issues for both parents and adult children. Many young adults in their 20s are choosing to return home and to live with their parents for longer periods. For these young adults, building a solid career identity is threatened by economic uncertainty, and the comforts of home are far more appealing than the substandard housing arrangements they typically can afford. Consequently, some young adults are postponing major life commitments, including marriage, children, and home ownership, because of declining job opportunities and rising costs of housing and education. Additionally, the time required to earn a college degree can be more than four years, as evidenced in the tee-shirt proclamation: "ECU, the best 5 or 6 years of my life."

For today's young adult, exercising the necessary self-discipline required for financial independence clearly is not easy. A generation ago, people bought only what they could afford because there were no financial structures to support other alternatives. Today's easy credit for purchases adults cannot really afford is creating a negative balance and significant debt, the magnitude of which is only beginning to be appreciated. The financial shortfall often is absorbed by parents, causing stress, anger, anxiety, and frustration for all concerned. Circumstances may warrant psychiatric intervention.

The Sandwich Generation

As more people live longer, adult children increasingly are called on to provide financial and other assistance to aging parents (Kingson et al, 1986; Aldwin et al, 1989). Actual physical care of the frail elderly creates an ongoing concern for those who cannot put an infirm parent in a nursing home for either financial or emotional reasons.

Women still remain the major caregivers to the elderly. Caught between two generations, both of which require care, many adults in midlife find it difficult to balance caregiving responsibilities. Teenagers require a different kind of parenting, and the frail elderly typically require the type of physical care accorded their children at an earlier age. Caregiving therefore requires a constant switching of gears. Moreover, caring for elderly parents is more difficult, first because the investment brings further dependence as the older adult becomes more frail and second because parenting the frail older adult necessarily entails role reversals. As Brody (1990) observes, "No matter how much care an older person needs, he or she does not become, and cannot become the child of the adult child in the feelings of either child or parent. Half a century or even more of a parent/child relationship cannot be discarded" (p. 87).

Unemployment

The pervasive fear of job loss—affecting blue-collar and white-collar workers alike—is becoming a powerful force. For U.S. workers, the 1990s have become the age of job insecurity. Each year, close to 2 million Americans permanently lose their jobs as companies "downsize" or "right size" to remain competitive. Furthermore, more than 20% of those who lose their jobs this year will be out of work for at least 6 months, according to Labor Department projections (*Washington Post*, 1994). Midlife layoffs in previously stable work situations create serious assaults on self-identity. Some people emerge stronger, but others are irreparably scarred. Being laid off invariably is experienced as a personal crisis of identity requiring significant attention to reframing one's sense of self in addition to the actual job search. From unskilled workers to corporate executives, employees increasingly are asking the same questions: Will the current wave of corporate restructuring that is shaping the economy affect me, and how will I cope if I lose my job?

Adding to the anxiety is the structural shift in the work force from permanent positions to a contingent work force that includes many employees who not part of the core establishment. New jobs often are temporary positions with little or no job security, and they often carry no benefits such as health insurance, pensions, and paid vacations. Contingent workers now make up more than 25% of the work force; they are part-time workers, temporary employees, and subcontractors. These structural changes have helped make the temporary services firm, Manpower, Inc., a company with twice as many employees as General Motors. Manpower is now the largest employer in the United States.

In the past, hard work and loyalty paid off (Morrow & McElroy, 1987). Economic security was based on constancy, seniority, and dedicated work. But this work ethic is fast becoming a relic of the past, replaced by structural changes in the work force that favor a temporary, or contingent, model. The use of consultants who are paid higher salaries but are not given benefits is becoming more and more prevalent. Companies choose to pay a little more for expertise in the short run, to be able to dismiss workers easily when company demands shift. The loyalty of the "company man" is evaporating, and work commitment is harder to sustain, as employees lose faith in their employer's ability to provide a caring, supportive work environment that rewards commitment.

Review of the literature reveals a higher incidence of mental health disruptions in the form of depression, loss of self-esteem, marital and family problems, and even suicide as correlates of job loss (Love & Torrence, 1989; Dooley & Catalano, 1991). Yet little is written about concrete preventive mental health strategies designed to help people cope with a job loss in a world where old paradigms about job search strategies no longer apply. A college degree no longer guarantees employment success, and career opportunities are far more competitive because of corporate restructuring, downsizing, and the automation of many skilled tasks once performed by human workers. Most companies are trying to do more with less, so that getting a job, regardless of age, is harder than it was even five years ago.

Getting another job becomes more difficult as one gets older. The U.S. Department of Labor identifies a mature worker as any employee age 40 or older. With the current restructuring of employment patterns, older workers report having a great deal of difficulty getting other jobs. Despite laws against discrimination of all types, age discrimination is a reality in today's job market. In 1989, the U.S. Senate Special Committee on Aging reported that more than a third of employers studied believed that age discrimination occurred on a regular basis. Older workers typically are stereotyped as being less creative or willing to find innovative solutions to challenging problems. They are viewed as less able to make quick decisions under pressure, as less interested in learning new technologies, and in some instances as untrainable. Many have made excellent salaries and earned management titles. Companies are hesitant to hire them because younger workers do not require the same salaries or entitlements and are willing to do the same jobs. Older workers report interview comments from potential employers such as, "You are overqualified for this job, and I don't think you would be really happy here" or "You have a lot of skills, but what we are looking for is someone who has this technical skill, which you don't seem to have." Issues such as retirement and health benefits also affect decisions about hiring the older worker because benefits most often are used by this age group and cost the company money without a commensurate return on investment. Characteristics associated with the successful older worker such as loyalty, expertise, and a record of steady performance get overlooked in today's unstable job market.

Many communities today are providing support for dislocated workers to learn the skills that will make them more competitive in the job market. Privately funded and volunteer organizations such as Forty Plus help the older worker find the necessary support and practical advice needed to negotiate today's uncertain job opportunities.

Adults as Lifelong Learners

Although adults now constitute approximately 50% of students in higher education (MacKinnon-Slaney, 1994), current theories to explain development in the adult learner pose more questions than provide answers. Adult learners come with a wide variety of life skills. Most are self-supporting. Most are looking for an educational experience that will build on their life experience and enhance the quality of their lives (Mezirow, 1990).

The characteristics and learning needs of the adult learner typically are much more diverse than they are for traditional college students in late adolescence and early adulthood (Bauer & Mott, 1990). Because of major differences in life experience, adults present a wider variation in their skill development and self-efficacy. The adult learner may have mastered life skills that will make learning tasks easier as the educational experience develops, but basic study skills and ability to organize content quickly typically benefit from having initial structural expectations and guidelines set forth by the instructor. Adult learners who have been out of school for a long time often lack confidence in their abilities to compete effectively in the classroom with younger students. Because adult learners are older and typically more experienced and self-motivated, their need for initial structure is often overlooked by instructors and frequently by the student as well. Basic assumptions relevant to the process of learning in adulthood are presented in Box 25–3.

The Future of Adult Development

In *A Tale of Two Cities,* the scene of an important social revolution several centuries ago, Charles Dickens begins with the line: "It was the best of times, it was the worst of times." As we approach the 21st century, we are arriving on the crest of unprecedented technological and sociological changes that will have important consequences for adult development. The technological revolution may indeed equal that of other social revolutions in its power. The potential for human development at the turn of the century to reach the best of times or the worst of times in large measure will depend on the judgments of its adult population. Maturity and level of mental health will affect important decisions.

New Theories Linked to Social Changes

Some developmental theorists link adult development more to maturational responses to life events and social relationships than to chronological age. These criteria may become more definitive ways to conceptualize developmental responses in a world of rapid social change, increasing focus on technology, and much less

BOX 25-3 Educating the Adult Learner

- We cannot teach another person directly; we can only facilitate his learning.
- A person learns significantly only those things which he perceives as being involved in the maintenance of, or enhancement of, the structure of self.
- Experience that is perceived as inconsistent with self can be assimilated only if the current organization of self is relaxed and expanded to include it.
- The educational situation that most effectively promotes significant learning is one in which the threat to the self of the learner is reduced to a minimum.

From *The adult learner: A neglected species* by Malcolm Knowles.

time for reflection. For example, genome therapy may dramatically improve life span, with projections that people could live to be 140 years old in the 21st century. How will this affect the staging of adult development? What will the quality of life be like? What are the implications for career development and personal relationships if the projection becomes a reality in the 21st century? Longevity is only one of the many changes tomorrow's adult can expect.

The process and outcome of change will greatly affect our understanding of self and other adults in the new era. From a practical perspective, negotiating adulthood in the 21st century may be a little like white water rafting. The waters will be swift, rapidly changing, and exciting, but potentially dangerous. Careful preparation for the trip helps ensure its success. People need to draw the map, develop perspectives on how to navigate the rapids, and identify the specific strengths and values one needs to bring as baggage on the kayak. Moreover, the white water rafter will need an experienced guide to direct the project and warn of potential dangers.

Adult travelers in the 1990s need to act as guides and mentors for the next generation of adults by linking together the past, present, and future in a meaningful way. Descriptions of human development in adulthood that blend the best of past traditions with the realities of the present and the trends of the future need to be carefully interwoven into the fabric of community life. Those adults who will enhance and even shape our lives in the next century need new explanations. The story of the adult traveler in the 20th century was of individualism and self-actualization, but as Keen (1991, p. 145) suggests:

> *. . . [R]ecently it has begun to look as if individualism is rapidly leading us into anarchy. What was once our strength is now tearing us apart. We are losing our moral consensus, our sense of community, our willingness to sacrifice for a shared ideal of the future, our understanding of what it is that gives dignity to the life of a man or woman.*

The turn of the century offers an opportunity to blend strong community values with those of individuals, to uphold and affirm the values of individualism as necessary and valid to full participation in the community. Perhaps then, the story of adulthood in the 21st century could be of community and of building a "just and loving society" (Bellah, 1985, p. 83).

Havighurst (1953; 1973) has suggested a number of problem areas that warrant research on personality through the life span. Among these areas for the study are career changes in relation to personality, age, and sex and the ways normal adults perceive the aging process as individuals, as family members, and as part of the wider community. Exploration of personality changes associated with alterations in physical vigor or health, the influence of leisure activities on adult personality development, documentation of human development in the 50s and 60s, attitudes toward death, and variables associated with development of dementia also are fruitful areas for inquiry into normal adult development.

Human Development as a Moral Imperative

Many of the decisions that technology and cost containment in health care have spawned will create moral dilemmas that focus on choice and responsibility. Human responses to these questions and decisions made will reside in the hands and souls of its adults in the 21st century. In an expanding concept of the meaning of adulthood, Tournier (1965, p. 49) notes that:

> *. . . [T]o speak of the person, and of respect for the person, is to speak, not of that man which is physical, psychological or intellectual, but of what is spiritual in him, his moral conscience, his sense of responsibility, his freedom of choice.*

Choice and responsibility will be key to strategies for promoting adult mental health at the turn of the century. Preventive psychiatry focused on reducing risk factors and strengthening protective factors will be of primary importance. To exercise their "response-ability" appropriately, adults will need to integrate biological, ethical, and social concerns as the building blocks of adult development in a new holistic paradigm. The means for this integration are education, values clarification, and social support to meet the challenge.

▶ Check Your Reading

3. How would you describe the impact of social changes in the last 35 years on mental health?
4. What are the differences between vertical and horizontal stressors in adult development?
5. What is meant by the sandwich generation?

PROMOTING THE MENTAL HEALTH OF THE ADULT TRAVELER

Bellah (1985) suggests that "if it is to provide any richness of meaning, the idea of a life course must be set in a larger generational, historical, and probably, religious context" (p. 82). Almost a century ago, Freud identified intrinsic personal fulfillment achieved through productive work and satisfying intimate relationships as the benchmark of adult mental health. These are likely to remain contemporary standards of adult maturity. Telling the story of adulthood at the turn of the century, however, is an art that needs to be firmly anchored in both objective and subjective definitions of roles and social institutions of the past and present and integrated with those needed to achieve the visions of the next millennium. An awesome undertaking, the story begins with this generation of adults. As Whitehead (1929) in his landmark book on education advises:

> *The mind is never passive: it is a perpetual activity, delicate, receptive, responsive to stimulus. You cannot postpone its life until you have sharpened it. Whatever interest attaches to your subject matter must be evoked here and now; whatever powers you are strengthening in the pupil must be exercised here and now; whatever possibilities of mental life your teaching should impart, must be exhibited here and now. That is the golden rule of education, and a very difficult one to follow (p. 18).*

Human Character Development

Human *character development* will become increasingly important in the next decade, primarily because of the crucial role these travelers will play at every stage of their psychological growth in shaping the new world. Adults in the next century will be called on to consider important ethical questions: end-of-life decisions, fetal tissue research, prophylactic surgery on well children and adults with genetic predispositions to cancer, access to care in a cost-containment health care environment, subsidized care and housing for migrant workers, and other social dilemmas. None of these issues has clear-cut answers. Yet all of them are being woven into the social fabric of the 21st century.

Ladner (1995) suggests that the solution to these problems lies in education:

> *Higher educational institutions are particularly suited to provide the leadership because they can link theory with practice and teach principle-centered leadership to today's college students. It doesn't matter whether one is a Republican, Democrat or independent: all students need to be guided by ethical imperatives if they are to be engaged in solving the problems of their generation (p. C2).*

Thus broad-based education for adult learners is based on a strong moral imperative. Practical strategies to cope successfully with a world these adults did not create will become a vital force in preventive adult mental health.

More than ever, tomorrow's adult will be a "tentative character type shaped by inherited values on the one hand and the challenges of the expanding frontier on the other" (Bellah, 1985, p. 39). For those dedicated to enhancing adult potential, the task is to preserve and integrate traditional values of responsibility, dedication to truth, and commitment as the cornerstone of adult maturity. Definitive educational strategies can support the learning needs of an increasingly diverse student population. At the same time:

> *There must be new flowerings, new prophets, new adventures—always new adventures—if the heart of man, albeit in fits and starts, is to go on beating (Tournier, 1965, p. 39).*

Education in Preventive Mental Health

Education will become increasingly important as a means of both shaping and telling the story of adulthood. Education acts as the gatekeeper, the first line of defense in reducing risk behaviors associated with mental illness and in promoting protective factors to enhance emotional health and well-being. Relevant curricula, however, need to support primary prevention. The current educational system also needs to reflect technical, social, and economic changes in society and to support purposeful character development. Formal and informal teaching methods related to health education should focus on the development of creative *processes* necessary to create a social environment, especially critical thinking and respect for diversity. Values clarification to improve the critical thinking and ethical decision-making abilities of adult travelers, combined with empowerment strategies, is a basic foundation for primary prevention mental health strategies in the 1990s and beyond. Broad-based curricula that integrate interventions supporting physical and emotional health can help alleviate many risk factors.

The restructuring of higher education also needs to account for the requirements of adult learners. Education should enhance personal development, thereby reducing unnecessary stress and frustration. Today's adult student population is much more diverse, with a tremendous range of interests, life experiences, maturity, and learning needs. Such diversity naturally affects students' approach to learning tasks and requires a broader educational mix of teaching strategies to support significant differences in student learning requirements. Granting course credit for comparable life experiences would make the curriculum more flexible and tailored to individual student needs. Redesigning courses that build on rather than repeat student experience would make the concept of the university as a community of scholars accessible to more students. Recognizing the complexity of student learning needs while balancing them with realistic expectations of academic performance are key elements in the restructuring of curriculum models to enhance student learning.

Values Clarification

We need to ensure that humanistic society not fall victim to the economic or technological tenor of the time. Thus, values clarification will become increasingly important as a preventive mental health strategy. Young and middle-aged adults will need to achieve a solid and recognizable identity as members of a humanistic community, embracing the notion of a shared, personal participation in life and attention to values and the moral domain. They will need to engage thoughtfully and compassionately in a continuous process of exploration, questioning and reflecting on critical matters, such as right to life, end-of-life decisions, access to health care, and care of the poor.

Young and middle-aged adult travelers will need to make difficult ethical decisions related to the goals and purposes of technological advances. Values clarification can help them sort criteria and look closely at relevant data from a more holistic perspective. Sharing common concerns and discussing differences become simpler when issues are named and more than one voice is heard. The process of inquiry should be personal and should include the spiritual, social, affective (emotional), and intellectual self in the full cognitive (mental) engagement of the individual. Respect for ideas presented by people with different backgrounds and beliefs and dissimilar ways of thinking is essential.

Technology in Preventive Mental Health

Technology is important in preventive mental health because of the possibilities technology offers for early diagnosis and health education and because of the problems it generates in using it wisely. Technological change is as dramatic as the development of books during the Renaissance. In fact, the computer is likely to become the "textbook of the future." The Internet has created an "information superhighway," allowing students to access vast amounts of information in a wide spectrum of formats. The classroom as we know it today has broadened, as the world shrinks through the creative use of technology. Today the instructor may be many miles away, as teaching is provided in "virtual reality classrooms" or at home, without a student ever having to put a foot in the classroom. Even surgery may be performed through interactive television.

Electronic interactive formats present a new, interesting, and informative way to enhance student learning. Interactive video presents material within a situational or interpersonal context. This format helps a student recognize that facts are embedded in larger situations. They can "see" and "hear" how people evaluate and respond effectively to complex situations. Computer-generated simulations can provide practical applications for problem-solving and allow more flexibility with differences in the time patterns some students need to maximize learning. Yet it is critical that technology support but not replace the spontaneous, reasoned human element in health education. Facts need a context and tone for a collective meaning. Human beings are meaning makers, and no matter how sophisticated a decision-making software package, it can never replace human dialogue. Consequently, modeling of behavior, development of social skills, and the relating of ideas to others must continue to be significant dimensions of health education.

The process of developing creativity is greater than the sum of its parts. The instructor must have the ability to understand and convey the social skills necessary to deal with the nuances, emotional sensitivities, and values of others in real-life situations. Personal encounters with the student about these matters are as important as mastering content. Fostering awareness of the human values and richness of shared discovery can occur only through ongoing conversations about meaning.

Empowerment Strategies

Most mentally healthy adults can generate their own answers and resolve their own problems in life with just a little support and guidance. Mentorship, particularly in novice adulthood, is an important element of preventive psychiatry (Levinson et al, 1978; Noe, 1988). Nurses can assist the adult traveler in learning assertive communication, negotiation, and conflict management strategies both spontaneously and in formal continuing education classes. Providing adults with information about the normal process of adult development and assisting them in the development of parenting skills, caring for aging parents, or surviving loss of a relationship or job in times of distress can reframe a crisis into a challenging possibility. Informal health teaching that assists adult travelers to find meaning in their current situations and plan for the future is a preventive strategy, easily accomplished without significant financial outlay. During times of transition, nurses can help adult travelers reclaim a sense of self-mastery through simple open-ended questions, such as:

- How are you adjusting to (identify the life transition: your job loss, having to care for your parents, death of a spouse, return to school)? Framing the question in this way suggests that the period of transition is one of temporary adjustment with a projected outcome that can be successful.
- What coping skills have you used in the past that have helped you? This question helps individuals identify productive coping skills that they may have forgotten, which can be used to negotiate the current transition successfully.

Social Support

Social support offers the adult opportunities to correct knowledge deficits, to develop networks that help enhance self-esteem, and to consider options for coping with difficult life problems. Primary prevention strategies in the form of stress management and coping skills, use of community resources, referral to appropriate support groups, and reading material on parenting are simple interventions. Crisis intervention (see Chapter 15) should be offered to those individuals and families presenting with inadequate coping skills, insufficient support systems, and perceived powerlessness to direct their lives. A related intervention is to provide sufficient time for personal reflection and subsequent human dialogue. As Wicks (1985) suggests, "use any technique necessary to slow yourself down so that you don't rush to the grave missing the scenery in your life along the way" (p. 142).

Support groups are an invaluable form of social support. As a primary therapeutic intervention or as an adjunct to other therapies, they provide emotional respite and direction for adult travelers. Nurses can help individuals and families find new meaning in uncertain times through referral to the many support groups serving the community for adults in crisis. (For a full discussion of the role of support groups see Chapter 17.)

One example of a support group is New Hope, a community-based job search group designed for people who have lost a job for any reason. The group has the collective purpose of helping the job seeker cope emotionally while looking for a new job, providing practical help and support with all aspects of the job search process, and offering an opportunity for networking among job seekers. Explicit norms include confidentiality, mutual respect, and commitment to the job search process. The clientele using the services of the group is mixed, with a heavier concentration of white-collar, male, and older workers displaced from the work force after many years of service.

New Hope's interactive process is based on an empowerment framework, defined as "the interpersonal process of providing the resources, tools and environment to develop, build and increase the ability and effectiveness of others to set and reach goals for individual and social ends" (Hawkes, 1992). To replace traditional paradigms of work efficacy and job security based on education, successful performance, and rational progression, the group has developed a different paradigm for the job search.

An explicit assumption is that workers face a new labor force paradigm of uncertainty and ambiguity in the workplace that applies to everyone, regardless of credentials and experience. Acknowledging this reality and developing initiatives to meet the challenge is an important group focus. Empowerment of self through personal responsibility is viewed as a primary strategy of effective job searching. Interventions are designed to help people identify their strengths and to recognize their value as individuals apart from their job. Clients are encouraged to accept ambiguity in work and to develop competencies related to versatility and networking in a time of turbulent economic change. Specific techniques include developing professional networks and cooperative human relationships, acceptance of feelings, sharing of job leads, action through knowledge, and the tools needed to understand and respond effectively in a rapidly changing job market.

People enter New Hope not knowing what to expect, usually experiencing diminished self-esteem and identity, anticipating changes in lifestyle, and feeling vulnerable about the future. Members of the group have identified the following helpful factors:

- Having a place to talk
- Finding that you are not alone
- Networking
- Maintaining motivation
- Developing concrete strategies in the job search
- Learning about resources
- Interest of other members

Participants in the group report the following outcomes as the result of group membership:

- Skills in networking
- Writing a résumé
- Interviewing skills
- Confidence building

New Hope offers a preventive mental health strategy to reduce anxiety, emotional pain, and loss while empowering people to negotiate a job search creatively. Similar support groups might promote empowerment and follow a similar format while helping individuals cope with divorce, death, illness, and many other vertical stressors that appear on the landscape of the adult journey.

▶ Check Your Reading

6. In what ways can education be considered as a primary means of preventive psychiatry?
7. How are support groups used as a tool to promote mental health?

The case study below presents a normal, predictable life crisis in the human journey of the adult traveler and suggests appropriate nursing interventions. For psychiatric conditions affecting adults, please consult Unit V.

CASE STUDY: DOROTHY

Dorothy is a 49-year-old executive secretary who lives in the Southwest. Her mother was diagnosed with lung cancer six months ago and is currently in the terminal stages. Her mother had a bilateral mastectomy four years ago for breast cancer. Two months ago, Dorothy divorced her husband of 25 years and is living alone in an apartment. Her two children are living on their own; one is in college, and one is married with two children. Her only sister lives on the West Coast and also works full-time. As of now, Dorothy's only social outlet is an occasional evening out with her friends from church.

Dorothy's mother asked her to promise her that she would not put her in a nursing home. Every evening after work Dorothy drives to her mother's home to check on her. Having Dorothy move in is not an option because her mother lives in a one-bedroom apartment. When Dorothy comes to the doctor's office for a check-up, she says that she is "exhausted, on edge and frustrated, and can't sleep through the night." She tells you that her mother is a strong person and she wants to abide by her wishes, but she isn't sure about what to do. When her father died several years ago, Dorothy was not there and still feels guilty. She also tells you that she is concerned that her mother's small savings will be gone soon.

ASSESSMENT

Assessment data are as follows:

- Insomnia
- Fatigue
- Anxiety
- Multiple personal stressors (divorce, multiple role changes)
- Financial concerns
- Perceived lack of support

DIAGNOSIS

***DSM IV* Diagnosis:** Adjustment Disorder, With Anxiety

Nursing Diagnosis: Caregiver Role Strain related to terminal illness of mother, financial concerns, and perceived lack of support evidenced by anxiety, insomnia, and feeling of extreme fatigue

OUTCOME IDENTIFICATION, PLANNING, AND IMPLEMENTATION

EXPECTED OUTCOME 1: By _____ the patient will obtain assistance with demands of caring for mother.

SHORT-TERM GOALS	NURSING INTERVENTIONS	RATIONALES
By _____ the patient will verbalize tasks that could be delegated.	1. Assist the patient in developing a list of the tasks necessary to care for her mother. 2. Have patient compile a list and review it with her.	1–2. A structured activity will help the patient focus on and complete a specific task.
	3. Help patient decide which items on the list could be delegated and which she needs to complete.	3. Patient will want to retain some tasks to remain a part of her mother's care, but delegating others will enable the mother to remain at home, which is what she asked of her daughter.
By _____ the patient will identify resource persons, both inside and outside the family, that could assist with her mother's care.	1. Identify possible caregiver resources for the patient.	1. Patient may be unaware of all the resources that are available.
	2. Develop possibilities for delegation of tasks that are within budgetary constraints.	2. Planning without considering finances is not time efficient.
	3. Discuss the concept of respite care with the patient.	3. Patient may be unaware of the concept of respite care.
	4. Assist patient and caregiver to develop a daily schedule of direct care activities.	4. A specific daily schedule will assist the patient in delegating activities.

EXPECTED OUTCOME 2: By _____ the patient will develop a support system with neighbors, family, and friends.

SHORT-TERM GOALS	NURSING INTERVENTIONS	RATIONALES
By _____ the patient will identify potential caregivers who could assist her.	1. Ask the patient to compile a list of potential caregivers from her neighbors, family, and friends. 2. Help patient to identify the type and source of support or care that would be most beneficial.	1–2. Actually putting the list on paper will assist the patient in completing the task.

SHORT-TERM GOALS	NURSING INTERVENTIONS	RATIONALES
By _____ the patient will ask a neighbor or church member to sit with her mother while she attends a church service on the following Sunday.	1. Further assess the patient's spiritual needs and previous attendance at a church. 2. Asking for the help of a church member will assure the patient that others are willing to help her during this time.	1–2. The spiritual comfort found in attending a church service will be particularly helpful to the patient at this time.
By _____ the patient will invite a former friend over for lunch or dinner.	1. Encourage the patient to socialize and build up a support network. 2. Continue to encourage the patient to make contact with former friends.	1–2. Friends and family are often willing to help, but do not know what would be helpful.

EXPECTED OUTCOME 3: By _____ the patient will verbalize the importance of self-care in maintaining the stamina needed to care for her mother.

SHORT-TERM GOALS	NURSING INTERVENTIONS	RATIONALES
By _____ the patient will develop and implement a plan for daily regular exercise.	1. Assist the patient in maintaining a daily log of exercise and sleep patterns. 2. Teach the patient about the correlation of sleep and exercise.	1–2. Regular exercise is a stress reducer and sleep enhancer.
By _____ the patient will develop and implement a plan for healthy eating.	1. Encourage the patient to keep a daily diary of food intake. 2. Teach the patient about the pyramid plan for healthy nutrition on a daily basis. 3. Assist the patient to begin a nutritional plan that will be based on her likes and dislikes.	1. It is important to assess both areas of dietary intake that are healthy and those that need improvement. 2. Patient may be unaware of what entails healthy nutritional status. 3. Compliance in changing behavior is more likely if the patient does not have to make radical changes, particularly during times of other personal stress.
By _____ the patient will make and keep appointment for yearly physical examination.	1. Assist the patient in arranging for a time when she can see her physician that fits into her schedule. 2. Remind the patient that maintaining her own health is of the utmost importance right now.	1–2. Multiple life stressors can lead to a breakdown in the immune system and ultimately cause illness. Regular monitoring of health status is important at this time.

Nursing Diagnosis: Altered Role Performance related to change in marital status and role reversal with mother evidenced by inability to accept new role or to ask for help from others

OUTCOME IDENTIFICATION, PLANNING, AND IMPLEMENTATION

EXPECTED OUTCOME 1: By _____ the patient will be able to function comfortably in new role.

SHORT-TERM GOALS	NURSING INTERVENTIONS	RATIONALES
By _____ the patient will specify behaviors to meet new role expectations.	1. Ask the patient to make a list of necessary behaviors to accomplish new role. 2. Offer suggestions such as assertiveness training. 3. Have the patient practice new behaviors with you in a role-play setting.	1–2. The patient may have some ideas in mind that would be helpful but may be so emotionally stressed that she is having difficulty generating new ideas for herself. 3. Initiating new behaviors is a difficult process. Practicing with someone who is accepting and encouraging fosters success.

SHORT-TERM GOALS	NURSING INTERVENTIONS	RATIONALES
By _____ the patient will discuss role performance with her sister and children and significant friends.	1. Have the patient delineate specific time frames for the change. 2. Assist the patient to express in behavioral terms what she expects from her sister and children.	1–2. Being specific in time frames and behavior will aid the patient in getting her needs met and is part of being an assertive person.
By _____ the patient will express satisfaction and acceptance with new role parameters.	1. Ask the patient to make a list of the pros and cons of her new role changes.	1. Actually writing down the changes will help the patient to quantify any difficult areas. Negative feelings usually indicate a form of resistance to change and may reveal some guilt about the change.
	2. Encourage the patient to talk openly about any negative feelings she continues to have with her change in behavior with her sister, children, and friends.	2. Talking about these feelings to an accepting person may help alleviate the guilt.

EXPECTED OUTCOME 2: By _____ the patient will be able to express ambivalent feelings of anger, guilt, fear, and sadness over the role changes that are necessary at this time in her life.

SHORT-TERM GOALS	NURSING INTERVENTIONS	RATIONALES
By _____ the patient will discuss a wide variety of feelings honestly and openly.	1. Ask the patient to keep track of feelings that occur in a 24-hour period. Provide her with a chart that describes feelings and feeling words.	1. The patient is probably being flooded with feelings and may be having difficulty distinguishing between them.
	2. Encourage the patient to make connections between strong negative feelings and bodily expressions. 3. Ask the patient to describe what bodily reaction she feels when she feels angry or fearful.	2–3. If the patient is unaccustomed to talking about or identifying feelings, making a connection with what is going on with her body will be helpful.
	4. Ask the patient to describe one or two things she feels hopeful about in the future.	4. It is important to focus not only on negative feelings but also on positive ones.
By _____ the patient will seek the help of clergy or therapist to help her with the grieving process.	1. Make the patient aware of all the grief she has experienced in the past year in regard to her divorce, her children leaving home, and her mother's history of poor health and impending death.	1. Often, patients are aware that they are experiencing a difficult time but do not have the necessary vocabulary to describe it. Labeling this process as the grief process and normalizing it for the patient may be helpful.
	2. Provide the patient with the names and phone numbers of nurse therapists or pastoral counselors who specialize in the grief process. 3. Encourage the patient to make the appointment within one week.	2. This patient has had considerable grief experiences in the past year, and working with a specialist in this area may prevent a delayed bereavement process.

EVALUATION

Formative Evaluation: Dorothy was able to meet each of the short-term goals in the time frames allotted. She developed strategies to provide respite from the constant care of her mother. Each week she appeared better able to ask for help and support from her friends and sister. She saw her physician and has taken steps to develop a more healthy lifestyle.

Summative Evaluation: Dorothy was able to meet all of the expected outcomes with the help and support of the nurse. She contacted a hospice and now has the support she needs to care for her mother. Dorothy states she feels she has regained balance in her life and no longer feels that her mother's care is a burden. In talking with her friends and reconnecting with her church, Dorothy has developed a strong support system that sustains her during this difficult time.

CONCLUSIONS

Adulthood encompasses a long stretch of the developmental journey. The story of human life is about a journey toward wholeness. We see the journey physically begin with conception and end with death. In between, life offers each individual multiple opportunities through their personalized attitudes and actions of integrity, courage, justice, and compassion to make meaningful contributions to life and to experience tremendous satisfaction from the effort and outcome. Although childhood and adolescence are significant periods in providing the foundation for adulthood, this next life stage is even more significant because in every society, the adults become the critics, architects, and change agents of their generation.

Sufficient raw data suggest that adult development in the 21st century will be quite different and that today's adults will play a critical role in shaping a new reality. The current generation of young adults will be called to solve complex social, economic, and moral problems that simply did not exist even a few decades ago. Ladner (1995) submits that today's youth are faced with a combination of such unprecedented social problems as teen pregnancy, violence, intergenerational poverty, and drugs. Although none of these problems is new, their combined prevalence among some groups and the extent of their impact are new phenomena. To these must be added the lack of access to health care (particularly for mental health), a graying population, dilemmas about end-of-life decisions, and high crime rates in virtually every segment of society. These external forces present mental health issues that require themes of exploration, risk-taking, and human character development combined in a completely different story of adult development. Successful negotiation of early and middle adulthood in the 1990s and beyond is both an awesome responsibility and a true adventure marked by personal challenge and opportunities for growth.

The tale of adulthood is experienced as an adventure in time and space. It typically begins when the traveler is ready to explore uncharted territory as an independent agent, with values as the compass, personal strengths as the tools, and mentors as guides along the way. Obstacles and detours emerge periodically in the landscape as unexpected crises, illness, and normative life events. The relevance of these crises is different for each traveler. Chance encounters also provide interruptions that affect the direction and meaning of the journey.

Atchley (1991) notes that "like a road map, the abstract concept of the life course in reality is composed of a great many alternative routes to alternative destinations" (p. 115). The adult traveler may take many possible paths and must choose among them. The choices determine in part whether or not the traveler reaches a worthy goal. Each decision influences normal career and relationship cycles related to various life stages. The excursion through this part of the life journey is a special but limited period accorded to each traveler in which to discover a deeper sense of self and to establish one's place in the larger scheme of life.

KEY POINTS TO REMEMBER

- Adult development is a dynamic life process characterized by responsibility and commitment.
- The experience of adulthood is different for men and women.
- In early adulthood, the focus is turned outward, toward meeting society's expectations. In midlife, the focus changes to an inward direction for meaning.
- Adults in their 20s are concerned with establishing a career, choosing a life mate, and selecting a mentor.
- Adults in their 30s consolidate and refine the commitments they made in their 20s.
- Physical, social, and emotional factors create a reevaluation of meaning in the 40s.
- A midlife crisis is a normal psychosocial event characterized by emotional upheaval but often resulting in a life that has more personal meaning.
- Adults in their 50s frequently experience a sense of renewal.

LEARNING ACTIVITIES

1. In a relaxed position, close your eyes. Think about what it means to be a woman (man) in today's society. What do you like best about being the sex that you are? How does your gender affect what you are doing? Now, think what it would be like to be a member of the opposite sex and ask yourself the same questions. Then ask yourself what are you missing by being a member of the opposite sex. Share your thoughts with your classmates, and discuss the implications of your choices.

2. Adulthood offers each person an opportunity to shape a creative identity with personal meanings reflective of personal choices. This exercise asks you to consider what essential values are needed in charting a direction for the future. Look over the following list and rank the words in order of importance, with the most important first. When you are finished, share your answers with a partner and discuss how you came to your decisions.

Physical appearance
Comfort
Money
Working conditions
Living conditions
Standard of living
Honesty
Caring
Flexibility
Motivation
Freedom
Choice
Autonomy
Equality
Articulateness
Innovation
Feelings
Teaching
Learning
Music and other arts
Religion
Politics

3. Reflect over the last 10-year period and identify the ways in which you have changed in your ideas, your outlook, and your feelings. Write a paragraph about how you see yourself today and another on how you were 10 years ago. Ask someone who knew you then how they would see you differently today. Share your observations with your small group and get their feedback.

4. Write a paragraph about how you see yourself in five years. What do you think might be different? What might stay the same? Share your observations with your small group and get their feedback.

CRITICAL THINKING EXERCISE

Kathy, a wife and mother of two college students and a teenager, has decided to return to college to finish nursing school. Her husband recently had surgery that kept him out of work for six weeks. Her husband has always been a good provider. Although their savings are adequate, his income is directly affected by his ability to work. When she informed her husband of her decision, he commented, "You don't have to do that, I'll be alright."

1. Under what assumptions do you think Kathy is operating in this story?

2. What do you think is her husband's point of view?

3. How would you check these assumptions by some simple inquiry?

Six months later, Kathy was talking to Danielle, a fellow nursing student with two grown children. Kathy told Danielle that since her husband had returned to work, he wanted her to travel with him to his next work assignment in France. The work assignment would be for two months in the early spring.

1. Make sense of this discussion.

2. Give a possible alternative interpretation of the situation that fits the facts.

3. What conclusions can you draw about Kathy's husband's point of view?

REFERENCES

Aldwin, C., Spiro, A., Lenenson, M., and Bosse, R. (1989). Longitudinal findings from the normative aging study: Does mental health change with age? *Psychology and Aging, 4,* 295–306.

Arnold, E. (1994). *Portrait of change: Women in the second half of life.* Paper presented at the American Psychological Association Conference on Psychosocial and Behavioral Factors in Women's Health: Creating an Agenda for the 21st Century, Washington, D.C., 1994.

Atchley, R. (1991). *Social forces and aging* (6th ed.). Belmont, CA: Wadsworth.

Baltes, P. (1987). Theoretical propositions of life-span developmental psychology: On the dynamics between growth and decline. *Developmental Psychology, 23,* 611–626.

Baltes, P., Reese, H., and Lipsitt, L. (1980). Life-span developmental psychology. *Annual Review of Psychology, 31,* 65–110.

Bandura, A. (1977). Self-efficacy: Toward a unifying theory of behavioral change. *Psychological Review, 84,* 191–215.

Baruch, G., Barnett, R., and Rivers, C. (1983). *Life prints: New patterns of love and work for today's women.* New York: McGraw-Hill.

Bauer, D., and Mott, D. (1990). Life themes and motivations of re-entry students. *Journal of Counseling and Development, 68,* 555–560.

Becker, H. (1960). Notes on the concept of commitment. *American Journal of Sociology, 66,* 32–40.

Bellah, R. (1985). *Habits of the heart: Individualism and commitment in American life.* New York: Harper & Row.

Bogin, B. (1988). *Patterns of human growth.* New York: Cambridge University Press.

Bowlby, J. (1977). The making and breaking of affectional bonds. Part I: Aetiology and psychopathology in the light of attachment theory. *British Journal of Psychiatry, 130,* 201–210.

Buhler, C., and Goldenberg, H. (1968). Structural aspects of an individual's history. In C. Buhler and F. Massarik (Eds.), *The course of human life: A study of goals in the humanistic perspective* (pp. 54–63). New York: Springer.

Burke, R., and McKeen, C. (1990). Mentoring in organizations: Implications for women. *Journal of Business Ethics, 9,* 317–332.

Caplan, G. (1981). Mastery of stress: Psychosocial aspects. *American Journal of Psychiatry,* 138, 413–420.

Carlsen, M. (1988). *Meaning-making: Therapeutic process in adult development.* New York: W. W. Norton.

Chinen, A. (1984). Modal logic—a new paradigm of adult development and late-life potential. *Human Development, 27,* 42–46.

Chiriboga, D. (1989). Mental health at the midpoint: Crisis, challenge or relief? In S. Hunter and M. Sandel (Eds.), *Midlife myths: Coping strategies.* Newbury Park, CA: Sage.

Clayton, V., and Birren, J. (1980). The development of wisdom across the life span: A reexamination of an ancient topic. In P. B. Baltes and O. G. Brim, Jr. (Eds.), *Life-span development and behavior* (Vol. 3). New York: Academic Press.

Commons, M., Sinnott, J., Richards, F., and Armon, C. (1989). *Adult development: Comparisons and applications of developmental models* (Vol. 1). New York: Praeger.

Cooper, K., and Gutmann, D. (1987). Gender identity and ego mastery style in middle-aged, pre– and post–empty nest women. *Gerontologist, 27,* 347–352.

Costa, P., and McCrae, R. (1994). Set like plaster? Evidence for the stability of adult personality. In T. Heatherton and J. Weinberger (Eds.), *Can personality change?* (pp. 21–40). Washington, D.C.: American Psychological Association.

Daniels, P., and Weingarten, K. (1982). *Sooner or later: The timing of parenthood in adult lives.* New York: W. W. Norton.

Dooley, D., and Catalano, R. (1991). Unemployment as a stressor: Findings and implications of a recent study. *WHO Region Publications European Series, 37,* 313–339.

Erikson, E. H. (1958). *Young man Luther: A study in psychoanalysis and history.* New York: W. W. Norton.

Erikson, E. H. (1969). *Gandhi's truth.* New York: W. W. Norton.

Erikson, E. H. (Ed.) (1978). *Adulthood.* New York: W. W. Norton.

Erikson, E. H. (1980). *Identity and the life cycle.* New York: W. W. Norton.

Erikson, E. H. (1982). *The life cycle completed.* New York: W. W. Norton.

Erikson, E. H., and Erikson, J. M. (1981). On generativity and identity: From a conversation with Erik and Joan Erikson. *Harvard Educational Review, 51,* 249–269.

Fiske, M., and Chiriboga, D. A. (1990). The interweave of societal and personal change in adulthood. In J. Munnichs, P. Mussen, M. Fiske, and D. Chiriboga (Eds.), *Change and continuity in adult life.* San Francisco: Jossey-Bass.

Gilligan, C. (1982). *In a different voice.* Cambridge: Harvard University Press.

Golombok, S., and Fivush, R. (1994). *Gender development.* New York: Cambridge University Press.

Gottfried, A., Gottfried, A. W., and Bathurst, K. (1988). Maternal employment, family environment and children's development: Infancy through the school years. In A. E. Gottfried and A. W. Gottfried (Eds.), *Maternal employment and children's development: Longitudinal research.* New York: Plenum.

Gould, R. (1975). Adult life stages: Growth towards self-tolerance. *Psychology Today, 8,* 74–78.

Gould, R. (1978). *Transformations: Growth and change in adult life.* New York: Simon & Schuster.

Haan, N. (1981). Common dimensions of personality development: Early adolescence to middle live. In D. H. Eichorn, J. Clausen, N. Haan, M. P. Honzik, and P. Mussen (Eds.), *Present and past in middle life.* New York: Academic Press.

Hammersjöld, D. (1964). *Markings.* Translated from the Swedish by L. Sjöberg and W. H. Auden. New York: Knopf.

Havighurst, R. (1953). *Developmental tasks and education.* New York: David McKay.

Havighurst, R. (1973). History of developmental psychology. In P.

Baltes and K. Schaie (Eds.), *Life span developmental psychology: Personality and socialization.* New York: Academic Press.

Hawkes, H. (1992). Empowerment in nursing education: Concept analysis and application to philosophy, education and instruction. *Journal of Advanced Nursing, 17,* 5, 609–618.

Hayes, R. (1994). The legacy of Lawrence Kohlberg: Implications for counseling and human development. *Journal of Counseling and Development,* 72, 261–267.

Hoffman, L. (1989). Effects of maternal employment in the two-parent family. *American Psychologist, 44,* 283–292.

James, W. (1981). *The principles of psychology* (Vol. 1). Cambridge: Harvard University Press. (Original work published 1890.)

Josselson, R. (1987). *Finding herself: Pathways to identity development in women.* San Francisco: Jossey-Bass.

Jung, C. G. (1969a). *The structure and dynamics of the psyche.* Princeton, NJ: Princeton University Press.

Jung, C. G. (1969b). The stages of life. In H. Read, M. Fordham, and G. Adler (Eds.), Hull RFC trans. *The collected works of C. G. Jung* (R. F. C. Hull, Trans.) (pp. 749–795). Princeton, NJ: Bollingen.

Kalish, R. (1989). *Midlife loss.* Newbury Park, CA: Sage.

Keen, S. (1991). *Fire in the belly: On being a man.* New York: Bantam Books.

Kelly, E., and Rasey, M. (1952). *Education and the nature of man.* New York: Harper & Brothers.

King, M. L., Jr. (1963). "I have a dream" [Speech]. Washington, D. C., August 23, 1963.

Kingson, E., Hirshorn, B., and Cornman, J. (Eds.) (1986). *Ties that bind: The interdependence of generations.* Washington, D.C.: Seven Locks Press.

Kitzinger, C. (1992). The individuated self concept: A critical analysis of social constructionist writing on individualism. In G. Breakwell (Ed.), *Social psychology of identity and the self concept.* London: Surrey University Press.

Kohn, M. (1980). Job complexity and adult personality. In N. J. Smelser and E. H. Erikson (Eds.), *Themes of work and love in adulthood.* Cambridge: Harvard University Press.

Kotre, J., and Hall, E. (1990). *Seasons of life.* Boston: Little, Brown and Company.

Ladner, T. (1995). Generation without a dream: What college students need to know about Martin Luther King, Jr. Outlook Section, *Washington Post.* January 15, 1995, p. C-z.

Lane, J. (1987). The care of the human spirit. *Journal of Professional Nursing, 3,* 332–337.

Lerner, R., and Hood, K. (1986). Plasticity in development: Concepts and issues for intervention. *Journal of Applied Developmental Psychology,* 7, 139–152.

Levinson, D., Darrow, C., Klein, E., Levinson, M., and McKee, B. (1978). *The seasons of a man's life.* New York: Knopf.

Lopata, H. (1975). Widowhood: Societal factors in life span disruption and alternatives. In N. Datan and L. H. Ginsberg (Eds.), *Life-span developmental psychology: Normative life crises.* New York: Academic Press.

Love, D., and Torrence (1989). The impact of worker age on unemployment and earnings after plant closings. *Journal of Gerontology, 44,* 190–195.

Lowenthal, M., Thurnher, M., and Chiriboga, D. (1975). *Four stages of life: A comparative study of women and men facing transitions.* San Francisco: Jossey-Bass.

Lowenthal, M., and Chiriboga, D. (1972). Transition to the empty nest: Crisis, challenge, or relief? *Archives of General Psychology, 26,* 8–14.

MacKinnon-Slaney, F. (1994). The adult persistence in learning model: A road map to counseling services for adult learners. *Journal of Counseling and Development,* 72, 268–275.

Maslow, A. (1969). Various meanings of transcendence. *Journal of Transpersonal Psychology,* 56–66.

McCrae, R., and Costa, P. (1983). Psychological maturity and subjective well-being: Toward a new synthesis. *Developmental Psychology, 19,* 243–248.

Mercer, R., Nichols, E., and Doyle, G. (1989). *Transitions in a woman's life: Major life events in developmental context.* New York: Springer.

Mezirow, J. (1990). *Fostering critical reflection in adulthood: A guide to transformative and emancipatory education.* San Francisco: Jossey-Bass.

Miller, W., and C'deBaca, J. (1994). Quantum change: Toward a psychology of transformation. In T. Heatherton and J. Weinberger (Eds.), *Can personality change?* Washington, D.C.: American Psychological Association.

Morrow, R., and McElroy, J. (1987). Work commitment and job satisfaction over three career stages. *Journal of Vocational Behavior, 30,* 330–346.

Murstein, B. (1985). *Paths to marriage.* Beverly Hills, CA: Sage.

National Center for Health Statistics (1987). Advance report of final marriage statistics. *Monthly Vital Statistics Report, 36,* 2.

Neugarten, B. (1969). Continuities and discontinuities of psychological issues into adult life. *Human Development, 12,* 121–130.

Neugarten, B. (1970). Adaptation and the life cycle. *Journal of Geriatric Psychiatry, 4,* 71–87.

Neugarten, B. (1977). *Middle age and aging.* Chicago: University of Chicago Press.

Neugarten, B., and Neugarten, D. (1986). Age in an aging society. *Daedalus, 115,* 1, 31–49.

Noe, R. (1988). Women and mentoring: A review and research agenda. *Academy of Management Review, 13,* 65–78.

Olshansky, E. (1994). Identity of self as infertile: An example of theory generating research. In P. Chinn P (Ed.), *Developing substance: Mid-range theory in nursing.* Gaithersburg, MD: Aspen. (Reprinted from [1987] *Advances in Nursing Science, 9,* 2, 54–63.)

Paludi, M. (1991). Sociophysiological and structural factors related to women's vocational development. *Annals of the New York Academy of Sciences,* 157–168.

Parse, R. R. (1981). *Man-living-health: A theory of nursing.* New York: Wiley.

Patterson, C. (1992). Children of lesbian and gay parents. *Child Development, 63,* 1025–1042.

Pearlin, L., and Schooler, C. (1978). The structure of coping. *Journal of Health and Social Behavior, 19,* 2–21.

Phoenix, A., Woollett, A., and Lloyd, (Eds.) (1991). *Motherhood: Meanings, practices and ideologies.* London: Sage.

Pierce, R., and Chiriboga, D. (1977). Dimensions of adult self-concept. *Journal of Gerontology.*

Reed, P. G. (1983). Implications of the life-span developmental framework for well-being in adulthood and aging. *Advances in Nursing Science, 6,* 18–25.

Reed, P. (1994). Toward a nursing theory of self-transcendence: Deductive reformulation using developmental theories. In P. Chinn (Ed.), *Developing substance: Mid-range theory in nursing.* Gaithersburg, MD: Aspen. (Reprinted from *Advances in Nursing Science,* 64–77.

Rogers, M. (1970). *An introduction to the theoretical basis of nursing.* Philadelphia: F. A. Davis.

Sheehey, G. (1976). *Passages: Predictable crises of adult life.* New York: Dutton.

Sheehey, G. (1981). *Pathfinders.* New York: Dutton.

Sheehey, G. (1993). *The silent passage: Menopause.* New York: Dutton.

Staube, J. (1981). *The adult development of C. G. Jung.* Boston: Routledge & Kegan Paul.

Thurnher, M. (1983). Turning points and developmental change: Subjective and 'objective' assessments. *American Journal of Orthopsychiatry, 53,* 52–60.

Tournier, P. (1957). *The meaning of persons.* London: SCM Publishers.

Tournier, P. (1960). *A doctor's case book in the light of the Bible.* New York: Harper & Row.

Tournier, P. (1965). *The adventure of living.* New York: Harper & Row.

Vaillant, G. (1977). *Adaptation to life.* Boston: Little, Brown and Company.

Vaughan, F. (1985). Discovering transpersonal identity. *Journal of Human Psychology, 25,* 3, 13–38.

Whitehead, A. N. (1929). *The aims of education.* New York: Macmillan.

Wicks, R. J. (1985). *Touching the holy: Ordinariness, self-esteem, and friendship.* Notre Dame, IN: Ave Maria Press.

Young-Eisendrath, P. (1985). Making use of human development

theories in counseling. *Counseling and Human Development, 17,* 1–12.
Younger, J. (1994). A theory of mastery. In P. Chinn (Ed.), *Developing substance: Mid-range theory in nursing.* Gaithersburg, MD: Aspen. (Reprinted from (1991). *Advances in Nursing Science, 14,* 1, 76–89.)

SUGGESTED READINGS

Bellah, R. (1985). *Habits of the heart: Individualism and commitment in American life.* New York: Harper & Row.
Gilligan, C. (1982). *In a different voice.* Cambridge: Harvard University Press.
Levinson, D., Darrow, C., Klein, E., Levinson, M., and McKee, B. (1978). *The seasons of a man's life.* New York: Knopf.
Sheehey, G. (1976). *Passages: Predictable crises of adult life.* New York: Dutton.

CHAPTER 26

THE ELDERLY TRAVELER

The heads of strong old age are beautiful

Beyond all grace of youth

—Robinson Jeffers

LEARNING OBJECTIVES

After studying this chapter, you should be able to:

1. Describe facts about the aging population.
2. Describe normal mental health in late life.
3. List age-related changes.
4. Recognize factors that affect mental health assessment of the elderly.
5. Discuss developmental tasks of late life.
6. Identify risks and signs associated with depression in the elderly.
7. Discuss the symptoms, causes, and differentiation of delirium and dementia.
8. Describe unique features of anxiety and schizophrenia in older patients.
9. List basic measures to promote mental health in late life.
10. Apply the nursing process to a patient experiencing normal changes associated with the aging process.

KEY TERMINOLOGY

Ageism
Delirium
Dementia
Developmental tasks
Old-old
Sundown syndrome
Young-old

More than 31 million Americans are over the age of 65 years, and most can be found living relatively normal lives in the community. They shop, maintain their households, pay their bills, and face the same stresses of daily life as adults of any age. They also face, to a greater degree than younger persons, added stresses such as the loss of loved ones, reduced income, forfeited roles, impaired function, and chronic illness. The road traveled in late life indeed can be a rocky one to navigate. But the roads already journeyed do give older travelers the added skill and strength required to face these challenges. Let us take a look at Mary Baxter's story for a glimpse of an elderly woman successfully navigating this part of life's journey.

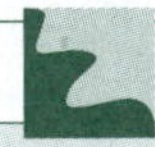

MARY'S STORY

Mary Baxter enjoys the warmth of the sun as she leisurely carries her groceries to the parking lot of the shopping center. She realizes that she once again has forgotten where she parked her car and wonders if this is a sign of a failing memory. "Well, I can't blame that on being 72," she chuckles to herself. "I've always had trouble remembering where I left the car."

This shopping trip was particularly enjoyable because she bought the foods to be used for the Sunday dinner she would prepare for her children and grandchildren. She has appreciated that her son and daughter live in communities that border the apartment complex in which she lives and that they feel free to drop in frequently. She has been equally glad to have her own space and to be able to spend time with her very active grandchildren on her own terms.

As she packs the groceries into her trunk, she notices a very impatient driver waiting for her parking space. Mary feels pressured and embarrassed that her lack of speed is causing inconvenience to another person. She nervously backs her car from the space at a faster pace than she would normally drive and is reminded of how she dislikes driving. Before her husband's death, four years ago, she always was the pampered passenger. Her husband used to preheat the car before she entered it, open and close her door, chauffeur her to the front door of her destination . . . these are the little niceties that she misses. They now serve as daily reminders of the caring relationship she and her husband shared. She is "getting on" with her life and adequately taking care of herself, but the little things that are no longer shared with her husband remind her of the void that no amount of bus trips or bridge games can fill.

Mary reflects on the "horrible year of existence," as she terms her first year of widowhood. Her husband's sudden death left her unprepared for the adjustments she would need to make after devoting 47 years to being a wife and mother. She recalls the emptiness in her heart that she was unable to express to anyone. The seemingly pointless act of preparing a meal for one caused her to skip meals and lose weight; rolling over in her sleep to find an empty space caused her to awaken and spend the remainder of the night watching television. Her physician saw the fatigue and weight loss and was quick to prescribe vitamins and sleeping pills, but the gnawing sadness and feeling that her life was in limbo did not leave her for over a year. She thinks of her 90-year-old mother, now living in a nursing home, who was widowed at age 45, and wonders how she coped. "Time heals all," she thinks.

Mary feels fortunate that except for a little arthritis and farsightedness, she has good health and can take care of herself. She wonders about her own death, weighing the benefits of a sudden death like her husband's to dying gradually over a long period as she observes her mother doing. She prays that God will spare her the agony of a long life filled with pain and dependency and allow her to leave this world with dignity and some control over her circumstances. In the interim, she faces life one day at a time.

FACTS ABOUT THE OLDER POPULATION

Mary Baxter is hardly an unusual example of today's older adult; however, today's elderly are a very diverse group. No longer do general descriptions about the "old population" apply. The old can encompass healthy, active people like Mary Baxter and frail, dependent individuals, such as Mary's mother. In fact, the older population is now divided into subpopulations: the **young-old**, who are under age 75, and the **old-old**, who are 75 and older. Each of these populations presents unique needs. For instance, the young-old may seek nursing assistance for guidance with health maintenance, retirement counseling, exercise programs, parent care, sexual adjustments, and selection of cosmetic surgeons. The old-old may desire assistance with administering medications, using assistive devices, selecting alternative housing, and thinking through advance directives. (Of course, as every good nurse understands, individual differences within each subgroup reinforce the importance of astute assessment.) The age-75 population has been the fastest-growing segment of the population, and this trend will continue, causing us to see more old-old people in society. The increasing prevalence of some mental illnesses with age speaks to the increased need for geropsychiatric nursing services in the future.

TABLE 26–1 Life Expectancy in Years

	White	Black
Female	78.9	73.8
Male	72.1	65.1

US Department of Commerce (1990). *Statistical abstract of the US* (110th ed.) (p. 72). Washington, D.C.: Bureau of the Census.

TABLE 26–2 Living Arrangements of Older Adults

	Male (%)	Female (%)
Living with spouse	75	39
Living alone or with nonrelative	18	43
Living with other relative	7	18

US Department of Commerce (1990). *Statistical abstract of the US* (110th ed.) (p. 3). Washington, D.C.: Bureau of the Census.

Although the average life expectancy is 75.5 years for the total population, differences do exist between the sexes and races. As Table 26–1 shows, women outlive men, resulting in a decrease in the ratio of males to females over the years. And although life expectancy has shown a steady increase for the white population, recent years have shown a substantial decrease in life expectancy for black males and, to a lesser extent, a decrease for black females also.

Like Mary Baxter, most older women are widowed, whereas most older men do have surviving spouses. The death of a spouse—and the emotional, financial, and sexual issues that result—offer opportunities for nursing intervention.

Women are more likely than men to be living alone, and a greater percentage of both sexes are living alone than with children (Table 26–2). About half of the elderly live within 25 miles of their children and have weekly contact with them. For both the elderly and their offspring, the arrangement of separate but close homes is preferable. Children do assist their elder parents with a variety of chores, and in turn they receive financial aid, child-rearing assistance, and emotional support.

Because of the "graying of America," more families are involved with caregiving of an elderly relative than ever before in history. An estimated 13.5 million, slightly over 7% of the adult population, have disabled elderly parents or spouses at home or in an institution; almost two million women who are both employed outside the home and caring for children at home are also involved with the care of an elder relative (Stone and Kemper, 1989). In every clinical setting, you will be involved with families of elders and must be prepared to offer interventions to promote the health of the entire family. (Please see Chapters 20 and 22 for more information on working with families.)

Although the rates for infections and injuries decline through the adult years, the rates of chronic illnesses significantly increase. In addition to the physical symptoms and caregiving demands imposed by these disorders, chronic illnesses can threaten mental health. For instance, the frustration of living with an incurable illness can cause depression. Uncertainty about the impact of the condition on roles, function, and life expectancy can produce anxiety. Furthermore, physiological disturbances caused by the illness can threaten homeostasis, resulting in delirium. The mind-body relationship is a significant concern for the chronically ill elderly. Psychiatric nurses must distinguish between common and pathological changes that occur with age (Table 26–3). You also need to identify unique symptoms (Box 26–1) and responses to treatment for physical health problems in the elderly.

▶ Check Your Reading

1. Why is it significant to subcategorize the elderly population?
2. What differences in life expectancy exist between the sexes and races?

TABLE 26–3 **Common Aging Changes**

Body System	Manifestations
Cardiovascular	Thickening and rigidity of heart valves Rise in aortic volume and systolic blood pressure Reduced cardiac output and efficiency Increased peripheral resistance Thickening and fragility of capillary walls
Pulmonary	Increased rigidity of lungs Decreased vital capacity and maximum breathing capacity Reduction in number and elasticity of alveoli Decreased ciliary activity Weaker thoracic muscles
Gastrointestinal	Increased prevalence of periodontal disease Reduced saliva production Increase in taste threshold, primarily affecting sweet and salty flavors Weaker gag reflex Reduced hunger contractions Decreased peristalsis
Genitourinary	Reduction in renal mass, glomerular filtration rate, renal blood flow, tubular function Decreased bladder capacity Hypertrophy of prostate gland Decreased testosterone production, sperm count, size of testes Decreased estrogen production, breast tissue, size of uterus Drier, more fragile vaginal canal
Musculoskeletal	Decreased muscle mass, strength, movement Increased brittleness of bones Deterioration of cartilage surface of joints
Neurological/Sensory	Decreased nerve cells, nerve conduction velocity, kinesthetic sense Presbyopia, narrowing of visual field, smaller pupil size, opacity and yellowing of lens Reduced lacrimal secretions Presbycusis Increased threshold for pain and touch Decreased olfaction
Integumentary	Reduced elasticity and moisture of skin Thinning of scalp, pubic, and axillary hair Slower growth of fingernails
Endocrine	Reduced weight and vascularity of pituitary gland Increased follicle-stimulating hormone (FSH) in women Decrease in plasma T_3 Lower basal metabolic rate Delayed release of insulin by beta cells of pancreas
Psychological	No change in personality Some decline in fluid intelligence; crystalized intelligence maintained Slower retrieval of information not used on daily basis Increased ease of distraction by stimuli Decreased vigilance performance

BOX 26–1 Differences in Presentation of Physical Illness in Late Life

Fever: lower basal metabolic rate causes lower normal body temperature; febrile conditions are apparent at lower levels than would occur with younger adults

Pain: altered pain sensations can result in little correlation between severity of problem and pain experienced; pain can be referred

Cough: reduced cough efficiency can result in significant accumulation of secretions in lungs without productive cough

Confusion: older adults are more likely to have impaired cognition as a result of many physical illnesses

DEVELOPMENTAL TASKS OF AGING

The path to old age is filled with unexpected twists and turns. Some parts of this adventurous journey are filled with delightful new experiences, such as becoming a grandparent and exploring creative interests. But this journey also includes obstacles and rocky roads, such as losing loved ones and adjusting to chronic illnesses. The challenges faced and adjustments made to achieve a sense of psychological and social well-being in late life are referred to as **developmental tasks**. Developmental tasks are part of an adult's continued growth through the lifespan and include (Eliopoulos, 1991):

- Coping with losses and changes: development of health problems, meeting demands of chronic illness, retirement, decreased income, death of loved ones, change in residence
- Establishing meaningful roles: redefining parent-child roles, entering a health care institution, grandparenting
- Exercising independence and control: maximizing capabilities in light of disabilities, making decisions regarding self, dependent loved ones, lifestyle, and plans for future
- Finding meaning in life: balancing current limitations against full life lived, reflecting on past accomplishments, leaving a legacy, connecting with others, growing spiritually

An outline of several theorists' views on development during aging is provided in Box 26–2.

You can facilitate good mental health in late life by assisting patients with the developmental tasks of aging. Some basic measures could be to

- Make a sincere effort to learn about the patient, including family background, work history, hobbies, achievements
- Listen with sincere interest
- Encourage discussions of past events
- Build on lifelong interests
- Offer suggestions for meaningful family activities
- Use humor therapeutically
- Personalize the caregiving environment
- Encourage maximum independence and decision-making
- Emphasize capabilities and minimize limitations

This act of recalling and reflecting on life experiences is a frequently observed behavior among older adults. Rather than an unhealthy "living in the past," reminiscing is considered to be a healthy and adaptive function in late life (Beadleson-Baird and Lara, 1988). Reminiscing can be used therapeutically to help older adults achieve a sense of psychosocial and spiritual well-being. You can help older people to

- Resolve unsettled issues
- Appreciate the significance of their lives
- Reaffirm their self-worth and identity

Often, current stresses can be put into perspective and managed effectively when seen in the context of one's total life.

The regular, direct contact that nursing staff members have with older adults puts them in an ideal position to use reminiscence as a psychosocial intervention. Often, reminiscence can be an approach to interactions rather than a time-specific intervention. During routine interactions with patients, you can

- Ask memory-evoking questions: What were styles like when you were young? What was it like for you to immigrate to America? What was the best holiday you can remember?
- Show sincere interest and listen when patients talk about the past
- Accept and validate feelings; for example, if someone like Mary Baxter becomes tearful discussing her husband's death, you might comment, "The loss of your husband must have been very painful for you." This statement could assist in triggering further reflection.

Chapter 10 can provide assistance with communication techniques to promote reminiscing.

NORMAL MENTAL HEALTH IN LATE LIFE

Most people do not become childlike, rigid, cantankerous, or mentally incompetent as they age. Nor do they become wise, sedate, or more creative. Generally, under normal circumstances, their mental status is a reflection of the lifelong pattern: those who demonstrated high intellectual function in youth are likely to be the elders who find pleasure in the *New York Times* crossword puzzles. Those who were loners when young are unlikely to be gregarious club joiners during their senior years. The mental profile of older adults is diverse. General intellectual capacity does not decline with age, although some specific functions do demonstrate change. Fluid intelligence, which controls emotions, retention of non-intellectual information, creativity, spatial perceptions, and aesthetic appreciation, is thought to decline with age. Crystalized intelligence, involving the use of past learning and experiences for problem-solving is maintained throughout adulthood.

Learning ability is maintained, although more time is needed for the early phases of the learning process. After a longer early phase, the elderly are able to learn at an equal pace with the young. Vigilance performance, the ability to retain information longer than 45 minutes, declines in old age. Older adults are more easily distracted by irrelevant information and stimuli and have a reduced ability to perform tasks that are complicated or demand simultaneous performance. Retrieval of information stored in long-term memory is slower. Pneumonic devices and other memory aids can improve some of this forgetfulness.

Drastic changes in personality are uncommon. If anything, people more openly express the personality they always had. Significant changes in personality can indicate pathology. Attitude, morals, and self-esteem tend to be stable through the lifespan.

The incidence of mental illness is higher among the old than the young. An estimated one fourth of the elderly in the community and one half of those in nursing homes have symptoms of mental illness (Eliopoulos, 1993). Almost 10% of the elderly have a problem with alcoholism. Approximately 65% of nursing home admissions are victims of Alzheimer's disease. Depression increases in prevalence with age, and suicide becomes a considerable risk: 25% of all suicides in the United States are committed by persons age 65 years and older.

▶ Check Your Reading

3. Describe the developmental tasks of late life.
4. What measures can you incorporate into routine nursing activities to facilitate reminiscence?
5. List major changes in mental function that occur with age.

PSYCHIATRIC DISORDERS IN THE ELDERLY

Depression

Depression increases in prevalence with age and is the most common psychiatric problem treated in the elderly. Obvious factors that cause the elderly to be at risk for

BOX 26-2 Major Developmental Theories of Aging

Erikson believed that individuals face stages of psychological development as they age:

- Trust versus mistrust
- Autonomy versus shame
- Initiative versus guilt
- Industry versus inferiority
- Identity versus identity confusion
- Intimacy versus isolation
- Generativity versus stagnation
- Ego integrity versus despair

The last stage, viewed as the task in old age, is to accept one's life as having been whole and satisfying to achieve ego integrity. Dissatisfaction and regrets with the life one has lived can lead to a sense of despair and disgust.

Peck identified three tasks faced in old age:

- **Ego differentiation versus work-role preoccupation:** to develop satisfactions from one's self as a person rather than through the work role
- **Body transcendence versus body preoccupation:** to find psychological pleasures rather than becoming absorbed with health problems or physical limitations imposed by aging
- **Ego transcendence versus ego preoccupation:** to feel pleasure through reflecting on one's life rather than dwelling on the limited number of years left to live

Havighurst has described tasks of aging individuals to include:

- Adjusting to decreased strength and health status
- Maintaining involvement with friends and society
- Establishing satisfactory living arrangements
- Readjusting one's lifestyle to reduced income and retirement
- Coping with the death of one's spouse

Butler views the major tasks of late life as:

- Adjusting to one's infirmities
- Developing a sense of satisfaction with the life that has been lived
- Preparing for death

Reprinted with permission from Eliopoulos, C. (Ed.). (1991). *Developmental tasks of aging. Long-term care educator.* Volume 2, Lesson 6, p. 4.

depression are the multiple losses experienced with age (e.g., of loved ones, income, roles, health, function, youthful appearance). Many chronic illnesses common among older persons are known to be accompanied by depression. These include cerebrovascular accident, chronic obstructive lung disease, Parkinson's disease, cancer, congestive heart failure, and multiple sclerosis. Drugs also may be a cause of depression. Some depressions may be associated with the age-related diminished production of mood-controlling neurotransmitters.

Signs of depression in the elderly are similar to those in younger adults (see Chapter 30). However, these signs may be undetected in the elderly. For example:

- The same poor grooming and dress habits that spark concern in younger adults may be accepted in the old.
- Slower movements and stooped posture can be misinterpreted as normal physical characteristics for an older person.
- Changes in sleep, appetite, elimination, and activity patterns can be attributed to physical health problems.
- Low mood, unclear thinking, and vegetative symptoms can easily be attributed to a dementia.
- Rather than complaints of a low mood, the elderly may present depression through somatic complaints (e.g., headaches, fatigue, pain).

Furthermore, caregivers may not take the time to identify depression. During the typical exchange between the busy health care provider and the patient, conversation may be limited to responses to specific questions (Did you have your MRI? Do you need your prescription refilled?) and discussions of certain topics (diet, treatments, follow-up appointments). Time may not be provided for the patient to describe symptoms and functional changes consistent with depression. Also, the patient may believe that a discussion of mood with the surgeon or cardiac nursing specialist is not appropriate.

You must be certain to recognize even subtle clues of depression in the elderly and refer the patient for psychiatric evaluation in a timely manner. The basic care of the older depressed individual is similar to that for depressed adults of any age. Treatment includes psychotherapy and antidepressants. You should ensure that older depressed patients are afforded the full range of treatment options available. Support groups, financial assistance, and other community resources can be especially helpful to patients with reactive depressions.

You can further assist older depressed patients by having frequent direct contact with them. Contact can be difficult because the behaviors of depressed patients—silence, slow response, pessimism, and irritability—can make caregivers uncomfortable. However, the need for human contact is especially important. Sitting in silence and using touch with depressed persons can be particularly important. Of course, you should encourage the open expression of feelings.

Monitoring the physical status of older depressed patients is particularly important because older persons have a smaller margin of safety in the development of complications. Areas to observe include food and fluid intake, bowel elimination, and quality and quantity of sleep. Weight should be assessed frequently; weight changes of 5% or greater are significant for older adults. Pay attention to promoting a good physical state, which strengthens the patient's ability to work through depression.

Because suicide is a significant risk to older depressed individuals, be alert to clues to suicide. Note any sudden interest in putting affairs in order, giving away possessions, self-neglect, hoarding medications, personality and behavioral changes, and comments alluding to ending life.

▶ Check Your Reading

6. List subtle clues of depression that the older patient can exhibit.
7. Describe physical care considerations for the older depressed individual.

Delirium and Dementia

In the past, confusion in older persons was not a cause for concern. Many practitioners considered a decline in intellectual function to be a normal outcome of aging and did nothing to evaluate or treat this finding. The result of this misunderstanding of confusion was that many older persons with reversible confusional states did not receive the benefit of treatment and were unnecessarily subjected to serious complications, low levels of function, and poor quality of life. Fortunately, today's practitioners now recognize confusional states to be associated with pathological conditions and manage this finding more competently. (See Chapter 38 for a comprehensive discussion of cognitive disorders.)

A variety of conditions can lead to **delirium**, an acute cognitive impairment. Many of the potential causes of delirium, such as dehydration and infection, are common among the elderly. Thus, delirium is not a stranger to geriatric practice. In fact, altered cognition can be the first symptom apparent with pneumonia, dehydration, and other health problems in old age. Symptoms of delirium in the elderly typically appear abruptly and include

- Disturbed intellectual function
- Disorientation
- Altered attention span
- Poor memory
- Labile mood
- Meaningless chatter
- Poor judgment
- Altered level of consciousness

Shortness of breath, fatigue, and slower psychomotor activities are some of the physical signs that can accompany behavioral changes. Disturbances in sleep-wake cycles also can occur.

Identification and correction of the cause are essential to correcting the delirium. Acute confusion is reversible if treated promptly. The risk is that signs of confusion in older patients can be accepted as "normal," thereby delaying diagnosis and treatment. Confusion is particularly common in the acute care setting; some studies have indicated that nearly 7 in 10 elderly patients who become confused while hospitalized do not have their confusion identified by physicians and nurses (Foreman, 1990). The problem is compounded if the symptoms rather than the cause are treated (e.g., administering a tranquilizer to a patient who is hypervigilant as a result of the delirium rather than correcting the disturbance that caused the delirium).

A good history and evaluation of cognitive function are essential to recognizing this acute mental disorder. Failure to recognize the underlying cause not only allows altered mental function to continue but also risks ignoring a physical condition that could seriously threaten the elder patient.

Dementia is a serious chronic mental disorder. You may play a significant role in ensuring that signs of confusion are recognized and evaluated in a timely manner. Upon first glance, patients with delirium and dementia appear to share similar symptoms. Both can demonstrate altered cognition and abnormal behaviors. Careful assessment, however, soon reveals the differences that separate these two conditions. Whereas the history of patients with delirium describes an abrupt onset of symptoms, the history of patients with dementia indicates subtle, progressive development of symptoms over a long period. Even close family members may report having missed clues of dementia for extended periods because they may have blamed forgetfulness, inattention to self-care, and eccentric behaviors on advanced age. Also, assessment will reveal some altered level of consciousness with delirium, whereas with dementia, level of consciousness is unchanged.

The nursing care of dementia patients is covered in Chapter 38. Here are some helpful tips for the care of the elderly with altered cognition. Many age-related changes (e.g., changes in vision and hearing, slower responses) increase the risk for accidental injuries of the elderly. This problem is significantly compounded when the older adult has impaired cognition. Be attentive to protecting the patient by ensuring that hazardous or noningestible substances and medications are kept out of the patient's sight. Ensure that doors are alarmed to signal the patient's exit. Cap electrical outlets and designate a supervised, safe area for walking and wandering.

Pay special attention to the basic physical needs of the elderly who experience altered cognition. Patients who are restless and who wander require a higher caloric intake to meet needs. Encouragement at mealtimes, nutritional supplements, and easy-to-eat foods can promote intake. Monthly weights should be obtained; weight losses greater than 5% of total body weight are significant and warrant daily weight monitoring. Elimination patterns also should be monitored. Patients with altered cognition are likely to be unreliable historians of their bowel elimination patterns, and feces could become impacted if such patients are left to report their own constipation. Because these patients are less likely to notice and report rashes, lesions, masses, and other problems, inspect their entire skin surfaces regularly.

Promoting maximum independence is a desirable caregiving goal in all circumstances but can be particularly challenging when patients are cognitively impaired. Maximize existing function through basic nursing measures:

- Affording ample time for the completion of tasks
- Breaking tasks into simple steps
- Guiding through activities by using one-stage commands
- Giving clear, simple directions
- Orienting to reality
- Adhering to a consistent routine
- Maintaining a stable environment

Some persons with impaired cognitive function display symptoms such as disorientation, agitation, and wandering as evening approaches, a condition referred to as **sundown syndrome** (because of its development when the "sun goes down"). Although the cause is not fully understood, factors that contribute to sundowner's syndrome include recent relocation (e.g., admission to a health care facility), dehydration, sensory overload or deprivation, sleep disturbances, and change in circadian rhythms. Reducing a pronounced transition from day to night by keeping the room lighted can aid in preventing this syndrome. Also, keep familiar objects in the patient's view, make frequent contact, offer toileting assistance, and provide ample fluids.

Families need instruction in basic care techniques. Do not assume family caregivers understand how to feed, lift, or control inappropriate behaviors safely.

An altered state of cognition jeopardizes the patient's ability to make competent decisions. Even when confusion is time limited, as when a delirium occurs secondary to an adverse medication reaction, the patient is unable to fully comprehend and make rational decisions. Ensure that patients do not grant consent or otherwise make decisions that affect their person or property. (See Chapter 38 regarding legal protection for the dementia victim's rights.)

▶ Check Your Reading

8. How does delirium differ from dementia?
9. What are the symptoms of sundown syndrome?

Anxiety

Estimates of anxiety suggest that it is present in 10% to 15% of the elderly (McCullough, 1992). Despite its common occurrence, anxiety is often undetected, primarily because the elderly tend to present somatic complaints (e.g., upset stomach, insomnia, urinary frequency, fatigue) that confuse the diagnosis. A thorough evaluation can assist in identifying anxiety and causative factors. Because chronic illnesses are highly prevalent in the elderly, consider the role of the medical condition in causing symptoms of anxiety. Conditions related to anxiety include hyperthyroidism, malnutrition, hypoglycemia, and cardiopulmonary disease. Also, sedatives, corticosteroids, over-the-counter cold and allergy medications, alcohol, and caffeine can cause symptoms of anxiety. Before treating anxiety as a psychiatric disorder, consider all other factors that could cause symptoms. (See Chapter 28 for generic information regarding care of the patient with anxiety.)

Schizophrenia

Schizophrenic elderly are few in number but pose caregiving challenges, partly because many older schizophrenics are in nursing homes. (The deinstitutionalization of these patients from mental hospitals a few decades ago has resulted in their reinstitutionalization in the nursing home setting!) Traditionally, nursing home staff have been ill prepared to care for the mentally ill. In addition to the basic care afforded any patient with schizophrenia (see Chapter 29), older schizophrenics need particular attention paid to their physical health. These patients are less likely to seek and accept medical care, may not verbalize pain associated with physical illness, and can derive secondary gains by causing or complicating physical health problems—for example, through self-mutilation or picking at a wound. The close and regular contact of nursing staff with patients allows nurses to detect these problems and refer patients for treatment as necessary.

Because knowledge regarding the effects of neuroleptics was scanty decades ago when many schizophrenic patients began using these drugs, tardive dyskinesia and other adverse reactions of neuroleptics are common findings among older schizophrenics. Even if their use of neuroleptics has been recent, older patients are at greater risk for developing tardive dyskinesia and experiencing more problems, such as respiratory infections and malnutrition. Make sure that adequate precautions are taken when neuroleptics are used and that the physical health of these patients is closely monitored.

▶ Check Your Reading

10. Why is anxiety often undetected in older adults?
11. What are some reasons for older schizophrenics to avoid seeking medical care?

PROMOTING MENTAL HEALTH IN LATER LIFE

Positive mental health throughout the lifespan builds a strong foundation for good mental health in old age. The development of meaningful roles and interests, methods to manage stress effectively, good communication skills, and problem-solving capabilities assist in promoting good mental health.

Identifying and Treating Physical Problems

The relationship of physical health to mental health is particularly significant in older patients. Cardiovascular disease, stroke, cancer, diabetes, and chronic obstructive pulmonary disease are among the chronic conditions, highly prevalent among the elderly, that can cause symptoms of mental illness or impairment of mental function. Identify and treat physical health problems early to prevent complications. Also, consider the impact of a mental illness on physical health status because older patients have a smaller margin of safety to protect their physical health. For instance, a depressed older person who does not eat properly will become malnourished faster and easier than a younger adult. Patients are well equipped to heal from a mental illness if they are in optimal physical condition.

Dealing With Losses

The losses faced in old age are many and at times can be overwhelming. Nurses can guide older patients in using internal and external resources to cope with these losses. Listening to patients and encouraging reminiscence can help them to identify strategies that have been effective in adjusting to change and coping with misfortune. Information can be shared regarding community resources and support services that can assist with specific needs.

As losses are faced, feeling a sense of purpose can be difficult. Older persons may be guided in identifying roles that have been valued and in developing ways to continue some degree of participation in these roles within any existing limitations. For instance, a recently retired schoolteacher who feels at a loss because of a lost work role can be encouraged to begin teaching a Sunday School class or to volunteer as a children's reading group leader at the local library. Hobbies and interests can be the source of new roles. For instance, the amateur toy train collector may find new opportunities in renting a table at a flea market to sell and trade collections or in giving lectures on collecting toy trains at the local community college. Of course, fulfillment and pleasure can be derived from exploring new interests and roles. A sense of integrity and productivity can be derived from purposeful activities.

The awareness of one's mortality is inescapable in old age. The frequently occurring death of loved ones and the development of serious illnesses themselves keep death a constant reminder. Cultural socialization and personal experience with death help determine the meaning that death holds for various individuals. For many people, spiritual beliefs provide an understanding of death and strength to accept the finiteness of life on earth. Great comfort can be obtained through the bond one possesses with a higher power. Older adults should be helped in obtaining spiritual support based on their personal belief systems. Be it attendance at a religious service, a bedside visit from clergy, or private time sitting in a garden, the need for nourishment of the soul must not be overlooked in care planning.

▶ Check Your Reading

12. What are some basic measures to promote mental health in old age?

NURSING PROCESS

ASSESSMENT

Assessment in the elderly requires knowledge of both psychological and physiological changes that place older adults at risk for dysfunction.

Interviewing the Elderly

Adjustments to the interview process with older adults can facilitate data collection. Unlike today's younger generations who are accustomed to openly discussing their finances, sexual practices, family conflicts, and bodily functions, the elderly are part of a generation who viewed these topics as private and, as a result, may be uncomfortable discussing these personal matters.

You can respect these feelings while reviewing essential history by

- Conducting the interview in a private area
- Establishing rapport and putting the patient at ease
- Explaining the type and purpose of the questions that will be asked and how this information will be used
- Informing the patient of the right to refuse to answer questions

Common aging changes also require adjustments to the interview. Increased opacity of the lens with age results in a sensitivity to glare, such as bright sunlight shining through a window or fluorescent lights, that may not present a problem to younger eyes. A preoccupation with glare and missed visual cues could interfere with the older adult's participation in the interview. Normal body temperature is lower in many older adults, and older persons are more sensitive to cold environmental temperatures that are not bothersome to younger persons. (This problem can be compounded when the patient is clothed only in an examination gown while the caregiver is wearing layers of street clothes.) Provide an environmental temperature of at least 75°F. Presbycusis is common in the elderly and interferes with the ability to adequately hear the interviewer's questions. Hearing competency should be evaluated before the interview and appropriate assistance (e.g., insertion of prescribed hearing aid, use of amplification device) provided to facilitate communication. The elderly patient's slower responses to stimuli can necessitate additional time for questions to be processed and responses formulated. Also consider the effects of illness and medications on such patients' abilities to participate in the interview.

Assessing Mental Status

Mental assessment in older adults involves some unique features. One important consideration is alteration in mental status as a result of physical illness. More likely than not, acute confusional states or delirium are the mental manifestation of physiological disturbances. Fluid and electrolyte imbalances, fever, hyperglycemia, hypoglycemia, hypoxia, dehydration, hypotension, anemia, and adverse drug reactions are only some of the physical health problems that can lead to delirium. Depression can result from physical illnesses such as anemia, hypothyroidism, congestive heart failure, and stroke. The relationship of physical and mental health demands that a thorough physical evaluation accompany every mental health assessment.

A thorough health history is essential. Remember that new signs can develop as a result of changes in long-term health conditions. Be careful not to overlook obvious causes for altered mental status. Laboratory tests can complement the physical examination and provide clues to potential disorders. Tests could include complete blood count, serum electrolytes, serological test for syphilis, blood urea nitrogen, blood glucose, bilirubin, blood vitamin level, sedimentation rate, and urinalysis. Electroencephalography, computed tomography, magnetic resonance imaging, and positron emission tomography are among the diagnostic tests that can be performed, depending on the suspected underlying cause.

Although an increasing number of practitioners are aware of the unique aspects of geriatric health problems, abnormal mental status in older adults still can be interpreted as a "normal" characteristic of old age. For instance, if Mary Baxter presented in an emergency room in a confused state, some staff could view her as a "confused old lady" and miss or postpone diagnosing the cause of her symptoms. Delayed treatment and the development of complications could result. You must ensure that the stereotype of **ageism,** which characterizes the elderly as incompetent, does not influence assessment and treatment decisions. Advocate for competent evaluation and care of older adults.

Assessing Medication Issues

Because of the increased risk of drugs causing adverse reactions, many of which are manifested through altered mental status, a review of all prescription and nonprescription drugs used by the patient is essential. In addition, an assessment of factors that can affect drug administration, absorption, metabolism, and excretion is essential to ensure that medications result in greater benefits than risks to the older patient.

Advanced age can contribute to unique problems in drug therapy and warrant special nursing intervention. Tablets and capsules can stick to the oral mucosa and not be swallowed as a result of drier mucous membranes of the oral cavity. If this occurs, not only does the drug not have the benefit of being absorbed but also it can dissolve and cause irritation in the mouth or throat. Suppositories can take longer to melt because of a general lower body temperature and decreased circulation to the lower bowel and vagina. The risk is that suppositories can be expelled undissolved. Reduced muscle mass and inactivity can interfere with the absorption of intramuscular medications. Intravenous administration of drugs carries a risk of circulatory overload due to reduced cardiac efficiency with age.

The less-acidic gastric environment common in old age can delay the absorption of drugs that require a low gastric pH. Reduced levels of serum albumin can create a problem when several protein-bound drugs (e.g., acetazolamide, amitriptyline, cefazolin, chlorpromazine, digitoxin, hydralazine, nortriptyline, phenytoin, salicylates, and warfarin) are administered together because less effective protein binding occurs. (This situation can be tricky in that if the serum albumin level is low, the patient can become toxic from protein-bound drugs despite having blood levels of the drugs within a normal or even low range.) Reduced numbers of functioning nephrons, decreased glomerular filtration rate, and less renal blood flow slow the filtration of drugs from the body and increase the ease with which drugs can reach toxic levels. Poor memory can interfere with the safe self-administration of drugs.

Special problems and risks associated with age-related changes should be considered and identified during the assessment. Plan interventions accordingly. Consider preventing drug-related problems by

- Ensuring that drug dosages are age adjusted (keep in mind that a dosage that was appropriate for a patient several years ago can now be too high because of changes in organ function with aging)
- Reviewing all drugs used for possible interactions
- Assisting patients in developing reminder systems and other means to promote safe self-administration of drugs
- Educating patients about the purpose, proper administration, side effects, and precautions of each drug administered
- Advising patients to drink fluids to moisten the oral cavity before swallowing a medication
- Inspecting the oral cavity after drug administration for patients who are demented or otherwise unable to detect the presence of capsules or tablets in their mouths
- Breaking large tablets for ease in swallowing (unless contraindicated)
- Reviewing drugs ordered for possible interactions
- Using the most muscular sites (e.g., upper outer quadrant of buttocks) for intramuscular injections
- Monitoring intravenous drip rates carefully
- Ensuring that serum albumin levels and blood levels of drugs are evaluated when protein-bound drugs are used
- Evaluating regularly that each drug used continues to be effective and needed

Certain drug groups are notorious for carrying a high risk of adverse reactions in the elderly. Common problems include the following:

- Delirium caused by anticholinergics, antihistamines, benzodiazepines, cardiac glycosides, cimetidine, ephedrine, muscle relaxants, nalidixic acid, narcotics, sedative-hypnotics, and urinary tract drugs
- Depression caused by indomethacin, muscle relaxants, nonsteroid antiinflammatory drugs, reserpine, and sedative-hypnotics
- Hallucinations caused by anticholinergics, general anesthetics, muscle relaxants, nalidixic acid, sympatholytics, and urinary tract drugs

Close monitoring and ongoing assessment of the appropriateness of dosage levels, effectiveness, and presence of adverse effects are crucial.

Assessing Cognitive Function

A baseline evaluation of cognitive function should be performed on every older adult regardless of the clinical setting or specialty in which service is obtained. However, results of the initial test of cognitive function must be carefully interpreted. Although impaired cognition is not a normal characteristic of old age, it can result from the multiple stresses and stimuli during assessment. For example, a perfectly mentally competent older adult may test poorly immediately after admission to a health care facility because of the overwhelming number of activities faced and anxiety about the situation. This same individual may score perfectly after having had several hours to adjust to the new environment. Labeling the person cognitively impaired on the basis of the intake assessment would be inappropriate and could risk biasing the care provided thereafter. When impaired cognition is observed during the initial assessment, repeated assessments are necessary.

Symptoms and observations noted during the assessment should be put in proper perspective before drawing conclusions about the older person's mental status. For instance:

- Inattention to self-care and grooming activities may be associated with arthritic fingers or fatigue secondary to anemia rather than a disturbance in mood or cognition
- Awakening from sleep at 3 a.m. every day could be caused by a sleep quota that has been fulfilled (about 5 to 7 hours of night sleep are adequate for most older adults) and may not be an indication of depression
- Grieving even though no loss of a significant person has occurred could be related to the loss of a beloved pet
- Suspiciousness about neighbors could be a valid perception of a crime risk rather than a manifestation of a paranoid disorder

Family and social history are therefore important to understanding mental status.

▶ Check Your Reading

13. What are some precautions that you must take to ensure an accurate mental status assessment?
14. Describe factors that can influence the validity of data obtained during an interview with the older person.

DIAGNOSIS

Analysis of the data will lead you to determine appropriate nursing diagnoses for the elderly. The diagnoses depend on the data collected. For instance, a depressed elderly person might have the nursing diagnosis of Hopelessness related to multiple losses evidenced by crying, sad affect, and expressions that life is not worth living. See chapters 28, 29, 30, and 38 for comprehensive listing of nursing diagnoses for elderly adults experiencing stress and anxiety, schizophrenia, a mood disorder, or cognitive disorder such as Alzheimer's disease.

OUTCOME IDENTIFICATION

The expected outcome depends on the diagnoses. For example, with a nursing diagnosis of Hopelessness related to multiple losses, the expected outcome might be expressed as follows: The patient will experience less sadness and crying, express that life continues to be meaningful, and invest self in pleasurable diversional activities.

PLANNING

The nursing plan focuses on establishing short-term goals that lead to the accomplishment of expected outcome and on determining who will perform which nursing interventions. For example, the expected outcome might be supported by the following short-term goals:

- The patient will discuss the multiple losses that have occurred.
- The patient will discuss the impact of these losses.
- The patient will express feelings of sadness.
- The patient will identify activities that give meaning to life.
- The patient will decide on one activity in which to invest self.
- The patient will explore spiritual issues surrounding losses.

Accomplishing these goals might be delegated to the nurse as well as an activity therapist, an occupational therapist, a nursing assistant, and a representative of the patient's faith tradition.

IMPLEMENTATION

Nursing interventions depend on the assessment, diagnoses, expected outcomes, and plan.

Interventions might include

- Administration of antidepressant medication
- Medication teaching
- Teaching regarding effects of loss
- One-to-one interpersonal relationship
- Interactions focusing on loss and meaning of loss
- Interactions focusing on what makes life meaningful
- Identification of pleasurable activities
- Commitment to invest time and energy in exploring activities that might give life continued pleasure
- Interaction with nurse, religious leader, or other staff regarding spiritual significance of multiple losses

For specific interventions related to stress and anxiety, schizophrenia, depression, and cognitive disorders, see Chapters 28, 29, 30, and 38.

EVALUATION

An evaluation includes a formative component, where you evaluate the ongoing process, and a summative evaluation, where you evaluate the overall effectiveness of the nursing care. Examine the comprehensiveness and accuracy of the assessment, the appropriateness of the nursing diagnoses and the expected outcome, as well as the specifics of the plan. Modifications are made throughout the entire process. The summative evaluation examines the achievement of the stated expected outcome. For example, if the patient experiences less crying and sadness, is able to see that life still has meaning, and is able to invest self in pleasurable activities, then the nursing care has been successful.

CASE STUDY: RICHARD

Richard is a 75-year-old retired mechanic who lives with his wife, Ruth. In July they celebrated 55 years of marriage. They have five children, 14 grandchildren, and two great-grandchildren. Richard is a devout practicing Catholic and has been able to find meaning in various life experiences. He is a healthy elder, and he and his wife enjoy traveling and spending time with their family. Working on the family genealogy on his home computer is one of his favorite hobbies.

Recently he developed painful arthritis in both of his hands that prohibits him from any activity that requires movement of his hands and wrists. Richard has had several major health problems during his lifetime, such as loss of the sight in one eye, basal cell carcinoma, hypertension, and mild diabetes. Both chronic conditions are controlled with diet and medication. He tells the nurse in the doctor's office that he cannot imagine continuing to live a productive life without the use of his hands and that he cannot tolerate the constant pain. The medication that the doctor prescribed for the pain and inflammation is contraindicated because he is taking warfarin (Coumadin), which could cause hemorrhage. His wife tells you she is very worried about him.

ASSESSMENT

Assessment data are as follow:

- Previously active elder
- Devout religious practice
- Ability to find solace in spiritual beliefs
- Chronic arthritic pain associated with loss of function
- Fear and apprehension
- Increased pulse and respiration and blood pressure
- Insomnia
- Good supportive network
- History of ability to cope with grief associated with loss of a body function

DIAGNOSIS

***DSM-IV* Diagnosis:** R/O Depression (300.4): Anxiety Disorder (300.02).

Nursing Diagnosis: Anxiety related to loss of control associated with inability to control pain and loss of previous level of functioning manifested by excessive worry, insomnia, and increased vital signs.

OUTCOME IDENTIFICATION, PLANNING, AND IMPLEMENTATION

EXPECTED OUTCOME 1: By _____ the patient will verbalize fear of loss of control associated with pain and decreased function.

SHORT-TERM GOALS	NURSING INTERVENTIONS	RATIONALES
By _____ the patient will verbalize three specific fears that relate to loss of control.	1. Using therapeutic communication techniques, encourage patient to verbalize subjective feelings such as anger and sadness.	1. These techniques will assist the patient in making the fear specific rather than general. This process will make the fear more manageable for the patient.
	2. Ask patient to locate these feelings in the body (e.g., shoulder, neck, stomach).	2. Identifying feelings is the first step in being able to work through them. Often, feelings are felt in the body, or somatized.
	3. Encourage patient to keep a record of feelings and associated fears. 4. Ask patient to share his feelings and fears with his spouse or a health care professional.	3–4. Recording fears and associated feelings is a therapeutic, effective way of working through them.

SHORT-TERM GOALS	*NURSING INTERVENTIONS*	*RATIONALES*
By _____ the patient will accurately describe current loss of function and how it has affected him.	1. Using therapeutic techniques, encourage patient to describe in detail current loss of function. 2. Ask the patient to describe specifically how the current loss of function is affecting him.	1–2. Having an empathic listener who will spend undivided time with the patient will aid in decreasing anxiety.
By _____ the patient will describe to the nurse a previous coping mechanism that worked for him when dealing with a fear associated with loss of function.	1. Ask the patient to describe a previous time in his life when he felt out of control. 2. Encourage the patient to describe his previous conquest over fear and anxiety regarding loss of function. 3. Validate the patient for being able to conquer this particular fear during his life journey.	1–3. Reminiscence empowers the patient to recognize previous coping mechanisms that work. The elderly have had many years of experience with loss, and these need to be validated.

EXPECTED OUTCOME 2: By _____ the patient will demonstrate relaxation techniques.

SHORT-TERM GOAL	NURSING INTERVENTIONS	RATIONALES
By _____ the patient will verbalize the rationale for and the components of a relaxation program.	1. Advise the patient regarding the relationship of anxiety, pain, and tension in the body. 2. Instruct the patient in deep breathing techniques.	1–2. Persons with increased anxiety tend to be shallow breathers.
	3. Teach the patient to achieve progressive muscle relaxation, focusing on a specific muscle group or the entire body, beginning with the hands and feet and moving progressively upward. 4. Have patient return a demonstration to ensure that he understands and is achieving relaxation. 5. Inform the patient that repeated practice will enhance efficacy of this technique.	3–5. Return demonstration and practice will ensure that the technique will become an integral component of the patient's lifestyle.

EXPECTED OUTCOME 3: By _____ the patient will experience reduced anxiety and improved sleep.

SHORT-TERM GOALS	NURSING INTERVENTIONS	RATIONALES
By _____ pulse and respiration rates will return to normal.	1. Monitor vital signs for any physical signs of returning anxiety.	1. The neuroendocrine system is activated during fear and anxiety, and any increase may indicate that the patient is hiding his fear.
	2. Encourage patient to eliminate any additional life stressors in his home environment.	2. Structure and safety in his home environment will assist this patient in reducing tension and anxiety.
By _____ the patient will sleep for at least four hours without being awakened by pain. By _____ the patient will verbalize being refreshed or rested upon awakening.	1. Have the patient avoid caffeine, alcohol, and strenuous activity four hours before sleep.	1. All of these factors are known to interrupt normal sleep patterns rather than induce sleep.
	2. Promote relaxation at bedtime (e.g., with back massage, progressive relaxation techniques).	2. Relaxation techniques are frequently helpful in attaining sleep.
	3. Encourage patient to sleep in comfortable environment that is conducive to sleep (e.g., with comfortable temperature, privacy, dimmed lights).	3. External stimuli are known to interfere with normal sleep patterns.
	4. Provide sedation, if necessary, but inform the patient that this is a temporary solution.	4. This measure will assist the patient in achieving sleep until a normal pattern can be attained.

EXPECTED OUTCOME 4: By _____ the patient will experience a decrease in pain and an increase in function.

SHORT-TERM GOALS	NURSING INTERVENTIONS	RATIONALES
By _____ the patient will describe increased mobility of the affected joints.	1. Encourage the patient to keep a record of the amount of joint movement that he has on a daily basis. 2. Encourage patient to expect a return to function that is reasonable considering the amount of dysfunction.	1–2. Empowers the patient to be an active participant in his own healing process and also helps the patient to be realistic in his recovery.
By _____ the patient will verbalize a decrease in joint pain.	1. Provide patient with a pain-rating scale and instruct him how to use it. 2. Ask patient to keep a record of measures used to decrease pain.	1–2. Rating the pain empowers the patient to be an active participant in his own pain control and enables the nurse to monitor the effectiveness of all measures used.
	3. Check with the patient's physician regarding the feasibility of adding an antidepressant medication such as amitriptyline to the patient's pain regimen.	3. Antidepressants in small doses are effective analgesics and could also assist the patient in improved sleep patterns.

Nursing Diagnosis: Potential for Enhanced Spiritual Well-Being related to patient's previous ability to cope with loss and ability to find solace in spiritual beliefs.

OUTCOME IDENTIFICATION, PLANNING, AND IMPLEMENTATION

EXPECTED OUTCOME 1: By _____ the patient will verbalize this episode of illness as one of the many opportunities he has experienced in his life to find meaning and inner strength.

SHORT-TERM GOALS	NURSING INTERVENTIONS	RATIONALES
By _____ the patient will make positive statements about his life and his relationship with God. By _____ the patient will verbalize that he is comfortable with his belief system.	1. Encourage and accept patient's verbalizations about his belief system. 2. Provide spiritual counsel and reading material congruent with patient's belief system.	1–2. A sense of integrity can result from being validated by caring professionals.
	3. Encourage patient to discuss these statements with his wife and children.	3. Relationship with significant others sustains a person's belief system during difficult times.

EXPECTED OUTCOME 2: By _____ the patient will verbalize a sense of hopefulness associated with his spiritual belief that pain and suffering are inevitable parts of the life cycle.

SHORT-TERM GOALS	NURSING INTERVENTIONS	RATIONALES
By _____ the patient will state that his depression has abated.	1. Encourage patient to articulate how this episode of chronic pain and discomfort was like others that he had in his lifetime. 2. Ask patient to help you understand the specific measures that worked for him this time.	1–2. These measures will enable the client to see how a strong belief system has helped him during his life.
	3. Encourage patient to self-monitor for signs of returning depression.	3. Encourages the patient to be an active participant in his overall health care.
By _____ the patient will express a desire to continue to enjoy his family and friends.	1. Ask patient what significant events are planned for his family (e.g., weddings, births, anniversaries). 2. Problem-solve with patient ways that he might be able to participate in these activities. 3. Encourage regular communication with children and grandchildren.	1–3. Hope often is associated with the desire to be a part of the future. The elderly often have to be reminded that they are an important part of the future for their family and friends. In this case study, the expected outcomes represent the summative evaluation criteria, and the short-term goals represent formative evaluation standards.

CONCLUSIONS

The developmental theorist Erik Erikson believed that late adulthood is a time in which mental health requires a sense of integrity. For the elderly, integrity means pride in the past and contentment with the present. Without this sense of integrity, an elderly person may experience despair, "feeling that the time is now short, too short for the attempt to start another life and try out alternate roads to integrity" (Erikson, 1963).

Nursing interventions can promote an elderly person's sense of integrity. Nurses need the time to spend with patients to help them validate their own experiences and belief systems. With integrity comes an ongoing commitment to life, however short the remaining time. For the elderly traveler, the last stage of the journey depends both on the road traveled and on a sense of self-worth, a belief that one's life will contribute to the future.

KEY POINTS TO REMEMBER

- Most older adults live normal lives in a community setting.
- The elderly are a highly diverse group encompassing the young-old who are under age 75, and the old-old who are age 75 years or older.
- Caregiving of elders by families is on the rise. Approximately 7% of the adult population cares for a disabled spouse or parent at home.
- Chronic illnesses are highly prevalent in late life and can threaten mental health.
- Older adults face developmental tasks—challenges and adjustments in response to life experiences—that assist in achieving a sense of psychological and social well-being.
- Reminiscence can be used therapeutically to help the elderly resolve unfinished business, appreciate the significance of their lives, and reaffirm self-worth and identity.
- When assessing the mental health of older adults, consider the impact of physical health on mental status.
- Normal aging does not result in a decline in mental function; signs of mental impairment warrant a thorough evaluation.
- Although most symptoms of mental illnesses are similar in older adults to those in younger adults, the risk exists that these symptoms can be overlooked and attributed to growing old.
- Closely monitor the impact of mental illness on physical health. Older adults have a smaller margin of safety in developing complications.
- Nurses must take an active role in advocating that older adults receive timely intervention for mental health problems and that the rights of this vulnerable group are protected.

LEARNING ACTIVITIES

1. Reminisce with a group of older adults and ask them to identify major stresses they faced in younger years. Ask them to discuss how these experiences helped them to cope with stresses they face currently.
2. Review the health histories of a group of patients. Identify physical conditions and medications that can cause or worsen mental health problems.
3. Examine several health care environments. Discuss components of the environment that facilitate or interfere with optimal mental function of the elderly.
4. Review the care plans of older adults who have mental illnesses. Determine if adequate consideration is given to their physical health needs; revise the care plan as needed.
5. Think about components of your own life that will provide strength and meaning to you as you age.

CRITICAL THINKING EXERCISE

Veronica, a student nurse, was assigned to Mrs. Donahue, a 70-year-old patient sitting in a geri-chair in the corner of the lounge on the inpatient psychiatric unit. While Veronica was doing a mini-mental status examination with Mrs. Donahue, she found out that she was a retired nurse who was going to be discharged to a nursing home. Mrs. Donahue complained about the loudness of the music on the unit and was sporting a black eye from a fall the night before when she attempted to walk to the dining room by herself.

1. What can you assume about Mrs. Donahue's condition?
2. What evidence supports your assumption(s)?
3. How could you find out if your assumptions are true?

As Veronica was talking to Mrs. Donahue, another patient approached Mrs. Donahue and began telling her about the medications she was taking. Mrs. Donahue promptly began to advise the other patient that she needed to take her meds with meals because they would upset her stomach. Mrs. Donahue also told the other patient to make sure that she reported any constipation.

1. Make sense of what might be happening.
2. What is the next thing you would say to Mrs. Donahue?
3. What is your purpose in responding in that way?

REFERENCES

Beadleson-Baird, M., and Lara, L. L. (1988). Reminiscing: Nursing actions for the acutely ill geriatric patient. *Issues in Mental Health Nursing 9*, 83–94.

Ebersole, P. (1989). *Caring for the psychogeriatric client.* New York: Springer.

Eliopoulos, C. (1991). Development tasks of aging. *Long-term care educator,* Volume 2, Lesson 6. Glen Arm, MD: Health Education Network.

Eliopoulos, C. (1993). *Gerontological nursing* (3d ed.) (p. 302). Philadelphia: J. B. Lippincott.

Eliopoulos, C. (1995). *Manual of gerontologic nursing.* St Louis: Mosby.
Erikson, E. (1963). *Childhood and society* (2nd ed.). New York: Norton.
Foreman, M. D. (1990). Complexities of acute confusion. *Geriatric nursing, 11*(3), 136.
Hosgtel, M. O. (1990). *Geropsychiatric nursing.* St Louis: Mosby.
Lowenthal, D. T. (1990). Clinical pharmacology. In W. B. Abrams, and R. Berkow (Eds.), *The Merck manual of geriatrics* (p. 181). Rahway, NJ: Merck Sharp and Dohme Research Laboratories.
McCullough, P. K. (1992). Evaluation and management of anxiety in the older adult. *Geriatrics, 47*(4), 35.
Stone, R. I., and Kemper, P. (1989). *Spouses and children of disabled elders: Potential and active caregivers.* Rockville, MD: National Center for Health Services Research and Health Care Technology Assessment.

SUGGESTED READINGS

Ebersole, P. (1989). *Caring for the psychogeriatric client.* New York: Springer.
Eliopoulos, C. (1991). Development tasks of aging. *Long-term care educator,* Volume 2, Lesson 6. Glen Arm, MD: Health Education Network.
Eliopoulos, C. (1995). *Manual of gerontologic nursing.* St Louis: Mosby.
Fidler, G. S. (1992). *Recapturing competence: A system's change for geropsychiatric care.* New York: Springer.
Hosgtel, M. O. (1990): *Geropsychiatric nursing.* St Louis: Mosby.
Lowenthal, D. T. Clinical pharmacology. In W. B. Abrams, and R. Berkow (Eds.), *The Merck manual of geriatrics* (p. 181). Rahway, NJ: Merck Sharp and Dohme Research Laboratories.

CHAPTER 27

LOSS ALONG THE JOURNEY

Loss is an inescapable part of being alive. It may not seem fair but it is real. The good news is you can get through a major loss experience and not be destroyed.

—Bob Diets

LEARNING OBJECTIVES

After studying this chapter, you should be able to:

1. Define loss and enumerate the types of losses people face in a lifetime.
2. Discuss the losses psychiatric patients face as a result of having mental health problems.
3. Name at least three people who have contributed to the work that has been done in the area of grief.
4. Describe the grief process: its length, stages, major tasks, and complications.
5. List several obstacles to grieving.
6. Describe the effects of loss and grieving upon the person with mental illness.
7. Outline several strategies that people use to cope with significant losses.
8. Discuss how to assist a psychiatric patient to cope with loss using the nursing process.

KEY TERMINOLOGY

Complicated grieving
Disenfranchised grieving
Grief
Grieving patterns
Grieving process
Loss
Survival guilt

Loss is a pervading theme in the life journey that all people undertake. Although loss is usually considered to be something very personal, the experience of loss is as universal as are the experiences of being born and dying. The life cycle is marked with advances, setbacks, changes, growth, and transitions, and amidst all of these is the experience of loss. People cope with their losses in very individual ways. Loss can be an opportunity for growth and transformation or it can be considered a curse upon one's life. Within this chapter you examine loss from a general perspective as well as from the perspective of the person who is battling mental illness; you explore the various ways that people cope with loss, how they choose to grieve their losses; and, how you can help psychiatric patients to survive losses, grieve adequately, and grow through the experience. Using the nursing process you journey with the psychiatric patient through her or his losses and help her or him discover ways of achieving a meaningful life, despite the losses faced. Let us take a look at Mary Ann's story to become acquainted with the experience of loss.

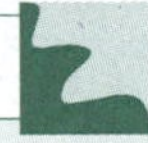

MARY ANN'S STORY

As Mary Ann sat in the warm sunshine, her heart was heavy and her thoughts confused. She had just written in her journal an account of the sad events that had occurred in her life a few short months ago. She wished she could escape the memories and painful feelings she was experiencing, but they just would not go away.... Mary Ann had dreamed of a beautiful marriage and a commitment that would last a lifetime. In its place she had a broken dream and only the memory of what could have been. She had met her husband just five years ago. For two years they knew the excitement of being in love. They enjoyed each other, and love gave new meaning and direction to their lives. They shared, planned, and prepared. Finally, they entrusted their lives and love to each other in marriage. They moved to the mountains of Vermont to build the home of their dreams. They worked hard but did not seem to mind. They had a goal and a dream that they both shared.

One year passed, and conflict began to occur. Undiagnosed and untreated mental health problems in Mary Ann's husband, linked with the usual struggles of marital adjustment, soon brought the couple to a marriage counselor. The professional help was too little, and perhaps too late, to remedy the many problems that existed. Mary Ann's spouse feared change and the challenge of growth; thus, he resisted and blocked the counseling.

This couple had hardly begun their journey in married life when obstacles fell in their path. Mary Ann tried harder than ever to move around them and to look beyond them. She felt, however, that she was alone in this work. Then, as would any weary traveler, she stopped, retraced her steps, and sadly realized that her life was going nowhere. Her energies were being robbed as a result of the constant struggles. Her peace was threatened. Her spirits were down, and she had lost her zest for living. Life was a burden. Her journey was taking her in directions she had not chosen.

The choices became clearer as time passed. She could give up the promises, the hopes, and the unrealized dreams or remain in the struggle. If she remained, it would mean a struggle for survival that could cost her her health, happiness, and well-being. She chose to let go of what was and to move in another direction. The new route was unclear and felt perilous at times. The pain, caused by the many losses she would incur because of her choice, sometimes felt unbearable. She was leaving the marriage and abandoning her dreams. Mary Ann felt lonely and afraid, yet resolute and assured of the rightness of her decision. As she wrote her farewell to the marriage dream that day, she had a keen sense of all that she had lost. What she was feeling was the pain of letting go and the experience of grieving.

DEFINITION OF AND RESEARCH ON LOSS AND GRIEF

Loss Defined

In defining **loss** within a broad context we might state that it is an event that involves the involuntary separation from something we have possessed and perhaps treasured. Loss requires that we give up that which is familiar, comfortable, and personal. In the introductory story, Mary Ann gave up her dream of a long happy marriage; she felt uncomfortable, in pain, and alone. She faced the challenge of adapting to a new set of circumstances and events in her life. Mary Ann's experiences with loss provide us a glimpse of how loss affects us all. Box 27–1 lists some general assumptions about loss.

BOX 27–1 General Assumptions About Loss

Loss is a universal experience among human beings.

Loss is painful because it implies separation.

Significant losses cause strong emotional responses.

Loss requires adjustment to what is unfamiliar, uncertain, and often unchosen.

The effects of a given loss can touch many lives.

Grief Defined

Someone you love has died. You are now faced with the difficult but important need to *grieve* or *mourn*, which involves the open expression of your thoughts and feelings regarding not only the death but also the person who has died. It is an essential part of healing. According to Wolfelt (1991a, pp. 11, 12), "You are beginning a journey that is often frightening, painful, overwhelming, and sometimes lonely."

Although grieving is most often linked with death experiences, it is a necessary process for all of the losses we face. The greater the commitment or investment we have in a person, object, project, or pursuit, the greater will be our sense of loss when it is gone. Significant losses are grieved intensely and for a longer period. Losses of lesser significance also are grieved, but usually for a shorter time and with less sadness and pain. Sudden, unexpected losses are difficult to face and often are grieved for a longer period of time. This is because of the lack of preparation for their occurrence.

The terms *grieving*, *mourning*, and *experiencing bereavement* refer to the same process and are used interchangeably in this chapter. Gyulay (1989, p. 2) defines **grief** as "a journey toward healing and recovering from the pain of a significant loss." This definition contains two important goals that are a part of the grief process: healing oneself and recovering from the loss. Gyulay indicates that experiencing grief is a blurred journey that does not necessarily follow a step-by-step sequence. Working through the grief that follows a loss does, however, lead to healing.

Clinical Work and Studies Done on Loss and Grief

Freud's Contributions

Freud (1959) attempted to explore normal and complicated grieving reactions in his classic work *Mourning and Melancholia*. Although he is widely quoted, Freud really wrote very little about mourning in comparison with the volumes he wrote on other topics. In his case studies of patients whom he was treating in therapy, Freud attempted to show the difference between normal grief responses and forms of mental illness like hysteria, neurosis, and melancholia.

Lindemann's Contributions

Eric Lindemann (1944) studied grief extensively during the 1940s. Through a series of interviews with grieving persons, he was able to record basic patterns of grief, physical symptoms that accompany it, and mental changes in people who had suffered significant losses. The study population that Lindemann used consisted of relatives of those who died in the armed forces, persons receiving psychiatric treatment who had lost a relative, and bereaved victims or relatives of victims who died in the Coconut Grove fire in Boston in the 1940s. Four major observations that Lindemann made in his pioneer studies of grief are shown in Box 27–2. (Also see Chapter 15.)

Engel's Contributions

George Engel (1964) built on the work of Lindemann. He identified the components of grief work to be

Freeing oneself from an inordinate attachment to the deceased
Readjustment to one's environment in which the deceased is no longer a part
Undertaking new relationships and social interactions

Bowlby's Contributions

During the 1960s, John Bowlby's (1969) work focused on describing mourning as a process that has three overlapping stages, including

Numbness and disbelief
Disorganization of the bereaved person's life and personality
The reorganization process

Bowlby researched the "separation response syndrome" in the 1960s and 1970s as he did work in the area of grief and attachment. *Separation anxiety* is considered a natural response to the threat of loss, and mourning is the expected response following a loss. He believed that the emotional distress of grief facilitated the breaking of attachment bonds (Bowlby, 1980).

BOX 27-2 Lindemann's Major Observations About Grief

- Acute grief is a definite syndrome with psychological and somatic symptoms.
- This syndrome may appear immediately after a crisis, it may be delayed, it may be exaggerated, or it may appear to be absent (pathological grief).
- In place of the typical syndrome, distorted pictures may appear, each of which represents one special aspect of the grief syndrome.
- By appropriate techniques, these distorted pictures of grief can be successfully transformed into a normal grief reaction.

Parkes's Contributions

Researchers focused strongly on grief in the 1970s, and this was paralleled with increased interest in death and dying. Among the noted authors and researchers in the areas of grief, death, and loss, we must mention Collin Murray Parkes (1972). He conducted a series of bereavement studies in the 1960s and 1970s examining the effects of loss upon the physical and mental health of persons during the first 6 to 12 months of their bereavement period. His studies revealed

An increase in visits to physicians
Multiple physical symptoms related to stress-related illnesses such as arthritis, hypertension, respiratory infections, and gastrointestinal malfunctioning
Psychological disturbances such as increased anxiety, depression, insomnia, and tiredness

Volkan's Contributions

Volkan (1970) described the distinctions between normal and pathological grief. Table 27–1 demonstrates these distinctions and is a reflection of the work of Volkan and other researchers on the topic of pathological grief.

Rando's Contributions

Theresa Rando's (1984, 1993) extensive work over the last 20 years focused on the areas of grief and death. She researched the course of the mourning process, the experiences of bereaved parents, and the increasing prevalence of complicated mourning. Other clinicians have used the terms *abnormal grief* or *pathological grief* to describe the same phenomenon. Rando believes that in all forms of **complicated grieving** the person attempts to do two things:

Deny, repress, or avoid aspects of the loss, its pain, and its repercussions for the mourner
Hold onto and avoid relinquishing what has been lost

In her latest work on complicated mourning (Rando 1993), Rando lists five factors that put a person at high risk for complicated mourning (Box 27–3).

Additional Contributions

A series of clinical studies addressing grief issues among parents who lost infants and young children were conducted in the late 1980s (Demi 1987; Hutti, 1988; Moore et al, 1988; Zambelli et al, 1988). Margaret Shandor Miles and Alice Sterner Demi have continued to do research in this area, focusing on dying children, parenting the child with a life-threatening illness, parental bereavement, survival guilt in bereaved parents and in those escaping natural disasters, and bereavement guilt after a suicide occurs (Miles and Demi, 1983–1984).

With the increased numbers of traumatic, unnatural, and premature deaths in our contemporary society, it is not unusual for people to be faced with multiple deaths to

TABLE 27–1 **Key Differences Between Normal and Pathological Grief**

Criteria	Normal Grief	Pathological Grief
Time since loss	Most intense reactions are seen before six months.	Intense reactions last longer than six months, with little sign of resolution or relief.
Reality testing of the loss	"Holding on" strategies: the person wants to believe the loss can be restored but knows it cannot. Reality-testing (after the initial phase of shock) is intact.	The person continues to operate as if the lost object were still there. Chronic, continuing hope for a return of the lost person or object. Refusal to actively test reality.
Preoccupation	Variable: can be intensely focused on the loss, or the person may be able to function. The person has an acute awareness of what happened at the time of the loss (emotionally, physically, and cognitively)	Active: seeking reunion with the lost object or person or a clear ongoing disruption and dysfunction in the daily routine; acute awareness of what happened at the time of the loss is usually cognitive only.
Dreams/imagery	The manifest content of dreams is variable but contains recognition of the absence of what has been lost.	The manifest content is focused on attempts to save or destroy what (who) was lost.
Approach/avoidance behaviors	The person is ambivalent about dealing with the loss but is willing to do so.	The person avoids situations that would remind him or her of the loss.
Intellectual/emotional integration	Intellectual and emotional awareness of the loss.	Intellectual awareness only or emotional awareness without linking to intellectual awareness.

Modified from Schneider, J. (1980). Clinically significant differences between grief, pathological grief, and depression. *Patient Counseling and Health Education*, Fourth Quarter.

mourn at a given time. This leads to what Kastenbaum calls *bereavement overload* (Kastenbaum 1977), which requires professional care and supportive assistance to allow the person to grieve adequately. Posttraumatic stress reactions caused by accidents, natural disasters, war, suicide, and the increasing number of homicides in our society can complicate grieving significantly. Problems usually arise when a person focuses on grieving without paying attention adequate to treating the posttraumatic stress as well.

During an interview conducted in 1991, Herman Fiefel, author of the book *The Meaning of Death*, reflected upon the stages of dying and phases of mourning outlined in literature and research. He warns about defining strict standards by which to plan care and provide support and instead advocates a focus on individual differences and personal choices (Corless et al, 1994). This is in keeping with the recent trends of working with grieving persons on a longer-term basis. Certainly when we consider the grieving psychiatric patient, it is essential that support is provided in a time frame that ensures his or her saftey and well-being.

▶ Check Your Reading

1. Define loss.
2. Define grief, or the grieving process.
3. What determines the length and intensity of grieving?
4. Identify three pioneers who did clinical work on loss and grieving.
5. What aspects of grief and mourning have been researched in the 1980s and 1990s?

BOX 27–3 Risk Factors for Complicated Mourning

- Sudden unanticipated death (death that is traumatic, violent, mutilating or random)
- Death from an overly lengthy illness
- Loss of a child
- A perception of the death as being preventable
- A premorbid relationship with the deceased marked by anger, ambivalence, or dependence
- Mourner liabilities like increased stresses, ungrieved losses, and mental health problems
- Lack of social support

From *Treatment of complicated mourning* by T. A. Rando, 1993, Champaign, IL: Research Press. Copyright 1993 by T. A. Rando. Adapted by permission.

LOSS

Loss and the Life Cycle

Loss is a common denominator throughout the life cycle. We each experienced our first loss when we were separated at birth from the warmth and safety of our mother's bodies and thrust into a world of noise, cold, brightness, and apparent confusion.

Losses in Childhood

Perhaps you can recall, at least once in your earlier years, losing your mother or some significant other in a crowd, in the supermarket, or at the beach. You probably remember the sense of panic caused by this temporary separation.

For some children, the first day of school or day care provokes an experience of loss and estrangement. Leaving the safe environment of home, where all is familiar, to enter a different environment filled with new faces and experiences is frightening.

Losses in Adolescence

Adolescence is a stormy time in the lives of many young people. Perhaps the experience of loss contributes to some of what the young person faces. Physiological changes, uncertainty about one's sense of identity, lack of ease in relationships, and concern regarding one's future life direction all bear the mark of having lost something, be it confidence, certainty, direction, or self-assurance.

Losses in Young Adulthood

Young adulthood is certainly a period of life in which each of us is confronted with new challenges and opportunities. We meet and relate to significant others as our friends, our mate, and our professional colleagues. We grow professionally, technically, and/or academically. As all of this occurs, we learn to give up selfish, personal pursuits to embrace corporate ideals, marital decisions, or business partnerships. We learn the process of give and take. This permits mutuality to occur within our close relationships. Linked with these experiences is the loss, in some sense, of what is solely "mine" so as to acquire what is "ours."

Losses in Parenthood

Parenthood makes its demands upon a young couple as they broaden mutual desires and goals to accommodate the desires and needs of their children. Personal freedom, time, and space become less available. It is not unusual during the parenting years for a mother or father to long for some of the independence and freedom once known and even to bemoan their loss.

Losses in Midlife

Midlife confronts us with the reality that time is speedily passing. Some of our goals and personal dreams may have been realized; others may never occur. Life opportunities come and go. Some are claimed, others are lost. The middle-aged person has accomplished and pursued and as a result of this has lost some of his or her vitality. By middle age, many people already have lost a parent or a trusted friend.

Losses in Older Adulthood

The golden years, so longed for in younger life because of the lure of retirement and the freedom to do as we choose, come sooner than we anticipate. Retirement is chosen by some and imposed upon others. If a person's identity intimately was related to her or his work, profession, or role, then a discontinuance of these can leave her or him feeling empty, estranged from self, and perhaps useless. This need not be the case, but frequently it is a sad reality for people who have never separated who they are from what they do.

Other losses faced by aging people are related to declining physical or mental health, decreased stamina, the experience of a sensory deprivation due to failing sight or hearing, and the death of a spouse or close friends.

Other Losses

Life events and circumstances also bring additional losses, including

The death of a pet, a friend, or a family member
Losses incurred because of geographic moves
Failure to obtain a given job, a promotion, a raise, or an A on an examination
Financial losses or bankruptcy
Loss of health, a body part, self-image, or self-worth

Westberg (1971, p. 16) states in a very practical manner that "A list of losses would be inexhaustible. We can lose our health, our eyesight, our hearing. We can lose our home through fire or tornado or through financial ruin. In some families grief comes with the loss of a pet which has been a part of everything that has gone on in that household for ten years or more. Any of these things, and many more, sets in motion a cycle of grief."

Getting in Touch with Loss

We have a tendency to underestimate the impact of loss experiences upon our lives. We try to move on with our lives as if the losses never occurred. We resist slowing down the pace of our rapidly moving lives to grieve our losses, or even to "count our blessings." The painful memories connected with loss are quickly repressed so that they will not interfere with our pursuits and undertakings. The tragedy of using repression is that the painful memories do not disappear. They are merely stored in the subconscious, to be dealt with at some later time. Stored grief and loss is cumulative and increases a person's vulnerability to experience a major grief reaction, triggered perhaps by a loss of lesser significance. The intensity of the grief reaction may lead the person to conclude that she or he has completely lost her or his emotional equilibrium. What she or he fails to realize is that she or he is grieving not one loss but a series of losses. Some may be more significant than others, but all may have been repressed for some time.

The *Diagnostic and Statistical Manual-IV (DSM-IV)* addresses the issue of grieving or bereavement by distinguishing symptoms related to "normal" bereavement from those of a major depressive disorder, exacerbated

MEDICAL DIAGNOSES AND RELATED NURSING DIAGNOSES — Grieving

***DSM-IV* Diagnosis:** Bereavement

Diagnostic Criteria

This category can be used when the focus of clinical attention is a reaction to the death of a loved one. As part of their reaction to the loss, some grieving individuals present with symptoms characteristic of a Major Depressive Episode (e.g., feelings of sadness and associated symptoms such as insomnia, poor appetite, and weight loss). The bereaved individual typically regards the depressed mood as "normal," although the person may seek professional help for relief of associated symptoms such as insomnia or anorexia. The duration and expression of "normal" bereavement vary considerably among different cultural groups. The diagnosis of Major Depressive Disorder is generally not given unless the symptoms are still present 2 months after the loss. However, the presence of certain symptoms that are not characteristic of a "normal" grief reaction may be helpful in differentiating bereavement from a Major Depressive Episode. These include (1) guilt about things other than actions taken or not taken by the survivor at the time of the death; (2) thoughts of death other than the survivor feeling that he or she would be better off dead or should have died with the deceased person; (3) morbid preoccupation with worthlessness; (4) marked psychomotor retardation; (5) prolonged and marked functional impairment; and (6) hallucinatory experiences other than thinking that he or she hears the voice of, or transiently sees the image of, the deceased person.

RELATED NURSING DIAGNOSES	DEFINITION	EXAMPLE
Dysfunctional Grieving	Extended, unsuccessful use of intellectual and emotional responses by which individuals attempt to work through the process of modifying self-concept based upon the perception of the loss	Dysfunctional Grieving related to the loss of a child

Diagnostic Criteria from American Psychiatric Association: *Diagnostic and Statistical Manual of Mental Disorders, Fourth Edition.* Washington, D.C., American Psychiatric Association, 1994; nursing diagnoses and definitions from North American Nursing Diagnosis Association (1994). *NANDA nursing diagnoses: Definitions and classification 1995–1996.* Philadelphia: NANDA.

perhaps by a loss experience (see "Medical Diagnoses and Related Nursing Diagnoses: Grieving").

In his book *Life After Loss* (Diets, 1988), Bob Diets writes "The only time you have to start working through your losses is today. Tomorrow will not be a better day to face up to the task. The only one who can make the journey through your grief is you. But as you make it, you will discover that you are equal to the challenge."

An excellent way to get in touch with losses experienced within your life is to use a personal survey or to prepare a loss inventory (Box 27-4). In doing this, you not only are able to recount loss events and their significance but also can recognize whether you adequately grieved these events.

Another exercise that is helpful in exploring issues of personal loss is to use a *loss time line.* To create a loss time line, randomly select a 5- or 10-year segment of your life. Then plot losses chronologically on a time line. As the events take shape graphically on the time line, the proximity of the losses and the number of losses experienced become clear. Case Example 27–1 tells the story of one woman's losses, and Figure 27–1 demonstrates the use of a loss time line to illustrate her losses.

Although it is helpful to recognize one's losses, it is equally important to look at how a person like Susan Smith has dealt with each loss. In Susan's case, the losses were significant, and her ability to cope was certainly taxed. Did Susan take the time to grieve each loss? Did one grief period blend into another? Did Susan emerge from the period of loss well, whole, and healed?

BOX 27-4 A Personal Loss Inventory

- The first significant loss I can remember in my life was ______________________
- The circumstances were ______________________
- My age was ______________________
- The feelings I had at the time were ______________________
- The first death that made its impact on my life was ______________________
- The thing I remember most about that experience was ______________________
- I coped with the loss by ______________________
- The most difficult death for me to face would be ______________________
- My primary style of coping with loss is ______________________
- I know my grief over a loss is resolved when ______________________

Case Example 27–1 Susan Smith's Story

Life was going well for 52-year-old Susan Smith. Although she had never had children, and although her marriage of 16 years had been rocky at times, she felt reasonably content with her lot in life. She had a well-paying job as an insurance executive, and she was in good health. Then, suddenly, her husband announced that he was leaving. He wanted a divorce.

After the divorce in 1976, Susan moved to an upscale apartment in Baltimore. She had barely settled into her new home when, on her way home from work, she was robbed at gunpoint. Susan lost her purse, her credit cards, and her wallet, but otherwise escaped unharmed.

Susan had purchased a new Oldsmobile after her divorce, and she felt proud of her ability, as a single woman, to afford such a prestigious car. However, in 1977, just six months after making her last payment on the car, local teens stole it and took it for a joyride, causing thousands of dollars of damage in the process.

Susan's life seemed to normalize in 1978, but by the end of that year, her father had become gravely ill with pancreatic cancer and had died.

After three years of uneventful living, Susan suddenly lost her job. Corporate reorganization and "downsizing" had left her with three options: take a major pay cut, take a lower-ranking position, or leave the company on severance pay. She chose the last option, and a long, tedious job search and a move to Colorado for a new job resulted.

Three and a half years later, Susan got a call from her gynecologist after a routine mammogram. A suspicious shadow showed up on the film, and a biopsy was necessary "just to be safe." Despite her doctor's cautious optimism, Susan feared the worst: breast cancer. After a wait that seemed like an eternity, Susan underwent the biopsy. The reports, thankfully, were negative. Susan did not have breast cancer.

Loss and the Psychiatric Patient

Loss issues are a concern as you journey with a person who struggles with mental illness. Dealing with losses or going through a grief reaction can even precipitate a crisis or a psychotic episode in someone whose mental health is already fragile. The psychiatric patient is vulnerable to the same losses as the person who is emotionally sound. Additionally, the psychiatric patient experiences losses directly related to mental illness, including

- Loss of job or career because of unstable mental health
- Loss of financial well-being due to hospital bills or the inability to work
- Loss of friends as a result of frequent hospitalizations or the inability to enter into meaningful relationships
- Loss of rootedness and a place called "home" as a result of the tendency to disengage from reality and the flow of human life

Less obvious but just as significant are the losses of a more personal and spiritual nature, including

- Loss of purpose and direction for life
- Loss of existential meaning
- Loss of health and wholeness
- Loss of hope, especially during periods of psychosis or depression
- Loss of grasp of what is real and true

Mental illnesses are chronic just like diabetes, heart disease, or hypertension. Some basic characteristics of chronic illnesses include

- That they progress over time
- That they are treated or ameliorated but not necessarily cured
- That periods of exacerbation can be triggered by stress and other circumstances
- That treatment is ongoing and lifelong

In light of these characteristics, the mentally ill experience certain additional losses, including

- Loss of physical and psychological stamina
- Loss of abilities
- Loss of health
- Loss of zest and joy for living

When the psychiatric patient becomes trapped in his or her flight from reality or intense state of self-

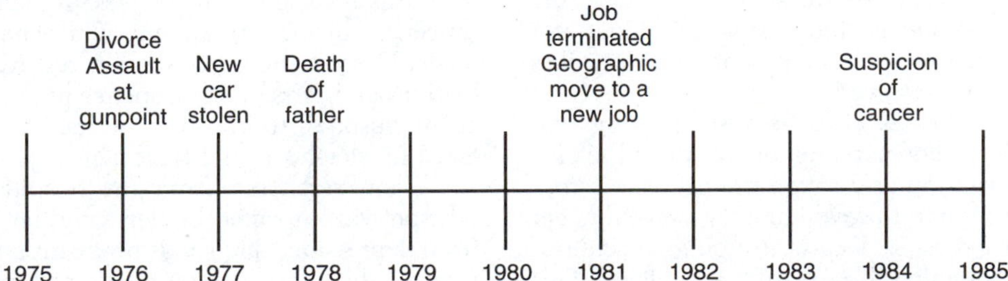

FIGURE 27–1
Example of a loss time line.

absorption, losses can be ignored easily. During periods of acute illness, losses cannot be fully perceived or grieved. The patient must experience emotional equilibrium before being able to process losses. During the time it takes for the psychiatric patient to regain emotional equilibrium, many losses may have occurred. Most significant of these losses are the deaths of parents, family members, close friends, or significant others. When mental health stabilizes, the person may be faced with many voids in her or his life, caused by the losses that have occurred. How then does she or he begin to grieve?

Similar is the plight of the person enmeshed in an addictive lifestyle. Years of events come and go without the addicted person being fully aware of or invested in these events. When the person begins a life of sobriety, he or she is faced with taking an inventory of all that has been missed, ignored, or avoided because of the addiction. Grieving these losses is a part of adjusting to a chemical-free lifestyle.

Your challenge involves helping the patient to reinvest in life once again through a recapturing of "what was" and a facing of "what is." Most certainly this process entails getting in touch with loss experiences that have occurred and discovering how they can be grieved. The work is slow and arduous. Your interventions must be gentle, directive, and well paced so as not to overwhelm the patient. The goal is to journey with the psychiatric patient toward wellness and healing as he or she grieves losses. Let us turn our attention to the process of grieving.

▶ Check Your Reading

6. What are some typical losses during young adulthood?
7. What are some disadvantages of using repression as a means of coping with loss?
8. How does the *Diagnostic and Statistical Manual-IV (DSM-IV)* differentiate a normal grief reaction from a major depressive episode?
9. What are some of the losses that people with mental illness face?

GRIEF

The Length of the Grieving Process

One of the major concerns regarding the **grieving process** is how long it will last. Many of us would just as soon grieve for a few days or weeks and then have the process completed—quickly and easily. This does not happen, primarily because grieving is a process that takes time to unfold and be resolved.

Diets (1988) indicates that because grieving and recovery from grief are demanding, people often look for any way to get out of going through the process. Before they finally go through it, they will first try to avoid it, get over it quickly, or detain it. To go through grief requires both stamina and an incredible amount of patience. This is especially so when one feels terribly sad, lost, lonely, angry, or all of these. To simply "wait it out" or "endure it" without any active participation in the process is counterproductive.

Experiencing the loss is the first step in letting go and moving beyond the loss experience (Carson, 1995). Lindemann (1944) indicates that experiencing the emotional pain of a loss is what many fear the most. This fear can block the grief process from unfolding or happening at all. "Getting on with one's life" is how some people refer to moving beyond a loss experience. Yet this can never happen unless the individual lets the grieving occur.

People grieve in different ways and at different rates. The important factor is that they grieve as soon after the loss as they can rather than postponing this necessary process for long periods of time (Bouvard, 1988). People usually grieve most intensely during the first months following their loss. By the end of the first year, persons who allowed the grieving to occur and who have had no complicating circumstances surrounding their grief process may be nearing some point of resolution (Caplan, 1974). We discuss the factors related to complicated grieving later in this chapter.

The length of the grief process is dependent upon

The significance of the lost object or person
The period of time that the person or object was known, loved, or cherished
One's preparation for the separation
The emotional strength and ability to cope possessed at the time of the loss

Mrs. Jackson's story (Case Example 27–2) demonstrates that grieving may be delayed because of particular circumstances.

Case Example 27–2 Mrs. Jackson's Story

Mrs. Jackson is a 42-year-old black female who has suffered with depressive episodes for 20 years of her life. She received some bad news from her 46-year-old husband one day. During his annual physical, something abnormal was seen on his chest x-ray. Mr. Jackson is the sole provider for his family of four, and he had to interrupt his work for an admission to the hospital. The couple live with their 16-year-old daughter and 17-year-old son in an apartment in the inner city, subsisting on a modest income.

Tests revealed that Mr. Jackson had inoperable lung cancer. Plans for treatment with chemotherapy were made. Despite the stress she felt regarding the failing of her husband, Mrs. Jackson spent a period of time each day at the hospital, trying to emotionally support him as he faced his diagnosis and treatment.

Upon returning from the hospital one day, Mrs. Jackson was informed by her daughter, who also suffers from depression, that she is pregnant and does not know what to do. Mrs. Jackson needs to look at options and make decisions, but concern over her husband's condition seems more immediate.

Treatment went poorly for Mr. Jackson—the tumor was not responsive to chemotherapy. His condition declined rapidly, and his wife was aware of this. While facing this dilemma, a call came from the school principal informing Mrs. Jackson that her son had been suspended from school for the possession and use of drugs. His admission back into school would be dependent upon the completion of a drug rehabilitation program.

As the days passed Mr. Jackson became weaker, and his death became more imminent. Mrs. Jackson kept news of problems at home from him. She was feeling more emotionally fragile as each day passed. She had always relied on her husband, and now he was no longer there for her.

Within days, Mr. Jackson died and his wife was faced with the loss of her husband, the funeral, loss of a source of income for the family, a son with a serious drug problem who was out of school, a daughter who was two months pregnant, her own failing mental health, the home, and financial affairs. Mrs. Jackson will deal with the immediate needs first. Her grieving process will be delayed until the urgent issues are resolved. The length of her grief process probably will be quite extensive because the acute phase of her grieving will be postponed for a considerable period. Her mental health will need attention before she is faced with another bout of major depression. Her financial problems and the needs of her son and daughter will be handled with the assistance of her sister. Much later, she will grieve the loss of her spouse.

Let us reflect for a moment upon the psychiatric patient who may be actively engaged in treatment for a psychotic episode or a progression of her or his particular form of mental illness. When a significant loss occurs during that period, several reactions can be expected. If the person is not in touch with reality at the time of the loss, the loss event will come and go without the person facing it. He or she even may go through the motions of attending a wake and funeral. Grieving will occur at some later time when the acute manifestations of the mental illness have been controlled by some form of treatment. On the other hand, news of a significant loss such as death, bankruptcy, or loss of job, can threaten an already weakened emotional state. This may result in a pathological grief reaction, a psychotic episode, flight from reality, or an acute depression with suicidal ideation. Mental illness may complicate or delay the grief reaction and may extend the period of grieving.

Stages of Grieving

The following sections describe the stages of grieving according to Kübler-Ross, Engel, Westberg, and Veninga. This information provides you with a broad picture of the various reactions to loss.

Kübler-Ross's Stages

Dr. Elisabeth Kübler-Ross (1969) identified five stages that a dying person experiences: denial, anger, bargaining, depression, and acceptance. These five stages can be applied to grief responses as well. Kübler-Ross suggests that people do not follow these five stages in an orderly pattern; rather, they move back and forth between the stages, experiencing them for varying periods of time.

Engel's Stages

George Engel (1964) indicated in his writings that successful grieving involves three phases: shock and disbelief, developing awareness, and restitution. In the phase of *shock and disbelief*, the person has a need to deny the loss to protect himself or herself from the painful feelings it evokes. The denial usually lasts for a short period of time (minutes to hours to days). During this time the bereaved person hopes against all hope that some mistake was made—that the loss never really happened. A lengthy period of denial signals an abnormal grief reaction and prevents the person from going forward in the grief process.

In the phase of *developing awareness*, the person realizes the emotional impact of the loss; the loss begins to penetrate consciousness. The bereaved becomes increasingly aware of the anguish created by the loss and has painful feelings of sadness and emptiness. Crying is one of the most evident activities in this phase of grieving. Somatic symptoms (e.g., a choking sensation, inability to eat or sleep, or shortness of breath), as well as strong emotional reactions (e.g., anger at the deceased, anger at persons deemed responsible for the loss, extreme helplessness, hopelessness, or guilt), are experienced.

In the phase of *restitution*, the task of mourning begins. In the case of a loss by death, the work of this stage can actually begin with the wake, funeral, and burial. Early in this stage, what was lost, whether it is an ideal, object, or person, is idealized. Nothing can replace it. The bereaved does not believe that life can go on or be the same without the lost object. In time, thinking becomes more realistic, and as the pain of the loss lessens, the bereaved begins to consider that he or she can find meaning and purpose for his or her life without the presence or possession of the lost object. The person begins to feel that he or she must go on with life.

Westberg's Stages

In his book *Good Grief*, Westberg (1971, p. 16) affirms that successful grieving after the small losses in our lifetime prepares us for grieving the more significant losses that we may come to face. He describes 10 stages of grieving, which include

State of shock
Expressing emotion
Depression and loneliness
Physical symptoms of distress
Panic

TABLE 27–2 **The Stages of Mourning**

Stages	Characteristics	Duration
Stage one: The bombshell	Shock, numbness, disbelief, denial; inability to make decisions; difficulty in carrying on conversations; short attention span, high anxiety; physical symptoms (e.g., nausea, vomiting, shortness of breath); not wanting help from others	Several hours, days, or weeks
Stage two: Deliberate activity, illusion of normalcy	Seems anesthetized; sets about reestablishing order, stabilizing his or her life; appears that all is as before; makes decisions, greets friends, shops, tries to fill the void	A few weeks
Stage three: Hitting rock bottom	Begins the painful journey into the darkest areas of life; expresses strong emotions (intense anger, intense loneliness, guilt); expresses four negative themes: "My life will never be the same," "I have let everybody down," "It is impossible to ever be happy again," "Others do not understand me." Each person reacts differently during this stage: stoically and logically—"You have to go on with living, and self-pity doesn't help," feel the hurt deeply and show it or dwell on the loss, counterattack to dispel the anger (e.g., join Mothers Against Drunk Driving), illness	Many months
Stage four: The awakening	Usually able to state a particular event that gave him or her hope that life could be happy again; forced to restructure his or her view of himself or herself and the world; the "shadows" begin to recede: a search for meaning begins; says something like "By God, I am going to make it!"	Many months
Stage five: Acceptance	Acceptance does not mean forgetting—as if to deny the significance of the heartbreak—nor does it imply glossing over the hurt; says "I realized I had to let go"; enters fully into life—whatever it offers; forgives himself or herself and others, expresses gratitude for what remains.	A year or two (maybe longer)

From *A gift of hope: How to survive our tragedies* by Robert Veninga. Copyright © 1985 by Robert L. Veninga. By permission of Little, Brown and Company.

Guilt feelings
Anger and resentment
Resistance
Hope
Affirming reality

Veninga's Stages

Table 27–2 demonstrates the stages of mourning as outlined in *A Gift of Hope: How to Survive Our Tragedies* (Veninga, 1985).

Major Tasks of Grieving

As shown in Box 27–5, a person faces four major tasks in any grief process (Worden, 1982). Each of these tasks is faced throughout the grief process. For example, in early grief, acceptance of the reality of the loss comes only when the shock and disbelief have passed. The reality of the loss is felt as acute pain, and energies are poured into coping with this reality. In the long midportion of the grief process (a period of 8 to 10 months or longer), acceptance of the reality of the loss and experiencing the pain of loss are accompanied by physical symptoms and strong emotional responses (Parkes, 1964). The person wonders whether he or she will ever feel better about the

BOX 27–5 The Four Major Tasks of Grieving

Task 1	Acceptance of the reality of the loss—believing that the loss has truly occurred, no mistake has occurred, the situation will not reverse itself, what one has lost is truly gone
Task 2	Experiencing the pain of the loss—knowing the disappointment, the loneliness, the absence, the emptiness; feeling the emotional pain that accompanies these realizations
Task 3	Adjustment to life and living without the "lost object"—recognizing that one's life is not over or totally destroyed by the loss; knowing that one can go on
Task 4	Reinvesting energies into new undertakings and relationships—letting go and moving on; discovering a new purpose and meaning for one's life

From Worden, W. (1982). *Grief counseling and grief therapy: A handbook for the mental health practitioner.* Springer Publishing Company, Inc., New York 10012, used by permission.

loss. As the months of grieving pass, the person begins to believe that he or she is adjusting to life without what was lost. However, the arrival and passing of a holiday or commemorative event may rekindle the pain and deep longing. The person questions whether any progress in grieving has been made. In time, the person realizes that he or she always will have some pain and regret connected with the loss, although they lessen significantly as time passes. Thus, in the last phase of the grief process, more emotional energy is available for meeting responsibilities, facing challenges, and accepting new undertakings. All of this is a part of the adjustment to life without the lost object. The person now has the energy to reengage in social activities, experiencing once again some degree of enjoyment. New relationships or projects may be pursued with some degree of enthusiasm.

Patterns of Grieving

As mentioned, many people would prefer not to grieve at all because the process is long, difficult, and emotionally draining. We now look at normal **grieving patterns** and contrast them with those that are abnormal. Much has been written on the topic of abnormal grieving (Schneider, 1980). It also is called complicated grief, morbid grief reactions, the pathological grief syndrome, distorted grief, and unresolved grief.

Normal Grieving

If grieving were regarded as an accepted social process, people would find the freedom to share their grief with others. When assisted in their grief work by caring others, people grieve more quickly and easily. Unfortunately, this is not the case in American society. Overt expressions of grief often are considered to be socially unacceptable. As death, the ultimate loss experience, continues to be regarded as something tragic, catastrophic, and unnatural, so too will grieving be regarded as something terribly painful, difficult, and counterproductive to the American way of life. If a person cannot freely grieve the loss of a significant other, much less is she or he free to grieve other losses.

Let us focus on what it feels like to grieve, as we discuss a normal grief reaction. The symptoms, experiences, and sensations felt during the grief process correspond in intensity and duration with the phase of grieving through which one is passing.

EARLY PHASE

The early phase of grieving, marked by disbelief, shock, and dismay, leaves a person feeling dazed, unproductive, and "mechanical" as he or she tries to function. This phase may last for hours, days, or weeks. The person may not remember much of what has happened during that period because of the psychological numbing caused by the loss experience.

MIDDLE PHASE

Following this, the longer, acutely painful, midportion of the grief process occurs. It extends over many months, depending on an individual's circumstances or need. This period includes reactions that are more intense in nature. In her book *Living Through Personal Crisis*, Ann Stearns (1984) addresses the physical expressions of loss. She writes "A wide range of marked physical changes can accompany an experience of loss. Not only through tears do we cry out our pangs of grief. Under the stress of what has been unrecoverably lost, our bodies have a dozen ways of weeping with us" (p. 16). Box 27–6 outlines some of the characteristics of normal grief reactions. These are experienced to a greater or lesser degree throughout the acute midphase of the grief process.

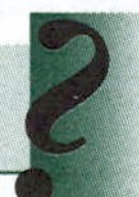

WHAT PATIENTS AND FAMILIES NEED TO KNOW **Grief**

Why do we grieve?
Grieving is our normal response to dealing with a loss. By working through the emotions of denial, anger, bargaining, depression, and acceptance, we are able to let go of the loss and focus on life, our relationships, and goals with renewed energy.

How do I know if I'm grieving?
You may experience a deep feeling of sadness and sorrow and sometimes guilt and anger about losing someone or something close to you. You may have physical symptoms such as muscle tension and weakness, a hollow feeling in the stomach, tightness in the chest, shortness of breath, or loss of appetite or overeating. In addition, you may have trouble sleeping and difficulty concentrating and making decisions. Sometimes you might feel you are going crazy, because you dream about the lost person or imagine that he or she is still alive. You might think that you hear or see the lost person in a crowd. All of this is normal and will lessen with the grieving process.

When does grieving become abnormal?
When grief does not follow the typical pattern and becomes incapacitating and of unusually long duration, it can be considered abnormal. If you feel your grief is abnormal, seek professional help.

What can I do to help someone grieve?
It is important to be a good listener and allow the grieving person to "retell" their loss over and over. Do not tell the person not to cry. He or she needs to get his or her feelings out. Grief affects all members of a family, so do not forget the children. They, too, experience grief. Encourage the grieving person to seek solace and spiritual comfort within his or her religious traditions. Remember, grief is self-limiting and will resolve over time. Tell the person to be patient with himself or herself.

BOX 27-6 Characteristics of Normal Grief Reactions

Feelings	A deep sadness, guilt, and self-reproach for somehow being responsible; loneliness; apathy; listlessness; yearning for a return of what was lost; blaming others for the loss; anger at self and others
Physical sensations	Hollowness in the stomach, tightness in the chest, oversensitivity to noise or the conversations of others, shortness of breath, muscle weakness, loss of appetite or a tendency to overeat, sleeplessness or sleeping long hours to cope, lack of energy, a sense of impending physical illness
Thought patterns	Difficulty concentrating, inability to make decisions, preoccupation with thoughts of the lost object, memory lapses, auditory or visual hallucinations in which one relates to the deceased, depression
Behavioral aspects	Absent-minded behavior, dreaming about what was lost, social withdrawal, restless overactivity, searching for the lost object, sighing in dismay, crying, lack of libido

Although what is felt as a person acutely grieves is considered a normal grief reaction, many people will feel that they are crossing over into the realm of mental illness. They may even begin to believe that they have lost their ability to cope and their grasp of reality (Carter, 1989). The fact that the symptoms, feeling, and sensations lose their intensity and become less frequent as time passes is a comfort to most.

LATE PHASE

The last phase of the grief process, called the awakening and acceptance stages by Veninga (1985) (see Table 27–2), is characterized by glimmers of hope. Over time, a person experiences new energy for coping, a returning sense of well-being, and a belief in self. However, it is not unusual for psychiatric patients to miss the experiences of awakening and acceptance.

Complicated Grieving

Grieving that is incapacitating, unusually long in duration, and that involves some disorganized, depressed behaviors falls into the category of complicated grieving. Persons predisposed to this kind of grief reaction are those with a history of

- Depressive reactions to transitions, crises, or misfortunes
- Psychiatric problems with periods of hospitalization
- Substance abuse, especially alcoholism
- Death of a parent or sibling during childhood or adolescence
- Prolonged conflict or marked dependency upon the deceased person
- Multiple deaths
- Posttraumatic stress

Professional help is always required when a person is trapped in complicated grief.

Eric Lindemann (1944) describes the characteristics of complicated grieving in the studies that he conducted. Calling it "morbid grief reactions," he described the following symptoms:

- Overactivity or agitation without a keen sense of one's loss
- Acquisition of symptoms experienced during the last illness of the deceased
- Exacerbation of a disease of a psychophysiological nature such as ulcerative colitis, rheumatoid arthritis, or asthma
- Alteration in relationships with friends and relatives, progressing to complete social isolation
- Repression of feelings and an absence of emotional display despite the significant loss
- Lack of initiative or poor decision-making, which leads to dysfunctional living patterns (e.g., poor grooming, not cooking or eating, not cleaning self or home)
- Loss of social status, professional standing, and financial well-being because of unwise or imprudent financial decisions
- Deterioration into a state of depression marked by agitation, insomnia, feelings of worthlessness, bitter self-accusation, the need for self-punishment (becoming dangerously suicidal)
- Extreme hostility toward persons held responsible for the loss

Along with the distorted responses seen in morbid grief reactions, other categories of complicated grief may be seen: absent grief, delayed grief, chronic grief, distorted grief, and converted grief (Wolfelt, 1991).

In *absent grief*, prolonged denial results from psychic numbing, which prevents a person from accepting the reality of a significant loss and from mourning that loss. The person experiencing absent grief is relatively unmoved and psychologically detached as he or she tells the story of the loss that has occurred. As mentioned earlier, persons actively pursuing an addictive lifestyle or caught in the throes of mental illness may exhibit absent grief, even when something or someone very treasured is lost. Absent grief may be present temporarily when uncertainties surround losses during wartime, natural disasters, or accidents. In most cases, grieving occurs when doubts are cleared and the extent of the losses is confirmed.

Delayed grief involves the postponement of grieving for weeks, months, or years. Delayed grief often can be abruptly ended by subsequent losses or by the losses of others that are similar to one's own ungrieved loss and may trigger grieving. Sometimes delays in grieving occur out of necessity, such as occurred in the case of Mrs.

Jackson in Case Example 27–2. If a significant period passes after an actual loss experience, during which a person cannot or will not grieve, these people have a tendency to repress rather than experience the grief response.

Chronic grief is a persistent pattern of grieving that tends to be exaggerated and does not reach resolution. It creates disabling symptoms, dysfunctional people, and irrational despair. Chronic grief related to death is characterized by attempts to keep the deceased person alive by talking about him or her frequently, maintaining his or her personal things intact, and expecting that the deceased will reenter the mourner's life.

Distorted grief is that type of grief that Lindemann called a morbid grief reaction. Anger and guilt are the two emotional expressions that become distorted in this type of grieving. The person is caught up in a state of emotional upheaval that inhibits him or her from effectively carrying out personal responsibilities and activities.

Converted grief can be referred to as "somatization disorder." It entails a preoccupation with physical or psychological symptoms that are not linked by the person to his or her loss.

Depression is often seen as a component of both normal and complicated grief reactions. The helplessness and hopelessness of depression often rob the grieving person of the emotional energy needed to do grief work. For a summary of the distinctions between grieving and depression see Table 27–3.

TABLE 27–3 **Differences Between Grieving and Depression**

Characteristic	Grieving	Depression
Loss	Bereaved has suffered a recognizable loss	Depressed, has suffered a recognizable loss, or the person may see the loss as punishment
Mood state	Bereaved quickly shifts from sadness to a more normal state in the same day	Person has variability in mood, psychomotor activity level, verbal communication, appetite, and sexual interest within the same day or week; sadness is mixed with anger
Energy level	Mourner feels tension or an absence of energy	Person feels consistent sense of depletion, psychomotor retardation, anorexia with weight loss, decreased interest in sex, decreased verbal communication, agitation, compulsive eating, sexuality or verbal output are diminished
Expression of anger	Griever shows open anger and hostility	Person has absence of externally directed anger and hostility
Expression of sadness	Griever weeps	Person has difficulty in weeping or in controlling weeping
Dreams, fantasies, and imagery	Mourner has vivid, clear dreams and fantasies; good capacity for imagery, particularly involving the loss	Person has relatively little access to dreams, low capacity for fantasy or imagery (except for self-punitive)
Sleep disturbance	Griever has disturbing dreams, episodic difficulties in getting to sleep	Person has severe insomnia, early-morning awakening
Self-concept	Person sees himself or herself as being to blame for not providing adequately for the lost object; has tendency to experience the world as empty; has preoccupation with the lost object or person	Person sees himself or herself as bad; has tendency to experience self as worthless; has preoccupation with self; has suicidal ideas and feelings
Responsiveness	Person responds to warmth and reassurance	Person responds to repeated promises, pressure, and urging or is unresponsive to most stimuli
Pleasure	Mourner has variable restrictions of pleasure	Person has persistent restrictions of pleasure
Reaction of others to the affected person	Others show tendency to feel sympathy for the person, to want to touch or hold the person	Others show tendency to feel irritation toward the person; others rarely feel like touching or reaching out to the person

From Schneider, J. (1980). Clinically significant differences between grief, pathological grief, and depression. *Patient Counseling and Health Education,* Fourth Quarter.

Grieving in Children

Children perceive loss and grieve differently than do adults. For instance, children under the age of three do not have a clear concept of the finality of death. The reactions of young children to loss is greatly affected by the sadness and seriousness of the adults around them who are grieving a recent loss. They come to understand that death involves leaving and separation. However, because they do not comprehend the finality of death, they may look for and talk about the deceased person as if he or she were coming back.

Children three to six years of age have a keener sense of loss experience. They know the experience of separation from a parent and the anguish this causes. They also may know what it is like to lose a pet or friend. Fear of having *caused* a significant loss by unacceptable behavior is very common. Trying to discuss ways of "undoing" a loss is also a preoccupation of the child.

As children reach the ages of six to nine years, they begin to realize that death is permanent and nothing will reverse it. In this age range, children have a lot of questions that they expect will be answered. Adults struggle with being candid when it comes to providing children with information about loss, separation, and death.

As children reach the ages of 10 to 12, death becomes a more familiar experience to them, as does loss. They may have lost in games and sporting events, had friends move away, and perhaps experienced the death of a child they knew. They come to realize that death can come to anyone at anytime.

Adolescents may vacillate between having a mature and a very childlike attitude toward death. Adolescents have a tendency to want to defy death and remain immune to it. They know about the losses one faces in life, but when it comes to accepting death as one of those losses, they show great resistance. Death to them is reserved for older people or for those who are very ill.

Obstacles to Grieving

Many obstacles to grieving exist. First, many people do not want to struggle with the pain of loss that grieving evokes. Second, grieving takes time, and some people do not want to put the time and energy into healing themselves after a significant loss. Various other factors may impede a person from expressing grief and from doing so in a timely manner. The following are some obstacles to grieving.

Living in a Modern Society

In 20th century America, life is generally fast paced, success oriented, goal seeking, and proficiency prone. Little recognition is given to the importance of grief work, and sufficient time to complete it may not be allowed. In addition, our society is very mobile. Many people find themselves without roots and a permanent place to call home because of their life circumstances. When faced with a significant loss, many find that they are geographically distant from family and relatives. This leads to a sense of being disconnected from one's former support system while facing the loss. The person may not yet have a community in the new place of residence in which to relate or from which to receive support. Thus, grieving is made more difficult.

Lack of Religious Rites and Rituals

Religious rituals and rites of passage, well supported and sanctioned by American society, can help people to mourn and undertake their process of grieving. The funeral provides loved ones with an opportunity to publicly and "reservedly" display their grief. Through the centuries, churches and religious institutions have offered support and comfort to persons who have faced losses. Through a ministry of prayer, consolation, and counseling, clergymen and -women have supported countless numbers of people in their grief process. A strong faith and deep religious principles have sustained many grieving persons during the long, hard months of grief. With the trend among younger Americans to withdraw from traditional church membership and participation, this vital source of strength and spiritual assistance often is lacking.

In light of the benefits that a funeral ritual provides to the grieving, we might question what happens when a person is cremated? Cremation has become a more common practice in our society, and it is a choice that many dying persons make. Cremation, without a memorial service to accompany it, can deprive grieving families and loved ones of the final act of separation from the deceased that funeral rites provide.

Social Norms for Grieving in Men

Men in our society have certain restrictions placed upon them with regard to grieving. This prevents healthy expression of grief and impedes the grief process. Wolfelt (1990) indicates that men are more likely to experience complicated grief processes, absent grief, delayed grief reactions, or any manifestation of abnormal grieving as a result of the socially dictated gender stereotypes. Wolfelt describes several factors that influence the manner in which men and boys grieve. These factors also affect their choice not to grieve (Table 27–4).

Unsanctioned Losses

Some losses are not validated or sanctioned by society (Doka, 1989). Included among these unsanctioned losses are the loss of a pregnancy through an abortion or a miscarriage; loss of a loved one by suicide; loss of someone with whom one had an extramarital affair, a homosexual relationship, or a nonmarital union (living together); bankruptcy; and the loss of one's job through dismissal with cause. Emotional, legal, and financial involvements related to these unsanctioned losses can compound the loss experience further. Psychiatric patients and drug abusers who attempt to flee from life and reality through failed suicide attempts face, together with their families,

TABLE 27–4 **Factors That Influence the Manner in Which Men and Boys Grieve**

Factor	Explanation
Social conditioning	Lessons given early in life teach that boys and men do not cry; acceptable feelings for men are fearlessness, aggressiveness, and defensiveness; unacceptable feelings are sadness, tenderness, and helplessness
Inability to seek support; need to be self-sufficient	Grieving requires a reaching out to caring others and a degree of dependence on them, in direct conflict with the societal norm that men be strong and independent; dependency creates anxiety, fear, and feelings of vulnerability in the "typical man"
Intolerance of slowing down to grieve	Grieving that terminates in growth and healing requires periods of quiet and time to process; masculinity is equated with striving, accomplishing, and producing; men in our society find difficulty in freeing themselves of their busy pursuits to engage in a period of grieving, slowing down to grieve is considered unmanly
Inability to acknowledge pain	Outwardly expressing the pain of loss is equated with weakness by men; since childhood they have learned that they must be strong; much emotional energy is used by men to repress sadness, loneliness, and the pain related to their losses

From Wolfelt, A. (1990). Gender roles and grief: Why men's grief is naturally complicated. *Thanatos*, Fall, 20–24.

an unsanctioned loss experience. Patients with AIDS have an increased risk for suicide (Marzak et al, 1988).

Disenfranchisement means being deprived of one's rights as a citizen. **Disenfranchised grieving** is a complicated form of grieving because it entails social stigma; difficulties with participation in mourning rites; delayed or private grieving; lack of social support systems; economic and legal problems; and the emotional burdens of guilt, shame, and blaming. According to Pine (1972), disenfranchised grievers are an underclass of grievers. They are shunted out of the mainstream because their relationships are socially unrecognized (e.g., with abortions or miscarriages), illegitimate (e.g., with an extramarital affair or a nonmarital union), or unsanctioned (e.g., a gay partner). The losses may not fit the norm of being appropriate or have societal approval. This is the case with suicide, bankruptcy, or being dismissed with cause from one's job.

With our economy being in a state of flux and decline, being dismissed from a job has become a more common occurrence. Perhaps it may even enter the category of sanctioned losses. Yet, the person involved may feel some degree of failure, culpability, or self-imposed stigma. Psychiatric patients who lose their job because of their illness also experience failure and stigma.

Other Obstacles to Grieving

Other obstacles to grieving include

- Inability to grieve because chemical dependence totally absorbs the person's life
- An altered state of physical or mental health that warrants the placement of energy on becoming physically or mentally well again
- Facing multiple losses, as in the case in a fire or natural disaster where possessions and loved ones are lost
- Uncertainty over the loss—circumstances prevent confirmation of the certainty of the loss, as is the case with victims of war and war prisoners
- Survivors find death from sudden illness (Saunders, 1982) or death in people with complicated interpersonal relationships (Steele, 1990) more difficult to resolve

Grieving and the Psychiatric Patient

Having looked at how people not suffering from mental health problems face the major tasks of grieving, let us now explore how the psychiatric patient faces these tasks. The psychiatric patient grieves to the degree that she or he has the emotional energy and a grounding in reality to do so. In undertaking the first task of grieving—accepting the reality of the loss—the person may enter into denial as a means of coping. He or she may believe that what has been lost will be returned. Some patients may become psychotic or immersed in depression (Kutsher, 1968). These circumstances inhibit any forward movement in accomplishing the task of grieving.

Psychiatric patients may avoid facing the pain of loss by developing somatic symptoms that distract from grieving and lead to a focus on physical illness. Some patients believe that they have acquired the same illness as their lost loved one. This may lead them to engage in an extensive diagnostic work-up. Lindemann (1994) describes this as symptom formation "by identification." Energies that could be spent on facing the pain of loss and adjusting to life without the lost object are spent on finding the cause of symptoms and controlling diseases that are thought to exist. The psychiatric patient can be supported in facing the emotional pain created by the loss, especially when the pain is recognized as being emotional or psychological as opposed to physical.

The third task of grieving—adjustment to life without the "lost object"—can be difficult for the psychiatric patient if the "lost object" is the person upon whom she or he depended for support, care, and supervision. The reality of the loss can create feelings of panic revolving around survival issues. It will be necessary to help the person to designate a substitute caregiver or a different support person for her or his life. The challenge lies in helping the person not to feel totally destroyed or hopeless because of this loss.

The fourth task of grieving—letting go and moving on—can happen if the psychiatric patient is supported in her or his grieving over a period of time. Assistance is given to help the patient process the significance of the lost person. Letting go and moving on require good-byes and reminiscence, coping with feelings of abandonment, and reaching out to others.

Significant losses may trigger intense feelings of shame, self-blame, diminished worth, and a more negative self-concept. Self-blame may be related to the belief that one is directly responsible for the major loss that has occurred. The intense feelings can precipitate a dysfunctional existence that may extend over a long period. In this case, the major tasks of grieving cannot be accomplished by the person without psychiatric assistance and guidance.

▶ Check Your Reading

10. How long do people usually grieve?
11. What is the initial reaction to loss in each theorist's classification of the stages of grief?
12. Name two of the four tasks of grieving.
13. Describe normal grieving.
14. Name three of the five categories of complicated grieving.
15. In what ways do children grieve differently than adults?
16. Identify four obstacles to grieving.
17. What problems does a psychiatric patient typically encounter as he or she tries to complete the tasks of grieving?

MOVING BEYOND LOSS AND GRIEF

In discussing some basic guidelines for doing grief work, Diets (1988) emphasizes the importance of believing that grief has a purpose and that it will have an end. So many people, including the psychiatric patient, get caught in the process of trying to discover why the loss occurred. This need for a logical explanation is a natural response to any crisis or tragedy. Individuals look at what happened and want to discover who is to blame. In addition, they review how the loss happened to find meaning in what occurred. Tragedies somehow seem easier to face if a "causative factor" can be pinpointed. Yet, with some losses the person cannot find clear reasons "why," persons to blame, or particular circumstances to which the losses relate. The truth is that loss and grief occur in our lives because we are mortal human beings who live in an imperfect world with other human beings. When individuals expend too much energy on the "whys" and "hows," they often delay or prolong their period of grieving needlessly. Energies spent on pursuits related to the loss can also delay effective grief work. For example, if a person who loses a loved one in an accident caused by someone who was driving under the influence of alcohol expends a significant amount of time and energy on bringing the perpetrator to justice, then grieving may be prolonged or prevented until legal and judicial processes are resolved. This may take months or even years.

Coping with loss can become more difficult when the elements of retribution become enmeshed in the process. Grieving persons easily can blame themselves, rightfully or erroneously, for a loss that has occurred. Self-recrimination and self-inflicted punishment in the form of guilt, shame, unforgiveness, or interminable sadness will complicate grieving or slow it down significantly. The death of an infant or child from causes such as sudden infant death syndrome (SIDS), a spontaneous abortion or stillbirth, or an accident can provoke the distraught parents to blame each other. This leads to marital strife, which makes coping with the loss much more difficult.

Guilt, shame, and self-recrimination also are seen in cases of suicide. It is difficult to face the haunting thought of being responsible for the death of a loved one. Sadness is mixed with feelings of negligence for being blind to or emotionally cut off from the person who just terminated his or her life. Grieving is very painful and intense, and moving beyond the grief seems impossible.

Religious issues also may become a point of focus following loss. By nature we are all spiritual beings. At our center is a yearning for association with and reliance upon a presence greater than we are. We come to know that presence as God, our higher power, or some spiritual, bonding force. Some people believe that their loss represents God's punishment for past wrongdoings. Others may feel betrayed or abandoned by God. It is not unusual to see persons cry out to God in dismay, "How could you do this to me?," "How could you let this happen?" Thus, God may be considered the direct cause of the loss and the pain. Some curse God as they curse their fate. Over time, many will find comfort and solace in their relationship with their God and their church. A spiritual crisis (spiritual distress) precipitated by a painful loss interferes with grieving. Such a crisis may lead to further alienation and isolation on the part of the grieving person or it may be resolved in time through a deeper bonding with his or her faith community and his or her God.

Coping mechanisms are learned patterns of behavior that permit us to deal with stressful situations or crisis moments. Their effectiveness is measured by their ability to bring some form of resolution to a stressful situation or by their ability to lower the feelings of distress being experienced. We learn to cope well or poorly, effectively or ineffectively. Our coping patterns can be changed or improved as necessity dictates. Box 27–7 provides a list of coping mechanisms classified into the categories of least effective, intermediately effective, and most effective. Some of these coping mechanisms provide short-term relief when used but do not lead to problem or crisis resolution. An example of this is a sense of humor. When situations are overwhelming, being able to smile or to laugh lightens the intensity of the pain. This enables improved coping until some form of resolution of the situation is achieved.

You are invited to explore which coping mechanisms you use most. Being in touch with how you cope, as well as how you grieve your losses, will help you to become more effective as a helping professional, change agent, companion, and fellow traveler to the psychiatric patient. You also assess coping patterns when you work with the grief-stricken mental health patient.

Diets (1988) writes of the need to make a decision to go on with one's life after a major loss. If grieving people wait until they "feel better" before undertaking their grief work, precious time will be lost. They can get trapped in their grieving. This will lead to stagnation and fixation on their state of misery and pain. This is a real danger for the psychiatric patient who is prone to periods of depression and hopelessness. He or she may have a desire to regress to a "safer way of being" where they have less chance of getting involved with the pressures and responsibilities of life.

BOX 27–7 Coping Mechanisms

Least Effective

Suppression (not worring, trying to forget)

Hypervigilance (expecting the worst, being unduly alert for "trouble")

Stoic submission (displaying unquestioning acceptance, being unmoved by the worst)

Passivity (thinking that others must help one, waiting to be directed or "saved")

Acting out (striking back, doing something . . . anything)

Blaming (faulting oneself, accusing others or circumstances)

Intermediately Effective

Humor (laughing it off, seeing the lighter side)

Tension reduction (eating, drinking, playing, working, smoking, or sleeping more)

Sharing responsibilities (delegating, relying on others)

Withdrawing (removing oneself for a while, stepping back to be objective)

Ventilating (unburdening periodically, discharging repressed emotions)

Most Effective

Confronting the issues (facing reality, problem-solving)

Seeking information (learning more, consulting the "experts")

Setting priorities (redirecting energies, focusing on important things)

Redefining goals (cultivating new dreams, rekindling hope)

Seeking support (sharing with friends, accepting encouragement and empathy)

▶ Check Your Reading

18. What makes it more difficult for couples to cope with and grieve the loss of a child?
19. Define coping mechanisms.

NURSING PROCESS

Let us return to the story of Susan Smith presented earlier in the chapter. When discussing loss as an experience of the human journey, it was suggested that a loss time line be used as a means of tracking loss experiences. An example was provided using a 10-year segment of time from Susan Smith's life (see Figure 27–1).

From 1975 to 1977, Susan faced three losses—a divorce, a physical assault, and the theft of her new automobile. The losses were close to each other in time. Strong emotional responses and some grieving occurred with each loss. The loss that was the most difficult for Susan to face, however, was the death of her father in 1978. She had been very close to him. His diagnosis of pancreatic cancer came as a shock to the whole family. At the end of a nine-month period, this 72-year-old man, once so vibrant and strong, had deteriorated physically and was in the terminal phase of his illness. Susan's father died in late October of 1978. In December of that year, just two weeks before Christmas, Susan was admitted to the psychiatric unit of a large teaching hospital in her city. Her admitting diagnosis was Bereavement. The psychiatric nurse assigned to be the primary nurse for Susan met with her the day of her admission.

ASSESSMENT

Susan did not communicate very much during the initial nursing assessment. The admission note of the attending physician indicated a history of chronic depression, as well as several short inpatient stays for treatment of the depression. Susan also had had six months of therapy following her divorce. The nurse performed a comprehensive assessment focusing on physical, emotional, social, and spiritual domains. Box 27–8 presents a summary of the assessment data obtained on Susan Smith.

BOX 27-8 A Summary of the Assessment Data on Susan Smith

Physical Status

The nurse observed a 52-year-old white female with an appearance that bespoke neglect. Susan's clothes were soiled, her hair uncombed. She wore no cosmetics, looked older than her age, and sat stooped in her chair with eyes cast down. Susan looked pale and thin. She complained of weight loss, poor appetite, and indigestion when she did eat. Susan indicated that she has not been able to sleep for the last month or so.

Emotional Status

She spoke little and seemed quite withdrawn. Her responses to questions were one- or two-word answers, unless prompted to be more specific. She showed very little emotion, especially when asked about her father's death. In a sad tone she spoke of how special she had always been to him. They had always done so many things together. She could describe the details of her father's illness and death, but she offered factual information that was devoid of any feeling component. Susan was agitated at times, looking toward the door as if she were eager to leave. Most of the time she stared at the floor, finding it difficult to make eye contact.

Social Status

From the medical history, the nurse learned that Susan had become a recluse during the last three weeks. When Susan was asked about her job, she informed the nurse that she resigned three weeks ago because the pressures were too great to handle. She indicated that she liked being alone and enjoyed spending her free time in her apartment. When asked about her friends, she stated that her best friend, her father, had died.

Spiritual Status

Susan grew up attending church services in the Lutheran church. She stated that after her marriage ended so painfully, she stopped going to church. She thought God would save her father from dying so soon of the cancer. "But he [God] failed to help me, just as he did when I was struggling in my bad marriage."

DIAGNOSIS

From the behaviors that Susan presented during the assessment, the psychiatric nurse identified the following nursing diagnosis:

> Dysfunctional Grieving related to a complicated grief reaction as evidenced by withdrawal, seclusion, absence of friends and support people, self-termination of employment, spiritual distress, and self-care deficits

OUTCOME IDENTIFICATION

The expected outcomes for Susan's care include the following:

- Susan will resolve the issues surrounding her complicated grief reaction.
- Susan will display behaviors indicative of successful grieving, including returning to work, reengaging in life's activities, and resuming self-care activities; behaviors indicative of spiritual well-being; and evidence of reconnection with others.

PLANNING

Having assessed Susan's present status, the psychiatric team members developed a plan of care to assist Susan in dealing with her sadness and to help her to get in touch with her most recent loss experience and its impact on her life. In addition, the plan included a focus on improving patterns of self-care; resolving somatic symptoms such as anorexia, insomnia, and weight loss; establishing needed support systems; and promoting spiritual well-being. The period of hospitalization would be approximately two to six weeks. The short-term goals, which represented a mutual effort by Susan and the staff, were as follows:

Expected Outcomes	Short-Term Goals
1. Susan will resolve the issues surrounding her complicated grief reaction.	1. Susan will participate in sessions held three times a week with her therapist so she can explore her recent significant loss. 2. Susan will attend group therapy twice weekly and be an active participant within the group. 3. Susan will begin to express the emotions she has surrounding the loss of her father. 4. Susan will report to her case manager, or to any nurse on duty, feelings of being out of control, hopeless, unable to go on, or intensely angry.

2. Susan will display behaviors indicative of successful grieving, including returning to work, reengaging in life's activities, and resuming self-care activities; behaviors indicative of spiritual well-being; and evidence of reconnection with others.	1. Susan will bathe, comb her hair, and dress in her own clothing each day. 2. Susan will spend two hours out of bed each morning, afternoon, and evening. 3. Susan will eat four smaller meals each day and report any symptoms of discomfort that occur as a result of eating. 4. Susan will use relaxation tapes at bedtime and report to the nurse each morning how well she slept. 5. Susan will participate in the unit social activities. 6. Susan will engage in interactions with others. 7. Susan will discuss her feelings of abandonment and anger at God. 8. Susan will plan for her return to work.

IMPLEMENTATION

Before looking at the interventions that the nurse chose to work with Susan, let us take a look at Box 27–9 for general nursing interventions that you will need in working with any grieving patient. Box 27–10 lists interventions to use with grieving children.

The general skills for adult patients guided the daily interactions between Susan and her psychiatric nurse and provided the foundation for a relationship of trust and respect. The mutual goals that had been established and identified as being feasible were reviewed daily. Thus, Susan was held accountable for her plan of care. Nursing interventions focused on present needs and the fulfillment of the mutual goals. The following nursing interventions were used in assisting Susan to deal with her bereavement:

- Encourage daily hygiene, grooming, and the wearing of personal clothing, as opposed to a hospital gown.
- Monitor food consumption at meal times.
- Provide a nutritious evening snack.
- Weigh the patient twice weekly.
- Teach Susan the basic concepts of relaxation therapy; provide a tape recorder and relaxation tapes at bedtime; monitor their effectiveness.
- Provide the medications prescribed for insomnia, depression, and gastric distress and note their effectiveness.
- Stimulate social interaction by encouraging walks to the day room and providing activities for increasing amounts of time spent there.
- Hold Susan responsible for participation in individual therapy sessions and biweekly group therapy.
- Engage the patient in conversation and encourage her to share how she is feeling at a given period of the day.
- Monitor for self-destructive tendencies.
- Observe the patient for changes in affect, statements of hopelessness or self-blame, increased depression or agitation, or threats of suicide.
- Be vigilant of the patient's safety by monitoring her whereabouts, removing sharp objects, and using 24-hour observation, as needed.
- Explore feelings of abandonment expressed by the patient, provide emotional support and availability.
- Encourage Susan to verbalize her feelings of abandonment by her father and by her God.
- Help Susan to explore her relationship with her father and the meaning of her life with and without him.
- Have Susan describe her spirituality and her present relationship to her God.
- Encourage Susan to write a farewell letter to her father in which she can express some of her feelings.
- Evaluate excuses for not being able to participate in therapy sessions.
- Monitor the effectiveness of Susan's mood-altering medications and communicate the need for dose adjustment.

EVALUATION

The formative evaluation of Susan's care took place in weekly evaluations of treatment progress made by the case manager and other team members. A team conference was held during the first week of admission. Susan's treatment course and progress were discussed. Revisions were made in the plan of care as needed. The evaluations of each team member were based upon whether progress was being made in decreasing Susan's depression; whether emotional, social, spiritual, and physical well-being were being established; and whether Susan was able to initiate grief work. Susan had engaged upon the journey toward wellness, assisted by caring and supportive mental health professionals.

At the end of four weeks, Susan was discharged. The summative evaluation indicated that her mood was brighter and her affect more pleasant; she had gained 4 lb and reported sleeping much better. Susan had begun to express her feelings of loss regarding her father. She had spoken to the nurse about her feelings toward God;

BOX 27-9 General Nursing Interventions for Grieving Patients

1. **Make contact and assess.**

   Reach out.

   Be present physically and emotionally.

   Give the person permission to grieve.

   Do not allow grievers to become isolated.

   Maintain a family systems perspective.

   Conduct an assessment of the mourner's grief.

   Determine which tasks of grief are incomplete.

   Ensure griever has appropriate medical attention, if needed.

2. **Maintain a therapeutic and realistic perspective.**

   Realize that you cannot take away the pain.

   Do not let your own sense of helplessness interfere.

   Expect to tolerate volatile reactions from the bereaved.

   Recognize the value of "the gift of presence."

   View the loss from the griever's unique perspective.

   Let your genuine concern and caring show.

   Do not let your own needs determine the griever's experience.

   Do not try to explain the loss in religious or philosophical terms too early.

   Do not tell grievers to "feel better because they still have other loved ones still alive."

   Do not try to "pretty up" the situation.

   Do not forget to plant the seed of hope.

   Do not encourage responses antithetical to appropriate grief.

   Maintain appropriate distance from the griever

   Hold out the expectation that griever will recover.

3. **Encourage verbalization of feelings and recollection of the deceased.**

   Help the bereaved to recognize, actualize, and accept.

   Listen nonjudgmentally with permissiveness and acceptance.

   Assist the griever in identifying, accepting, and expressing feelings.

   If the griever is resisting the grief process, explore defenses to discover reasons behind it.

   Allow crying, talking, and reviewing without interruption except to ask for clarification.

   Do not be surprised if the griever talks about same things repeatedly.

   Do not be afraid to mention the dead person.

   Encourage the griever to realistically review his or her relationship with the deceased.

   Help the griever identify and resolve secondary losses and unfinished business.

4. **Help the griever identify current and potential secondary losses.**

   Help the griever identify any unfinished business.

   Look for appropriate ways to facilitate closure.

   Assist the griever to recognize the need to grieve for lost dreams, fantasies, and expectations.

5. **Support the griever in coping with the grief process.**

   Design interventions using the griever's positive coping skills.

   Help compensate for deficient coping skills.

   Provide the griever with normative information about the grief process.

   Make sure the griever understands that his or her reactions will be unique.

   Communicate your understanding of the pain and the wish to avoid it.

   Help the griever recognize that he or she must yield to the painful process.

   Make it clear that grief affects all areas of one's life.

   Assist the griever with appropriate time and course expectations.

   Encourage the griever to be patient and not to expect too much of self.

   Encourage the griever to give self respite times from grief.

   Help the griever find a variety of ways to replenish self.

   Suggest some form of physical activity to release feelings.

   Help the griever maintain good physical health.

   Do not support flight.

   Help the griever to deal with practical problems.

6. **Help the griever accommodate to the loss.**

   Assist in achieving appropriate perspective on meaning of resolution.

   Help the griever recognize that a major loss always changes us.

   Help the griever discover his or her new identity and the social roles he or she must assume or relinquish.

   Assess which roles and skills must be assumed and work to accomplish this.

   Help the griever form a healthy new relationship with the deceased.

   Ask how he or she will keep the deceased's memory alive.

   The griever should not be made to feel that the amount of grieving is a testimony to the deceased.

   Assist the griever to reestablish a system of belief or meaning.

7. **Work with the griever to reinvest in a new life.**

   Encourage the griever to find rewarding new things and people in which to invest.

   Do not push into new relationships.

   Help the griever identify the gain he or she has derived from the loss.

From *Grief, Dying, and Death: Clinical Interventions for Caregivers* by T. A. Rando, 1984, Champaign, IL: Research Press.

BOX 27-10 Interventions to Use With Grieving Children

- Talk, talk, talk with openness and honesty; use "teachable moments" such as the death of a pet, changing seasons, or television programs to discuss death with children.
- Assure them of their safety and physical well-being.
- Assure them of being loved.
- Explain and let them see feelings of grief; in the long run, it is best to err on the side of too much disclosure of feelings than too little.
- Assure them of the normalcy of their feelings. Let them know that loss engenders intense feelings that must be dealt with.
- Include them in rituals of mourning.
- Recognize that mourning comes and goes for them (in part, this is a denial and/or coping mechanism).
- Help the very young to remember the deceased through pictures, stories, and memories.
- Look for "magical thinking" regarding a return of the lost object.
- Recognize that children will "grow up" with their grief and so will have different experiences of the death as they mature.
- Make sure changing roles of children are appro priate for their age level.
- Recognize that children are not born afraid of death—they learn to be afraid of it.
- Know that their grief will be expressed through play, art work, and other behaviors, rather than predominantly through verbalization.

From *Grief, Dying, and Death: Clinical Interventions for Caregivers* by T. A. Rando, 1984, Champaign, IL: Research Press. Copyright 1984 by T. A. Rando. Adapted by permission.

however, she was not willing to talk to a clergy person and indicated that she still felt very angry toward God. The psychiatric team strongly advised Susan that although she had made tremendous progress, more work still needed to be accomplished. Susan was encouraged to join a support group designed for persons who have lost loved ones, as well as to continue to see an outpatient therapist.

► Check Your Reading

20. Identify at least one expected outcome in working with a patient with a nursing diagnosis of Dysfunctional Grieving.
21. Identify four interventions that you would use with a grieving adult.
22. Identify four general interventions that you would use with a grieving child.

CASE STUDY: JOSIE

Josie is a 45-year-old nurse entrepreneur who has been feeling sad and guilty that she has been unable to spend time (due to a busy, traveling schedule) with her mother, who lives in another state and is dying with cancer. Two years ago, her mother, age 68, was diagnosed with adenocarcinoma of the colon. After Josie's mother recovered from the colon resection, she underwent weekly chemotherapy treatments for 18 months.

Although Josie was able to be with her mother for the surgery and visited her several times during the 18 months of chemotherapy, she tells her friends that over the past two years, she has felt helpless to assist her family because she lives out of state. Josie has experienced episodes of crying when driving her car and chokes up when she talks to friends about her mother. Recently, she has experienced a lack of interest in sex and increasing conflict with her spouse, who seems less than supportive, and she has lost interest in attending her exercise class and has stopped attending church. On her last visit with her mother, arrangements were made for her mother to enter a local hospice program.

ASSESSMENT

Assessment data are as follows:

- Guilt, sorrow, choked feelings, and altered libido
- Change in activity level—not attending exercise class
- Feelings of helplessness and spiritual distress noted in Josie's behavior

DIAGNOSIS

***DSM-IV* Diagnosis:** Adjustment Disorder

Nursing Diagnosis: Anticipatory grieving related to anticipated loss of mother (and spouse) as evidenced by feelings of guilt, sorrow, altered libido, change in activity level, "choked" feelings, and denial and minimization of situation by spouse

OUTCOME IDENTIFICATION, PLANNING, AND IMPLEMENTATION

EXPECTED OUTCOME 1: By _____ Josie will identify and express feelings appropriately about the anticipated loss of her mother.

SHORT-TERM GOAL

By _____ the patient will identify and express feelings to self and others.

NURSING INTERVENTIONS

1. Provide an open, accepting environment so Josie feels free to discuss feelings and concerns.
2. Listen to Josie's perceptions of the situation by using therapeutic communication skills, active listening, silence, and acknowledgment.

RATIONALES

1. Accept all grief behavior—the response is highly individual, as no two people experience or behave in the same way or at the same rate.
2. Any type of meaningful loss (e.g., loss of parent, body part, role, or functioning) will precipitate a reaction that will follow the general stages or patterns of the grief response.

EXPECTED OUTCOME 2: By _____ the patient will return to previous level of functioning.

SHORT-TERM GOAL

By _____ the patient will resume normal activity within 3 weeks.

NURSING INTERVENTIONS

1. Encourage Josie to attend exercise class and discuss problems related to activity level, sexual desire, and role performance.
2. Assist in the use of creative visualization and relaxation skills for family members.
3. Provide teaching on common symptoms of grief, the strong emotional responses that can occur, and the importance of taking special care of herself during this period prior to and following a major loss.
4. Discuss control issues with family members; determine what is within the person's power to change and what is beyond her control.

RATIONALES

1–2. During the grief process, changes may occur in self-care, appetite, and activity levels, which are normal and similar to anxiety responses.

3. The availability of support persons facilitates the resolution of grief. Avoid reinforcing the belief that holding in feelings is a sign of emotional strength.

4. Feelings of control and ineffective coping skills contribute to a failure to resolve grief.

EXPECTED OUTCOME 3: By _____ the family will demonstrate acceptance of the need for counseling and hospice services support.

SHORT-TERM GOAL

By _____ the family will seek assistance during the grief process by participating in hospice care.

NURSING INTERVENTIONS

1. Encourage family members to utilize the services provided by hospice.
2. Refer to other resources such as clergy, religious affiliation, counseling, psychotherapy, and support groups as needed.
3. Incorporate family members in problem solving, supporting, and assisting the mother to deal with the situation.
4. Encourage family members to become involved in activities unrelated to the anticipated loss.

RATIONALES

1–3. The availability of support persons facilitates the resolution of grief. A strong religious faith may assist family members in dealing with loss.

4. Rational thinking and involvement in everyday activities facilitates grief resolution. Cultural and social practices support individuals adjusting to separation and loss.

Nursing Diagnosis: Spiritual Distress related to anticipated loss of mother evidenced by feelings of helplessness and separation from church ties and support

OUTCOME IDENTIFICATION, PLANNING, AND IMPLEMENTATION

EXPECTED OUTCOME 1: By _____ the daughter will verbalize spiritual concerns and feelings about anticipated loss.

SHORT-TERM GOAL	NURSING INTERVENTIONS	RATIONALES
By _____ the patient will verbalize feelings about spiritual crisis.	1. Encourage Josie to discuss what has triggered feelings of helplessness. Discuss differences between grief, guilt, and helplessness, and assist Josie to identify and deal with each.	1. Often feelings of helplessness may be triggered by false guilt. Grief occurs as a response to a loss. Guilt is about not doing something you feel you should have. Feeling helplessness occurs as response to feelings of powerlessness and loss of control over a situation.
	2. Focus on short-term, concrete goals that the patient can do now (being with her mother when she can, telephoning frequently, arranging business travel to stay over one or two days with her mother).	2. Patients may experience fewer feelings of hopelessness and helplessness if they can feel as though they are making progress in some small area.
	3. Incorporate family members in problem-solving, supporting, and assisting the mother to deal with the situation.	3. The availability of support persons facilitates the resolution of grief. A strong religious faith may assist family members in dealing with loss.
	4. Encourage family members to become involved in activities unrelated to the anticipated loss.	4. Rational thinking and involvement in everyday activities facilitates grief resolution. Cultural and social practices support individuals adjusting to separation and loss.

EVALUATION

Formative Evaluation: Josie met all of her short-term goals. She had begun to share her feelings with one of her close girlfriends and her spouse. She stated that even though she did not feel like exercising, she was making the effort, and once she got to exercise class, she felt better. While visiting her mother, she accompanied her father to church, which made her feel better and supported her father.

Summative Evaluation: Josie met all of the expected outcomes. She was able to be with her mother when hospice care was initiated. She felt very good about the hospice nurse who was to take care of her mother. As for dealing with her guilt about not spending "enough" time with her mother and not always being available to her, Josie stated, "I am aware of what is going on. I need to allow myself time to feel sad." I suggested to Josie that she work with her business partner to have some time off in the next month and to not schedule any extra activities, as her mother's condition was deteriorating. Her ongoing plan of care was continued during this process.

CASE STUDY: CAMILLA

Camilla is a 28-year-old mother who lost her three-month-old son to sudden infant death syndrome (SIDS) two years ago. Since then, she has lost over 50 pounds and is very frail in appearance, with her current weight at 99 lb on her 5′6″ frame. She has lost total interest in work and has been on leave for the past two weeks because of constant crying spells, which have interfered with customer relations at her place of employment. Her husband reports that she has lost interest in sex and becomes agitated when he suggests they try and have another child.

ASSESSMENT

Assessment data are as follows:

- Excessive crying, altered libido, lack of interest in work
- Weight loss of 50 lb over past two years
- Lack of resolution of normal grieving response

DIAGNOSIS

***DSM-IV* Diagnosis:** Adjustment Disorder

Nursing Diagnosis: Dysfunctional grieving related to lack of resolution of unresolved issues of son's death two years ago as evidenced by excessive crying, weight loss, decreased libido, and lack of interest in normal work activities

OUTCOME IDENTIFICATION, PLANNING, AND IMPLEMENTATION

EXPECTED OUTCOME 1: By _____ the patient will have 2- to 3-lb weight gain.

SHORT-TERM GOAL	NURSING INTERVENTIONS	RATIONALES
By _____ the patient will identify the weight loss as an issue related to the loss of her son and begin to gain weight by eating normally.	1. Discuss the symptom of weight loss and how it relates to the grieving process.	1. Accept all grief behavior—the response is highly individual, as no two people experience or behave in the same way or at the same rate.
	2. Motivate the patient to assume responsibility for self-care and well-being. 3. Explore with the patient fears associated with loss, particularly those related to loss of control.	2. Any type of meaningful loss (e.g., loss of parent, body part, role, or functioning) will precipitate a reaction that will follow the general stages or patterns of the grief response.

EXPECTED OUTCOME 2: By _____ the patient will work through the phases of grieving by expressing feelings about the loss of the infant to SIDS.

SHORT-TERM GOAL	NURSING INTERVENTIONS	RATIONALES
By _____ the patient will verbalize behaviors associated with the normal stages of grief.	1. Identify which stage of grief that the patient is stuck in or what is being expressed.	1. Often patients are fixed or stuck in the anger stage of the grieving process, where the anger is directed inward and toward the self. An assessment of where the patient is in the grieving process is necessary to plan effective care.
	2. Provide information about the normalcy of grieving and the typical feelings and actions associated with each of the stages of grief.	2. Knowledge of the stages of grieving may assist the patient in understanding the normal process of loss. The more significant the loss to the person, the more time is required for and the more severe the grief reaction.
	3. Encourage the patient to verbalize feelings and explore the reality of the loss and the means of resolution so she can move on with her life.	3. Verbalizing feelings in a nonthreatening, supportive environment provides the basis for the patient to deal with the reality of loss. This will assist the patient in recognizing her position within the grief process and help her come to terms with unresolved issues related to the loss.
	4. Encourage the patient to review the loss in terms of the relationship and meaning it has in her life. When necessary, point out distortions and misinterpretations of the reality of the situation.	4. Families (especially mothers) who have lost a child to SIDS often have unresolved guilt issues—they feel they could have "done something" to prevent the death of their infant. Accurate information and identification of the reality of the situation and acknowledgment of the feelings of guilt may assist the patient to begin to resolve the grief.

EXPECTED OUTCOME 3: By _____ the patient will participate in work activities and verbalize a sense of progress toward resolution of the grief and hope for the future.

SHORT-TERM GOALS	NURSING INTERVENTIONS	RATIONALES
By _____ the patient will begin to resume normal activities and return to work.	1. Assist the patient with identifying methods for more adaptive coping with the loss of her son by focusing on assets and strengths.	1. Focusing on strengths and assets promotes self-esteem, encourages repetition of desirable behaviors, and aids in assisting the patient to cope with the situation.
	2. Refer the patient to self-help groups for parents who have lost a child to SIDS (e.g., Compassionate Friends, SIDS Support Groups, National Sudden Infant Death Resource Center, SIDS Alliance).	2. Community outreach programs and groups are helpful in preventing prolonged grieving responses by providing immediate support and referral in the critical period after the death. Later, these self-help groups provide the opportunity for parents to draw support from other parents of SIDS infants.
By _____ the patient will begin to express feelings of hope for the future and a sense of control over her life situation.	1. Encourage the patient to find ways to experience pleasure as grief subsides and reinforce any experiences of pleasure.	1. Grief inhibits feelings of pleasure and joy in living.
	2. Support and encourage by reinforcing any creative efforts.	2. Creative efforts can assist the patient in discovering a new purpose in life.
	3. Encourage the use of self-affirmations.	3. Self-affirmations enhance self-esteem.

EVALUATION

Formative Evaluation: Camilla met all of the short-term goals except the last one. She stated that it was hard for her to find joy in her life at this time; however she did not feel as saddened and depressed over the situation.

Summative Evaluation: Camilla achieved all of her expected outcomes. By the end of a month, she had gained 10 pounds and was able to go back to work. She stated, "I feel better knowing that I didn't do something to cause my son's death. I carried such a burden, thinking that I did something wrong. It feels much better to know that there was nothing I could have done to cause or prevent what occurred." To help her work on feeling more pleasure and joy in her life, I encouraged her and her husband to identify those activities that they enjoyed doing when they first met. She expressed that she thought that she would feel more pleasure in time. I modified her plan of care to give her additional time to integrate pleasurable activities and actions into her future.

CONCLUSIONS

In helping patients move beyond grief and loss, we help them to realize that they are and can continue to be stronger people for having faced the challenge of grieving. People facing losses so often assume responsibilities that they may never have thought themselves capable of assuming. Circumstances require much of them. When helped to look back at how far they have come in the journey through grief, they realize that they have grown as they have moved forward. Building upon newly found strength that comes as they pass through the grief process, they can dare to dream new dreams, set new goals, foster new relationships, and pursue new undertakings.

Sandra L. Bertman (1991, p. 200), in her book *Facing Death*, writes about grieving and its effects:

Grief is not a disease. It is love not wanting to let go. It can be likened to a blow or a cut in which the wound gradually heals. For a while, one is acutely vulnerable, physically and emotionally. Though grief can be temporarily disabling, working through it ultimately brings strength.

How do you know when the psychiatric patient has completed the journey through grief and loss? The patient provides you with the information. She or he will feel and look better. Symptoms that seemed so frightening months back will be gone. Behavioral changes such as resocialization, new energy, a return to religious practices, and a new enthusiasm about being alive will be observable. As you journey with the patient through grief, you will find that the process becomes less taxing and more rewarding. Both who have journeyed together through the dark times will gain a real sense of satisfaction. Both find light, direction, purpose, and meaning.

We end this chapter with the biblical text from the book of

Ecclesiastes (3:1–8). The text fosters a sense of hope as it captures the journey of life:

There is an appointed time for everything, and a time for every affair under the heavens.
A time to be born, and a time to die; a time to plant and a time to uproot the plant.
A time to kill, and a time to heal; a time to tear down and a time to build.
A time to weep and a time to laugh; a time to mourn, and a time to dance.
A time to scatter stones, and a time to gather them; a time to embrace and a time to be far from embraces.
A time to seek, and a time to lose; a time to keep, and a time to cast away.
A time to rend, and a time to sew; a time to be silent, and a time to speak.
A time to love, and a time to hate; a time of war and a time of peace.

KEY POINTS TO REMEMBER

- Loss accompanies all human beings in their life experiences from the moment of birth to death.
- Loss is an event within the life of a person that involves giving up that which is familiar, comfortable, and personal.
- Grief is a natural response to having lost something of significance in one's life. Grief involves feelings of sadness, emptiness, longing, pain, helplessness, and sometimes despair.
- Some people have a tendency to repress loss experiences rather than to face the emotional pain of grieving them.
- A way to get in touch with losses experienced in one's life is to do a loss inventory. A part of that process requires that one explore how losses were grieved after they happened.
- Psychiatric patients know the losses that come with their mental illness. These might include poor health, frequent hospitalizations, a meager support system because of the illness, inability to maintain steady employment, lack of purpose in life, and an inadequate grasp of what is real.
- According to cultural standards maintained in our American society, to grieve freely and openly is to demonstrate some degree of weakness.
- Eric Lindemann is a pioneer in the area of grief work. He did studies on grief and loss as early as the 1940s.
- John Bowlby described mourning as a process with three overlapping stages: numbness and disbelief, disorganization, and the reorganization of one's life and person.
- Therese Rando did significant clinical work in the areas of grief and complicated grief during the 1980s and 1990s.
- People grieve in individual ways and for varying lengths of time. The grief process may extend from 12 to 24 months.
- Factors affecting a person's grief are the significance of what one has lost, the period of time it was possessed, the preparation one has had for the loss, and the emotional strength or ability to cope possessed at the time of the loss.
- Significant losses may precipitate a major grief reaction with depression and the exacerbation of the mental health problems already being treated.
- Major tasks of grieving include acceptance of the reality of the loss, experiencing the pain of loss, adjusting to life without what one has lost, and a reinvestment of energy into going on with one's life.
- "Normal" grief reactions affect the feelings, behaviors, thought patterns, and physical well-being of a person. Symptoms lose their intensity as time passes.
- Persons predisposed to encounter an abnormal or complicated grief response are the chemically addicted; psychiatric patients; those facing sudden, violent, or mutilating deaths; victims of multiple, unresolved losses or multiple deaths; parents losing a child; and those with an unhealthy or dependent relationship to the deceased.
- Treating the grief of the psychiatric patient usually requires a period of hospitalization, the use of medications, and psychotherapeutic interventions.
- Chronic grief can be characterized by attempts to keep the deceased alive by talking about him or her frequently, maintaining his or her personal things intact, or expecting that the deceased will reenter the mourner's life.
- Obstacles to grieving include societal norms about grieving patterns, gender roles and expectations, uncertainty about the loss, intolerance of slowing down to grieve, and unsanctioned losses.
- Unsanctioned losses are those losses related to situations that are not always socially acceptable, such as losses connected to abortion, suicide, divorce, nonmarital unions, extramarital affairs, homosexuality, bankruptcy, and drug abuse.
- Tragedies and losses seem easier to cope with if a "causative factor," a "why," can be identified.
- Coping with loss can become more difficult if the elements of blame and retribution become enmeshed in the process.
- It is necessary to help psychiatric patients recognize that growth and new strength for living can be the positive outcome of grieving their losses adequately.
- Helping people to say good-bye in some meaningful, creative manner will help them to let go and move on.

LEARNING ACTIVITIES

1. Prepare a loss time line covering the last five years of your life. Consider the kinds of losses you have experienced, how many you had, and whether you took some time to grieve those losses.
2. Write in your journal about losing a special person in your life. Describe what impact this has had upon you. What do you miss the most about that person? Are there some things you wish you would have said to him or her? Write about these things.
3. Read a book or some journal articles about the effects that the death of children, be they well children or sick children, have upon their parents. How do the parents usually cope?
4. What are your thoughts about suicide? If you need to, read more about its occurrence among people with mental health problems and problems with addictions. Talk with a friend about this topic.
5. Plan how you would help a patient deal with the losses in life faced because of mental health problems. Consider how mental illness has affected his or her life and well-being. Make your plan holistic.

CRITICAL THINKING EXERCISE

Mrs. Naver, a 26-year-old mother of two children in her third month of pregnancy, was admitted to the obstetrical unit with vaginal hemorrhaging at 1:00 a.m. By 7:00 a.m., it was clear that she was having a miscarriage. As Nurse Anders gently approached Mrs. Naver to assess her condition, the patient in a tearful, soft-spoken voice stated, "Why do those babies have to cry so loud, they kept me awake all night."

1. What assumption(s) can you make about Mrs. Naver?
2. How would you test these assumptions?
3. What inferences can you draw about the approach Nurse Anders should use?

As Nurse Anders is about to respond to Mrs. Naver's comment, Nurse Barr, a married nurse without children, comes into the room and tells the patient that she officially had a miscarriage and needs to have a surgical procedure to remove the remaining contents of her uterus. As the patient begins to sob loudly, Nurse Barr states, "At least you have two other children."

1. How do you think Mrs. Naver responded to Nurse Barr's comment?
2. What assumption(s) is Nurse Barr making?
3. How might she determine if her assumptions are faulty?

REFERENCES

American Psychological Association. (1994). *Diagnostic and statistical manual, fourth edition.* Washington, D. C.: American Psychological Association.

Averill, J. R. (1979). The functions of grief. In C. E. Izard (Ed.), *Emotions and personality and psychopathology.* New York: Plenum Press.

Bertman, S. L. (1991). *Facing death.* New York: Taylor and Francis Publishers.

Bouvard, M. (1988). *The path through grief.* Wellesley, MN: Brewer Press.

Bowlby, J. (1969). *Attachment and loss.* Vol. I. New York: Basic Books.

Bowlby, J. (1980). *Attachment and loss. Vol. III. Loss, sadness, and depression.* New York: Basic Books.

Caplan, G. (1974). Forward. In I. Glick, R. Weiss, and C. M. Packer (Eds.), *The first year of bereavement.* New York: Wiley and Sons.

Carson, V. (1995). Losses and endings in the nurse-patient relationship. In E. Arnold, and K. Bogg (Eds.), *Interpersonal relationships: Professional communication skills for nurses* (2nd ed.). New York: W. B. Saunders.

Carter, S. (1989). Themes of grief. *Nursing Research,* November/December, *38* (6), 354–358.

Catholic Biblical Association. (1983). *The new American Bible.* New York: Thomas Nelson.

Corless, I. B., Germino, B. B., and Pittman, A. (1994). Attitudes toward death: A personal perspective. In *Death, dying and bereavement.* Boston: Jones and Bartlett.

Corey, G. (1977). *Theory and practices of counseling and psychotherapy.* Belmont, CA: Brooks-Cole.

Demi, A. S., et al. (1987). Relationship of parental grief to sibling grief. *Archives of Psychiatric Nursing,* Sec. 1 (6), 385–391.

Diets, B. (1988). *Life after loss.* Tucson, AZ: Fisher Books.

Doka, K. (1989). *Disenfranchised grief—Recognizing hidden sorrow.* Washington, D. C.: Lexington Books.

Engel, G. (1964). Grief and grieving. *American Journal of Nursing, 64,* (7), 93–96.

Fiefel, H. (1959). The meaning of death. New York: McGraw-Hill.

Firth, R. (1964). *Elements of social organization.* Boston: Beacon Press.

Freud, S. (1959). *Mourning and melancholia.* In Collected Papers. Vol. 4. New York: Basic Books.

Gyulay, J. E. (1989). Grief responses. *Issues in Comprehensive Pediatric Nursing, 12,* 1–31.

Hutti, M. H. (1988). A quick reference table of interventions to assist families to cope with pregnancy loss or neonatal death. *Birth,* March, *15* (1), 33–35.

Kastenbaum, R. (1977). Death, society and human experience. C. V. Mosby.

Klepsen, M. (1978). How long does grief go on? *American Journal of Nursing, 78* (3) 420–421.

Krauss, P., and Goldfischer, M. (1988). *Why me?—Coping with grief, loss, and change.* New York: Bantam Books.

Kübler-Ross, E. (1969). *On death and dying.* New York: Macmillan.

Kutscher, A. (1968). Psychiatric implications in bereavement. In *Death and Bereavement.* Springfield, IL: Charles C Thomas.

Lindemann, E. (1944). Symptomatology and management of acute grief. *American Journal of Psychiatry,* #101, 141–148.

Marzuk, P. M., Tierney, H., Tardieff, K., Gross, E. M., Morgan, E. B., Hsu, M., and Mann, J. J. (1988). Increased risk of suicide in persons with AIDS. *Journal of the American Medical Association, 259,* 1333–1337.

Miles, H. S., and Demi, A. C. (1983–1984). Toward the development of a theory of bereavement guilt. *Omega, 14* (4), 299–314.

Moore, I. M., et. al. (1988). Psychosomatic symptoms in parents two years after the death of a child with cancer. *Nursing Research,* March–April, *37* (2), 104–107.

Parkes, C. M. (1972). *Bereavement: Studies of grief in adult life.* New York: International Universities Press.

Parkes, C. M. (1964). Recent bereavement as a cause of mental illness. *British Journal of Psychiatry, 110,* 198–204.

Parkes, C. M., and Weiss, R. (1983). *Recovery from bereavement.* New York: Basic Books.

Pine, V. (1972). Social organization and death. *Omega, 3* (2), 149–153.

Rando, T. (1984). *Grief, dying and death: Clinical interventions for caregivers.* Champaign, IL: Research Press.

Rando, T. (1993). *Treatment of complicated mourning.* Champaign, IL: Research Press.

Sanders, C. (1982). Effects of sudden versus chronic illness death on bereavement outcome. *Omega, 13* (2), 227–241.

Schneider, J. (1980). Clinically significant differences between grief, pathological grief, and depression. *Patient Counseling and Education,* Fourth Quarter, 267–275.

Stearns, A. (1984). *Living through personal crisis.* Chicago: The Thomas Moore Press.

Steele, L. L. (1990). The death surround: Factors influencing the grief experience of survivors. *Oncology Nursing Forum, 17* (2), 235–241.

Veninga, R. (1985). *The gift of hope: How we survive our tragedies.* New York: Little, Brown and Company.

Volkan, V. (1970). Typical findings in pathological grief. *Psychiatric Quarterly, 44,* 231.

Westberg, G. (1971). *Good grief.* Philadelphia: Fortress Press.

Wolfelt, A. (1991a). Helping yourself heal when someone loved dies. *Thanatos,* Spring, 11, 12.

Wolfelt, A. (1991b). Toward an understanding of complicated grief: A comprehensive overview. *The American Journal of Hospice and Palliative Care,* March/April, 28–30.

Wolfelt, A. (1990). Gender roles and grief: Why men's grief is naturally complicated. *Thanatos,* Fall, 20–24.

Worden, W. (1982). *Grief counseling and grief therapy—A handbook for the mental health practitioner.* New York: Springer Publishing.

Zambelli, G. C., et al. (1988). An interdisciplinary approach to clinical intervention for childhood bereavement. *Death Studies,* January–February, *12* (1), 41–50

SUGGESTED READINGS

Diets, B. (1988). *Life after loss.* Tucson, AZ: Fisher Books.

Rando, T. (1993). *Treatment of complicated mourning.* Champaign, IL: Research Press.

Worden, W. (1982). *Grief counseling and grief therapy—A handbook for the mental health practitioner.* New York: Springer Publishing.

Westberg, G. (1971). *Good grief.* Philadelphia: Fortress Press.

UNIT V
THE WOUNDED TRAVELER

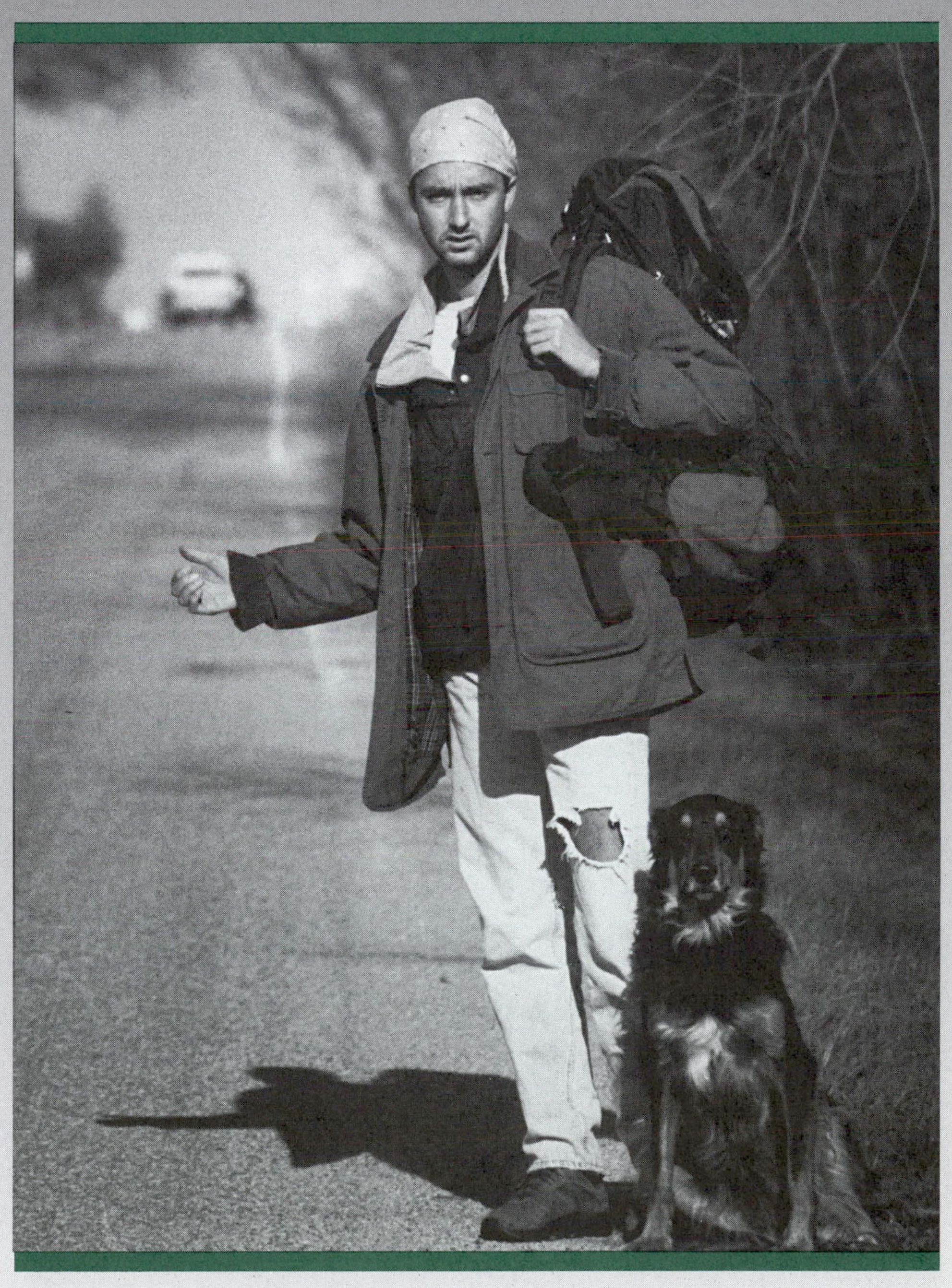

CHAPTER 28

THE JOURNEY THREATENED BY STRESS AND ANXIETY DISORDERS

This is, I think, very much the Age of Anxiety, the age of neurosis, because along with so much that weighs on our minds there is perhaps even more that grates on our nerves.

—Louis Kronenberger

LEARNING OBJECTIVES

After studying this chapter, you should be able to:

1. Recognize signs and symptoms of anxiety.
2. Identify various defense mechanisms.
3. Recognize coping behaviors.
4. Differentiate between defense mechanisms and coping behaviors.
5. Conceptualize effective nursing strategies to decrease the identified signs and symptoms of anxiety overload.
6. Apply the nursing process to a patient with an anxiety disorder.
7. Discuss the effect of stress on a patient's journey.

KEY TERMINOLOGY

Agoraphobia
Anxiety
Anxiety disorders
Anxiolytic
Coping
Defense mechanism
Generalized anxiety disorder
Obsessive-compulsive disorder
Panic disorder
Posttraumatic stress disorder
Social phobia
Specific phobia
Stress

Maturation is the task of a lifetime. It is known that growth and development do not begin at birth or end at a definitive age but that progressive unfolding is a journey traversing all the years of a person's life. In all lives, periods of contentment, sadness, and curiosity lead to growth, happiness, and sometimes despair. Life is sometimes in balance and sometimes not. During those parts of the journey that are not balanced, people tend to be more vulnerable to **anxiety,** the feeling of alertness and concern that prepares the person to take action of some kind. Anxiety, in normal proportions, is a trigger that is helpful to growth. Normal anxiety is short term and of low to moderate intensity. Sometimes anxiety balloons to greater proportions in which it is not useful. Sometimes it is transformed into crippling physical or psychological symptoms. This chapter is about those occurrences.

Mild to moderate feelings of vague unease are felt by almost everyone during periods of unrest throughout the life journey. Frequently these periods precede growth-producing events, such as learning to walk, going to nursery school for the first time, leaving grade school for junior high, going away to college, getting ready for one's wedding and for one's first child, retirement, and planning care for one's aged parents.

Feelings ranging from severe anxiety to panic are experienced by between 3% and 8% of the general population. **Anxiety disorders** are characterized by symptoms of anxiety and by efforts to avoid those symptoms. The latter are behavioral efforts at avoidance or transformation of anxiety into physical complaints.

Acute anxiety is an unbearable feeling. It includes sensations of physiological arousal. Perceptual capacities are narrowed. Cognitive abilities are significantly reduced as the person focuses intently on the identified trigger (stimulus) for the response. Anxiety is considered abnormal when reasons for it are not evident or when manifestations are excessive in intensity and duration (Hoehn-Saric, 1979; Brown et al, 1994). The manifestations of anxiety are felt holistically. Box 28–1 shows the range of physical, emotional, cognitive, and spiritual signs and symptoms of anxiety.

Research suggests that anxiety may arise from neuronal activity in the limbic system of the brain. Also indicated are such neurotransmitters as norepinephrine and serotonin, which are the stimulating neurotransmitters within the central nervous system. Gamma aminobutyric acid (GABA) is the major inhibitory central nervous system neurotransmitter. The discovery of stimulatory and inhibitory neurotransmitters led to the hypothesis that a possible interaction between the neurotransmitters may lead to the modulation of anxiety and the effects of drugs, called **anxiolytics**, that decrease anxiety (Hill, 1991).

The following story depicts the plight of Susan, a moderately anxious woman, who has partially transformed her anxiety into a symptom on which she focuses to the exclusion of her underlying problem.

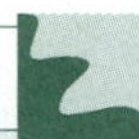

SUSAN'S STORY

I don't think that you can help me but I came anyhow... It's my last hope. I know that there is something terribly wrong with me because I keep having awful thoughts that get into my head and I don't know how long it will be before I start saying things that I am ashamed of. I don't want you to ask me about them because I am too embarrassed to tell you. I want you to help me to control myself. I am not that kind of person. I can't understand myself because I am really shy and terribly conservative. But something is so terribly wrong with me. These thoughts are really crazy. I don't know where they come from. I can be in the middle of the market, or waiting in line to buy a ticket to the movies, or even at my typewriter on the job and the thoughts just pop up. I try to make myself think of other things, but the more I try to think differently, the more I think of the bad thoughts. I feel desperate. I don't know what to do to shut my brain down. I know that something in me wants to blurt everything out and that someday I won't be able to control it. If I ever do that, I shall have to kill myself because I wouldn't be able to stand my shame.

► Check Your Reading

1. Define anxiety.
2. What is the difference between "normal" and "abnormal" anxiety?
3. What is the category of medication that is frequently used to treat anxiety?

The group of disorders characterized by intense anxiety or efforts to alter that experience include panic disorder (with and without agoraphobia—fear of being in an area with no escape), the phobic disorders (irrational and paralyzing fears), obsessive-compulsive disorder (OCD), generalized anxiety disorder, posttraumatic stress disorder (PTSD), anxiety associated with a medical condition, and substance-induced anxiety. All of these conditions are described in the American Psychiatric

BOX 28-1 Physical, Emotional, Cognitive, and Spiritual Signs and Symptoms of Anxiety

Physical

Dry mouth

Elevated vital signs

Diarrhea

Increased urination

Nausea

Diaphoresis

Hyperventilation

Fatigue

Insomnia

Sexual dysfunction

Irritability

Tenseness

Emotional

Fear

Impending doom

Helplessness

Insecurity

Low self-confidence

Anger

Guilt

Cognitive

With mild anxiety, increased awareness and problem-solving abilities

With anxiety increased above mild, narrowed perceptual field, missed details, diminished problem-solving skills

Deteriorated logical thinking

Spiritual

Hopelessness

Feeling of being cut off from God

Anger at God for allowing the anxiety

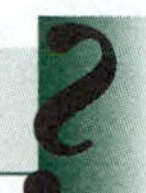

WHAT PATIENTS NEED TO KNOW **Anxiety**

What is anxiety?
Anxiety is a diffuse response to a vague threat. Fear, on the other hand, is an acute response to a clear-cut external threat.

What are the symptoms of anxiety?
Because anxiety symptoms are vague, it is often more difficult to describe accurately. The physical symptoms of anxiety include an increase in blood pressure and heart rate. The palms become sweaty and the pupils dilate. The feelings that are involved during an anxiety attack are guilt, grief, and anger. Intellectual symptoms include an altered perception of events, inability to concentrate, indecisiveness, inability to learn or reason, and worry. Social symptoms include talkativeness or extreme quietness, apprehension with groups of people, and fear of losing control in social situations. In addition, the person who experiences anxiety may describe spiritual symptoms such as fear of death, failure, or the future; feelings of hopelessness and despair; and the inability to find meaning in life.

What are the different levels of anxiety?
The four levels of anxiety range from mild to severe. Mild anxiety is common and can be beneficial. Persons who experience mild anxiety are alert, aware, and able to problem-solve. With moderate anxiety, people experience tension and fear and a greater increase in the physical symptoms such as blood pressure and heart rate. They have a sense of helplessness and also an ability to increase a focus in one area and to shut out irrelevant data. With severe anxiety, the physical symptoms are exaggerated and the person is obviously distressed. He or she has a fear of going crazy or of losing control and greatly diminished perception. During a panic level of anxiety, continued physical arousal occurs, and the person is emotionally overwhelmed. At this point, he or she responds only to internal distress and feels as if he or she is going to die.

What can be done to alleviate anxiety?
Many medications can be used to treat anxiety. In addition, forms of behavioral therapy that include systematic desensitization, relaxation, and guided imagery are very effective. Support and encouragement are also helpful when used with therapy that focuses on understanding and on the internal conflicts that produce anxiety.

Association's *Diagnostic and Statistical Manual of Mental Disorders–IV (DSM-IV)*, published in 1994.

Anxiety disorders are common in the modern world. Indeed, the years since World War II have been termed the "Age of Anxiety." A large scale study found a one-month prevalence of 7.3% for anxiety disorders and a lifetime prevalence of 14.6% (Schatzberg, 1991). In general, anxiety disorders are far more common in women than in men.

THEORIES OF ANXIETY

Several categories of theories concern the etiology of anxiety, including the psychobiological, psychodynamic, and behavioral. We examine these three.

Psychobiological Theories

The Limbic System and Anxiety

In the laboratory setting, it has been revealed that a definite anatomical pathway through the *limbic system* underlies the experience of anxiety. The limbic system is composed of a group of structures that form a border separating the structures of the brain stem (pons and medulla) from the major sensory systems of the cortex. The *first limbic pathway* includes the *hypothalamus* and *thalamus*.

The hypothalamus is especially important to the regulation of endocrine functions. It receives impulses from all limbic structures and is the major output pathway of the limbic system. The *second circuit* of the system contains the *amygdala* and *hippocampus*. These structures are involved with memory and evaluation of sensory information. Research findings suggest that the association of prior experiences converges with sensory input within the hippocampus and amygdala and influences the degree of hypothalamic responses. The *third limbic pathway* is the *cingulate gyrus/septal circuit*. Stimulation of this area, also known as the pleasure zone, elicits sexual functions and social behaviors. This area forms a transitional space between the cortex and limbic structures and sends signals from the cortex to the lower limbic structures (Hill, 1991; Brown et al, 1994).

Neurotransmitters and Anxiety

The anatomical pathways of anxiety provide the structures and pathways that electrical impulses traverse to receive input or to affect a response. Chemical actions provided by the neurotransmitters and their receptors inhibit, stimulate, or modulate the activities of the limbic system. The monoamine and GABA receptors are the primary chemical regulators of anxiety. The monoamine, or catecholamine, neurotransmitters include epinephrine, norepinephrine, dopamine, and serotonin. These neurotransmitters are involved in emotion, attention, and visceral regulation. Their receptors are found in blood vessels, heart, and lung tissue. Over 50% of the brain's norepinephrine-producing neurons are located in the locus coeruleus, a dense group of neurons within the fourth ventricle.

Research suggests that norepinephrine plays a role in anxiety and may be responsible for its amplification. GABA is the most abundant neurotransmitter in the brain. Its concentration is 200 to 1000 times greater than that of norepinephrine or serotonin. GABA's action seems to be completely inhibitory and involves 30% to 50% of all neurons. GABA is thought to be involved in the modulation of sleep, lowering muscle tone, and reduction of anxiety (Hill, 1991). The therapeutic effect of anxiolytics on anxiety occurs through the decrease of activity of serotonin or the enhancement of GABA.

► **Check Your Reading**

4. What neurotransmitters are the prime regulators of anxiety?
5. Where are the monoamine neurotransmitters found?
6. What role does the limbic system play in the development of anxiety?
7. Compare the action of norepinephrine and GABA in modulating anxiety.
8. How do the therapeutic effects of the anxiolytic drugs occur?

Psychodynamic Theories

Sigmund Freud, the father of psychoanalysis and himself a neurologist of the 19th century, postulated that anxiety resulted from a failure to repress painful memories, impulses, or thoughts. He believed that some of the symptoms of the anxiety disorders were actually the memories, impulses, or thoughts that broke into consciousness in disguised forms. The psychodynamic theories suggest that anxiety is the result of an intrapsychic struggle between id and superego to hold in (repress) conflicted impulses or to have them emerge into consciousness through the ego.

Behavioral Theories

Most behaviorists, such as Watson and Skinner, believe that anxiety is the outcome of conditioning. That is, anxiety is a learned response. They theorize that a person must experience the physiological symptoms of anxiety to be conditioned to an event that is then recognized as the psychological or subjective response that is called "anxiety." This theory is the basis for biofeedback treatment, in which the patient is taught to regulate various physiological processes that cause his or her symptoms. For a fascinating account of the research underlying biofeedback, see Restak's (1980) *The Brain: The Last Frontier*.

► **Check Your Reading**

9. According to Freud, what causes anxiety?
10. What do the behaviorists say about anxiety?
11. How does biofeedback treatment relate to anxiety's being a conditioned response?

STRESS

It is almost impossible to discuss anxiety without also exploring **stress**. (See also Chapter 37.) In the complex, technological climate of the 20th century world in which we live, stress is ubiquitous. No one is insulated from its effects, which include anxiety. Contemporary research has revealed that the stress response is a prolonged psychophysiological reaction. Its initial phase manifests itself through perceived anxiety. The stress response is set into motion at any time that an individual is affected by an event that is perceived as threatening to the self. Such an event may be the presence of another person or that person's statements; it may be a natural disaster; or it may be nothing more problematic than a cold. A person defines and responds to a stressor based on the meaning that it holds for him or her. Because of individual interpretation, stressors are frequently person specific. However, major stressors, such as illness, accidents, and catastrophic events, are almost universally recognized as tremendously distressing. According to Lazarus and Folkman (1984), psychological stress "is a particular relationship between the person and the environment that is appraised by the person as taxing and/or exceeding his or her resources and endangering his or her well being." This appraisal is succeeded by a series of physiological responses that can be categorized within a temporal context. A stress response has three phases: immediate, intermediate, and long term.

The Immediate Stress Response

In the immediate response, the autonomic nervous system is activated after the person perceives a threat or taxing demand from the environment. The body prepares for "fight or flight." The effects of sympathetic stimulation occur within two to three seconds and last between 5 and 10 minutes. Sympathetic nerve fibers release the catecholamines epinephrine and norepinephrine. At this point, anxiety is experienced and can be observed both through the individual's verbal report and through clinical signs, including perspiration, tremulousness, and rapid pulse and breathing. The *DSM-IV* identifies Acute Stress Disorder as a new disorder with diagnostic criteria occurring over more than two days and no more than a month in connection with a traumatic event. The diagnostic criteria for this disorder are presented in the Medical Diagnoses and Related Nursing Diagnoses box on page 710.

The Intermediate Stress Response

During the intermediate response, which begins within two to three minutes after the presentation of the stressor, stimulation continues via the neurotransmitters, which have triggered the end organs. Gluconeogenesis is also triggered, which provides the body with additional energy (Robinson, 1990).

The Long-Term Stress Response

The long-term response involves the endocrine system, which has multiple effects, such as elevating blood pressure and altering the breakdown of fats and proteins for energy.

▶ **Check Your Reading**

12. What is the relationship between stress and anxiety?
13. In what ways are stressors "person specific?"
14. Describe the characteristics of the immediate stress response.
15. When does the intermediate stress response occur?
16. What is the long-term stress response?

The Relationship Between Anxiety and Stress

Anxiety is one dimension of the broader stress response. Anxiety is a felt psychological state that has a definable physiological component. It is a sensation triggered by a perceived threat, and it is experienced in a range of feelings, from mild anxiety through panic. Anxiety is not always bad. In the healthy range it alerts the person to danger, enabling preparation for survival. Without the alerting levels of mild anxiety, people would not be able to ready themselves for protective action. On the other hand, at the panic end of the spectrum, preparation for organized protective action usually is not possible. It is important for you to assess an anxious patient's level of response to design nursing care to bring that anxiety into the normal, healthy range, so that the patient can more effectively cope with perceived stressors. Table 28–1 summarizes the characteristics of the four levels of anxiety.

Mild anxiety, which is useful in preparing to protect self, is evident in persons facing a routine visit to the dentist or on a short jog to the bus stop to avoid being late for work. At this level, patients are alert and able to concentrate and solve problems. Such persons feel "ready to go." They do not require intervention, although supportive statements are useful. In the hospital setting, when you observe that a preoperative patient is mildly anxious, you might tell the patient that most people feel a little jittery before their operations, but that the surgery will soon be over. Concentrating on the passage from going to sleep to awakening in the recovery room provides a time frame to the patient that helps to anchor the person in a familiar or at least an understandable context. Having an end point that limits the unknown of the surgical experience and loss of awareness through anesthesia may help to keep anxiety within healthy limits.

Moderate anxiety causes subjective symptoms that interfere with coping and problem-solving. The person is more focused on the stressful issue but less able to attend to other events: the perceptual field is narrowed. The person is aware of physiological changes such as sweating of hands and feet, dry mouth, tense muscles, slight tremor of extremities, and decreased appetite. The moderately anxious person may report feeling hot, sick, shaky, and unable to sit still.

Moderate anxiety might also be felt after a narrow escape from a traffic accident or while expecting criticism from a perceived authority figure. Patients experiencing this level of anxiety can be helped by a variety of interventions that create distraction or calming (Box 28–2). Although the interventions in Box 28–2 are useful in promoting distraction and relaxation, they cannot be used to teach. Box 28–3 demonstrates how to teach relaxation by means of guided imagery.

Severe anxiety and *panic* are infrequently observed outside of the emergency department or psychiatric unit. In this state, patients are unable to think clearly because attention and concentration are markedly reduced. Sym-

TABLE 28–1 Characteristics of the Four Levels of Anxiety

Level	Physiological	Emotional	Cognitive	Subjective
Mild	Increase in pulse, B/P, and heart rate due to sympathetic arousal	Affect positive	Alert; aware; able to problem-solve	Attentive
Moderate	Muscle tension; diaphoresis; pupils dilated; increased pulse, B/P, and breathing rate; peripheral vasoconstriction	Tension, fear	Attention focused on issue of concern; able to shut out irrelevant data	Sense of helplessness; apprehensive expectation; sweating of palms; vigilance and irritability
Severe	"Fight or flight" responses; generalized sympathetic nervous system response; dry mouth; numbness of extremities	Distress, trembling	Sensory perception greatly reduced; person can focus only on small details; learning cannot occur	Dyspnea, dizziness; fear of going crazy; visual disturbances; motor tension with hyperactivity
Panic	Continued arousal	Emotionally overwhelmed; may regress to primitive coping behaviors	Responds only to internal distress	Feelings of impending doom or death; chest pain or discomfort

BOX 28-2 Nursing Strategies to Reduce Patient Anxiety

- Active listening to show acceptance
- Honesty; answering all questions at the client's level of understanding
- Clearly explaining procedures, surgery, and policies and giving appropriate reassurance based on data
- Acting in a calm, unhurried manner
- Speaking clearly, firmly (but not loudly)
- Giving information about laboratory tests, medications, treatments, rationale for restrictions on activity
- Setting reasonable limits and providing structure
- Encouraging patients to explore reasons for the anxiety
- Encouraging self-affirmation through positive statements, such as "I will," "I can"
- Using play therapy with dolls, puppets, games, drawing for young patients
- Using touch, giving warm baths, back rubs
- Initiating recreational activities, such as physical exercise, music, card games, board games, crafts, reading
- Teaching breathing and relaxation exercises
- Using guided imagery
- Practicing covert rehearsal

Data from Gerrard, B., Boniface, W., and Love, B. (1980). *Interpersonal skills for health professionals.* Reston, VA: Reston Publishing.

pathetic nervous system stimulation has caused increased blood pressure, pulse, and respirations. Subjective reports might include a felt inability to sit down, nausea, agitation, shortness of breath, and panicky statements such as "I am going to pass out" or "I am going to die" or "I am going crazy." Clearly, such patients require immediate nursing intervention. Severe anxiety has caused decompensation of ego functions so that the patient is overwhelmed with feeling and has a significant lessening of the capacity to think and problem-solve. This extreme reaction might be observed in persons involved in a major automobile accident, in a patient who has just been told about a terminal illness, or in one who is reacting to bad news about a significant other. Such a patient requires the immediate psychological and sometimes physical support of the nurse. The patient should not be left alone. His or her deficits in focused thinking, affect modulation, and problem-solving require the capacities of the nurse as an "alter ego" whose functions have not been impaired by anxiety. Such patients need specific instructions if task completion is required. In some cases, anxiolytic medication may be appropriate.

Mild to moderate anxiety is experienced by almost everyone. Most individuals have used conscious (voluntary) behaviors to alter the unpleasant experience. These behaviors are called **coping**. Examples of the use of coping to reduce anxiety include distraction, avoidance, and seeking information.

Preconscious and unconscious (involuntary) processes used to alter anxiety are called **defense mechanisms**. Their use permits the person to avoid the painful experience of anxiety or to transform anxiety into a more tolerable symptom. Defense mechanisms include, but are not limited to, repression, suppression, projection, introjection, reaction formation, undoing, displacement, denial, and regression (Box 28–4).

Your recognition of defense mechanisms and coping behaviors is a signal that the patient feels anxious. Two broad categories of response exist. The first is to help the patient to feel less anxious. You might administer a PRN anxiolytic drug, involve the patient in distracting or calming activities, or facilitate avoidance of the threat. The second option is to facilitate the patient's exploration of the cause of that anxiety. That choice necessitates purposive interviewing. The patient needs to be made aware that he or she is experiencing anxiety. Then, the interview is used to explore the basis of the patient's experience. If the patient feels moderate to severe anxiety, nursing care should be focused on anxiety reduction. Only if the patient is experiencing mild, well-controlled anxiety should its cause be probed.

BOX 28-3 Teaching Relaxation by Means of Guided Imagery

Place the patient in a quiet, calm environment that is free from other distractions such as noise, strong light, or extraneous conversation. You might choose to sit away from the direct gaze of the person and ask him or her to select a place that has been conducive to rest and peace in the past. Then, ask the patient to close his or her eyes, if desired, and to imagine that peaceful place. Ask the patient to describe the place in terms of its appearance, its odors if appropriate, and other sensual characteristics such as its temperature. Use a quiet, subdued tone of voice to avoid interrupting the mood that is being established. Should the patient identify a place such as the beach, you can prompt responses with such nonthreatening questions as "What does the sky look like? What color is it? Is the air warm? How does the warm sand feel to your body? Are you alone on the beach?" You also could say "Tell me how the water feels to your foot. Tell me more about the things that you think and do at the beach." All of these questions require that the patient focus on the place that is being described. Gradually, his or her focus on the stressful event is weakened, resulting in a temporary diminution of anxiety. Relaxation occurs as a result of associations with the nonthreatening and calming beach.

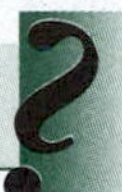

WHAT PATIENTS NEED TO KNOW Panic Attacks

What is a panic attack?
A panic attack is a specific period of intense fear or discomfort that is accompanied by at least four of the following symptoms: palpitations, pounding heart, or increased heart rate; sweating; trembling or shaking; sensations of smothering or difficulty breathing; feeling of choking; chest pain; nausea; feeling dizzy or faint; feeling of unreality, losing control, or going crazy; numbness; and chills or flushes. People who are having panic attacks often fear they are having a heart attack and have the desire to run away.

What causes them?
The most current research indicates that an underlying chemical imbalance causes a panic attack. It is also thought that the tendency to experience panic attacks can be inherited.

How are panic attacks treated?
Tricyclic antidepressant medications are very effective in treating panic attacks, but they may require several weeks of use before they are effective. Other types of medication may be needed during an acute attack. Assuring the person that he or she is not dying is very important. It is equally important that you remain calm and move the person to a quiet area.

What can I do to help myself if I feel an approaching panic attack?
It is important to reinterpret the symptoms you are feeling as anxiety and not as a heart attack or impending death. When you feel the symptoms of panic beginning, breathe into a paper bag until you begin to calm down. This type of treatment is very effective and works much of the time.

BOX 28-4 Defense Mechanisms

Repression

This is the most basic of defense mechanisms. Components of it are present in many of the more complex defenses. In repression, whatever is a threat to the ego is banished from awareness. For instance, a person with multiple personalities is unaware of the alter egos because they are banished from awareness through repression.

Suppression

This mechanism is similar to "forgetting." The individual does not have recall for the threatening event but if cued is capable of remembering. Through suppression, threats to the ego are avoided.

Projection

The utilization of this mechanism causes threats to the ego to be disavowed by perceiving them to be outside of the self. Thus, the person who is angry assumes the object of the anger to be angry at him or her. This is a transformation of the anger, which is a threat to the ego.

Introjection

The process of taking in characteristics of others begins early in life. In its healthy form, children adopt morals and values from parents through this process. Introjection is related to three defenses: *identification*, *imitation*, and *incorporation*. Identification and imitation are more mature defenses, while incorporation is one that is primitive, e.g., it develops in infancy and involves the taking in of whole aspects of the parent or other model.

Reaction Formation

This mechanism disguises the person's actual feeling that is too threatening to experience. Thus, the person is aware of the opposite of his or her actual feeling, while the real, underlying feeling is repressed.

Undoing

With this mechanism, a thought or action is utilized to negate an anxiety-provoking experience. For instance, the person with obsessive-compulsive traits might keep several scheduling books to hold in check the impulse to be free of social restraints.

Displacement

This is a commonly used mechanism that alters the object of threatening feelings. For instance, a child might be angry at the teacher but instead picks a fight with a peer on the playground at recess.

Denial

Two forms of this mechanism exist: one is denial of a fact, and the other is denial of the significance of the fact. The first form is the more serious because it alters reality. The second alters one's response to that reality. As an example, denial is used when a patient does not accept that he or she has a drinking problem. An example of the less serious form of denial is seen when a person is persistently late for a scheduled class because that person is actually very fearful of the topic.

Regression

This mechanism makes it possible for the threatened person to move backward developmentally to a place where he or she is more secure. One who feels tense in social situations might physically lean on a partner and be quieter than usual. That person might also become uncharacteristically boisterous as in earlier adolescence. An example of regression in its most malignant form is when psychiatric patients who are acutely ill give up all social graces such as wearing clothes and using the toilet and eating, necessitating complete nursing care that mimicks the parenting provided when the patient was an infant.

As you read the following pages, you will explore the major categories of anxiety disorders described in the American Psychiatric Association's *Diagnostic and Statistical Manual of Mental Disorders–IV (DSM-IV)*. You also will learn about the therapeutic strategies used to treat these conditions and how to apply the nursing process to anxiety disorders. In the *DSM-IV*, the anxiety disorders (or anxiety and phobic neuroses) are categorized as follows:

- Panic Disorder Without Agoraphobia
- Panic Disorder With Agoraphobia
- Agoraphobia Without History of Panic Disorder
- Specific Phobia
- Social Phobia
- Obsessive-Compulsive Disorder
- Posttraumatic Stress Disorder
- Acute Stress Disorder
- Generalized Anxiety Disorder
- Anxiety Disorder Due to . . . [general medical condition]
- Substance-Induced Anxiety Disorder
- Anxiety Disorder Not Otherwise Specified

In this chapter, we focus on generalized anxiety disorder, panic disorder with and without agoraphobia, obsessive-compulsive disorder, posttraumatic stress disorder, specific phobia, and social phobia. While learning about these disorders, keep in mind that the underlying problems for the patient are the *experience* of anxiety and the *behaviors* used to control or to disguise the anxiety to minimize pain in his or her journey.

▶ Check Your Reading

17. Differentiate among mild, moderate, severe, and panic levels of anxiety.
18. What is the difference between coping and defense mechanisms?
19. At which level of anxiety do people think more clearly?
20. At which level of anxiety do people begin to experience physiological responses?
21. At which level of anxiety is it possible to use guided imagery?
22. Describe guided imagery.
23. Name two distracting techniques that may facilitate lowering anxiety.

ANXIETY DISORDERS

Generalized Anxiety Disorder

Background

According to the *DSM-IV*, the essential feature of **generalized anxiety disorder** is unrealistic or excessive anxiety and worry about two or more life circumstances. The patient who experiences this disorder is anxious and exhibits motor tension, autonomic hyperactivity, vigilance, and scanning behavior. Motor tension symptoms include trembling, twitching or feeling shaky, muscle tension, aches or soreness, restlessness, and easy fatigueability. Symptoms of autonomic hyperactivity include shortness of breath, palpitation, sweating, cold clammy extremities, dry mouth, dizziness, nausea, diarrhea, flushes or chills, frequent urination, and possibly a "lump in the throat." Symptoms of scanning include feeling on edge, having an exaggerated startle response, having difficulty concentrating or having the mind go blank because of anxiety, experiencing a sleep pattern disturbance, and feeling irritable. Patients who are so diagnosed experience chronic anxiety for at least six months. Their excessive concerns revolve around two or more life circumstances, such as finances, a child's welfare, or health. The latter is a prominent concern in anxiety in the elderly (Brawman-Mintzer et al, 1994).

Social and occupational functioning may be compromised. Patients diagnosed with generalized anxiety disorder tend to be chronically worried. Case Example 28–1 illustrates a patient with generalized anxiety disorder.

Case Example 28–1 Joan's Story

Joan is a 37-year-old school teacher. She is physically attractive except for her habitual scowl and the facial lines carved downward around her mouth. She rarely smiles to relieve her expression of intense thought and concern. If queried about her thoughts, she admits to being worried about the demands of her job or her children's whereabouts. She knows that her children either are in school or have gone home and then out to play with their neighborhood friends, but Joan is always vigilant and wondering. At times when events at school become overwhelming, Joan loses her cordial facade and becomes irritable and jittery. She eschews counseling because it is "too expensive."

Etiology

Psychodynamic theory suggests that children learn to repress "unacceptable" thoughts because they have learned that those thoughts are not approved by significant others. When these children mature, the same thoughts occur in real or symbolic form at a conscious or preconscious level. Anxiety erupts and whatever strategy is used to manage that sensation is also ellicited. *Behavioral theory* suggests that anxiety disorders are learned responses. A painful experience conditions the person to avoid similar experiences that cause anxiety. Lipsitz et al (1994) contend that childhood separation anxiety is a sufficiently painful experience to lead to multiple anxiety disorders in adulthood, including generalized anxiety disorder.

Recent nursing research suggests that adult children of alcoholics (ACOAs) may be particularly vulnerable to severe anxiety disorders (Haack and Alim, 1991). Although the cause is not yet known, it is well established that this group frequently experiences psychological stressors such as explosive relationships, family strife, and unstable environments. Studies of correlates of anxiety in ACOAs identified divorce, separation, spousal abuse, and poor parental modeling as common stressors. The children of alcoholics may come from poor, financially unstable homes and experience undersocialization. These conditions are difficult on children and may lead to negative self-concepts. A longitudinal study of ACOAs from birth to 18 years of age reported that those who developed serious problems as adults had experienced more stressful life events in their first two years of life.

Treatment

Anxiety disorders are amenable to therapy with both drugs and supportive psychotherapy. Reassurance, being available to listen to the patient, behavioral exercises for relaxation, group therapy, and stress management classes are all helpful. The drugs for anxiety disorders include the benzodiazepines and a recently released nonbenzodiazepine drug called buspirone (Buspar).

The benzodiazepines alleviate anxiety by facilitating the inhibitory actions of the neurotransmitter gamma aminobutyric acid (GABA) in the brain. Some of the shorter-acting anxiolytics are oxazepam (Serax), midazolam (Versed), alprazolam (Xanax), and lorazepam (Ativan). The longer-acting benzodiazepines are diazepam (Valium), clorazepate (Tranxene), chlordiazepoxide (Librium), and prazepam (Centrax).

Buspirone has a slow onset of therapeutic effect. Optimal effects usually are not obtained before four to six weeks. The site of action is not known but is suspected to be serotonin receptors. The advantage of this drug versus the benzodiazepines in treating anxiety is its low abuse and dependence profile (Porterfield, 1991).

Nursing Implications

Benzodiazepines must be administered with care in patients who are taking central nervous system depressants, including alcohol, barbiturates, anticonvulsants, and hypnotics. Therefore, a careful history must be developed focusing on the patient's use of other drugs. (See Chapter 31 for discussion of cross-tolerance.) Their usage may not be revealed during initial history-taking but may come up in more informal, relaxed interactions with the patient.

Patients also need reassurance that the risk of drug dependence with appropriate treatment is low (although patients with a history of drug abuse are at risk). When appropriate, gradual reductions in drug dosage will prevent symptoms of drug withdrawal.

You should monitor vital signs before and after administration of any intravenous or intramuscular anxiolytic for hypotensive reaction. Doses of these drugs should be the lowest possible for elderly patients because they have altered metabolism and take longer to excrete drugs. Patients should be cautioned that these drugs impair coordination and diminish reflexes, making driving cars or operating equipment dangerous. Additionally, intravenous benzodiazepines can induce significant amnesia. Patients may not recall conversations with family or care providers following drug administration.

▶ Check Your Reading

24. What is generalized anxiety disorder?
25. What is the relationship between generalized anxiety disorder and ACOAs?
26. How do the benzodiazepines alleviate anxiety?
27. What advantage does buspirone have over the benzodiazepines?

Panic Disorder With and Without Agoraphobia

Background

The essential features of **panic disorders** are discrete periods of intense fear or discomfort that are recurrent. Panic attacks usually last minutes, although some may be longer. They are unexpected and do not occur immediately before or on exposure to a definable stimulus. The unexpected aspect of the panic attack is a prominent feature of this disorder. Panic attacks begin with the sudden onset of intense apprehension, fear, or terror. Frequently the person has a feeling of impending doom. The symptoms experienced during an attack include dizziness, unsteady feelings, faintness, choking, palpitations or accelerated heart rate, trembling, sweating, nausea or abdominal distress, depersonalization, numbness, flushes or chills, chest pain, fear of dying, and fear of going crazy or of doing something uncontrolled during the attack.

In many cases, the person who has experienced recurrent panic attacks develops some signs of **agoraphobia.** The latter is the fear of being in places or situations from which escape might be difficult or embarrassing or in which help might not be available in the event of an attack of anxiety. Frequently agoraphobia includes fear of being outside the home alone, being in a crowd of people, standing in a waiting line, or traveling (Hunt, 1988; Danton et al, 1994).

Physical disorders, including hypoglycemia, pheochromocytoma, and hyperthyroidism, must be considered before a diagnosis of panic disorder is assigned. Panic disorder is differentiated from generalized anxiety disorder by the lack of focus on an object of concern. It is differentiated from posttraumatic stress disorder by the lack of a traumatic event in the patient's past history. It is estimated that 3% to 10% of the population have had recurrent or isolated panic attacks. They usually begin in the person's 20s and are rare after age 40 (Flint, 1994). Women appear to be twice as prone to the disorder as men. Panic disorder is associated with significant functional impairment. If untreated, patients face an increased risk of alcohol and other drug abuse because they may rely on these substances to calm and treat their condition. They alter social relationships in an effort to prevent and to hide their attacks. Marital relationships also suffer. If untreated, these patients are at risk for suicide (Johnson et al, 1990).

Etiology

An increasing body of research literature suggests that an underlying neurochemical dysfunction is the basis of panic disorder. Attacks are characterized by increases in blood norepinephrine levels and heart rate. Blood epinephrine levels remain elevated between attacks. Investigators theorize that symptoms are the result of central nervous system dyscontrol of the locus coeruleus, the small area at the base of the fourth ventricle that is packed with norepinephrine-containing neurons. Evidence suggests that electrical and pharmacological stimulation of that area produces anxiety. Other neurotransmitters, in particular serotonin and GABA, also may be implicated (Katon et al, 1988). A hereditary vulnerability to this disorder through alteration of chromosome 16 also has been conjectured. Vulnerability also may be carried on chromosome 6 (Crowe et al, 1980).

Researchers have found that panic attacks can be induced by a biological agent. For example, in a study, patients with a history of panic attacks were hooked up to an intravenous line. Sodium lactate, a chemical that normally produces rapid, shallow breathing and heart palpitations, was slowly infused into their bloodstreams. Within a few minutes, about 60% to 90% of these patients experienced a panic attack. Normal controls, those with no history of panic, rarely had panic attacks when infused with lactate (Seligman, 1994). Additionally, the PET scan, a technique that looks at how much blood and oxygen different parts of the brain use, shows that patients who panic from the infusion of lactate have higher blood flow and oxygen use in relevant parts of their brains than patients who do not panic.

A genetic component to panic disorders also exists. In identical twins, if one has panic attacks, so will the other in 31% of cases. But in fraternal twins, if one has panic attacks, the other twin has the same chance as any other blood relative of developing the disorder.

Clark (Seligman, 1994) contends that rather than being biological, panic represents a severe cognitive distortion. He believes that patients misinterpret symptoms of anxiety as symptoms of impending death, and it is this misinterpretation that leads to a full-blown panic attack.

Treatment

One of the most effective therapies for panic disorder is imipramine, a tricyclic antidepressant. This finding is surely related to the theorized alterations of neurotransmitters in the brain and, in particular, in the locus coeruleus. Clinical trials reveal that therapeutic effects tend to require several weeks of treatment. As with all of the tricyclic antidepressants, imipramine has anticholinergic, antihistaminic, and postural hypotensive effects. Monoamine oxidase (MAO) inhibitors are also useful. However, postural hypotension and hypertensive reactions occur with administration of these drugs. MAO, which inactivates biogenic amines, is blocked in all tissues by the MAO inhibitors. A disadvantage of this category of drugs is that the patient must be disciplined and reliable concerning dietary alterations. Tyramine-containing foods such as beer, most cheeses, smoked fish, and red wine must be restricted. Also, other drugs with sympathetic or sympathomimetic action, such as over-the-counter stimulants or ephedrine, must not be used because of the risk of a hypertensive crisis, which may occur because the action of the MAO inhibitors decreases the level of inactivation of these compounds (Lader, 1994; Seligman, 1994).

Seligman (1994) reports a technique developed by Clark to treat panic attacks that is disarmingly simple. Patients are told that panic results when they mistake normal symptoms of mounting anxiety for symptoms of heart attack, going crazy, or dying. Anxiety itself, patients are informed, produces shortness of breath, chest pain, and sweating. Furthermore, they are told that as soon as they misinterpret these bodily sensations as an imminent heart attack, their symptoms become even more pronounced because the misinterpretation changes their anxiety into terror. A vicious circle culminates in a full-blown panic attack.

Patients are taught to reinterpret the symptoms realistically as mere anxiety symptoms. They practice dealing with the physical symptoms of anxiety by breathing rapidly into a paper bag, which causes a build-up of carbon dioxide and shortness of breath, mimicking the sensations that provoke a panic attack. The therapist points out that the symptoms the patient is experiencing—shortness of breath and heart racing—are harmless, simply the result of overbreathing and not a sign of a heart attack. The patient learns to reinterpret the symptoms correctly. Clark (Seligman, 1994) reports that this simple and brief form of therapy, which has no side effects, has a 90% cure rate.

Nursing Implications

Patients present in the emergency department certain that they are dying of a heart attack. Once a physical examination rules this out, the patient is vigorously reassured that death is not imminent. Teaching about panic attack is a valuable means of reassurance that the patient's condition is not terminal.

After the patient has been medicated with a rapidly absorbed benzodiazepine, you should move the patient to a quiet room and remain nearby. Communication is couched in clear, short, and simple statements, and your voice should be low and calm.

Before leaving the emergency department, the patient is linked to a psychotherapist, preferably a psychiatrist because the patient is to remain on medication for at least several months. If the patient is opposed to such care or has difficulty understanding the psychobiological nature of the diagnosis, you will have to help the patient to understand the disorder. If the patient is resistant to psychotherapy, you must clarify the nature of the patient's biases.

Another consideration in caring for a patient diagnosed with a panic disorder is the need to teach the patient about the deleterious effects of caffeine on anxiety. During a study on the effects of caffeine on sleep, Uhde (Brown et al, 1994) reported that not only did caffeine induce a restless sleep in the volunteers but it also produced a panic attack in the volunteer receiving the largest amount of caffeine—about 500 mg. Uhde states that 60% of those who suffer from panic attacks suffer the attacks while they are sleeping. Uhde hypothesized that caffeine intake may be a strong contributory factor in nighttime panic attacks.

The strategy developed by Clark described here is an appropriate approach for nurses who frequently focus on a psychoeducational approach with patients. Case Example 28–2 describes Mike's journey with panic disorder.

Case Example 28–2 Mike's Story

Mike Samuels was transported by ambulance to the hospital. He is a 28-year-old married graduate student at a local university. He had been mowing his lawn when suddenly he had felt crushing chest pain. He experienced difficulty breathing, diaphoresis, nausea, and weakness. His legs felt rubbery, but he managed to get himself into the house, where he collapsed in a chair. He was sure that he was having a heart attack. He desperately wished for his wife, who had gone to the campus to do some library work. Knowing that she was gone for an indefinite time, he called 911, seeking an ambulance to take him to the hospital. The emergency crew noted his symptoms, responded with their standing orders, and transported him. Mike was terrified! He wondered if he would ever see his wife or his parents again. He wondered if he would live until the hospital came into sight. He wondered what would be done if he did reach the hospital alive. Along the way, the pressure in his chest began to subside. In the emergency department, a stat EKG was done. Blood was drawn, and a physician examined him. Very shortly Mike's wife arrived. Together they prepared for bad news. When the physician arrived, he said, "Mr. Samuels, I have good news for you. . . . You have not had a heart attack." Mike could hardly believe what he was hearing. "I haven't had a heart attack? Are you sure? How can that be? What about the pain I had? And not being able to breathe?"

"I know that it felt like a heart attack and that it must have been very frightening. But your tests are all negative. Your heart is fine," said the physician.

"Then what is wrong with him?" asked Mike's wife.

"We cannot be absolutely sure without further tests," responded the physician, "but I think that your husband has just experienced a panic attack." Turning to Mike, he continued, "The symptoms and test results suggest that. I am going to give you some medicine to help you calm down, and tomorrow I want you to go to the university clinic for further blood work. I am also going to give you the names of several psychiatrists. I want you to call one of them tomorrow for an appointment."

"But I'm not crazy," Mike protested.

"No. You certainly are not. You have had some sort of a brain event that has caused a sudden alteration in your central nervous system. We are medicating you with drugs that are best managed by a psychiatrist. You need to stay on this medication for several months. You may never have another attack. And then again, you might. In the meantime, the psychiatrist is the best person to give you some help. . . ."

Mike listened. He felt relief that he had escaped death and worried that maybe this doctor was wrong. "You are quite sure that I do not have anything wrong with my heart?"

"Quite," responded the doctor.

A nurse interrupted the conversation to give Mike his medicine. After Mike became calm and drowsy, the nurse engaged his wife in a discussion of panic disorder, answered her questions, and got a commitment from her to support her husband in the therapy that lay ahead.

▶ Check Your Reading

28. What is a panic disorder?
29. What is agoraphobia?
30. What do most patients who experience a panic attack erroneously conclude is happening to them?
31. What is the most effective medication in the treatment of panic attacks?

Obsessive-Compulsive Disorder

Background

Obsessive-compulsive disorder (OCD) was thought to be a rare condition, but recent epidemiological studies have proved that wrong. In fact, the rates are about 25 to 60 times greater than previously thought. A 1988 study revealed a lifetime prevalence rate ranging from 1.9% to 3.3%. The disorder affects approximately four million people (Karno et al, 1988).

Obsessive-compulsive disorder is reflected in ritualistic behavior, which may occur in thought or action. Because of the recurrent, time-consuming nature of the behavior, its victims may be unable to hold jobs, to maintain social relationships, or to participate in other areas of their lives. Persons with OCD are quite aware of the irrationality of their symptomatic behavior, but they are unable to control it: they are, in effect, prisoners of themselves!

Obsessions are persistent thoughts, ideas, impulses, or even images that are experienced as intrusive and senseless. Frequently occurring obsessions include thoughts of violence or contamination and doubt about one's own performance.

Compulsions are repetitive behaviors that follow an obsession. The behavior is performed in a particular order or in a stereotyped manner. The behavior is designed to neutralize or to prevent some dreaded event or situation.

The act is not realistically connected to the event or situation. Typically, it is viewed by the patient as excessive, irrational, and shameful, despite its tension-relieving role. Common compulsive behaviors include hand-washing, counting, checking, and touching. When the person tries to resist the compulsion, anxiety increases and is relieved only by completion of the ritual.

This disorder usually begins in early adolescence, but it may start in childhood. Because of the disruptions in lifestyle, such as problems in relationships and possible impairment in job performance, persons with this disorder often experience increased anxiety or depression. Sometimes its victims abuse drugs or alcohol in an effort to control their symptoms.

In about one half of all cases, the course of the illness may be chronic and unremitting. Life stress has been noted to increase symptoms in some persons; however, it is associated with a decrease in symptoms in others (most notably, if the stressor is external, such as war or a natural disaster). Treatment success is variable.

Etiology

As with other anxiety disorders, several psychological theories, mainly psychoanalytic, explain the meaning of OCD. However, contemporary biological theories seem to better explain the problem and offer a rational explanation for its symptoms. The most promising neurotransmitter theory has developed from clinical observations that antidepressants that are highly specific serotonin reuptake inhibitors are effective in treating OCD. Some evidence also shows dopaminergic involvement in patients with OCD who have tic disorders. Response to a psychotropic drug does not necessarily imply etiology. Rather, the changes in any neurotransmitter system associated with a drug response may be directly or indirectly related to the primary cause of the disorder (Zetin and Kramer, 1992). Brain imaging studies, neuropsychological examination, and lesion studies also have revealed abnormalities that may be related to OCD.

Treatment

Psychotherapy, behavioral therapy with familial involvement, and pharmacotherapy have all been useful in treating OCD. Supportive psychotherapy with a focus on patient and family education about the disorder is useful. Zetin and Kramer (1992) indicate that "the usual psychoanalytic approach is notoriously ineffective in resolving the symptoms of obsessive-compulsive disorder and may needlessly prolong the patient's suffering."

A combination of behavioral and pharmacotherapy usually is effective. In behavioral therapy of compulsions, the patient is exposed to progressive degrees of the stressor and asked to respond in a controlled environment with a modified, and perhaps delayed, behavior. Pleasurable activities and relaxation are encouraged by the therapist to replace unhealthy responses to anxiety with effective, goal-directed ones. This type of therapy is called *desensitization therapy*. For a more complete discussion, see Chapter 18.

Long-term treatment with medications appears to be necessary for most OCD patients. Therapeutic response occurs over a one- to two-month period after treatment is begun. Clomipramine (Anafranil) is the drug of choice. This drug is a tricyclic, relatively new in the United States but used for many years abroad. It causes obsessive thoughts to grow weaker and allows the patient to fight the urge to carry out ritual behaviors. The blunting or removal of obsessions or compulsions is caused by the effect of the drug on serotonin receptors in the brain. Because clomipramine is a tricyclic antidepressant, the side effects are similar to those of other drugs in this category: dry mouth, fatigue, drowsiness, constipation, tremor, decreased libido, impotence, and diaphoresis (Wright et al, 1994).

Patients with OCD usually progress unevenly. Periods of regression occur in the face of stressors. During certain intervals, the patient is able to control unwanted thoughts or behaviors. Of most importance is the long-term goal of the patient's being able to work, play, and maintain relationships.

Nursing Implications

Patients with OCD who are in residential treatment settings need to be taught about their medications. They need to learn to take the drugs in the evening shortly before sleep if they are troubled by side effects of fatigue or drowsiness. They should be supported as drug therapy is initiated and helped to be hopeful about the effects of pharmacotherapy. If their ritual behaviors involve excessive hand-washing, they need to be taught how to safeguard their skin with special preparations that will replace the natural oils that are being removed in washing. If patients are discharged without referral, they may benefit from finding behavior therapists through the Association for Advancement of Behavior Therapy. This national organization supplies referral lists of behavior therapists for particular geographic areas. Another national organization, the OCD Foundation, can put patients and their families in touch with local OCD support groups.

▶ Check Your Reading

32. What is an obsession?
33. What is a compulsion?
34. What is the drug treatment of choice for OCD?
35. What would a nurse teach a patient who engages in excessive hand-washing?

Posttraumatic Stress Disorder

Background

Posttraumatic stress disorder (PTSD) is a maladaptive set of responses to an event that has been overwhelmingly distressing. (See Chapter 41 for more details.) The stressor that has triggered this set of responses is typically outside of the range of usual human experience. The person reacts to it with intense fear, terror, and helpless-

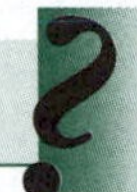

WHAT PATIENTS AND FAMILIES NEED TO KNOW — Obsessive-Compulsive Disorder

What is obsessive-compulsive disorder (OCD)?
Obsessions are intrusive, irrational thoughts—unwanted ideas or impulses that repeatedly well up in a person's mind. Again and again, the person experiences disturbing thoughts such as "My hands must be contaminated; I must wash them." On one level, the sufferer knows these obsessive thoughts are irrational. But on another level, he or she has a great fear that these thoughts might be true. Trying to avoid such thoughts creates great anxiety.

Who gets OCD?
People of all ages and from all walks of life can be afflicted with OCD. It strikes both males and females of all ethnic groups. Symptoms typically begin during the teenage years or young adulthood.

What causes OCD?
Evidence suggests that OCD results from a chemical imbalance in the brain. For years, mental health professionals assumed that OCD resulted from bad parenting or personality defects. This theory has been disproved over the past 20 years.

How is OCD treated?
Since the discovery that OCD results from a chemical imbalance, medication frequently is indicated for treatment. Numerous drugs are on the market, and one that is used specifically for OCD is clomipramine (Anafranil). Various forms of behavioral and cognitive therapies also are used. Reducing anxiety and improving self-esteem are two main goals of therapy.

How can family and friends help someone who has OCD?
Continue to be caring and avoid interrupting the ritualistic behaviors, because this only increases the anxiety. Help the person find alternative ways of controlling anxiety and support any efforts in doing so. Remember that the person is not engaging in ritualistic behavior because he or she consciously wants to; he or she often is equally disturbed by the ritualistic behaviors and wishes he or she could stop.

ness. The kinds of overwhelming events that are associated with PTSD include natural disasters, such as hurricanes and floods, and disasters caused by people, such as the Coconut Grove fire (a fire in a Boston nightclub where hundreds of patrons were trapped and burned). Other incidents that trigger PTSD include horrifying events in wartime (such as the observation of or participation in the napalming of Vietnamese natives), rape, and catastrophic accidents. Some candidates for PTSD include

- Burn victims who must undergo repetitive painful treatments, such as tubing, débridement, and dressing change for extended periods (the PTSD can result from the trauma of the fire or, later, from repetitive traumatic treatments for the burn)
- Paramedics who are repeatedly exposed to horrific situations
- Nurses who practice in critical care areas for long periods where they are exposed to serial deaths, trauma, and mutilation, and where they frequently have demands placed upon them that they cannot possibly meet

Psychic trauma occurs when a person observes or is part of a terrible event that is beyond his or her control. On the basis of clinical data, it is theorized that the lack of control causes neurobiological and behavioral changes. Because of these changes, sudden and severe loss of psychological integrity and cohesiveness results. The *Diagnostic and Statistical Manual of Mental Disorders-IV (DSM-IV)* identifies three dimensions of the resulting syndrome:

Reexperiencing the trauma
Avoidance or numbing
Physiological symptoms of arousal

The primary defining feature of PTSD is reexperiencing of the event through intrusive and unbidden thoughts or nightmares. Without this feature, a diagnosis of anxiety, depression, or adjustment disorder would be made. Likewise, for the diagnosis of PTSD to be made, an identified precipitating event must have occurred.

A person who is so diagnosed becomes preoccupied with the traumatic event. Memories of it invade his or her awareness at random times. The person struggles with obsessive thoughts about what was done and what was not done. Fear is experienced about the possibility of the event's occurring again because it was not in the person's control the first time. Some victims may have no memories of the trauma for unpredictable periods of time. For some, diminished responsiveness to external events is reflective of "psychic numbing." The victim may complain of feeling detached or separate from others and of losing the ability to enjoy pleasurable events. The process of ruminating over the event is an effort to work through the trauma. Anger, sadness, rage, depression, and stoicism all may be demonstrated. In cases in which the victim actually has been a participant in violent acts, as with veterans of war, changes may occur in aggression: some may fear losing control. More severely affected victims may have a reduced capacity for modulation of affect, which is expressed in unpredictable explosions of aggressive behavior or an inability to express angry feelings.

Persistent states of arousal are evidenced by difficulty in falling asleep or remaining asleep. The latter may be associated with recurrent nightmares in which the traumatic event is relived. Hypervigilance as well as an exaggerated startle response may be observed. Some persons experience difficulty in concentrating or in task completion.

Both psychological and physiological symptoms may be intensified or precipitated when the person is exposed to situations that resemble or symbolize the original trauma. The duration of the symptoms is at least one month, and the syndrome can emerge many months, or even years, after exposure to the traumatizing event. In the latter case, however, efforts to avoid remembering usually have been present.

Etiology

Posttraumatic stress disorder is qualitatively different from the other anxiety disorders in that its cause is a real and devastating event in the person's life. It can be argued that PTSD is not really an illness but a maladaptive means of coping. On the other hand, some theorists believe that biological changes occur as a result of the stressor's impact.

Mardi Horowitz has developed a theory based on his research that serves as a conceptual framework for further research and treatment of PTSD (1986). Horowitz views trauma as a stressor that has an impact on the person's information-processing capacity. He notes that all people who survive a traumatic event have a "completion tendency," an unconscious tendency to think about the experience in an attempt to understand what has happened. Although Horowitz does not identify the completion tendency as spiritual, the desire to find meaning in events is always a spiritual task. The victim of PTSD attempts to integrate feelings about the traumatic event into the inner working model of self. The victim ruminates about memories until the related emotions and behaviors are understood. Intrusion and avoidance are major components of the process. As the victim reacts, involuntary and intrusive thoughts and images of the event emerge. Nightmares, flashbacks, and uncontrollable waves of emotion threaten the victim's sense of cohesiveness. Horowitz views behavioral attempts at avoidance, such as dissociation, repression, and denial, as attempts to defend against the avalanche of uncontrollable feelings associated with memories of the event. He proposes that PSTD develops when integration of painful feelings and thoughts about the event does not occur. Table 28–2 shows the phases of normal and pathological responses to PTSD.

Some theorists consider PTSD to be a biological disorder with changes to be found in the hormones and cerebral cortex of both animals and humans exposed to aversive events. Kolb (1987) has noted that persons exposed to stressful events showed an increased responsiveness with sympathetic nervous system activity, increased plasma catecholamine levels, and elevated urinary epinephrine and norepinephrine levels. He theorizes that after repeated exposure to stress, persons such as battle-scarred soldiers show signs of posttraumatic stress disorder (PTSD) and lose their physiological control of incoming stimuli. Cortical neurons become vulnerable to neuroendocrine disturbance. This results in the loss of inhibitory cortical control (Norman, 1989).

Van der Kolk and colleagues (1984) theorize that massive amounts of endorphins are released when persons are affected by traumatic events. The endorphins produce an analgesic needed to survive the ordeal. When the trauma ends, endorphin levels decrease. They theorize that PTSD symptoms occur in response to the decrease in endogenous opioids like endorphins. Van der Kolk and associates have noted that symptoms such as hyperalertness, irritability, and anxiety, which they have observed in laboratory animals, are equivalent to the symptoms seen in traumatized humans.

Treatment

Both pharmacotherapy and psychotherapy are used in the treatment of PTSD. Because of the patient's level of distress, psychotropic drugs may be the first line of therapy. Excessive arousal of the sympathetic nervous system causes neurochemical changes that are related to learning and habituation. It becomes difficult for the person to discriminate perceptual cues, especially as they pertain to the traumatic event. Excessive arousal pushes the victim into reactive, emotional states. Tricyclics (antidepressants) may be utilized for symptoms of reexperiencing and numbing, as well as for hyperalertness, memory difficulties, and sleep disturbance. Amitriptyline (Elavil) has been proven to be helpful with nightmares

TABLE 28–2 The Phases of Normal and Pathological Responses to Traumatic Stress

Normal Response	Pathological Response
1. Outcry: Fear, sadness, rage	1. Being overwhelmed and disorganized by the reaction
2. Denial: Refusing to explore memories of the event	2. Panic or exhaustion secondary to the emotional reaction
3. Intrusion: Involuntary thoughts of the event	3. Extreme avoidance: Use of alcohol or other drugs and acting-out to deny distress
4. Working through: Exploration and integration of the traumatic event and its meaning	4. Flooding: Disturbing, persistent images and thoughts of the event
5. Completion: Reengagement and commitment to ongoing life	5. Psychosomatic responses: Bodily complaints developing in response to incomplete processing of the event
	6. Character distortions: Persistent changes in thoughts and behavior that evolve as defenses, causing chronic alterations in lifestyle

Modified from Horowitz, M. (1986). *Stress response syndromes* (2nd ed.). New York: Aronson.

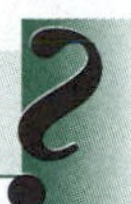

WHAT SOCIETY NEEDS TO KNOW **Posttraumatic Stress Disorder**

What is posttraumatic stress disorder (PTSD)?

Posttraumatic stress disorder is the development of some specific symptoms after exposure to an extreme traumatic stressor. This involves direct personal experience of an event that involves actual or threatened death or serious injury or the witnessing of or learning about an event that causes death, injury, or the threat to the physical integrity of another person.

Who is affected by PTSD?

Examples of traumatic events that one might experience directly include military combat, violent personal assault, being kidnaped or taken hostage, terrorist attacks, natural or other disasters, severe automobile accidents, and learning that one has a life-threatening illness. Any major trauma that a person may have witnessed or learned about also can trigger the symptoms of PTSD.

What are the symptoms?

Symptoms of PTSD include recurrent flashbacks and dreams of the event and attempts to avoid thoughts, feelings, activities, people, and places associated with the event. The person also may experience difficulty sleeping, an inability to have loving feelings, irritability, difficulty concentrating, hypervigilance, and an inability to recall specific aspects of the trauma.

How prevalent is this condition?

In the general population, the incidence of PTSD is relatively rare, but when high-risk populations are studied (combat veterans, natural disaster survivors, or populations with a high rate of criminal violence), the percentage is often over 50% of the studied population.

What causes PTSD?

Several theories exist. Some researchers do not consider it an illness at all but a maladaptive way of coping. Some researchers do believe that biological changes occur as a result of the stressor's impact. Others note that an acute trauma interrupts the person's ability to process information and results in a need to make some sense of the trauma and to integrate thoughts and feelings.

How is PTSD treated?

Medications and various psychotherapies are used in the treatment of PTSD. Medications may be used initially to help with the overt symptoms of anxiety and to enable the person to sleep. During therapy, the person needs to be assisted to integrate the trauma experience into his or her overall life. This process frequently takes considerable time and often becomes a spiritual journey for the patient. Group therapy is very effective, particularly when the group members have suffered similar trauma experiences.

and flashbacks. Imipramine (Tofranil) was found helpful in relieving intrusive symptoms. The monoamine oxidase (MAO) inhibitors have been helpful with outbursts of aggression or high levels of anxiety.

The outcome of psychotherapy, as well as the process, is dependent on certain characteristics unique to each patient:

- The nature of the traumatic event
- The patient's support system prior to the trauma
- The patient's personality prior to the trauma
- The time that has elapsed since the event

The severity of PTSD may be associated with the degree of loss and life threat in the traumatizing event. Younger and older persons are reported to be more susceptible because the young have less experience and lower neuron level activities and older people have neural inactivation associated with aging (Beigel and Berren, 1985; Scurfield, 1985; Kolb, 1987; DiNartdo and Barlow, 1988). People who have been previously traumatized or who have other psychopathology are theorized to have greater vulnerability to PTSD. Likewise, the manner in which a person appraises an event may be affected by his or her preexisting personality. If that person tends to perceive situations with anxiety, vulnerability to PTSD will increase.

The role taken by a survivor of trauma affects later psychopathology. If the survivor was a victim or aided other victims during the traumatizing event, these factors will alter not only the symptoms but also the recovery phase. It has been demonstrated that those who have helped during a disaster are better able to cope. Finally, it has been observed that disasters caused by humans are more emotionally devastating than natural disasters. Victims of natural disasters do not feel the same sense of responsibility as with disasters caused by humans because natural disasters are out of their control. Violent crimes, including deaths and mutilation through drunk driving, are particularly traumatizing because they violate human justice.

Scurfield (1985) has defined five aspects of treatment for those experiencing PTSD:

1. Developing trust within the therapeutic relationship
2. Educating the patient about the recovery process
3. Stress management
4. Helping the patient to regress or reexperience the trauma
5. Integrating the trauma experience

Victims of trauma lose the trust they previously felt in their own capacities to survive and in God's ability to protect them. Previously embraced views of the world as a safe and rational place, as well as beliefs about the imperviousness of the self, are reviewed and reworked. The process takes time and much cognitive restructuring. It is a time of introspection as the trauma victim faces a period of personal chaos. Therapy helps the victim to make peace with the behavior at the time of the trauma and to view that behavior as reasonable and moral considering the available options. The person must achieve a new balance with self related to the past and to the present. Many Vietnam War veterans who experienced PTSD found that the integration happened only when they began to believe that the trauma that they suffered caused God to suffer as much, if not more, than they did, but because of God's gift to each of us of free will, He cannot arbitrarily step in and stop us from hurting each other.

▶ **Check Your Reading**

36. Identify the symptoms of PTSD.
37. What must have occurred in the patient's history to justify the diagnosis of PTSD?

Nursing Implications

One of the major issues in nursing care of PTSD is to encourage patients to talk about their painful stored memories. The only way that patients will be able to engage in healthy relationships is to first share the horror associated with past events, to let go of the feelings attached to these events, and to move on with life. The process of sharing, letting go, and moving on is a difficult one that produces feelings of dread, terror, and helplessness, as well as physiological responses such as cardiac palpitations and shortness of breath. Your ability to teach the patient adaptive coping skills, such as slow, deep breathing and relaxation techniques, may make the difference between whether or not the patient is able to move on successfully.

Phobias

Specific Phobia

The most prominent feature of the **specific phobia** is severe and persistent fear of clearly identifiable objects or situations. When the patient is exposed to the latter, an immediate anxious response is elicited. The diagnosis is made only if the patient avoids the feared object or endures it with dread. Additionally, the avoidance, fear, or dread must interfere significantly with the patient's daily life. Adolescents and adults with this disorder usually recognize that their reactions are excessive or irrational. However, they cannot alter the horror that they feel in response to the phobic object. The *Diagnostic and Statistical Manual of Mental Disorders-IV (DSM-IV)* subdivides the specific phobias into the following categories:

- Animal type, such as dogs or snakes
- Natural environment type, such as thunder and lightning or heights
- Blood-injections-injury type, including administration of intramuscular medication and various endoscopic procedures
- Situational type, such as flying and public transportation
- Other type, such as choking or vomiting

Patients with these specific phobias are infrequently admitted to the hospital because they tend to have insight and seek outpatient treatment, usually including anxiolytics as needed, possibly relaxation, education about their conditions, and cognitive therapy.

Social Phobia

The essential symptom of **social phobia** is a profound and enduring fear of social or performance situations where embarrassment could occur. Exposure to the phobic situation causes an immediate anxiety attack that may reach the proportions of panic. The diagnosis is made only if the person's daily activities in school, social life, or work are severely modified by the symptom. In the affected parameters of the person's life, she or he is fearful that others will judge her or him to be stupid, crazy, or particularly undesirable. Social situations are avoided to avoid exposure to the expected reaction from others. The particular social situation that is feared may be public speaking, eating in a restaurant, or giving an artistic performance, such as singing or dancing. Persons with social phobia usually recognize that their reactions are excessive. Sometimes they try to endure the feared situation because of this realization, but inevitably their worst concerns are realized. The person who fears eating out will accidentally overturn a water glass and others will stare; the singer will have stage fright; or the speaker will forget a portion of the speech or lose his or her place in the document from which he or she is reading (Seligman, 1994; Stein et al, 1994). These experiences only reinforce the phobia. Epidemiological and community-based studies indicate that this disorder is more common in women than in men. In clinical studies, these findings are reversed.

Treatments for this condition include those already outlined for the other anxiety disorders plus the use of medications known as beta blockers. Beta blockers include propranolol, metaprolol, and atenolol. It is necessary to obtain a careful evaluation of blood pressure, pulse rate, heart, and lungs before initiating the use of beta blockers. A history of congestive heart failure, cardiac arrhythmia, or chronic obstructive pulmonary disease with asthma poses contraindications to treatment with beta blockers (Keltner and Folks, 1993).

▶ **Check Your Reading**

38. What is a phobia?
39. What is the difference between a social and a specific phobia?
40. What is the classification of medications that are very effective in treating social phobias?

NURSING PROCESS

ASSESSMENT

The symptoms of anxiety tend to be self-evident in those experiencing it because of the person's maladaptive or ineffective behaviors that have been employed to alter or to deny the original distressing experience. Four behavioral patterns are commonly used for coping with anxiety:

1. An adaptive, growth-producing behavior that incorporates problem-solving and uses anxiety to learn positive adaptive behaviors
2. Withdrawal and avoidance
3. Acting out
4. Somatization

The latter three groups of behaviors are maladaptive because they do not facilitate the person's management of anxiety but actually only avoid it at the expense of reality and growth.

Assess for defining characteristics of anxiety and for its severity, as well as for the impact of the symptoms of anxiety on the daily life of the patient. This includes the patient's capacity:

To work
To recreate
To eat
To sleep
To parent
To relate to others

In the intake interview, ask about medical conditions that might be associated with anxiety. The history includes information about the patient's childhood, family issues, marital issues, sleep problems, somatic complaints, drug and alcohol use, current medications, prior psychiatric illnesses, social and occupational functioning, and the patient's relationship with his or her personal God.

Several assessment tools specific to anxiety disorders are available. These include the Anxiety Disorders Interview Schedule–Revised (ADIS-R) (Hoover and Parnell, 1984), the Sheehan Patient-Rated Anxiety Scale and the Modified Anxiety Scale, and the Modified Spielberger State Anxiety Scale (Spielberger, 1984). These paper-and-pencil assessment tools are easily administered and scored. Once these data are available, along with the history and physical examination, you can identify the nursing diagnosis and, with the patient, plan for intervention.

▶ Check Your Reading

41. What are the four behavioral patterns commonly used to cope with anxiety?
42. Of those four behavioral patterns, which one is adaptive?
43. In conducting an assessment on a patient experiencing anxiety, what should you ask about in the history?
44. Identify two standardized anxiety rating scales that are used to evaluate anxiety.

DIAGNOSIS

To establish medical and nursing diagnoses, the interdisciplinary treatment team analyzes the patient's assessment data. *DSM-IV* psychiatric diagnoses and North American Nursing Diagnosis Association (NANDA) nursing diagnoses for patients with anxiety disorders are shown in the Medical Diagnoses and Related Nursing Diagnoses box.

OUTCOME IDENTIFICATION

The expected outcomes for a patient depend on the specific medical and nursing diagnoses. For a patient with a nursing diagnosis of anxiety, for example, expected outcomes might include

- The patient will demonstrate techniques to reduce his or her own anxiety.
- The patient will be free of anxiety attacks.
- The patient will be safe.
- The patient will report a significantly decreased anxiety level.

For a patient with a nursing diagnosis of Ineffective Individual Coping, expected outcomes might include

- The patient will demonstrate alternative ways of coping with stress, including problem-solving and relaxation techniques.
- The patient will identify plans for future handling of stressful events.

For a patient with a nursing diagnosis of Post-Trauma Response, expected outcomes might include

- The patient will begin the grieving process.
- The patient will express feelings directly and openly in a healthy, nondestructive manner.
- The patient will experience an increased ability to deal with stress.
- The patient will integrate the trauma into her or his life and be able to articulate a personal meaning that gives comfort and peace.
- The patient will express her or his feelings to God, thus experiencing resolution of the spiritual conflict and restoration of his or her relationship with God.

PLANNING

The short-term goals that you plan for a patient depend on the specific medical and nursing diagnoses, and they flow from the expected outcomes that you identified previously. For a patient with a nursing diagnosis of

Text continued on page 713

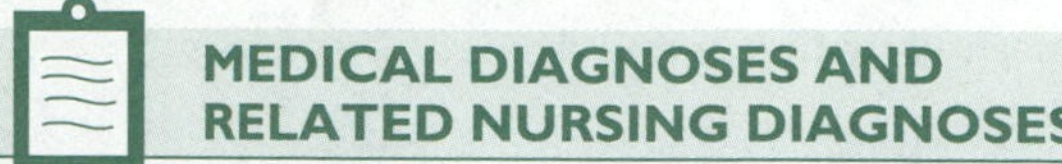

***DSM-IV* Diagnosis:** Panic Disorder Without Agoraphobia

Diagnostic Criteria

A. Both (1) and (2).
  (1) Recurrent unexpected Panic Attacks.
  (2) At least one of the attacks has been followed by 1 month (or more) of one (or more) of the following.
    (a) Persistent concern about having additional attacks.
    (b) Worry about the implications of the attack or its consequences (e.g., losing control, having a heart attack, "going crazy").
    (c) A significant change in behavior related to the attacks.
B. Absence of Agoraphobia.
C. The Panic Attacks are not due to the direct physiological effects of a substance (e.g., a drug of abuse, a medication) or a general medical condition (e.g., hyperthyroidism).
D. The Panic Attacks are not better accounted for by another mental disorder, such as Social Phobia (e.g., occurring on exposure to feared social situations), Specific Phobia (e.g., on exposure to a specific phobic situation), Obsessive-Compulsive Disorder (e.g., on exposure to dirt in someone with an obsession about contamination), Posttraumatic Stress Disorder (e.g., in response to stimuli associated with a severe stressor), or Separation Anxiety Disorder (e.g., in response to being away from home or close relatives).

***DSM-IV* Diagnosis:** Panic Disorder With Agoraphobia

Diagnostic Criteria

A. Both (1) and (2).
  (1) Recurrent unexpected Panic Attacks.
  (2) At least one of the attacks has been followed by 1 month (or more) of one (or more) of the following.
    (a) Persistent concern about having additional attacks.
    (b) Worry about the implications of the attack or its consequences (e.g., losing control, having a heart attack, "going crazy").
    (c) A significant change in behavior related to the attacks.
B. The presence of Agoraphobia.
C. The Panic Attacks are not due to the direct physiological effects of a substance (e.g., a drug of abuse, a medication) or a general medical condition (e.g., hyperthyroidism).
D. The Panic Attacks are not better accounted for by another mental disorder, such as Social Phobia (e.g., occurring on exposure to feared social situations), Specific Phobia (e.g., on exposure to a specific phobic situation), Obsessive-Compulsive Disorder (e.g., on exposure to dirt in someone with an obsession about contamination), Posttraumatic Stress Disorder (e.g., in response to stimuli associated with a severe stressor), or Separation Anxiety Disorder (e.g., in response to being away from home or close relatives).

***DSM-IV* Diagnosis:** Agoraphobia Without History of Panic Disorder

Diagnostic Criteria

A. The presence of Agoraphobia related to fear of developing paniclike symptoms (e.g., dizziness or diarrhea).
B. Criteria have never been met for Panic Disorder.
C. The disturbance is not due to the direct physiological effects of a substance (e.g., a drug of abuse, a medication) or a general medical condition.
D. If an associated general medical condition is present, the fear described in Criterion A is clearly in excess of that usually associated with the condition.

***DSM-IV* Diagnosis:** Specific Phobia

Diagnostic Criteria

A. Marked and persistent fear that is excessive or unreasonable, cued by the presence or anticipation of a specific object or situation (e.g., flying, heights, animals, receiving an injection, seeing blood).
B. Exposure to the phobic stimulus almost invariably provokes an immediate anxiety response, which may take the form of a situationally bound or situationally predisposed Panic Attack. **Note:** In children, the anxiety may be expressed by crying, tantrums, freezing, or clinging.
C. The person recognizes that the fear is excessive or unreasonable. **Note:** In children, this feature may be absent.
D. The phobic situation(s) is avoided or else is endured with intense anxiety or distress.
E. The avoidance, anxious anticipation, or distress in the feared situation(s) interferes significantly with the person's normal routine, occupational (or academic) functioning, or social activities or relationships, or there is marked distress about having the phobia.
F. In individuals under age 18 years, the duration is at least 6 months.
G. The anxiety, Panic Attacks, or phobic avoidance associated with the specific object or situation is not better accounted for by another mental disorder, such as Obsessive-Compulsive Disorder (e.g., fear of dirt in someone with an obsession about contamination), Posttraumatic Stress Disorder (e.g., avoidance of stimuli associated with a severe stressor), Separation Anxiety Disorder (e.g., avoidance of school), Social Phobia (e.g., avoidance of social situations because of fear of embarrassment), Panic Disorder With Agoraphobia, or Agoraphobia Without History of Panic Disorder.

Specify type:
Animal Type
Natural Environment Type (e.g., heights, storms, water)
Blood-Injection-Injury Type
Situational Type (e.g., airplanes, elevators, enclosed places)
Other Type (e.g., phobic avoidance of situations that may lead to choking, vomiting, or contracting an illness; in children, avoidance of loud sounds or costumed characters)

***DSM-IV* Diagnosis:** Social Phobia

Diagnostic Criteria
A. A marked and persistent fear of one or more social or performance situations in which the person is exposed to unfamiliar people or to possible scrutiny by others. The individual fears that he or she will act in a way (or show anxiety symptoms) that will be humiliating or embarrassing. **Note:** In children, there must be evidence of the capacity for age-appropriate social relationships with familiar people and the anxiety must occur in peer settings, not just in interactions with adults.
B. Exposure to the feared social situation almost invariably provokes anxiety, which may take the form of a situationally bound or situationally predisposed Panic Attack. **Note:** In children, the anxiety may be expressed by crying, tantrums, freezing, or shrinking from social situations with unfamiliar people.
C. The person recognizes that the fear is excessive or unreasonable. **Note:** In children, this feature may be absent.
D. The feared social or performance situations are avoided or else are endured with intense anxiety or distress.
E. The avoidance, anxious anticipation, or distress in the feared social or performance situation(s) interferes significantly with the person's normal routine, occupational (academic) functioning, or social activities or relationships, or there is marked distress about having the phobia.
F. In individuals under age 18 years, the duration is at least 6 months.
G. The fear or avoidance is not due to the direct physiological effects of a substance (e.g., a drug of abuse, a medication) or a general medical condition and is not better accounted for by another mental disorder (e.g., Panic Disorder With or Without Agoraphobia, Separation Anxiety Disorder, Body Dysmorphic Disorder, a Pervasive Developmental Disorder, or Schizoid Personality Disorder).
H. If a general medical condition or another mental disorder is present, the fear in Criterion A is unrelated to it, e.g., the fear is not of Stuttering, trembling in Parkinson's disease, or exhibiting abnormal eating behavior in Anorexia Nervosa or Bulimia Nervosa.
Specify if:
Generalized: If the fears include most social situations (also consider the additional diagnosis of Avoidant Personality Disorder)

***DSM-IV* Diagnosis:** Obsessive-Compulsive Disorder

Diagnostic Criteria
A. Either obsessions or compulsions.
Obsessions as defined by (1), (2), (3), and (4)
(1) Recurrent and persistent thoughts, impulses, or images that are experienced, at some time during the disturbance, as intrusive and inappropriate and that cause marked anxiety or distress.
(2) The thoughts, impulses, or images are not simply excessive worries about real-life problems.
(3) The person attempts to ignore or suppress such thoughts, impulses, or images, or to neutralize them with some other thought or action.
(4) The person recognizes that the obsessional thoughts, impulses, or images are a product of his or her own mind (not imposed from without as in thought insertion).
Compulsions as defined by (1) and (2)
(1) Repetitive behaviors (e.g., hand-washing, ordering, checking) or mental acts (e.g., praying, counting, repeating words silently) that the person feels driven to perform in response to an obsession, or according to rules that must be applied rigidly.
(2) The behaviors or mental acts are aimed at preventing or reducing distress or preventing some dreaded event or situation; however, these behaviors or mental acts either are not connected in a realistic way with what they are designed to neutralize or prevent or are clearly excessive.
B. At some point during the course of the disorder, the person has recognized that the obsessions or compulsions are excessive or unreasonable. **Note:** This does not apply to children.
C. The obsessions or compulsions cause marked distress, are time consuming (take more than 1 hour a day), or significantly interfere with the person's normal routine, occupational (or academic) functioning, or usual social activities or relationships.
D. If another Axis I disorder is present, the content of the obsessions or compulsions is not restricted to it (e.g., preoccupation with food in the presence of an Eating Disorder; hair pulling in the presence of Trichotillomania; concern with appearance in the presence of Body Dysmorphic Disorder; preoccupation with drugs in the presence of a Substance Use Disorder; preoccupation with having a serious illness in the presence of Hypochondriasis; preoccupation with sexual urges or fantasies in the presence of a Paraphilia; or guilty ruminations in the presence of Major Depressive Disorder).

continued

E. The disturbance is not due to the direct physiological effects of a substance (e.g., a drug of abuse, a medication) or a general medical condition.
Specify if:
With Poor Insight: If, for most of the time during the current episode, the person does not recognize that the obsessions and compulsions are excessive or unreasonable.

***DSM-IV* Diagnosis:** Posttraumatic Stress Disorder

Diagnostic Criteria
See Chapter 41.

***DSM-IV* Diagnosis:** Acute Stress Disorder

Diagnostic Criteria
A. The person has been exposed to a traumatic event in which both of the following were present.
(1) The person experienced, witnessed, or was confronted with an event or events that involved actual or threatened death or serious injury, or a threat to the physical integrity of self or others.
(2) The person's response involved intense fear, helplessness, or horror.
B. Either while experiencing or after experiencing the distressing event, the individual has three (or more) of the following dissociative symptoms.
(1) A subjective sense of numbing, detachment, or absence of emotional responsiveness.
(2) A reduction in awareness of his or her surroundings (e.g., "being in a daze").
(3) Derealization.
(4) Depersonalization.
(5) Dissociative amnesia (i.e., inability to recall an important aspect of the trauma).
C. The traumatic event is persistently reexperienced in at least one of the following ways: recurrent images, thoughts, dreams, illusions, flashback episodes, or a sense of reliving the experience; or distress on exposure to reminders of the traumatic event.
D. Marked avoidance of stimuli that arouse recollections of the trauma (e.g., thoughts, feelings, conversations, activities, places, people).
E. Marked symptoms of anxiety or increased arousal (e.g., difficulty sleeping, irritability, poor concentration, hypervigilance, exaggerated startle response, motor restlessness).
F. The disturbance causes clinically significant distress or impairment in social, occupational, or other important areas of functioning or impairs the individual's ability to pursue some necessary task, such as obtaining necessary assistance or mobilizing personal resources by telling family members about the traumatic experience.
G. The disturbance lasts for a minimum of 2 days and a maximum of 4 weeks and occurs within 4 weeks of the traumatic event.
H. The disturbance is not due to the direct physiological effects of a substance (e.g., a drug of abuse, a medication) or a general medical condition, is not better accounted for by Brief Psychotic Disorder, and is not merely an exacerbation of a preexisting Axis I or Axis II disorder.

***DSM-IV* Diagnosis:** Generalized Anxiety Disorder

Diagnostic Criteria
A. Excessive anxiety and worry (apprehensive expectation), occurring more days than not for at least 6 months, about a number of events or activities (such as work or school performance).
B. The person finds it difficult to control the worry.
C. The anxiety and worry are associated with three (or more) of the following six symptoms (with at least some symptoms present for more days than not for the past 6 months). **Note:** Only one item is required in children.
(1) Restlessness or feeling keyed up or on edge
(2) Being easily fatigued
(3) Difficulty concentrating or mind going blank
(4) Irritability
(5) Muscle tension
(6) Sleep disturbance (difficulty falling or staying asleep, or restless unsatisfying sleep)
D. The focus of the anxiety and worry is not confined to features of an Axis I disorder, e.g., the anxiety or worry is not about having a Panic Attack (as in Panic Disorder), being embarrassed in public (as in Social Phobia), being contaminated (as in Obsessive-Compulsive Disorder), being away from home or close relatives (as in Separation Anxiety Disorder), gaining weight (as in Anorexia Nervosa), having multiple physical complaints (as in Somatization Disorder), or having a serious illness (as in Hypochondriasis), and the anxiety and worry do not occur exclusively during Posttraumatic Stress Disorder.
E. The anxiety, worry, or physical symptoms cause clinically significant distress or impairment in social, occupational, or other important areas of functioning.
F. The disturbance is not due to the direct physiological effects of a substance (e.g., a drug of abuse, a medication) or a general medical condition (e.g., hyperthyroidism) and does not occur exclusively during a Mood Disorder, a Psychotic Disorder, or a Pervasive Developmental Disorder.

MEDICAL DIAGNOSES AND RELATED NURSING DIAGNOSES

Stress and Anxiety

***DSM-IV* Diagnosis:** Anxiety Disorder Due to . . . [a General Medical Condition]

Diagnostic Criteria

A. Prominent anxiety, Panic Attacks, or obsessions or compulsions predominate in the clinical picture.
B. There is evidence from the history, physical examination, or laboratory findings that the disturbance is the direct physiological consequence of a general medical condition.
C. The disturbance is not better accounted for by another mental disorder (e.g., Adjustment Disorder With Anxiety in which the stressor is a serious general medical condition).
D. The disturbance does not occur exclusively during the course of a delirium.
E. The disturbance causes clinically significant distress or impairment in social, occupational, or other important areas of functioning.

Specify if:
With Generalized Anxiety: If excessive anxiety or worry about a number of events or activities predominates in the clinical presentation.
With Panic Attacks: If Panic Attacks predominate in the clinical presentation.
With Obsessive-Compulsive Symptoms: If obsessions or compulsions predominate in the clinical presentation.

***DSM-IV* Diagnosis:** Substance-Induced Anxiety Disorder

Diagnostic Criteria

A. Prominent anxiety, Panic Attacks, or obsessions or compulsions predominate in the clinical picture.
B. There is evidence from the history, physical examination, or laboratory findings of either (1) or (2).
(1) The symptoms in Criterion A developed during, or within 1 month of, Substance Intoxication or Withdrawal.
(2) Medication use is etiologically related to disturbance.
C. The disturbance is not better accounted for by an Anxiety Disorder that is not substance induced. Evidence that the symptoms are better accounted for by an Anxiety Disorder that is not substance induced might include the following: the symptoms precede the onset of the substance use (or medication use); the symptoms persist for a substantial period of time (e.g., about a month) after the cessation of acute withdrawal or severe intoxication or are substantially in excess of what would be expected given the type or amount of the substance used or the duration of use; or there is other evidence suggesting the existence of an independent non–substance-induced Anxiety Disorder (e.g., a history of recurrent non–substance-related episodes).
D. The disturbance does not occur exclusively during the course of a delirium.
E. The disturbance causes clinically significant distress or impairment in social, occupational, or other important areas of functioning.

Note: This diagnosis should be made instead of a diagnosis of Substance Intoxication or Substance Withdrawal only when the anxiety symptoms are in excess of those usually associated with the intoxication or withdrawal syndrome and when the anxiety symptoms are sufficiently severe to warrant independent clinical attention.

Specify if:
With Generalized Anxiety: If excessive anxiety or worry about a number of events or activities predominates in the clinical presentation.
With Panic Attacks: If Panic Attacks predominate in the clinical presentation.
With Obsessive-Compulsive Symptoms: If obsessions or compulsions predominate in the clinical presentation.
With Phobic Symptoms: If phobic symptoms predominate in the clinical presentation.

Specify if:
With Onset During Intoxication: If the criteria are met for Intoxication with the substance and the symptoms develop during the intoxication syndrome.
With Onset During Withdrawal: If criteria are met for Withdrawal from the substance and the symptoms develop during, or shortly after, a withdrawal syndrome.

continued

MEDICAL DIAGNOSES AND RELATED NURSING DIAGNOSES

Stress and Anxiety

RELATED NURSING DIAGNOSES	DEFINITION	EXAMPLE
Anxiety	A vague, uneasy feeling whose source is often nonspecific or unknown to the individual	Anxiety related to beginning new job
Impaired Verbal Communication	The state in which an individual experiences a decreased or absent ability to use or understand language in human interaction	Impaired Verbal Communication related to cultural differences
Decisional Conflict (Specify)	The state of uncertainty about course of action to be taken when choice among competing actions involves risk, loss, or challenge to personal life values	Decisional conflict related to perceived threat to value system
Ineffective Family Coping: Compromised	A usually supportive primary person (family member or close friend) is providing insufficient, ineffective, or compromised support, comfort, assistance, or encouragement that may be needed by the client to manage or master adaptive tasks related to his or her health challenge	Ineffective Family Coping: Compromised related to multiple situational crises
Hopelessness	A subjective state in which an individual sees limited or no alternatives or personal choices available and is unable to mobilize energy on own behalf	Hopelessness related to long-term stress
Ineffective Individual Coping	Impairment of adaptive behaviors and problem-solving abilities of a person in meeting life's demands and roles	Ineffective Individual Coping related to recent unemployment
Parental Role Conflict	The state in which a parent experiences role confusion and conflict in response to crisis	Parental Role Conflict related to perceived inability to meet child's psychological needs
Altered Parenting	The state in which a nurturing figure(s) experiences an inability to create an environment that promotes the optimum growth and development of another human being	Altered Parenting related to chronic stress experienced by parents
Post-Trauma Response	The state of an individual experiencing a sustained painful response to an overwhelming traumatic event(s)	Post-Trauma Response related to terrorist attack
Powerlessness	Perception that one's own actions will not significantly affect an outcome; a perceived lack of control over a current situation or immediate happening	Powerlessness related to inability to deal with anxiety
Chronic Low Self-Esteem	Long-standing negative self-evaluation/feelings about self or own capabilities	Chronic Low Self-Esteem related to inability to problem-solve daily situations effectively
Impaired Social Interaction	The state in which an individual participates in an insufficient or excessive quantity or ineffective quality of social exchange	Impaired Social Interaction related to self-imposed isolation
Social Isolation	Aloneness experienced by the individual and perceived as imposed by others and as a negative or threatened state	Social Isolation related to inability to engage in satisfying personal relationships
Spiritual Distress (Distress of the Human Spirit)	Disruption in the life principle which pervades a person's entire being and which integrates and transcends one's biological and psychosocial nature	Spiritual Distress related to intense suffering
Risk for Violence: Self-Directed or Directed at Others	A state in which an individual experiences behaviors that can be physically harmful either to the self or to others	Risk for Violence: Self-Directed related to unrelenting course of anxiety disorder

Diagnostic criteria from American Psychiatric Association. (1994). *Diagnostic and statistical manual of mental disorders, fourth edition.* Washington, D.C.: American Psychiatric Association. Nursing diagnoses and definitions from North American Nursing Diagnosis Association. (1994). *NANDA Nursing diagnoses: Definitions and classification 1995–1996.* Philadelphia: NANDA.

Anxiety, for example, short-term goals for the identified expected outcomes might include

Expected Outcome	Short-Term Goals
1. The patient will demonstrate techniques to reduce his or her own anxiety.	The patient will demonstrate deep breathing. The patient will demonstrate progressive relaxation.
2. The patient will be free of anxiety attacks.	The patient will take medications as prescribed. The patient will state the importance of taking medications in preventing anxiety attacks.
3. The patient will be safe.	The patient will state that his or her anxiety is under control.
4. The patient will report a significantly decreased anxiety level.	The patient will keep a daily journal to monitor his or her levels of anxiety.

For a patient with a nursing diagnosis of Ineffective Individual Coping, short-term goals for the identified expected outcomes might include the following:

Expected Outcome	Short-Term Goals
1. The patient will demonstrate alternative ways of coping with stress, including problem-solving and relaxation techniques.	The patient will state the steps of the problem-solving process. The patient will demonstrate progressive relaxation.
2. The patient will identify plans for future handling of stressful events.	The patient will state the importance of setting priorities in dealing with stress. The patient will state the importance of monitoring negative thoughts when confronted with stress.

For a patient with a nursing diagnosis of Post-Trauma Response, short-term goals for the identified expected outcomes might include the following:

Expected Outcome	Short-Term Goals
1. The patient will begin the grieving process.	The patient will acknowledge his or her loss. The patient will state the importance of allowing himself or herself to grieve.
2. The patient will express feelings directly and openly in a healthy, nondestructive manner.	The patient will allow himself or herself to cry. The patient will talk about his or her feelings concerning the loss.
3. The patient will experience increased ability to deal with stress.	The patient will report effective use of his or her new coping skills.
4. The patient will integrate the trauma into his or her life and be able to articulate a personal meaning that gives comfort and peace.	The patient will write about the trauma in his or her journal. The patient will identify in what ways the trauma has affected his or her life in a meaningful way.
5. The patient will express his or her feelings to God, thus experiencing resolution of the spiritual conflict and restoration of his or her relationship with God.	The patient will verbalize his or her feelings toward God. The patient will articulate spiritual conflicts. The patient will begin to pray again. The patient will talk with his or her member of the clergy.

▶ Check Your Reading

45. Identify at least four nursing diagnoses that might be appropriate for a patient suffering with an anxiety disorder.
46. Identify at least one expected outcome for each of the nursing diagnoses that you just listed.

IMPLEMENTATION

This section discusses therapy for the anxiety disorders in two practice settings, residential and outpatient. It is assumed that, for the most part, the severely disabled patient will be treated in a residential service; the less severely impaired patient will be seen in the community. It is further assumed that the residentially treated patient will receive nursing care both from psychiatric nurses who are generalists and from some with advanced preparation. Nursing care in the community is more likely to be provided by psychiatric nurses with clinical specialty preparation or by generically prepared nurses who receive supervision from clinical specialists.

Residential Treatment Setting

Patients who are severely distressed will likely be placed on anxiolytic drug therapy in combination with cognitive and/or behavioral therapies, individual supportive therapy, and group psychotherapy.

Your first nursing concern is the *safety of the patient.* The highly anxious patient is one whose condition is more labile and whose behavior reflects this rapidly changing status. It is imperative that any changes in the patient's status be promptly documented and any necessary changes in the care plan be made. You are legally responsible for provision of a safe patient environment.

Anxiety in substance abuse patients is a situation in which you are particularly vulnerable legally. Such patients are at much greater risk for elopement, drug diversion, and misuse of heparin locks. (Elopement refers to the patient's leaving the unit or hospital without permission, drug diversion refers to using drugs for other than prescribed purposes, and misuse of heparin locks refers to opening the heparin lock wide for direct access to the vein.) Because they succeeded previously in their attempts to make themselves less uncomfortable with drugs, they try to repeat this behavior with drugs that are found in the hospital or they attempt to elope in order to locate a "fix." If you are assigned to such a patient you are responsible for that person at all times during your shift. You need to know where that patient is and what she or he is doing.

Safety also encompasses the awareness that some of the patient's somatic complaints might be cardiovascular in nature. When severely distressed anxious patients present in the emergency department and are diagnosed, you may have a tendency to be less vigilant with them. Such patients need careful monitoring, and new complaints reported by them must be taken seriously and not assumed to be the somatization associated with acute anxiety. Less accurate assessment could result in overlooking actual cardiovascular problems.

Decreasing anxiety is your second nursing concern. In the ongoing nursing care of hospitalized patients, the calm, quiet voice of the nurse helps the patient to modulate his or her own affect. Help to objectify the patient's symptoms and to bring them under his or her control by asking questions to focus the patient on examining felt anxiety. Such questions can get the patient to recognize stimuli that trigger anxiety and to rank the intensity of it. Questioning the patient's experience can facilitate the patient's deciding on self-initiated behaviors to reduce anxiety, such as pacing, talking to the nurse or other patients, or asking for medication as needed.

It is important to provide the patient with the tools necessary to experience some control over symptoms. Therefore *teaching is the third nursing concern.* You can teach patients about a variety of anxiety-reducing tools and strategies, including:

Guided imagery (see Box 28–3)
Progressive relaxation
Controlled breathing
Physical exercise
Proper nutrition

Box 28–5 provides the directions for progressive relaxation.

You also can teach patients how to use controlled breathing to relieve anxiety. When people are in emotional distress, oxygen levels decrease. Breathing tends to become erratic and slow. Patients may begin to breathe too fast or might even stop breathing altogether for brief periods . . . all without realizing it. These are unhealthy breathing patterns. The exercise shown in Box 28–6 practiced for three to five minutes, can result in a feeling of calm, as well as relax and loosen muscles.

Teaching patients the benefits of physical exercise, particularly aerobic types, provides them with yet another tool to deal with anxiety. Exercise discharges the "fight or flight" energy associated with anxiety without harming personal relationships or the body. The benefits of

BOX 28–5 Directions for Progressive Relaxation

When your muscles are tense, movement is limited and energy flow is constricted. Muscles receive decreased blood circulation and oxygenation while accumulating waste products such as lactic acid and carbon dioxide. The following exercise, performed with or without soothing music, facilitates relaxation:

- Lie in a comfortable position. Allow your arms to rest at your sides, palms down, and exhale slowly and deeply with your eyes closed.
- Become aware of your feet, ankles, and legs. Notice if these parts of your body have any muscle tension or tightness. If so, breathe deeply and concentrate on that part of your body until you feel it relax. Release any anxious feelings with your breathing, continuing until the feelings begin to decrease in intensity and fade.
- Next, move your awareness into your hips, pelvis, and lower back. Breathe deeply until you feel them relax. Release any negative emotions as you breathe in and out.
- Focus on your abdomen and chest. Notice any anxious feelings located in this area and let them drop away as you breathe in and out.
- Finally, focus on your neck, arms, and hands. Note any tension in this area and release it. With your breathing, release any negative feelings blocked in this area until you cannot feel them any more.
- When you have finished releasing tension throughout the body, continue breathing deeply and relaxing for another minute or two. At the end of this exercise, you should feel lighter, more energized, and in control. Your body is relaxed and calm, and more important, no longer primed for an anxiety attack.

BOX 28–6 Directions for Controlled Breathing

- Lie flat on your back and pull your knees up. Keep your feet slightly apart and try to breathe in and out through your nose.
- Inhale deeply. As you breathe in, allow your stomach to relax so the air flows into your abdomen. Your stomach should balloon out as you breathe in.
- Visualize your lungs filling up with air so that your chest swells out.
- Imagine that the air you breathe is filling your body with energy.
- Exhale deeply. As you breathe out, let your stomach and chest relax. Imagine the air being pushed out, first from your stomach and then from your lungs.

exercise include improved oxygenation and blood circulation to tight muscles and organ systems; more efficient removal of wastes such as carbon monoxide, lactic acid, and other metabolic byproducts; the lowering of acidity of the blood to an optimal range; and the production of energy by the cells becoming more efficient.

Another way that exercise helps to reduce anxiety is through the action of hormones called beta endorphins. Beta endorphins, which are thought to be responsible for the "runner's high" experienced by marathon runners, are increased as much as five times by brisk exercise like running, cycling, walking, or swimming. Patients for whom anxiety is accompanied by significant muscle tightness and tension should also include activities that promote muscular flexibility, such as stretching exercises (Lark, 1994).

Proper nutrition is still another avenue that needs to be explored with patients. For instance, caffeine, as well as other stimulants such as diet pills and decongestants, foods high in refined sugar, and alcohol should be avoided by all patients who suffer from anxiety. Other foods such as dairy products, wheat, and gluten-containing grains may prove problematic for nutritionally sensitive patients and can exacerbate symptoms of anxiety as well as depression. Just as some foods should be avoided, others are beneficial in reducing anxiety. These include vegetables and fruits, legumes, gluten-free grains, whole grains, and seeds and nuts (Communication Channels, Inc., 1994; Lark, 1994).

Hoover and Parnell (1984) report on an inpatient educational group on stress and coping. Although the length of stay using their format would not be possible in the current health care environment, the tools for self-control that the authors offered the group are still of value. First, they provided handouts on the nature of stress and coping. They also asked their group members to complete a questionnaire on their coping methods. They used the group format to have patients share their perceptions of the meaning of stress. They also used the group format to provide some information in lecture format about other aspects of stress and its management. "Homework" assignments were used to help patients relate their own problems to the theoretical material that had been presented. In another session, patients were given materials on various kinds of relaxation methods. It is known that prayer, soothing music, progressive relaxation, guided imagery, and meditation are all useful tools for persons who tend to be tense; however, their usefulness increases only when patients have acquired the skills necessary to carry out the relaxation method without intense concentration on the technique. Thus, the methods themselves might not be optimally useful in the hospital setting while patients are learning, but if the patients could be exposed to the methods and persuaded to learn them while hospitalized, the skills could then be used after discharge.

The group discussed type A (uptight and driven) and type B (relaxed and calm) personalities and behaviors. They also were exposed to tenets of rational-emotive therapy (RET). They learned that a person's emotions and behaviors (C) are not caused by the events (A) that happen to them, but by the beliefs (B) that they hold about the events. To arrive at a different emotional effect (E) to the events, one must dispute (D) the "irrational beliefs" that cause the disturbance. This material led to examining individually held irrational beliefs and the substitution of rational ones. The last group session targeted the development of individual coping plans in which patients utilized the information about stressors, rational and irrational beliefs, tension-reducing behaviors, and coping to design a plan for their own rehabilitation. Homework assignments were given between sessions so patients could think about and list information that they needed for development of their own rehabilitation plans (Hoover and Parnell, 1984).

Medication teaching is the last issue that you must address with patients. The medications that are used to treat anxiety disorders include the anxiolytics, buspirone, antidepressants, and beta blockers. These medication teaching issues are addressed under nursing implications throughout the chapter.

The residential treatment setting is used to protect the patient, assess immediate needs, and begin pharmacotherapy, psychotherapy, and education. Before discharge, it is your legal responsibility to ensure that the patient has comprehended the material that was taught. Comprehension should be tested through instructions repeated by the patient or by return demonstrations. If the patient has not mastered that content, other alternatives need to be tried, such as inclusion of a significant other or family member in specified classes, provision of a review after discharge, or, if necessary, delay of discharge.

▶ Check Your Reading

47. Name three of the content areas that would be covered in an inpatient group focused on stress and coping.
48. What is the purpose of homework assignments for patients participating in a group on stress and anxiety?
49. What precautions are necessary if you are assigned to a patient who suffers from both extreme anxiety and a substance abuse problem?
50. What are the tenets of rational-emotive therapy?

Community Setting

The community as a practice setting is more frequently used by advanced psychiatric nurse practitioners. In that setting, pharmacotherapy can be continued with the patient's taking responsibility for necessary medical monitoring. For panic-related disorders, a combination of cognitive therapy, behavioral therapy, and pharmacotherapy has proved most useful in management of anxiety. Cognitive therapies are based on the assumptions that thinking mediates behavior and that thinking must change if behavior is to follow suit.

One well-researched technique is cognitive restructuring, in which negative statements about self are first identified. Their role in self-concept, behavior, and mood is acknowledged. Then the negative statements are replaced with positive statements about self that suggest the patient's ability to control and take care of himself or herself.

Behavioral therapies include planned and progressive exposures to the phobic stimulus under supervision. With support, systematic desensitization is accomplished through imagery and gradual presentation of scenes from the hierarchy in order of increasing difficulty. Flooding is another technique that involves the presentation of high-intensity aversive, anxiety-producing stimuli, either through imagery or in vivo without relaxation or pause until the anxiety is extinguished.

For obsessive-compulsive disorder (OCD), the combination of behavioral therapy and medication also is the best choice. You and the patient must take the time to properly assess the nature of the rituals and when they occur. You need to ask the patient to keep a diary initially to ascertain data concerning when, where, and for how long the ritual behavior(s) occurs. Research has supported the importance of using response recognition and delay as opposed to response prevention to reinforce the idea of reasonable behavior. The goal is for the patient to learn to delay the behavior(s) until an appropriate time rather than to prevent the behavior(s).

In behavioral therapy, key elements are realistic exposure to trigger situations and follow-up sessions to reinforce the behavioral changes. When behavioral modification is used, the patient learns to substitute positive, anxiety-reducing behaviors such as physical exercise and other pleasurable activities for ritualistic behaviors such as hand-washing or house-cleaning. It is important, however, to substitute varied behaviors so that one ritual is not substituted for another. For instance, it would not be helpful if the patient received a behavioral prescription to jog each time that the urge to wash his or her hands emerged. When working with a patient with OCD, you must evaluate the patient's daily life. When appropriate, you teach about leisure in a healthy lifestyle and the need for relaxation and pleasure. Overall, the goal is to reduce anxiety and to learn to delay ritualistic behavior. Anxiety management strategies may include talking about feelings with a trusted friend, physical activity, other individualized hobbies, utilizing the support of spiritual conviction, prayer, spiritual and/or religious reading, and possibly guided imagery.

The drug of choice for OCD is clomipramine (Anafranil). About 70% of patients in clinical trials of this drug get some relief from it.

For the patients who do not achieve reduction of their anxiety and ritualistic behavior, the risk of suicide should never be overlooked, especially in patients who come from families in which other members carry the same diagnosis. It is difficult enough to manage one's own distress. It is even more difficult to undergo trials of therapy, hoping for relief and finding none. Experiencing these problems and anticipating a future based on observations of older family members with unremitting OCD must be extremely difficult to bear.

For the patient who is severely impaired—whose daily life is dictated by ritualistic behavior—the chronic nature of the illness is not unlike other physical chronic illnesses. Depression sometimes evolves. Some of the most effective long-term interventions are spiritual in nature. Interventions that focus on meaning and on the needs of others and less on self and that encourage a patient to choose to participate in activities that are other directed provide hope and give purpose to life. You must be alert to changes in the patient's affect and mood. If suicidality is suspected, you assess for it just as you would in the case of a depressed patient without OCD.

▶ Check Your Reading

51. What is flooding, and when would it be used?
52. What is the treatment goal for a patient who suffers from OCD?
53. Why is suicidality a risk for a patient suffering from OCD?

EVALUATION

Once you have identified the patient's problem through thorough and accurate data collection in the assessment phase, you devise a plan for intervention that addresses deficits or appropriate alterations that are needed. The treatment plan is devised with the patient and any others that will be involved in the plan. Conceptualizing the plan in terms of expected initial and long-term outcomes for the patient makes later evaluation uncomplicated. You return to the baseline data from the initial interview. The formative evaluation compares the patient's state along the dimension(s) that were targeted. You modify the outcomes and plan as new data emerge. The summative evaluation compares the patient's state along those targeted dimension(s) at the conclusion of nursing care. Positive changes, as well as negative alterations and dimensions that have not changed from the baseline data, are noted.

CASE STUDY: TRAN

Tran is 28 years old and came to the United States from Vietnam 10 years ago. He is married and has two small children. Tran is employed as a manicurist and tells you that he lived in California for eight years but moved to the Midwest after a major earthquake two years ago. As a result of the earthquake, Tran and his wife Kim lost all of their possessions. He comes to the clinic today because he is having difficulty sleeping. He frequently experiences flashbacks and often has difficulty falling asleep. He tells you that he tries not to think about the earthquake, but that sometimes, "I see things in my mind as if they were real. I see dead bodies, people crying because they can't find their children or family." Tran tells you that when the thoughts come, he cannot rid his mind of them. His wife tells you that she is concerned because he will not leave the children out of his sight and is worried that another tragedy will befall their family. He used to laugh often and enjoy his work and now receives little enjoyment from any activity that previously brought him pleasure.

ASSESSMENT

Assessment data are as follows:

- Insomnia
- Flashbacks of earthquake
- Hypervigilant parenting
- Unable to experience pleasure
- Concerned wife

DIAGNOSIS

***DSM-IV* Diagnosis:** Posttraumatic Stress Disorder

Nursing Diagnosis: Post-Trauma Response related to survival of major earthquake as evidenced by flashbacks, sleep disturbance, hypervigilant parenting, fear of impending doom, and inability to find pleasure in daily activities.

OUTCOME IDENTIFICATION, PLANNING, AND IMPLEMENTATION

EXPECTED OUTCOME 1: By _____ the patient will begin the grieving process.

SHORT-TERM GOALS

By _____ the patient will talk about the traumatic event.

By _____ the patient will verbalize his need to grieve losses associated with the trauma.

NURSING INTERVENTIONS

1. Approach the patient in a nonthreatening and nonjudgmental manner; convey acceptance.
2. Listen attentively to the patient's story.
3. Allow the patient to describe in detail the losses associated with the earthquake.
4. Educate the patient about the grief process and the importance of working through all the thoughts and feelings associated with the loss.
5. Assess the patient's use of chemical substances to help repress or release emotions.

RATIONALES

1–2. Your manner displays respect and allows the patient to feel safe in your presence.

3. Retelling the experience to a trusted person helps the patient clarify reality and any misconceptions.

4. Grieving is a universal phenomenon, and knowing that it is normal and healthy to grieve losses will help the patient through the process in a more adaptive way.

5. It is not uncommon for patients to abuse chemicals in an attempt to blunt the feelings associated with the grieving process.

EXPECTED OUTCOME 2: By _____ the patient will express feelings directly and openly in a healthy, nondestructive manner.

SHORT-TERM GOAL

By _____ the patient will be able to identify basic feelings of anger, fear, guilt, sadness, shame, and happiness.

NURSING INTERVENTIONS

1. Educate the patient about the importance of paying attention to feelings as they occur and that all feelings are acceptable.
2. Encourage the patient to label the feelings for himself and to name what he thinks the feeling is, not what another person says he is feeling.

RATIONALES

1. Identifying and expressing feelings are central to the process of working through the grief process.

2. Feelings are very subjective and it is important for the patient to identify what he is feeling. Also, many cultures are taught to disregard feelings.

SHORT-TERM GOAL	NURSING INTERVENTIONS	RATIONALES
	3. Encourage the patient to acknowledge feelings for one week and to keep a daily record of these feelings in a journal.	3. Actually writing the feelings down on paper makes them real and more acceptable.
	4. Ask the patient to share these feelings with you or another trusted person or a support group when he is ready.	4. The patient needs to know that his feelings are acceptable to others and can be shared. Participating in a group will enable the patient to know that many others share his experience, which will help to alleviate his guilt.
	5. If the patient is unable to talk through his feelings or write about them because of a language barrier or cultural barrier, encourage expression in any way that is acceptable to the patient, such as physical release or crying.	5. It is important to individualize the treatment plan to allow for individual differences.
	6. Be aware of your own feelings as the patient experiences the intense rage, anger, and guilt associated with Posttraumatic Stress Disorder.	6. It is important in working with patients experiencing intense feelings that you do not project feelings on the patient that you have not acknowledged or avoid issues that you have not addressed yourself.

EXPECTED OUTCOME 3: By _____ the patient will experience increased ability to deal with stress.

SHORT-TERM GOAL	NURSING INTERVENTIONS	RATIONALES
By _____ the patient will establish an adequate balance of sleep, rest, and activity.	1. Ask the patient to keep a record of sleep patterns. 2. Educate the patient about the natural methods to induce sleep; if these do not work after one week, consider asking the physician to prescribe a sleeping medication.	1–2. Sleep often is disrupted in patients with Post-Trauma Response, and it may be necessary to intervene with pharmacotherapeutics.
	3. Assist the patient in structuring time for basic needs, such as hygiene, grooming, rest, and nutrition.	3. These measures will increase self-esteem and promote health and safety.
	4. Determine if the patient has a healthy balance of work and leisure time.	4. Workaholism is a common avoidance behavior associated with inability to process grief.

EXPECTED OUTCOME 4: By _____ the patient will integrate the trauma into his life and be able to articulate a personal meaning that gives comfort and peace.

SHORT-TERM GOALS	NURSING INTERVENTIONS	RATIONALES
By _____ the patient will recognize the need to understand the trauma in a context of meaning for him on his life's journey. By _____ the patient will use spiritual resources to seek comfort and relieve the distress he is feeling.	1. Encourage the patient to verbalize how he "makes sense" of his trauma in regard to his overall life journey. 2. Determine how the patient's religious beliefs affect his overall resolution of the trauma. 3. Determine if the patient participates in some type of organized religion.	1–3. Guilt and forgiveness are typically spiritual issues for the patient. If he is active in a church, the clergy and church members will be assets in his healing.
	4. Encourage the patient to make realistic plans for the future. 5. When the patient has worked through the anger and sadness of the grief process, ask him to verbalize the significance of the trauma on his life's journey.	4–5. Making realistic plans for the future and recognition of the survival of his wife and children enable him to have hope and to gain acceptance of the trauma.

EXPECTED OUTCOME 5: By _____ the patient will express his feelings to God and experience a resolution of his spiritual conflict.

SHORT-TERM GOALS	NURSING INTERVENTIONS	RATIONALES
By _____ the patient will recognize the anger and disappointment towards God for not protecting him and his family from the earthquake.	1. Encourage the patient to express any anger he may be feeling towards God and convey acceptance and understanding that this is a normal part of the grieving process.	1–2. It often is difficult for patients to feel and express anger toward God. Your gentle acceptance will enable the feelings to surface.
By _____ the patient will verbalize hope that his situation will improve.	2. Explain to the patient that all events in our lives, even painful and traumatic ones, have significance.	
	3. Periodically ask the patient if he feels any hope for the future.	3. Expressing hope indicates acceptance of the trauma and spiritual resolution.

EVALUATION

Formative Evaluation: Tran met each of the short-term goals except that he continued to have difficulty keeping a healthy balance between work and leisure. With the help of the nurse he found a support group for dealing with grief issues at his church. He decided to stay in the group for at least one year to gain additional support from the group members in maintaining a healthy balance in his life.

Summative Evaluation: After six months Tran was beginning to see some hope for the future but continued to have some difficulty with integrating the trauma into his life's journey. He continued to be angry about having to start over and continued to worry about his children's future. The nurse encouraged him to remain in a support group to continue to process these issues with others who experienced similar trauma.

CASE STUDY: ANNETTE

Annette is a 35-year-old woman whose husband, Jim, brought her to the clinic because she has been acting "strange" for the past several months. Jim tells you that for the past several months Annette has not been willing to leave the house and has been having attacks of anxiety and fear. Annette tells you that she has a fear of being closed in. She tells you that she is particularly fearful of tunnels and elevators. Jim is concerned because they are planning a driving trip soon.

Upon further questioning, Annette tells you that at least once a day she has "fear attacks." She says that during these episodes her heart pounds and beats very fast, her head hurts, she gets sick to her stomach, and she feels like she is going to die. She says that she has difficulty falling asleep and has nightmares. You notice that Annette seems tense, with sweaty palms and a fixed, anxious facial expression. Her heart rate is 120 and her respirations are 28.

ASSESSMENT

Assessment data are as follows:

- Daily panic attacks
- Anxious
- Unable to leave house
- Sleep disturbance
- Increased pulse and respirations, sweaty palms
- Supportive, concerned husband

DIAGNOSIS

***DSM-IV* Diagnosis:** Panic Attack With Agoraphobia

Nursing Diagnosis: Anxiety related to perceived threat of death and potential exposure to phobic stimulus evidenced by verbalizations of daily panic attacks, fear of leaving her house, and physical manifestations of anxiety (tense facial expression and increased vital signs).

OUTCOME IDENTIFICATION, PLANNING, AND IMPLEMENTATION

EXPECTED OUTCOME 1: By ____ the patient will demonstrate a significant decrease in symptoms of anxiety.

SHORT-TERM GOALS	NURSING INTERVENTIONS	RATIONALES
By ____ the patient will be able to verbalize a significant decrease in physical manifestations of anxiety.	1. Approach the patient in a calm, relaxed manner. 2. Listen actively to the patient's fears and anxieties, regardless of how irrational they may seem. 3. When the patient is able to tolerate it and adequate trust is established, ask her to describe physiological responses to anxiety. 4. Ask the patient to keep a written record for one week of any physical responses to anxiety. 5. Administer an anxiolytic per physician's order.	1–2. This helps the patient gain control and be able to accept help from the nurse. 3. Assisting the patient to recognize autonomic responses to anxiety helps her acknowledge feelings rather than deny or avoid them. 4. This empowers the patient in gaining some sense of control over anxious situations. 5. These medications are very effective when used to relieve the patient's immediate symptoms of anxiety.
By ____ the patient will be able to anticipate an impending anxiety attack.	1. Encourage the patient to share with you her written record of feelings and responses in the body. 2. Teach the patient to distinguish between anxiety that can be connected to a specific situation and anxiety for which no specific source is present. 3. Teach the patient to be able to tolerate mild levels of anxiety without having them escalate into an anxiety attack.	1–2. Being able to verbalize and clarify specific versus nonspecific anxiety helps the patient to control the response and accept times when anxiety-reduction strategies may be effective and when they may not be. 3. Anxiety is a part of human existence and can be both protective and constructive.

EXPECTED OUTCOME 2: By ____ the patient will actively employ measures to control anxiety.

SHORT-TERM GOALS	NURSING INTERVENTIONS	RATIONALES
By ____ the patient will demonstrate an ability to employ learned relaxation techniques.	1. Instruct the patient in the following relaxation techniques: progressive relaxation, slow, deep-breathing exercises, and visual imagery. 2. Have the patient practice these exercises with you or refer to a practitioner who will work with the patient. 3. Have the patient practice one or more of these techniques for one week and keep a journal of the effects.	1. These techniques help the patient using the principles of distraction and focused attention. 2–3. This enables the patient to determine what is effective and what does not work as well, incorporates behavioral modification in altering the patient's behavior, and requires the patient to be an active participant rather than a passive one.

SHORT-TERM GOALS	NURSING INTERVENTIONS	RATIONALES
By _____ the patient will verbalize the safe use of anxiolytic, tricyclic, and beta blocker medications for use in conjunction with behavioral and cognitive methods of anxiety control.	1. Teach the patient safe use of prescription for anxiolytics, tricyclics, and beta blockers and the potential dangers of addiction, especially for benzodiazepines. 2. Instruct the patient to keep a record of any medication that she takes for anxiety, noting the response and any side effects.	1. Patients should be taught the uses, side effects, and potential abuses of all pharmacological interventions. 2. Patients need to take an active part in the management of their anxiety.
By _____ the patient will be able to utilize functional coping strategies to assuage anxiety.	1. Using a nonjudgmental approach, determine previous coping strategies used by the patient to manage anxiety. 2. Encourage the patient to adopt more favorable strategies to manage anxiety, such as suppression and displacement. 3. Give the patient concrete examples of new ways to cope. For example, encourage her to say, "I choose not to talk about my fear about going outside right now—I will talk about it tomorrow."	1. Some of the patient's previous strategies for coping have worked. The patient needs to be validated for this success and then will perhaps be open and willing to learn additional strategies. Helps to maintain personal integrity. 2. Suppression and displacement are effective when used as temporary measures. 3. One or two concrete examples rather than a long list of nonspecific suggestions are more likely to ensure success.

EXPECTED OUTCOME 3: By _____ the patient will demonstrate a marked reduction in avoidance behavior when confronted with feared situations—tunnels, bridges, and social outings.

SHORT-TERM GOALS	NURSING INTERVENTIONS	RATIONALES
By _____ the patient will be able to verbalize an understanding of activities that precipitate a panic attack.	1. Ask the patient to identify specific factors that increase or decrease phobic responses. 2. Encourage collaboration with you in making a decision about the patient's approach to the phobia. For example, the patient may choose to work on issues and circumstances related to agoraphobia and not address the phobias associated with bridges and tunnels.	1. Recognizing precipitating factors is the first step in teaching the patient to interrupt escalating anxiety. 2. This allows the patient some control in the decision-making process. Unless the phobia is affecting the patient significantly, it may be more appropriate to work on only one phobia at a time. If the patient never goes through a tunnel except on vacation, this issue can be delayed.
By _____ the patient will limit intake of caffeine, nicotine, and other central nervous system stimulants that produce physiological manifestations of anxiety.	1. Determine the extent of use of central nervous system stimulants by the patient. 2. Inform the patient of the effects of caffeine and nicotine on the central nervous stimulation and elicit cooperation from the patient in reducing the intake of these substances.	1–2. Reduction of the intake of these substances will rule out their impact on the patient's anxiety.
By _____ the patient will actively participate in a planned program to desensitize phobic responses.	1. When the patient is ready, have her participate in a planned desensitization program. 2. Expose the patient to the feared object or situation progressively and monitor response. 3. Offer positive reinforcement whenever the patient is able to confront the phobic situation with a minimum of anxious behaviors.	1–2. Patients who are gradually exposed to a feared object or situation will eventually become desensitized. This is a form of behavior modification. 3. Positive statements that are truthful help convey confidence and help restore previous coping skills.

EXPECTED OUTCOME 4: By _____ the patient will express hopeful, futuristic plans.

SHORT-TERM GOAL	NURSING INTERVENTIONS	RATIONALES
By _____ the patient verbalizes a sense of control over her behavior and management of care.	1. Encourage the patient to verbalize the meaning and significance of her anxiety and agoraphobia in relation to the rest of her life and her future.	1. This helps the patient to make some sense of this event as one of many in a full life experience.
By _____ the patient is able to view this event as one of many on her journey in life.	2. Ask the patient to describe an event in the future that the patient is anticipating.	2. This enables the patient to have hope that this treatment approach will be effective.
	3. Encourage the patient to share this hope for the future with significant others in her life.	3. By verbalizing her hopes to significant others, she strengthens her own position and allows others to affirm her positive thinking.

EVALUATION

Formative Evaluation: Annette met each of the short-term goals in the time frames that were allotted except for learning relaxation exercises. She stated that she would keep trying but that she was still having difficulty with relaxation.

Summative Evaluation: With the help of the nurse and Annette's husband, Annette was able to meet all of the expected outcomes. Two months after her initial visit to the clinic, she and her husband were planning a car trip, and Annette was confident that she would complete the trip without an anxiety attack.

CONCLUSIONS

Both residential and community nursing care of patients with anxiety disorders is challenging and ultimately satisfying. Anxiety disorders tend to be amenable to treatment with anxiolytic drugs, supportive psychotherapy, and behavioral and cognitive therapies. As you care for patients with anxiety, notice how readily anxiety is shifted to other patients and to the staff. Take measures to prevent that process by identifying the source of the anxiety and to whom it belongs. It is also imperative that you correctly assess the patient's level of anxiety and that you take measures to bring distress to manageable levels. Finally, it will be your responsibility to provide and maintain a safe environment for the patient, to determine when the patient may be at greater risk for self-injury or suicide, and to communicate those findings to the appropriate resources.

KEY POINTS TO REMEMBER

- Anxiety is a feeling of alertness and concern that prepares a person to take action of some kind. Anxiety in normal proportions is a trigger that is helpful to growth. Normal anxiety is short term and of low to moderate intensity.
- Anxiety disorders are characterized by symptoms of anxiety and efforts to avoid those symptoms.
- Anxiety affects the body, mind, spirit, and emotions.
- Anxiolytics are the drugs that usually are used to reduce anxiety.
- The etiology of anxiety is theorized to be in psychobiological, psychodynamic, and behavioral terms.
- Stress is the broader response of which anxiety is one dimension.
- Stress is examined in terms of its immediate, intermediate, and long-term responses.
- Anxiety occurs along a continuum ranging from mild, to moderate, to severe, to panic.
- People cope with anxiety using either conscious coping mechanisms or preconscious or unconscious processes called defense mechanisms.
- Generalized anxiety disorder is characterized by unrealistic or excessive anxiety and worry about two or more life circumstances.
- Generalized anxiety disorders usually respond to benzodiazepines, as well as buspirone.
- Nursing implications for a patient diagnosed with generalized anxiety disorder include medication teaching and monitoring.
- Panic disorder is characterized by discrete periods of intense fear or discomfort that are recurrent.
- Panic disorder may exist with or without agoraphobia.
- Imipramine is one of the most effective medications in treating panic disorders.
- Patients experiencing panic attacks usually present in the emergency department.
- Obsessive-compulsive disorder (OCD) is reflected in ritualistic behaviors that may occur in thought or action.
- Obsessions are persistent thoughts.
- Compulsions are repetitive behaviors that follow an obsession.

- Clomipramine is the drug of choice in treating OCD.
- Posttraumatic stress disorder (PTSD) is a maladaptive set of responses to an event that has been overwhelmingly distressing.
- PTSD presents with physiological as well as psychological symptoms.
- Both pharmacotherapy and psychotherapy are used in the treatment of PTSD.
- Phobias are irrational fears. Specific phobia includes severe fear of clearly identifiable objects or situations; social phobia is a profound and enduring fear of social or performance situations where embarrassment could occur.
- Assessment of a patient with an anxiety disorder identifies the pattern used by the patient to cope with the anxiety.
- Assessment focuses on the defining characteristics of anxiety and its severity and the impact of the symptoms of anxiety on the patient's life.
- Nursing diagnoses for anxiety disorders include Anxiety, Fear, Social Isolation, Ineffective Individual Coping, High Risk for Self-Directed Violence, and Post-Trauma Response.
- Expected outcomes include a decrease in the feelings of anxiety and increased coping abilities in dealing with anxiety.
- Nursing strategies vary whether the patient is in residential or community-based treatment.
- Evaluation includes a formative and summative focus.

LEARNING ACTIVITIES

1. Observe yourself the next time you are anxious. What behaviors are you exhibiting?

2. Write down the behaviors you use to cope with anxiety. Which are most effective?

3. Read *The Boy Who Couldn't Stop Washing* by Rappoport (1989). What impact do you think having OCD has on a patient's journey?

4. Observe your behavior with your peers, patients, and others. Are you able to calm others when they are anxious? If so, what behaviors are you using that are effective? If people become more "uptight" in your presence, examine what behaviors are causing them to escalate in their anxiety.

5. Observe someone who you think is very effective with patients. What strategies do you observe the person doing?

CRITICAL THINKING EXERCISE

Mrs. Peterson, a 45-year-old patient on the psychiatry unit, approaches the nurse's station clutching her chest, gasping for air. Nurse A, a new nurse to the unit, does not know this patient's history. She asks the patient to sit down while she takes her vital signs. Nurse B, who knows that Mrs. Peterson has a history of anxiety attacks, tells Nurse A that the patient just wants attention and to ignore her hysteria.

1. What assumption is Nurse B making?

2. If Nurse A follows Nurse B's advice, what assumption is Nurse B making?

3. What other evidence is needed to determine the appropriate intervention?

Nurse A decides to consider an alternative approach. She notes that the patient's husband and a female visitor have just left the unit. She asks Mrs. Peterson about the intensity, duration, and severity of her pain. The patient reports that the pain started when her husband told her he has filed for divorce and does not want her to return to the house. When asked what would help her feel calmer, the patient states that Valium helps. Nurse A decides to give the patient Valium and observe her frequently for the next hour.

1. What could have happened if Nurse A had not considered an alternative approach?

2. If Nurse B interacted with the patient, what else could have happened as a result?

3. What is an alternative to the above approaches?

REFERENCES

American Psychiatric Association. (1994). *Diagnostic and statistical manual of mental disorders–IV.* Washington, D.C.: American Psychiatric Association.

Beigel, A., and Berren, M. (1985). Human induced disasters. *Psychiatric Annals, 15* (3), 143–150.

Brawman-Mintzer, O., Lydiard, R. B., Crawford, M. M., Emmanuel, N., Payeur, R., Johnson, M., Knapp, R. G., and Ballenger, J. C. (1994). Somatic symptoms in generalized anxiety disorder with and without comorbid psychiatric disorders. *American Journal of Psychiatry, 151* (6), 930–933.

Brown, T. A., Barlow, D. H., and Liebowitz, M. R. (1994). The empirical basis of generalized anxiety disorder. *American Journal of Psychiatry, 151* (9), 1271–1281.

Communication Channels, Inc. (1994). Fertility and anxiety affected by caffeine. *Better Nutrition for Today's Living, 56* (9), 22, 23.

Crowe, R., Pauls, D., and Slymen, D. (1980). A family study of anxiety neurosis: Morbidity risk in families of patients with and without mitral valve prolapse. *Archives of General Psychiatry, 37,* 77–79.

Danton, W. G., Altrocchi, J., Antonuccio, D., and Basta, R. (1994). Nondrug treatment of anxiety. *American Family Physician, 49* (1), 161–167.

DiNartdo, P., and Barlow, D. (1988). Anxiety disorders interview schedule revised (ADIS-R). Albany: Phobia and Anxiety Disorders Clinic, University of Albany, State University of New York.

Flint, A. J. (1994). Epidemiology and comorbidity of anxiety disorders in the elderly. *American Journal of Psychiatry, 151* (5), 640–650.

Haack, M., and Alim, T. (1991). Anxiety and the adult child of an alcoholic: A co-morbid problem. *Family Community Health, 13* (4), 49–60.

Hill, L. (1991). The neurophysiology of acute anxiety: A review of the literature. *CRNA: The Clinical Forum for Nurse Anesthetists, 2* (2), 52–61.

Hoehn-Saric, R. (1979). Anxiety—normal and abnormal. *Psychiatry Annals, 9,* 447–449.

Hoover, R., and Parnell, P. (1984). An inpatient educational group on stress and coping. *Journal of Psychosocial Nursing, 22* (6), 17–22.

Horowitz, M. (1986). *Stress response syndromes* (2nd ed.). New York: Aronson.
Hunt, D. (1988). *No more fears.* New York: Warner Books.
Johnson, J., Weissman, M., and Klerman, G. (1990). Panic disorder, comorbidity, and suicide attempts. *Archives of General Psychiatry, 47,* 805–808.
Karno, M., Golding, J., Sorenson, S., and Burnam, M. (1988). The epidemiology of obsessive-compulsive disorder in five US communities. *Archives of General Psychiatry, 45,* 1094–1099.
Katon, W., Sheehan, T., and Uhde, T. (1988). Panic disorder: A treatable problem. *Patient Care,* March 30, 149–154.
Keltner, N. L., and Folks, D. G. (1993). *Psychotropic drugs.* St. Louis: Mosby-Year Book.
Kolb, L. (1987). Neuropsychological hypothesis explaining posttraumatic stress disorder. *American Journal of Psychiatry, 144* (8), 989–995.
Lader, M. (1994). Treatment of anxiety. *British Medical Journal, 309* (6950), 321–325.
Lark, S. M. (1994). Strike back at anxiety: Natural ways to stay calm in stressful times. *Vegetarian Times,* #198, 90–93.
Lazarus, R., and Folkman, S. (1984). Stress, appraisal and coping. New York: Springer.
Lipsitz, J. D., Martin, L. Y., Mannussa, S., Chapmann, T. F., Liebowitz, M., Klein, D. F., and Fyer, A. J. (1994). Childhood separation anxiety disorder in patients with adult anxiety disorders. *American Journal of Psychiatry, 151* (6), 927–930.
Norman, E. (1989). Analysis of the concept of posttraumatic stress disorder. *Journal of Advanced Medical Surgical Nursing, 1* (4), 55–64.
Porterfield, L. (1991). Update on anxiolytics. *Advancing Clinical Care,* September/October, 14, 15.
Rappoport, J. (1989). *The boy who couldn't stop washing.* New York: E. P. Dutton.
Restak, R. (1980). *The brain: The last frontier.* New York: Warner Books.
Robinson, L. (1990). Stress and anxiety. *Nursing Clinics of North America, 25* (4), 935–943.
Schatzberg, A. (1991). Overview of anxiety disorders: Prevalence, biology, course, and treatment. *Clinical Psychiatry, 52* (7), 5–8.
Scurfield, R. (1985). Post-trauma stress assessment and treatment: Overview and formulations. In C. R. Figley (Ed.), *Trauma and its wake* (pp. 219–256). New York: Brunner/Mazel.
Seligman, M. E. P. (1994). What you can change & what you cannot change. *Psychology Today, 27* (3), 34–47.
Spielberger, C. (1984). *State Trait Anxiety Inventory.* Palo Alto, CA: Consulting Psychologists Press, Inc.
Stein, M. B., Walker, J. R., and Forde, D. R. (1994). Setting diagnostic thresholds for social phobia: Considerations from a community survey of social anxiety. *American Journal of Psychiatry, 151* (3), 408–413.
Van der Kolk, B., Boyd, T., and Krystal, J. (1984). Posttraumatic stress disorder as a biologically based disorder: Implications of the animal mode of inescapable shock. In B. van der Kolk (Ed.), *Posttraumatic stress disorder: Psychological and biological sequelae.* Washington, D. C.: American Psychiatric Press.
Wright, N., Caplan, R., and Payne, S. (1994). Community survey of long term use of benzodiazepines. *British Medical Journal, 309* (6946), 27–29.
Zetin, M., and Kramer, M. (1992). Obsessive-compulsive disorder. *Hospital and Community Psychiatry, 43* (7), 689–699.

SUGGESTED READINGS

Lark, S. M. (1994). Strike back at anxiety: Natural ways to stay calm in stressful times. *Vegetarian Times,* #198, 90–93.
Rappoport, J. (1989). *The boy who couldn't stop washing.* New York: E. P. Dutton.
Robinson, L. (1990). Stress and anxiety. *Nursing Clinics of North America, 25* (4), 935–943.
Zetin, M., and Kramer, M. (1992). Obsessive-compulsive disorder. *Hospital and Community Psychiatry, 43* (7), 689–699.

CHAPTER 29

THE JOURNEY CONTROLLED BY THOUGHT DISORDERS

True—nervous—very, very dreadfully nervous I had been and am!—not destroyed—not dulled then. Above all was the sense of hearing acute. I heard all things in the heaven and in the earth. I heard many things in hell. How, then, am I mad? Harken! and observe how healthily—how calmly—I can tell you the whole story.

—*Edgar Allan Poe*

LEARNING OBJECTIVES

After studying this chapter, you should be able to:

1. Describe the hallucinatory experiences that affect the journey of the schizophrenic patient.
2. Give examples of affective disturbance, disordered association of thought, autism, and ambivalence.
3. Define first-rank and second-rank symptoms, Bleuler's four As, and positive and negative symptoms that describe the schizophrenic's journey.
4. Discuss potential causes for the journey of schizophrenia.
5. Describe the nurse's role in facilitating the journey of the schizophrenic patient and the family.
6. Identify the role of psychotropic medications in schizophrenia.
7. Identify assessment strategies for collecting data on a patient with schizophrenia.
8. Identify appropriate nursing diagnoses for a patient with schizophrenia.
9. Identify expected outcomes when working with a patient with schizophrenia.
10. Apply the nursing process to a patient with schizophrenia.
11. Describe schizophrenic patients' vulnerabilities to abusing substances and strategies to prevent frequent relapse.

KEY TERMINOLOGY

Biological vulnerability
Delusions
Delusions of grandeur
Delusions of persecution
First-rank symptoms
Formal thought disorder
Hallucinations
High expressed emotion
Ideas of reference
Illusions
Loose association
Negative symptoms
Neuroleptic medication
Paranoid personality disorder
Personal vulnerability
Positive symptoms
Psychoeducation
Schizophrenia
Schizotypal personality disorder
Second-rank symptoms
Word salad

"Schizophrenia is to psychiatry what cancer is to medicine: a sentence as well as a diagnosis" (Hall et al, 1985, p. 3). **Schizophrenia** is the most disabling of major mental disorders. An estimated 180,000 patients are hospitalized each year in the United States with schizophrenia. When undiagnosed, untreated, and ambulatory patients are added to this number, the number of schizophrenic patients tops half a million people. In 1994, the cost of treating schizophrenia in the United States was $33 billion a year, with 25% of hospital beds occupied by schizophrenics (NAMI Advocate, 1994). Hospital costs are estimated to exceed $100,000 annually for chronic inpatient treatment and up to $10,000 per relapse.

Typically, schizophrenia begins in late adolescence or early adulthood, usually appearing before age 30 and appearing in men earlier than in women. The onset may be abrupt or insidious. First signs are often gradual social withdrawal, loss of interest in school or work, unusual behavior, and angry outbursts. The disease occurs across all races around the world.

Most schizophrenics become chronic victims of the illness. Their symptoms persist for at least 6 months and generally for a lifetime. The most disturbed of these individuals are tortured by voices and other personal "demons." The stress of caring for such a disturbed family member may strain a marriage, interfere with social life, and drain the family's resources. The cost of suffering to families cannot be estimated; a lifetime commitment to caring for a chronically ill family member carries with it a considerable cost to families (Winter, 1990).

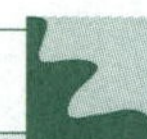

MARK'S STORY

In the 1970s, Mark Vonnegut, son of author Kurt Vonnegut, traveled toward a simpler life in Vancouver, B.C., leaving the staidness and conservatism of the East Coast. At the end of his journey, because of his own personal vulnerabilities, he became frankly psychotic. His first-person account, *Journey to Eden* (1975), is filled with descriptions from the ill person's perspective.

"By this time the voices had gotten very clear. At first I'd had to strain to hear or understand them. They were soft and working with some pretty tricky codes. Snap-crackle-pop, the sound of the wind with blinking lights and horns for punctuation. I broke the code and somehow was able to internalize it to the point where it was just like hearing words. In the beginning it was mostly nonsense, but as things went along they made more and more sense. Once you hear the voices, you realize they've always been there. It's just a matter of being tuned into them" (p. 106).

As Mark traveled with his friends and began homesteading with them in Vancouver, he began to experience more and more of the perceptual difficulties and misinterpretation of reality common to those experiencing their first psychotic break. Perhaps because he was living with such an "anti-establishment" group, the early clues to his psychotic disintegration were ignored or otherwise explained away. Eventually, though, even his tolerant group of friends recognized his need for psychiatric treatment. They could see that his bizarre behavior was causing him great distress and pain.

DIFFERENTIATING NORMAL PERCEPTIONS FROM PSYCHOSIS

In Edgar Allan Poe's "The Tell-Tale Heart" (1843), the main character, sensitive to his companion's "pale blue eye" with its film over it, is filled with horror and dread. The "madman" attaches great significance to this "evil eye" and believes it has great power to control him: It makes his "blood run cold." He concocts a murder plan to rid himself of the old man and the image forever. The protagonist, probably having lapsed into some sort of schizophreniclike condition, states, "Have I not told you that what you mistake for madness is but overacuteness of the senses?" In a clear description of a psychotic person's subjective experience, this character is tormented by the loud beating of the old man's heart. "Meanwhile, the hellish tattoo of the heart increased. It grew quicker and quicker, and louder and louder every instant . . . I thought the heart must burst," until he finally kills him and stuffs him under the floor. Obviously, in the "real" world, people's hearts do not beat loudly enough to be heard thumping through the floorboards, especially after a person has been killed. In this chilling description of the character's torment, however, Poe has placed his finger on a central theme of madness: the alteration of the senses so especially prominent in the early stage of schizophrenia.

This story told by Poe is frightening and unfortunately reinforces many cultural stereotypes about mental illness—especially that of the dangerous maniac who will misinterpret what we say and act to harm us. Actually, few schizophrenics commit violent crimes, although those who do certainly receive a lot of publicity. The misperception or heightened sense of reality experienced by the schizophrenic, however, may be far more common than we realize.

The whole disease process of "madness" is foreign to us. We find it difficult to sympathize with people who act bizarrely, say strange things, withdraw from us, or even threaten to harm us. This person is not the one we have known and we cannot understand why he or she is acting as he or she is. Inability of outsiders to understand the subjective experience of madness increases the suffering of the schizophrenic. Families and health care providers have difficulty reaching out to the person suffering with a "brain playing tricks on itself," hearing unseen voices, unable to feel emotions or to reason logically.

Bleuler (Kaplan and Sadock, 1989) has pointed out that nearly all schizophrenic mechanisms—daydreams, for example, and the bizarre and disjointed symbolism often found in dreams—can be found in normal people. What separates the person with schizophrenic disease is the inability to distinguish between the two realities—that of the internal world and that of the objective world. The psychosis associated with schizophrenia is defined as loss of contact with reality. Imagine waking from a terrifying nightmare to be still in it.

Normal and Enhanced Perceptions

We know the world around us by the ability of our senses—seeing, hearing, tasting—to take in information and interpret it according to our previous learning. Even an infant gradually sorts through the perceptual bombardment of stimuli to organize the world to have most basic needs met. Understanding "what to expect" when we notice our environment interferes with the freshness with which we view the world.

People have long searched for ways to counter the "filtering" effect that gives the world order and predictability by expanding and enhancing sensory perception. Writer Aldous Huxley experimented with mescaline (1956) and reported, "Mescaline raises all colors to a higher power and makes the person aware of innumerable fine shades of difference, to which, at ordinary times, he is completely blind." Others have sought these "peak experiences" through physical challenge, art, or religious experiences. These peak experiences are those times when we experience colors, sounds, or tastes acutely: Our attention is fully directed toward that object outside ourselves. Csikszentmihalyi (1990) describes these "optimal experiences" as ". . . what the sailor holding a tight course feels when the wind whips through her hair, when the boat lunges through the waves like a colt—sails, hull, wind, and sea humming a harmony that vibrates in the sailor's veins. It is what a painter feels when the colors on the canvas begin to set up a magnetic tension with each other, and a new thing, a living form, takes shape in front of the astonished creator."

Sensory Alterations

The early prepsychotic experiences of the schizophrenic are not much different from these peak experiences. Some studies state that perceptual dysfunction occurs in almost two thirds of patients becoming psychotic. Most patients cannot describe these sensual alterations until they have recovered from a psychotic episode. The alterations can be either enhancement (most common) or blunting of any or all of the senses. Initially, before more complete disorganization occurs, the sensations can be quite pleasant, as Vonnegut (1975, p. 74) describes:

Things were still unbearably beautiful. I got this giddiness in my stomach and walked around completely overwhelmed by the incredible loveliness of the trees and the sky and the moss, infinitely delicate worlds within worlds, and people's faces and the way they moved and my own body and what a perfect machine it was and the stove and our funky house. Everything fit together so perfectly. It wasn't just in the way things looked. It was in the sounds of the wind and the stream and the way things felt, the ground gushing ever so slightly under my feet, the way everything smelled.

Closely related to the experience of overacute sensation is the flooding of the senses with stimuli. Not only do the senses become sharper, but they are also unable to filter anything out (Torrey, 1988). Normally, we can concentrate our attention on whatever we choose. Persons with schizophrenia, unable to filter and select stimuli, experience flooding of their brains. The initially pleasant hyperawareness gradually or suddenly becomes uncomfortable and confusing.

Sensory modalities other than hearing and vision may also be affected. Pain may be misperceived, and the person may find the touch of a health care provider excruciatingly unpleasant. Sensations can be blunted as well as enhanced in schizophrenia, more often in the later course of the illness. The blunting is described as if a "heavy curtain were drawn over his mind; it resembled a dead thickening cloud that prevented the free use of his senses" (Torrey, 1988). Blunting of pain may have dramatic consequences for the patient who is not aware of physical symptoms, such as broken bones or fingertips burned with cigarettes. Psychotic patients are at risk for self-mutilation in response to voices commanding them to harm themselves, and they may not feel pain.

Sexual feelings may be heightened, as Mark Vonnegut (1975) describes:

I was electric with sexuality. Breathing gave me orgasm upon orgasm. I can't begin to describe what dancing with angels was like. Occasionally the puritan in me would try to worry about having to pay for this some day, but the pleasure was so all-engulfing there was very little room for second thoughts.

Because of the breakdown of the brain's "filter," presumed to originate in the limbic system, the brain may also be flooded with thoughts that cannot be sorted and that decrease the ability to concentrate. It is as though the mind is flooded with stimuli from both outside (sensual perception) and inside (thoughts and memories). Some people feel that others are putting thoughts in their heads.

A fundamental defect of the schizophrenic's brain is a frequent inability to sort, interpret, and respond, perhaps because of a deficiency in the limbic system (see Chapter 7). Although this is often described as a **formal thought disorder,** more than just thoughts are involved. Visual and auditory stimuli are misarranged in similar ways, much as if a switchboard operator were plugging wires into the wrong connection. The operator (i.e., the brain) is receiving all of the input (i.e., sensory stimuli, thoughts, emotions, memories, and ideas) and is unable to sort them automatically into a pattern of coherent thought that allows for logical responses, as Case Example 29–1 shows.

Case Example 29–1 Rick's Story

One hot night in the summer of 1976, I was driving my father's Volkswagen, and I had a psychotic episode behind the wheel. I ended up in Dundalk, going down a one-way street, when a policeman pulled me over. He questioned me about my actions. I was together externally at first: I gave him my license and waited to get my ticket. But I was scared, like a paranoid schizophrenic. While the cop looked at the license, I pulled off down the one-way street, driving like mad.

Six police cars chased me. They finally got me on a field and pulled me out of the car. They hit me with a stick; I got beat up. I had a gash in my forehead and I was taken to a special police hospital to have stitches put in. Using substances led to some weird things.

This incident led to my first hospitalization at Provident Medical Center. A counselor I was seeing and my parents decided I needed hospitalization. I remember how alienated and alone I felt, and how the patients were abusive. One fellow there was court committed. He had stolen some furs, and he was acting like he was king of the place and we were his servants.

I lied and told the staff I wasn't on any drugs, but they must have found out—they did blood tests. For treatment they put me on medication: Haldol, then Thorazine. It was pretty strange—Haldol is a very powerful antipsychotic. It was a different kind of feeling; I don't want to say a different high—by no means are these medications a high. I felt bad but they stabilized me for a period of time, till I could go out and get more drugs.

In the hospital I thought I was an extra-terrestrial. I had read a lot about extra-terrestrials from occult scientists. We were here to usher in a new age and help mankind. Since I was from another planet, I thought I had special powers. Sometimes, I could pick up universal vibrations that would help me to play music. I would see trees move and when I'd see a certain flight pattern of birds I would think a certain way. You start putting that together day after day, week after week, and you begin to think that you have control over nature and man.

I became telepathic; I could listen to anything, even plants and trees. The birds in the trees would have a voice. With me musing in my thoughts, I would have a conversation. "Hi, how are you doing, a sunny day isn't it?" The birds would say, "Fine, it's a nice day." They would reflect my thoughts. I would talk to my plants too. It's a fine line between reality perception and fantasy because a lot of people talk to their plants and they do grow better. I still talk to my plants, and they grow pretty good.

From Suska, M. A. (1991). *Cry of the invisible* (pp. 19–20). Baltimore: Conservatory Press.

▶ Check Your Reading

1. How are the perceptual experiences of a schizophrenic similar to a peak experience?
2. What is a thought disorder?
3. What area of the brain is thought to be defective in filtering sensory stimuli?

The Schizophrenic's Journey and the Role of Nursing

Patients with schizophrenia demand the best skills that you have. Because of the difficulties these patients experience with communication and relatedness, you are challenged to reach out without being threatening and to be natural and honest while maintaining a professional role. Empathic understanding of the patient's experience is essential. To approach and develop a relationship with a person who may be misinterpreting the environment, you must be sensitive to the psychotic person's difficulties. To employ the therapeutic use of self, you must be aware of the process of a thought disorder while showing respect for the patient as a person. For example, you assess the patient's perceptual differences by asking the patient about hallucinations and by observing behaviors that might indicate the patient is either responding or attending to internal stimuli. You ask the patient to describe experiences and note the degree to which this description differs from the your perception of the environment. Case Example 29–2 describes a schizophrenic person's perception of reality.

Case Example 29–2 Don's Story

SOMEONE'S SCREAMING,
BUT THERE IS NO SOUND

By Don Shack

Someone's screaming, but there is no sound.
Flames of fury which blaze within the innermost soul,
extinguished by reality.

A night with no darkness,
like a grain of sand trapped in time,
on the beaches of reality.

A sunrise with no morning.
Castles built of dreams,
which are washed away by the flow of reality.

A love with no regret,
awash on a tempestuous sea of reality.
Crying, but not with tears.
Scared, but there are no fears.
Getting older, but not in years.
Could it be that no one hears?

And as the end draws near,
Listen hard, and I think you'll hear
someone screaming. Is it you?

So take my hand and follow me,
and as we drift across that stormy sea,
maybe we'll lose reality.

And if we don't,
we'll both wake up in the morning.
So stop screaming—now I can hear you.

But, can I reach you?

From Suska, M. A. (1991). *Cry of the invisible* (p. 67). Baltimore: Conservatory Press.

▶ Check Your Reading

4. Why does the schizophrenic patient pose a challenge to the psychiatric nurse?
5. How do you assess whether or not a person is experiencing hallucinations?

DEFINITIONS OF SYMPTOMS AND DISEASE

As early as 1400 B.C., a condition described in Hindu literature was thought to be brought on "by devils," in which the afflicted person was "gluttonous, filthy, walks naked, has lost his memory, and moves about in an uneasy manner." Soranus, in the 2nd century A.D., described delusions of grandeur of patients who believed themselves to be God or were afraid to urinate because they would cause a new deluge. Until the 18th century, people with mental disorders were simply contained or hidden rather than treated because many believed that insanity resulted from possession by the devil or evil spirits or indicated some punishment by the gods. The insane were feared and stigmatized until the concept of "moral treatment," which resembles today's milieu therapy and other social therapies, was applied widely to hospitalized psychotics in the United States in the 19th century. Unfortunately, with the establishment of large mental hospitals in the late 1800s, personal approaches to individual patients were lost. Only in the early 1900s did the scientific community begin to experiment and speculate about treatment for the insane.

Even today, recognition of schizophrenia as a disease entity continues to be the subject of much confusion and debate. With considerable overlap among symptoms of different mental disorders, schizophrenia is probably more than one disease entity, with different types, subgroups, and brain dysfunctions. Psychotic symptoms also do not always indicate schizophrenia. Symptoms can be caused by metabolic abnormalities as well as other neurological diseases. For example, a person experiencing the sensation of bugs crawling over the skin could be suffering from a psychosis caused by alcohol withdrawal or even exposure to some toxic drug or chemical. Persons suffering from an acute episode of schizophrenic illness could also experience some of the same symptoms as a person experiencing drug withdrawal, usually accompanied by other symptoms, such as hearing voices.

Symptomatic definitions of mental states or disorders are imprecise, yet an accurate diagnosis is of utmost importance. The diagnosis determines the type of treatment. For instance, if the symptoms are a result of schizophrenia, antipsychotic medication is prescribed; if the symptoms result from drug withdrawal, benzodiazepines are the medication of choice.

▶ Check Your Reading

6. Give two historical examples of how schizophrenia was viewed.
7. Why is it difficult to diagnose schizophrenia on the basis of psychotic symptoms alone?
8. Why is it important to differentiate schizophrenia from another disorder that might produce similar psychotic symptoms?

Kraepelin's Understanding of Schizophrenia

The term *demence precoce* was first introduced by Morel in 1856, the time of the first distinctions between early defects and "idiocy" as congenital and "dementia" as acquired or reversible defects (Kaplan and Sadock, 1989). Kraepelin, a European physician who worked in a number of mental institutions, attempted to identify the syndrome of schizophrenia in 1896. He classified psychoses into *dementia* (a progressive intellectual deterioration), *dementia praecox* (early onset), and *manic-depressive psychosis*, recognizing their similarities and lack of external causes. Kraepelin believed that dementia praecox was a sort of early senility with organic origin, was degenerative, and always ended in a state of disorganization after a chronic and deteriorating course. Persons afflicted with this illness, he assumed, never returned to their baseline level of functioning after becoming ill (Torrey, 1988). He also noted its occurrence in young, previously healthy persons.

Bleuler's Understanding of Schizophrenia

Bleuler, also a European physician, attempted to identify the behaviors typical of schizophrenia. He renamed the illness *schizophrenia* instead of dementia praecox, deriving the name from the concept of "splitting," meaning that the patient is split off from reality, not that the person has a "split personality." The concept, however, is much misunderstood by the lay public. In this split from reality, thoughts and associations are fragmented and without meaning. The person's expressed emotions or facial expressions are not adequate or appropriate to the situation. Bleuler is best known for identifying the "four As" associated with schizophrenia (Box 29–1).

The schizophrenic person's *affect* is disturbed, often blunted, so that there is a minimal change in facial expression and the consistent use of a monotonous tone of voice. Patients are typically described as having a flat affect, unable to joke or be engaged in conversation. The person may become hostile when threatened. Sometimes the person's affect is incongruous to the topic discussed; for example, the person describing some impulse to harm a family member may giggle.

Association between thoughts may be disrupted, providing the basis for describing this disturbance as a *thought disorder.* Sometimes *thought blocking* may occur, as evidenced by a person's difficulty in articulating a response to a question or simply stopping midsentence. The person may also lose track of a statement's meaning after starting a sentence, with resultant **loose associations** (e.g., "Look at my blue veins. I asked a Russian woman to make them red.").

The person may appear to be *autistic*, preoccupied with self and inner experiences only, unable to relate to stimulation from the surrounding environment. It is not uncommon to see ill or untreated schizophrenic patients

BOX 29-1 Bleuler's "Four As" of Schizophrenia

- Affective disturbance
- Disordered association of thought
- Autism
- Ambivalence

sitting on sofas or the floor of inpatient recreation rooms, rocking, holding themselves, or appearing oblivious to the surrounding confusion and noise of the television and other patients arguing with one another.

The fourth "A" identified by Bleuler is *ambivalence*, meaning that the person simultaneously experiences strong positive and negative feelings, making it nearly impossible to make decisions. For instance, a person may be unable to decide to take medication, simultaneously believing that the drug could be "poison" as well as a necessary treatment to relieve disturbing hallucinations (Kaplan and Sadock, 1989). Case Example 29–3 represents one person's experience with schizophrenia.

Case Example 29–3 Cathy's Story

LADY SCHIZOPHRENIA

You are my real mother.
Your breast is filled with sweet poison milk.
I suck desperately to save my life.
I cannot live without you.
If I leave you for a moment
you destroy the world around me;
if I cling to you
your poison invades my body.
You are everywhere.
I have fought you, begged you,
bargained with you, flirted with you,
tried to be your friend,
and still my greatest dread has come to pass;
I have become you.

THE ANGELS OF MERCY
MEET LADY SCHIZOPHRENIA

We know you
and are not afraid.
We see you
among your masks
and we see your victim
though she cannot
see herself.
We will protect her
beneath our wings
and be light shining
through your dark veils.
We will let her choose—
something you have
never done.
We will lend our
eyes and ears
until she is
her own.
She will tame you.
You will let yourself
be chained
and she will go free.

by Cathy King

From Suska, M. A. (1991). *Cry of the invisible* (p. 79). Baltimore: Conservatory Press.

▶ Check Your Reading

9. What was Kraepelin's contribution to our understanding of schizophrenia?
10. What are Bleuler's four "As"?

Schneider's First-Rank and Second-Rank Symptoms

Another attempt describing symptoms, which continues to be used today, was developed by Schneider (1959). He divided symptoms into first-rank and second-rank symptoms. Schneider emphasized that none of these behaviors is absolutely indicative of schizophrenia. The presence of several of these symptoms and the absence of any other identifiable pathological conditions, however, makes the diagnosis of schizophrenia probable. Schneider's **first-rank symptoms** include

- The hearing of one's thoughts spoken aloud.
- Auditory hallucinations that comment on the patient's behavior.
- Somatic hallucinations.
- The experience of having one's thoughts controlled (thought insertion).
- The spreading of one's thoughts to others (thought broadcasting).
- Delusions.
- The experience of having one's actions controlled or influenced from the outside (passivity experiences) (Kaplan and Sadock, 1989, p. 439).

Second-rank symptoms include

- Other forms of hallucinations.
- Depression.
- Euphoria.
- Perplexity as disorders of affect and emotional blunting (Kaplan and Sadock, 1989).

▶ Check Your Reading

11. What are first-rank symptoms?
12. What are second-rank symptoms?

International Pilot Study of Schizophrenia

In 1965, the World Health Organization initiated the International Pilot Study of Schizophrenia (IPSS) in an effort to obtain new knowledge about the epidemiology of the illness. One of the major objectives of the IPSS was to develop and standardize diagnostic criteria that could be used in all nine countries in the study: Denmark, India, Colombia, Nigeria, England, the Soviet Union, Taiwan, the United States, and Czechoslovakia. A major problem in cross-cultural epidemiological studies has always been doubt that similar diagnostic criteria had been used to identify illness. For example, schizophrenia is diagnosed at much higher rates in the United States than in Great Britain and Europe.

A 12-point diagnostic system, shown in Box 29–2, was derived from the work of the IPSS. The IPSS

BOX 29-2 12-Point Diagnostic System of the IPPS for Schizophrenia

- Restricted affect
- Poor insight
- Hearing one's thoughts spoken aloud
- Absence of early waking
- Poor rapport
- Lack of depressed facial expression
- Lack of elation
- Widespread delusions
- Incoherent speech
- Unreliable information given
- Bizarre delusions
- Nihilistic delusions

represented a major advance in the epidemiological study of mental illness, providing valuable information about the course of illness across nine cultures. One interesting conclusion from the study was that subjects who live in developing nations seemed to do better than those from more highly developed societies. This determination followed a two-year study of subjects who were interviewed a second time. This study laid the groundwork for future epidemiological research.

▶ **Check Your Reading**

13. What was the purpose of the IPSS?
14. Describe the 12-point diagnostic system derived from the work of the IPSS.

DSM-IV Diagnosis and the Journey of Schizophrenia

Under the revised diagnostic criteria of the *DSM-IV*, a diagnosis of schizophrenia is made when strict criteria are fulfilled. These include the stipulation that the person must have exhibited symptoms for at least six months. In the past, failure to consider the six-month duration of symptoms probably led to overdiagnosing of schizophrenia in the United States.

DSM-IV describes the essential features of schizophrenia as the presence of characteristic psychotic symptoms during the active phase of the illness with functioning below the highest level previously achieved lasting at least six months. The illness may include characteristic prodromal or residual symptoms (American Psychiatric Association, 1994, p. 187). At some phase, the illness always involves delusions, hallucinations, or certain characteristic disturbances, both in affect and in form of thought. An organic factor must not be responsible for the disorder, and these symptoms must not be due to a mood disorder (see Chapter 30) or schizoaffective disorder. *Schizoaffective disorder* is defined as one period of illness with symptoms of major depression or mania along with the symptoms of schizophrenia, including for some period delusions or hallucinations (American Psychiatric Association, p. 292). Tables 29–1 and 29–2 list specific diagnostic criteria and categories of schizophrenia. The *DSM-IV* addresses the course of the illness by dividing it into five subcategories, which include: catatonic, undifferentiated, disorganized, residual and paranoid.

▶ **Check Your Reading**

15. How does the *DSM-IV* address the course of schizophrenia?
16. How many types of schizophrenia does the *DSM-IV* identify?

THE CAUSE OF SCHIZOPHRENIA

With the explosion of research in the neurosciences, knowledge about the cause of schizophrenia is continuing to expand. Yet scientists still do not know precisely what causes schizophrenia. Some established facts are shown in Box 29–3.

Although schizophrenia was once classified as a *functional* disorder (one with psychological origins), evidence supports the position that the brains of persons who have schizophrenia are different from those of persons who do not have this disease. The differences can be measured by gross pathology, by microscopic pathology, by neurochemistry, by cerebral blood flow and metabolism, electrically, neurologically, and neuropsychologically (Torrey, 1988, p. 132).

▶ **Check Your Reading**

17. Describe the facts of schizophrenia.
18. Why is schizophrenia no longer considered a functional disorder?

Brain Structure and Function

Since 1976, CT scans and nuclear MRI scans have been used to study structural differences of patients with schizophrenia. Before this, study of brain differences was limited to postmortem studies. The following abnormalities have been consistently reported:

- Enlargement of the lateral ventricles or the third ventricles.
- Atrophy of a portion of the cerebellum.
- Abnormalities in brain density.
- Increased markings on the surface of the brain, suggesting loss of brain tissue.
- Abnormalities in brain asymmetry.

TABLE 29–1 Characteristics of Schizophrenia

Type of Schizophrenia	Characteristics
Catatonic type	Catatonic stupor (marked decrease in reactivity to the environment and/or reduction in spontaneous movements and activity) or mutism Catatonic negativism (an apparently motiveless resistance to all instructions or attempts to be moved) Catatonic rigidity (maintenance of a rigid posture against efforts to be moved) Catatonic excitement (excited motor activity, apparently purposeless and not influenced by external stimuli) Catatonic posturing (voluntary assumption of inappropriate or bizarre posture)
Undifferentiated type	Prominent delusions, hallucinations, incoherence, or grossly disorganized behavior Lack of criteria for paranoid, catatonic, or disorganized type of disorder
Disorganized type	Incoherence, marked loosening of associations, or grossly disorganized behavior Flat or grossly inappropriate affect Lack of criteria for catatonic type of disorder
Residual type	Absence of prominent delusions, hallucinations, incoherence, or grossly disorganized behavior Continuing evidence of the disturbance, as indicated by two or more of the residual symptoms as listed in Box 29–2
Paranoid type	Preoccupation with one or more systematized delusions or with frequent auditory hallucinations related to a single theme None of the following: incoherence, marked loosening of associations, catatonic or grossly disorganized behavior

Data from American Psychiatric Association (1994). *Diagnostic and statistical manual of mental disorders fourth edition. Washington, D.C.: American Psychiatric Association.*

Always consider two major factors in interpreting reported biological differences in schizophrenia:

- What a *biological abnormality* signifies. Such an abnormality is, at most, a correlation and should not be assumed to be a causal factor.
- Whether the abnormality is related to the disease process itself or to treatment, especially antipsychotic medication. This determination is often difficult.

In the studies reported, the brain changes are apparently not due to medication and are not limited to schizophrenia. They are also evident in patients with manic-depressive illness and other brain diseases (Andreasen et al, 1986; Breier et al, 1992; Wolkin et al, 1992; Pettegrew et al, 1993; Utas and Cotman, 1993).

Suddath and colleagues (1990) studied brain structure in twins, one of whom had schizophrenia and one of whom did not. They found evidence of anatomical changes in the brains of the schizophrenic twins. The fact

TABLE 29–2 Differences in the Course of Schizophrenia

Subchronic	The time from the beginning of the disturbance, when the person first began to show signs of the disturbance (including prodromal, active, and residual phases) more or less continuously, is less than 2 years but at least 6 months
Chronic	Same as above but more than two years
Subchronic with acute exacerbation	Reemergence of prominent psychotic symptoms in a person with a subchronic course who has been in the residual phase of the disturbance
Chronic with acute exacerbation	Reemergence of prominent psychotic symptoms in a person with a chronic course who has been in the residual phase of the disturbance
In remission	When a person with a history of schizophrenia is free of all signs of the disturbance Differentiating schizophrenia in remission from no mental disorder requires consideration of overall level of functioning, length of time since the last episode, total duration of the disturbance, and whether prophylactic medication is being given
Unspecified	

that the twins could be differentiated on the basis of structural differences probably meant that the cause of the underlying neuropathological process was not completely genetic.

▶ **Check Your Reading**
19. What have MRI and CT scans demonstrated about the brains of schizophrenics?
20. What have twin studies demonstrated?
21. What are the two major cautions when interpreting brain studies?

The Limbic System

Abnormalities in the limbic system in animals produce profound changes in emotion, inappropriate behavior, and an impairment in the animal's ability to screen out multiple visual stimuli. In humans, diseases of the limbic system are likely to produce schizophreniclike symptoms. Many researchers have debated the location of the primary brain lesion that affects the development of schizophrenia. Many believe the spot may be the limbic system (Torrey, 1988, p. 140).

That pathology has been identified in one area, however, does not mean that the primary area of pathology has been defined. For example, identification of the limbic system as the site of pathology could be caused by some hyperactive input from some other region of the brain. Also, a single pathological process in the brain can cause a wide range of phenomena in different patients, and a single specific abnormality in the brain can have many different causes. Parkinson's disease, for example, can have idiopathic, infectious, traumatic, or toxic causes (Kaplan and Sadock, 1989).

BOX 29-3 Established Facts About Schizophrenia

- Schizophrenia is a brain disease. The brain does not appear to be functioning normally, but abnormalities in structure are debatable. Brain chemicals appear to be functioning abnormally.
- The limbic system and its connections are primarily affected.
- Schizophrenia often runs in families. In the past, various types of family influences were proposed, such as deprivation or abnormalities in early mother-child relationships, but well-controlled studies have failed to identify any particular environmental factors in this regard. Stress does seem to have something to do with aggravating the illness in vulnerable individuals.
- The brain damage may occur early in life. Factors such as inheritance, development before birth, and early trauma are thought to play a part in predisposing a person to schizophrenia (Torey, 1988).

▶ **Check Your Reading**
22. Why is the limbic system important in understanding the symptoms of schizophrenia?
23. Why are researchers cautious about concluding that the limbic system is the site of the primary cause for schizophrenia?

Genetic Factors

It is generally acknowledged that schizophrenics inherit a genetic vulnerability to the disease rather than the disease itself. Evidence supporting inheritance shows that relatives of schizophrenics have a greater chance of developing the disease than the general population. Most researchers concur about the familial aggregation of schizophrenia (Baron et al, 1985, p. 447). One percent of the general population develops schizophrenia, whereas 10% of first-degree relatives (parents, siblings, children) of schizophrenics are diagnosed during their lifetimes (Benes, 1993).

The data also suggest that schizotypal and paranoid personality disorders are genetically related to schizophrenia. **Schizotypal personality disorder** is a lifelong pattern of social detachment and inability to form relationships as well as cognitive or perceptual distortions and eccentricities in behavior (American Psychiatric Association, 1994, p. 641). The salient feature of **paranoid personality disorder** is a lifelong suspiciousness of others that is unrelated to a full-blown schizophrenic disorder (American Psychiatric Association, 1994, p. 634).

▶ **Check Your Reading**
24. What do genetics suggest to us about schizophrenia?
25. What are the relationships of schizotypal and paranoid personality disorders to schizophrenia?

Dopamine Theories

One of the most extensively studied theories related to the underlying biochemical basis of schizophrenia is related to the brain's use of dopamine. Dopamine is one of the brain's neurotransmitters that assists in the transmission of information between nerve cells. The drugs that reduce schizophrenic symptoms have been studied to determine their dopamine activity. The dopamine hypothesis is that schizophrenia may be related to overactive neuronal activity. There appears to be excessive dopamine levels in persons with schizophrenia.

Pharmacological research demonstrates that drugs, such as amphetamines, that increase dopamine activity worsen schizophrenic symptoms, and drugs that decrease dopamine activity alleviate symptoms. The neuroleptic medications phenothiazine and the butyrophenones (e.g., Haldol) have been extensively studied. Although these classes of drugs are chemically quite different, they both block dopamine receptors and decrease schizophrenic symptoms. Speculation suggests that neuroleptic drugs act at the nerve synapse by binding dopamine receptor sites. The cause of excessive dopamine activity in schizophrenics is not known, and it is impossible to conclude that schizophrenia is caused by excessive dopamine. Symptoms could come from increased numbers of or activity of receptors.

▶ **Check Your Reading**

26. What is the theoretical significance of dopamine to schizophrenia?

Viral Theories

Since 1929, some most interesting studies have reported that more schizophrenics are born during the winter and early spring than during other seasons. The viral hypothesis of psychosis thus suggests that major environmental determinants lead to the onset of psychosis. Observations further suggest that schizophrenic psychoses sometimes occur in relation to infective illness (Menninger, 1926). The hypothetical conclusion is that birth season prevalence may be somehow related to a viral infection, but whether schizophrenia could be due to an unidentified agent, perhaps interacting with a genetic predisposition, remains an open question (Crow, 1991; Butler et al, 1993; Crow, 1993).

Crow (1991, 1993) believes that direct evidence for viral involvement is lacking and so has formulated more elaborate hypotheses regarding the type of virus that might be present. He proposes that the viral agent may be acting by altering neuronal systems in such a way as to produce changes consistent with the dopamine hypothesis of schizophrenia.

Evidence has begun to accumulate that schizophrenia may be caused by a virus, but the evidence is far from definitive. Crow has found that the cerebrospinal fluid of one third of patients with schizophrenia has viral-like activity suggesting the presence of a virus. Three studies have demonstrated that during periods in which more individuals who eventually developed schizophrenia were in utero, viral illnesses were especially prevalent. This finding may or may not be related to season of conception. Boyd and colleagues (1986) find substantial evidence that schizophrenics are more likely to be born in the winter than in other seasons, even in the Southern Hemisphere, where the winter months are June, July, and August. Some evidence also suggests that patients with bipolar mood disorder are more likely to be born in winter months (Torrey et al, 1993).

If a seasonal factor damages the central nervous system during fetal development and thereby predisposes the fetus to later development of schizophrenia or other major mental illness, we might expect to find the subgroup of schizophrenics exposed to that seasonal factor different from other schizophrenics. Yet despite the limited number of studies investigating these characteristics, some evidence suggests that winter-born schizophrenics are more likely to have a better prognosis, less genetic risk for schizophrenia, and an earlier age of onset of the disorder (Boyd et al, 1986; Torrey et al, 1993).

▶ **Check Your Reading**

27. What is the viral theory?
28. In what ways are schizophrenics exposed to a seasonal factor different from other schizophrenics?

Influence of the Family on Illness Development

The family environment has a powerful influence on the course of illness in a patient with a thought disorder, so much that researchers once believed family environment was a causative factor in schizophrenia. Bateson (1956), family therapist and communication theorist, described a family situation called the *double bind*, in which a child must make a choice between two alternatives, both of which are unbearably confusing for the child. Bateson suggested this situation as a cause for development of schizophrenia. There were no control studies of this theory, and it was never statistically tested (Bateson et al, 1956). Sullivan concluded from his clinical investigations that some schizophrenic patients had been made anxious as infants by their anxious mothers. Anxiety, he concluded, caused the disintegration of ego function seen in the disorder.

Unfortunately, Bateson's work as well as Sullivan's and others came to signify "blaming" the family for the schizophrenic's illness because these researchers went beyond commenting on family communication patterns. The terms *schizophrenogenic* mother and family were coined by Bateson and his group and adopted by the lay public. Such erroneous conclusions further added to the stress, shame, stigma, and guilt that families of the mentally ill endure. These conditions, in turn, led family to mistrust health practitioners. Today we know that communication patterns in the family do not "cause" schizophrenia to develop in a person.

Current research focuses on the quality of the family's relationships with its schizophrenic loved one. The goal is to determine ways in which these relationships protect against or contribute to the course of illness. Researchers have extended the scope of research beyond the husband-wife and parent-child relationships to encompass sibling relationships as well. Gerace and colleagues (1993) found that siblings identify their involvement in the care of a schizophrenic sibling in three ways:

- Collaborative. The sibling shared the care-taking responsibilities with the parents and other family members and was actively involved in collaboration with the health team.
- Crisis oriented. The sibling's involvement was situation specific with no carryover between crises. In these family situations, virtually no long-term planning decreased the incidences of crises.
- Detached concern. The sibling is involved indirectly and attempts to create distance between self and the ill brother or sister and sometimes between self and the entire family.

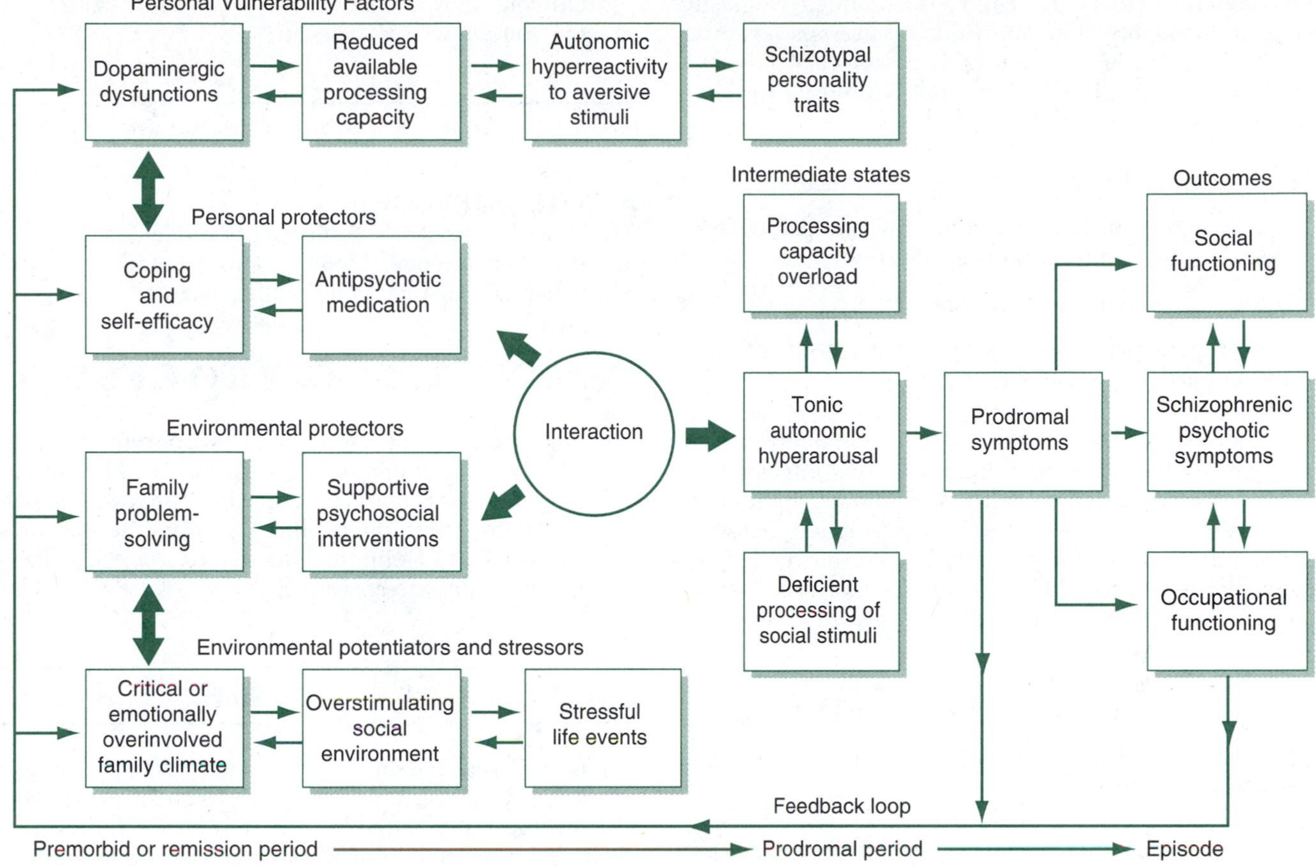

FIGURE 29–1

The stress-vulnerability model of schizophrenia. (From Nuechterlein, K. H., et al. [1985]. *Schizophrenia Bulletin, 11*. Published by the U.S. Public Health Service, National Institute of Mental Health, Rockville, MD.)

The focus on siblings is significant because it directs attention to another area of potential support for the schizophrenic. It also increases sensitivity to the needs of families who care for a schizophrenic family member daily.

▶ **Check Your Reading**

29. What did Sullivan say about the role of anxiety in causing schizophrenia?

30. What impact did the theorists such as Bateson and Sullivan have on perceptions of families with schizophrenic members?

The Stress-Vulnerability Model

The stress-vulnerability model of schizophrenia (Figure 29–1) identifies personal and environmental factors that contribute to relapse or to minimizing schizophrenic symptoms. The model also attempts initially to identify individuals who may be more vulnerable to developing the disorder. Earlier perspectives viewed schizophrenia as a chronic disorder attributable to a particular biological or environmental cause. This model emphasizes a permanent vulnerability to schizophrenia. Although some vulnerable individuals may never experience a psychotic episode, others have periodic episodes over many years (O'Connor, 1991).

The stress-vulnerability model integrates many biological and social stress theories. **Biological vulnerability** may inhibit the individual's ability to cope with even minor stressors, and stressful family relationships may be potentiators of the disorder. Children with two schizophrenic parents have a 35% to 46% risk of developing the disorder compared with a 1% to 2% risk in the general population. Children with one schizophrenic parent have a lifetime risk of 12%. One major limitation in studying the offspring of schizophrenics is that 85% to 90% of schizophrenic persons do not have a schizophrenic parent. It is unclear whether vulnerability markers derived from this high-risk sample can reliably be generalized to samples of those who lack this family history. Some signs of neurointegrative and social dysfunction appear in infancy studies, but the patterns become clearer and more pronounced in middle childhood and adolescence. There is little evidence, however, that the attention and information-processing tasks deficits are markers for biological vulnerability. More comparisons are needed with children whose parents have not manifested a schizophrenic disorder (Goldstein, 1987).

Current thinking in developmental psychology reflects a more sophisticated view of the transaction. It is now recognized that every child has a unique biologically based individuality. This individuality exerts a powerful impact on the type of parenting behavior elicited by the child (Goldstein, 1987). **Personal vulnerability** thus includes factors such as

- Brain biochemistry (dopaminergic dysfunction).
- Dysfunction in attention and information processing (reduced available processing capacity).
- Autonomic nervous system hyperactivity.
- Certain personality traits (schizotypal personality disorder, in particular) (Goldstein, 1987).

The second part of the stress-vulnerability model attempts to identify stressful life events that interact with indices of personal vulnerability. This model implies that researchers must investigate the interaction between intrafamilial relationships and indices of vulnerability to a specific psychiatric disorder. Studies of family factors have identified two types of stresses in vulnerable offspring:

- Disordered communication among family members.
- Negative affective climate in the family, termed **high expressed emotion** (Lefley, 1992).

These factors have also been indicated as factors in relapse for schizophrenic patients.

The stress-vulnerability model is complex and demands sophisticated research strategies to uncover factors associated with healthy or psychopathological development (Dworkin et al, 1993). Case Example 29–4 describes some of the complexities that a schizophrenic experiences.

Case Example 29–4 Lynn's Story

Do you know what it is like to go mad
Fading in and out of reality
Not remembering the memories you've had
One minute you're there, one minute you're not
It's not as if you're a fatality
You're body lingers on to rot
Do you know what it's like to be lost
The fog in your mind covers your eyes
And the tears that tear through the body are the cost
But you see I don't feel all that sad
It's a beautiful world in all those lies
Do you know what it's like to be mad?
Do you know what it's like to see yourself
disappearing
And the labels they've stuck on you can't
keep you around
All those who seem to help are only learning
While I build a guilty mound
That will be my burial ground
Do you know if it's better to be dead or mad?
Do you know

by Lynn

From Suska, M. A. (1991). *Cry of the invisible* (p. 47). Baltimore: Conservatory Press.

▶ Check Your Reading

31. Describe the stress-vulnerability model.
32. What are biological vulnerability factors?
33. What are personal vulnerability factors?

NURSING PROCESS

Nursing care for the person with schizophrenia requires an understanding of the patient's experience. The schizophrenic's journey is marked by specific symptoms, which both diagnose the illness and describe the person's perceptions. Case Example 29–5 is one story of schizophrenia and supportive care.

Case Example 29–5 Bill's Story

Bill is a 27-year-old single white man. He was brought into the psychiatric Emergency Department for evaluation by the police after he was observed standing and pacing near the railing of a bridge, muttering to himself. A bag of torn clothing and papers, a Bible, and half a bottle of Haldol were found near him and brought to the Emergency Department. Initially, he was not cooperative with the questioning from the nurse and psychiatrist, and he accused them of trying to take thoughts from his head. The name of his therapist was on the bottle of pills, and he was contacted by phone.

The therapist told the health care personnel that he was concerned because Bill's mother had reported that Bill, concerned about side effects of Haldol, had stopped taking his medication. Bill had left his mother's home to wander and had not been seen for several days. Bill did accept a dose of his regular medication, and he revealed some time later that he had been hearing voices inside his head telling him to jump from the bridge. He said in a soft voice over and over "I am what I am," and said that he saw the world with "deep eyes" and could feel the pain of others' poverty, hunger, and drug abuse. He felt pain in his body, "the pain of bullets," and expressed a desire to solve the world's problems. He believed he had a special gift, "mind throwing," through which he could control the thoughts of others. His repetition of the phrase "I am what I am" seemed related to his belief that he was the founder of a new religion.

When Bill accepted the Haldol, he was also given a dose of benetropine (Cogentin) to prevent side effects from the neuroleptic. Routine blood tests included electrolytes and serum and urine toxicology tests. Toxicology studies were negative, and serum sodium was slightly elevated but not dangerously so, probably indicating that he had not been drinking enough fluids during the time he had been living on the street. He agreed to voluntary admission to the short-term psychiatric unit to prevent himself from harming himself and to restabilize him on medications.

ASSESSMENT

Assessment of patients with schizophrenia occurs at the individual, family, and environmental levels. You must be aware of changes not only in the patient's physiological, psychological, and perceptual condition, but also in the patient's personal life. Factors to consider include living situation, family support, and stresses. Such an assessment is consistent with the stress-vulnerability model of schizophrenia. You assume that changes in any aspect of the schizophrenic's life influence potential for relapse.

Clinical Signs and Symptoms

Three key issues should be considered when assessing the symptoms of the schizophrenic or thought-disordered patient. The first is that no clinical sign or symptom is seen only in schizophrenia. Every sign or symptom can also be seen in other psychiatric and neurological disorders. To diagnose schizophrenia, a clinician must consider both a mental status examination or examination of the person's presenting appearance and a history.

The second key issue is that the symptoms of the patient change over time. Symptoms depend on the course of illness and response to somatic therapy.

The third issue is educational level. Intellectual ability and cultural background of the patient must be taken into consideration (Kaplan and Sadock, 1989).

Patients with schizophrenia describe *positive* and *negative* symptoms. Although Kraepelin and Bleuler did not use these terms, they still divided symptoms into categories that roughly correspond to these two concepts (Kaplan and Sadock, 1989). **Positive symptoms** are present in the schizophrenic but absent in normal individuals. These symptoms generally respond well to medications. They include hallucinations, delusions, and disordered thinking such as loose associations.

Negative symptoms are altered emotional responses that respond less successfully to medication. These include apathy, social withdrawal, poverty of thoughts, blunting of emotions, slow movement, and lack of drive. These negative symptoms can severely compromise a patient's ability to enter into a therapeutic relationship, inhibiting receptivity to compliance with prescribed medication regimens (Case Example 29–6). The symptoms caused by the illness thus also inhibit a patient's ability to get well.

Crow (1980) have argued that patients with predominantly positive symptoms (called type I, florid) have less structural damage to the brain, a better response to antipsychotic drugs, and a better prognosis. Those with predominantly negative symptoms (type 2, defect) have more structural brain damage as seen on CT scans, a poorer response to drugs, and a worse prognosis (Andreasen et al, 1986). Whether the two types represent two different causes of schizophrenia, however, is still unknown (Kay et al, 1989; Kay, 1990; McGlashan and Fenton, 1993; Erlenmeyer-Kimling et al, 1993).

Case Example 29–6
One Schizophrenic's Story

I didn't have a nervous breakdown, I just started to hear voices. They were obnoxious, insulting, like "You're no good" and allusions to my sex life. They said things that would make anyone's anger flare up. The voice itself was a "translucent acoustical sound within a sound." I would hear the whining of wheels on a forklift, and sub-sounds would occur at points within the whine. The voices were high pitched, but frustratingly complacent and calm. They provoked me to anger. At first, I controlled my anger and did the natural thing, which was to escape. Sometimes I would yell and destroy my things.

When I discovered that the voices were a negative occurrence, making me unhappy, I quit my job. I think the voices came from sexual frustration—my lack of experience with the opposite sex—and evil spirits. The voices sounded evil. I start talking with them sometimes because there's nobody to keep company with. Loneliness is a function of it.

From Suska, M. A. (1991). *Cry of the invisible* (p. 37). Baltimore: Conservatory, Press.

Crow (1980) speculated that positive symptoms that are primarily biochemical in origin and not related to structural abnormalities tend to respond better to **neuroleptic medication.** These medications exert their therapeutic effect through blockage of dopamine transmission. As yet, positron emission tomography studies of never-medicated schizophrenics (perhaps the most powerful techniques for studying the mechanisms that mediate abnormal mental phenomena) have not shown any specific relationship between abnormal elevations in dopamine transmission as measured by D_2 receptor density and prominent positive symptoms (Wong et al, 1986; Farde et al, 1987; Kay et al, 1989; Kay, 1990; McGlashan and Fenton, 1992, 1993; Erlenmeyer-Kimling et al, 1993). See Box 29–6.

DESCRIBING POSITIVE SYMPTOMS

Illusions and Hallucinations

Both illusions and hallucinations are positive symptoms. **Illusions** occur when the patient misperceives or exaggerates stimuli in the environment. Schizophrenics may see objects and people change their dimensions, their outline, and their brightness from minute to minute, as Mark Vonnegut so vividly described in *Journey to Eden.* Sometimes these perceptual changes can signal the prodromal phase of schizophrenic illness. At other times, they can be part of the florid psychosis. At times, the patient may perceive a mirrored self-reflection change into a monster.

Hallucinations are sensory experiences of perceptions without corresponding stimuli in the environment (Table 29–3). They can occur in any sensory modality, but auditory hallucinations, or "hearing voices," are most common in the schizophrenic's experience. The voices can be those of God, the devil, relatives, neighbors, or persons unknown to the patient. Auditory hallucinations often begin with friendly voices and progress to threatening, persecutory, and frightening messages and commands as the person decompensates. As the illness progresses, the patient is at risk to act on the voice commands. The voices are generally described as being "outside" and not merely thoughts spoken aloud. In Case Example 29–5, Bill was at serious risk to harm himself in response to command hallucinations that told him to jump from the bridge. Another vivid hallucinatory experience is the beating heart in Poe's (1927) story:

> *No doubt I grew very pale;—but I talked fluently, and with a heightened voice. Yet the sound increased and what could I do? It was a low, dull, quick sound—much such a sound as a watch makes when enveloped in cotton. I gasped for breath—and yet the officers heard it not. I talked more quickly—more vehemently; but the noise steadily increased. . . . I swung the chair upon which I had been sitting, and grated it upon the boards, but the noise arose over all and continually increased. It grew louder—louder—louder! And still the men chatted pleasantly, and smiled. Was it possible they heard not? Almighty God!—no, no! They heard!—they suspected—they knew!—they were making a mockery of my horror!*

You might ask Bill about the voices and what he is experiencing, but you should expect that Bill may not be forthcoming about his internal experience. If Bill appears distracted, glances up at the ceiling for extended periods, appears to be talking to himself, yet denies hearing voices, record these observations. They may be evidence that Bill is hearing voices.

TABLE 29–3 **Types of Hallucinations**

Hallucination	Example
Auditory	Hearing choirs of angels inside one's head
Visual	Seeing a monstrous glowing face on the wall
Olfactory	Smelling acrid poison gas coming from a radiator
Gustatory	Tasting sharp lemon in absence of food
Tactile	Feeling small insects crawling under one's skin
Somatic	Sensing that a tunnel runs through one's head
Altered sense of self	Confusing one's self with a doll or another person

Visual hallucinations occur less frequently in schizophrenic patients, but they are not rare. When they occur in the absence of auditory hallucinations, they usually indicate a concurrent organic problem, such as alcohol withdrawal or drug toxicity.

Hallucinations must always be evaluated in their cultural context. In medieval times and today among some religious groups, visual hallucinations do not necessarily suggest mental illness. Arieti (1976) proposes the following criteria to distinguish religious hallucinations from the schizophrenic's hallucinations:

- Religious hallucinations are usually visual.
- Religious hallucinations usually involve benevolent guides or advisors.
- Religious hallucinations are usually pleasant.

Tactile (touch), olfactory (smell), and gustatory (taste) hallucinations are less common. They are usually unpleasant.

Delusions

Delusions are false fixed beliefs that cannot be corrected by reasoning. They may be simple and focused or detailed and involved. They are sometimes difficult to elicit on first encounter, although some patients have chronic fixed delusions and may describe them easily. The schizophrenic's delusions tend to be grotesque; loosely organized; and centered on themes of persecution, grandiosity, sex, bodily functioning, and control by others (Hagerty, 1984).

Delusions of persecution are most frequent and are the key symptom of paranoid schizophrenia. Individuals believe they are being persecuted by powerful agencies such as the FBI or specific persons such as a neighbor who can control them through walls and sometimes pipe in dangerous gases. Delusions of persecution may be more subtle. In Case Example 29–5, Bill's suspicion that the psychiatrist and nurse might be trying to harm him in their initial psychiatric interview was a delusion. The feeling of being controlled by some unseen mysterious force that exerts its power from afar occurs in most schizophrenics at one time or another. Many schizophrenics believe their minds are controlled by telepathy or hypnotism. The modern schizophrenic could be preoccupied by x-rays, space ships, or atomic power that affect the mind and could take over the world. **Delusions of grandeur,** in which the patient assumes the identity of a famous individual such as Napoleon, Christ, or the president, are seen in schizophrenia as well as in mood disorders (see Chapter 30).

In identifying delusional thinking, consider the method you use to collect data. In Case Example 29–5, Bill did not trust the nurse or psychiatrist. This lack of trust interfered with Bill's ability to express his internal experiences freely. You therefore assess delusions by inquiring about their content while accepting the patient's perceptions: "You say people are following you . . . Who is following you? Do you have any thoughts about why they are following you?"

Initially, assess the delusional content to understand the patient's concerns. If you continue to focus attention on the delusion, however, you may inadvertently reinforce false beliefs. Be careful neither to argue with the patient over the delusions nor to condone them. Rather, listen to them, validate that you are correctly understanding the patient's perception of reality, and refocus the direction of the interview into reality. You can show understanding of the patient's perception and simultaneously introduce reality. For example, "I can see you are frightened and believe that the FBI is looking for you, but I have no reason to believe the FBI is after you."

Ideas of reference are delusional ideas wherein schizophrenic people believe that the actions of others are directed toward them. The patient may believe that the television announcer is referring to something the patient must do, or songs on the radio may have special significance. Some patients believe that others can read their thoughts or can put thoughts into their heads. One schizophrenic patient showed the nurse a photograph of a pair of shoes leaning against a pillow. "Look, here is the evidence! The toes point toward the window where prostitutes walk up and down the street and call to my husband!"

Formal Thought Disorder

Both the content of thought and the form of thought are disturbed in the schizophrenic. This formal thought disorder is different from the content disturbance in delusional thinking. The most common example of formal thought disorder is loosening of associations, in which ideas shift from one subject to another, completely or only marginally related. The person appears unaware that the topics are disconnected. Statements having no meaningful relationship may be contained in the same expressed thought, or the person may shift from one frame of reference to another. When loosening of associations is severe, the person may become incoherent, with speech described aptly as **word salad.**

Interviewing a patient with a thought disorder is difficult. Keep the interview short. Focus on current issues. Patients think and reason on the basis of their own intricate private rules of reason. Thought processes do not lead to conclusions based on reality or universal logic. Thinking is said to be concrete, so that people may be unable to abstract when given a proverb to interpret. The expression "people in glass houses shouldn't throw stones," for example, might come to mean that "people who live in houses made of glass might break windows if they threw stones out of them." The schizophrenic also may consider things to be identical merely because they share some properties. For example, "the Virgin Mary was a virgin. I'm a virgin; therefore I'm the Virgin Mary" (Kaplan and Sadock, 1989). The patient thus loses the ability to generalize correctly.

The schizophrenic tends to include many irrelevant items in thought and speech. Because of increased arousal level, schizophrenics show greater responsiveness to irrelevant stimuli and less responsitivity to relevant stimuli than normal persons. Consequently, irrelevant stimuli become incorporated into thought and speech.

The person may experience *thought blocking*, in which thoughts and psychic activity unexpectedly cease. This can be a fleeting experience or can sometimes last for longer periods. Patients may appear perplexed and express the belief that someone has taken thoughts out of their heads.

The schizophrenic has difficulty with *concreteness and symbolism.* Preoccupation with invisible forces, witchcraft, religion, and philosophy is common. Schizophrenic thinking is characterized by being overly symbolic as well as overly concrete.

The language of the schizophrenic may be difficult to understand. Because of the autistic nature of the illness, language becomes for the schizophrenic more a tool of self-expression than a tool of communication. Sometimes the person may create *neologisms*, or completely new words.

▶ Check Your Reading

34. What is a positive symptom? Give three examples.
35. What is a negative symptom? Give two examples.
36. What is the difference between an illusion and a hallucination?
37. What is a delusion?
38. What are ideas of reference?

DESCRIBING NEGATIVE SYMPTOMS

Part of the constellation of symptoms descriptive of schizophrenia are those labeled negative. These deficit symptoms can include affective flattening or blunting, poverty of speech or speech content, thought blocking, poor grooming, social withdrawal, lack of motivation, anhedonia (inability to take pleasure in activities or other people), and cognitive and attentional deficits.

When these symptoms occur during an initial breakdown, they often suggest the outcome of the disease and can be used as predictive factors. Catatonic symptoms (marked motor psychomotor disturbance) and paranoid symptoms (suspicions) are often thought to be associated with better long-term outcomes. The predominance of negative symptoms such as flattening of emotions and social withdrawal are considered to be predictive of a poor outcome. Patients with negative symptoms tend to respond less well to medication and often have a history of poor adjustment before the onset of illness. They require an extensive support network to remain long-term in a community setting.

Social withdrawal, sloppiness about dress and hygiene, and loss of motivation and judgment are all common in schizophrenia. Schizophrenics may sit silently while others converse, and families may express concern about the time a person spends alone. Some schizophrenic persons do nothing for extended periods, or they engage in pointless or repetitive activity. They may lose interest in their surroundings, become seclusive, lose all initiative, and even refuse to leave their own rooms. Researchers believe that this withdrawal may be a reaction to overstimulation, an adaptive response to a world the person experiences as too full of stimuli and too complex. Alternatively, withdrawal may be a response to understimulation. Close relationships may seem too frightening, and low self-esteem and feeling devalued by others add to the person's social withdrawal.

Whether a predominance of negative symptoms represents a different type of schizophrenia is still under discussion. Social withdrawal as a symptom of the illness has important implications in nursing treatment issues and family education.

▶ Check Your Reading

39. What are two different explanations for why schizophrenics withdrawal from social interaction?

Assessing the Family Environment

The family environment and the family's ability to provide support have a powerful impact on the schizophrenic's ability to function independently. Although no longer seen as the "stimuli" to mental illness, families are called to adapt to an immensely difficult situation. Keep this focus in mind when assessing family functioning. The family assessment includes the following:

- *Any history of mental illness in the patient's family*, especially schizophrenia, mood disorders, or substance abuse. History of any of these disorders may indicate a genetic predisposition toward development of illness. Mental illness in other family members also directly affects the family's ability to provide long-term support to a schizophrenic family member.
- *Family communication patterns.* Although research on this issue is inconclusive, family communication patterns may determine the type of intervention needed. The family may need assistance in responding to the ill family member, who may be speaking in a thought-disordered way. Or the family may need assistance in modifying an overstimulating or high-demand environment, which research has demonstrated to be particularly toxic for persons with schizophrenia (Lefley, 1992, Miklowitz, 1994).
- *The environment.* To determine support and services available, look beyond the patient and immediate family. Consider community groups and organizations such as Alliance for the Mentally Ill, a national family support system network with local chapters.
- *Family stress and cohesion.* Chronic schizophrenia in a family member creates long-term stress in the family and can be associated with considerable psychological distress. Behaviors that families identify as stressful are gross deficits in task functioning, failure to take care of personal needs, difficulties in handling money, an inability to plan for the future, and episodic eruptions of deviant and sometimes threatening behavior (Hatfield and Lefley, 1987).

Assess and document the patterns of family interaction and, in the inpatient setting, note the effects of family visits on the patient (Case Example 29–7).

Case Example 29–7 Win's Story

We walk on stiff dry grass, bare trees motionless, pointing to a near-perfect blue sky. The only stir is the rustling of the dry leaves beneath our feet. I listen to her and think: *Oh God, the pain. I had closed it off so well since the last time . . .*

(Like Grendel, it crouches there on the fringe of my consciousness, waiting for precisely the right moment to slouch in and mar all the perfect blue domes and scorch the whole brown earth to black.)

"The staff is nice to us, very courteous and polite. The food's not bad." She kicks a stone in her path. "But they don't let us have seconds on meat or dessert. We get fresh fruit everyday, and with Christmas coming we'll get special things."

I glance sidelong at her, my sometime daughter, so beautiful, even in her sickness unto death. *Surely you've made a mistake, God, not her . . .*

I say nothing, merely look at my feet as I walk and wait for her to speak again. I pray her words won't come out chaotic and irrelevant. Sometimes, I want to grab what she says out of midair and shove it back in her mouth, demand that she retract what she's saying and tell her, "No, no! You don't mean that!" But when I think it, the darkness around her eyes reproaches me. *Stop*, they say, *You don't know what you're asking. I've been there, I know.*

"It's really not bad here. Marie and I are good friends. She gave me a martini last night. She mixed it in a shampoo bottle."

Outdoors, with night coming on, I'm grateful that here, at least, there is a semblance of order and predictability without the incoherent mumblings and uncoordinated movements and stares of nonrecognition.

You've got it all wrong, God, she doesn't belong here! You've made a mistake! She's intelligent . . . she's artistic . . . she's got talent . . .

. . . On Tuesdays, she paints ceramic ashtrays in the shape of hearts and stars . . .

With some animation, she tells me about her courses at the "University-Without-Walls." She is very tired, she says, because she was up late the past few nights studying and practicing chords on the piano, 156 of them. She has to be able to identify any one of them for her final exam. She expects to pass, even though she's never played the piano.

We trudge down the hill to the gardens. Amid the flowerless shrubs, standing tall, defiant against last week's freezing rain that bends them to the ground, is a quiescent waterfall and fish pond; the water runs empty except for soggy black leaves. "One of the patients here designed this park, but I think he's gone now." I notice her left foot dragging slightly. It does that when she gets tired. I suggest we start back to her unit.

Retracing our steps back up the hill, something comes to me, something I have denied for 9 years. Not the pain—no, no denying that—but the fact that she may not leave here this time. Before, I had *known* she would get better, and she did. But each time it has taken longer for her to recoup her losses—more medication, more effort—and this time, she seems not so fervent or angry or committed to her cause. She seems, in fact, quite content. Her hallucinations aren't nearly so bothersome as they once were; they're not *all* bad, she assures me, some quite pleasant, actually.

I reckon that now she has crossed over the line that once she drew between herself and "the dopies and the droolies and the druggies." I brood that maybe there is nothing in my world to draw her back. Heretofore, when the "real world" had become too much for her, she would "dip in and out of psychosis"—or so her therapist said. But now her stays in the never-never land seem to be growing longer and the drugs and psychotherapy less effective. Someday, I feel sure, she will slide irretrievably into the world of her own making and not come back—and what will I tell myself then? The time, the effort, the expertise that has gone into her care and keeping—it was all for naught?

She leads me to what she calls her favorite place, a slab of concrete with a dozen picnic tables stacked away for the season, echoes that there once was a summer. She stops to extract a cigarette from the pocket of her jacket, but she has no match. She stops a fellow patient passing by for a light.

Why does her madness repel me? Why do I ache at the thought of her slipping into an oblivion where I cannot follow? She functions well here. She has everything she needs: food, shelter, friends, caretakers. Why can't I let her go? She's better off here, without me. They can give her everything I can . . . and more. They can give her what I and the world can't: permission to be crazy.

Clouds to the west mount as the sun hides just beyond the horizon. The air is as still and cold as the stone steps leading to the residence hall. She says something about the job she might get when she graduates to the halfway house. But there is no future in her voice. And as I have no future to offer her either, we turn toward the place from whence we came.

Here in the usually noisy and always smoke-filled C-2 recreation room, I deposit her, a fragment of my loss and helplessness, and then I walk to my car. I bury whatever grief I can in the night and the cold, knowing it will be resurrected the next time I come—just as surely as the picnic tables will be spread out in the spring and the waterfall will be turned on.

From Winship, W. (1993). First person account: How do I let go? *Schizophrenia Bulletin, 19* (4), 853–854.

▶ Check Your Reading

40. What is included in a family assessment?
41. What are the issues that families have the most difficulty with in dealing with a schizophrenic loved one?

Assessing Spiritual and Religious Issues

Frequently, schizophrenics experience delusions and hallucinations with religious content, and some health care providers tend to dismiss religious or spiritual verbalizations as psychotic murmurings. This response is unfortunate but may be changing; the DSM-IV included religious and spiritual problems under additional conditions that may be a focus of clinical attention (American Psychiatric Association, 1994, p. 24). Studies have shown that schizophrenics who have a religious foundation have fewer exacerbations of the illness and spend less time hospitalized. Similar findings have been demonstrated when the caregiver of the schizophrenic is religious and views the caretaking role as a ministry and not a burden (Larson and Larson, 1991).

You need to ask about religious commitment, religious practices, and spiritual issues, such as the meaning of the meaning of the illness to the person, the role of God, and sources of hope and support. These may be sources of great comfort to the patient and need to be encouraged, not denied (Larson and Larson, 1991; Carson, 1994). Leon, in Case Example 29–8, in the midst of active delusions of persecution, maintained his lifelong habit of reading Scripture every night.

Case Example 29–8 Leon's Story

"You asked me why I read the Bible every night. Well, I have done it as long as I can remember. My favorite passage is Psalm 23. I read that one every night before I go to bed. Even when I am really sick and hearing voices, I still read Psalm 23. I know that the Lord is not going to take away this schizophrenia . . . I wish He would . . . but He gives me strength . . . and I know that one day all my suffering will be over and I will be with Him. Reading the Bible reminds me that I am never alone."

▶ Check Your Reading

42. What do you assess in regard to spiritual or religious issues?
43. State two findings that support the positive role of religion in the life of the schizophrenic.

Assessing the Variability of Schizophrenia Over a Lifetime

Approximately 200,000 new cases of schizophrenia are diagnosed each year in the United States, with approximately 2 million worldwide. Diagnosis of schizophrenia before age 10 or after age 50 is unusual.

AGE OF ONSET

As Case Example 29–5 indicates, onset of the illness is usually during adolescence or early adulthood. The disorder may, however, begin in middle or late adult life. Onset in males may be somewhat earlier than in females. Peak age in men is between age 15 and 25 and in women between 25 and 35.

Young Adults and Schizophrenia

The first "life break" or acute episode of the illness most frequently occurs to young adults or to those individuals just beginning to leave home and establish some sort of independence. Because of the dependence associated with any chronic illness, the timing of this "first break" may make the normal separation and individuation issues of late adolescence especially difficult to achieve.

Schizophrenic patients are more likely to have a good outcome if they were considered relatively normal before getting sick. Thus, if as children they were able to make friends with others, did not have major problems with delinquency, and achieved successfully in school according to their intelligence level, their outcome is likely to be good.

Torrey (1988) reflects that the young adult chronic population so publicized today are simply more visible and not confined to institutions as they were years ago. He believes that 40 years ago, young adults with schizophrenia were hospitalized, usually for many years, during which time they were "socialized" to their disease. Most learned to expect little from life and to respect mental health personnel. When they were finally released into the community, these people were usually docile.

Young adults with schizophrenia today face much different circumstances. They are often hospitalized for two to three weeks at a time and are then followed in community mental health clinics. By growing up around "normal" adolescents and young adults, they have different expectations—to be rid of their symptoms and lead a normal life. It is difficult to convince a young adult who sees an entire life stretching ahead that life will probably be a journey with chronic illness and that some sort of medication or at least monitoring will always be necessary. Because they are living in the community, these young people have access to alcohol and drugs, which they use just as their nonschizophrenic peers do (Nuechterlein et al, 1992).

Dealing with repeated episodes of schizophrenia and surviving the impact of the illness are a difficult struggle. Much energy is spent coping with the illness, severely reducing opportunities to accomplish normal developmental tasks that young adults face, such as finding a partner and raising a family. Some patients even with prolonged and episodic illnesses, however, do experience some recovery and may lead far richer, less chaotic, and more complex lives than the mental health system once imagined they could.

▶ Check Your Reading

44. What is the usual age of onset for schizophrenia?
45. How is life today different for the young schizophrenic than it was years ago?
46. Cite two factors that predict a good outcome for an individual diagnosed with schizophrenia.

First-Time Symptoms in the Elderly

It is estimated that around 10% of first admissions to a psychiatric hospital after age 60 exhibit schizophrenic symptoms of late onset. The typical patient in this age group has a mixture of paranoid delusions and auditory hallucinations. Intellect and personality typically appear intact, in contrast to symptoms in young adults. Most studies indicate that women are more prone than men to develop late-onset schizophrenia (Castle and Murray, 1993). Several studies have indicated that patients with late-onset schizophrenia have a family history of psychoses rather than mood disorders.

A number of researchers have argued that sensory impairment, specifically deafness, may be a general risk factor for the development of hallucinations and delusions in later life. When present, deafness often precedes the development of schizophrenic symptoms by many years. Visual impairment has also been implicated by several authors as a risk factor. The mechanism by which sensory deficit leads to schizophrenic symptoms is poorly understood but may be the "final straw" for a socially isolated and predisposed individual (Prager and Jeste, 1993).

The biochemistry of the mechanisms underlying late-onset schizophrenia might be a reversal of normal aging processes (i.e., increased dopamine). This process may produce an increased vulnerability to environmental stressors and sensory deficits that sometimes accompany aging (Caligiuri et al, 1993; McDowd et al, 1993).

Determining that a person has schizophrenia rather than a dementing illness such as Alzheimer's disease, in which persecutory delusions also occur, is difficult. In fact, there are many causes for the development of hallucinations and delusions in the elderly population. Remember that schizophrenia is a possibility in the elderly and that the hallucinations and delusions apparently respond well to small doses of neuroleptic medication.

▶ Check Your Reading

47. What is the role of sensory deficits in developing late-onset schizophrenia?
48. Cite one diagnosis that occurs in the elderly that makes differential diagnosis for schizophrenia difficult.

COURSE OF ILLNESS

A diagnosis of schizophrenia requires that continuous signs of the illness have been present for at least six months. This period always includes an active phase with psychotic symptoms (e.g., hallucinations, delusions, formal thought disorder). The development of an active phase of the illness is usually preceded by a *prodromal* phase with clear deterioration from the previous level of functioning. This phase may be marked by social withdrawal, poor hygiene, blunted affect, perceptual changes, and changes in usual interests and energy. The prodromal phase is extremely variable in length, and prognosis is especially poor when the person has had a slow downhill course for many years (American Psychiatric Association, 1994).

During the *active* phase, psychotic symptoms are prominent. Such symptoms might include hallucinations, delusions, and formal thought disorder and must persist for at least one week, unless they are successfully treated. A *residual* phase usually follows the active phase of the illness. It is similar to the prodromal phase except that affective blunting and problems in role functioning are more prominent. The person may still experience hallucinations and delusions but is not so disturbed by them.

The person may return to the preillness level of functioning. The most common course is one of acute illness episodes with some residual impairment between episodes. During the initial years of the disorder, the residual impairment often increases.

There are few reports of complete recovery. In an autobiographical article, Frese (1994) describes his life with schizophrenia. Frese is the Director of Psychology at a large state mental institution. In this position, he is involved in the care of many chronic schizophrenics. He describes his own 12 steps to recovery from schizophrenia:

- Denial is part of the illness and must be addressed early. Without acceptance that the person has a mental illness, there can be no healing.
- Education about the illness is vitally important.
- Medications are usually necessary to stabilize the biochemical imbalance in the brain, but street drugs and other chemicals serve only to destabilize a schizophrenic.
- Delusional thinking can be seductive. Each individual needs to identify how delusions are patterned.
- Circumstantiality, or the tendency to stray from a train of thought, is common. Patients need to teach themselves to stay on target in conversations.
- Rehearsing in the form of talking to self is a common pattern. Patients need to learn to limit this activity to private times.
- Immediate memory and decision-making abilities are often impaired. The schizophrenic needs to remember these limitations and be cautious when making decisions. Also important are developing coping strategies to augment problems with memory and letting others know that information processing occurs slowly.
- Because the facial expressions of the schizophrenic tend to be delayed in responding to conversations with others, the other person may be uneasy. In close relationships, it is important for the schizophrenic to discuss this response pattern.
- Stress-relieving hobbies such as playing, listening, or dancing to music; gardening; exercising; shopping; and reading are all essential to staying well.
- Problems of stigma, discrimination, and ostracism are serious problems that need to be addressed carefully and systematically.
- Making the decision to tell others about the schizophrenia is difficult. Explaining lost time spent in a hospital for crisis-oriented stabilization requires tremendous creativity.
- Because loneliness is a serious problem for persons suffering with schizophrenia or other psychoses, networking with others who have similar problems is important. Organizations like the Alliance for Mentally Ill and the National Mental Health Consumers' Association are wonderful resources (Frese, 1994, p. 24).

Research has shown considerable differences in the long-term course of schizophrenia. The variations in course may be different types of schizophrenia. In the period preceding the onset of frank psychosis, patients vary as to rapidity of onset, social withdrawal, and the presence or absence of perceptual changes. The active phase of hallucinations may be episodic or continuous and may or may not include negative symptoms. In late adult life, patients vary in the presence or absence of an improvement in psychosis and social capability (Carpenter and Kirkpatrick, 1988). Between episodes of illness, the extent of disability may range from none to disability so severe that institutional care is required.

The life expectancy of people with schizophrenia is shorter than that of the general population because of an increased suicide rate and death from a variety of other causes. Forty years ago, when most patients were kept indefinitely on locked hospital wards, suicide was not a significant problem. Estimates now suggest that 10% of all schizophrenic patients commit suicide; schizophrenics kill themselves within the first 10 years of their illness, and about three quarters of all suicides are men. Those at highest risk have a relapsing course of illness, good insight (i.e., they know they are sick), and a poor response to medication. They are also socially isolated, hopeless about the future, and perceive gross discrepancies between their earlier achievements in life and their current level of functioning (Torrey, 1988). Bill, in Case Example 29–5, is at high risk for suicide. Continual assessment of his suicidal ideation is important. Occasionally persons with schizophrenia commit suicide accidentally while in an acute stage of psychosis; they might, for example, not know they are unable to fly and may jump off a building.

▶ Check Your Reading

49. What characterizes the prodromal, active, and residual phases of schizophrenia?
50. Identify at least five of Frese's suggestions to schizophrenics for staying well.
51. What subgroup among schizophrenics is at greatest risk for suicide?

COMORBIDITY OF SCHIZOPHRENIA WITH SUBSTANCE ABUSE

Substance abuse has been identified increasingly as a source of vulnerability and cause for relapse for schizophrenic patients. Between 20% and 25% of psychiatric patients admitted with a diagnosis of schizophrenia report recent substance abuse (Norris and Naegle, 1990) and higher proportions of substance abuse can be uncovered if patients are laboratory tested. These patients are referred to as the dually diagnosed.

Use of illicit substances does not produce the mental illness of schizophrenia, as defined by DSM-IV, although hallucinations, delusions, and paranoia can be a side effect of alcohol and cocaine abuse.

Drug abuse of PCP can trigger a drug-induced psychosis, indistinguishable in many ways from schizophrenia. Treating schizophrenics with substance abuse problems requires an approach different from treating patients with strictly substance abuse problems. Substance abuse treatment programs, with their heavy emphasis on vigorous and dramatic confrontation, may produce too much anxiety for the recovering schizophrenic. Most treatment centers do not usually wish to be burdened by the special needs of this population.

Patients with a primary diagnosis of substance abuse need to experience directly the devastation they are bringing on themselves so that they can counteract the addiction. The interactions in these programs through peer group confrontation lead to extremely high levels of expressed emotion, and one of the most significant findings in psychosocial investigations of the course of schizophrenia is that an environment with high expressed emotion (i.e., an environment rated high for criticism, intrusiveness, and hostility) is strongly associated with psychotic relapse (Koenigsberg and Handley, 1986).

▶ Check Your Reading

52. What can be the impact of traditional confrontational drug treatment programs on the patient who is dually diagnosed with both substance abuse and schizophrenia?
53. What is the impact of the use of illicit substances on the course of schizophrenia?

DIAGNOSIS

Medical diagnoses are descriptive, so that a minimum number of symptoms meeting a minimal level of severity lead to a medical diagnosis. Symptoms listed in the DSM-IV form the constellation of medically relevant symptoms. Nursing diagnoses, in contrast, describe the quality, content, or context of the patient's health concern and its relationship to contributing factors.

You do not wish to duplicate the medical diagnosis but must use the language of medicine to describe symptoms. Both symptoms and their severity are then included in the nursing diagnosis. Clear descriptions of psychiatric symptoms are essential to assess the effects of medication as well as the patient's potential for self-harm. Patients who are admitted to the hospital in an acute crisis, such as Bill in Case Example 29–5, are responding to vivid auditory hallucinations and require restabilization on higher-than-normal doses of medication. Therefore, in arriving at a nursing diagnosis, you must describe accurately what you observe as well as what the patient describes (Table 29–4). Standardization of nursing actions and common terminology are an important foundation for the provision of nursing care and are provided through the nursing diagnosis, which, of course, is the basis for the nursing care plan. Certain nursing diagnoses are common to individuals with specific psychiatric disorders (Box 29–4). Nursing diagnoses with schizophrenic patients focus on alterations in the pattern of activity, cognition, emotional processes, interpersonal processes, and perception.

▶ Check Your Reading

54. What do the nursing diagnoses provide that the medical diagnoses do not provide?
55. Cite two appropriate nursing diagnoses for a schizophrenic patient.

TABLE 29–4 Nursing Diagnosis: Altered Thought Processes

Type of Thought	Definition	Example
Paranoid delusions	Belief that others are trying to harm the individual	A man notices a woman on the street and believes she is going to kill him
Grandiose delusions	Belief that one has special powers or is a special person	A man believes he has the power to control the weather or is Jesus
Erotomania	Belief that another person is deeply in love with one (usually famous)	A woman believes she is engaged to Senator E. Kennedy, although they haven't met
Thought broadcasting	Belief that one's thoughts can be heard by others	A man believes his thoughts are broadcast over TV
Somatic delusions	Belief that one's body is altered from normal structure or function	A woman believes that her bowels are filled with cement and refuses to eat
Ideas of reference	False belief that public events are related to the individual	A man believes he has caused the bombing of Beirut

BOX 29-4 Medical and Nursing Diagnoses Related to Caring for the Patient with a Thought Disorder

Medical Diagnoses (DSM-IV)

Schizophrenia
- Paranoid type
- Catatonic type
- Disorganized type
- Undifferentiated type
- Residual type

Nursing Diagnoses (NANDA)

Impaired Verbal Communication
Family Coping, Ineffective
Individual Coping, Ineffective
Personal Identity Disturbance
Altered Role Performance
Impaired Social Interaction
Self-Care Deficit
Self-Esteem Disturbance
Sensory/Perceptual Alteration
Social Isolation
Altered Thought Processes

OUTCOME IDENTIFICATION

You must be careful to set realistic outcomes for patients with schizophrenia, as with any chronic illness. Unfortunately, deterioration in all aspects of functioning is part of the illness. The most troublesome areas of patient functioning should be the focus of expected outcomes, setting incremental, short-term outcomes that can set the stage for achieving more long-term outcomes. For example, you might expect a patient experiencing hallucinations to define and test reality at the time of discharge. For a patient exhibiting delusional thinking, you might expect the patient to distinguish between the delusions and reality.

PLANNING

As you plan for the care of a schizophrenic, there are multiple considerations beyond that of initial stabilization. These considerations include discharge planning that focuses on community-living options and the availability of crisis-oriented inpatient treatment.

Role of the Nurse in Discharge Planning

From the moment of admission to the inpatient system, you need to assess factors related to the precipitating crisis and relapse with the purpose of formulating the discharge plan. Establishing a working relationship with the patient and family should lay a foundation for the entire process of treatment as early as possible during acute psychosis. A working alliance needs to be developed between the nurse and the patient and family so that family strengths are maximized and resources identified. Be careful not to focus on weaknesses and deficits. In the initial encounter, which lays the foundation for discharge planning, you need to gain an understanding of life experiences that might contribute to the stress level of a patient or other family members. Identify primary support people. A contract that establishes rules and expectations of treatment with specific, attainable, and mutually agreed-upon goals helps target discharge criteria. Explore issues that contributed to the present hospitalization. Ask questions such as

- Were there factors in the patient's life that helped the patient to fail? If so, what can be done to eliminate or mediate those factors?
- Were the problems related to substance abuse, for example, not taken into account when the person was last in the hospital or last in contact with an outpatient therapist?
- Was there a change in social support that increased the patient's stress level?

Community-Living Options

Until the mid-1950s nobody worried about community aftercare for psychiatric patients because almost no schizophrenic patients left the mental hospitals. The current trend in the treatment of the severely ill thought-disordered patient involves a variety of community-based treatment approaches. This trend has resulted in shorter periods of hospitalization, with inpatient care only for the acute phase of illness, and increased dependence on a wide assortment of aftercare and rehabilitation services. Community-based treatment has also resulted in large numbers of psychiatrically impaired persons returning to their families. Many live with their families throughout their adult lifetimes; in fact, a number of studies have reported that from 25% to 60% of deinstitutionalized patients return to their families (Torrey, 1988).

Crisis-Oriented Inpatient Treatment

Patients need to be hospitalized during an acute phase of their illness, when they are no longer able to live in the community or with their loved ones. They may enter the health care system by seeing their regular outpatient therapist or a community outreach worker on a mobile treatment team, or the family may bring a patient into a hospital's Emergency Department for evaluation. Depending on local regulations, families dealing with an ill family member who appears to be losing control at home may seek an emergency petition requiring the police to bring the person to the local hospital for evaluation. If the person is not living with family, a landlord or caretaker

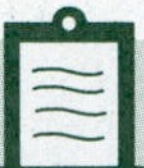

MEDICAL DIAGNOSES AND RELATED NURSING DIAGNOSES

Schizophrenia

DSM-IV **Diagnosis:** Schizophrenia

Diagnostic criteria

A. *Characteristic symptoms:* Two (or more) of the following, each present for a significant portion of time during a one-month period (or less if successfully treated):
   (1) delusions
   (2) hallucinations
   (3) disorganized speech (e.g., frequent derailment or incoherence)
   (4) grossly disorganized or catatonic behavior
   (5) negative symptoms, i.e., affective flattening, alogia, or avolition
   Note: Only one Criterion A symptom is required if delusions are bizarre or hallucinations consist of a voice keeping up a running commentary on the person's behavior or thoughts, or two or more voices conversing with each other.

B. *Social/occupational dysfunction:* For a significant portion of the time since the onset of the disturbance, one or more major areas of functioning such as work, interpersonal relations, or self-care are markedly below the level achieved before the onset (or when the onset is in childhood or adolescence, failure to achieve expected level of interpersonal, academic, or occupational achievement).

C. *Duration:* Continuous signs of the disturbance persist for at least six months. This six-month period must include at least one month of symptoms (or less if successfully treated) that meet Criterion A (i.e., active-phase symptoms) and may include periods of prodromal or residual symptoms. During these prodromal or residual periods, the signs of the disturbance may be manifested by only negative symptoms or two or more symptoms listed in Criterion A present in an attenuated form (e.g., odd beliefs, unusual perceptual experiences).

D. *Schizoaffective and Mood Disorder exclusion:* Schizoaffective Disorder and Mood Disorder With Psychotic Features have been ruled out because either (1) no Major Depressive, Manic, or Mixed Episodes have occurred concurrently with the active-phase symptoms; or (2) if mood episodes have occurred during active-phase symptoms, their total duration has been brief relative to the duration of the active and residual periods.

E. *Substance/general medical condition exclusion:* The disturbance is not due to the direct physiological effects of a substance (e.g., a drug of abuse, a medication) or a general medical condition.

F. *Relationship to a Pervasive Developmental Disorder:* If there is a history of Autistic Disorder or another Pervasive Developmental Disorder, the additional diagnosis of Schizophrenia is made only if prominent delusions or hallucinations are also present for at least a month (or less if successfully treated).
   Classification of longitudinal course (can be applied only after at least one year has elapsed since the initial onset of active-phase symptoms):
   Episodic With Interepisode Residual Symptoms (episodes are defined by the reemergence of prominent psychotic symptoms); *also specify if:* **With Prominent Negative Symptoms**
   Episodic With No Interepisode Residual Symptoms
   Continuous (prominent psychotic symptoms are present throughout the period of observation); *also specify if:* **With Prominent Negative Symptoms**
   Single Episode In Partial Remission; *also specify if:* **With Prominent Negative Symptoms**
   Single Episode In Full Remission
   Other or Unspecified Pattern

RELATED NURSING DIAGNOSIS	DEFINITION	EXAMPLE
Sensory/Perceptual Alteration: Auditory/Visual	Condition in which sensory stimuli are not experienced realistically or are misinterpreted	Sensory perceptual alteration: Auditory related to schizophrenia as evidenced by auditory hallucinations and subjective complaints about internal voices.
RELATED NURSING DIAGNOSIS	**DEFINITION**	**EXAMPLE**
Altered Thought Processes	Condition in which an individual's thought processes are interrupted or not based in reality	Altered Thought Processes related to schizophrenia as evidenced by delusional thinking; inability to concentrate; altered attention span; misinterpretations of reality; hypervigilance; impaired ability to make decisions, solve problems, reason, abstract, conceptualize, or calculate; inappropriate social behavior

Diagnostic criteria from American Psychiatric Association (1994). *Diagnostic and statistical manual of mental disorders, fourth edition.* Washington, D.C.: American Psychiatric Association; nursing diagnoses and definitions from North American Nursing Diagnosis Association. (1994). *NANDA nursing diagnoses: Definitions and classification 1995–1996.* Philadelphia: NANDA.

can petition the court to seek an evaluation. Patients can sometimes become violent, especially as they misperceive cues from others. In these instances, or in instances in which persons may be at risk of imminently harming themselves, police can usually bring the person to a hospital for psychiatric evaluation.

In contrast to most chronic illnesses, such as diabetes, in which investigation has identified the early warning signs of being out of control, schizophrenia and the early warning signs of relapse have been identified only through systematic study. The outcome of most studies of schizophrenia is that the illness is primarily one characterized by exacerbations and remissions. The most common outcome after an acute psychotic episode is a nonpsychotic deficit characterized by blunted affect, low energy levels, social withdrawal, and increased vulnerability to stress (Herz et al, 1990; Frese, 1994).

▶ Check Your Reading

56. Identify two aspects of the nurse's role in discharge planning.
57. Why are community living options an important consideration in discharge planning for the schizophrenic?

IMPLEMENTATION

Specific interventions depend on both the medical and the nursing diagnoses. General guidelines are listed in Boxes 29–5 and 29–6.

Medication

Psychotropic medications play an important part in the treatment of schizophrenic disorders. Drugs do not cure but control symptoms—just as they do the symptoms of diabetes. These drugs are also called neuroleptics or major tranquilizers, but *antipsychotic* is the most descriptive name because their goal is not to produce tranquilization but reduction and control of psychotic symptoms. Chapter 23 provides an in-depth discussion of the medications used in treating schizophrenia.

BOX 29–5 Interventions for a Patient with Altered Thought Processes

- Convey acceptance of patient, but do not confuse delusion with reality.
- Do not argue or deny the belief. Denial may impede the development of a trusting relationship.
- Reinforce and focus on reality in the here and now.
- Assist and support patient in an attempt to verbalize feelings of anxiety, fear, and so on.

BOX 29–6 Interventions for a Patient with Auditory/Visual Sensory/Perceptual Alteration

- Observe the patient for signs of hallucinations. Early intervention may prevent aggressive behavior as a result of misperception of stimuli or response to command hallucination.
- Avoid touching the patient. Touch may be perceived as threatening or could be sensorially painful.
- Do not validate the hallucination but accept that the patient is having the experience.
- Try to connect the occurrence of hallucinations with times of increased anxiety.
- Involve the patient in interpersonal activities that could provide distraction and bring the patient back to reality.
- Medicate with antipsychotic drugs as prescribed.

The goals of antipsychotic therapy are

- To enable the patient to exert self-control (as contrasted with using the drug to control the patient).
- To relieve specific symptoms of psychosis.
- To improve the patient's self-care ability.

Negative symptoms—apathy, withdrawal, loss of motivation, lack of social competence, blunted affect—respond poorly to medication (Harris, 1988; Gournay, 1993; Littrall and Magill, 1993; Marder and Meiback, 1994).

The antiparkinsonian drugs, or anticholinergics, include benztropine (Cogentin), biperiden (Akineton), and trihexyphenidyl (Artane). Because of the known ability of anticholinergics to block dystonic reactions, they have been used in conjunction with antipsychotic drugs since the antipsychotic drugs were introduced. They are also used to treat tremors and akathisia caused by antipsychotic drugs. The general practice today is to use them prophylactically, even before side effects appear, especially in patients who are younger or male, in whom dystonic symptoms are more common.

▶ Check Your Reading

58. What are the purposes of antipsychotic treatment?
59. What are the antiparkinsonian drugs used to treat?

Teaching Patients to Identify and Manage Symptoms

Persons with schizophrenia who receive neuroleptic medication and basic supportive care have been shown to relapse at the rate of 20% to 40% during the first year after hospitalization (O'Connor, 1991). Recognizing early signs of relapse can help reverse the pattern. According to the stress-vulnerability perspective, the onset of psychotic

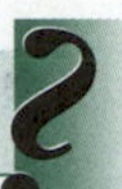

WHAT PATIENTS NEED TO KNOW Schizophrenia

What causes schizophrenia?
The cause of schizophrenia is not precisely known, but the following are generally accepted facts: (1) The brain's chemicals appear to be functioning abnormally; (2) development before birth, early trauma, and inheritance are believed to be predisposing factors; and (3) relatives of schizophrenics have a greater chance of developing the disease than the general population.

Are there different types of schizophrenia?
There are five types of schizophrenia: paranoid (characterized by extreme suspiciousness, delusions of grandeur, and delusions of persecution), catatonic (characterized by a stuporous condition associated with rigidity, posturing, and waxy flexibility), disorganized (characterized by flatness of affect, silliness, incoherence), undifferentiated (characterized by symptoms found in more than one type), and residual (characterized by absence of delusions, hallucinations, or grossly disorganized behavior). Specific symptoms are diagnosed with each type. Symptoms must be present for at least six months to be labeled schizophrenic.

What happens if I don't take my medications?
It is important to take both the antipsychotic and the antiparkinsonian medications to control the symptoms. If the medications are stopped, a recurrence of the symptoms is likely.

What if the symptoms reappear?
Symptoms can recur, even with medication therapy and supportive care. Early recognition of signs such as social withdrawal, sleep changes, increased anxiety, and stress may be observed. It is important to understand the relationship between stress and relapse. Relying on family members and friends is important during a relapse.

Will I always have schizophrenia?
Yes, it is a disease process, one in which controlling the symptoms and living with the illness are important. There is no cure, but medications, community and family support, and therapy can be helpful.

episodes results from interactions among four factors: basic vulnerabilities, environmental stress, personal factors, and environmental protectors (Goldstein, 1987). Because of the multiple factors involved in this dynamic system, the degree of change in stressors or protectors that begin the trend toward relapse cannot be predicted.

Becoming aware of early prodromal signs that signal the beginning of a relapse facilitates efforts to initiate restabilization. People with schizophrenia and their families typically are able to describe symptoms that are very individual. Often, sleep changes, anxiety, and depression as well as general social withdrawal are the first signs the person or family notices. Although these signs can sometimes be subtle, helping the family and patient to identify the individual pattern and notify the outpatient therapist early can prevent relapse. Evidence indicates that most psychotic relapses are preceded by at least two weeks of prodromal symptom increases (O'Connor, 1991). The high rate of restabilization with early intervention suggests that if clinicians respond to all increases in early signs with increased surveillance and support, reduction of stimulation, and perhaps a temporary increase in medication, many relapses can be averted.

The goal of teaching is to identify *target* symptoms that are reliably associated with significant worsening of symptoms for a particular patient and not present at other times. Sometimes early signs subside without deliberate intervention. By involving both patients and their families in the process of routine symptom monitoring, the burden can be lessened. It is important to develop an anticipatory plan that delineates the steps to be taken when family members identify symptomatic changes believed to signal exacerbation. It is also important that patients and families understand the relationship between stress and relapse. When stressful events occur or accustomed supports are lost, informed patients and families recognize the need for especially vigilant monitoring.

► Check Your Reading

60. What are the benefits of teaching patients and families to identify the early signs of illness exacerbation?
61. What interventions can be instituted to prevent relapse when prodromal signs are identified?

Supportive Counseling

Schizophrenics respond best to supportive counseling that focuses on strengths, increasing coping and problem-solving skills and offering affirmation, long-term concern, hopefulness, and commitment. Analytic insight-oriented therapy is too stressful for the schizophrenic and is inappropriate because the illness is biologically based. Case Example 29–9 expresses the need of the schizophrenic for kindness and love.

Case Example 29–9 Elaine's Story

KINDNESS

You seek kindness in these prison hallways,
in the laugh of a nurse
like a light through fog,
in rooms hungry for love. Trees blow in a wind
you do not hear. Now you know

the monotony of dry toast
caught in your throat, stale coffee
in your cup, the pride that even God
did not break down, like a property

you try to save. You crave kindness
like a drunkard his bottle,
you who are abandoned,
left in the middle of the road,
an animal cry darkening the morning.
You remember how summer closed down
city streets, trees bowed with heat,
a rock tune winding down
through an open window. You pray

for a miracle, remembering
how you poured out your heart to someone,
how rain drippling from branches
turned to dogwood blossom.

Elaine Erickson

From Suska, M. A. (1991). *Cry of the invisible* (p. 114). Baltimore: Conservatory Press.

▶ Check Your Reading

62. What are the functions of supportive counseling with the schizophrenic?
63. Why is insight oriented counseling inappropriate for the schizophrenic?

Family Support and Education

STRATEGIES

Two types of clinical programs, psychoeducation and support groups, are reported strategies to help families cope with the problems posed by the symptoms of psychiatric illness. The support group consists of nonstructured discussions usually led by family members to provide social support. A **psychoeducation** group is usually conducted by mental health professionals. The group has an organized, structured format designed to educate families about mental illness and its treatment. The thrust of the family education and management strategy is to lower the emotional climate of the home while maintaining reasonable expectations for patient performance, that is, striking a balance between overstimulation and understimulation. The interventions attempt to

- Increase the stability and predictability of family life by decreasing the family's guilt and anxiety.
- Increase self-confidence.
- Provide a sense of cognitive mastery through the provision of information concerning both the nature and the course of schizophrenia as well as specific management strategies thought to be helpful in coping with schizophrenic symptoms on a day-to-day basis.

When this family education process is effective, it decreases the intensity of interaction between the patient and family members and diminishes the possibility of patients' being overstimulated by even the simplest elements of family life (Hogarty et al, 1990).

Both psychoeducational programs and support groups appear to be helpful to families, and it is unclear whether one modality is more helpful than the other (Wiedemann et al, 1994). The information provided by a psychoeducation group may make patient behavior more understandable and less bothersome to family members. In addition, because of the emphasis on communication and problem-solving in the psychoeducation model, relationships with relatives and friends may improve, contributing to a feeling of increased social support. Some find the organized structure of the psychoeducation group comforting, whereas those with a higher tolerance for ambiguity might favor the free-flowing discussions of the support group. Psychoeducation groups usually cover the following topics in four sessions:

- Schizophrenia
- Medication side effects and communication
- Communicating negative feelings and problem-solving
- Reducing stress and managing disruptive behavior.

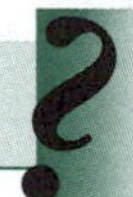

WHAT FAMILIES NEED TO KNOW **Schizophrenia**

Will my family member ever be cured?
Schizophrenia is a chronic disease, which similar to other chronic diseases, has early warnings signs of being out of control. It is important to know that this disease is characterized by exacerbations and remissions. Often, when the symptoms of an acute episode subside, the person has blunted affect, has a low energy level, and may withdraw from social and family situations.

What can I do to help my family member?
It is helpful for the family to become aware of the individual pattern of early signs of relapse that the ill family member may feel. Learning how to identify these target symptoms and routine symptom monitoring by both patient and family can assist in restabilization with early intervention. Most of the time a one- to two-week period of prodromal symptoms, such as sleep changes, depression, anxiety, and social withdrawal, precedes a period of exacerbation.

What resources are available?
Several programs are available to assist the family with support and educational information. Joining a support group with members who have the same experience as yourself can be helpful in providing social and emotional support in dealing with schizophrenic behavior. Education programs in both the community and the hospital can provide necessary important information on medication and side effects, communication techniques for dealing with negative feelings, and managing disruptive behavior.

▶ **Check Your Reading**

64. What are two of the purposes of family education regarding schizophrenia?

65. Identify two topics covered in a psychoeducation group.

TREATING A COEXISTING SUBSTANCE ABUSE PROBLEM

When a patient presents with both schizophrenia and a substance abuse problem, treatment must be directed toward both conditions. For instance, the patient may need to undergo detoxification from the abused substance(s) before adequate, appropriate medication can be prescribed. Once the patient is receiving neuroleptic medications for schizophrenia, consideration must be given to appropriate and concurrent substance abuse treatment, including attendance at a 12-step program and a substance abuse education group. Treating only the schizophrenia and ignoring the substance abuse problem sets the patient up for failure. Both issues require treatment.

Programs that treat psychiatric patients often experience difficulty in treating patients with substance abuse problems because they may have little expertise with drug withdrawal protocols and do not have a well-planned psychosocial approach to treatment of schizophrenia and substance abuse together. Because of the high rates of relapse of substance-abusing psychiatric patients and the common feelings that the patient is deliberately sabotaging treatment, health care providers and family may have a vehement negative response to the patient or feel hopeless and demoralized. It is important that this dual diagnosis problem is faced squarely and programmatically, to avoid these countertherapeutic reactions.

You need to realize the importance of a strong therapeutic alliance to successful outcomes of treatment. You may need to function more as a coach to the patient in a nonjudgmental relationship, working to build adaptive behaviors and extinguish maladaptative ones, focusing on positive steps the patient has made. Patients should be encouraged and admired for their constructive alternative behaviors.

A group psychoeducation approach, with combined education and support about schizophrenia and the complications of substance abuse, may be useful. Group support can be helpful for a patient trying to make behavioral changes and may help reduce loneliness and provide concrete encouragement. It may also provide education and support for families and health care providers, who are the necessary psychosocial link to a schizophrenic recovery.

▶ **Check Your Reading**

66. What are the components of an effective treatment program for dually diagnosed patients?

67. What is the purpose of a psychoeducation group for the dually diagnosed patient?

Spiritual Interventions

Your interventions must include a spiritual component. This component focuses on the meaning of the illness to the patient as well as the patient's relationship with God. Sometimes the patient's behavior during exacerbation is so bizarre that health care providers forget that what is being observed are symptoms. The patient is not the symptoms, and the patient is not the illness. When a patient is viewed as the illness, any attempts to understand the suffering and the existential meaning of the illness generally cease. Likewise, efforts to focus on the patient's strengths and supports, including the patient's relationship with God, are ignored. Jean Vanier, founder of L'Arche movement in which mentally handicapped people, once institutionalized, are given homes in the community, emphasizes the spiritual aspect of care (quoted in Susko, 1991, p. 328):

> *There are three gifts of growth: one is community, a network or covenanted relationships. You would not have chosen some of them. There's a mystery of community, a discovery of forgiveness. The community is to encourage growth, to confirm and challenge. But it can only challenge if it comforts and confirms.*
>
> *There is no community without prayer. Prayer is to say Father, which says I trust. The first part of prayer is the cry, the cry of the wound. The second part of prayer is the prayer of rest, of bridegroom and lover. The cry leads to rest. Prayer finally leads to an offering. Prayer becomes the sacrament of the poor.*

▶ **Check Your Reading**

68. Why is it essential to provide spiritual interventions in the care of the schizophrenic?

EVALUATION

To complete the nursing process, evaluate changes in patient status and behavior in response to nursing interventions. Evaluation criteria are linked to nursing goals and an understanding of the limitations and vulnerabilities of the schizophrenic patient based on a biopsychosocial and spiritual perspective.

The formative evaluation looks at the short-term goals identified for the patient and makes necessary adjustments as the patient's situation changes. The database is continually updated, the nursing diagnoses revised, and expected outcomes modified to meet changes in the patient. For instance, the formative evaluation looks at the patient's immediate response to antipsychotic medication, response to the caregiver, increasing ability to manage personal care, and any changes in symptoms, such as hallucinations or delusions. The summative evaluation reviews the entire nursing process and draws conclusions about the effectiveness of nursing interventions in meeting the expected outcomes. Issues such as community placement, successful acclimation to a psychosocial program, long-term compliance with medications, and resolution of family concerns are addressed in the summative evaluation.

It is important when evaluating the effectiveness of care provided to the chronically ill patient, such as the schizophrenic, that an exacerbation of the illness is not viewed as a treatment failure. Chronic illnesses are episodic, with remissions and exacerbations. Schizophrenics need the freedom to "get sick" without the burden of being blamed as if they have failed the treatment team.

▶ Check Your Reading

69. How should recognition that schizophrenia is a chronic illness affect the evaluation process?

CASE STUDY: ERNIE

Ernie is a 55-year-old white man who has been a salesman in the auto industry for the past 30 years. Over the past few months, Ernie's sales have declined significantly. Recently, his coworkers reported to their boss that Ernie has been behaving in a peculiar fashion. Each morning he would arrive at his office, pick up his telephone, and look under it and unscrew the face plate to check for a microphone. Ernie was sure that someone was tapping his telephone to sabotage his sales. Ernie's usual attire and appearance had also become increasingly untidy and unkempt. He complained to coworkers about having difficulty sleeping.

During the nursing admission, Ernie states, "My coworkers are plotting against me." The nurse notes that Ernie is very cautious and anxious about signing the insurance and admission forms. During the entire process, he sits on the edge of his chair, answers questions evasively, and avoids direct eye contact with the nurse.

ASSESSMENT

Assessment data are as follows:

- Extreme anxious suspicion of coworkers and nurse
- Poor personal hygiene
- Hypervigilance and hyperalertness

DIAGNOSIS

***DSM-IV* Diagnosis:** Schizophrenia, paranoid type

Nursing Diagnosis: Altered Thought Processes related to delusional thinking as evidenced by verbalizations that coworkers are plotting against patient, extreme suspicion, and anxiety.

OUTCOME IDENTIFICATION, PLANNING, AND IMPLEMENTATION

EXPECTED OUTCOME 1: By _____ the patient will be able to distinguish between situations that arouse suspicion and delusional thinking and situations that reflect reality.

SHORT-TERM GOAL	NURSING INTERVENTIONS	RATIONALES
By _____ the patient will have improved reality testing and decreased delusional thinking.	1. Accept patient, by letting him know you respect his feelings and point of view, even though you do not share them.	1. This approach promotes an unconditional acceptance that will be helpful in developing basic trust with the patient.
	2. Do not deny or say directly that the patient's thinking or belief is wrong.	2. This type of confrontation may escalate the patient's anxiety further because he may feel threatened, or confrontation may lead to counterarguments with more delusional details.
	3. Assess patient's delusions and ability to test reality daily. Do not dwell on delusions once the assessment is done; refocus back to reality.	3. Ongoing assessment provides data to determine if treatment (therapy, medication) is making any progress in alleviating the altered thinking processes.

SHORT-TERM GOAL	NURSING INTERVENTIONS	RATIONALES
	4. Reframe frightening delusional system of thinking. Assess for events that increase patient's anxiety and determine what triggers delusions. 5. Assist patient to affirm self as a worthy human being who finds meaning in relatedness with others.	4–5. Persecutory delusions can arise from spiritual distress associated with a negative, hopeless view of life. As the patient begins to value himself, he will convey a positive self-concept.
	6. Administer antipsychotic medications.	6. Medication therapy relieves target symptoms of psychosis (delusions). It does not cure but controls symptoms.

EXPECTED OUTCOME 2: By _____ the patient will identify trusting characteristics in a relationship and begin to develop a relationship with at least one other person during hospitalization.

SHORT-TERM GOALS	NURSING INTERVENTIONS	RATIONALES
By _____ the patient will develop a therapeutic relationship with the nurse.	1. Make short, frequent visits or contact with patient. 2. Avoid whispering around patient and arguing. 3. Inform patient of anticipated schedule changes. 4. Maintain a concerned but not overly concerned attitude toward patient.	1–4. This is a most helpful approach for establishing trust with a patient.
	5. Be aware it is difficult for the patient to be self-aware and that self-disclosure is often uncomfortable.	5. Pushing or pressuring patient may cause an increase in anxiety. Allow patient to set the pace in the relationship.
By _____ the patient will increase social skills.	1. Encourage patient to participate in activities when he feels comfortable in doing so. 2. Provide feedback on behavior, reinforce strengths, and build on them.	1–2. Sharing experiences and participating in activities is a way for the patient to validate thoughts and feelings and receive feedback.

Nursing Diagnosis: Self-Care Deficit related to altered thought processes and anxiety as evidenced by difficulty in dressing appropriately and maintaining personal hygiene.

EXPECTED OUTCOME 3: By _____ the patient will perform self-care at highest level of functioning and ability.

SHORT-TERM GOAL	NURSING INTERVENTIONS	RATIONALES
By _____ the patient will dress appropriately and maintain personal hygiene.	1. Provide a quiet, nonstimulating environment. 2. Give positive feedback for efforts to dress appropriately and maintain grooming.	1–2. Excessive anxiety and preoccupation with safety and delusions contribute to a lack of attention to personal hygiene and appearance. Positive feedback promotes self-esteem and a sense of control.

EVALUATION

Formative Evaluation: Ernie met each of his short-term goals. He immediately began to attend to appropriate personal hygiene practices, and his appearance during the first few days of treatment dramatically improved because of the therapeutic effect of antipsychotic medication. Ernie was able to establish a trusting relationship with the nurse but was not comfortable sharing his feelings in a group setting.

Summative Evaluation: Ernie achieved all of the expected outcomes except that he continued to have difficulty thinking about returning to work. Assisting Ernie to develop and increase his social skills required giving him additional time to meet this goal. Ernie was able to state how ashamed he felt about his behavior at work and did express a considerable amount of apprehension as to how his coworkers might view him. Ernie's ability to begin to share his feelings with the group was an initial step for him to begin to reestablish his relationships with his coworkers. To continue to reinforce and strengthen Ernie's efforts to recognize his sense of self-worth, the treatment team made positive comments. Further therapy revealed that Ernie's father was very authoritarian and critical, while his mother was domineering and argumentative. Ernie began to understand how this type of parenting style lead to his forming a negative view of life with a general mistrust of others and lack of security while growing up.

CASE STUDY: CINDY

Cindy, age 20, has been diagnosed schizophrenia, undifferentiated type. She has shared little of her family background with her college roommate, preferring instead to be alone rather than talk. For the past month, her roommate has noticed that Cindy seems to be off in her own world. She has noticed Cindy "talking to someone" even when there was no one in the room. During the admission interview, Cindy sat quietly and seemed to be listening and watching as if someone were talking to her. She was totally unaware of her surroundings and seemed preoccupied. Occasionally, she would laugh, look up at the ceiling, and nod her head as if in agreement.

ASSESSMENT

Assessment data are as follows:
- Acting as if she is listening to sounds—auditory hallucination
- Looking up at ceiling and nodding head—visual hallucination
- Unawareness of surroundings
- Laughing at inappropriate intervals

DIAGNOSIS

***DSM-IV* Diagnosis:** Schizophrenia, undifferentiated type

Nursing Diagnosis: Sensory/Perceptual Alteration: Hallucinations, Auditory and Visual related to social withdrawal as evidenced by listening to sounds, looking up and nodding to the ceiling, and laughing at inappropriate intervals.

OUTCOME IDENTIFICATION, PLANNING, AND IMPLEMENTATION

EXPECTED OUTCOME I: By _____ the patient will be able to define and test reality, eliminating the occurrence of hallucinations.

SHORT-TERM GOAL	NURSING INTERVENTIONS	RATIONALES
By _____ the patient will have improved reality testing.	1. Evaluate and observe for hallucinations. Redirect the patient back to reality by distracting her with conversation.	1. Early assessment may prevent escalation of behavior into aggression.
	2. Avoid touching patient. Reduce environmental stimuli.	2. Distortion of reality may lead to misinterpretation of a physical touch along with excessive environmental stimuli, which can increase the patient's anxiety and precipitate a hallucination.
	3. Administer antipsychotic medications as ordered.	3. Neuroleptic (antipsychotic) agents reduce psychotic symptoms such as hallucinations.
	4. Determine when anxiety increases. Stay with patient to ensure safety.	4. Escalating anxiety often precedes hallucinations.

SHORT-TERM GOALS	NURSING INTERVENTIONS	RATIONALES
By _____ the patient will interact with others without hallucinating.	1. Assist patient to increase social interaction gradually, starting first with one-to-one interaction and then progressing to small groups. 2. Be available in a consistent, no-demand supportive relationship.	1–2. Social isolation and lack of interpersonal relationships contribute to the use of hallucinations as a substitute for human interaction. A slow, gradual approach of interaction allows the opportunity for some desensitization because interpersonal contacts often precipitate anxiety.
By _____ the patient will be able to understand the hallucinatory experience and how it relates to stress and anxiety.	1. Investigate with patient sources of stress and explain relationship of anxiety and stress on the hallucinations. 2. Teach patient to verbalize fears and methods to manage anxiety and stress constructively.	1. Hallucinations can be reduced by taking medications and reducing stress. 2. Verbalization of fears reduces anxiety. Alternative coping methods may help patient manage anxiety.

EVALUATION

Formative Evaluation: Cindy met all of the short-term goals. Her hallucinations stopped after her medication was stabilized.

Summative Evaluation: Cindy achieved the expected outcome of being able to test reality. With time, she was able to refrain from responding to external visions and voices. She understood the importance of taking her medication and was hopeful that it would control her symptoms. Her roommate remained supportive to her during the entire hospitalization process. Cindy learned not only to listen to her own feelings, fears, and concerns, but also to share with her roommate (who had some of the same fears) some of her fears about college and "being on her own."

CONCLUSIONS

Schizophrenia is a terrible disease. Although our understanding of the disease has increased, we still know very little. Present treatments are directed at controlling symptoms and somehow learning to live with the illness. No current treatment even hints at curing the illness. Although we need to support continuing research directed at identifying specific causes and effective treatments, our attentions must equally be directed to the caring aspect of treatment. Instead of stigmatizing and blaming the schizophrenic and family, we need to develop programs that decrease family burden, to recognize the commitment to care made by families, and to reach out with compassion to the suffering individual. The psychiatric nurse, who frequently has extensive contact with patients and their families over a long period, knows these problems and needs to be a voice for improved care of the mentally ill.

KEY POINTS TO REMEMBER

- Schizophrenia is to psychiatry what cancer is to medicine. The toll is tragic in patients, families, and society as a whole.
- Schizophrenia typically strikes in late adolescence or early adulthood.
- Most schizophrenics become chronic victims of the disease.
- In schizophrenia, normal perceptions of reality become distorted, resulting in auditory, visual, olfactory, or gustatory hallucinations; delusions; illusions; and a variety of other symptoms.
- Schizophrenics experience a defect in the limbic system of the brain resulting in an inability to filter and select stimuli.
- Schizophrenia is considered a formal thought disorder, although more than thoughts are involved in the illness.
- Because of the schizophrenic's difficulties in communicating and relating, these patients pose a challenge to the psychiatric nurse.
- Kraepelin distinguished the symptoms of schizophrenia from manic-depressive psychosis.
- Bleuler identified the four "As" of schizophrenia: affect, association, autism, and ambivalence.
- Schneider identified first-rank and second-rank symptoms of schizophrenia.
- The IPSS identified a 12-point diagnostic system that standardized diagnosis of schizophrenia across nine cultures.
- The *DSM-IV* identifies specific symptoms that must be met in diagnosing schizophrenia and specifies that the symptoms must have been present for at least 6 months.
- The *DSM-IV* classifies schizophrenia according to course and subtype.
- Current research into the cause of schizophrenia has focused on the structure and function of the brain and the role of the limbic system, genetic factors, dopamine, and viral transmission.
- Early theories of causation of schizophrenia focused on the communication patterns in families and the role of the mother. Today we know that the schizophrenogenic mother is a myth.

• The stress-vulnerability model explains schizophrenia according to biological vulnerability and personal vulnerability factors.

• Assessment of the patient with schizophrenia involves assessing positive and negative symptoms, psychosocial and family support, spiritual and religious issues, variability over the life span, and comorbidity with substance abuse.

• Nursing diagnoses use the symptom descriptions provided by medical diagnoses but expand those descriptions to include the patient's response to symptoms.

• Expected outcomes and short-term goals for a schizophrenic must be realistic and allow for periods of exacerbation.

• Implementation includes medication issues, teaching the patient and family to identify and manage symptoms, supportive counseling, psychoeducation and support for families, managing a coexisting substance abuse problem, and spiritual interventions.

• Evaluation includes focusing on the immediate stabilization of a schizophrenic in the midst of an acute exacerbation as well as the long-term adjustment of the patient.

LEARNING ACTIVITIES

1. Read Edgar Allan Poe's "The Tell-Tale Heart" or Mark Vonnegut's *Journey to Eden*. What impressions do you get about schizophrenia? How does what you read challenge your stereotypes of schizophrenia?

2. Research your community's resources. What is available for the long-term support of the schizophrenic patient and the family?

3. Ask five people what they know about schizophrenia. Compare what they tell you with the facts about schizophrenia. How does lack of knowledge contribute to stigma and discrimination?

4. Try to imagine yourself with a disease such as schizophrenia. Your brain no longer works the way that it used to or the way that it should, but you still have the same needs for love, companionship, friendship, and understanding. How do you think you would be treated? What do you think and feel about your own answer?

5. Reflect on the impact of advances in brain research into the causes of schizophrenia on stigma and discrimination. How might new knowledge change public perception of mental illness?

6. Identify something you can do to reduce stigma. How might you implement this action?

CRITICAL THINKING EXERCISE

Mr. Rhodes, a 39-year-old male patient who was due to be discharged from the mental health unit in two days, watched the nurses discussing the flow of patient activity on the unit. About 20 minutes later, as he was approached by the nurse to plan for discharge, Mr. Rhodes said to the nurse, "You put thoughts into my head, didn't you?"

1. What assumption is the patient making?

2. What evidence suggests that the patient's conclusion may be faulty?

3. What inference(s) can the nurse draw from the patient's statement?

Based on her keen observational skills and her knowledge of patients with thought disorders, the nurse responded, "Mr. Rhodes, I did not put any thoughts in your head. It sounds like it is a very frightening experience for you. Tell me about it."

1. What conclusions has she drawn about the patient's thought system?

2. What is the style of intervention?

3. What are alternative approaches that the nurse might use?

REFERENCES

American Psychiatric Association (1994). *Diagnostic and statistical manual of mental disorders* (4th ed.). Washington, D.C.: American Psychiatric Association.

Andreasen, N., Nasrallah, Dunn, V., et al (1986). Structural abnormalities in the frontal system in schizophrenia. *Archives of General Psychiatry, 43*, 136–144.

Anscombe, R. (1987). The disorder of consciousness in schizophrenia. *Schizophrenia Bulletin, 13* (2), 241–259.

Antai-Otong, D. (1989). Concerns of the hospitalized and community psychiatry patient. *Nursing Clinics of North America, 24* (3), 665–673.

Arieti, S. (1976). *Creativity: The magic synthesis* (p. 251). New York: Harper Colophon.

Baron, M., Gruen, R., Rainer, J., et al (1985). A family study of schizophrenia and normal control probands: Implications for the spectrum concept of schizophrenia. *American Journal of Psychiatry 142*, 4, 447–455.

Bateson, G., Jackson, D., Haley, J., and Weakland, J. (1956). Towards a theory of schizophrenia. *Behavioral Science, 1*, 251–264.

Benes, F. M. (1993). Neurobiological investigations in cingulate cortex of schizophrenic brain. *Schizophrenia Bulletin, 19* (3), 537–550.

Boyd, J., Pulver, A., and Stewart, W. (1986). Season of birth: Schizophrenia and bipolar disorder. *Schizophrenia Bulletin, 12* (2), 173–186.

Breier, A., Buchanan, R. W., Elkashef, A., Munson, R. C., Kirkpatrick, B., and Gellad, F. (1992). Brain morphology and schizophrenia. *Archives of General Psychiatry, 49*, 921–926.

Brooker, C. (1990). The health education needs of families caring for a schizophrenia relative and the potential role for community psychiatric nurses. *Journal of Advanced Nursing, 15*, 1092–1098.

Butler, L. D., and Stieglitz, T. L. (1993). Contagion in schizophrenia: A critique of Crow and Done (1986). *Schizophrenia Bulletin, 19* (3), 449–454.

Caligiuri, M. P., Lohr, J. B., Panton, D., and Braff, D. L. (1993). Extrapyramidal motor abnormalities associated with late life psychosis. *Schizophrenia Bulletin, 19* (4), 747–754.

Carpenter, W. (1987). Approaches to knowledge and understanding of schizophrenia. *Schizophrenia Bulletin, 13* (1), 1–7.

Carpenter, W., and Kirkpatrick, B. (1988). The heterogeneity of the long-term course of schizophrenia. *Schizophrenia Bulletin, 14* (4), 645–652.

Carson, V. B. (1994). Spiritual issues in the care of the mentally ill. *DRADA Newsletter, January*, 2.

Castle, D. J., and Murray, R. M. (1993). The epidemiology of late-onset schizophrenia. *Schizophrenia Bulletin, 19* (4), 691–700.

Crow, T. J. (1980). Molecular pathology of schizophrenia: More than one disease process? *British Medical Journal, 280,* 66–68.

Crow, T. J. (1991). The virogene hypothesis of psychosis: Current status. In E. Kurstak (Ed.), *Psychiatry and biological factors* (pp. 9–21). New York: Plenum.

Crow, T. J. (1993). Should contagion be resurrected?—a response to Butler and Stieglitz. *Schizophrenia Bulletin, 19* (3), 455–460.

Csikszentmihalyi, M. (1990). *Flow: The psychology of optimal experience.* New York: Harper & Row.

Dworkin, R. H., Cornblatt, B. A., Friedmann, R., Kaplansky, L. M., Lewis, J. A., Rinaldi, A., Shilliday, C., and Erlenmeyer-Kimling, L. (1993). Childhood precursors of affective vs social deficits in adolescents at risk for schizophrenia. *Schizophrenia Bulletin, 19* (3), 563–578.

Erlenmeyer-Kimling, L., Cornblatt, B. A., Rock, D., Roberts, S., Bell, M., and West, A. (1993). The New York high-risk project: Anhedonia, attentional deviance, and psychopathology. *Schizophrenia Bulletin, 19* (1), 141–152.

Frese III, F. J. (1994). A calling. *Second Opinion, 19* (3), 11–25.

Gerace, L. M., Camilleri, D., and Ayers, L. (1993). Sibling perspectives on schizophrenia and the family. *Schizophrenia Bulletin, 19* (3), 637–648.

Goldstein, M. (1987). Psychosocial issues. *Schizophrenia Bulletin, 13* (1), 157–167.

Gournay, K. (1993). Trends in managing schizophrenia. *Nursing Standard,* 7 (12), 31–36.

Hagerty, B. (1984). *Psychiatric mental health assessment.* St. Louis: C. V. Mosby.

Hall, W., Andrews, G., Goldstein, G. (1985). Cited in Torrey, E. F. (1988). *Surviving schizophrenia: A family manual.* New York: Harper & Row.

Harris, E. (1988). The antipsychotics. *American Journal of Nursing, Nov.,* 1508–1512.

Hatfield, A., and Lefley, H. (Eds.) (1987). *Families of the mentally ill: Coping and adaptation.* New York: Guilford Press.

Herz, M., Keith, S., and Docherty, J. (Eds.) (1990). *Psychosocial treatment of schizophrenia* (Vol. 4). Amsterdam: Elsevier.

Hogarty, G., Anderson, C., Russ, D., Korblith, S., Greenwald, D., Javna, C. (1990). Family psychoeducation, social skills training and maintenance chemotherapy in the aftercare of schizophrenia. *Archives of General Psychiatry, 43,* 633–642.

Huxley, A. (1956). *The doors of perception.* New York: Harper & Row.

Kane, C., Dimartino, E., and Jimenez, M. (1990). A comparison of short-term psychoeducational and support groups for relatives coping with chronic schizophrenia. *Archives of Psychiatric Nursing, 4* (6), 343–353.

Kaplan, H. and Sadock, B. (1989). *Comprehensive textbook of psychiatry.* 5th ed. Baltimore: Williams & Wilkins.

Kay, S. R. (1990). Significance of the positive-negative distinction in schizophrenia. *Schizophrenia Bulletin, 16* (4), 635–652.

Kay, S. R., Opler, L. A., and Lindenmayer, J. P. (1989). The positive and negative syndrome scale (PANSS) rationale and standardization. *British Journal of Psychiatry, 155* (suppl. 7), 59–65.

Kety, S. (1985). Schizotypal personality disorder: An operational definition of Bleuler's latent schizophrenia? *Schizophrenia Bulletin, 11* (4), 590–594.

Koenigsberg, H. W., Handley, R. (1986). Expressed emotion: From predictive index to clinical construct. *American Journal of Psychiatry, 143,* 1361–1373.

Kurstak, E. (Ed.) (1991). *Psychiatry and biological factors.* New York: Plenum.

Larson, D. B., and Larson, S. S. (1991). Religious commitment and health: Valuing the relationship. *Second Opinion, 17* (1), 26–40.

Lefley, H. (1992). Expressed emotion: Conceptual, clinical, and social policy issues. *Hospital and Community Psychiatry, 43* (6), 591–598.

Littrall, K., and Magill, A. M. (1993). The effect of clozapine on preexisting tardive dyskinesia. *Journal of Psychosocial Nursing and Mental Health Services, 31* (9), 14–18.

Marder, S., and Meibach, R. (1994). Risperidone in the treatment of schizophrenia. *American Journal of Psychiatry, 151,* 6, 825–835.

McDowd, J. M., Filion, D. L., Harris, J., and Braff, D. L. (1993). Sensory gating and inhibitory function in late-life schizophrenia. *Schizophrenia Bulletin, 19* (4), 733–746.

McGlashan, T. H., and Fenton, W. S. (1993). The positive-negative distinction in schizophrenia. *Archives of General Psychiatry, 49* (1), 63–72.

Menninger, K. A. (1926). Influenza and insanity. *American Journal of Psychiatry, 5,* 469–529.

Miklowitz, D. (1994). Family risk indicators in schizophrenia. *Schizophrenia Bulletin, 20* (1), 137–146.

Moller, M., and Wer, J. (1989). Simultaneous patient/family education regarding schizophrenia: The Nebraska Model. *Archives of Psychiatric Nursing, 3* (6), 332–337.

NAMI Advocate (January, 1994)

Norris, E., and Naegle, M. (1990). The complexities of treating the dually diagnosed substance abuser. *Addictions Nursing Network, 2* (4), 4–7.

Nuechterlein, K. (1987). Vulnerability models for schizophrenia: State of the art. In H. Hafner, W. F. Gattax, and W. Janzarik (Eds.), *Search for the causes of schizophrenia* (pp. 296–316). Heidelberg: Springer-Verlag.

Nuechterlein, K. H., Dawson, M. E., Ventura, J., Goldstein, M. J., Snyder, K. S., and Mintz, J. (1992). Developmental processes in schizophrenic disorders: Longitudinal studies of vulnerability and stress. *Schizophrenia Bulletin, 18* (3), 387–424.

O'Connor, F. (1991). Symptom monitoring for relapse prevention in schizophrenia. *Archives of Psychiatric Nursing, 5* (4), 193–201.

Pettegrew, J. W., Keshaven, M. S., and Minshaw, N. J. (1993). 31 P nuclear magnetic resonance spectroscopy: Neurodevelopment and schizophrenia. *Schizophrenia Bulletin, 19* (1), 35–53.

Prager, S., and Jeste, D. V. (1993). Sensory impairment in late-life schizophrenia. *Schizophrenia Bulletin, 19* (4), 755–772.

Poe, E. A. (1927). The tell-tale heart. In *The best known works of Poe.* Cornwall, N.Y.: Cornwall Press.

Savage, P. (1991). Patient assessment in psychiatric nursing. *Journal of Advanced Nursing, 16,* 311–316.

Schneider, K. (1959). *Clinical psychopathology* (M. W. Hamilton, Trans.). New York: Grune & Stratton.

Simpson, R. (1989). Expressed emotion and nursing the schizophrenic patient. *Journal of advanced nursing,* (14), 459–466.

Suddath, R., Christison, G., Torrey, E. F., et al (1990). Anatomical abnormalities in the brains of monozygotic twins discordant for schizophrenia. *New England Journal of Medicine, 322* (12), 789–794.

Sullivan, H. S. (1952). *The interpersonal theory of psychiatry.* New York: Norton.

Suska, M. A. (1991). *Cry of the Invisible.* Baltimore: Conservatory Press.

Tamminga, C., and Schulz, S. C. (Eds.) (1991). *Schizophrenia research.* New York: Raven Press.

Torrey, E. F. (1988). *Surviving schizophrenia: A family manual.* New York: Harper & Row.

Torrey, E. F., Bowler, A. E., Rawlings, R., and Terrazas, A. (1993). Seasonality of schizophrenia and stillbirths. *Schizophrenia Bulletin, 19* (3), 557–562.

Utas, J., and Cotman, C. W. (1993). Excitatory amino acid receptors in schizophrenia. *Schizophrenia Bulletin, 19* (1), 105–117.

Vonnegut, M. (1975). *The Eden express.* New York: Praeger.

Walker, E. (Ed.) (1991). *Schizophrenia: A life-course developmental perspective.* San Diego: Harcourt Brace Jovanovich.

Wiedemann, G., Hahlweg, K., Hank, G., Feinstein, E., Muller, U., and Dose, M. (1994). Deliverability of psychoeducational family management. *Schizophrenia Bulletin, 20* (3), 547–544.

Winter, D. (1990). Questions and answers about schizophrenia. *Journal of Psychosocial Nursing, 29* (8), 7.

Wolkin, A., Sanfilipo, M., Wolf, A. P., Angrist, B., Brodie, J. D., and Rotrosen, J. (1992). Negative symptoms and hypofrontality in chronic schizophrenia. *Archives of General Psychiatry, 49,* 959–965.

Wong, D., Wagner, H., Tune, L., et al (1986). Positron emission tomography reveals dopamine receptors in drug-naive schizophrenics. *Science, 234,* 1558–1562.

SUGGESTED READINGS

Frese III, F. J. (1994). A calling. *Second Opinion, 19* (3), 11–25.

Simpson, R. (1989). Expressed emotion and nursing the schizophrenic patient. *Journal of Advanced Nursing,* (14), 459–466.

Suska, M. A. (1991). *Cry of the Invisible.* Baltimore: Conservatory Press.

Winter, D. (1990). Questions and answers about schizophrenia. *Journal of Psychosocial Nursing, 29* (8), 7.

CHAPTER 30

THE JOURNEY COLORED BY MOOD DISORDERS

Perhaps the blackest moment of all came when a friend, a dear and usually understanding person, said, "You've changed, you're not the same as you were," and said it in a tone not only of puzzlement but of rebuke. Anyone who has suffered from a depression will know how I felt. Of course I've changed, you scream inwardly, I've got a depression, you know that. I can't, I can't, can't "snap out of it"....

—Sheila Bovell

LEARNING OBJECTIVES

After studying this chapter, you should be able to:

1. Define terms such as depression, mania, affective, bipolar, hypomania, dysthymia, and cyclothymia.
2. Discuss the current research related to pharmacological, neurochemical, endocrinological, and genetic causes of mood disorders.
3. Discuss the association of depression with other medical conditions.
4. Describe the importance of family involvement in the treatment of patients with mood disorders.
5. Describe the emotional, psychological, and spiritual components to consider throughout the nurse-patient journey characterized by mood disorders.
6. Identify expected outcomes for patients with depression and mania.
7. Discuss the treatment options available to patients experiencing mood disorders.
8. Describe the nursing role in each treatment option available to patients experiencing mood disorders.
9. Identify the nursing interventions for assisting families of patients with mood disorders.
10. Apply the nursing process to a patient diagnosed with depression and a patient diagnosed with bipolar disorder mania.

KEY TERMINOLOGY

Affect
Bipolar disorder
Cyclothymia
Depression
Dysthymia
Empowerment
Euthymia
Hypomania
Longitudinal course specifiers
Mania
Mixed episode
Mood
Postpartum depressive pattern
Rapid cycling
Seasonal affective pattern
Self-attitude
Vital sense

The mood disorders are characterized by disturbance in mood (profound sadness or apathy, irritability, or elation). This group of disorders is distinguished by two important facts: (1) They rank among the most serious health problems in the United States, and (2) they are among the most poorly diagnosed and treated of the health problems in the United States.

No one is immune from the mood disorders. They are common in men, women, adolescents, and children. Mood disorders affect the way people feel about themselves and the world in which they live. People with **depression** experience feelings of unbearable sadness or irritability, despair, and hopelessness. They frequently desire suicide. In addition, depression carries with it disturbances in emotional, cognitive, behavioral, somatic, and spiritual dimensions of the individual. People with **mania** experience feelings of excitement, elation, or extreme irritability. Mania also carries disturbances in emotional, cognitive, behavioral, somatic, and spiritual dimensions. Both depression and mania include the possibility of psychotic behavior. All of the mood episodes and mood disorders involve variations of or combinations of depression and mania.

Estimates are that up to 15% of the adult population at any given time suffers with a mood disorder. Approximately 2% of adolescents and adults (more than 4 million people) in the United States are currently suffering from a major depressive disorder. The mood disorders are more widespread than coronary heart disease (7 million) or cancer (6 million). These illnesses most often strike during a person's most productive years—nearly 70% of adults with depression are below the age of 45, and 72% of those are in the labor force. Although the mood disorders can have their onset at any age, major depressive disorder usually begins in the 20s and 30s. **Bipolar disorder** usually begins in the 20s. As many as half of the people who experience serious depressions also have episodes of mania. Women are twice as likely than men to experience an episode of depression and several times more likely to seek or accept treatment (*Depression in primary care* . . . , 1993). Women and men are equally affected with bipolar disorder.

These illnesses are relapsing, episodic conditions, although their pattern varies with each individual. About 70% of patients who have suffered from depression can expect to face the illness again. The median number of recurrences during a lifetime is four. Despite the wide reach of the mood disorders, research demonstrates that artistic individuals (especially poets) are particularly vulnerable to the disorders. Among this notable group of artists are Vincent van Gogh, Virginia Woolf, Ernest Hemingway, Edgar Allan Poe, and Robert Schumann. In addition to the suffering caused by attacks of mania and depression, the natural course of the mood disorders, if left untreated, worsens over time. Attacks become more frequent and severe (Jamison, 1993).

PETER'S STORY

April 4, 1983, was a gorgeous spring day. The banners were waving in a balmy breeze, and short sleeves were the order of the day. I was excited and excitable, hopeful and expectant—certainly, a man at ease in his surroundings. In this setting my experience with manic-depressive illness began.

It was the opening-day game for the Baltimore Orioles, a team I have followed religiously for years. Better yet, "The Birds," as true fans call them, were ahead. Normally, I would hav e been overjoyed by a win in the home opener. But in the sixth inning, in the midst of celebrating with friends and my favorite sports team, I began to feel fuzzy, blurry-eyed, unsure of myself, afraid of the crowd, uneasy about the height of our seats over the field. I became very quiet.

My friends noticed the change in my mood on the way home: my short answers, the lack of life in my voice, my pregame excitement extinguished. I recall telling them that I felt that my mind was tired, but now I know that on that day I came face-to-face with my first biochemical depression.

Recognition of Illness

I was born and live today in a small town in West Virginia where I practice medicine. I am fortunate to have a loving, caring wife who is also my best friend. We have three children, ages 12, 6, and 4. The 6-year-old is a boy, surrounded by his sisters in age.

Looking at my family tree, I should not have been surprised to have psychiatric illness at some point in my life. My great-grandfather exhibited times of great activity and great melancholy, according to my grandmother's writings. She herself was diagnosed with manic-depressive illness, but she was never treated. My father was an alcoholic who died as a result of his drinking. His life included great business successes and failures, several divorces, and frequent depressions.

With what I suppose was an inherited predisposition, I met with several stresses during the months before the Orioles' opening day. My grandmother, with whom I enjoyed a very close relationship all my life, passed away. In the same month, my father died. My wife and I were expecting a new baby at the end of April. My work weeks at my office climbed to 75 hours.

The low and fearful mood I experienced at the game was just the beginning. For weeks, I progressively lost more and more motivation, curiosity, and creativity. My appetite waned, and my sleep was disturbed. At first, I sought relief in my office and tried, literally, to work through it. I realized that this was not a solution when one morning I could not force myself to get out of bed and go to work.

Treatment

I saw a doctor and got medication, but it seemed to work too well, and I became manic. I became oblivious to reason and experienced extreme financial difficulties as a result of spending sprees. Delusions of grandeur, sexual indiscretions, and extreme irritability threatened my marriage.

For five months, I experienced cycles of mania and depression every ten days. My doctor tried changing the dosage of my medication. My wife, Karen, and I both knew what was sure to follow with each new cycle, and the feeling was oppressive. We were unable to count on anything enjoyable in the future, knowing that I would be unreachably high, severely depressed and anxious, or in transition from one to the other.

When I look back on that period of several months, I wonder at the fact that my wife stayed with me. I am thankful that she was able to remember things about me when I was well that helped to carry her through this low point of our time together.

Still seeing no improvement, I became a research volunteer at the National Institute of Mental Health (NIMH) on September 14, 1983. As time passed, a more effective medication for my particular brand of bipolar disorder was found; the proper dosage was determined, and I improved immediately. While it was extremely difficult being away from my family and my work during my stay at the NIMH, I had many introspective moments to think about piecing my life back together.

Story from DePaulo, J. R. Jr., and Ablow, K. R. (1989). *How to cope with depression: A complete guide for you and your family* (pp. 41–43). New York: McGraw-Hill.

Rehabilitation

Before I returned home, I began to carefully rebuild my marriage, faith, friendships, and business. My wife never wavered, nor, at its foundation, did my faith. Former friends looked askance, as if they could not believe that I was now "normal" after being on a "psych ward." Present friends were happy for my health and interested in the new genetic principles behind the biochemistry of my illness. I called each of my own patients to inform them of my renewed well-being and to assess their intentions. This was an incredibly difficult experience, but it was central to my plans to reestablish myself professionally.

Today I continue to take only lithium carbonate. Minor mood swings still come and go with this medication, but not of a severity near that which I experienced during 1983. I have not missed a day of work or of active living since March 26, 1984, when I first returned to the practice of dentistry. I complain at times about the increased appetite, some weight gain, and the occasional fatigue that I experience with the medication, but I continue to take it. Staying well is so important to me.

I went trout fishing recently—one of the few things I love more than the Orioles. When I returned home, Karen told me, as she often does, how happy she was to have me healthy. I was happy to hear that and to feel that. The baby I mentioned as an added stress in 1983 is a beautiful little girl named Erica Marcia. She was five years old on May 1, 1988.

I reflect often on the five years since her birth and am thankful we are all together. I don't know whether we need to be concerned about Erica or our other children having this illness. I hope and pray always that the researchers working on affective disorders have continued success. In the meantime, we all need to help educate Erica and others and give them hope for the future. There is a great deal more to be done in the world.

OUR UNDERSTANDING OF MOOD DISORDERS

Almost 90 years ago, Emil Kraeplin best described manic and depressive conditions as two parts of a "single disease process." He also reported that he found nothing wrong in the brains of *affectively ill* (referring to mood disorders) patients who had died and that he could offer no truly effective treatments. As a result, there was doubt that these conditions were bodily diseases. The doubt about a physiological explanation gave greater credence to psychoanalytical theory as a treatment to the mentally ill. Before long, however, psychiatrists using psychoanalysis realized how ineffective it was with most severely depressed or manic patients. As a result, for many years the most seriously ill individuals were not treated (DePaulo and Ablow, 1989).

Within the past 50 years, new medical treatments have evolved that are helpful and safe in the treatment of serious mood disorders. The development of these treatment tools supports the view that major forms of mental illness not only can be distinguished from each other, but also respond to specific medical treatments (DePaulo and Ablow, 1989). Most of the research interest and funding have focused on discovering better treatments for the disease. Little attention has been paid to the emotional, psychological, and spiritual aspects and origins of mood disorders.

The Impact of Mood Disorders on the Journey

Unfortunately, diagnosis of mood disorders is hampered by our inability to describe moods and changes in mood. This imprecision limits our ability to understand mood problems in a "medical sense." It is not an easy task to discuss basic but complex feelings the same way we talk about physical pain. We can usually describe physical pain by its location, intensity, and beginning.

Mood symptoms are generally more difficult to pinpoint. For instance, the word *depression* is often used to describe unpleasant feelings such as sadness, loss, or nostalgia, which are normal feelings of living. This usage complicates the process of distinguishing the disease of depression, which is a more fundamental and pervasive experience. Depression goes beyond sadness. It seriously affects an individual's feelings about the future and erodes the most basic attitudes about self. Sometimes this depression can deepen and widen to poison self-attitude and feelings about life, creating despair, hopelessness, and spiritual distress.

Mood refers to an individual's pervasive feeling state. A *normal* mood, also referred to as **euthymia,** refers to what is usual, common, or expected in a given situation (Figure 30–1). For example, when good things happen to us, we find ourselves in a good mood. When we have problems, disappointments, and setbacks, it is normal to be in a bad mood, or to experience **dysthymia.** Normal moods are reactive. Our moods respond and react to situations, to what happens to us, and to what is important to us. Normal mood changes in proportion to life situations. For example, the normal change in mood after the death of a loved one is usually severe and markedly different from the mood change following the loss of an inanimate object. Based on our own experience and observations, we have an intuitive sense of normal direction and degree of mood change in specific situations (Mondimore, 1993).

Affect is a term closely related to mood. **Affect** refers to the feelings that are reflected on our faces, in our expressions, and by our demeanor. Affect is fleeting. The full range of affect indicates normal changes that occur in our facial reflection of feelings. Flat affect indicates no changes in our facial reflection of feelings. Blunted affect indicates minimal changes in our facial reflection of feelings.

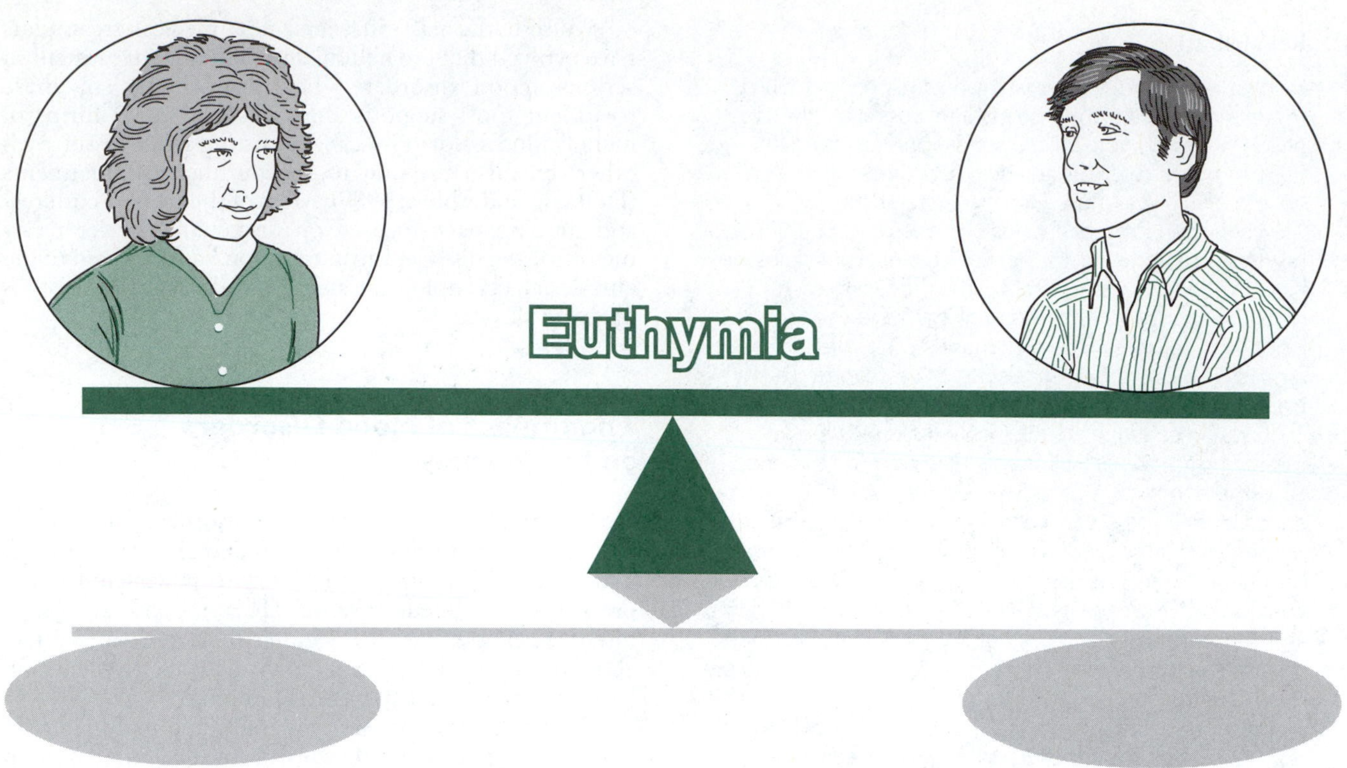

FIGURE 30–1
The term *euthymia* refers to a *normal* mood—what is usual, common, or expected in a given situation.

Cooccurrence of Mood Disorders with Other Disorders

Complicating the course of the mood disorders is a high rate of comorbidity (cooccurrence) with other psychiatric disorders. These include anxiety disorders, substance-related disorders, eating disorders, obsessive-compulsive disorders (OCD), somatization disorders, and personality disorders. In addition, mood disorders have a high rate of cooccurrence with other general medical conditions. These include stroke, dementia, diabetes, coronary artery disease, cancer, chronic fatigue syndrome, and fibromyalgia.

Cooccurrence with Other Psychiatric Disorders

Severe forms of anxiety—phobias, panic attacks, obsessions, and compulsions—may occur alone or as a part of depression. People with panic attacks have been found to have a higher-than-expected number of relatives who suffer from a major depressive disorder. Data on eating disorders, anorexia nervosa and bulimia nervosa, suggest that depression is common in young women who suffer from dysregulation of food intake. Data also suggest that focus on the eating disorder, not the depression, is usually the most efficacious approach to treatment. Eighty percent to 100% of patients who are diagnosed with OCD also experience symptoms of depression. In these patients, the OCD is the focus of treatment. Patients who do not have OCD but present with severe depression often experience problems with obsessive thoughts. In these patients, the depression is the focus of treatment. Depressed patients often see their primary physicians with complaints of aches and pains. Primary physicians often focus entirely on the patient's somatic complaints to the exclusion of the depression. It is vital to recognize and assess somatic symptoms as possible indicators of depression. Another classification of psychiatric disorders that occur with depression are personality disorders. Generally, when depression is complicated by a personality disorder, the course is more complicated, with increased rates of suicide attempts and self-harm (*Depression in primary care* . . . , 1993).

Additional problems are created by the use of substances such as alcohol, cocaine, nicotine, and prescribed or street drugs. People appear to use these and other drugs to medicate depression or to induce the elevated moods associated with bipolar disorder. The relief provided by these substances is described by some patients as a "calming effect" or by others as "instant energy." Although these drugs may produce short-term relief of the symptoms of depression and mania, they lead to long-term problems of addiction. William Styron describes the advent of his most menacing forms of depression after he was forced to give up his alcohol addiction (Styron, 1990) (see Chapter 31).

Cooccurrence with Medical Conditions

Many general medical conditions are risk factors for depression. In fact, clinical depression is present in approximately 12% to 36% of patients with another nonpsychiatric, general medical condition (*Depression in primary care . . .*, 1993). For instance, many stroke patients experience depression believed to be causally related to the injury in the brain. Dementia is another medical condition in which depression often coexists. Patients with diabetes frequently develop depression, perhaps as a reaction to the management issues that surround diabetes. In each of these medical conditions, stroke, dementia, and diabetes, treatment of the depression is advisable.

Because of a strong correlation between depression and higher mortality and morbidity rates in post–myocardial infarction patients as well as coronary artery disease patients without myocardial infarction, patients with either of these medical conditions should be carefully screened and treated for depression. Depression also coexists with cancer and occurs in about 25% of all cancer patients. Therefore, every cancer patient should be screened for depression and, if necessary, treated.

Patients with depression characteristically complain of fatigue and lack of energy. The complaint of chronic fatigue is not sufficient to meet the criteria for chronic fatigue syndrome. If both depression and chronic fatigue syndrome are present, however, the patient is treated for depression. Patients diagnosed with fibromyalgia have higher lifetime rates of major depressive disorder than do rheumatoid arthritis patients (Hudson et al, 1985). When fibromyalgia coexists with depression, the depression is treated.

Implications of Mood Disorders

The journey toward wellness for individuals with mood disorders involves acceptance that the mood disorder is a medical illness requiring aggressive treatment. These illnesses bring untold misery, along with wasted days, months, and even years of impaired functioning at work and in personal life. Loss of productivity and its economic cost to society affect business at a cost of about $43.7 billion annually, over half of which is paid directly by American business (Greenberg et al, 1993).

These diseases have a frightening mortality rate. Suicide is the most serious complication. In fact, suicide is one of the top 10 causes of death at all ages and the third leading cause of death in teenagers and young adults. The most serious symptoms of depression are hopelessness, despair, and a sense of spiritual emptiness. Those who feel that life is meaningless and that God has abandoned them consider suicide a viable option.

As common and as potentially serious as the mood disorders are, one would expect that physicians would be vigilant regarding the diagnostic possibility of a mood disorder. Yet these illnesses are misdiagnosed by physicians, misunderstood by the lay public, and too often ignored or considered a character weakness or a temporary difficulty that an individual can just "snap out of." The lack of acceptance by the medical community as well as by the general public increases the difficulty the patient experiences in accepting the illness. Yet acceptance of the illness is a prerequisite for the patient to benefit fully from all available treatment. Only through acceptance can the individual learn to exert control over the illness and to make responsible decisions related to coping with the illness on a daily basis.

Mood disorders are holistic. They affect physical, emotional, cognitive, social, occupational, and spiritual dimensions. Peter describes his personal experience with **bipolar disorder** (a mood disorder characterized by extreme shifts in mood from sadness to either elation or irritability). Peter's story is a glimpse into the life of one person with a mood disorder.

▶ Check Your Reading

1. What are the symptoms of depression?
2. What are the symptoms of mania?

DEFINING MOOD DISORDERS

Included in mood disorders are mood episodes. These include major depressive, manic, mixed, and hypomanic episodes, which are not disorders in themselves but provide the building blocks for the major disorders. Mood disorders are further categorized into depressive disorders (also referred to as unipolar disorders) and bipolar disorders. Depressive disorders include major depressive disorder, dysthymic disorder, and depressive disorder not otherwise specified. Bipolar disorders include bipolar I and bipolar II disorders, cyclothymic disorder, and bipolar disorder not otherwise specified (Figure 30–2). Tables 30–1, 30–2, and 30–3 provide the definitions of the mood episodes, depressive disorders, and bipolar disorders. Note that some of these conditions involve milder symptoms than those seen in major depressive disorder or bipolar disorder. **Hypomania,** for example, is a manic state not severe enough to impair functioning. **Cyclothymia** involves relatively mild depressive symptoms.

Diagnostic Symptoms

A limitation of the DSM-IV or any other checklist of symptoms is that it does a better job of deciding who should be called depressed or manic than it does describing the ill person's experience. Emphasis is on the patient's sadness, not on the potentially devastating effects of hopelessness and isolation (DePaulo and Ablow, 1989). For instance, knowing that Peter was diagnosed with bipolar disorder provides no information regarding his suffering, the struggles that he experienced in his move toward stability, the personal trials and tribulations he endured, or the support that he received from his wife, Karen. Nursing diagnoses, in contrast, do more to describe the person's experiences.

In diagnosing a mood disorder, the clinician assesses presenting signs and symptoms, the patient's history and prior response to treatment, and the family's history. The central issues are whether the patient is experiencing a persistent change in mood, **self-attitude** (self-esteem or self-confidence), and **vital sense** (physical and bodily health). In Peter's story, all of these symptoms were present. He described "feeling fuzzy, blurry eyed,

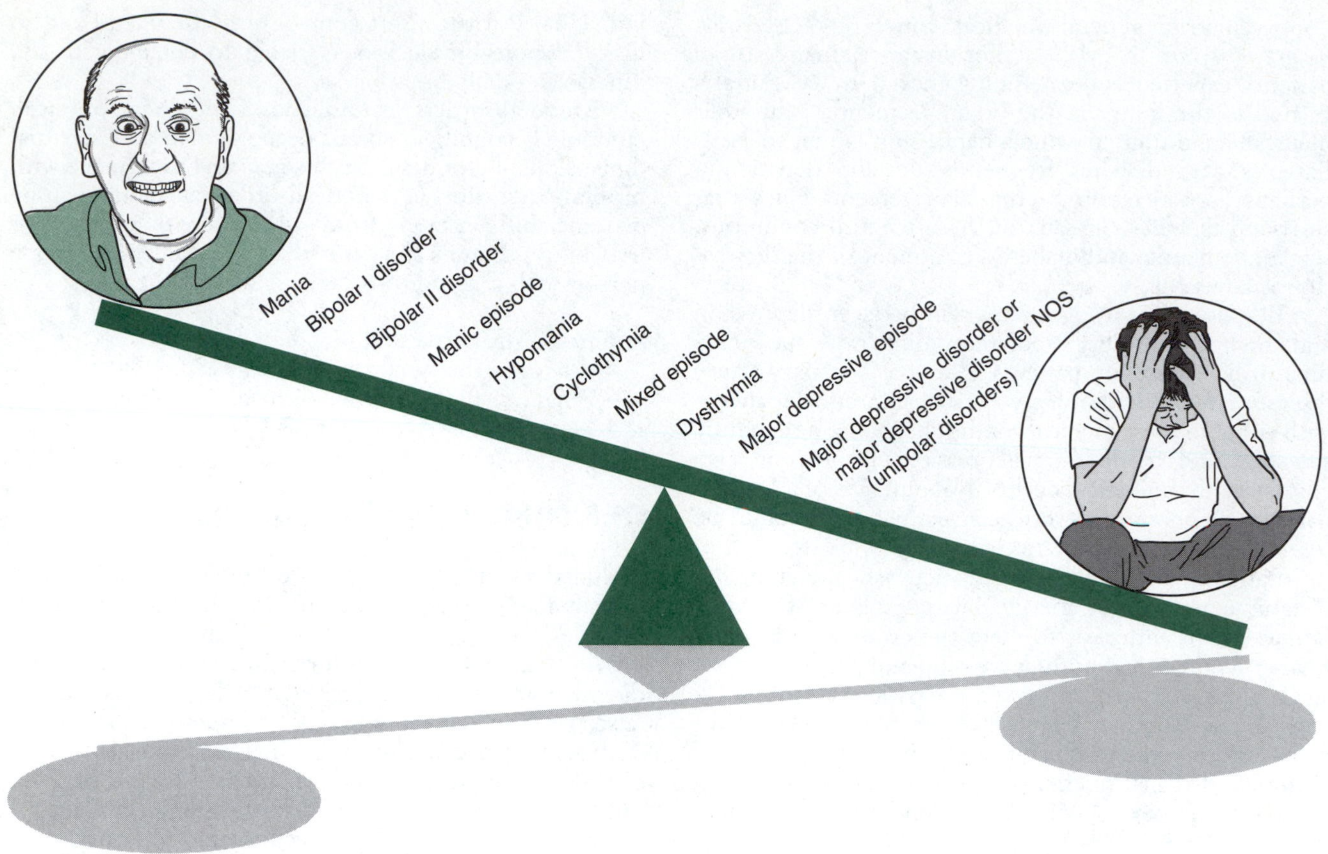

FIGURE 30–2
The see-saw continuum of mood disorders.

unsure of myself, afraid of the crowd, uneasy about the height of our seats over the field. I became very quiet and withdrawn." Peter noted that he had a genetic background that made him vulnerable to developing a mood disorder. His story illustrates the dramatic swing between depression (the feelings that began while watching the baseball game) and the severe symptoms of **mania:** "I became oblivious to reason and experienced extreme

TABLE 30–1 Definitions of Mood Episodes

Major depressive episode	Characterized by feelings of either depression or the loss of interest in nearly all activities. Symptoms must last at least two wk. At least four other symptoms from the following list must be present: changes in appetite or weight, sleep, or psychomotor activity; feelings of worthlessness and guilt; difficulty concentrating or making decisions; recurrent thoughts of death or suicidal ideation, plans, or attempts
Manic episode	Characterized by a period in which there is a dramatic change in mood; either elation and expansiveness or irritability is present. This change in mood must last at least one wk (less if hospitalization is required). At least three other symptoms from the following list must be present: inflated self-esteem or grandiosity, decreased need for sleep, pressured speech, flight of ideas, distractibility, increased involvement in goal-directed activities or psychomotor agitation, and overinvolvement in pleasurable activities with potentially damaging consequences (e.g. hypersexuality, impulsive spending)
Mixed episode	Characterized by rapidly changing alternating moods (sadness, irritability, euphoria) accompanied by symptoms from both manic and depressive episodes lasting at least one wk. Disturbance severely affects functioning, may require hospitalization, and may result in the emergence of psychotic behaviors
Hypomanic episode	Characterized by at least four d of abnormally and persistently elevated, expansive, or irritable mood accompanied by at least three additional symptoms seen in a manic episode. Disorder is not severe enough to impair functioning seriously or to require hospitalization. Disorder does not involve psychotic behavior

TABLE 30–2 Definitions of Depressive Disorders

Major depressive disorder	A major mood disorder characterized by one (single) or more (recurrent) episodes of major depression, with or without full recovery between episodes
Dysthymic disorder	A mood disorder characterized by depressed mood and loss of interest or pleasure in activities of life, with some additional signs and symptoms of depression present most of the time for at least two y. Many patients with dysthymia go on to develop major depressive episodes
Depressive disorder not otherwise specified	A category of mood disorder characterized by specified depressive features that do not meet the criteria for major depressive disorder, dysthymic disorder, adjustment disorder with depressed mood, or adjustment disorder with mixed anxiety and depressed mood

financial difficulties as a result of spending sprees. Delusions of grandeur, sexual indiscretions, and extreme irritability threatened my marriage." The primary risk factors for depressive disorder are shown in Box 30–1.

Variations of Mood Disorders

As you can see in Tables 30–1, 30–2, and 30–3, mood episodes and disorders are all characterized by a dysfunctional regulation of mood. For example, in the mixed affective disorder, or **mixed episode,** symptoms of depression and mania occur together. The two most common mixed states are dysphoric (unhappy) mania and exalted depression. In dysphoric mania, individuals have high energy levels, racing thoughts, and pressured speech. Instead of being in an elated mood, however, they report feeling irritable, fearful, or unhappy. Exalted depression is also characterized by depressed mood but is accompanied by grandiose delusions. For example, one patient believed that she was a prophet condemned for having failed to save the souls of others with her powers (DePaulo and Ablow, 1989).

In addition to the diagnoses seen in Tables 30–1, 30–2, and 30–3, the DSM-IV specifies criteria for a patient's most recent mood episodes as

- Mild, moderate, or severe without psychotic features; severe with psychotic features; in partial remission; or in full remission. These criteria apply to major depressive episode, manic episode, and mixed episode.
- With catatonic features
- With melancholic features
- With atypical features
- With postpartum onset

DSM-IV also specifies the course of recurring episodes as

- Longitudinal course specifiers (with or without full interepisode recovery)
- With seasonal pattern
- With rapid cycling

TABLE 30–3 Definitions of Bipolar Disorders

Bipolar I disorder	A major mood disorder characterized by episodes of major depression and mania or hypomania. The diagnosis of bipolar I disorder requires one or more episodes of mania
Bipolar II disorder	A major mood disorder characterized by the occurrence of one or more major depressive episodes accompanied by at least one hypomanic episode. The presence of a manic episode or a mixed episode excludes the diagnosis of bipolar II disorder
Cyclothymic disorder	A mood disorder of at least two years duration characterized by numerous periods of mild depressive symptoms not sufficient in duration or severity to meet the criteria for major depressive episodes interspersed with periods of hypomania. Some view this as a mild form of bipolar disorder
Bipolar disorder not otherwise specified	A mood disorder characterized by bipolar features that do not meet the criteria for any specific bipolar disorder

BOX 30-1 Risk Factors for Depression

- Prior episodes of depression
- Family history of depressive disorder
- Prior suicide attempts
- Female gender
- Age of onset under 40
- Postpartum period
- Medical comorbidity
- Lack of social support
- Stressful life situations
- Current alcohol or substance abuse

Postpartum depressive pattern describes mood disturbance that can be applied to any of the mood disorders when the onset is within 4 weeks after the delivery of a child. For instance, a woman could be diagnosed with major depressive disorder with postpartum onset or bipolar disorder with postpartum onset. Symptoms of depression seem to be exacerbated in some women during times of dramatic hormonal events—the premenstrual period, the postpartum period, and possibly the menopausal period. Although some women experience a major depressive disorder with postpartum onset, many others experience only transient mood changes (apparently due to hormonal changes). Women with histories of mood disorders before pregnancy are more likely to suffer more severely during the postpartum period and are also at greater risk of developing a mood disorder unrelated to childbirth later in life (DePaulo and Ablow, 1989).

Beck's (1993) study of postpartum depressive pattern cited loss of control as the basic sociopsychological problem. One mother stated, "I had absolutely no control, and that was the scariest thing because I always had control." Women with postpartum depression lack control over their emotions, thought processes, and actions. As one mother described, "I just couldn't get out of the pain. It's like you hurt so bad, and you don't want to be that way, and yet you lose all control of everything." The major problem related to these disorders is delayed recognition and treatment, which affects not only the depressed mother but also her infant and the rest of her family. "When I was sick, I didn't want my baby. I didn't love my husband. I didn't want to work. I hated everything. When I got better, it all melted away" (Beck, 1993, p. 47).

Longitudinal course specifiers are used to characterize the course of illness in patients who experience recurrent major depressive disorder, bipolar I disorder, or bipolar II disorder. These specifiers are applied to the period between the two most recent episodes. There are four longitudinal course patterns:

- Recurrent, with full recovery between episodes and with no dysthymic disorder.
- Recurrent, without full recovery between episodes and with no dysthymic disorder.
- Recurrent, with full recovery between episodes, superimposed on dysthymic disorder.
- Recurrent, without full recovery between episodes, superimposed on dysthmic disorder.

Seasonal affective pattern describes a variation of mood disorder typically characterized by depression occurring in the fall and winter and normal moods in the spring and summer. Less commonly reported are patients with recurrent summer episodes of depression. The disease has been referred to as seasonal affective disorder (SAD). Although the depression in SAD meets all the diagnostic criteria for major depression, several mood symptoms seem to be more common. As in any major depressive disorder, people with SAD have changes in appetite and sleep patterns. The SAD patient, however, almost always has an increase in sleep, complaints of chronic winter fatigue, an increase in appetite, and a craving for sweets and other carbohydrates. Seasonal depressions tend to be less severe than many episodes of major depression (Rosenthal, 1989).

Seasonal variations of mood are believed to be determined by the amount of time exposed to light rather than by temperature changes. Apparently, melatonin, a hormone produced by the pineal gland, is strongly influenced by light exposure. Each night, like clockwork, the pineal gland releases melatonin into the bloodstream in minute quantities and continues to do so until dawn. Although it is unclear whether melatonin is instrumental in causing seasonal changes in humans, the research in this area may prove critical in understanding and treating SAD.

Treatment of SAD with light is still being refined. Four to six hours of bright light each day seems necessary. The light must be five to 10 times brighter than ordinary room light, about the same brightness as can be seen looking out a window on a sunny spring day. Patients sit a few feet from the special fluorescent bulbs and read, sew, or do paperwork. They must keep their eyes open and are instructed to glance directly into the light for a few seconds every minute or so. A SAD patient treated with light notices an improvement within three or four days (Rosenthal, 1989).

The characteristics of **rapid cycling** include four episodes of a mood disturbance occurring in the previous 12 months and meeting the criteria for major depressive disorder, manic episode, mixed episode, or hypomanic episode. The episodes are delineated by either partial or full remission of at least two months or by a switch to an episode of the opposite mood (e.g., major depressive episode switches to manic episode). Peter described rapid cycling of his bipolar illness.

▶ Check Your Reading

3. Define mood.
4. Define affect.
5. What are the central issues when diagnosing a mood disorder?

6. What is the difference between bipolar I disorder and bipolar II disorder?
7. What is a seasonal affective pattern?
8. What does rapid cycling mean?

CAUSE OF MOOD DISORDERS

There are many theories regarding the causation of depression. Research supports the influence of many factors.

Sleep and Its Effects

Research demonstrates a relationship between sleep and mood disorders. One of the hallmarks of major depression is sleep disturbance. Depressed individuals typically have EEGs with abnormalities in the duration and intensity of REM sleep. These findings however, lack the consistency necessary to use the EEG as a diagnostic tool.

Deprivation of sleep in the latter part of the night, when more time is spent in REM sleep, correlates with improvement in patients' moods. Although the improvement lasts in a few patients, most have a relapse of their depressed mood as soon as they get some sleep. Research also demonstrates that sleep deprivation can precipitate manic episodes in patients with bipolar illness. This finding is important because it suggests that by observing regular bedtimes, bipolar patients may reduce their risk of an episode of mania (Mondimore, 1993). As with seasonal depressions, research seems to indicate a connection between mood regulation and an internal clock. Future research may show us ways to manipulate this clock and relieve symptoms more quickly.

Pharmacological Factors

While scientists observed that reserpine, the antihypertensive medication, caused symptoms of major depression, they also recognized that this medication depleted the neurotransmitter norepinephrine in nerve cells. The tendency to trigger symptoms of major depression is shared by many drugs used to treat high blood pressure. Of particular interest is that the tricyclic antidepressants and the monoamine oxidase (MAO) inhibitors used to treat depression *increase* the availability of norepinephrine (DePaulo and Ablow, 1989).

Steroids are a large group of medications that can cause mood changes in either direction, depression or mania. Oral contraceptives are related to steroids. These too cause depression. Sedatives and minor tranquilizers, used to treat anxiety symptoms and to induce sleep, frequently cause mood symptoms and are prone to abuse, thereby causing further complications. In addition, poisons such as lead at low levels of exposure can cause depression (Mondimore, 1993). Table 30–4 lists many classifications of drugs that may induce depression.

Neuronal Factors

Abnormalities of the nervous system result from bodily disturbances that involve injury or malfunction to the brain. Huntington's disease, for example, is a rare genetic condition in which an adult experiences a decline in intellectual abilities and an inability to control movements. Interestingly, symptoms of bipolar illness often appear early in the course of Huntington's disease. Parkinson's disease is another, more common abnormality, in which movement disorders result from the death of nerves connecting two regions within the brain. These nerves use the neurotransmitter dopamine to communicate with one another. People with Parkinson's disease often suffer from depression. Their mood disturbances are treated with accepted antidepressant interventions.

Another neuronal cause of depression is a cerebrovascular accident, or stroke, which is characterized by the

TABLE 30–4 **Drugs That May Induce Depression**

Classification	Drug Name
Analgesics and nonsteroidal antiinflammatory agents	Indomethacin
Antihypertensives	Reserpine Methyldopa (Aldomet) Clonidine Guanethidine Propranolol (Inderal) Hydralazine
Antimicrobial	Co-Trimoxazole Sulfonamide Cycloserine Gram-negative agents
Antiparkinsonian drugs	L-Dopa Amantadine
Antipsychotic drugs	Enanthate/decanoate Haloperidol Fluphenazine
Cardiovascular agents	Digitalis Procainamide
Sedatives and antianxiety drugs	Benzodiazepines Barbiturates Choral hydrate Ethanol
Steroids and hormones	Corticosteroids Estrogen Progesterone Oral contraceptives
Stimulants and appetite suppressants	Amphetamine Fenfluramine Phenmetrazine

Data from Frederick, P. (1989). Southwestern Internal Medicine Conference: Depression and medical illness. Am J Med Sci *298*, 64; and Derogatis, L. R., and Wise T. N. (1989). *Anxiety and depressive disorders in the medical patient* (p. 125). Washington, D.C.: American Psychiatric Press. From Neese, J. B. (1991). Depression in the general hospital. *Nursing Clinics of North America, 26* (3), 619.

sudden interruption of the blood supply to the brain. Studies show that among patients who suffer strokes, about 25% develop major depressions. Robinson and colleagues (1985) found that these injuries to the brain might cause depression by destroying nerves that use the catecholamine neurotransmitters. They observed that the location of the injury within the brain predicts both the likelihood and the severity of depression. A stroke in the left front quadrant of the brain carries a 60% chance that the individual will experience a major depressive disorder, a significantly greater chance than if the stroke is in any of the other quadrants of the brain (Robinson et al, 1985).

Ample evidence supports the role of neurotransmitters in the cause of depression (Jacob, 1994). Antidepressant medications actually target specific neurotransmitter systems. (For more about the role of neurotransmitters, see Chapter 7.)

Endocrinological Factors

The endocrine system is another physiological system linked with mood disorders. The endocrine system contains the body's network of glands that release hormones into the bloodstream affecting every organ of the body. The thyroid gland is a major part of the endocrine system. When too little thyroid hormone is released into the blood, hypothyroidism results. In addition to causing muscle aching, hair loss, constipation, and diminished hearing, too little thyroid hormone also causes depression.

Cushing's disease, another endocrine abnormality, results from excessive stimulation of the adrenal glands by the pituitary gland. This overstimulation causes the adrenals to produce too much of the hormone cortisol. People suffering from Cushing's disease often have round, moonlike faces and rotund abdomens. Many suffer from diabetes and high blood pressure. Some of these patients also develop symptoms of mania and depression (DePaulo and Ablow, 1989).

Genetic Factors

As Peter noted, his family tree should have prepared him for his mood disorder. Mood disorders do run in families, and patients are usually anxious about the chances of passing the disorder on to their offspring. People who have a first-degree relative (parent, sibling, or child) with a major depressive disorder are 1.5 to 3 times as likely as the general population to have the same disorder. Up to 25% of those with a major depressive disorder have a relative with a mood disorder of some kind. The hereditary occurrence of bipolar illness is even more striking. Up to 50% of those with bipolar illness have a relative with some mood disorder, 10 to 20 times the rate in the general population (Mondimore, 1993).

Studies of identical twins, whose genes are exactly the same, show that if one twin suffers from depression or bipolar illness, the chance that the other twin will develop the illness is 50% to 90%. If only one gene were involved and if there were no environmental contribution, we would expect a 100% concordance rate for these disorders in identical twins (DePaulo and Ablow, 1989). These findings, however, indicate that although there is a strong genetic influence in the development of mood disorders, other influences are important contributors. One important factor could be that the disorder in the affected twin is the result of a nongenetic cause, possibly neuronal, endocrinological, or pharmacological. A second explanation could be that only a vulnerability to the mood disorders is passed through the genes and that environmental factors may trigger a genetic predisposition in the individual. Environmental factors could include difficult relationships, financial trouble, legal problems, and the medications and medical conditions related to mood disorders.

Adoption studies also support the view that depressive illnesses are inherited. Children of affectively ill parents who are adopted into families having no history of these illnesses still show three times as many depressive disorders as the biological children in the same families (DePaulo and Ablow, 1989). With currently available methods and cooperative families, research can be expected to identify the location of the genes on the 23 pairs of chromosomes that are linked to these illnesses. So far, regions of chromosomes 6, 11, and X have been linked to bipolar illness in several families. More study is needed to generalize these results to other families.

The role of genetics versus environment is often debated among mental health professionals as well as the lay public. Rather than a competition between genetics versus environment or "nature versus nurture," an interrelationship is likely. The relationship is probably "nature *and* nurture." Genetic research should eventually identify environmental factors in the prevention and treatment of mania and depression.

The complexities surrounding the search for the genes responsible for depression and bipolar illness are enormous. It is highly unlikely that only one gene is involved, and even if an individual carries the gene or genes, there is no guarantee that person will become ill. Interactions with the environment might precipitate the first manic or depressive episode (for example, sleep reduction, drug or alcohol intake, childbirth). Other genes might either trigger or protect against the disease. Physical and psychological factors also clearly play an important (although currently unidentified) role in the triggering and maintaining or protecting against an underlying genetic predisposition to these illnesses (Jamison, 1993). Spiritual factors may also play a role in promoting resiliency against mood disorders.

Psychodynamic Causes

A variety of psychodynamic theories address the causes of mood disorders. *Psychoanalytical theory*, developed by Freud, seeks to uncover unconscious conflicts that contribute to psychiatric symptoms. Freud emphasized the importance of unresolved trauma or difficulties in the cause of psychiatric illnesses. Depression, for example, is sometimes understood in psychoanalysis as anger turned inward after a real or perceived loss. Working in therapy to uncover the sources of the anger enables the individual to face inner conflicts and early life experiences that created the symptoms (DePaulo and Ablow, 1989; Mondimore, 1993).

In bipolar illness, psychodynamic theories describe the patient's abnormal character development and inability to maintain good relationships. These features, coupled with an ongoing sense of impending loss of objects, produce a rageful stance toward these objects and their inability to gratify self-centered demands (Freud, 1917). Fromm-Reichmann (1949) similarly described a "lack of subtlety," a "lack of any close interpersonal relatedness," and a tendency to exaggerate the intensity of interactions with other people as characteristics of patients with bipolar illness. Studies of families with a high incidence of bipolar illness have demonstrated the importance of rigid role conformity within the family system. Speculation suggests that the combination of a domineering parent and unrealistically high expectations led to a "walled-in existence" and deep hostility later manifested as depression or mania (Finley and Wilson, 1951).

Communication patterns between spouses have proven to be critical to childrearing practices. Mayo and coworkers (1979) found that many of the spouses of patients viewed manic or depressive episodes as willful acts of irresponsibility or manifestations of weakness of character and self-indulgence that had to be met with a firm display of power and control. The unspoken but powerfully communicated message to children is that mommy (or daddy) is "sick" through some personal fault. Such a message places children in a conflictual position between the parents. The child may view the "sick" parent as lovable but irresponsible and the well parent as responsible but feared. A pattern develops in which caretaking roles are vague, loyalties tenuous, and affection and approval dependent on a family member's degree of health and responsibility. This pattern disrupts unity and closeness of family members.

The *cognitive model* provided therapies that were shorter-term than the years of therapy so common to psychoanalysis. The most important cognitive theories relate to depression. These include Beck's cognitive model and Seligman's learned helplessness model.

The basic premise of Beck's cognitive model is that depressed persons think and process information in negative ways, even in the midst of contradictory evidence (Calarco and Krone, 1991). This thinking develops over time as the individual experiences stress in life. Early stress seems to shape the development of cognitive patterns in a negative self-referring manner. These negative patterns are believed to remain dormant until they are activated by stressful environmental experiences (Beck et al, 1979).

The *learned helplessness theory* postulates that depression occurs in people who perceive their own behavior out of control and feel helplessness (Seligman, 1975). Seligman's original theory was modified to include a cognitive dimension suggesting that the cognitive interpretation of what happens is critical. Therefore, attributions that people make about particular events and the degree of importance that they attach to these events are believed to be central to the development of depression (Abramson et al, 1978).

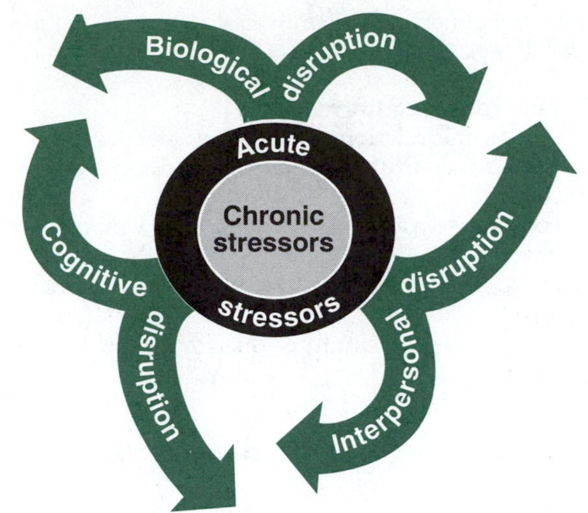

FIGURE 30–3
Calarco and Krone's integrated model of depressive behavior. (From Calarco, M., and Krone, K. [1991]. An integrated nursing model of depressive behavior in adults: Theory and implications for practice. *Nursing Clinics of North America, 26* [3], 573–583.)

The *interpersonal psychotherapeutic model* explains depression (Klerman et al, 1984). Central to this model is the belief in a relationship between depression and current interpersonal functioning. Multiple interpersonal factors are important in the development of depression. These include unsatisfactory early interpersonal experiences, stresses in current interpersonal relationships, and lack of supportive relationships.

Given the need for integration of the medical and the understanding of the human response to the depressive experience, Calarco and Krone (1991) developed an integrated model of depressive behavior (Figure 30–3). This model reflects interaction among the variables of cognition, interpersonal response, and biological response. In addition, this interaction is affected by both acute and chronic stressors that affect a person's thoughts about self, relationships with others, and biological integrity. The center of this model reflects the critical component of acute and chronic stressors that may influence depression and mania. The cognitive component of the model addresses the negative view of self and the future as well as the cognitive disruptions (i.e., decreased concentration, decreased decision-making and problem-solving ability, and short-term memory deficits) seen in many who suffer from depression. The biological component reflects the physiological symptoms of depression, such as sleep disruption, appetite changes, and fatigue, as well as the biochemical changes in the brain and hormonal changes. The interpersonal component reflects the social withdrawal and isolation common in depression as well as the helplessness, frustration, and anger often generated in family and friends (Calarco and Krone, 1991).

▶ Check Your Reading

9. What is the relationship between sleep and mood?
10. Name three drugs that are implicated in causing depression.
11. According to psychoanalytical theory, what causes depression?
12. According to the cognitive model, what causes depression?
13. According to the interpersonal model, what causes depression?

NURSING PROCESS

ASSESSMENT

Because mood disorders are holistic, you are concerned with much more than just an assessment of mood. You are also concerned with an assessment of self-attitude (feelings of self-worth) and vital sense (sense of physical well-being). The typical physical signs of mood disorders include eating and sleep disturbances as well as changes in sexual interest and activity. Boxes 30–2 and 30–3 outline the areas of concern in assessing depression and mania. A number of effective scales are available to quantify the degree of both depression and mania (see Chapter 13).

In addition to the areas of assessment listed in Boxes 30–2 and 30–3, you need to collect data concerning

- The patient's feelings, attitudes, and knowledge about the illness.
- The degree and intensity of suicidal thinking and the potential risk for suicide.
- The family's feelings, attitudes, and knowledge about the illness.
- Issues of powerlessness.
- Spiritual concerns such as hopelessness.
- Social isolation.

Patient's Feelings, Attitudes, and Knowledge

Patients with mood disorders express a wide variety of negative feelings. These include shame, humiliation, fear of reprisals if others find out, denial, anger, fear of

BOX 30–2 Indicators of Depression

Signs of Low Mood

- Withdrawal: A person suffering from depression may lose interest in activities that once gave him or her pleasure and may participate less in social interactions
- Negativism: A person who is usually tolerant of many different viewpoints may become excessively skeptical when depressed. He or she may stubbornly resist the suggestions, orders, or instructions of others
- Unhappiness: A depressed person may experience persistent sadness or frequent crying

Signs of Lowered Self-Attitude

- Self-deprecating, guilty, or self-blaming comments: When depressed, a person may put himself or herself down with comments such as "I'm such a failure; I wonder how you stay with me." A depressed person may also accept blame for problems that do not exist or are clearly not his or her fault
- Expressions of hopelessness: In depression, a person may experience unusually persistent pessimism and may express despair in suicidal statements or acts

Signs of Decreased Vital Sense

- Decreased attentiveness to oneself or to one's tasks: A depressed person may neglect his or her appearance and let assignments at school, housework at home, or projects at work slide
- Decreased energy: A person with depression may complain of fatigue and lack of energy or "motivation." He or she may have particular difficulty getting activities started, especially in the early morning hours
- Decreased ability to concentrate: Depression often makes it difficult for a person to think through a problem and, thus, to initiate and complete a complex mental task. A usually avid reader may begin to read many books but may not finish them. A faithful correspondent may be unable to write
- Excessive indecisiveness: A depressed person may vacillate between choices to an unusual degree and may defer decision-making to others. This may be true even for simple decisions that were previously made routinely

Additional Signs

- Change in weight or in eating patterns: Decreased appetite leading to weight loss is a common symptom of depression. In some depressives (especially those whose depressions come during a particular season of the year), appetite and weight increase
- Change in sleep patterns: Characteristically a depressed person's sleep is interrupted, especially in the early morning hours (2 to 6 a.m.), but in some depressives sleep is excessive and waking is difficult
- Change in sexual interest and activity: Characteristically, sexual interest and performance are decreased in a depressed person

From DePaulo, J. R. Jr., and Ablow, K. R. (1989). *How to cope with depression: A complete guide for you and your family.* New York: McGraw-Hill. Reproduced with permission of McGraw-Hill, Inc.

BOX 30–3 Indicators of Mania

Signs of Elevated or High Mood

• Excessive cheerfulness: A manic person may be unusually elated

• Irritability: A person with mania may become irritable even over small matters, especially when one attempts to "reason" with him or her

• Anger beyond irritability: When suffering from mania, a person may develop a haughty or superior stance that is not usual for him or her

Signs of Increased Self-Attitude

• Expressions and acts of unusual optimism: These can show poor judgment. Unfortunately the overconfident, manic person's energy is often channeled into inappropriate, dangerous, or indiscreet behavior. A normally conservative person may undertake foolish or risky business ventures, may engage in sexual indiscretions, or may speak in overly critical or judgmental terms, often at inappropriate times and about sensitive subjects

Signs of Increased Vital Sense

• Increased energy: A person with mania may appear tireless in the face of physical and mental efforts that would greatly tax an unaffected person. He or she may feel completely refreshed after just a few minutes or hours of sleep

• Increased activity: The increased energy of mania often translates to a host of new projects at work, a seemingly insatiable desire to socialize, or greatly increased participation in sexual activities

• Excessive talking: A person with mania may seem to talk endlessly, sometimes jumping haphazardly from idea to idea. Alternatively a manic person may adopt an unusually abrupt and short or clipped manner of speaking to others

Additional Signs

• Change in eating patterns: A manic person may have a voracious appetite or may be too busy to eat

• Change in sleep patterns: When suffering from mania, a person feels less need for sleep, so sleep is usually decreased

• Change in sexual interest: Sexual interest is often increased in a manic person

From DePaulo, J. R. Jr., and Ablow, K. R. (1989). *How to cope with depression: A complete guide for you and your family.* New York: McGraw-Hill. Reproduced with permission of McGraw-Hill, Inc.

experiencing a relapse, fear of passing the disorder onto their children, and fear of rejection by significant others. The *feelings of shame and humiliation* derive from the belief that the patient is to blame for the illness and somehow should have been able to control it. These feelings are compounded if the patient has experienced a psychotic episode. Recollections about inappropriate or bizarre behavior, embarrassing actions, or financial problems lead the patient to further shame. The self-blame and sense of personal inadequacy go beyond feeling responsible for the illness and extend to therapy itself. Some patients, believing if they just worked harder in therapy they would feel better, are hesitant to bring up their mood problems with their therapists. Admitting to feelings of depression or elation is like admitting that the therapy is a failure or that they themselves are a failure at therapy.

The *fear of reprisal if others find out about the illness* is a strong barrier effectively blocking both women and men from seeking treatment. People prefer suffering in isolation to the anticipated reactions of others' knowing that they are suffering with a "mental illness." Fear of losing employment, employee benefits, and social stature are just a few of the concerns that patients with mood disorders confront.

Denial, another common response of the patient with a mood disorder, is normal when people are confronted with painful and destructive life events. Denial allows slow assimilation of thoughts and feelings that are initially overwhelming, even devastating, to accept (Goodwin and Jamison, 1990). Denial was described by Endler (1990, p. 148), a psychologist writing about his illness and the effect on those around him (Case Example 30–1).

Case Example 30–1 Norman's Story

When I first started getting depressed, not only did I deny it to myself but so did my friends and colleagues. My gradual withdrawal from interaction, my lack of cheerfulness, and my quietness were interpreted by them as anger at something they had done wrong. My children said nothing to me. My colleagues said nothing to me, and the professionals that I worked with said nothing to me. I'm sure that some, if not most of them, must have noticed that something was wrong with me.

From Endler, N. (1990). *Holiday of darkness: A psychologist's personal journey out of his depression.* Toronto: Wall & Emerson, Inc.

In manic-depressive illness, which often involves a psychotic diagnosis, an uncertain course, and a lifetime sentence of medication, *anger* is a common reaction. Although the anger is an understandable response, it often leads patients irrationally to reject an effective treatment or to vent their anger on the clinician.

Another issue for people recovering from mood disorders is *fear of relapse or recurrence.* A patient describes this feeling: "I think a person who's had a history of depression always fears that the bottom's going to fall out and they are going to get depressed again." The poet Robert Lowell (1977, p. 31) wrote a similar description of depressed individuals: "If we see a light at the end of the tunnel, it's the light of an oncoming train." Several questions form the crux of patients' concerns. Will there be further episodes? How frequently? Will they be debilitating? Will I be able to work, earn a living, occupy myself, and fulfill my responsibilities? These questions reflect the long-term meaning of the illness to patients. Related to the fear of recurrence of illness, patients agonize over the possibility that their children will *inherit the mood disorder.*

The *fear of rejection by significant others* is of great consequence. Part of the symptom profile of the mood disorders is their ability to disrupt interpersonal relationships with coworkers, family, and friends. Widely varying reactions to the patient may include anger, concern, withdrawal, unrealistically low or high expectations, rejection, and denial of the illness (Goodwin and Jamison, 1990). Negative reactions of others affect the patient's already diminished sense of self.

A *patient's information needs* are another vital area to assess. For instance, distinguishing between normal and abnormal moods can be quite confusing for patients. The patient who is angry, irritable, a little down, or even feeling especially good may worry that these feelings are not part of the normal range of human emotion but early symptoms of depression or hypomania (Dowling, 1993). Goodwin and Jamison (1990) note: "These overlapping emotions can be confusing and arouse anxiety in many patients who may then question their own judgment and become unduly concerned about recurrences of their affective illness" (p. 732).

Patients need information about the following:

- The nature and causes of mood disorders.
- The treatment options including the value of psychotherapy used in conjunction with medications.
- The actions and side effects of medications.
- The importance of social support.
- The need to take control of decisions related to the illness.
- The importance of spiritual support.
- The need to manage stress, which can be a precipitant of both mania and depression.

The better an individual is able to manage life stress, the better the chance of leading a relatively stable life.

Suicidality

Suicide assessment is critical with depressed patients. Assess whether or not the patient is currently suicidal. Ask the patient, "Have you thought of hurting yourself? Are you presently considering hurting yourself? If you have been thinking about suicide, do you have a plan? What is the plan? Have you thought about what life would be like if you were no longer a part of it?" These questions are essential for identifying suicidal ideation and the lethality of any plan.

Consider a patient's prior history of suicide attempts and depression to be clear indicators that the patient is at high risk in the present for attempting suicide. A patient whose depression is lifting is at higher risk for suicide than a severely depressed individual. Increased energy occurs as the depression lifts. The energy is not enough to make the patient feel good or hopeful, but it is enough to carry out a suicidal plan. (Chapter 36 presents a comprehensive review of suicide.)

Family's Feelings, Attitudes, and Knowledge

Include the reactions of family and friends in the assessment. Unfortunately, many of those closest to the patient mistakenly believe that depression is a self-induced illness. These individuals provide well-intentioned but inaccurate advice to the depressed individual to "pull yourself up by the bootstraps," meaning "avoid giving in to the depression." Ironically, in depression it is the bootstraps that are defective, and no amount of effort can "snap the individual out of the depression."

The illness affects the patient's working, playing, thinking, feeling, and communicating. Family members and friends may operate under the misconception that they have somehow caused the illness. The truth is that they could not have caused this kind of depression, and they cannot make it go away. Common-sense solutions such as logic, advice, reassurance, and sympathy all miss the mark in helping the person; family and friends begin to feel that they are failures. Feelings such as helplessness, anger, frustration, guilt, irritability, fearfulness, hopelessness, and being tired of hearing all of the depression problems are understandable reactions of the patient's loved ones (Frank, 1988).

Although this array of feelings sounds like a listing of symptoms of depression, it is actually a list of feelings of family members trying to help, live with, and cope with a person who has a depressive illness. The husband of a 37-year-old woman with recurrent depression describes his reactions like this: "I've always felt like I was walking on eggs, but no matter how softly I walked, they broke. I often thought, 'I don't know this person.' When you're constantly being the provider and not receiving any support or comfort, you become very discouraged. Eventually, I felt lost and unsuccessful" (Frank, 1988, p. 1). This man expresses the sense of burden and responsibility that many family members experience—feeling that they ought to be able to "succeed" by knowing what to do to help.

In manic-depressive illness, in which psychosis is often a component of the symptoms, the patient is frequently hospitalized. The psychosis transforms the patient into a stranger whose bizarre behavior betrays the intimacies shared within the family. Often the stranger is angry and does not respond to love or acceptance. It is not surprising that relatives react with withdrawal, denial, and an inability to comprehend what has happened.

In working with depressed patients, recognize that depression is an illness that can cause marked changes in a person's mood, thinking, bodily functions, and behaviors. Many people, including health care providers, associate only sadness or suicidal thinking with depression. It is important for you to assess the family's level of understanding about the mood disorder.

Norbeck and colleagues (1991) studied the needs of family caregivers in different age groups and found that the most frequently identified need by family members was for information about the illness, behavior management, coping, and making decisions. These needs probably stem from the ambiguous nature of mood disorders, which may develop insidiously and unpredictably, leaving families without the clear explanations or directives that they desire. It may also reflect the relatively new focus on educating and informing the general public about mental illnesses and specifically involving families more collaboratively in care (Weiss, 1986).

Issues of Powerlessness

As you get to know the patient, you also gather information about the patient's perceived sense of powerlessness. When illness develops, the sense of control over one's life may be threatened. People's responses to the stress of illness depend on personal characteristics and social resources. These responses significantly affect the individual's health and well-being. Feelings of powerlessness stem from the unpredictability of the mood disorders as well as some of the treatment issues.

For instance, taking medications, feeling unsure about the prognosis of the disorder, and fearing the possibility of future exacerbations leave the individual feeling totally vulnerable. Patients frequently express dissatisfaction over taking medications, particularly if the medications have annoying side effects. Complaints about medication may represent covert expressions of powerlessness to control the illness and to prevent it from recurring. Some patients may feel that by taking the medical approach they have abdicated all control to others. These feelings can lead to rejection not only of medication, but also of therapy. A comprehensive assessment identifies feelings of powerlessness and considers the resolution of these feelings in the plan of care.

Spiritual Issues

The many spiritual side effects of depressive illness warrant assessment. Experiences common to depressive illness, such as marital and family problems, divorce, and sudden unemployment, contribute to the downward spiral of negative self-reflections. The depressed person thinks in negative ways about self, the environment, and the future, resulting in a loss of faith in self, others, life, and ultimately God (Carson, 1994; Kerr, 1987–1988). The sense that God ceases to care and is removed is probably one of the most devastating symptoms of depression. Once this sense of separation has occurred, individuals often consider suicide a viable option to end the pain of the illness. The sense of aloneness and abandonment in a hostile world is unbearable (Miller, 1987).

You need to inquire about spiritual issues. Ask questions such as

- What role has God played in your illness?
- What role do you think God will play in your healing?
- What significance are your religious beliefs and practices?
- What are your sources of hope and comfort?
- What is your God like?
- What can I do to assist you in meeting your spiritual needs?

The answers to these questions allow you to address spiritual issues adequately in the plan of care.

Social Isolation

The amount of social support available to the patient is important. Individuals suffering with mood disorders frequently experience disruptions in their relationships with others. Depression causes loss of interest in activities that were formerly pleasurable and satisfying. The result is withdrawal from friends, family, and other sources of social support. In mania, the individual displays a superior sense of self and is irritable, argumentative, and rigid, thus creating a wall between self and others. Frequently the patient's perception of isolation is painfully and objectively true.

▶ Check Your Reading

14. Identify at least five areas to assess in a patient with a mood disorder.
15. Identify at least three of the negative feelings expressed by patients suffering with mood disorders.
16. What do you assess in regard to suicide risk?
17. Why is powerlessness an important issue?

DIAGNOSIS

Arriving at nursing diagnoses in mood disorders demands that you understand the complex interplay of concepts such as self-concept, anxiety, and hostility. The nursing diagnoses provide a way of attributing meaning to the information gained in the assessment. By linking behaviors, nursing diagnoses facilitate understanding of the patient's problems. For patients diagnosed with a mood disorder, the following are primary nursing diagnoses in establishing the plan of care:

- Anxiety
- Impaired Verbal Communication

- Ineffective Individual Coping
- Hopelessness
- Risk for Injury
- Altered Nutrition
- Powerlessness
- Self-Care Deficit
- Self-Esteem Disturbance
- Sexual Dysfunction
- Sleep Pattern Disturbance
- Social Isolation
- Spiritual Distress
- Altered Thought Processes
- Risk for Self-Directed Violence

OUTCOME IDENTIFICATION

The expected outcomes for a patient experiencing indicators of either depression or mania (see Boxes 30–2 and 30–3) are shown in Box 30–4. Remember that outcomes, like your assessment, need to include family members affected by the illness.

PLANNING

In addition to the expected outcomes, establish short-term goals with the patient. These goals vary according to whether the patient is being treated in an outpatient or an inpatient setting. Hospitalization implies that the illness is more serious. In general, whether the symptoms are depression or mania, the patient needs the structure provided by an inpatient setting. Review the expected outcomes. The short-term goals directly relate to these outcomes. Box 30–5 shows short-term goals appropriate for inpatient care.

▶ Check Your Reading

18. Identify at least five nursing diagnoses that might be appropriate for a depressed patient; a manic patient.
19. Identify three expected outcomes for a patient with depression; with mania.
20. Identify three short-term goals for a patient with depression; with mania.

IMPLEMENTATION

Nurse as a Counselor

Many of the feelings and attitudes that patients are confronted with are issues that you will deal with in your role as counselor. Therefore, your interpersonal and communication skills are essential when assisting the patient with a mood disorder. For instance, a generalist in psychiatric nursing

- Spends time with the patient to provide support and a reminder of reality.
- Approaches the patient using a moderate, level tone of voice, avoiding appearing overly cheerful.
- Uses active listening to indicate concern for the patient and to show that the patient is worthwhile.
- Communicates using simple, direct sentences, avoiding complex sentences or directions.
- Avoids asking too many questions or questions that are too probing.
- Encourages the patient to talk about feelings in whatever way that the patient is comfortable doing so.
- Establishes contract with patient. If, for example, negativism dominates the patient's conversation, limit the focus on negativity to an agreed amount of time, after which the patient agrees to discuss other topics.
- Allows and encourages crying.
- Avoids cutting off the patient's conversation with false reassurance and platitudes.
- Provides positive feedback as the patient achieves goals of treatment.
- Explores the patient's strengths and coping responses.

Many patients diagnosed with mood disorders are also in therapy, which is conducted by psychiatrists, advanced-practice certified psychiatric-mental health nurses, psychiatric social workers, or psychologists. Psychotherapy alone may treat mild and some moderate forms of depression. In patients with major depressive disorder or bipolar disorder, however, the combination of psychotherapy and medications has been proven to be more effective than either treatment alone (Hollon et al, 1991; Weissman et al, 1987).

Psychotherapy serves a number of purposes. First, it teaches a person alternative ways to handle stresses. Second, it helps explore how the illness affects the individual's life. Therapy helps patients in "learning to unravel what is normal personality from what the illness has superimposed upon it—turbulence, impulsiveness, lack of predictability, and depression" (Goodwin and Jamison, 1990, p. 732). Third, psychotherapy deals with denial. Denial is diminished by exploring the meaning of the illness with the patient. The natural course of the illness, its high relapse rate, and risks and benefits of medications are discussed. Fourth, psychotherapy provides a safe place to express feelings of anger and shame and have them accepted. Fifth, therapy allows for the conceptualization of mood disorders as fundamentally medical. This determination decreases stigma; provides effective, specific treatment; and minimizes family and

MEDICAL DIAGNOSES AND RELATED NURSING DIAGNOSES **Depression**

***DSM-IV* Diagnosis:** Major depressive disorder, single episode

DIAGNOSTIC CRITERIA

A. Presence of a single Major Depressive Episode.
B. The Major Depressive Episode is not better accounted for by Schizoaffective Disorder and is not superimposed on Schizophrenia, Schizophreniform Disorder, Delusional Disorder, or Psychotic Disorder Not Otherwise Specified.
C. There has never been a Manic Episode, a Mixed Episode, or a Hypomanic Episode. **Note:** This exclusion does not apply if all of the manic-like, mixed-like, or hypomanic-like episodes are substance or treatment induced or are due to the direct physiological effects of a general medical condition.

Specify (for current or most recent episode):
Severity/Psychotic/Remission Specifiers
Chronic
With Catatonic Features
With Melancholic Features
With Atypical Features
With Postpartum Onset

***DMS-IV* Diagnosis:** Major depressive disorder, recurrent

DIAGNOSTIC CRITERIA

A. Presence of two or more Major Depressive Episodes. **Note:** To be considered separate episodes, there must be an interval of at least 2 consecutive months in which criteria are not met for a Major Depressive Episode.
B. The Major Depressive Episodes are not better accounted for by Schizoaffective Disorder and are not superimposed on Schizophrenia, Schizophreniform Disorder, Delusional Disorder, or Psychotic Disorder Not Otherwise Specified.
C. There has never been a Manic Episode, a Mixed Episode, or a Hypomanic Episode. **Note:** This exclusion does not apply if all of the manic-like, mixed-like, or hypomanic-like episodes are substance or treatment induced or are due to the direct physiological effects of a general medical condition.

Specify (for current or most recent episode):
Severity/Psychotic/Remission Specifiers
Chronic
With Catatonic Features
With Melancholic Features
With Atypical Features
With Postpartum Onset
Specify:
Longitudinal Course Specifiers (With and Without Interepisode Recovery)
With Seasonal Pattern

Box continued on following page

individual responsibility as the cause of the illness. The therapist, however, needs to avoid focusing on the medical approach to the exclusion of all else. Such an approach might mean that significant life issues and problems adjusting to the illness may be ignored.

One of Goodwin's patients differentiates the role of different treatments by saying, "No pill can help me deal with the problem of not wanting to take pills; likewise, no amount of analysis alone can prevent my manias and depressions. I need both" (Goodwin and Jamison, 1990, p. 725). Research indicates that several forms of short-term psychotherapy, such as supportive, cognitive, and interpersonal, are effective in treating depression.

SUPPORTIVE PSYCHOTHERAPY

The objectives for supportive psychotherapy are

- To promote the patient's best psychological and social functioning.
- To bolster self-esteem and self-confidence.
- To make the patient aware of what can and cannot be achieved, both personal limitations and the limitations of treatment.
- To prevent undue dependence on professional support and unnecessary hospitalizations.
- To promote the best use of available support from family and friends (Bloch, 1979).

Supportive psychotherapy with medication treatment is most appropriate for patients with severe forms of depressive illness. For those whose abilities to understand the illness are impaired, the therapist provides concrete explanations about depression or mania. Therapists continually encourage patients and convey optimism about the future. Patients require frequent repetition of the message of optimism before they derive any benefit. Recovered patients often report that the persistent

MEDICAL DIAGNOSES AND RELATED NURSING DIAGNOSES **Depression** *Continued*

RELATED NURSING DIAGNOSES	DEFINITION	EXAMPLE
Risk for Self-Directed Violence	A state in which an individual experiences behaviors that can be physically harmful either to self or to others	High Risk for Self-Directed Violence related to depressed mood and feelings of worthlessness as evidenced by verbalization of suicidal ideation or pain or both
Self-Esteem Disturbance	Negative self-evaluation or feelings about self or self capabilities, which may be directly or indirectly expressed	Self-Esteem Disturbance related to negative view of self as evidenced by expressions of worthlessness
Powerlessness	Perception that one's own actions will not significantly affect an outcome; a perceived lack of control over a current situation or immediate happening	Powerlessness related to belief that agreeing to take medications or participating in therapy relinquishes control of illness to others as evidenced by refusal to participate in treatment program
Spiritual Distress	Disruption in the life principle that pervades a person's entire being and that integrates and transcends one's biological and psychosocial nature	Spiritual Distress related to sense of despair and feelings of abandonment by God as evidenced by inability to pray or practice other meaningful spiritual activities
Social Isolation	Aloneness experienced by the individual and perceived as imposed by others and as a negative or threatened state	Social Isolation related to feelings of inadequacy in social interactions as evidenced by withdrawal, problematic interactions with others, and seeking to be alone
Altered Thought Processes	A state in which an individual experiences a disruption in cognitive operations and activities	Altered Thought Processes related to neurobiological changes as evidenced by delusions, confusion, and impaired problem-solving
Altered Nutrition: Less than Body Requirements	A state in which an individual experiences an intake of nutrients insufficient to meet metabolic needs	Altered Nutrition, Less than Body Requirements related to depressed mood, loss of appetite or lack of interest in food as evidenced by weight loss, weakness, poor muscle tone, and poor skin turgor
Sleep Pattern Disturbance	Disruption of sleep time causes discomfort or interferes with desired lifestyle	Sleep Pattern Disturbance related to depressed mood, anxiety, and fears as evidenced by difficulty falling asleep, early morning awakening, and complaints of feeling tired
Self-Care Deficit	A state in which the individual experiences an impaired ability to perform self-care activities	Self-Care Deficit related to depressed mood as evidenced by disheveled clothing, offensive body odor, failure to brush teeth, and uncombed hair

Diagnostic Criteria from American Psychiatric Association (1994). *Diagnostic and statistical manual of mental disorders, fourth edition.* Washington, D.C.: American Psychiatric Association; nursing diagnoses and definitions from North American Nursing Diagnosis Association (1994). *NANDA nursing diagnoses: Definitions and classification 1995–1996.* Philadelphia: NANDA.

hopefulness of their therapist and others kept them from giving up before treatment worked or before the illness remitted on its own. The truthful message to be communicated is that success is almost always the outcome of determined treatment. Even if the patient's disorder cannot be helped with current medical treatments, new treatments are always being developed.

Supportive psychotherapy for manic patients can be particularly difficult. Patients with mania usually have difficulty accepting that they suffer from a disease requiring immediate medical treatment. They may need supervision in spending their money or their time, and they cannot trust their confident and cheerful feelings to lead them to rational actions. Often, supportive therapy of a manic patient takes the form of finding any area of mutual understanding that allows a short-term agreement about treatment. These agreements can "carry" the patient, family, friends, and clinician until a more normal mood returns (DePaulo and Ablow, 1989).

COGNITIVE AND INTERPERSONAL PSYCHOTHERAPIES

Studies conducted by the National Institute of Mental Health show that in outpatients with mild and moderate depressions, cognitive and interpersonal short-term

MEDICAL DIAGNOSES AND RELATED NURSING DIAGNOSES

Mania

***DMS-IV* Diagnosis:** Bipolar I disorder, single manic episode

DIAGNOSTIC CRITERIA

A. Presence of only one Manic Episode and no past Major Depressive Episodes. **Note:** Recurrence is defined as either a change in polarity from depression or an interval of at least 2 months without manic symptoms.

B. The Manic Episode is not better accounted for by Schizoaffective Disorder and is not superimposed on Schizophrenia, Schizophreniform Disorder, Delusional Disorder, or Psychotic Disorder Not Otherwise Specified.

Specify:
Mixed: if symptoms meet criteria for a Mixed Episode
Specify (for current or most recent episode):
Severity/Psychotic/Remission Specifiers
With Catatonic Features
With Postpartum Onset

***DSM-IV* Diagnosis:** Bipolar I disorder, most recent episodic mania

DIAGNOSTIC CRITERIA

A. Currently (or most recently) in a Manic Episode.

B. There has previously been at least one Major Depressive Episode, Manic Episode, or Mixed Episode.

C. The mood episodes in Criteria A and B are not better accounted for by Schizoaffective Disorder and are not superimposed on Schizophrenia, Schizophreniform Disorder, Delusional Disorder, or Psychotic Disorder Not Otherwise Specified.

Specify (for current or most recent episode):
Severity/Psychotic/Remission Specifiers
With Catatonic Features
With Postpartum Onset
Specify:
Longitudinal Course Specifiers (With and Without Interepisode Recovery)
With Seasonal Pattern (applies only to the pattern of Major Depressive Episodes)
With Rapid Cycling

RELATED NURSING DIAGNOSES	DEFINITION	EXAMPLE
Risk for Injury	A state in which an individual is at risk of injury as a result of environmental conditions interacting with the individual's adaptive and defensive resources	Risk for Injury related to extreme hyperactivity as evidenced by increased agitation and lack of control over behavior
Risk for Violence: Self-Directed or Directed at Others	A state in which an individual experiences behaviors that can be physically harmful to either self or others	Risk for Violence: Self-Directed or Directed at Others related to degree of manic excitement, delusional thinking, and hallucinations as evidenced by threats to self and others and impulsive and volatile behaviors
Altered Nutrition: Less than Body Requirements	The state in which an individual experiences an intake of nutrients insufficient to meet metabolic needs	Altered Nutrition: Less than Body Requirements related to inability to sit still long enough to eat as evidenced by weight loss
Sensory/Perceptual Alterations	A state in which an individual experiences a change in the amount or patterning of oncoming stimuli accompanied by a diminished, exaggerated, distorted, or impaired response to such stimuli	Sensory/Perceptual Alterations related to possible sleep deprivation as evidenced by auditory and visual hallucinations
Impaired Social Interaction	The state in which an individual participates in insufficient or excessive quantity or ineffective quality of social exchange	Impaired Social Interaction related to narcissistic behavior as evidenced by inability to sustain relationships
Sleep Pattern Disturbance	Disruption of sleep time causes discomfort or interferes with desired lifestyle	Sleep Pattern Disturbance related to excessive hyperactivity and agitation as evidenced by difficulty falling asleep and sleeping for only short periods

Diagnostic Criteria from American Psychiatric Association (1994). *Diagnostic and statistical manual of mental disorders, fourth edition.* Washington, D.C.: American Psychiatric Association; nursing diagnoses and definitions from North American Nursing Diagnosis Association (1994). *NANDA nursing diagnoses: Definitions and classification 1995–1996. Philadelphia: NANDA.*

psychotherapies are helpful. Both of these approaches can be used alone or in conjunction with pharmacological approaches.

The goal of *cognitive psychotherapy* is to correct negative thinking that determines feelings and behavior. For example, depressed patients frequently view life through gray-tinted glasses. They expect the worst from themselves, from others, and from the environment. They view the future as hopeless. They predict that these inadequacies and this current pain will continue indefinitely. "Everything I do turns out badly" is a characteristic self-evaluation of a depressed patient. The expectation of failure paralyzes the individual from initiating new behaviors. The therapist, using verbal procedures and behavior modification techniques, works with the patient to

- Teach the patient to recognize automatic negative thoughts and to change them.
- Identify distortions in the patient's self-image and view of the world.
- Identify and correct dysfunctional beliefs about events.

Consider a depressed person whose mood plummets when her spouse failed to compliment her on her appearance. She reported thinking, "He is not attracted to me anymore because I am ugly." She also reported feeling down when a friend talked to her for only five minutes in the grocery store. "She would want to spend more time with me if I weren't so dull." Through dialogue, therapist and patient identify the silent assumption, "If others don't attend to me, it is disturbing and it happens because there is something wrong with me." The therapeutic process identifies assumptions from themes in negative automatic thoughts (Jarrett and Rush, 1989).

Interpersonal therapy focuses on the patient's relationships with others. The emphasis is on the "here and now" and on current problems. Interpersonal therapy differs from other psychotherapies in that it is time-limited and focuses primarily on both the patient's current symptoms

BOX 30-4 Expected Outcomes for Patients Experiencing Depression or Mania

Depression

The patient will

- Remain free from self-inflicted harm
- Be free of psychotic symptoms
- Demonstrate functional behavior in activities of daily living
- Maintain balanced physiological functioning
- Demonstrate an increased ability to deal with feelings of sadness, anxiety, or frustration
- Demonstrate behaviors indicative of improved self-esteem
- Demonstrate increased spiritual well-being
- Demonstrate increased understanding of illness
- Demonstrate increased understanding of treatment options
- Identify a support system in the community

The family will

- Demonstrate increased understanding of depression and its symptoms
- Verbalize the recognition that the family is not responsible for the cause or the healing of the depression
- Demonstrate increased understanding of the treatment issues in depression
- Identify a support system in the community
- Demonstrate increased spiritual well-being

Mania

The patient will

- Remain free from self-inflicted harm
- Be free of restlessness, hyperactivity, and agitation
- Be free of threatened aggression toward others
- Demonstrate behaviors indicating feelings of self-worth
- Demonstrate appropriate appearance and behavior
- Be free of psychotic symptoms
- Demonstrate functional behavior in activities of daily living
- Maintain balanced physiological functioning
- Demonstrate increased spiritual well-being
- Demonstrate increased understanding of illness
- Demonstrate increased understanding of treatment options
- Identify a support system in the community

The family will

- Demonstrate increased understanding of mania and its symptoms
- Verbalize the recognition that the family is not responsible for the cause or the healing of the mania
- Demonstrate increased understanding of the treatment issues in mania
- Identify a support system in the community
- Demonstrate increased spiritual well-being

BOX 30-5 Planning Short-Term Goals for Hospitalized Patients Who Are Depressed or Manic

Depression

The patient will

- Be free of self-inflicted harm
- Be oriented to person, place, and time
- Express feelings
- Communicate with congruent verbal and nonverbal messages
- Express anger or hostility outwardly in a safe manner
- Participate in activites
- Verbalize feelings of self-worth
- Verbalize hopefulness

Mania

The patient will

- Be free of self-inflicted harm
- Refrain from harming others
- Be oriented to person, place, and time
- Eat enough to maintain energy needs
- Restore balance in rest and activity
- Engage in therapeutic interactions

Case Example 30–2 Joe's Story

I had been feeling pretty bad for almost a year. Looking back on that time, I know that I was depressed. After a year, it wasn't getting better. In fact, there were mornings when I contemplated ways to end my life. I can hardly believe that I actually felt that despairful. One of the most important factors in my seeking treatment was my sister-in-law's constant teaching and encouragement. She is a psychiatric nurse, and I guess it was pretty obvious to her that I was sick. She always asked me how I was doing, which reminded me that she cared. But what really helped was her teaching. She would "bring up" a psychiatric patient she was working with in a general way, and then she would use this to lead into a discussion of depression, its symptoms, and the effectiveness of treatment. Then I remember her saying things like, "Some people feel that if they accept help, then that proves that they are weak. Can you believe what society has done to people suffering from psychiatric disorders? Somehow we convince them that it is their fault and deny them the very thing that would alleviate their suffering." I know now that she was saying these things to me in the only way that I could hear them. Had she been direct with me I would have vigorously denied that I had a problem. One morning I cried like a baby; I just couldn't get out of bed. I knew I couldn't go on like this. My wife said, "Call Vickie; she'll know what to do." So I did. She gave me the name of a wonderful psychiatrist and a nurse psychotherapist. The doctor started me on Prozac (fluoxetine), which has worked wonders in my life. I feel better than ever! But the nurse is helping me to look at some negative thinking patterns that have always kept me from getting the most out of life. I am so grateful to Vickie. I think she may have saved my life.

of depression and the interpersonal context associated with the depression.

Nurse as Teacher to Patient and Family

An essential nursing role is that of a teacher. Many people lack understanding about the causes, characteristics, and appropriate treatments for the mood disorders. Because of this knowledge deficit, patients tend to blame themselves for their illness, and others do the same. When people understand all of the components of the mood disorders, they are less frightened and are more hopeful (Schoenbeck et al, 1992). The teaching role is built into every nurse-patient interaction. Frequently, opportunities present themselves quite informally, so that you can speak to issues such as the biological basis for depression or mania or the importance of treatment. In Case Example 30–2, Joe benefited from his sister-in-law's persistence, support, and encouragement. But most of all, her constant nonthreatening approach to teaching broke Joe's resistance and opened him to the possibilities of treatment.

You may also teach in formal ways, perhaps to groups of patients or families as well as to the community at large. Formal presentations provide the opportunity to educate a large number of people. Ideally, such presentations are followed by time for individual counseling. This allows people who are reticent to speak in a large group; to have their questions answered; and to seek advice, referrals, or support on a one-on-one basis. Formal presentations can effectively eliminate or reduce stigma by providing accurate information.

Included in the topics that you can address are medication issues along with other strategies to deal with stress and stay well. In addition, teach the patient about the importance of social support and the significance of spirituality to healing. Patient teaching also focuses on assisting the patient to communicate explicitly and honestly regarding needs. For example, the patient might say, "I know you mean well, but please don't do that." Another helpful thing for patients to recognize and be able to communicate to family members is that needs may change as the episode improves or worsens. The patient might say, "Something that isn't helpful to me today doesn't mean I might not want it tomorrow." The patient can learn to communicate gratitude even when the help offered is not what is needed. The patient in this situation might say, "I know you mean well by trying to talk to me, but I just can't talk right now." Clear feedback helps family members and others close to the patient remain long-term resources for the patient.

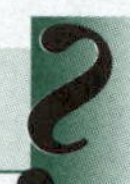

WHAT PATIENTS AND FAMILIES NEED TO KNOW — Symptoms of Mania

What is mania?
Mania is the term used to describe an elevated or "hyper" mood. Mania can range from mild symptoms to symptoms severe enough that the afflicted person requires hospitalization. Symptoms of mania include an exaggerated feeling of importance, increased activity, poor judgment, distractibility, decreased need for sleep, and racing thoughts and speech.

Can some people have symptoms of both mania and depression?
A person can have both manic symptoms and depressive symptoms; this condition is termed bipolar disorder or mixed affective disorder. The symptoms range from mild to severe. Switching from manic symptoms to depressive symptoms can occur quickly or be independent of each other for a longer period.

What causes a person to become manic?
Considerable research on mania and depression over the past several years indicates that mania is the result of a chemical imbalance. It is also well known that a manic episode can be precipitated by a loss or a major stressor.

How is mania treated?
Because mania is biochemical, medications are effective in helping the symptoms subside. Lithium carbonate, a mineral, is one of the major drugs used. It works by stabilizing the extremes of low or high moods. Research has found several other mood stabilizers to be effective. Often, it may take a combination of two or more medications to stabilize the mood.

Will I need to be on medication for the rest of my life?
In many instances, people with symptoms of mania need to be on medications for the rest of their lives. Just as people who develop diabetes need to take insulin on a daily basis, people with bipolar disorder frequently need some type of medication to maintain a balance. When taking medications to treat mania, it is necessary to monitor blood levels and be under the supervision of a physician.

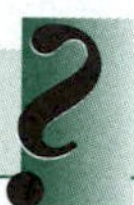

WHAT SOCIETY NEEDS TO KNOW — Symptoms of Depression

How would I recognize depression in someone?
There are many indicators that a friend or family member may be suffering from depression. Often when a person is grieving a major loss, the term "depressed" is used to define normal sadness and pain. With the illness of depression, however, the sadness is overwhelming, and the person feels hopeless, helpless, and irritable. There is a noticeable change in eating habits and sleeping patterns, either sleeping too much or inability to feel rested after sleep. A person with depression loses energy and is unable to enjoy activities that previously brought pleasure. The person often cannot think or concentrate. A person who describes recurring thoughts of death or suicide needs to be seen by a physician immediately.

What are the major causes of depression?
There is no one single cause for depression. Researchers have found that depression tends to run in families. Also, some type of chemical imbalance frequently is present. Neurotransmitters are substances in the brain that allow brain cells to communicate with others. In depression, the deficiency in these chemicals causes insomnia, irritability, anxiety, fatigue, and lack of energy. Researchers do not know if these imbalances cause the disease or if the illness gives rise to the imbalances. It is not uncommon for major losses or stressors to precipitate a depressive illness.

How many people have depression?
Depression is the most common of all mental illnesses and often goes untreated because well-meaning family and friends advise the depressed person to "snap out of it." It is estimated that in any six-month period, 9.4 million Americans suffer from depression. Depression is more common in women but does affect both genders and all age groups.

What can be done to treat depression?
Because a chemical imbalance is frequently the cause of depression, medications are typically indicated for treatment. These medications do not solve the stressors and problems that may have precipitated the symptoms, but they provide a person with the energy to deal with the issues. Antidepressants work by altering the brain's response to certain chemical reactions. Because these medications take about four to six weeks before they are fully effective, psychotherapy is usually recommended. Medications or psychotherapy or a combination of both usually relieves the symptoms of depression in weeks.

From American Psychiatric Association (1994). *Let's talk about depression.* Washington, D.C.: American Psychiatric Association.

Nurse as Protector from Self-Injurious Behavior

Protecting patients from harming themselves or others is a priority in dealing with patients diagnosed with mood disorders. The nursing interventions include the following:

- Establish a written no-suicide contract with the patient.
- Make sure safety of patient is ensured, whether patient is experiencing suicidal ideation or also has intent and a plan. For a patient with ideation, intent, and plan, one-on-one contact with a staff member at *all times* (even when sleeping and in bathroom) is necessary. The patient is restricted to the hospital unit and is permitted nothing that could cause self-harm (sharp objects, a belt). A patient who poses a less serious threat is assigned one-on-one contact with a staff member at all times but may go off the unit to attend activities while continuing one-on-one supervision. For a patient who expresses ideation and no plan, knowing the whereabouts of the patient at all times is sufficient. The patient may be accompanied by a staff member while off the unit, but one-on-one supervision is not required.
- Explain suicidal precautions to the patient.
- Be aware of potentially dangerous objects in the environment such as sharps, matches, lit cigarettes, glass containers. These items should not be in the patient's possession.
- Check the environment to ensure that windows in the room are locked and are not accessible to the patient.
- Observe the patient, frequently observing behavior patterns. Note the patient's response to different activities on the unit, various staff members, and participation in tasks and activities.
- Be aware of relationships the patient may be forming on the unit. Be especially alert to relationships with other patients who may be manipulated into cooperating with patient's suicide plan.
- As the patient takes medication, watch carefully to ensure that the patient is not cheeking and saving it.
- Observe any changes in the patient's mood.
- Encourage the patient to discuss feelings. Do not reinforce dwelling on previous suicide attempts or the details of such events.
- Communicate that the patient is a worthwhile human being and that there is always hope.
- Attempt to determine what keeps the patient "hanging on" and then reinforce that issue. For instance, if a patient says the only thing that keeps her from committing suicide is her children, reinforce how important it is for her to remain alive for them.
- Explore spiritual issues with the patient. Make a referral to clergy if necessary.
- Encourage the patient's expression of anger.
- Assist the patient to examine life, including the home environment and relationships outside of hospital.
- Help the patient to identify situations and feelings that precipitate suicidal ideation. Assist the patient to plan how to deal with these feelings and situations to avert a disaster.

Nurse as Collaborator with Patient and Family

Your work in assisting family members to know how to help the patient is essential. When family members feel that they are partners in the health team, they can be not only useful, but also a long-term resource. To partner with a family, you need to assist family members to pull together. Your communication, interpersonal, and counseling skills are essential. You affirm family efforts on behalf of the patient, make suggestions for continued well-being, provide information so that family members can be more effective, and invite them to collaborate in planning the patient's care. Such an approach presents a unified, supportive, and realistically hopeful environment in which the patient can begin the healing process.

In the "old" psychiatry, the relationship between the patient and physician or therapist was a privileged and confidential relationship. It was strictly forbidden that a family member be informed about anything that was going on between the physician and patient. Fortunately that has changed. If collaboration with the family is permitted by the patient, more complete information is brought to the clinician and can greatly influence both the patient's diagnosis and the treatment. Most experienced clinicians recognize that a concerned family member can be the best support for both clinician and patient.

This partnership can be used to develop a plan to prevent relapses. Discuss the individual's symptoms, learn to recognize early warning signs of the illness as well as potential stressors that may precipitate an episode of illness. Sometimes the patient and family member can contract regarding the family member's role in helping the patient stay well. This supportive relationship, with the clinician as coach and facilitator, recognizes the family and patient as the vital motivators of maintaining wellness and support. This position is empowering for both the patient and the family and facilitates success.

Logan, a practicing internist, offers this advice to other family members from his experience during his wife's depressive illness: "Listen and reassure! Listen to the patient agonize over her condition and then respond with reassurance. Remember that episodes of depression are temporary in most cases. With proper treatment, you will soon notice improvement and ultimately help contribute to a full recovery" (Logan, 1988, p. 41).

You can teach the family the importance of decreasing the focus on the patient and trying as much as possible to "normalize" family routines. If the family is to remain intact, family members must avoid becoming dominated by the depressed person's needs. This is tremendously hard because even a depressed person who cannot speak or move and is immobilized by depression is a kind of magnetic focus for everyone in the family. Maintaining normal levels of socializing with family and friends is important. Obtaining support from others assists the family members to try not to feel guilty and avoid taking responsibility for the illness.

Nurse as Facilitator of Empowerment

You can be of great assistance to the patient struggling for control and acceptance of the inevitable changes that come with illness. Using empowerment strategies, you can function in the role of facilitator and resource person, recognizing that self-awareness, self-growth, and resources are the tools that facilitate empowerment (Gibson, 1991).

Gibson (1991) defines **empowerment** as a social process of recognizing, promoting, and enhancing people's abilities to meet their own needs, solve their own problems, and mobilize necessary resources to take control of their own lives. In helping people assert control over their health, you are not only a resource person, but also a mobilizer of resources. You need to facilitate access to both personal and environmental resources that foster a sense of control and self-efficacy and support health (Jones and Meleis, 1993).

Power, a component of the word empowerment, is synonymous with energy. Natural power is the capacity of acting or being active. Other synonyms are strength, efficacy, and effectiveness, implying "power to." Empowerment can occur when you and the patient are mutually active, respecting one another's needs and working together to achieve a result.

An implication of this shared control is the mutual responsibility for the nurse-patient relationship. Both nurse and patient bring to the situation what each is authentically able to give. This process creates meanings that promote better outcomes (Benner and Wrubel, 1988). The patient gains efficacy in coping with concerns. You experience efficacy in providing genuinely helpful care (Marck, 1990). The empowering process does not result in the patient gaining power while you lose it. Rather the patient is empowered by you; you are equally empowered by the ability to care, support, advise, and assist the patient. The patient gains self-esteem, mutual regard, and family respect and is perceived to cope well with life problems. Empowered individuals form a new network of community support, replacing fragile or lost supportive resources (McKay et al, 1990).

McKay and colleagues (1990) identify three components of mutual empowerment for patient and nurse: knowledge, confidence, and communication skills. The patient requires knowledge about the illness, and you need to be able to admit any knowledge deficits and find what the patient needs to know. The patient and nurse need to be able to listen and understand each other and effectively share information. The patient needs to experiment with information and advice given and confidently apply this knowledge to personal health care. You also need to be aware of the patient's understanding of the information provided and the extent of the patient's ability to cope through help and support rather than control and direction. Both you and the patient need confidence in each other to form a successful relationship. Figure 30–4 illustrates empowerment in nursing.

Nurse as Facilitator of Spiritual Growth

Nurses are in a unique position to understand the body, mind, and spirit relationship. The depressed person's spirit is oppressed. The mind is filled with thoughts of despair. The body is sluggish, dull, and unalive. Through understanding these factors, you can help the patient alter his or her perception of life. Through treatment, the individual may achieve a higher level of wellness and understanding than before the illness began.

Continue to pursue treatment that works, but in the meantime, encourage and support an individual's faith and convictions about life and God and, above all else, the will to live. The individual may emerge from the painful experience having found knowledge and meaning and feels that this experience has been growth producing. Thurman provides a glimpse of such hope: "The roots are silently at work in the darkness of the earth against the time when there shall be new leaves, fresh blossoms, green fruit. Such is the growing edge" (Miller, 1987).

The search for spirituality in our society is expressed individually as well as collectively through religious practices and convictions. Despite the erosion of the spirit during episodes of depressive illness, individuals are still drawn toward God and spiritual practices. Sometimes the spirituality and the beliefs of others serve to anchor a person in the present and provide hope that is so lacking internally. Although spirituality is a private affair, a matter of the heart, it is enhanced when intimacy and caring are part of a person's experience. The patient's spirituality may be bolstered by loved ones who continue to be faithful in their prayers, in their religious practices, and in the encouragement they offer the patient that things will get better (Carson, 1994). There is a strong connection among healthy, caring communities, healing, and spirituality (Wuthnow, 1994). Ralph Waldo Emerson describes the spirit: "It is one of the most beautiful compensations of life that no man can seriously help another without helping himself." Figure 30–5 illustrates the Calarco and Krone (1991) model modified to include the spiritual dimension.

Nurse as a Referral Source for Social Support

In an effort to connect with one another in the search for spirituality, self-help or mutual support groups have developed as an important adjunct to treating individuals with mood disorders and family members. Members come to meetings to share feelings and experiences with other people who have also experienced illness. They go away feeling satisfied that they may have helped another with their sharing. To qualify as a participant, an individual has to have the illness and be willing to use the

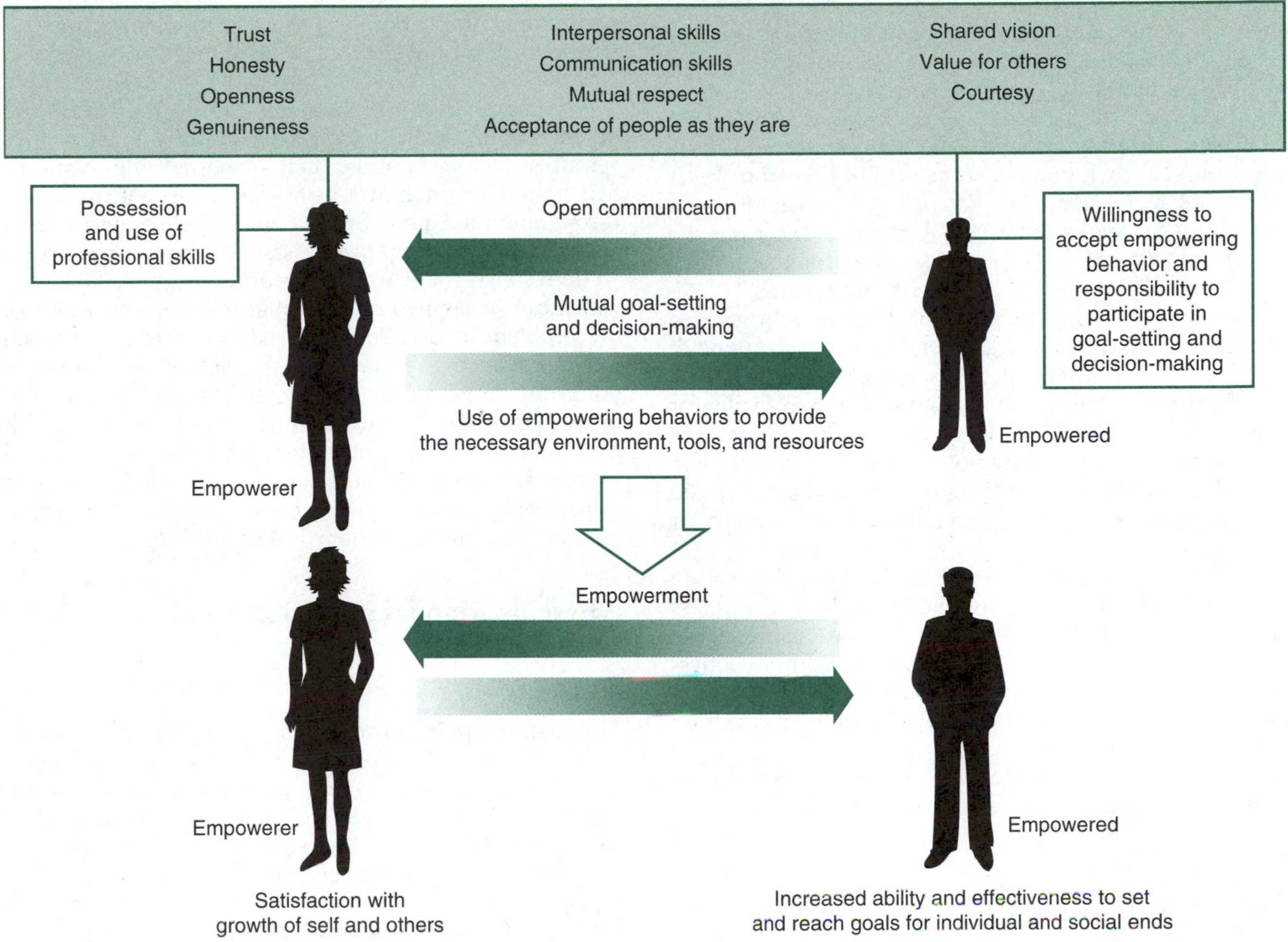

FIGURE 30–4

Empowerment in nursing. (From Hawks, J. [1992]. Empowerment in nursing education: Concept analysis and application to philosophy, learning and instruction. *Journal of Advanced Nursing, 17,* 613. Reprinted by permission of Blackwell Scientific Publications, Oxford, England.)

experience to help others. Meetings are run by and for members (Silverman and Murrow, 1976).

Although the term *self-help* is traditionally used in the literature, *mutual help* connotes the reality of these meetings as members struggle together to find solutions to problems related to illness. In mutual help groups, people experience the support and validation of others in similar situations. This process helps to decrease the social isolation so often experienced by both the patient and family members. William Styron writes about his friend who had also experienced depression, "His support was untiring and priceless. It was he who kept admonishing me that suicide was 'unacceptable,' and it was also he who made the prospect of going to the hospital less fearsomely intimidating. I still look back on his concern with immense gratitude. The help he gave me, my friend later said, had been a continuing therapy for him, thus demonstrating that, if nothing else, the disease engenders lasting fellowship" (Styron, 1990).

Studies have shown that breast cancer patients who attended mutual help groups lived longer, regardless of the stage of their cancer or their treatment regimens. Support groups enhance the effectiveness of the medical treatment. Patients attending support groups are less depressed, fatigued, and confused and are actively coping better than those not in support groups (Support groups lengthen your life, 1990). Apparently sharing experiences, feelings, and fears with others reduce anxiety and promote constructive behavior.

Skovhold (1974) summarized the benefits of this "helper therapy" principle. First, the effective helper often feels an increased level of interpersonal competence as a result of making an impact on another individual's life. Second, the effective helper often feels a sense of equality in giving and taking. Third, the effective helper is often the recipient of valuable personalized learning acquired while working with someone in need. Finally, the effective helper often receives social approval from the people he helps. It has been hypothesized that all four factors, rather than any one, make helper therapy potent (Gartner and Reissman, 1984).

Members of a mutual help group for people with affective disorders reflect on their experience of belonging in a group facilitated not by professionals but by people who are affected by the illness themselves. "I wept when I first met Bob. I couldn't believe there was anyone else like me." Another group member describes the experience, "It gives you a marker. If you see others worse than yourself, then you get some idea of how you are. It makes me feel I can't be that bad if I managed to do something for somebody else." A member expresses the long-term value of the group: "I see the group as a safety net. I can go back to it if my depression returns."

The role for the nurse in the mutual help groups, evolves from generator, organizer, and catalyst to one of less direct involvement, perhaps as an advisor (Gartner and Reissman, 1980). You may function as a facilitator initially and gradually pursue other organizational and educational interests meaningful to the group. For example, you might train group leaders and assist in the development of group projects related to outreach or advocacy.

Through supplying information, you can be an important resource regarding questions about the illness and dissemination of written material that ensures accuracy about mood disorders. As individuals with the illness and family members gain confidence in their knowledge and understanding of the illnesses, they will be less afraid to confront the stigma.

According to Silverman (1978), nurses collaborate with mutual help groups in at least four ways:

- Making referrals
- Serving on professional advisory boards
- Serving as consultant to existing groups
- Initiating and working on the development of new mutual help groups

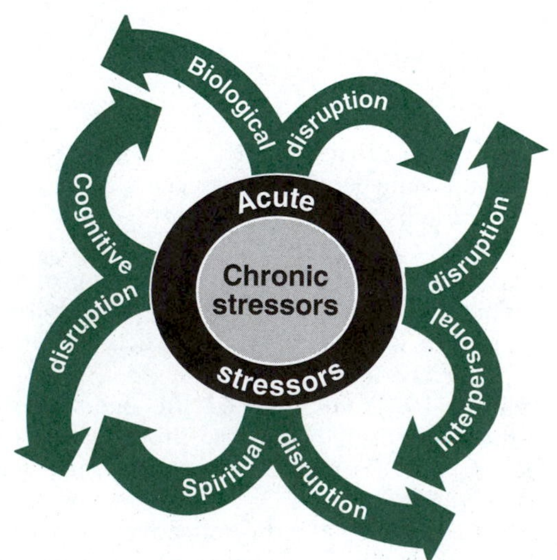

FIGURE 30–5
Calarco and Krone's integrated model of depressive behavior, modified to include the spiritual dimension. (Modified from Calarco, M., and Krone, K. [1991]. An integrated nursing model of depressive behavior in adults: Theory and implications for practice. *Nursing Clinics of North America, 26* [3], 573–583.)

Nurses can recruit patients, family members, and other mental health professionals into collaborative ventures such as mutual help groups. The National Self-help Clearinghouse provides a list of resources throughout the United States that can help in networking and providing consultative assistance. Another resource is "The Manual for Affective Disorder Support Groups," which can be applied to any support group regardless of the problem or disease addressed. The Depression and Related Affective Disorders Association (DRADA), a nonprofit organization composed of individuals with mood disorders, family members, and mental health professionals, offers information, education, referral, and support services to people nationwide. DRADA sponsors a nationally renowned training program for group leaders. The phone number is 410-955-4647.

Nurse as Manager of Biological Interventions

MEDICATIONS

Although Chapter 23 provides a comprehensive review of the medications that are used in the treatment of mood disorders, there are still medication-related issues for the nurse to address. Research indicates that the most effective treatment for mood disorders includes both medication and psychotherapy. Not only will psychotherapy make it more likely for someone to stay on medication, but also medication will make it more likely that the individual stay in psychotherapy.

The medication-related issues to address are

- Establishing open and honest communication with the patient.
- Dealing with stigma associated with taking medications.
- Providing accurate information about medications, actions, and side effects.
- Teaching the patient to address medication issues with the prescribing physician assertively.

The nurse needs to understand accurately what the patient is experiencing as a result of the medications. For instance, patients may withhold information about side effects they are experiencing, the lack of effectiveness of the medication, or the fact that they have stopped taking the medication. Factors that may precipitate the patient's "noncompliance" with antidepressant therapy include

- An attitude that the medication is a crutch.
- Feelings of guilt and worthlessness.
- Fears of drug dependency and addiction (Dowling, 1993).

• Lack of acceptance that the mood disorders are really a medical illness.

• Feelings of shame, embarrassment, and stigma attached to mental illness and the idea of being "crazy."

Even when they are helped by medication, people may continue to believe they should have been able to handle the illness without medication. They may feel that if they tried a little harder or had done this or that differently, they would not have become ill. When faced with disagreement in their choice of treatment by their friends or family, the struggle is all the more difficult without a supportive therapist (Dowling, 1993).

Adequate teaching cannot occur unless you have established an environment in which the patient can honestly discuss feelings about medication. You must fully understand how the patient thinks and feels about medication. You must be cognizant of the patient's right to choose medications as part of treatment. Common nursing reactions to a patient's noncompliance are anger and frustration and a sense that the patient is rejecting interventions. You must guard against letting these feelings limit the exploration of a patient's choice to stop taking medications.

ELECTROCONVULSIVE THERAPY

Electroconvulsive therapy (ECT) induces a seizure by applying electric current. ECT provides the most rapid relief of any treatment for severe depression. Most of the severely ill patients who fail to respond to medication respond to ECT. This form of treatment should be considered when drug therapy has failed, when the patient is at high risk for suicide or starvation, or when depression is judged to be overwhelmingly severe. It is also particularly useful when the depressed person is troubled by delusions or hallucinations (DePaulo and Ablow, 1989).

ECT was discovered in the mid-1930s. At that time, it was the only treatment available and was frequently used and misused. In the mid-1960s the use of general anesthesia and a muscle relaxant, most commonly succinylcholine, became a clinical standard for use with ECT. Since then, the frequency of adverse effects related to the seizure have essentially become nonexistent (Abraham et al, 1991).

ECT treatments are given three times a week, with an average series involving 8 to 12 treatments and a duration of two to four weeks. How ECT works is still not clear. It appears to alter receptors for the catecholamine neurotransmitters in a way similar to that of the tricyclic antidepressants. The most common side effects are amnesia of events occurring near the period of the treatment and the potential for transient confusion as a result of the seizure and the barbiturate anesthetic.

Following the course of ECT, patients may have some memory deficits for the period before ECT was begun. These memory deficits tend to disappear with time, and in most cases patients suffer little long-term memory loss. Measuring the extent of memory loss is complicated because depression itself impairs concentration and memory. The memory deficits of which the patient complains may be the product not of the ECT but of the preexisting depression (Klein and Wender, 1988). Sensitive testing of memory has revealed minor defects after three months, but these resolve within six months (DePaulo and Ablow, 1989).

Most patients who have had repeated episodes of depression are started on antidepressants after the course of ECT is completed. These act as an added precaution against the return of symptoms. A few patients do need a prolonged course of ECT. Those with severe major depression that does not respond to medications may be prescribed what has been called "maintenance ECT" (Mondimore, 1993). These patients receive a regular course of ECT and then continue their treatments on a reduced schedule, often on an outpatient basis, for several months. They may have one treatment a month or be treated less often. Table 30–5 outlines the nurse's responsibilities monitoring the patient receiving ECT treatment.

▶ Check Your Reading

21. In the role of counselor, identify five things that you would do.
22. Name two areas that you would teach the patient and family.
23. How do you collaborate with the patient and family?
24. What is empowerment?
25. Identify three ways that you can be a facilitator of empowerment for the patient.
26. How can you facilitate spiritual growth in the patient?
27. Identify at least two ways that nurses collaborate with support groups.
28. Name two things that you would teach a patient who was preparing to have ECT.

EVALUATION

If you have established clear goals with the patient and the family, you can easily determine whether the plan needs to be modified or continued. The formative evaluation addresses such questions as the following:

• Has the patient remained safe? Has the patient made suicide attempts? If so, how does the plan need to be modified to ensure the patient's safety?

• Has the patient "connected" with a caring professional while in the hospital?

• Has the patient reestablished balance in eating, sleeping, and activity?

• Is the patient feeling better? Is there a noticeable improvement in mood, sociability, energy level, and interest in life?

• Has there been a significant improvement in the patient's score on the standardized depression inventory?

• Does the patient verbalize understanding of medication issues?

TABLE 30–5 **Nursing Interventions for the Patient Receiving Electroconvulsive Therapy**

Before Treatment	During Treatment	After Treatment
Provide teaching for the patient and family regarding the risks and benefits of ECT. Include the rationale for ECT, how ECT works, side effects of ECT, ECT procedures, activity after ECT and ECT outcomes Offer handouts that might include a guide to ECT Make a videotape available that might outline the necessary information about ECT. Use this as a follow-up to your explanation to reinforce teaching or to stimulate questions and discussion Whenever possible, encourage the exchange of information between patients and family members about their experiences with ECT	Before the procedure, check emergency equipment Keep NPO several hours before the treatment Remove potentially harmful objects, such as jewelry, dentures Check vital signs Maintain patent airway Position on side until alert Assist with ambulation Offer analgesic or antiemetic as needed	Reorient the patient Be with the patient for comfort and support Assist family members to understand behavior associated with confusion or memory loss Discuss with the patient and family how ECT has affected them and the effect it has on the patient's individual symptoms of depression

ECT = Electroconvulsive therapy; NPO = nothing by mouth.

- Does the patient verbalize understanding of illness issues?
- Is the patient participating in therapy?
- Is family involved in care?
- Has the patient begun to address the spiritual components of the illness?

The summative evaluation deals with issues such as discharge planning, referral to a support group, continuation of therapy, and the patient's ability to establish realistic goals.

▶ **Check Your Reading**

29. Identify at least five areas that you would review in a formative evaluation.
30. What would be important to consider in a summative evaluation?

CASE STUDY: WANDA

Wanda is a 45-year-old African-American woman who was admitted to the psychiatric hospital yesterday because she was no longer able to work or care for herself or her family. Her 25-year-old daughter, Laronda, became worried when she noticed that her mother was sleeping all the time, was not eating, and talked about "ending it all because life is just too difficult." Laronda is present with her mother during the admission process.

When you interview Wanda for the first time, you find that she is the single mother of three children. Laronda is also a single mother of two children and is attending community college, sharing the care of the two children with her mother. A son, James, is 23, works in a restaurant, and is also a part-time student. When Wanda speaks of her youngest son, Jesse, you notice that tears begin to well up in her eyes. She shares that Jesse, who is 20, became involved in drugs and gang activity several years ago and is currently serving a 10-year prison term for possession of drugs and armed robbery. He was incarcerated six months ago, and Laronda tells you her mother hasn't been the same since. Laronda is concerned because her mother has lost interest even in her grandchildren and going to church. Wanda tells you, "I know that God left me; I am such a bad person—nothing I do is right."

ASSESSMENT

The assessment data are as follows:

- Insomnia
- Sad affect

- Decreased appetite
- Verbalizations of despair: "Life is just too difficult."
- Loss of interest in previously enjoyable activities
- Verbalizations of shame and guilt: "I am a bad person."
- Verbalizations of abandonment by God: "I know God has left me."

DIAGNOSIS

***DSM-IV* Diagnosis:** Major depressive disorder, single episode

Nursing Diagnosis: Hopelessness related to long-term stress and loss of belief in God, evidenced by vegetative symptoms of depression and verbalizations of despair and abandonment by God

OUTCOME IDENTIFICATION, PLANNING, AND IMPLEMENTATION

EXPECTED OUTCOME 1: By _____ the patient will be free of suicidal and depressive symptoms.

SHORT-TERM GOALS	NURSING INTERVENTIONS	RATIONALES
By _____ the patient will sleep uninterrupted for at least six hours, and her appetite will return to normal.	1. Monitor and assess patient's sleeping and eating patterns. 2. Administer prn medication for sleep if patient is unable to gain restful sleep. 3. Determine patient's food preferences. 4. Encourage socialization while eating as the patient is ready.	1. Before intervention, it is important to establish a baseline. 2. If the patient's sleep has been disturbed for a long period, it may be necessary to intervene chemically initially. 3–4. Promote compliance and provide for decreased alienation.
By _____ the patient will report a mood change consistent with hopefulness.	1. Conduct a suicide assessment and initiate appropriate staff supervision depending on the level of risk. 2. Administer antidepressant medications as ordered. 3. Teach patient individually or in a group setting specifically how antidepressant medications alleviate the symptoms of depression.	1. Hospitalization for depression usually indicates that the patient is at high risk for suicide. 2. To stabilize the mood and promote sleep, medications are often indicated when persons are hospitalized. 3. Teaching the patient about the physiological action of medications ensures compliance.
By _____ the patient will be able to verbalize feelings associated with depression.	1. In group therapy or individually, encourage the patient specifically to verbalize the feelings associated with hopelessness. 2. As trust is developed, encourage open expression of patient's feelings about her son's incarceration. 3.Remain nonjudgmental and accepting.	1. Patients are often reluctant to talk about negative feelings because of the fear of overwhelming emotional pain. 2–3. There is shame associated with incarceration, and the patient may have been reluctant to share her feelings with anyone.

EXPECTED OUTCOME 2: By _____ the patient will participate willingly in daily activities on the unit and engage in self-care behaviors.

SHORT-TERM GOALS	NURSING INTERVENTIONS	RATIONALES
By _____ the patient will initiate self-grooming activities.	1. Offer genuine praise for patient's efforts for goal setting, grooming, and other self-care activities.	1. Genuine, specific praise promotes continuance of positive behaviors. Patients tend to refute any praise that is general, such as "You look nice today."

SHORT-TERM GOALS
By _____ the patient will willingly attend all unit functions.

NURSING INTERVENTIONS
2. Encourage the patient to participate in all activities that promote positive thoughts, feelings, and validation, such as recreational therapy, communication with her daughter, and perhaps a grief group.

RATIONALES
2. These activities foster inclusion and decrease the alienation associated with hopelessness.

EXPECTED OUTCOME 3: By _____ the patient will demonstrate hopefulness regarding future life.

SHORT-TERM GOAL
By _____ the patient will (on three separate occasions) state something that she is hopeful about.

NURSING INTERVENTIONS
1. Encourage the patient to express negative feelings of hopelessness, despondency, and alienation.
2. Identify positive parts of the patient's existence, such as the loving support of her two older children and her grandchildren, her participation in a group, and something she has accomplished on the unit.
3. Help the patient identify behaviors that promote hopelessness, such as not attending group activities, eating alone, or ruminating about events over which she has little or no control.
4. Educate the patient about positive thinking and how to create a place of safety in her mind to combat hopelessness.

RATIONALES
1. This process allows the patient an opportunity to ventilate feelings that have been pent up for a long time.
2. Helping the patient see positive people and situations promotes the expectation that hope is possible.
3. This process enables the patient to recognize experiences that precipitate feelings of hopelessness.
4. Feelings of hopelessness will inevitably reappear, and it is important that the patient is ready to deal with these feelings rather than perceive she has no control over them.

EXPECTED OUTCOME 4: By _____ the patient will find hope and meaning in her relationship with God.

SHORT-TERM GOALS
By _____ the patient will make a positive statement about God.

By _____ the patient will verbalize how the events in her life, particularly her son's incarceration, have affected her on her life's journey.

NURSING INTERVENTIONS
1. Provide models of persons from literature or the Bible who have overcome misfortune.
2. Encourage the patient to discuss these situations and attempt to relate them to herself.
3. Ask the patient to think about how this situation relates to her situation and how they are alike.
4. Explain to the patient the importance of attempting to find meaning in all of life's events, even the most difficult ones.
5. Ask the patient if there are any spiritual resources that would be helpful to her at this time. Ask if there is something that you could do to respond to her distress.

RATIONALES
1–3. Knowing that others have been able to overcome painful and shameful situations is often comforting.
4. Finding spiritual meaning in pain and trauma helps the process of grieving and acceptance.
5. Assisting the patient in rekindling her relationship with God is a loving and compassionate act because the patient is vulnerable and unable to do this for herself at this time.

Nursing Diagnosis: Chronic Low Self-Esteem related to long-standing history of minimal accomplishments and losses, evidenced by self-negating verbalizations and feelings of shame, guilt, and despair.

OUTCOME IDENTIFICATION, PLANNING, AND IMPLEMENTATION

EXPECTED OUTCOME 1: By _____ the patient will demonstrate behavior consistent with increased self-esteem.

SHORT-TERM GOALS	NURSING INTERVENTIONS	RATIONALES
By _____ the patient will verbalize feelings of self-worth. By _____ the patient will demonstrate absence of self-negating statements. By _____ the patient will actively engage in group therapy and activities on the unit.	1. Encourage the patient to engage in self-care grooming activities.	1. Attending to grooming is often an initial step in feeling better about one's self.
	2. Honestly praise the patient for all observable accomplishments.	2. Patients with low self-esteem do not benefit from flattery or insincere praise. Honest positive feedback enhances self-esteem.
	3. Begin with simple recreational activities or art projects and proceed to more complex situations in a group context.	3. Initially the client may be too overwhelmed to engage in activities with more than one person.
	4. If the patient persists in negativism about self, place a limit on the length of time you will be able to listen to negativity. For example, agree to 10 minutes of negativity followed by 10 minutes of positive comments.	4. Time limits allow the client a safe time and place to ventilate negative feelings and demonstrate thought stopping, the conscious interruption of negative thoughts.
	5. Explore with the patient her personal strengths and suggest making a written list to use as a reminder when negativity returns.	5. Having a written list to review can help the patient during difficult times after discharge, when the support of hospital staff is not there.

EXPECTED OUTCOME 2: By _____ the patient will demonstrate understanding of the effect of negative self-talk and irrational belief systems.

SHORT-TERM GOALS	NURSING INTERVENTIONS	RATIONALES
By _____ the patient will verbalize realistic statements about self and others. By _____ the patient will accept praise from the staff without self-negating comments.	1. Listen and accept the patient's irrational beliefs and feelings without judgment. 2. Respectfully confront persistent irrational beliefs, such as "I am a bad person," or "all or nothing" thinking.	1–2. When the patient perceives your listening and confronting as a caring intervention, she will be better able to accept what you are intending her to hear.
	3. Encourage thought-stopping and thought-substituting techniques.	3. This technique enables the patient to replace irrational thoughts with rational ones.
	4. Give patient positive affirmation when she is able to accept praise verbally or nonverbally.	4. Positive feedback encourages positive behavior.

EXPECTED OUTCOME 3: By _____ the patient will accept suggestions from the staff for increasing self-esteem and assertiveness.

SHORT-TERM GOAL	NURSING INTERVENTIONS	RATIONALES
By _____ the patient will practice suggestions for increasing esteem and will request support from the staff and peers.	1. Encourage the patient to be proactive and assertive.	1–3. Becoming proactive and assertive is a skill and requires coaching.
	2. Teach necessary assertive skills and help the patient distinguish between assertiveness and aggressiveness. 3. Have patient practice new behaviors with the staff and her peers.	2. It is not unusual for people with passive personalities to become aggressive because they have allowed transgressions to occur for a long time.
	4. Encourage the patient to identify her own needs and to practice asking for what she needs.	4. Part of being assertive is becoming aware of your own needs and asking for help when necessary.

EXPECTED OUTCOME 4: By _____ the patient will verbalize a desire to live and develop realistic plans for the future.

SHORT-TERM GOAL	NURSING INTERVENTIONS	RATIONALES
By _____ the patient will verbalize a desire to live by identifying daily goals and at least one long-term goal.	1. As the depression lifts, encourage the patient to set a daily goal and to put it in writing. An example is to call her daughter or write her son a letter. 2. Once daily goals are achieved and the patient has experienced some success, assist the patient in formulating long-term goals such as a change in career, financial goals, interpersonal goals, or goals related to her health.	1–2. Writing both daily goals and long-term goals enables the patient to begin to believe in herself. Having a plan for the future is a proactive way of combating depression.

EVALUATION

Formative Evaluation

Wanda met all of her short-term goals. She said that she wasn't aware of how depressed she had become. She had always been a person with a strong drive and ambition, and this episode of depression took her by surprise. Wanda realized that the low self-esteem was not new but resolved to continue to work on feeling better about herself.

Summative Evaluation

Wanda also met all of the stated long-term goals. At the time of discharge, the staff told Wanda that they were concerned for her regarding continued support. Wanda was a compliant patient and responded well to the structure provided by the hospitalization and the caring and concern of the treatment team. Wanda's typical role is to be a caretaker, and she was just beginning to learn to accept praise and genuine concern from others without negating it. The treatment team recommended that Wanda see a psychotherapist either individually or in a group for at least six months.

CONCLUSIONS

Mood disorders are common and are frequently overlooked by some health professionals and misunderstood by others. The challenge for the nurse is to recognize the often misleading symptoms of depressive illnesses and assist the patient through diagnosis and treatment. Assessment of individual, family, spiritual, and environmental factors are important in planning for the patient's care. You need to address the impact of the illness on the patient's self-perception and sense of control over life. Through empowerment, you can encourage and develop a collaborative approach to helping, so important to preventive health. With this approach, the patients are assisted in taking responsibility and control of their own health care decisions. Additionally, family members need to be included as caregivers in the process. Provide them with the necessary preparation and support.

Both patients and family members need access to reliable written information and teaching about the illness. You need to be familiar with community resources that can help patients and families. You need to have a good working knowledge of the mutual help groups available and use them as referral sources. These groups assist individuals to prevent or recover from illness and to attain their optimal level of health and independence. The stigma associated with mood disorders must be addressed through education and research efforts. Increased knowledge of the biological and genetic influences leads to a better understanding of how physical and psychosocial stressors may influence these illnesses. With more specific and accurate information to give people about depression and manic-depressive illnesses, fear and stigma can be reduced.

Mood disorders are treatable diseases. William Styron (1990) shares this message:

> *For those who have dwelt in depression's dark wood, and known its inexplicable agony, their return from the abyss is not unlike the ascent of the poet, trudging upward and upward out of hell's black depths and at last emerging into what he saw as "the shining world." There, whoever has been restored to health has almost always been restored to the capacity for serenity and joy, and this may be indemnity enough for having endured the despair beyond despair (p. 84).*

KEY POINTS TO REMEMBER

- Mood disorders affect the way people feel about themselves. The impact of these disorders is holistic.
- Depressed people tend to be sad, irritable, despairful, hopeless, and suicidal.

- Manic people tend to be excited and elated or extremely irritable.
- All the mood disorders involve variations of or combinations of depression and mania.
- Mood disorders affect as many as 10% to 15% of Americans. They affect a person's most productive years. They are relapsing, episodic, and if left untreated, become more frequent and severe.
- Mood disorders have a high rate of cooccurrence with other disorders.
- Mood disorders have a high mortality rate. Suicide is the most common complication.
- Diagnosis of mood disorders is hampered by our inability to describe moods and changes in moods.
- Mood refers to a person's pervasive feeling state. A normal mood is euthymia; a bad mood is dysthymia; a high mood is elation.
- Affect refers to the fleeting feelings that show on our faces.
- Diagnosis of mood disorders looks at whether the patient is experiencing a persistent change in mood, self-attitude, and vital sense.
- The cause of mood disorders is most likely due to multiple factors, including sleep alterations; pharmacological interventions; and neuronal, endocrinological, genetic, and psychodynamic causes.
- Assessment of a patient with a mood disorder involves collecting data regarding the patient's mood, self-attitude, and vital sense. In addition, standardized depression inventories are frequently used. In addition, information is collected regarding suicidal ideation, intent, and plan; the family's feelings, attitudes, and knowledge; issues of powerlessness, spiritual concerns, and social isolation.
- There are many nursing diagnoses appropriate for the patient with a mood disorder.
- Expected outcomes focus on the patient's safety, normalization of mood, return of energy level to normal, and functional improvement.
- Implementation involves multiple roles, including counselor, teacher, protector, collaborator, facilitator of empowerment, facilitator of spiritual growth, referral source for social support, and manager of biological interventions.
- Evaluation examines the assessment data and the original short-term goals and expected outcomes. If the patient has made progress toward goal achievement, the plan is continued; if the progress has not been made, the plan is modified.

LEARNING ACTIVITIES

1. Monitor your own moods for a week. How would you describe your mood changes? Is there wide variability in your moods? What affects your own changes? When you feel "blue," what helps you to feel better?

2. Read William Styron's account of his depression. Write your reactions to his story in your journal.

3. Individuals who suffer with mood disorders are afraid that if others know the diagnosis, they will be stigmatized. What do you think about people who have mood disorders? Would you want to work with a person who suffers with periodic depressions? How do you think people who have mood disorders should be treated? Ask five other people (a mix of health professionals and non–health professionals) what they think about people with mood disorders. From these interviews and your own reactions, how real is the issue of stigma? How can stigma be countered?

CRITICAL THINKING EXERCISE

Mrs. Buzzer, a 30-year-old woman, was brought to the crisis unit after she was found directing rush hour traffic wearing red leotards, a see-through bathing suit top, and a bright green feather in her safari hat. When she spoke to the nurse on the unit, she stated, "I am the Amazon queen of all people." Mrs. Buzzer asked the nurse if she could call her sister to bring other clothes for her to wear. The nurse debated whether to allow this request.

1. What assumptions can be made about Mrs. Buzzer's behavior?

2. What evidence suggests that the nurse should deny or approve the request?

3. What might happen if she denies the request?

The following afternoon, Mrs. Buzzer's husband called the unit stating that he had received a call from a department store telling him that his wife had charged $500.00 on their credit card to buy shoes and dresses. She told the salesgirl that she was on her way to Africa to hunt baboons.

1. Make sense of the information.

2. What conclusion can be made about whether the nurse denied or approved the request?

3. What evidence leads you to draw this conclusion?

REFERENCES

Abraham, I., Neese, J., and Westerman, P. (1991). Depression: Nursing implications of a clinical and social problem. *Nursing Clinics of North America, 26*(3), 527–535.

Abramson, L., Seligman, M., and Teasdale, J. (1978). Learned helplessness in humans: Critique and reformulation. *Journal of Abnormal Psychology, 87*, 49–74.

American Psychiatric Association (1994). *Diagnostic and statistical manual of mental disorders* (4th ed.). Washington, D.C.: American Psychiatric Association.

Beck, A., Rush, A., Shaw, B., et al (1979). *Cognitive theory of depression.* New York: Guilford Press.

Beck, C. (1993). Teetering on the edge: A substantive theory of postpartum depression. *Nursing Research, 42*(1), 42–47.

Benner, P., and Wrubel, J. (1988). *The primacy of caring, stress and coping in health and illness.* Canada: Addison-Wesley.

Bloch, S. (1979). Supportive psychotherapy. In S. Bloch (Ed.), *An introduction to the psychotherapies* (pp. 196–220). New York: Oxford University Press.

Calarco, M., and Krone, K. (1991). An integrated nursing model of depressive behavior in adults: Theory and implications for practice. *Nursing Clinics of North America, 26*(3), 573–583.

Carson, V. B. (1989). *Spiritual dimensions of nursing practice.* Philadelphia: W. B. Saunders.

Carson, V. B. (1994). Spirituality and depression. *Smooth Sailing: DRADA Newsletter, January,* 3–4.

DePaulo, R., and Ablow, K. (1989). *How to cope with depression: A complete guide for you and your family.* New York: McGraw-Hill.

Depression in primary care: Vol. 1. Detection and diagnosis. Clinical Practice Guideline, No. 5. (1993). Rockville, Md.: U.S. Department of Health and Human Services, Public Health Service, Agency for Health Care Policy and Research. AHCPR Publication No. 93-0550.

Dowling, C. (1993). *You mean I don't have to feel this way?: New help for depression, anxiety, and addiction.* New York: Bantam Books.

Endler, N. (1990). *Holiday of darkness: A psychologist's personal journey out of his depression.* Toronto: Wall & Thompson.

Finley, C., and Wilson, D. (1951). The relation of the family to manic-depressive psychosis. *Diseases of the Nervous System, 12,* 39–43.

Frank, E. (1988). *Family interrelationships.* University of Pittsburgh School of Medicine, Western Psychiatric Institute and Clinic. In lecture notes given at National Depressive and Manic Depressive Association, Fifth Annual Convention.

Freud, S. (1917). Mourning and melancholia. In W. Gaylin (Ed.), *The meaning of despair: Psychoanalytic contributions to the understanding of depression.* New York: Science House.

Fromm-Reichmann, F. (1949). Intensive psychotherapy of manic-depressives: A preliminary report. *Confina Neurologica, 9,* 158–165.

Gartner, A., and Reissman, F. (1980). *A working guide to self-help groups.* New York: Viewpoints/Vision Books.

Gartner, A., and Reissman, F. (1984). *The self-help revolution.* New York: Human Services Press.

Gibson, C. (1991). A concept analysis of empowerment. *Journal of Advanced Nursing, 16,* 354–361.

Goodwin, F., and Jamison, K. (1990). *Manic-depressive illness.* New York: Oxford University Press.

Greenberg, P., Stiglin, L., and Finkelstein, S. (1993). The economic burden of depression. *Journal of Clinical Psychiatry, 54* (11), 406–418.

Hollon, S. D., Shelton, R. C., and Loosen, P. T. (1991). Cognitive therapy in relation to pharmacotherapy in depression. *Journal of Consulting Psychology, 59,* 88–99.

Hudson, J. L., Hudson, M. S., Pliner, L. F., Goldenberg, D. L., and Pope, H. G., Jr. (1985). Fibromyalgia and major affective disorder: A controlled phenomenology and family history study. *American Journal of Psychiatry, 142* (4), 441–446.

Jacob, B. L. (1994). Serotonin, motor activity and depression-related disorders. *American Scientist, 82,* 456–463.

Jamison, K. (1993). *Touched with fire: Manic-depressive illness and the artistic temperament.* New York: The Free Press.

Jarrett, R., and Rush, J. (1989). Cognitive-behavioral psychotherapy for depression. In *Treatments of psychiatric disorders: A task force report of the American Psychiatric Association.* Washington, DC: American Psychiatric Association, (pp. 1834–1846).

Jones, P., and Meleis, A. (1993). Health is empowerment. *Advances in Nursing Science, 15(13),* 1–13.

Kerr, N. (1987–1988). Signs and symptoms of depression and principles of nursing intervention. *Perspectives in Psychiatric Care, 14* (2), 48–63.

Klein, D., and Wender, P. (1988). *Do you have a depressive illness?: How to tell, what to do.* New York: New American Library.

Klerman, G., Weissman, M., Rounsaville, B., and Chevron, E. (1984). *Interpersonal psychotherapy of depression.* New York: Basic Books.

Logan, R. (1988). Helping a spouse over a major depression. *Medical Aspects of Human Sexuality, May,* 34–41.

Lowell, R. (1977). *Day by day.* New York: Farrar, Straus and Giroux.

Marck, P. (1990). Therapeutic reciprocity: A caring phenomenon. *Advances in Nursing Science, September,* 49–59.

Mayo, J., O'Connell, R., and O'Brien, J. (1979). Families of manic-depressive patients: Effects of treatment. *American Journal of Psychiatry, 136,* 1535–1539.

McKay, B., Forbes, J., and Bourner, K. (1990). Empowerment in general practice: The trilogies of caring. *Australian Family Physician, April,* 513–520.

Miller, L. (1987). Spiritual aspects of depression. *Friends Journal, September 1 and 15,* 6–8.

Mondimore, F. (1993). *Depression: The mood disease.* Baltimore: The Johns Hopkins University Press.

Neese, J. (1991). Depression in the general hospital. *Nursing Clinics of North America, 26* (3), 613–621.

Norbeck, J., Chaftez, L., Skodol-Wilson, H., and Weiss, S. (1991). Social support needs of family caregivers of psychiatric patients from three age groups. *Nursing Research, 40* (4), 208–213.

Robinson, R., Lipsey, J., and Price, T. (1985). Diagnosis and clinical management of post-stroke depression. *Psychosomatics, 26,* 769–778.

Rosenthal, N. (1989). *Seasons of the mind: Why you get the winter blues and what you can do about it.* New York: Bantam Books.

Schoenbeck, S., Trujillo-Stanley, J., and Lokken, M. (1992). Helping the patient and their family understand depression. *The Journal of Practical Nursing, September,* 35–38.

Seligman, M. (1975). *Helplessness.* San Francisco: Freeman Press.

Silverman, P. (1978). *Mutual help groups: A guide for mental health workers.* Publication ADM 78-646. Rockville, Md.: National Institute of Mental Health.

Silverman, P., and Murrow, H. (1976). Mutual help during critical transitions. *Journal of Applied Behavioral Science, 12,* 411–418.

Skovhold, T. (1974). The client as a helper: A means to promote psychological growth. *Counseling Psychology, 4,* 58–64.

Story, M., and Anderson, G. (1992). Assessment and treatment strategies for depressive disorders commonly encountered in primary care settings. *Nurse Practitioner, June,* 25–36.

Styron, W. (1990). *Darkness visible: A memoir of madness.* New York: Random House.

Support groups lengthen your life. (1990). *Johns Hopkins Medical Letter, 2,* 9.

Terry, M., and Anderson, G. (1992). Assessment and treatment strategy for depressive disorders encountered in psychiatric care centers. *Nurse Practitioner, 17(6),* 34.

Weiss, S. (1986). Consensual norms regarding patient involvement. *Social Science and Medicine, 22,* 489–496.

Weissman, M., Jarrett, R., and Rush, J. (1987). Psychotherapy and its relevance to the pharmacotherapy of major depression: A decade later 1976–1985. In H. Y. Meltzer (Ed.), *Psychopharmacology: The third generation of progress* (pp. 1059–1069). New York: Raven Press.

Wuthnow, R. (1994). *Sharing the journey: Support groups and America's new quest for community.* New York: The Free Press.

SUGGESTED READINGS

Abraham, I., Neese, J., and Westerman, P. (1991). Depression: Nursing implications of a clinical and social problem. *Nursing Clinics of North America, 26*(3), 527–535.

Beck, C. (1993). Teetering on the edge: A substantive theory of postpartum depression. *Nursing Research, 42*(1), 42–47.

Gibson, C. (1991). A concept analysis of empowerment. *Journal of Advanced Nursing, 16,* 354–361.

Jones, P., and Meleis, A. (1993). Health is empowerment. *Advances in Nursing Science, March, 15(13),* 1–13.

Story, M., and Anderson, G. (1992). Assessment and treatment strategies for depressive disorders commonly encountered in primary care settings. *Nurse Practitioner, June,* 25–36.

CHAPTER 31

THE JOURNEY ANESTHETIZED BY SUBSTANCE USE

She [Helen of Troy] threw into the wine which they were drinking a drug which takes away grief and passion and brings forgetfulness of all ills.

—Homer, *Odyssey*

LEARNING OBJECTIVES

After studying this chapter, you should be able to:

1. Discuss the historical context of substance use disorders
2. Define substance use disorders and related terminology
3. Identify two theoretical perspectives on the cause of substance use disorders
4. Discuss the four primary drug classifications
5. Describe the nurse's role in the treatment of patients with substance use disorders
6. Identify populations with special needs
7. Survey the family implications of substance use disorders

KEY TERMINOLOGY

Addiction
Alcoholics Anonymous
Blackouts
Central nervous system stimulant
Cocaine blues
Codependency
Craving
Cross-tolerance
Delirium tremens
Denial
Dependence
Detoxification
Dual diagnosis
Enabling behaviors
Flashback
Halfway house
Hallucinogens
Hypnotic sedative
Intoxication
Kindling effect
Korsakoff's syndrome
Narcotic analgesic
Physical dependence
Polydrug dependence
Projections
Psychoactive substances
Psychological dependence
Rationalization
Recovery
Reinforcing properties
Relapse prevention
Substance abuse
Substance dependence
Tolerance
Toxicity
Wernicke's encephalopathy
Withdrawal

Chapter 31 tells the story of the human journey anesthetized by the routine use of a psychoactive substance. A person's life journey, obscured from personal awareness by alcohol or other **psychoactive substances,** is a static one. The traveler and those closest to him or her are immobilized by the alcohol or drug use, unable to move forward or fully process what is happening around them because of their single-minded focus on its use. As a result, the story of the journey stops midstream as if stuck in time and space, as a nonconsecutive chapter in the book of life because its author has lost his or her voice.

Substance use disorders are unlike any other, replete with paradoxes and social, moral, and legal overlays. Although the disorder is self-inflicted, it develops without the full awareness or consent of its victims. Although the disorder directly affects the diagnosed patient, it can have equally devastating effects on family members who never ingest a psychoactive substance. The disorder is classified as a medical disorder; however, many consider it a social, moral, and behavioral disorder. It is the only medical disorder for which one can be jailed rather than being treated medically. Understanding the complex interrelationships among the physical, psychological, spiritual, and social dimensions of substance use disorders is the first step in developing a comprehensive treatment plan applicable to the needs of affected patients and their families. These understandings can help you to draw those suffering with substance use disorders to consider the potential of leading a richer human existence without drugs or excessive use of alcohol. We begin with Joe's story, a professional young man with a future who sees only the benefits of drug use and none of its disadvantages. To him as to so many others, recreational drug use is harmless. This chapter argues the point that this assumption simply is not true for far too many people.

JOE'S STORY

I first tried hallucinogens in college after having smoked pot for a few years in high school. I guess it was both intense curiosity and part peer pressure from the guys in the dorm that led me to try mescaline and then LSD later on. The first sensation is a temporary nausea and an extremely heightened sense of awareness, as if I have had many cups of coffee and things have sped up dramatically. Light is much brighter, colors are more vivid, and my hearing is much more keen, with music being especially pleasurable. All the senses are more intense and seem to blend together, mixing with thoughts and emotions. These thoughts, feelings, and perceptions sweep together and seem to drift and pull me away as if I am floating so that I can literally get swept away in thoughts that seem to last forever. At times I can be talking a lot, laughing and then minutes later, I am anxious and scared. Sometimes I would cry with overwhelming waves of emotion. The crying can be primal and hurting and healing all at once. The feelings of ecstasy have an "electric" quality as if one were having sex with the brain. Sometimes a feeling of being "at one with the universe" and with people around me is comforting and is very magical. It also is rather fleeting.

After many experiences with LSD, I would say that the environment and my underlying emotional state were *key to how the trip would go*. If I had already been elated or happy-go-lucky, it would be an overall intensely pleasurable experience. If I had any doubts about myself or if I was under a lot of pressure or turmoil, it was like experiencing a really bad nightmare yet I was awake. I soon learned that I had to be careful when I chose to take LSD, the dosage was critical, and I had to try to steer myself toward a good mood if I decided I was going to trip.

I go back to it from time to time, especially if I am going to an intense jazz or rock concert like the Grateful Dead. Although it is mostly uplifting and freeing to my spirit, it is still very mysterious to me. It is as if I am unlocking the door to my closet and seeing myself and people without masks—a little scary at times. Even if I go through an hour or so of hell with bad emotions, paranoia, and painful memories, it is so cathartic. I feel as if I have had an intense spiritual reawakening, as if being reborn. To be able to really understand suffering and the peace that follows that experience is very comforting and humbling. This, I think, is one of the attractions to LSD: to be able to be free, uninhibited, and even to cry like a baby and to comfort myself! Did I ever get enough consoling or relief as a child? This could be the real unanswered question here.

This story was written by Joe approximately 3 weeks after a very bad "trip" on lysergic acid diethylamide (LSD) in which he was almost mugged and spent the night sleeping in a doorway. Although Joe was badly frightened by his experience and its potential to harm him, the draw of hallucinogenic drugs was just as strong 3 weeks later, as it was before his bad experience with the voluntary use of LSD. It was almost as if the bad effects of his last "trip" were erased from memory.

Joe's selective memory and euphoric recall of the positive aspects of his drug experience are not unusual, and his rationalization of the negative consequences are common. In large part, they derive from the substance's effects on the brain.

HISTORICAL PERSPECTIVE

A detailed historical context provides the background to understand the multifaceted nature of substance use disorders. The human evolution of our understanding of drug-taking behaviors began many centuries ago with the use of mind-altering **psychoactive substances** as pain relievers, medicinal agents, and a welcome accompaniment to the success of recreational events and religious ceremonies.

Early Understandings of Psychoactive Substances

Naturally occurring psychoactive agents such as opiates and alcohol were used to stimulate euphoria and a sense of well-being, with the earliest known consumption of alcohol dating back to 4000 B. C. Early Indians routinely chewed coca leaves in the Andes Mountains in South America more than 3000 years ago (Carroll, 1977). In the middle ages, alcohol was referred to as "aqua vitae" (the water of life), a term also used as the Gaelic derivative for whiskey. Jesus marked his coming of age by turning water into wine when it ran out at a wedding, symbolically signaling its importance to the success of a social event. Bacchus, revered as the god of pleasure, was draped with symbols of wine during pagan times, and Native Americans had a long-held tradition of using "peyote buttons" to enhance the feeling of celebration in their religious ceremonies. So popular was cocaine as a mild euphoric agent in the late 1800s that it was found in the first composition of Coca-Cola, hence the inclusion of the word "coca" in the full name of the drink. Freud enthusiastically endorsed the use of cocaine, used it himself, and prescribed it for several of his patients until the destructive effects of the drug with one of his patients became obvious to him. He described its use in detail, as being a mood elevator and as having an energizing effect that began within 10 to 20 minutes of ingestion and lasted for as long as 4 to 5 hours.

The healing and pain-reduction capabilities of psychoactive substances received early recognition in many societies. Cannabis was identified as a Chinese herbal as early as 2700 B. C. In the late 1800s, powdered morphine sulfate and other opiates were prescribed routinely by physicians to treat a variety of physical and nervous symptoms in respectable middle-class citizens. Morphine was used extensively for pain relief during the civil war, and its addictive behaviors were aptly called the "soldiers' disease" (Kleber, 1990). Overt addictive behaviors were overlooked because the patients taking them were judged to be the pillars of the community or they were attributed to a logical aftermath of prescribed pain treatment. It was quite fashionable for dentists and physicians in the same time period to use cocaine as a local anesthetic.

Despite the duly noted positive effects of psychoactive substances, their destructive elements also were known in early civilization. Silverstein (1990) noted that "part of the code of Hammurabi of Babylonia, written in 1700 BC, limits the sale and drinking of alcohol. In ancient China drunkards were executed" (p. 22). The laws of Romulus in early Roman times specifically banned women from drinking alcohol; they could be starved or stoned to death for drinking alcoholic beverages (Johnson, 1990). Newlyweds in early Greek cultures were cautioned to avoid drinking alcoholic beverages on their wedding night because they might conceive a defective child (Streissguth, 1986).

Classification as a Medical Disorder

In 1956, alcoholism was labeled officially as a medical disease by the American Medical Society, and 4 years later, the classification of alcoholism as a treatable medical disease received further credibility with the publication of Jellinek's classic text *Disease Concept of Alcoholism*. Jellinek argued that alcoholism should not be considered a uniform disorder, suggesting that the cause and effects of the disorder on a given individual are variable and multifactored. This was a new concept that significantly changed the perception of the disorder from a personal one to a highly interactive one with a polygenic mode of transmission affected by context and other personalized variables (Figure 31–1).

The first attempt to classify alcoholism as a medical disease was in 1785 in a classic work by Dr. Benjamin Rush entitled *An Inquiry Into the Effects of Ardent Spirits Upon the Human Body and Mind, With an Account of the Means of Preventing and of the Remedies for Curing Them.* Unfortunately, Rush's efforts to reframe alcoholism as a medical disease in need of a medical treatment were largely discounted by the medical community. It was not until 1804, when Dr. Thomas Trotter reintroduced the disease concept, that the voice was heard (Jellinek, 1941). Initial attempts to treat alcoholism started with the Washington Home for the Treatment of Alcohol Abuse in 1841, and by 1900 there were 50 public or privately owned centers for the medical treatment of alcoholism.

Legal Interpretations

A narrowed focus on alcohol as primarily a social-behavioral problem continued despite the more enlightened view of it as a medical disorder, peaking in the early 1900s as society sought to deal with the issue by making psychoactive substance use a criminal activity (Kleber, 1990). In 1914, passage of the Harrison Narcotic Act mandated that narcotics be identified as controlled substances that could be dispensed only for medical reasons after stringent legal guidelines. The implications of this act automatically transformed an identified disease process into a criminal act on paper and also, more importantly, in the eyes of the society who voted it into law. The law provided a statute for prosecuting individuals for possession and distribution of drugs, but so many people were jailed for a drug-related offense that they overflowed the prisons.

In addition to legal condemnation of psychoactive substance use, there were strong moral admonitions against alcohol use. Drug abuse was thought to be an offense against society, so on January 6, 1919, the 18th ammendment to the U.S. constitution specifically prohibited alcohol consumption in the United States. This began the Prohibition era. Passage of the law satisfied the proliferation of temperance and prohibition groups, who hoped to eliminate the problem of alcoholism by making the selling or consumption of alcohol illegal. Initially, the law significantly reduced alcohol consumption, but within 10 years, alcohol consumption equaled pre-Prohibition levels. The prohibition amendment was repealed in 1933 largely because it was ineffective. One positive effect was that it drew the nation's attention to the presence of a serious social problem in search of a more effective treatment approach. With the prisons overflowing with recalcitrant alcoholics, it was clear that incarceration was an insufficient deterrent to addictive behavior. As a result, two federal prison hospitals were specifically designated for the care and drug treatment of inmates. Patients were admitted voluntarily to these experimental treatment programs, one near Lexington, Kentucky, and the other in Fort Worth, Texas.

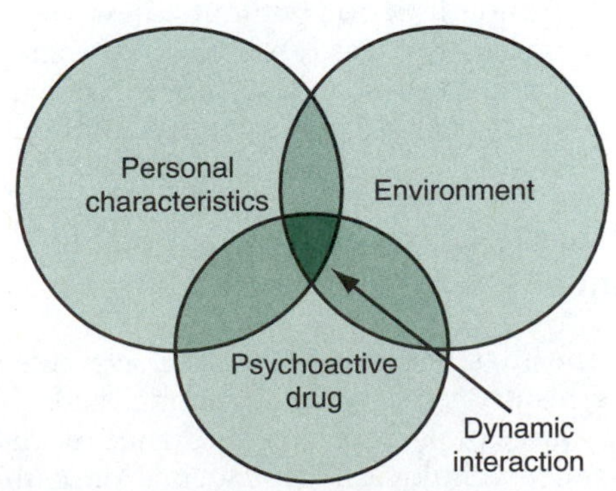

FIGURE 31–1
The polygenic model of transmission of substance use disorders.

TABLE 31–1 **Controlled Substances Act (CSA) Classification***

Drug	CSA* Schedule	Medical Use
Narcotics		
Opium	II, III, IV	Analgesic, antidiarrheal
Morphine	II, III	Analgesic, antitussive
Codeine	II, III, V	Analgesic, antitussive
Heroin	I	None
Hydromorphone (Dilaudid), Meperidine (Demerol, Mepergan)	II	Analgesic
Depressants		
Chloral hydrate	IV	Hypnotic
Barbiturates	II, II, IV	Anesthetic, anticonvulsant, sedative
Benzodiazines	IV	Antianxiety, anticonvulsant, sedative
Methaqualone (Quaalude)	I	Hypnotic sedative
Stimulant		
Cocaine	II	Local anesthetic
Amphetamines	II	Attention deficit disorders, narcolepsy, weight control
Phenmetrazine (Preludin)	II	Weight control
Methylphenidate (Ritalin)	II	Attention deficit disorders, narcolepsy, weight control
Hallucinogens		
Lysergic acid diethylamide (LSD)	I	None
Mescaline and peyote	I	None
Phencyclidine	I	None
Marijuana	I	None
Tetrahydrocannabinol (THC)	I, II	Cancer chemotherapy antinauseant
Hashish	I	None
Hashish oil	I	None

*CSA criteria:
Schedule I, No recognized medical use, high abuse potential; Schedule II, some medical use, high abuse potential; Schedule III, medical use, moderate to high abuse potential; Schedule IV, medical use, low abuse potential; Schedule V, medical use, very low abuse potential.

In 1970, again in response to a dramatic increase in drug-taking behaviors, Congress passed the Comprehensive Drug Abuse Prevention and Control Act, more commonly referred to as the Controlled Substances Act. This legislation assigned commercial use of psychoactive substances to one of five categories reflecting a balance between medical use and potential for abuse (Table 31–1). Those assigned to Schedule I are not available commercially even with a prescription. Written prescriptions are required for Schedule II drugs. Schedule III and IV drugs can be obtained with oral or written prescriptions, but there is a limit on how often the prescription can be refilled in a 6-month period without a new prescription. Schedule V drugs are easily obtainable, some in low quantities without a prescription. There are harsh legal penalties for dispensing drugs in violation of this act.

Synthetically Derived Psychoactive Substances

In 1903, the first barbiturate became available and so began the history of sedative, hypnotic, and anxiolytic abuse as a source of psychoactive substance use disorders. Physical and psychological dependence on natural and synthetic hypnotics developed with alarming frequency as drug experimentation became commonplace with the recreational use of marijuana, cocaine, LSD, and phencyclidine (PCP). It peaked during the 1960s and 1970s with a decline in use over the past two decades (U.S. Department of Health and Human Services, 1990).

The benzodiazepines were developed in the 1960s as synthetic minor tranquilizers to replace the more dangerous barbiturates to reduce anxiety. Initially, these drugs were thought to be nonaddictive and were prescribed with impunity. These drugs were added to the list of controlled drugs in the 1970s when their physically addictive properties became apparent.

Hallucinogenic drugs also were introduced in the 1960s and achieved peak popularity in the 1970s. However, the "bad trips," unpredictability of effects, and notoriety associated with people diving out of windows under the influence of a **flashback** shortened their popularity (Strassman, 1984). PCP became the hallucinogenic drug of choice shortly afterward. A relatively cheap drug to synthesize, PCP also is one of the most dangerous, capable of producing irreversible neuropsychological damage. Cannabis (marijuana), always a favorite with adolescents, has continued its strong status as the most frequently used illicit drug, although it became less popular when cocaine began to dominate the drug scene in the last decade. Over the past decade there has been a decline in illicit drug use from the 1960s and 1970s, but it still remains a major focus for treatment planning in the year 2000 (U.S. Department of Health and Human Services, 1990).

Establishing a Treatment Focus

Establishing a realistic and compassionate treatment plan for substance use disorders received a strong boost from the efforts of Bill W. and Dr. Bob, the original founders of **Alcoholics Anonymous**. In 1935, these two men, abandoned by the medical community as hopeless, untreatable drunks, developed a lay fellowship organization dedicated to providing support for recovering alcoholics who wished to become and remain sober (Marron, 1993). The basic 12-step program they developed formed an important foundation for the therapeutic modification of alcoholism and associated **codependency** behaviors in family members. This model is used worldwide not only for the treatment of alcoholism but also for the treatment of many other addictive behaviors. Basically, the 12-step program and 12 traditions are guidelines for healthy living.

From the initial two founding members, Alcoholics Anonymous has grown to have worldwide membership of more than 1.5 million recovering alcoholics. For the first time, alcoholics received respect for their efforts to remain sober as well as encouragement and hope from others who had successfully mastered their addictive behaviors, often on a daily basis. There is no direct cost to join, and members can receive lifelong support if needed. Active and ongoing involvement with Alcoholics Anonymous or Narcotic Anonymous still remains one of the most effective treatments and adjuncts to therapy for substance use disorders.

In 1970, the Hughes Act (P.L. 91-616) created the National Institute of Alcohol Abuse and Alcoholism as an independent institute within the National Institute of Mental Health. This act gave formal recognition to the importance of the issue as a public and social phenomenon, distinguishable from other mental illnesses. The institute was charged with developing comprehensive programs for the prevention and treatment of alcoholism. Major initiatives included the Employee Assistance Programs, which are state and federal programs for education about and treatment of drug abuse, primary prevention, and enhancement of third-party insurance plans for treatment coverage.

In the early 1980s, the American Nurses' Association (ANA) established addictions as an independent area of specialized nursing practice. Since that time, the ANA, the Drug and Alcohol Nurses Association, and the National Nurses Society on Addictions have joined forces to develop standards of nursing practice and appropriate prevention strategies to address primary, secondary, and tertiary prevention of addictions (ANA, 1988; NNSA, DANA, ANA, 1987). Their goal is to develop an understanding of patterns of abuse and addiction and to develop a comprehensive treatment approach to one of the most complex mental health problems of our century.

Recognizing the theoretical paradox of psychoactive substances being simultaneously useful as medicinal agents and highly destructive as recreational drugs is important because it helps the nurse understand the confusion that continues to exist about the most appropriate treatment for substance use disorders. As we enter the next century, new federal guidelines for the treatment of alcohol abuse have been passed into law and are meeting with some success. People with a drug abuse problem can no longer be discriminated against in work and educational settings. Despite significant advances, there is more work to be done because a legalistic treatment approach to a medical disorder persists. Viewing substance use disorders as a weakness of character and addressing them as a moral-legal issue remains a popular but single-minded approach to a very complex problem. In fact, no other mental or physical disorder carries quite the same moral and legal stigma consistently associated with psychoactive substance use disorders.

The use of legal constraints is not without merit, but it complicates treatment in many cases. As a deterrent to drug abuse and a motivator for treatment, legal consequences for drug abuse play an important role in prevention and treatment. More often than not, it is to avoid or comply with legal consequences of drug abuse that the person with a substance use disorder first enters treatment. These same legal consequences, however, make pregnant women reluctant to admit to drug use and family members uneasy about reporting drug use among their sons and daughters. Equally detrimental to a therapeutic approach are the moralistic attitudes of health professionals and the general public regarding the role of will power in the development of a substance use disorder.

With the emergence of a resource-driven health care delivery system, insurance companies are limiting third-party reimbursement for drug treatment and rehabilitation. There is irony in the paradox of mandating employers and schools to recognize substance use disorders as a medical disability and to support treatment efforts for its victims while limiting treatment for a chronic disorder. In practical terms, the cost containment measures for treatment of substance use disorders make it financially unavailable for a significant portion of the population who desperately needs such services.

DEFINITION

Substance use disorder is a broad, generic diagnostic term used by the medical community to describe a predictable, composite set of physical symptoms and behavioral patterns associated with the voluntary ingestion of a psychoactive substance. The symptom pattern of the disorder is characterized by ongoing compulsive use of one or more psychoactive substances. Consumption continues as a compelling drive despite increasingly negative life consequences and adverse social responses from significant others regarding drug-taking behaviors.

The term **psychoactive substances** refers to any mind-altering agent capable of modifying a person's behavior, mood, thinking, arousal level, state of consciousness, and perceptions. Changes in behavior occur because of the drug's effect on the normal synaptic transmission of internal messages in the brain, with special attention given to the role of acetylcholine, norepinephrine, dopamine, and serotonin (Leccese, 1991). Although virtually all medications are capable of producing neuropsychological effects, with many having the potential for creating abuse and dependence, substance use disorders are concerned primarily with the use of distinctly psychoactive substances voluntarily ingested for other than medical purposes. These substances, commonly referred to as drugs rather than as medications, include a number of legally sanctioned drugs such as alcohol, benzodiazepines, narcotics, caffeine, and nicotine. The list of illegal drugs used for recreational use includes the hallucinogens, phencyclidine, cocaine, opiates, amphetamines, barbiturates, and volatile solvents.

Related Terminology

Other terms used to describe the behaviors associated with substance use disorders include drug addiction, drug abuse, and chemical dependency. The World Health Organization (WHO) defined **addiction** as "a state of chronic intoxication produced by the repeated consumption of a drug (natural or synthetic)." Characteristics include (1) an overpowering desire or need (compulsion) to continue taking the drug and to obtain it by any means; (2) a tendency to increase the dose; (3) a psychic (psychological) and generally a physical dependence on the effects of the drug; and (4) a detrimental effect on the individual and/or society" (Kleber, 1990, p. 59).

Substance (drug or chemical) abuse is another term frequently used to describe substance use disorders. The term refers to the nontherapeutic use of psychoactive agents or the illicit use of a prescribed drug on a regular, binge, or episodic basis. To meet *Diagnostic and Statistical Manual of Mental Disorders* (fourth edition) *(DSM-IV)* criteria for substance abuse, the patients must have gone for at least a month, or frequently over a longer period of time, without meeting the criteria for psychoactive substance dependence, which involves physical dependence and withdrawal symptoms.

Box 31–1 presents a broad glossary of terms related to substance use disorders. Distinctions among misuse, drug habituation, and drug abuse are also important in a discussion of drug-taking behaviors. Substance misuse embraces a wide spectrum of drug-taking behaviors. Examples include taking a legitimate drug prescription in a nonprescribed manner, obtaining it in an unlawful way or without a legitimate medical reason, and giving a prescribed medication to a friend. Substance (drug) habituation refers to regular use without developing physical dependence. This term is used by many substance users to describe the recreational use of marijuana or LSD. The distinction in many cases is one of semantics; the line between drug dependency and recreational use of drugs on a regular basis is a relatively thin one.

BOX 31–1 A Glossary of Terms Related to Substance Use Disorders

Psychoactive Substance: Any mind-altering agent that alters a person's mood, behavior, perceptions, thinking, arousal level, or state of consciousness.

Substance Abuse: Nontherapeutic use of psychoactive drugs or illicit use of a prescribed drug.

Tolerance: Decreased sensitivity to drug with chronic use that allows a person to increase the dosage of a psychoactive drug without suffering toxic effects.

Physical Dependence: Withdrawal syndrome of physical symptoms that occur when the drug is withdrawn and persist until system functioning readapts to the predrug state.

Withdrawal: Physical symptoms directly related to the abrupt termination of the psychoactive drug.

Overdose: Physical and potentially life-threatening symptoms directly related to drug ingestion.

Detoxification: Medically supervised elimination of the drug from the body.

Recovery: Sobriety; comfortable abstinence from drug.

Relapse: Reemergence of symptoms associated with substance abuse disorders.

Drug Addiction: Compulsive use of a drug that produces a state or period of chronic intoxication.

Substance Use Disorder: Mental disorder characterized by pathological use of a psychoactive drug over a significant period of time that interferes with physical stability, emotional, social, or occupational functioning.

Cross-Tolerance: Capacity of psychoactive drugs with similar pharmacological properties to produce the same adaptive changes as the original drug, making them interchangeable in effects on the brain.

Psychological Dependence: Craving or insatiable hunger for a drug even after successful detoxification.

Reinforcing Properties: Positive behavioral effects of drug taking and negative memories of withdrawal reactions.

Potentiate: The capacity of two psychoactive drugs to produce psychological and physical effects greater than the sum of two agents; also referred to as "synergistic" effects.

Flashbacks: Reexperiencing of emotions and behavioral effects of drug without further drug intake and after the drug has cleared the body.

Kindling Effect: Reexperiencing of drug behaviors without the ingestion of a psychoactive substance.

Blackouts: Amnesia for events and conversations despite appearing normal and engaging in conversation of which there is no memory later.

Substance (chemical) dependence is the pathological use of a psychoactive drug over a significant period of time with symptoms of physical and psychological addiction to the drug such that it interferes with physical, social, or occupational functioning. Evidence of sustained pathological use includes an inability to control use of the drug despite clear knowledge of the problems associated with its use and the development of craving and physical symptoms when the drug is withdrawn. A primary distinction between drug abuse and chemical dependency is that the former represents a voluntary behavior and the latter does not. With drug abuse, a person voluntarily ingests a psychoactive substance as a free and conscious act, whereas with chemical dependence, although the person voluntarily ingests the substance, his or her action is compulsive.

Difficulty in Establishing a Common Definition

Establishing a commonly held definition for substance use disorders has proven difficult for the medical community because it is such a complex disorder. The National Commission on Marijuana and Drug Use in 1973 noted that "drug using behavior is described by such an array of non-specific, unscientific and judgmental terms that it is often difficult to ascertain who is being described and what behavior is being evaluated" (p. 73). Although the official classification of substance use disorders is a medical one, if you were to seek a sample of definitions from the general public, you would be more likely to hear moral, social, and behavioral definitions. Many would define it as a lack of will power, a societal problem associated with poverty, deprivation, and homelessness, or a response to parental neglect or training. Some view it as a criminal problem in which young people are seduced into drug-taking behaviors by hardened criminals intent on making a fortune without actually working for it. All of these definitions fit some aspect of the meaning of a substance use disorder. All are incomplete explanations. Regardless of how it is defined, substance use disorders represent a multifactorial behavioral syndrome with physical, social, spiritual, and psychological consequences for the individual, family, and society. As Hughes (1989) suggested, "addiction is more than a toxic state, a criminal offense, a disease, a mental health problem, or an unhealthy habit. It also is a social problem that affects every aspect of life—physical, psychological and interpersonal" (p. 10). To this must be added the profound effect of substance use disorders on the spiritual life of the patient, family, and community. This diagnosis usually entails a serious loss of contact with the inner spirit of the person intrapersonally and interpersonally, leaving the perception of almost everything other than the drug use completely devoid of meaning. The loss of a loved one in a random alcohol-related accident and the human suffering this disorder causes others bring to mind the senselessness of drug-induced behaviors on innocent victims.

THEORETICAL MODELS

Theoretical models traditionally provide a way of making sense of a phenomenon and offer a map to understanding the relationships within it. Two of the more popular explanations of substance abuse disorders center on alcoholism as a prototype and describe a disease model and a model of faulty adaptation. There is persuasive evidence for a genetic predisposition to the development of alcoholism in some individuals (Stone and Gottesman, 1993). Among identical twins (monozygotic) the concordance rate for the development of alcoholism was much greater than for fraternal twins (dizygotic) in a number of research studies (Merekangas, 1990). Other studies of familial predisposition strongly implicate the role of genetics in the development of alcoholism, because having a first-degree blood relative increases the incidence of alcoholism from two to four times the probability in the normal population (Milkman and Shaffer, 1983).

Several studies point to the possible role of dopamine in the reinforcing effects of several types of drug classifications, again suggesting a biological explanation for the development of chemical dependency (Stone and Gottesman, 1993). Most studies suggest that a genetic biochemical susceptibility combined with the learned behaviors developed through living in a dysfunctional family place the affected individual at high risk for the development of chemical dependency (Goodwin, 1979). After an extensive review of the literature, Stone and Gottesman (1993) concluded that

- Genetic factors contribute to the development of alcoholism, but their precise levels of influence differ related to gender, age of onset, and severity of the disorder. There is more evidence of genetic contributions with males, early onset, and severe drinking patterns.
- No single gene and no single biochemical or structural defect is likely to mediate the disorder. Instead there appears to be a multifactorial polygenic mode of transmission related to the development of alcoholism.

By contrast, the adaptive model suggests that substance use disorders occur as a socially caused phenomenon, the result of learned social coping strategies based on substance use. Proponents of this model cite addictive behaviors learned in the family of origin as primary etiological factors. These adaptive models fault sociocultural factors that allow children early access and role modeling of drug behaviors by adults and peers as causative agents and suggest that for children who are exposed to drugs as a way of earning money, coping with stressful situations, and achieving acceptance in a social group, it is difficult to consider other alternative options. For children growing up in a drug culture, smoking pot, drinking alcohol, and using intravenous (IV) drugs, drug-taking behaviors are normal and living without the drug is intolerable.

Most theoretical explanations today suggest a polygenic mode of transmission, which consists of the dynamic relationship among the individual's unique psychobiological make-up, genetic and environmental factors, and the effects of the particular psychoactive substance on that person's physical and emotional system. A multimodal framework helps explain why two individuals with similar genetic backgrounds may turn out quite differently and likewise why two individuals from very different family backgrounds can have similar problems with chemical dependence. Considering the context for drug-taking behaviors provides an explanation for the many different types of responses a single drug can have on a person.

▶ **Check Your Reading**

1. In what ways do drug abuse and chemical dependency differ?
2. How does the historical context of substance use disorders contribute to our current understanding of substance use disorders?
3. How would you describe the role of genetic factors in the development of alcoholism?

COMMON PROPERTIES OF PSYCHOACTIVE SUBSTANCES

A number of common properties associated with all psychoactive substances bear mention before discussing the individual drug classifications. These include acute and chronic structural and functional changes in the brain associated with drug intake, variable effects on the person taking them, and the concept of **recovery** and **relapse** prevention after cessation of drug intake. The concepts of dependence, **tolerance**, and **reinforcing properties** are unique properties of most psychoactive substances and are not found in other pharmacological classifications.

Changes in Brain Structure and Function

Psychoactive drugs act directly on one or more of the delicate electrochemical neurotransmitters in the brain that convey information and regulate mood. Their differential actions alter the normal electrochemical circuits in the brain and interfere with the normal biochemical balance of the body. Even single doses can dramatically disrupt the intricate internal biochemical processes in the brain that influence behavioral response. Prolonged or chronic use can reset the body's internal biochemical response system in a new homeostatic but distinctly abnormal pattern. Paradoxically, over time, the drug abuser's behavior may appear more "normal" while on the drug and may look bizarre when the drug is withdrawn precipitously. Moreover, chronic drug use affects not only the chemistry in the brain but indirectly or directly many critical body systems. Cardiovascular damage, coma, seizures, respiratory collapse, hepatic failure, renal failure, hemorrhagic disorders, transient psychosis, and nutritional deficiencies are serious secondary medical consequences of prolonged psychoactive drug abuse. Psychoactive drugs lower resistance to infection and many are immunosuppressive. Unintentional suicides, automobile accidents, physical injuries, and homicides occur more often under the influence of psychoactive drugs.

Variable Effects

Substance use disorders are much more complicated to understand and treat than other mental disorders because they can have multiple and variable physical effects on different persons and on the same person under different circumstances. Unlike other medications, psychoactive substances produce unexpected effects that vary with the dosage of the drug, the environmental context in which the drug was taken, and the person's mood at the time of ingestion. Alcohol, for example, produces an initial euphoria in which the affected person feels more socially competent and lighter in mood. At a higher dosage, however, sedation and central nervous system depression occur. Cocaine has local anesthetic properties as well as powerful central nervous system stimulant actions (Jones, 1984). Some alcoholics do not show any changes on physical examination. Although they are in the minority, their testimony to the lack of ill effects associated with their disorder is unsettling because it encourages others to assume that excessive alcohol intake is not dangerous. Other factors such as the person's body weight and musculature, rate of metabolism, food consumed before drug ingestion, mood at the time of ingestion, other drug use, tolerance variability, and mode of administration also affect the way in which the brain responds to the presence of a psychoactive substance.

Dependence

In 1964, the WHO identified dependence as the distinguishing characteristic of sustained abnormal drug use. **Dependence** is defined as "a state of psychic or physical dependence or both, on a drug, arising in a person following administration of that drug on a periodic or continuous basis. The characteristics of such a state will vary with the agent involved" (Kleber, 1990, p. 60). A chemical dependence derives from structural and functional changes in the brain as the brain adapts to the chronic presence of a psychoactive substance such that the adaptation requires continued ingestion of the drug to prevent unpleasant withdrawal symptoms. There are two types of dependence, both of which are important to the understanding of substance use disorders: physical and psychological dependence. Persons who are considered to have a substance use dependency are sometimes referred to as being chemically dependent.

Physical Dependence

Physical dependence is described as a physical need for the psychoactive substance such that the person suffers marked physiological symptoms when the drug is withdrawn and is directly related to the drug of use or its interaction with other psychoactive substances. All of the hypnotic sedative and narcotic analgesic pharmacological classifications can create physical dependencies. Abrupt, unsupervised withdrawal from these drugs in heavy consumers can result in respiratory collapse and sudden death.

Intoxication occurs with clinically significant signs and symptoms associated with recent ingestion of a psychoactive substance not attributable to any other medical or psychological condition. A person can be intoxicated without suffering the withdrawal effects of a chronic condition, or the intoxication can be superimposed on a drug dependency, resulting in acute symptoms.

Withdrawal describes the spontaneous removal of the drug from the body system as either an unplanned event or a gradual tapering of the drug under medical supervision. Symptoms from unintended or unsupervised withdrawal can cause death. Without a secure environment and medical supervision, withdrawal symptoms are so uncomfortable that they act as a reinforcement for further drug use.

Detoxification refers to a medically supervised withdrawal process over a prescribed time period, ranging from 7 to 28 days. Observation and treatment of medical complications, short-term use of pharmacological agents to reduce patient discomfort, and intense motivational-educational therapeutic approaches are used to quickly reestablish a drug-free state in the chemically dependent patient.

Toxicity (overdose) refers to toxic physiological symptoms caused by taking too much of a drug or mixing drugs that "potentiate" and enhance the physical effects of each primary drug. People can become comatose, suffer cardiac arrhythmias or respiratory collapse, and die quickly from overdose. Overdoses can occur in first-time users who have not built up a tolerance to heavy doses of a drug. Chronic drug abusers can experience a toxicity with the administration of a purer form of a drug that has not been cut or with the ingestion of more than one drug simultaneously.

Tolerance

Tolerance is a common property of psychoactive substance disorders and a precursor of chemical dependence. Tolerance refers to the body's need for larger amounts of a psychoactive substance to achieve the same effects previously obtainable with less of the drug. Ingestion of increasingly greater amounts has no toxic effects as the neurotransmitters in the brain begin to adapt to biological alterations created by the presence of the drug. This increases the likelihood of greater drug use and eventual dependence.

Tolerance varies from individual to individual so that not everyone who takes the same amount of a drug responds in a similar fashion. For example, some people can drink large amounts of alcohol without ill effects, whereas others can consume very little and experience hangover symptoms. In general, people with a low tolerance to a drug are at a lower risk for developing a substance use disorder because the effects are so uncomfortable.

Cross-tolerance is the term used to describe (1) the capacity of other psychoactive substances in the same drug classification to enhance (potentiate) the effects of the primary abused drug and (2) the ability of the primary drug to expand similar behavioral responses to other psychoactive substances after repeated exposure to a single drug. Because most persons diagnosed as having a substance use disorder are in reality polydrug users, understanding the mechanisms of cross-tolerance is critical for effective nursing care.

Most central nervous stimulants, hypnotic sedatives, and benzodiazepines potentiate or enhance the effects of each other and alcohol. The additive effects of the drug combinations can kill the drug user, whereas each drug taken individually would not have had the same consequence. A popular combination of drugs with potentially lethal effects for the user is excessive alcohol and benzodiazepines. Cross-tolerance also has implications for medicating patients requiring a narcotic analgesic for pain relief (e.g., surgical and hospice patients). Because of cross-tolerance, almost anyone with a history of or a current substance use disorder will require larger doses of narcotic analgesics, even if they have not used drugs for many years.

Psychological Dependence

Some psychoactive substances do not establish a physical tolerance. Instead, they create a **psychological dependence** in which obsessive thinking about the drug causes the person to repeatedly seek drug relief despite the inevitable compromise of personal values, violation of conduct codes, and negative consequences of drug-taking behaviors. Drugs identified with a heavy incidence of psychological dependence among chronic abusers include cocaine, marijuana, and the hallucinogens. Because of its reinforcing properties, psychological dependence can be as debilitating as physical dependence in the persistence of a substance use disorder (Adams and Durrell, 1984).

Reinforcing properties refers to the positive or negative behavioral effects of self-administered psychoactive substances that serve to intensify desire or hunger for the drug. Psychological dependence is always associated with reinforcing properties, the most significant of which is **craving**, whereby the person experiences an insatiable compulsive desire for a particular psychoactive substance accompanied by vivid remembrances of either the good feelings the drug produces or the relief of anxiety and mood swings. Although exactly how it works is not fully understood (see Chapter 7 for physiological explanation), the **kindling effect** also is an intrinsically psychological reinforcing property of addictive drugs in which the memory of pleasure exerted by the drug reactivates the addict's desire for the drug. This euphoric recall (Bluhm, 1987) permits the substance abuser to selectively remember the feelings with no linkage to the potential self-destructive effects of the drug, much as Joe relates earlier in his story.

Positive reinforcing properties consist of the initial mood elevation associated with effects of the drug on dopaminergic synapses, implicated in the brain reward circuitry. Activation of the natural brain reward system may provide immediate relief from anxiety, temporary pain relief, a natural euphoria, and increased energy (Wise, 1984). Negative reinforcing properties include the dysphoric or depressed mood that occurs in many substance users after the drug effects wear off. Usually the unpleasant feelings create such emotional discomfort that quick relief from further ingestion of the drug is sought. Thus painful memories of the withdrawal syndrome may provide the most powerful reinforcers for psychoactive substance addiction.

Recovery and Relapse Prevention

Two other common properties of substance use disorders relate to the treatment process involving concepts of recovery and relapse prevention. Because these disorders represent a chronic disease condition, the word "cure" is not used even years after the last ingestion of a psychoactive drug. Instead, the American Medical Society (1982) defined **recovery** in substance use disorders as a psychologically comfortable abstinence from other alcohol and other dependency-producing drugs. Recovery continues throughout life, and persons in the rehabilitative phase identify themselves as recovering alcoholics and recovering addicts. This psychological reframing cues the person to remember that recovery requires a daily effort to remain abstinent.

The other concept deemed important in the understanding and treatment of drug dependencies is **relapse prevention.** Relapse occurs when the symptoms of a disease reappear after a period of improvement. Many substance users will require more than one treatment episode because substance use disorders are chronic disorders. When the patient relapses, it is as if he had never stopped using drugs. Although discouraging, this fact does not preclude active intervention brought to bear on the symptoms as quickly as possible.

Relapse prevention includes a wide variety of nursing strategies that help recovering addicts develop meaningful life goals without the use of a psychoactive drugs, find new support systems, and learn new coping strategies. Relapse prevention is particularly important during the first few months after intensive treatment and during stressful times. One way to guard against recividism is to help the patient develop a written prevention plan and to work with others in the patient's life to empower them to assist the patient in achieving the goal of abstinence. Active involvement in Alcoholics Anonymous, Cocaine Anonymous, or Narcotics Anonymous also can be life saving in helping the person with a substance use disorder maintain his or her resolve (see Case Example 31–2, later in this chapter).

TRAJECTORY OF THE JOURNEY INTO SUBSTANCE USE DISORDERS

Understanding the sequential pattern of behaviors associated with addiction provides the nurse with a firm knowledge base and credibility in helping patients constructively confront the magnitude of their problem. Clearly, there is a defined developmental path associated with substance use disorders that begins with social or medical use of a psychoactive substance and ends with the consistent presence of addictive behaviors. Usually the road to chemical dependency begins innocently enough, and the point at which voluntary use becomes involuntary cannot be readily identified. Many factors such as drug availability, personality factors, genetic predisposition, exposure to stressful situations, and environmental support conspire to produce substance use disorders.

First-time use of a psychoactive substance for young people typically occurs within the context of a person's social and developmental peer group, as Joe related in his story. Alternatively, it can develop from the use of medically prescribed drugs to reduce anxiety, relieve physical pain, or promote sleep. The drugs help people feel better, and they begin to depend on them for relief from minor emotional and physical discomfort. No one would identify the possibility of addiction as a consequence of regular ingestion of psychoactive substances. If you asked novice drug takers why they take drugs, use pot, drink alcohol, or snort cocaine, they would tell you "to relax," "as part of having a good time," "it makes me feel good," "it gets me more in touch with myself," or "simply out of curiosity because their parents or peers use them." Others would describe the "thrill-producing" effects of the drug experience. They would suggest that the drugs stimulate a sense of spontaneous awareness, oneness with the world, and self-confidence while diminishing boredom, tension, and meaninglessness.

The cross-over from experimental, recreational use to habitual use is subtle. Solitary use, hiding the habit, and growing tolerance are definitive signs of growing dependence. Many people also have help in establishing habitual use in a drug supportive environment. The drugs are readily available and often are offered free or at very low fee to the potential consumer. Once the drug habit has taken effect, full price is charged and the person has become enslaved in the drug-taking behavior.

As the habit increases, faith in the drug to relieve stress begins to replace trust in other interpersonal relationships. New friends interested in similar drug experimentation crowd out old relationships, and an extraordinary loyalty builds up among them, fueled by a secret that they all share and must protect: their use of psychoactive drugs (Case Example 31–1).

Case Example 31–1 Dana's Story, Part 1

I never grew up wanting to be a drug addict or alcoholic. In fact, I was always taught in school and by my parents that drugs were bad and bad things could happen to you if you used them. So I really grew up afraid of them. I think the reason I picked up my first drink and later my first drug was as for most people, because of peer pressure. I saw all my friends doing it and they weren't jumping off buildings or wanting to fly, and nobody was dying or freaking out. I didn't see any bad things happening to them. In fact, nothing but good things were happening. They were more popular than me; they were being invited on dates and I wasn't. I guess after a while, I wanted to do drugs so I could be like them. Some people's theory about people on drugs or alcohol is that there is a void in their lives, a hole in their gut they can't seem to fill, or a lack of self-esteem. That was true with me. I didn't have enough self-esteem to stand on my own two feet and not "follow the crowd." I didn't know I was okay just the way I was. I needed acceptance from these people I thought were my friends. I didn't think I was pretty, I thought I was fat, and I just didn't think I was good enough. But when I was drinking or on drugs, well that's a different story. I was pretty, thin, funny, life of the party, cracking jokes. Everybody noticed me and liked me. If feeling like that meant that I had to drink, well so be it. I was having the time of my life. That feeling lasted about 3 to 4 years. Then I started feeling not good enough again. I guess there were always periods of feeling like that when I was by myself, but now the feelings started coming back even when I was out with my friends, cracking jokes and being the life of the party. Everyone else still seemed to like me except me. So those awful feelings that drugs at one time suppressed came back even stronger. Because this time, the feelings were not only of not being good enough, but also of fear that I was going to get caught soon if I kept it up, either by my parents or the police. I guess some people would call that paranoia. I also had feelings of guilt that I treated my family badly, that I wasn't there for them. It was more important for me to be out with my friends than to talk with them or help my mom out. At family functions I would try to slip away to smoke a joint or make an excuse not to go so I could go out with people who didn't care about me. I guess I started realizing these people were not my friends when I started to see how they behaved not only toward me but toward other people. I saw them doing raunchy things to people, fighting and making fun of them because they were too drunk or messed up to do any better. The stealing, the lies, the manipulation, the schemes really bothered me. Of course at this point, I really didn't think any of this had to do with drugs. I blamed it on everyone and everything else.

Denial and rationalization provide structure and meaning to drug-taking behaviors. In the patient's mind, personal reverses are associated with a problem boss or the wife's nagging despite what everyone in close contact with the patient can observe: that the problems exist in relation to the effects of a psychoactive substance. Physical evidence of organ system involvement appears in the form of physical disorders and neurological impairment. Frequently, those most intimately involved with the effects of dependency behaviors shake their heads in amazement that chemically dependent persons cannot distance themselves from a chemical that literally is destroying them and everything that is important to them. Without treatment, substance dependence inevitably leads to personal, marital, financial, and job-related reverses directly attributable to the effects of the disorder. Death and impoverishment, the loss of everything that is meaningful, and often serious harm to others are potential outcomes.

DIAGNOSTIC CLASSIFICATIONS

Diagnostic and Statistical Manual of Mental Disorders, fourth edition General Classification

The *DSM-IV* (American Psychiatric Association, 1994) made several changes from the DSM III-R related to dependence replacing the earlier stipulation that the disorder must have persisted for at least a month with symptoms occurring at any time in the last 12 months (Ghodse, 1995, p. 160). The intent was to make the category more inclusive. The *DSM-IV* also distinguishes between psychoactive substance–induced organic mental disorders and those that clearly evidence abuse and dependency without definitive organic sequelae. The diagnostic manual does not make generic distinctions related to the specific drug causing the disorder. **Polydrug dependence** (304.90) involves the regular use of three or more psychoactive substances over a period of at least 6 months (Kaplan and Sadock, 1988).

The rationale for classifying psychoactive substance disorders within a generic category of substance use or substance dependence relates to commonalities in psychological behavioral patterns across drug classifications. Regardless of specific cause (which is important in treating toxicity and withdrawal), it is the outcome of psychoactive drug use, shared in common by all drug classifications, that are most likely to account for the problems associated with the disorder (Wise, 1984). With the exception of the acute withdrawal stage, the medical treatment and rehabilitation of any drug dependency are similar in approach and not dependent on a precise knowledge of the causative agent. Considering all psychoactive substance disorders collectively as a primary medical phenomenon rather than focusing on the specific drug is useful in an age when most substance abusers use more than one psychoactive substance (Kaufman, 1982). The *DSM-IV* classification of substance abuse and substance dependence disorders is presented in "Medical Diagnoses and Related Nursing Diagnoses." For a complete descriptive analysis of the diagnostic criteria applied to the substance use and substance-related disorders, please consult the *DSM-IV* chapter on substance-related disorders.

Nursing Diagnoses

The nursing diagnoses for substance use disorders refer to the functional patterns a patient presents. Management of acute symptoms relate to the specific differential classification of the disorder. In the rehabilitative phase,

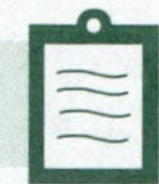

MEDICAL DIAGNOSES AND RELATED NURSING DIAGNOSES — *DSM-IV* Diagnostic Criteria for Substance-Related Disorders

DEPENDENCE AND ABUSE

Substance Dependence

A maladaptive pattern of substance use, leading to clinically significant impairment or distress, as manifested by three or more of the following occurring at any time in the same 12-month period:

1. Tolerance, as defined by either of the following:
   (a) Need for markedly increased amounts of the substance to achieve intoxication or desired effect
   (b) Markedly diminished effect with continued use of the same amount of the substance
2. Withdrawal, as manifested by either of the following:
   (a) The characteristic withdrawal syndrome for the substance (refer to criteria A and B of the criteria sets for withdrawal from the specific substances)
   (b) The same (or closely related) substance is taken to relieve or avoid withdrawal symptoms
3. The substance is often taken in larger amounts or over a longer period than was intended
4. A persistent desire or unsuccessful efforts to cut down or control substance use
5. A great deal of time is spent in activities necessary to obtain the substance (e.g., visiting multiple doctors or driving long distances), use the substance (e.g., chain smoking), or recover from its effects
6. Important social, occupational, or recreational activities given up or reduced because of substance use
7. Continued substance use despite knowledge of having had a persistent or recurrent physical or psychological problem that was likely to have been caused or exacerbated by the substance (e.g., current cocaine use despite recognition of cocaine-induced depression, or continued drinking despite recognition that an ulcer was made worse by alcohol consumption)

Specify if:
With Physiological Dependence: Evidence of tolerance or withdrawal (i.e., either item (1) or (2) is present).
Without Physiological Dependence: No evidence of tolerance or withdrawal (i.e., neither item (1) nor (2) is present).
There are modifiers that address the issue of course. First, it is most important to recognize that once a person has ever had a pattern of substance use that meets criteria for dependence, the person can no longer qualify for a diagnosis of abuse for that substance. However, the patient may meet criteria for early remission, full or partial, or sustained remission, full or partial. There is a modifier that applies to a patient who is **on agonist therapy,** such as methadone maintenance or nicotine replacement, when the agonist medication is not being abused. There is also a modifier that applies to a patient who is **in a controlled environment** for one month or longer where no criteria for dependence or abuse are met, but the person is in an environment where controlled substances are highly restricted, such as locked hospitals, therapeutic communities, or substance-free jails.

Substance Abuse

A. A maladaptive pattern of substance use leading to clinically significant impairment or distress, as manifested by one or more of the following occurring at any time during the same 12-month period:
   1. Recurrent substance use resulting in a failure to fulfill major role obligations at work, school, or home (e.g., repeated absences or poor work performance related to substance use; substance-related absences, suspensions, or expulsions from school; neglect of children or household)
   2. Recurrent substance use in situations in which it is physically hazardous (e.g., driving an automobile or operating a machine when impaired by substance use)
   3. Recurrent substance-related legal problems (e.g., arrests for substance-related disorderly conduct)
   4. Continued substance use despite having persistent or recurrent social or interpersonal problems caused or exacerbated by the effects of the substance (e.g., arguments with spouse about consequences of intoxication, physical fights).

B. Has never met the criteria for Substance Dependence for this class of substance.

SUBSTANCE INTOXICATION AND SUBSTANCE WITHDRAWAL

Substance Intoxication

The development of a reversible substance-specific syndrome due to recent ingestion of (or exposure to) a substance. (Note: different substances may produce similar or identical syndromes.)

Substance Withdrawal

The development of a substance-specific syndrome due to the cessation of, or reduction in, substance use that has been heavy and prolonged.
The substance-specific syndrome causes clinically significant distress or impairment in social, occupational, or other important areas of functioning.
Not due to a general medical condition and not better accounted for by another mental disorder.

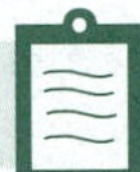

MEDICAL DIAGNOSES AND RELATED NURSING DIAGNOSES ***DSM-IV*** **Diagnostic Criteria for Substance-Related Disorders** *Continued*

RELATED NURSING DIAGNOSIS	DEFINITION	EXAMPLE
Ineffective coping, individual	The state in which an individual experiences or is at risk of experiencing an inability to manage internal or environmental stressors adequately because of inadequate resources (physical, psychological, behavioral)	Ineffective coping, individual related to substance use evidenced by using drugs to relieve anxiety
Ineffective denial	The state in which an individual minimizes or disavows symptoms or a situation to his or her detriment of health	Ineffective denial related to substance use evidenced in refusal to admit problem

Diagnostic criteria from American Psychiatric Association (1994). *Diagnostic and statistical manual of mental disorders, fourth edition.* Washington, DC: Author. Nursing diagnoses and definitions from North American Nursing Diagnosis Association. (1994). *NANDA nursing diagnoses: Definitions and classification 1995–1996.* Philadelphia: NANDA.

however, the nurse will see similar functional patterns in need of nursing intervention across all pharmacological categories, a strong representative sample of which is provided in Box 31–2.

Differential Classification

In addition to making general diagnostic distinctions among substance intoxication, abuse, and dependence, the *DSM-IV* further categorizes psychoactive substance use disorders according to their general pharmacological effects on the brain and central nervous system. Four primary classifications cover most of the illicit drug use responsible for the diagnosis of substance use disorders: (1) sedative hypnotics, (2) hallucinogens, (3) narcotic analgesics, and (4) central nervous system stimulants and two additional categories for over-the-counter drugs and volatile solvents (Box 31–3).

Alcohol Use Disorders

Alcohol is a central nervous system depressant derived from the "fermentation of sugar, starch or other carbohydrates" (Matuschka, 1985, p. 50). The drug is rapidly metabolized, appearing in the bloodstream within five minutes and affecting the higher cortical functions in the brain almost immediately. Most people can metabolize approximately 1 ounce per hour. Milk and fatty foods delay the absorption rate. With consistent use, alcoholics can metabolize liquor more quickly, leading to the assumption that they can handle their liquor better. What

BOX 31-2 Nursing Diagnoses for Patients With Substance Use Disorders

Biological Responses

- Sensory/Perceptual Alteration
- Self Care Deficit
- Injury, potential for
- Sexual Dysfunction
- Infection, potential for
- Sleep Pattern Disturbance
- Nutrition, Altered: Less than Body Requirements
- Pain
- Growth and Development, Altered

Cognitive Responses

- Knowledge Deficit
- Thought Processes, Altered
- Noncompliance (specify)

Psychosocial Responses

- Impaired Verbal Communication
- Ineffective Individual Coping
- Social Isolation
- Anxiety
- Family Processes, Altered
- Parenting, Altered
- Violence, potential for
- Growth and Development, Altered

Spiritual Responses

- Spiritual Distress
- Powerlessness
- Hopelessness
- Dysfunctional Grieving

Modified from American Nurses' Association (1988). Standards of addictions nursing practice with selected diagnoses and criteria. Kansas City, MO: ANA.

actually happens is they develop greater tolerance for the substance. Another common myth is that the percentage of alcohol accounts for drug dependency. Many people naively think that if they drink beer or wine they will not become alcoholics. Unfortunately, this simply is not true and many alcoholics drink only beer or wine. The standard beverage equivalency is as follows: one beer equals 4 ounces of whiskey and one glass of wine equals 1 to 1.5 ounces.

Alcohol has the unique distinction among abused psychoactive substances of being legally sanctioned, easily obtainable and at a relatively low cost, and actually promoted by advertising in the media (Gualtieri, 1990). Anyone 21 years or older can purchase alcohol legally over the counter, and even the most rural communities possess a liquor store. Liquor stores are looked on as social gathering sites and reservoirs of information about the community in many urban settings, particularly in less affluent neighborhoods. In some communities, liquor stores are willing to cash paychecks, thus implicitly encouraging people to spend at least part of their paycheck on liquor.

Society actively supports the use of alcohol in moderation. Socially, it not only is acceptable to drink but in many circles it is expected. How many parties have you attended where alcohol was not served? If it was not served, you probably heard some derogatory comments about its absence. Often there is a special table or area set aside for alcoholic beverages. Other party edibles do not enjoy a similar emphasis. There is little question that alcohol enlivens parties and social gatherings by producing a temporary state of lightheartedness and a reduction of self-consciousness, particularly in people who feel insecure about themselves. Taken in excess, alcohol inevitably leads to trouble, destroying the life of the party and in some instances taking the life of a partygoer through overdose or accident.

Television portrays social drinking as both normal and desirable (Cafiso et al, 1982). Only within recent years have drug prevention messages been portrayed with any regularity in television spots. Interestingly, these advertisements target the adolescent. Drug problems among adults and the elderly usually are addressed in documentaries, but rarely are they addressed as issues in preventive messages seen on television.

The incidence and prevalence of alcohol use as a mind-altering drug provide staggering evidence of the magnitude of the problem. As the most frequently used and abused psychoactive substance in the United States, alcohol often is the first psychoactive drug used by potential polydrug abusers. Up to 20 million Americans could be diagnosed as having a major problem with alcohol, and approximately 40% of the population have lived some part of their lives in alcoholic families (Robertson, 1993).

Alcohol has been identified as both a cause and an effect of homelessness, placing the homeless individual at risk for infection, AIDS, tuberculosis, victimization, and hypothermia (U.S. Department of Health and Human Services, 1990). According to government studies, alcohol claims up to 100,000 lives per year. It is a factor in more than half of the reported automobile accidents and emergency room admissions and an underlying dynamic in many medical conditions. Moreover, alcoholism accounts for up to 50% of the violence between spouses and is a contributing factor in one third

BOX 31-3 Classification of Commonly Abused Drugs

Drug Classifications

Central nervous system sedatives, hypnotics, and anxiolytics

- Barbiturates (Luminal, Amytal, Nembutal, Seconal, Pentothal)
- Alcohol
- Meprobamate, Miltown
- Benzodiazepines (Librium, Valium, Xanax, Halcion, Dalmane)

Stimulants

- Amphetamines (Benzedrine, Dexedrine)
- Cocaine
- Caffeine

Narcotic analgesics: opiates

- Opium
- Heroin
- Morphine
- Codeine
- Methadone
- Other synthetic analgesics (Dilaudid, Percodan, Darvon, Talwin, Demerol)

Hallucinogens, psychedelics

- Lysergic acid diethylamide (LSD)
- Cannabis, marijuana, hashish
- Mescaline, peyote
- Phencyclidine (PCP), angel dust

Over-the-counter drugs

- Drugs containing atropine, scopolamine, antihistamines

Solvents

- Aerosol sprays, glue, gasoline, paint thinner, nail polish remover

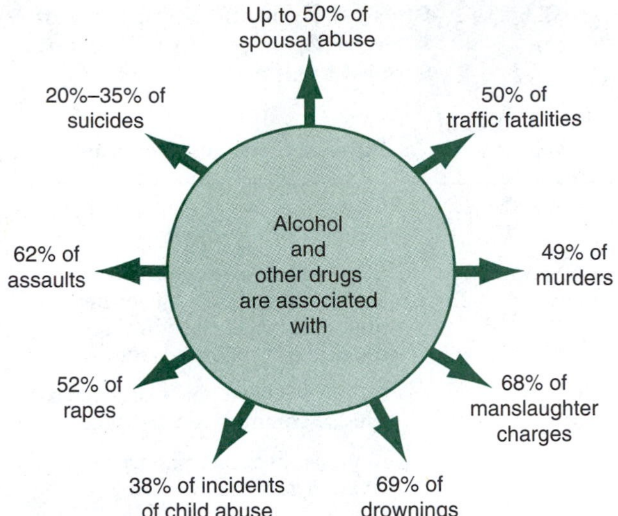

FIGURE 31–2
The social implications of alcohol abuse. (From *The fact is... OSAP responds to national crisis* [MS400]).

of child molestation cases (Silverstein, 1990). The costs to the American public related to alcohol problems were estimated to exceed $70 billion per year.

Alcoholism is listed as the third leading cause of death, and cirrhosis, its most common sequela, is the fifth leading cause of death in the United States. Because the range between a nontoxic dose of alcohol and a lethal dose is relatively narrow, death can occur with little warning and with no intent. The lifespan of the alcoholic is shortened by approximately 12 years (Moore, 1986). Figure 31–2 provides some of the data related to the far-reaching social implications of alcohol abuse.

Physical Symptoms

Physically, chronic alcoholism affects every organ in the body. Alcohol contains calories, but they are empty calories. Missing essential amino acids, vitamins, and minerals, a typical alcoholic who consumes up to 50% of caloric intake in the form of alcohol develops a severe nutritional deficiency. Malnutrition and irritation of the intestinal mucosa create a lack of thiamine (vitamin B_1), leading to numbness, changes in gait, and pain in the extremities associated with peripheral neuritis. Pancreatitis, cirrhosis of the liver, and diabetes occur with greater frequency in alcoholics and, untreated, can lead to death. Many alcoholics also demonstrate a low-grade hypertension. Some of the more common effects of chronic alcohol use on body systems are presented in Box 31–4.

Psychological Symptoms and Behavior Patterns

Psychological markers of alcoholism are overuse of defensive mental mechanisms to explain drug use, most prominently, denial, rationalization, and projection. **Denial** is apparent in the alcoholic's insistence that he does not have a problem despite concrete evidence of significant interference with normal life patterns directly attributable to his drug habit such as missed days at work, traffic tickets for alcohol-related behaviors and automobile accidents, the obvious concerns of others, and related physical ailments. Statements such as "I don't have a problem; it's your attitude that's a problem" or "I can stop any time I want to" are strong indicators of denial. **Rationalization** appears in the form of self-imposed rules that explain the person's drinking habits as legitimate. Sample statements include "I'm not an alcoholic because I just drink on weekends" or "I limit myself to beer; none of the hard stuff for me." **Projection** is evidenced in the blaming of external forces (e.g., nagging wife, an impossible boss, a stressful job) for stimulating the need to drink.

The alcoholic's use of these mental mechanisms is not a conscious effort to conceal the truth. Rather, it stems from self-deception, the direct result of the reinforcing properties of the drug, and **blackouts**, which erase the alcoholic's memory of self-destructive behaviors while under the influence. Breaking through this denial system is essential in supporting self-diagnosis, the cornerstone of successful rehabilitation in alcoholism.

Establishing the Diagnosis

Major symptoms supportive of a diagnosis of alcohol dependency include the following:

- Withdrawal symptoms and significant interference with psychosocial functioning in family and job relationships
- Tolerance, as evidenced by the ability to consume the equivalent of a fifth of liquor or a blood level of 100 dL or greater
- Indiscriminate or regular drinking in spite of social or medical contraindications
- Blackouts

In making a differential diagnosis of alcoholism, the nurse would look for a family history, history of drug use, and

BOX 31–4 Common Effects of Chronic Alcohol Use on Body Systems

- Polyneuropathy
- Chronic gastritis
- Cardiomyopathy
- Increased incidence of cancer (mouth, esophagus, pharynx, liver, larynx)
- Teratogenic fetal effects
- Cirrhosis
- Permanent brain damage
- Decreased immunity to infection

the behavior patterns described previously, which usually can be ascertained on interview. This information also yields data about preexisting mental disorders, metabolic conditions, other medications, or head injuries whose symptoms sometimes mimic acute intoxication or withdrawal symptoms. Often the nurse can smell alcohol on the patient's breath.

Two of the most common assessment tools used to establish a definitive diagnosis are the MAST Alcohol Screening Guide and the CAGE questionnaire. The MAST assessment guide consists of 23 questions that provide fairly reliable data about the drug habit (see Appendix). The CAGE questionnaire is composed of four questions:

Have you felt the need to *c*ut down on your drinking?
Have you been *a*nnoyed by criticism of your drinking?
Have you felt *g*uilty about your drinking?
Have you ever had a morning *e*ye opener after a night of drinking?

Two or more positive answers suggest a diagnosis of substance use disorder and three or more confirm it. The CAGE instrument obviously is easier but slightly less reliable because it is more prone to answers reflecting social desirability.

Treatment for alcoholism is primarily psychosocial and educational, following the mandated general pattern presented later in the chapter for acute and rehabilitation phases of all substance use disorders. Disulfiram (Antabuse) is sometimes used in the treatment of alcoholism during the rehabilitation phase to reinforce the alcoholic's desire to stop drinking. The drug acts as an antagonist to alcohol by blocking its breakdown of acetaldehyde, which in turn results in the development of acute physical distress. When the person on disulfiram takes an alcoholic drink, within 5 to 10 minutes, systemic symptoms begin to appear known as the "acetaldehyde syndrome" (Leccese, 1991). Flushing, a throbbing headache, nausea, vomiting, muscular aches, weakness, difficulty breathing, and chest pains ensue. It usually takes 5 days for the system to clear the disulfiram out of the system, a fact the recovering alcoholic needs to understand. Patients on disulfiram require close medical supervision and education about the danger of taking alcohol concurrently.

Toxicity

Physical signs and symptoms of alcohol toxicity with different blood levels are presented in Table 31–2. Combined with other hypnotic sedatives, the merged synergistic effects of alcohol and a benzodiazepine or barbiturate can prove fatal. Suicide and accidental death from overdose or lethal toxic combinations with other psychoactive drug substances make alcohol abuse one of the most dangerous preoccupations known to humankind.

Psychological symptoms associated with toxicity include marked alterations in sensory perceptions, which can resemble psychosis. The alcoholic presents with an agitated state and experiences extrasensory input from strange voices, sounds, or shadows. Auditory and visual hallucinations usually are menacing, often taking the form of rats or snakes. By contrast, with a schizophrenic psychotic episode, the patient retains orientation to self, place, and time but little else.

TABLE 31–2 **Physical Signs and Symptoms of Alcohol Toxicity With Different Blood Levels***

Blood Alcohol Level	Physical Signs and Symptoms
20–99 dL	Changes in mood, impaired judgment, muscle incoordination
100–199 dL	Marked cognitive impairment, pronounced muscle incoordination, prolonged reaction time; should not be allowed to drive
200–299 dL	All of the above plus marked ataxia, nausea, vomiting, slurred speech
300–399 dL	Amnesia, hypothermia, tremors, severe dysarthria
400–700 dL	Coma, respiratory failure, death

*A person is considered legally drunk with a blood alcohol level of greater than 100 mg/dL.

One of the most serious effects of chronic alcohol abuse is the development of irreversible brain damage. Occurring in chronic alcoholics after the age of 40 years, **Wernicke's encephalopathy** is characterized as the early stage of the more chronic and serious organic brain dysfunction associated with Korsakoff's syndrome. Symptoms of Wernicke's encephalopathy occur as a result of thiamine deficiency and are reversible with treatment in most cases. They include mental confusion, ataxia, gaze disturbance, and significant memory loss. Alcohol abstinence combined with heavy administration of thiamine has been used with excellent success in the treatment of this disorder. **Korsakoff's syndrome** is a serious organic disorder marked by dementia symptoms. Essentially, brains cells have been destroyed by the alcohol. Memory is grossly impaired, especially short-term memory, and the person exhibits confabulation and gait disturbances. The computed tomographic (CT) scan reveals profound brain atrophy, and there is no treatment available to reverse the dementia with Korsakoff's syndrome.

Withdrawal

Alcohol **withdrawal** symptoms can include diaphoresis, tachycardia, tremors, nausea and vomiting, temporary hallucinations, and heightened anxiety. The most serious form of withdrawal is known as **delirium tremens,** which occurs as a result of acute central nervous system irritability. Characterized by coarse tremors, tachycardia, marked increase in blood pressure, grand mal seizures, and fever, its victims sometimes will die from the condition even if medical treatment is instituted. Death occurs from cardiac or respiratory failure.

Dual Diagnosis

Alcoholism can be superimposed on a psychiatric disorder, and many people self-medicate themselves to reduce feelings of inferiority, depression, and anxiety. There are those who believe that alcoholism is related to deep-seated psychopathology. Others insist that alcoholism must be considered as a primary disorder and treated as separate from any underlying personality dynamics. For the former, there is a natural tendency to look for underlying psychopathology as "causing" the need to take drugs. The latter belief leads the clinician to treat the alcoholism as if it had no relation to the presence of any other psychiatric disorder. **Dual diagnosis** is a major emerging problem, as evidenced by current estimates suggesting that up to 60% of persons with substance use disorders also have a dual psychiatric diagnosis. Many patients use alcohol or other psychoactive drugs to forestall depressive symptoms, alleviate anxiety, stop frightening hallucinations, or express anger. The most common dually diagnosed psychiatric disorders are depression, panic disorder, antisocial personality disorder, and eating disorders. Developing knowledge about dual diagnosis suggests the need for a coordinated treatment approach with these patients (McKelvy et al, 1987).

Most clinicians believe that it is important to treat alcoholism as a primary disease process while recognizing and handling the coexistence of other mental disorders in the rehabilitative phase. The rationale for treating the substance use disorder first is that the drug use typically interferes with an accurate assessment of the underlying psychiatric disorder. What looks like a serious personality disorder or depression can clear or improve when the alcohol or drug abuse is modified. The person under the influence of drugs cannot even begin to address underlying psychological issues while the psychoactive properties of the drug are affecting effective thought processing and decision making.

Treatment of the coexisting psychiatric disorder begins as soon as initial detoxification is complete. It is a critical component of aftercare because many patients use psychoactive substances instead of appropriate medication to self-medicate their anxiety and depressive symptoms. Using prescribed antipsychotic or antidepressant medication and developing different coping strategies through long-term supportive or insight psychotherapy may be crucial to the success of treatment for the substance dependency.

Sedative, Hypnotic, or Anxiolytic Use Disorders

Psychoactive drugs in this psychopharmacological classification include benzodiazepines, barbiturates, and minor tranquilizers such as meprobromate (Equanil) and oxazepam (Serax). They act as central nervous system depressants and, in low doses, relieve anxiety and relax inhibitions. Psychological relief is obtained rapidly after ingestion, because hypnotic sedatives produce a short-term sense of euphoria and well-being with few side effects at low doses. With high doses, however, hypnotic sedatives can depress vital central nervous system functions, particularly those involving respiratory centers. All of the hypnotic sedatives can be obtained legally, and they are all capable of producing psychological and physical dependence.

BENZODIAZEPINE USE

The benzodiazepines are the most commonly prescribed anxiolytic (antianxiety) medications for treatment of insomnia and mild tension states. Listed as Schedule IV drugs, they are highly effective as short-term treatment for anxiety related to situational circumstances. Diazepam (Valium) and chlordiazepoxide (Librium) also have an important medical use in treating the withdrawal symptoms of alcohol and other psychoactive substances predisposing an individual to violent behaviors. Usually, 50 to 100 mg is given intramuscularly and repeated every 4 to 6 hours until the acute effects are under control. Thereafter, the drug is given orally and tapered slowly. Beyond this time period, these drugs should be given with great care, if at all, to reduce the anxiety of the recovering alcoholic because of their addictive properties. This pharmacological classification is more likely to be the drug of choice for older adults, who typically are not thought to have a substance use disorder. The problem arises when benzodiazepines are prescribed without regard for careful monitoring.

Toxicity

The rationale for providing close monitoring of these drugs stems from the fact that, although moderate and long-acting benzodiazepines have a wider threshold of safety than other sedatives, they are potentially lethal in combination with other psychoactive drugs (Ghodsey, 1994). Cross-tolerance to other hypnotic sedatives is high, and lethal overdoses occur when benzodiazepines are ingested with other psychoactive drugs. Oversedation or respiratory depression occur in the elderly, and the benzodiazepines are a major contributing factor in psychiatric emergencies and unintentional death.

Withdrawal

Compared with the other drugs in this classification, the benzodiazepines have a relatively long half-life of the drug in the bloodstream. Consequently, onset of withdrawal to intermediate and long-acting benzodiazepines occurs within 3 to 5 days after cessation of the drug. Often the cause-and-effect relationship between drug withdrawal and emergence of symptoms is not always recognized because withdrawal symptoms are not abrupt (Mondanaro, 1990). Shorter-acting benzodiazepines such as triazolam (Halcion), alprazolam (Xanax), Lorazepam (Ativan), and oxazepam (Serax) produce more severe withdrawal symptoms that begin soon after the drug is withdrawn. Treatment consists of gradual withdrawal of the drug, psychotherapy, and skill development of different, more effective coping strategies.

BARBITURATE USE

Barbiturates derive from barbituric acid and produce pharmacological effects similar to those of alcohol. They are frequently the drug of choice among the middle class, who initially use them primarily as a prescribed drug from their physician to relieve insomnia or minor anxiety. Mode of administration is usually oral, with IV use by serious drug abusers. IV use of barbiturates is popular because it is financially easier to support than a heroin addiction.

Barbiturates also are used frequently in conjunction with other drugs to enhance euphoric effects or to help avoid the intensity of withdrawal symptoms. Barbiturate intoxication is associated with poor judgment, exaggeration of sexual and aggressive tendencies, sluggishness, and psychomotor impairment. It is frequently associated with unintentional overdose in children and is the drug classification most frequently implicated in adult attempted suicides (Kaplan and Sadock, 1988). Barbiturates potentiate the effects of alcohol, and death occurs with the characteristic pattern of seizures and cardiorespiratory collapse. Withdrawal symptoms are severe and include agitation, tremors, delirium, and convulsions.

A major problem with barbiturate addiction is its legal availability through medical prescription. The addiction may go undiscovered because the abuser often can receive several prescriptions for the same drug from different physicians to support an undiagnosed habit.

Hallucinogen Use Disorders

The **hallucinogens** are a unique classification of psychoactive drugs for two reasons: (1) There are marked differences in the ways people experience them, ranging from no effect whatsoever to profound changes in perception, as described in Joe's story, and (2) there are no distinct physical withdrawal effects. Naturally occurring hallucinogens include mescaline or peyote taken from the cactus plant and psilocybin derived from mushrooms and marijuana. Synthetically derived hallucinogens include LSD, and PCP, among others. The exact mechanism by which synthetic psychedelic drugs interact with the central nervous system is not readily identified, although LSD appears to interfere with the serotonin receptors of the neurons (Buskist and Gerbing, 1990). The blocking of important receptors of neurons frees the neurons and gives rise to the out-of-body and intense emotional feelings experienced by the user; hence the typing as psychedelic drugs. Mode of administration is oral, usually as a tasteless powder that the person licks from a small blotter-type paper or swallowed in pill form.

The hallucinogens involve sensory perceptual changes with a characteristic intense emotional experience and heightened awareness. When perceptual changes occur, the range can vary from having the experience of a freeing, pleasurable trip to greater perception to primary effects of an intensely dysphoric mood and paranoid ideation. They also vary from situation to situation so that the same person can experience "good" or "bad" trips from ingestion of the drug at different times. Flashbacks, which represent a reexperiencing of the intense feelings associated with a previous drug-taking episode *without further drug ingestion*, can create a severe panic attack or psychotic behavior. They are sometimes activated with cannabis ingestion in the LSD user (Ghodse, 1995).

PHENCYCLIDINE USE

Phencyclidine (PCP, angel dust) became popular in the late 1950s but lost its popularity two decades later because of its potential to cause psychosis and violence. This drug sometimes is classified as a hallucinogen because the pharmacological effects of the drug produce similar dramatic subjective effects and perceptions. PCP affects the opiate receptors associated with motivation and emotion (Buskist and Gerbing, 1990). The drug stimulates the release of dopamine, and, taken in large doses, can precipitate a schizophreniclike disorder. PCP stimulates paranoid ideation, auditory hallucinations, and a highly inconsistent pattern of behavior in users ranging from excitement to catatonic stupor.

Toxicity

PCP toxicity is most likely to present as a medical or psychiatric emergency in the form of an acute psychosis, and a person taking PCP is capable of sudden violent, impulsive behavior. They should be considered dangerous until proven otherwise. Luisada (1978) described rageful delusions in which the person on PCP images himself as having superhuman strength. During a bad trip, a person can experience panic attacks, and many former PCP users are found among the homeless or on chronic psychiatric units with a drug-induced psychosis.

Complications of Chronic Use

Chronic PCP use can result in permanent neurological and cognitive changes evidenced in loss of memory and impulse control, slowed thinking, dulled reflexes, and difficulty concentrating. Unfortunately, the strong feelings of invincibility, power, and strength are pleasurable enough that giving it up is difficult for most serious PCP abusers.

Cannabis Use Disorders

Of all the illicit drugs, cannabis is the most commonly used, especially by adolescents. Marijuana and its close cousins, hashish and tetrahydrocannabinol (THC), are derived from an Indian hemp plant, cannabis sativa. The gummy resin covering the flowering tops and upper leaves contains the psychoactive agents responsible for the mind-altering properties of the drug. THC is the primary active ingredient in marijuana. Over the years, marijuana has been classified as a stimulant and more recently as a hallucinogen. Medically, THC has been used successfully in the treatment of glaucoma and in the relief of the nausea associated with cancer chemotherapy.

The most common route of administration for marijuana is into the lungs via smoking, which produces almost immediate effects. Some users ingest marijuana orally but because three times as much of the drug must be taken to achieve the same effects, this mode of administration is less favored (Abel, 1985). Drug effects are almost immediate. For most users, there is a sense of euphoria and a feeling of serenity. Time either is suspended or accelerated, depending on the overall mood of the user. There are marked perceptual changes in vision, hearing, taste, touch, and smell. With some people, visual and auditory perceptions are not pleasant; they are frightening and accompanied by a sense of depersonalization. A user described it as follows: "I felt as though I was going to die. My heart pounded and I could hear the clock ticking as though it was part of me. Everything was swimming around me and I thought someone was going to kill me." The drug remains in the body for up to 6 weeks after smoking it.

Relatively inexpensive and easily accessible, marijuana's initial euphoria and later the euphoric recall make it difficult for patients to give it up in favor of working through difficult problems without its support. One patient describes it as follows: "When things get really overwhelming, I can tune out with pot. It dulls the sensation and I think things are manageable again. I know it won't last, but for the moment, I can pretend, and I feel like I can cope. It doesn't help in the end, but I can't stand feeling that I have no control over what's happening to me."

Another reason for its popularity is the general belief that marijuana is not harmful. As one young man expressed it, "give me one good reason why I shouldn't smoke it. It doesn't hurt me and it doesn't impact on anyone else like alcohol and other drugs do. Why shouldn't I use it?" Unfortunately, there are reasons why regular use of marijuana is harmful to the self as well as to others. The most commonly observed developmental pattern of drug abuse follows an ordered sequence of alcohol, cigarettes, and marijuana (Yamaguchi and Kandel, 1984). There is slim but growing evidence of teratogenic effects on the fetus with prolonged marijuana use.

Marijuana clearly is a *gateway* drug in the typical progression to chronic use and IV administration of hard drugs. Many people use the drug to self-medicate dysphoric mood and depressive symptoms. The quick "high" marijuana creates allows the person to feel in control again and to avoid painful emotional realities by slipping past them into the oblivion of the drug effects. Long-term use of the drug seems associated with a lack of motivation or initiative. Known as the "amotivational syndrome," individuals with a history of long-term marijuana use demonstrate a characteristic aimlessness and lack of realistic goal attainment. Sometimes it is difficult to follow their conversation, and there is a tendency for the person to focus only on tangential parts of difficult reality circumstances.

In a few cases, a functional psychosis from chronic use can develop, lasting for a few hours or days and characterized by deep confusion, depersonalization, and hallucinations. The symptoms resolve quickly with antipsychotic medication but can reappear with resumption of marijuana use. The "cannabis psychosis" is more prevalent in countries with extremely heavy use (e.g., the West Indies and parts of Asia). Although marijuana toxicity can produce serious psychological symptoms and paranoia, the drug does not appear to have the fatal potential of overdose associated with other psychoactive substances.

Opioid Use Disorders

The narcotic analgesics are opioid agonists consisting of heroin, morphine, fentanyl, codeine, and methadone. With the exception of heroin, all of these drugs have significant medical value in regulated dosage for pain relief, and codeine is used as an active ingredient in medications for cough suppression. The opioids stimulate the neural activity of the opiate receptors and bind with various opioid receptors, thereby giving these narcotics their deserved reputation as effective pain killers. Reinforcing effects of this pharmacological drug classification appear to be related to their effect on dopaminergic pathways, particularly along the mesocorticolimbic circuits believed to be the reward and pleasure centers of the brain (Jaffe and Martin, 1990). In addition to providing physical relief from pain, the opioids suppress emotional tensions. Reduction of emotional pain and anxiety allows the heroin abuser to assume a passive adaptation to painful inner pressures.

Heroin, with no medical value, is a depressant drug and the most widely misused. Street names for heroin include H, Harry, horse, or China white. High-grade heroin finds its way into this country from Southeast Asia, an area that includes Myanmar, Thailand, and Laos. Heroin is illegally transported in false-bottom suitcases, in passenger bags, and even in the stomachs of airline passengers who swallow rubber pouches filled with the drug; the incidence of heroin smuggling has increased dramatically within the last few years.

Opiates usually are taken orally and through IV injection. Because IV injection produces the most intense and immediate effects, most serious narcotic addicts prefer "mainlining" as mode of administration. The disadvantages of IV drug administration are related to infections and vein collapse with frequent use. Fever of unknown origin in any drug abuser should raise suspicion of endocarditis, or "cotton fever," a condition brought about by the direct IV injection of small particles or bacteria into the bloodstream. Novice narcotic abusers frequently use intramuscular or subcutaneous injections, referred to as "skin popping," before moving into IV modes of administration.

Complications of Chronic Use

Organ system complications associated with heroin abuse include endocarditis, pulmonary edema, and pulmonary fibrosis caused by the insoluble materials used to cut the drug for IV administration that collect in the lung. The most serious effects of heroin abuse are acute respiratory depression and pulmonary edema, which not infrequently result in cardiorespiratory arrest and the rather quick death of the victim.

Hepatitis is a frequent medical complication; IV drug use can account for up to 80% of hospitalizations for this disorder (Levine et al, 1995). Septic conditions contribute to bacterial meningitis and skin lesions. Opiates create a state of chronic constipation, with the onset of diarrhea and abdominal cramping occurring symptomatically with withdrawal. Finally, susceptibility to infection and the development of hyperplastic nodes ("addicts' nodes") offer clear indication of the immunosuppressive qualities of heroin dependency (Donohoe, 1988).

Toxicity

Opiate overdose constitutes a medical emergency requiring immediate recognition and treatment. It is characterized by pinpoint pupils, depressed respiration, cardiac arrhythmias, convulsions, and coma. Death can result from pulmonary edema (Schuckit, 1995). Treatment consists of administering an opioid antagonist (naltrexone) that can reverse the symptoms in a relatively short time. An adverse reaction can occur, however, in the form of withdrawal symptoms. Clonidine, alone and in combination with naltrexone, also has proven effective in detoxification protocols with heroin addicts (Charney et al, 1986).

Withdrawal

Although withdrawal symptoms do not constitute a medical emergency, they are extremely uncomfortable for the patient. Because of the discomfort involved, many patients seek immediate relief from the drug, and it is difficult for them to remain drug free. Characteristic symptoms include delusional thinking, nightmares, severe tremors, diaphoresis, frequent yawning, abdominal pain, muscle spasm, and tearing. Withdrawal symptoms can be reversed with tapered doses of methadone. This drug acts as a heroin agonist, having analgesic effects without producing the high typically associated with heroin.

TABLE 31–3 Using the Nursing Process in Detoxification With Methadone

Step	Drug Administration
Assessment	
1. Obtain complete assessment data regarding heroin use	
2. Establish a diagnosis of opiate dependence based on intravenous use, urine screens, naloxone testing	
Planning	
1. Gain patient's cooperation	
2. Provide information regarding methadone, mechanism of action, side effects, and so on	
Implementation	
1. Administer medication	10 mg
2. Observe for signs of opiate intoxication, withdrawal	
3. Monitor vital signs	
4. Establish methadone maintenance dosage once patient is stabilized (24–48 h)	20–30 mg/d
5. Reduce methadone dosage by 5 mg/d	
6. Use supportive counseling and education during withdrawal	Detoxification can be completed in 7–14 d
7. Reassure patient that withdrawal symptoms are normal even with methadone and will diminish.	

Methadone Treatment

Methadone was the first drug used for the treatment of heroin addiction. Although marked differences exist between the natural and synthetic chemical bases for the opiates, their effects on the neurotransmitter system in the brain are similar. Because of their close resemblance to each other, administering controlled doses of methadone to heroin addicts has received support from both the medical and legal communities as a safe, long-term treatment for heroin dependency. First prescribed in 1965, administration of the synthetically developed methadone seems to correct the unyielding chemical imbalance in brain metabolism related to chronic use of heroin. Heroin addicts receiving oral methadone in controlled dosages do not seem to experience the euphoria or withdrawal symptoms associated with heroin dependency or the damaging toxicological side effects associated with heroin consumption (Table 31–3).

In 1972, the Federal Drug Administration reclassified methadone in a special drug category that would allow medically supervised administration of the drug to addicts with chronic, intractable addictions to heroin. Drug addicts requiring detoxification are entitled to methadone treatment for up to 21 days. Federal guidelines for inclusion in a maintenance treatment protocol include a history of opiate dependency of more than 2 years and evidence of physical withdrawal symptoms associated with this drug classification. The only exception to this rule is the administration of methadone to a drug addict who is hospitalized for an illness other than drug dependency for more than 21 days. Methadone can be given to the patient until recovery from the illness is complete to curb withdrawal symptoms (Fultz et al, 1980).

The expected outcomes of methadone maintenance are twofold: (1) to reduce illicit use of heroin and the criminal behaviors used by heroin addicts to sustain their habit and (2) to improve the psychological well-being and social productivity of the heroin addict (Gerstein and Harwood, 1990). Clinical efficacy is demonstrated in the marked decrease in criminal activities and social rehabilitation attributable to maintenance treatment programs for hard-core heroin addicts.

Sympathomimetic Use Disorders

Drugs pharmacologically classified as central nervous system stimulants (amphetamines, cocaine, nicotine, and caffeine) act on catecholamine neurotransmitters, serotonin, norepinephrine, and dopamine in the brain.

AMPHETAMINE USE

The most commonly used amphetamines include dextroamphetamine (Dexedrine), methamphetamine, methylphenidate (Ritalin), and Benzedrine. Amphetamines originally were used as an appetite suppressant for weight loss. Because of their energizing effects, this class of drugs also is used by athletes and long-distance truck drivers to increase energy and counteract fatigue. Medically, the drug classification is sometimes used in the treatment of depression, particularly when associated with narcolepsy. Ritalin is a very effective medication used to offset the symptoms of hyperactive attention deficit disorder, and Benzedrine inhalers are used in the treatment of asthma.

COCAINE USE

Cocaine has emerged as the signature drug of the central nervous system stimulants and cocaine abuse has increased with alarming frequency over the past decade. Nuckols and Greeson (1989) noted that up to 5000 people use cocaine for the first time each day, and a startling jump in the prevalence of people who had tried cocaine at least once from 5.4 million in 1977 to 21.6 million in 1982. Adams and Durrell (1984) suggested that, because cocaine is a drug of choice among higher socioeconomic groups, the true incidence of cocaine use may be underreported.

Cocaine is derived from a plant, Erythroxylon. Cocaine alkaloid can be broken up into smaller pieces referred to as "crack," so named because of the crackling sound of the substance when heated. Compared with the cost of powdered cocaine, crack is cheap, purer, and more available in individual doses. Crack is free based, a term used to describe taking the pure cocaine alkaloid and smoking it in a pipe or sprinkling it on a marijuana joint.

Like heroin, the drug is smuggled into the United States and Canada from foreign sources, chiefly from Columbia, South America, where the plant grows well. Pharmacologically, cocaine affects the metabolism of dopamine, norepinephrine, acetylcholine, and serotonin. Of primary importance in understanding the action of cocaine on the brain is its effect on the dopaminergic system. The action of this psychoactive substance in the brain is that it "prolongs the activity of dopamine in the synapse by blocking the dopamine reuptake mechanism (which usually inactivates the transmitter by removing it from the proximity of its synaptic targets)" (Wise, 1984, p. 27). This action, according to Wise, is responsible for its strong reinforcing properties. Cocaine has definite stimulant properties; it produces euphoria, increased energy, improved performance, loss of fatigue, and a sense of well-being and freedom from boredom.

Cocaine is a short-acting drug, particularly when injected or smoked as "crack" (American Psychiatric Association, 1994). This makes it particularly attractive as a mood-altering drug because it also produces a sense of power unparalleled to other psychoactive drugs. There is an almost instantaneous positive sense of well-being, heightened sense of competency, and increased sex drive. Although some consumers experience an initial nausea, it is transitory and usually does not detract from the enhanced sense of well-being and self-esteem that accompanies cocaine. The euphoric effects of the drug block out or "numb" uncomfortable emotional pain and counteract the boredom and emptiness of life.

Modes of administration vary; insufflation (snorting or inhalation) and IV injection are used with traditional cocaine powders. With insufflation, the drug is inhaled into the lung and transported almost immediately to the brain via the circulatory system. Less frequently used methods include oral ingestion and chewing coca leaves much as one would chew tobacco. Cocaine also can be injected subcutaneously or intramuscularly.

The pattern of cocaine abuse is different from that of other psychoactive drugs in that abusers are "binge" rather than "maintenance" abusers, with binges lasting from several hours to several days. Nightclubs are fertile grounds for the habit. In between binges, the cocaine addict may be drug free. Because it is a short-acting drug, physical tolerance does not develop in the same manner as with other psychoactive substances (Jones, 1984).

Complications of Chronic Use

The crack or cocaine abuser often presents in the emergency department as acutely anxious, possibly combative, and paranoid. Potentially violent behavior is always a possibility with a person under the influence of cocaine. The patient has a tendency to misinterpret the environment, which heightens the potential for violence. The cocaine addict responds best to a quiet and soothing environment with sufficient space and openness in communication and gestures.

Extensive use can produce nasal ulcerations, chronic cough or sore throat, malnutrition, and insomnia. Significant "snorting" can irrevocably affect the nasal mucosa, and chronic use can stimulate characteristic repetitive behaviors such as picking at the skin. Some patients experience psychotic symptoms such as auditory and tactile hallucinations (coke bugs) and paranoid ideation.

Although ingestion of cocaine produces euphoric effects that are very intense and rapid, they are followed by an equally intense emotional low, and this may account for the strong psychological dependence on cocaine. Dackis and Gold (1985) suggested that the rapid, cycling bipolar effects of excitement and depression may be the result of the temporary dopamine increase noted with acute cocaine administration followed by a dramatic decrease in dopamine level found with repeated administration. The fact that the dysphoric symptoms can be corrected with subsequent cocaine administration increases the likelihood of persistent psychological dependence.

Of particular clinical concern is the development of **cocaine blues,** a sequela of drug cessation that consists of a dysphoric mood having clinical significance and suicidal ideation. The deep depression that often accompanies cocaine withdrawal makes the client a strong suicidal risk and increases the desire for the drug to relieve the overwhelming dysphoric mood and associated feelings.

Typically, the cocaine addict is a polydrug user, which further complicates treatment initiatives. This may occur because cocaine produces such an uncomfortable level of stimulation that alcohol, marijuana, and other hypnotic sedatives are used to equalize the stimulating effects of the drug. A favored combination of many cocaine abusers is IV injection in combination with heroin, known as "chasing the dragon." Cocaine provides the "high," and heroin helps to "mellow" the sharper stimulating effects of cocaine that can be troublesome. Cocaine also is used by heroin addicts to provide energy and sometimes the courage needed to perform criminal acts to sustain the heroin habit. Referred to as "speedballing," many heroin addicts list heroin as their primary drug and cocaine as secondary.

Toxicity

Cocaine toxicity was the second most frequent cause of death reported to the American Association of Poison Control Centers in 1988. Although chronic use can lead to toxic overdose, it is not necessary to be a long-time abuser to suffer significant side effects. Death can result in first-time users as well as in those severely addicted to cocaine. Toxicity and potential for overdose are greater with this particular drug because the purity of the drug can be as much as 90%; in addition, because it is free based, it enters the brain with minimal alteration in concentration. Overdose can produce severe systemic responses, including respiratory collapse and sudden death. Thus, death can be instantaneous as it was for Len Bias, an otherwise healthy athlete. Other signs and symptoms of cocaine toxicity include acute anxiety, extreme agitation, seizures, cardiac arrythmias, and pulmonary edema. Unfortunately, there are no drug antagonists to arrest the toxic effects of cocaine overdose. Naloxone is given to reduce the concurrent toxic effects of other narcotic drugs in the victim's body systems.

Central nervous system stimulant toxicity in nonlethal situations usually is self-limited. Delusional symptoms are treated symptomatically with supportive measures. Antipsychotic medication is given when warranted, and diazepam is used in the first few days of treatment to reduce agitation. A peculiarity of cocaine is its natural sedative effect as it wears off; it is important not to oversedate the cocaine patient because this can heighten the possibility of respiratory depression with drug cessation.

Withdrawal

Patients experiencing withdrawal symptoms complain of headache, lethargy, craving, muscle pain, eating disturbance, alterations in sleep patterns, irritability, paranoid, and delusional thinking. In describing these characteristic symptoms of withdrawal from cocaine, Jones (1984) argued that "these symptoms must be more than simply the consequence of what traditionally has been termed 'psychological dependence.' When listening to descriptions of this state by cocaine-using patients, these dysphoric and often dramatic symptoms must be viewed as negative reinforcers" (p. 47).

Treatment Considerations

Cocaine addiction is difficult to treat because of its rewarding or "reinforcing" properties. Wise (1984) suggested that, "of the habit forming drugs, cocaine and heroin stand out as perhaps the most powerful reinforcers as defined by the rapidity of acquisition of self-administration" (p. 15). To neutralize the effects of craving, part of the treatment process for cocaine abusers is deliberate exploration of the positive effects of the drug with an eye to substitution. Finding other ways to feel good and to feel more sexual and competent is a necessary part of an effective treatment program (Mondanaro, 1990).

Generally, hospitalization is needed to provide the setting required for drug abstinence and rehabilitation. More often than not, cocaine addictions coexist with other psychiatric disorders, the most common being major or bipolar depression, panic disorder, and attention deficit disorder (Miller et al, 1990). Thus, the underlying disorder must also be treated simultaneously. Antidepressants and lithium have been used with some success in reducing the craving and dysphoric mood associated with cocaine addiction withdrawal.

CAFFEINE AND NICOTINE USE

Caffeine and nicotine are not always thought of as drugs of abuse because they do not present the same destructive clinical impairment associated with substance abuse or dependence. Yet both are capable of producing tolerance and withdrawal symptoms with excessive, chronic use, and both are found in the new DSM-IV classification. Caffeine is found in a number of drinks, including coffee, tea and soft drinks, some analgesics, diet aids, and cold medications. Toxicity is characterized by increased anxiety, irritability, psychomotor agitation, diaphoresis, and tinnitus. In a small number of cases, excessive caffeine can result in cardiac arrhythmias, grand mal seizures, and respiratory collapse. Caffeine is known to exacerbate peptic ulcers and circulatory failure. Women can sometimes decrease the symptoms of premenstrual syndrome by eliminating caffeine from their diet 2 weeks before the menses. Drowsiness, depression, headache, irritability, and dysphoric mood often are signs of caffeine withdrawal.

Nicotine typically does not create the social problems that other forms of dependence create. What it does generate is a serious health risk not only for smokers but also for those most intimately involved with them. Cancer of the lung, larynx, throat, and mouth, emphysema and other lung conditions, cardiac and circulatory problems, and low birth weight in infants have been observed with heavy use of nicotine. Inhalation of passive smoke by nonsmokers can produce similar symptoms in people who have never smoked. Women who smoke frequently have low-birth-weight infants. For all of these reasons, habitual use of nicotine is a major health hazard.

Nicotine withdrawal occurs within 24 hours of cigarette stoppage. Symptoms include irritability, insomnia, tension, and decreased heart rate. Weight gain and oversensitive, peevish behaviors are characteristic of deliberate smoking cessation. The undesirable withdrawal symptoms and craving for cigarettes that remain long after cigarette smoking has stopped reduce the success rate. Those who wake up to a cigarette and who crave it when ill or who are willing to stand outside in the bitter cold to have a cigarette have the most difficulty giving it up. There is a high incidence of nicotine dependence among the mentally ill and those with other substance use disorders. Treatment for dependence consists of a variety of measures ranging from self-hypnosis to a nicotine patch, family support, and self-help groups.

Volatile Solvent Use Disorders

Within the last decade, it has become fashionable for adolescents to inhale volatile solvents such as glue, gasoline, paint thinners, cleaners, and other propellants for their stimulant effects. The substances are inhaled through the nose and mouth via a cloth or a plastic bag saturated with the substance or are sprayed directly from the can into the nose or mouth. The effects of the drug are immediate, and intoxication can result in a number of signs and symptoms, among them changes in lethargy, psychomotor retardation, and generalized muscle weakness. Some of the propellants in particular can freeze the larynx or cause respiratory and cardiac depression. Toxicity can lead to cirrhosis or renal failure. The expected outcome of treatment, as in other dependencies, is complete abstinence. The same supports, however, are not available for the treatment of this dependence compared with other types of substance use disorders.

▶ Check Your Reading

4. What are the distinguishing characteristics of substance dependence?
5. How does alcohol compromise a person's life journey?
6. What role does craving play in cocaine addiction?

NURSING PROCESS: ACUTE PHASE

Treatment of substance use disorders generally is broken down into two phases. The first is the acute phase, in which the nurse assesses and treats the medical, toxic, or withdrawal symptoms associated with the disorder. This phase typically lasts a short time and culminates in the medical stabilization of the patient's condition. This is followed by a much longer phase of treatment—rehabilitation—lasting months, years, or, with most people having this disorder, a lifetime.

The acute phase consists of all of the nursing interventions associated with the medical stabilization of the patient's symptoms. Patients demonstrating acute toxicity or withdrawal symptoms require *immediate triage*. A full psychosocial assessment is deferred until the patient can be stabilized medically. The nurse elicits information related to amount and type of drug taken within the last 48 hours and routes of administration. This information is used to determine whether lavage is necessary and as a basis to administer drug antagonists, if appropriate. Relevant nursing diagnoses can include one or more of the following:

Injury: Potential for
Altered Nutrition: Less than Body Requirements
Sleep Pattern Disturbance
Impaired Gas Exchange
Fluid Volume Deficit
Cardiac Output, Altered
Self Care Deficit: Feeding, hygiene, toileting
Thought Processes, Altered
Sensory/Perceptual Alterations: Visual, auditory, tactile
Violence, Potential for Self-Directed or Directed at Others
Breathing Pattern, Ineffective
Communication, Impaired Verbal
Self-Concept, Disturbance in: Personal Identity

Expected treatment outcomes relate to the restoration and maintenance of physiological and psychological stability. Treatment is largely symptomatic and immediate. Depending on the nature and severity of the emergency situation, nursing interventions to meet any and all of the treatment goals listed next are appropriate.

- Prevention of cardiovascular collapse
- Support of the respiratory system
- Identification of psychoactive drugs and removal, if ingested orally
- Administration of narcotic antagonist, if appropriate
- Treatment of hypotension or hypertension
- Prevention-treatment of seizures
- Prevention of aspiration
- Treatment of hypothermia or hyperthermia
- Protection from self-inflicted or other-directed injury

Monitoring vital signs, establishment of an adequate airway, administration of oxygen if needed, and use of IV fluids are first-priority nursing interventions. If the patient is an IV drug abuser, the likelihood of cotton fever, thrombophlebitis, endocarditis, hepatitis, and bacteremia are considered. Look for needle marks over veins, indicative of recent injection, and signs of hyperthermia. Fever of unknown origin may be the only indicator of endocarditis, persisting even in the absence of positive cultures. Look for other evidence of drug complications such as electrolyte-nutritional deficiencies. These observations offer more precise data about the type of intervention needed. For example, recent oral ingestion of drugs can be reversed with proper administration of emetic medications. Routine measurement of intake-output and frequent vital signs is imperative because the patient's condition can change quickly. Urine and blood toxicology tests help determine drug toxicity levels, which are needed to make a differential diagnosis from psychosis and as the basis for deciding on immediate treatment options. Most psychoactive drugs and their metabolites will clear the body system within 48 hours unless the client is a chronic abuser of the drug. The benzodiazepines take longer to clear the system, and the toxic effects of chlordiazepoxide will not peak until 5 to 7 days after ingestion.

While under the acute influence of drugs, the patient is likely to be a danger to self or others. Thus, a second-order assessment is for potential for violence or suicide related to sensory perceptual deficits created by the drug toxicity. If this potential is noted, the nurse needs to take appropriate measures taken to ensure patient and nursing personnel safety (see Chapter 38 for treatment of delirium).

TABLE 31–4 **A Mini-Care Plan for the Acute Phase of Treatment of Substance Use Disorder**

Expected Outcome	Nursing Actions
Long term Patient will maintain psychological and physiological stability.	
Short term Patient will maintain physical homeostasis.	1. Monitor vital signs every 15 min until stabilized. 2. Administer oxygen and other medications as needed. 3. Observe and report signs of impending seizure. 4. Monitor and report intake, output and critical laboratory values 5. Use intravenous therapy or oral fluids to correct nutritional deficiency.
Patient will verbalize orientation to person, place, and time.	1. Speak to the patient in a calm voice and use short sentences. 2. Orient patient to unit, and explain all procedures. 3. Administer antianxiety medications as ordered.
Patient will remain injury free during detoxification.	1. Establish a calm environment with low lights and minimal stimuli. 2. If restraints are necessary, explain their use in simple terms and reassure patient they will be removed when the patient is no longer a danger to self or others. 3. Stay with patient if agitated or confused. 4. Institute seizure precautions if needed.

Once the patient's immediate life-threatening needs are under control, the nurse turns his or her attention to simplifying the patient's environment. Placing the patient in a quiet, well-lit room, orienting the patient, and providing information about necessary procedures help decrease patient anxiety. Seizure precautions minimize chances of injury from seizure activity. Table 31–4 presents a minicare plan for the following common nursing diagnoses found in the acute phase of treatment of substance use disorder:

- Injury: Potential for related to substance abuse toxicity
- Cardiac output decreased related to effects of substance abuse toxicity
- Altered Thought Processes related to drug toxicity

NURSING PROCESS: REHABILITATION PHASE

The rehabilitative treatment of substance use disorders requires an integrated psychopharmacological and behavioral psychiatric approach for successful outcome; family therapy also is appropriate when the family unit is intact. Schuster and Snyder (1990) noted that, "just as insulin will not save a diabetic who cannot change his diet and life style, medications to treat drug addiction will not work by themselves. They must be part of a comprehensive treatment program that gives addicts the capabilities to achieve a life without drugs" (p. 72). A critical part of the treatment process for chronic substance use disorders is the development of a new lifestyle completely devoid of old patterns and in most cases of past drug-using companions.

ASSESSMENT

The rehabilitative phase begins with education about the nature of addictive behaviors and a comprehensive personal assessment of past and present drug use. The information sought includes a history of the drinking or drug abuse pattern, social functioning, resources, and level of basic skill development. A complete history of the patient's drug abuse pattern includes age of onset, types of substances abused (including alcohol), mode of administration, usual conditions or situations in which drug-taking behaviors occur, previous treatment attempts, and medical treatments for secondary symptoms. Employment history, legal status, and family history provide an insight into the level of disruption in the chemically dependent person's life related to substance abuse. Mental status and questions about disturbances in mood elicit important information about associated psychiatric problems that may compound the drug abuse. Questions to include in a substance abuse history are presented in Figure 31–3.

Interviewing family members has two purposes: (1) It helps to verify the substance user's historical perspective, supplying missing details and modifying information in joint consultation with the patient, and (2) it provides an opportunity to observe the interactions between the patient and family members. The latter offers important clues about behaviors that may be reinforcing or enabling the disorder to continue without treatment.

Questions to Include in the Substance Abuse History

History of substance use	History of experimentation with any drugs in childhood. Any current recreational drug or alcohol use (obtain the following information for each drug used [e.g., nicotine, alcohol, cocaine] including drug of choice). • Age of first use. Duration of use, method of use (e.g., intravenous injection, snorting, smoking). Last use. • Amount and cost of drug used per day or week. Patterns of binge use, amount used during a binge. • Method used to support habit (e.g., stealing, prostitution, employment, Aid to Dependent Children checks). • History of needle sharing (if intravenous drug user).
Presence of withdrawal symptoms	Alcohol—morning shakes, seizures (if pertinent, last seizure, and type of seizure), hallucinations (visual, auditory, or tactile). Opioids—nausea, vomiting, abdominal pain/cramps, diarrhea, chills, runny nose and eyes, sweating, bone or muscle pain. Cocaine—depression, suicidal thoughts (if pregnant, contractions, hyperactive baby).
Substance-related illnesses	Hepatitis, pancreatitis, gastrointestinal bleeding, heart complications, frequent bronchitis or pneumonia, positive HIV test (date of last test), cellulitis, frequent sexually transmitted disease and treatment dates.
Treatment history	Attempts at self-detoxification and outcome, names of treatment programs and dates, length of stay, and drug-free period after each treatment. Longest drug-free period, activities during that time.
Past medical history	Admissions for liver disease, peptic ulcers, heart attack, surgical procedures, history of diabetes, hypertension.
Medications	Prescribed and over the counter—usual dose, amounts actually used.
Family history	History of substance abuse. (Go back at least two generations and include current close relatives.)
Childhood history	Problems growing up, history of physical/sexual/emotional abuse, family relationships.
Consequences of substance use	Losses (jobs, property, relationships, children, self-respect, health).
Legal history	Arrests, incarcerations, current status (e.g., parole, probation).
Psychiatric history	Admissions, any known diagnoses, medications, history of suicide attempts or thoughts.
Social history	Marital status, number of children, ages and whereabouts, living situation and source of support, level of education and work history.
Sexual history	Sexual orientation, history of multiple partners, use of safe sex methods, history of rape, problems with impotence or other sexual dysfunction.
Gynecological history	Last menstrual period, irregularities, birth control method, gravidity, parity, abortions, miscarriages, ectopic pregnancies, complications during pregnancy, source of prenatal care, history of drug use during pregnancy, health of newborns.
Review of systems	Evaluate present status, whether intoxicated or in withdrawal at time of visit.

From Caulker-Burnett, I. (1994). Primary Care Screening for Substance Abuse. *Nurse Practitioner 19(6)*, 46.

FIGURE 31–3
Questions to include in the substance abuse history. (From Caulker-Burnett, I. [1994]. Primary care screening for substance abuse. *Nurse Practitioner, 19(6)*, 42–48.)

For example, the discovery that family members have been covering for the substance user so that he or she will not lose his job is an invaluable source of information about enabling behavior.

Although the primary diagnosis may be the substance use disorder, evidence of an underlying untreated psychiatric disorder may interfere with the patient's ability to engage fully in the rehabilitation process. Thought disturbances and tangential thinking may suggest a secondary problem with psychosis, whereas lack of anxiety and disregard for the rights of others may indicate an underlying personality disorder. When circumstantiality, perseveration, and disordered thinking are marked during the intake interview, an organic component should be considered. Evaluation of impulse control yields information about the patient's need for structure in planning treatment. Those with poor impulse control will need a stronger treatment structure and more personalized support to remain with the treatment program.

Self-diagnosis and *motivation for treatment* form the cornerstone of successful treatment. Motivation to change is perhaps the most important aspect of a favorable prognosis, and self-diagnosis of the problems created by substance use allows the substance user to take responsibility for his actions. In addition to providing an accurate database, the assessment process forms an important bridge to engaging the patient in the treatment process and the encouragement of self-diagnosis.

When a patient lacks motivation for treatment, as many do initially, therapeutic confrontation is a strategy often used to break through denial of the disorder's impact on the chemically dependent person's life and those most important to him or her. The family, with the treatment team's help, present the substance user with irrefutable evidence of behaviors related to chemical abuse or dependency with a firm call for treatment. This strategy is likely to have the greatest impact on patient readiness, particularly if coupled with realistic consequences for noncompliance. Another benefit is that it engages family cooperation from the outset of treatment.

Johnson (1990) defined a therapeutic confrontation as "meaningful people presenting reality to a person in a receivable way" (p. 3). Family members prepare for the confrontation in much the same way as a student would prepare for an important class presentation. Specific relevant data are presented in a logical and meaningful way so that the person receiving the information can easily comprehend it. The presented data include external problems (marital, social, occupational, financial) and personal problems such as physical impairments that are explicitly linked to specific substance use activities. Each person presents how the behavior he or she describes affects them personally. Factual information about the progression, treatment, and consequences of substance abuse is presented in a nonemotional, supportive manner. Attempts by the substance user to divert attention from the discussion or to make excuses without relating them to the problem of substance abuse are not accepted. Only the behaviors, and not the motivations, are up for consideration. Several pertinent behavioral examples are hard to refute even by the most hard-core chemical dependent. Implementable consequences of noncompliance are identified, and the person is advised that the decision to seek treatment is no longer an option.

Arrangements for immediate detoxification have been made before the confrontation, and, in many cases, a professional specially trained in therapeutic confrontations for addictive behaviors is present. The family must be willing to follow through on the consequences identified in the confrontation, and often the family will need a significant time beforehand to work through feelings about participating in it. Nevertheless, it is a powerful tool that has been used successfully as a motivator for treatment.

Nursing diagnoses relevant to the rehabilitation phase may include one or more of the following:

Ineffective Individual Coping
Altered Family Processes
Coping, Ineffective Family, compromised, dysfunctional
Knowledge Deficit
Social Isolation
Spiritual Distress
Self Care Deficit: Feeding, bathing/hygiene, dressing/grooming, toileting
Self-Concept Disturbance in: Self-esteem, personal identity, role performance
Powerlessness

OUTCOME IDENTIFICATION

The expected outcomes of treatment are simple to identify and difficult to implement:

- The patient will remain drug free.
- The patient will establish and maintain a productive and satisfying lifestyle.

Short-term goals consistent with the patient's nursing diagnoses are mutually defined so that they are acceptable to the chemically dependent and the family. This helps promote ownership of treatment goals and motivation to achieve them. In most instances, goal achievement will require a total commitment and daily effort. Setting goals one day at a time that are action oriented, realistic in scope, and achievable increases self-awareness and self-confidence.

PLANNING

Figure 31–4 presents the continuum of treatment options for drug abuse. Inpatient treatment of substance use disorders has been severely curtailed in a climate of restricted health benefits for mental disorders. Nevertheless, a variation on the Minnesota model, originally developed by three treatment Centers in Minnesota—Pioneer House, Hazelden, and Wilmar—continues to be operative in the treatment of substance use disorders. The Minnesota model uses the 12 steps of Alcoholics Anonymous (AA) (Box 31–5) as the foundation for treatment,

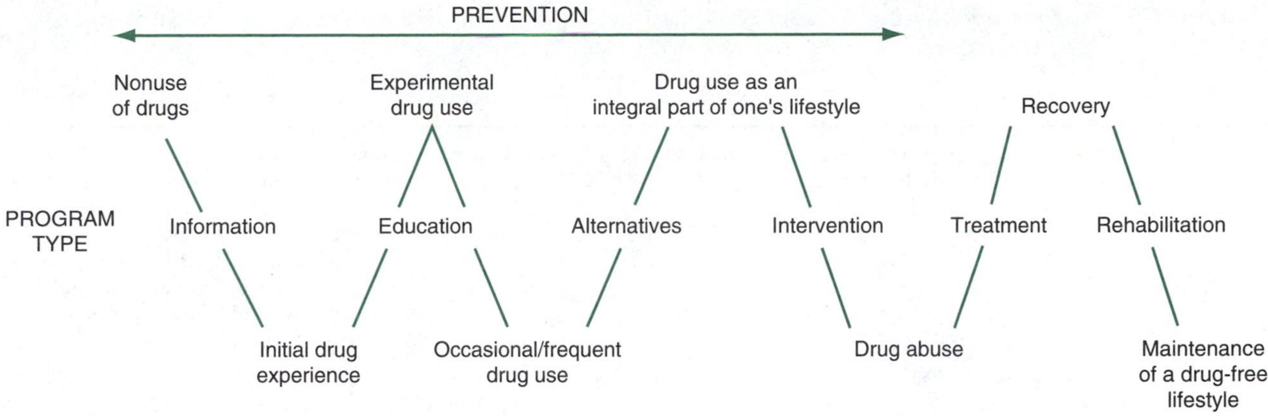

FIGURE 31–4
The continuum of treatment options for substance use disorders. (From French, J. F., and Kaufman, N. J. [1981]. *Handbook for prevention evaluation*. Rockville, MD: National Institute on Drug Abuse.)

BOX 31–5 The Twelve Steps of Alcoholics Anonymous*

1. We admitted we were powerless over alcohol—that our lives had become unmanageable.
2. Came to believe that a Power greater than ourselves could restore us to sanity.
3. Made a decision to turn our will and our lives over to the care of God *as we understood Him*.
4. Made a searching and fearless moral inventory of ourselves.
5. Admitted to God, to ourselves and to another human being the exact nature of our wrongs.
6. Were entirely ready to have God remove all these defects of character.
7. Humbly asked Him to remove our shortcomings.
8. Made a list of all persons we had harmed, and became willing to make amends to them all.
9. Made direct amends to such people wherever possible, except when to do so would injure them or others.
10. Continued to take personal inventory and when we were wrong promptly admitted it.
11. Sought through prayer and meditation to improve our conscious contact with God, *as we understood Him*, praying only for knowledge of His will for us and the power to carry that out.
12. Having had a spiritual awakening as the result of these steps, we tried to carry this message to alcoholics, and to practice these principles in all our affairs.

*The Twelve Steps are reprinted with permission of Alcoholics Anonymous World Services, Inc. Permission to reprint the Twelve Steps does not mean that A.A. has reviewed or approved the contents of this publication, nor that A.A. agrees with the views expressed herein. A.A. is a program of recovery from alcoholism *only*—use of the Twelve Steps in connection with programs and activities which are patterned after A.A., but which address other problems, or in any other non-A.A. context, does not imply otherwise. From Alcoholics Anonymous. (1955). *Twelve steps*. New York: Alcoholics Anonymous World Services.

and the staff usually consists of recovering addicts as well as health professionals specially trained in the treatment of addictive disorders. The treatment protocol involves an admission to a residential treatment facility with a heavy emphasis on self-diagnosis, intensive group counseling, educational lectures, and mandatory AA attendance. Table 31–5 provides suggested nursing actions for inpatient treatment or day treatment of substance use disorder. After discharge, the patient continues with an outpatient group for a few weeks or months as needed. The goal of this progressive treatment approach is to help the patient in the rehabilitative phase develop self-confidence and make needed connections in the community for continued aftercare.

IMPLEMENTATION

Nursing intervention strategies for the patient with a substance use disorder tend to be highly structured with an emphasis on self-diagnosis, limit setting, group therapy, skill development, and family treatment.

Self-Diagnosis

Self-diagnosis forms the cornerstone of treatment, and it is not easy for someone locked in a rigid world in which emotional reactions, mental processes, and spiritual values were controlled by a psychoactive substance for a long time. As the initial euphoria about taking the first step toward abstinence subsides, there is an awareness of the radical lifestyle changes required to maintain it. Old routines and personal habits that activate alcoholic or drug-taking behaviors have to be replaced with new and productive patterns of behavior; long-standing angers and resentments need a different outlet and resolution. These changes go to the very core of a person's self-concept, and the former substance user must now confront many painful attitudes and emotional responses. On a daily basis, the recovering addict must accept self and others as imperfect human beings living in an imperfect world, without the use of a psychoactive substance to dull the reality. There is the knowledge that in times of stress the person will be drawn once again to the landscape of substance use because this is familiar territory, whereas working through difficult life problems without alcohol

TABLE 31–5 **Suggested Nursing Actions for Inpatient Treatment or Day Treatment of Substance Use Disorder**

Expected Outcome	Nursing Actions
1. Client will verbalize that he is a chemical dependent and is powerless over his drug habit.	1. Assess current knowledge base. 2. Encourage ventilation of feelings related to substance abuse. 3. Describe natural progression of the disorder. 4. Identify resources for support and information. 5. Give positive reinforcement for self-diagnosis and assumption of personal responsibility for treatment. 6. Encourage involvement of significant others in treatment.
2. Client will participate in all treatment activities.	1. Assess client's motivation to change. 2. Establish schedule with client and hold client accountable for attendance. 3. Enforce agreed-on contingencies for manipulative and acting-out behaviors. 4. Encourage and reinforce acceptance of responsibility. 5. Mutually identify problems in coping and help client develop prevention plan. 6. Refer to community agencies and Alcoholics Anonymous before discharge. 7. Arrange for aftercare and easy revisiting of therapeutic community for discharged client.

or drugs is not as well known. There are many blanks in the patient's mental map, for which one must make amends. The recovering addict must discover the precise details that fill in the puzzle of the past and develop a new set of puzzle pieces. The human context against which the map of life will be drawn must be fluid enough to provide meaningful choice and fixed enough to provide the structure necessary for survival.

Rehabilitative efforts begin with helping the patient self-diagnose situations and feelings likely to get in the way of developing a different drug-free self-identity. Breaking through the denial is a necessary first step in the recovery process for the patient and family members. This can be accomplished in a number of ways, and the process usually begins with education. Providing basic information about the nature and development of the

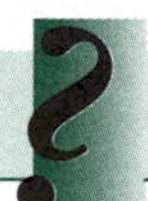

WHAT SOCIETY NEEDS TO KNOW **Alcoholism, cocaine addiction, and heroin addiction**

What is alcoholism?
Alcoholism is a term that applies to end stage of the continuum of nonuse versus addiction to alcohol. Addiction implies complete loss of control and drinking in spite of alcohol-related problems that involve social and occupational functioning. Alcoholism usually develops over many years of heavy drinking when the patient experiences a physiological and psychological dependence. With physical dependence tolerance develops (drinking more and more to achieve the same effect) and withdrawal (increased heart rate and blood pressure, irritability, and possible seizures). Psychological dependence involves compulsive use and craving.

What is cocaine addiction?
Cocaine is a naturally occurring stimulant extracted from the leaf of the coca bush. Cocaine affects the central nervous system and changes the way a person thinks, feels, and behaves. Dependence on this drug develops very quickly. The initial high (lasting 15 to 30 minutes) is followed by a deep depression. This reinforces the addictive nature of cocaine. Long-term chronic users have violent temper outbursts, disturbed thinking, and paranoia. Effects on the heart can lead to cardiac failure and death.

What is heroin addiction?
Heroin is an illegal street drug; therefore, addiction to heroin usually entails some type of antisocial or criminal behaviors. Heroin intoxication is manifested by constricted pupils, decreased breathing, drowsiness, lowered blood pressure, and slurred speech. There is often an initial euphoria and impaired memory and judgment. Withdrawal from heroin is similar to a bad case of influenza and is not life threatening. To recover from heroin addiction, methadone substitution is often used along with counseling and job training.

What does recovery from these three conditions entail?
Abstinence from the mood-altering chemical is usually necessary along with the continued, sustained support of a 12-step program. Certainly, there must be a desire to change behavior. In some instances such as with heroin addiction, a therapeutic community is necessary to maintain abstinence. At one time it was believed that a person had to "hit bottom" to recover. Today, with the help of professionals, interventions for each of these addictions can occur at an earlier point in the progression of the illness.

disorder offers hope and help with the realization that substance use disorders are treatable. An educational format provides a nonthreatening way to deliver emotionally charged information about a disorder that is difficult to understand and accept. Providing opportunities for patients to learn about the disease surprisingly provides information he or she has never heard before. Intensive group discussion of feelings expressed in the educational segment is an invaluable tool for breaking through the denial.

Group Therapy

Group therapy and self-help groups focused on abstinence and the behaviors needed to achieve it are the treatment of choice for alcoholics and drug abusers (Galanter et al, 1991). This is so for several reasons. First, groups provide a social network for the patient. Many will need this because without the bond of drinking or drug abuse, the patient has no friends. Other group members also provide consensual validation for the patient's experience and challenge any deceptions. They provide a powerful mechanism for breaking through the patient's denial because they have been there and know exactly how to get at the truth. At the same time, the group can support the patient's efforts to remain abstinent, and this is highly reinforcing. There is an opportunity to share the pain, shame, and small triumphs with others who understand. Group confirmation of similar feelings and experiences allows maladaptive behaviors and feelings to be normalized rather than repressed or exaggerated. Reality testing is practiced by sharing with others having similar experiences, finding self-confidence in the confrontations and problem-solving strategies. The acceptance that comes from other group members who like you just the way you are and yet who encourage you to become all that you are capable of is very empowering.

Behavioral Therapy

The behavioral component of the intervention (limit setting) is designed to help patients respond constructively to the ongoing stresses of everyday life in a self-disciplined way. Part of the behavior pattern seen frequently with substance use disorders is the avoidance of responsibility for common life tasks coupled with excuses for dealing with unmet obligations. Correction of the attitudes and behaviors that support a lifestyle of denial and rationalization is difficult but necessary. Mixed with the behaviors are unresolved negative attitudes and feelings of alienation, anger, loneliness, and self-doubt that form the underpinnings of resumption of drug-taking behaviors. Patients have learned to repress feelings and bottle them up inside until they explode often with disastrous results or until these feelings are acted out with the help of a psychoactive drug. Clear, consistent limits provide the external structure many patients need to internally respond effectively to their environment. Over time, these limits help the patient to internalize the process of setting limits on his or her own behavior in line with the needs of self and others. To be effective, the recovering substance user should participate actively in setting his or her own behavioral expectations. This helps ensure ownership.

The steps in a behavioral approach to treatment are as follows:

- Identify the rule, behavior, or emotion that is the focus of the intervention.
- Ask the patient to express feelings about it and possible alternative solutions.
- Agree on a behavioral expectation(s).
- Identify mutually defined natural and realistic consequences of noncompliance.
- Explain in what ways consequences for rule violations will be applied and when.
- Ask the patient for cooperation with protocol.
- Use a written contingency contract if needed.
- Develop criteria for termination of the consequence.
- Use agreed-on consequences immediately and without exception in a matter of fact but supportive way for infractions.

Following these steps often is difficult for the beginning practitioner who has established a relationship with the patient and wants to focus on a person's effort as well as outcome. To apply a consequence when the patient slips seems unfair because the patient appears to be trying so hard and reasons given for noncompliance are so plausible. Remembering that the nature of the disease is built on excuses provides the basis for understanding that the patient must accept full responsibility for mistakes. It is critical to the treatment process that the patient acknowledge full accountability for the natural consequences of his or her behavior. Thus, all caregivers should remain firm in using agreed-on consequences for seemingly minor infractions that ordinarily would escape notice in other patients.

Developing Social Skills

Social skill development is a critical aspect of successful treatment. Skill development related to basic management of uncomfortable emotions (e.g., anger) and the ability to recognize the situations that provoke them occur in small-group sessions. Identifying feelings of anger, fear, and vulnerability are frightening to people for whom emotions are not an acceptable part of life. Seeing others link behaviors to feelings as a norm of the group encourages the likelihood of similar effort on the patient's part. During this process, the patient learns to identify internal warning signs, leading to potential relapse. Signs of increasing stress that require attention include

- Increased desire for sugar or food binges
- Inability to concentrate
- Sleep disturbances

- Mood swings
- Increased stress

Patients will be more susceptible to the devitalizing effects of stress until they learn effective coping strategies to reduce it (Gorski, 1986). A compassionate, goal-directed approach helps the patient assume accountability for thoughts and feelings. Keeping the patient on track and clarifying roles and expectations aid in building needed trust and self-confidence. Broad guidelines to help the patient develop more effective patterns without drug use are presented in Box 31–6.

Another strategy in the early stages of supportive intervention is accomplished through cognitive restructuring (see Chapter 16). Cognitive restructuring involves becoming aware of faulty thinking patterns, validating perceptions and feelings with others, and practicing adaptive responses and behaviors. Restructured phrases remind the patient to "live and let live," to live "one day at a time," and that "easy does it," all slogans of AA. Living these platitudes provides a format for living in the present and taking responsibility for one's own needs as well as those of others.

BOX 31–6 Guidelines to Help Patients Develop More Effective Social Patterns Without Drug Use or Alcohol

Phase I: Self-Diagnosis

Identifying problem situations

Identifying feelings associated with need for drugs

Linking feelings with problem situations

Phase II: Self-Awareness

Identifying fears and vulnerabilities

Linking behaviors and feelings

Identifying behaviors needing change

Developing insight into impact of behaviors on self and others

Phase III: Self-Change

Identifying alternative constructive changes

Expressing feelings and needs to others

Establishing realistic daily goals and meeting them

Making amends when appropriate

Managing difficult emotions productively

Anticipating difficult situations

Phase IV: Integrating Gains

Developing a written prevention plan

Identifying and contacting outside resource supports

Providing Structural Supports

For those who need it, a drug-free therapeutic community in a hospital, day treatment setting, or halfway house offers a safe place where chemically dependent persons can develop skills needed in the larger community of life. The amount of help each person needs varies depending on their premorbid functioning, social support, and a host of other variables. Some patients can manage with little structure and a strong focus on developing adaptive skills in managing emotions. Others will need a defined environmental or treatment structure for a period of time to resume responsibility and develop increased independence in conducting a life without drugs. With some, strict limit setting, privileges systems, and an uncompromising program schedule provide the basic foundation for psychosocial skill development and gradual integration back into the community and family as a responsible, drug-free person.

Halfway houses are communal living situations that provide structure and support for those recovering addicts who lack family support and who cannot live on their own. Each halfway house has its own set of rules and expectations for those living in the house, with regular group meetings to discuss relevant issues. Housed in the community, the recovering patient can attend school or work during the day and return to a supportive environment each evening for meals and emotional sustenance. Usually the stay ranges from 1 to 4 months. Halfway houses provide an effective transitional bridge from the therapeutic inpatient community to the outside community, especially when coupled with outpatient treatment.

Aftercare

Patterns leading to substance use disorders are hard to erase, and recovering from a substance use disorder involves more than simply abstinence. Although it is easier for the patient in a detoxification program to feel confident about resisting the temptation to use drugs as a coping mechanism, this can lead to a false sense of confidence. Stresses are reduced, and the patient has a structure to his or her daily routine. The resolve may be there, but, once discharged, the stresses return and the old companions are available. Faulty thinking patterns of relying on the drug rather than other people, of not asking for help, or sharing important feelings are well ingrained. Without ongoing external support and structure, the patient's coping mechanisms may be too fragile to withstand the chronic daily stresses that occur in everyone's life, particularly when drug availability presents itself as an easy out. Thus, *ongoing aftercare is an essential part of the rehabilitative recovery process in the treatment of substance use disorders.*

Aftercare takes a variety of forms. It often includes a structured plan for relapse prevention, active participation in continuing treatment and self-help groups, and access to the original professional treatment center as needed. Education and support are provided in equal proportion. Patients need to understand that the pathological physiology developed in their systems with chronic drug use will persist throughout their lifetime. This means they cannot use drugs again. If they do, the drug effects are reactivated as if they had never stopped taking it. Staying off drugs when this has been a way of life will require intense effort, one day at a time, and for some, the craving will never disappear completely.

Developing Realistic Community Supports

For many patients, significant changes in their external world are needed because it is not unusual for some to have entered treatment with the loss or threat of loss of employment as the primary motivating factor. Returning to the work place is frightening as well as a bench mark of recovery that can lead to a different and balanced sense of identity. Counseling and role playing related to explaining their recovery process, responding to the discomfort of others who do not know how to react to them, and the need to prove oneself in the work place are practical interventions needed for return to the workplace. Unfortunately, many times these issues do not receive the attention they should with the recovering patient.

Most urban communities have Employee Assistance Programs (EAPs) and vocational rehabilitation for those who will have difficulty returning to the work force. Helping the patient seek another career when the original one is not conducive to recovery or is no longer available is also an important aspect of the recovery plan. Vocational and educational counseling, legal counseling, marital counseling, and development of realistic support systems in the community require a collaborative interdisciplinary approach to be successful.

Referral to Self-Help Groups

Referral to self-help groups in the community may be an important element of the rehabilitative process, particularly in a resource-driven health care system that no longer pays for the ongoing treatment many patients need. Groups such as Alcoholics Anonymous, Cocaine Anonymous, and Narcotics Anonymous use the 12-step program summarized in Box 31–5 to help those afflicted with substance use disorders develop a different lifestyle. The recovering addict typically is introduced to the group as a mandatory part of the treatment plan, or they go because someone else thinks it is a good idea. Hearing the facts from those who have been there and who are willingly making the commitment to achieve a drug-free lifestyle is a particularly effective part of the chemical dependent person's education.

Alcoholics Anonymous (AA) is the prototype for all support groups dedicated to the treatment of substance use disorders. It consists of "a fellowship of men and women who share their experience, strength and hope with each other that they may solve their common problem and help others to recover from alcoholism. The only requirement for membership is a desire to stop drinking" (AA World Services, 1955, p. 564). Led by fellow alcoholics, the AA organization provides formal meetings and informal support to those alcoholics who wish to become and remain sober. There are both open and closed meetings. Open meetings generally have a few designated speakers who tell the group about how AA has benefited them in their recovery process. In addition to these larger speaker meetings, there are smaller closed-group meetings with opportunities to discuss more personal issues with others and step meetings for more complete discussion of ways to meet the 12 steps needed for recovery. Groups for special needs (e.g., gays, women, minorities, professionals) are available in most larger urban communities. AA also provides an important informal network of support to those in need through its sponsorship component. Each new member who desires it is paired in a one-to-one relationship with a person who has been sober for some time. This person usually is of the same sex to forestall development of difficult intimate relationships. The sponsor is always available to the new member by telephone for encouragement, for clarification, and as a sounding board, particularly during the early stages of recovery. Vulnerable periods are the first month and after the first anniversary. Milestones are marked publically in the meeting with a token, speech, and sometimes refreshments.

The effectiveness of the 12-step program and its influence in reducing the incidence of recidivism with substance use disorders are indisputable, as described in Case Example 31–2.

Case Example 31–2 Dana's Story, Part 2

Narcotics Anonymous really changed my life. I got into it in the following way. I was visiting my aunt in the hospital. My cousin was there, and we had partied together before. The subject of drugs came up, and she mentioned that she had quit and she did it through Narcotics Anonymous. Well, I thought that was great for her; she had finally gotten her life together; I was forgetting, of course, to look at my own life. She offered to take my sister and I to a meeting with her. My sister went, but I passed. A couple of weeks later, I decided to go really just out of curiosity. I didn't like my first meeting, I think, because I was so preoccupied with looking around to see if anyone was looking at me and just feeling very uncomfortable. It also wasn't exciting enough for me. I guess when you live in the fast lane long enough, sitting in a room with people and having everything that goes on be organized takes a little getting used to. I was real scared and couldn't wait to get out of there. I have no idea what made me do it, but I went to another meeting later that week. I felt more comfortable and met a lot of real good people I guess because I wasn't in a race to get out the door. I started to go regularly and someone told me, "Just try it for 30 days and if you don't like it, the drugs aren't going anywhere." So that's what I did and I've been there ever since. That was 3 years ago.

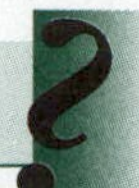

WHAT PATIENTS AND FAMILIES NEED TO KNOW 12-step programs

What do you mean by a 12-step program?
A 12-step program is a fellowship of men and women who have a common problem (alcoholism, substance abuse, relationships, overeating, gambling, and so on). The only requirement for membership is the desire to stop a behavior that has become unmanageable. Twelve-step programs are not allied with any sect, denomination, political affiliation, religious institution, or organization. These programs will not endorse or oppose any causes and are completely based on voluntary membership and are totally self-supporting.

Where did 12-step programs originate?
In 1935 Bill W. and Dr. Bob founded the original 12-step support group for alcoholics. Shortly thereafter, Al-Anon was founded by Lois Wilson, the wife of Bill W. Since that time hundreds of 12-step support groups have begun that follow the model of Alcoholics Anonymous.

How are 12-step programs helpful?
Twelve-step programs provide an anonymous setting in which people with similar problems can share experience, strength, and hope. People who attend these meetings on a regular basis find a sense of community and are able to find acceptance and unconditional love and support. The 12 steps are "worked through" with the help of the members or a sponsor. The essence of the steps entails admitting that you have a problem, acknowledging that you are in need of a power greater than yourself to stop the behavior, admitting strengths and weaknesses, making amends to others you have offended as a result of the problem, and helping others through the same process. Twelve-step members do not actively solicit members but are always available when a potential member asks for help.

Isn't it necessary to have professional help when you have a substance abuse disorder?
To help an addicted person with the potentially harmful symptoms of withdrawal, medical attention is often necessary because death can be a complication of improperly managed withdrawal. In some cases in which there is a dual diagnosis (an addictive process and a mental illness) present, professional help is indicated. Otherwise, programs like Alcoholics Anonymous have helped millions of people worldwide.

I am now 21 years old and live in my own apartment that I share with a girl I met in the program. I'm taking risks, like moving out, buying a car, looking into college, and getting involved with different causes and movements I believe in. I'm doing things I wouldn't have done before, like sticking up for myself and not accepting unacceptable behavior. Narcotics Anonymous and the people in it taught me that I am someone, that I am pretty, and that I am important. They try to show you and to help you to live life on life's terms, which isn't always easy whether you use drugs or you don't. It wasn't hard for me to give up my old friends, because once I stopped getting high most of them really didn't want me around anyway. They told me in NA that if I missed my friends to just stick around and they would come back if they didn't die first. Now a lot of people I used to party with are with me in the rooms of Narcotics Anonymous. Narcotics Anonymous has definitely given me back respect for myself. They gave me back a chance at life and trying to be the best person I can be.

EVALUATION

The evaluation criteria are directly linked to achievement of the patient outcomes identified earlier in the chapter. What you should look for is evidence that the patient is taking steps to reduce risk factors for potential relapse. The recovering substance user should be able to verbalize and demonstrate lifestyle changes needed to achieve and maintain abstinence from psychoactive substances. Successful treatment results are seen in the patient's ability to cope with life situations in a realistic way without drug use. This person is able to acknowledge and work through difficult feelings and to seek support from people and God rather than drugs in times of distress. Specific examples of evaluation criteria applications are presented in the case study. Indicators of potential difficulty maintaining abstinence care include insomnia/hypersomnia, racing thoughts, increased irritability or agitation, social isolation and withdrawal.

VULNERABLE POPULATIONS AND SUBSTANCE USE DISORDERS

Although substance use disorders cross all social and economic groups, certain populations are at higher risk for experiencing the disorder or present special needs associated with their substance use. For example, cultural differences in drinking patterns and whether or not the unfavorable behavioral effects of alcoholic behavior are tolerated by the society play a role (Helman, 1990). Ethnic cultures that support controlled drinking in moderation as a normal part of life while strongly disapproving of any forms of intoxication or deviant behavior associated with drinking are less likely to experience significant problems. Thus, Italians and Orthodox Jews who incorporate moderate intake of alcohol into mealtimes and social religious functions have significantly lower rates of alcoholism.

Extremes in attitudes about drinking seem to produce the negative drinking patterns likely to lead to alcoholism. In the Irish culture, there is no one dependable attitude toward drug consumption. Large quantities of alcohol consumption are encouraged at social functions, and yet alcohol consumption is strongly disapproved of as a regular part of life. The alcoholism rate among the Irish is higher than normal. Other cultures that specifically condemn alcohol use on religious grounds—Mormons, certain Muslim cultures, and Baptists, for example—have a slightly higher than normal incidence of deviant drinking patterns.

Disadvantaged minority groups have a proportionately higher incidence of chemical dependency than the dominant culture for another social reason. The instant money, lure of excitement, and comraderie of seemingly self-made, confident individuals in control of life and the people around them are powerful seducers of the young and poor living in substandard conditions with little promise of a better life. The power of such enhancements is hard to eradicate. Alcoholism is identified as one of the leading health problems in the black ghetto community activated by informal structures of unemployment, availability of alcohol, peer pressure, and social norms that support drinking as an important part of life (Rouse, 1989). Hispanics and Native Americans have similar issues of deprivation, availability, and social support of drug-taking behaviors that make them high risk for drug abuse. Among Native Americans, the second leading cause of death in young men is alcohol abuse, and it is estimated that "95% of American Indian families are affected either directly or indirectly by a family member's alcohol abuse" (U.S. Department of Health and Human Services, 1990, p. 39).

Women

Finnegan and Kandall (1992) estimated that women account for approximately 34% of those diagnosed with substance use disorders. Yet addiction in women is largely hidden because it carries an even greater stigma than for men. Social conditioning about the role of women, even in an era of women's liberation, does not allow for the same type of understanding accorded her male counterpart. Yet women typically experience symptoms of alcoholism at a faster rate than men do, and there is a stronger link between stress and development of symptoms (Quinby and Graham, 1993). Substance use disorders are often associated with secondary social problems for women, with a higher reported incidence of abuse, incest, and exploitation among women diagnosed as chemically dependent (Senay, 1983). Instead of turning to crime to support their drug dependency, women are more likely to become prostitutes. This increases the risk of AIDS and other sexually transmitted diseases in this population.

Treatment issues for women also are more complicated as physicians tend to overlook substance use disorders as a primary diagnosis in women. They are more likely to treat their signs and symptoms of alcoholism as secondary to a woman's presenting psychological and medical symptoms or as reflecting self-medication for such symptoms. These women are more likely to be found in general mental health treatment centers being treated for a depressive disorder rather than in chemical dependency programs, where their substance use disorder could be addressed (Mondanaro, 1989). Nurses can become strong advocates for these women, who frequently lack the judgment or skills to act in their own best interest.

Adolescents

Shiff and Cavarola (1988–1989) estimated that 1 of every 10 adolescents will graduate from high school with a pattern of psychoactive substance abuse. Adolescence is a time of rapid transition of biological and psychological changes unparalleled in most other life stages. Adolescents are prone to explore different life experiences, among them experimentation with drugs. In fact, 47% of high school graduating seniors in the United States admitted to illicit drug use (Muramoto and Leshau, 1993).

For teenagers, the first drink or experiment with psychoactive drugs often signifies "risk taking," doing what adults do. "Binge" drinking at parties and smoking pot with friends at school are tolerated without significant stigma attached. Peer pressure and a desire to appear successful with friends take precedence in activity choices without the reflective thinking that would look at the more adverse consequences of such risk-taking behavior.

Because drug abuse retards attainment of developmental milestones, the adolescent literally suffers from developmental arrest at the point that the chemical dependency begins. Thus, the 18-year-old adolescent who began drinking at age 12 years developmentally stopped maturing at age 12 years and frequently has the psychosocial skills of a beginning adolescent when chemical dependency is brought under control. The phenomenon of developmental arrest with psychoactive disorders is important in treatment and discharge planning. Otherwise, the recovering adolescent is thrown into social situations that chronologically he or she should be able to handle without much guidance but developmentally cannot without assistance and support. Dana's story describes a typical chain of events associated with substance use disorders in adolescence; a typical trajectory from simple recreational use to a full-blown addiction marked with denial, rationalization, and projection. Dana did not see that she was in trouble until it was almost too late. Dana was lucky because her story has a happy ending. She found Narcotics Anonymous and through this group eventually found herself.

Some adolescents are more at risk than others for the development of a substance use disorder. A number of studies have identified difficult family situations, interpersonal skill deficits, early delinquent behaviors, and exposure to psychoactive drugs as strong predictors of adolescent chemical dependency (Dishion and Lober, 1985; Patterson, 1982). Family discord in the form of bitter custody battles, inconsistent rules, splitting of child-rearing approaches that leave the child in the middle, and lack of supervision contribute to a higher incidence of substance abuse disorders in these adolescents. Adolescents introduced to drug use by their parents or significant others in the home are particularly at risk for the development of chemical dependency (Shiff and Cavarola, 1988–1989). So are adolescents who do not fit into their peer group because of differences in cognitive, attentional, behavioral control, or peer relations skills (Chaudron and Wilkenson, 1988). Social and intellectual differences become more apparent during pubescence and with the added stress of moving from junior high to high school. The combination of easy availability of drugs and a need to belong is particularly dangerous for insecure adolescents. In many instances, boredom and low self-esteem heighten the prevalence of drug abuse among disenchanted adolescents. When life does not have much to offer, and psychoactive drugs can transform that reality into a more pleasant one, drug-taking behaviors become commonplace. Other social factors that influence drug-taking behaviors revolve around the lifestyles of high school dropouts and unemployed youth with easy access to drugs, higher levels of stress, and lower conformity to social norms. Chemical dependency in the adolescent progresses more rapidly than in adults. An adolescent can become an alcoholic with 6 months of heavy drinking.

The Unborn

All psychoactive drugs cross the placenta, and most are capable of causing serious teratogenic effects in the fetus. In the United States, it is estimated that 2.6 million of infants born each year will have had significant exposure to alcohol through maternal abuse, and approximately 1 in 100 will demonstrate clinical teratogenic effects as a result (Finnegan and Kandall, 1992). Heavy drinking increases the risk of miscarriage and stillbirth. Excessive use of alcohol during pregnancy can lead to the development of fetal alcohol syndrome (FAS) in the newborn infant. Alcohol passes through the placenta from the mother to the fetus, and the amount of alcohol consumed by the fetus equals that consumed by the mother. Approximately 5000 infants are born each year with FAS (Streissguth, 1986).

The incidence of FAS is higher among certain ethnic groups. For example, it occurs 33 times more often in Native Americans and 6.7 times more often in the black population than in whites. The probability of having a second FAS child increases for women who have one FAS infant (Dorfman, 1989).

Fetal alcohol syndrome presents with a distinctive pattern of physical and mental defects. It is one of the three most prevalent causes of mental retardation in the newborn (Johnson, 1990). Infants born with this condition suffer gross structural malformations. They appear retarded with abnormally small heads and a higher incidence of microcephaly. There is a distinctive narrowing of the eyes and low nasal bridge. Almost half of the infants born with FAS have a heart defect, and many suffer defects in their joints and have low birth weight. There is a correlation of severe mental deficiency in infants with noticeable physical defects. Such children are prone to behavioral problems and characteristically demonstrate short attention spans, nervousness, and poor coordination (Finnegan and Kandall, 1992). There is no treatment for FAS.

Cocaine dependency in the mother can cause serious problems in pregnancy. Women who consistently use cocaine are at risk for miscarriage and premature birth. There is evidence that regular cocaine use contributes to the development of abruptio placentae, a condition in which the placenta breaks away from the uterine wall, causing excessive bleeding and possible termination of the pregnancy. Newborns subjected to the cocaine dependence of their mothers demonstrate withdrawal symptoms after birth. Frequently, they are jittery, irritable, and difficult to comfort (Finnegan and Kandall, 1992). Because of their drug-related personality characteristics and the drug dependency of the mother, children of cocaine addicts are at increased risk for child abuse.

Opiates are appetite suppressants, often compromising the birth weight of the infant as well as the mother. Prenatal sedative and opiate dependence can endanger the birth process and create serious problems for the newborn. Passive heroin addiction can be fatal for the newborn cut off from maternal supply source at birth when the umbilical cord is cut. Withdrawal symptoms include high-pitched cry, central nervous system excitability, poorly coordinated sucking-swallowing reflex, muscle hypertonicity, and hyperirritability. If the mother has an opiate dependency, there is a 60% chance that the infant will suffer withdrawal symptoms once the cord is cut (Finnegan, 1988).

The problem of passive drug addiction in the newborn is further complicated by associated sociomedical complications (e.g., polydrug use, poor nutrition, heavy smoking, and inadequate prenatal care). Hospitals are experiencing a marked increase in the number of seriously ill and "boarder" infants associated with maternal substance abuse. The expanding population of passively addicted boarder infants, abandoned by mothers incapable of caring for them, creates a unique health care challenge and suggests the need for nontraditional models of intervention and innovative ways to engage and treat substance-abusing adolescents in the community. Allowing grandparents to assume custody for the infant can be a faulty solution because problems with drug abuse and dysfunctional family patterns often are prevalent in the grandparents' household as well. Even after successful detoxification, children exposed to psychoactive drugs in utero experience a higher incidence of developmental delays and significant behavioral problems in childhood and adolescence. Table 31–6 summarizes the teratogenic effects of psychoactive substances.

The Elderly

Substance use disorders in the elderly has been called the "hidden addiction" because one does not usually think of the elderly as having drug problems. The problem becomes increasingly more prevalent as more people are living longer (Buys and Saltman, 1982). Psychoactive drug use in the elderly is most likely to involve alcohol or benzodiazepines prescribed for mild tension or sleeplessness. In general, psychoactive drugs, as with most other drugs administered to the elderly, are metabolized much more slowly than they are at an earlier stage of life, and individual responsiveness to drug actions is more variable in the elderly than at any other stage of life. As a result, the effects of the drug occur with greater intensity and last longer. Prescriptions to relieve sleeping problems and undiagnosed depression in the elderly may actually intensify rather than treat the underlying problem.

Treatment of the elderly follows therapeutic approaches similar to those used for other chemically

TABLE 31–6 **Teratogenic Effects of Psychoactive Substances**

Psychoactive Substance	Medical Use	Teratogenic Effects
Alcohol	Formerly used to stop contractions in premature labor	Weak to strong teratogenic effects Fetal alcohol effects Low birth weight Central nervous system dysfunction Learning disability Decreased maternal folate levels Retardation
Benzodiazepines	Short-term treatment of alcohol withdrawal; anxiolytic	Transient fetal tachycardia Neonatal withdrawal effects First trimester—cleft palate
Barbiturates	Seizure control in epilepsy	May decrease fetal movement resulting in malpresentation during birth Anomalies similar to fetal alcohol syndrome Neonatal toxicity: poor sucking reflex, hypotonia Neonatal withdrawal: restlessness, irritability, hyperreflexes, disturbed sleep patterns
Cocaine	None	Constricts placental and umbilical blood vessels Fetal hypoxia Intrauterine growth retardation Premature labor Neonatal withdrawal: irritability, hypertonicity, tremor Increased incidence of childhood behavior problems, attention deficit disorder
Opiates	None	Spontaneous miscarriage Higher incidence of stillbirth Intrauterine growth retardation Higher incidence of toxemia Low birth weight Neonatal withdrawal: impaired sucking, hyperactivity, hypertonicity, vomiting, sleep disturbances, diarrhea, and tremors Childhood behavior problems

dependent populations with regard to detoxification, family interventions, and the need for long-term follow-up. Additionally, lack of family and occupational supports, lost as the person ages, may require a greater emphasis on social, financial, and medical support services in the community as part of the treatment plan.

People with Acquired Immunodeficiency Syndrome

Intravenous drug abuse has played a major role in the spread of the AIDS virus; IV drug abusers form the second largest primary risk group for development of the disorder. Secondary victims include newborn infants and nonabusing heterosexual or homosexual partners. According to the Centers for Disease Control (CDC), more than 25% of AIDS cases are attributable to IV drug abuse. Not counted in this assessment are homosexuals who also are IV drug abusers. The CDC classifies these individuals as homosexuals only. IV drug use accounts for 52% of the cases in women (Amsel, 1990). Further complicating the picture is the long prodromal period possible between time of initial exposure to HIV and development of diagnosable symptoms. At special risk are minority populations, Puerto Ricans, and blacks, who have a proportionately higher incidence of AIDS by contrast with their numbers in the general population.

Chronic substance use suppresses the immune system. In particular, alcohol, amphetamines, and marijuana actively compromise the effectiveness of the body's immune system. Drug abuse contributes to the spread of AIDS in two ways: (1) through IV drug use with contaminated needles among drug abusers who share needles and (2) through "survival sex" in which teenagers and adults prostitute themselves to obtain the money to buy drugs. Their anonymous and often multiple sex partners are frequently infected with the AIDS virus (Kerr, 1989). Prevention programs need to address high-risk sexual behaviors as well as drug abuse in a combined format because they are so closely interrelated in women of childbearing age (Box 31–7).

Acquired immunodeficiency syndrome in children of drug-abusing parents is a serious and growing threat to society. More than 50% of the infants born to women who test seropositive are affected by the virus, and there is no known way to prevent maternal transmission. Indirect or direct IV drug abuse is a major factor in the transmission of this fatal disease.

▶ **Check Your Reading**

7. What are the implications for women of having a substance use disorder?
8. What role does substance use play in pregnancy and neonatal care?
9. What are important considerations in the nursing care of adolescents with substance use disorders?

SUBSTANCE USE DISORDERS AND THE FAMILY

Chemical Dependency Is a Family Disease

The nature of the disorder makes it a psychodynamic force in the family with adaptive properties that influence how the family system functions. No one in close contact with a substance-dependent person can escape being touched by the disease process. Dependency on drugs or alcohol takes first priority so that little if any emotional support is available to family members. In response, family members develop defensive styles of relating, conflict management, and rules for handling behaviors associated with the substance use disorder. The spouse generally is the most keenly aware of the pathological substance use pattern and its implications for family functioning. One woman described it as like having her husband's mistress living in the house, so great was her husband's attachment to the bottle. The frequent visits to the basement for the purpose of drinking and returning with a lie to cover for the time spent struck her as analogous to the sneaking around that people with external relationships engage in with their spouses. Yet although these behaviors would never be tolerated with an actual mistress, frequently they are endured with someone having equally heavy involvement with a psychoactive substance.

Anxiety, anger, and resentment are powerful emotions experienced by most family members coping with a family member on drugs. Anxiety in the spouse and children about excessive drug use in a family member creates its own set of problems in which each feels guilty, angry, and responsible for each other's response in addition to the feelings associated with the identified patient. For example, the children may blame the mother for allowing their father to drink and abuse the family. The wife may resent the inability of the husband to be a good father. A child may feel that he or she is responsible for his or her father's unpredictable moods while under the influence of the psychoactive substance. Anger at not having appropriate role models and grief for the loss of the parent who should be present but is not are very normal feelings. Children often feel resentment at having to take the role of the parent when the parent cannot assume this role because of the disorder. The focus on the drug-taking behavior and patterns becomes as obsessive for the family as it does for the drug abuser. Although the reasons are different, the outcome is the same. There is little time for anything else other than the incessant call of the psychoactive substance.

Without treatment, family members usually are unable to disengage themselves with overconcern for the patient's behavior. Like the identified patient, they too give up their self-respect, often their possessions, and everything that is important to them in response to the addiction. In every story of a substance use disorder, there is a parallel family story with recurring themes of the family's hopelessness and anger about the patient's unpredictability in emotional response, the lack of sensitivity the person under the influence of psychoactive drugs displays, and the sheer terror that those closest to the chemically dependent person experience, sometimes on a daily basis. Control is a constant underlying dynamic. The chemical-dependent substance user lacks control over the psychoactive agent; the family seeks to control the use of the drug. For this reason, the family members are referred to as codependents.

BOX 31-7 What Women Should Know About Pregnancy and Acquired Immunodeficiency Syndrome (AIDS)

- Seventy-three percent of AIDS cases are attributed to maternal transmission during pregnancy.
- A seropositive woman does not need to be sick with AIDS to transmit it to her fetus.
- Fifty to 60% of children born to seropositive mothers will be infected.
- There is no way to prevent the fetus from becoming infected if the mother is infected.

Adapted from Mondanaro J. (1990). Community-based AIDS prevention interventions: Special issues of women intravenous drug users. In U.S. Department of Health and Human Services (Ed.), *AIDS and intravenous drug use: Future directions for community-based prevention research*, (NIDA Research Monograph, p. 7893). Washington, DC: U.S. Department of Public Health and Human Services.

Codependency

The term *codependency* was developed in the 1970s to describe a predictable pattern of behaviors in family members characterized by overfunctioning, a lack of objectivity, powerlessness, and the need to control another's behavior (Fig. 31–5). Those closest to the patient try in every way possible to orchestrate a relationship that is meaningful. It is a hopeless task accompanied by hypervigilance and feelings of intense loneliness, self-doubt, resentment, and anger, which preoccupy the codependent and influence his or her behavior. There is a wish to retaliate, generally with the knowledge that it will have no effect. According to Johnson (1990) the self-destructive patterns presented by the substance user that are most likely to stimulate a strong desire to retaliate in the codependent include the following:

- Breaking family commitments, both major and minor
- Spending more money than planned

Overview of Codependence Development: From the Precious to the Adapted Child into the Adult State of "Dis"-ease

Authenticity (Real Self)	Adaptation (Loss of Self)	Adult Codependence (Primary Symptoms)	Related Problems (Secondary Symptoms)
Child abuse —causes→	Shame issues —which generate→	Powerlessness —related to→	Unmanageability
1. Valuable (precious)	1. Less than vs better than	1. Self-esteem issues	1. Negative control issues
2. Vulnerable (protection)	2. Too vulnerable vs invulnerable	2. Boundary issues	2. Resentment issues
3. Imperfect (reality)	3. Bad or rebellious vs good or perfect	3. Reality issues	3. Spirituality issues
4. Dependent (needs/wants)	4. Too dependent vs anti-dependent or needless/wantless	4. Dependency issues	4. Addiction issues; physical illness; mental illness
5. Immature (age-specific)	5. Super-immature or no control vs super-mature or in control	5. Moderation issues	5. Intimacy issues

FIGURE 31–5
Overview of codependence development. (Copyright © 1988 by Pia Mellody, P.O. Box 1739, Wickenburg, Arizona 85358.)

- Driving while intoxicated and getting arrested
- Making inappropriate statements to friends, family, and coworkers
- Arguing, fighting, and other antisocial actions (p. 203)

Although the family confronts the patient in anger about these breaches of contract or expectations, typically the confrontation fails to achieve its desired purpose of changing the addict's behavior. Reflex confrontations stemming from anger and resentment over behaviors suffered while under the influence increase the individual's painful feelings of shame and guilt, stimulating further substance use.

The need to rescue others, to make everything okay, and not to stir the waters to avoid stimulating further drug use and the wish to construct a world in which everything is predictable, black or white, and thus controllable become defining characteristics for codependency. Ironically, these behaviors enable the identified patient to continue substance use by allowing this person to escape the consequences of his or her behavior and in many cases by providing a legitimate rationale for downplaying the seriousness of the problem.

Enabling behaviors refer to actions designed to protect the chemically dependent from the consequences of the dependency either by covering for them or by denying their personal uneasiness about the addictive behavior (Pires, 1989). The behaviors represent an unspoken pact between the patient and family member to protect the patient from being embarrassed outside of the home by behaviors related to their substance use. This conspiracy of silence stems from the family's insecurity about themselves and a desire to protect their reputation in the community. It is not uncommon for family members to feel that if only they were different—more loving, a different personality, less angry, or more understanding—the chemically dependent person would stop using drugs. Guilt about their inability to be whatever it is they think they should be so the person would not use drugs and shame about what is occurring within the family compel them to assume responsibility for controlling a living environment that is not controllable. The "enabler" colludes with the substance user in avoiding responsibility for his or her actions by shielding him or her from suffering the painful consequences of the dependency needed for recovery.

Recovery

In many instances, family members feel that unless the person with the substance use disorder seeks treatment, there is little purpose in engaging in treatment themselves. This is not true. Without external support, the family becomes so emeshed in trying to control the dependency or in reacting reflexively to the behaviors of the person under the influence that they unconsciously "enable" the individual to deny the dependency.

The importance of a family focus should not be underestimated; the constructive support of the immediate family is identified as the single most important variable in preventing relapse. Often affected family members enter treatment with the idea that the chemically dependent person is the problem in the family dynamics, and they see their role as being of help to this person. Effective treatment of codependency requires an attitudinal change for the family. The primary goal in initial encounters with the family is to establish a therapeutic tone and to broaden the focus from the identified patient to include the entire family, particularly those who have power and influence.

Expected outcomes of codependency treatment are the reestablishment of personal boundaries, development of a strong sense of personal identity, and, in many instances, the restructuring of a life without a primary focus on substance use. Recovery from codependency begins when other family members begin to reorganize their lives in spite of, and not around, the problem. Group formats benefit codependents, and there are many community resources (Al-Anon, Ephesians) available to help family members gain the proper perspective and knowledge of substance use disorders. These groups offer a safe place to explore feelings. People with similar issues provide guidance and support related to skill development, identifying and reinforcing personal boundaries and the balance needed for a satisfying, productive life. They assist each other in developing a healthy productive sense of self-identity that does not ignore the existence of their life problem but rather emotionally detaches from accepting responsibility for it.

In individual formats, a family genogram (see Chapter 20) often provides important access into the various family member's experiences in their family of origin and provides beginning data that invariably are relevant to the patient's current situation. This information serves as the basis for understanding present relationship problems and how historical data relate to it. Other assessment data helpful in the treatment of the family unit consist of the following:

- Physical and psychological isolation
- Degree of insight
- Types of enabling behaviors
- Capacity to form intimate relationships
- Financial or marital problems
- Self-esteem
- Degree of blame and hostility
- Capacity to express deep personal feelings
- Presence of related physical and psychological disorders
- Communication patterns
- Family strengths and support systems

Communication patterns in families coping with substance use disorders generally are negative and related to a number of family issues: (1) responsibility, (2) control, (3) adequacy, (4) self-esteem, and (5) trust. In many families, the person diagnosed with the disorder actually performs a very important function by maintaining family homeostasis. Without the chemical dependence, family communication might be nonexistent. Discussions about the substance user's behavior form the content for most interactions. Abstinence frees the mind to engage in active dialogue with significant others, and it liberates the family from its constant vigilance of the substance use. Often, however, there is nothing to take its place. This is where a problem arises. For a significant period of time, the person and the family have maintained a psychological distance from each other's world, and now each needs to reestablish emotional connections. Each needs to reexplore the heart of his or her own center for its meaning and to develop a new family history built around family strengths rather than a psychoactive substance. However, usually there is much anger and resentment, which needs a safe repository. Moreover, the family dream of a meaningful family life will take time to cultivate. For those who have lived anesthetized with a psychoactive substance for a significant period of time, there has been little exposure to the types of values, skills, and attitudes required to live a meaningful life. Communication becomes the means by which families rediscover the possibilities of a life without psychoactive drugs. Once the psychoactive substance is no longer the center of discussion, families need help in developing functional communication patterns.

Psychological treatment consists of helping families identify and correct dysfunctional communication patterns. Interventions build on family strengths, and each family member is expected to assume responsibility for modifying his or her part in the dysfunctional process. Family treatment often includes multifamily group support. Not all families embrace with enthusiasm the idea of multifamily groups. The nurse can be an important resource in giving families permission to just listen until they feel comfortable participating. This simple intervention often is all that is needed. The common bond of chemical dependence in the family serves as a powerful source of identification as families support each other's efforts to express powerful feelings and to develop effective coping strategies. Seeing oneself in relation to peers with similar experiences and hearing how others perceive them can destroy the tendency to see everything in one's own family as all good or all bad. The group format allows family members to test out their ideas with other parents, spouses, and siblings rather than comparing themselves only in relation to their own family.

Treatment for Children

Children of chemically dependent parents experience long-lasting effects of substance use disorders even if they never ingest a psychoactive substance. Although they directly experience the effects of the disorder in the form of abuse or neglect, these children have an added disadvantage. They often have difficulty establishing normal behavioral standards for themselves because they lack the necessary role models and life experiences that could guide them appropriately. Normal emotions that should alert the child to danger, pleasure, and basic needs are overshadowed by the need to cope with the erratic and irrational behaviors of one or both parents. Instead, the child learns to suppress normal emotions and to "control" his or her inner conflict and chaos by pleasing others, staying out of the way, and repressing legitimate feelings of grief, anger, and resentment. These children learn mistrust, shame, and guilt instead of trust and self-confidence. The fear and emotional trauma of living in a dysfunctional home also manifest themselves in childhood nightmares, perfectionism, behavioral problems, poor school performance, and passive withdrawal from life.

Children of drug-dependent parents frequently overfunction or act out their distress. Having limited life experience, the child imagines that he or she is in some way responsible for the development of the chemical dependency. The child incorporates this information into his or her memory bank. There it lies dormant but is seen as an underlying dynamic in the child's trying to please everyone and erupting from time to time in the form of panic attacks and depressive symptoms. What logically follows for the child from this faulty line of reasoning is that, if one creates the problem, it also is within one's power to fix the problem. Often the youngster takes on responsibilities that should not be expected of a child to counteract feelings of helplessness. The child literally does not have a childhood experience, which further sabotages normal growth and development.

Many of these children doubt their own reality and do not realize that their family life is different in critical and damaging ways until they leave home. They avoid bringing other children home either because of the condition of the house, the unpredictability of the chemically dependent parent, or the wishes of the codependent parent to keep things at an even keel so as to avoid the possibility of stimulating drinking or abusive behavior. Ala-Teen and Ala-Tot groups provide ongoing support for children and help reduce the feelings of isolation and family sabotage that children experience on a daily basis in chemically dependent families. School counselors are an invaluable resource for children coping with chemical dependency and dysfunctional behaviors in their families. As a nurse, you will need to become acquainted with the professional services and community support opportunities available for children living in dysfunctional, chemical dependent households. The approach to the child needs to be proactive because the child's cry for help often is weak and indirect. Often school or behavioral problems are the first indicator of severe dysfunction within the family. The child frequently will not request assistance. However, if it is offered, usually they will be highly receptive to understanding intervention.

Treatment for Adult Children of Alcoholics

Growing up in a dysfunctional home leads to significant problems in adulthood, as research is just beginning to demonstrate. So much emotional energy goes into hiding the family secret of addiction, helping to maintain the false sense of normalcy, and the squelching of legitimate feelings that adult children of alcoholics (ACOAs) may have no memory for significant portions of their childhood. ACOAs are more likely to become substance abusers themselves, because this is the only life pattern they know, or to marry a chemically dependent person. Often they have trouble recognizing and expressing feelings in constructive ways. In varying degrees they experience emotional over- or underreactions to stressful and emotional situations. It is hard for many ACOAs to trust their own reality or to consider their opinions valid. Growing up with a consistent pattern of unpredictable human responses keeps the developing child off balance, storing up memories that are reactivated in uncertain stressful situations as an adult. There is no solid base to draw from so that previous maladaptive coping styles are carried into adult life, usually with limited awareness of how they restrict the development of intimacy and the normal give and take required of mature, adult relationships. For some, these attitudes are well ingrained because they have been passed on in the form of negative perspectives and feelings for generations. The repetitive intergenerational transmission of addictive behaviors and ways of responding to them occur without anyone's deliberate intent or awareness.

Adult children of alcoholics frequently complain that they feel as though they do not belong. Sudden outbursts or overreactions are remnants of a previous inability to make sense of a chaotic childhood superimposed on a current life event. Unfortunately, the spouse, coworker, or boss does not know the script and interprets the behavior negatively. Those who have grown up in a chemically dependent household often need to reconstruct new and different developmental memories that incorporate the reality of the dysfunctional family experiences, while developing a realistic and loving sense of self in relation to others. Usually, supportive or insight therapy is needed to achieve these objectives. Treatment focuses on identifying feelings and accepting their legitimate role in one's life, releasing anger, and separating

BOX 31-8 Guidelines for Empowering Adult Children of Alcoholics

Analyze the appropriateness of an emotional response

Feel the feelings

Create your own reality as one that is supportive and nurturing

Release shamebound feelings by:

Talking about them with a supportive person

Claiming your emotions as your own and no longer governed by your parents' rules

Cognitive restructuring

Use positive self-talk to reestablish perspective

Take actions that support your positive self-analysis

Seek support from significant others to reinforce the new behaviors

feelings from past relationships from present relational circumstances. Guidelines for empowering adult children of alcoholics to try out new behaviors are presented in Box 31–8. Self-help groups designed to meet the needs of adult children of alcoholics are available in most communities.

CASE STUDY: THE MILLER FAMILY

As a case manager in the trauma unit of a local emergency room, you are assigned to Sam Miller, a 49-year-old business executive, who sustained a fractured femur when he was in a motor vehicle accident yesterday. The emergency room report indicates that, at the time of the accident, Sam's blood alcohol level was 0.15 dL. When you enter the room, you find his wife standing at the bedside. She communicates with you in short, terse sentences and appears to be unaffected by her husband's serious condition. While gathering a family history, you find that Sam has been drinking heavily (a 12-pack of beer or 2 liters of wine daily for the past 10 to 15 years). He is currently on probation for driving under the influence. Susan, his wife of 28 years, tells you that she is aware that Sam drinks a lot but hopes that someday he will come to his senses and stop drinking. She tells you that he drinks daily and gets really "drunk" at least once or twice a week. Sam tells you, "My wife is exaggerating the amount I drink and I can quit drinking any time I want to: I have just been under a lot of pressure." You notice considerable tension between the couple. You find out that Sam and Susan have three children, Sarah, age 18 years, Trisha, age 16 years, and Judd, age 13 years. Trisha and Judd seem worried about their father, but Sarah tells you she is "fed up." She says, "I think my father is an alcoholic and I am tired of it; I wish he would stop drinking." You find that Sarah is an honor student, whereas Trisha and Judd are both experiencing difficulty in school. Trisha tells you she wants to run away.

ASSESSMENT

Assessment data are as follows:

- Blood alcohol level on admission 0.15 dL (legal for intoxication in most states)
- Automobile accident related to excessive alcohol ingestion
- Minimization of alcoholism symptoms by patient and wife
- Tension and stress between couple
- Varying levels of denial among family members regarding father's drinking
- Inadequate understanding or knowledge of alcoholism among family members
- Verbalizations of anger and resentment by Sarah: "I'm fed up . . . I wish my father would stop drinking"
- School problems apparent for Trisha and Judd
- Trisha wants to run away
- Family members unable to relate to each other for mutual support, love, and affection

***DSM-IV* Diagnosis:** Alcohol dependence (husband), Adjustment disorder with depressed mood (wife)

Nursing Diagnosis: 1. Family Processes, Alcoholism, Altered related to long-term patterns of denial, rationalization, and enabling behaviors evidenced by behavioral problems in the children, marital discord, lack of knowledge of the disease process of alcohol dependence, and inability to relate to each other for mutual support, love, affection, and spiritual needs.

OUTCOME IDENTIFICATION, PLANNING, AND IMPLEMENTATION

EXPECTED OUTCOME 1: By _____ the family will acknowledge the dysfunctional behavioral dynamics present in the family system.

SHORT-TERM GOALS	NURSING INTERVENTIONS	RATIONALES
By _____ family members will admit the alcohol abuse problem of the patient to a trusted friend (minister, nurse, or member of a self-help group).	1. Assess the family members for factors that would keep them from accepting help such as shame, guilt, or excessive denial. 2. Provide an opportunity for the family members to discuss their experiences of living with the disabling effects of alcoholism. 3. Listen; be genuine, and nonjudgmental. 4. Educate the family about the effects of alcoholism on the family, including roles of enabler, hero, scapegoat, lost child, and mascot.	1. Helps determine the best approach and types of referrals. 2–3. Assists you in joining with the family and validates their experience. 4. Encourages family members to have a realistic appraisal of their family dynamics and dispel myths and guilt.
By _____ the family members will strongly encourage the patient to enter a treatment facility.	1. Provide the family with a list of services and treatment options available. 2. Outline the benefits of a professional intervention or confrontation. 3. Assess the family's potential strength or desire to participate in an intervention or confrontation.	1–2. Ensures the family's continued support and helps them from returning to their previous state of denial. 3. To benefit the greatest from an intervention, family members need to be in agreement of the necessity for it.
By _____ the family members will cease to protect (enable) the patient.	1. Define the term *enabling* for family members. 2. Encourage each family member to delineate at least one time when they enabled the patient. 3. Offer family members alternative choices to enabling and have them practice what they will say and do when a situation arises.	1–2. Reframing "helping" behavior as enabling behavior is often necessary. 3. Changing previously entrenched patterns of behavior requires practice and feedback. During times of anxiety, it is normal to return to previous ways of responding.

EXPECTED OUTCOME 2: By _____ the parents will verbalize the need to resolve the discord in the marital relationship.

SHORT-TERM GOAL	NURSING INTERVENTIONS	RATIONALES
By _____ the parents will openly acknowledge the long-term discord in their marriage with a trusted professional.	1. Encourage the couple to begin to talk about resentments and regrets that have occurred as a result of the alcoholism. 2. Have patient and his wife each write out specific resentments that occurred as a result of the alcoholism. 3. Have couple share these feelings in the presence of a therapist. 4. Teach the couple how to listen and attend to each other by not interrupting or defending while the other person is speaking. 5. Encourage marital counseling after discharge.	1. After many years of denial, it is important to begin to talk about feelings that have been buried. 2. Writing out the resentments and regrets before verbalization allows the couple to stay structured and specific rather than generalized (i.e., "You ruined my life"). 3–4. A professional would act as a mediator in this instance and will begin to teach the couple how to communicate without blaming, a common dynamic in alcoholic marriages. 5. To continue the support, this couple will need to change entrenched behaviors.

EXPECTED OUTCOME 3: By _____ the family will acknowledge the need to relate to each other for their needs for mutual support, love, affection, and spirituality.

SHORT-TERM GOALS	NURSING INTERVENTIONS	RATIONALES
By _____ the family will maintain appropriate roles with each other.	1. Continue to inform the family how roles have changed within their family system as a result of the alcoholism. 2. Have each family member identify which role they have taken on (i.e., enabler, hero, scapegoat, lost child, or mascot). 3. Assess individual family members' readiness for "letting go" of their individual roles.	1. Teaching may need to be repeated on the basis of individual's family members' readiness to learn. 2–3. Helps family members to break through denial and to begin the grieving process.
By _____ the family members will be able to verbalize their support and caring for each other.	1. Encourage family to identify what they need from each other. 2. Help family members realize that caring about each other is different than enabling or protecting.	1. Social and emotional isolation and denial of needs are common for alcoholic families. 2. Enabling behaviors are often intended to be caring behaviors.
By _____ the family will acknowledge the lack of spirituality in their daily lives and verbalize their need for spiritual nurturing.	1. Ascertain from each family member the degree of spiritual bankruptcy present. 2. Encourage family members to talk about their needs regarding spirituality and the presence of the God of their understanding in their lives.	1–2. Feeling hopeless and abandoned by God is not uncommon in alcoholic families.

EXPECTED OUTCOME 4: By _____ the family will willingly attend support group meetings such as Alcoholics Anonymous, Al-Anon, and Alateen.

SHORT-TERM GOAL	NURSING INTERVENTIONS	RATIONALES
By _____ the family will agree to attend a support group meeting.	1. Encourage the mother to attend an Al-Anon meeting while the husband is still hospitalized. 2. If the wife is resistant to attending a meeting for herself, encourage her and the children to attend an open Alcoholics Anonymous (AA) meeting. 3. Assure the wife and children that anonymity is present at AA meetings.	1. In alcoholic families, once a crisis is over, it is not unusual to return to previous levels of denial. 2. Attending an open AA meeting will aid in breaking through denial that alcoholism affects all age and socioeconomic groups. 3. Alcoholic families are often shame based and have concerns about being exposed.

Nursing Diagnosis: 2. Denial, ineffective related to a lifestyle of denial and rationalization evidenced by unrecognized guilt and shame, a knowledge deficit regarding the negative effects of alcohol abuse, and minimization of the symptoms of alcoholism.

OUTCOME IDENTIFICATION, PLANNING, AND IMPLEMENTATION

EXPECTED OUTCOME 1: By _____ the patient will admit that his drinking is out of control and his life has become unmanageable.

SHORT-TERM GOALS	NURSING INTERVENTIONS	RATIONALES
By _____ the patient will willingly participate in a treatment program.	1. Approach the patient in a direct, genuine, nonjudgmental manner. 2. With a positive, supportive attitude, help the patient to see the need for treatment.	1–2. Approach gains the trust of the patient to begin a therapeutic relationship and shows genuine concern for the patient.

SHORT-TERM GOALS	NURSING INTERVENTIONS	RATIONALES
	3. Encourage the patient to self-admit to an alcohol treatment program.	3. Self-admittance is preferred because the element of denial has been addressed to a certain degree.
	4. Assure the patient that alcohol dependence is a physiological problem and not a moral one.	4. Shows the patient that you are not judging his character; let him know that you believe he has an illness, not a moral problem.
By _____ the patient will verbalize the deleterious physiological and psychological effects of excessive alcohol use.	1. Encourage the patient to compile a written list of the deleterious consequences of excessive alcohol use he has experienced in the past 10 years. 2. Have the patient present this list to a nurse on the unit and to his peer group.	1–2. Both of these interventions assist with breaking through the denial associated with the illness.

EXPECTED OUTCOME 2: By _____ the patient will abstain from alcohol.

SHORT-TERM GOALS	NURSING INTERVENTIONS	RATIONALES
By _____ the patient will verbalize all situations that could lead to a relapse.	1. Ask the patient to compile a list of situations that influenced excessive drinking (i.e., social situations, work-related affairs, after work). 2. Offer suggestions for engaging in these situations without drinking.	1–2. To help the patient avoid relapse, it is important to know what situations triggered excessive drinking in the past.
By _____ the patient and treatment team will draft a plan for prevention of relapse after discharge.	1. Encourage attendance at AA meetings while in treatment. 2. Help patient to recognize his strengths and abilities. 3. Have patient agree to attend AA and aftercare when discharged.	1–3. Sobriety is easier to maintain in a structured setting such as a treatment facility; a strong support group is necessary after discharge.

EXPECTED OUTCOME 3: By _____ the patient will acknowledge how the absence of a higher power has affected him on his life's journey.

SHORT-TERM GOALS	NURSING INTERVENTIONS	RATIONALES
By _____ the patient will openly discuss any shame or guilt that he feels as a result of his drinking behavior.	1. Educate the patient about shame and guilt and how they fit into the cycle of abuse. 2. Encourage the patient to vent feelings of shame and guilt related to drinking.	1–2. Once the patient is sober, it is not uncommon to feel negative feelings that have been numbed for along time. Venting these feelings in a safe place is very therapeutic.
By _____ the patient will admit that a power greater than himself will be able to help him maintain sobriety and heal broken relationships.	1. Encourage the patient to begin talking about the God of his understanding. 2. Inquire about any specific religious practices that would bring solace to the patient. 3. Ask the patient how he views his acceptance of the disease of alcoholism as part of his life's spiritual journey.	1–2. It is not unusual for an alcoholic to have abandoned all spiritual practices because of low self-esteem. 3. As the patient gains progress toward spiritual wholeness, he will be able to place his alcoholism in perspective.
By _____ the patient will engage in daily meditation to obtain spiritual nurturing and solace.	1. Encourage the patient to begin a process of daily meditation while in treatment. 2. Ask the patient whether there are any spiritual resources that you can provide for him.	1–2. To maintain sobriety, it is important for the alcoholic to abstain from mood-altering chemicals one day at a time; therefore, it is important to begin the practice of grounding oneself spiritually on a daily basis.

EVALUATION

Formative Evaluation: The family met many of the short-term goals. They were able to confront their father and help him get treatment, but they were unable to "let go" of their firmly entrenched roles in the family system. Susan and Sarah were able to nurture and support each other, but Trisha and Judd remained on the outside. Sam and Susan openly acknowledged their marital conflict and were willing to continue in marital therapy. Susan and the three children attended three open AA meetings. Sam met all of the short-term goals that were intended for him. He was able to talk about his need for spirituality. The three children and Susan, however, did not want to talk about a lack of spirituality in their lives.

Summative Evaluation: The family achieved each of the expected outcomes, except the need for relating to each other for mutual support, love, affection, and spirituality. I encouraged the family to continue with family therapy after discharge. Each individual family member had wounds to heal. I encouraged each of them to attend a 12-step support program where they felt comfortable and to also find a sponsor to work with them individually. Family members do not heal at the same rate, and it is difficult to support other family members when you are not feeling supported yourself. Sam met each of the expected outcomes intended for him. He said, "I know I am an alcoholic and I am grateful that my higher power did not leave me. With the help of my higher power, my family's support, and my sponsor, I know I can stay sober."

CONCLUSIONS

Chemical dependency has reached epidemic proportions within the last few years. Chemical dependency was identified as the nation's number one health problem in the late 1980s; funding for research related to drug abuse and treatment has increased dramatically in the last few years. Research initiatives in the 21st century will reflect new possibilities for diagnosis and direction for treatment.

With the current focus on genome therapy, researchers will continue to look for genetic factors in the development of substance use disorders. Other research will search for cellular and biochemical explanations related to the effects of psychoactive drugs on the brain, especially those involved with the reinforcing properties of substance use dependence. For example, what is the effect of drug activity on the γ-aminobutyric acid (GABA) neurotransmitter system, and what are the psychophysiological processes responsible for craving a psychoactive substance? Other important areas of research will center on understanding the interrelationships of the chronic effects of alcohol on the central nervous system and other organ systems.

Primary prevention strategies when National Institute on Alcohol Abuse and Alcoholism established a prevention research branch to address strategies that might be effective in preventing drug problems (U.S. Department of Health and Human Services, 1990). Of particular concern are certain subpopulations vulnerable to substance use disorders with special treatment needs: adolescents, women, children, certain ethnic groups, the homeless, and the elderly, and so on.

Relevant research questions related to primary prevention would include the following:

- What is the role of peer pressure on the drug-taking behaviors of high school and college students?
- What is the effect of parent skills training on the prevention of substance use disorders?
- What strategies of community intervention are most effective in meeting the specific prevention-treatment needs of Native Americans, women, and the homeless?
- What structural characteristics of the work situation enhance or prevent the development of substance use disorders?
- What is the relationship between life stressors and the development of substance use disorders?
- What is the role of social supports in the prevention of substance use disorders?

Research on secondary prevention of substance use disorders could focus on identifying the following:

- What type of treatment protocols are most effective in treating patients with different drug abuse typologies?
- What are the criteria for matching a chemically dependent person's need with appropriate treatment in different subpopulations (adolescent, women, maternal, elderly)?

Research related to tertiary prevention of substance use disorders could consider the following:

- What is the efficacy of using family (or behavioral) therapy approaches in the treatment of substance use disorders?
- What are the factors (personal, social, spiritual) most consistently related to recidivism in substance use disorders?

There is a need to develop better assessment tools for diagnosis. Improvement of current tools and formulation of more precise diagnostic tools for early detection of substance use disorders in general community and medical situations would enhance treatment initiatives. Developing better methods for the identification of persons at risk for the disorder also is warranted.

KEY POINTS TO REMEMBER

- Psychoactive substances refer to any mind-altering drug capable of modifying a person's behavior.
- Substance use disorders is a medical term used to describe a predictable set of physical and psychological symptoms associated with the voluntary ingestion of a psychoactive substance.
- Current etiological models suggest a polygenic mode of transmission consisting of a dynamic interaction among physical, psychological, social, and situational factors.
- Common properties of substance use disorders are tolerance, physical and psychological dependence, reinforcing properties, concepts of relapse, and recovery.
- The *DSM-IV* distinguishes between substance abuse and substance dependence as the generic descriptors for all drug classifications.
- The primary drug classifications include alcohol, hypnotic sedatives, hallucinogens, narcotic analgesics, central nervous system stimulants, and volatile solvents.
- Persistent use of psychoactive drugs leads to physical and emotional symptoms that in the extreme can cause death.
- Treatment for substance use disorders has an acute phase and a rehabilitative phase.
- The treatment goals for the acute phase relate to stabilizing the patient's medical status.
- Rehabilitation focuses on helping chemically dependent persons develop new coping skills needed for a life without drugs.
- Self-help groups (Alcoholics Anonymous, Cocaine Anonymous, and Narcotics Anonymous) provide the fellowship and information chemically dependent persons and their families need for abstinence.
- Certain populations (women, infants, cultural groups, adolescents, and elderly) are at risk for the disorder or have special treatment needs.
- Substance use disorders affect the family as well as the identified patient.
- Codependency is a term used to describe maladaptive behaviors in family members that occur as a result of a personal response to substance use.

LEARNING ACTIVITIES

1. Attend an open Alcoholics Anonymous or Narcotics Anonymous meeting. Report on your experience to the class.
2. Write down everything you have heard about the cause of substance use disorders and how they should be treated. Include your own thoughts as well. Share your observations with your classmates. Have a class discussion about the paradoxes associated with substance use disorders.

CRITICAL THINKING EXERCISE

The high school nurse had just arrived in her office when a male junior student raced into her office informing her that his classmate, John, had just collapsed outside the rest room. When she reached his side, she observed a young man who appeared very sleepy with pinpoint pupils and breathing with depressed respirations. His pulse was 50 beats per minute, and he did not respond to her verbal questions. Several of the male students nearby told her that the patient and several other boys had just been in the rest room. Another student reported that he had fallen outside and banged his head against the door.

1. What evidence suggests that John's problem may be drug related?
2. What other evidence do you need to support this point of view?
3. What are possible alternate explanations for these symptoms?

Because of his poor vital signs, the nurse made arrangements to have John admitted to the emergency room of the nearby hospital. Later that day, John's sister came into the nurse's office crying. She expressed great concern about her brother's behavior since their parent's divorce.

1. What other information would you want to know from John's sister?
2. Suggest alternative possibilities.
3. How would you check your assumptions about John's symptoms?

REFERENCES

Abel, E. (1985). Effects of prenatal exposure to cannabinoids. In T. Pinkert (Ed.), *Current research on the consequences of maternal drug abuse* (NIDA Research Monograph 59). Washington, DC: U.S. Department of Health and Human Services.

Adams, E., and Durell, J. (1984). Cocaine: A growing public health problem. In J. Grabowski (Ed.), *Cocaine: Pharmacology, effects and treatment of abuse* (NIDA Research Monograph 50). Washington, DC: U.S. Department of Health and Human Services.

Alcoholics Anonymous. (1955). *Twelve steps*. New York: AA World Services.

American Nurses Association. (1988). *Standards of addictions: Nursing practice with selected diagnoses and criteria*. Kansas City, MO: American Nurses Association.

American Psychiatric Association. (1994). Substance-related disorders. In: *Diagnostic and statistical manual of mental disorders* (4th ed., pp. 175–272). Washington, DC: Author.

Amsel, Z. (1990). Introducing the concept of "community prevention." In *AIDS and intravenous drug use: Future directions for community-based prevention research* (NIDA Research Monograph 93). Washington, DC: U.S. Department of Health and Human Services.

Andreasen, N., and Black, D. (1991). *Introductory textbook of psychiatry* (p. 311). Washington, DC: American Psychiatric Press, Inc.

Black, C. (1981). *Children of alcoholics: "It will never happen to me."* New York: Ballantine Books.

Bluhm, J. (1987). *When you face the chemically dependent patient: A practical guide for nurses*. Maryland Heights, MO: Ishiyaku EuroAmerica.

Bowen, M. (1984). Alcoholism as viewed through family systems theory and family psychotherapy. *Annals of the New York Academy of Sciences, 133*, 115–122.

Busch, D., McBride, A., and Benaventura, L. M. (1986). Chemical dependency in women: The link to OB/GYN problems. *Journal of Psychosocial Nursing and Mental Health, 24*(4), 26–30.

Buskist, W., and Gerbing, D. (1990). *Psychology: Boundaries and frontiers* (pp. 106–103). Glenview, Il: Scott, Foresman.

Buys, D., and Saltman, J. (1982). *The unseen alcoholics—The elderly*. New York: Public Affairs Pamphlet.

Cafiso, J., Goodstadt, M. S., Garlington, W. K., (1982). Television portrayal of alcohol and other beverages. *Journal on Studies on Alcohol, 43*, 964–989.

Carroll, E. (1977). Coca: The plant and its use. In R. Petersen and R. Stillman (Eds.), *Cocaine* (NIDA Research Monograph 13, pp. 35–46). Washington, DC: U.S. Government Printing Office.

Caulker-Burnett I. (1994). Primary care screening for substance abuse. *Nurse Practitioner, 19(6)*, 42–48.

Charney, D. S., Heninger, G., and Kleber, H. (1986). The combined use of clonidine and naltrexone as a rapid, safe and effective treatment of abrupt withdrawal from methadone. *American Journal of Psychiatry, 143*, 831–837.

Chasnoff, I. J., Burens, W. J., Schroll, S. H., and Burns, K. A. (1985). Cocaine use in pregnancy. *New England Journal of Medicine, 313*(11), 666–669.

Chaudron, C. D., and Wilkenson, D. A. (Eds.). (1988). *Theories on alcoholism*. Toronto: Addiction Research Foundation.

Cole, J., and Chiarello, R. (1990). The benzodiazepines as drugs of abuse. *Journal of Psychiatric Research, 24*(2); 135–144.

Dackis, C., and Gold, M. (1985). New concepts in cocaine addictions: The dopamine depletion hypothesis. *Neuroscience Biobehavioral Review, 9*, 469–477.

Dishion, T. J., and Lober, R. (1985). Male adolescent marijuana and alcohol use: The role of parents and peers revisited. *Journal of Alcohol and Substance Abuse, 11*(1, 2); 11–25.

Donohoe, R. (1988). Opiates as immunocompromising drugs: The evidence and possible mechanisms. In Harris L (Ed.), *Problems of drug dependence* (NIDA Monograph 90). Washington, DC: U.S. Department of Health and Human Service.

Dorfman, A. (1989, August 28). Alcohol's youngest victims. *Time, 134*(9), 60.

Finnegan, L. (1988). Management of maternal and neonatal substance abuse problems. In L. Harris (Ed.), *Problems of drug dependence* (NIDA Monograph 90). Washington, DC: U.S. Department of Health and Human Service.

Finnegan, L., and Kandall, S. (1992). Problems in pregnancy. In Lowenson J, Ruiz P, Millman R (Eds.), *Substance abuse: A comprehensive textbook* (2nd ed.). Baltimore, MD: Williams & Wilkins.

Fossum, M. A., and Mason, M. J. (1986). *Facing shame: Families in recovery*. New York: Norton.

Fultz, J., Senay, E., Pray, B., and Thornton, W. (1980). When a narcotic addict is hospitalized. *American Journal of Nursing, 80*(3), 478–481.

Galanter, M., Castaneda, R., and Franco, H. (1991). Group therapy and self-help groups. In R. Frances, S. Miller (Eds.), *Clinical textbook of addictive disorders* (pp. 430–451). New York: Guilford Press.

Gerstein, D., and Harwood, H. (1990). *Treating drug problems: Volume I*. Washington, DC: National Academy Press.

Ghodse A. H. (1994). Combined use of drugs and alcohol. *Current Opinion in Psychiatry, 7(3)*, 249–251.

Ghodse A. H. (1995). *Drugs and addictive behavior: A guide to treatment* (2nd ed.). Oxford: Blackwell Science Ltd.

Gomberg, E. S. L. (1986). Women and alcoholism: Psychosocial issues. In *Women and alcohol: Health related issues.* (Research Monograph 16).

Goodwin, D. W. (1979). Alcoholism and heredity: A review and hypothesis. *Archives of General Psychiatry*, 36, 57–61.

Gorski, T. (1986). Relapse prevention planning: A new recovery tool. *Alcohol, Health and Research World*, 6–11.

Grabowski, J. (1984). *Cocaine: Pharmacology, effects and treatment of abuse* (NIDA Research Monograph 50). Washington, DC: U.S. Department of Health and Human Services.

Gualtieri, T. (1990). The neuropharmacology of inadvertent drug effects in patients with traumatic brain injuries. *Journal of Head Trauma Rehabilitation, 5*(3), 32–40.

Helman, C. (1990). *Culture, health and illness: An introduction for health professionals* (2nd ed.). London, England: Wright.

Hughes, T. (1989). Models and perspectives of addiction: Implications for treatment. *Nursing Clinics of North America, 24*(1), 1–12.

Jaffe, J. H., and Martin, W. R. (1990). Opioid analgesics and antagonists. In A. Gilman, T. Rall, A. Nies, and P. Taylor (Eds.), *Goodman and Gilman's Pharmacological Basis of Therapeutics* (8th ed., pp. 485–522). New York: Pergamon Press.

Jellinek, E. M. (1941). An early medical view of alcohol addiction and its treatment: Dr. Thomas Trotter's essay, medical, philosophical and chemical, on drunkenness. *Quarterly Journal of Studies on Alcohol, 2*, 584–591.

Jellinek, E. M. (1960). *The disease concept of alcoholism*. New Haven, CT: Hillhouse.

Johnson, V. (1990). *Intervention: How to help someone who doesn't want help*. Minneapolis: Johnson Institute.

Jones, R. (1984). The pharmacology of cocaine. In J. Grabowski (Ed.), *Cocaine: pharmacology, effects and treatment of abuse* (NIDA Research Monograph 50). Washington, DC: U.S. Department of Health and Human Services.

Kaplan, H., and Sadock, B. (1988). *Clinical psychiatry*. Baltimore: Wilkins & Wilkins.

Kaufman, E. (1982). The relationship of alcoholism and alcohol use to the abuse of other drugs. *American Journal of Drug and Alcohol Abuse, 9*(1), 1–17.

Kerr, P. (1989, August 11). Crack and resurgence of syphilis spreading AIDS among the poor. *New York Times*, pp. 1, 17.

Kinney, J., and Leaton, G. (1986). *Loosening the grip* (3rd ed.). St. Louis: Times Mirror/Mosby.

Kleber, H. (1990). The nosology of abuse and dependence. *Journal of Psychiatric Research, 24*(2), 57–64.

Kurtz, E. (1981). Shame and guilt: Characteristics of the dependency cycle. In *Professional Education* 7. Hazelden Foundation.

Kurtz, E. (1982). Why AA works. *Journal of Studies on Alcohol, 43*(1), 40–80.

Leccese, A. (1991). *Drugs and society: Behavioral medicines and abusable drugs* (5th ed.). Englewood Cliffs, NJ: Prentice-Hall.

Lettieri, D. J. (1985). Drug abuse: A review of explanations and models of explanation. *Advances in Alcohol and Substance Abuse, 4*, 9–40.

Levine, O. S., Vlahov, D., Koehler, J., et al. (1995). Seroepidemiology of hepatitis B virus in a population of injecting drug users. *American Journal of Epidemiology, 142*(3), 331–341.

Luisada, P. (1978). The phencyclidine psychosis: Phenomenology and treatment. In R. Peterson, R. Stillman (Eds.), *Phencyclidine (PCP) abuse: An appraisal* (1978 Monograph 21, pp. 19–43). Washington, DC: National Institute on Drug Abuse Research.

Mallinson, M. (1990). Nursing at the front—of the cocaine wars. *American Journal of Nursing, 4*, 7.

Marrow, J. (1993). The twelve steps: A pathway to recovery. *Primary Care 20(1)*, 107–119.

Matuschka, P. (1985). The psychopharmacology of addiction. In T. Bratter and G. Forrest: Alcoholism and substance abuse: Strategies for clinical intervention (pp. 49–73). New York: The Free Press.

McKelvy, M. J., Kane, J., and Kellison, K. (1987). Substance abuse and mental illness: Double trouble. *Journal of Psychosocial Nursing, 25*(1), 21–25.

Milkman, H., and Shaffer, H. (1985). *The addictions: Multidisciplinary perspectives and treatments*. Lexington, MA: Heath.

Miller, N., Mahler, B., Belkin, M., and Gold, M. (1990). Psychiatric diagnosis in alcohol and drug dependence. *Annals of Clinical Psychiatry, 3*(1), 79–89.

Mondanaro, J. (1990). Community-based AIDS prevention interventions: Special issues of women intravenous drug users. In US Department of Health and Human Services (Ed.), *AIDS and Intravenous Drug Use: Future Directions for Community-Based Prevention Research* (NIDA Research Monograph 93). Washington, DC: U.S. Department of Health and Human Services.

Moore, D. (1986). Reversal of alcohol effects: Acute and chronic conditions. *Alcohol and Research World*, 52–59.

Muramoto M., and Leshau L. (1993). Adolescent substance abuse: Recognition and early intervention. *Primary care, 20(1)*, 141–152.

National Commission on Marijuana and Drug Abuse. (1973). *Drug use in America: Problem and perspective*. Washington, DC: U.S. Government Printing Office.

National Institute of Drug Abuse. (1982). *Population projections, based on the National Survey on Drug Abuse 1982*. Washington, DC: U.S. Government Printing Office.

NNSA, DANA, ANA. (1987). *The care of clients with addiction: Dimensions of nursing practice*. Kansas City, MO: American Nurses Association.

Patterson, G. R. (1982). *Coercive family process*. Eugene, OR: Castalia.

Pires, M. (1989). Substance abuse: The silent saboteur in rehabilitation. *Nursing Clinics of North America*, *24*(1), 291–296.

Quinby, P. and Graham A. (1993). Substance abuse among women. Primary Care *20(1)*, 131–139.

Rinaldi, R. C., Steindler, E. M., and Wilford, B. B. (1988). Classification and standardization of substance abuse terminology. *Journal of the American Medical Association*, *259*, 555–557.

Rouse, B. (1989). Drug abuse among racial/ethnic minorities: A Special Report. Rockville, MD: National Institute of Drug Abuse.

Schuckit, M. A. (1995). A theory of alcohol and drug abuse: A genetic approach. In D. J. Lettieri, M. Sayers, H. W. Pearson (Eds.), *Theories on drug abuse* (NIDA Research Monograph 30). Washington, DC: U.S. Department of Health and Human Services.

Schuckit, M. A. (1995). *Drug and alcohol abuse: A clinical guide to diagnosis and treatment* (4th ed.). New York: Plenum Press.

Schuster, C., and Snyder, M. (1990). NIDA's medication development program—1989. In U. S. Department of Health and Human Services (Ed.), *Problems of drug dependence 1989* (Research Monograph Series 95). Washington, DC: U.S. Department of Health and Human Services.

Senay, E. (1983). *Substance abuse disorders in clinical practice*. Boston, MA: John Wright.

Shiff, M., and Cavarola, A. (1988–1989). Adolescents at risk for chemical dependency: Identification and prevention issues. *Journal of Chemical Dependency Treatment*, 25–47.

Streissguth, A. P. (1986). Fetal alcohol syndrome: An overview and implications for patient management. In N. Estes, and M. E. Heinemann (Eds.), *Alcoholism: Development, consequences, and interventions* (3rd ed.). St. Louis: Mosby.

Stone, W., and Gottesman, I. (1993). A perspective on the search for the causes of alcoholism: Slow down the rush to genetic alcoholism. *Neurology, Psychiatry and Brain Research*, (1), 123–132.

Strassman, R. (1984). Adverse reactions to psychedelic drugs: A review of the literature. *Journal of Nervous Mental Disorders*, *172*, 577–595.

U.S. Department of Health and Human Services. (1990). *Healthy people 2000: National health promotion and disease prevention objectives* (Publication No. [PHS] 91-50212). Washington, DC: U.S. Department of Health and Human Services.

Valliant, G. E. (1983). *The natural history of alcoholism: Causes, patterns and paths to recovery*. Cambridge, MA: Harvard University Press.

Wise, R. (1984). Neural mechanisms of the reinforcing action of cocaine. In J. Grabowski (Ed.), *Cocaine: Pharmacology, effects, and treatment of abuse* (NIDA Research Monograph 50, pp. 15–33). Washington, DC: U.S. Department of Health and Human Services.

Yamaguchi, K., and Kandel, D. B. (1984). Patterns of drug use from adolescence to young adulthood: III. Predictors of progression. *American Journal of Public Health*, *74*, 673–681.

SUGGESTED READINGS

Alcoholics Anonymous. (1955). *12 Steps*. New York: AA World Services.

American Nurses Association. (1988). *Standards of addictions: Nursing practice with selected diagnoses and criteria*. Kansas City, MO: American Nurses Association.

American Psychiatric Association. (1994). Substance-related disorders. In: *Diagnostic and statistical manual of mental disorders* (4th ed., pp. 175–272). Washington, DC: Author.

Black, C. (1981). *Children of alcoholics: "It will never happen to me."* New York: Ballantine Books.

Johnson, V. (1990). *Intervention: How to help someone who doesn't want help*. Minneapolis: Johnson Institute.

Lettieri, D. J. (1985). Drug abuse: A review of explanations and models of explanation. *Advances in Alcohol and Substance Abuse*, *4*, 9–40.

Mallinson, M. (1990). Nursing at the front—of the cocaine wars. *American Journal of Nursing 4*, 7.

McKelvy, M. J., Kane, J., and Kellison, K. (1987). Substance abuse and mental illness: Double trouble. *Journal of Psychosocial Nursing*, *25*(1), 21–25.

Millam, J., and Ketcham, K. (1981). *Under the influence: A guide to the myths and realities of alcoholism*. New York: Bantam Books.

Naegle, M. (1988). Substance abuse among women: Prevalence, patterns and treatment issues. *Issues in Mental Health Nursing*, *9*, 127–137.

Powell, A. (1988). Alcohol withdrawal syndrome. *American Journal of Nursing*, *3*, 313–315.

CHAPTER 32

THE JOURNEY TROUBLED BY BEHAVIORAL DISORDERS

Assuming that our capacity for self-perception outweighs that of self-deception, we will find that our thoughts and feelings have described a constant (more or less intense, more or less eccentric) seesaw toward and away from a state of fantasies concerning things which we wish we could do or wish we had done.

—Erik Erikson

LEARNING OBJECTIVES

After studying this chapter, you should be able to:

1. Identify three factors that constitute a healthy personality.
2. Identify three factors that identify an individual with a personality disorder.
3. Distinguish among the three clusters of personality disorders described in the *Diagnostic and Statistical Manual of Mental Disorders-IV (DSM-IV).*
4. List three features and behavior patterns associated with each personality disorder.
5. For each personality disorder, identify two behaviors that affect the individual's relationships with family, friends, and caregivers.
6. Discuss three nursing diagnoses appropriate for each axis II cluster.
7. Identify three patient outcomes appropriate for nursing diagnoses related to personality disorders.
8. Identify two interventions for each patient outcome.
9. Identify two medications useful when treating patients with personality disorders.
10. Discuss spiritual issues that affect patients with personality disorders.
11. Discuss spiritual issues that affect nurses who care for patients with personality disorders.

KEY TERMINOLOGY

Antisocial personality disorder
Avoidant personality disorder
Borderline personality disorder
Cluster A disorders
Cluster B disorders
Cluster C disorders
Dependent personality disorder
Histrionic personality disorder
Narcissistic personality disorder
Object constancy
Obsessive-compulsive personality disorder
Paranoid personality disorder
Personality disorder
Schizoid personality disorder
Schizotypal personality disorder
Splitting
Transitional object

One of our greatest challenges in psychiatric nursing is in relating effectively to patients who are "difficult to work with." Facing this challenge is necessary to study personality disorders. As we journey with patients who have behavioral disorders, we sometimes see similar conduct in ourselves. This awareness can be not only frightening but also enlightening as we gain deeper understanding of our ability to relate to others and define our own sense of self.

Difficulties arising when dealing with individuals having personality disorders are the tendency to judge or label unusual or dramatic conduct as abnormal rather than analyzing factors that cause these behaviors. Judging patients interferes with forming therapeutic alliances. It increases the psychological and spiritual distress of the patient, and it leads to emotional frustration and spiritual distress for the nurse confronted with an inability to understand the "why" behind the patient's behavior and to respond to the patient in a loving manner.

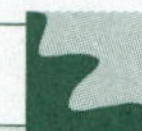

JEFF'S STORY

Jeff is 40 years old, single, and living alone. He leads a quiet life and has no friends or associates. Jeff works as a mail sorter for the post office. He is known as a loner, rarely talking to his coworkers. He has never married, and his family states that he has never dated. His free time is spent alone, building model airplanes, reading science fiction and fantasy novels, and watching action movies on his video machine. He has minimal interactions with anyone, including his parents and his brother.

He visits his family only when invited, usually during holidays such as Thanksgiving and Christmas. His mother states, "Jeff has always been quiet, to himself, doesn't need much, doesn't ask for much, and is a loner. I don't understand how he got like that, except maybe he is like his dad's brother who has schizophrenia. You know, I've never seen him angry, or happy, or emotional in any way, even if his football team wins a close game. He doesn't say much. I don't know what he even thinks about. I do know he takes care of his bills and is responsible for what he says he will do."

A HEALTHY PERSONALITY

How do you know when someone has a healthy personality? What is a personality disorder? Individuals with healthy personalities can

- Identify "self" as the total of strengths and weaknesses
- Identify the types of interactions or thoughts that create joy, sadness, anger, love, hate, and other strong emotions
- Relate to others without expecting others to meet all their needs
- Define where they end and another person begins
- Balance work and play
- Express spirituality
- Identify goals accomplished through discipline and creativity (Erikson, 1963; Maslow, 1968).

Case Example 32–1 illustrates Janet, a woman with a healthy personality. Janet can receive love and trust from her family members and demonstrates these same qualities back to them.

Case Example 32–1 Janet's Story

Janet has very close relationships with her mother, her husband, and her two children. She can identify her strengths as a loving wife and as a mother who loves her children and encourages them to express their individuality. "My mother enjoyed my curiosity and ability to ask questions and learn new things. I know Mom is interested in fashion. I'm interested in music. We make a good pair. My daughter writes poetry. My son is like my husband, interested in woodwork."

▶ Check Your Reading

1. Identify three behaviors necessary to a healthy personality.

PERSONALITY DISORDERS DEFINED

Personality disorders, are listed on axis II of the *Diagnostic and Statistical Manual of Mental Disorders–IV* (1994) *(DSM-IV)*. A personality disorder is defined as "an enduring pattern of inner experience and behavior that deviates markedly from the expectations of the individual's culture, is pervasive and inflexible, has an onset in adolescence or early adulthood, is stable over time, and leads to distress or impairment (*DSM-IV,* 1994, p. 629).

You can ascertain these behaviors by observing how the individual relates to others. Watch the person's perception of surroundings and ability to solve problems. Mansfield (1992) states that personality disorders reflect deficiencies in how a person identifies feelings, and in the ability to experience "self" as unique. The individual with a personality disorder does not look within to locate feelings or make decisions but instead looks outside the self for evaluations, directions, rules, or opinions.

PERSONALITY DEVELOPMENT: A VIEW FROM PSYCHOLOGY AND BIOLOGY

Understanding "why" something happens helps us to accept difficult situations and improves our problem-solving. Such understanding is especially important when caring for individuals with personality disorders. If you can understand "why" a behavior pattern exists, you will be better prepared to develop expected outcomes and treatment interventions.

Margaret Mahler: Contributions to Object Relation Theory

To develop a model for the early phases of infant development, Margaret Mahler and her colleagues observed infants and their mothers. She distinguished the psychological birth of the infant (when the child has a beginning sense of being an individual, or self) from the biological birth. She theorized that the child passes through phases, or maturational events, to develop a separate and unique sense of being (Mahler, 1963, 1971, 1972a, 1972b; Akhtar, 1992, 1995; Cauwels, 1992). Mahler's phases are as follows:

1. *Autistic phase.* Mahler theorized that the neonate (one to two months old) was encased in a self-absorbed barrier with no recognition of others.
2. *Symbiotic phase.* The infant (four to five months old) begins to recognize the mother, becomes enmeshed with the mother's self, and perceives the mother as an extension of her or his own self.
3. *Separation-individuation phase.* The third phase is subdivided into four overlapping subphases:

   • *Differentiation subphase* (five to eight months). The child becomes aware of people other than the mother and can distinguish them. The child learns psychological separateness from the mother by beginning to explore both the body and the environment.

   • *Practicing subphase* (8 to 16 months). The child becomes more mobile, is able to crawl and toddle away from the mother, and "checks in" with the mother frequently.

   • *Rapprochement subphase* (16 to 25 months). The child increasingly differentiates self from mother and mother's environment; begins to learn that her or his separateness, autonomy, and motor abilities are limited; realizes that the self is no longer the center of the universe, and feels very small in a larger world. These feelings are exhibited by anxiety and ambivalent clinging and darting away from mother when she tries to confine or hold the child, who learns that the mother will be there for emotional support but is a separate being. The child begins to tolerate the mother's absence. The child who works through the conflicts in this subphase learns to deal with love and trusting of parents and how to view relationships with other people realistically.

   • *Object constancy subphase* (25 to 36 months). **Object constancy** is reached when one can evoke the memory of a significant other (or a parent, in the child's case), which assures the child that he or she is loved. During this subphase, the child learns to tolerate long separations from the mother by use of **transitional objects** (objects such as teddy bears, dolls, or blankets that remind the child of the mother). These objects are soothing to the child during times of stress or insecurity. Another task accomplished during this subphase is that the child learns to cope with intense emotions, such as ambivalence, frustration, and rage. The child forms a realistic view of self by internalizing a loving image and attitude of the mother and working through the powerful emotions of frustration and rage with the positive parental image intact.

Throughout the separation-individuation phase, the child has to work through the conflicts between autonomy and dependence, as well as fears of engulfment and abandonment by the mother. The child learns that when the mother leaves, the absence is temporary, and the mother will continue to exist when the child cannot see her. The child also discovers that the mother will return (i.e., object constancy). During this phase, the child works through the tendency to see the mother as either all good, therefore meeting all needs or all bad, not meeting needs.

Mahler and colleagues hypothesized that borderline personality disorder and other severe personality disorders developed during the rapprochement subphase of the separation-individuation phase of development. The cause of these disorders, these researchers suggested, is a mother who is either too emotionally distant from the child or excessively clinging to a child who needs to explore the environment.

▶ Check Your Reading

2. What is the autistic phase of development described by Mahler?
3. Why did Mahler and associates identify the rapprochement subphrase an important stage in the development of borderline personality disorder?

The Biological View

Since the 1970s, biological studies have been performed on patients with an Axis I diagnosis. In the last several years, some of these biological tests have been applied to people with Axis II personality disorders. Although this research is in the early phases, it will be useful in furthering knowledge about the biological etiology of personality disorders, assisting in the accurate labeling of the disorders, and promoting psychopharmacological agents to decrease symptoms. Research now focuses on cognitive-perceptual organization, affective regulation, impulse control, and anxiety/social inhibition (Kavoussi and Siever, 1991).

Genetics

Some reports (Mann et al, 1986; Coryell and Zimmerman, 1989) of genetic and family studies suggest causal factors for the development of a personality disorder. Siever (1992) reports that schizotypal personality disorder is more prevalent in relatives of schizophrenic individuals than in relatives of patients with other psychiatric disorders. Genetic studies suggest that schizotypal traits occur more frequently than chronic schizophrenia in relatives of chronic schizophrenic patients. Schizotypal traits therefore may be a more common manifestation of the schizophrenogenic genotype than chronic schizophrenia. Some family studies suggest that paranoid personality disorder may be slightly more common in relatives of schizophrenic patients than in controls. More research is needed to determine what part of the etiology of personality disorders is genetic.

Neurotransmitters

Dopaminergic dysfunction, as measured by cerebrospinal fluid and plasma levels of the dopamine metabolite homovanillic acid, has showed differences from the norm that correlate to psychotic symptoms in schizophrenia (Siever, 1985; Davidson and Davis, 1988). Siever and Davis (1991) demonstrated an increase in cerebrospinal and plasma homovanillic acid in preliminary studies of schizotypal patients. This finding correlates with positive schizotypal symptoms of magical thinking, illusions, and ideas of reference.

Several studies demonstrate serotonergic subsensitivity in impulsive behaviors of aggression and self-destruction (Brown and Linnoila, 1990). Brown et al (1982) found that aggressive and suicidal behaviors in individuals with personality disorders correlated inversely with cerebrospinal fluid levels of 5-hydroxyindoleacetic acid (5-HIAA), a major metabolite of serotonin. Some evidence links low levels of serotonin with suicidal behavior (Roy, 1989). Stanley and Stanley (1990) have studied concentrations of serotonin and 5-HIAA in postmortem receptor-binding studies. They note changes in both pre- and postsynaptic serotonergic binding sites in people who have been examined after suicide as opposed to the postmortem studies of the control group.

Although some biological studies have been done on patients with panic disorder, they are not applicable to patients with cluster C personality disorders (described later in the chapter). More research is necessary to study the biological factors underlying the anxiety traits of patients with personality disorders.

Because many prison inmates are diagnosed with antisocial personality disorder, considerable research has focused on this population. Many of these people had attention deficit disorder in childhood. They also display a high rate of nonspecific EEG abnormalities. Their autonomic nervous systems are characterized by high arousal states, and the most recent research demonstrates that many of them have a depletion of serotonin and 5-HIAA. Such a deficiency has been linked to aggression in mammals.

▶ Check Your Reading

4. What areas of study are currently being undertaken to understand the implications of biology in the etiology of personality disorders?
5. What have researchers found when studying 5-HIAA levels on individuals who have completed suicide?

DESCRIPTIONS OF PERSONALITY DISORDERS

The authors of the *Diagnostic and Statistical Manual of Mental Disorders-IV (DSM-IV)* define general diagnostic criteria for all personality disorders that specify that the person must demonstrate an enduring pattern of inner experiences and behavior that deviates from the person's cultural expectations. These patterns are evident in two or more of the following areas:

- Cognition, or thought pattern. The person has different ways of perceiving and interpreting self, others, and events in the environment.
- Affect. The person displays a range, intensity, lability, and appropriateness of emotional response different from those of others in the same cultural group.
- Interpersonal functioning. Individuals with personality disorder experience more difficulty socializing and maintaining friendships, work relationships, and marital relationships than others in their cultural group.
- Impulse control. People with personality disorders may be more impulsive, aggressive, or self-destructive than the norm.

These inflexible and enduring patterns are present across a broad range of personal and social situations. For example, a person may have the same problems with different bosses at several different work sites throughout a work history. This person probably is unable to recognize the pattern of inflexible behavior that was similar in each job. This inability leads to clinically significant distress in social, occupational, or other important areas of functioning. A person may have difficulty maintaining a friendship because the friend is expected to meet most of his or her emotional needs but the person does not reciprocate.

These behavioral and thought patterns exist over a long period. They generally begin in adolescence or early adulthood. They are not manifestations of any other psychiatric illness, nor are they due to direct physiological effects of a substance (such as alcohol or a medication) or a general medical condition (such as a head trauma).

▶ Check Your Reading

6. What is meant by "an enduring pattern of inner experience and behavior that deviates markedly from the expectations of the individual's culture"?
7. What are three behavioral or thought patterns exhibited by individuals with a personality disorder?

CLUSTERS OF BEHAVIORS

Personality disorders are grouped by common behavior patterns into three clusters on the Axis II part of the *DSM-IV.* Although the three clusters are useful in aiding clinicians with diagnosis of personality disorders, overlapping of behaviors, points to the need for more research to differentiate one disorder from another. The first group, **cluster A disorders,** includes paranoid, schizoid, and schizotypal personality disorders. A common trait among patients with these disorders is that they often appear odd or eccentric. The second group, **cluster B disorders,** includes antisocial, borderline, histrionic, and narcissistic personality disorders. These patients typically exhibit dramatic, emotional, or erratic behaviors. The third group, **cluster C disorders,** includes dependent, avoidant, and obsessive-compulsive personality disorders. These patients characteristically display anxious or fearful behaviors.

Cluster A Personality Disorders

Paranoid Personality Disorder

The essential feature of a **paranoid personality disorder** is a pattern of mistrust and suspiciousness of others, beginning by early adulthood. The person with this disorder believes that others have malevolent motives for every interaction. In addition, people with this condition display at least four of the following:

- Suspicion that others are exploiting, harming, or deceiving them
- Preoccupation with doubts about the loyalty or trustworthiness of others
- Reluctance to confide in others, worry that others will later use this information against them
- Perception of hidden demeaning or threatening meanings into benevolent remarks made by others
- Grudges held against others who are perceived to be insulting or injurious
- Perception of attacks on character or reputation, with quick, angry reactions
- Suspicion regarding the fidelity of a spouse or sexual partner

Schizoid Personality Disorder

The essential feature of **schizoid personality disorder** is a pervasive pattern of detachment from social relationships and a restricted range of expression of emotions, particularly in interpersonal settings, beginning by early adulthood. Jeff, for example, manifests behavioral patterns consistent with this disorder. The person with a schizoid personality disorder displays at least four of the following:

- Lack of desire for or enjoyment of any close relationships, including being part of a family
- Consistent choice of solitary activities
- Little interest in a sexual relationship
- Little pleasure in any activities
- No close friends other than first-degree relatives
- Indifference to praise or criticism from others
- Emotional coldness or detachment and a flat affect

Schizotypal Personality Disorder

The essential feature of **schizotypal personality disorder** is a pervasive pattern of social and interpersonal deficits marked by acute discomfort with and a reduced capacity for close relationships. The condition begins by early adulthood. The person displays at least five of the behaviors identified in the *DSM-IV.*

▶ Check Your Reading

8. Describe two ways in which the schizotypal personality might be considered odd.
9. What is the essential feature or pattern of behavior for the individual with a paranoid personality disorder?
10. What is the essential feature or behavioral pattern for the individual with schizoid personality disorder?

Cluster B Personality Disorders

Antisocial Personality Disorder

The essential feature of **antisocial personality disorder** is a pervasive pattern of disregard for and violation of the rights of others. An individual with an antisocial personality disorder does not exhibit any sense of guilt and often is very manipulative. To make the diagnosis of antisocial personality disorder, the individual must be at least 18 years old and must have shown evidence of conduct disorder before the age of 15. Antisocial personality disorder—which used to be called psychopathic disorder, sociopathic disorder, or moral insanity—affects approximately 3% of American men and 1% of American women. These individuals do to not seek psychiatric treatment unless they also have an Axis I diagnosis or are remanded by the courts for evaluation of their mental status because of criminality and/or substance abuse. Much is written about this disorder in the forensic literature.

The Diagnostic and Statistical Manual of Mental Disorders-IV (DSM-IV) states that a diagnosis of antisocial personality disorder should be made if the person satisfies at least three of the behaviors identified in the *DSM-IV.*

Borderline Personality Disorder

The essential feature of **borderline personality disorder** is a pervasive pattern of unstable interpersonal relationships, difficulty defining self and determining self-image, labile affects and/or mood, and marked impulsive behavior, beginning by early adulthood. This disorder is more pervasive in women than in men. In Case Example 32–2, Joanne demonstrates behavior patterns consistent with borderline personality disorder. The behavior of people with this disorder includes at least five of the behaviors identified in the *DSM-IV.*

Case Example 32–2 Joanne's Story

Joanne is 30 years old and has been married for seven years to a man who is quiet and passive. They have no

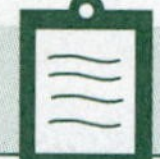

MEDICAL DIAGNOSES AND RELATED NURSING DIAGNOSES — Cluster A Personality Disorders

***DSM-IV* Diagnosis:** Schizotypal Personality Disorder

A. A pervasive pattern of social and interpersonal deficits marked by acute discomfort with, and reduced capacity for, close relationships as well as by cognitive or perceptual distortions and eccentricities of behavior, beginning by early adulthood and present in a variety of contexts, as indicated by five (or more) of the following:
   (1) Ideas of reference (excluding delusions of reference)
   (2) Odd beliefs or magical thinking that influences behavior and is inconsistent with subcultural norms (e.g., superstitiousness, belief in clairvoyance, telepathy, or "sixth sense"; in children and adolescents, bizarre fantasies or preoccupations)
   (3) Unusual perceptual experiences, including bodily illusions
   (4) Odd thinking and speech (e.g., vague, circumstantial, metaphorical, overelaborate, or stereotyped)
   (5) Suspiciousness or paranoid ideation
   (6) Inappropriate or constricted affect
   (7) Behavior or appearance that is odd, eccentric, or peculiar
   (8) Lack of close friends or confidants other than first-degree relatives
   (9) Excessive social anxiety that does not diminish with familiarity and tends to be associated with paranoid fears rather than negative judgments about self

B. Does not occur exclusively during the course of Schizophrenia, a Mood Disorder With Psychotic Features, another Psychotic Disorder, or a Pervasive Developmental Disorder.

Note: If criteria are met prior to the onset of Schizophrenia, add "Premorbid," e.g., "Schizotypal Personality Disorder (Premorbid)."

RELATED NURSING DIAGNOSES	DEFINITION	EXAMPLE
Impaired Social Interaction	The state in which a person participates in an insufficient or excessive quantity or ineffective quality of social exchange	Impaired Social Interaction related to magical thinking and anxiety when in a social situation as evidenced by thoughts that the patient can feel a "sixth sense" when in a social environment, verbalizations regarding increased anxiety in a social setting, and statements that the patient experiences ideas of reference in social settings

Diagnostic criteria from American Psychiatric Association: *Diagnostic and Statistical Manual of Mental Disorders, fourth edition.* Washington, D.C., American Psychiatric Association, 1994; nursing diagnoses and definitions from North American Nursing Diagnosis Association (1994). *NANDA nursing diagnoses: Definitions and classification 1995–1996.* Philadelphia: NANDA.

children. Joanne is often impulsive, angry, emotional, and critical of others. She has a history of seeking revenge when angry. She is currently having an affair with a man she met at an Alcoholics Anonymous (AA) meeting. She feels "happy with Carlos" (her lover) and thinks her marriage with Jack is over. She is afraid to leave her husband because she feels Carlos, although fun, would never be able to support them financially.

Joanne does not work and perceives the work world as threatening and scary. Joanne has been clean and sober from alcohol and benzodiazepines for the last seven months. She is going to AA meetings to see Carlos, but she does not have a sponsor and does not feel comfortable discussing her issues in the "open."

Joanne has attempted suicide several times in her life. Two of the three overdose attempts were in response to termination of a relationship with a lover. She attempted suicide when, at age sixteen, she found her father with another woman. She told the therapist at the time, "If Mom leaves Dad, I'd be all alone. I was so upset by that prospect, I became overwhelmed with grief and took a razor to my wrist."

Joanne has had stormy relationships with women who tried to befriend her. "They were jealous of my talents; they really did not want to be my friend; they really wanted to learn how to sew." Joanne is estranged from her family and discusses her anger at her mother and two sisters when asked why she has not maintained contact. Joanne also has a stormy relationship with God, fluctuating between intense love for Him and intense hatred. She feels alone much of the time.

People with borderline personality disorders frequently engage in a manipulative behavior referred to as **splitting**, which "pits" people against one another. Because of their tendency to view people as "all good" or "all bad," those with this disorder frequently are disillusioned when family, friends, or professional caregivers fail to be perfect. For instance, a hospitalized patient diagnosed with borderline personality disorder might tell one staff person that she is the best nurse, the only one who understands the patient, but at the same time the patient paints a very negative picture of another staff member's behavior. If staff members are unaware of the patient's splitting behavior, contention and inconsistency in the patient's plan of treatment may develop.

Histrionic Personality Disorder

The essential feature of **histrionic personality disorder** is excessive emotionality and attention-seeking behavior, beginning by early adulthood. People with this disorder feel uncomfortable or unappreciated when they are not the center of attention and therefore behave in a manner to glean this attention. People with a histrionic personality disorder also display at least five of the behaviors identified in the *DSM-IV.*

Narcissistic Personality Disorder

The essential feature of **narcissistic personality disorder** is the pattern of grandiosity, need for admiration, and lack of empathy toward others, beginning by early adulthood. This tendency is manifested in five or more of the following:

- A grandiose sense of self-importance. Achievements and talents are often exaggerated. The person often expects recognition as a superior performer without the commensurate achievements.
- Preoccupation with fantasies of unlimited success, power, brilliance, beauty, or ideal love.
- Belief that he or she is "special" and unique and can associate only with others who are also special and have a high status.
- Need for an excessive amount of admiration.
- An unrealistic sense of entitlement.
- Interpersonal exploitation and taking advantage of others to meet personal goals.
- Lack of empathy, as this individual is unwilling to recognize or identify with the feelings or needs of others.

MEDICAL DIAGNOSES AND RELATED NURSING DIAGNOSES **Cluster B Personality Disorders**

DSM-IV **Diagnosis:** Antisocial Personality Disorder

Diagnostic Criteria

A. There is a pervasive pattern of disregard for and violation of the rights of others occurring since age 15 years, as indicated by three (or more) of the following:
  (1) Failure to conform to social norms with respect to lawful behaviors as indicated by repeatedly performing acts that are grounds for arrest
  (2) Deceitfulness, as indicated by repeated lying, use of aliases, or conning others for personal profit or pleasure
  (3) Impulsivity or failure to plan ahead
  (4) Irritability and aggressiveness, as indicated by repeated physical fights or assaults
  (5) Reckless disregard for safety of self or others
  (6) Consistent irresponsibility, as indicated by repeated failure to sustain consistent work behavior or honor financial obligations
  (7) Lack of remorse, as indicated by being indifferent to or rationalizing having hurt, mistreated, or stolen from another

B. The individual is at least age 18 years.

C. There is evidence of Conduct Disorder with onset before age 15 years.

D. The occurrence of antisocial behavior is not exclusively during the course of Schizophrenia or a Manic Episode.

RELATED NURSING DIAGNOSES	DEFINITION	EXAMPLE
Ineffective Individual Coping	Impairment of adaptive behaviors and problem-solving abilities of a person in meeting life's demands and roles	Ineffective Individual Coping related to lifestyle of defensive behaviors as evidenced by the patient's mistrust and suspicious statements directed toward others, aggressive behavior that is justified in the patient's mind as retaliatory, and blaming of others for own behavior
Ineffective Denial	The state of a conscious or unconscious attempt to disavow the knowledge or meaning of an event to reduce anxiety or fear, to the detriment of health	Ineffective Denial related to the patient's impaired ability to accept consequences for own behavior as evidenced by continuing the same pattern of rage and aggression, blaming others for own aggressive behavior, and refusing to acknowledge own contribution to arguments

Continued

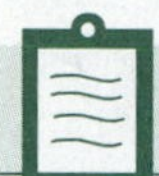

MEDICAL DIAGNOSES AND RELATED NURSING DIAGNOSES **Cluster B Personality Disorders** *Continued*

***DSM-IV* Diagnosis:** Borderline Personality Disorder

Diagnostic Criteria

A pervasive pattern of instability of interpersonal relationships, self-image, and affects, and marked impulsivity beginning by early adulthood and present in a variety of contexts, as indicated by five (or more) of the following:

(1) Frantic efforts to avoid real or imagined abandonment. **Note:** Do not include suicidal or self-mutilating behavior covered in Criterion 5.

(2) A pattern of unstable and intense interpersonal relationships characterized by alternating between extremes of idealization and devaluation.

(3) Identity disturbance: markedly and persistently unstable self-image or sense of self.

(4) Impulsivity in at least two areas that are potentially self-damaging (e.g., spending, sex, substance abuse, reckless driving, binge eating). **Note:** Do not include suicidal or self-mutilating behavior covered in Criterion 5.

(5) Recurrent suicidal behavior, gestures, or threats, or self-mutilating behavior.

(6) Affective instability due to a marked reactivity of mood (e.g., intense episodic dysphoria, irritability, or anxiety usually lasting a few hours and only rarely more than a few days).

(7) Chronic feelings of emptiness.

(8) Inappropriate, intense anger or difficulty controlling anger (e.g., frequent displays of temper, constant anger, recurrent physical fights).

(9) Transient, stress-related paranoid ideation or severe dissociative symptoms.

RELATED NURSING DIAGNOSES	DEFINITION	EXAMPLE
Ineffective Individual Coping	Impairment of adaptive behaviors and problem-solving abilities of a person in meeting life's demands and roles	Ineffective Individual Coping related to inadequate psychological resources, poor self-esteem, and excessive negative thoughts about self as evidenced by impulsive alcohol consumption and sexual promiscuity, labile emotional states of anger and crying, and verbalization of feelings of being overwhelmed, alone, without support, and unable to identify the reasons for these feelings
Risk for Violence: Self-Directed	A state in which a person experiences behaviors that can be physically harmful to either self or others	Risk for Self-Directed Violence related to history of cutting self when highly emotional as evidenced by the patient's expressed fears of being abandoned by a significant other and sense of unreality
Self-Esteem Disturbance	Negative self-evaluation or feelings about self or self-capabilities, which may be directly or indirectly expressed	Self-Esteem Disturbance related to the patient's relationship problems with spouse as evidenced by the patient's describing self as unable to deal with conflict in the marriage, expressing guilt and feelings of shame about marital discord, and extreme sensitivity to criticism by spouse and other family members

- Envy of others and belief that others are envious of him or her.
- Arrogance and haughtiness in behavior and attitude.

▶ Check Your Reading

11. State the essential feature demonstrated by the person with antisocial personality disorder and borderline personality disorder.

12. What common psychiatric problem often seen in the emergency department is part of the behavior exhibited by a person with borderline personality disorder?

Cluster C Personality Disorders

Avoidant Personality Disorder

The essential feature of **avoidant personality disorder** is a pervasive pattern of social inhibition, feelings of inadequacy, and hypersensitivity to negative evaluations from others, beginning by early adulthood. Individuals diagnosed with this personality disorder display at least four of the characteristics identified in the *DSM-IV.*

MEDICAL DIAGNOSES AND RELATED NURSING DIAGNOSES — Cluster B Personality Disorders *Continued*

***DSM-IV* Diagnosis:** Histrionic Personality Disorder

Diagnostic Criteria

A pervasive pattern of excessive emotionality and attention-seeking, beginning by early adulthood and present in a variety of contexts, as indicated by five (or more) of the following:

(1) Is uncomfortable in situations in which he or she is not the center of attention
(2) Interaction with others is often characterized by inappropriate sexually seductive or provocative behavior
(3) Displays rapidly shifting and shallow expression of emotions
(4) Consistently uses physical appearance to draw attention to self
(5) Has a style of speech that is excessively impressionistic and lacking in detail
(6) Shows self-dramatization, theatricality, and exaggerated expression of emotion
(7) Is suggestible, i.e., easily influenced by others or circumstances
(8) Considers relationships to be more intimate than they actually are

RELATED NURSING DIAGNOSES	DEFINITION	EXAMPLE
Self-Esteem Disturbance	Negative self-evaluation or feelings about self or self-capabilities, which may be directly or indirectly expressed	Self-Esteem Disturbance related to the patient's relationship problems with spouse as evidenced by the patient describing self as unable to deal with conflicts in the marriage, expressing guilt and feelings of shame about marital discord, and extreme sensitivity to criticism by spouse and other family members

Diagnostic criteria from American Psychiatric Association: *Diagnostic and statistical manual of mental disorders, fourth edition.* Washington, D.C., American Psychiatric Association. 1994; nursing diagnoses and definitions from North American Nursing Diagnosis Association (1994). *NANDA nursing diagnoses: Definitions and classification 1995–1996.* Philadelphia: NANDA.

MEDICAL DIAGNOSES AND RELATED NURSING DIAGNOSES — Cluster C Personality Disorders

***DSM-IV* Diagnosis:** Avoidant Personality Disorder

Diagnostic Criteria

A pervasive pattern of social inhibition, feelings of inadequacy, and hypersensitivity to negative evaluation, beginning by early adulthood and present in a variety of contexts, as indicated by four (or more) of the following:

(1) Avoids occupational activities that involve significant interpersonal contact, because of fears of criticism, disapproval, or rejection
(2) Is unwilling to get involved with people unless certain of being liked
(3) Shows restraint within intimate relationships because of the fear of being shamed or ridiculed
(4) Is preoccupied with being criticized or rejected in social situations
(5) Is inhibited in new interpersonal situations because of feelings of inadequacy
(6) Views self as socially inept, personally unappealing, or inferior to others
(7) Is unusually reluctant to take personal risks or to engage in any new activities because they may prove embarrassing

RELATED NURSING DIAGNOSES	DEFINITION	EXAMPLE
Anxiety	A vague, uneasy feeling whose source is often nonspecific or unknown to the individual	Anxiety related to fear that no one will accept the patient in a social setting as evidenced by preoccupation with potential embarrassing incidents that may occur, verbalizations of feelings of inferiority, fear, and apprehensiveness

Continued

MEDICAL DIAGNOSES AND RELATED NURSING DIAGNOSES **Cluster C Personality Disorders** *Continued*

***DSM-IV* Diagnosis:** Dependent Personality Disorder

Diagnostic Criteria

A pervasive and excessive need to be taken care of that leads to submissive and clinging behavior and fears of separation, beginning by early adulthood and present in a variety of contexts, as indicated by five (or more) of the following:

(1) Has difficulty making everyday decisions without an excessive amount of advice and reassurance from others.
(2) Needs others to assume responsibility for most major areas of his or her life.
(3) Has difficulty expressing disagreement with others because of fear of loss of support or approval. **Note:** Do not include realistic fears of retribution.
(4) Has difficulty initiating projects or doing things on his or her own (because of a lack of self-confidence in judgment or abilities rather than a lack of motivation or energy).
(5) Goes to excessive lengths to obtain nurturance and support from others, to the point of volunteering to do things that are unpleasant.
(6) Feels uncomfortable or helpless when alone because of exaggerated fears of being unable to care for himself or herself.
(7) Urgently seeks another relationship as a source of care and support when a close relationship ends.
(8) Is unrealistically preoccupied with fears of being left to take care of himself or herself.

RELATED NURSING DIAGNOSIS	DEFINITION	EXAMPLE
Fear	Feeling of dread related to an identifiable source, which the person validates	Fear related to the anticipated loss of a parent as evidenced by increased questioning of the medical staff as to when the parent may die, hypervigilance about the parent's vital signs, refusal to leave the parent's side, and statements of concern regarding self-care after parent's death
Self-Esteem Disturbance	Negative self-evaluation or feelings about self or self-capabilities, which may be directly or indirectly expressed	Self-Esteem Disturbance related to relationship problems with spouse as evidenced by the patient describing self as unable to deal with conflict in the marriage, expressed guilt feelings and shame about marital discord, and extreme sensitivity to criticism by spouse and other family members
Personal Identity Disturbance	Inability to distinguish between self and nonself	Personal Identity Disturbance related to recent breakup of relationship with a significant other as evidenced by constant statements like "I'm nothing without him" and difficulty discussing self without mentioning the significant other as if he or she were part of self

Diagnostic criteria from American Psychiatric Association: *Diagnostic and statistical manual of mental disorders, fourth edition.* Washington, D.C., American Psychiatric Association, 1994; nursing diagnoses and definitions from North American Nursing Diagnosis Association (1994). *NANDA nursing diagnoses: Definitions and classification 1995–1996.* Philadelphia: NANDA.

Dependent Personality Disorder

The essential feature of **dependent personality disorder** is the excessive need to be taken care of by others, which leads to submissive, clinging behavior and fear of separation, beginning by early adulthood. Individuals with a dependent personality disorder exhibit at least five of the characteristics identified in the *DSM-IV.*

Obsessive-Compulsive Personality Disorder

The essential feature of **obsessive-compulsive personality disorder** is a preoccupation with orderliness and perfectionism developing by early adulthood. People with this disorder exert emotional as well as interpersonal control in relationships, at the expense of flexibility, openness, and efficiency. In Case Example 32–3 Martin demonstrates behavioral and emotional traits consistent with obsessive-compulsive personality disorder.

Additionally, people with this disorder exhibit at least four of the following behaviors:

- Preoccupation with details, rules, lists, order, organization, or schedules, to the extent that the major reason for an activity is lost.
- Perfectionism that interferes with task completion. A student who has difficulty completing papers in a

timely fashion because she or he expects herself or himself to read every available reference is demonstrating perfectionism that interferes with task completion.

- Excessive devotion to work and productivity to the exclusion of leisure activities and friendships.
- Overconscientious, scrupulous, and inflexible belief system about morality, ethics, or values that is not part of the person's cultural or religious affiliation.
- Inability to discard worn-out or worthless objects even when he or she has no reason (such as sentimental value) to hold on to these objects.
- Reluctance to delegate tasks or to work with others unless they acquiesce to doing the assignment exactly as directed.
- Hoarding money for the future and frugality when spending money on self or others.
- Rigidity and stubborn thoughts and behavior.

Case Example 32–3 Martin's Story

Martin is a 33-year-old computer programmer. He is known for being accurate, a perfectionist, and a person who is detail oriented. He often is critical of others as well as himself and believes that criticism "drives progress and competence." Martin spends most of his time at work because he is concerned about doing a superior job and because of the nature of his work (he says "one cannot do a half-baked job").

Martin has a girlfriend, Lilly, a nurse he met when he was working on a program for the local hospital's computer information department. Lilly claims that Martin is stingy with his time and financial resources; "He saves everything; he doesn't spend on himself either." Lilly complains that Martin and she have never had a vacation, as Martin can never see the "right" break in his work projects to get away. "I can barely get him to relax on a Saturday evening!"

Martin's subordinates say he "micromanages" their projects. His behavior causes resentment, and at times they "forget to do part of the project, because Martin will only do it over; let him do it in the first place!" Martin does not spend much time with his family. He feels out of place, as he views his siblings and parents as "emotionally charged." Martin feels the best way to deal with feelings is to think through the issues and "go on with life." Martin follows the rules of his religion but expresses no emotional commitment, nor does his spirituality seem to provide him with a sense of joy—only boundaries.

▶ Check Your Reading

13. State one characteristic of each of the cluster C personality disorders.

NURSING PROCESS

ASSESSMENT

When working with patients who have personality disorders, the assessment must include questions regarding the patient's perception of self and others, expression of emotions, interaction with others, and patterns of relating, emotions, behavior, and thought. You need to determine whether these patterns occur over time and are a stable part of the patient's responses to the world. Behavior patterns and examples of assessment questions appear in Box 32–1.

In addition to the questions that specifically identify a personality disorder, also assess the patient spiritually to determine if the patient is able to gain a sense of meaning out of life's experiences. Does the patient believe that life has purpose? Does the patient have a relationship with God? How does this relationship affect daily life? Does the patient experience comfort from spiritual beliefs? If so, what beliefs? Does the patient interpret failures and interpersonal difficulties according to a relationship or lack of relationship with God? Does spirituality assist the patient in dealing with life's difficulties? Is there anything that you might assist with in addressing spirituality for this patient?

DIAGNOSIS

Diagnostic and Statistical Manual of Mental Disorders-IV (DSM-IV) diagnoses suggest patterns in cognition, affect, interpersonal functioning, and impulse control that determine related nursing diagnoses. A patient with dependent personality disorder, for example, is likely to experience fear related to possible loss.

▶ Check Your Reading

14. State one question that you could ask a patient regarding his or her perception of self and others?
15. How would you determine that a patient demonstrated an enduring pattern of inflexible behavior?
16. Give one example of an assessment question that you might ask to determine the quality of a patient's relationships.

OUTCOME IDENTIFICATION

Expected outcomes are based on nursing diagnoses. Examples of outcomes and goals are listed in Table 32–1.

PLANNING

The planning phase of the nursing process consists of several parts: selecting the nursing interventions to meet the identified goals and collaborating with everyone involved in the patient's care to ensure consistency and commitment to the treatment plan. In planning interventions for the patient with a personality disorder, note that behaviors are stable and of long duration. Change does not occur overnight. Rather, it is gradual and characterized by an uneven course. Patience, forbearance, tolerance, and perseverance are prequisites when you work with a patient who has a personality disorder.

▶ Check Your Reading

17. Identify one patient outcome for Case Examples 32–1 and 32–2.
18. When planning interventions for patients with personality disorders, what must you consider?

IMPLEMENTATION

Interventions for the patient with a personality disorder include counseling, which includes contracting with the patient for behavioral change and providing consistent limit-setting; health teaching regarding issues such as social skills, problem-solving, and risks of promiscuous behaviors; milieu therapy; and psychobiological interventions.

Counseling and Health Teaching

Developing a therapeutic relationship with the patient is very challenging, sometimes exasperating, yet absolutely essential. These patients can change if they experience care in the context of a relationship with clear boundaries, defined and reinforced limits, and praise. You need to confront manipulation and deal with behavior matter of factly rather than punitively. Patients must know that they are valued. Box 32–2 lists general nursing strategies that are part of counseling the patient with a personality disorder.

Health teaching is an important strategy. Frequently,

BOX 32–1 Questions for Assessing Patients With Behavior Disorders

Thinking and Views of the World

Do you often find that you have different views of the world than most people? What are those ideas?

Suspiciousness

Do you ever think that others are trying to harm you in some way? Do you think that you are always the one getting the bad end of the bargain?

Affect—Anger

Are you often angry? What is your behavior like when you are angry? Do you become aggressive and at times get into physical fights? Do you ever feel like hurting or killing anyone? Have you ever been in trouble with the law?

Affect—Expression

Are you often very emotional? Has anyone ever told you that you are cold and do not show any emotions? Has anyone ever told you that you are seeking attention?

Impulsive Behavior

Do you ever become impulsive and maybe drink to excess, use illegal substances, or have sex on impulse with someone you do not know well?

Suicidal or Self-Mutilating Behavior

Have you ever been suicidal? Are you suicidal now? Have you ever hurt yourself by cutting or burning yourself? Do you do that now? When does this occur?

Relationships—Significant Other

Tell me about your relationships with others. Are you married, or do you have a significant other? What is that relationship like? Are you able to make decisions jointly? Do you often have arguments? What are these arguments about? Do you have any fears that your spouse or partner will have an affair? Do you ever think about having an affair?

Relationships—Family

What is your relationship like with your family? How do you get along with your children? How often do you see your parents and siblings? What is your relationship like with your parents and siblings?

Relationships—Work

How do you get along with your boss? Do you have any friends at work?

Relationships—Friends

Do you have any friends? How often do you visit with them? What activities do you do together?

Socialization

What types of socializing do you do? Do you enjoy these events, or do you become anxious and unable to participate comfortably?

Recurrent Patterns of Behavior

Do you find that you have had some of the same problems over the years? What have these problems been like? When did they start? Do you identify any patterns to these problems?

TABLE 32–1 Nursing Process Related to Findings Common in Personality Disorders

Nursing Diagnosis	Expected Outcomes	Short-Term Goals	Interventions
Anxiety related to fear that no one will accept the patient in a social setting as evidenced by preoccupation with embarrassing incidents that may occur, verbalized feelings of inferiority in social settings, and signs of fear and apprehension	Patient will experience less anxiety.	Patient will be able accurately to interpret environmental stimuli in a social setting.	Assist the patient to interpret the environmental stimuli in the therapy room. Ask the patient to pick another place, one with greater comfort. Ask the patient to interpret the environmental stimuli in that setting. Ask the patient to identify some of the similarities and differences in these environments. Ask the patient to compare similarities and differences between the comfortable setting and the social setting most feared. Teach the patient strategies such as deep breathing and relaxation techniques to decrease anxiety.
		Patient will be able to recognize events that increase the feelings of apprehension and fear.	Ask the patient to list several events in social settings that cause anxiety and fear. Discuss each incident to determine what the patient is thinking while experiencing anxiety. Teach the patient that negative thoughts increase feelings of anxiety and fear. Discuss other thoughts that could be used to assist the patient in feeling less anxious (e.g., use of positive affirmations). Discuss the benefits of spiritual interventions to decrease anxiety and fear.
		Patient will identify examples of embarrassing incidents and will plan methods to cope with these possible events.	Assist the patient to list examples of embarrassing incidents feared in a social setting. Discuss how these incidents may occur. Discuss methods to avoid the embarrassing incidents. Discuss new ways to deal with embarrassing incidents that might occur. Teach the patient to recognize how negative thinking patterns may inflate perceptions of the incident. Use affirmations or prayer when these negative thought patterns occur.
Risk for Violence: Self-Directed related to history of cutting self when highly emotional as evidenced by patient's verbalization that she has been abandoned by her boyfriend and her verbalization that she is experiencing feelings of unreality	The patient will no longer self-mutilate.	The patient will be able to identify cues that usually occur before her self-mutilating behavior.	Discuss how the patient self-mutilates, how long she has been doing this, and how she feels before and after cutting herself. Ask the patient to keep a journal and write her thoughts and feelings about subjects that are important to her emotionally. Ask her to include any thoughs or feelings that occur before self-mutilation. Discuss whether the patient becomes "spacey" or "numb" before cutting herself. Examine the patient's feelings of abandonment by her boyfriend.
		The patient will identify support systems that can assist her to prevent self-mutilating behavior.	Help the patient identify being with another person as a way of decreasing the urge to self-mutilate. Help patient state that she can call a friend when feeling upset or "numb." Contract with the patient about going to a friend or family member's house when disturbed to defuse the intensity of the feelings.

Table continued on following page

TABLE 32–1 Nursing Process Related to Findings Common in Personality Disorders *Continued*

Nursing Diagnosis	Expected Outcomes	Short-Term Goals	Interventions
			Encourage the patient to take a bath to soothe self and as a means of decreasing the urge to self-mutilate. Contract with the patient for safety so that the patient will call the nurse if she is unable to decrease the urge to self-mutilate.
Risk for Violence: Directed at Others related to patient's history of aggression, physical fights with others, and use of a weapon as evidenced by lack of remorse and verbalizations that he is justified in wanting to hurt his coworker for getting a raise and a promotion	The patient will not harm self or others.	The patient will identify alternatives to violence.	Contract with the patient that he will use neither verbal nor physical threats while receiving treatment. Contract with the patient so that the patient will isolate himself in a safe room and try to determine other means of communicating his needs rather than verbal or physical aggression. In his next counseling session, discuss any verbally aggressive incidents with the patient.
		The patient will give his gun to an exchange program (e.g., Guns for Money).	Locate an exchange program offered by the local police or a local business. If there is no program, have the patient agree to give any weapons to a significant person for safe keeping until he can locate a program.
		The patient will identify other nonviolent behaviors that he can use when he feels like harming others.	Discuss using a quiet but safe room to "cool off." Identify thought patterns that maintain the patient's anger. Discuss alternative thoughts the patient may use when he realizes he is ruminating about the situation that caused him to feel like harming someone. Assist the patient to think of new ways to voice his needs rather than using aggressive means.

the patient does not know how to interact appropriately. Patients may misread social cues and respond in ways that increase their social isolation. Modeling desired behaviors provides concrete examples. The patient may be engaging in dangerous activities such as excessive alcohol intake, drug use, or promiscuous sexual behavior. Your teaching focuses not only on the risks associated with these behaviors but also on strategies to change these potentially destructive ways of being. Table 32–1 lists appropriate counseling and teaching interventions related to specific nursing diagnoses.

Milieu Therapy

When working with a person who has a personality disorder, you need to maintain not only a structure of activities but also your own personal and professional boundaries. Boundary maintenance is especially important with individuals having antisocial personality disorder, borderline personality disorder, histrionic personality disorder, and narcissistic personality disorder. Patients with these conditions may test your boundaries. For example, a patient might ask for a special favor or request that you "bend the rules" of the unit. Recognizing that the request may not be appropriate, you set a limit on the patient's behavior. If the limit-setting is done with respect and a rationale is offered, the effort may assist the patient to explore a lifelong behavioral pattern. The fact that the patient is momentarily angered by your insistence on realistic boundaries does not mean that he or she is incorrect. Patients need truth with empathy to begin to establish internal boundaries for themselves. If, however, limit-setting is perceived as punitive, rigid, or controlling, the patient will not learn from the experience and will repeat the behavior at another time.

Another important issue is the provision of safety, not only for the patient but also for other patients and staff members. Personality disorders most likely seen in inpatient settings include borderline, antisocial, and paranoid personality disorders. Each of these has the potential to cause upheaval, disruption, and even violence on a unit.

BOX 32-2 General Nursing Strategies Necessary in Counseling Patients With Personality Disorders

- Constant awareness of your own reactions to patient's behavior
- Supervision to deal with your feelings toward the patient
- Patience, persistence, consistency, flexibility, and trust
- A direct and matter-of-fact approach in confronting behavior
- Modeling appropriate problem-solving, interpersonal, and social skills
- Reinforcing appropriate behaviors
- Setting clear limits
- Encouraging verbal expression of feelings
- Encouraging responsibility and accountability
- Assisting the patient to delay gratification
- Establishing clear rules, regulations, and consequences
- Contracting for behavioral changes

Psychobiological Interventions

Psychobiological interventions involve a collaborative relationship with a physician who may prescribe medications to help patients with personality disorders. The pharmacotherapeutic treatment of a patient with a personality disorder is symptomatic. Soloff and coworkers (1991) studied the use of psychotropic agents with patients diagnosed with borderline personality disorder, schizotypal personality disorder, and both disorders in a mixed presentation. The researchers found that haloperidol was helpful in improving global functioning; in decreasing schizotypal symptoms, depression, and hostility; and in improving impulse control. Unstable patients with borderline personality disorder demonstrated a strong response to amitriptyline for hostility and lack of impulse control, with a near significant effect on subjective feelings of depression (Soloff et al, 1991).

For patients demonstrating out-of-control or violent behavior, Keltner and Folks (1993) suggest either an oral anxiolytic or a medication from the sedative-hypnotic class. If the patient cannot take an oral agent, these clinicians recommend intravenous or intermuscular sedative-hypnotics, such as barbiturates, benzodiazepines such as diazepam, or antipsychotics such as haloperidol. Patients who exhibit agitated or psychotic behavior may respond to a neuroleptic medication.

Patients who demonstrate depression as well as a personality disorder may benefit from either a tricyclic antidepressant or a selective serotonin reuptake inhibitor (SSRI). The SSRIs are more expensive than the tricyclics, and the cost may be prohibitive to some patients. Monitor a patient on an antidepressant for suicidal ideation and the possibility of an overdose. The probability of completed suicide with an overdose of an SSRI is lower than that with a tricyclic; a tricyclic overdose could cause cardiac toxicity.

Your role is to monitor patients on medications for side effects and to teach patients about medications. This education assists in patient compliance. If the medications are an adjunct to psychotherapy, patients with personality disorders can become more functional.

▶ Check Your Reading

19. Give an example of counseling as a nursing intervention.
20. How can limit-setting encourage patient learning?

EVALUATION

The evaluation stage of the nursing process helps you to determine if the patient has achieved the expected patient outcomes. The formative evaluation involves examining each short-term goal and comparing the patient's current thought pattern and behavior to the outcome criteria. For example, if the expected outcome is that the patient will determine other nonviolent behaviors that he can use when feeling like harming his coworkers, the current patient status might demonstrate that the patient has discussed with his boss going on a work detail or obtaining a transfer to another department. Or the patient might have chosen to stay away physically from his coworker, especially if the patient originally worked in the health care system, to prevent an aggressive act toward his coworker. If this patient decides on a strategy he can feel comfortable executing, he will successfully avoid an aggressive confrontation with his coworker. This process allows you to conclude in the summative evaluation that the expected outcome was achieved.

If, however, the formative evaluation demonstrates that the short-term goals and expected outcomes were not accomplished, you are motivated to revisit the entire nursing process. Ask yourself whether the assessment was complete, the diagnoses accurate, and the plan adequate to achieve the identified outcomes. If not, modifications are made, and the process continues.

NURSING'S JOURNEY WITH PATIENTS HAVING PERSONALITY DISORDERS

As you work with patients diagnosed with personality disorders, you may find yourself questioning your own skills, abilities, and the limits of your tolerance for difficult patients. Feelings of frustration are to be expected when you work with this population. Such feelings, however, need to be dealt with through supervision, if you are to remain a caring and holistic provider.

Your own spirituality can be affected when you work with patients who challenge your sense of competence. You may struggle with finding the answer to "why" you are not as effective as you would like to be with these patients. Talking about your own feelings, your frustrations, and your insecurities defuses your tension and allows you to stay connected to the patient and maintain your own spiritual well-being. You may find that spiritual interventions such as prayer help you to keep your perspective on healing. You are not responsible for a patient's healing. You are responsible for caring and providing the best that you have to offer. You can act as a healing presence and guide in a life troubled by personality disorder; you cannot accept responsibility for how the person chooses to conduct his or her journey.

CASE STUDY: NANCY

Nancy, a 25-year-old single female, is admitted to the inpatient psychiatric unit where you work because she recently lost her job and told her psychotherapist that she was going to kill herself. She lives alone in an apartment, has minimal support systems, and in the past few weeks began cutting on her wrists. Nancy has two younger sisters. She reports that she was sexually abused by her father when she was in her teens and that her mother is a drug addict. Her parents divorced 15 years ago.

While taking her history, you find that Nancy has a long history of mental illness. When she was 13 years old, she was first admitted to an adolescent psychiatric unit and had two other admissions since that time. Nancy is visibly upset about this hospitalization and says to you "I am a failure; I can't do anything right."

Within a few days, the staff observes that the self-mutilation behavior has escalated; so have the verbalizations of suicide. During a staff meeting you find that the unit manager and many of the nurses and the mental health technicians are very sympathetic with Nancy, while the psychiatrist and social workers and some of the nurses consider her behaviors manipulative.

The evening staff nurse reports that Nancy and one of the male patients, Jimmy, are spending all their free time together. Nancy tells you that she is in love with Jimmy, even though they have known each other for a short time. You also note that her emotions range widely within a span of a few moments, from being elated and laughing to crying hysterically.

ASSESSMENT

Assessment data are as follows:

- Suicidal ideation
- Self-mutilation behavior (cutting wrists)
- Splitting behaviors evidenced by staff's reaction to patient
- Development of impulsive, intense relationship with male patient
- Minimal support system
- Emotional instability
- Verbalizations of failure

DIAGNOSIS

***DSM-IV* Diagnosis:** Borderline Personality Disorder

Nursing Diagnosis 1: Ineffective Individual Coping related to sudden loss of job and minimal support system as evidenced by staff-splitting behaviors, verbal manipulation, and self-destructive behavior

OUTCOME IDENTIFICATION, PLANNING, AND IMPLEMENTATION

EXPECTED OUTCOME 1: By ____ the patient will be able to express a consistent, congruent response to staff with no evidence of splitting (idealizing or devaluing staff members).

SHORT-TERM GOALS	NURSING INTERVENTIONS	RATIONALES
By ____ the patient will demonstrate significant reduction in extreme responses toward staff.	1. Convey an accepting attitude to the patient. Be honest and keep promises.	1. Trust is an issue for clients with borderline personality disorder; congruence in the nurse's behavior is of paramount importance.
	2. Gently challenge the patient's idealistic views with realistic responses.	2. Challenging the patient in a gentle manner will help correct distortions and decrease the incidence of splitting.
	3. Encourage the patient's participation in therapeutic groups.	3. In light of their inherent nature and purpose, groups decrease splitting because it will be confronted as the group works through the stages of group process.
By ____ the patient will express a realistic view of the staff and significant others in her life.	1. Challenge the patient's tendency to devalue others by setting firm limits similar to parents' need to set loving, firm limits for their children. 2. Encourage the patient to look for positive and negative features in staff and significant others.	1–2. Patients often need assistance in the form of firm limit-setting to change an entrenched behavior.
	3. Encourage the patient to share observations in a group setting. 4. Teach the patient ways of centering self so that feedback can be nonthreatening.	3–4. Group formats can help the patient develop more constructive responses to significant others in her life.

EXPECTED OUTCOME 2: By ____ the patient will verbalize a desire to curtail manipulation as a way of getting needs met.

SHORT-TERM GOALS	NURSING INTERVENTIONS	RATIONALES
By ____ the patient will express needs directly.	1. Give the patient support for direct, clear communication.	1. Patients are often rewarded for manipulative communication in their families of origin; positive support leads to an increase in positive behaviors.
	2. Assign the same staff members each shift and encourage all staff members to follow the treatment plan.	2. Consistent staff assignment will sharply decrease the patient's ability to split staff.
	3. Do not argue, rationalize, or bargain with the patient.	3. The patient may invite this behavior by her actions, but you are the professional and are expected to be an expert in clear, congruent communication.
	4. Do not assume that all physical complaints are necessarily invalid.	4–5. The patient may have legitimate complaints, and they must be thoroughly evaluated, but continuing to engage in discussion regarding invalid complaints will negatively reward the patient.
	5. Investigate any medical complaints; if they are invalid, redirect the patient. 6. Assure the patient that her needs will be met without resorting to manipulation.	5. This will reduce the incidence of manipulative behaviors.

By _____ the patient will exhibit congruent verbal and nonverbal messages.	1. Have the patient practice clear, nonmanipulative communication with staff and group members. 2. Give the patient feedback regarding your observations. 3. Be consistent in your own verbal and nonverbal messages. 4. Praise the patient for engaging in behaviors that are free from manipulation and that indicate consideration and respect for others.	1–2, 4. Behaviors that are positively reinforced are likely to be repeated. 3. It is important for the nurse to provide mature role modeling.

EXPECTED OUTCOME 3: By _____ the patient will verbalize a desire to continue on her life journey and cease verbalizations of self-destructive behavior.

SHORT-TERM GOALS	NURSING INTERVENTIONS	RATIONALES
The patient will remain safe while in the hospital.	1. Assess degree of suicidality. 2. Implement suicide precautions—create a safe environment for the patient.	1–2. Safety is a number-one priority for any patient with suicidal ideation.
	3. Formulate a short-term contract with the patient stating that she will not harm herself. 4. Renew contract as necessary.	3–4. Patients often are relieved to discuss suicidal feelings openly and feel supported by the strength of the staff member. Contracting to ask for assistance from a trusted staff member will decrease ambivalence and promote the decision to live rather than to die.
	5. Have the patient promise that she will seek out a staff member if the desire to harm herself arises.	5. This action further supports the notion that the patient is a valued human being.
By _____ the patient will verbalize hope for her future.	1. Spend uninterrupted time with the patient and *listen* to her. 2. Encourage verbalization of honest feelings.	1–2. Patients who have enough emotional pain to consider suicide benefit from uninterrupted time with a caring person.
	3. Ask the patient what has kept her from hurting herself in the past.	3. This question assists the patient in remembering her strengths and support system.
	4. Encourage the patient to express any angry feelings and to get to the true source of her feelings.	4. Suicide and other self-destructive behaviors often are considered a result of anger turned inward.

Nursing Diagnosis: Risk for Self-Directed Violence related to history of sexual and emotional abuse as evidenced by cutting on wrists, inability to cope, and widely fluctuating emotions

OUTCOME IDENTIFICATION, PLANNING, AND IMPLEMENTATION

EXPECTED OUTCOME 1: By _____ the patient will verbalize that her desire to self-mutilate has subsided.

SHORT-TERM GOAL	NURSING INTERVENTIONS	RATIONALES
By _____ the patient will be able to identify and label positive and negative feelings.	1. Listen and encourage the patient to express her feelings openly and honestly. 2. Educate the patient that feelings are neither right nor wrong, good nor bad.	1–2. Patients often feel overloaded with all their feelings and need to learn ways to recognize basic feelings of sadness, happiness, pain, fear, and anger.
	3. Encourage the patient to identify feelings of anxiety.	3. Self-mutilating behaviors often are accompanied by high levels of anxiety.

SHORT-TERM GOAL	NURSING INTERVENTIONS	RATIONALES
By _____ the patient will be able to connect the desire to self-mutilate with escalating anxiety levels.	1. Have the patient keep a journal of feelings or ask staff members for help when anxiety begins to escalate. 2. Encourage the patient to employ diversional measures such as journal-writing, walking, or anger work to deal with the desire to self-mutilate.	1–2. When the desire to self-mutilate occurs, engaging in some type of therapeutic activity is important.
	3. If the patient does engage in any form of self-mutilation, care for the wounds in a matter-of-fact manner.	3. Lack of attention to the maladaptive behavior may decrease its use as a coping mechanism.
	4. Administer antianxiety medications as needed.	4. Antianxiety medications are an appropriate short-term measure to deal with disabling anxiety and will foster patient compliance in the treatment plan.
By _____ the patient will be able demonstrate two new methods to reduce anxiety.	1. Teach at least four stress-reduction measures and have the patient demonstrate them.	1. The patient needs some alternative measures other than manipulation or self-mutilation for dealing with overwhelming feelings.
	2. Share the patient's accomplishments with other members of the team through the care plan.	2. All staff members need to reinforce positive behaviors.

EXPECTED OUTCOME 2: By _____ the patient will sign a contract not to engage in any further self-mutilating behavior.

SHORT-TERM GOALS	NURSING INTERVENTIONS	RATIONALES
By _____ the patient will agree to talk to a staff member if the desire to self-mutilate arises.	1. Observe the patient's behavior frequently, but avoid appearing suspicious. 2. Secure a verbal contract from the patient indicating that she will talk to a staff member before engaging in any self-mutilating behavior. 3. Remove all dangerous objects from the patient's environment.	1–3. Patient safety is always a nursing priority. Verbal contracts support the patient's need to take positive action rather than engaging in a self-destructive act.
By _____ the patient will acknowledge the need to work through memories of childhood abuse to assist in decreasing painful repressed memories.	1. As the patient is ready, encourage her to share painful, repressed memories of abuse.	1. Sharing painful memories often decreases anxiety.
	2. Remain nonjudgmental and nonreactive in your response to the patient when she is sharing.	2. Overreacting to the patient's pain, either positively or negatively, may affect her perception.
	3. Inform the patient that it is not necessary to recover every detail to feel better and that, if remembering is more distressing than not remembering at this time, she should trust her own judgment.	3. Always afford a patient the opportunity to maintain defenses; the patient must be psychologically ready to be vulnerable and should be allowed to learn to trust herself.

Nursing Diagnosis: Impaired Social Interaction related to disturbance of self-concept and absence of available significant others as evidenced by impulsive intense relationship with a male patient on the unit and a diminished ability to set personal boundaries

OUTCOME IDENTIFICATION, PLANNING, AND IMPLEMENTATION

EXPECTED OUTCOME 1: By _____ the patient will express feelings toward her male friend that are realistic, with the absence of intense emotions.

SHORT-TERM GOAL	NURSING INTERVENTIONS	RATIONALES
By _____ the patient will demonstrate calm, consistent emotions when interacting with other patients.	1. Gently confront the patient's beliefs that intense feelings are a necessary part of a relationship. 2. Help the patient understand that intense, violent emotions are more harmful than beneficial to a relationship.	1–2. This patient grew up in a home in which emotions were particularly intense. She needs to know that relationships can thrive in the absence of intensity.

SHORT-TERM GOAL	NURSING INTERVENTIONS	RATIONALES
	3. Teach the patient ways to increase the time between stimulus and response, such as counting to 10 or slow, deep breathing.	3. This will provide the patient with an opportunity to choose a different, more acceptable response.

EXPECTED OUTCOME 2: By _____ the patient will be able to set personal boundaries.

SHORT-TERM GOALS	NURSING INTERVENTIONS	RATIONALES
By _____ the patient will be able to verbalize the need for boundaries.	1. Educate the patient about personal boundaries. 2. Demonstrate how to set boundaries with the patient by maintaining a professional relationship.	1. Setting boundaries requires discipline and practice, and encouragement is needed. 2. Patients with borderline personality disorder frequently will encroach upon the boundaries of professionals by asking for extra time or special favors.
By _____ the patient will be able to demonstrate setting boundaries on the unit (both with staff and with other patients).	1. Observe the patient's response in all group interaction on the unit and with her boyfriend. 2. Give the patient feedback about setting realistic boundaries with others.	1. It is not unusual for patients who are not used to setting boundaries to be very rigid with them initially. 2. Give realistic positive feedback for efforts to maintain boundaries.

EXPECTED OUTCOME 3: By _____ the patient will verbalize three community support systems that will be available to her upon discharge.

SHORT-TERM GOAL	NURSING INTERVENTIONS	RATIONALES
By _____ the patient will have contacted at least one community agency.	1. Have the patient talk with a social worker and her previous therapist to investigate suitable outpatient options. 2. Have the patient place the calls to the identified agencies and set up the appointments.	1. The patient will need help initially in knowing what is available in the community. 2. This will discourage dependence upon the staff members.

EVALUATION

Formative Evaluation: Nancy met all of her short-term goals while in the hospital except in regard to her relationship with her boyfriend. He was discharged before her and came to see her every day. She said she was going to move in with him and that he was the "man of her dreams." On occasion, she continued to press the personal boundaries of staff members and showed little evidence of ability to set personal boundaries with her boyfriend.

With the help of group and individual therapy, Nancy stopped using manipulation to get her needs met and no longer engaged in staff-splitting behavior. With the help of antianxiety medication and staff support, Nancy stopped the self-mutilation. After one week of hospitalization, she no longer talked of suicide, and Nancy began to express hope for the future. Nancy did acknowledge her need to work through her memories of childhood sexual abuse and had contacted her previous therapist and set up an appointment before discharge.

Summative Evaluation: By discharge, Nancy had met all expected outcomes except those concerning her relationship with her boyfriend. Her feelings continued to be intense and unrealistic. She fantasized that he was going to take care of all of her problems. The treatment team was concerned that if the relationship began to falter, Nancy would be at risk for self-destructive behaviors again. They recommended she stay in weekly individual therapy.

CONCLUSIONS

Working with people with personality disorders is both challenging and rewarding. People who have personality disorders have significant relationship difficulties, including difficulty relating to the psychiatric nurse. Understanding the pattern of the person's behavior provides you insight into the best plan and intervention for the patient. The thoughts and behavior patterns of these patients are long standing. Therefore, you should expect change to occur slowly.

It is critical that you monitor your response to these people. People with these disorders often are very angry, critical, manipulative, and distant in their interactions. If you react to these affective states emotionally, you may feel devalued and angry. When you intervene from an emotional foundation of anger and a sense of inadequacy, you fail to provide the patient with the opportunity for a different affiliation, a professional relationship based on empathy, problem-solving, and learning new ways of dealing with old issues.

KEY POINTS TO REMEMBER

- A person with a healthy personality can relate to others even during periods of stress, frustration, and anger without devaluing the relationship. This person can describe self, identify likes and dislikes and strengths and weaknesses, and experience strong emotions such as joy, happiness, love, anger, and sadness.
- A person with a personality disorder has an enduring pattern of inner experience and behavior that is markedly different from those of that person's culture. This pattern is demonstrated in different ways of perceiving and interpreting self and others.
- In a person with a personality disorder, the range, intensity, lability, and appropriateness of emotional responses differs from the emotions expressed by most people.
- Individuals with personality disorders have problems relating to others, manifested by relationship difficulties with home, work and the community.
- Impulse control is sometimes difficult for people with personality disorders, particularly those who have dramatic personality disorders.
- Mahler identified developmental tasks in relationship to the caretaker. She studied infants and mothers. Current discussions about the development of a personality disorder focus on Mahler's separation-individuation phase of development.
- Research currently is under way to understand the biological components of personality disorders. From that research, new treatment strategies may emerge.
- *The Diagnostic and Statistical Manual of Mental Disorders-IV (DSM-IV)* has defined the personality disorders on Axis II. These have been separated into clusters of similar types of personality disorders. Cluster A includes odd or eccentric personality disorders such as paranoid, schizoid, and schizotypal personality disorders. Cluster B includes dramatic, emotional, or erratic behaviors exhibited by people with antisocial, borderline, histrionic, or narcissistic personality disorders. Cluster C includes anxious or fearful behavior manifested by people with dependent, avoidant and obsessive-compulsive personality disorders.
- The nursing process is a cognitive structure that is helpful for preventing the nurse from becoming emotionally reactive to the behavior of a patient with a personality disorder.

LEARNING ACTIVITIES

1. Read a novel involving characters who have personality disorders. Examples are Sylvia Plath's *The Bell Jar* and Judith Rossner's *Looking for Mr. Goodbar.* Such reading can provide you with insight into the perspective of a person with such a disorder.

2. Read a theoretical book such as Jerold Kreisman and Hal Staus's *I Hate You—Don't Leave Me: Understanding the Borderline Personality* and Janice Cauwel's *Imbroglio: Rising to the Challenges of Borderline Personality Disorder.* These books provide understanding of the person with borderline personality disorder. They are written in language that is easy to understand and are helpful to share with patients to assist them in identifying with those having similar behaviors, areas of distress, and the need for interventions promoting positive change.

3. Watch a movie such as *Shoot the Moon* (featuring a man who has borderline personality disorder and alcoholism and a stormy relationship with his wife) or *Fatal Attraction* (featuring a woman with borderline personality disorder who is having an affair with a married man). These stories are helpful in observing how a negative style of relating to others, extreme emotionality, and destructive and possessive behavior cause problems that are chaotic and destructive, both to the person with the disorder and to others.

4. Watch a daytime drama and identify characters who exhibit signs of personality disorders.

CRITICAL THINKING EXERCISE

Jean is a 29-year-old graduate student in criminal justice. While visiting her Aunt McDougal, she slashed her left wrist several times. Frightened, her aunt rushed her to the local hospital's emergency department. There, the nurse's assessment of the lacerations showed several superficial wounds and a laceration that required two stitches. No arteries were punctured. During the interview, Jean told the nurse that she was very upset with her psychotherapist and that she had left therapy after 10 years. She was convinced that the fact that her therapist went on vacation was evidence that he did not care about her and was only interested in her money. After the lacerations were sutured, Jean was discharged.

1. What do you think the nurse assumed about Jean's behavior?

2. Suggest possible reasons why Jean was discharged.

3. What are alternative possibilities, besides suicide, to explain Jean's behavior?

When she arrived at her Aunt McDougal's home, she cried to her and said "Those doctors are just like the others, they don't believe me that I really want to die." Upset, Mrs. McDougal called a nurse therapist to talk to Jean. Mrs. McDougal was aware that this was not the first time Jean had attempted suicide. After the nurse therapist saw Jean, she spoke with Mrs. McDougal about her concerns.

1. Put yourself in the nurse therapist's place. What would you tell Mrs. McDougal?

2. What assumption(s) is Jean making about other people's responses to her cutting attempts?

3. What conclusions can you draw about Jean's behavior?

REFERENCES

Akhtar, S. (1992). *Broken structures: Severe personality disorders and their treatments*. Northvale, NJ: Aronson.

Akhtar, S. (1995). *Quest for answers: A primer of understanding and treating severe personality disorders*. Northvale, NJ: Aronson.

American Psychiatric Association (1994). *Diagnostic and statistical manual of mental disorders, fourth edition*. Washington, D.C.: American Psychiatric Association.

Brown, G. L., Ebert, M. H. M., Goyer, P. F., et al (1982). Aggression, suicide and serotonin relationships to CSF amine metabolites. *American Journal of Psychiatry, 139*, 741–745.

Brown, G. L., and Linnoila, M. I. (1990). CSF serotonin metabolite (5-HIAA) studies in depression, impulsivity, and violence. *Journal of Clinical Psychiatry, 51* (Suppl. April), 31–43.

Carpenito, L. J. (1992). *Nursing diagnosis: Application to clinical practice*. Philadelphia: J. B. Lippincott.

Cauwels, J. M. (1992). *Imbroglio: Rising to the Challenges of borderline personality disorder*. New York: Norton.

Coryell, W. H., and Zimmerman, M. B. A. (1989). Personality disorder in the families of depressed, schizophrenic, and never-ill probands. *American Journal of Psychiatry, 146* (April), 496–502.

Davidson, M., and Davis, K. L. (1988). A comparison of plasma HVA concentrations in schizophrenia patients and normal controls. *Archives of General Psychiatry, 45*, 564–567.

Erikson, E. H. (1963). *Childhood and Society*. New York: Norton.

Houseman, C. (1990). The paranoid person: A biopsychosocial perspective. *Archives of Psychiatric Nursing, 5* (6), 176–181.

Kaplan, H. I., and Sadock, B. J. (1990). *Pocket handbook of clinical psychiatry*. Baltimore: Williams and Wilkins.

Kavoussi, R. J., and Siever, L. J. (1991). Biologic validators of personality disorders. In J. M. Oldham (Ed.), *Personality disorders: New perspectives on diagnostic validity*. Washington, D.C.: American Psychiatric Press.

Keltner, N. L., and Folks, D. G. (1993). *Psychotropic drugs*. St. Louis, MO: Mosby-Year Book.

Kreisman, J. J., and Straus, H. (1989). *I hate you—don't leave me: Understanding the borderline personality*. Los Angeles: The Body Press.

Lencz, T., Raine, A., Scerbo, A., Redmon, M., Brodish, S., Holt, L., and Bird, L. (1993). Impaired eye tracking in undergraduates with schizotypal personality disorder. *American Journal of Psychiatry, 150* (1), 152, 153.

Mahler, M. S. (1963). Thoughts about development and individuation. *Psychoanalytic Study of the Child, 18*, 307–324.

Mahler, M. S. (1971). A study of the separation-individuation process and its possible application to borderline phenomena in the psychoanalytic situation. *Psychoanalytic Study of the Child, 26*, 403–424.

Mahler, M. S. (1972a). On the first three subphases of the separation-individuation process. *International Journal of Psychoanalysis, 53*, 333–338.

Mahler, M. S. (1972b). Rapprochement subphase of the separation-individuation process. *Psychoanalytic Quarterly, 41*, 487–506.

Mann, J. J., Stanley, M., McBride, P. A., et al (1986). Increased serotonin-2 and beta-adrenergic receptor binding in the frontal cortices of suicide victims. *Archives of General Psychiatry, 43*, 954–959.

Mansfield, P. (1992). *Split self split object: Understanding and treating borderline, narcissistic, and schizoid disorders*. Northvale, NJ: Aronson.

Marin, D., De Meo, M., Frances, A., Kocsis, J., and Mann, J. (1989). Biological models and treatments for personality disorders. *Psychiatric Annals, 19* (March), 143–146.

Maslow, A. (1968). *Toward a psychology of being* (2nd ed). Princeton, NJ: Norstrand Reinhold.

Plath, S. (1971). *The bell jar*. New York: Harper and Row.

Rossner, J. (1975). *Looking for Mr. Goodbar*. New York: Pocket Books (division of Simon and Schuster).

Roy, A. (1989). Suicide. In H. I. Kaplan, and B. J. Sudock (Eds.), *Comprehensive Textbook of Psychiatry* (5th ed). Baltimore: Williams & Wilkins.

Siever, L. J. (1985). Biologic markers in schizotypal personality disorder. *Schizophrenic Bulletin, 11*, 564–575.

Siever, L. J. (1992). Schizophrenia spectrum personality disorders. In A. Tasman, and M. B. Riba (Eds.), *American Psychiatric Press Review of Psychiatry*. Vol. 11. Washington, D.C.: American Psychiatric Press.

Siever, L. J., and Davis, K. L. (1991). A psychobiological perspective on the personality disorders. *American Journal of Psychiatry, 148* (12), 1647–1658.

Soloff, P. H., George, A., Cornelius, J., et al. (1991). Pharmacotherapy and borderline subtypes. In J. M. Oldham (Ed.), *Personality disorders: New perspectives on diagnostic validity*. Washington, D.C.: American Psychiatric Press.

Stanley, M., and Stanley, B. (1990). Postmortem evidence for serotonin's role in suicide. *Journal of Clinical Psychiatry, 51* (Suppl. April), 22–27.

Steele, R. L. (1993). Staff attitudes toward seclusion and restraint: Anything new? *Perspectives in Psychiatric Care, 29* (July–September), 23–28.

Townsend, M. C. (1994). *Nursing diagnoses in psychiatric nursing: A pocket guide for care plan construction* (3rd ed). Philadelphia: F. A. Davis.

Tyson, P., and Tyson, R. (1990). *Psychoanalytic theories of development and integration*. New Haven: Yale University Press.

Valente, S. M. (1991). Deliberate self-injury management in a psychiatric setting. *Journal of Psychosocial Nursing, 29* (December), 19–25.

SUGGESTED READINGS

Coryell, W. H., and Zimmerman, M. B. A. (1989). Personality disorder in the families of depressed, schizophrenic, and never-ill probands. *American Journal Psychiatry, 146* (April), 496–502.

Houseman, C. (1990). The paranoid person: A biopsychosocial perspective. *Archives of Psychiatric Nursing, 5* (6), 176–181.

Lencz, T., Raine, A., Scerbo, A., Redmon, M., Brodish, S., Holt, L., and Bird, L. (1993). Impaired eye tracking in undergraduates with schizotypal personality disorder. *American Journal of Psychiatry, 150* (1), 152, 153.

Marin, D., De Meo, M., Frances, A., Kocsis, J., and Mann, J. (1989). Biological models and treatments for personality disorders. *Psychiatric Annals, 19* (March), 143–146.

Steele, R. L. (1993). Staff attitudes toward seclusion and restraint: Anything new? *Perspectives in Psychiatric Care, 29* (July–September), 23–28.

Valente, S. M. (1991). Deliberate self-injury management in a psychiatric setting. *Journal of Psychosocial Nursing, 29* (December), 19–25.

CHAPTER 33

THE JOURNEY COMPARTMENTALIZED BY DISSOCIATIVE DISORDERS

The goal of the hero's journey is yourself, finding yourself.

—J. Campbell

LEARNING OBJECTIVES

After studying this chapter, you should be able to:

1. Describe the concept of dissociation as a continuum.
2. Identify events in everyday life that are examples of dissociation.
3. Discuss major categories of dissociative disorders and theories of cause.
4. Identify nursing behaviors necessary to work effectively and therapeutically with the patient who demonstrates dissociative psychopathology.

KEY TERMINOLOGY

Amnesia
Childhood trauma
Depersonalization
Derealization
Dissociation continuum
Fugue
Hypnosis
Identity alteration
Identity confusion

When we perceive ourselves as being in a state of well-being, peaceful, or mentally healthy, there is a sense of unity of self as a human being with a basic personality. Our thoughts, feelings, and actions seem both connected and to have a sense of continuity (at least, most of the time). Thus, we have a perception of being integrated or whole. Persons with dissociative disorders experience gaps in memory, confusion, and, often, a sense of compartmentalization. This chapter focuses on some of the types of dissociative disorders, associated problematic behaviors, and nursing interventions.

The following example is based on the experiences of a woman manifesting a specific type of dissociative disorder.

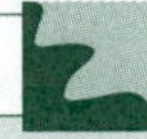

CHARLOTTE'S STORY

A young woman appearing to be in her late 20s or early 30s was brought to the emergency unit of a county hospital by police officers who had found her wandering the streets in the downtown area of a large city. The initial concern of the officers was promoted by the woman looking rather dazed and being unaccompanied in a section of streets known for high crime activity. On questioning the woman concerning her activities, the officers were met with a blank stare along with assertions of being not only unaware of where she was, but also of who she was. No objections were voiced by this individual about being taken to the county hospital.

In the triage area, the woman was dubbed "Madame X" by an attendant who admitted to believing the patient was "faking" or was simply on some kind of drugs. Interestingly the label remained, and Madame X seemed rather to like the diminutive—later introducing herself in like manner to others on arriving on the psychiatric unit. During the assessment by the professional staff, she was alert and cooperative. Additionally, Madame X claimed to have completely lost her memory for all details of her life. Although appearing quite perplexed, she did not give the impression of being distraught.

After admission to the psychiatric unit, she appeared fairly comfortable in the milieu. After two days on the unit, Madame X was still amnesic; additionally, all laboratory tests were within normal limits, and her drug screen was negative except for the presence of nicotine and caffeine. Because the patient appeared to be in excellent health and had not responded to verbal interventions, a sodium amytal interview was recommended by a consulting psychiatrist. Madame X readily gave her consent to this procedure and it was scheduled for the following day. The next morning the patient's primary nurse accompanied her to the treatment room to offer support and a familiar face. During the interview, the patient responded openly to the questions posed by the psychiatrist. She revealed that her name was Charlotte S. and that she was 32 years old. For the last four years she had been living in a common-law relationship with a man several years older, about whom she had mixed feelings. Although he could be extremely physically and verbally abusive at times, there were other occasions when he was very "loving." Charlotte remembered her childhood, adolescence, and young adulthood as being very deprived—financially, socially, and emotionally. Her father had deserted the family when she was in the first grade, and she had been told many times by her mother that she was responsible for driving him away because she was such an evil girl who had been "shamed by God." The mother had multiple psychiatric hospitalizations over the years, and Charlotte recalled no social support from relatives or others, describing herself as "alone" and "never good enough for anyone to care about." All of her relationships with men had been short-lived, but she had believed this last one to be destined to last, admitting that she felt no significant anger about the physical, sexual, and verbal abuse she had tolerated from her "lover." About five days ago, he had announced that he no longer cared for her, had found another woman he preferred, and was moving out of the apartment they had shared for the past four years. "I remember feeling in a state of shock—like why was he doing this to me? I think I cried and begged him not to leave, but he did anyway and wouldn't even look at me. I kept hearing these voices inside my head telling me how I was no good and everything was my fault. I think I left the apartment—maybe to look for him, but I don't remember much else about the police and the hospital."

Charlotte was suffering from a dissociative disorder referred to as *psychogenic amnesia*, most likely precipitated by what would be an event of devastating trauma to her—that of abandonment by someone whom she desperately wanted to believe cared about her. Both her recent and long-term memory were retrieved during the interview, and she experienced no lapses of memory while in the hospital. The major issues that emerged were a rather severe depression which had been dormant for many years, fueled by her low self-esteem.

THE CONCEPT OF DISSOCIATION

Although there was considerable interest in the concept of dissociation as a major defense mechanism in the 19th century, especially before the influence of Freud, a decreased concern in dissociative processes seemed to occur between about 1920 and 1970 (Greaves, 1980). As a concept for observation and scientific study, dissociation was first formulated by the French physician Pierre Janet. He viewed dissociation as the primary phenomenon that explained the symptoms of hysteria, which typically involved somatic complaints and symptoms that were not supported by physical findings. With the dominant influence of Freudian theory in the latter part of the 19th and most of the 20th century, however, dissociation has been relegated to the position of a secondary defense mechanism to repression—as have all other ego defense mechanisms. In fact, Freud (1962) viewed dissociation as simply a type of repression employed in the excision of threatening or unacceptable mental contents from conscious awareness. Although Janet pioneered the study of dissociative behaviors in the 1890s, there is little that is definitively known about this mechanism by behavioral scientists today. Opinions vary as to whether dissociation should always be classified as a psychopathological defense. In 1887, Janet first used the term *dissociation* as it is used today. Working primarily with "hysterical" female patients, presenting with a myriad of somatic symptoms expressed in a highly dramatic fashion, he asserted the mechanism always to be pathological. In Janet's practice, he discovered that his patients often possessed a multiplicity of "egos" or "personalities" that coexisted within individual women and that these "personalities" were able to function separately from each other. He described this phenomenon as a dissociative process, occurring because of a "weakening of the synthesizing power of the psyche" (Crabtree, 1992). Other emerging authorities in the field, however, did not agree with him unanimously. For example, James (Taylor, 1983), Prince (1907, 1914), and Myers (1903) all held that dissociation was a normal human function and that multiplicity, as described by Janet, was simply a fact of everyday life, to varying degrees. Indeed, Myers insisted in his writings in the 1880s and the 1890s that what is thought of as normal "consciousness" is only a small part of the human psyche. Both Myers and James believed that the future of psychological research would be focused on exploring the parts of the human mind that are typically dissociated from our daily consciousness—which were considered the repository of the true richness of human nature.

▶ Check Your Reading

1. Who first coined the term *dissociation*?
2. How did Freud describe dissociation?

THE DISSOCIATION CONTINUUM

Some contemporary theorists view this ego defense as a **dissociation continuum** that ranges from minor dissociations of everyday life, such as daydreaming, to the florid symptoms of identity alteration as experienced by Charlotte in the background story. As students in nursing school and other educational settings, most of us have probably experienced the pleasures of daydreaming to escape the drudgery of a boring lecture. Only when we were called on to answer a question were we jolted to the realization that a total lack of knowledge existed as to the content presented in the last few minutes or even the last hour, although we were physically present in the classroom.

The argument for the adaptive value of dissociation has been promoted by several contemporary theorists, e.g., Braun and Sachs (1985), Kluft (1984), and Spiegel (1984). An idea central to the construct of dissociation as an adaptive entity is that it exists on a continuum and becomes maladaptive only when it surpasses certain limits in frequency or intensity or occurs in inappropriate contexts that may be harmful to the individual or others. Hilgard (1977) has been an instrumental modern figure advocating the existence of a dissociation continuum—ranging from the normal to the pathological. He strongly promotes the idea that everyday life is full of small dissociations if we but look for them.

Putnam (1989) sees dissociation as pathological when the individual's sense of consciousness, behavior, and identity is fragmented. Contrast this fragmentation of the sense of self with the temporary alteration in consciousness that occurs in daydreaming, "tuning out" of conversations, and "highway hypnosis." These examples on a continuum are supported by surveys conducted by Bernstein and Putnam (1986), using the Dissociative Experiences Scale (DES). The DES is a brief, self-administered questionnaire that asks one to estimate, by marking on a 100-mm-line visual analog scale, the frequency with which specific dissociative experiences occur (see Appendix). This instrument has demonstrated a high degree of reliability and validity when scores of normal controls, people with occasional dissociative episodes, and patients with severe dissociative disorders were compared.

Vaillant (1986) classifies dissociation as one of the "neurotic" defenses that are seen in adults under stress and are frequently used by obsessive-compulsive and hysterical persons. His definition of dissociation is:

A temporary but drastic modification of character or sense of personal identity to avoid emotional distress; it includes fugue states and hysterical conversion reactions.

Sullivan placed much credence in the dissociative processes in development of the personality or the *self-system*. Theoretically the development of self-esteem begins in a fairly sequential pattern. What Sullivan referred to as the *good-me* evolves from positive appraisals by others, such as "Johnny is a good boy" or "Jenny is a smart girl." If the child hears genuine favorable comments often and is provided with tenderness and appreciation, these positive appraisals become a significant part of the sense of self. Conversely the *bad-me* reflects negative appraisals by others that are accompanied by increasing levels of anxiety. If barraged with comments such as "You're such a dummy" or "Why are you such a bad girl?" accompanied by varying degrees of rejection and other punishment, these views are also incorporated into one's sense of self. *Not-me* (not of me) is evidenced in *dissociated* behavior, which can be manifested in everyday lapses of consciousness (e.g., daydreaming) or in naturally occurring trance states—such as occurs when one drives alone for long stretches on a road surrounded by monotonous terrain (previously referred to as "highway hypnosis"). Most of us have experienced the operation of not-me processes following a nightmare. When one awakens, one may not know who or where he or she is. The self-system usually responds quickly, however, and soon the person regains the normal state of consciousness. Viewed on a continuum, the not-me in a more pathological form is experienced in severe mental disorders, including, but not limited to, the dissociative disorders.

In much of the contemporary literature, dissociation is conceptualized as a posttraumatic defense, energized by the patient as protection from catastrophic trauma and pain. The tendency to detach oneself from memories, consciousness, and sense of identity is considered a natural response to repeated physical, verbal, and sexual abuse. It is also a frequent response to other overwhelming traumas—including rape, combat, and other life-threatening situations (Steinberg, 1993). Because dissociative experiences can and do occur within a number of psychiatric syndromes, including anxiety, mood disorders, and substance abuse disorders, it is essential that you have a conceptual understanding of dissociation in the journey with the patient, regardless of the path taken.

▶ Check Your Reading

3. Give one example of a minor dissociation associated with normal life.
4. What is the name of the scale used to determine the degree of dissociation used by a particular individual?
5. Identify at least two other psychiatric illnesses that may include dissociative experiences.

THE DETOUR OF PATHOLOGICAL DISSOCIATION

Steinberg (1993) notes that few topics in the mental health–mental illness spectrum have experienced as great a renewal of interest and investigation as the field of dissociation. In the past few years, there has been an accumulating number of clinical reports and research studies in this area. Also, the increased attention given to the range of childhood abuses, resulting in cognitive and affective impairments, has provided impetus for the development of specialized treatment units for patients with dissociative disorders.

Although the dissociative disorders have historically been considered rare, research has refuted this position (Coons et al, 1988; Franklin, 1990; Putnam, 1989). If anything, the number of patients suffering from these disorders is probably underreported because the symptoms frequently elude detection for two major reasons. First, dissociative manifestations may be indistinguishable from symptoms of other psychiatric syndromes—including those of the psychotic, mood, and anxiety disorders; second, dissociative symptoms frequently are difficult for the patient to verbalize clearly because the patient is detached from his or her memories and sense of identity (Steinberg, 1993). For these reasons, it is especially important for you to be attuned to the presence of *five* symptoms considered a hallmark of dissociative disorders, although variations of these behaviors can occur in persons with other mental health problems or in individuals subjected to overwhelming traumas.

Symptoms of Pathologic Dissociation

Amnesia

Amnesia is usually defined as memory loss related to personal data or events occurring during a specific period of time or even a loss of all past memories. Table 33–1 presents the characteristics of the five major types of amnesia. Some people with severe amnesia related to dissociative disorders frequently experience recurrent memory gaps. Other people are unable to remember their name, age, or activities occurring during specific hours, days, or longer. For example, a young woman in her 20s stated that her life was a "complete blank" between the ages of 9 and 12. It is crucial to distinguish between the description of amnesia given here and the amnesic behavior or syndrome attributed to specific pathophysiological factors, the most common of which is chronic heavy alcohol abuse. In the latter type, these individuals often confabulate responses to questions, as if to deny any problems with their mental faculties. A careful observer, however, can usually note a pattern of vagueness to many of their responses to questions that call for dates or other historical details. With patients experiencing a dissociative amnesia, there is typically no attempt to cover up the memory loss. As one patient, a successful graphic artist with her own business, stated:

It's scary as hell to realize all of a sudden that today is Thursday, and I don't remember a thing since coming home from the office on Monday night. Where did those two days go? I look at my calendar and see that appointments were scheduled with clients. Did I keep any of the appointments? I have no idea. Someone is going to notice that I "space out" and think I'm going crazy. Maybe I am.

Derealization

Derealization occurs when objects in the external world take on a quality of unreality and estrangement. Thus, familiar people and places are perceived as unfamiliar or unreal. This symptom exists on a continuum from mild, brief feelings associated with anxiety to more severe manifestations, as in the example of Charlotte. Nothing about her surroundings was recognizable to her, although she had lived in the same city for a number of years. Other patients experiencing a high degree of derealization have described feeling that family members (e.g., a parent or spouse) were difficult to recognize as being their own. On the other end of the continuum, most of us have had temporary episodes of perceiving a familiar setting, such as a classroom or shopping mall, as being somewhat alien. This experience occurs most frequently when one's anxiety has shifted from moderate to severe—in which we may be able to focus only on scattered details of the perceptual field. As one patient described it: "The neighborhood where I had lived for years looked like a two-dimensional stage set."

Depersonalization

Depersonalization is viewed as an alteration in the perception or experience of the self; one's usual sense of relatedness to the rest of the world is temporarily lost or changed. Some individuals describe feeling detached, being in a dreamlike state, or feeling like outside observers of their own minds and bodies. Although *derealization* concerns perception of external objects, *depersonalization* is related more to the experience of self

TABLE 33–1 Types of Amnesia

Type	Characteristics
Localized	Inability to recall events that occurred for a short period of time (a few hours to a few days); the most common type of amnesia. *Example:* Inability to recall events occurring during and following a burglary in one's home
Generalized (global)	Loss of memory for a whole lifetime of experience, including one's personal identity; considered to be rare
Selective (systematized)	Failure to recall some but not all events during a short period; continuous failure to recall specific events occurring after a specific time up to and including the present. The person forgets each successive event as it occurs, although is clearly alert and aware of what is happening at the time. *Example:* Not remembering anything about a burglary, but remembering when the police arrived
Anterograde	Amnesia for short-term memory, although remote memory remains intact; present in blackouts; a common symptom of alcohol abuse; difficulty in learning new information
Retrograde	Loss of memory about events that occurred before the amnesia-producing event

and is perhaps more limited in scope—and possibly more distressing to the individual because the nature of one's existence is in question. One patient described feeling like a robot, experiencing his arms and legs as being mechanically controlled. Although he knew this not to be the case, the feeling persisted. Thus, reality testing is intact and people experiencing depersonalization are not delusional. Similar to derealization, depersonalization may be experienced in milder degrees when "normal" people are highly anxious or stressed in other ways. As another patient expressed the depersonalization experience for herself:

I'm sitting on the couch but I feel invisible—and yet I see myself from another part of the room. At least I think it's me, whatever me *is. My body looks the same as it always did—and yet it doesn't seem to be a part of that "me" I was talking about. If this isn't crazy, I don't know what is.*

Identity Confusion

Identity confusion has been defined as a subjective sense of conflict, puzzlement, or uncertainty in relation to one's identity, usually accompanied by significant distress. Comments such as "I don't know who I am" are typical. Some patients arrive at clinics, hospitals, and emergency rooms claiming *global amnesia* or some other form of amnesia. If a medical/neurological work-up is negative, further assessment of the patient is necessary.

> Although Charlotte did not believe she had ever experienced a full-blown amnesic episode before, she later recalled that there seemed to be an ongoing inner struggle in which she doubted her identity. "It's like my insides are a boxing ring with two opponents. There's a fight going on and someone's going to get knocked out—but I don't know which one. It's real scary sometimes."

Identity Alteration

Identity alteration is evidenced as an organized shift in one's personality, including the way one relates to others, character traits, knowledge, and preferences. Although similar to other dissociative symptoms, identity alteration usually occurs without the individual's awareness. It may be masked or overshadowed by more overt and commonly described symptoms such as anxiety and depression. Persons with what has traditionally been referred to as *multiple personality disorder* undergo severe identity alteration. Additionally, they are often amnesic for their behavior or experiences during the altered identity state. This symptom can be assessed indirectly by questioning the patient about new objects in his or her possession, observing skills about which the patient was unaware, and acquiring reports from others about the person's behavioral inconsistencies (Steinberg, 1993). One patient was noted to play the piano beautifully, particularly Chopin études, and kept a collection of musical scores. When she shifted periodically to an altered identity, she could do little more than "chopsticks" awkwardly with two fingers, claimed that she could not read music, and was totally uninterested in the piano. She would giggle in a childlike manner and insist, "We don't really like music that much."

Cause of Pathologic Dissociation

According to Nemiah (1989), biological researchers have attempted to define dissociative symptoms in terms of the ascending reticular activating system, thalamocortical projections, and other neurological pathways. Information currently available related to neurophysiological processes, however, is too limited to provide explanatory concepts that are useful in application with patients. As psychobiological research continues in this decade, it is imperative that nurses stay abreast of these activities. It is not inconceivable that, at some point, underlying brain mechanisms will be discovered that mediate certain types of dissociative symptoms.

Current views of cause relate more to psychosocial factors as being the major causative elements of these disorders—particularly, severely traumatic experiences, whether having occurred recently or in the past. An analysis of possible causative factors is included in the discussion of the specific disorders later in this chapter.

Classification of Pathologic Dissociation

Currently the *DSM-IV* recognizes *five* dissociative disorders:

- Dissociative amnesia
- Dissociative fugue
- Depersonalization disorder
- Dissociative identity disorder (DID)
- Dissociative disorder not otherwise specified (DDNOS)

In the past, these disorders were classified as hysterical neuroses of the dissociative type. Memory disturbances often affect one's sense of identity—which may be manifested by changes in psychomotor behavior and affect. One or two of these functions may cease to work in concert (or be integrated) with the others. The behavior of some persons experiencing this "dis-integrity" of consciousness, memory, or identity appears bizarre. Other persons, however, present themselves as alert, lucid, and generally appropriate. These same individuals may be totally unable to recall their names, addresses, or occupations.

Dissociative Amnesia

A person suffering from this disorder is plagued with the sudden inability to access information that has already been stored in one's memory bank. This inability is not due to ordinary forgetfulness, and there is no evidence indicative of an underlying brain disorder (Kaplan et al, 1994). These individuals retain the capacity to learn new information; thus, they do not manifest what is termed *continuous amnesia*. Contrasted with patients with organically induced amnesias, in which one sees confused and disorganized behavior, these persons appear intact and coherent.

Dissociative amnesia is generally considered to be the most common type of dissociative disorder—occurring more frequently in women than in men. Often a thorough assessment uncovers a precipitating emotional trauma charged with conflict and painful feelings, as in the description at the beginning of this chapter. Charlotte's sudden abandonment by her lover triggered traumatic childhood conflicts related to being abandoned and unloved. This disorder generally begins abruptly, and patients are aware of their memory loss. Some people may be distraught regarding the memory loss; others may seem indifferent. Thus, during an initial assessment, it is important for nurses to evaluate the patient's affective state. As previously noted, most patients are alert before and after amnesia occurs. Some report a slight clouding of consciousness, however, during the brief interval immediately surrounding the amnesic period. Amnesia may have a primary or secondary gain. In the example of Charlotte, a primary gain was achieved by the amnesia protecting her from painful memories and emotions. A secondary gain was experienced in the caring and concern she received from the emergency room and hospital staff.

The specific treatment varies with individual attributes, such as motivation and level of anxiety. If careful interviewing leads to no clues related to the traumatic precipitant and the patient remains amnesic, other approaches may be considered. As with Charlotte, sodium amytal given intravenously may be facilitative in recovery of memories. Other individuals may respond favorably to hypnosis. Once the buried memories are retrieved, psychotherapy may be helpful to assist the person to cope with the painful feelings and depression that may follow.

Dissociative Fugue

A person with dissociative **fugue** wanders, sometimes far from home, and may assume a completely new identity for an indefinite period of time—days, weeks, or longer. The individual's travel and behavior appear more purposeful than the confused wandering that may be seen in dissociative amnesia (American Psychiatric Association, 1994). As with other dissociative disorders, fugue states are considered rare in the general population. In contrast to the person with dissociative amnesia, the individual in a fugue is unaware of having forgotten anything. Following recovery, there is no recollection of activities that occurred during the fugue.

An interesting case illustrating psychogenic (dissociative) fugue occurred in New England during the 1880s (Case Example 33–1).

Case Example 33–1 Ansel Bourne's Story

On January 17, 1887, the Reverend Ansel Bourne withdrew over $500 from a bank in Providence, Rhode Island, with which to purchase a lot of land nearby. He left in a carriage that morning, did not return home that night, and nothing was heard of him for two months. On the morning of March 14, however, in Norristown, Pennsylvania, a man calling himself A. J. Brown, who had rented a small shop six weeks ago, stocked it with stationery, confectionery, fruit, and small articles and began to conduct business. He carried on his quiet trade without seeming eccentric or unnatural to anyone.

One day, however, he woke up in a fright. He called in the people of the house, urging them to tell him where he was. He claimed that he was Ansel Bourne, that he knew nothing about Norristown, and that he was totally ignorant about shopkeeping. The last thing he remembered—it seemed only yesterday—was drawing the money from the bank in Providence. He could not believe that two months had elapsed. After returning to Providence, he had complete amnesia for the two months of his absence.

This historic case of the Reverend Bourne is a fairly typical example of fugue episodes as they are reported in contemporary times. Some persons predisposed to fugue states have a history of heavy alcohol abuse, but this behavior certainly does not always occur. Sometimes the fugue is less elaborate than that of Ansel Bourne's and may involve little more than brief, seemingly purposeful travel. In these instances, social contacts are usually minimal or avoided entirely. Reports of violent outbursts have been cited in reports of some persons; these outbursts are thought to be related to fear of unknown circumstances surrounding emergence from the fugue state. Unless the fugue is particularly prolonged, the most useful approach is to provide the patient with a safe, supportive environment with a low level of stimulation. Nurses can assume an especially important role by teaching nonprofessional staff to avoid overly friendly, probing behaviors with these patients because such approaches may precipitate agitation, leading to aggressive behavior.

Depersonalization Disorder

This disorder is characterized as a recurrent or persistent change in the quality of self-awareness. One's own sense of reality may be temporarily lost. Some persons may describe themselves as being mechanical, detached from their bodies, or in a dream. These experiences are referred to as *ego-dystonic*, in that the individual realizes the bizarreness or unreality of the symptoms. As mentioned previously, *depersonalization* concerns feelings that one's own body or self is unreal or strange; *derealization* relates to the perception of objects in the external world as being in some way strange or unreal.

Persons experiencing this disorder usually seem to be markedly distressed and intact reality testing is maintained. The onset is rapid, but disappearance is usually gradual (American Psychiatric Association, 1994). It is currently believed that depersonalization disorder is associated with an array of precipitants, including psychological, neurological, or systemic diseases. Certain drugs, such as alcohol, barbiturates, benzodiazepines, scopolamine, marijuana, and others, have been determined to be contributory. At this time, depersonalization is most often viewed as a *symptom* occurring in association with anxiety, depression, and schizophrenia. Ostensibly, it is quite rare as a pure disorder (Kaplan et al, 1994).

Dissociative Identity Disorder

Considered one of the most controversial of all psychiatric disorders, this syndrome has achieved increasing notoriety in the past few years. Previously known as multiple personality disorder, DID is characterized by the existence of two or more personality states that can take full control of the person's behavior accompanied by an inability to remember significant personal information. This inability of recall is too pervasive to be explained by ordinary forgetfulness. This new name highlights the failure of personality integration that is a central feature of this phenomenon in many patients. Although it is extremely difficult to obtain statistics as to the prevalence of this disorder, it is believed to occur much more frequently than was previously thought. The majority of these patients report histories of severe trauma during childhood, including physical, sexual, and even ritual cult abuse by some. Although DID is not usually diagnosed until adulthood, dissociative episodes are often experienced by patients initially at an early age, although they are not recognized as such at the time. The essence of multiplicity has probably eluded many clinicians; it is likely that many so-called "multiples" in the past were inaccurately diagnosed as being schizophrenic.

DID is considered the ultimate dissociative phenomenon—containing all the elements of the other disorders in this class. Patients with this syndrome, on occasion, manifest amnesia, fugue, and profound depersonalization. Without effective treatment, DID appears to be a lifelong process; however, it may present itself differently over a period of time (Kluft, 1985).

Although a number of cases of DID have been chronicled in the historical literature, the ones most likely familiar to contemporary readers through written accounts are *Sybil* (Schreiber, 1973) and *When Rabbit Howls* (Chase, 1987). The book *The Three Faces of Eve* (Thigpen and Cleckley, 1957) was made into what is now considered a classic film starring Joanne Woodward. The story follows "Eve" and her discovery of her three separate personalities as she works with her therapist to understand her strange behavior. The book *Sybil* described the psychotherapy as well as the memories of a young woman who, as a child, had been emotionally, physically, and sexually abused by a schizophrenic mother and who, as a result, had developed 15 separate personalities. *When Rabbit Howls* was supposedly autobiographical, as opposed to being the report of a professional journalist or psychotherapist. In this account, the different personalities, termed as *alters*, numbered over 90 and were referred to as The Troops. The major character, Truddi, had been subjected to horrendous sexual abuse by the stepfather as far back as two years of age. As is usually the case, many of the Troop members served protective functions.

The best times growing up were when I was totally alone, at the rock in the back field of the second farmhouse. The rock was huge; it had a deep indentation in the middle, so deep you could barely see over the edge. I hated the snakes. They lay around on the rim of the rock, basking in the sun. Once you made it to the center of the

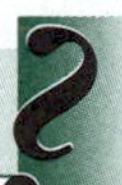

WHAT SOCIETY NEEDS TO KNOW — Dissociative Disorders

What are dissociative disorders?
Dissociative disorders involve a temporary loss or disturbance of the ability to integrate memory, consciousness, identity, and sometimes motor behavior. Individuals who are diagnosed with a type of dissociative disorder will experience amnesia or memory loss that ranges from mild to severe and could include recent or past events. These disturbances can appear suddenly or gradually and can be chronic. Dissociative experiences appear on a continuum from daydreaming or "tuning out" to a complete fragmentation of self into a different personality.

What causes dissociative disorders?
In recent years, renewed interest in the study of dissociative disorders has been seen. Many of the current researchers are making a connection between dissociative experiences and repressed trauma and/or acute or long-term stress. Many mental health professionals consider the ability to detach oneself from memories, consciousness, and sense of identity to be a normal or natural response to repeated trauma or abuse.

How are dissociative disorders treated?
These conditions are treated with long-term psychotherapy. It is generally thought that it is better to allow memories to return when the person is psychologically ready, rather than to attempt to force or rush the return.

What is multiple personality disorder?
Once considered a rare condition, Multiple Personality Disorder (recently classified as Dissociative Identity Disorder) is now recognized as a more common entity. In this condition, patients have more than one distinct personality. They usually have a core personality, but the personality who goes to the doctor for treatment is often an alter or subpersonality. Changing from one personality to another can occur within seconds, or one personality may remain dominant for days. One common characteristic of patients diagnosed with this condition is that they were sexually abused as children. Most people diagnosed with this disorder are female, and their history may reveal suicide attempts, substance abuse, and self-mutilation.

BOX 33–1 Some Signs and Symptoms of Dissociative Identity Disorder

- Inconsistencies in accounts of elapsed time
- A history of several medical and psychiatric diagnoses
- Inconsistencies in physical behaviors, such as switching right-handedness or left-handedness, voice changes, or marked differences as in clothing and hairstyles on different occasions
- Psychophysiological complaints, such as severe headaches, chest pain, or a fluctuation in pain threshold
- Hearing voices inside one's head talking to one another or to the person
- Reference to oneself as "we" rather than "I"

rock, you kept an eye out for the snakes and any human being sneaking up on you from the house at the other end of the farm.

In the previous quote from *When Rabbit Howls*, the extreme hypervigilance is apparent. To relieve the frightened, exhausted child in her quest for a safe place, different Troop members (alters) would take over to protect her from the perpetrator. In Truddi's case, the melding of all personalities (integration) was not seen as a realistic goal.

Owing to the extreme complexity of this disorder, some cases may remain completely undetected, whereas others may be misdiagnosed. Nurses working in all settings need some knowledge of signs and symptoms manifested by patients with DID (Box 33–1). For example, many individuals present with complaints of physical problems that tend to be vague and unsupported by laboratory tests and other medical findings. Depression, mood swings, self-mutilative behavior, and suicidal ideation are often present in at least one personality. Additionally, sleep disturbances, similar to those noted in posttraumatic stress disorder (PTSD), are common and should always be included in the assessment interview (Putnam, 1989). Particularly significant are reports of "time loss," which some patients are reluctant to admit, along with fears of "going crazy." Phobic anxiety and substance abuse are not uncommon. Hallucinations are often present and frequently denied initially. Auditory hallucinations often discuss the patient in the third person or may argue among themselves. In contrast to hallucinatory experiences in schizophrenia, these "voices" are heard within the patient's head and are heard clearly and distinctly (Coons, 1984). Additionally, many DID patients refer to themselves as "we" rather than "I."

If the DID patient requires hospitalization because of direct or indirect self-destructive behavior, milieu management is a critical factor in safe and therapeutic care (Stafford, 1993). The inability to trust others, frequency of self-mutilative episodes, and manipulative "borderline" behaviors pose a challenge to the clinical nurse specialist. The novice nurse needs additional education and ongoing supervision to work effectively with these individuals. Many of these patients have an Axis II diagnosis of borderline personality disorder, posing an additional challenge to the nurse in dealing therapeutically with divisive, manipulative behaviors.

It is not uncommon for these individuals initially to have a "favorite" nurse, until that nurse inadvertently displeases the patient in some way. At that point, the formerly trusted nurse is seen as "all bad" or as an enemy. Part of therapeutic nursing intervention is to maintain acceptance of the patient and to avoid taking rebuffs personally. Additionally, maintaining a safe environment is critical because these individuals frequently exhibit self-mutilative behavior, such as cutting or puncturing the skin with sharp objects, head banging, and a variety of other self-destructive behaviors. Before hospitalization, many DID patients have engaged in abuse of alcohol, other drugs, and illicit substances. Eating disorders are not uncommon.

The nature of the traumas associated with DID poses an array of problems. Tessier (1992) avows that we know exceedingly more about the physical, social, and psychological aftermath of childhood sexual abuse than we do of the spiritual consequences. She further asserts that our Western culture's norms of encouraging the victim to put the past behind one is destructive because healing cannot occur before the extensive damage to the spiritual part of the person is acknowledged. Thus, nurses, clergy, and other health professionals should focus on the healing aspects of treatment with caution. Although it is essential to forgive the perpetrator, this usually cannot be done immediately or before the victim is allowed to work through anger and feelings of betrayal. As every case is unique, so is the extent of devastation to the human spirit. The decision to forgive the perpetrator(s) is a process that would seem best left to the victim as he or she traverses in the journey toward being a survivor.

Dissociative Disorders Not Otherwise Specified

The NOS category is a residual one for disorders in which the primary feature is a dissociative syndrome that does not meet the criteria for one of the previously described types. Data from studies in which these patients were compared with persons diagnosed with DID (Briere and Runtz, 1990; Chu and Dill, 1990; Ross et al, 1990), however, have consistently supported the assertion that the dissociative disorders exist on a spectrum of increasing severity and complexity, with DID at the extreme end of the continuum. The most current research evidence supports the position that DDNOS is simply a milder variant of DID with less severe trauma and symptoms. From reviewed studies, it would appear that DID is the prototype human response to chronic, severe, childhood trauma.

▶ Check Your Reading

6. What are the five hallmark symptoms of dissociative disorders?
7. Describe each of the five symptoms.
8. Describe the characteristics of the dissociative disorders.
9. Which dissociative disorder is considered to be the most controversial of all psychiatric disorders?

NURSING PROCESS

Effective use of the nursing process with these patients requires a working knowledge of the continuum of dissociative experiences and the accompanying mild to severe symptoms.

ASSESSMENT

Assessment of the patient with a possible dissociative disorder uses strategies emphasized in Chapter 13 for evaluating mental status. Some of the specific assessment skills involve detection of dissociative symptoms, particularly those that relate to disturbances in *memory*, *consciousness*, and *sense of identity*. The nurse should be observant for any of the five cardinal symptoms of dissociative disorders: *amnesia*, *derealization*, *depersonalization*, *identity confusion*, and *identity alteration*. Although these symptoms may be present, to some degree, in many individuals under stress or with other psychiatric problems, they are particularly suggestive of a disturbance on the continuum of dissociative responses. Amnesia may be experienced in a global sense or in a milder degree, such as of events surrounding one event, for instance, an automobile accident. It is extremely important to listen carefully to the patient for *subjective data*, which typically take the form of a personal attribution statement in which the patient presents herself as a "nonknowing" person. The following examples are congruent with a dissociative state: "I don't know why I'm here." "The police brought me to the hospital."

Regardless of the setting, it is critical to assess the perception of reality of the individual who may be experiencing a dissociative episode. In dissociative amnesia states, the *objective data* are also critical. How upset does the patient appear? A careful physical assessment is essential because some persons' amnesia may have a specific pathophysiological cause. For example, transient global amnesia (TGA), often caused by transient ischemic attacks, migraine headaches, sedative-hypnotic drugs, or seizures, can mimic psychogenic (dissociative) amnesia. The personal identity of the patient with psychogenic amnesia is lost, however, whereas that of the individual with transient global amnesia is retained. Table 33–1 identifies the behaviors associated with various types of amnesia.

In the assessment of a patient who may be experiencing (or may have recently experienced) a fugue state, the situation becomes complex. These individuals are rarely brought to emergency departments or hospitals or to the attention of mental health professionals, because they typically do little to attract attention. Perhaps the most frequent reason for their entry into the system is an aggressive outburst against property or other persons.

Subjective data may be difficult to obtain because these patients are unaware that they have forgotten anything. Objective data should also include a thorough physical assessment because temporal lobe epilepsy may also involve episodes of travel, although a new identity is not assumed. Also, episodes of temporal lobe epilepsy are not thought to be heralded by psychosocial stress, as is often the case with dissociative fugues. In terms of subjective and objective data, DID is more likely to be confused with other psychiatric disorders. As previously mentioned, depersonalization may occur as a symptom in numerous other psychiatric syndromes. It is sometimes the earliest presenting symptom of a person with a neurological disorder. Thus, symptoms of depersonalization should be observed carefully.

However the subjective and objective data are obtained, it is essential to remember that accurate problem identification and interventions depend on the quality of the data collected. Additionally, although nurses must be knowledgeable about disease processes and specific disorders, the major purpose of the assessment phase always is to collect information needed to care for the patient in a holistic manner—regardless of the medical or psychiatric diagnosis.

DIAGNOSIS

A critical analysis of the assessment data leads to clearer definitions of patient problems and decisions related to therapeutic nursing interventions. *DSM-IV* diagnoses for the patient with a dissociative disorder, and a related NANDA diagnosis, are presented in "Medical Diagnoses and Related Nursing Diagnoses." Additional nursing diagnoses that may be appropriate for the patient with a dissociative disorder are as follows:

- Altered Role Performance
- Spiritual Distress
- Risk for Violence: Self-Directed
- Risk for Violence: Directed at Others
- Hopelessness
- Anxiety

Return now to the case of Charlotte, to see how the process of diagnosis worked in her case.

Charlotte was diagnosed as suffering from dissociative amnesia, according to the *DSM-IV* criteria. In reviewing the limited data initially obtained, however, it was apparent that many knowledge gaps existed regarding the unique nature of this person. For example,

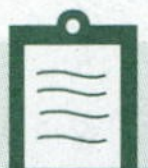

MEDICAL DIAGNOSES AND RELATED NURSING DIAGNOSES

Dissociative Disorders

***DSM-IV* Diagnosis:** Dissociative Amnesia

Diagnostic Criteria

A. The predominant disturbance is one or more episodes of inability to recall important personal information, usually of a traumatic or stressful nature, that is too extensive to be explained by ordinary forgetfulness.
B. The disturbance does not occur exclusively during the course of Dissociative Identity Disorder, Dissociative Fugue, Posttraumatic Stress Disorder, Acute Stress Disorder, or Somatization Disorder and is not due to the direct physiological effects of a substance (e.g., a drug of abuse, a medication) or a neurological or other general medical condition (e.g., Amnestic Disorder Due to Head Trauma).
C. The symptoms cause clinically significant distress or impairment in social, occupational, or other important areas of functioning.

***DSM-IV* Diagnosis:** Dissociative Fugue

Diagnostic Criteria

A. The predominant disturbance is sudden, unexpected travel away from home or one's customary place of work, with inability to recall one's past.
B. Confusion about personal identity or assumption of a new identity (partial or complete).
C. The disturbance does not occur exclusively during the course of Dissociative Identity Disorder and is not due to the direct physiological effects of a substance (e.g., a drug of abuse, a medication) or a general medical condition (e.g., temporal lobe epilepsy).
D. The symptoms cause clinically significant distress or impairment in social, occupational, or other important areas of functioning.

***DSM-IV* Diagnosis:** Dissociative Identity Disorder

Diagnostic Criteria

A. The presence of two or more distinct identities or personality states (each with its own relatively enduring pattern of perceiving, relating to, and thinking about the environment and self).
B. At least two of these identities or personality states recurrently take control of the person's behavior.
C. Inability to recall important personal information that is too extensive to be explained by ordinary forgetfulness.
D. The disturbance is not due to the direct physiological effects of a substance (e.g., blackouts or chaotic behavior during Alcohol Intoxication) or a general medical condition (e.g., complex partial seizures). *Note:* In children, the symptoms are not attributable to imaginary playmates or other fantasy play.

***DSM-IV* Diagnosis** Depersonalization Disorder

Diagnostic Criteria

A. Persistent or recurrent experiences of feeling detached from, and as if one is an outside observer of, one's mental processes or body (e.g., feeling like one is in a dream).
B. During the depersonalization experience, reality testing remains intact.
C. The depersonalization causes clinically significant distress or impairment in social, occupational, or other important areas of functioning.
D. The depersonalization experience does not occur exclusively during the course of another mental disorder, such as Schizophrenia, Panic Disorder, Acute Stress Disorder, or another Dissociative Disorder, and is not due to the direct physiological effects of a substance (e.g., a drug of abuse, a medication) or a general medical condition (e.g., temporal lobe epilepsy).

***DSM-IV* Diagnosis:** Dissociative Disorder Not Otherwise Specified

RELATED NURSING DIAGNOSES	DEFINITION	EXAMPLE
Ineffective Individual Coping	Impairment of adaptive behaviors and problem-solving abilities of a person in meeting life's demands and roles	Ineffective Individual Coping related to confusion about self

Diagnostic criteria from American Psychiatric Association (1994). *Diagnostic and statistical manual of mental disorders, fourth edition.* Washington, D.C.: American Psychiatric Association; nursing diagnoses and definitions from North American Nursing Diagnosis Association. (1994). *NANDA nursing diagnoses: Definitions and classification 1995–1996.* Philadelphia: NANDA.

was she able to support herself financially? If not, was she motivated for vocational training? Did she have spiritual concerns? As mentioned previously, the most consistent message Charlotte had received from her mother was that she was a "bad" person, whose badness drove her father and others away. She had subsequently experienced disruptive, chaotic relations with others. Based on an appraisal of assessment data, her initial nursing diagnosis was Ineffective Individual Coping related to altered self-concept as evidenced by amnesia.

OUTCOME IDENTIFICATION

The primary expected outcome for a patient with a dissociative disorder is that the patient will develop new, more adaptive ways of coping with stress.

PLANNING

Based on the identified expected outcomes, the nurse and patient, working together with the interdisciplinary treatment team, jointly establish short-term goals, such as the following:

Expected Outcome	Short-Term Goals
The patient will develop new, more adaptive ways of coping with stress.	1. The patient will participate in life skills assessment group. 2. The patient will contact state agency regarding job training skills. 3. The patient will review transferable skills with a counselor.

Return now to Charlotte, to see how her plan of care unfolded.

The plan for Charlotte, and other patients diagnosed with a dissociative disorder, includes trying to establish some degree of rapport, considered especially important on her arrival on the psychiatric unit. Although Charlotte's history was sketchy and although there were no family or friends to provide additional data, the nursing staff were careful not to overwhelm the patient with questions she could not answer. She was initially engaged in occupational therapy and other milieu activities, based on the rationale that recall of the past might occur during activities that simulate life experiences. Because these treatment modalities did not seem to promote recall, the staff planned an amytal interview. As Charlotte's life sketch was filled in with more details, the nursing staff formulated the following additional nursing diagnoses:

- Altered Role Performance related to chaotic style of living and lack of involvement in the pursuit of productive work and healthy relationships
- Spiritual Distress related to feelings of being "evil" invoked by early childhood experiences related to abandonment by father and verbal abuse by mother.

At this point, the treatment team reviewed Charlotte's progress, and Charlotte and her treatment team jointly established the following short-term goals:

- During and after participation in individual and group psychotherapy, Charlotte will assess her goals for a more satisfying lifestyle in relation to interpersonal and vocational experiences.
- Charlotte will begin to verbalize her self-perception of being "evil," "immoral," "whorish," and so forth as perceptions that she does not have to own because they were projected onto her by a mentally unstable mother.
- Charlotte will report feeling a brightening in her mood, as evidenced by increased interaction with peers, social smiling, and normal sleep patterns.
- After participation in a psychoeducation group, Charlotte will state the major actions and potential side effects of her antidepressant medication.

The issues of implementation in Charlotte's care after her memory was regained involved:

- Coordinating individual and group psychotherapy.
- Administering the prescribed antidepressant medication and arranging a teaching session regarding both therapeutic and potential side effects of the drug.
- Arranging for consultation with a hospital chaplain when this intervention was requested by the patient.
- Providing opportunities in the milieu for Charlotte to experience success in completion of tasks and in interaction with peers.

Because most patients with dissociative disorders have experienced physical and psychological trauma, it may be difficult to establish rapport or trust with them or even to collect admission data. If the patient is experiencing some form of amnesia, it is important to provide a safe, supportive environment and not push the patient for information. As with any other patient-nurse situation, the qualitative aspects of the relationship are of central importance: establishing rapport and developing trust.

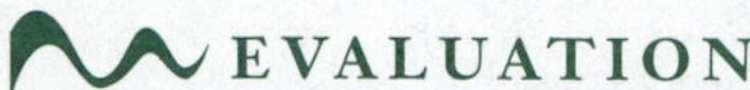

EVALUATION

Evaluation of patient care occurs ideally throughout the nursing process. Treatment is considered effective when a patient not only regains memory for past events, but also experiences an improved quality of life in interpersonal relationships and demonstrates an ability to plan for immediate and future needs. A necessary step is to look back at the goals to see if they were realistic under the circumstances. Should some modifications be made? Few phenomena occur in a totally linear fashion, and the nursing process is no exception.

▶ Check Your Reading

10. Identify four areas to be assessed in dissociative disorders.
11. Identify at least two nursing diagnoses appropriate to a patient with a dissociative disorder.
12. What is the most important outcome when working with a patient who has a dissociative disorder?
13. Identify at least two interventions used with a patient with a dissociative disorder.

CASE STUDY: CINDY

Cindy is a 35-year-old file clerk who lives alone in an apartment in a major northern city. You are a home health nurse assigned to visit Cindy while she is recuperating from major abdominal surgery. On one of the visits, Cindy confides in you that she fears she is going insane. She tells you that for the past two years she has experienced increasingly frequent episodes of feeling "outside herself." Cindy says that during these episodes she feels like parts of her body are dead and she frequently loses her balance.

Cindy tells you that since her surgery she is experiencing these episodes more frequently, and each episode lasts three to four hours. She confides that you are the first person she has ever shared this information with and asks you to help her. She is markedly distressed and has difficulty sleeping. A mental status examination reveals that she is oriented to time, place, and person and has intact memory and good judgment. She tells you that she is concerned that she will lose her job if she does not get back to work soon. Cindy's parents were killed in an automobile accident when she was 14, and her only brother died of AIDS three years ago. She was raised as a Methodist but has not been to church since her parents were killed.

You refer Cindy to a psychiatrist, who diagnoses her with Depersonalization Disorder and asks you to continue seeing her once a week, because Cindy seems to trust you.

ASSESSMENT

Assessment data are as follows:

- Persistent, recurrent feeling of being detached from self
- Loss of balance during dissociative episode
- Insomnia
- No support system in place
- History of trauma and loss
- Fear of losing job and going insane
- Marked distress

DIAGNOSIS

***DSM-IV* Diagnosis:** Depersonalization disorder

Nursing Diagnosis 1: Personal Identity Disturbance related to history of severe, traumatic interpersonal experiences and current stressor of severe illness evidenced by dissociative experiences, marked distress, insomnia and fear of losing job

OUTCOME IDENTIFICATION, PLANNING, AND IMPLEMENTATION

EXPECTED OUTCOME 1: By _____ the patient will report a marked reduction in dissociative experiences.

SHORT-TERM GOAL	NURSING INTERVENTIONS	RATIONALES
By _____ the patient will report one dissociative experience per week.	1. Continue to work on the trusting relationship that has been initiated. 2. Convey interest and caring.	1–2. Trust is the basis of a therapeutic relationship and is especially important for a patient who is not grounded in reality.
	3. Help the patient determine what is real and what is not real. Validate what is real and gently correct misperceptions.	3. As with a patient who is hallucinating, it is important not to reinforce what is not real.
	4. Encourage the patient to limit her external environment.	4. This will foster psychological safety.
	5. Ask the patient to keep a record of any dissociative experiences she is having and share them with you at your next visit.	5. Actually recording the dissociative experiences aids in reinforcing reality.

EXPECTED OUTCOME 2: By _____ the patient will verbalize absence of distress and fear of going insane.

SHORT-TERM GOALS	NURSING INTERVENTIONS	RATIONALES
By _____ the patient will sleep at least six hours without interruption	1. Educate the patient about the importance of sleep.	1. Dissociative experiences are known to occur more frequently when a patient is sleep deprived.
	2. If the patient is unable to gain restful sleep via natural methods, consider sleeping medications until a pattern is established.	2. If normal sleeping patterns have been interrupted for a long period of time, it is often necessary to intervene with medication.
	3. Have the patient keep a record of her sleep pattern.	3. Recording information helps the patient distinguish between reality and unreality.
By _____ the patient will report a significant reduction in anxiety.	1. Educate the patient about stress reduction measures such as meditation, writing, taking a warm bath, or talking to a friend. 2. Encourage the patient to try at least one new stress reduction measure each week.	1–2. Dissociative experiences are likely to be increased when the patient is anxious. Employing measures to reduce anxiety will aid in reducing the frequency of dissociation.

Nursing Diagnosis 2: Risk for Loneliness related to lack of support system, history of multiple losses, and the physical isolation necessitated by her current illness evidenced by lack of support system, marked distress, and fear of going insane.

OUTCOME IDENTIFICATION, PLANNING, AND IMPLEMENTATION

EXPECTED OUTCOME 1: By _____ the patient will report a desire to rekindle a sense of spirituality.

SHORT-TERM GOAL	NURSING INTERVENTIONS	RATIONALES
By _____ the patient will openly acknowledge her estrangement from the God of her understanding.	1. Encourage the patient to talk about her earlier relationship with God. 2. Offer to get the patient reading materials or to be available to listen.	1–2. Being available to listen and to broach the subject of spirituality is an important part of healing for many patients with psychiatric conditions, especially when they have been spiritually bankrupt for a long time.
	3. Remain supportive and nonjudgmental if the patient describes anger toward God.	3. When patients have had multiple, profound losses, it is not unusual for them to be angry at God for "letting it happen."
	4. Ask the patient to describe times in her life when she found solace and comfort in her spiritual beliefs.	4. This intervention shifts the focus and helps the patient get in touch with the self-nurturing aspect of a strong spiritual belief system.

SHORT-TERM GOAL	NURSING INTERVENTIONS	RATIONALES
By _____ the patient will report a desire to join a local church group.	1. Discuss with the patient the advantage of joining a church group. 2. Encourage the patient to be proactive in acknowledging her need for love and support and spirituality. 3. Honor the patient's initial reluctance in joining a group. 4. Continue to support growth, even though the patient may experience setbacks.	1–4. Even though the notion of joining a group may be appealing for many reasons, it is not unusual for patients to be reluctant. Framing this reluctance as fear rather than oppositional behavior will enable the nurse to continue to be supportive through any setbacks.

EXPECTED OUTCOME 2: By _____ the patient will acknowledge the need to grieve the loss of her brother and her parents.

SHORT-TERM GOALS	NURSING INTERVENTIONS	RATIONALES
By _____ the patient will discuss the anger and sadness related to the loss of her brother and parents.	1. Identify the functions that pent-up anger and sadness serve for the patient. 2. Explain the behaviors associated with normal grieving. 3. Encourage the expression of these feelings in a safe manner. 4. Encourage the expression of rage though participation in large motor activities, such as physical exercise, walking, or jogging. 5. Encourage the patient to also focus on the sad feelings that have been buried and convey to her that you are not uncomfortable with the expression of deep sadness.	1–3. Knowledge of the acceptable feelings associated with normal grieving may aid in relieving some of the guilt and shame that inhibits resolution. 4. This encourages the patient to be proactive and direct in processing negative feelings, in lieu of having them appear in a more pathological form. 5. Patients sometimes refuse to share their deepest feelings because they are trying to protect the nurse.
By _____ the patient will agree to pursue additional counseling for her issues surrounding loss.	1. Provide the patient with a list of grief groups available in the community. 2. Also provide the patient with a list of sliding scale community counseling centers. 3. Encourage the patient to continue on the path to good mental health.	1–2. Providing the patient with multiple options may make her feel more comfortable initially in individual therapy. 3. Patients who have been isolated for a long period of time need a strong patient advocate.

EVALUATION

Formative Evaluation

Cindy met each of the short-term goals. The dissociative episodes were dramatically reduced, and she reported being able to sleep. Within two months, she decided to contact the minister of the local Methodist church and begin attending services. This church also has a grief group, which Cindy will begin attending.

Summative Evaluation

All of the expected outcomes were also met. Within three months, Cindy reported no further dissociative experiences. She was close to completing her grief group and was attending church services on a regular basis. She told the nurse she was so grateful to feel whole again and to know she was not crazy.

CONCLUSIONS

A renewed interest in the phenomena of dissociation and dissociative disorders has undeniably occurred in the past 20 or so years. A number of factors have contributed to this rebirth of interest. The suffering of many people from posttraumatic syndromes has been one phenomenon that has increasingly called attention to the power of dissociative states. The plight of Vietnam veterans and, more recently, veterans of other international wars and disasters has called national attention to reactions of survivors—which typically include dissociative symptoms. Also in recent years, the concurrence of borderline psychopathology with dissociative symptoms and a history of incest among women has been increasingly noted (Gartner and Gartner,

1988). This finding serves as an additional factor that has contributed to heightened involvement in research and treatment of dissociative disorders. Finally, public awareness of severe child abuse, a major causative factor in chronic dissociative pathology, has dramatically increased within the past few years. It is imperative that professional nurses in all settings be attuned to detect dissociative symptoms and have a conceptual understanding of their mechanism. Otherwise, the symptoms may go unrecognized and untreated, and patients will be denied the care that they need to help them in their journey toward healing.

KEY POINTS TO REMEMBER

- Persons with dissociative disorders experience gaps in memory, confusion, and often a sense of compartmentalization.
- Theorists have been divided as to whether dissociation is a pathological process or a part of normal human activity.
- Freud viewed dissociation as a form of the defense mechanism, repression.
- Janet was the first theorist to use the term *dissociation.*
- Dissociation occurs along a continuum ranging from the mildest forms of dissociation, which include daydreaming, to the most serious form of dissociation, which is dissociative identity disorder.
- The DES is a scale that measures how frequently an individual experiences dissociation.
- Sullivan conceptualized dissociation as an expression of *not-me behavior.*
- Pathological dissociation is associated with five hallmark symptoms: amnesia, derealization, depersonalization, identity confusion, and identity alteration.
- The *DSM-IV* recognizes five dissociative disorders: dissociative amnesia, dissociative fugue, depersonalization disorder, dissociative identity disorder, and dissociative disorder not otherwise specified.
- Assessment of dissociative disorders includes collecting data about memory, consciousness, and sense of identity, in addition to the five hallmark symptoms.
- There are several appropriate nursing diagnoses for patients with dissociative disorders. The most important, however, is: Ineffective Individual Coping related to. . . .
- Goals for a patient with a dissociative disorder include participating in individual and group psychotherapy, verbalization of self-concept, improvement in mood, knowledge of medication, and improvement in coping skills.
- Implementation includes (1) coordinating individual and group psychotherapy, (2) administering the prescribed antidepressant medication and arranging a teaching session regarding both therapeutic and potential side effects of the drug, (3) dealing with spiritual issues, and (4) providing opportunities in the milieu.

LEARNING ACTIVITIES

1. Complete the Dissociative Experiences Scale on yourself. What is your reaction to your score?
2. In the next week, try to be aware of the times you use dissociation as part of your normal activities of daily life.
3. What do you think about the importance of forgiveness to the patient who has suffered childhood abuse? Do you think that the ability to forgive is a decision or a process that occurs over time as the individual heals? Should the patient be encouraged to forgive his or her abuser? Give a rationale for your answer.

CRITICAL THINKING EXERCISE

Molly is a 27-year-old African-American woman who was admitted to the dissociative disorder unit two weeks previously. She was diagnosed with a multiple personality disorder. During her stay on the unit, the nurses were able to assess at least 10 different personalities. Among these personalities were a destructive female, a frightened child, a seductive teenager, a soft-spoken young woman, and an angry male. At 7:30 p.m., the nurse supervisor, Miss Yeager, responded to an emergency call about Molly. When Miss Yeager arrived on the unit, she saw Molly crouched in a fetal position hiding under a table in the dining room area. As soon as any staff members tried to touch her, she began to scream in a high-pitched shrill voice.

1. If you were Nurse Yeager, what would you need to know before you approached Molly?
2. What knowledge about multiple personality disorder would help you to determine your intervention?
3. Suggest possible interventions.

After about 45 minutes, the staff members finally were able to make some interventions that attended to Molly's needs. Then a nurse overheard two staff members talking about Molly. They were unhappy with Molly's manipulation of the staff and failure to take responsibility for her actions. Both of them were convinced that Molly was acting.

1. What assumptions have the two staff members made about multiple personality disorder?
2. How might these assumptions affect their interactions with Molly?
3. What are possible ways they could test whether their assumptions are faulty?

REFERENCES

American Psychiatric Association (1994). *Diagnostic and statistical manual of mental disorders* (4th ed.). Washington, D.C.: American Psychiatric Association.

Bernstein, E., and Putnam, F. W. (1986). Development of reliability and validity of a dissociation scale. *Journal of Nervous and Mental Disease, 174*(12), 727–735.

Braun, B. G., and Sachs, R. G. (1985). The development of personality disorder: Predisposing, precipitating, and perpetuating factors. In R. P. Kluft (Ed.), *The childhood antecedents of multiple personality.* Washington, D.C.: American Psychiatric Press.

Briere, J., and Runtz, M. (1990). Augmenting Hopkins SCL scales to measure dissociative symptoms: Data from two non-clinical samples. *Journal of Personality Assessment, 55,* 376–379.

Chu, J. A., and Dill, D. L. (1990). Dissociative symptoms in relation to childhood physical and sexual abuse. *American Journal of Psychiatry, 147,* 887–892.

Coons, P. M. (1984). The differential diagnosis of multiple personality: A comprehensive review. *Psychiatric Clinics of North America, 7,* 51–65.

Coons, P. M., Bowman, E., and Milstein, V. (1988). Multiple personality disorder: A clinical investigation of 50 cases. *Journal of Nervous and Mental Disease, 176*(5), 519–527.

Crabtree, A. (1992). Dissociation and memory: A two-hundred-year perspective. *Dissociation, 5*(3), 150–154.

Franklin, J. (1990). The diagnosis of multiple personality disorder based on subtle dissociative signs. *Journal of Nervous and Mental Disease, 178,*(4).

Freud, S. (1962). The neuro-psychoses of defense. In J. Strachey (Ed.), *Standard edition of the complete psychological works of Sigmund Freud, vol. 3.* London: Hogarth Press. (Original work published 1894.)

Gartner, A., and Gartner, J. (1988). Borderline pathology in post-incest female adolescents. *Bulletin of the Menninger Clinic, 52,* 101–113.

Greaves, G. B. (1980). Multiple personality: 165 years after Mary Reynolds. *The Journal of Nervous and Mental Diseases, 168,* 577–596.

Hilgard, E. R. (1977). *Divided consciousness: Multiple controls in human thought and action.* New York: Wiley.

Janet, P. (1907). *The major symptoms of hysteria.* New York: Macmillan.

Kaplan, H. I., Sadlock, B. J., and Grebb, J. A. (1994). Dissociation disorders. In H. I. Kaplan and B. J. Sadlock (Eds.), *Synopsis of psychiatry* (6th ed.) Baltimore: Williams & Wilkins.

Kluft, R. P. (1985). The natural history of multiple personality disorder. In Kluft, R. P. (Ed.), *The childhood antecedents of multiple personality disorder.* Washington, D.C.: American Psychiatric Press.

Kluft, R. P. (1984). Aspects of the treatment of multiple personality disorder. *Psychiatric Annals, 14,* 51–55.

Myers, T. (1903). *Human personality and its survival of bodily death,* vol. I and II. London: Longman, Green, and Co.

Nemiah, J. C. (1989). Dissociative disorders (hysterical neuroses, dissociative type). In H. P. Kaplan and B. J. Sadlock (Eds.), *Comprehensive textbook of psychiatry,* vol. I (5th ed.). Baltimore: Williams & Wilkins.

Osborn, D. (1991). *Reflections on the art of living. A Joseph Campbell companion* (p. 154). (Selected and edited by Diane Osborn). New York: HarperCollins.

Prince, M. (1907). A symposium on the subconscious. *Journal of Abnormal Psychology, 2,* 67–80.

Prince, M. (1914). *The unconscious: The fundamentals of human personality, normal and abnormal.* New York: Macmillan.

Putnam, F. W. (1989) *Diagnosis and treatment of multiple personality disorder.* New York: Guilford Press.

Ross, C. A., Anderson, G., Heber, S., and Norton, G. R. (1990). Dissociation and abuse among multiple personality disorder patients, prostitutes, and exotic dancers. *Hospital and Community Psychiatry, 41,* 328–330.

Spiegel, D. (1984). Multiple personality as a post-traumatic stress disorder. *Psychiatric Clinics of North America, 7,* 101–110.

Stafford, L. L. (1993). Dissociation and multiple personality disorder: A challenge for psychosocial nurses. *Journal of Psychosocial Nursing and Mental Health Services, 31*(1), 15–20.

Steinberg, M. (1993). Advances in detecting dissociation. *Psychiatric Times, 10*(4), 20–23.

Taylor, E. (1983). *William James on exceptional mental states: The 1986 Lowell lectures.* New York: Charles Scribner's Sons.

Tessier, L. J. (1992). Women sexually abused as children: The spiritual consequences. *Second Opinion, 17*(3), 11–23.

Vaillant, G. (Ed.) (1986). *Empirical studies of ego mechanism and defense.* Washington, DC: American Psychiatric Press.

SUGGESTED READINGS

Coons, P. (1984). The differential diagnosis of multiple personality: A comprehensive review. *Psychiatric Clinics of North America,* 1, 51–65.

Kaplan, H. I., Sadlock, B. J., and Grebb, J. A. (1994). Dissociation disorders. In H. I. Kaplan and B. J. Sadlock (Eds.), *Synopsis of psychiatry* (6th ed.). Baltimore: Williams & Wilkins.

Stafford, L. L. (1993). Dissociation and multiple personality disorder: A challenge for psychosocial nurses. *Journal of Psychosocial Nursing and Mental Health Services, 31* (1), 15–20.

CHAPTER 34

THE JOURNEY UNDERMINED BY PSYCHOSEXUAL DISORDERS

For what I want to do I do not do, but what I hate I do. For what I do is not the good I want to do; no, the evil I do not want to do—this I keep on doing.

—Romans 7:14, 19

LEARNING OBJECTIVES

After studying this chapter, you should be able to:

1. Discuss how sexuality changes across the life span.
2. Discuss the phases of the sexual response cycle.
3. Discuss abnormalities that occur across the phases of the sexual response cycle.
4. Describe the process for conducting a sexual assessment.
5. List and describe sexual deviations.
6. Discuss the spiritual aspects of normal and abnormal forms of sexual expression.
7. Apply the nursing process to patient situations in which there is either a sexual dysfunction or a sexual deviation.
8. Identify your own attitudes and biases about sexuality.

KEY TERMINOLOGY

Anorgasmia
Dyspareunia
Exhibitionism
Fertility
Fetishism
Frotteurism
Gay
Gender
Gender dysphoria
Gender identity
Homosexuality
Human sexual response cycle
Impotence
Lesbian
Masochism
Orgasm
Paraphilia
Premature ejaculation
Sadism
Sex
Sexual identity
Sexuality
Sexual tension
Transsexualism
Transvestic fetishism
Vaginismus
Voyeurism

As we journey through life, each of us becomes increasingly aware of ourselves as sexual beings. This awareness is far broader than our recognition of lovemaking behaviors; it encompasses our views of ourselves as men and women, as mothers and fathers, as generative individuals who create and give to society in multiple ways. Our views are shaped by societal attitudes and mores, which seem to change with each generation. These shifting cultural pressures, however, are not the only determinant of sexual beliefs, attitudes, and behaviors. Parental views, spiritual and religious teaching, socioeconomic status, and education all greatly affect our sexual behavior.

In our time, women's expressions of sensuality and sexuality have perhaps undergone the greatest transformation. Women are increasingly viewed by society as fully sexual beings who possess the right to say no to unwanted sexual advances. Courts have decided that married women can be victims of marital rape and their spouses punished accordingly. The whole issue of what constitutes consent to engage in sexual activity is brought to the courts with greater frequency.

Another issue that has undergone reconsideration is the diagnostic dilemma regarding whether homosexuality is an abnormal behavior or a variation of normal behavior. With the current epidemic of sexually transmitted diseases, the issue of sex education is more vital than ever, yet the debate continues over who should teach safer sex practices and at what age level.

These issues have an impact on psychiatric nursing. It belongs within the purview of all nurses to assess patients' sexual practices and be prepared to educate, dispel myths, assist with values clarification, refer to appropriate care providers when indicated, and share resources. Health promotion and prevention is a key role for nurses. It alleviates or decreases patient illness and suffering and reduces health care cost. As a student of nursing, you are introduced to the complex issue of sexual behavior to facilitate thoughtful discussion of the topic and to develop personal belief systems that consider the broader perspective of sexual issues as they exist in contemporary society.

The goals of this chapter are to provide enough knowledge about normal and abnormal human sexuality for you to conduct a sexual assessment, to understand what is meant by human sexuality and the sexual response cycle, and to be able to recognize sexual dysfunctions that can occur at different stages of the cycle. You will be able to identify deviations from normal sexual behaviors and recognize nursing implications, formulate interventions, and state the rationale for planned therapeutic interventions. You will not be prepared to be a sex therapist.

To accomplish these goals, you must first explore personal sexual biases and knowledge deficits. You need to develop a degree of comfort when discussing sexual issues to put the patient at ease, thereby facilitating a candid dialogue. A basic knowledge of sexual anatomy and physiology, although essential, is insufficient for an appreciation of the complex nature of sexual development and behavior. Box 34–1 provides questions to encourage self-awareness about sexuality.

This chapter provides definitions of important terms, a review of the sexual response cycle and problems associated with normal sexual response, an overview of the major sexual disorders, and an examination of your role in responding to sexual disorders through the modality of the nursing process. First, let's review John's story.

JOHN'S STORY

I call myself John, but maybe I should have chosen a less gender-specific name, like Chris. My appearance may confuse some people. It confuses me! I feel like I've spent my entire life trying to make the inner me match the outer me. Since I was young, I've felt this way, like somebody made a terrible mistake that I now have to try to correct. I was never like my sisters. They were sweet and delicate and played typical little girl games. I always knew that I was different . . . not a tomboy . . . but different—like I was molded into the wrong body. I felt that God had made a major mistake with me; he put me into the wrong body. My parents recognized that I wasn't like my sisters, despite their best efforts to get me to conform. It never worked, so finally they gave up. I think I'm an embarrassment to them. They don't know how to explain me to their friends.

BOX 34-1 Questions to Encourage Sexual Self-Awareness

As you answer these questions, be aware of how you feel.

Am I at ease? uncomfortable? embarrassed?
Am I comfortable being a woman (man)? When I consider my own sexuality, what do I mean? What behaviors and roles do I associate with my sexuality? Have I examined my own attitudes, feelings, and beliefs about sexual issues, such as:

Gender roles

Life cycle changes, including menstruation, pregnancy, and menopause

Sexually transmitted diseases, including AIDS

All forms of sexual activity, including masturbation/self-pleasure, homosexual activity, bisexual activity, fellatio, cunnilingus, anal intercourse, sexual activity with multiple partners, nonmarital sexual activity

Sexuality across the life cycle; i.e., in children, adolesents, elderly

Sexuality in handicapped persons or in the mentally retarded

Lubrication, orgasm, ejaculation

Nudity (my own and others), touching my own body or another's body

Frequency of intercourse, positions for intercourse

Abortion, contraception

Talking about sexual issues, talking about sexual issues with patients

As I look at my own attitudes, feelings, and beliefs, can I identify the sources of these? What part of my own attitudes, feelings, and beliefs can I attribute to my early upbringing? to my culture? to my religious beliefs? to my own sexual experiences?
Am I aware of what "turns me on" sexually? Conversely, what "turns me off" sexually?
Am I able to accept myself as a sexual human being? What about patients?
Am I willing to have my own beliefs challenged by learning accurate information regarding sexual issues?
Am I willing to increase my self-acceptance and my acceptance of others' sexuality?

I feel like an outcast, never fitting into any group. For the past three years, I've dressed in male garments or unisex clothing. My hair is cut by a barber in a contemporary male style, and I drive a "macho" car. At the nursing home where I work, I do maintenance jobs such as washing and waxing floors. The nature of the job allows me to keep to myself, so I can avoid getting into personal conversations. After three years of hormone therapy, my appearance is more masculine, although my voice hasn't dropped as low as I had hoped it would. I'm more pleased with my outer appearance than I used to be, and I really feel great when someone addresses me as "mister" or "sir." Seeing myself undressed is still disturbing, and I can't go to places like the beach. My breasts are the biggest problem. I wear a binder all the time to try to get them as flat as possible.

Sex change surgery is extremely expensive, and it isn't easy to find surgeons who are experienced with the types of procedures involved. When you can find a surgeon, then you have to be able to convince him or her that you are not crazy for wanting to have these body-altering procedures, because they are concerned that the person requesting the surgery will, at a later time, regret the decision. I don't ever expect to have a penis surgically constructed, but it would be nice to be able to stand at a urinal like other men, instead of using a stall. Penile construction involves a whole series of operations, and I could never afford them on my salary. I'm just hoping to find a surgeon who would be willing to remove my breasts. That would be enough to make me feel more like the man I was supposed to be. I'm not looking for surgery to make me attractive to females; for me, this isn't just "cosmetic" surgery. Loneliness is a problem—I admit that. And I would eventually like to have a relationship with a woman. But for now, my goal is simply to be more comfortable with me.

John's story provides a glimpse into the suffering experienced by an individual whose journey is marked by feeling as if she was born into the wrong body; she has the body of a woman, but the inner sense that she is a man. John suffers from gender dysphoria.

DEFINITIONS

Because there is considerable confusion regarding terms such as *sex*, *gender*, *sexual identity*, *gender identity*, *gender dysphoria*, *transsexualism*, and *homosexuality*, some definitions are presented (Stuntz, 1983).

The term **sex** refers to whether the person is anatomically male or female. This determination is based on the person's inherited biological endowment, that is, the vagina, ovaries, uterus, and 46XX karyotype or the penis, testicles, and 46XY karyotype.

Gender identity is the earliest acquisition of the basic sense of maleness or femaleness, which occurs normally during the first 18 months of life. It develops along with the sense of being a self separate from mother and all others. Gender identity thus is a part of self-identity, which in the normal course of personality development comes to include sexual identity. **Gender** refers to the person's psychological reaction to or sense of being male or female. A person has an inner conviction about being a boy or a girl, a man or a woman. Normally sex and gender are the same, i.e., "I have a vagina and I am a woman," or "I have a penis and I am a man." When sex and gender differ, however, the individual suffers from **gender dysphoria.** Such a person might have a physically normal female reproductive tract and yet have the "sense" that she is a male and might describe herself as "I am a man trapped in a woman's body." This is an example of the most extreme gender dysphoria, called **transsexualism.**

The identification of oneself as being male or female, the process of developing traits of masculinity or femininity, and the unfolding of the appropriate eroticism result in **sexual identity.** The majority of people develop a *heterosexual identity;* that is, they are sexually attracted to the opposite sex. A percentage of people in all cultures, however, develop a *homosexual identity*, wherein they express a sexual preference for persons of the same gender. Homosexuals can be either ego-syntonic, in which the person is emotionally comfortable with his or her sexuality, or ego-dystonic, in which the person is emotionally distressed by the same-sex attraction. Homosexual men are frequently referred to as **gay** and homosexual women as **lesbian.**

In addition some people are not exclusively heterosexual or homosexual but are attracted to members of both genders. These persons are *bisexual* in their sexual identity. Although sexual identity normally is believed to develop between the ages of three and five, it is continually reworked and reinforced psychologically through adolescence and probably continues to develop in some measure throughout life. In the normal adult, the terms *gender identity* and *sexual identity* are synonymous; however, the gender-dysphoric person describes these terms as being at odds. Most such persons describe their anatomy as being irrelevant to their sense of self (Stuntz, 1983).

▶ Check Your Reading

1. Define the term *sex.*
2. What is the difference between sexual identity and gender identity?
3. What does it mean if an individual is gender dysphoric?
4. To what does gender refer?

SEXUAL DEVELOPMENT ACROSS THE LIFESPAN

Just as people are holistically physical, spiritual, and social beings, they are also sexual beings. Awareness and

TABLE 34–1 **Stages of Human Psychosexual Development**

Stage	Characteristics
Prenatal stage	Chromosomal and hormonal factors influence the gender of the fetus. The gender of the fetus is determined by the seventh week.
Birth through 2 years	Gender assigned at birth Societal influence reinforces the child's sexual identity. Oral phase of development Infants exhibit reflexive signs of sexual arousal Physical affection toward the child is essential for normal psychosocial development
2 to 5 years	Anal phase of development, characterized by learning sphincter control The concept of privacy is manifested. Self-exploration of genitals Awareness and mimicking of sex-role behaviors Association between genitals and pleasure begins. The child has an attraction to the opposite-sex parent.
5 to 12 years	Sex play between age-mates Curiosity about reproduction Friendship predominately with same-sex age-mates
13 to 20 years	Sexual self-consciousness Increased sexual fantasy Dating the opposite sex Concern about the physical changes of the body Menarche, breast enlargement, development of underarm and genital hair, and widening of the hips in females Nocturnal emissions, broadening shoulders, increase in muscle mass, and development of body hair in males Masturbation, petting, and intercourse
Young adulthood	Learning how to handle sexuality responsibly Sexual experimentation and focus on sexual technique Establishment of long-term relationships Pregnancy and childbearing
Middle adulthood	Self-acceptance Decreased performance anxiety Decreased frequency of intercourse Hormonal changes—menopause Decrease in secondary sex characteristics Change in erectile potential in males
Late adulthood	Sexual activity focused on intimacy rather than intercourse Sexual accommodation for physical handicaps Decrease in the frequency of intercourse

expression of sexuality change across the lifespan as the person grows and matures in all other domains. Sexuality encompasses the whole person. Physically, **sexuality** refers to appearance and physical expressions, such as kissing, hugging, embracing, fondling, and sexual intercourse. Socially, sexuality usually involves another person for full expression. Spiritually, sexuality includes a sense of connectedness and creativity. Table 34–1 illustrates the changes in sexual function, sexual self-concept, and sexual roles and relationships across the lifespan.

SEXUAL RESPONSE CYCLE

To evaluate sexual complaints in a scientific manner, you need knowledge of normal sexual functioning as well as deviations from the norm. Sexuality is a relational process that develops between two individuals of the same or opposite gender or between one person and his or her fantasy world. Physical and emotional intimacy is shared with the desire to relieve physical and emotional tension, in a manner that is described by most people as being supremely pleasurable.

One may think of "having sex" as being something like playing a violin. There are many parts of the violin, all of which must be in place and in working condition to allow the production of sound. That is, no music could be obtained without the neck, the pegs, the strings, the finger board, the sounding chamber with the "f"-shaped soundholes, and, of course, the bow. The similarities seem obvious. A woman interested in sexual activity must have the appropriate anatomy in working condition, normal hormones present in adequate amounts, a responsive and integrated nervous system, and, finally, to correspond with the "bow," an available and erect penis. Certainly, it is possible to produce excellent and intense sexual "music" without a partner and without relying either on the "bow" penis or the "violin" vagina, but for most individuals the truly soaring sensual experience requires the violin and the bow, the penis and the vagina.

Reproduction depends (in most cases) on the sexual act, which results in the pooling of male and female genetic material. This act of contributing genetic material toward the production of a fetus has been named *sexual,* and because of its overriding importance to the survival of the species, all societies have attempted to control sexual behavior in some manner. These societal constraints, sometimes in the form of religious dogma or moral teachings, introduce psychological tensions, which materially affect the manner of sexual expression and which, in turn, may produce symptoms of psychological illness. This is a more formal way of stating that beliefs, attitudes, and experience in regard to sexuality may influence the way people function and interact with other people.

An understanding of what is normal and expectable in the sexual response cycle is a prerequisite to recognizing what is "out of order." The research of Masters and Johnson (1963) provides an understanding of the sexual response cycle. Masters and Johnson are attributed with dividing the **human sexual response cycle** into four phases: excitement, plateau, orgasm, resolution. Kaplan (1979) later added the concept of a desire phase, which precedes the excitement phase and resumes following the end of the resolution phase.

Stuntz (1988) built on the antecedent work of Masters and Johnson and Kaplan to describe a model of the human sexual response cycle that he named the D-E-P-O-R-D (Desire, Excitement, Plateau, Orgasm, Resolution, Desire) model (Figure 34–1). The actual dimensions of sexual tension are difficult to measure empirically because there are few indicators, other than self-report. Also, the total elapsed time of each phase of the cycle as well as of the cycle as a whole varies with each person and with each sexual encounter. All complete normal human sexual response cycles pass consecutively through each of these phases, however, and therefore the model is consistent with, but not necessarily identical with, the sexual experiences of those persons, men or women, whose sexual encounters involve normal response cycles. This model, in general, is descriptive of the normal sexual response cycles of both men and women, although it is probable that sexual tension in women usually takes longer to rise through the excitement phase as well as longer to descend through the resolution phase.

Desire Phase

About 40% of the people applying to the Marriage Council of Philadelphia for help with their sexual problems described their difficulties as having to do with the desire for sexual activity (Leif, 1977). Many factors in one's life may affect the interest in sexual activity, including but not limited to age, both physical and emotional health, availability of a sexual partner, and the context of the individual's life (Chandraiah et al, 1991; Currier and Aponte, 1991; Williams, 1991; Dunning, 1993). In fact, in a number of individuals, the lack of sexual desire is not a source of distress either to themselves or to their partners; in that situation decreased or absent sexual desire would not be thought of as an "illness."

Excessive sexual desire becomes a problem when this creates difficulties for the individual's partner or when such excessive desire drives that person to demand or force sexual compliance from unwilling partners.

The so-called "male" hormone *testosterone* (which is present in the circulation of both normal human women and men but in a much higher level in men) appears to be a prerequisite for sexual appetite in both men and women. Men who, for one reason or another, have lost the ability to produce testosterone describe the change in their sexual feelings in such terms as "I still have the basic inclination for sex but do not seem to have the energy to put it into effect." In some of these men, replacing their testosterone appears to restore their "sexual energy."

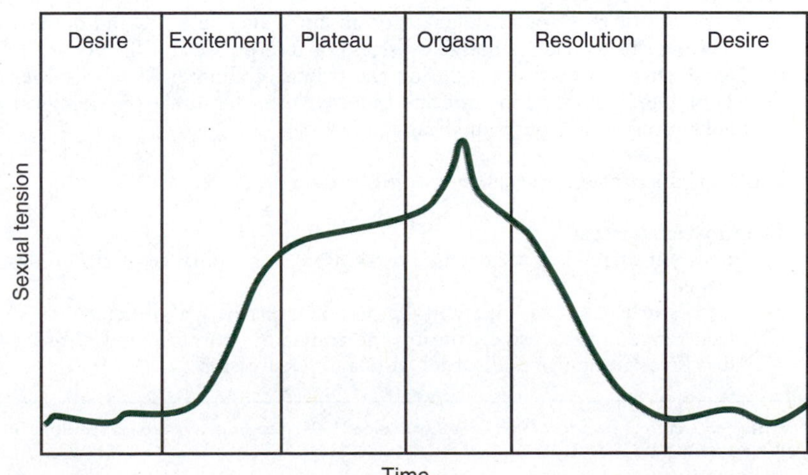

FIGURE 34–1
Stuntz's DEPORD model of the human sexual response cycle. (Redrawn from Stuntz, R. [1988]. Assessment of organic factors in sexual dysfunction. In R. Brown, and J. Field [Eds.]. Treatment of sexual problems in individual and couples therapy (pp 188–201). Dana Point, CA: PMA Publishing.)

Testosterone appears to have a positive effect in increasing interest in sexual activity in women. A serendipitous finding confirmed this when, many years ago, postmenopausal women with cancer of the breast were given testosterone to slow the rate of the cancerous growth. Many of these women reported strong and unusual interest in sexual activity, including fantasies, dreams, and urges to become sexually involved, none of which they had entertained for many prior years. Although testosterone has been used frequently to increase sexual desire in postmenopausal women, there have been no well-designed treatment outcome studies, but there have been many case reports such as Ella's story (Case Example 34–1).

Case Example 34–1 Ella's Story

Ella is a 67-year-old woman, widowed many years, who has just been approached by a 75-year-old widower with a marriage proposal. Ella is concerned about the sexual implications of a marriage so late in life. She confided in her nurse practitioner, "I really haven't even thought about sex for so many years. I know Joe is just an old goat. He's always after me to take my clothes off." After discussing the possibility of a physiological cause for her lack of interest in sex, Ella's nurse practitioner gave her small doses of testosterone. Within a remarkably short time, Ella stopped talking about Joe as "an old goat" and began talking again about "how great life can be if you have the right partner."

There does not appear to be a direct relationship between the "female" hormone *estrogen* and sexual desire in women. A secondary effect, however, may be present in the requirement of estrogen for the maintenance of the normal vaginal distensibility and lubrication. If these functions are lost secondary to estrogen deficiency, as may occur in some postmenopausal women or in younger women who have had their ovaries removed, **dyspareunia** (painful coitus) and **vaginismus** (spasm of the vagina) may be the result. In addition to estrogen deficiency, there are other physical factors, such as vaginal infections and lesions to name a few, that can lead to dyspareunia and vaginismus. Once these occur, however, the causes then include a psychological anticipation of pain. At that point, the experience of painful coitus and the expectation of further coital discomfort may be hard to separate from the perceived lack of sexual desire. After all, no one, once burned, enjoys even the idea of putting their hand back on the hot stove.

In evaluating a patient with a sexual desire disorder, the physical assessment, including laboratory studies, would be performed before exploring psychological factors, such as emotional factors, life situation, and experiences (Leiblum, 1992; Jensen, 1992; Alexander, 1993; Patterson, 1993). The *DSM-IV* diagnostic criteria for desire phase disorders are shown in "Medical Diagnoses: Sexual Desire Disorders."

Excitement Phase

The excitement phase of the normal human sexual response cycle is that period of time during which sexual tension rises from the preceding level of sexual desire to the relatively high sexual tension levels that merge into

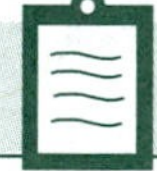

MEDICAL DIAGNOSES Sexual Desire Disorders

***DSM-IV* Diagnosis:** Hypoactive Sexual Desire Disorder

Diagnostic Criteria

A. Persistent or recurrently deficient or absent sexual fantasies and desire for sexual activity.
B. The disturbance causes marked distress or interpersonal difficulty.
C. Occurrence not exclusively during the course of another Axis I disorder (other than a Sexual Dysfunction), such as Major Depression, and is not due exclusively to the direct physiological effects of a substance (drug of abuse or medication) or a general medical condition.

***DSM-IV* diagnosis:** Sexual Aversion Disorder

Diagnostic Criteria

A. Persistent or recurrent extreme aversion to, and avoidance of all, or almost all, genital sexual contact with a sexual partner.
B. The disturbance causes marked distress or interpersonal difficulty.
C. Occurrence not exclusively during the course of another Axis I disorder (other than a Sexual Dysfunction), such as Obsessive-Compulsive Disorder or Major Depression.

Diagnostic criteria from American Psychiatric Association (1994). *Diagnostic and statistical manual of mental disorders, fourth edition.* Washington, D.C.: American Psychiatric Association.

TABLE 34–2 Physiological Changes Accompanying the Normal Excitement Phase

Changes in Women	Changes in Men
Swelling of the vagina	Penile erection
Lubrication of the vagina	Nipple erection (two thirds of men)
Enlargement of the clitoris in diameter	
Nipple erection (two thirds of women) and darkening of the areolae	

the following plateau phase. Traditionally, penile erection and vaginal lubrication have been used as indicators of the presence or development of sexual excitement. If erection or lubrication does not occur in what, for that individual, is a sexually stimulating and appropriate situation, in that instance there has been an inhibition of sexual excitement, regardless of the causative factors. No other valid markers of sexual excitement occur except for the individual's self-report. For example, no physiological way exists to measure whether sexual excitement is experienced by a man who cannot obtain an erection or a woman who cannot become vaginally lubricated.

Finally a few words about the difference in female and male sexual functioning. Pleasure aside, the female vagina can function purely as a physical receptacle for the erect male penis whether or not the woman feels sexual desire or excitement. This difference makes it possible for women to have intercourse without sexual feelings. The man must be able to demonstrate sexual excitement with a penile erection for him to be able to participate in coital activity. This is an absurdly simple but amazingly important difference in sexual functioning that is frequently overlooked or perhaps not fully appreciated. This difference is basic to the understanding of how men and women relate to each other sexually.

The physiological changes that accompany the normal excitement phase are shown in Table 34-2.

The *DSM-IV* diagnostic criteria for excitement phase disorders are shown in "Medical Diagnoses: Sexual Arousal Disorders."

Plateau Phase

As sexual tension continues to escalate, the plateau phase emerges out of the excitement phase at high levels of sexual tension. Sexual tension continues to increase but at a reduced rate until a level of orgasmic inevitability is reached, which marks the onset of the following orgasmic phase. The plateau phase can be understood as a waiting period between the development of sexual excitement and the onset of orgasm, which most people perceive as extremely pleasurable and which sexually competent couples may wish to prolong until orgasm becomes inevitable. The physiological changes that accompany the normal plateau phase are shown in Box 34–2. The *DSM-IV* does not recognize any specific disorders or dysfunctions related primarily to the plateau phase.

Orgasm Phase

The orgasmic phase of the human sexual response cycle is attained only at high levels of sexual tension in both women and men. **Sexual tension** (also described as sexual arousal) is produced by a combination of mental activity, including thought, fantasy and dreams, and erotic stimulation of erogenous areas, which may be more or less specific for each individual. Most men require some penile stimulation and most women some clitoral stimulation, either directly or indirectly, to produce the high levels of sexual tension necessary for orgasm to occur. **Orgasm** may be described purely based on its physical characteristics as a neurophysiological event with accompanying release of erotic tension. Orgasm is considered by most individuals who have experienced that event as being the acme of pleasure. Comparisons have been made of orgasm descriptions made separately by women and by men. When references concerning the gender of the author or of the genitalia being stimulated are removed, it is impossible to determine whether the description was written by a man or by a woman. This suggests either that orgasm is not gender specific, that is, that men and women enjoy a similar sensation, or that it is impossible to describe sensations accurately (Musher, 1990; Lawrence and Madakasira, 1992).

There is at least one major gender difference concerning orgasm: Most women who have experienced one orgasm may have repeated orgasms during the continuation of the same sexual activity. This occurrence depends on the maintenance of high levels of sexual tension through continued stimulation. Men, once they ejaculate as a part of their orgasm, go through a refractory period during which they cannot again ejaculate. The refractory period refers to the time required to produce another ejaculate and varies primarily according to age, with a young man measuring this refractory period in minutes, while an older man may require several hours. **Premature ejaculation** refers to the sudden release of semen with little or no penile stimulation. The inability to sustain high levels of sexual tension without ejaculating can seriously compromise the sexual act as a source of pleasure for both partners. Women, because they do not produce an ejaculate, do not have a comparable refractory period. The normal physiological changes occurring during the orgasm phase are shown in Table 34–3. The *DSM-IV* diagnostic criteria for dysfunctions associated with the orgasm phase are shown in "Medical Diagnoses: Orgasmic Disorders."

MEDICAL DIAGNOSES **Sexual Arousal Disorders**

***DSM-IV* Diagnosis:** Female Sexual Arousal Disorder

Diagnostic Criteria

A. Persistent or recurrent inability to attain or to maintain until completion of the sexual activity an adequate lubrication-swelling response of sexual excitement.
B. The disturbance causes marked distress or interpersonal difficulty.
C. The sexual dysfunction is not better accounted for by another Axis I disorder (except another Sexual Dysfunction) and is not due exclusively to the direct physiological effects of a substance (e.g., a drug of abuse, a medication) or a general medical condition.

***DSM-IV* Diagnosis:** Male Erectile Disorder

Diagnostic Criteria

A. Persistent or recurrent inability to attain or maintain an erection until completion of the sexual activity.
B. The disturbance causes marked distress or interpersonal difficulty.
C. The sexual dysfunction is not better accounted for by another Axis I disorder (except another Sexual Dysfunction) and is not due exclusively to the direct physiological effects of a substance (a drug of abuse, a medication) or a general medical condition.

Diagnostic criteria from American Psychiatric Association (1994). *Diagnostic and statistical manual of mental disorders, fourth edition.* Washington, D.C.: American Psychiatric Association.

BOX 34-2 Physiological Changes Accompanying the Normal Plateau Phase

Increases in muscle tone, heart rate, blood pressure, and respiratory rate
Appearance of a sex flush (in some people), which spreads across the upper body and face and resembles a measles rash without the itch

Resolution Phase

During this phase, sexual tensions developed in prior phases subside to baseline levels presuming that sexual stimulation has ceased. The physiological changes that developed during the earlier phases of the response cycle now tend to dissipate. This is a period of psychological vulnerability and either may be a period of pleasurable "afterglow" or may be described by some as being "uncomfortably emotionally exposed." With the restoration of normal physiological pulse, respiratory rate, and blood pressure, individuals frequently experience markedly increased perspiration. The *DSM-IV* does not recognize any specific resolution phase diagnoses.

▶ Check Your Reading

5. What characterizes the desire phase?
6. What physiological changes occur during orgasm?
7. Define the plateau phase.
8. What are the dysfunctions that can occur during the desire phase?

SEXUAL DYSFUNCTIONS

A few of the sexual dysfunctions are discussed in detail.

Sexual Arousal Dysfunction

Men who experience erectile dysfunction may have feelings of embarrassment, guilt, or anxiety (Case Example 34–2). These psychological stressors may make it difficult for the individual to ask for help. Ego strength in men appears to be closely associated with the ability to perform sexually and to be attractive to the opposite sex. When a man decides to seek treatment for the complaint of erectile dysfunction, which may commonly be referred to as **impotence,** he may not know from which specialist he should seek treatment. If there is a family physician or medical generalist, they might be the first medical professionals that are consulted. Other specialists that are sought out for the treatment of erectile dysfunction include urologists, psychiatrists, psychologists, and sex therapists. In many cases, patients who experience difficulties achieving and maintaining erections may already be in the care of a physician because many medical conditions and their treatments cause or contribute to erectile difficulties.

Case Example 34–2 Bill's Story

Bill is a 46-year-old unemployed salesman who was referred to the inpatient substance abuse program by his family physician. He is complaining of abdominal pain, loss of appetite, and low mood. A full health history revealed a pattern of heavy alcohol consumption over the past four years.

"I feel stressed out all the time," said Bill. "First it was job stress, then marital problems. Sales work is incredibly competitive; quotas and deadlines hang over me all the time. After work, I wind down at the bar and then go home where I have a few more drinks. After a while, our life really began to change. My wife said she felt left out, and the kids said I wasn't fun to be around anymore. When I tried to get close to my wife, I couldn't . . . you know . . . perform, and that made me feel even worse. I feel like such a loser. My wife thinks this program might save our marriage, but I'm afraid that I might not ever be the man I was."

You need to know how to assess a patient's complaint of impotence and should have a clear understanding of your educational role about the sequelae of medical and surgical conditions in regard to sexual functioning. You have a primary responsibility to educate patients about medications and their side effects. For this reason, it is necessary to be informed about and comfortable with the topic of erectile dysfunctions. The patient may not independently introduce the topic of sexual functioning, fearing the discomfort of the discussion. It is incumbent on you to ask questions about sexual functioning in a manner that allows the patient to speak candidly.

When a patient complains of impotence, a full assessment is carried out to determine the nature of the complaint. It is important to understand what the patient means when he says he is impotent. It is useful to have the patient explain what he is experiencing in his own words. If you do not understand the patient's vocabulary, it is important to encourage the patient to describe what happens or does not happen when he tries to perform sexually. Some patients equate impotence with infertility, so it is important to clarify terms throughout the assessment, that is, explaining the difference between inability to achieve and maintain an erection adequate for intercourse and fertility. **Fertility** refers to the viability of the sperm cells and their ability to reach and penetrate the ovum. The patient with erectile dysfunction can father a child through the aid of artificial insemination techniques, if treatment cannot restore functioning.

According to Greenblatt and coworkers (1972), the incidence of impotence increases with age, with 50% of men reporting impotence by the age of 75. Kinsey's research found 27% of white men to be impotent by 75 years of age (Kinsey et al, 1988). Other causes for impotence include medical illness, surgery, injury, anatomical defects, acute infection, medication side effects, and psychological causes. Davidson (1986) states that 50% of patients seen for the complaint of impotence have an organic cause.

Organic causes include prescribed or illicit drug use; acute or chronic medical illness, such as diabetes, hypertension, cardiac disease, infection, or neurological disorders; surgical procedures; structural defects of the genitalia; and hormonal disturbances. In a study of 314 patients with diabetes, 160, or 51%, had a disturbance in sexual functioning (Schoffling, 1980). Another study by Kolodny and colleagues (1980) found 49% of 175 randomly selected male, diabetic patients to be impotent.

When assessing the complaint of impotence, there are several etiologic considerations. A sexual assessment tool, medical and psychiatric history, laboratory studies, and physical examination are used to identify the probable cause of the dysfunction. Treatment is guided by whether the cause is of an organic, psychological, or mixed type.

▶ Check Your Reading

9. Identify three causes of erectile dysfunction.
10. What is the difference between impotence and infertility?
11. What feelings are typically associated with erectile dysfunction?
12. Name three medical conditions associated with impotence.

Anorgasmia

Case Example 34–3 Patricia's Story

Patricia is a 25-year-old, married grade school teacher who has been admitted to an acute care psychiatric unit

TABLE 34–3 Physiological Changes Accompanying the Normal Orgasm Phase

Changes in Women	Changes in Men
A sudden surge of sexual tension	Pooling of seminal fluid in the proximal urethra caused by contractions of the prostate, seminal vesicles, and vas deferens
An equally sudden release of sexual tension	A sensation of ejaculatory inevitability
Simultaneous rhythmic contractions of the uterus, perivaginal muscles, and rectal muscles	Simultaneous contractions of the prostate, the perineal muscles, and the shaft of the penis propel a bolus of semen down the urethra

MEDICAL DIAGNOSES Orgasmic Disorders

***DSM-IV* Diagnosis:** Female Orgasmic Disorder

Diagnostic Criteria

A. Persistent or recurrent delay in, or absence of, orgasm in a woman following a normal sexual excitement phase during sexual activity that the clinician judges to be adequate in focus, intensity, and duration. Some women are able to experience orgasm during noncoital clitoral stimulation but are unable to experience it during coitus in the absence of manual clitoral stimulation. In most of these women, this represents a normal variation of the female sexual response and does not justify the diagnosis. In some of these women, however, this does represent a psychological inhibition that justifies the diagnosis. This difficult judgment is assisted by a thorough sexual evaluation, which may even require a trial of treatment.

B. The disturbance causes marked distress or interpersonal difficulty.

C. The orgasmic dysfunction is not better accounted for by another Axis I disorder (except another Sexual Dysfunction) and is not due exclusively to the direct physiological effects of a substance (e.g., a drug of abuse, a medication) or a general medical condition.

***DSM-IV* Diagnoses** Male Orgasmic Disorder

Diagnostic Criteria

A. Persistent or recurrent delay in, or absence of, orgasm in a man following a normal sexual excitement phase during sexual activity that the clinician, taking into account the person's age, judges to be adequate in focus, intensity, and duration.

B. The disturbance causes marked distress or interpersonal difficulty.

C. The orgasmic dysfunction is not better accounted for by another Axis I disorder (except another Sexual Dysfunction) and is not due exclusively to the direct physiological effects of a substance (e.g., a drug of abuse, a medication) or a general medical condition.

***DSM-IV* Diagnosis:** Premature Ejaculation

Diagnostic Criteria

A. Persistent or recurrent ejaculation with minimal sexual stimulation before, on, or shortly after penetration and before the person wishes it. The clinician must take into account factors that affect the duration of the excitement phase, such as age, novelty of the sexual partner or situation, and frequency of sexual activity.

B. The disturbance causes marked distress or interpersonal difficulty.

C. The premature ejaculation is not due exclusively to the direct effects of a substance (e.g., withdrawal from opioids).

Diagnostic criteria from American Psychiatric Association (1994). *Diagnostic and statistical manual of mental disorders, fourth edition.* Washington, D.C.: American Psychiatric Association.

following an overdose of sedatives. On admission, she reported feeling depressed and generally unhappy with herself. Patricia and her husband of three years do not have children despite a shared desire to become parents. Patricia describes her husband as hard-working, loyal, and affectionate, yet Patricia says that she feels uncomfortable with the intimacy of marriage.

According to Patricia, the marriage was consummated on the wedding night, but Patricia was unable to achieve orgasm at that time or ever since, although she is able to achieve it with self-stimulation. Patricia's perceived inability to share herself intimately left her feeling like a failure as a wife. She increasingly avoided sexual activity, fabricating excuses when the opportunity for sexual intercourse presented itself.

Patricia never talked about her sexual concerns with her husband and had no close friends. Her mother, her closest relative, lived more than 200 miles away.

During the psychiatric assessment, Patricia revealed that she had come from a poor family and was an only child. To make ends meet, her mother worked as a store cashier in the evenings, while her father provided child care. Patricia's father was therefore the one to bathe her and to supervise other bedtime routines.

Patricia recalled that her father had started fondling her genitals while she was still a young child and proceeded to have intercourse with her when she was between the ages of 12 and 14. Patricia says that she initially responded to this abuse with fear that she might be physically harmed. Later, her father threatened to abandon the family if Patricia shared their "secret."

The abuse stopped when Patricia's father was killed suddenly in a car accident. It was the father's insurance money that afforded Patricia the opportunity to go to college and pursue a teaching degree. Patricia never did tell her mother about her father's behavior, thinking that she might be blamed in some way.

As a young adult, Patricia began to feel an intrusive anger toward herself and both of her parents. Patricia hoped that by accepting a marriage proposal, she could get on with her life and put her past behind her.

In this story, Patricia would not have what Masters and Johnson (1970) termed primary orgasmic dysfunction. The diagnosis of primary anorgasmia is used only when the patient has never experienced orgasm, either during intercourse of adequate duration or during masturbation.

Complaints of anorgasmia are not uncommon in patients with a history of sexual abuse. Maltz (1988) observed that incest is commonly identified by many therapists as the primary cause of a host of psychosocial problems, including sexual dysfunction. The degree of emotional distress and the form of the sexual dysfunction vary with the type of sexual abuse, that is to say, which body parts were fondled and whether there was penetration. Factors that affect the patient's resilience after the abuse include age, maturity, coping skills, personality traits, supportive relationships, the duration and frequency of abuse, and degree of violence. Therapy involves helping the patient to deal with guilt, anger, low self-esteem, helplessness, and trust. Maltz (1988) believes that the final stage of treatment should focus on resolving the negative feelings directed at the abuser. She suggests that the patient confront the abuser directly, through face-to-face contact or by letter or indirectly through an unmailed letter or in therapeutic role playing. Box 34–3 provides guidelines for helping a patient to disclose incest.

Anorgasmia is usually psychogenic in origin, although there can be a physiological basis, such as fatigue, acute illness, medication, decreased perineal musculature, or neurological and vascular conditions. Psychological factors that affect orgasmic potential include societal mores as they relate to women's sexual roles, family attitudes, childhood experiences, sex education or lack of it, and religious beliefs.

The evaluation of anorgasmia includes the patient's medical and psychiatric history, sexual history including current pattern of sexual functioning, physical examination, and laboratory studies. The sexual pattern of functioning includes questions about the use of foreplay before coitus and the duration of coitus. Women require a longer period of time to become fully aroused to achieve orgasm. Therefore, it is important to ascertain if one or both partners would benefit from sex education. The nonsexual aspects of the relationship with the sexual partner also affect their ability to enjoy intimacy; therefore, the relationship itself should be explored. Discord or displeasure with a partner has a physiologically inhibiting quality. Likewise, unresolved psychological conflict may continue to intrude on sexual functioning.

Treatment of anorgasmia by trained professionals includes psychoanalysis, psychoanalytically oriented psychotherapy, and behavior modification. For patients who

BOX 34-3 Guidelines for Helping a Patient to Disclose Incest

Responding to Patient Needs During Counseling

Reassure the patient that
- You believe and do not blame the patient
- The responsibility for incest belongs with the offender
- The patient did the best she could to survive the circumstances
- As a child, she was not in control of the situation
- The details of the counseling will remain confidential
- Victims of incest are "survivors" and recover from their victimization
- Patients can get over their feelings of shame
- Your feelings toward the patient will not change as a result of hearing about the incest

Encourage and validate that
- The patient may temporarily feel worse about disclosure before starting to feel better
- The patient has the right to feel anger and grief
- The patient has the right to have positive feelings toward the offender
- The patient did not deserve the abuse
- The patient is making gains despite how small the gains seem
- The patient is an important and intelligent person
- You see the patient's coping mechanisms as "survivor skills" and adaptive

Addressing Incest During Counseling

Elicit disclosure by
- Asking directly if sexual abuse occurred during childhood
- Using a structured questionnaire, such as an intake form, to receive a complete early sexual history
- Mentioning that the symptoms that the patient is describing have been related to histories of sexual abuse in other patients
- Defining incest for the patient
- Asking about best and worst experiences during childhood
- Being persistent in probing histories of sexual abuse

Once disclosure takes place
- Identify incest as a primary cause of the patient's difficulties
- Acknowledge and validate the significance of the incest
- Relate specific difficulties in adult life to coping skills developed to survive incest
- Do not minimize incest even if it occurred infrequently
- Encourage the patient to be fully aware of her own reactions to hearing about incest

Reprinted from Josephson, Fong-Beyette (1987). Factors assisting female clients' disclosure of incest during counseling. *Journal of Counseling and Development, 65*, pp. 475–478.

are diagnosed as having primary anorgasmia, masturbation therapy can be an effective adjunct to traditional modes of treatment. Cognitive therapies may be helpful, and in many cases, sex education is used to correct misinformation.

Sex education is in the domain of nursing and can take the form of didactic teaching, dispelling myths, facilitated discussion, charts, anatomical models, or other audio-visual aids. Other methods to assist the patient to cope with sexual dysfunction can take the form of values clarification, conflict resolution, roleplaying, communication skills, and, in some cases, relaxation techniques.

You also identify the stage of psychosocial development in which the patient seems to be stalled. In the case of Patricia, childhood sexual abuse resulted in difficulties in trust. A review of Erikson's stages of psychosocial development may be helpful in understanding what the patient is experiencing (see Chapters 6 and 8). You reassure the patient that these psychological issues do not resolve overnight and may take patience over time to be resolved. You facilitate the patient's receptivity to exploring sexual issues and support the patient during periods of crisis. Increasing the patient's ability to cope with stress is a critical component of the nursing care plan. It is important to include both the patient and the partner in some, but not necessarily all, sessions because sexual functioning is a shared problem.

If you are providing care to the patient complaining of anorgasmia, you need to be a good listener. Sexual problems are usually difficult to discuss, so the slow-paced interview allows time for the patient's story to unfold. Care of the anorgasmic patient involves sensitivity, emotional support, and encouragement. You can act as a resource person by offering to make referrals to other health care professionals.

▶ Check Your Reading

13. What is primary anorgasmia?
14. What is secondary anorgasmia?
15. What is the most common cause of primary orgasmia?
16. What are two interventions used to treat anorgasmia?

SEXUAL DISORDERS

People do not decide voluntarily what arouses them sexually. Rather, in maturing, they discover the nature of their own sexual orientation and interests. Individuals differ from one another in terms of

- The types of partners whom they find to be erotically appealing
- The types of behaviors that they find to be erotically stimulating

They also differ in intensity of sexual drive, in the degree of difficulty that they experience in trying to resist sexual temptations, and in their attitudes about whether or not such temptations should be resisted. The sexual disorders include many forms of **paraphilia,** a term used to identify repetitive or preferred sexual fantasies or behaviors that involve preference for use of a nonhuman object, repetitive sexual activity with humans involving real or simulated suffering or humiliation, and repetitive sexual activity with nonconsenting partners. Most paraphiliacs are men, and about 50% of those individuals develop the onset of their paraphilic arousal before age 18.

Paraphilias

There are eight distinct types of paraphilias (Table 34-4). The *DSM-IV* diagnostic criteria for paraphilias are shown in "Medical Diagnoses and Related Nursing Diagnosis: Paraphilias."

Cause

Case Example 34–4 illustrates how paraphilias manifested in two patients, Michael and Steve. There are a number of explanations for the causes of paraphilias (Brown, 1983). Various studies have implicated biological factors. These factors include abnormalities in the limbic system and temporal lobes of the brain. Abnormal levels of androgens have also been implicated. Kafka (1991) categorized sexual disorders of nonparaphilic men as well as paraphilic men as being reflective of sexual dysregulation disorders associated with a primary mood disorder. The psychoanalytical explanation is that the individual failed to resolve the oedipal crisis and identifies with the parent of the opposite gender or selects an inappropriate object for libido focus. The behavioral model hypothesizes that whether the individual participates in paraphilic behavior or not depends on the type of reinforcement he receives following the behavior. The first act may be committed for a variety of reasons (e.g., modeling the paraphilic behavior of others, mimicking sexual behavior depicted in the media). But once the initial act has been committed, a conscious evaluation of the behavior occurs, and a decision is made of whether or not to repeat it. The last model to posit causative explanation is the transactional model of stress adaption. This model suggests that most likely the cause of pharaphilias is influenced by multiple factors.

Case Example 34–4 The Stories of Two Paraphiliacs

Michael's Story

Michael is a 26-year-old single white man who has reported an eight-year history of exhibitionistic behavior

TABLE 34–4 Types of Paraphilias

Type of Paraphilia	Definition/Characteristics
Exhibitionism	Characterized by recurrent, intense, sexual urges and sexually arousing fantasies involving the exposure of one's genitals to a stranger
Fetishism	Involves recurrent, intense sexual urges and sexually arousing fantasies involving the use of nonliving objects (e.g., bras, underpants, stockings)
Frotteurism	A recurrent preoccupation with intense sexual urges or fantasies involving touching or rubbing against a nonconsenting person
Pedophilia	Involves recurrent sexual urges and sexually arousing fantasies involving sexual activity with a prepubescent child
Masochism	Involves recurrent, intense sexual urges and sexually arousing fantasies involving the act (real or simulated) of being humiliated, beaten, bound, or otherwise made to suffer
Sadism	Involves recurrent, intense sexual urges and sexually arousing fantasies involving the act (real or simulated) of inflicting psychological or physical suffering (including humiliation) on someone else
Transvestic fetishism	A persistent association in a heterosexual man, lasting a total of at least 6 mo, between intense sexual arousal or desire and acts, fantasies, or other stimuli involving cross-dressing
Voyeurism	Involves recurrent, intense sexual urges and sexually arousing fantasies involving the act of observing unsuspecting people, usually strangers, who are naked, in the process of disrobing, or engaging in sexual activity
Paraphilia not otherwise specified (NOS)	Paraphilias that do not meet the criteria for any of the specific categories
Telephone scatologia	A desire to place obscene phone calls
Necrophilia	A sexual attraction to corpses
Partialism	An exclusive sexual focus on parts of the body
Zoophilia	A sexual attraction to animals
Coprophilia	A sexual focus on feces
Klismaphilia	A sexual focus on enemas
Urophilia	A sexual focus on urine

From American Psychiatric Association (1994). *Diagnostic and statistical manual of mental disorders, fourth edition.* Washington, DC: American Psychiatric Association.

that increased at times of stress, anger, and depression. His sexual fantasies focus on power, dominance, and exposing himself. When Michael is not exposing himself, he spends hours driving around bus stops and masturbating while making verbal remarks to women waiting for buses.

Steve's Story

Steve is a 30-year-old single African-American man who has reported a compulsion that he has had since early adolescence: to view photographs of young boys between the ages of 11 and 15 and to masturbate while viewing these pictures. While masturbating, he would fantasize about oral-genital sexual activity as well as anal penetration. He also describes urges to rub against young boys while in swimming pools or at sporting events. He reports that he engages in these fantasies and behaviors at least four times a week or when the opportunity presents itself.

Treatment

The treatment is effected by the explanatory model for paraphilias. For example, a biological model might include blocking or decreasing the level of circulating androgens or treating with an antidepressant such as fluoxetine (Prozac) or a mood stabilizer such a lithium (Kafka, 1991). The psychoanalytic model would assist the patient to identify unresolved conflicts and traumas from early childhood, thus resolving the anxiety that prevents him or her from forming appropriate sexual relationships. In the behaviorist model, the patient would be subjected to aversion techniques, such as the use of electric shock and chemical induction of nausea and vomiting in combination with exposure to photographs depicting the undesired behavior. These techniques have been successfully used to modify the undesirable behavior of the paraphiliac.

▶ Check Your Reading

17. What is a paraphilia?

18. Name three of the eight different types of paraphilias.
19. State two possible causative explanations for the paraphilias.
20. What treatment is used for the paraphilias when the cause is considered to be physiological?

Gender Identity Disorder

Childhood and adolescent gender identity disorders have four main characteristics (American Psychiatric Association, 1994). First, the person has a strong and persistent cross-gender identification. This identification is not merely a desire for any perceived cultural advantages of being the other sex. In children, this cross-gender identification is manifested by four or more of the following:

- A repeatedly stated desire to be, or insistence that he or she is, the opposite sex
- In boys, a preference for cross-dressing or simulating female attire; in girls, an insistence on wearing only stereotypically masculine clothing
- Strong, persistent preferences for cross-sex roles in make-believe play or persistent fantasies of being the opposite sex
- An intense desire to participate in the stereotypical games and pastimes of the opposite sex
- A strong preference for playmates of the opposite sex

In adolescents and adults, this cross-gender identification is manifested by statements of a desire to be the opposite sex, frequent masquerading as the opposite sex, a desire to live or be treated as the opposite sex, and the conviction that they have the typical feelings and reactions of the opposite sex. Second, the person has persistent discomfort with her or his sex or a sense of inappropriateness in the gender role of that sex. In children, this persistent discomfort with one's sex is manifested by any of the following:

- In boys, assertions that their penis or testes are disgusting or will disappear or that it would be better not to have a penis; aversion to rough-and-tumble play; and rejection of stereotypically male toys, games, and activities
- In girls, rejection of urinating in a sitting position, assertions that they will grow a penis, assertions that they do not want to grow breasts or menstruate, and marked aversion toward normative female clothing

This persistent discomfort with one's sex is manifested by preoccupation with getting rid of primary and secondary sex characteristics (e.g., requests for hormones, surgery, or other procedures to alter sexual characteristics physically to simulate the other sex) or by the belief that they were born the wrong sex. Third, the disturbance is not concurrent with a physical intersex condition. Finally, the disturbance causes clinically significant distress or impairment in social, occupational, or other important areas of functioning.

MEDICAL DIAGNOSES AND RELATED NURSING DIAGNOSIS — Paraphilias

***DSM-IV* Diagnosis:** Pedophilia

Diagnostic Criteria:

A. Over a period of at least six months, recurrent, intense sexually arousing fantasies, sexual urges, or behaviors involving sexual activity with a prepubescent child or children (generally age 13 years or younger.)
B. The fantasies, sexual urges, or behaviors cause clinically significant distress or impairment in social, occupational, or other important areas of functioning.
C. The person is at least 16 years old and at least five years older than the child or children in criterion A.

RELATED NURSING DIAGNOSIS	DEFINITION	EXAMPLE
Altered Sexuality Patterns	The state in which an individual expresses concern regarding his or her sexuality.	Altered Sexuality Patterns related to conflict with preference of partner; knowledge/skill deficit about alternative responses to health-related transitions; altered body function or structure; illness or medical condition; lack of privacy; lack of significant other; ineffective or absent role models; conflicts with sexual orientation; fear of pregnancy or of acquiring a sexually transmitted disease; impaired relationship with a significant other.

Diagnostic criteria from American Psychiatric Association (1994). *Diagnostic and statistical manual of mental disorders, fourth edition.* Washington, D.C.: American Psychiatric Association; nursing diagnoses and definitions from North American Nursing Diagnosis Association (1994). *NANDA nursing diagnoses: Definitions and classification 1995–1996.* Philadelphia: NANDA.

▶ **Check Your Reading**
21. Identify two characteristics of childhood gender identity disorder.
22. Identify two characteristics of adolescent gender identity disorder.
23. Identify two characteristics of adult gender identity disorder.

HOMOSEXUALITY

Homosexuality is defined as sexual or erotic attraction to members of one's own sex. There are two types of homosexuality: obligatory and situational. In obligatory homosexuality, erotic and sexual desires are uniformly directed toward members of the same sex. In situational homosexuality, erotic and sexual desires are directed toward members of the same sex only in certain situations (for example, long-term confinement in same-sex institutions such as prison).

Much controversy exists over whether homosexuality is a normal variant of human sexuality or whether it is a gender disorder. Although the percentage of people with a homosexual orientation in any population is difficult to determine, sexual activity between people of the same sex has occurred throughout history and across regional, national, social, and cultural boundaries. It occurs in animals as well as humans. Although homosexual expression of human sexuality has been considered normal and acceptable in various times, places, and cultures, it has nevertheless been considered inappropriate by much of society through the ages. Throughout history, religious leaders, legislators, and society at large have therefore sought to eliminate sexual activity between people of the same sex.

To date, psychiatry, biomedical science, religion, government, and society as a whole still have not come to terms with whether sexual activity between people of the same sex is a normal variant of human sexuality, a manifestation of a gender disorder, or a moral problem (see Chapter 42 for further discussion of this issue). In 1974, however, the Board of Trustees of the American Psychiatric Association decided to label homosexuality a gender disorder only when the homosexuality is ego-dystonic. That is, homosexuality would be considered a gender disorder only when a person's homosexual orientation causes him or her marked distress.

A number of theories exist about why some people develop a homosexual orientation. Some medical researchers believe that intrauterine levels of sex steroids may play a role. They believe that the androgen levels to which a fetus is exposed in utero may affect not only the anatomical differentiation of males and females, but also psychosexual orientation. There is also some preliminary research to indicate a tendency for homosexual orientation to be inherited genetically.

Some subscribe to a psychodynamic explanation of homosexuality. Freud (1978) wrote that homosexuality represents an arrested level of psychosexual development. "Homosexuality," wrote Freud, "is assuredly no advantage, but nothing to be ashamed of, no vice, no degradation; it cannot be classified as an illness: we consider it to be a variation of the sexual functions produced by a certain arrest of sexual development." Freud considered heterosexual development to be the positive outcome of resolution of the oedipal conflict.

Bieber (1962) suggested a dysfunctional family pattern as the underlying factor leading to homosexuality in males. According to Bieber, the typical mother of a boy who grows up with a homosexual orientation dominates both father and son; is overprotective, possessive, and seductive in her interactions with her son; and is demeaning toward the father. The typical father of a boy who grows up with a homosexual orientation, according to Bieber, is passive, distant, and a covertly or overtly hostile figure in the boy's life.

Because the medical profession and society as a whole have not reached definitive conclusions about whether homosexual orientation is a valid lifestyle alternative, a psychiatric illness, or a moral issue, you will encounter many different approaches to helping patients with a homosexual orientation.

For those mental health professionals who see a homosexual orientation as a normal variant of human sexuality, therapeutic efforts likely focus on helping patients to deal with the social stigma associated with homosexual behavior, exploring psychological conflicts, helping patients foster healthy relationships, teaching patients how to avoid infection with HIV and other sexually transmitted organisms, and generally facilitating the efforts of patients to live emotionally satisfying lives (Saghir and Robins, 1978).

For those mental health professionals who see a homosexual orientation as a gender disorder, therapeutic efforts are aimed at exploring the root causes of the patient's sexual orientation and working with the patient to modify deeply ingrained feelings and behaviors.

Regardless of how a homosexual orientation develops, and regardless of whether homosexuality is a normal variant or a gender disorder, many patients with a homosexual orientation come to therapy bearing a heavy load of pain. The person with a homosexual orientation frequently experiences profound shame and well-justified fears of stigmatization and hostility and sometimes even physical harm. As a nurse, it is vital that you demonstrate compassion in the face of such pain. Such compassion is at the core of a theistic world view, and it is the hallmark of the profession of mental health nursing.

▶ **Check Your Reading**
24. What is obligatory homosexuality?
25. What is situational homosexuality?
26. Discuss the biological theory of homosexuality.
27. According to Bieber, what role does the mother play in the development of male homosexuality?
28. What are the usual goals of treatment when homosexuals seek therapy?

OTHER SEXUAL PROBLEMS

Sexual problems can also result from head trauma, chromosomal abnormalities, and psychosis.

Sexual Problems Resulting from Head Trauma

Patients who have experienced head trauma with damage to the frontal lobe of the brain may display symptoms of promiscuity, poor judgment, inability to recognize triggers that set off sexual desires, and poor impulse control.

Sexual Problems Resulting from Chromosomal Abnormalities

Klinefelter's syndrome, a condition that is found on genetic examination, occurs when instead of the normal XY genetic coding for male gender, the patient has an extra X as his genetic makeup. These patients frequently present with immature genitalia and not uncommonly have schizophrenic symptoms.

Sexual Problems Resulting from Psychosis

Sexual functioning may be adversely affected any time there is a disturbance in an individual's ability to develop and maintain stable relationships. This is especially true for schizophrenic patients, who have difficulty coping with stress, a decrease in reality-based orientation to the world, and defense mechanisms that lead to withdrawn behavior (Case Example 34–5).

Case Example 34–5 Josephine's Story

Josephine has been admitted for inpatient psychiatric care after treatment on a medical unit for injuries sustained when she was struck by a car while wandering in the street. Josephine is well-known to the staff and has had many previous admissions to stabilize her schizophrenia. Referral to a community mental health center had been only partially successful, in that Josephine did not return for treatment after the last discharge. She had been doing fairly well until three weeks before the automobile accident, when her purse containing her medication was stolen. Instead of going to the health center to get a new prescription, she went to a bar and drank heavily. This pattern continued for three weeks, during which time the auditory hallucinations that Josephine had experienced in the past returned.

Josephine has been hearing a male voice telling her she was God's gift to men. These hallucinations, coupled with the effects of her heavy alcohol intake, led her into promiscuous behavior, soliciting sex with men in bars and proclaiming that she was doing "the Lord's work." Josephine's behavior put her into conflict with bar owners, and frequently she was asked to leave. On the night of the accident, after such an episode, Josephine ran out of the bar and into the street and was hit by a passing car. She fell to the pavement complaining of leg pain. An ambulance brought her to the hospital, and x-rays showed that her leg was not broken. She was fully conscious and oriented but had no recall of the accident. The mental status examination revealed auditory hallucinations consisting of commands to share herself with men and become "the mother of the Earth."

A review of Josephine's prior admissions showed that fluphenazine (Prolixin) was effective in controlling her symptoms of schizophrenia. A treatment plan was formulated to begin Josephine on oral fluphenazine and later change to fluphenazine decanoate (administered intramuscularly) to ensure better compliance. Hospital staff contacted the mental health center that would follow up on Josephine's progress, and the center approved of the plan. Josephine accepted the plan because she was afraid that she would come to harm again and because she trusted the staff.

The challenge to the nursing staff was to prevent Josephine from engaging in inappropriate sexual behavior while the hallucinations were still present. To facilitate this goal, female nurses cared for Josephine whenever possible. When male nurses had to care for Josephine, they set limits with her when she became seductive. Another intervention to reduce the risk of inappropriate sexual behavior was to place Josephine in a room closer to the nurse's station, for closer monitoring. If these measures were not adequate, Josephine would be placed on close observation status (one nurse assigned to stay near Josephine at all times).

The policy on the unit was to have the hall monitored during the night so that patients did not have access to the rooms of other patients. Additionally, all patients were informed on admission that visiting in the rooms of other patients was not allowed. The unit rule also stated that physical contact between patients was against policy and would result in discharge.

Because Josephine's sexually inappropriate behavior was driven by her command hallucinations, the staff expected that as the hallucinations resolved, the behavior would stop. Because compliance with an oral medication regimen had been a problem for Josephine, the staff expected that the change in the form of Josephine's medication would result in improved compliance.

Other issues of concern to the nurses were the patient's lack of "safer sex" practices, her lack of use of birth control, her lack of information about sex, and her need for screening for sexually transmitted diseases. At a point when Josephine was able to hold a conversation free from the effects of her thought disorder, the staff initiated discussions with her about these issues. They provided Josephine with a referral to the gynecology clinic while she was still an inpatient.

The last issue of concern to the nurses was Josephine's self-esteem. As Josephine's symptoms abated, the behaviors that she had exhibited during her illness were a source of great embarrassment to her. The nurses responded to Josephine's embarrassment by being supportive, by being good listeners, and by encouraging her. The nurses frequently reminded Josephine that her behaviors were symptoms of an illness—not manifestations of a character weakness.

The schizophrenic patient's sexual drive may be altered only during the acute phase of illness or it may be of an ongoing nature. This could depend partially on the severity of the illness. Additionally, patients with chronic schizophrenia have difficulty communicating their needs and concerns to others. For the schizophrenic patient, self-concept and ego strength deteriorate over time, further decreasing the patient's ability to develop or maintain intimate relationships.

Schizophrenia is not necessarily associated with sexual dysfunction or deviant sexual behavior, but the symptoms of schizophrenia and even the treatment with neuroleptic medications (Patterson, 1993) may make the patient vulnerable to disturbances in sexual functioning and often childlike and passive in relationships. The primary goal of the treatment team in the patient psychiatric setting is the control of acute symptoms. Sometimes the acute symptoms present as delusions. These delusions can be sexual in form, or they can be of a paranoid type that drives the patient away from meaningful relationships and produces a sexual problem from the resulting alienation. Delusions may also be of a grandiose nature in that the patient may believe himself or herself to be a great lover or have a "special mission" of a sexual nature.

Sexually inappropriate or dangerous behaviors that are of a delusional origin are noted during the initial psychiatric assessment. Even if the patient does not initially share these thoughts, they could emerge later in treatment as you develop rapport with the patient. Most patients respond to treatment with neuroleptic medications, and the inappropriate sexual behaviors resolve as the delusion subsides. Conversely the patient who does not have delusions primarily of a sexual nature may, in the course of the hospitalization, be willing to discuss issues of daily living that might include relationships and sexuality. A third type of patient would be the schizophrenic who is admitted for control of acute symptoms but who additionally has a sexual problem that is not associated with the primary diagnosis. This problem may be detected by the patient's self-report, the physician's physical examination, or the nursing assessment.

Some sexual problems require immediate interventions, such as alleviating the sexual symptoms caused by side effects of medications or controlling inappropriate sexual behavior. Other sexual problems are better managed through interventions as identified in the long-term goals. These might include helping the schizophrenic to develop social skills that increase the probability of forming relationships. This may be accomplished by referring the patient to a psychosocial rehabilitation program. Some sexual problems can be remedied by achieving short-term goals that use education as a nursing intervention. Frequently, sexual myths and misinformation can be corrected, giving the patient almost instant relief from perceived problems. For instance, some people continue to believe that there is a connection between masturbation and becoming "crazy." All patients can benefit from an assessment of their sexual knowledge. Sexual hygiene, methods of birth control, and sexual health are important issues, as is the patient's understanding of sexual anatomy and physiology. Although these topics may not be the initial focus of nursing interventions, they become important at some point in the course of the hospitalization. You assess the patient's sexual functioning and offer information when indicated. All patients on a psychiatric inpatient unit should be informed on admission about unit rules regarding personal contact between patients and between patients and staff. Limit setting is done consistently when indicated.

▶ Check Your Reading

29. What is the connection between head trauma and sexual problems?
30. What impact does psychotic behavior have on sexuality?
31. What is Klinefelter's syndrome?

YOUR RESPONSE TO SEXUAL DISORDERS AND OTHER SEXUAL ISSUES

When making judgments regarding sexual behavior, it is important for you to appreciate the state of mind that contributed to the individual's behavior. Inappropriate sexual behaviors can occur for a variety of reasons. For example, a person with schizophrenia may behave in a particular way in response to hallucinations, whereas the alcoholic's behavior may be a reflection of diminished judgment secondary to intoxication. A mentally retarded individual may become involved with a child (who may be of the same approximate mental age as he) because of the lack of availability of adult partners and the lack of capacity to appreciate and understand fully the wrongful nature of his actions.

It is also important when discussing sexual deviations to differentiate between an individual's sexual orientation and interest and the individual's temperament and traits of character, such as kindness versus cruelty, caring versus uncaring, sensitivity versus insensitivity, conscientiousness versus lacking in conscience, and so on. Imagine the emotional and spiritual distress experienced by a pedophile who is unhappy with his sexual orientation. A person diagnosed with a sexual disorder may be a more concerned person dealing less than successfully with sexual temptations of a sort that are foreign to most individuals.

It is easy for a nonsmoker to argue that any smoker could stop if he or she really wanted to; in the case of the pregnant smoker, if not for her own sake, then surely for the sake of not damaging her unborn child. It is easy for a nonobese person to argue that successful dieting can be accomplished through willpower alone. Similarly, it is easy for a person who is not tempted by inappropriate sexual thoughts or behaviors to argue that any sex offender could have stopped the behavior if he really wanted to and would simply make up his mind to do so. When it comes to appetites or drives, such as hunger, thirst, pain, the need for sleep, or sex, however, biological regulatory systems may exist that can cause an individual to experience desires to satisfy those hungers in ways that cannot be successfully resisted by willpower alone. People can become so discomforted by cravings related to such appetites that they feel compelled to act in ways that diminish their discomfort.

When a person falls deeply in love with another person, be it a child or an adult, it becomes easy for that person to convince himself or herself that the relationship is good and healthy and not harmful or wrong. One of the major issues in trying to understand human behavior relates to where the line should be drawn between considering a person to be the passive product of life experiences and biological make-up and considering him or her (by virtue of having subjective consciousness) to be an active agent capable of transcending prior determinants.

NURSING PROCESS

ASSESSMENT

Caring for patients with sexual complaints requires that you are proficient in the science as well as the art of the profession. Sexual issues are assessed scientifically by understanding the biological process of the reproductive system. The manner in which you develop a helping relationship with the patient is more akin to an art in that it is tempered by compassion and empathy.

The sexual assessment includes both subjective and objective data. Many psychiatric hospitals use a nursing history tool that is biologically oriented but may have a few questions on sexual functioning. Health history questions pertaining to the reproductive system may be limited to menstrual history, parity, history of sexually transmitted diseases, method of contraception, and questions regarding "safer" sex practices. There may be some vague questions about sexual functioning or sexual concerns. You may be uncomfortable exploring sexual issues with your patients for fear that you or the patient will be embarrassed or that you will not know what questions to ask or why you should ask them. Patients themselves may sense your discomfort with the topic, or they might also be uncomfortable when discussing sexual issues.

There are many tools available for conducting a sexual assessment that can supplement the basic health history, but forms and tools in themselves are impersonal and do not provide a good format for dialogue. An awareness of the content of a complete sexual assessment tool may, however, give you a fuller appreciation of the scope of questions to be asked and acquaint you with a conceptual framework. In psychiatric hospitals that provide care to patients that come specifically for the treatment of sexual disorders, an assessment tool that evaluates sexual dysfunction or deviation is useful for the systematic collection of data for research purposes. The GRISS Questionnaire (female or male version) is frequently used to evaluate sexual dysfunctions. It is also helpful as a method of orienting new staff to the assessment process. See the Appendix for female and male versions of the GRISS Questionnaire.

Guidelines for Conducting a Sexual Assessment

The sexual history captures not only the patient's physiological functioning, but also behavioral, emotional, and spiritual aspects of sexuality. It also includes cultural and religious beliefs in regard to sexual behavior and sexual knowledge base. During the assessment, both you and the patient are free to ask questions and to clarify information. It is reasonable to defer lengthy sexual health assessment when acute psychiatric symptoms preclude a calm, thoughtful discussion. As symptoms subside and rapport is developed, the assessment may be resumed. With experience, you will be able to identify those patients that are at a greater risk for difficulties in sexual functioning. Key indicators might include patients with a history of medical problems such as diabetes, multiple sclerosis, history of myocardial infarction, Parkinson's disease, epilepsy, or surgical procedures (Walbroehl, 1992; Aass et al, 1993; Corney et al, 1993; Meyer-Bahlburg et al, 1993); those requiring maintenance medications (Balon et al, 1993); or those patients that are experiencing relationship difficulties. Table 34–5 lists drugs known to have side effects that can disturb sexual function.

The initial sexual assessment may be a basic screening to detect areas of concern. It should be incorporated into the general physical assessment, which includes questions of a demographic nature, such as age, sex, marital status, religion, and educational level. The review of systems may reveal medical diagnoses that could have an impact on sexual functioning. The reproductive history is a logical place in history taking to introduce nonthreatening questions of a sexual nature. In the psychiatric setting, many patients have illnesses that prevent them from developing relationships, yet they still have a need for

TABLE 34–5 **Drugs Known to Have Side Effects That Can Disturb Sexual Function**

Drug	Effect on Sexual Function
Antianxiety	Decreased libido
Anticholinergics	Erectile dysfunction
Antidepressants	
Tricyclics	Decreased libido
MAO inhibitors	Ejaculation difficulties Erectile dysfunction
Selective serotonin re-uptake inhibitors	Decreased libido Erectile dysfunction
Antihistamines	Decreased libido Erectile dysfunction
Antihypertensives	
Diuretics	Erectile dysfunction
Centrally acting sympatholytics	Decreased libido Erectile dysfunction
Alpha- and beta-adrenergic blockers	Erectile dysfunction Ejaculation difficulties
Ganglion blockers	Erectile dysfunction Ejaculation difficulties
Sympathetic nerve terminal agents	Decreased libido Erectile dysfunction Ejaculation difficulties
Nonadrenergic vasodilators	Decreased libido Erectile dysfunction
Antipsychotics	
Phenothiazines	Decreased libido Erectile dysfunction Ejaculation difficulties
Butyrophenones	Erectile dysfunction Decreased libido
Narcotics	Decreased libido Erectile dysfunction Ejaculation difficulties
Cocaine	Decreased libido Ejaculation difficulties
Alcohol	Decreased libido Erectile dysfunction Ejaculation difficulties
Sedative-hypnotics	Decreased libido Erectile dysfunction Ejaculation difficulties
Marijuana	Decreased libido Erectile dysfunction
Amphetamines	Erectile dysfunction Ejaculation difficulties

Data from *The Johns Hopkins Medical Journal,* 151(4), 1982, *The Medical Letter* 25(641), 73–76, 1983.

sexual expression. If there appears to be an indication for a fuller assessment, you may want to use a complete sexual assessment tool (such as the GRISS Questionnaire) as a reference from which to compile a more patient-specific interview. The complete assessment includes questions about the patient's family, relationship between the parents, acquisition of sexual information (both formal and informal), gender roles, toilet training history, and attitudes about sexuality and sexual expression.

An important issue to explore is the relationship of spirituality or religious belief to sexuality. An individual may experience acute spiritual distress related to his or her choice of sexual expression. This distress may originate in religious dogma or tenets of moral behavior. Imagine the spiritual distress of a prominent religious leader accused of being a pedophile. The significance and meaning of sexuality to the individual is far-reaching and is as important to understanding the individual's journey as the physical and psychological aspects of the assessment.

Settings for a Sexual Assessment

When you conduct a sexual interview, provide a setting that allows for privacy and an absence of distractions. Although note taking may be necessary for the beginner, it can be distracting to the patient and interrupt the flow of the interview. When necessary, it should be kept brief and unobtrusive. When you master the content of the sexual assessment, the questions will flow in a logical sequence. You conduct the interview free from personal biases and judgmental attitudes that would impede open discussion of sexual issues. Body language communicates openness and receptivity. Good eye contact, relaxed posture, and friendly facial expressions facilitate the patient's comfort.

Conducting the Interview

First introduce yourself to the patient and then explain the purpose of the sexual assessment. Inform the patient that confidentiality is strictly maintained. Questions should proceed from least intrusive to more intrusive. The interview should be efficient but not hurried. A directive approach can be used for data gathering that is less personal, whereas a less directive approach provides more information by allowing the patient to express feelings and beliefs freely. Accepted medical terminology should be used when discussing sexual issues, but you must also have knowledge of commonly used slang expressions to understand what the patient is saying. In the process of using medically correct terminology, the patient-nurse therapeutic relationship is maintained, and the patient learns a way of communicating that is less embarrassing. Table 34–6 presents some common slang expressions related to sexuality and their corresponding medical terms. You may find it helpful to share this information with patients.

TABLE 34–6 Some Common Slang Expressions Related to Sexuality

Medical Term	Slang Expression(s)
Breasts	Tits, sacks, front, headlights, knockers, boobs, bosom, bonkers, bust, jugs, buds
Climax	Come, go off, shoot cream, blast off
Clitoris	Bed fellow, little gem, badge of shame, gaiety, madness, narrow strip
Cunnilingus	Eating it, going down, eating pussy
Erection	Hard on, stiff, bone, boner, hot rocks, lover's nuts
Fellatio	Going down, sucking, blowing, getting a blow job, giving head, cocksucking
Homosexual	*Male:* Fairy, fag, faggot, gay, queen, nellie, homo, swish, pervert, pansy, back door artist *Female:* Lez, sister, lesbo, dyke, bull dyke
Hymen	Cherry, membrane, maidenhead
Impotence	Couldn't get it up, couldn't get a hard-on
Intercourse, coitus	Make love, screw, fuck, get down, ball, make it, get laid, mess around, score, bang, jive, frig, get a piece, sleep with, get some tail, hook up
Masturbation	Jack off, jerk off, pocket pod, hand fuck, circle jerk, beat the meat, hand job
Menstruation	Curse, monthly period, devil's making ketchup, red-bearded cousin from the south, the flag's up, on the rag
Mutual oral-genital stimulation	Sixty-nine
Orgasm	Come, climax
Penis	Joystick, worm, dick, prick, stick, peter, rod, john, third leg, middle leg, joint, glans, cock, organ, thing
Pubic hair	Beaver, bush, pubes
Semen	Come, juice, egg white, gizzum
Sexual choice	Straight (heterosexual), gay (homosexual), AC-DC (bisexual)
Sexual desire	Horny, cold fish (decreased libido), nympho (increased libido)
Testes	Balls, nuts
Vagina	Pussy, hole, cunt, cat, pocketbook, treasure, twat, furburger, box, beaver, snatch, tunnel

Adapted from Green, R. (1975). *Human sexuality: A practitioner's text.* Baltimore: Williams & Wilkins.

Throughout the interview, it is important to note the patient's body language. Decreased eye contact, fidgeting, turning away from the interviewer, and hesitancy in answering questions may indicate an area of concern for the patient. Box 34–4 lists patient cues that may indicate concerns about sexuality.

At this point, you may choose to ask the patient if there is discomfort in the area of sexual functioning. Generally, it is more comfortable for the patient first to be asked questions in a general manner and then to proceed to the patient's experience. For example: "Some people who are prescribed this medication find it difficult to achieve an erection. Have you had this problem?" This allows the patient to feel that he or she is not alone in what he or she is experiencing. Table 34–7 provides facilitative statements for the interviewer conducting a sexual assessment. Table 34–8 provides some interviewing do's and don't's to follow when obtaining sexual information.

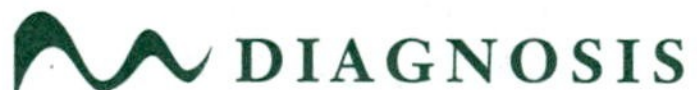

DIAGNOSIS

A comprehensive sexual assessment reveals areas of sexual concern and dysfunction for the patient. These data are analyzed to determine the appropriate medical and nursing diagnoses. A sample nursing diagnosis might read: "Sexual dysfunction related to marital problems evidenced in painful intercourse and inability to have orgasm."

OUTCOME IDENTIFICATION

The expected outcomes for a patient with a sexual problem vary with the medical and nursing diagnoses. The following are examples of expected outcomes for patients with sexual problems:

- The patient will resolve marital difficulties and resume a satisfying sexual relationship with her spouse.
- The patient will cease drinking and experience the ability to achieve an erection.
- The patient will no longer experience pain while engaging in sexual intercourse.

PLANNING

Based on the identified expected outcomes, the nurse and patient, working together with the interdisciplinary team, jointly establish short-term goals, such as the following:

Expected Outcomes	Short-Term Goals
The patient will resolve marital difficulties and resume a satisfying sexual relationship with her spouse.	1. The patient will identify her feelings toward her spouse. 2. The patient will communicate her feelings toward her spouse taking an "I" stance rather than a "blaming" stance. 3. The patient will participate in homework that focuses on small steps in achieving sexual satisfaction.
The patient will cease drinking and experience the ability to achieve an erection.	1. The patient will agree to attend AA meetings. 2. The patient will work with a sponsor who will help him to remain sober. 3. The patient will not drink. 4. The patient will resume sexual activity.
The patient will no longer experience pain while engaging in sexual intercourse.	1. The patient will demonstrate relaxation exercises that she will use before sexual intercourse. 2. The patient will practice thought-stopping techniques to control her *anticipatory fear* that she will experience pain with sexual intercourse. 3. The patient will use a lubricant such as K-Y Jelly before engaging in sexual intercourse.

BOX 34-4 Patient Cues That May Indicate Concerns About Sexuality

Nonverbal Behaviors

- Showing discomfort through blushing, looking away, tight fists, fidgeting, crying
- Openly engaging in overt sexual behaviors, e.g., touching own body parts, masturbating, exposing genitals, placing nurse's hand on genitals, making sexually suggestive sounds

Verbal Behaviors

- Telling sexually explicit jokes
- Making sexual comments about the nurse
- Asking inappropriate questions about the nurse's sexual activity
- Discussing sexual exploits
- Asking the nurse to perform sexual acts
- Expressing concern about relationship with partner
  "I don't feel the same about my partner"
  "My partner doesn't feel the same about me"
  "We're not as close"
  "Our relationship is changed"
  "My personal life has changed"
- Expressing concern that sexuality has been diminished, e.g., feeling less of a man, less of a woman
  "I've lost my manhood"
  "I'm not as desirable as I once was"
- Expressing concern over lack of sexual desire
  "I'm not horny anymore"
  "My desire has changed"
  "I'm not the man/woman I used to be"
  "We don't click anymore"
- Expressing concern over sexual performance
  "I don't get wet"
  "I've lost my power"
  "Will I still be able to get hard?"
  "What will happen to my ability to perform?"
  "I can't perform like I used to"
- Expressing concern about one's love life
  "My love life has changed"
  "The spark has worn off"
- Expressing concern over the sexual impact of drugs, surgery, or some other medical issue
  "Will this drug interfere with my sex life?"
  "Will I still be able to perform sexually after surgery?"

TABLE 34–7 **Facilitative Statements for the Interviewer Conducting a Sexual Assessment**

Purpose	Facilitative Statement
To give a rationale for a question	As a nurse, I'm concerned about all aspects of your health. Many individuals have concern about sexual matters, especially when they are sick or when they are having other health problems.
To give statements of "generality" or "normality"	Most people are hesitant to discuss . . . Many people worry about feelings . . . Many people have concerns about . . .
To identify sexual dysfunction	Most people have difficulties sometime during their sexual relationships. What have yours been?
To obtain information	The degree to which unmarried persons have sexual outlets varies considerably. Some have sexual partners. Others have none. Some relieve sexual tension through masturbation. Others need no outlet at all. What has been your pattern?
To identify sexual myths	While growing up, most of us have heard some sexual myths or half-truths that continue to puzzle us. Are there any that come to mind?
To identify feelings about masturbation	Many of us grown-ups have heard a variety of stories about masturbation and what problems it supposedly causes. This can cause worry even into adulthood. What have you heard?
To determine whether homosexuality is a source of conflict	Some say homosexuality is a mental disorder, others an emotional block, others a crime or sin. What is your attitude toward your homosexual orientation?
To identify an older person's concerns about sexual function	Many people, as they get older, believe or worry that this signals the end of their sex life. Much misinformation continues this myth. What is your understanding about sexuality during the later years? How has the passage of time affected your sexuality (sex life)?
To obtain and give information (miscellaneous areas)	Frequently people have questions about . . . What questions do you have about . . . What would you like to know about . . .
To close the history	Is there anything further in the area of sexuality that you would like to bring up now? I hope that if questions or concerns do come to mind in the future we'll be able to discuss them.

Adapted from Green, R. (1975). *Human sexuality: A health practitioner's text.* Baltimore, Williams & Wilkins.

IMPLEMENTATION

A decision tree is helpful for determining the appropriate course of treatment for a person with a sexual complaint, even if it will not be you who actually carries out the treatment (Figure 34–2). Although most nurses will never be sex therapists, all nurses need to know when and to whom to refer the patient with a sexual complaint. Depending on the nature of the problem, the patient may need a referral to such professionals as a marital counselor, psychiatrist, gynecologist, urologist, clinical nurse specialist, or pastoral counselor.

Many nursing interventions have already been discussed along with specific deviations. Appropriate strategies for intervening include milieu therapy, education, behavioral therapy, medication, and psychotherapy. Although psychotherapy alone has not been helpful in stopping the deviant sexual behavior, it does provide an adjunct support. Psychotherapy is used to assist the patient in identifying triggers that set off the inappropriate sexual behavior (Kaplan, 1975, 1979). Once the triggers have been identified, alternative coping skills are discussed. These alternative coping skills include thought blocking and thought changing.

Covert sensitization, a behavioral technique, is a widely used procedure in the treatment of inappropriate sexual behaviors. Covert sensitization may act as a self-control technique whereby the individual uses the aversive cue to control the inappropriate behavior.

Medication is the last treatment intervention to be addressed. There is insufficient research and data to conclude that this intervention could be used independently as a treatment without the other interventions. The drug that is frequently used in treating sexual deviations, however, is medroxyprogesterone acetate (Depo-Provera). Medroxyprogesterone acetate, in both men and women, in sufficient quantity decreases sexual urges and assists in controlling the offending sexual behavior (Berlin, 1985).

EVALUATION

Evaluation of expected outcomes and achievement of short-term goals relate to the level of control and personal satisfaction that is achieved. Acceptance of sexual dysfunctions, such as impotence, as being a part of, but not necessarily the defining characteristic of, sexual behavior can result in greater satisfaction. The degree to which negative attitudes about sex are no longer problematic also is important.

▶ Check Your Reading

32. Describe the setting for a sexual assessment.
33. Identify one nursing diagnosis for a sexual dysfunction.
34. What medication is used with sexual disorders such as pedophilia?
35. Identify two interventions used with patients with sexual disorders.

TABLE 34–8 Do's and Don't's to Follow When Obtaining Sexual Information

Do	Don't
Obtain information about all areas of need	Focus only on sexuality Obtain information when others are present or take copious notes
Strive for an unhurried atmosphere	Check your watch, tap your foot
Maintain an attitude that is frank, open, warm, objective, empathetic	Project discomfort, become defensive
Use nondirective techniques when possible	Ask many direct questions
Have a prepared introduction to the stated purpose of interview	Be vague about the purpose of interview
Use appropriate vocabulary	Use street terms
"Check out" words to ensure that patient understands	Assume the patient understands what you're saying
Adjust the order of questions according to patient's needs	Follow a rigid form
Give the patient time to think and answer questions	Answer questions for the patient
Recognize signs of anxiety	Focus on getting information without recognizing patient's feelings
Give permission not to do something	Have preset expectations of the patient's sexual activity
Listen in an interested but matter-of-fact way	Overreact or underreact
Identify your attitudes, values, beliefs, and feelings	Project your concerns or problems onto the patient
Identify significant others	Assume that no one else is involved in the patient's sexual concerns
Identify philosophical, religious beliefs of patient	Impose your moral judgments on the patient
Acknowledge when you don't have an answer to a question	Pretend you know when you don't

From Hogan, R. (1980). *Human sexuality: A nursing perspective,* (p. 246). New York: Appleton-Century-Crofts.

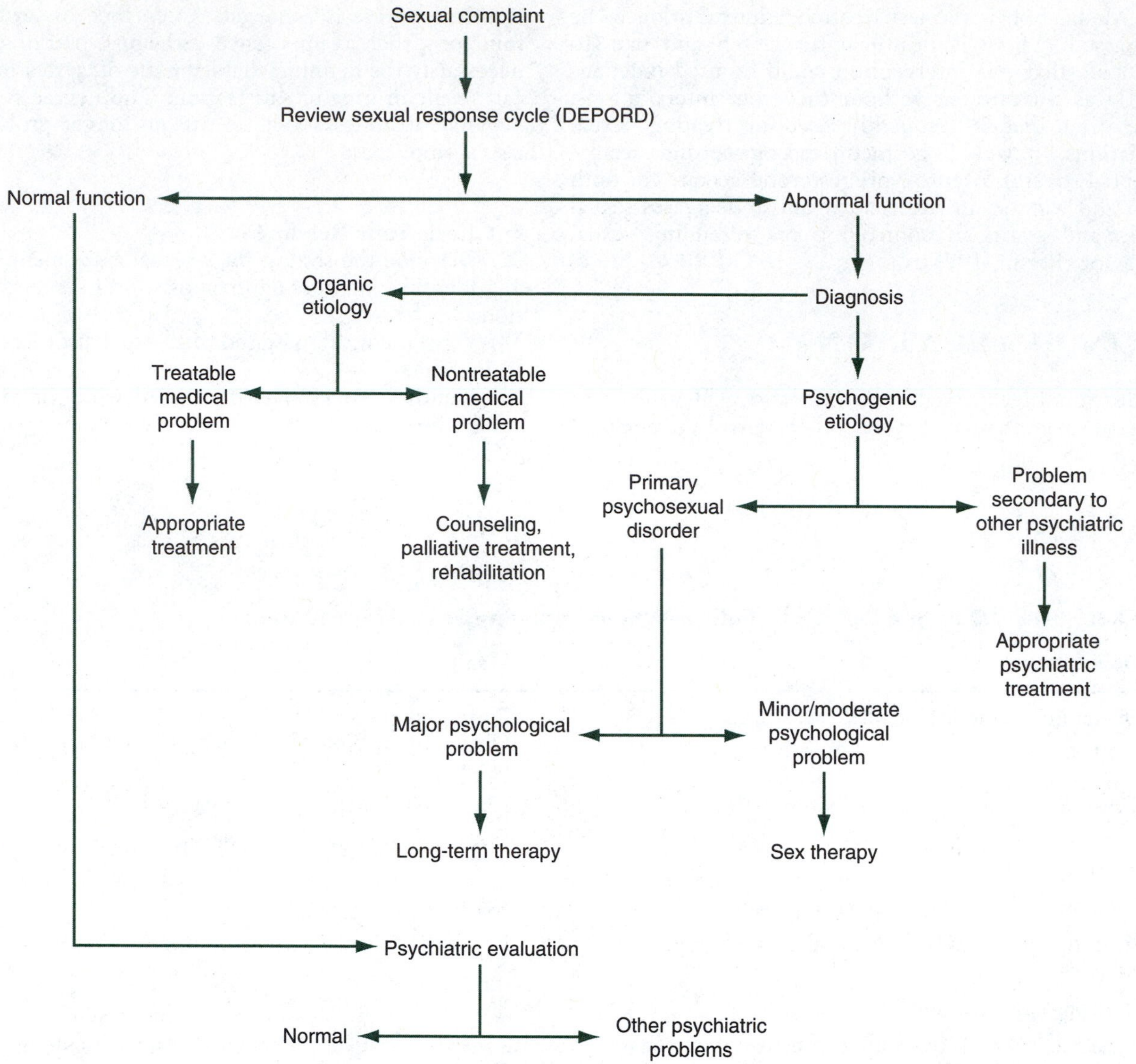

FIGURE 34–2
A decision tree used to help determine what interventions are appropriate for a patient with a sexual disorder.

CASE STUDY: ALEXIA

Alexia is a senior in college who lives at home with her mother. Alexia's mother has been married twice and divorced twice; during Alexia's high school and college years, her mother has had numerous sexual partners, some of whom have lived with them for a time.

Until her high school senior prom, Alexia had remained a virgin. Then, on prom night, Alexia had her first sexual experience with her boyfriend of nine months. Alexia enjoyed the experience, and she felt okay about it. She continued to have sexual relations with her boyfriend. Then, suddenly, he broke off the relationship. Alexia was devastated—depressed and desperately lonely. She felt as though she were the only teen in the world without a boyfriend.

Eager to replace that relationship, Alexia quickly resumed dating. She dated a number of young men. With her newfound freedom to engage in sexual relationships and her heightened interest in sex, Alexia readily had intercourse with the young men she dated. Although her much-longed-for romantic relationship never materialized, Alexia found the variety of sexual experiences exciting.

A week ago, however, Alexia noticed several small painful growths on her labia and several wartlike lesions near her anus. Concerned over these growths she quickly overcame her anxiety and went to see her gynecologist. The gynecologist told Alexia that the labial lesions were genital herpes and that the warts were genital warts (condylomata acuminata). Those terms meant little to Alexia until the gynecologist told her that they were sexually transmitted diseases. Alexia was stunned.

Still reeling with shock and embarrassment, Alexia began a course of treatment for the condition. The gynecologist dealt with the physical problem in a matter-of-fact manner, paying little attention to Alexia's emotional and spiritual reactions to the condition. Over the next few weeks, however, Alexia stopped dating. Soon, she even began to avoid talking with men, associating only with her girlfriends, to whom she expressed a total lack of interest in sex.

One of her friends suggested that she seek treatment at a Christian nurse-managed clinic. At first opposed to the idea because of her promiscuity, Alexia remembered the comfort she had early in life attending Sunday school. She agreed to go to a clinic and was seen on a weekly basis by a nurse clinical specialist in adult mental health.

ASSESSMENT

Assessment data are as follows:
- Presence of genital herpes and genital warts
- Shame and anxiety
- Lack of sexual desire
- Numerous sexual partners, lack of stable relationships
- Parental role model that did not model responsible sexuality

DIAGNOSIS

***DSM-IV* Diagnosis:** Sexual aversion disorder

Nursing Diagnosis: Sexual Dysfunction related to the acute effects of two sexually transmitted diseases (STDs) as evidenced by withdrawal from relationships with men and lack of sexual desire

OUTCOME IDENTIFICATION, PLANNING, AND IMPLEMENTATION

EXPECTED OUTCOME 1: By _____ the patient will recognize the link between her search for meaningful relationships with men and her willingness to engage in sexual intercourse.

SHORT-TERM GOALS	NURSING INTERVENTIONS	RATIONALES
By _____ the patient will discuss her feelings about her family situation.	1. Help Alexia to complete a family genogram.	1. A family genogram is a nonemotional method of diagraming and examining family patterns.
	2. Teach Alexia about family patterns—how behaviors and attitudes are transmitted from one generation to another, how events such as a divorce affect the whole family; teach her about family triangles. 3. Help Alexia to recognize the patterns of relationships in her family—in particular the relationships Alexia's mother had with men.	2–3. A family approach to Alexia's problem provides her with a way of analyzing and problem-solving about her own situation. By examining what has happened in her family, Alexia can understand her own behavior, not only as learned from the modeling of her mother but also as her own response to the intense anxiety and sense of loss that she must have felt within her family.
By _____ the patient will identify the impact of her family situation on her feelings and behaviors.	1. Encourage Alexia to identify and discuss her feelings about the divorce of her parents and the subsequent relationships her mother had with men.	1. By recognizing and discussing her own feelings, Alexia is taking the first step toward changing her own behavior. Unrecognized and unnamed feelings usually result in reactive and impulsive behaviors that are often self-destructive.

SHORT-TERM GOALS	NURSING INTERVENTIONS	RATIONALES
By _____ the patient will discuss the connection between her own lack of a stable, loving relationship with a father figure and her willingness to become intimately involved with many men.	1. Encourage Alexia to identify and discuss her feelings about the many losses she has experienced with men throughout her life. 2. Encourage Alexia to examine and discuss her own behaviors related to intimate relationships with men with what she observed and learned as a child growing up.	1–2. By understanding the deep losses that she experienced, Alexia is better able to understand her present behavior, to forgive herself, and to seek forgiveness from her God.
By _____ the patient will identify other alternatives to this pattern of behavior and relating to men.	1. Encourage Alexia to identify alternative ways of interacting with men in meaningful ways but without premature intimacy.	1. Identifying alternative modes of behaving before a situation presents itself is an empowering strategy. If Alexia waits to think through alternatives when she is confronted with the difficult situations, she may find that the old patterns of feeling and behaving overpower her ability to effectively problem-solve.

EXPECTED OUTCOME 2: By _____ the patient will identify practices and coping patterns that will help her to achieve meaningful relationships with men and restoration of sexual desire.

SHORT-TERM GOALS	NURSING INTERVENTIONS	RATIONALES
By _____ the patient will identify the behaviors she currently exhibits when relating to men.	1. Encourage the patient that it is possible for her to change unhealthy patterns of behaving; just as she learned destructive patterns, she can relearn healthy patterns of relating. 2. Encourage the patient to role-play various scenarios in which she interacts with men. 3. Ask the patient to look at her behavior in these scenarios; to analyze her speech, her nonverbal behavior, her dress, and her feelings as she acts out these scenarios.	1. Patients are often discouraged about the prospects of changing patterns of behavior that seem deeply ingrained; encouragement provides hope for pursuing change. 2. By asking the patient to role-play, you are allowing her to see her own behaviors in a different and more objective way. 3. By asking her to identify each of her behaviors, you are putting her in charge of identifying her problematic behaviors and conveying confidence in her ability to find a solution to her problems.
By _____ the patient will examine these behaviors to determine which, if any, are sexually provocative behaviors or that invite intimacy before a sound relationship has developed.	1. Ask the patient to analyze the responses to her behavior that she receives from men. Ask her if the responses she is receiving are sexual. Do the responses indicate a premature or inappropriate level of intimacy, given the stage of the relationship? 2. Ask the patient to categorize which of her own behaviors provoke these responses in men and which of her behaviors reinforce and encourage these responses in men.	1–2. By asking her to categorize her own behaviors, you are recognizing that not everythng that she does needs to change. This is affirming to the patient. By asking her to examine the impact of her behaviors on men, you are affirming her responsibility and her role in the relationships that she develops; you are affirming her not as a "victim" but as someone who has the ability to take charge and to change.
By _____ the patient will examine behaviors that she needs to develop to really get to know and form meaningful relationships with men.	1. Explore alternative behaviors; ways of acting that are friendly and interested, but with clear boundaries of sexual involvement. 2. Role-play various scenarios in which the patient "tries out" these new behaviors. Reanalyze the responses she receives. 3. Give homework assignments in which the patient keeps a journal of her interactions with men; ask her to analyze these interactions and to "try on" her new behaviors.	1. By establishing realistic boundaries, you are helping the patient to assume control over her body and sexual activities. 2. By role-playing different behaviors, you are allowing the patient to try out new ways of behaving in a safe, protected environment. 3. The journal entries keep the patient focused on the areas she is targeting for change; she is an active participant in the change—continually recording and evaluating her own responses.

SHORT-TERM GOALS	NURSING INTERVENTIONS	RATIONALES
By _____ the patient will identify strategies to cope with feelings that interfere with her development of meaningful relationships with men.	1. Ask the patient to keep a record of her feelings as she interacts with men. These recordings can be discussed within the therapy session to facilitate the patient's understanding of her own relationship patterns.	1. The ongoing recording and follow-up discussion of her feelings expand her awareness and understanding of her own patterns of behavior; greater understanding and awareness lead to greater control.

EXPECTED OUTCOME 3: By _____ the patient will state an understanding of her medical condition and its treatment and identify practices to prevent the contraction or spread of STDs.

SHORT-TERM GOALS	NURSING INTERVENTIONS	RATIONALES
By _____ the patient will verbalize accurate information about her STD and STDs in general.	1. Teach the patient the facts about STDs—the methods of contracting the diseases, the available treatments, and the risks. 2. Provide written information on this topic. 3. Assess the patient's understanding of the information presented.	1. People frequently have inadequate or inaccurate information about sexual issues. 2. Written information allows the patient to review the material in privacy. 3. It is important that you ask the patient to discuss the information you have presented. The patient may say that she understands or that she already knew the information to avoid the embarrassment of talking about a sensitive issue.
By _____ the patient will verbalize the risks of multiple sexual relationships and will state that condom use does not afford 100% protection against the risk of contracting all STDs.	1. The patient will verbalize an understanding that the only 100% guarantee of protection against STDs is abstinence from questionable sexual relationships, and that even protected sexual activity (sexual activity with the use of either a male or female condom) carries some risk of contracting STDs.	1. Patients frequently have inaccurate or inadequate information about the protection offered by condom use. If patients choose to engage in risky behavior, it is important that they have accurate information upon which to base their decisions.

EXPECTED OUTCOME 4: By _____ the patient will state the meaning that she has found in the experience of having contracted a STD and will find spiritual comfort.

SHORT-TERM GOALS	NURSING INTERVENTIONS	RATIONALES
By _____ the patient will verbalize the significance of the STD on her life's journey.	1. Discuss the meaning of sexually expression. 2. Discuss the spiritual significance of sexuality.	1. Sexual expression is an intimate way of relating to another in a committed relationship. Sexual expression disconnected from a committed relationship often leaves the participants feeling used and unfulfilled. 2. Sexuality is an expression of our spirituality, in that sexuality transcends the individual and is creative. For many people, sexual intimacy outside of a marital relationship carries with it guilt and remorse for violation of religious beliefs.
By _____ the patient will utilize spiritual resources to alleviate the spiritual distress she is feeling.	1. Discuss with Alexia the spiritual resources (prayer, meditation, clerical counsel, reading of scripture or other inspirational materials) that might be helpful and supportive to her. 2. Ask how you might support Alexia in her efforts to attain comfort and consolation.	1. Alexia may find spiritual support and strength from these resources. 2. Offering the self is a caring therapeutic modality that shows support and help for the patient who is spiritually distressed.

EVALUATION

Formative Evaluation: Alexia met all of the short-term goals. She was able to examine her family situation, and she easily recognized that her pattern of relating to men was linked to her early family experiences and the behavior modeled by her mother. Alexia was able to identify that she engaged in a pattern of sexually flirtatious behavior and that she really never attempted to get to know a man before she had sex with him. She began to look at the behaviors she uses to make friends with women and to transfer these behaviors to situations in which she found herself with men. Furthermore, Alexia became increasingly aware of her feelings of insecurity when she interacted with men and her overwhelming desire to be taken care of by them. She identified these feelings as being rooted in the many early losses she experienced. Alexia was knowledgeable about her own STDs as well as STDs in general. She sought the spiritual support of her clergy person and found solace in prayer and scripture reading.

Summative Evaluation: Alexia met all of the expected outcomes. She developed friendships with two young men that involved social activities with groups of friends rather than sexual relationships. She expressed that "I feel like I am just learning how to be a friend to a guy." She was able to forgive herself for having an STD and to seek a committed relationship with a special person before engaging in sexual activity.

CONCLUSIONS

Sexuality is as much a part of who we are as our personality, our intelligence, and our physical appearance. Normal sexuality imbues our journeys with both creative and generative desires. When there are dysfunctions in sexuality, individual journeys can be painful. It is part of the nurse's role to understand and assess sexuality, to recognize when there are problems related to sexuality, to teach about it, and to offer empathy and concern to patients whose journeys are affected by sexual dysfunctions or disorders.

KEY POINTS TO REMEMBER

- Sexual attitudes and behaviors are affected by multiple factors, including shifting cultural mores, religious teachings, parental role modeling, age, developmental stage, socioeconomic status, health, and education.
- It is essential for the nurse to examine personal attitudes and values concerning sexuality.
- The term *sex* refers to whether one is anatomically male or female.
- *Gender identity* refers to the earliest sense of maleness or femaleness acquired by an individual.
- *Gender* refers to the psychological reaction to or sense of being a male or female.
- *Gender dysphoria* refers to a sense of discomfort experienced when one's sex and gender differ.
- Transsexualism is the most common type of gender dysphoria.
- *Sexual identity* refers to the identification of oneself as male or female.
- *Heterosexual identity* means that the individual is attracted to individuals of the opposite sex.
- *Homosexual identity* means that the individual is attracted to individuals of the same sex.
- Sexual development continues over the life span.
- The sexual response cycle has six phases: desire, excitement, plateau, orgasm, resolution, and desire. Each phase is characterized by predictable behavioral and emotional responses.
- *Dyspareunia* refers to painful intercourse or coitus.
- The *DSM-IV* includes diagnostic criteria for disorders occurring during the various phases of the sexual response cycle.
- Erectile dysfunction can result from organic as well as psychogenic causes.
- Anorgasmia, or the inability to achieve an orgasm, is common in patients with a history of sexual abuse.
- The causes of anorgasmia include psychogenic trauma, medical problems, illness, medication, neurological conditions, or vascular conditions.
- Sexual disorders include paraphilias and gender identity disorders.
- There are many theories regarding the cause of homosexuality.
- Only when homosexuality is ego dystonic is it considered to be a psychiatric illness.
- Head trauma that results in damage to the frontal lobe of the brain may result in promiscuous behavior, poor judgment, and poor impulse control.
- Klinefelter's syndrome is a genetic abnormality that produces sexual deviations.
- Psychoses can have an impact on sexual behavior and functioning.
- Sexual assessment must be holistic to understand fully the patient's situation.
- Sexual assessment collects data regarding medications that the patient is presently taking; many medications are associated with sexual dysfunction.

- A structured sexual assessment tool may assist the novice nurse to gather comprehensive sexual data.
- The setting for the sexual assessment should be private and quiet.
- The nurse needs to have an awareness of slang expressions used for sexual terms.
- Patients communicate nonverbally that they are uncomfortable with the sexual assessment.
- Interventions for sexual dysfunctions and disorders include medication, psychotherapy, behavioral therapy, teaching, and milieu therapy.

LEARNING ACTIVITIES

1. Reflect on the sexual disorders presented in the chapter. What are your attitudes and beliefs about patients with paraphilias? Are you sympathetic? Do you believe they are in control and responsible for their behavior? What do you think society's view should be—punishment or treatment?

2. Complete the questions asked in Box 34–1. What do your answers tell you about yourself? Regarding sexuality, are you comfortable with your own sexuality? With that of others? Are you judgmental? Could you be helpful to someone who had a sexual disorder?

3. What factors have influenced your beliefs and values regarding sexuality?

4. What do you think is the impact of sexually explicit television, music videos, and movies on an individual's attitudes, values, and beliefs regarding sexuality?

CRITICAL THINKING EXERCISE

Miss Jennifer Hines, a 24-year-old student nurse in her psychiatric nursing clinical experience, was assigned to Miss Gloria Thomas, a 27-year-old patient admitted with alcohol abuse. During one of the counseling interviews related to Miss Thomas's options when she left the detoxification unit, the patient told Miss Hines that she was gay and that she was sexually attracted to Miss Hines. When Miss Hines asked her why she felt this way, Miss Thomas said, "You must like me also, you treat me differently than you treat the other patients."

1. What assumption(s) is Miss Thomas making about Miss Hines's behaviors?

2. What evidence might suggest to Miss Thomas that her assumption is faulty?

3. What might happen if Miss Hines's response were different?

After Miss Thomas was discharged, she called Miss Hines at home to invite her to a party that she was having. She stated that a lot of Miss Hines's friends would be there.

1. Make sense of this information.

2. Consider alternate explanations.

3. What conclusion(s) can be drawn about the nurse-patient relationship?

REFERENCES

Aass, N., Grunfeld, B., Kaalhus, O., and Fossa, S. D. (1993). Pre- and post-treatment sexual life in testicular cancer patients: A descriptive investigation. *British Journal of Cancer, 67*(5), 1113–1117.

Alexander, B. (1993). Disorders of sexual desire: Diagnosis and treatment of decreased libido. *American Family Physician, 47*(4), 832–838.

American Psychiatric Association. (1994). *Diagnostic and statistical manual of mental disorders* (4th ed.). Washington, D. C.: American Psychiatric Association.

Balon, R., Yeragani, V. K., Pohl, R., and Ramesh, C. (1993). Sexual dysfunction during antidepressant treatment. *Journal of Clinical Psychiatry, 54*(6), 209–212.

Berlin, F. S. (1985). Pedophilia: Medical castration and group counseling session help to modify this type of sexual behavior. *Medical Aspects of Human Sexuality, 19*(8), 79–88.

Brown, J. C. (1983). Paraphilias: Sadomasochism, fetishism, transvestism, and transsexuality. *British Journal of Psychiatry, 143*, 227–231.

Chandraiah, S., Levenson, J. L., and Collins, J. B. (1991). Sexual dysfunction, social maladjustment, and psychiatric disorders in women seeking treatment in a premenstrual syndrome clinic. *International Journal of Psychiatry in Medicine, 21*(2), 189–204.

Corney, R. H., Crowther, M. E., Everett, H., Howells, A., and Shepherd, J. H. (1993). Psychosexual dysfunction in women with gynecological cancer following radical pelvic surgery. *British Journal of Obstetrics and Gynaecology, 100*(1), 73–78.

Currier, K. D. and Aponte, J. F. (1991). Sexual dysfunction in female adult children of alcoholics. *International Journal of Addiction, 26*(2), 195–201.

Davidson, J. (1986). Androgen replacement therapy in a wider context: Clinical and basic aspects. In L. Dennerstein & I. Fraser (Eds.), *Hormones and behavior* (p. 434). Amsterdam: Excerpta Medica.

Freud, S. (1978). Letter to an American mother (1951). *American Journal of Psychiatry, 107*, 786–787. Cited in J. Marmor and R. Green. *Homosexual behavior.* In J. Money & H. Mustapha (Eds.), *Handbook of sexology* (p. 1060). New York: Elsevier.

Greenblatt, R., Jungck, E., and Blum, H. (1972). Endocrinology of sexual behavior. *Medical Aspects of Human Sexuality, 6*, 110–131.

Haber, C. H. (1991). The psychoanalytical treatment of a preschool boy with a gender identity disorder. *Journal of the American Psychoanalytic Association, 39*(1), 107–129.

Harbert, T. L., Barlow, D. H., Herses, M., and Austin, D. B. (1974). Measurement and modification of incestuous behavior: A case study. *Psychological Reports, 34*, 79–86.

Jensen, S. B. (1992). Sexuality and chronic illness: A biopsychosocial approach. *Seminars in Neurology, 12*(2), 135–140.

Kafka, M. P. (1991). Successful antidepressant treatment of nonparaphilic sexual addictions and paraphilias in men. *Journal of Clinical Psychiatry, 52*(2), 60–65.

Kaplan, H. S. (1975). *The illustrated manual of sex therapy.* New York: The New York Times Book Co.

Kaplan, H. S. (1979). *Disorders of sexual desire and other new concepts and techniques in sex therapy.* New York: Brunner/Mazel, Inc.

Kinsey, A. C., Pomeroy, W., and Martin, C. (1988). Sexual behavior in human males (1948). Cited in R. Brown and J. Field (Eds.), *Treatment of sexual problems in individual and couples therapy* (p. 236). Dana Point, CA: PMA Corp.

Lawrence, J. S., and Madakasira, S. (1992). Evaluation and treatment of premature ejaculation: A critical review. *International Journal of Psychiatry in Medicine, 22*(1), 77–97.

Leiblum, S. R. (1992). The sexual difficulties of women. *Journal of the Medical Association of Georgia, 81*(5), 221–225.

Leif, H. (1977). What's new in sex research. *Medical Aspects of Human Sexuality*, 7, 94–95.

Maltz, W. (1988). Identifying and treating the sexual repercussions of incest: A couple approach. *Journal of Sex and Marital Therapy*, *14*, 142–169.

Masters, W. H., Johnson, V. E. (1970). *Human sexual inadequacy.* Boston: Little Brown.

Meyer-Bahlburg, H. F., Nostlinger, C., Exner, T. M., Ehrhardt, A. A., Gruen, R. S., Lorenz, G., Gorman, J. M., el-Sadr, W., and Sorrell, S. J. (1993). Sexual functioning in HIV+ and HIV– injected drug-using women. *Journal of Sex and Marital Therapy*, *19*(1), 56–68.

Morhr, J. W., Turner, R. E., and Jerry, M. B. (1964). *Pedophilia and exhibitionism: A handbook.* Toronto: University of Toronto Press.

Musher, J. S. (1990). Anorgasmia with the use of fluoxetine (letter). *American Journal of Psychiatry*, *147*(7), 948.

North American Nursing Diagnosis Association (1994). *NANDA nursing diagnoses: Definitions and classification 1995–1996.* Philadelphia: NANDA.

Patterson, W. M. (1993). Fluoxetine-induced sexual dysfunction (letter). *Journal of Clinical Psychiatry*, *54*(2), 71.

Rooth, F. G. (1973). Exhibitionism outside Europe and America. *Archives of Sexual Behavior*, *2* 351–363.

Saghir, M., and Robins, E. (1978). *Male and female homosexuality* (1973). Cited in J. Money & H. Mustapha (Eds.), *Handbook of sexuality* (p. 1062). New York: Elsevier.

Stuntz, R. (1983). Gender dysphoria and dyssocial behavior. In L. B. Schlesinger & E. Revitch (Eds.), *Sexual dynamics of anti-social behavior* (pp. 88–89). Springfield: Charles C Thomas.

Stuntz, R. (1988). Assessment of organic factors in sexual dysfunction. In R. Brown & J. Field (Eds.), *Treatment of sexual problems in individual and couples therapy* (pp. 188–201). Dana Point, CA: PMA Publishing Corp.

Walbroehl, G. S. (1992). Sexual concerns of the patient with pulmonary disease. *Postgraduate Medicine*, *91*(5), 455–460.

Williams, W. (1991). Male sexuality. *Medical Journal of Australia*, *155*(2), 101–104.

Wise, T. N., Epstein, S., and Ross, R. (1992). Sexual issues in the medically ill and aging. *Psychiatric Medicine*, *10*(2), 169–180.

SUGGESTED READINGS

Dewis, M. E., and Thornton, N. G. (1989). Sexual dysfunction in multiple sclerosis. *Journal of Neuroscience Nursing*, *21*(3), 175–179.

Dunning, P. (1993). Sexuality and women with diabetes. *Patient Education and Counseling*, *21*(1–2), 5–14.

Hook, M., Guevarra, J., Perce, M. K., and Scott-Sorenson, N. (1989). Critical care voices: Including sexual counseling in clinical practice, *Dimensions of Critical Care Nursing*, *8*(6), 375.

Shell, J. A. (1990). Sexuality for patients with gynecologic cancer. *NAACOGS Clinical Issues in Perinatal and Women's Health Nursing*, *1*(4), 479–494.

CHAPTER 35

THE JOURNEY CHALLENGED BY EATING DISORDERS

An eating disorder may be defined simply as an obsession with eating in the midst of an abundance of food. (Eating disorders rarely occur in countries where there is a scarcity of food supplies or among people who must worry where their next meal is coming from.)

—*R. Epstein*

LEARNING OBJECTIVES

After studying this chapter, you should be able to:

1. Discuss at least three important roles that food plays in life's journey.
2. Describe anorexia nervosa.
3. Describe bulimia nervosa.
4. Define binge eating disorder.
5. Discuss the causes of eating disorders from a biological, psychological, sociocultural, and spiritual perspective.
6. State at least four defining characteristics of anorexia nervosa, bulimia nervosa, and binge eating disorder.
7. Identify at least three factors you would assess in anorexia nervosa, bulimia nervosa, or binge eating disorder.
8. State at least three possible nursing diagnoses for a patient diagnosed with anorexia nervosa, bulimia nervosa, or binge eating disorder.
9. State at least two expected outcomes for a patient diagnosed with anorexia nervosa, bulimia nervosa, or binge eating disorder.
10. Discuss at least two treatment approaches for the patient with either anorexia nervosa or bulimia nervosa.
11. Discuss the psychiatric nurse's challenge when journeying with a patient with an eating disorder.

KEY TERMINOLOGY

Anorexia nervosa
Binge eating disorder
Binging
Bulimia nervosa
Purging

The journey marked by eating disorders begins with the role of food in our lives—a role that has always been and will always be a crucial one. Primarily, we need food for nourishment so that our bodies grow and develop during childhood years and remain healthy as we mature and grow older. In each of our journeys, however, food plays roles other than nourishment. These roles are worth pondering as we begin to understand eating disorders.

Food is often used as a reward or punishment for children's behaviors. Adults, too, use "dinners out" as celebrations for job promotions, birthdays, and so forth. Not only are business or "working" lunches to discuss professional concerns common, but in some professions they are the only way business is conducted. Holidays are distinguished from one another by the kinds and types of food served: ham at Easter, turkey at Thanksgiving, matzo at Passover, and candy canes at Christmas. Abstaining from food is an important practice of many of the world's religions on certain holy days. Additionally, Christian, Jewish, and Muslim rituals such as communion, Passover, and Ramadan are commemorated with special foods.

Other than food's essential relationship to our health, the most important relationship, and the one that wields the most power, is the one tied to our appearance. You only need to read a fashion magazine or watch television to be aware of the pressure placed on young women (and to a lesser degree, young men) to be thin. Many young people believe that they are defined by their weight and "can never be too thin." Anorexia nervosa and bulimia nervosa, both of which are characterized by disturbances in the person's perception of body shape and weight, may be the responses of young people to this irrational pressure to be thin.

Food is used to meet other emotional needs, such as needs for comfort, security, and love. The binge eating disorder may represent a person's response to these unmet needs. Table 35–1 provides an overview of the three types of eating disorders: anorexia nervosa, bulimia nervosa, and binge eating disorder.

Anorexia nervosa and bulimia primarily affect white women, 12 to 22 years of age, in the middle and upper socioeconomic groups in industrialized countries such as the United States, Europe, Canada, Japan, Australia, and South Africa. Typical onset of anorexia nervosa is between 12 and 14 years of age and bulimia is between 16 and 20 years of age. Males, representing between 0.4% and 10% of cases of anorexia nervosa and bulimia, fall into the same age group and cultures. Western cultures have been singled out because of their shared emphasis on dieting, weight, and body shape. Current estimates place the prevalence of eating disorders at 1 of 100 American women and girls with signs of anorexia nervosa and 2% to 8% of adolescent and college women with signs of bulimia (Love and Seaton, 1991). Members of professions that emphasize physical appearance and weight standards, such as dancers, flight attendants, athletes, actors, and models, are at especially high risk for eating disorders. This pathology has been found to begin after people have entered these professions, which discounts the supposition that only thin people pursue these types of occupations (White, 1992). The incidence of binge eating disorder is less researched. In samples drawn from weight control programs, however, the overall prevalence ranges from 15% to 50% with a mean of 30% (Miller, 1991; deZwaan and Mitchell, 1992). Women experience this disorder approximately 1.5 times more often than men.

As nurses we need to be aware of eating disorders, not only because of their increasing frequency but also because of their potentially fatal outcomes. Anorexia nervosa is reported to have a mortality rate of 5% to 18% (Kaplan and Sadock, 1991). Bulimia nervosa is also associated with life-threatening consequences, including severe electrolyte imbalances such as hypokalemia, which can lead to cardiac arrhythmias and cardiac arrest (Johnson and Pure, 1986; Laraia and Stuart, 1990). However, obesity is also associated with multiple physical and psychological problems.

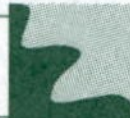

CARRIE'S STORY

On the icy highway, Carrie applied the brake and the car spun forward, missing another vehicle by inches. She panicked, wrenched the wheel, and barely missed a truck coming from the opposite direction. A few seconds later Carrie managed to stop the car. With her hands shaking and her voice trembling, she turned to her friend and said, "I'm hungry."

"Hungry? Who thinks of food at a time like this?"

"I do," Carrie answered. "I think about food all the time."

Story from Billigmeier, S. (1991). *Inner eating.* Nashville: Oliver Nelson.

HISTORICAL BACKGROUND

Evidence exists that problems in the regulation of food intake are not just common to 20th century life. In first century Rome, vomitoriums were invented as a means to relieve bloated stomachs from the food orgies that were common. These rooms, built expressly for the partygoer to vomit and then return to the banquet room to gorge once more, were socially acceptable. It was not until the Middle Ages, however, that any illness resembling an eating disorder was documented.

Although Richard Morton in 1694 is credited with first describing anorexia's cause as "arising in underlying sadness and anxious cares" (Patton, 1992, p. 281), it was not until 1873 that both an English physician and a French physician first documented series of cases of

TABLE 35–1 Overview of the Three Types of Eating Disorders

Disorder	Characteristics
Anorexia nervosa	Refusal to maintain a minimally normal body weight. The anorexic may control weight by either severely restricting caloric intake or engaging in a binge-purge cycle of eating. Binge-purge eating occurs when a person eats a large amount of food over a short period of time and follows the eating with purging
Bulimia nervosa	Repeated episodes of binging and purging through self-induced vomiting; misuse of laxatives, diuretics, or other medications; fasting; or excessive exercise. (Binging refers to overeating; purging refers to voluntarily vomiting or using methods to stimulate defecation.)
Binge eating disorder	Excessive intake of calories without effort to prevent weight gain. The person feels that she has no control over her eating. The behaviors include eating very rapidly, eating until uncomfortably full, eating excessive amounts of food, and eating alone. The person feels guilty, disgusted, embarrassed, and depressed. It is important to be aware that not everyone who is obese engages in binge eating and not everyone who is diagnosed with a binge eating disorder is obese

Adapted from American Psychiatric Association (1994). *Diagnostic and statistical manual of mental disorders, fourth edition.* Washington, D.C.: American Psychiatric Association.

BOX 35-1 Characteristics of Anorexia Nervosa

- Refusal to eat
- Emaciation
- Amenorrhea
- Hypothermia
- Hyperactivity
- Hypotension

anorexia. Sir William Gull, a physician to England's Royal Family, described anorexia as a disease separate from hysteria or biological eating problems. Because he viewed the disease as distinct, he did not prescribe the standard treatment of the day, which was imprisonment in an insane asylum.

At the same time in France, Charles Lasegue, a French psychiatrist, saw anorexia as a form of rebellion found in wealthy children who were stressed by all the dinner table rules and regulations. Lesegue further suggested that anorexia was connected with suffocating and manipulative parental love. The characteristics of anorexia, first cited in 1873, are still relevant (Box 35–1).

During the 1800s, the ideal woman was thought to be "perfectly" devout so that her spiritual beauty shone brightly. The ability to refuse food was viewed as an excellent form of self-discipline that translated into spiritual discipline—the mark of a devout woman. This ideal consumed the thinking of much of the upper classes because they had access to unlimited quantities of food. Thinness in the poor, however, was not viewed as a symbol of restraint but rather a reflection of their lower state in life. "Thinness was therefore socially desirable to the upper class, just as robust health was considered a mark of the lower classes. Thus, morally, spiritually, and socially it was considered desirable for Victorian women to refuse food, even before the dictates of 20th century fashion and advertising" (Epstein, 1990, p. 37).

At the turn of the century, Freud linked anorexia with emotional and sexual conflicts. Pierre Janet, a French psychiatrist in the early 1900s, agreed with Freud but also connected this obsession to the spiritual issues of the Victorian age. It was not until the 1930s, however, that psychiatry had enough credibility for psychiatric views to be respected and incorporated into the treatment of anorexia.

▶ Check Your Reading

1. Identify three characteristics of anorexia nervosa.
2. Identify three roles that food plays in our lives.
3. Describe bulimia nervosa.
4. Describe binge eating disorder.
5. What are the life-threatening consequences of anorexia? Of bulimia?

CAUSES

Eating disorders share multifactorial causes, including biological factors, psychological factors, sociocultural factors, and spiritual factors. Each of these factors is discussed.

Biological Factors

Genetic Factors

Although the evidence linking genetics with eating disorders is far from conclusive, some support exists for this link. For instance, twin studies demonstrate a higher incidence of eating disorders in monozygotic twins than in dyzygotic twins. Furthermore, mothers and sisters of anorexics have a higher incidence of anorexia than sisters of controls. Major mood disorders such as depression and bipolar disorder seem to be prevalent in first-degree family members of anorexics (Kaplan and Sadock, 1991). In bulimic families, however, the parents are frequently obese. Bulimics frequently suffer from major depression.

Neurochemical Factors

ROLE OF SEROTONIN

Again, the research linking neurotransmitters to eating disorders is equivocal. However, evidence exists of a fundamental problem in the hypothalamus, which regulates appetite through the control of neurotransmitters, hormones, and neuromodulators. Serotonin is the specific neurotransmitter that seems most important in this process. Serotonin inhibits food intake and acts as a satiety agent. In fact, when the first selective serotonin reuptake inhibitor (SSRI) antidepressant, fluoxetine (Prozac), was developed, the manufacturer considered marketing it as a dietary medication because of its satiety affect. Serotonin, however, does not work in isolation. Research has demonstrated that when the byproduct of serotonin, 3-methyl-4-hydroxyphenylglycol (MHPG), is reduced in urine and spinal fluid, it decreases the activity of the neurotransmitter norepinephrine (Brownell, 1986).

ROLE OF ENDOGENOUS OPIOIDS

Another line of biological research into the cause of eating disorders focuses on the observation that binge eaters prefer concentrated sweets and other carbohydrates during periods of binging. This observation has led to the hypothesis that people who binge on sweets are deficient in endogenous opioid activity. To compensate, they crave food with a high concentration of sugar; this stimulates beta-endorphin activity and can lead to overeating (Fava et al, 1989; Laraia and Stuart, 1990).

Conversely the anorexic compensates for low levels of endogenous opioids with intensive physical exercise, which increases the amount of endorphins in the brain by twice the amount that existed before exercise. This gives the anorexic a euphoria similar to the commonly described "runner's high" and reinforces the pattern of starvation and exercise (Epstein, 1990).

ROLE OF STARVATION

Self-starvation as a form of stress reduction has a physiological basis and therefore may be reinforced on a physiological as well as psychological level. "Biologically there is an increase in metenkephaline in some patients who mutilate or engage in self-destructive behaviors. It is speculated that self-destructive behaviors that release neurotransmitters may reduce anxiety and stress" (Riley, 1991, p. 718).

Psychological Factors

Current thinking favors psychological and personality factors as critical in the development of both anorexia and bulimia. The journey of eating disorders has at its psychological base the issues of self-esteem and perfectionism (Case Examples 35–1 and 35–2). Perceptions about self-identity and fitting in to family, social circles, and society, in turn, affect views on body image ". . . [T]he primary problem is not with food, but with issues of control, self-esteem, depression, difficulty with intimate relationships, and developmental expectations. The excessive regulation and usage of food and behaviors associated with these disorders are an expression of the individual's difficulties in those areas" (Riley, 1991, p. 715).

Case Example 35–1 Veronica's Story

But thinness itself didn't matter to me as much as people's responses to it. . . . Every flattering comment was an affirmation of success. Since I came from a family which valued other people's opinion more than our own, I constantly sought the approval of others. . . . My thin figure gave me my only sense of worth. Until this time I never thought I could do anything well; staying thin was a major accomplishment. As much as I hated bulimia, I loved the self-esteem that being thin gave to me.

From Ault, M. (1990). I am a Christian bulimic. *Journal of Christian Nursing, 7*(1), 5–8.

Case Example 35–2 Renee's Story

I have so many rules, I can't live with anyone. They couldn't stand it. Everything I do has to be perfect. I know some of the things I feel I have to do don't make sense, but I am compelled to do them and get very anxious if I am not allowed to do things my way. I have rules for everything: how I exercise, how I dress, how I clean, even how I study. I have got to have control of everything.

From Flood, M. (1989). Addictive eating disorders. *Nursing Clinics of North America, 24*(1), 45–53.

Although multiple factors may be responsible for causing these emotional problems, food for these people takes on the role of "counselor." "Willful starvation for whatever reason is always a powerful interpersonal statement and may be used to express anger or elicit concern" (Hsu, 1990, p. 102). By focusing attention on food, the patient's time is consumed, and this allows him or her to avoid making decisions and to reduce challenges. The person usually becomes the center of the family's attention. At the same time, this focus on food decreases obvious secondary sex changes. With adolescence being the prime time for an eating disorder to appear, the body changes at puberty influence some girls to start dieting as a means of controlling the increasingly rounded hips, developing breasts, and all-around increase in body fat that is the mark of the menarche.

Family factors, such as mother-daughter and parental relationships, as well as the role the eating-disordered person plays in the family, have an impact on the development and maintenance of the eating disorder. It has been noted that anorexics' mothers may be intrusive, whereas bulimics' mothers do not give them the attention they crave, and so, in both cases, patients' relationships with their mothers are less than ideal. The eating disorder seems to be the remedy for the young woman's emotional stresses. Other family problems, such as alcohol or substance abuse, rape, incest, verbal abuse, or neglect, are common in the backgrounds of people with eating disorders. Food, or lack thereof, becomes the mechanism to deal with anger, hurt, and frustration.

The psychological characteristics of a woman whose journey is marked by anorexia include that she is

- Well behaved
- Eager to please
- Not consciously willing to be singled out for attention
- A perfectionist
- Poor in self-image
- Dependent on the opinions of others at the expense of her own
- Dependent

Curiously, as the anorexic loses weight, the fear of fatness increases. He or she loses the ability to read his or her body signals. Although these patients are not classified as delusional, no conclusive explanation has been found for the grossly distorted body image that develops (Hsu,

1990). Body image disturbance appears to be a critical factor.

People with bulimia tend to be of normal weight but often feel tense and anxious before they binge. The binging brings a sense of relief with no anxious or negative thoughts. After the binge, the anxiety begins again to mount, until the individual purges. With purging, a release of tension occurs, as weight gain has once again been averted. As with anorexic patients, bulimics also fear fatness, but it is accompanied by an irresistible urge to binge and purge (Hsu, 1990). "Due to its highly ritualized and repetitive nature, a binge can be used to organize thoughts and behavior" (Brownell and Forey, 1986, p. 457). Bulimia has also been seen in combination with borderline personality and with symptoms of mood lability, impulsivity, explosive interpersonal relationships, and self-mutilation (Hsu, 1990).

Compulsive overeaters eat to soothe themselves and may never be truly "hungry" because they graze all day long. Because food is used as a substitute for relationships that are not working or do not exist, the overeater can attain some sense of comfort and well-being from gorging on the food. Food becomes a companion, and the binging temporarily gives the binger a "lift" or "high" that he or she feels cannot be obtained through conventional means. In a study designed "as exploration of thoughts, moods and physiological sensations associated with binge eating in a non-purging population," 19 obese women were questioned. "While nearly half the participants reported awareness of being hungry before binging, when asked to rate the importance of hunger relative to other factors, it emerged as least important. It appears that while this population experiences hunger prior to a binge, it is not hunger itself that brings about the binge" (Arnow et al, 1992, p. 163). The following quote describes a binger's response to stress (Billigmeier, 1991, p. 140):

When you can't accomplish your too high goals, you eat.
When things don't go right, you eat.
When people don't do what they should, you eat.
When events don't run smoothly, you eat.
When people don't like your behavior, you eat.

In the case of anorexia nervosa, the previous statements would all be finished with "you don't eat." Not eating for anorexia patients becomes the control mechanism by which they order their lives into "perfection" even though outward circumstances beyond their control appear to be "out of control" to them. This form of self-"discipline" reinforces the idea that they are "good" at something even though that something is starvation. Essentially, this self-destructive behavior is a form of stress control for anorexic patients.

Sociocultural Factors

"It is difficult to watch television without being confronted by advertisements for both high-caloric foods as well as the latest diet plans. The social (and usually family) pressures are also contradictory: you must eat everything other people give you but you must not get fat" (Abraham and Llewellyn-Jones, 1990, p. 27; Fontaine, 1991).

Socially the anorexic is

- Introverted
- Emotionally reserved
- Socially insecure
- Self-denying
- Deferential toward others
- Overly compliant

Although the outward behavior of an anorexic woman may reflect the "good little girl," her body is paying for every act of compliance by the brutality of starvation. The praise of initial weight loss makes the anorexic feel good and gives her something she desperately seeks: the attention and approval of others. This attention she desires is not in the form of others prying into her eating habits or preoccupation with weight, but rather in the end result, which she perceives as "required" to be accepted.

The bulimic is also socially isolated because of the nature of the binging/purging ritual. There exists a deep fear of being rejected by others if they discover the patient's binging/purging ritual.

Compulsive overeaters share many of the bulimic and anorexic personality traits with the major difference involving social concerns. Compulsive overeaters primarily use food as a replacement for relationships. Also, the extra weight gives the overeater added social protection. In contrast to those who suffer with bulimia or anorexia, the compulsive overeater does not seem to have the same obsessive preoccupation with becoming fat. This extra weight provides the overeater with an insulation from others, especially from the harmful words or abuse others might heap on them (Case Example 35–3).

Case Example 35–3 Bernadette's Story

Bernadette, a student nurse who was hospitalized for an acute schizophrenic episode and who had grown quite fat, was observed to eat ravenously whenever she had an argument or felt threatened. Eventually she gave an explanation. She was afraid that the hostility of others and their angry words would rattle around inside her and keep wounding her. By stuffing herself with food, Bernadette would cover her "sore" inside, as with a poultice, and she would not feel the hurt so much.

Spiritual Factors

For some anorexics, because of their overly rigid and stereotypical thinking, religious influences such as the following verses from the Bible may accentuate their drive to be perfect:

> Be perfect, therefore, as your heavenly Father is perfect (Matthew 5:48).
>
> You must be blameless before the Lord your God (Deuteronomy 18:13).

If an anorexic sees perfection as a spiritual goal, he or she might—tragically—see weight loss as an act of devotion to God. Spirituality and fasting have always had a strong relationship, so the anorexic patient may rationalize his or her behavior as a spiritual act of devotion superior to what other mortals can accomplish. Despite these lofty thoughts, however, anorexia produces not spiritual fulfillment but rather a profound, overwhelming physical and spiritual emptiness.

The bulimic patient tends to be a superstitious and insecure thinker, and this spills over into his or her view of spirituality. Because of the need to purge himself or herself of food, it has been equated in some patients as a spiritual cleansing of evil. The "evil" that lurks within may be seen as bad attitudes, impatience, or unhappiness with how his or her life's journey is unfolding. Anderson (1993) reports that many eating-disordered persons he has worked with feel the need to purge themselves of evil forces they believe live within them. He also states that along with purging, some patients also cut themselves, describing the same spiritual cleansing rationales. "One young lady was taking seventy-five laxatives a day. . . . When I talked with her I asked, 'This has nothing to do with eating, does it?' 'No,' she responded. 'You're defecating to purge yourself from evil, aren't you?' She nodded in agreement" (Anderson, 1993, p. 87).

Compulsive overeaters use eating as a coping mechanism to deal with the emptiness or absence of a spiritual reality in their lives. Food is expected to fill that emptiness; it cannot meet this expectation, and the person is left with a painful void that refuses to be filled.

From the Victorian age to the present, the journey marked by eating disorders has linked spiritual to perfectionism ideals. The aforementioned Bible verses, when studied from the Greek (Matthew) and Hebrew (Deuteronomy), actually refer to obedience to God rather than human efforts at living lives without error or flaw. The interpretation of these verses, however, may be distorted to focus on the person's need to be perfect. Such perfection includes total control of anger. For the eating-disordered person, it may involve suppression of all angry feelings.

▶ Check Your Reading

6. What is the hypothesized role of serotonin in anorexia?
7. What evidence is there for a genetic link to the eating disorders?
8. Cite one psychological issue that may be part of the cause of anorexia; of bulimia; of binge eating disorder?
9. How do spiritual issues play into the cause of eating disorders?
10. What are two of the family issues in eating disorders?

RELATIONSHIP TO OTHER PSYCHIATRIC PROBLEMS

Depression is seen across the board in all eating disorders. A study by Walsh and colleagues (1985) indicates lifetime prevalence of major depression at 71% for those with eating disorders. The long-term outcome is poor for as many as 40% of patients with eating disorders because of the co-occurrence of depression (Silverstone, 1992). Major depression or dysthymia is reported in as many as 50% to 75% of anorexics. Obsessive-compulsive disorder also is seen in 10% to 15% of anorexics.

Bulimia studies report that as many as 40% of these patients show signs of clinical depression: increased rates of anxiety (45%), substance abuse disorders (49%), and bipolar illness (12%). Bulimia also seems to have high coincidence (as high as 60%) with borderline personality disorder. Binge eating disorder is also associated with increased rates of psychiatric illness, including major depression, panic disorder, and borderline and avoidant personality disorders (Yanovski et al, 1993).

NURSING PROCESS

ASSESSMENT

It is essential for the patient with an eating disorder to receive a comprehensive assessment, including physical, psychological, sociocultural, family, and spiritual assessment. A psychiatric history, a developmental history, and a history of substance abuse are also necessary (see Chapter 13).

Physical Assessment

Because eating disorders are associated with such high mortality and morbidity, the physical examination is extremely important. Begin by taking a full set of *vital signs.* The anorexic patient frequently has bradycardia, lowered body temperature, amenorrhea, and hypotension. It is important to assess how much the patient weighs, what is his or her normal weight, how much he or she has gained or lost, and in what time frame the weight loss occurred. While you are weighing the patient, ask what he or she thinks of his or her body; is his or her weight change related to mood or to external circumstances?

Assess the patient's *eating habits.* What is the pattern of the patient's eating? Where does he or she eat? Does the patient engage in binge/purge cycles of eating? If so, how does he or she feel about this pattern? Where does he or she binge? Where does he or she purge? Does he or she eat, binge, and purge in secret? Does the patient fast? How often does he or she engage in these behaviors? Does the patient take amphetamines, diet pills, or caffeine pills to lose weight?

Assess the patient's *activity*. Does the patient engage in excessive exercise? How does it make him or her feel? Is there a pattern to the patient's excessive exercise?

Assess for *other physical signs* of eating disorders. Anorexic patients frequently have significant hair loss; yellowish, dry, atrophic skin; lanugo; cessation of menses; cachexia; cyanosis of the extremities; and peripheral edema. Bulimic patients frequently display hoarseness, parotid gland enlargement (giving them a chipmunk appearance), dental damage caused by regurgitation of stomach acid, electrolyte imbalances, and dehydration.

Finally, assess the patient's *elimination habits*. Does the patient use laxatives or diuretics to lose weight? If so, how many are used and how often?

Psychological Assessment

Anorexic and bulimic patients have a core of psychological characteristics in common. These are shown in Box 35–2. The anorexic tends to use greater denial than the bulimic—not only denying hunger, but also denying that there is a problem at all. The bulimic is usually aware of his or her problem and distressed about it.

Sociocultural Assessment

It is important to inquire about the patient's belief system about what is "normal" weight and what is "normal" eating. Is there pressure on the patient to be thin? Does he or she feel that his or her acceptance and love are conditional, based on weight? How much has he or she integrated society's message that "you can never be too thin"? It is important to look at the quality and extent of the patient's support system. The anorexic tends to be introverted and isolated; the bulimic may appear extroverted, engaging in sexually promiscuous behaviors, drug use, stealing, and suicidal gestures.

BOX 35–2 Psychological Characteristics Common to People with Anorexia Nervosa and Bulimia Nervosa

- Low self-esteem
- Suppression of feelings, especially anger
- Perfectionism
- Reliance on schedules, lack of spontaneity
- Obsession with body size and food
- Sexual problems
- Identity crises
- Lack of autonomy
- Immaturity, "black-and-white" thinking
- Depression

Family Assessment

An assessment of family function often reveals significant differences between the anorexic and the bulimic. The family environment of the anorexic patient is more controlled, rigid, and marked by less overt discord. The family environment of the bulimic patient is marked by conflict and chaos, with violence and substance abuse the norm.

It is also important to assess the eating patterns of the family. Questions focusing on the family's approach to mealtimes might include:

- Who plans the meals in your family?
- Who cooks the meals in your family?
- What are mealtimes like in your family?

Spiritual Assessment

In conducting a spiritual assessment, ask about the patient's view of himself or herself in relation to God. Does the patient feel that he or she is "not good enough"? Is there a need to strive for perfection? Does the patient believe that he or she measures up only when he or she weighs a certain amount? Does the patient use spiritual rationalization to explain eating behaviors (e.g., "fasting makes me stronger")?

Additional Areas to Assess

As you gather data from the patient and other reliable resources, include a variety of dimensions to help identify and clarify specific contributing factors for each patient. Love and Seaton (1991) list the following dimensions as important aspects of the assessment for patients with eating disorders:

- Alliance building
- Motivation for treatment
- Coping strategies

▶ Check Your Reading

11. What impact does anorexia have on blood pressure; on pulse?
12. Identify at least two areas where anorexics and bulimics differ.
13. What would you want to know about a bulimic's eating patterns?
14. What impact does society's pressures have on individuals with eating disorders?

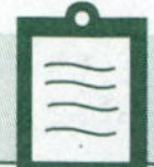

MEDICAL DIAGNOSES AND RELATED NURSING DIAGNOSES — Eating Disorders

***DSM-IV* Diagnosis:** Anorexia nervosa

DIAGNOSTIC CRITERIA

A. Refusal to maintain body weight at or above a minimally normal weight for age and height (e.g., weight loss leading to maintenance of body weight less than 85% of that expected; or failure to make expected weight gain during period of growth, leading to body weight less than 85% of that expected).
B. Intense fear of gaining weight or becoming fat, even though underweight.
C. Disturbance in the way in which one's body weight or shape is experienced, undue influence of body weight or shape on self-evaluation, or denial of the seriousness of the current low body weight.
D. In postmenarcheal females, amenorrhea, i.e., the absence of at least three consecutive menstrual cycles. (A woman is considered to have amenorrhea if her periods occur only following hormone, e.g., estrogen, administration.)

Specify type:

Restricting Type: During the current episode of Anorexia Nervosa, the person has not regularly engaged in binge eating or purging behavior (i.e., self-induced vomiting or the misuse of laxatives, diuretics, or enemas).

Binge Eating/Purging Type: During the current episode of Anorexia Nervosa, the person has regularly engaged in binge eating or purging behavior (i.e., self-induced vomiting or the misuse of laxatives, diuretics, or enemas).

***DSM-IV* Diagnosis:** Bulimia nervosa

DIAGNOSTIC CRITERIA

A. Recurrent episodes of binge eating. An episode of binge eating is characterized by both of the following:
   (1) Eating, in a discrete period of time (e.g., within any 2-hour period), an amount of food that is definitely larger than most people would eat during a similar period of time and under similar circumstances.
   (2) A sense of lack of control over eating during the episode (e.g., a feeling that one cannot stop eating or control what or how much one is eating).
B. Recurrent inappropriate compensatory behavior to prevent weight gain, such as self-induced vomiting; misuse of laxatives, diuretics, enemas, or other medications; fasting; or excessive exercise.
C. The binge eating and inappropriate compensatory behaviors both occur, on average, at least twice a week for 3 months.
D. Self-evaluation is unduly influenced by body shape and weight.
E. The disturbance does not occur exclusively during episodes of Anorexia Nervosa.

Specify type:

Purging Type: During the current episode of Bulimia Nervosa, the person has regularly engaged in self-induced vomiting or the misuse of laxatives, diuretics, or enemas.

Nonpurging Type: During the current episode of Bulimia Nervosa, the person has used other inappropriate compensatory behaviors, such as fasting or excessive exercise, but has not regularly engaged in self-induced vomiting or the misuse of laxatives, diuretics, or enemas.

DIAGNOSIS

Medical and nursing diagnoses for the patient with an eating disorder are shown in "Medical Diagnoses and Related Nursing Diagnoses: Eating Disorders."

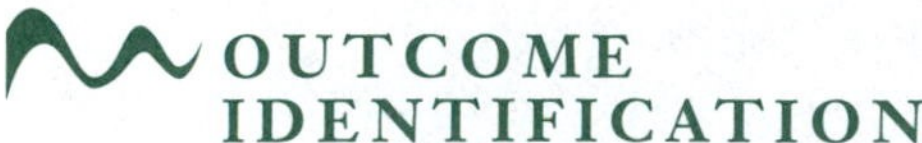

OUTCOME IDENTIFICATION

The expected outcomes for a patient with an eating disorder are as follows:

- The patient will achieve and maintain his or her weight within normal parameters for his or her age and size.
- The patient's fluid and electrolyte balance will be within normal parameters, and the patient will no longer engage in binge/purge eating.
- The patient will express an accurate appraisal of body size and body weight.

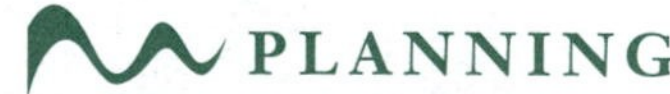

PLANNING

The short-term goals for a patient with an eating disorder are as follows:

Expected Outcome	Short-Term Goals
The patient will achieve and maintain his or her weight within normal parameters for his or her age and size.	1. The patient will participate in treatment. 2. The patient will acknowledge having an eating disorder. 3. The patient will state the components of a balanced diet.

MEDICAL DIAGNOSES AND RELATED NURSING DIAGNOSES Eating Disorders *Continued*

***DSM-IV* Diagnosis:** Binge eating disorder

DIAGNOSTIC CRITERIA

A. Recurrent episodes of binge eating. An episode of binge eating is characterized by both of the following:
   (1) Eating, in a discrete period of time (e.g., within any 2-hour period), an amount of food that is definitely larger than most people would eat in a similar period of time under similar circumstances.
   (2) A sense of lack of control over eating during the episode (e.g., a feeling that one cannot stop eating or control what or how much one is eating).

B. The binge eating episodes are associated with three (or more) of the following:
   (1) Eating much more rapidly than normal.
   (2) Eating until feeling uncomfortably full.
   (3) Eating large amounts of food when not feeling physically hungry.
   (4) Eating alone because of being embarrassed by how much one is eating.
   (5) Feeling disgusted with oneself, depressed, or guilty after overeating.

C. Marked distress regarding binge eating is present.

D. The binge eating occurs, on average, at least 2 days a week for 6 months.
   Note: The method of determining frequency differs from that used for Bulimia Nervosa; future research should address whether the preferred method of setting a frequency threshold is counting the number of days on which binges occur or counting the number of episodes of binge eating.

E. The binge eating is not associated with the regular use of inappropriate compensatory behaviors (e.g., purging, fasting, excessive exercise) and does not occur exclusively during the course of Anorexia Nervosa or Bulimia Nervosa.

RELATED NURSING DIAGNOSES	DEFINITION	EXAMPLE
Altered Nutrition: Less than Body Requirements	The state in which an individual experiences an intake of nutrients insufficient to meet metabolic needs	Altered Nutrition: Less than Body Requirements related to insufficient intake of calories evidenced by weight 20% less than normal
Body Image Disturbance	Disruption in the way one perceives one's body image	Body Image Disturbance related to fear of weight gain evidenced by preoccupation with being fat
Fluid Volume Deficit	The state in which an individual experiences vascular, cellular, or intracellular dehydration	Fluid Volume Deficit related to purging activities evidenced by abnormal blood chemistry values
Self-Esteem Disturbance	Negative self-evaluation/feelings about self or self capabilities, which may be directly or indirectly expressed	Self-Concept Disturbance: Self-Esteem related to feelings of inadequacy evidenced by self-derogatory statements

Diagnostic criteria from American Psychiatric Association (1994). *Diagnostic and statistical manual of mental disorders,* Fourth Edition. Washington, D.C.: American Psychiatric Association; nursing diagnoses and definitions from North American Nursing Diagnosis Association (1994). *NANDA nursing diagnoses: Definitions and classification 1995–1996.* Philadelphia: NANDA.

	4. The patient will eat a balanced diet. 5. The patient's nutritional status will be stabilized. 6. The patient will participate in an appropriate level of daily exercise.		4. The patient will discuss alternatives to binging/purging. 5. The patient will discuss feelings experienced before and after a binge/purge cycle.
The patient's fluid and electrolyte balance will be within normal parameters, and the patient will no longer engage in binge/purge eating.	1. The patient will agree to talk about his or her urges to binge and purge. 2. The patient's nutritional intake will restore normal fluid and electrolyte balance. 3. The patient will discuss the destructive results of binging/purging.	The patient will express an accurate appraisal of body size and body weight.	1. The patient will accurately describe his or her body shape. 2. The patient will accurately state his or her ideal body weight. 3. The patient will identify the cognitive distortions that support an inaccurate appraisal of body image and weight.

The plan defines not only short-term goals but also the intensity of treatment. Whether treatment is offered in an outpatient or an inpatient setting depends on the severity of the patient's physical and psychiatric condition. For instance, the following physical findings would warrant inpatient treatment:

- Weight loss greater than 30% of body weight over three months
- Heart rate less than 40 beats per minute
- Temperature less than 96.8°F
- Systolic blood pressure less than 70 mm Hg
- Serum potassium less than 2.5 mEq/L
- Severe dehydration

The psychiatric findings warranting inpatient treatment include the following:

- High risk for suicide
- Self-mutilating behaviors
- Severe depression
- Inability to comply with treatment plan
- Inadequate response to treatment
- Psychotic behavior

Inpatient treatment provides the support, safety, physiological monitoring, and psychological care supportive of behavioral change offered by the 24-hour availability of nursing staff. The inpatient care of patients with eating disorders requires interdisciplinary planning and collaboration to deal with the manipulation and "splitting" behaviors often displayed by the patients.

Nevertheless, outpatient treatment of people with eating disorders is generally preferred. It is certainly the least restrictive. It relies on the patient to exercise self-control. Finally, it calls for the active support and involvement of family members. The success of outpatient treatment depends on the patient's commitment and motivation.

Regardless of the setting for treatment, the treatment team mutually develops a treatment plan with the patient and family, including expectations for weight gain, fluid and electrolyte balance, and decreased binging and purging. It is also essential for you to engage the patient in a therapeutic alliance and to seek the patient's commitment to treatment. The therapeutic alliance frequently includes a written and signed contract in which the patient agrees to specific goals of the treatment plan.

▶ Check Your Reading

15. Identify one expected outcome for an eating-disordered patient.
16. Identify one short-term goal to support the expected outcome that you identified in question 15.
17. Identify two physical and two psychiatric symptoms that would lead to inpatient treatment of an anorexic.
18. Identify one benefit of outpatient therapy for an eating-disordered patient.
19. Identify one nursing diagnosis that might be applied to an eating-disordered patient.

IMPLEMENTATION

The aim of treatment for the patient with an eating disorder varies with the type of eating disorder. For the anorexic patient, weight gain is essential. The bulimic patient needs to organize his or her eating habits better. The compulsive overeater needs to control his or her impulse to eat too much. Underlying all of these physical needs, however, are the root causes of the particular disorder.

There are five major methods of treatment for all eating disorders:

- Behavior modification
- Inpatient psychotherapy
- Outpatient psychotherapy
- Psychopharmacology
- Family therapy

Patients always are the focus of care. Nursing care is affected, however, by your perspective about a patient's diagnosis as well as your personal beliefs and values. Realizing this, it is essential for each of us to step back and evaluate, before caring for patients with eating disorders, our own ideas, values, opinions, and beliefs not only regarding people with eating disorders, but also caring for patients on the journey marked by eating disorders.

The first step involves identifying your own beliefs and values regarding body shape and weight. Culture and society at large daily affects and subtly shapes our thoughts and ideas. Only after you have taken a serious look at your own values, biases, and beliefs regarding this issue can you provide genuine care to patients with eating disorders. The question each of us must answer is: "Whose eyes am I looking through—my own or the eyes of society?" We need to ask ourselves further: "Am I making judgments about personal worth based on a person's body weight, shape, or size? Have I bought into cultural stereotypes, such as losing weight will solve all of life's problems or having a thin body will guarantee a happy-ever-after life?" These beliefs can attack the core of a person with an eating disorder. The patient's sense of happiness, self-worth, and value as a human being are challenged if such stereotypes are believed.

As we care for overweight patients, it is important to realize that these people do not have more emotional problems than normal weight people. Much of the emotional trauma they experience is most likely the result of prejudice and stigma and the cultural pressure to lose weight (Fontaine, 1991).

Nursing collectively must be willing to challenge these cultural stereotypes. This challenge begins with each nurse determining how to view a sense of worth. Do we as nurses believe "Beauty is in the eye of the beholder" or are we too busy "judging the book by the cover"? Nurses stand at the door of opportunity; the question is will we stand or walk through the door? Nurses must be proactive when caring for patients with eating disorders. We must become leaders in this arena by "fostering a humane approach to body size" (Fontaine, 1991, p. 675).

Behavior Modification

Behavior modification techniques are widely accepted as a form of treatment with eating-disordered patients. The key is to implement the behavior modification program in such a way that the patient perceives he or she is in control. Control is a foundational component in the mind of the patient with an eating disorder, so the success of this treatment depends largely on this issue.

The patient contracts with the staff and participates in deciding the goals as well as rewards for achievement of goals, such as weight gained, exercise, and vomiting or not. The hospital setting is much more likely to be the treatment setting for the anorexic patient than the bulimic or compulsive overeater, so the behavior modification techniques would vary.

The anorexic patient, in an inpatient setting, would naturally be more closely monitored and perhaps have peer as well as caregiver support to enhance his or her goal-keeping. For the bulimic or compulsive overeater, the behavior modification techniques used may consist of keeping a daily self-monitoring diary, limiting amount of food per meal, limiting high-carbohydrate foods in the home, and limiting unstructured time. (See Chapter 18 for behavioral strategies.)

Inpatient Psychotherapy

Most inpatient treatment of eating disorders is with anorexia nervosa patients because the starvation state is life-threatening. Bulimia patients are hospitalized usually when severely depressed or suicidal. Individual therapy involves delving into the root issues of self-esteem, independence, sexuality, and perfectionism, as discussed earlier. Cognitive therapy is an important modality in addressing the cognitive distortions that the patient holds regarding eating (see Chapter 16). The fear of fatness has been relabeled by some clinicians as a phobia of adolescent weight (Crisp, 1967; Crisp et al, 1980). Developmental issues are also discussed with the female patient as a means of understanding herself in relationship to the world as she transcends from girl to woman (Nusbaum and Drever, 1990). In male anorexics, the issues of masculinity and all that it signifies is explored.

Refeeding as a form of nutritional treatment is used with anorexic patients in most hospital settings. Your role is to be present during meals to encourage and reassure the patient that he or she will not get fat from meals and explain the feeling of fullness after eating to calm the anxiousness commonly felt by the patient (Hsu, 1990).

Outpatient Psychotherapy

These patients include those who are not binging, purging, or emaciated to a life-threatening degree. Inpatient goals are still valid except there is not the same level of supervision. Some suggest that families involved in family therapy be responsible for weight gain by anorexia nervosa patients, and this has shown signs of success (Dare, 1983). The best approach to outpatient treatment is multifaceted and includes individual, family, nutritional, and group therapies (Hsu, 1990; Titus and Smith, 1992). Support groups such as Overeaters Anonymous are helpful to many. Accountability works well in group counseling or peer support groups and provides healthy interactions with others so as to help build self-esteem and feelings of worthiness so often lacking in patients with eating disorders.

Psychopharmacology

Although antidepressants such as fluoxetine (Prozac) have shown decreased depression and increased weight gain in anorexic patients as well as decreasing by 50% bulimic binge episodes, the long-term effects of these drugs is unclear. Most studies have shown that antidepressants do improve the mood of the eating-disordered patient. This improvement may result in the patient being better able to address the psychological impetus for his or her eating disorder. Therefore, the physician who has taken a thorough psychological and family history of the patient may be able to prescribe an antidepressant as an adjunct to addressing the underlying problems affecting or initiating the eating disorder.

Family Therapy

Minuchin and colleagues see the anorexic patient as the symptom of a family problem. The goal in family therapy

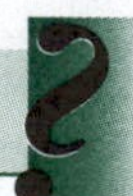

WHAT PATIENTS NEED TO KNOW Eating disorders

Why do I need to sign a contract?
A contract is a written set of rules, consequences, and rewards that both you and the treatment team have agreed on. It can be renegotiated as progress is made. It serves as a guideline for identifying prohibited as well as desired behaviors. Items that are typically negotiated relate to meals; privileges such as TV watching, radio playing, and trips off unit; and weight gain.

What is healthy eating or "gentle" eating?
These are new behaviors to help you prepare and eat foods to achieve weight gain and weight stabilization goals. Some of the following eating behaviors are encouraged: eat food slowly, chew thoroughly, put utensils down between bites, do not eat while doing other activities, eat in a specific place at home (dining room), and sit down while eating at prescribed times.

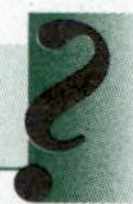

WHAT PATIENTS AND FAMILIES NEED TO KNOW — Bulimia nervosa

How is bulimia nervosa different from anorexia nervosa?
Bulimia is a separate and different condition from anorexia nervosa and compulsive eating. Most often the bulimic patient is of normal weight or only slightly overweight who binges and purges to maintain or lose weight. Also, anorexics who have lost their rigid control over fasting or not eating may purge as an attempt to gain some type of control. Sometimes, anorexics may have been bulimic before the onset of anorexia nervosa. It is estimated that bulimia may occur in as many as 40% of college women.

What is the binge-purge cycle?
This compulsive cycle is characterized by a total loss of control over consuming thousands of calories (binge), which are high-calorie (candy bars) and high-carbohydrate (potato chips, cookies, cake) foods taken with lots of fluids (soft drinks, juices), followed by a purge. The cycle interferes with normal daily functioning to the extent often seen with alcoholics or drug addicts. The bulimic becomes so preoccupied with binge-purge behavior that job and relationships suffer as the patient becomes more isolated and depressed.

What are the different forms of purging?
There are various forms of purging, such as self-induced vomiting; use of diuretics, laxatives, and enemas; or strict dieting or fasting. Excessive or vigorous exercise is also a form of purging, especially if it is done to prevent weight gain.

What can I do to stop the binge-purge cycle?
Seek professional help. It is difficult to stop the cycle. You have probably made promises to yourself every morning to stop binging and purging and then feel guilty when it happens. Having this sense of loss of control about eating may make you feel depressed and anxious. These are normal feelings when you feel powerless and unable to enjoy or take charge of your life.

is "to transform the issue of an anorectic patient to the drama of a dysfunctional family" (Minuchin et al, 1978). Characteristics of a family that reinforce anorexia are enmeshment, rigidity, overprotectiveness, lack of conflict resolution, and involvement of the sick child in unresolved parental conflicts (Minuchin et al, 1978). Opening up family communication is a goal in family therapy with an anorexic patient.

Although many clinicians view family process as important to the cause of the eating disorders, family therapy has not proven to be any more effective than individual therapy in the treatment of bulimia (Hsu, 1990). Bulimic patients tend to be older and therefore not living at home. Separation and individuation issues are commonly addressed in individual therapy sessions.

Spiritual Aspects of Care

The previously discussed interventions are considered traditional and provide an overall framework in identifying and caring for patients with eating disorders. The authors believe these interventions are necessary to implement but do not believe they provide a holistic approach to patient care. The focus of this chapter is holistic—considering the physical, psychosocial, and spiritual dimension of an individual. With this as the foundation, the aspect not addressed in the previously mentioned interventions is the spiritual dimension. All people, whether or not they are practicing a particular formal religion, have a spiritual component (Carson, 1989). The person's spiritual nature must be considered

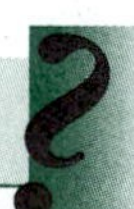

WHAT FAMILIES NEED TO KNOW — Anorexia nervosa

What do I need to know about anorexia nervosa?
Anorexia nervosa is a potentially life-threatening illness in which adolescent girls (or boys) literally starve themselves to death. These young people have an intense fear of becoming fat, relentlessly pursue thinness, and often have a delusion about their body image. The self-starvation is not only the absence of eating or the ingesting of low-calorie foods, but also may involve purging, which includes behaviors such as self-vomiting; taking diuretics, laxatives, or enemas; and excessively exercising to the point of exhaustion.

What should I do about cooking or preparing meals?
Often, anorexics have a personal "food list" of items they will eat. They will go to extreme lengths to avoid foods not on their list. You may begin noticing your adolescent hiding food, eating alone, or giving food to others or to household pets. Sometimes the adolescent gets involved with cooking rich, high-calorie meals for the family but will not even taste her or his own cooking.

What can I do to help my child?
Family therapy and intervention are key aspects to the long-term care and management of the anorexic patient. Understanding and family education are important aspects to assist parents to gain insight into what is happening within the family. Early recognition of recurrence of self-starvation behavior is important. Medical treatment should be sought when a 10% to 15% weight loss occurs, rather than waiting longer, when the patient becomes more debilitated and dehydrated as weight loss approaches 20% to 25% of normal body weight.

as part of their total care, along with the physical and psychosocial components (Carson, 1989; Wald and Bailey, 1990).

Research shows that people tend to experience lower levels of anxiety when they exhibit higher levels of spiritual well-being (Kaczorowski, 1989). Spiritual activities, for many people, provide and serve as direct coping actions (Sodestrom and Martinson, 1987). Case Example 35–4 illustrates the role of spiritual activities in a patient with anorexia nervosa.

Case Example 35–4 Ella's Story

Within my being there are two separate entities warring one with another. The stronger denies my need for nourishment during the waking hours. I pictured food as a dragon spitting tongues of flame trying to draw out the "fat" person hiding inside of my frail body. I would go to sleep at night feeling superior toward mere humans who gorged themselves on a regular basis. I took extreme precautions to keep the "night monster" under control. I plastered my home with notes reminding me that to eat would make me a "bad person." I'd lock and barricade myself in the bedroom. I was addicted to popcorn. I would get out of bed to eat. I'd meticulously clean all signs of this unconscious eating. When I woke in the morning, I had no memory of what I'd done during the night. Somewhere deep inside of the me who told the world I could "live on air," there was just a spark crying out to be loved and nurtured.

From Flood, M. (1989). Addictive eating disorders. *Nursing Clinics of North America, 24*(1), 45–53.

Feelings such as being out of control or feeling unloved or unaccepted can lead to feelings of hopelessness, helplessness, or lack of meaning in one's life. These feelings are reflective of spiritual distress. If you are committed to providing holistic care, you must address these spiritual issues with the eating-disordered patient. All the behavioral contracts, medications, and therapy will not succeed if the patient continues to feel unloved and unimportant. Addressing these issues goes right to the person's spirit.

▶ Check Your Reading

20. Identify two of the intervention strategies used with eating-disordered patients.
21. Identify one psychotropic medication used in the treatment of anorexia.
22. What is the goal of family therapy with the eating-disordered patient?

EVALUATION

The plan of care needs to be continually evaluated to ensure that goals set are realistic and success adequately measured. The formative evaluation looks at short-term goals initially set for a patient with an eating disorder to see if these goals need to be modified. Perhaps the goals did not include a focus on decreasing the anxiety experienced by the patient before mealtime. Modifying the plan might include teaching the patient relaxation techniques to make mealtimes more pleasurable. The summative evaluation examines the patient's physical, emotional, and spiritual state as treatment ends. The summative evaluation answers the following questions:

- Has the patient gained or lost weight (depending on the goal)?
- Is the patient's fluid and electrolyte balance restored?
- Is the patient articulating a normal body image?
- Is the patient feeling as if his or her life matters? Is he or she feeling loved?

CASE STUDY: JENNY

Jenny, a 13-year-old white girl, has been admitted to the psychiatric unit. According to her parents, her normal weight is 100 pounds and she has rapidly lost 20 pounds over the past month on a strict diet. Her mother states that she is very proud of Jenny, especially when she finishes first in the competitive gymnastic program she is involved with. Jenny believes that losing weight will help her improve her skills, so that she can attain a better score and stay at the top competitively at the next regional gymnastics meet. Jenny's mother said that she was a "straight A student in school" and was the "perfect, obedient" child. Lately, her parents stated they were exasperated with her dieting and refusal to eat even her favorite foods. On admission, Jenny's weight is 80 pounds, and her height is 5 feet and 5 inches. Her mother reported that Jenny started her menses at age 11, but she has not had a period for the past year.

Jenny remained quiet and withdrawn during the interview and glared at her parents while avoiding eye contact with the nurse. The nurse noted that her skin was cool to touch and was slightly yellow with a fine covering of lanugo. Her mother stated that Jenny would often say to her gymnastics coach that she was fat.

ASSESSMENT

Assessment data are as follows:

- Emaciated, sallow skin color
- 20% body weight loss
- Amenorrhea for past 12 months
- Appearance of lanugo
- Overachiever, "perfect, obedient" child

DIAGNOSIS

***DSM-IV* Diagnosis:** Anorexia Nervosa

Nursing Diagnosis: Altered Nutrition: Less than Body Requirements related to self-starvation behaviors as evidenced by 20-pound weight loss, amenorrhea, lanugo, and emaciated appearance

OUTCOME IDENTIFICATION, PLANNING, AND IMPLEMENTATION

EXPECTED OUTCOME 1: By _____ the patient's weight will be within safe limits.

SHORT-TERM GOAL	NURSING INTERVENTIONS	RATIONALES
By _____ the patient will establish a minimum weekly weight gain (0.5–1.5 kg per week).	1. Provide nutrition consultation to facilitate weight gain.	1. Medical and nutritional management is needed to provide for a safe regimen of weight gain in patient's debilitated state. The patient is more likely to eat foods she has a choice in selecting.
	2. Initiate eating contract that specifies three meals per day to be eaten with other patients and staff.	2. Contract negotiation fosters the patient's independence and provides for positive reinforcement of appropriate eating behavior.
	3. Observe patient during and after eating noting any rituals or signs of purging.	3. During early hospitalization, some deception as well as a need to feel in control of the environment and food intake occurs. Purging may occur as a response to weight gain.
	4. Maintain a regular weighing schedule (usually one to three times per week) with patient in light clothing. May have patient weigh with back to scale in some situations (to prevent patient from knowing actual weight, especially in extreme obsession cases).	4. Limited weighing focuses on issue of trust and minimizes patient's obsessing about weight gain or loss.

EXPECTED OUTCOME 2: By _____ the patient will demonstrate minimal complications from nutritional imbalances.

SHORT-TERM GOAL	NURSING INTERVENTIONS	RATIONALES
By _____ the patient will exhibit a minimum of adverse side effects caused by refeeding schedule.	1. Monitor vital signs and observe for adverse side effects to refeeding. 2. Check laboratory values.	1–2. Patient is at risk for arrhythmias, bradycardia, hypotension, electrolyte imbalance (especially hypokalemia), and hypothermia.
	3. Begin refeeding schedule slowly.	3. Other problems may occur with too rapid weight gain, including congestive heart failure, abdominal discomfort, edema, and gastric dilation.

Nursing Diagnosis: Body Image Disturbance related to inaccurate perception of self and dysfunctional family system as evidenced by statements of being fat despite thinness, emaciated appearance, and controlling behavior of parents

PLANNING, OUTCOME IDENTIFICATION, AND IMPLEMENTATION

EXPECTED OUTCOME 1: By _____ the patient will establish a more realistic body image.

SHORT-TERM GOAL	NURSING INTERVENTIONS	RATIONALES
By _____ the patient will have a realistic perception of her body image.	1. Explore need to excel at gymnastics and possible feelings of inadequacy.	1. Feelings of inadequacy, loneliness, or need to be perfect within the family system need to be examined.
	2. When unrealistic statements are made with regards to body size, gently confront patient with reality. 3. Assist the patient to identify manageable goals related to gymnastics and self. 4. Encourage acceptance of shortcomings as well as strengths.	2–4. Self-deprecating comments and an inability to see self as someone unique and distinct within the family are important. Often, the patient feels helpless in family situations and finds comfort in control of eating behavior because parents may not control this aspect of life.

EXPECTED OUTCOME 2: By _____ the patient will verbalize feelings and acknowledge self by taking responsibility for actions.

SHORT-TERM GOAL	NURSING INTERVENTIONS	RATIONALES
By _____ the patient will verbalize feelings with nurse and members on the unit.	1. Encourage comments.	1. Therapeutic communication and unconditional positive regard promote feelings of trust, which are necessary before patient will verbalize feelings.
	2. Listen nonjudgmentally and without criticism. 3. Avoid overreacting when patient has deceived staff, e.g., hidden food or purging.	2–3. Patients often come from rigid family environments in which the parents (usually mother) make all their decisions and expect them to be perfect in everything they do.

EVALUATION

Formative Evaluation: Jenny did not meet her weekly weight gain contract for the first 2 weeks of hospitalization. She would hide food and secretly purge. The contract was renegotiated and the expectations of weight gain were reduced to weight maintenance for 1 week, to which she agreed. During that time, Jenny was able to talk about the expectations of weight gain, which made her feel powerless and helpless, plus the feelings of fullness in her stomach. She was beginning to understand the family dynamics and needed the unhurried, unconditional acceptance by the nurse during the early phase of her treatment. A supportive, nonrigid, forgiving atmosphere was the important milieu setting for Jenny to work on her family and spiritual needs.

Summative Evaluation: By discharge, Jenny had gained 15 pounds and was feeling in better control of her own life. She decided to take a short break from gymnastics until she could rebuild her strength. Her mother was upset that she would not make the gymnastic competition. Jenny was able to express her feelings to her mother about the pressure she felt from the comments that were made. She was beginning to feel more in touch with who she really was, a young beautiful child of God who didn't have to prove anything to be accepted in His love. Jenny had not mentioned how "fat she was" during her last 3 weeks of hospitalization. An outpatient family therapy program was negotiated, which Jenny and her parents agreed to attend. It was reported that Jenny began to be involved with the youth group at her church.

CONCLUSIONS

Eating disorders stem from a variety of psychological issues and are a form of addiction, such as alcoholism or drug abuse. Behavioral changes necessary to conquer this addiction, however, are not found in avoidance as in alcohol or drug addictions. Rather, the patient with an eating disorder must redefine his or her relationship with food. He or she must explore the reasons he or she has turned to food to solve problems. In closing, we would like to quote from a nurse who identifies herself as a recovering bulimic (Ferraro, 1990, p.2):

The pursuit of help by a closet bulimic nurse can be further hampered by nurses' self-care styles. In general, nurses historically are "other-focused," always trying to ease the burden of patients and families. Daily we push ourselves to give the best possible care even when under tremendous time constraints. When and how can we stop long enough to care for ourselves? Perhaps, too, some of those nurses who speak negatively of bulimic patients do so because they see a little of themselves in these patients. If we do not invest the time and effort required to maintain our own health, how can we expect to continually assist others in maintaining theirs?

KEY POINTS TO REMEMBER

- Food plays several important roles in our lives: to provide nutrition; to reward achievement and punish misbehaviors; and to comfort, support, and love. Also, it is intricately tied to the impressions we have of ourselves in terms of our body image and self-esteem.
- Anorexia nervosa and bulimia affect young, white women in the middle to upper socioeconomic groups in Western countries.
- Eating disorders are associated with significant medical consequences, including life-threatening conditions.
- Problems with food regulation have a historical basis.
- Anorexia nervosa is a disorder characterized by the refusal to maintain a normal body weight; this is done through strict dieting or engaging in a binge/purge cycle of eating.
- Bulimia nervosa is characterized by repeated episodes of binging and purging.
- Binge eating disorder is characterized by excessive intake of calories.
- The cause of eating disorders is believed to be multifactorial with significant roles played by biological, psychological, sociocultural, and spiritual issues.
- There is a significant co-occurrence of psychiatric problems, such as depression, obsessive-compulsive disorder, panic disorder, and personality disorders, along with eating disorders.
- The assessment for eating disorders must include a comprehensive physical examination along with a focus on mental status and family, psychological, sociocultural, and spiritual issues.
- There are many nursing diagnoses appropriate to the eating disorders, including Nutrition, Alteration In: Less than Body Requirements, Fluid Volume Deficit, and Self-Concept Disturbance in Body Image; Self-Esteem.
- The identified outcomes focus on restoring nutritional and fluid and electrolyte balance as well as achieving normal weight.
- The nursing interventions focus on behavioral modification, inpatient psychotherapy, outpatient psychotherapy, psychotropic medications, family therapy, and spiritual interventions.

LEARNING ACTIVITIES

1. Reflect on the following questions in your journal: What do I think about weight? Do I link my own self-worth with my weight? Do I link the value of others to their weight? Do I give preferential treatment to people whose appearance is more pleasing to me? How much is my thinking affected by social stereotypes about weight and body shape?

2. Watch television one night and keep track of how many commercials or television programs extoll the value of thinness and the desirability of fast food. What impact does this have on young people's attitudes toward food? Toward diet? Toward what is good and desirable in relationship to body size and shape?

3. Survey one fashion magazine. How many advertisements do you see that "push" the idea that a woman's or man's self-worth is tied to outward appearance? When you look at advertisements showing very slim models, how do you react?

CRITICAL THINKING EXERCISE

Terri Mader, a 5 foot, 9 inch, 16-year-old high school swimmer, was admitted to the eating disorder unit weighing 98 lb. Her father was her swim coach and traveled with her to tournaments, while her mother, an executive, stayed home to care for her brother who was 13 years old. She was referred to the eating disorder unit by the physician who examined her following a fainting episode before her last swim meet when she lost consciousness for several minutes. She told the referring physician that she had been taking laxatives to keep her weight down.

1. What assumptions do you think Terri is operating under?
2. What evidence suggests that she may be anorexic?
3. What other possibilities might explain Terri's behavior?

One week following admission, Terri asked the nurse for her prn laxative. The nurse, aware of her abuse of laxatives, refused to give it to her. One hour later, her attending psychiatrist called the nurse on the unit stating, "I just received a call from my patient that you will not give her medication. I order you to give it to her now."

1. What is the psychiatrist's point of view?
2. Give an alternative viewpoint of the situation.
3. What conclusion(s) might be drawn about the relationship between the nurse, the patient, and the psychiatrist?

REFERENCES

Abraham, S., and Llewellyn-Jones, D. (1987). *Eating disorders: The facts* (2nd ed.). Oxford: Oxford University Press.

American Psychiatric Association (1994). *Diagnostic and statistical manual of mental disorders* (4th ed.). Washington, D.C.: American Psychiatric Association.

Anderson, N. T. (1993). *Released from bondage.* Nashville: Thomas Nelson, Inc.

Arnow, B., Kenardy, J., and Agras, W. S. (1992). Binge eating among the obese: A descriptive study. *Journal of Behavioral Medicine, 15,* 161–163.

Ault, M. (1990). I am a Christian bulimic. *Journal of Christian Nursing,* 7(1), 5–8.

Billigmeier, S. (1991). *Inner eating.* Nashville: Oliver Nelson, div. of Thomas Nelson.

Brownell, K. D., and Foreyt, J. P. (Eds.) (1986). *Handbook of eating disorders: Physiology, psychology, and treatment of obesity, anorexia, and bulemia.* New York: Basic Books, Inc.
Bruch, H. (1973). *Eating disorders.* New York: Basic Books, Inc.
Carson, V. B. (1989). *Spiritual dimensions of nursing practice.* Philadelphia: W. B. Saunders.
Crisp, A. H. (1967). Anorexia nervosa. *Hospital Medicine, 1,* 713–718.
Crisp, A. H., Hsu, L. K., and Harding, B. (1980). The starving hoarder and voracious spender: Stealing in anorexia nervosa. *Journal of Psychosomatic Research, 24,* 225–231.
Dare, C. (1983). Family therapy for families containing an anorectic youngster. In D. E. Redfern (Ed.). *Understanding anorexia nervosa and bulimia.* Columbus: Ross Laboratories.
deZwaan, M., and Mitchell, J. E. (1992). Binge eating in the obese. *Annals of Medicine, 24,* 303–308.
Epstein, R. (1990). *Eating habits and disorders.* New York: Chelsea House.
Fava, M., Copeland, P. M., Schweiger, U., and Herzog, D. B. (1989). Neurochemical abnormalities in anorexia nervosa and bulimia nervosa. *American Journal of Psychiatry, 146* (6), 963.
Ferraro, A. R. (1990). Bulimia: A look from within. *Pediatric Nursing, 16* (2), 187–191.
Flood, M. (1989). Addictive eating disorders. *Nursing Clinics of North America, 24* (1), 45–53.
Fontaine, K. L. (1991). The conspiracy of culture. *Nursing Clinics of North America, 26* (3), 669–675.
Hsu, L. K. G. (1990). *Eating disorders.* New York: The Guilford Press.
Johnson, C., and Pure, D. L. (1986). Assessment of bulimia: A multidimensional model. In K. D. Brownell and J. P. Foreyt (Eds.). *Handbook of eating disorders* (pp. 121-142). New York: Basic Books, Inc.
Kaczorowski, J. M. (1989). Spiritual well-being and anxiety in adults diagnosed with cancer. *The Hospice Journal, 5* (3/4), 105–115.
Kaplan, H. I., and Sadock, B. J. (1991). *Synopsis of psychiatry* (6th ed.). Baltimore: Williams & Wilkins.
Laraia, M. T., and Stuart, G. W. (1990). Bulimia: A review of nutritional and health behaviors. *Journal of Child and Adolescent Psychiatry, 3,* 91–96.
Love, C. C., and Seaton, H. (1991). Eating disorders: Highlights of nursing assessment and therapeutics. *Nursing Clinics of North America, 26* (3), 677–680.
Miller, K. D. (1991). Compulsive overeaters. *Nursing Clinics of North America, 26* (3), 699–701.
Minuchin, S., Rosman, B. L., and Baker, L. (1978). *Psychosomatic families.* Cambridge: Harvard University Press.
Nusbaum, J. G., and Drever, E. (1990). Inpatient survey of nursing care measures for treatment of patients with anorexia nervosa. *Issues in Mental Health Nursing, 11,* 175–184.
Patton, G. C. (1992). Eating disorders: Antecedents, evolution and course. *Annals of Medicine, 24* (4), 281–285.
Riley, E. A. (1991). Eating disorders as addictive behavior—Integrating 12-step programs into treatment planning. *Nursing Clinics of North America, 26* (3), 715–718.
Silverstone, P. H. (1992). Is chronic low self-esteem the cause of eating disorders? *Medical Hypotheses, 39* (4), 311–315.
Sodestrom, K. E., and Martinson, I. M. (1987). Patients' spiritual coping strategies: A study of nurse and patient perspectives. *Oncology Nursing Forum, 14* (2), 41–46.
Titus, M. A., and Smith, W. H. (1992). Contemporary issues in the psychotherapy of women. *Bulletin of the Menninger Clinic, 56,* 48–61.
Wald, F. S., and Bailey, S. S. (1990). Nurturing the spiritual component in care for the terminally ill. *Caring Magazine, 9* (11), 64–68.
Walsh, B. T., Roose, S. P., Glassman, A. H., Gladis, M., and Sadik, C. (1985). Bulimia and depression. *Psychosomatic Medicine, 47,* 123–131.
White, J. H. (1992). Women and eating disorders, Part I: Significance and sociocultural risk factors. *Health Care for Women International, 13,* 351–362.
Yanovski, S., et al (1993). Association of binge eating disorder and psychiatric comorbidity in obese subjects. *American Journal of Psychiatry, 150,* 1472.

SUGGESTED READINGS

Ferraro, A. R. (1990). Bulimia: A look from within. *Pediatric Nursing, 16* (2), 187–191.
Flood, M. (1989). Addictive eating disorders. *Nursing Clinics of North America, 24* (1), 45–53.
Fontaine, K. L. (1991). The conspiracy of culture. *Nursing Clinics of North America, 26* (3), 669–675.
Love, C. C. (1991). Eating disorders: Highlights of nursing assessment and therapeutics. *Nursing Clinics of North America, 26* (3), 677–680.
White, J. H. (1992). Women and eating disorders, Part I: Significance and sociocultural risk factors. *Health Care for Women International, 13,* 351–362.

CHAPTER 36

THE JOURNEY SCARRED BY SUICIDE

The wind comes over the Carrico Dam
And falls a mile below
I stand looking over the edge
And I feel the steady blow

The friendly faces looking my way
Not one knows who I am
I see them search for strength in my eyes
But I'm leaning toward the Dam

I've tried to be what others want
To follow what they've planned
I wish I was as strong in my heart
As I am in my hand

I will leap without a word
Flying like a bird
Falling like a star, falling like a star
The wind comes over the Carrico Dam

And I feel it on my face
Now every step I took in my life
Is ended in this place

Oh, the Carrico Dam
Is not where I should be
Oh, the Carrico Dam
Will be the death of me

—Susan Graham White

LEARNING OBJECTIVES

After studying this chapter, you should be able to:

1. Discuss one fact related to the history of suicide.
2. Describe three examples of the theoretical foundations for the study of suicidal behavior.
3. List five questions used to assess the level of lethality of a patient's suicide potential.
4. Identify two clinical variables that influence a patient's suicidal behavior.
5. List two symptoms that are present when a patient is at risk for self-mutilation.
6. Identify three behavior patterns that would indicate that a patient is at risk for a lethal suicidal attempt.

7. Identify two nursing interventions for a patient who exhibits self-mutilative behavior.

8. Discuss three nursing interventions for a patient who has made a serious suicide attempt.

9. Identify two methods to help you with your own feelings, beliefs, and behaviors resulting from working with suicidal or self-mutilating patients.

10. Discuss two reasons for continuing to evaluate the nursing care provided for suicidal patients.

KEY TERMINOLOGY

Alexithymia
Completed suicide
Direct self-destructive behavior
Every-15-minute checks
Indirect self-destructive behavior
Level of lethality
Life balance
One-to-one supervision
Self-mutilation
Suicidal ideation
Suicide
Suicide attempt
Suicide gesture

Life is an unpredictable journey. In life, we all encounter problems, both minor and major, and we all come face to face with the reality that life is a hazardous journey. For a time, we may drive along smooth, sunlit roads, but eventually we all encounter potholes, fallen branches, and washed-out bridges.

We all face choices about how we will cope with these hazards. We make some of these choices consciously and others unconsciously. Whether conscious or unconscious, however, these choices depend on our individual coping style, our faith in our ability to change, our world view, and our skill in maintaining a life balance.

The term **life balance** refers to the interaction among the physical, psychological, social, and spiritual variables in each of our lives that keeps us feeling well and that allows us to believe that life is generally good and worth continuing. An important component of life balance is the spiritual component. For example, a person with a theistic world view is likely to believe that physical life is a precious gift from the Creator and that it is not ours to terminate at will. Also consistent with a theistic world view is the perspective that physical life is only a part of life and that there is a spiritual afterlife.

When a person's life balance becomes so seriously disturbed that he or she loses the belief that the journey has meaning and is worth continuing, the person may engage in suicidal behavior. Suicidal behavior may be a desperate person's last message—that life's journey is unbearable and that the person sees ending physical life as the only way to end the pain.

CHARLES THOMAS'S STORY

Charles Thomas is a 55-year-old white married man who had been relatively free of physical and emotional problems most of his adult life. He has always prided himself on his ability to handle whatever problems he encountered—until the day he was seen in the emergency department for a psychiatric evaluation at the recommendation of his internist.

In the emergency department, Mr. Thomas related the following story to the psychiatric liaison nurse:

"I own my own business—in fact I have run it by myself for 25 years. Over the last five years I've tried to get my wife interested in learning the business, so she could take part in it with me, but she hasn't been interested. Eventually, I wanted my son to take over the business."

Problems Begin to Mount

"Then, two years ago, I started having problems with my youngest son. He started to use drugs and even ended up arrested a few times for stealing. During the past year I started to have financial problems with my business; I was forced to lay off one of my employees. God knows how hard that was for me! My daughter is away at college; my oldest son is married and lives out of state."

Feeling Alone

"For the first time in my life, I felt alone. I knew that, because of his drug problems, I couldn't count on my youngest son to help with the business. My wife didn't seem to understand that I needed help. I felt myself becoming more and more overwhelmed and depressed."

Crisis

"Now I worry all the time about losing my business, even though my accountant keeps assuring me that it's fine. This morning I told my wife that I couldn't go on; I told her that I wanted to die. I know I must have frightened her. She immediately called my doctor, who told her to bring me here for evaluation. To tell you the truth, I was too tired and worn out to even resist."

Assessing the Scope of the Problem

The psychiatric liaison nurse noted that Mr. Thomas was tearful. He said that he had not been able to sleep for the past week. He felt that he had no support from his family and stated that he did not want to go on with his life. Mr. Thomas told the nurse that he felt he was a total failure, both in running his business and in taking care of his family, and that he felt hopeless about making any changes in his situation.

Mr. Thomas said that he could not concentrate and was losing or forgetting things he needed to do at work. He was experiencing a lack of drive and energy; he was withdrawn and had begun to isolate himself from his friends and family, and he no longer enjoyed activities that he used to find pleasurable, including sex. He related that his appetite was poor; in the past six weeks, he has lost 20 pounds.

A Suicide Plan Revealed

Mr. Thomas also admitted to the psychiatric liaison nurse that he had formulated a suicide plan: He had been practicing how to knot a strong rope that he had bought in order to hang himself. He had checked his insurance policy to see what coverage his family would receive on his death, but then he had begun to wonder whether his family would receive *any* of the money if he were to hang himself.

Crisis Averted, Healing Begun

When he began to realize the seriousness of his thoughts, he decided to talk to his wife one more time before implementing his plan. That was when she called the family internist for help.

After a full psychiatric evaluation, Mr. Thomas was diagnosed as having *major depression with suicidal ideation* and was hospitalized to prevent suicide as well as to begin treatment for the depression.

This chapter will help you to explore why people like Charles Thomas attempt and often successfully complete suicide, what factors influence a person's decision to take his or her own life, the influence of maintaining a positive life balance on the risk of suicide, and what you can do to help prevent suicides.

DEFINITIONS RELATED TO SUICIDE

When we think of the term **suicide,** we usually think of a conscious attempt to kill oneself. Suicidal behavior, however, occurs on a continuum, so some important terms related to suicide are defined here:

Indirect self-destructive behavior
Direct self-destructive behavior
Suicide attempt (suicide gesture)
Suicidal ideation
Completed suicide
Lethality of suicide threat

Indirect self-destructive behavior refers to activities that are potentially detrimental to a person's physical, psychological, social, and spiritual well-being. These behaviors *may* result in death but without the person's conscious intent or awareness. Examples of these behaviors include anorexia, bulimia with purging, use of alcohol or other drugs of abuse, and engaging in unprotected sex with multiple partners.

Direct self-destructive behavior involves activities that signal that a person intends to cause self-harm or death. The person has an awareness of the desired outcome, with a cognitive component of a self-destructive plan. Examples of self-destructive behaviors include wrist slashing, self-mutilation, buying a gun and munitions for the purpose of ending life, and taking an overdose of prescribed medications.

A **suicide attempt** or **suicide gesture** is the use of direct self-destructive behavior for the express purpose of killing oneself. The term **suicidal ideation** refers to a person's thoughts about suicide. The term **completed suicide** refers to willful, self-inflicted, life-threatening acts that result in death. Finally, the term **level of lethality** of suicide threat refers to the seriousness of a suicide threat—the degree to which it is likely to result in death.

▶ Check Your Reading

1. Define the concept of life balance.
2. What is indirect self-destructive behavior?
3. How is indirect self-destructive behavior different from direct self-destructive behavior?
4. How does suicidal behavior relate to indirect and direct self-destructive behavior?

EPIDEMIOLOGY OF SUICIDE

Suicide is not something unique to 20th century life; there have always been people who out of hopelessness have committed suicide to end the pain of living. The attitude of society toward suicide has ranged from mild disapproval to outright condemnation. St. Thomas Aquinas (1225–1274) argued against suicide by claiming that suicide was a violation of love—love of self, neighbor, and society. He stated that committing suicide represented a breach of God's sovereignty over us. St. Thomas Aquinas described suicide in terms of theft; suicide steals God's gift of life and so misappropriates the property that rightfully belongs to God.

In the United States, there has been public debate as to whether there are some situations when suicide is acceptable. For instance, a Michigan physician, Dr. Kevorkian, has assisted people who are terminally ill to commit suicide. These assisted suicides challenged the Michigan law that governs this practice. The Hemlock Society publishes literature on the "how to's" of completing a suicide. In 1994, Oregon state passed a bill that allows physicians and pharmacists to prescribe and dispense lethal doses of a pain medication to terminally ill patients who choose to end their lives.

PREVALENCE OF SUICIDE

The National Center for Health Statistics in 1990–1991 ranked suicide as the eighth cause of death in the United States, with 13.6 persons per every 100,000 population completing a suicidal act. Busch and colleagues (1993) report that of the 30,000 suicides that occur in the United States each year, 5% to 6% take place in an inpatient psychiatric hospital. These statistics are, however, at best, estimates of suicides. Sometimes physicians, coroners, and police are reluctant to cite a death as a suicide because of variances in criteria that would indicate a completed suicide (Sainsbury, 1986). It is likely that some deaths that are the result of "accidents" such as drowning, car wrecks, gunshot wounds, drug abuse, and self-poisoning may actually be suicides but are missed in the count. According to Durkheim, the term *suicide* should be applied to all cases of death that result either directly or indirectly from the positive or negative acts of the victim himself and in which the victim knows the consequences of the acts (Durkheim, 1951 [1897]).

Suicide ends all kinds of human journeys; it is not bounded by culture, age, class, religion, or socioeconomic status. Although women tend to make more suicide attempts than men, more men complete the suicidal act (National Center for Health Statistics, 1989).

White men are the highest risk group for completing suicide, followed by Native Americans, African-Americans, Hispanics, and Asians. More men who complete suicide are single, followed by widowed, separated, and divorced men (Forster, 1994). Table 36–1 presents statistics on completed suicides by age group, and Table 36–2 summarizes the myths and realities of suicide.

▶ **Check Your Reading**

5. What is the eighth cause of death in the United States?
6. Who makes more suicidal gestures, men or women?
7. Who is more likely to complete a suicidal act, a single white man, a Hispanic woman, or an adolescent Asian?

TABLE 36–1 **Completed Suicides by Age Group**

Age Group	Percentage of Completed Suicides
15–24 y	11.9
25–34 y	14.4
35–44 y	14.4
45–54 y	14.6
55–64 y	14.0
65–74 y	19.9
75–84 y	29.2
85 y and older	27.6

The age group most at risk according to this study are people who are between 75 and 84 years old.

Data from U.S. Department of Health and Human Services, National Center for Health Statistics. (1992). *Vital statistics report, 40, 1990–1991.* Hyattsville, MD: Public Health Service.

SUICIDE AS A SYMPTOM OF PSYCHIATRIC ILLNESS

Suicide is one of the outcomes of untreated depression. Fifteen percent to 20% of all patients diagnosed with major depression complete suicide (Robins, 1986). Additionally, patients with psychotic depression have a high risk for completing suicide. This is due to the combination of symptoms including:

Depression
Delusions
Guilt
Paranoid thoughts
Social withdrawal

Psychotic patients have a tendency to withdraw from seeking adequate psychiatric intervention and often use violent methods to commit suicide (Forster, 1994).

Wolfersdorf and coworkers (1990) identified a suicidal depressive syndrome. They describe patients with major depression to be at the highest risk, especially those patients who have feelings of worthlessness, anxiety, depressive delusions, sleep disturbances, and a history of past suicidal behavior. William's story illustrates the potential for a suicide attempt resulting from a major depression (Case Example 36–1).

Case Example 36–1 William's Story

William had a history of dysthymia, a long-term depression. He had been placed on Prozac 20 mg twice a day. During the course of treatment, he was laid off from work. He became depressed, he was unable to get out of bed in the morning, his energy had decreased, and he had difficulty concentrating. Often, he would feel like yelling about being laid off; other times, he felt tearful. He felt no one understood how much work meant to him; not just to pay bills, but that it gave a purpose to his life. William was afraid to share his feelings of loss with his girlfriend, for fear she would leave him. He felt his parents would be critical. He had not told his therapist how depressed he felt because he was afraid he would be hospitalized, as he was when he was younger. William's depression became worse; he began to question the value of his life. He started to plan for what he could do to end his life and therefore his misery. His girlfriend noticed he had become more preoccupied; he did not call her as often as he used to. She asked him to "level with her, as she felt scared she was going to lose him." He did tell her he was feeling hopeless and a burden. She encouraged him to tell his therapist how he was feeling so he could get better.

TABLE 36–2 **Myths and Realities of Suicide**

Myth	Reality
Only psychotic people commit suicide	Suicide can be a choice made by a sane and moral person
Suicidal persons are fully intent on dying	Most persons who think about suicide have mixed feelings about dying
Suicide is an impulsive act	The suicide act may be impulsive, but usually suicide has been carefully thought out
The chance of suicide lessens as depression gets better	When a person's depression is lifting, he or she has more energy to carry out a previously considered suicide plan
Suicide can be an inherited trait	Although alcoholism and depression are most likely genetic, and having a relative who has committed suicide is a risk factor, no known genetic markers for suicide exist
Most suicidal persons give no warning	About 75% of people who attempt or commit suicide give definite clues about their intent
If you suspect suicidal ideation, do not bring the subject up; it might make the person kill himself or herself	Open talking is most often a relief to the suicidal person. Talking actually decreases the risk of suicide
All nonwhite persons have a lower suicide rate than whites	Except for young African-American men, all nonwhites have a lower suicide rate than whites
Professionals such as doctors, lawyers, dentists, police officers, and air traffic controllers have a low suicide rate	Professionals such as those listed have a higher suicide rate than the general population
People who are psychotic have the greatest chance of killing themselves among those with psychiatric illnesses	Although risk increases with psychosis, among people with serious mental illness, those with alcoholism and depression are most at risk for suicide
Only people with serious problems, mental illness, or physical illness think about suicide	At one time or another, almost everyone contemplates suicide
People who just want attention use suicide threats to manipulate others	*All* suicide threats should be taken seriously. Even if a suicide threat is manipulative, the person may inadvertently commit suicide
People who go from "rags to riches" are less likely to commit suicide than those who lose their money	People with a sudden change in fortune (success, riches, acclaim) are also at risk for suicide

Several other psychiatric disorders are associated with suicidal behavior, such as bipolar disorder, schizophrenia, and substance abuse disorders. Patients who have bipolar disorder are at the greatest risk for suicide when they are depressed. Schizophrenic patients have a 10% to 13% rate of completed suicide (Forster, 1994). Many of these patients experience hopelessness about the chronicity of their illness and do not always communicate their suicidal intent or plan. Because of these factors, they are at high risk and require a thorough assessment. Another psychiatric disorder often associated with completed suicide is alcohol and substance abuse. Alcohol is associated with 25% to 50% of all completed suicides (Forster, 1994). The risk increases dramatically when the patient suffers from major depression along with alcoholism (Cornelius et al, 1995).

Self-mutilation, or intentional self-destructive behavior that destroys or alters body tissue, occurs in an estimated 24% to 40% of psychiatric patients and approximately 750 per 100,000 of the general population (Favazza, 1987). Self-mutilating behavior has a different psychological intention than a suicidal gesture. Patients who self-mutilate often have a history of being neglected as well as sexually and physically abused as children (Goodwin, 1989; Herman, 1992; Barstow, 1995).

Self-mutilation often occurs when patients have **alexithymia,** or the inability to identify and put words to the experience of emotional feelings. The American Psychiatric Association (1984) identifies alexithymia as a disturbance in affective and cognitive functioning in which emotions are experienced mostly in physical form. Patients with alexithymia identify body sensations as emotional feelings and frequently use actions to express emotions. People who have alexithymia have a disturbed communication style in which the emotional and the symbolic functions are strained. Their fantasy life is impoverished, and their interpretation of life's events is concrete and literal (Wheeler and Broad, 1994). Often when patients self-mutilate, they are angry, lonely, scared, and fearful of abandonment.

Van der Kolk (1987) discusses an animal model in which self-mutilation was observed. Using Harlow's work with monkeys, which studied monkeys' reactions to receiving "nurturing" from a wire monkey as opposed to a mother monkey, responses were observed regarding issues such as separation from mother and peers, the effect on socialization, and parenting future generations. The monkeys that were separated from the mother monkey during the first year of life demonstrated abnormal social and sexual behavior. These monkeys did not mate, and if a female monkey in this group was artificially inseminated, this monkey mutilated or killed her babies. Young monkeys who were removed from their mothers demonstrated socially withdrawn or aggressive behaviors. These monkeys developed self-destructive and self-stimulating behaviors such as huddling, self-clasping, self-sucking, and self-biting. Animal behavior, particularly primate behavior, can assist in understanding human behavior. If monkeys self-mutilate in reaction to a separation from their mothers, self-mutilation behaviors observed in humans may also be tied to early deprivation.

▶ Check Your Reading

8. Why do you need to do a suicide assessment on a patient who is diagnosed with schizophrenia?
9. What is the relationship between alcohol use, depression, and suicide?
10. Why do some patients self-mutilate?

CAUSE OF SUICIDE

No one theory adequately explains suicidal or self-destructive behavior or guides clinical practice. Biological, psychological, sociocultural, and spiritual factors may all contribute to self-injury.

Physical Factors

Biological studies have found that neurotransmitters, such as dopamine, serotonin, and endogenous opioids, influence self-injury, but the actions of these biochemical agents are poorly understood. There is some evidence to indicate that low levels of serotonin are present in some people who have attempted suicide (Roy, 1989). Stanley and Stanley (1990) have studied concentrations of serotonin and 5-HIAA (a serotonin metabolite) in postmortem receptor binding studies. They note changes in both presynaptic and postsynaptic serotoninergic binding sites in suicides who have been examined postmortem as opposed to the postmortem studies of the control group.

The relationship between self-injury and the endogenous opioids was discovered serendipitously. Naloxone, a blocker of opioid effects, was administered to several developmentally delayed patients, and the incidence of self-injury decreased significantly (Favazza, 1989).

Psychological Factors

Psychological theories suggest that self-destructive behavior may have its roots or beginnings in early interpersonal trauma. These theories focus on the role of aggression and the inner world of the suicidal person.

According to Freud (1964 [1933]), the act of suicide represents a conflict between the instincts for life and death. Suicide apparently occurs when the wish for death predominates, and the patient no longer is able to maintain a life balance on his or her journey. Menninger (1938) suggested that the individual turns aggression that is intended for others inward against the self. According to Adams (1985), the "aggression turned inward" theory may be a way of understanding suicide as well as other self-destructive behaviors, such as self-mutilation, eating disorders, and smoking, and other indirect self-destructive behaviors, such as self-neglect, compulsive gambling, alcohol and drug abuse, selling drugs, and taking other extreme risks.

Some common psychological antecedents to self-destructive behaviors are depression; eating disorders; drug and alcohol dependency or abuse; bipolar disorder; personality disorders, such as borderline personality disorder, narcissistic personality disorder, antisocial personality disorder, and histrionic personality disorder; cognitive mental disorders; and psychoses, particularly with command hallucinations, cultural expectations, and religious rites (Barstow, 1995).

Filstead (1980) states that despair is usually present when indirect self-destructive behavior occurs. He further describes despair as "a psychosocial state that people experience when they are trying to resolve what has become a serious personal problem . . . and realize that there does not appear to be any way to resolve it." The self-destructive behavior may serve as a personal, albeit ineffective, defense against the sense of despair (Case Example 36–2).

Case Example 36–2 Mary's Story

Mary often feels lonely, isolated, and depressed because she believes no one cares for her. She frequents a local bar in an effort to meet an available man. Mary usually drinks a few beers and then "hard liquor" as the night progresses. She flirts with several men and sometimes goes home with one of them. She wakes up feeling alone and scared and often has a hangover. Her sense of self is negative; she says she is "a low-life." Mary's problems with low self-esteem, difficulty relating to others, and aloneness are not solved by her current behavioral pattern. Her actions lead only to self-defeat and worsening feelings about the self, with greater dissatisfaction. Mary's despair increases, and, along with it, the risk for suicidal behavior also increases.

According to Beck (1963), hopelessness and negative expectations are psychological variables that may be used to predict suicide. He states that hopelessness plays a critical role in suicide and is illustrated in the sequence of events that leads a depressed person to commit suicide. The person believes there is no way out, that the existing problems are insoluble ones, and he or she anticipates disastrous outcomes (Beck, 1967). In a 10-year prospective follow-up study looking at the relationship between hopelessness and suicide, 165 patients were hospitalized with suicide ideation. Out of 11 patients who committed suicide, 10 (90.9%) had scored nine or greater on the Beck Hopelessness Scale. One patient (9.1%), who ultimately committed suicide, had scored lower than a nine (Beck et al, 1985).

People with a diminished capacity to cope are at increased risk for suicidal behavior. Folkman and Lazarus (1984) define coping as thoughts and actions that are flexible, solve problems, and reduce stress. The more flexible and varied an individual's coping repertoire is, the better able the person is to deal successfully with the challenges that appear in every life's journey. It is important to note, however, that even the best coping skills can be taxed to their limit by too many stressors at one time or stressors that are too intense and demanding.

Social Factors

The social and cultural context in which a person lives also influences the expression of suicidality (Adams, 1985). Durkheim (1951 [1897]) describes four types of suicide that are integrally linked to the quality of community life:

Egotistical
Anomic
Fatalistic
Altruistic

In an *egotistical suicide*, a person's ties to the community are too loose or tenuous, the person is not invested in maintaining his or her relationship with the community, the person has no close relationships, and the person does not respond to the usual social constraints on behavior.

In an *anomic suicide*, the person experiences the aloneness or estrangement that occurs as a result of a precipitous deterioration in his or her relationship with society (e.g., loss of a job, a close friend, a parent).

In a *fatalistic suicide*, the person feels that he or she is excessively regulated; there is no personal freedom or hope for obtaining it.

In *altruistic suicide*, rules or customs demand suicide under certain situations; in these situations, self-inflicted death is viewed as honorable. Altruistic suicides may be seen in time of war, such as the kamikaze attacks by Japanese pilots on American ships in World War II.

Racism is also linked with suicide. Durkheim (1951 [1897]) suggests that any group that is denied society's usual privileges and rights experiences an increased risk for alienation and anomic suicide. Studies of African-American populations indicate that there has been a dramatic increase in the suicide rate in young African-American men (Davis, 1982).

Spiritual Factors

In a theistic world view, our spirits are seen as eternal. There are times in each of our lives, however, when we deny the existence of our spirit, when we refuse to rely on our spirit, and when we seem to ignore the importance of our spirit to our overall health and well-being. It is essential for you to assess each patient's spirituality to assist the patient to recognize and use spirituality to maintain a positive life balance and improve coping skills.

According to Vanzant (1992), "spirit is the life essence which is covered and protected by the skeletal frame we call the body. . . . Spirit has only one purpose and mission, which was determined by God at the time of creation. . . . Everything that has life, can create life, nurtures life or serves a purpose in life, is spirit."

Frankl (1964) was acutely aware of the importance of spirit operating in people as he observed his own behavior and responses and those of fellow prisoners during his confinement in a Nazi concentration camp. He observed that spirit was intricately tied to meaning and purpose in life as well as hope. Frankl observed that when people find life meaningless and without purpose and God seems distant and uncaring, there is no reason to live. He believed that suffering is a requisite ingredient of living; and that finding meaning in that suffering is an important ingredient for survival. Frankl wrote that if a person succeeds in discovering a "why" for the suffering, he or she will continue to grow despite all indignities (Frankl, 1964).

Frankl (1964) also viewed hope as an expression of a healthy spirit and a prerequisite to survival. Conversely, Frankl believed that hopelessness, an expression of a depleted spirit, could be fatal. Frankl cited the case of a prisoner who pinned his hopes on being rescued from the concentration camp on a certain date. When it became clear that the rescue operation would not occur on the expected date, the man died within a matter of hours.

Nurses are in an extraordinary position to encourage patients to reestablish their purposes in life, to renew their hopes, and to tap into their own spirituality. Some patients may have lost their faith in God or have felt an alienation from their own values or from other people. These people experience life as no longer having any meaning or purpose, and they may find it too painful to continue (Pallikkathayil and McBride, 1986). In essence, these people have lost hope. It is possible through a comprehensive nursing assessment and intervention that hope can be restored; patients may feel a sense of connectedness to their own values, to themselves, to their God, and to others.

▶ Check Your Reading

11. Explain the "aggression turned inward" theory. Why does this theory provide a way of understanding suicide as

well as other self-destructive behaviors, such as self-mutilation?
12. How does the social and cultural context in which a person lives contribute to an understanding of suicidal behavior?
13. What is meant by the "spirit of life," and how does that relate to understanding life's purpose?

DYNAMICS OF SUICIDE

The suicide of a patient, the premature end of a journey, because of its finality, is perhaps the most devastating experience in the practice of psychiatry and psychiatric nursing. Through the act of suicide, the individual communicates his or her final message to others. The person may view suicide as a way to escape life's suffering or a way to get away from situations that are viewed as intolerable, such as a loss of a spouse, a difficult relationship, loss of a series of jobs, or a terminal illness. Different people meet adversity with their own styles of coping, depending on personal problem-solving skills, self-esteem, ability to relate to others, and defense mechanisms. A person who has a poorly integrated personality may respond to stress by committing suicide.

As a result of studying suicide notes and conducting discussions with people who have attempted suicide, many theorists have begun to understand the emotional components of suicide. Suicidal patients characterize their emotional states as feeling:

Intense anger
Devastating depression
Profound feelings of hopelessness
A loss of life's meaning and purpose

Often the suicidal person expresses ambivalence about completing the act; while wishing to be dead, this individual sometimes has a desire to be saved or rescued. Mintz (1971) stated: "...[I]t is a clinical fact that the suicidal person is usually highly ambivalent about committing suicide. None would seek help if this were not true." This ambivalence provides the opportunity to intervene and attempt to convince despairing people that suicide is not the answer.

NURSING PROCESS

When providing care for the suicidal patient and the family, you can use your knowledge of the epidemiology, cause, and dynamics of suicidal behavior as a guide. This knowledge has an impact on the effectiveness of the nursing process.

ASSESSMENT

To perform a comprehensive assessment, you must focus on the physical, psychological, social, and spiritual domains that represent the foundation of human functioning (Cardell and Horton-Deutsch, 1994). An important consideration is to determine the patient's positive or negative life balance. This is assessed by observing the patient's adaptive or maladaptive behavior when the patient is confronted with a problem. Does the patient use positive physical, psychological, social, and spiritual means of examining the problem to determine healthful options, or is the patient using negative physical, psychological, social, or spiritual options toward problem solving? See Chapter 13 for in-depth assessment information.

Severity Index for Risk of Suicide

Another consideration is whether or not the patient is in a high-risk group for suicide (Box 36–1). Box 36–2 identifies questions to ask and observations to make when assessing a person's risk of suicide. Box 36–3 provides clues to suicidal ideation.

Green and coworkers (1995) identified a severity index useful in assessment of risk. The patient's severity is conceptualized as a continuum ranging from *no suicidal ideation* to a patient with a *severe level of suicidal risk.* Using the severity index assists you to plan the intensity and type of care the patient requires to prevent a suicidal gesture (Figure 36–1).

Assessment of the Physical Domain

It is helpful to determine if the patient has any signs or symptoms of a physical illness. Does the patient focus on body sensations, particularly if he or she has chronic pain?

BOX 36–1 Groups at High Risk for Suicide

- People with a family history of suicide
- People with a previous history of having attempted suicide
- Psychotic patients, especially those with command auditory hallucinations
- Depressed people (including those who are terminally ill)
- People who are overwhelmed or under great stress
- Patients with personality disorders, such as schizoid, schizotypal, histrionic, borderline, and antisocial
- People addicted to alcohol or other drugs
- People who experience extreme guilt and shame
- Adolescents who suffer with a major depression or have friends or family members who have completed suicide
- People with early-stage organic brain syndrome or AIDS dementia

BOX 36-2 Questions to Ask and Observations to Make When Assessing a Person's Risk of Suicide

Questions to Ask

- How much are you thinking about suicide or harming yourself?
- Do you have a plan? (If yes: "Could you tell me about your plan?")
- Have you ever attempted to harm yourself before? (If yes: "Could you describe what happened?")
- Do you have any idea what might have triggered your thoughts about harming yourself?

Observations to Make

- Is there a weapon or a method available to the patient?
- Observe the verbal and nonverbal clues that the patient is giving about her plan to commit suicide or to do self-harm. Is the patient feeling as though she is a burden that her family would do better without? Has she given away valuable items? Has she checked her will or life insurance policy?
- Does the patient comprehend his degree of risk for suicide or self-harm? Does he verbalize a fear of being alone?
- What is the level of knowledge of the patient or significant other about depression (or any other psychiatric or physical disorder the patient may have) and about suicidal ideation?
- Assess the patient for abuse of alcohol or other drugs.
- Assess the patient's ability to function in her roles at work, at home, and in the community. How does the patient view her purpose in life?
- Determine the patient's ability to interact with others. Can the patient ask for help when feeling overwhelmed? Is the patient isolated from others?
- How supportive and available to the patient are the family or significant other(s)?
- Does the patient feel abandoned? Does the patient make statements of loss?
- Is the patient experiencing rage?
- Determine the patient's degree of depression and anxiety.

From Green, E., Katz, J., and Marcus, P. (1995). Practice guidelines for suicide/self harm prevention. In E. Green and J. Katz (Eds.), *Clinical practice guidelines for the adult patient* (pp. 250-1–250-21). St. Louis: Mosby-Year Book.)

Does the patient experience the pain as more excruciating when overwhelmed with emotional issues? Is the patient experiencing the neurovegetative signs of depression, such as difficulty concentrating, changes in appetite, decreases in energy, decreases in libido, or changes in sleep pattern? You might want to ask:

- What are your thoughts about your illness? What impact has this illness had on your life?
- How would you describe your pain? Are there times when the pain is more difficult to handle?

BOX 36-3 Clues to Suicidal Ideation

Direct Statements

- "I can't take it anymore."
- "Life isn't worth living anymore."
- "I wish I were dead."
- "Everyone would be better off if I died."

Indirect Statements

- "It's okay now, soon everything will be fine."
- "Things will never work out."
- "I won't be a problem much longer."
- "Nothing feels good to me anymore, and probably never will."
- "How can I give my body to medical science?"

Behaviors

- Giving away prized possessions
- Writing farewell notes
- Making out a will
- Putting personal things in order

Physical Clues

- Headaches
- Muscle aches
- Trouble sleeping
- Constipation
- Change in appetite
- Weight loss

Emotional Clues

- Social withdrawal
- Feelings of hopelessness
- Feelings of helplessness
- Confusion
- Irritability
- Feeling exhausted

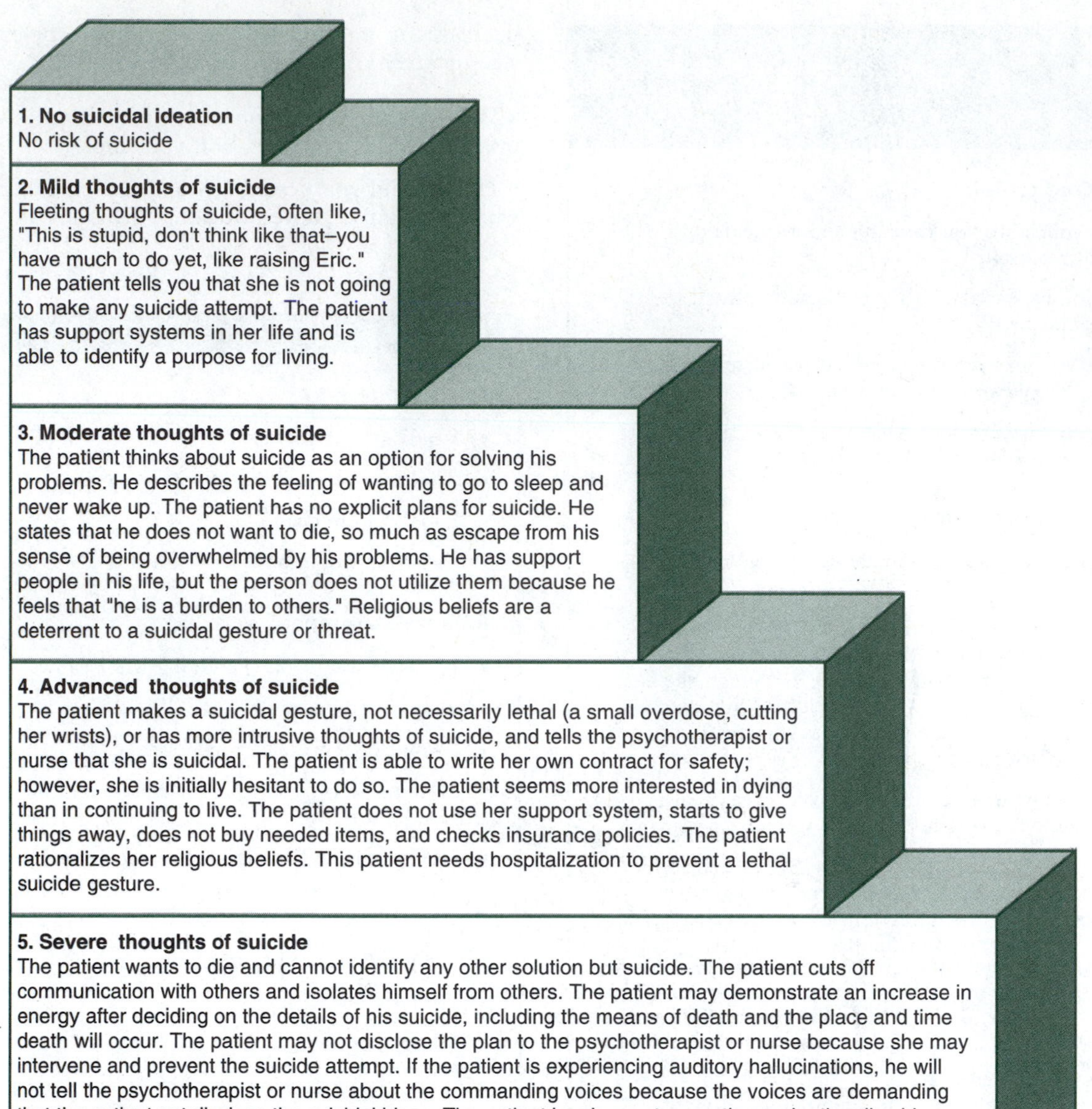

FIGURE 36–1
Severity index for suicide risk. (Data from Green, E., Katz, J., and Marcus, P. [1995]. Practice guidelines for suicide/self harm prevention. In E. Green and J. Katz [Eds.], *Clinical practice guidelines for the adult patient* [pp. 250-1–250-21]. St. Louis: Mosby-Year Book.)

• Have you noticed changes in your concentration? Your appetite? Your energy level? Your interest in sex? Or your need for sleep?

Assessment of the Psychological Domain

ASSESSMENT OF THE EMOTIONAL DOMAIN

When a patient is experiencing suicidal thoughts, he or she is also having problems in the emotional domain and is usually experiencing feelings of despair and hopelessness. These feelings are expressed through a suicide plan (Sanger et al, 1988). To assess the emotional domain thoroughly, you must ask the patient directly: "Have you ever had, or are you now having, thoughts of hurting yourself?" Box 36–4 offers suggestions for talking to a patient who has suicidal ideation. If the patient answers in the affirmative, you continue to inquire about the presence of a plan and the lethality of the plan. *Lethality* refers to seriousness of the suicide threat, including the means that the patient plans to use to commit the suicide and the availability of those means. You might ask: "Do you have a plan? If so, could you describe it to me? Do you have a weapon? Is it readily available to you?" If the patient responds, "I do not really have a plan. . . . I just think that life would be better if I were gone. And besides . . . my religion strictly forbids suicide," the patient is experiencing *suicidal ideation*, does not have a lethal plan, and is experiencing strong religious constraints against committing suicide. Your nursing response would affirm the patient's religious constraints and encourage the patient to sign a no-harm contract stating that she will not harm herself.

If the patient responds: "I think about suicide all the time. . . . It scares me so much I don't want to be alone. I have a loaded gun in the drawer of my bedside table. So far I haven't had the courage to use it . . . but I think it's just a matter of time. Things seem so hopeless. I really believe that everyone would be better off if I were dead," the response indicates not only the presence of serious and persistent suicidal ideation, but also a highly lethal plan. The patient knows exactly how she will commit suicide and has the weapon available to her. In this case, the patient requires inpatient care to ensure her safety.

You must also determine if the patient has a history of a previous suicide attempt(s) or if anyone in the patient's family has ever attempted or completed a suicide gesture (Cugino et al, 1992). You need to inquire: "Have you written a suicidal note? What does the note say? Where is the note? What do you think will happen when you die? Have you given any thought about what will happen to your family and friends when they learn of your suicide?" You need to determine whether the patient is depressed and how the patient views the depression. Does the patient express hope for the future? Has the patient told anyone about his suicidal thoughts or plans? How does the patient see herself as having any worth or value? See Chapter 15 for further guidelines on how to respond to a patient with suicidal ideation.

BOX 36-4 Suggestions for Talking to a Patient Who Has Suicidal Ideation

- Ask: "How are you feeling?"
- Ask: "Are you still having thoughts about hurting yourself?"
- Ask: "Have your thoughts changed?"
- Ask: "Do you have a plan to hurt yourself?"
- Ask: "If you have a plan, would you tell me about it?"
- Never tell the patient: "You shouldn't feel that way." Instead say: "It must be painful to feel that way."
- If you are unsure what to say, continue to listen in attentive silence, encouraging the patient to speak by using open-ended statements such as, "And then what happened?" "Uh huh . . ." "Tell me more about . . ."

ASSESSMENT OF THE COGNITIVE DOMAIN

Implementing a suicidal gesture is part of the cognitive domain. To assess the cognitive domain, it is important to determine how often the patient thinks about suicide or a suicide plan:

- Is the patient preoccupied with himself?
- What is the patient's view of the problems that are overwhelming her? Does the patient have insight into these problem areas or her behavior?
- Is the patient's judgment clouded with intrusive thoughts of suicide?
- Does the patient experience voices telling him to commit suicide (command auditory hallucinations)? Is the patient able to tell you about these hallucinations, or is the patient being directed by these auditory hallucinations not to talk to others?
- Does the patient focus on negative themes to the exclusion of other, more positive thoughts?

Assessment of the Social Domain

Often people who are suicidal feel a lack of social support. You should assess the social domain to determine the patient's perception of her support network. Is the patient interacting with family, friends, boss, and coworkers in the usual manner? If the patient is in a hospital or a Day Treatment Center/Partial Hospitalization program, is this individual participating with patient peers and staff in the milieu? Has the patient eliminated social activities that were once a pleasurable and meaningful part of life?

Assessment of the Spiritual Domain

According to Green and coworkers (1995), when you assess the spiritual domain, it is important to ask the following questions:

- What is the patient's relationship with a deity or higher power?
- Does the patient have a sense of purpose in life?
- Does the patient have hope that his or her problems will have a meaningful resolution?
- Has the patient begun to question the role of his or her spiritual beliefs in light of the current crisis?
- Is the patient angry with God, or does the patient feel that God is angry with him or her?
- Does the patient believe that God is using the current difficulties as a means of punishment?
- Is the patient connected with his faith community, either through a spiritual leader or through members of his or her religious group?

• Does the patient experience meaning through participation in religious rites, rituals, and other religiously oriented activities?

▶ Check Your Reading

14. What questions would you ask a patient to determine if there is a risk in the physical domain?
15. What questions in the emotional domain give information about the lethality of the patient's suicidal plan?
16. What questions in the cognitive domain are helpful to determine the extent of the patient's suicidal plan?
17. Why are the questions in the social domain important to determine the patient's level of suicidal ideation?
18. What three indicators are present when a patient has severe thoughts of suicide?

DIAGNOSIS

The next step in providing care is to identify the appropriate medical and nursing diagnoses. Case Example 36–3 illustrates a patient for whom Risk for Self-Mutilation would be an appropriate nursing diagnosis.

Case Example 36–3 Janice's Story

Janice is a recovering alcoholic currently in therapy to explore issues related to a history of incest. During the course of therapy, Janice revealed to her mother that her father's best friend sexually molested her. Janice's mother did not display the emotion that Janice expected after the disclosure. Janice became very emotional and then cut herself with a sharp knife. She claimed she felt relief. While exploring this incident in therapy, she remembered that she has been cutting herself since her adolescence. She began to explore whether there might be a correlation between her tendency toward self-mutilation and her history of sexual abuse. An appropriate nursing diagnosis for Janice is Risk for Self-Mutilation related to unresolved grief, inability to express feelings, fears of abandonment, and fears that her mother will be unsupportive as evidenced by Janice's past self-mutilative behaviors when experiencing these same reactions.

For Charles Thomas, the patient whom we met at the beginning of the chapter, an appropriate nursing diagnosis might be Risk for Violence: Self-Directed related to numerous perceived failures, feelings of abandonment by his significant others, depressed mood, and feelings of hopelessness as evidenced by verbalizations of suicidal thoughts to his wife.

OUTCOME IDENTIFICATION

The expected outcomes for a patient with a nursing diagnosis of Risk for Violence: Self-Directed or Risk for Self-Mutilation are as follows:

• The patient will remain free from self-harm while maintaining the highest degree of autonomy that is possible.

• The patient will not exhibit suicidal or self-mutilative behaviors.

PLANNING

When planning care for a suicidal patient, it is important to take into account the following factors:

• The patient's past and present history of emotional and physical illnesses

• The patient's life experiences

• The patient's cultural, ethical, and religious or spiritual background

Based on the identified expected outcomes for the patient at risk for suicide or self-mutilation, the nurse, the patient, and the interdisciplinary care team jointly establish short-term goals, such as the following:

Expected Outcomes	Short-Term Goals
1. The patient will remain free from self-harm while maintaining the highest degree of autonomy that is possible.	1. The patient will sign a no-harm contract.
	2. The patient will agree to talk to a staff member if he experiences a change in suicidal thinking.
2. The patient will not exhibit suicidal or self-mutilative behaviors.	1. The patient will participate in the unit activities.
	2. The patient will discuss his self-destructive feelings rather than act on them.
	3. The patient will participate in efforts to understand the crises that lead to his suicidal or self-mutilative behaviors.
	4. The patient will turn over to the staff any objects that could be used to harm himself.

Return now to the case of Charles Thomas, to see how care planning worked in his case.

To address Mr. Thomas's diagnosis of Risk for Violence: Self-Directed, Mr. Thomas's nurse, working together as part of the interdisciplinary care team and together with the patient, established the following expected outcome: "Mr. Thomas will remain free from self-harm while maintaining the highest degree of autonomy that is possible." Specific short-term goals related to this expected outcome were as follows:

- Mr. Thomas will remain free from harm while in the hospital.
- Mr. Thomas will seek out staff for support if he feels an increase in the urge to harm himself.
- Mr. Thomas will contract for safety with the nursing staff as a means of demonstrating impulse control.

▶ Check Your Reading

19. Identify a nursing diagnosis that might be appropriate for a patient who has threatened to slash his wrists.
20. Identify two expected outcomes for the patient who is at risk for self-mutilation or suicide.
21. State a short-term goal for a patient whose expected outcome is that he "will remain free from self-harm while maintaining the highest degree of autonomy that is possible."

IMPLEMENTATION

Once you have identified short-term goals for the patient at risk for suicide or self-mutilation, you are ready to plan appropriate interventions to help the patient meet his or her goals. The following strategies should be part of the plan of care for any patient at risk for suicide or self-harm.

Handle Suicide Threats as Emergencies

Consider any case of attempted suicide a serious psychiatric emergency. Conduct a full assessment to determine the appropriate interventions. Does the patient require inpatient care, or is outpatient care adequate? If the patient is stable enough to go home, with whom should the patient go home? Sometimes patients deny suicidal ideation to gain the freedom to go home to make a more serious suicide attempt or to please a family member or staff person. Therefore, ask repeatedly during your interaction with the patient whether the patient has thoughts of and plans for harming himself or herself.

In your interview, include questions about future plans, including plans for the day of the evaluation, plans for the next few days, plans for the weekend, and longer-term plans. If the patient is unable to make future plans, assess this issue further. If the patient cannot engage in problem-solving, including not being able to structure time effectively for meaningful activity, this is a signal that the patient may require a hospital stay to support him or her in problem-solving to deal with the factors that caused the suicidal ideation.

Determine the Patient's Level of Lethality

In an inpatient setting, determine the patient's level of lethality (Box 36–5). This determination helps the interdisciplinary team to determine whether the patient should be on a "suicide watch."

There are two types of suicide watches: *every-15-minute checks* and *one-to-one supervision.* For instance, if the patient demonstrates less lethal thoughts of suicide, with no explicit plan, and is still able to engage in problem-solving, every-15-minute checks would be appropriate.

In **every-15-minute checks,** a staff member checks on the patient every 15 minutes to ensure patient safety. Also, the patient takes an active part in the suicide watch by agreeing in writing, in the form of a no-harm contract (Figure 36–2), to inform the staff if he or she has any changes in suicidal ideation. If the patient can write his or her own no-harm contract, the patient experiences increased ownership of impulse control. While awake on every-15-minute checks, the patient is responsible for notifying staff members of changes in suicidal ideation.

If the patient has a suicide plan, has been thinking about a note that he or she wants to leave behind, has a means to carry out the suicide plan, has no plans for the future, and is hesitant to write a no-harm contract or will not sign a no-harm contract, *one-to-one supervision* is probably appropriate. In **one-to-one supervision,** staff members monitor the patient constantly, without interruption, until the patient presents a less lethal suicide risk.

For any patient on a suicide watch, observe the patient to see whether he or she experiences a reduction in suicidal ideation and an increase in problem-solving ability. If you determine that the patient feels more in control of his or her impulses and the issues related to his

BOX 36–5 Determining the Suicidal Patient's Level of Lethality

- How specific are the details of the plan? Has the person worked out the specifics? Where? How? When?
- How lethal is the proposed method? High-risk methods include using a gun, jumping, hanging, poisoning with carbon monoxide, and engineering an automobile accident. Examples of low-risk methods are slashing the wrists, inhaling house gas, and ingesting pills.
- Are the means available? A person who says that he will shoot himself and has a loaded gun in a bedside stand is in grave danger of committing suicide. Likewise, a person who states he will jump to his death and has access to a high building is at serious risk.
- Is the person psychotic? People who are psychotic are at high risk regardless of the specificity of the details, lethality of method, and availability of means. Their impulse control, judgment, and thinking are so impaired that they are at risk.

I, ______________________________, promise not to harm myself for the next 24 hours. I commit myself to tell the nursing staff of any change in my thinking regarding the infliction of self-harm. That is, I will tell them of any increase in the frequency or intensity of thoughts about injuring myself, or any change in the seriousness of my potential plan for harming myself. I will cooperate with the staff to preserve my own well-being.

SIGNED: ______________________________

WITNESSED: ______________________________

DATE: ______________________________

FIGURE 36–2
A sample no-harm contract.

or her problem areas, consult the other members of the interdisciplinary team, including the attending psychotherapist or psychiatrist, before reducing the level of suicide watch. If the patient seems to be feeling more depressed and hopeless, continue to determine the level of suicidal lethality and consult the interdisciplinary team, including the attending psychotherapist or psychiatrist. Placing the patient on a more restrictive suicide watch may be appropriate.

To reduce a patient's risk, remove the patient from any immediate danger to a physically safe environment and remove all harmful objects, including drugs. Assign the patient to a room that is easily accessible and can be observed closely.

Identify the Underlying Crisis

Try to identify the crisis that led to the episode of suicide or self-harm, and help the patient identify options for dealing with the issues behind the crisis (Badger, 1995). If the patient cannot identify any options, hospitalization is indicated to prevent a suicide attempt. Ask the patient with a history of suicide attempts if this crisis is similar to others in the past when he or she felt suicidal. Hospitalization is indicated in this situation as well. Patients with a history of suicide attempts often repeat such behavior as a means of problem-solving. During each session with a hospitalized patient, discuss options for dealing with the underlying issues.

Ask the Patient to Sign a No-Harm Contract

Ask the patient to sign—or, ideally, to write and sign—a no-harm contract. Milieu therapy, individual psychotherapy, family psychotherapy, problem-solving groups, art therapy, and movement therapy are important aspects of an inpatient hospital stay for helping to prevent the patient from carrying out suicidal impulses. During each therapy session, evaluate the degree to which the patient is complying with the contract and the degree of suicidal intent.

Engage the Patient's Support Network

If the patient identifies a key support person, ask the patient to contact this person, to tell him or her about the seriousness of the problem, and to request support. If the patient cannot identify any support network, hospitalization is indicated. If the patient is hesitant to involve a support person, hospitalization is also appropriate. When a patient is suicidal, he or she feels totally alone and worthless. A supportive friend or family member can reinforce the patient's worth. It is important to encourage the patient to allow support people to be integrated into treatment (Mullis and Byers, 1987).

Monitor Your Own Feelings

It is important that you continually assess your own feelings about suicide and suicidal ideation in patients. If you find that you tend to discount the suicidal threats of patients as "acting out," "attention-seeking," or "manipulation," you may miss a potentially lethal suicide threat. If you have such thoughts about patients with suicidal ideation or patients who self-mutilate, seek clinical supervision to help you understand the patient's desperation.

When there are several suicidal or self-mutilative patients on the unit at the same time, a staff meeting to discuss each patient's care and the feelings of staff members about the behavior of the patients may be helpful (Gallop, 1992). Staff members who maintain a positive life balance by integrating work, play, spiritual beliefs, and exercise in their lives are better equipped to deal with patients who are chronically depressed and hopeless about the quality of their lives (Badger, 1995).

Return now to the story of Charles Thomas, to see how the mental health team intervened to help him meet his short-term goals.

A thorough assessment to determine Mr. Thomas's suicidal intent reveals that Mr. Thomas has advanced suicidal ideation. The nursing staff therefore encourage Mr. Thomas to write a no-harm contract in his own words, and they ask Mr. Thomas to seek them out every 15 minutes to demonstrate a commitment that he would not harm himself. While Mr. Thomas is on 15-minute checks, the nursing staff assess Mr. Thomas's level of safety.

During his hospitalization, Mr. Thomas is encouraged to attend all milieu groups to increase his repertoire of options for problem-solving and to increase his level of social interaction. The nursing staff also request an evaluation for antidepressant medications to help Mr. Thomas to feel more energetic, to sleep better, to have a better appetite, to concentrate for longer periods, and to feel an increase in libido. After a psychiatrist prescribes an antidepressant medication for Mr. Thomas, the nursing staff begin to teach the patient about the role that medication will play in his recovery. They monitor side effects and medication compliance.

Once Mr. Thomas's condition improves, he begins attending a stress reduction group that is co-led by the staff occupational therapist, and the nursing staff teach him relaxation exercises to use when business worries intrude on his thoughts.

▶ Check Your Reading

22. What are the indications for hospitalization for a patient with suicidal ideas?
23. When is it appropriate to use every-15-minute checks?
24. When is it appropriate to place a patient on one-to-one supervision?
25. How can you avoid becoming "drained" by patients who are suicidal or self-mutilate?

EVALUATION

As we implement care for the patient who uses self-injury or suicide to problem-solve, it becomes important to evaluate the process of this care. The formative evaluation provides us with information about the patient's progress as well as information about the deficiencies and reasons the patient may not have benefited from the implementation of the plan. Questions for further clinical research in nursing can grow out of a thorough summative evaluation as we explore more effective ways to deliver nursing care to the suicidal patient.

One issue that is important to examine during the evaluation phase of the nursing process is when the plan of care is not working (Case Example 36–4).

Case Example 36–4 Anne's Story

Anne continued to cut herself no matter what the nursing staff did. The staff were feeling demoralized. "We have tried everything—what else can we do? She just keeps cutting!" The case was reviewed by a nurse from another unit who was not familiar with Anne, but who was interested in providing nursing care to patients who self-mutilate. The nurse from the other unit asked the staff if they had worked with Anne to determine thoughts she may have before the self-mutilating. This nurse provided the nursing staff with several questions that may assist Anne to learn if she dissociates before self-mutilating or if she is using the self-mutilation to punish herself or to deal with overwhelming feelings. The nurses on the unit felt better after the consultation because they now had a new direction in which to proceed.

Another example that points out the need for an ongoing evaluation of care would be a patient whose suicidal ideation is lethal, and the nursing staff members fail to recognize the seriousness of this ideation. In this situation, the formative evaluation identifies the deficiencies in the care that was given (Case Example 36–5).

Case Example 36–5 John's Story

John had been hospitalized for two days after he came to the emergency department reporting feeling suicidal. He is well known to the staff and frequently comes through the emergency department for a brief hospitalization after telling the staff in the emergency department that he is suicidal. The psychiatric nursing staff members feel John abuses the system, as he is a known alcoholic and drug abuser who "manipulates" a hospital stay by saying he is suicidal. This time John left the hospital and within 24 hours shot himself in the head with a hand gun. The psychiatric staff were upset; some sad, some angry, some questioning their care. After evaluating the overall care, the deficit cited was that the staff did not perform an in-depth suicidal evaluation before John's discharge. One nurse claimed, "He looked like his usual self—I thought he was just going to get his booze and he'd be back." Another nurse asked, "How do we know when someone is being manipulative?"

In Case Example 36–5, the nursing staff's belief that they knew the patient's next move got in the way of a comprehensive evaluation that may have prevented John's suicide. Evaluating the care delivered to the patient on a routine basis decreases mistakes or omissions made owing to predictions of the patient's behavior based on the nurses' emotional response to the patient behavior. In the practice of psychiatric nursing, it is important to monitor any emotional response you may have toward a patient's behavior to prevent nursing judgment errors. Because hospital stays are short, evaluations of the patient care need to be done daily and communicated during change of shift report.

The evaluation stage in the nursing process provides opportunities for new strategies in providing comprehensive care. If the nursing staff members become "stuck" in an intervention cycle that is not successful, a peer review by a nurse who is interested in the patient's problem may be helpful. Receiving clinical supervision from a certified clinical specialist also assists the nursing team to determine patient outcomes and interventions that are within the patient's capacity. Additionally, using the current literature to assist with planning and implementation of the nursing care is also helpful.

▶ Check Your Reading

26. When is it appropriate to evaluate the nursing care of a patient who is suicidal or self-mutilating?
27. How often should this evaluation take place?
28. What can you do when the nursing interventions are not helping the patient achieve the desired patient outcomes?

CASE STUDY: MARK

You are a psychiatric clinical nurse specialist working in the emergency department of a large metropolitan hospital in the southwest. The staff nurse asks you to consult with Mark, a 23-year-old male who attempted suicide last evening, and his mother, Jane, a 49-year-old elementary school teacher. When you arrive, Mark is unconscious, and his mother tells you that he took a bottle of over-the-counter sleeping pills and drank a large quantity of alcohol. She is distressed but also seems to be coping well. Upon interviewing her, you find that Mark has a long history of problems, and this episode is not a complete surprise to her. Mark's parents divorced when he was 18 years old. His two older sisters are both in college and doing well. His father is a recovering alcoholic who has remarried. Mark quit school at age 15 and has not been able to cope with life in an effective manner since that time.

Jane has an active support group and a strong spiritual base. She tells you that she is concerned that Mark will never mature to adulthood because he has made so many poor choices in his life. You discover that he has a criminal record for unauthorized use of a vehicle when he was 18. Jane tells you that she feels guilty because she did not encourage Mark to go to church and receive the sacraments of First Communion and Confirmation when he was a young boy.

When Mark awakens from his semicomatose state the next day, he tells you that he was concerned that his girlfriend was pregnant and felt life was not worth living anymore. He says, "I don't think there is a God or anyone who loves me; everyone would be better off if I were dead." As soon as he is recovered physically, Mark is moved to the psychiatric unit.

ASSESSMENT

Assessment data are as follows:

- Serious suicide attempt
- Poor coping skills
- Hopelessness
- History of criminal activity
- Verbalizations of despair regarding perceived loss of God's love and family support
- Supportive mother
- Lack of attainment of educational goals or job training skills

DIAGNOSIS

***DSM-IV* DIAGNOSIS:** Major Depressive Disorder, Single Episode, Severe without Psychotic Features

Nursing Diagnosis 1: Risk for Violence: Self-directed related to feelings of worthlessness and hopelessness as evidenced by serious suicide attempt, poor coping skills, and history of criminal activity

OUTCOME IDENTIFICATION, PLANNING, AND IMPLEMENTATION

EXPECTED OUTCOME 1: By _____ the patient will no longer verbalize thoughts of suicide or self-destruction.

SHORT-TERM GOALS	NURSING INTERVENTIONS	RATIONALES
By _____ the patient will seek out staff members when feeling the urge to harm himself.	1. Determine appropriate level of suicide precautions. 2. Assess the patient's level of suicidal potential and reassess daily. 3. Initiate suicide precautions as warranted by current level of suicidality.	1–3. Providing a safe environment for the patient is a number one priority.
	4. Convey warmth and unconditional acceptance of the patient.	4. This conveys the message to the patient that he is a worthwhile person, even though his behavior may not be acceptable.
	5. Monitor closely for any changes in mood or temperament.	5. Once medications are beginning to take effect, the patient may have enough energy to take his life.
By _____ the patient will make a short-term verbal contract not to harm himself.	1. Initiate a 24-hour verbal contract with the patient stating that he will not harm himself. 2. Be caring but firm in requesting the contract.	1–2. Discussing suicidal feelings with a caring person provides the patient with a sense of security and provides some relief that the professional will be able to protect him from his negative feelings.
	3. Involve the patient in as much of the treatment planning as possible.	3. Assists in making the patient more responsible for his health and well-being.

EXPECTED OUTCOME 2: By _____ the patient will demonstrate three new coping mechanisms.

SHORT-TERM GOAL	NURSING INTERVENTIONS	RATIONALES
By _____ the patient will verbalize at least four alternative ways of coping with stress.	1. Educate the patient about ways to reduce stress, such as meditation, guided imagery, engaging in physical activity, and journaling.	1. The patient needs to develop skills that will replace the tendency to turn to self-destructive behavior for relief.
	2. Remain an active listener and spend time with the patient.	2. The patient may feel shame about the suicide attempt and may have difficulty sharing honestly.
	3. Encourage the patient to express anger and to attempt to get to the source of anger.	3. Self-destructive behavior is often seen as anger turned inward. Venting the anger in a productive way can be very therapeutic.

EXPECTED OUTCOME 3: By _____ the patient will be connected with two outside community resources for assistance with any suicidal ideation after discharge.

SHORT-TERM GOAL	NURSING INTERVENTIONS	RATIONALES
By _____ the patient will contact an outside agency for support upon discharge.	1. As soon as the patient is physically able, provide him with a list of outside agencies. 2. Continue to encourage the patient.	1–2. Increasing the patient's support system will lessen the tendency toward suicidal behavior. Social isolation always increases the risk of suicide.
	3. Consider a family therapy session with the patient's mother.	3. The mother wants to be supportive and will need assistance in this process. An attempted suicide is a very traumatic event.

SHORT-TERM GOAL	NURSING INTERVENTIONS	RATIONALES
	4. Clarify the relationship between the patient and his girlfriend.	4. The possibility of the girlfriend's pregnancy was the trigger event for the suicide attempt and should not be ignored at this time.

Nursing Diagnosis 2: Spiritual Distress related to perception of loss of God's love and support from nuclear family as evidenced by suicide attempt, verbalizations of lack of spiritual presence, and hopelessness

OUTCOME IDENTIFICATION, PLANNING, AND IMPLEMENTATION

EXPECTED OUTCOME 1: By _____ the patient will improve overall spiritual well-being.

SHORT-TERM GOALS	NURSING INTERVENTIONS	RATIONALES
By _____ the patient will make positive statements about his life.	1. Engage in active listening and convey a caring, genuine attitude.	1. Attempting suicide is indicative of low self-worth; this patient needs to know that he is a worthwhile human being.
	2. Provide examples from literature, the Bible, and life experiences of people who have overcome great difficulties.	2. Helps the patient to see that much can be learned from experiencing hardships, and many others have overcome great personal tragedy and have a stronger spiritual self because of it.
	3. Encourage and accept verbalization of all feelings; gently help patient access hidden anger.	3. Depressed persons often bury feelings, especially anger, and need encouragement to verbalize them.
	4. Encourage the patient to remember a time in his life when he felt nurtured, loved, and accepted.	4. Enables the patient to shift the focus from negativity to remembering the unconditional love and acceptance that comes from a strong sense of spirituality.
By _____ the patient will articulate a belief system he finds acceptable.	1. Provide spiritual reading material consistent with the patient's spiritual beliefs.	1–2. These interventions assure the patient of your continued caring and concern and interest in his spiritual growth.
	2. Offer to pray with or for the patient.	
	3. Use guided imagery, prayer, and/or music to aid in healing past hurts.	3. Getting in touch with one's spiritual self can be accomplished in many ways other than traditional "talk therapy."
	4. Encourage the patient to try new religious exercises gradually and more than one time.	4. Spiritual well-being or distress will vary from day to day. Letting the patient know this is normal will keep him from getting discouraged.

EXPECTED OUTCOME 2: By _____ the patient will develop a support system with a church or self-help group.

SHORT-TERM GOALS	NURSING INTERVENTIONS	RATIONALES
By _____ the patient will initiate a healthy relationship with a person who has a well-developed sense of spirituality.	1. Educate the patient about healthy relationships.	1–3. This patient has a long history of difficult relationships.
	2. Use role-playing to prepare the patient for new relationships.	
	3. Explore with the patient the negative aspects of previous relationships.	
	4. Observe the patient in therapy groups and gently give the patient feedback about your observations.	4. The patient may be unaware of how his actions and reactions invite negative or undesirable behavior in others.

SHORT-TERM GOAL	NURSING INTERVENTIONS	RATIONALES
	5. Ask the patient to talk about three adults he knows who have a well-developed sense of spirituality. 6. Encourage the patient to contact one of these persons for support after he is discharged.	5. This exercise helps provide the patient with mental role models. 6. Supports the patient in being assertive in meeting his spiritual goals.
By _____ the patient will participate in group activities at a church or self-help group.	1. Encourage participation in prayer, social, and athletic groups while in the hospital. 2. Remain an advocate for the patient and do not be discouraged by setbacks.	1. By their very nature, groups foster learning about oneself in relationship to others. 2. This patient has a long history of setbacks, and expecting perfection in following the treatment plan would be self-defeating and feed into the patient's "all or nothing" thinking patterns.

EXPECTED OUTCOME 3: By _____ the patient will find a job, engage in job training skills, or begin an educational program.

SHORT-TERM GOALS	NURSING INTERVENTIONS	RATIONALES
By _____ the patient will articulate goals in life.	1. Support the patient in exploring both short-term and long-term goals. 2. Give the patient feedback about the realistic completion of his goals.	1. This patient has a history of impulsive activity. Setting goals will give the patient some hope for the future. 2. If goals are too global, the patient will experience failure again.
By _____ the patient will obtain a job and/or educational counseling.	1. Refer the patient to a vocational counselor or social worker. 2. Remain an advocate for the patient in this process.	1. This patient needs to begin to feel good about himself. Being successful in a job that uses his natural talents will foster self-esteem. 2. Suicidal, depressed patients have a high degree of negativity and need a great amount of support.

EVALUATION

Formative Evaluation Mark met all of the short-term goals except initiating a healthy relationship with a person who has a well-developed sense of spirituality. He did not contact anyone while he was in the hospital and had difficulty in identifying three people whom he knew who had a strong sense of spirituality. Prior to hospitalization, Mark was isolated socially except for his relationship with his girlfriend. Mark did agree to return for aftercare therapy groups at the hospital and to participate in individual therapy. He was able to commit to a verbal contract not to harm himself. He also contacted the local rehabilitation agency to begin working on vocational training. He said that his real dream was to go to college, but did not think that was realistic right now.

Summative Evaluation Mark met all of the expected outcomes regarding suicidal behavior but was still having difficult outcomes related to spiritual distress. His overall sense of spiritual well-being was dramatically improved by discharge, but he continued to experience difficulty with finding a support system. He says that he grew up feeling that he did not "fit in." The staff recommended that Mark remain in outpatient therapy and aftercare for at least a year because he does remain vulnerable to returning thoughts of suicide.

CONCLUSIONS

Providing nursing care for a patient who is suicidal is a complex issue. The idea that someone wants to end his or her life generates feelings in the nurse that need to be acknowledged to provide care that is thoughtful. A suicidal patient may not disclose suicidal feelings and thoughts in order to complete the act. When a patient is successful in committing suicide, the nursing staff have to evaluate the care delivered without blaming one another.

The key to providing comprehensive care to the patient who is suicidal is to perform an in-depth assessment regularly until the patient has a decrease in suicidal ideation. Determining whether the patient is *not at risk* for suicide or a *severe suicidal risk* using the continuum described in the chapter can guide whether the patient requires hospitalization, *every-15-minute checks*, or *one-to-one*. Questions that relate to the patient's ability to control his or her impulses to commit suicide are important in determining the intensity of care. Asking the patient to write his or her own contract for safety and placing that document in the chart is helpful in deciding whether the patient is joining with the care team to prevent a suicidal gesture. Assisting the patient to think through other options to problem-solve the crisis that was perceived as overwhelming and precipitated the suicidal thoughts can provide hope for the patient. Encouraging the patient to use his or her support system can reinforce the patient's value to others and may decrease the feelings of isolation. Assisting the patient to think through his or her spiritual beliefs by providing linkages with clergy and church members may assist the patient to use this powerful mechanism to regain a sense of purpose. It is important to assist the patient to understand his or her depression or other psychiatric illness that may have played a part in the feelings of wanting to die. By providing psychoeducation about the illness and the treatment, the nurse is promoting hope for a future.

Patients who self-mutilate have different psychodynamics than suicidal patients. Some patients have symptoms of self-mutilation and are *moderately to severely suicidal*. It is important to assess the patient who self-mutilates for suicidal ideation as well as dissociation, rage reactions, alexithymia, and feelings of worthlessness and shame. This patient has difficulty relating to others and is often socially isolated. It is important to assist the patient to link the act of self-mutilation with causal factors by assisting him or her to identify the thoughts that preceded the action. The patient who self-mutilates often feels shame about the self-injury. By providing the patient with appropriate medical care for the injury and a thoughtful approach for exploring the psychodynamics, the nurse can help the patient reduce this self-mutilating behavior.

The nursing care of this population of patients is potentially draining for the nurse. It is important to be aware of your own feelings about the patient and to receive clinical supervision or time away from the patient if you are feeling overwhelmed by your negative feelings toward the patient. Maintaining your own positive life balance is a worthy investment for your own mental health, especially when working with patients who are suicidal or who self-mutilate.

KEY POINTS TO REMEMBER

• The National Center for Health Statistics in 1990–1991 ranked suicide as the eighth cause of death in the United States, with 13.6 persons per every 100,000 population completing a suicidal act. Of the suicides that occur in the United States, 5% to 6% take place in an inpatient psychiatric hospital.

• Suicidal ideation and completion is not bounded by culture, age, class, religion, or socioeconomic status. Women tend to make more suicide attempts than men; however, more men complete the suicidal attempt. White men are the highest risk group for completing suicide, especially if the man is single and between the ages 75 to 84 years old.

• Suicide is one of the outcomes of untreated depression. There are several other psychiatric disorders that are associated with suicidal behavior, such as bipolar disorder, schizophrenia, and substance abuse disorders.

• Self-injury or intentional self-destructive behavior that destroys or alters body tissue occurs in an estimated 24% to 40% of psychiatric patients. Self-mutilating behavior has a different psychological intention than a suicidal gesture. Patients who self-mutilate have often had a history of child abuse, sexual abuse, and neglect. Self-mutilation often occurs when patients have alexithymia, or the inability to identify and put words to the experience of emotional feelings.

• There is no one theory that adequately explains suicidal or self-destructive behavior or can guide clinical practice. Biological, psychological, sociocultural, and spiritual factors may all contribute to self-injury.

• A comprehensive suicide assessment must include the physical, emotional, cognitive, social, and spiritual domains that represent the foundation of human functioning. An assessment also includes evaluating the patient to determine whether he or she is in the high-risk group.

• Patients who pose a threat to themselves through the use of a suicidal gesture or self-mutilation have a *risk for* nursing diagnosis.

• A severity index can be used when determining the nursing diagnosis and plan for a patient who is suicidal. This severity index is conceptualized as a continuum of the patient with *no suicidal ideation* to a patient with a *severe level of suicidal risk*. This information can assist the nurse to plan what type of care the patient requires to prevent a suicidal gesture.

• The overall goal for the patient is to protect the patient from self-harm while assisting him or her to maintain the highest degree of autonomy that is possible with a predicted outcome that the patient will no longer display suicidal or self-mutilative behavior.

• If a patient is successful in committing suicide, the nursing staff have to evaluate the care delivered without blaming one another.

LEARNING ACTIVITIES

1. Role play performing a suicide assessment interview. During this exercise, instruct the "patient" to play varying levels of suicidal lethality. The "nurse" determines the nursing care of the "patient," who then responds to the planning and implementation by getting better or more suicidal. During this role-playing exercise, the "patient" shares with the "nurse" why he or she got better or worse.

2. Attend a support group for suicide survivors in the community. Write your thoughts and feelings about this experience.

3. Read the book *The Bell Jar* by Sylvia Plath, who writes about her difficulties relating to others, her depression, and her suicidal thoughts and feelings. Sylvia Plath did commit suicide. Discuss your reactions in class.

4. View a documentary (PBS) on Van Gogh, whose paintings depicted his psychological pain from bipolar disorder; he died from suicide. Discuss your reaction in class.

CRITICAL THINKING EXERCISE

Jane Bayer, school nurse, is one of four members of the high school crisis team that evaluates high-risk students for potential self-destructive behaviors. Today the student under review is Peter. Peter lives with his parents and two sisters. He has a 3.8 grade-point average and has just been accepted to Harvard University as a chemistry major. He has come to the attention of the team because of an incident in gym class during which he "accidentally" cut his wrists. At that time, the nurse was told by Peter that his parents were getting a divorce and that his father was not sure he could afford to pay Peter's college tuition.

1. What assumptions can you make about Peter's behavior?
2. How would the team check their assumptions?
3. What further evidence would you need, if any?

The team decided to call Peter in to talk to him about his plans. Peter told the team that he was looking forward to college and had bought a new car and a new computer that he had lent to his girlfriend. He seemed in very high spirits and thought that the team was overreacting to his sisters' call to the counselor about his moodiness.

1. Do you have evidence that suggests that the team needs to act immediately?
2. If the team assumed that an immediate intervention was needed, what else could happen as a result?
3. Would that necessarily happen or only probably happen?

REFERENCES

Adams, K. S. (1985). Attempted suicide. *Psychiatry Clinics of North America, 8,* 183–203.

American Psychiatric Association (1984). *The American Psychiatric Association's Psychiatric Glossary.* Washington, D.C.: American Psychiatric Press.

Badger, J. (1995). Reaching out to the suicidal patient. *American Journal of Nursing, 95,* 24–32.

Barstow, D. (1995). Self-injury and self-mutilation: Nursing approaches. *Journal of Psychosocial Nursing and Mental Health Services, 33,* 19–22.

Beck, A. T. (1963). Thinking and depression: Idiosyncratic content and cognitive distortions. *Archives of General Psychiatry, 9,* 324–325.

Beck, A. T. (1967). *Depression: Clinical, Experimental and Theoretical Aspects.* New York: Harper Row.

Beck, A. T., Brown, G., Berchick, R. J., Stewart, B. L., and Steer, R. A. (1990). Relationship between hopelessness and ultimate suicide: A replication with psychiatric outpatients. *American Journal of Psychiatry, 147,* 190–195.

Busch, K. A., Clark, D. C., Fawcett, J., and Kravitz, H. M. (1993). Clinical features of inpatient suicide. *Psychiatric Annals, 23,* 256–262.

Cardell, R., and Horton-Deutsch, S. (1994). A model for assessment of inpatient suicide potential. *Archives of Psychiatric Nursing, 8,* 366–372.

Cornelius, J. R., Salloum, I. S., Mezzich, J., Cornelius, M., Fabrega, H., Ehler, J. G., Ulrich, R. F., Thase, M. E., and Mann, J. J. (1995). Disproportionate suicidality in patients with comorbid major depression and alcoholism. *American Journal of Psychiatry, 152,* 358–363.

Cugino, A., Markovich, E. I., Rosenblatt, S., Jarjoura, D., Blend, D., and Whittier, F. C. (1992). Searching for a pattern: Repeat suicide attempts. *Journal of Psychosocial Nursing, 30,* 23–25.

Davis, R. (1982). Black suicide and social support system: An overview and some implications for mental health practitioners. *Phylon, 43,* 304–314.

Durkheim, E. (1951). *Suicide.* Glencoe, Ill.: The Free Press. (Originally published as *Le Suicide,* 1897.)

Fauman, M. A. (1989). Quality assurance monitoring in psychiatry. *American Journal of Psychiatry, 146,* 1121–1130.

Favazza, A. R. (1987). *Bodies under siege: Self mutilation in culture and psychiatry.* Baltimore: Johns Hopkins University Press.

Favazza, A. R. (1989). Why patients mutilate themselves. *Hospital and Community Psychiatry, 40,* 137–145.

Filstead, W. J. (1980). Despair and its relationship to indirect self-destructive behavior. In N. L. Farberow (Ed.), *The many faces of suicide: Indirect self-destructive behavior.* New York: McGraw-Hill.

Folkman, S., and Lazarus, R. (1984). *Stress, appraisal, and coping.* New York: Springer.

Forster, P. (1994). Accurate assessment of short-term suicide risk in a crisis. *Psychiatric Annals, 24,* 571–578.

Fortinash, K. M., and Holoday-Worret, P. A. (1991). *Psychiatric nursing care plans.* St. Louis: Mosby-Year Book.

Frankl, V. E. (1964). *Man's search for meaning.* New York: Washington Square Press.

Freud, S. (1964). New introductory lectures on psychoanalysis: Lecture XXII. In *Anxiety and instinctual life.* Hogarth. (Originally published 1933.)

Gallop, R. (1992). Self-destructive and impulsive behavior in the patient with a borderline personality disorder: Rethinking hospital treatment and management. *Archives of Psychiatric Nursing, 6,* 178–182.

Goodwin, J. M. (1989). *Sexual abuse: Incest victims and their families* (2nd ed.). Chicago: Year Book Medical Publishers.

Green, E., Katz, J., and Marcus, P. (1995). Practice guidelines for suicide/self harm prevention. In E. Green and J. Katz (Eds.), *Clinical practice guidelines for the adult patient* (pp. 250-1–250-21). St. Louis: Mosby-Year Book.

Herman, J. L. (1992). *Trauma and recovery.* New York: Basic Books.

Kuperman, S., Black, D. W., and Burns, T. L. (1988). Excess suicide among formerly hospitalized child psychiatry patients. *Journal of Clinical Psychiatry, 49,* 88–93.

Menninger, A. (1938). *Man against himself.* Orlando, FL: Harcourt Brace.

Mintz, R. S. (1971). Basic considerations in the psychotherapy of the depressed patient. *American Journal of Psychotherapy, 2,* 56–72.

Mullis, M. R., and Byers, P. H. (1987). Social support in suicidal inpatients. *Journal of Psychosocial Nursing, 25,* 16–19.

National Center for Health Statistics (1989). *Vital statistics for the United States: 1987, deaths for selected causes.* Rockville, MD: National Center for Health Statistics.

Pallikkathayil, L., and McBride, A. B. (1986). Suicide attempts: The search for meaning. *Journal of Psychosocial Nursing, 24,* 13–17.

Robins, E. (1986). Psychosis and suicide. *Biological Psychiatry, 21,* 665–672.

Roy, A. (1989). Suicide. In H. I. Kaplan and B. J. Sadock (Eds.), *Comprehensive textbook of psychiatry* (5th ed.). Baltimore: Williams & Wilkins.

Sainsbury, P. (1986). The epidemiology of suicide. In A. Roy (Ed.), *Suicide.* Baltimore: Williams & Wilkins.

Sanger, E., Thomas, M. D., and Whitney, J. D. (1988). A guide for nursing assessment of the psychiatric inpatient. *Archives of Psychiatric Nursing, 2,* 334–338.

Stanley, M., and Stanley, B. (1990). Postmortem evidence for serotonin's role in suicide. *Journal of Clinical Psychiatry, 51,* 22–28.

U.S. Department of Health and Human Services, National Center for Health Statistics (1992). *Vital statistics report, 40, 1990–1991.* Hyattsville, MD: Public Health Service.

van der Kolk, B. A. (1987). *Psychological trauma.* Washington, D.C.: American Psychiatric Press.

Vanzant, I. (1992). *Tapping the power within.* New York: Harlem River Press.

Wheeler, K., and Broad, R. D. (1994). Alexithymia and overeating. *Perspectives in Psychiatric Care, 30,* 7–10.

Wolfersdorf, M., Hole, G., Steiner, B., and Keller, F. (1990). Suicide risk in suicidal versus nonsuicidal depressed patients. *Crisis, 11,* 85–97.

SUGGESTED READINGS

Badger, J. (1995). Reaching out to the suicidal patient. *American Journal of Nursing, 95* 24–32.

Buchanan, D. M. (1991). Suicide: A conceptual model for an avoidable death. *Archives of Psychiatric Nursing, 5,* 341–349.

Cardell, R., and Horton-Deutsch, S. (1994). A model for assessment of inpatient suicide potential. *Archives of Psychiatric Nursing, 8,* 366–372.

Roy, A. (1989). Suicide. In H. I. Kaplan and B. J. Sadock (Eds.), *Comprehensive textbook of psychiatry* (5th ed.). Baltimore: Williams & Wilkins.

CHAPTER 37

THE JOURNEY EMBEDDED IN PSYCHOPHYSIOLOGICAL DISORDERS

For this is the great error of our day, that physicians separate mind from body.

—Socrates

LEARNING OBJECTIVES

After studying this chapter, you should be able to:

1. Recognize the impact of psychophysiological illness on routine health care.

2. Describe the contributions that Descartes, Cannon, and Selye have made to the recognition of the stress response.

3. Describe an interactive model of stress and physical illness.

4. Describe the components of a complete psychophysiological and spiritual assessment.

5. List the five pain-producing structures of the back.

6. List the factors contributing to the poor description of most pelvic pain.

7. List the factors contributing to the development of irritable bowel syndrome.

8. Describe the two major psychophysiological theories related to development of hypertension.

9. Describe the role of serotonin and norepinephrine in the development of a migraine headache.

10. Identify the physical and psychological factors that contribute to the development of temporomandibular disorder.

11. Describe the common characteristics of somatoform disorders.

12. List the differentiating characteristics of each of the seven somatoform disorders.

13. Identify expected outcomes of working with a patient diagnosed with a psychophysiological disorder.

14. Identify expected outcomes of working with family members of a patient diagnosed with a psychophysiological disorder.

15. Describe the use of the nursing process in the holistic care of a patient with low back pain.

16. Describe the holistic treatment of each of the psychophysiological illnesses discussed.

17. Identify how research has clarified the relationships among the physical, psychological, and spiritual components of health.

KEY TERMINOLOGY

Body dysmorphic disorder
Chronic back pain
Chronic pelvic pain
Conversion disorder
Hypertension
Hypochondriasis
Irritable bowel syndrome
La belle indifference
Migraine headache
Pain disorder
Primary gain
Psychophysiological assessment
Psychophysiological illness
Secondary gain
Somatization disorder
Somatoform disorder not otherwise specified
Somatoform disorders
Temporomandibular disorder
Undifferentiated somatoform disorder

It has been estimated that as many as 70% to 80% of all visits to internists and family practice physicians are made by persons suffering from **psychophysiological illness** (Corbin L., et al, 1988). Increasingly we recognize the psychological dimension of these illnesses; clearly, psychological issues interrelate with the body in such an intimate manner that we cannot separate one from the other and still do justice to alleviating the patient's problem. We have been much slower to recognize the importance of the spiritual dimension. No research looks at the role that spiritual distress plays in the etiology of psychophysiological illnesses or at the role of spiritual well-being in the healing of patients diagnosed with these illnesses. Although the research to support the role of spirituality is lacking, we must use a holistic approach that addresses spirituality or we do a disservice to our patients. Patients suffering with these illnesses need care that addresses physical, psychological, spiritual, cognitive, and social issues; anything less brings them only partial healing.

In this chapter you are introduced to the most prevalent psychophysiological illnesses: chronic pain (back and pelvic), hypertension, irritable bowel syndrome (IBS), migraines, and temporomandibular disorder (TMD). In addition, you are presented with information about the seven types of somatoform disorders: body dysmorphic disorder, conversion disorder, hypochondriasis, somatization disorder, pain disorder, undifferentiated somatoform disorder, and somatoform disorder not otherwise specified. Each diagnosis is discussed in holistic terms, beginning with the epidemiology, etiology, psychological and spiritual factors, and treatment. The nursing process is applied to the journey of Monica, a young woman who suffers from chronic back pain. Some of the contributing factors of Monica's story are generic to all psychophysiological illnesses.

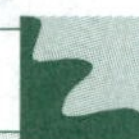

MONICA'S STORY

I am a 28-year-old woman with a Master's degree in math. My car was hit in the rear when I was driving to work on a snowy afternoon two years ago. My initial diagnosis was acute muscle spasm of the back and neck. I was seen by my internist, who prescribed Flexeril and hot compresses and told me to rest. I followed the treatment and returned to work as a computer programmer three days after my injury. I could not sit without discomfort. I was sleeping poorly and had no appetite.

The Problem Escalates

I continued to have shooting pain in my back and arms. I could not stand, sit, or lie down for more than 30 minutes without experiencing increased pain. I also lost six pounds. I went back to my internist, and he discontinued the Flexeril and ordered Darvocet for pain. With the Darvocet, I could manage to sit at my computer for almost a complete day, but I continued to lose weight and could not sleep.

My parents, who lived out of state, insisted that I come home for a visit. This entailed a six-hour car ride. I complied with their wishes, although I knew I could not sit still for more than a few hours without experiencing increased pain. I arrived at my parents in acute distress. I had never told them about the accident, and I did not tell them during the visit. I slept on a pull-out bed, which was very soft and did not support my back and neck. I left my parents in excruciating pain; when I got home, I called my doctor, who prescribed Fiorinal with Codeine No. 3. This did little to relieve my pain during the day, but I began to sleep a little better.

Surgery Becomes an Option

I could not work the following week because of muscle spasms in my back. I called my doctor multiple times in pain. He insisted that I now consult an orthopedic surgeon. The surgeon diagnosed me as having facet injury and recommended extensive surgery. My husband was pressuring me to have the surgery because we had not been able to be intimate since before the accident because of my back and neck pain.

I wanted a second opinion before surgery. The second physician suggested I try physical therapy and counseling before surgery. I felt it was important to try the more conservative treatment before resorting to surgery. I chose a certified specialist in adult psychiatric nursing for my counselor. When I talked to her on the phone, she encouraged me to begin a holistic approach to my problems. She said that I needed to deal with the components of my life that contribute directly to my physical pain and my inability to recover from the accident.

A Psychophysiological Approach

I see my counselor once a week, and I go to physical therapy three times a week. In therapy I have learned to control my pain with deep breathing and imagery. I practice every day. I take deep breaths and imagine myself at my grandfather's farm. I pretend to go there as I did as a child. I walk through the fields and visit with the animals. It was a safe, secure place for me, and now I revisit it in my mind daily. I have stopped taking the Fiorinal with Codeine No. 3, and I just take two to four ibuprofen a day to help ease the muscle spasms. The physical therapist has taught me to do stretching exercises, and I do them daily also.

A New Approach to Life

In counseling I also have learned to accept myself as a person who has been in an accident and now has pain. I have told my boss that I cannot do overtime for now and that I must stretch every hour. I find that I am more productive when I rest. This was a hard lesson for me—I felt like I was giving up and allowing my pain to rule my life. I also have been more honest with my parents and my husband. My parents just cannot seem to understand that I cannot drive to their house and that they will have to visit me. They call me selfish and refuse to visit. It's difficult not seeing my parents; even though they are in good health they have never been to my home. I am learning in counseling that always doing what another person wants is "codependent behavior." My husband has been more understanding. He has learned to listen to me, and we have been able to resume a different but in some ways more satisfactory sexual relationship.

My injury will be with me the rest of my life. It has taught me a valuable lesson in taking care of myself and being honest about my feelings. Spiritually, I have developed a very strong personal connection with God. I am learning to depend on Him. I realize that I can still be a "good person" without overfunctioning in my relationships. I also feel I am taking better care of myself. This injury has taught me to ask for the things I need. I wish my back would just be better, but it is not; however, I can live a full, healthy life if I allow myself.

HISTORICAL OVERVIEW

The Mechanistic View

The modern medical model is based on the philosophy of René Descartes. In 1637, Descartes described the human body as a machine that operates on scientific principles. This mechanistic view of the body split the mind and spirit from the body (Descartes, 1967). Even today, many health care practitioners treat the patient's body and not the whole person.

The Theory of Homeostasis

Claude Bernade's (1957) theory of homeostasis described the body as a self-regulating machine which is kept in balance through feedback from one organ to another. Bernade's model has made explorations about the links between mind, body, and spirit in health and illness almost impossible to consider. Viewing the body as a machine, it is impossible to consider how the lifestyle, emotions, and spirituality affect this machine that is the person and contribute to health and illness.

Psychophysiology describes an illness as an interaction between the mind, body, and spirit. Almost all physical problems are affected by the mind and spirit. Stress is generally accepted to play a part in most illnesses.

The Theory of Stress

The theory of stress and how it affects the body began with the work of Walter Cannon (1929). Cannon elucidated the body's capacity to fight or flee during stress. The "fight or flight" response is a sympathetic nervous system reaction that causes the release of epinephrine and norepinephrine to most major organ systems. This response is adaptive for a short period of time and mobilizes the body for intense exertion. However, these responses can be maladaptive and lead to disease if they continue for a prolonged period.

Hans Selye (1956) described the general adaptation syndrome (GAS). Selye reported a triad of pathological consequences to prolonged stress: adrenal gland enlargement, thymus involution, and gastrointestinal ulceration. Current research indicates that Selye's GAS was not completely correct. In a series of classic studies, Mason (1968, 1971) refined the stress response and demonstrated that it is more specific than originally described by Selye.

A stress is a stimulus that is either consciously or unconsciously perceived by the person. To be viewed as stressful, this stimulus must be perceived to be a threat to the person. The person also must feel that the demand made by the stress is beyond his or her ability to cope. This threat sets off a series of physiological responses. Repeated and prolonged episodes of arousal in the absence of active movement toward resolution of the conflict set up the pathway for physical illness (Sterling and Eyer, 1981; Allen, 1983; Lowery, 1987). Figure 37–1 presents an overview of the factors that affect the relationship between stress and physical illness.

Factors within the person (age, sex, socioeconomic status, occupation, education, and fitness) all interact to either decrease or increase this response. Behaviors of the person also modify the stress response (smoking, alcohol, and drug use and abuse, eating habits, and exercise). Mediating factors either diminish (coping, economic resources, and social support) or attenuate (conflict and abusive relationships) the person's responsiveness. The person's coping abilities, spiritual support, economic resources, as well as "people" resources, such as family and friends, modify reactivity. Conflict and abusive relationships intensify reactivity.

► Check Your Reading

1. What does the theory of homeostasis say about the body?
2. What is the General Adaptation Syndrome?
3. Identify two factors within the person that either decrease or increase the individual's responsivity to stress.
4. Identify two mediating factors that either diminish or attenuate responsivity to stress.

DIAGNOSIS

Diagnosis begins with a multifaceted **psychophysiological assessment.** The clinical history is focused on the whole person, the person's story, and not just the physical symptom. A careful social, educational, occupational, spiritual, and family history can elucidate the relationships between the person's presenting problem and the rest of her or his life.

Use of Psychometric Instruments

The use of psychometric instruments can answer specific questions regarding the psychological status of the patient. The instruments selected for review here are only a small number of those available for use.

State-Trait Anxiety Scale

The State-Trait Anxiety Scale (STAI) (Speilberger et al, 1970) is a 40-item tool that contains self-report scales for measuring two different types of anxiety, state and trait. The STAI trait scale contains 20 statements that ask respondents to describe how they usually feel. The state scale also contains 20 items but asks for a description of how the respondent feels at a specific point in time. The STAI is a very popular tool for assessing anxiety; it is convenient, reliable, grounded in psychological theory, and able to be used in many contexts.

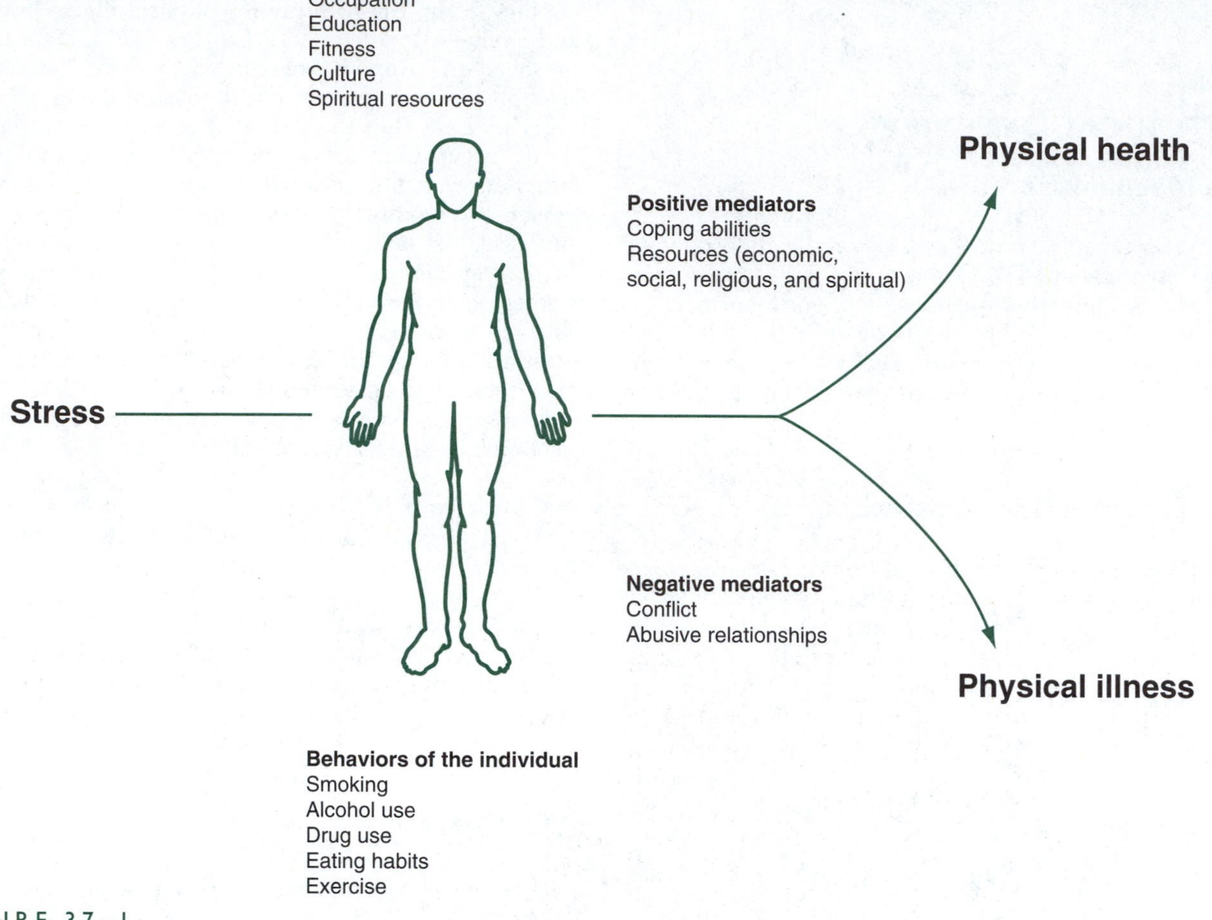

FIGURE 37–1
An overview of the factors that affect the relationship between stress and physical illness.

Beck Depression Inventory

The Beck Depression Inventory (BDI) (Beck, 1972) is an instrument that approximates clinical judgments of depression. The inventory is composed of 21 multiple-choice items that reflect specific behavioral signs of depression. The behavioral signs are weighted in severity from 0 to 3. The Beck Depression Inventory is widely used in both research and clinical situations.

Life Experience Survey

Sarason et al (1978) developed the Life Experience Survey (LES) to assess a person's assessment of life stresses experienced during the preceding year. The LES is a 57-item self-report inventory. The respondent is asked to identify which events were experienced during the past year, whether the event was viewed as positive or negative on a seven-point scale, and what was the perceived impact of the event rated on a seven-point scale. A higher score on the LES is indicative of increasing life stress.

Symptom Check List 90

This is a 90-item self-report symptom inventory (Derogatis, 1977). Each item is rated on a five-point scale from "not at all" to "extremely." The responses are then interpreted along nine symptom dimensions: somatization, obsessive-compulsive, interpersonal sensitivity, depression, anxiety, hostility, phobic anxiety, paranoid ideation, and psychoticism. Scoring requires adding specific items for each of the nine dimensions to obtain distress scores. This test briefly evaluates a broad range of symptoms. It can serve as a screening tool and guide the practioner to further evaluation.

Minnesota Multiphasic Personality Inventory

This is a 566-item true-false questionnaire. The MMPI inventory has 10 basic clinical scales: hypochondriasis, depression, hysteria, psychopathic deviance, male sexual introversion, paranoia, psychasthenia, schizophrenia, hypomania, and social introversion. Scores are transformed into profiles reflecting each of the scales. This tool is extremely comprehensive but requires at least one hour to an hour and a half to administer (Dahlstrom et al, 1972).

Sarason Social Support Questionnaire

Sarason's Social Support Questionnaire (SSQ-6) (Sarason et al, 1986; Sarason et al, 1987) consists of six items, each of which presents a given set of circumstances that require social support. The tool then asks on whom the respondent could rely in that situation and how satisfied they are with that support. The number of supports are quantified. In addition, the individual's satisfaction with support is measured by the use of a six-point scale.

Spiritual Well-Being Scale

Most psychophysiological assessments do not include the spiritual dimension. This is a serious oversight leading to an incomplete database. Ellison (1983) and Paloutzian's Spiritual Well-Being Scale could appropriately be used, along with additional interview questions, to assess spiritual health. The instrument consists of two subscales, the Religious Well-Being and the Existential Well-Being subscales. The Religious Scale measures the individual's well-being in relationship to God; the Existential Scale measures the individual's well-being in relationship to a personal sense of life's meaning and significance. Each of the subscales has 10 items rated on a Likert scale of 0 to 6.

Other Psychometric Instruments

Many other specific tools can be used to evaluate the various psychophysiological disorders. The Jenkins Type A Scale is useful for cardiac patients. The McGill Pain Questionnaire is standard for the evaluation of chronic pain. Visual Analogue Scales and Pain Drawings are frequently used for a subjective evaluation of chronic pain. Diaries often are important to document the patient's symptoms and drug use (Green, 1985).

Use of Measures of the Stress Response

The final aspect of assessment is a psychophysiological measurement of stress response. The measurement of temperature, heart rate, and blood pressure responses during a discussion of a stressful event provides documentation of physiological reactivity. Twenty-four–hour monitoring of heart rate and blood pressure along with a diary of daily events contributes an overview of cardiovascular reactivity.

▶ Check Your Reading

5. Why does the assessment include the use of psychometric instruments?
6. What is the Life Experience Survey used to evaluate?
7. What is the Minnesota Multiphasic Personality Inventory?
8. What are the two components of the Spiritual Well-Being Scale?

CHRONIC LOW BACK PAIN

Eighty percent of Americans experience low back pain at least once in their life, and the majority resolve this pain in less than two months (Rowlingson, 1993). Monica in the opening story is one of the 10% to 40% of all patients with back injuries who go on to develop a chronic pain disorder (Philips et al, 1991). **Chronic back pain** is defined as pain that persists for more than six months and results in the need for long-term treatment. A total of 1% to 2% of low back pain is caused by disc herniation. Postural and muscular low back pain account for 80% to 90% of all complaints. Chronic back pain imposes not only the physical impact of the pain but also the emotional, spiritual, and occupational effects as well. For this reason, this physical disorder has significant implications as a mental health issue.

In a holistic approach to chronic back pain, the definition of pain is made by the patient. The patient describes where the pain is, what exacerbates the pain, and what relieves it. Although no anatomical or physiological basis for the pain which the patient describes may be known, the pain is accepted as described by the patient. The inability to define the precise cause of the patient's pain may be due to our poor understanding of the mechanisms of pain development (Burckhardt, 1990).

Source

We do know that five pain-producing structures exist in the lower back (Box 37–1). Under normal circumstances, the anterior spinal column with its vertebrae and discs performs the weight-bearing functions of the body. Trauma, dysfunction, or degeneration of the anterior spinal column trigger pain, which causes increased curvature in the lumbar lordotic region. Reflex muscle spasm then occurs in an attempt to stop the motion and decrease irritation of the tissues. These spasms shift the spine and move the weight-bearing functions to the more delicate posterior elements. The facet joints are stressed, the alignment is distorted, and more pain and muscle spasm occur (Rowlingson, 1993).

BOX 37–1 Pain-Producing Structures in the Lower Back

Posterior longitudinal ligaments

Interspinous ligaments

Nerve roots and dorsal coverings

Facet joints

Deep muscles

Specific Diagnoses

Many specific diagnoses for low back pain reflect the area of dysfunction. *Posterior facet syndrome* is caused by a rotational strain to both the facet joints and the annulus fibrosis. *Myofascial syndrome and piriformis syndrome* are caused by spasms and changes in the muscles of the lower back. These syndromes can progress into facet-disc pain with sustained contractions of the muscles. *Sacroiliac syndrome* is a common chronic condition in which the exact pathological lesion is obscure, but it involves the muscles and joint of the lower back and hip. As the diagnostic procedures for low back pain are further refined, even more specific diagnosis will evolve.

Psychological and Spiritual Responses

Depression, along with significant spiritual distress, and even drug abuse are very common concurrent issues with chronic back pain and may contribute to the person's assuming a sick role. The loss of occupational and family roles may contribute to the person's depression and sense of despair. Spiritually, the patient may wonder "Why did God let this happen to me?," "Why doesn't He make me better?," and "Does He have a purpose for my suffering?" The answers to these questions contribute to his or her ability to accept and cope with the chronic back pain. Sometimes the excessive use of pain medications, including narcotic analgesics, results in drug abuse. Alcohol is frequently consumed in greater quantities in an effort to reduce the pain. Withdrawal from pain medication or alcohol can complicate the treatment process.

BOX 37-2 An Overview of Chronic Low Back Pain

Characteristics

Affects 40% of the population

Treatment

Medical
- Aspirin
- Nonsteroidal antiinflammatory drugs
- Muscle relaxants
- Tricyclic antidepressants

Cognitive-behavioral
- Biofeedback
- Relaxation
- Diet
- Physical therapy/exercise

Spiritual
- Helping others
- Inspirational reading
- Journaling
- Music
- Meditation
- Prayer

Treatment

The treatment of chronic back pain emphasizes the management of the pain and the accompanying dysfunction. Three broad categories of treatment exist: medical management, cognitive-behavioral treatments, and spiritual intervention.

Medical Treatment

Aspirin and other nonsteroidal antiinflammatory drugs help to decrease the inflammation and should be prescribed. Muscle relaxants reduce the reflex muscle spasms. Tricyclic antidepressants decrease the underlying depression and promote sleep.

Cognitive-Behavioral Treatment

Cognitive-behavioral treatments include biofeedback, relaxation, exercise, and diet. These techniques can be used to help decrease anxiety and muscle spasm (Rowlingson, 1993). Exercise and weight loss are important components in reducing low back pain. Many patients require a referral to physical therapy to be taught appropriate exercises. Daily stretching and muscle toning exercises strengthen the muscles and decrease pain. Losing weight, especially in the abdominal region, decreases the strain on the back.

Spiritual Intervention

Spiritual intervention includes encouraging the patient to use spiritual resources that have been meaningful in the past and to consider trying new ones. Asking the patient about the significance of the pain to her or his life and what meaning the pain has are ways to focus the patient on the important spiritual task of providing an acceptance to the new limitations imposed by this chronic illness.

▶ Check Your Reading

9. Name one reason why depression often accompanies lower back pain.
10. What are included in cognitive-behavioral treatments?

CHRONIC PELVIC PAIN

Chronic pelvic pain is defined as nonmenstrual pelvic pain of greater than six months duration. It may be intermittent or continuous. Chronic pelvic pain is a major diagnosis for women, accounting for 10% of outpatient visits and up to 25% of diagnostic laparoscopies. It is the third most common indication for hysterectomy and accounts for approximately 78,000 hysterectomies annually. The average age of patients with chronic pelvic pain is 30 years (Reiter et al, 1991).

Diagnosis

Traditionally, the diagnostic laparoscopic procedure has been used to evaluate the patient with chronic pelvic pain. It has been assumed that if all visible intrapelvic abnormalities have been excluded by the laparoscopy, the cause of the pain is psychogenic. A substantial body of controlled investigations shows that the laparoscopic examination, although it can identify the presence of adhesions and endometriosis, cannot differentiate which patients will experience pelvic pain (Reiter et al, 1991).

The Nature of the Pain

The pain experienced by women who suffer from chronic pelvic pain is poorly localized because the parenchyma of the internal pelvic organs do not contain pain receptors. The arterial walls in the peritoneum are richly innervated. Pain from the pelvic organs often is perceived at a site far from the source. Pain from the fundus of the uterus is perceived as lower midline abdominal pain. Pain from the ovaries only occurs when stretching of the surrounding peritoneum and vascular structures occurs; therefore, the description of pelvic pain can be vague and seemingly anatomically incorrect (Lichter and Laff, 1993).

Psychological and Spiritual Responses

Studies have documented that patients whose journey is complicated by chronic pelvic pain are significantly more likely to develop depression, somatization, substance abuse, and sexual dysfunction (Reiter et al, 1991). All of these psychological complications carry a high rate of spiritual distress as well.

Individuals with chronic pelvic pain have a tendency to "doctor shop" in an effort to obtain relief from their pain. The use of analgesic drugs to control pain over an extended period contributes to the risk of drug addiction or dependency.

Treatment

A comprehensive, multidisciplinary approach that addresses the physiological aspects of the pain as well as the psychological and spiritual needs of the patient is necessary.

Medical Treatment

Medications traditionally prescribed include hormones and nonsteroidal antiinflammatory drugs. Frequently these women have had several surgeries. One third of all chronic pelvic pain patients will have already undergone a complete abdominal hysterectomy. Conservative surgical approaches may be considered to relieve pain. These include removal of endometrial implants and presacral neurectomies and lysis of adhesions (Kames et al, 1990).

Psychological and Spiritual Care

The psychological and spiritual components of a comprehensive treatment approach include stress management, relaxation, cognitive therapy, spiritual support, and sexual education. The treatment focuses on all aspects of the person's life, including family, social, spiritual, occupational, and sexual functioning. The treatment for

BOX 37-3 An Overview of Chronic Pelvic Pain

Characteristics

Average age of patient—30 years

Poorly localized

High rates of depression, somatization, substance abuse, sexual dysfunction, history of sexual abuse

"Doctor-shopping"

Drug dependency

Treatment

- Medical
  - Medications
    - Hormones
    - Nonsteroidal antiinflammatory drugs
  - Surgeries for symptom relief
- Psychological
  - Stress management
  - Relaxation
  - Cognitive therapy
  - Sexual education
- Spiritual
  - Helping others
  - Inspirational reading
  - Journaling
  - Music
  - Meditation
  - Prayer

patients with chronic pelvic pain must be supportive and empathetic (Kames et al, 1990).

▶ Check Your Reading

11. Define chronic pelvic pain.
12. Name two of the psychiatric disorders that are commonly associated with chronic pelvic pain.
13. What does the psychological treatment for chronic pelvic pain include?

IRRITABLE BOWEL SYNDROME

The current diagnostic criteria for **irritable bowel syndrome** (IBS) state that continuous or recurrent symptoms of abdominal pain that is relieved with a bowel movement or is associated with a change in either the frequency or texture of the stool must occur. These symptoms must be present for at least 3 months to make the diagnosis of IBS. Individuals with IBS report an irregular bowel pattern at least 25% of the time. The bowel pattern includes two or more of the following (Drossman et al, 1990; Phipps et al, 1995):

- A change in the frequency of bowel movements, with diarrhea alternating with constipation
- A feeling of bloating or abdominal distension
- Passage of mucus

IBS is characterized by inflammation of the gastrointestinal tract, which contributes these symptoms. Additional symptoms include fever, anorexia, nausea, vomiting, and weight loss (Lewis, 1988). The pain associated with IBS is chronic and is located in either the right or left lower abdomen. Eating usually causes the pain, and bowel movements usually relieve it.

The development of IBS generally is unexpected and occurs most commonly in young adults between 20 and 40 years of age and often in children under 15 (Lewis, 1988). IBS is diagnosed in 10.4% of patients seen by gastroenterologists (Everhart and Renault, 1991).

Physiological Basis

The physiological mechanism for IBS symptoms appears to be abnormal pain perception. Several studies have demonstrated that patients with IBS report low pain thresholds when a balloon is inflated in various areas of the digestive tract, with an increased sensitivity to pain in the abdomen. These same individuals do not have a decreased tolerance for painful stimuli on the skin, nor is their pain response correlated with an abnormal psychological profile (Whitehead, 1992).

Psychological and Spiritual Responses

A study by Drossman and colleagues (1988) compared psychosocial profiles of three groups: (1) normal people, (2) people who had not consulted a physician but who had symptoms compatible with IBS (nondiagnosed), and (3) people who had a medical diagnosis of IBS (diagnosed). The subjects were given a group of standard psychometric tests (McGill Pain Questionnaire, Minnesota Multiphasic Personality Inventory, Profile of Mood States, Life Expectancy Survey, and an Illness Behavior Questionnaire). Results of the studies demonstrated that the diagnosed people were psychosocially different from the nondiagnosed people with IBS and from the normal people. For those people who suffered from IBS but had not consulted a physician, scores fell between those of the people diagnosed with IBS and the normal people; however, their scores were closer to those of normal people. The nondiagnosed IBS group had better coping abilities, perceived their illness as less disruptive to their lives, and used less psychological denial than those diagnosed with IBS. This would suggest that patients who experience both IBS and psychological symptoms are more likely to consult a health care provider than are patients with IBS symptoms only.

The role of psychological stress in IBS is further documented in a study reported by Whitehead and colleagues (1988). A community sample of approximately 400 women was divided into three groups:

- Normal subjects
- Those who met strict criteria for IBS but had not consulted a physician
- Those with the abdominal pain who had sought help

All subjects were assessed every three months for both bowel symptoms and for stressful life events. Results demonstrated that those women with IBS symptoms who had not consulted a health care provider reported no more symptoms of psychological distress than did those who were normal subjects. Those women who had sought assistance with their physical symptoms demonstrated significantly more psychological symptoms than those with bowel symptoms who had not sought the interventions of a health care provider. These studies demonstrate that both physical and psychological symptoms must be treated in these patients. The health care provider must assess and assist the patient to deal with the psychosocial factors that are contributing to their symptom pattern. Although this study did not include spiritual well-being as a variable, one might wonder if differences in spiritual well-being occur across patients with IBS and what those differences might suggest.

Data suggest that childhood trauma may be related to IBS later in life. For instance, parental loss through death or divorce, a situation that causes profound psychological and spiritual distress in children, has been reported more frequently by IBS patients than by healthy control subjects. It also has been reported that 53% of medical clinic patients with gastrointestinal disorders reported being abused sexually as a child, compared with 37% of medical clinic patients with other organic diseases (Whitehead, 1992).

BOX 37-4 An Overview of Irritable Bowel Syndrome

Characteristics

Onset between 20 and 40 years of age

Sudden onset

Low pain threshold

Possible childhood trauma

Symptoms

Change in bowel pattern

Bloating/abdominal distention

Mucus passage

Fever

Anorexia/nausea

Vomiting/weight loss

Pain in the lower abdomen

Treatment

Medical therapy in conjunction with psychotherapy

Stress management/relaxation

Cognitive-behavioral therapy

Spiritual resources

- Helping others
- Inspirational reading
- Journaling
- Music
- Meditation
- Prayer

Treatment

Numerous controlled studies have demonstrated that a combination of psychological treatment approaches with standard medical therapy provides more benefits for IBS patients than medical therapy alone (Rowlingson, 1993). These treatment approaches include strategies such as insight-oriented psychotherapy (Svedlund et al, 1983), relaxation-based stress management training (Lynch and Zamble, 1989; Guthrie et al, 1991; Blanchard et al, 1992), cognitive-behavioral therapy (Guthrie et al, 1991), and hypnosis (Harvey et al, 1989; Whorwell et al, 1984). Stress management training and psychotherapy seem to offer more promise for the relief of symptoms of irritable bowel syndrome (IBS) than does the direct modification of physiological activity with biofeedback. No promising evidence exists at present that psychological interventions are effective at improving physical symptoms in IBS, although these interventions are related to improvement in the patient's subjective sense of well-being. No mention is made in the literature of spiritual interventions, but holistic care demands that spiritual issues be addressed.

▶ Check Your Reading

14. Name two of the symptoms of IBS.
15. What role does psychological stress play in the etiology and recurrence of IBS?
16. Name two of the treatment approaches used with IBS patients.

HYPERTENSION

Hypertension is a multifactorial psychophysiological illness. The most consistent and profound response during stress is elevation of blood pressure (Boone, 1991). Hypertension is a life-threatening disorder and a significant risk factor for the development of coronary artery disease and cerebral vascular disease. Over 16 million Americans have high blood pressure. Hypertension is twice as frequent among African-Americans (Calhoun, 1992). African-American women have an incidence of hypertension four and a half times higher than that of Caucasian women. The incidence of hypertension is greater for men than women until women reach menopausal age when women surpass men. (American Heart Association, 1992).

Hypertension is defined by the World Health Organization as chronically elevated blood pressure exceeding 160/95 mmHg. Borderline hypertension is defined as blood pressure above 140/90 mmHg. The risk of developing fatal or nonfatal end organ damage is correlated with the amount of rise in blood pressure over 160/95 mmHg (American Heart Association, 1992).

Causes

Physiological Causes

The cause of essential hypertension is unknown, and the pathophysiological mechanisms vary among individuals. High blood pressure may result from increased cardiac output, increased peripheral resistance, and increased blood volume due to decreased sodium and water excretion (Guyton, 1995). Multiple behavioral, psychological, social, dietary, and other factors influence blood pressure and contribute to the development of essential hypertension.

Two major psychophysiological theories relate behavioral factors to the development of essential hypertension: the hyperreactivity theory and the symptoms specificity theory. The *hyperreactivity theory* states that excessive reactivity in blood pressure to all environmental stimuli initiates and maintains essential hypertension. The *symptom specificity theory* states that a consistent reactivity in blood pressure to specific environmental stressors initiates and maintains essential hypertension. Increased cardiovascular reactivity is seen in children of hypertensive parents and in borderline hypertensive persons. This provides support for the theory that increased reactivity is a precursor to essential hypertension (Fredrickson, 1991).

Psychological and Social Causes

Socioeconomic status and stressors, including poverty, low occupational and educational status, and high stress levels, are related to essential hypertension (Calhoun, 1992). Anger, both suppressed and expressed, is positively related to hypertension (Niaura and Goldstein, 1992). Verbal communication also is related to increased blood pressure reactivity and/or hypertension. Talking for two minutes increases blood pressure from 10% to 50% above resting baseline, and the higher the resting blood pressure, the greater the increase during talking (Lynch, 1985). The faster an individual speaks, the greater the increase in blood pressure (Thomas and Friedmann, 1994). Speaking to a person of perceived higher status causes significantly greater increases in blood pressure than speaking to a person of the same status (Long et al, 1982).

BOX 37-5 An Overview of Hypertension

Characteristics

Gender

- Male
- Female (postmenopausal)

Culture: African-Americans twice as likely to get hypertension as whites

Course: Chronic blood pressure greater than 160/95 mmHg

Treatment

Medical: Pharmacological agents

Psychosocial

- Behavior modification
- Relaxation
- Biofeedback
- Diet and exercise

Spiritual

- Helping others
- Inspirational reading
- Journaling
- Music
- Meditation
- Prayer

Treatment

The medical management of hypertension has been refined in recent years. The use of pharmacological agents to reduce blood pressure is generally accepted. For further discussion of drug treatment of hypertension, the reader is referred to general medical-surgical and pharmacology texts.

Dietary interventions include weight reduction, limited use of alcohol and caffeine, low-salt diets, and reduction of fats and cholesterol. Moderate to excessive use of alcohol is related to increased hypertension. Exercise has been demonstrated to reduce blood pressure. In general, a healthy diet low in fats and salt and a consistent exercise regimen are beneficial in reducing blood pressure (Boone, 1991).

Behavioral and psychological treatments of hypertension include psychotherapy, relaxation, and biofeedback. Biofeedback and relaxation seem to be most effective when combined with pharmacological treatment. These behavioral interventions may permit reduction of medication dose and may decrease end-organ damage (Lynch, 1985, Niaura and Goldstein, 1992).

▶ Check Your Reading

17. What does the theory of hyperreactivity say about hypertension?
18. What is the relationship of anger to hypertension?
19. What is the effect of speech on blood pressure?
20. Name two of the behavioral and psychological approaches to the treatment of hypertension.

MIGRAINE

Approximately 16 to 18 million people suffer from *migraine headaches* throughout their life journeys. Diagnosis of a migraine rests on the presence of characteristic symptoms in the patient's history. Migraine headaches usually begin in adolescence, although they may begin in childhood. They rarely begin after age 40. Four times as many women are treated for migraines than men. The headache presents with a pulsating quality that is usually, but not always, unilateral. The headache lasts from two hours to days. Migraines occur most frequently upon awakening but may occur at any time of day. Diamond and Dalessio (1986) reported that migraines are more common on weekends and vacations; however, this finding was refuted by Morrison (1990). On average, migraines occur one to three times a month and are recurrent.

Symptoms

The *prodrome* is the period of time preceding the migraine that occurs hours to days before the headache. The prodrome may include subtle symptoms (e.g., change in mood, irritability, fatigue) or specific symptoms (e.g., blurring of vision, increased sensitivity to sound, inability to tolerate bright lights). If the patient with migraines learns to recognize their specific prodrome pattern, his or her ability to abort the migraine increases. Patients suffering with migraines usually have low blood pressure and high heart rates. Their extremities generally are vasoconstricted, causing them to have cold hands and feet. During the migraine, they experience vasodilatation, and their hands, feet, and body become warm. Anorexia, nausea, vomiting, and diarrhea usually accompany the migraine, along with increased urinary frequency. Often these patients experience increased sensitivity to light, sound, movement, and smell. They complain of tenderness and sometimes swelling on the side of the skull where the headache is experienced. After the headache leaves, patients may feel either euphoric or depressed. Feelings of fatigue may last several days after the headache (Gallagher, 1990).

Classification

The classification of migraines recently has been revised. Now, migraines generally are divided into two types: migraine with aura and migraine without aura. The migraine with aura was the former classic migraine. An *aura* is a group of neurological symptoms that precedes the headache by 5 to 20 minutes. The most common symptoms of the aura are visual disturbances (Saper et al, 1993). Once the aura begins, the physiological pattern of the migraine is initiated.

Precipitants

Migraines can be precipitated by many factors, including the menstrual cycle, stress, physical activity, caffeine, certain foods, and alcohol. Some women have migraines only during menstruation. Migraines usually decrease or cease after menopause. During pregnancy, migraines usually stop (Gallagher, 1990).

Migraines occur after periods of stress when the person relaxes (Benedittis et al, 1990). This may account for the association of migraines with weekends and vacations. Variations in sleeping patterns, hot weather, and humidity also may precipitate a migraine. Chronic use of daily headache medicines may cause rebound headaches (Gallagher, 1990).

Mechanism

The precise mechanisms involved in the production of migraine headaches are unknown. Vascular, neural, and biochemical factors are involved in migraines. For instance, metabolic factors such as estrogen, tyramine, and tyrosine play a role in many migraine headaches. These factors, in combination with internal and external stress, initiate a cascade of physiological changes (vascular and neural) that produce the headache. The aura is produced by either a cortical vasospasm or a spreading depression of neural activity. Pain is inhibited during the aura. After the aura fades, a vasodilatation occurs. This eliminates the pain inhibition, and the migraine headache begins (Solomon and Lipton, 1990).

Vascular Factors

During a migraine headache, scalp vessels dilate. The aura of the migraine is caused by vasospasm followed by a reactive vasodilatation during the headache. The dilatation is associated with increased blood vessel permeability and the release of bradykinin and proteolytic enzymes. However, recent evidence shows that the decrease in cerebral blood flow is insufficient to cause neural ischemia and that the subsequent increase in blood flow does not always correlate with the onset of the headache. Increased platelet adhesiveness occurs during a migraine. Most researchers think that platelets play a secondary role in the headache. The increased platelet activity could contribute to the impaired circulation during the migraine. Free fatty acids mobilized by norepinephrine may activate the platelets to release serotonin. Bradykinin, histamine, and other polypeptides may act in concert with serotonin in increasing the vascular wall sensitivity to pain (Solomon and Lipton, 1990).

Neural Factors

Neural theories of migraines propose that the decreased cerebral blood flow in migraines is a consequence of decreased metabolic demands and spreading depression of the cortex. It is still unknown whether vascular or neural mechanisms are the primary causal factor in migraines (Solomon and Lipton, 1990).

Biochemical Factors

Biochemicals such as serotonin and norepinephrine are the mediators of neural transmission and vascular reactivity. Serotonin levels fall during a migraine. The action of serotonin varies with the size of the blood vessel. It causes constriction of large vessels in the external carotid tree and dilatation of small vessels. Serotonin also promotes platelet aggregation (Solomon and Lipton, 1990).

Norepinephrine levels rise during a migraine, causing vasoconstriction in the peripheral vascular bed. Patients with migraines have elevated sympathetic activity and higher norepinephrine levels when compared with people without headaches. The rise may be a response to the physiological stress of the migraine and may be a consequence rather than a precipitating factor.

Other Factors

Seventy-five percent of all patients with migraines have a first-degree relative with migraines. The personality of migraine patients has been described as hard working, hard driving, and perfectionistic. Symptoms of depression with insomnia, anorexia, constipation, lack of libido, and feelings of hopelessness are frequently reported (Diamond and Dalessio, 1986).

BOX 37-6 An Overview of Migraines

Characteristics

Onset between adolescence and age 40 years

Affects women more frequently than men

Pulsating pain

Pain lasts two hours to days

Pain occurs on awakening

Relative with history of migraine

Symptoms of depression and despair

Insomnia, anorexia, constipation

Symptoms

Premigraine

- Prodrome
- Low blood pressure and high heart rate
- Cold hands and feet

During migraine

- Extremities become warm
- Nausea, vomiting, diarrhea
- Sensitivity to light, sound, smell, and movement
- Tenderness on skull

Postmigraine

- Feeling of euphoria or depression
- Fatigue

Treatment

Medical: Multiple pharmacological agents

Psychological

- Relaxation with biofeedback
- Stress management

Spiritual

- Helping others
- Inspirational reading
- Journaling
- Meditation
- Prayer

Foods and beverages that cause vasodilatation are associated with migraine headaches. Alcoholic beverages, processed foods containing nitrates, and monosodium glutamate are common triggers. Hard cheeses, beer, and red wine are high in tyramine. Phenylethylamine in chocolate may provoke a headache. Caffeine in food and drinks also may cause vasoconstriction and precipitate a migraine (Saper et al, 1993).

Treatment

Many drugs are used for the prevention and treatment of migraine headaches. The reader is referred to Saper and colleagues (1993) for further information regarding drug treatment of migraines.

The most widely used nonpharmacological treatment is relaxation training combined with thermal biofeedback. A recent metaanalysis evaluating the use of propranolol and the effectiveness of biofeedback and relaxation training concluded that these two very different treatments have similar results. Both treatments were associated with a 45% decrease in headaches (Holroyd and Penzien, 1990).

A patient with migraines is encouraged to avoid foods and beverages that might trigger a headache (Saper et al, 1993) and to engage in daily exercise as a preventative strategy for migraines. Exercise causes vasodilation, which reduces the risk of developing a migraine.

▶ Check Your Reading

21. Name two precipitants of migraine headaches.
22. What happens to levels of serotonin during a migraine?
23. What happens to levels of norepinephrine during a migraine?
24. What is the most widely used nonpharmacological treatment for migraine headaches?
25. Name two foods that are associated with migraines.

TEMPOROMANDIBULAR DISORDER

Temporomandibular disorder (TMD) has been defined as chronic or intermittent pain in the face, neck, and/or ears that is the result of a problem in the mandible joint caused by a variety of muscular, nerve, and dental problems. Symptoms can occur alone or with other problems (Aghabeigi et al, 1992). A great deal of research has documented that TMD is stress related (Lefer, 1966; Fine, 1971; Feinmann and Harris, 1984).

Several theories have attempted to explain the cause of TMD. Early theories suggested a displacement of the condyle within the temporomandibular joint. This later was demonstrated to be anatomically impossible. Later, it was proposed that most of the pain associated with TMD did not come from the joint but from the muscles of mastication. Stress leads to clenching the jaw and "grinding" or bruxing teeth and has been found to be the origin of the pain associated with TMD (Diamond and Dalessio, 1986). Recently, orthodontic treatment has been implicated as a cause of some cases of TMD (Just et al, 1992). Another cause of TMD is removal of upper and lower molars, which can result in misalignment of the jaw, placing a strain or pressure on the mandibular joint. The patient will complain of clicks or pain. However, a significant number of patients with mandibular joint pain have normal temporomandibular joints. In addition, patients with molars removed and misalignment of the jaw do not always report joint pain (Peatfield, 1990).

It is estimated that between 50% and 60% of the general population have experienced one or more of the symptoms of TMD. Women report TMD more frequently than do men, and the symptoms seem to increase with age. TMD frequently is first reported in people in their 30s and 40s (Buxbaum and Myslinski, 1993; White, 1993).

BOX 37-7 An Overview of Temporomandibular Disorder

Characteristics

Affects women more frequently than men

Onset between 30 and 40 years of age

History of depression or stress

Signs and Symptoms

Clenching jaw

Grinding teeth

Misalignment of jaw

Normal joint

Treatment

Physical
- Dental appliances
- Antiinflammatory drugs
- Muscle relaxants
- Physical therapy
- Soft diet

Psychological
- Behavior modification
- Relaxation therapy
- Biofeedback

Spiritual
- Helping others
- Inspirational reading
- Journaling
- Music
- Meditation
- Prayer

As was mentioned, a great deal of research has documented that TMD is stress related (Lefer, 1966; Fine, 1971; Feinmann and Harris, 1984). In a study conducted by Aghabeigi and colleagues (1992) of 34 patients experiencing chronic TMD, it was found that 50% of the subjects suffered from major depression and 15% suffered from Posttraumatic Stress Disorder.

In assessing the patient for TMD pain and dysfunction, the health care professional cannot assume that it is the result of only mechanical or neuromuscular problems. Sufficient research data suggest that stress also is a factor.

The conservative approach to treating TMD has been found to be the most effective in the majority of cases. The objective of treatment is to rest the joint and relax the muscles. This can be accomplished through the use of local heat; soft diet; use of nonsteroidal antiinflammatory and muscle-relaxing drugs; joint exercises; and behavioral, relaxation, and biofeedback therapy. Patients with TMD often benefit from dental appliances (occlusal therapy), which have as their goal the realignment of the joint and the restoration of the normal range of movement of the jaw. Surgical procedures should be avoided except in extreme circumstances (Saper et al, 1993; White, 1993). For those patients not responding to standard treatment, appropriate cognitive-behavioral counseling, biofeedback, and the use of spiritual resources is critical to their improvement.

▶ **Check Your Reading**

26. What is TMJ?
27. What is the relationship between stress and TMJ?
28. Name two of the treatment approaches used with TMJ.

SOMATOFORM DISORDERS

Somatoform disorders are defined as a group of disorders in which the person presents with physical symptoms suggesting a physiological etiology. However, after an in-depth assessment and diagnostic testing, no organic disease or physiological abnormalities are found. Because no positive evidence of physical problems is able to be identified, the presumption is made that the physical problems of substance abuse, or of other mental disorders (e.g., anxiety attacks), are psychological in origin. A variety of physical symptoms are not under the control of the patient. This group of disorders is so widespread that it may involve 30% to 40% of the medical patients seen in general and family practice settings (Fava, 1992). Somatoform disorders are classified as psychiatric disorders.

Under the heading of Somatoform Disorders, the *Diagnostic and Statistical Manual-IV* (*DSM-IV;* American Psychiatric Association, 1994) lists several distinct and yet

BOX 37-8 An Overview of the Somatoform Disorders

- Physical symptoms with no disease or abnormalities
- Physical symptoms worsen during crisis
- "Doctor-shopping"
- Unwarranted surgical procedures
- Substance abuse
- Avoidance of social or work activities
- Obsessive-compulsive or depressive personality
- Refusing referral for mental health care
- Symptoms not intentional (not under conscious control)

possibly related disorders. They differ from the category Psychological Factors Affecting Medical Conditions because no medical conditions exist in a somatoform disorder. The new *DSM-IV* category Psychological Factors Affecting Medical Conditions may be useful with patients experiencing psychophysiological disorders. The essential feature of this condition is the presence of one or more specific psychological or behavioral features that negatively affect a general medical condition. It could be used in a patient with low back pain who insists upon doing activities that aggravate the pain.The seven disorders listed are Body Dysmorphic Disorder, Conversion Disorder, Hypochondriasis, Somatization Disorder, Pain Disorder, Undifferentiated Somatoform Disorder, and Somatoform Disorder Not Otherwise Specified. The person diagnosed with one of these disorders often has physical symptoms that worsen during life crisis, but she or he is unaware of the relationship between the symptoms and stressful events. Evidence of "doctor-shopping" and of strained doctor-patient relationships often is seen. Persons with somatoform disorders may submit to unnecessary or unwarranted surgical procedures. In addition, because the health care providers are looking for the organic cause of specific symptoms, true pathology may be overlooked. The possibility exists among this group of patients of psychoactive substance abuse because of overuse of prescribed medications.

Many of these patients report a history of avoiding social or occupational activities. Often an obsessive-compulsive personality trait or depression is seen in these patients. These patients experience spiritual distress. They are likely to resist referral for mental health care. The intensity of the symptoms often decreases with support from a concerned health care provider.

Body Dysmorphic Disorder (Dysmorphophobia)

Body dysmorphic disorder is the preoccupation with an imagined flaw in appearance in a normal-appearing person. These patients most frequently focus on a facial

MEDICAL DIAGNOSES AND RELATED NURSING DIAGNOSES **Body Dysmorphic Disorder**

***DSM-IV* Diagnoses:** Body Dysmorphic Disorder

Diagnostic Criteria

A. Preoccupation with an imagined defect in appearance. If a slight physical anomaly is present, the person's concern is markedly excessive.

B. The preoccupation causes clinically significant distress or impairment in social, occupational, or other important areas of functioning.

C. The preoccupation is not better accounted for by another mental disorder (e.g., dissatisfaction with body shape and size in Anorexia Nervosa).

RELATED NURSING DIAGNOSES	DEFINITION	EXAMPLE
Body Image Disturbance	The person experiences or is at risk to experience an alteration in how one perceives one's body. The person expresses (verbally or nonverbally) a negative response to a perceived change in structure or function of the body.	A person has obsessive concern over a small freckle.
Self-Esteem, Chronic Low	A person experiences long-standing negative self-evaluations about his or her appearance or capabilities. The person expresses shame or guilt, feels unable to deal with new events or situations, rejects positive feedback, and exaggerates negative feedback about self.	A man who refuses to accept a compliment related to his appearance.

Diagnostic criteria from American Psychiatric Association: *Diagnostic and statistical manual of mental disorders, fourth edition.* Washington, D. C., American Psychiatric Association, 1994; nursing diagnoses and definitions from North American Nursing Diagnosis Association (1994). *NANDA nursing diagnoses: Definitions and classification 1995–1996.* Philadelphia: NANDA.

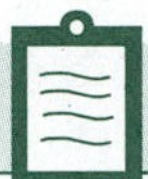

MEDICAL DIAGNOSES AND RELATED NURSING DIAGNOSES **Conversion Disorder**

***DSM-IV* Diagnosis:** Conversion Disorder

Diagnostic Criteria

A. One or more symptoms or deficits affecting voluntary motor or sensory function suggest a neurological or other general medical condition.
B. Psychological factors are judged to be associated with the symptom or deficit because the initiation or exacerbation of the symptom or deficit is preceded by conflicts or other stressors.
C. The symptom or deficit is not intentionally produced or feigned (as in Factitious Disorder or Malingering).
D. The symptom or deficit cannot, after appropriate investigation, be fully explained by a general medical condition, by the direct effects of a substance, or as a culturally sanctioned behavior or experience.
E. The symptom or deficit causes clinically significant distress or impairment in social, occupational, or other important areas of functioning or warrants medical evaluation.
F. The symptom or deficit is not limited to pain or sexual dysfunction, does not occur exclusively during the course of Somatization Disorder, and is not better accounted for by another mental disorder.

Specify type of symptom or deficit:
With Motor Symptom or Deficit
With Sensory Symptom or Deficit
With Seizures or Convulsions
With Mixed Presentation

RELATED NURSING DIAGNOSES	DEFINITION	EXAMPLE
Physical Mobility, Impaired	The person experiences limitations of physical movement but is not immobile. The person has decreased ability to move purposefully, decreased muscle strength or control.	A person who is depressed or who has experienced a traumatic event.
Individual Coping, Ineffective	The person is not able to manage internal or environmental stressors adequately because of inadequate resources (psychological, behavioral, or cognitive). The person is able to state that he or she cannot cope with the situation, uses defense mechanisms inappropriately, and is not able to meet expectations of his or her life roles.	When a person has difficulty adapting to stressful events, the usual coping mechanisms which have been successful in past similar situations may be ineffective.

Diagnostic criteria from American Psychiatric Association: *Diagnostic and statistical manual of mental disorders, fourth edition.* Washington, D. C., American Psychiatric Association, 1994; nursing diagnoses and definitions from North American Nursing Diagnosis Association (1994). *NANDA nursing diagnoses: Definitions and classification 1995–1996.* Philadelphia: NANDA.

defect and less commonly are concerned about physical deformity in other parts of their bodies. The patients may focus on this defect for hours a day, and these thoughts may dominate their lives with resulting impairment in social work roles. The social isolation and depression related to their physical appearance may lead to repeated hospitalizations, suicide attempts, and completed suicides. The key to the identification of a body dysmorphic disorder is the patient's *excessive* concern over the perceived physical defect. Individuals with this problem present as early as the teen years through the 20s. These patients often seek plastic surgery, which will not correct the distorted ideation. No familial pattern or predisposing factors have been identified. It is reported equally in males and females. Body dysmorphic disorder is a chronic condition that usually persists for several years. The diagnostic criteria for body dysmorphic disorder are given in "Medical Diagnoses and Related Nursing Diagnoses: Body Dysmorphic Disorder."

Conversion Disorder

Conversion disorder is the presentation of an alteration or loss of a sensory-motor function that is not the result of a physiological disorder. Conversion disorders develop in response to a catastrophic event such as threat of loss or harm, which results in the development of physical symptoms. The resulting symptoms lead to serious deficits in functioning. Although conversion disorders are rarely reported today, this was a common diagnosis 20 years ago. The most common conversion symptoms include paralysis, seizure, disturbance in coordination, or blindness. However, these patients may present with the complete array of neurological symptoms.

The symptoms experienced by the patient are serious but not intentionally produced. The key to the identification of a conversion disorder is that the person appears calm although the symptoms are serious. This calmness and relative lack of concern is referred to as **la belle**

indifference. The patient may also present his or her symptoms in a dramatic manner.

Adolescence and early adulthood is the most common age of onset, although a conversion disorder may appear at any age. Conversion disorder is more common in women than in men, and some data suggest a familial pattern. Commonly, a predisposing physical illness with similar symptoms has occurred either in the patient or in someone who is close to that person (APA, 1994). It has been reported more frequently in rural populations and in people with lower socioeconomic and educational status.

People who experience a conversion disorder derive **primary gain,** i.e., the stress they experienced from the trauma is no longer felt; **secondary gain** also is derived—because of the conversion symptoms, the person no longer has to participate in distasteful or stressful activities, e.g., a soldier who develops paralysis of his arm can no longer hold a gun and is therefore removed from combat. The diagnostic criteria for conversion disorder are given in "Medical Diagnoses and Related Nursing Diagnoses: Conversion Disorder."

Hypochondriasis

Hypochondriasis has four major criteria:

- The patient is preoccupied with bodily functions (frequently focusing on heartbeat, breathing, or digestion, or on a minor physical ailment such as a small scratch or cough).
- The patient interprets the symptoms as indicative of a serious illness.
- A comprehensive physical examination will not find evidence of a physical disorder.
- The fear of having a serious illness continues despite medical reassurance that this is not the case.

The beliefs are not delusional, in that the patient can acknowledge the possibility that he or she is exaggerating the extent of the disease or that disease may not be present (APA, 1994). This concern, however, causes clinically significant problems and negatively affects social and work roles.

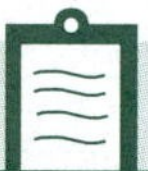

MEDICAL DIAGNOSES AND RELATED NURSING DIAGNOSES — Hypochondriasis

DSM-IV **Diagnosis:** Hypochondriasis

Diagnostic Criteria

A. Preoccupation with fears of having, or the idea that one has, a serious disease based on the person's misinterpretation of bodily symptoms.
B. The preoccupation persists despite appropriate medical evaluation and reassurance.
C. The belief in Criterion A is not of delusional intensity (as in Delusional Disorder, Somatic Type) and is not restricted to a circumscribed concern about appearance (as in Body Dysmorphic Disorder).
D. The preoccupation causes clinically significant distress or impairment in social, occupational, or other important areas of functioning.
E. The duration of the disturbance is at least six months.
F. The preoccupation is not better accounted for by Generalized Anxiety Disorder, Obsessive-Compulsive Disorder, Panic Disorder, a Major Depressive Episode, Separation Anxiety, or another Somatoform Disorder.

Specify if:

With Poor Insight: If, for most of the time during the current episode, the person does not recognize that the concern about having a serious illness is excessive or unreasonable.

RELATED NURSING DIAGNOSES	DEFINITION	EXAMPLE
Fear	A feeling of physiological or emotional disruption related to an identifiable source which is perceived as dangerous. The person has feelings of apprehension, behaviors of avoidance, and deficits in attention, performance, or control.	The person may feel that he or she is critically ill and will die.
Role Performance, Altered.	The person experiences a disruption in how he or she perceives his or her life roles. There is a conflict within the person related to his or her ability to carry out one or more of life's roles (social, work, family).	The person is so preoccupied with his perception of having a serious disease that he is not able to perform his role as parent, breadwinner, church member.

Diagnostic criteria from American Psychiatric Association: *Diagnostic and statistical manual of mental disorders, fourth edition.* Washington, D. C., American Psychiatric Association, 1994; nursing diagnoses and definitions from North American Nursing Diagnosis Association (1994). *NANDA nursing diagnoses: Definitions and classification 1995–1996.* Philadelphia: NANDA.

MEDICAL DIAGNOSES AND RELATED NURSING DIAGNOSES — Somatization Disorder

***DSM-IV* Diagnosis:** Somatization Disorder

Diagnostic Criteria

A. A history of many physical complaints beginning before age 30 years that occurred over a period of several years and resulted in treatment being sought or significant impairment in social, occupational, or other important areas of functioning.

B. Each of the following criteria must have been met, with individual symptoms occurring at any time during the course of the disturbance:

(1) *Four pain symptoms:* A history of pain related to at least four different sites or functions (e.g., head, abdomen, back, joints, extremities, chest, rectum, during menstruation, during sexual intercourse, or during urination).

(2) *Two gastrointestinal symptoms:* A history of at least two gastrointestinal symptoms other than pain (e.g., nausea, bloating, vomiting other than during pregnancy, diarrhea, or intolerance of several different foods).

(3) *One sexual symptom:* A history of at least one sexual or reproductive symptom other than pain (e.g., sexual indifference, erectile or ejaculatory dysfunction, irregular menses, excessive menstrual bleeding, vomiting throughout pregnancy).

(4) *One pseudoneurological symptom:* A history of at least one symptom or deficit suggesting a neurological condition not limited to pain (conversion symptoms such as impaired coordination or balance, paralysis or localized weakness, difficulty swallowing or lump in throat, aphonia, urinary retention, hallucinations, loss of touch or pain sensation, double vision, blindness, deafness, seizures; dissociative symptoms such as amnesia; or loss of consciousness other than fainting).

C. Either (1) or (2):

(1) After appropriate investigation, each of the symptoms in Criterion B cannot be fully explained by a known general medical condition or the direct effects of a substance (e.g., a drug of abuse, a medication).

(2) When a related general medical condition is present, the physical complaints or resulting social or occupational impairment are in excess of what would be expected from the history, physical examination, or laboratory findings.

D. The symptoms are not intentionally produced or feigned (as in Factitious Disorder or Malingering).

RELATED NURSING DIAGNOSES	DEFINITION	EXAMPLE
Pain, Chronic	A person experiences pain which is intermittent or persistent and lasts for more than six months. The person may be angered, frustrated, or depressed because of the situation.	A person demonstrates depressive behaviors because she is not able to be free of pain.
Management of Therapeutic Regimen, Ineffective	The person experiences difficulty integrating a program of treatment into his or her daily life because he or she does not receive relief. He or she may state that he or she would like to incorporate the regimen but has difficulty doing so. He or she may choose inappropriate methods for meeting the treatment regimen.	Because of frustration due to no relief from multiple symptoms, "doctor-shopping" occurs and different regimens are used.

Diagnostic criteria from American Psychiatric Association: *Diagnostic and statistical manual of mental disorders, fourth edition.* Washington, D. C., American Psychiatric Association, 1994; nursing diagnoses and definitions from North American Nursing Diagnosis Association (1994). *NANDA nursing diagnoses: Definitions and classification 1995–1996.* Philadelphia: NANDA.

Hypochondria most commonly occurs between age 20 and 30, although it may appear at any age. It is equally common in males and females, and no familial pattern exists. Predisposing factors include stress and past experience with the presenting symptoms. Usually hypochondria is chronic, with remission and exacerbation of the symptoms. The problem must be present for at least six months and is not better accounted for by other mental or somatoform disorders. It is most important in the diagnosis that the early stages of a medical condition not be overlooked. Doctor-shopping is common because patients cannot get the answer they want. These patients resist referral to mental health practitioners (APA, 1994). The diagnostic criteria for hypochondriasis are given in "Medical Diagnoses and Related Nursing Diagnoses: Hypochondriasis."

Somatization Disorder

Somatization disorder is the presentation of many physical complaints that occur with no identified organic basis for the complaints. The identification of somatization must include four pain symptoms in differing sites or functions. The distinction between somatization and conversion disorders is based mainly on the number of signs and symptoms; somatization disorder includes multiple physical symptoms in several body systems. The most frequent complaints are pseudoneurological, gastrointestinal, female reproductive, psychosexual, pain, and cardiopulmonary. Many of these patients are anxious or depressed (APA, 1994).

Symptoms of somatization disorders begin during the teen years and occasionally in the 20s. Menstrual difficulties are often one of the earliest complaints in females. Younger patients may present a variety of initial complaints such as abdominal pain, depression, headaches, or seizures. This diagnosis is rare in males. A familial tendency can be seen with somatization disorders. Somatization disorder is a chronic problem; the patient's symptoms vary in seriousness, but it is rare for a year to pass without the patient seeking medical attention (APA, 1994). The diagnostic criteria for somatization disorder are given in "Medical Diagnoses and Related Nursing Diagnoses: Somatization Disorder."

Pain Disorder

The patient with *pain disorder* is preoccupied with pain when no physical findings account for the pain or for its intensity. Psychological factors play a definite role in the

MEDICAL DIAGNOSES AND RELATED NURSING DIAGNOSES **Pain Disorder**

***DSM-IV* Diagnosis:** Pain Disorder

Diagnostic Criteria

A. Pain in one or more anatomical sites is the predominant focus of the clinical presentation and is of sufficient severity to warrant clinical attention.
B. The pain causes clinically significant distress or impairment in social, occupational, or other important areas of functioning.
C. Psychological factors are judged to have an important role in the onset, severity, exacerbation, or maintenance of the pain.
D. The symptom or deficit is not intentionally produced or feigned (as in Factitious Disorder or Malingering).
E. The pain is not better accounted for by a Mood, Anxiety, or Psychotic Disorder and does not meet criteria for Dyspareunia.

Code as follows:

307.80 Pain Disorder Associated With Psychological Factors: Psychological factors are judged to have the major role in the onset, severity, exacerbation, or maintenance of the pain. (If a general medical condition is present, it does not have a major role in the onset, severity, exacerbation, or maintenance of the pain.) This type of Pain Disorder is not diagnosed if criteria are also met for Somatization Disorder.

Specify if:

Acute: Duration of less than 6 months.

Chronic: Duration of 6 months or longer.

307.89 Pain Disorder Associated With Both Psychological Factors and a General Medical Condition: Both psychological factors and a general medical condition are judged to have important roles in the onset, severity, exacerbation, or maintenance of the pain. The associated general medical condition or anatomical site of the pain (see below) is coded on Axis III.

Specify if:

Acute: Duration of less than 6 months.

Chronic: Duration of 6 months or longer.

Note: The following is not considered to be a mental disorder and is included here to facilitate differential diagnosis.

Pain Disorder Associated With a General Medical Condition: A general medical condition has a major role in the onset, severity, exacerbation, or maintenance of the pain. (If psychological factors are present, they are not judged to have a major role in the onset, severity, exacerbation, or maintenance of the pain.) The diagnostic code for the pain is selected based on the associated general medical condition if one has been established or on the anatomical location of the pain if the underlying general medical condition is not yet clearly established—for example, low back (724.2), sciatic (724.3), pelvic (625.9), headache (784.0), facial (784.0), chest (786.50), joint (719.4), bone (733.90), abdominal (789.0), breast (611.71), renal (788.0), ear (388.70), eye (379.91), throat (784.1), tooth (525.9), and urinary (788.0).

RELATED NURSING DIAGNOSES	DEFINITION	EXAMPLE
Chronic Pain	See Somatization	The person has significant pain that lasts longer than six months (chronic back pain).
Role Performance, Altered	See Hypochondriasis	Because of the pain, the person must take several breaks during the work day to change position and exercise.

Diagnostic criteria from American Psychiatric Association: *Diagnostic and statistical manual of mental disorders, fourth edition.* Washington, D. C., American Psychiatric Association, 1994; nursing diagnoses and definitions from North American Nursing Diagnosis Association (1994). *NANDA nursing diagnoses: Definitions and classification 1995–1996.* Philadelphia: NANDA.

MEDICAL DIAGNOSES AND RELATED NURSING DIAGNOSES **Undifferentiated Somatoform Disorder**

***DSM-IV* Diagnosis:** Undifferentiated Somatoform Disorder

Diagnostic Criteria

A. One or more physical complaints (e.g., fatigue, loss of appetite, gastrointestinal or urinary complaints).

B. Either (1) or (2):
   (1) After appropriate investigation, the symptoms cannot be fully explained by a known general medical condition or the direct effects of a substance (e.g., a drug of abuse, a medication).
   (2) When a related general medical condition is present, the physical complaints or resulting social and occupational impairments are in excess of what would be expected from the history, physical examination, or laboratory findings.

C. The symptoms cause clinically significant distress or impairment in social, occupational, or other important areas of functioning.

D. The duration of the disturbance is at least six months.

E. The disturbance is not better accounted for by another mental disorder (e.g., another Somatoform Disorder, Sexual Dysfunction, Mood Disorder, Anxiety Disorder, Sleep Disorder, or Psychotic Disorder).

F. The symptom is not intentionally produced or feigned (as in Factitious Disorder or Malingering).

RELATED NURSING DIAGNOSES	DEFINITION	EXAMPLE
Role Performance, Altered	See Hypochondriasis	Because of excessive fatigue, a mother is unable to care for her children.
Ineffective Individual Coping	See Conversion Disorder	Mechanisms used in past situations do not help the person adjust in this situation.

Diagnostic criteria from American Psychiatric Association: *Diagnostic and statistical manual of mental disorders, fourth edition.* Washington, D. C., American Psychiatric Association, 1994; nursing diagnoses and definitions from North American Nursing Diagnosis Association (1994). *NANDA nursing diagnoses: Definitions and classification 1995–1996.* Philadelphia: NANDA.

beginning or worsening of pain. This pain is not voluntarily produced, and the diagnosis is not appropriate if the pain is better accounted for by another mental disorder. Pain disorder usually begins during the 30s and 40s, although it can occur at any age. This diagnosis occurs more frequently in females, particularly with headache and musculoskeletal pain, and some evidence of a familial pattern has been found (APA, 1994).

The patient reports a history of excessive analgesic use with no pain relief and frequently requests surgery. It is not unusual for a patient to have adopted the lifestyle of an invalid. Patients who are also depressed or who have pain related to terminal illness are at increased risk for suicide attempts. The patient with pain disorder resists the possibility that psychological factors may be involved in the complaints of pain and may spend considerable time and energy searching for care. In many patients, the diagnosis of major depression is also appropriate (APA, 1994). The diagnostic criteria for pain disorder are given in "Medical Diagnoses and Related Nursing Diagnoses: Pain Disorder."

Somatoform Disorder Not Otherwise Specified

Somatoform disorder not otherwise specified includes disorders with somatoform symptoms that do not meet the criteria for any specific somatoform disorder. Some of these disorders are: pseudocyesis, which is a false belief accompanied by physical signs of pregnancy; a disorder with nonpsychotic hypochondriacal symptoms of less than 6 months duration; and a disorder involving unexplained physical complaints such as fatigue or body weakness of less than 6 months' duration that are not due to another mental disorder (APA, 1994).

Undifferentiated Somatoform Disorder

Undifferentiated somatoform disorder is when the patient's symptoms and physical findings do not meet the description of somatoform disorder. The patient has fewer physical complaints or symptoms, and the symptoms are not voluntarily produced. The symptoms are unlike the multiple exaggerated complaints seen in somatoform disorders. As in many of the somatoform disorders, the symptoms cannot be explained by physical abnormalities after medical examination and are thought to be psychological in origin. In addition, the patient's complaints occur without the diagnosis af another somatoform or psychotic disorder. No data suggest that this diagnosis is more common in one gender or has common predisposing factors or familial tendencies. Many patients with this disorder are anxious and depressed, but they have fewer physical and social limitations than those with somatoform disorder. The course of the disease is variable (APA, 1994). The diagnostic criteria for undifferentiated somatoform disorder are given in "Medical Diagnoses and Related Nursing Diagnoses: Undifferentiated Somatoform Disorder."

Treatment

Treatment of somatoform disorders traditionally has been limited to insight-oriented psychotherapy; the success of this approach has been limited. Therefore, a holistic framework is more appropriate in conditions where it is difficult to ascertain a physiological basis. Although patients usually resist suggestions that they may have psychological reasons for these disorders, they respond to a caring environment where they are respected and not dismissed as "crazy" or "neurotic." When the clinician seriously considers the patient's expressions of pain, other symptoms, and in fact the patient's whole story, the clinician is providing holistic care. In such cases, the patient and the health care provider are more likely to engage and begin effective work toward recovery (Corbin et al, 1988; Cohen, 1986; Goldberg et al, 1992). Table 37–1 summarizes important characteristics of somatoform disorders.

TABLE 37–1 **Important Characteristics of the Somatoform Disorders**

Disorder	Description	Age	Gender	Predisposing Factors
Body dysmorphic disorder	*Excessive* attention to imagined flaws in appearance, usually on an exposed body part	Teens to 30s	No gender differences	None
Conversion disorder	The person is *calm* while experiencing symptoms such as paralysis, seizures, or blindness	Teens to early adulthood	More frequent in females	Catastrophic event (war or disaster); the person may have been exposed to a disease with similar symptoms
Hypocondriasis	Preoccupation with body function (heart rate, breathing); the person is convinced that he or she has a serious illness but can acknowledge that he or she may be exaggerating	20 to 30	No gender differences	Stress and past experience with symptoms
Somatization disorder	Expression of several symptoms in several body systems	Teens to 20	More common in females than in males	Menstrual difficulties, abdominal pain, depression, headache
Pain disorder	Preoccupation with pain, with no real physical cause identified	Any age	More common in females than in males	History of use of analgesics, The patient typically denies the possibility of psychological involvement Major depression may be present
Undifferentiated somatoform disorder	Fewer physical symptoms than above; no physical cause can be found	None identified	No gender differences	None identified
Somatoform disorder not otherwise specified	Somatoform symptoms that do not meet the criteria for any specific somatoform disorder	None identified	No gender differences	None identified

▶ Check Your Reading

29. What does *la belle indifference* mean? In what somatoform disorder is this symptom commonly seen?
30. What is a conversion disorder?
31. What are the characteristics of somatoform disorder?
32. What is body dysmorphic disorder?

NURSING PROCESS

The focus of care for patients with psychophysiological disorders is holistic, taking into account physical, psychosocial, and spiritual sources for the behavior which is being demonstrated.

ASSESSMENT

Assess the whole person—mind, body, and spirit—rather than just the signs and symptoms of the disease. Keep in mind that multiple causes for the presenting signs and symptoms may exist. Understanding this will help you to perform a comprehensive assessment in which you collect physical, psychosocial, and spiritual data about the patient and family that may have an impact on the patient's care.

DIAGNOSIS

Specific nursing diagnoses are based on the assessment of the patient and her or his presenting behaviors. Although two patients may have the same psychophysiological illness and display similar signs and symptoms, the nursing diagnoses for these two patients may be quite different because of the uniqueness of each patient (Carpenito, 1993).

When developing nursing diagnoses for patients with psychophysiological disorders, it also is important that the diagnoses describe not only the patient's physiological problems but also his or her psychosocial and spiritual problems. Nursing diagnoses for patients with psychophysiological problems therefore truly run the gamut from A (activity intolerance) through S (social isolation). For example, for the patient with irritable bowel syndrome, appropriate diagnostic labels addressing physical problems might include Pain and Diarrhea. Likewise, appropriate diagnostic labels addressing psychosocial and spiritual problems might include Anxiety, Knowledge Deficit, Self-Esteem Disturbance, and Altered Role Performance.

Spirituality is a significant aspect of any chronic illness, because of its wearing and relentless nature. (Carpenito, 1993). The spiritual components of the patient's life should be thoroughly reviewed.

Let us look now at how a specific diagnostic label, Ineffective Individual Coping (a label that could well apply in any psychophysiological disorder), might apply to a patient with chronic back pain:

> Ineffective Individual Coping related to frequent and intense pain, as evidenced by weight loss, fatigue, and poor judgment related to decisions or activities.

OUTCOME IDENTIFICATION

The expected outcomes for a particular patient depend on the specific psychophysiological illness and nursing diagnoses. For the patient with chronic back pain whose diagnosis we just examined, an appropriate expected outcome might be as follows:

> The patient will experience significant relief and improved management of pain from her back pain.

PLANNING

The short-term goals for a particular patient depend on her or his medical diagnosis, her or his nursing diagnoses, and the expected outcomes flowing from those diagnoses. For our patient with back pain, short-term goals might be as follows:

Expected Outcome	Short-Term Goals
The patient will experience significant relief and improved management of pain from back pain.	The patient will verbalize feelings of stress, fear, or anger.
	The patient will express her feelings in a nondestructive manner.
	The patient will verbalize the connection between stress and pain.
	The patient will participate in the treatment program designed to decrease or control the chronic back pain.
	The patient will use problem-solving to identify positive alternative coping strategies.
	The patient will demonstrate alternative coping strategies for dealing with pain, stress, and emotional problems.
	The patient will verbalize an understanding of the relationships among stress, lifestyle issues, exercise, and the occurrence of back pain.
	The patient will verbalize an understanding of the relationship between spirituality and physical health.
	The patient will develop plans for follow-up therapy to maintain and continue her progress.

IMPLEMENTATION

Direct your nursing interventions first toward the patient and second toward the patient's family. For our patient with chronic back pain and a nursing diagnosis of Ineffective Individual Coping related to frequent and intense pain, the interventions used to meet the short-term goals with the patient would include:

- Focusing care on both physical problems and psychosocial and spiritual problems.
- Discussing with the patient the relationships among physical, psychosocial, and spiritual issues.
- Asking the patient about her perceptions of the back pain. How does she understand this back pain? What does she think causes her pain? What does she think will help the pain?
- Asking the patient to identify goals for the care she is receiving. Enlist the full engagement of the patient in the healing process by using open-ended questions, encouragement, and active listening.
- Helping the patient to complete a stress inventory of her lifestyle, support systems, dependency needs, expression of emotions, and spiritual supports. Encourage the patient to identify areas where change is needed.
- Discussing with the patient the results of the stress inventory. The patient may be unaccustomed to making links between lifestyle issues, sources of stress and satisfaction, spiritual resources, and the development of physical symptoms.
- Providing positive feedback when the patient begins to express her feelings about emotional issues.
- Role-playing to build the patient's confidence in her abilities to express her feelings verbally, especially with her parents.
- Teaching the patient stress management strategies, such as meditation, thought-stopping techniques, deep breathing and relaxation, and rehearsal of stressful interpersonal situations. These strategies are all effective at managing and defusing stress; the more effective the patient is at managing stress, the less she will express the stress somatically.
- Gradually making the link between emotions and physical expressions. Positively reinforce the patient's growing awareness of this link.
- Teaching the patient the use of the problem-solving approach. The patient may never have learned a logical, step-by-step approach to dealing with problems.
- Teaching the patient about the importance of lifestyle changes in managing stress. Good nutrition, eliminating caffeine and alcohol from the diet, regular exercise, and adequate rest are essential parts of this teaching.
- Teaching the patient about the significance of spirituality in healing; the importance of finding balance in meeting physical, emotional, and spiritual needs; and the importance of finding time for God (however the individual defines God) and spiritual practices.
- Teaching the patient about the importance of follow-up treatment to serve as a check on progress made and to help her modify strategies that need fine tuning.

For this same patient, the family interventions used to meet the short-term goals would include:

- Teaching the family the concept of psychophysiological illness and the relationship between stress and physical signs and symptoms.
- Involving the family in teaching stress management techniques. Family members can be a powerful support if they are knowledgeable about what is helpful to the patient.
- Involving the family in teaching about lifestyle issues. Again, the support of a family in changing diet, exercise, and rest patterns can make the difference between success and failure.
- Talking with the family or significant other to determine whether they are communicating that *only physical symptoms are acceptable*, and that verbal expression of feelings is unacceptable. If this is the message being received by the patient, the patient's continued improvement is in question.

EVALUATION

Evaluation involves returning to the expected outcomes and short-term goals. Looking at the short-term goals is the formative aspect of the evaluation and tells the nurse whether the plan is "on the right track." If the short-term goals are not being met, review the interventions and the assessment data to determine whether the assessment was complete and whether the interventions were appropriate and adequate. For instance, the nurse caring for our patient with chronic back pain might evaluate that the patient experienced difficulty in verbalizing the relationship between stress and physical symptoms. During the teaching intervention, the nurse observed that the patient was a very concrete learner. This was not part of the initial data assessment. The nurse then modified the intervention to use a different teaching technique. Apply this process to every short-term goal and make appropriate modifications.

The summative evaluation focuses on the expected outcomes. In the example that we have been using, the nurse caring for the patient with back pain would ask, "Is the patient experiencing significant relief and improved management of the pain from chronic back pain?" If the answer is yes, then the nurse can conclude that the plan was effective; if the answer is no, then the nurse reviews the whole process, from assessment to interventions, to determine the appropriate modifications.

▶ **Check Your Reading**

33. What are the three areas to assess in patients with psychophysiological illnesses?

The case study approach for outcome identification planning and implementation in Monica's case might read as follows:

ASSESSMENT

Assessment data are as follow:

- Chronic back and neck pain described as increasingly intolerable since auto accident
- Guarded body movements
- Fatigue and feelings of despair in life situation
- Social withdrawal from usual activities and friends
- Pain increases with stress
- Spiritual distress results from her emotional and physical problems

DIAGNOSIS

***DSM-IV* Diagnosis:** Chronic Pain

Nursing Diagnosis: Chronic Pain related to back and neck injury for past two years as evidenced by statements of pain and guarded body movements

OUTCOME IDENTIFICATION, PLANNING, AND IMPLEMENTATION

EXPECTED OUTCOME 1: By _____ the patient will achieve a satisfactory measure of pain control and engage in activities of daily living without preoccupation of pain.

SHORT-TERM GOAL	NURSING INTERVENTIONS	RATIONALES
By _____ the patient will accept some pain and learn how to cope more effectively with it.	1. Acknowledge and validate patient's experience of pain.	1. All pain experiences are real. Pain always has a cause, either physical or psychological in origin.
	2. Encourage the patient to identify situations that influence the occurrence and severity of pain.	2. Pain assessment is paramount to understanding the nature of pain. Pain is individualized—personal meanings and situations that evoke emotional responses influence the expression of pain.
	3. Involve the patient in setting goals for establishing pain management.	3. Involving the patient increases her feelings of autonomy and control by her participating actively in her pain-control program.
	4. Provide for adequate rest.	4. Fatigue will increase patient's perception of pain.

EXPECTED OUTCOME 2: By _____ the patient will use noninvasive pain relief measures, including diversional and recreational activities.

SHORT-TERM GOAL	NURSING INTERVENTIONS	RATIONALES
By _____ the patient will use two noninvasive pain relief measures.	1. Teach the patient ways to manage pain such as biofeedback, relaxation, meditation, skin stimulation (heat or cold), massage, imagery, music, and recreational and diversional activities (crafts, painting).	1. This encourages the patient to take responsibility for treatment of pain and allows her the opportunity to select which noninvasive method works best.
	2. Give positive feedback on efforts to share feelings and to use pain relief measures.	2. Encouragement helps the patient receive support.

Nursing Diagnosis: Spiritual Distress related to chronic neck and back pain as evidenced by withdrawal from social functions, church activities, and friends, along with feelings of despair

OUTCOME IDENTIFICATION, PLANNING, AND IMPLEMENTATION

EXPECTED OUTCOME 1: By _____ the patient will participate in social and recreational functions that add positive quality to her life.

SHORT-TERM GOAL	NURSING INTERVENTIONS	RATIONALES
By _____ the patient will look forward to pleasurable, social activities as a time out from pain.	1. Explore with the patient the specific meaning the pain has in her life.	1. Support the patient's endeavors to find meaning and understanding in her pain suffering.
	2. Encourage the patient to experience life, endure some pain, and to learn ways to move beyond the pain experience.	2. Hopefully this will add quality to the patient's life situation, prevent despair, and help her cope more effectively.
	3. Provide reassurance to both patient and family as she works through issues and finds meaning in her pain.	3. Supportive therapy is important during this time and assists both the patient and her family to cope.
	4. Provide activities the patient can do with others and enlarge her support system.	4. This will provide her the opportunity to be with others and experience pleasure and prevent a sense of aloneness.
	5. Encourage participation in social church functions.	5. Choosing activities that build on the patient's interests and personal strengths fosters greater participation.

EVALUATION

Formative Evaluation: Monica achieved all of the short-term goals. She began to understand that her unresolved issues with her family contributed to her back pain experience. She found that church groups and meditation were helpful therapies to deal with her pain.

Summative Evaluation: Monica achieved all of the expected outcomes through outpatient counseling. She became active in her church and her husband reported they were beginning to make contact with their old set of friends. She still experienced back pain but was able to use relaxation, meditation, and imagery to respond and deal with the pain at work and at home, which strengthened her self-esteem and promoted a more satisfying life. Support from her husband helped her recovery.

CONCLUSIONS

Psychophysiological disorders are the underlying cause of the majority of visits to internists and family practice physicians. Because psychological and spiritual components affect the patient's physical symptoms, it is important that this group of patients be treated in a holistic manner. Many illnesses belong to this diagnostic category; the chapter presents only the most prevalent. Nurses need to remember that there are multiple causes for presenting symptoms.

KEY POINTS TO REMEMBER

- René Descartes viewed the body as a machine, totally separate from mind and soul.
- Cannon was the first to identify the body's capacity to fight or flee during stress.
- Hans Selye described the general adaptation syndrome.
- Stress is a stimulus perceived by the person as a threat that exceeds his or her coping abilities.
- An interaction occurs among stress, factors within the patient, behaviors of the patient, and mediators that influence the development of illness.
- Multiple psychometric instruments are used to assess the psychological functioning of the patient.
- A psychophysiological measurement of stress response is obtained through temperature, heart rate, and blood pressure responses during the discussion of a stressful event.
- Chronic back pain can originate in five pain-producing structures in the lower back.
- Treatment for chronic back pain includes the use of medications as well as cognitive-behavioral treatments.
- Chronic pelvic pain is highly correlated with depression,

somatization, substance abuse, sexual dysfunction, and sexual abuse.

• Treatment of chronic pelvic pain includes medications as well as stress management, relaxation, cognitive therapy, and sexual education.

• Irritable bowel syndrome (IBS) involves continuous or recurrent symptoms of abdominal pain relieved with a bowel movement; the symptoms also may be associated with a change in either the frequency or texture of the stool.

• The physiological mechanism for IBS seems to be abnormal pain regulation.

• Stress plays a significant role in IBS.

• Treatment of IBS involves medical management as well as a variety of psychological strategies.

• Essential hypertension is a life-threatening disorder with multifactorial causes.

• The cause of hypertension is unknown, but it is known that factors such as stress, poverty, anger, talking, and educational status can adversely impact on blood pressure.

• The hyperreactivity theory states that excessive reactivity in blood pressure to all environmental stimuli initiates and maintains essential hypertension.

• The symptoms specificity theory states that a consistent reactivity in blood pressure to specific environmental stressors initiates and maintains essential hypertension.

• Treatment for hypertension includes medication, behavioral and psychological interventions, and lifestyle changes.

• Migraine headaches produce pain that can be incapacitating.

• A prodrome is the period preceding the migraine and occurs hours to days before the headache. The prodrome includes many symptoms such as change in mood, irritability, fatigue, blurring of vision, and increased sensitivity to sound.

• Migraines are divided into two types: migraine with aura and migraine without aura.

• An aura is a group of neurological symptoms that precede a headache by 5 to 20 minutes.

• Migraines can be precipitated by stress, caffeine, certain foods, and alcohol, as well as by the menstrual cycle.

• Serotonin plays a role in migraine headaches; serotonin falls during a migraine and promotes platelet aggregation that may contribute to the decrease in cerebral blood flow during a headache.

• Norepinephrine levels rise during a migraine, causing vasoconstriction in the peripheral vascular bed.

• Treatment of migraine headaches includes medications, as well as relaxation training combined with thermal biofeedback.

• Temporomandibular disorder (TMD) is defined as chronic or intermittent pain in the face, neck, and/or ears that is the result of a problem in the mandible joint caused by a variety of muscular, nerve, or dental problems.

• TMD has a strong stress component in its etiology.

• The treatment of TMD includes medication, joint exercises, relaxation training, and biofeedback therapy.

LEARNING ACTIVITIES

1. Keep a lifestyle journal for a week. Write down your activity, how you are feeling about doing the activity, and any bodily responses you have to doing this activity.

2. Review your journal. Did your bodily responses correpond with physical problems you might have? For example, did you feel tightness in your head? If so, are you prone to headaches? What feelings were being expressed through your pain?

3. Pay attention to what mediates or lessens your body's response to stress. Do you use any strategies that could be generalized to dealing with stress in a healthy manner?

4. Review the guidelines for relaxation, controlled breathing, and guided imagery that appear in Chapter 28. Practice these over the next week while you monitor your body's response to stress. Note any change. If a change occurs, note what it is.

CRITICAL THINKING EXERCISE

Veronica is a 10th grader at Barton High. She visits the nurse's office weekly with somatic complaints such as stomach aches, menstrual cramps, headaches, and sore throat. She tells the nurse that she lives with her father and uncle. Most of the time she visits the nurse during the second class period, gym class. The gym teacher is concerned that Veronica is trying to avoid gym. When Veronica does go to gym class, she refuses to shower with the other girls. In consulting the nurse, the gym teacher has requested that Veronica be returned to class as soon as possible when she sees the nurse. She wonders "out loud" if Veronica might have some other problem.

1. What does the gym teacher seem to be assuming?

2. Give an alternative viewpoint that could be plausible and fits the facts.

3. Under what assumptions do you think Veronica is operating?

After one month, the nurse asks Veronica why she visits the office so frequently. Veronica starts to cry, stating that she does not like to exercise because it hurts her back. The nurse makes an appointment with the doctor to examine Veronica's back. On the day of the appointment, Veronica is absent.

1. What can the nurse infer from Veronica's behavior?

2. Make sense of the data.

3. What conclusions, if any, can you draw from the given evidence?

REFERENCES

Aghabeigi, B., Feinmann, C., and Harris, M. (1992). Prevalence of post-traumatic stress disorder in patients with chronic idiopathic facial pain. *British Journal of Oral & Maxillofacial Surgery, 30,* 370–374.

Allen, R. (1983). *Human stress: Its nature and control.* Minneapolis: Burgess Publishing Company.

American Psychiatric Association. (1994). *Diagnostic and statistical manual of mental disorders—Fourth edition.* Washington, D. C., American Psychiatric Association.

American Heart Association. (1992). *1993 Heart and stroke facts statistics.* Dallas, TX: American Heart Association.

Beck, A. (1972). *Depression: Causes and treatment.* Philadelphia: University of Pennsylvania Press.

Benedittis, G., Lorenzetti, A., Pieri, A. (1990). The role of stressful life events in the onset of chronic primary headache. *Pain, 40,* 65–75.

Bernard, C. (1957). *An introduction to the study of experimental medicine* (1865). New York: Dover Publications.

Blanchard, E., Schwarz, S., Suls, J., Gerardi, M., Scharff, L., Greene, B., Taylor, A., Berreman, C., and Malamood, H. (1992). Two controlled evaluations of a multi-component psychological treatment of irritable bowel syndrome. *Behavior Research and Therapy, 2,* 175–189.

Boone, J. (1991). Stress and hypertension. *Primary Care, 18,* 623–649.

Burckhardt, C. (1990). Chronic pain. *Nursing Clinics of North America, 25,* 863–870.

Buxbaum, J., and Myslinski, N. (1993). Headache associated with temporomandibular dysfunction. In C. Tollison, and R. Kunkel (Eds.), *Headache diagnosis and treatment.* Baltimore: Williams & Wilkins.

Calhoun, D. (1992). Hypertension in blacks: Socioeconomic stressors and sympathetic nervous system activity. *American Journal of Medical Sociology, 304,* 306–311.

Cannon, W. (1929). *Bodily changes in pain, hunger, fear and rage: An account of recent research into the function of emotional excitement* (2nd ed.). New York: Appleton.

Carpenito, L. (1993). *Nursing diagnosis: Application to clinical practice* (5th ed.). Philadelphia: J. B. Lippincott.

Carson, V. B. (1989). *Spiritual dimensions of nursing practice.* Philadelphia: W. B. Saunders.

Cohen, S. (1986). Somatoform disorders: Symptoms and psychiatric implications. *Hospital Practice,* June 15, 165–198.

Corbin, L., Hanson, R., Happ, S., and Whitby, A. (1988). Somatoform disorders. *Journal of Psychosocial Nursing, 26,* 31–34.

Dahlstrom, W., Welsh, G., and Dahlstrom, L. (1972). *An MMPI handbook.* Vols. I,II. Minneapolis: University of Minnesota Press.

Derogatis, L. (1977). *SCL-90-R.* Baltimore: Johns Hopkins University Press.

Descartes, R. (1967). *Philosophic works of Descartes.* Vol. 2. E. Haldane and G. Ross [Trans]. Oxford: Oxford University Press.

Diamond, S., and Dalessio, D. (1986). *The practicing physician's approach to headache* (4th ed.). Baltimore: Williams & Wilkins.

Drossman, D., McKee, D., Sandler, R., Mitchell, C., Cramer, E., Lowman, B., and Burger, A. (1988). Psychosocial factors in the irritable bowel syndrome. A multivariate study of patients and non-patients with irritable bowel syndrome. *Gastroenterology, 95,* 701–708.

Drossman, D., Thompson, W., Talley, N., Funch-Jensen, P., Janssens, J., and Whitehead, W. (1990). Identification of subgroups of functional gastrointestinal disorders. *Gastroenterology International, 3,* 159–172.

Ellison, C. W. (1983). Spiritual well-being: Conceptualization and measurement. *Journal of Psychology and Theology, 11* (4), 330–340.

Everhart, J., and Renault, P. (1991). Irritable bowel syndrome in office-based practice in the United States. *Gastroenterology, 100,* 998–1005.

Fava, G. (1992). The concept of psychosomatic disorder. *Psychotherapy Psychosomatic, 58,* 1–12.

Feinmann, C., and Harris, M. (1984). Psychogenic facial pain. *British Dental Journal, 156,* 205.

Fine, E. (1971). Psychological factors associated with nonorganic temporomandibular joint dysfunction syndrome. *British Dental Journal, 131,* 402.

Fredrickson, M. (1991). Psychophysiological theories on sympathetic nervous system reactivity in the development of essential hypertension. *Scandinavian Journal of Psychology, 32,* 254-274.

Gallagher, R. M. (1990). Precipitating causes of migraine. In Diamond, S. (ed.). *Migraine headache prevention and management* (pp. 1–30). New York: Dekker.

Goldberg, R., Novack, D., and Gask, L. (1992). The recognition and management of somatization. *Psychosomatics, 33,* 55–61.

Green, C. (1985). The use of psychodiagnostic questionnaires in predicting risk factors and health outcomes. In P. Karoly (Ed.). *Measurement strategies in health psychology.* New York: John Wiley & Sons.

Guthrie, E., Creed, F., Dawson, D., and Tomenson, B. (1991). A controlled trial of psychological treatment for the irritable bowel syndrome. *Gastroenterology, 100,* 450–457.

Guyton, A. (1996). *Textbook of medical physiology* (9th ed.). Philadelphia: W. B. Saunders.

Harvey, R., Hinton, Gunary, R., and Barry, R. (1989). Individual and group hypnotherapy in treatment of refractory irritable bowel syndrome. *Lancet, i,* 424–425.

Holroyd, L., and Penziero, D. (1990). Pharmacological versus non-pharmacological prophylaxis of recurrent migraine headache: A meta-analytic review of clinical trials. *Pain, 42,* 1–13.

Jenkins, C., Zyzanski, S., and Roseman, R. (1970). *Jenkins activity survey manual.* New York: Psychological Corp.

Just, J., Perry, H., and Greene, C. (1992). Treating TM disorders: A survey on diagnosis, etiology and management. *JADA, 122,* 55.

Kames, L., Rapkin, A., Naliboff, B., Afifi, S., and Ferrer-Brechner, T. (1990). Effectiveness of an interdisciplinary pain management program for the treatment of chronic pelvic pain. *Pain, 41,* 41–46.

Lefer, L. (1966.). A psychoanalytic view of a dental phenomenon. *Contemporary Psychoanalysis, 2,* 135.

Lewis, M. (1988). Attribution and illness. *Journal of Psychosocial Nursing, 26,* 14–21.

Lichter, E., and Laff, S. (1993). Pelvic pain. In C. Warfield (Ed.). *The principles and practices of pain management* (pp. 147–151). New York: McGraw-Hill.

Long, J., Lynch, J., Machira, N., Thomas, S., and Malinow, K. (1982). The effect of status on blood pressure during verbal communication. *Journal of Behavioral Medicine, 5,* 165–172.

Lowery, B. (1987). Stress research: Some theoretical and methodological issues. *Image: Journal of Nursing Scholarship, 19,* 42–46.

Lubkin, I. (1990). *Chronic illness: Impact and interventions* (2nd ed.). Boston: Jones and Bartlett.

Lynch, J. (1985). *The language of the heart: The human body in dialogue.* New York: Basic Books.

Lynch, P., and Zamble, E. (1989). A controlled behavioral treatment study of irritable bowel syndrome. *Behavior Therapy, 20,* 509–523.

Mason, J. (1968). Organization of endocrine mechanisms. *Psychosomatic Medicine, 30,* 565.

Mason, J. (1971). An evaluation of the concept of nonspecifity in stress theory. *Journal of Psychiatric Research, 8,* 32,33.

Morrison, D. P. (1990). Occupational stress in migraine: Is weekend headache a myth or reality? *Cephalalgia, 10,* 189–193.

Niaura, R., and Goldstein, M. (1992). Psychological factors affecting physical conditions: Cardiovascular disease literature review, part II. *Psychosomatics, 33,* 146–155.

Peatfield, R. C. (1990). Migraine—Unproven therapeutic measures. In S. Diamond (ed.). *Migraine headache prevention and management.* New York: Marcel Dekker.

Philips, H., Grant, L., and Berkowitz, J. (1991). The prevention of chronic pain and disability: A preliminary investigation. *Behavior Research Therapy, 29,* 443–450.

Phipps, W. J., Sands, J., Lehman, M. K., and Cassmeyer, V. (1995). *Medical-surgical nursing: Concepts and clinical practice* (5th ed.). St. Louis: Mosby-Year Book.

Reiter, R., Shakern, L., Gambone, J., and Milburn, A. (1991). Correlation between sexual abuse and somatization and nonsomatic chronic pelvic pain. *American Journal of Obstetrics and Gynecology, 165,* 104–109.

Rowlingson, J. (1993). Low back pain. In C. Warfield (Ed.). *The principles and practices of pain management* (pp. 129–140). New York: McGraw-Hill.

Saper, J., Silverstein, S., Gordon, C., and Hamel, R. (1993). *The handbook of headache management.* Baltimore: Williams & Wilkins.

Sarason, I., Johnson, J., and Siegel, J. (1978). Assessing the impact of life changes. *Journal of Consulting and Clinical Psychology, 46,* 932–946.

Sarason, I., Sarason, B., and Shearin, E. (1986). Social support as an individual difference variable: Its stability, origins and relational aspects. *Journal Personality and Social Psychology, 50,* 845–855.

Sarason, I., Sarason, B., and Shearin, E. (1987). A brief measure of social support: Practical and theoretical implications. *Journal of Social and Personal Relations, 4,* 497–510.

Selye, H. (1956). *Stress of life.* New York: McGraw-Hill.

Solomon, S., and Lipton, R. (1990). Diagnosis and pathophysiology of migraine. In S. Diamond (Ed.). *Migraine headache prevention and Management* (pp. 1–30). New York: Dekker.

Speilberger, C., Gorsuch, R., and Lushene, R. (1970). *The State-Trait Anxiety Inventory Manual.* Palo Alto, CA: Consulting Psychologists Press.

Sterling, P., and Eyer, J. (1981). Biological basis of stress-related mortality. *Social Science and Medicine, 153,* 3–42.

Svedlund, J., Sjodin, I., Ottosson, J., and Dotevall, G. (1983). Controlled study of psychotherapy in irritable bowel syndrome. *Lancet ii,* 589–592.

Thomas, S., and Friedmann, E. (1994). Cardiovascular responses during verbal communication: Effect of rate of verbalization in blood pressure and heart rate responses of Type-A and Type-B cardiac s. *Journal of Cardiovascular Nursing, 9*(1), 16–26.

White, P. (1993). Pain management. In C. Warfield (Ed.). *The principles and practices of pain management* (pp. 27–39). New York: McGraw-Hill.

Whitehead, W., Bosmajian, L., Zonderman, A., Costa, P., and Schuster, M. (1988). Symptoms of psychologic distress associated with irritable bowel syndrome. Comparison of community and medical clinic samples. *Gastroenterology, 95,* 709–714.

Whitehead, W. (1992). Behavioral medicine approaches to gastrointestinal disorders. *Journal of Consulting and Clinical Psychology, 60,* 605–612.

Whorwell, P., Prior, A., and Faragher, E. (1984). Controlled trial of hypnotherapy in the treatment of severe refractory irritable-bowel syndrome. *Lancet. ii,* 1232–1234.

SUGGESTED READINGS

Burckhardt, C. (1990). Chronic pain. *Nursing Clinics of North America, 25,* 863–870.

Lowery, B. (1987). Stress research: Some theoretical and methodological issues. *Image: Journal of Nursing Scholarship, 19,* 42–46.

Reiter, R., Shakern, L., Gambone, J., and Milburn, A. (1991). Correlation between sexual abuse and somatization and nonsomatic chronic pelvic pain. *American Journal of Obstetrics and Gynecology, 165,* 104–109.

Rowlingson, J. (1993). Low back pain. In C. Warfield (Ed.). *The principles and practices of pain management* (pp 129–140). New York: McGraw-Hill.

Saper, J., Silverstein, S., Gordon, C., and Hamel, R. (1993). *The handbook of headache management.* Baltimore: Williams & Wilkins.

CHAPTER 38

THE JOURNEY CLOUDED BY COGNITIVE DISORDERS

No theory of medicine can explain what is happening to me. Every few months I sense that another piece of me is missing. My life... my self... are falling apart. I can only think half thoughts now. Someday I may wake up and not think at all... not know who I am. Most people expect to die someday, but who ever expected to lose their self first?

—*Cohen*

LEARNING OBJECTIVES

After studying this chapter, you should be able to:

1. Characterize the historical perspective of cognitive disorders.
2. Identify the defining characteristics of acute cognitive disorders (delirium).
3. Describe the treatment and nursing care of acute cognitive disorder.
4. Contrast the different types of dementia as chronic cognitive disorders.
5. Identify the defining characteristics of dementia.
6. Describe current theories related to the cause of Alzheimer's disorder.
7. Apply the nursing process at different stages of dementia.
8. Describe family caregiver issues and related nursing interventions to support the caregiver.
9. Identify legal and ethical issues related to the care of patients with cognitive disorders.

KEY TERMINOLOGY

Acetylcholine
Agnosia
Alcohol-induced persisting amnestic disorder
Alzheimer's disease
Anomia
Aphasia
Apraxia
Ataxia
Brain stem
Catastrophic reactions
Conservatorship
Creutzfeldt-Jakob disease
Crystallized intelligence
Delirium
Dementia
Disorientation
Dysphagia
Durable power of attorney
Emotional disinhibition
Global memory loss
Huntington's disease
Lewy body dementia
Limbic system
Living will
Normal-pressure hydrocephalus
Parkinson's disease
Pick's disease
Plasticity
Pseudodementia
Remote memory
Short-term memory
Sundown syndrome
Vascular dementia

The clarity and purpose of each individual's personal journey depend on an individual's ability to reflect on its meaning. Cognition represents a fundamental human feature that distinguishes living from existing. This mental capacity has a distinctive, personalized impact on the individual's physical, psychological, social, and spiritual conduct of life. For example, the ability to "remember" the connections between related actions and how to initiate them depends on cognitive processing. Moreover, this cognitive processing has a direct relationship to activities of daily living. Although primarily an intellectual and perceptual process, cognition is closely integrated with an individual's emotional and spiritual values. When human beings can no longer understand facts or connect the appropriate feelings to events, they have trouble responding to the complexity of life's many challenges. Emotions take a back seat to profound disturbances in cognitive processing that either cloud or destroy the meaning of the journey. The labyrinth of current knowledge about cognitive disorders requires a compassionate understanding of the patient and family from both a medical and a human perspective. Nursing interventions involve three therapeutic goals: protecting patient dignity, preserving functional status, and promoting quality of life for cognitively impaired patients.

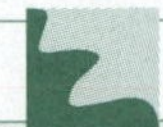

FRANCIS'S STORY

For over 30 years, Francis was a well-known corporate attorney who took pride in his ability to cite relevant law cases from memory. The first signs of his failing memory came when he could no longer connect the appropriate citation with his current law cases. An avid pinochle player, Francis gradually forgot how to play cards. Other subtle signs were present long before he received the official diagnosis. For example, when he visited his daughter, he occasionally turned to the cellar door instead of the bathroom. His family attributed his behavior to benign forgetting and unfamiliarity with a new setting, but elusive personality changes alarmed Mrs. Michaels. Francis would get angry over simple things. His outbursts, however, were transitory and episodic. It was hard to pinpoint the meaning of his emotional blankness around issues he would once have had strong opinions about.

Francis was a quiet man, so only Mrs. Michaels had a true awareness of his growing deficits in communication. In simple social situations, his speech seemed normal. Other people didn't seem to notice the personality change. Without validation from her husband or others, Mrs. Michaels had trouble trusting her own judgment and growing fear of changes in her husband's behavior. She would get angry with him but was unsure when her anger did not produce familiar responses. Francis now had two responses, both out of character with his past decisive and collaborative behavior in the marriage. He would get angry and frustrated, or he would withdraw emotionally. It pained Mrs. Michaels to see her husband, with whom she had a close relationship and on whom she depended for major decisions affecting every aspect of their lives, unable to connect at any meaningful level with her. At times he was more lucid, and the "old Francis" seemed to emerge, but these times grew fewer, gradually replaced with confusion and growing agitation.

Francis's Diagnosis

Francis received the medical diagnosis of dementia in the summer of 1990, after laboratory studies and a computed tomography (CT) scan failed to reveal other causes. In some ways, his wife was relieved to have his condition labeled. The physician advised Mrs. Michaels to seek legal advice regarding a living will, estate planning, protection of financial assets, and a durable power of attorney. Again she had trouble accepting the need to take these actions. After all, her husband was a lawyer himself. She felt her husband would be insulted by the suggestion of going to an outside lawyer, and indeed he was. As the physician explained, however, unless the family attended to legal matters while Francis still knew what he was signing, the document would not hold up legally. In such instances, the family needs to have the patient declared mentally incompetent by a court, and for most families this is an extremely painful alternative.

Francis was still driving and resisted giving up his car keys. His wife was reluctant to force the issue because she felt so bad for him. Moreover, her previous pattern of relating to him was through acquiescence, and she couldn't bring herself to cross him. In some ways, taking the actions needed to stop his driving also acknowledged a painful reality she was not quite willing to accept. Finally, the possibility of his being involved in an accident or hurting himself or others because of his condition motivated her to take the necessary steps. Mrs. Michaels introduced the topic of driving and legal alternatives when her husband seemed less agitated, and in time she achieved the necessary cooperation.

Francis wanted to do more than he was capable of doing, and he became frustrated when he was unable to accomplish simple tasks. He blamed his wife for his inability to find things. Mrs. Michaels could see he was responding to his failing abilities rather than attacking her reliability. Her love for him and her sadness about his condition allowed her to accept his outbursts without retaliation, but his behavior affected the way she felt about herself. Fortunately, Francis did not seem fully aware that his accomplishments were much more modest than before, although his limitations were painfully obvious to Mrs. Michaels. He could still enjoy simple family and commonplace social interactions, but he became agitated in unfamiliar social situations. Uncomplicated excursions to see a parade or a birthday party would bring delight; activities that demanded a complex social response served to frustrate or silence him.

Francis's Progressing Disease

As the disease progressed to the middle stage, Francis lost the power to express his thoughts and feelings verbally. This loss was the worse part for his wife. Later, she would comment that there were two deaths she experienced with Francis: the death of communication with the person she knew as her husband and his actual death. The first death was the worst.

As Francis became nonverbal, touch became an important vehicle of communication. When he became agitated, sitting quietly with him and holding his hand seemed to calm him. Mrs. Michaels found that praying with him was a form of communication they could still share. The familiar prayers were an automatic rather than recent memory, and he seemed to find comfort in remembering them.

Care in the middle stages was constant and intense because Francis was unable to complete even the simplest activities of daily living without massive external support. His table manners disintegrated. He either stared at his food or grabbed it with his hand, shoving it in his mouth. Mealtime required constant supervision to make sure that Francis ate properly and to prevent his choking. Francis needed full assistance with dressing, and he could no longer bathe himself. Incontinence and mobility became issues that required consistent attention. In many ways, however, coping with the physical care was easier than responding to the growing emotional dependence and lack of communication. Francis followed his wife everywhere, allowing no more than 12 inches between them. To Francis, Mrs. Michaels represented his only security in an increasingly alien world, although he no longer seemed to know who she was or how she fit into his life. Reconciling the "before" and "now" portraits of Francis was particularly painful but even more so was her growing inability to connect with him as a person.

Caring for Francis day in and day out was physically and emotionally wearing. Mrs. Michaels coped with the problem by engaging a nurse's aide to come in the evening to bathe and put him to bed. The aide could get up at night with him if he wandered, and Mrs. Michaels could finally get the sleep she needed. With the help of the aide and the support of her adult children, Mrs. Michaels kept her husband at home until he died four years later. Caring for him at home was her choice, and she had the financial means to accomplish it. It is not every family's choice or realistic option.

Francis's Death

Toward the end of his life, Francis had trouble swallowing, and he experienced significant weight loss. Only the physical shell of the man remained, a frail shadow of his former physical body. He could no longer even respond with the interactive ability of a young infant. There were few connections between Francis and his environment. He responded to music and prayer but to little else. Finally, Francis found release through death from the imprisonment of a mind that no longer served him as a source of information. His wife experienced sadness and relief but also a significant void. Her total caregiving, consuming every moment of her life for so many years, had left little time for the development of other relationships. Now, her role as caregiver suddenly terminated. The void left an empty hole in the fabric of her life that required time to "reweave."

HISTORICAL PERSPECTIVES ON COGNITIVE DYSFUNCTION

Greek philosophers recognized the power of the mind as the conductor and regulator of human behavior long before the common era (see Chapter 6). In ancient times, the mind, commonly acknowledged as the center of thought and emotion, was subdivided into different regions in the brain. Their biological aspects, however, were not well described until the 19th century.

Understanding of Dementia

Dementia was the first identified psychiatric disorder, described by an Egyptian prince in 3000 B.C. (Mack et al, 1994). A few centuries later, Hippocrates included *phrenitis* as one of six types of mental disorders. This disorder presented as "an acute mental disturbance with fever" (Mack et al, 1994, p. 516). Today, similar symptoms would be classified as febrile delirium.

In the 18th century, dementia was described as "a disease consisting in a paralysis of the spirit characterized by abolition of the reasoning faculty . . . abolition may follow: (1) damage to the brain caused by excessive usage, congenital causes, or old age; (2) failure of the spirit; (3) small volume of the brain; (4) violent blows to the head causing brain damage; (5) incurable diseases, such as epilepsy, or exposure to venoms (Diderot and d'Alembert, 1765, cited in Berrios, 1994, p. 6). Today, we would call the "abolition of the reasoning faculty" and "failure of the spirit" the loss of self.

By the 19th century, most clinicians thought of dementia as the product of "brain softening" resulting in cognitive impairment. They believed that cerebral arteriosclerotic hardening of the arteries, together with biological risk factors such as syphilis, alcohol, hypertension, and the aging process, caused dementia (Berrios, 1994). Even in the earlier parts of this century, cognitive disorders traditionally have been thought of as "senility," a common and perhaps standard part of the aging process. In fact, the word *senile* derives from the Latin, *senilis*, meaning "pertaining to old age."

In 1907, Alois Alzheimer presented his findings of presenile dementia based on observations of a 51-year-old woman with severe memory loss. His work represented the first definitive description of dementia as an organic behavioral syndrome. Alzheimer was intrigued that a woman so young could have such profound memory loss, and he followed the course of her dementia until she died at the age of 56. Alzheimer proposed that her symptoms were consistent with a diagnosis of progressive neurological dysfunction. He described symptoms related to cognitive impairment, delusional thinking, and hallucinations. Over time, his patient became mute and was bedridden. On autopsy, Alzheimer found concrete evidence of neuritic plaques and neurofibrillary tangles in the woman's brain. He described his observations: "Scattered through the entire cortex, especially in the upper layers, one found miliary foci that were caused by the deposition of a peculiar substance in the cerebral cortex" (Alzheimer, 1907; 1987). The substance Alzheimer found in his patient's brain is referred to today as beta-amyloid protein.

Today, it is clear that the lesions Alzheimer originally described at the turn of the century are consistent with the distinctive structural and biochemical changes in the brains of patients with Alzheimer's disease. This scientific understanding accounts for the prevailing classification of cognitive disorders as organic behavioral syndromes and the current research on their neurological and biological markers. Contemporary research has established that the brain operates as a biological unit, with each of its three principal regions—cerebral cortex, limbic system, and brain stem—responsible for different functions.

The cerebral cortex is commonly associated with cognitive processes, the limbic system with emotional processes, and the brain stem with basic life processes such as breathing and temperature regulation. A wide variety of lesions, structural and metabolic disturbances in the brain, can cause significant changes in cognitive and behavioral functioning. Some of these determinants are reversible, and others are not, at least within our current scope of knowledge.

Changes in the *DSM-IV*

In all previous categorization of cognitive disorders, delirium and dementia were considered *organic brain disorders*. In the fourth edition of the *Diagnostic and Statistical Manual (DSM-IV)*, published and presented to the American Psychological Association in 1994, however, the classification of organic mental disorders has disappeared, and a new category of *cognitive disorders* takes its place. The change occurred in response to current research in the "decade of the brain," which clearly established the presence of organic factors in traditionally described functional psychiatric diagnoses (Wilson and Skodol, 1994). Thus, the term *organic brain syndrome* applies to most major mental disorders. The new classification reflects the primacy of the definitive cognitive deficit, which is common to the clinical features of all cognitive disorders. Box 38–1 presents the process by which this change occurred.

BOX 38–1 Fate of Organic Mental Disorders in *DSM-IV*

Problem

Framers of *DSM-IV* acknowledged that the organic-nonorganic dichotomy in *DSM-III-R* was obsolete, given new knowledge about the contribution of organic factors to the development of functional diagnoses.

Challenge

The challenge to the American Psychiatric Association Organic Mental Disorders Work Group was to deal with both the traditional organic disorders, such as delirium, dementia, and amnesia, and with the more circumscribed *DSM-III-R* organic categories, such as organic anxiety disorder, organic hallucinosis, and organic delusional disorder.

Options

Numerous options included grouping these disorders together as cognitive function disorders or cognitive impairments, but this option was discarded as inappropriate because cognitive impairment presents as a symptom in other disorders, such as schizophrenia.

Outcome

Ultimately the Work Group's decision was twofold: Traditional organic mental disorders are now grouped as delirium, dementia, and amnestic, and other cognitive disorders. Greater specificity in identifying causative factors is possible—for example, substance intoxication or substance withdrawal delirium and dementia of the Alzheimer's type or vascular dementia. When delirium is superimposed on a dementia disorder, it is possible to identify this circumstance. Organic anxiety or organic delusional disorders appear under the appropriate category, such as anxiety disorder due to a general medical condition or psychotic disorder due to a general medical condition.

Summary of key points from Wilson, H., and Skodol, A. (1994). Special report: DSM-IV: Overview and examination of major changes. *Archives of Psychiatric Nursing, VIII*,(6; December); 344.

BRAIN FUNCTION AND COGNITIVE DISORDERS

Normal Brain Functioning

The central nervous system (CNS) carries messages from the brain to different areas of the body, which act in concert to negotiate life tasks effectively. When the physiological changes in brain tissue associated with cognitive disorders occur, the brain can no longer send messages, despite having an intact CNS. It is as if the telephone is off the hook. All of the structural elements are still in place, but the connection between the wiring and phone receiver is broken. Messages can be neither transmitted nor received until the "phone" connection is restored.

The brain has a certain amount of **plasticity,** so that when one area of the brain is damaged, other areas can reorganize and partially compensate for the injury. For example, as the brain struggles with a small cerebral vascular accident, other parts of the brain can take over the functions of the damaged area. Unfortunately the progressive degeneration of brain tissue associated with Alzheimer's disease and loss of acetylcholine, a neurotransmitter, eliminates plasticity (see Chapter 7 for a more detailed explanation of the neurotransmitter and a more complete discussion of neurophysiology).

Regions of the Brain

Cognitive disorders affect one or more of the brain regions, most typically the cerebral cortex and then the limbic system. As the disease progresses, global involvement occurs in all three regions, resulting in profound neurovegetative signs and symptoms and eventual death.

Cerebral Cortex

The *cerebral cortex*, often referred to as the information-processing center of the brain, receives, retrieves, and processes information that becomes the basis for making decisions. Voluntary motor functions occur under the direction of the cerebral cortex. Memory, recall, visuospatial functions, and the ability to calculate and construct complex data into a meaningful whole are associated with higher cortical functioning. Damage to the cerebral cortex results in language impairment. Complex cortical functions in the brain regulate the integrated mental activities involved in perception, thinking, speaking, comprehension, and listening. They play an important role in communication, allowing a person to understand and respond verbally and nonverbally to another person's communication. With loss of communication ability, the individual's capacity to make sense of the journey or to share its meaning with another is lost.

When damage is localized, it is more indicative of vascular dementia. Two areas of the brain, named after the investigators who discovered them, are particularly important in language deficits. These deficits may occur as a primary diagnosis or may be superimposed on a multiinfarct or dementia of the Alzheimer's type. In 1865, a French physician, Paul Broca, discovered that damage to the left frontal lobe resulted in an impaired use of expressive language. When damage occurs in this region of the brain (causing *Broca's aphasia*), an individual struggles to form words without much success. Interestingly, patients who have an inability to formulate the same words in intentional meaningful sentences can sing familiar songs with ease.

In 1874, a German researcher, Carl Wernicke, described damage to the left temporal lobe resulting in a person's inability to understand language and to use words in a meaningful way. Left temporal lobe damage is known as *Wernicke's aphasia*, or receptive aphasia. Here the normal connections allowing the patient to understand and respond appropriately to verbal messages are lost. Sentence structure is no longer connected to symbolic meanings, so that although a person tries to communicate through words, the message expressed is meaningless babble. Often the listener's inability to make sense of patients' messages becomes so frustrating to patients that they stop talking.

From a behavioral perspective, the higher cortical functions act together as a highly complex conceptual organizer of information. They allow people to gather and interpret data about their world, to make observations, to problem-solve, and to draw valid conclusions. Human beings rely on their ability to think (cognition) in a variety of interrelated ways. First, cognitive processes integrate and connect the self with human experience by acting as the bridge between reality and its personalized meaning. When the connections are broken, cognitive deficits directly affect a person's ability to complete behavioral tasks. The capacity to process perceptual data cognitively and make sense of it directly influences an individual's reasoning skills and the appropriateness of judgments. Resourceful living typically reveals an individual's ability to make clear decisions about what is occurring and to plan for the future. Dementia gradually robs an individual of cognitive processing abilities, and others must act on behalf of the patient.

Limbic System

The **limbic system** regulates emotional arousal, memory, and basic drives such as aggression, food, and sex. Patients with damage to the limbic system display significant personality alterations. They have little control over the expression of their emotions. Some become apathetic and emotionally disengage from their environment. Others become emotionally labile, with episodic crying, laughing, and anger appearing with close approximation. These rapid changes in emotions are seemingly unrelated, in many cases, to external stimuli. The patient with limbic system involvement displays little control over sexual and anger expression. This lack of discretion is called **emotional disinhibition.** The patient may appear physically able. Those unfamiliar with the behavioral changes associated with cognitive impairment may not realize that the patient has a cognitive deficit governing his or her emotional responses.

The **brain stem,** the brain's innermost region, controls basic life functions. Damage to the brain stem region affects heart beat and breathing and ultimately human survival.

Multiple Causes

Cognitive disorders originate from multiple causes. For this reason, current thinking considers cognitive disorders a syndrome rather than a specific disease. Jacques (1992) defines a syndrome as "a characteristic pattern of clinical features—the symptoms and signs—which can be caused by one or other of a number of illnesses" (p. 2). The customary clinical features of a behavioral syndrome help define the nature of the deficit and point to its central pathology. General agreement exists about the nature of cognitive impairment regardless of cause.

Delirium is the name given to the acute forms of cognitive dysfunction resulting from secondary changes in brain metabolism. **Dementia** is the term used to describe chronic exemplars of cognitive disorders. Acute cognitive disorders represent a separate category and are represented as quite distinct from chronic forms, rather than viewed on a continuum of cognitive dysfunction. The *DSM-IV* criteria describe the basic defining characteristics of both acute and chronic cognitive disorders, each as a streamlined unit, with delirium due to multiple causes and dementia due to multiple causes. The intent of the current nomenclature is to classify each as an explicit syndrome of behaviors rather than as a single disease.

Acute cognitive disorders (delirium) can occur as a primary syndrome; as the corollary of excessive use of alcohol; and as a result of a host of structural, metabolic, and infectious causes. Delirium can be superimposed on chronic cognitive disorders, increasing the confusion and cognitive impairment the individual already suffers. This distinction is important because the physiological management of delirium symptoms can sometimes restore the dementia patient to a higher level of functioning (Katz, 1993).

By whatever name the disorder is known, to lose one's cognitive functioning, whether temporarily or permanently, is one of the most horrifying circumstances an individual can ever experience. It affects every aspect of what we do and who we are. The Lears (1980, p. 217) poignantly describe its impact on their lives in the novel *Heartsounds:*

The most painful thing was what happened to my mind. Nothing in my life was ever worse than that, or ever will be (p. 222) . . . (And his wife observes), It was not, of course, no memory. It was damaged memory. Of all his disabilities, this was the most devastating. He had always taken memory so far for granted. Who does not when it works? He had no awareness how paralyzed one might be without it. Now he understood the obvious as philosophers do, profoundly. He understood that without memory, life was not human life but vegetation. Without memory, one could not tie a shoe.

▶ Check Your Reading

1. How would you describe the differences between Wernicke's aphasia and Broca's aphasia?
2. Why would the nurse consider dementia a syndrome?
3. What are the significant changes in the *DSM-IV* classification of cognitive disorders, and why are they important in mental health nursing?

ACUTE COGNITIVE DISORDERS: DELIRIUM

Delirium represents a group of acute cognitive disorders directly attributable to diagnosable neurological, metabolic, and toxic conditions that influence brain function. Gomez and Gomez (1987) describe the primary clinical features of delirium as "a clouded state of consciousness," which causes the patient to "become disconnected from immediate surroundings, misinterpret reality, and experience perceptual distortions. The condition worsens as the patient's level of anxiety increases" (p. 330). Regardless of the cause, delirium creates a marked disturbance in consciousness.

Although extreme confusion is a key symptom, the precise presentation of symptoms varies, reflecting the specific underlying physical disturbance. Some patients become stuporous; others become agitated. In most cases, the patient's presenting behavior is bizarre and dramatic. Delirious patients also can experience significant perceptual changes as hallucinations, illusions, and disorientation. Hallucinations, when they occur, typically are visual. A patient may report having "night visitors" or seeing a vision of a deceased family member. Illusions take the visual form of misinterpreting staff as police or a piece of medical equipment as a lethal weapon. Shadows on the wall appear as monsters. **Disorientation,** defined as an inability to know who one is, where one is, or what the time or date is, is a common occurrence. In contrast to patients with psychotic disorders, most delirious patients are oriented to person; they know their names. But they experience difficulty with time and date, and they have trouble identifying their current circumstances appropriately.

Nursing Care for Delirium

Delirium represents a state of acute physical and psychological urgency. Accurate assessment is perhaps the most critical element of effective nursing care; it can mean the difference between life and death. Typically, delirious patients present in the emergency room in a state of acute confusion and usually not of their own volition.

Emergency Triage

Emergency medical triage of the delirious patient is a primary nursing intervention. Patients with suspected delirium should receive treatment as a medical emergency first and then from a psychiatric treatment perspective. Autonomic symptoms, such as elevated blood pressure, tachycardia, fever, excessive perspiration, and constricted pupils, provide evidence of an acute medical emergency. Clearly, vital signs and assessment of physical symptoms take priority, and symptoms of cardiopulmonary instability require immediate stabilization (Kaplan and Sadock, 1993).

Besides assessment for emergency physical conditions, evaluation of the patient's mental status is critical. Patients with acute cognitive impairment often are a danger to themselves or others. The threat they pose depends on the nature of the cognitive deficit and its underlying pathology, particularly if drug induced. Until proven otherwise, suicide/homicide potential is always a possibility with delirious patients. (See chapters 17 and 36 for further detail on assessment and treatment.) With these patients, you must decide quickly whether the patient's symptoms warrant immediate physical or psychological intervention or a combination of modalities.

Establishing the Diagnosis

Once you address the emergency aspects of the patient's condition, the next step is to confirm the diagnosis of delirium through patient history, observation of symptoms, and laboratory and other diagnostic tests. Patients with delirium rarely are good historians. Even with periods of relative lucidity, delirious patients are unable to give accurate, coherent information because the psychoactive substance, infection, imbalance, or injury remains operative in their brains. Typically, direct patient interviews are postponed until the delirium symptoms have cleared. When the patient is the only available informant, having the same interviewer and keeping careful notes are important. These patients may appear cognitively intact during one interview and quite confused at a second interview the same day. Comparison data are essential to the development of an accurate diagnosis and appropriate treatment. Usually, seeking information from the person accompanying the patient elicits the most accurate data during the assessment and acute treatment phase.

BOX 38-2 Common Features of Delirium

- Reduced ability to maintain attention to external stimuli (e.g., questions must be repeated because attention wanders) and to shift attention appropriately to new external stimuli (e.g., perseverates answer to previous question)
- Disorganized thinking, as indicated by rambling, irrelevant, or incoherent speech
- At least two of the following:
  - Reduced level of consciousness (e.g., difficulty keeping awake during examination)
  - Perceptual disturbances: misinterpretations, illusions, or hallucinations
  - Disturbance of sleep-wake cycle with insomnia or daytime sleepiness
  - Increased or decreased psychomotor activity
  - Disorientation to time, place, or person
  - Memory impairment (e.g., inability to learn new material, such as the names of several unrelated objects after five minutes, or to remember past events, such as history of current episode of illness)
  - Clinical features develop over a short period of time (usually hours to days) and tend to fluctuate over the course of a day
- Either of the following:
  - Evidence from the history, physical examination, or laboratory tests of a specific organic factor (or factors) judged to be causatively related to the disturbance
  - In the absence of such evidence, a presumed organic factor if the disturbance cannot be accounted for by any nonorganic mental disorder (e.g., manic episode accounting for agitation and sleep disturbance)

Adapted from American Psychiatric Association (1994). *Diagnostic and Statistical Manual of Mental Disorders, fourth edition.* Washington, D.C.: American Psychiatric Association.

Box 38–2 lists characteristics common to delirium. Obtaining a complete history, particularly with symptom onset and behavioral change, is essential to developing an appropriate treatment plan. Those in close contact with the patient usually can report a distinct change in behavior. Critical data include identification of precipitating factors, such as medications the patient currently is taking; blows to the head or falls; drug use, particularly as it relates to the past few days; recent illness; and changes in environment. If the patient has suffered a recent blow to the head, the area needs to be identified. Information about past treatment for emotional and physical illness is important, and you need to document history of drug use, including polydrug use (e.g., cocaine and benzodiazepines). Abrupt withdrawal from alcohol, barbiturates, or benzodiazepines can lead to episodic symptoms of delirium. Moreover, the cross-tolerance effects of past drug abuse can influence the choice of medication to reduce delirium symptoms. The agitation, explosive anger, and clouded consciousness associated with other psychiatric disorders such as bipolar disorder and psychosis can mimic delirium. Thus, data about past psychiatric treatment can be helpful in establishing a differential diagnosis of delirium rather than mania or psychosis. Table 38–1 summarizes differences in the differential diagnosis of delirium and dementia.

Observation of individuals with suspected delirium reveals a characteristic constellation of behavioral symptoms. Patients may appear stuporous or in a state of high agitation. Patients may shift rapidly between the two states. Memory for immediate and recent events is difficult to elicit (Marachlewski, 1994). The patient's speech may be incoherent, rambling, and at complete odds with reality. Seriously affected patients may indicate visceral effects, such as the sensation of bugs crawling under their skin. Patients also may demonstrate a compulsive reflex, picking at bed covers or clothing (Haller & Binder, 1995).

Other observations relate to the patterning of symptoms. With delirium, symptoms present a distinctive configuration. Symptoms appear suddenly, often beginning at night, and they present a fluctuating course of symptom exacerbation and remission. Florid cognitive symptoms and explicit behavior changes noted over a short period suggest a delirium rather than dementia. The cognitive symptoms, although intense, usually last no more than a few hours or days and rarely longer than a month. Once the underlying pathology is recognized, the symptoms can be reversed quickly and dramatically.

Finding the cause of the delirium obviously forms the foundation for decisions about primary treatment. Delirium in the elderly is particularly important to assess because these patients are less likely to be substance abusers and may have underlying dementia. Keith (1994) suggests that "delirium is frequently superimposed on dementia in up to 40% of hospitalized demented patients and complicating the differential diagnosis of the two conditions, which are by no means mutually exclusive" (p. 42).

Gomez and Gomez (1987) note that most physical illnesses, medications, drugs, or alcohol have the potential to cause delirium in the elderly (Table 38–2). Other possible causes include congestive heart failure, malnutrition, dehydration, diabetes, hypoxia affecting cerebral blood flow, pneumonia, and hypokalemia. Drug toxicity, particularly with anticholinergic or arrhythmia drugs, is particularly dangerous in the elderly because of the slower metabolic rate that allows medication buildup in these patients (Ross, 1991). Patients with premorbid organic brain disease are at highest risk for the development of

TABLE 38–1 Differential Diagnosis of Delirium and Dementia

Feature	Delirium	Dementia
Onset	Acute, often at night	Insidious
Course	Fluctuating, with lucid intervals during the day; worse at night	Stable over the course of the day
Duration	Hours to weeks	Months or years
Awareness	Reduced	Clear
Alertness	Abnormally low or high	Usually normal
Attention	Lacks direction and selectivity; distractibility; fluctuation over the course of the day	Relatively unaffected
Orientation	Usually impaired for time; tendency to mistake unfamiliar for familiar places and persons	Often impaired
Memory	Immediate and recent impaired	Recent and remote impaired
Thinking	Disorganized	Impoverished
Perception	Illusions and hallucinations, usually visual and common	Often absent
Speech	Incoherent, hesitant, slow, or rapid	Difficulty in finding words
Sleep-wake cycle	Always disrupted	Fragmented sleep
Physical illness or drug toxicity	Either or both present	Often absent, especially in Alzheimer's disease

From Lipowski, Z. (1990). *Delirium: Acute Confusional States* (p. 192). New York: Oxford University Press.

TABLE 38–2 Underlying Mechanisms of Medication-Induced Mental Changes

Mechanism of Action	Medication Examples
Anticholinergic interactions	Atropine, scopolamine, antihistamines, antipsychotics, antidepressants, antispasmodics, antiparkinsonian agents
Decreased cerebral blood flow	Antihypertensives, antipsychotics
Depression of respiratory center	Central nervous system depressants
Fluid and electrolyte alterations	Diuretics, alcohol, laxatives
Altered thermoregulation	Alcohol, psychotropics, narcotics
Acidosis	Diuretics, alcohol, nicotinic acid
Hypoglycemia	Hypoglycemics, alcohol, propranolol
Hormonal disturbances	Thyroid extract, corticosteroids

From Miller, C.A. (1995). *Nursing Care of Older Adults: Theory and Practice* (2nd ed.) (p. 441). Philadelphia: J.B. Lippincott.

anticholinergic symptoms, characterized by confusion, agitation, visual hallucinations, disorientation, incoherence, stupor, and bizarre behavior.

Delirium in the young is associated most frequently with drug toxicity, head trauma, infection, and brain tumors. The violent behaviors associated with delirium are particularly dangerous with young adults having drug toxicity or head trauma. These patients have greater physical capacity to harm themselves and others. In young adults presenting with violent behavior, organic brain disease should be considered until it is ruled out. Table 38–3 summarizes common causes of delirium.

Determination of underlying pathology causing the delirium requires a thorough physical assessment, appropriate laboratory tests, and other diagnostic assessments, such as MRI, angiogram, and CT scan. Table 38–4 lists common laboratory tests and their clinical applications. Testing should be completed as quickly as possible because the data become the basis for treatment decisions. For example, patients can achieve symptom relief quickly with the discontinuation or dose reduction of the drug responsible for the delirium. Sometimes, restoration of fluid or electrolyte balance clears the delirium. Immediate blood and toxicologic screening tests can save an individual's life and often mandate the prompt need for surgery, gastric lavage, intubation, or transfer to the intensive care unit. Fever suggests an infectious origin, whereas abnormally elevated pulse and blood pressure suggest drug withdrawal. Tests such as the Glasgow Coma

Scale and CT scan of the head can reveal subdural hematomas. Other common tests used in differential diagnosis include MRI, positron emission tomography scan, and angiogram.

Patient Care Guidelines

The first nursing intervention is to stabilize the patient medically. Once the patient's physical condition is secure, nursing interventions are oriented toward behavior and symptom reduction. No single nursing intervention is

TABLE 38–3 Common Causes of Delirium

Condition	Manifestations
Vascular insufficiency	Thrombosis or embolism, transient ischemic attacks, hypoxia
Cerebral vascular accident	Subdural hematoma, intracranial hemorrhage, ruptured aneurysm
Tumors	Primary malignant, metastatic, benign
Electrolyte imbalances	Hyper/hypokalemia, chloremia, natremia, glycemia
Fluid volume depletion	Diuretics, inadequate fluid intake
Postsurgery, intensive care unit psychosis	Physiologic or psychological stress
Infections	Viral, bacterial, meningitis, brain abscess
Drug toxicity	Virtually any drug, steroids, digitalis, beta blockers, anticholinergics, amphetamines
Drug withdrawal	Barbiturates, alcohol, benzodiazepines, sedative-hypnotics
Nutritional deficiencies	Vitamin B_{12}, niacin, thiamine

TABLE 38–4 Suggested Laboratory Tests for Patients Presenting with Cognitive Disorders

Test	Clinical Application
Complete blood count: white blood count with differential; sedimentation rate	Presence of infection
Blood chemistry Blood urea nitrogen Creatinine	Renal failure
Glucose	Diabetes, hypoglycemia
Trilodothyronine, thyroxine	Thyroid disease
Electrolytes (Na^+, K^+, Ca^{++}, Cl^-, PO_4)	Electrolyte imbalance
Serum folate level	Liver disease or failure
Vitamin B_{12} level	Nutritional deficits
SGOT, SGPT	Liver disease or failure
VDRL	Syphilis
Drug blood levels	Drug toxicity for therapeutic drugs, e.g., steroids, digitalis toxicity; nonprescribed drugs, such as barbiturates, cocaine, phenodiazepines, alcohol
Urinalysis, glucose, acetone	Diabetes
Albumin	Renal failure
Porphyria screen	Renal failure
Leukocytes	Infection
Urine toxicology (barbiturates, phenodiazepines, cocaine)	Drug toxicity
Computed tomography, positron emission tomography, magnetic resonance imaging	Brain tumor, subdural hematoma, brain hemorrhage, infection

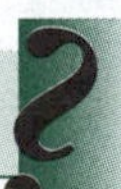

WHAT FAMILIES NEED TO KNOW — Delirium

Delirium is an acute, reversible problem that can be frightening, as extreme confusion leads to symptoms that are bizarre and dramatic. Hallucinations, delusions, disorientation, and extreme anxiety may occur, which can lead to the possibility of the person harming himself or herself or others. These symptoms appear quite suddenly, and once the cause is treated, the symptoms subside as rapidly as they occurred. You might be asking yourself, "What causes delirium?" Many different causes of delirium exist including most physical illnesses, medications, drugs, or alcohol. In young adults and children, delirium is more often associated with drug toxicity, head trauma, infection, and brain tumor.

It is most important to remember that seeking medical attention is of an urgent nature when delirious symptoms appear. Take your loved one or family member immediately to an emergency care setting. The sooner medical intervention occurs, the quicker the cause can be determined and the symptoms treated. Your quick response in this type of emergency can literally mean life or death for the delirious patient.

equally effective in all cases. Instead, nursing interventions are specifically tailored to meet the needs of the individual patient and the specific demands of the situation.

Most delirium patients respond best to one-to-one clinical supervision from a single caregiver because the ability to shift attention from one person to another in a meaningful way diminishes in direct proportion to the brain pathology. Establishing eye contact and identifying the purpose of the interview offer a significant landmark when sensory input threatens the patient's security. Receiving all information from this person also reduces the chance of misinterpretation, a significant problem with delirium patients (Hall and Buckwalter, 1987).

Patients with acute confusional states lack the concentration needed to follow a discussion. Expecting them to follow a complicated conversation increases anxiety. Instead, one directive at a time, delivered in calm, yet decisive tones, provides the structure a patient needs when the objective world does not make sense. Additionally, nurses may have to identify themselves at regular intervals, orienting the patient to the setting and what will happen next. Lack of environmental cues increases anxiety, whereas information needed for familiarization with the environment calms the anxious patient. As the patient's condition improves, the level of intervention lessens to adapt to the patient's growing awareness and responsiveness to environmental cues.

You also may choose to limit the number of people present. Patients with acute cognitive deficits overreact to almost any stimulus. Asking those who seem to agitate the patient to leave for a short time can go a long way in reducing patient frustration. If this is done tactfully, most significant others are grateful that you have taken charge of the situation. Explaining that patients with delirium act irrationally toward those they care about helps soften the perception of rejection.

CONTAINING PATIENT ANXIETY

Delirious patients are acutely anxious, and their tension level is contagious. Staff and other patients often have difficulty maintaining calm around the patient in an acute confusional state. Yet what the patient needs most are clear boundaries and someone to take charge of the situation. Staff attitude is important. All personnel involved with the patient should have a thorough understanding of delirium, which allows them to maintain a nonanxious presence and a consistent approach. Using a minimum of simple, concrete words spoken in a calm, low, but authoritative voice can calm patients much more easily than trying to reason with them.

REDUCING ENVIRONMENTAL STIMULI

Inadvertent actions taken by others, even if totally unrelated to the patient, are sources of distraction. Environmental noises often increase agitation. Ideally, you will have the option of placing the delirious patient in a quiet room, with the door closed, apart from the mainstream of activity. This measure helps reduce sensory incitement. If this is not possible, the patient needs to have the curtains drawn around the bed. Lighting is important because a poorly lit room, glare, and reflections can stimulate illusions and other perceptual distortions. Because many patients are both physically and emotionally exhausted from the effects of their delirium, a quiet environment provides a needed respite. This nursing intervention has a complementary therapeutic effect in that it expands the patient's cognitive functioning capacity.

MINIMIZING PERCEPTUAL DISTORTIONS

Spatial/perceptual distortions found in acute confusional states often lead to significant misinterpretations of people, space, objects, or directives. For example, patients may misinterpret nurses moving toward them as huge malevolent persons out to kill them. Remember that delirious patients typically have limited ability to interpret accurately and respond to environmental, physical, or emotional stimuli because of neurobiochemical changes in the brain. Repeated explanations and orientation to the setting provide a flow of orienting and calming sensory and informational inputs (Lipowski, 1990).

GIVING MEDICATION

Medication may be necessary if the patient is out of control. Preferably, it is given before the patient is ready to hurt someone. Indications for immediate medication management of anxiety include significant paranoid tendencies, combative gestures, intense anger, threats, and threatening body language. If the patient is highly agitated, small doses of a high-potency neuroleptic, such as haloperidol, are administered, generally in doses of 0.25 to 5.0 mg intramuscularly, to reduce tension. A neuroleptic such as haloperidol has fewer sedative, cardiotoxic, hypotensive, and anticholinergic side effects (Gomez and Gomez, 1987, p. 332).

Moreover, these medications are less likely to decrease the seizure threshold than lower-potency neuroleptics, and they tend to have a lessened adverse effect on the patient's cognitive functioning. Repeat administration of the antipsychotic medication is appropriate after 30 minutes, when indicated. The addition of a benzodiazepine (Lorazepam) is helpful if previous treatment with the antipsychotic medication proves ineffective (Kaplan and Sadock, 1993). When administering medications, avoid a scene and supervise the medication administration when it is taken orally to ensure that the medication is swallowed. You need to record the patient's response to the medication and to report any adverse effects.

ELIMINATING CAUSATIVE FACTORS

Elimination of the causal factors is central to the nursing management of patients with delirium. Following identification of the cause, appropriate medication, nutrition, and electrolyte support are aimed at restoring the patient to premorbid functioning and providing for the comfort and safety of the patient. Because causative agents vary, so does the treatment. Obviously, antibiotics for patients with infectious disorders, such as meningitis or encephalitis, are appropriate. Correction of malnutrition, dehydration, electrolyte imbalance, and vitamin deficiencies can reduce the severity and continuation of delirium symptoms related to these contingencies. If medication toxicity is suspected—for example, steroids, lithium, or digitalis toxicity—the implicated drug should be discontinued immediately. Some drug toxicities, such as barbiturates, require gradual discontinuance. They cannot be withdrawn precipitously without significant adverse effects. Such patients must be weaned gradually from drugs. They are given titrated doses of the drug until the symptoms are brought under control, and then the drug is gradually removed.

Patients who require immediate stabilization with medication exhibiting cross-tolerance behaviors typically receive benzodiazepines to minimize withdrawal symptoms. For example, the acute symptoms of alcohol withdrawal respond well to temporary administration of a benzodiazepine. Virtually all of the drugs in this classification are useful in reducing the seizures and the acute confusional states associated with alcohol withdrawal. The most frequently used, however, are "chlordiazepoxide, diazepam, oxazepam, and lorazepam" (Katz, 1993, p. 70). (See chapter 31 for more information regarding cross-tolerance.)

When analyzing causal factors as the foundation for treatment decisions, realize that several contributing factors can coexist in creating the patient's delirium. For example, an elderly patient may simultaneously suffer from dehydration, drug toxicity, infection, and electrolyte imbalance. Unless all causative factors are addressed, the patient's delirium may not resolve (Lipowski, 1990).

MANAGING AGGRESSIVE BEHAVIOR

The primary treatment goal in the management of aggressive behavior is to prevent its escalation into actual violence toward self, others, or objects in the environment. In addition to using medication for tension relief, staff attitude is critical. Close but relaxed supervision is a key strategy in preventing the escalation of aggressive behavior among patients with organic brain dysfunction. Moving the patient out of the area into a quiet, nonstimulating environment is crucial because delirious patients lack the capacity to do this on their own. Kaplan and Sadock [1993] also suggest isolating the patient from the source of anger. Removal of objects is appropriate. If the patient is expressing anger toward a particular staff member, it may be appropriate to have another staff member be the primary contact. The same holds true for family members.

The way in which staff approach patients and the number of demands placed on them affects physical and verbal aggression. For example, moving toward the patient with arms at one's side and using the patient's name with simple directives is less threatening than quick or random movements.

Providing patients with choices is a useful intervention as long as the patient is not completely out of control, and the choices do not compromise the rights of others. Statements such as "I'd like to ask you to come with me to the room down the hall where we can talk about this with less distraction," said in a quiet, firm voice is more effective than a sudden show of force. When needed however, a calm but decisive show of force, delivered verbally with uncomplicated direct language, often decreases patient anxiety and encourages cooperation. Never turn your back to a delirious patient, and never try to subdue a patient without sufficient personnel.

In the event of escalating aggression, staff members need to act decisively and deliberately, with physical force if necessary. One person explains the purpose of each movement in advance, in a composed voice. Seclusion and restraints need application with compassion and respect for the patient's dignity as a human being. Chapter 15 also provides more guidelines for anticipating and handling violent behavior.

Follow-Up Care

Many patients lack insight related to an association among lifestyle factors, drug abuse, past hospitalizations for mental illness, past trauma, and current circumstances, even after the immediate medical condition has stabilized. Nevertheless, including patients in treatment planning, to whatever extent possible once their symptoms are under control, usually is beneficial. Follow-up referral for treatment of drug abuse or medication monitoring can prevent further episodes of delirium.

▶ Check Your Reading

4. How would you describe the common characteristics of delirium?
5. Why is an accurate diagnosis so important?
6. What interventions would the nurse use to contain the delirium patient's anxiety?
7. What medication is the most useful with delirium patients? Why?

CASE STUDY: RANDY

Randy is a 17-year-old high school senior who is admitted into the intensive care unit after smoking crack cocaine at a friend's party. He is delirious and confused as to how he ended up in the emergency department. His friends report that he had smoked two to three rocks of crack during the evening. They became alarmed when they found him in the shower with all of his clothes on with the shower running. As he sat in the shower, he was formulating sentences using nonsensical terms while crying and laughing. He became combative when his friends tried to take him out of the shower. They called 911 for assistance.

ASSESSMENT

Assessment data are as follows:

- Delirious and confused
- Impaired cognition
- Combative
- Rapid mood swings

DIAGNOSIS

***DSM-IV* Diagnosis:** Delirium

Nursing Diagnosis: Acute Confusion related to delirium as evidenced by use of nonsensical terms, fluctuations in mood, agitation, and impaired cognition

OUTCOME IDENTIFICATION, PLANNING, AND IMPLEMENTATION

EXPECTED OUTCOME 1: By _____ the patient will have safely detoxified from crack.

SHORT-TERM GOALS	NURSING INTERVENTIONS	RATIONALES
By _____ the patient will have safely detoxified from crack.	1. Monitor vital signs. 2. Check level of consciousness. 3. Decrease environmental stimuli.	1–3. Detoxification can lead to alterations in normal vital signs; it is especially important to monitor for cardiac arrhythmias and seizure activity.
	4. Administer medications as ordered.	4. Medications typically ordered are antipsychotics, sedatives, antiarrhythmics, and anticonvulsants. Psychotropic medication can decrease symptoms and agitated behavior.
By _____ the patient will have a premorbid level of cognitive functioning.	1. Encourage Randy to do as much as possible for self after detoxification phase.	1. Active participation in own care assists the patient to maintain self-esteem and independence, which are important developmental issues for an adolescent.
	2. Provide orientation to environment, present new information slowly. 3. Talk to Randy about mutual areas of interest, i.e., friends at school, sports, hobbies.	2–3. After a period of acute confusion, a slow process of orientation will support memory and orientation for the patient.
By _____ the patient will demonstrate socially acceptable behavior.	1. Discuss with Randy the crack episode. Determine if this was one-time experimentation or a pattern of abuse.	1–3. Early assessment and intervention are important components in planning nursing care for an adolescent using drugs.
	2. Encourage Randy to ventilate his feelings, especially any shame or embarrassment over drug use. 3. Refer Randy to drug rehabilitation program.	2. Shame and guilt accompany actions that are socially unacceptable, i.e., taking a shower with all your clothes on.
By _____ the patient will participate in activities and with others at a socially acceptable level.	1. Encourage Randy to participate in unit activities.	1. Participation in unit activities is a socially acceptable type of behavior that encourages a sense of belongingness.
	2. Assess level of confusion and watch for return to normal functioning.	2. Delirium confusion is marked by an acute onset and usually is temporary once the underlying cause is treated (i.e., drug use).

EVALUATION

Formative Evaluation: Randy met each of the short-term goals. He was a very pleasant adolescent and participated readily in the therapeutic milieu. He admitted to a one-time experimentation with crack, stating that everyone was trying it, and he wanted to "see what it was like."

Summative Evaluation: Randy achieved all of the expected outcomes. He decided to attend an outpatient support group that supported a "just say no" attitude toward drugs. He verbalized on several occasions how lucky he was to have survived his drug experimenting and how fortunate he was to have friends who promptly sought medical help for him.

CHRONIC COGNITIVE DISORDERS: DEMENTIA

Edwards (1993) defines dementia, the term used for chronic cognitive disorders, as "a set of conditions, medically diagnosed, and leading to recognized and measurable behavioral changes in an individual" (p. 6). By contrast with delirium, which responds to treatment, dementia is a degenerative neurological disorder that invariably worsens and always ends in death. There is no known cure.

Chronic cognitive disorders have a slow insidious onset, with gradual deterioration of cognitive, mental, and physical neurological systems. The conditions comprising the chronic cognitive disorder classification include primary dementia, dementia with extrapyramidal symptoms, dementia caused by brain lesions, dementia associated with other conditions, and pseudodementia. Common features of dementia, encompassing all chronic cognitive disorders, regardless of cause, are presented in Box 38–3. Distinguishing among the different types can be important for diagnosis. All patients need a comprehensive neurological assessment to rule out reversible causes of dementia, to provide treatment direction, and to establish parameters for families regarding genetic implications. For example, treatment of underlying hypertension can offset further insults to brain tissue in some cases, whereas this would not be the case for the Alzheimer's disease patient. Familial Alzheimer's and Huntington's disease raise questions in first-degree relatives about their chances of contracting the disorder and are important determinants of future family genetic decisions.

Primary Dementia

Alzheimer's disease

Clinicians consider **Alzheimer's disease** a *primary dementia* because the syndrome occurs with distinctive brain lesions and without any known physiological basis. The disorder is classified as a neurological brain disease with multifactorial cause (O'Brien, 1994). Alzheimer's disease affects between 2 and 4 million people, making it the most common neuropsychiatric illness in the elderly. The actual course of the disorder follows a predictable pattern of early, middle, and late stages, each displaying characteristic behaviors and requiring a different focus of treatment. Yi and coworkers (1994) refer to the early stage as the amnestic stage, the middle stage as the dementia stage, and the late stage as the vegetative stage.

Morphologically, Alzheimer's disease patients develop neurofibrillary tangles and neuritic plaques, which take up space in the brain as lesions, replacing normal tissue in the cell body of the neuron (Edwards, 1993). There is a global decline in cortical functioning, particularly during the middle stages, that affects not only cognitive functioning, but also the voluntary exercise of bodily functions. As the disease progresses, patients lose control over their bladder and bowel functions and later over swallowing. Other signs of increased neurological

BOX 38–3 Common Features of Dementia

- Impairment in short-term and long-term memory
- One of the following
  - Impairment in abstract thinking: inability to find similarities and differences between related words, trouble defining related words
  - Impaired judgment: inability to make plans, hiding money, giving money or possessions away, accusing spouse of infidelity, acting out sexually
  - Disturbances of higher cortical functioning: aphasia (disturbance in language), apraxia (inability to carry out motor activities), agnosia (failure to recognize objects or people), constructional difficulty (inability to copy figures or assemble blocks or put things together in a logical way)
  - Personality: changes or inappropriate accentuation of personality traits
  - Known organic cause or determination that the disorder is not a mental disorder

Adapted from American Psychiatric Association (1994). *Diagnostic and Statistical Manual of Mental Disorders, fourth edition.* Washington, D.C.: American Psychiatric Association.

TABLE 38–5 **Terms Related to Neurological Deficits Found in Dementia**

Term	Definition
Agnosia	Inability to recognize mirror image, familiar others, or everyday objects
Agraphia	Inability to write
Apraxia	Inability to carry out purposeful motor functions, despite intact structural musculature and sensory functions
Akathisia	Extreme motor restlessness and inability to remain seated
Anomia	Difficulty in associating the right word with an object
Aphasia	Inability to communicate verbally and/or understand verbal communication. Receptive aphasia refers to being unable to comprehend what one has heard; expressive aphasia refers to being unable to express oneself verbally, despite understanding the message; global aphasia refers to a combination of the two, i.e., the patient can neither comprehend messages nor verbally respond
Ataxia	Difficulty walking and with fine motor coordination
Carphologia/floccillation	Purposeless picking at bedcovers or clothes
Constructional difficulty	Inability to put objects together, or to copy complex figures
Dysarthria	Slurred speech, difficulty in articulating words
Dysphagia	Difficulty swallowing
Echolalia	Repeating words or questions without being able to respond appropriately
Formication	Illogical sensation of bugs crawling under one's skin
Mutism	Patient does not communicate verbally despite intact physical structural ability to speak
Paraphasia	Substituting a word or describing rather than naming an object

deficit appear as an inability to walk. Seizures are common. Death inevitably occurs as a result of neurological complications imposed by the brain lesions.

Alzheimer's disease represents the clinical prototype for chronic cognitive disorders (Berrios, 1994). It is the most common form of dementia, and the care given to dementia patients regardless of cause is essentially the same, particularly in the middle and late stages of the disorder. Although classified as a single disorder, Yi and coworkers (1994) suggest that Alzheimer's disease represents a syndrome of related disorders with multiple origins.

The cognitive symptoms of dementia involve serious memory impairment and significant alterations in language, perceptual acuity, ability to abstract, ability to problem-solve, and ability to make appropriate judgments. Patients ultimately experience **global memory loss** (loss of all memory), and **aphasia** (loss of meaningful verbal communication). Noncognitive behavioral symptoms can be just as profound. They include significant personality changes, purposeless movements, agitation and aggression, overreaction to situations, irritating behavior, and emotional disinhibition. Medical terms related to the neurological, language, and behavioral deficits found with dementia are presented in Table 38–5.

Pick's Disease

Pick's disease occurs most often between the ages of 40 and 60, striking less than 1% of the population. Although the symptoms of Pick's disease resemble Alzheimer's disease in many ways, the changes in the brain differ. With Pick's disease, there is a characteristic shrinkage of brain tissue, particularly in the frontal and temporal lobes. Consequently, behavioral changes inconsistent with the level of cognitive deficit (language, memory, visuospatial skills) are early diagnostic signs (Keith, 1994). Emotional disinhibition, evidenced in hypersexuality and exhibitionism, can appear as a dominant behavioral symptom. Patients with Pick's disease typically display greater emotional apathy, irritability, or mood disturbance. Patients with this disorder may exhibit excessive ritualistic picking, scratching, licking, or sucking. Diagnosis of Pick's disease is based on results of CT imaging. There is no known cure for the disorder, and most of these patients die within six years of diagnosis (Edwards, 1994).

Creutzfeldt-Jakob Disease

Creutzfeldt-Jakob disease is an extremely rare brain disorder that causes dementia, occurring in approximately 1 of every million people (Edwards, 1994). The cause of the disorder is a slow-acting virus that has existed in the patient's body long before it manifests itself symptomatically. Symptoms are more varied than with Alzheimer's disease. They include psychotic behavior; loss of muscular function; and muscle spasms, seizures, and visual symptoms beyond memory loss. These patients show heightened emotional lability, and behavioral reactions can appear quite extreme (Edwards, 1994). Again, there is no known cure for the disorder, and patients typically die within a year of diagnosis.

Dementia of the Lewy Body Type

Lewy body dementia is a chronic cognitive disorder associated with subcortical pathology and the presence of Lewy body substance formation in the cerebral cortex. Similar to Alzheimer's disease, abnormal brain matter is found at autopsy. Although the Lewy body substance appears with senile neuritic plaques, the customary neurofibrillary tangles associated with Alzheimer's disease are scant or absent. Current findings suggest that dementia identified with this cause may be much more prevalent than originally suspected (Keith, 1994).

Consistent with a diagnosis of Lewy body dementia is a greater fluctuation of cognitive impairment with episodic periods of confusion and lucid intervals, similar to that seen with delirium. In contrast to the patient with delirium, however, the fluctuating symptom pattern persists over a significant period. Eventually the symptom pattern presents with the sustained serious neurological deficits associated with end-stage dementia. These patients show a toxic effect to neuroleptic medications, reacting with profound rigidity and immobility, and the course of their disease is more rapid than that seen with Alzheimer's disease. They are more likely to experience paranoid delusions, vivid hallucinations, unexplained falls, and transient disturbances in consciousness (Keith, 1994).

Dementia with Extrapyramidal Symptoms: Huntington's Disease

Huntington's disease, also known as Huntington's chorea and St. Vitus' dance because of its characteristic involuntary jerking movements, is an inherited progressive neurological disease. Huntington's disease is transmitted as an autosomal dominant trait (Keith, 1994). If one parent has the disorder, there is a 50% probability of it occurring in the child. Although the disease is present at birth, the symptoms manifest themselves in affected adults between the ages of 35 to 45.

Many but not all patients with the disorder eventually develop dementia. Huntington's disease affects reasoning abilities. Individuals with the disorder become poor problem-solvers, typically displaying impoverished judgment. Patients gradually lose their ability to converse intelligently and later to speak. Emotional disinhibition and aggressive behavior are common (Keith, 1994). Patients with Huntington's disease are at risk for suicide because of the depression often associated with the disorder and the knowledge that most of them have about the course of their disease. This disorder also presents with marked disturbances in motor abilities, particularly with abnormal random movements of the extremities and lower part of the body. Although the disorder can be diagnosed early, there is no cure. The prognosis is for a vegetative existence, and early death.

Dementia Due to Brain Lesions

Foci of Lesions

Anything that takes up space in the brain (subdural hematoma, intracranial neoplasm, aneurysm, benign cysts) can create cognitive changes. With a brain lesion, the patient initially presents with a sudden onset of symptoms and with a focal presentation of signs and symptoms related to the precise area of damaged brain tissue. Well-localized signs and symptoms always warrant CT scan and MRI and sometimes cerebral angiography to rule out possible brain lesions as part of the assessment protocol.

Vascular Dementia

Vascular dementia, the second most common chronic cognitive disorder, is a broad term used to describe dementia symptoms secondary to vascular disease of which there are many varieties. Multi-infarct dementia occurs most often. Consequently, many people refer to all types of vascular dementia as multi-infarct dementia when, in fact, there are many other subtypes. Multi-infarct dementia is associated with small cerebral vascular accidents (strokes), which cause cell destruction and death of brain tissue. Although a major stroke can represent a life-threatening event resulting in paralysis, coma, and death, smaller infarcts can affect speech, thought patterns, memory, and behavior. Cerebral emboli, more common with atherosclerosis, create a similar symptom pattern.

Brain imaging through a CT scan or MRI pinpoints the affected area and the extent of brain damage. Neurological examination includes level of consciousness, sensory evaluation, reflexes, and pain perception to verify the diagnosis. The degree of recovery from each infarct varies greatly, with some patients responding to medication and stabilizing at a relatively high level of cognitive functioning. Others show little or no recovery.

A history of hypertension (Forette and Boller, 1991) predisposes a person to the development of multi-infarct dementia, as does a history of hyperlipidemia, diabetes mellitus, cigarette smoking, and excessive alcohol consumption. Differential diagnosis is important for several reasons. First, medications can reduce hypertension and prevent new clots from forming. Second, surgery for clogged arteries is an option in some cases, with rapid recovery from dementia symptoms.

Any type of vascular impairment can destroy brain tissue. For example, a blood clot can block a cerebral artery, cutting off the supply of oxygen to the brain. A ruptured blood vessel in the brain can result in a hemorrhagic stroke. Brain tissue in the affected area dies within a few minutes of oxygen deprivation. From that point forward, the parts of the body controlled by those brain cells can no longer function properly.

There is little question that an accurate diagnosis and prompt treatment to minimize permanent brain damage are essential components of effective nursing care. With vascular dementia, the onset is more abrupt, and the patient displays a fluctuating course of symptom development. There is likely to be evidence of focal neurological signs and symptoms. Vascular dementia presents with a distinctive progression pattern. It manifests a less rapid and more stepwise mental decline than other forms of dementia. The progression of behavioral symptoms tends to plateau after each infarct, with each episode creating a deeper level of dysfunction (Hamdy et al, 1994). As the number of vascular insults increases, so does the level of cognitive deficit. Dementing signs and symptoms appear as patchy rather than global dysfunction. There is less evidence of the inclusive cortical dysfunction characteristic of Alzheimer's disease. Many of these patients retain intact functioning in some areas of daily self-care, while displaying significant deficits in others until the disorder is well advanced. Death often occurs from cardiac rather than neurological causes.

Another type of vascular dementia is called *Binswanger's disease*, named for Binswanger, who originally described it in 1894 as a chronic, progressive encephalitis. It is associated with persistent severe hypertension and systemic vascular disease. It presents as a degenerative subcortical vascular disorder with symptoms of dementia, focal neurological signs and symptoms, and significant motor deficits, including pseudobulbar palsy. The patient experiences aphasia, hemiplegia, and sensory disturbances consistent with subcortical infarctions involving the basal ganglia and thalamus. Diagnosis by CT scan and MRI is correlated with a decrease in the density of hemispheric white matter and significantly enlarged ventricles.

Dementia Associated with Other Physical Conditions

Normal-Pressure Hydrocephalus

Normal-pressure hydrocephalus is a reversible form of dementia that accounts for about 10% of cases. It occurs in elderly patients, as the brain atrophies, and additional fluid forms to fill the spaces in the ventricles. The patient typically presents with a triad of symptoms: memory loss, physical gait disturbances, and urinary incontinence. An early appearance of problems with gait or urinary incontinence suggests a differential diagnosis of normal-pressure hydrocephalus. Dementia symptoms can be completely reversed or significantly diminished with ventricle shunts inserted in the brain. Under sterile conditions, the surgeon inserts a plastic tube in the brain to reroute the fluid into the jugular vein. It is a procedure with significant risk to patients, but it offers them a temporary opportunity to reduce the impact of symptoms. Over time, the symptoms of dementia return and usually become permanent.

Alcohol-Induced Persisting Amnestic Disorders

Chronic use of alcohol can result in loss of brain cells and dementia. Without proper nutrition to provide needed vitamins, "slow starvation of brain cells may result" (Edwards, 1994, p. 69), and the person can develop dementia. **Alcohol-induced persisting amnestic disorder** or Korsakoff's syndrome, occurs because of a thiamine deficiency. The deficiency affects cortical functioning. If a person drinks enough over a significant period, there is brain cell destruction, accompanied by significant deficits in recent and remote memory. By contrast with the dementia associated with Alzheimer's disease, in which the progression is consistently downhill, the Korsakoff patient demonstrates fluctuation in symptoms and changes in personality. The symptoms are more compatible with the pathophysiological changes secondary to excessive alcohol abuse. Such patients may demonstrate consistent difficulty with abstract thinking and calculations and impaired judgment. They do not, however, show the progressive intellectual deterioration associated with the diffuse neurological signs of Alzheimer's disease or the stepwise progression of a multi-infarct dementia.

AIDS Dementia Complex

AIDS dementia complex is a behavioral syndrome that can appear as an isolated symptom set or with other CNS complications of the AIDS virus. Symptoms reflect global cognitive impairment. Patients have **ataxia** (lack of motor coordination), memory disturbances, and an inability to concentrate. Typically, motor problems precede other cognitive symptoms. Once begun, however, the course of the syndrome can be rapid, "characterized by severe dementia with mutism that occurs within a few weeks or months, or it can be a milder, less precipitous one that lasts many months or longer than a year" (Hamdy et al, 1994, p. 55). Typically the patient loses memory for recent events and is unable to carry out activities of daily living without considerable assistance.

Parkinson's Disease

The development of **Parkinson's disease** appears to be associated with a deficiency of dopamine, a neurotransmitter in the brain needed for controlling complex muscle function. Parkinson's disease can produce dementia symptoms, particularly if the disorder develops later in life.

Dementia symptoms occur in approximately 30% to 40% of patients with Parkinson's disease, and more subtle cognitive changes are noted in an additional 40% (Keith, 1994; Cummings, 1988). For this reason, these patients need to have a good neurological assessment at regular intervals. Another reason for a good differential diagnosis of signs and symptoms associated with dementia is the higher-than-normal incidence of depression in Parkinson patients. Depressive symptoms respond to antidepressant medication.

The disease itself typically appears in middle adulthood (45 to 65 years), and progressive neurological deterioration occurs over many years. Typically the dementia associated with Parkinson's disease takes the form of a marked difficulty with language function and abstract thinking rather than significant memory loss (Edwards, 1994). Patients experience dysarthria and impaired ability to retrieve information. Although less able to process information, they typically do not seem to have the same level of aphasia and agnosia experienced by Alzheimer's disease patients. Parkinson's disease and Alzheimer's disease can occur together, thus complicating the diagnostic picture (Keith, 1994).

Multiple Sclerosis

Patients with advanced multiple sclerosis can demonstrate dementia symptoms secondary to multiple sclerosis. The course of the disease is quite similar to that of Parkinson's disease but is related to CNS demyelination (Absher and Cummings, 1994). Additionally, significant personality alterations appear, typically apathy or mood swings. Patients do not display the behavioral problems associated with other forms of dementia.

Depressive Disorder

Depressive disorder in the elderly frequently presents with symptoms characteristic of irreversible dementia. Some people call this a reversible dementia, or **pseudodementia,** because although the symptoms are similar, the disorder is treatable. In reality, depression in the elderly is neither a reversible nor a pseudo form of dementia. It is a mood disorder presenting with marked vegetative symptoms and acute confusion that mimic the chronic cognitive disorder. It is treatable in many cases with appropriate antidepressants.

There are several important differences that can aid the clinician in making a differential diagnosis. There are significant differences in the patient's history and in the way patients express themselves about their symptoms. Answers to assessment questions reflect a personal or family history of depressive disorder. The patient expresses feelings of worthlessness, hopelessness, or anhedonia. A rapid onset, particularly if associated with a life event or situation, suggests a differential diagnosis of depressive disorder. Usually the depressed patient recognizes that something is wrong with concentration or memory. The dementia patient typically does not display a similar awareness. These patients sense that there is something wrong, but they seem less concerned and are unable to pinpoint the nature of their difficulty—for example, in concentrating.

Depression can be a clinical feature superimposed on early dementia because the signs and symptoms of chronic cognitive disorders tell only one part of the dementia story: Inevitably the human story line of dementia is about loss. Personal losses suffered with chronic cognitive disorders are profound, multidimensional, and progressive for patients even in the early stage. Antidepressant medications can relieve depressive symptoms, although they cannot retard the progression of the neurological symptoms.

Treatment of depressive symptoms is an option for the caregiver. Although not a part of the patient picture, clinical depression is a common finding among caregivers, particularly those with limited options and sources of social support. As the story of the journey clouded by cognitive disorder unfolds, everyone involved encounters, with shattering clarity, the meaning of *person,* the challenge of compassion, and the limits of medical knowledge. The recognition of the losses involved—self, role, value, dignity, and personal meaning for the victim and loss of freedom and status for the caregiver—are inevitable.

▶ Check Your Reading

8. What would be the first nursing action in the treatment of delirium? Why is this action important?
9. How can the nurse distinguish between the symptoms of delirium and dementia?
10. What are the primary differences between Alzheimer's disease and vascular dementia?

Incidence and Prevalence of Dementia

Alzheimer's disease, the most common cause of dementia, accounts for 60% to 80% of dementia cases (Weiler, 1994). Treatment costs range from $80 to $90 billion a year (Hamdy et al, 1994). The disorder is age related because the prevalence and incidence of the disorder increase sharply with age. These data are consistent worldwide (Rocca, 1994). Alzheimer's disease, however, is not a normal process of aging. Healthy older adults do not experience profound cognitive deficits as they age. They may demonstrate a gradual decline in recall and recognition memory, but healthy older adults retain **crystallized intelligence,** found in the individual's commonsense judgments, creativity, and wisdom. This form of cognitive growth continues to develop, reflecting the elder's broad life knowledge and experience (Miller, 1990).

The incidence of dementia is on the increase. People are living longer, and past the age of 70, the frequency of a dementia diagnosis jumps substantially. Moreover the elderly represent the most rapidly growing segment of the population in the United States. By the year 2050, approximately 67 million Americans will be 65 or older, and of this number, approximately 14 million will develop dementia.

Dementia affects women more often than men. Other demographic variables, such as occupation, marital status, or living arrangements, do not appear greatly to affect the development of the disorder. Research findings supporting an association between level of education are mixed, with some studies demonstrating increased frequency in subjects with less education. Other studies, however, failed to confirm this finding (Beard et al, 1992). Some studies suggest a higher incidence of dementia among patients with previous head trauma, particularly associated with loss of consciousness (Chandra et al, 1989).

Speculation About Causes of Dementia

Theories about the causes of dementia of the Alzheimer type are many and varied. To date, however, researchers have been unable to pinpoint the precise cause of dementia. Currently, there is no known therapeutic treatment to stop the progression of neurological deficit symptoms. Common theories include the following speculations.

Increased Aluminum

Elevated trace levels of aluminum have been found in the brain tissues of Alzheimer's victims (Cooke and Gould, 1991). Aluminum exists free floating in the atmosphere, however, and is found routinely in many commonly used deodorants, some antacids such as Tums, and other substances. People with cancer of the digestive tract who cannot metabolize aluminum, and consequently may have elevated levels of the metal, do not develop dementia.

Genetic Loading

Certain family genograms demonstrate a high familial incidence, with specific clinical features of early onset and rapid progression in a larger-than-normal percentage of first-degree relatives (Breitner and Folstein, 1984). In these families, more than 50% of clinically diagnosed dementia patients have at least one first-degree relative with the disorder. Evidence of a genetic abnormality on chromosome 14 is associated with the disorder. Genetic mapping may provide some clues to familial occurrence in Alzheimer's disease.

One of the strongest arguments for a genetic formulation of the disorder is its connection with Down's syndrome. Scientists have identified gene sites on chromosome 21 for the amyloid protein precursor of Alzheimer's disease. Alzheimer's disease is more prevalent in families with Down's syndrome. Of patients with Down's syndrome who live much past the age of 35, a large percentage develop symptoms of dementia (Edwards, 1994).

Decreased Acetylcholine

The role of acetylcholine in the development of dementia has been studied extensively (Hamdy et al, 1994). **Acetylcholine** is a neurotransmitter judged essential in message transmission by "carrying the electrical impulse across the synapse from the axon of one cell to the dendrite of another" (Edwards, 1993, p. 69). Abnormally low levels of the neurotransmitter have been found in the brain tissue of patients with dementia. Researchers had hoped that by giving dementia patients lecithin, a food substance containing choline, the precursor of acetylcholine, and hydrogine, a medication with similar properties, they might be able to stimulate memory and retard memory loss. Attempts to treat patients clinically using this drug have, however, proven uneventful, despite clear evidence that a significant loss of the transmitter occurs with dementia.

The Food and Drug Administration has approved a new drug, tetrahydroaminoacridine (THA), known by the trade names Tacrine and Cognex, for use with patients with early dementia. This drug, marketed by Parke Davis, works by inhibiting the breakdown of acetylcholine. Although this drug does not modify the overall progression of the disorder, it appears to have a delaying effect on the memory loss in the beginning stages in some patients. The predominant potential side effect is liver toxicity. Careful weekly monitoring of SGOT for liver toxicity should accompany administration of this drug. Other relevant side effects include gastrointestinal distress ranging from nausea to diarrhea and abdominal pain.

Slow-Acting Virus

Some researchers believed that a slow-acting virus created the neurofibrillary tangles in the brain associated with dementia, but reports of studies designed to isolate the virus or to replicate the symptoms in animals have failed to verify an association (Rocca, 1994).

Care of the Dementia Patient

The staging of dementia is important because the symptoms and related levels of nursing care differ so dramatically in each stage. Care begins as supportive for the patient and educative for the family in the early stage. In the middle stage, nursing care is largely oriented toward behavior management. The nurse or primary caregiver provides total care for patients in the late stage. These stages in the course of a dementing illness, although fluctuating in duration, are so consistent that they provide a suitable framework for considering the comprehensive care of the dementia patient from diagnosis to death.

Three goals, referred to as the 3 Ps (protecting, preserving, promoting) govern the care of the dementia patient from initial diagnosis to death (Table 38–6).

TABLE 38–6 **Goals for Care of the Patient with Cognitive Disorders: The Three Ps**

Goal	Related Intervention
Protecting the dignity of the patient	Referring to the patient by name Individualizing nursing actions Incorporating cultural standards Providing privacy
Preserving functional status	Providing a structured environment Working from the patient's strengths Encouraging socialization Providing boards and cues for reality orientation Making routines of care consistent
Promoting quality of life	Stating advance directives Supporting losses Encouraging family interaction

Protecting the Dignity of the Patient

Patients with dementia lose all defining characteristics of self, but they should never have to lose their right to dignity as unique human beings. You can protect the dignity of the patient in many ways. Some actions are quite simple. Referring to the patient by name each time you enter the room acknowledges the patient as a person. Avoid calling the patient "honey," "baby," or "sweetie," and hence recognize the person with dementia as an adult, not a child, even though behaviors are not those of an adult.

Related to acknowledging the patient's name is recognizing the patient's presence, even when the individual is unable to participate fully in the discussion. More often than not, health care conversations take place in the presence of the dementia patient, but they occur almost as if the patient were not physically present. The staff talk to the family without ever looking at or verbally acknowledging the patient's presence. Regardless of the patient's mental condition, the nurse can protect the person's dignity with a simple introduction. Identifying the purpose of the consultation in simple words places the patient as part of the conversation and provides important orienting cues. Modest eye contact and body movements that include the patient in the conversation can occur with little effort, without distracting from the information given to family members.

For example, a physician assigned to Paul Noble, a patient with suspected dementia, came into the room and began examining him without an introduction. The physician talked across the hospital bed, to the family but not to Paul, about the diagnostic testing he was proposing. At one point in the conversation, Paul said, "I'm Paul Noble, and I didn't catch your name." The physician then introduced himself. This patient was sufficiently alert to call attention to the physician's lack of acknowledgment and join the discussion that directly affected his health care. When this is not possible, *you* need to call explicit attention to the patient's dignity as a human being.

Responding to communication efforts, rather than dismissing them as irrelevant or correcting them as untrue, recognizes the patient's attempt to connect through words. For example, one patient consistently greeted his nurse with "Hi, Sally, how are the kids?" In this situation, an appropriate response might be "Mr. Jones, tell me about Sally. It sounds like she was someone special in your life." A little later, the nurse might add, "I think I may remind you of someone else, but my name is Mrs. Allen, and I will be your nurse for the day." Making an issue of the patient's confusion through direct confrontation and immediate correction of a cognitive error rarely is useful. Entering the patient's life and stating the person's name at the beginning of the conversation fosters social bonding.

Individualized physical and socially oriented nursing actions that acknowledge the unique humanness of the dementia patient concurrently reinforce the patient's dignity. For example, considering the patient's cultural standards and religious preferences in planning care can answer fundamental social and spiritual needs. Individualizing basic nursing actions can be as simple as providing the patient with privacy for intimate examinations, toileting, bathing, and dressing. That the patient is unaware of nakedness is unimportant. Even if the patient cannot fully appreciate your efforts, the family usually is grateful for respect shown a dementing relative's personhood. You are often an innocent but important role model of respect for family and ancillary personnel taking care of the patient. Nursing actions to show respect take little additional time or skill. Yet each time you confirm the value of the dementia patient as a person through words, actions, and touch, caring in the true sense of the word occurs.

Preserving Functional Status

Preserving functional status is particularly important during the early stage because cognitive deficits are mild. Again the interventions are simple caring actions that require only time, patience, and imagination. Most people, including dementia patients, perform more effectively when they are acting on their personal strengths and preferences. Detailed information regarding previous functioning and behavior, likes and dislikes provides a baseline for choosing nursing interventions that best support the patient's independent functioning. Dementia patients frequently have difficulty staying involved with daily activities and taking charge of their lives without cues even in the early stage. Although they continue to participate in planned activities, these patients frequently need some assistance with structuring their free time. They also may need reminders to complete tasks and verbal cues on how to accomplish them.

In the middle stage of progressive dementia, you have to look for patient strengths, but they are still there. Hall and Buckwalter (1987) propose a stress reduction model for behavioral management of dementia patients based on supporting patient strengths and reframing patient losses. For example, you can recast the incessant pacing of the patient as getting rid of excess energy. Although the patient's behavior remains the same, its meaning is different. Once the family (and you) can see a positive aspect to the patient's annoying behavior, it becomes easier to tolerate.

Once the patient enters the late stage of dementia and assumes a vegetative state, little functional ability remains. You can still, however, support the little that is left. For example, offering the patient juices, using the patient's hand to guide a spoon, and stroking the throat while telling the patient to swallow fulfill this function.

Personal strengths of individual and collective family members also are important to assess and reinforce because the patient's quality of care ultimately depends on the family's investment. These can include a strong faith, a loving relationship with the patient, financial resources, and a good sense of humor. Each of these personal assets can lend resiliency to the caregiving role and ultimately benefit the patient.

Promoting Quality of Life

It is not easy to watch a person deteriorate neurologically and change from a functional adult to a vegetative state,

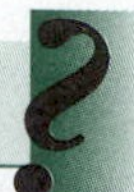

WHAT FAMILIES NEED TO KNOW — Dementia

How do I know if my family member has dementia?
Some of the early signs family members notice are a change in cognitive functioning or personality. Short-term memory impairment occurs with a noticeable loss of the ability to remember activities of daily living, including carrying on a meaningful conversation. The most disturbing and troubling symptoms are related to personality changes. A lower frustration level, a lack of interest, and a decreased attention span are among the early changes noted. Restlessness and rapid mood changes may occur, followed by periods of blank facial expression. In the early stage, the patient may be aware that something is wrong with his or her mind and how it's working.

What can I do to help?
No known cures for dementia exist. Learning about the disease process of dementia is important. The National Alzheimer's Association is an excellent source of education and support. Most cities have local chapters and may provide a hotline for assistance.

unable to communicate and incapable of even simple personal care. Quality-of-life issues begin to emerge with diagnosis, and the family must move quickly on the patient's behalf to maximize quality of life later. For example, financial and legal planning should be enacted early, when patients are still aware of what their decisions mean. Eventually the patient will lose the mental capacity to handle money matters, make decisions about property, and implement advance directives legally. Advise patients to protect assets through a **durable power of attorney,** which designates a decision maker, and to initiate **living wills,** which describe a patient's wishes, early in the disease process, when patients know what they are signing. Having these documents can prevent later problems.

Throughout the illness, professional and family caregivers can provide for the patient's quality of life by anticipating and responding to patient distress in a compassionate, knowledgeable manner. Education and emotional support for family members helps caregivers take the necessary actions to enhance the quality of the patient's life and their own lives.

Quality of life becomes particularly important in the late stage of dementia, creating significant ethical dilemmas for many families. Family members often are in a quandary about whether to provide nutrition and hydration when the patient can no longer function as a human being. Use of intravenous lines to support hydration is a question when the quality of life is so limited. The desirability of prolonging life is a common source of conflict. Ideally, these decisions related to care are made before the need presents itself because discontinuance of extraordinary measures is difficult once they are initiated. Hospice services can provide significant comfort and family support during the terminal stages of the illness. Pointing this resource out may be necessary because many families do not think of hospice as a resource for the dementia patient.

Implementation: Levels of Care

Early Stages of Dementia

The elusive and varied presentation of Alzheimer's disease in the early stage makes it difficult for families to recognize the problem as dementia. From a medical perspective, signs and symptoms reflect the number of neurofibrillary tangles and neuritic plaques found in focal areas of brain tissue destruction. Later the destruction of brain tissue becomes global, affecting all areas of the brain and human functioning. But the effects of dementia are more complicated and puzzling, particularly in the initial stage. Although subtle signs of memory loss and personality changes suggest that something is wrong, most early-stage patients display fragmentary cognitive decline, with many areas remaining cognitively intact. Thus, brief visits with the patient do not reveal significant changes that alert the observer to dementia. These patients can rally cognitive functions for short periods and appear quite normal. Only if visitors stay for a while, usually for more than a few days, is it possible to see the full extent of the problem. Clarifying with family members that this is a common occurrence often is helpful for them because it is easy to doubt one's own reality in the beginning stages of a dementia.

Often family members, living on a daily basis with patients in the early stage, are not fully aware of the bit-by-bit cognitive or personality losses associated with dementia. Emotionally wanting the patient to be the same can blind the caregiver to the possibility of a significant cognitive deficit. Often, they doubt their own perceptions, much as Mrs. Michaels did. Their relative typically retains superficial social skills and many automatic functional abilities. Physical appearance does not change dramatically. Although patients may appear emotionally distant in many social situations, they generally can respond appropriately when addressed by others. Sometimes, it takes a visit from an adult child or old family friend to call attention to the patient's cognitive decline.

Nursing care of patients in the early stage typically takes place in the home, unless the patient is admitted for diagnostic studies or another reason. (See Chapter 44 for more on home health assessment.) The nurse's role is primarily educational when the nurse is called for other medical reasons or at a community health presentation. Care in the early stage centers on the following critical care issues:

- Obtaining a differential diagnosis
- Family education

- Patient safety
- Conservation of functional ability
- Legal protection

DIFFERENTIAL DIAGNOSIS

Obtaining an accurate differential diagnosis of dementia is essential. Alzheimer's disease is basically a **rule-out disorder;** that is, the diagnosis is made after family history, laboratory tests, and brain imaging eliminate other disorders with similar cognitive deficits from active consideration. A differential diagnosis to rule out toxic or metabolic causes is extremely important. Some forms of dementia are reversible or controllable with medication. Kaplan and Sadock (1991) estimate that up to 20% of individuals presenting with dementia symptoms have a reversible form of the disorder, and another 20% can experience symptom reduction. For the limited percentage of patients with a reversible cognitive disorder, these figures have significant clinical value.

Sources of information needed to make a differential diagnosis of dementia include a full neurological assessment, laboratory tests to rule out metabolic factors (see Table 38–4), family history of the patient's past behavior and symptom progression, mini-mental status examination (see Chapter 13), and functional assessment of activities of daily living. A CT scan identifies structural deficits. Brain imaging with positron emission tomography provides the clinician with information about changes in the metabolic activity and neurochemical characteristics associated with dementia.

If medical test findings fail to account for the cognitive changes, the differential diagnosis is Alzheimer's disease. Typically, testing of patients in the early stage reveals a normal EEG, CT, and MRI. Findings from laboratory tests are within normal range. Guidelines for a multidisciplinary psychiatric assessment are presented in Table 38–7. Extensive psychotherapy is not indicated in the care of dementia patients, but supportive interventions may help alleviate depressive symptoms in the early stage.

Nursing diagnoses are expressed in functional terms and reflect the patient's ability to meet basic needs. Sample nursing diagnoses describing the patient may include

- Altered Thought Processes related to dementia
- Impaired Physical Mobility related to compromised cortical functioning
- Alteration in Nutrition, less than body requirements, related to neurological deficits in swallowing

TABLE 38–7 Psychiatric Assessment of the Patient with Alzheimer's Disease

Purpose	Assessment of primary and secondary psychiatric manifestations of Alzheimer's disease and differential diagnosis from Psychosis Depression Anxiety and phobias Behavioral disturbances Rule out delirium Assess needs and strengths of patient, caregiver, and family Treatment planning Educate caregivers
Areas assessed	Family history (dementing illness, psychiatric disease, neurologic disease, substance abuse) Social history (education, past level of functioning per occupational history, close relationships, current living situation) Medical history (all past and present medical illnesses; past surgeries; past trauma, especially head; allergies; medication) Psychiatric history (psychotic illness, depressive illness, other psychiatric illnesses, psychiatric symptoms, past and current treatments, hospitalizations, suicide, violence) Present illness (length of cognitive loss, other presenting problems, physical symptoms, functional deficits, psychiatric symptoms) Mental status (appearance, behavior, speech, mood, hallucinations, delusions, anxiety, phobias, cognition) For delirium: medical evaluation For behavioral disturbances: environment
Process	History of patient, caregiver, and family Mental status examination Medication review
Sources of information	Patient, caregiver, and family Past medical and psychiatric records Multidisciplinary team

From Abraham, I., Holroyd, S., Snustad, D., Manning, C., Brashear, H., Deamond D, and Thompson-Heisterurau, A. (1994). Multidisciplinary assessment of patients with Alzheimer's disease. *Nursing Clinics of North America, 29*(1), p. 120.

BOX 38-4 Behavior Patterns Found in the Early Stage

- Initial variance according to which part of the brain is most affected
- Forgetfulness
- Trouble concentrating, carrying on an in-depth conversation
- Trouble coping with everyday events, particularly unstructured
- Change in personality, most commonly apathy, irritability, or sudden temper outbursts
- Language disturbance
- Limited problem-solving ability, ability to learn new things

- Ineffective Individual Coping related to cognitive deficits
- Self-Care Deficit related to cognitive deficits around bathing, grooming, eating

Nursing diagnoses involving the family may include

- Ineffective Family Coping related to care of the dementia patient
- Knowledge Deficit related to the disease and care of the dementia patient
- Spiritual Distress related to caregiver burden associated with dementia
- Caregiver Role Strain related to 24-hour care
- Social Isolation related to 24-hour care of the dementia patient

Altered Role Performance is a relevant diagnosis for both patient and caregiver, as is Powerlessness related to the diagnosis of a terminal illness.

Because dementia is basically a rule-out disorder, an accurate history of past performance and functioning is of primary importance. Edwards (1993) notes that "dementia expresses itself by interfering with the normal or usual pattern of behavior demonstrated by the individual in the past" (p. 55). A detailed history of the individual's behavioral changes from those who are most familiar with the patient's normal behavior is invaluable. In fact, some geropsychiatric researchers consider this historical data the most important aspect of the assessment process (Matzo, 1990). The focus of the family history interview is on identifying the ways in which the patient's behaviors disrupt current functioning and noting changes from past performance. Box 38–4 summarizes behaviors characteristic of the early stage.

Ask questions about past psychiatric history, particularly depression and chemical dependence, head trauma, and recent stressful events. Data about sleeping and eating patterns, level of supervision required, availability of care, and financial resources help the clinician understand the nature and depth of the cognitive deficit. Box 38–5 is an assessment guide outlining areas of psychosocial concern with potential behavioral descriptors. You can use this guide or a similar format to develop and document baseline behavioral data from the assessment interview.

APPEARANCE

Although few changes in physical characteristics are visible to the casual observer, the family may have noticed a distinct change in the patient's attention to dress and cleanliness. Lack of interest in hygiene is common. A problem less frequently talked about involves the cleanliness of patients living alone. With dementia, the sense of smell diminishes, so the patient may have a strong urine smell from not bathing or wiping correctly without being aware of it. Most patients, even in the early stage, may need gentle encouragement to shower daily and to use good oral hygiene.

MEMORY DEFICITS

Memory impairment during the early stages involves the storage and retrieval of new information. The patient's recent memory loss is not a simple forgetting of objects such as a pocketbook or an appointment. Rather it is for common activities of daily living that the individual was able to recall without any difficulty. **Short-term memory** (immediate and recent memory) for things that happened that day, or even a few minutes ago, is impaired, whereas in most instances **remote memory** for events in the past is preserved. Thus, these patients typically can recall what happened 10 years ago but cannot tell the interviewer what they just had for breakfast or whether it was raining yesterday.

Learning new information is no longer possible because the short-term memory required to process and synthesize new information misses a meaningful connection with the current situation (Hamdy et al, 1994). Memory loss creates demonstrable problems with initiating and sustaining conversations. Patients evidence constructional difficulty and cannot put discrete pieces of data or objects together in a meaningful whole.

PERSONALITY CHANGES

Ironically, often the personality changes accompanying memory loss rather than the loss itself cause family members to seek a definitive diagnosis for their relative. Common personality changes involve low tolerance for normal frustration and oversensitivity to the remarks of others. Family members complain of their relative's lack of initiative, decreased attention span, and diminished emotional presence. They describe declining self-awareness as: "He just doesn't seem interested anymore." "He seems to get angry over things that never bothered him before." "She just seems so self-absorbed, not at all like her old self."

Emotional lability and restlessness are other characteristic behaviors. A dementia patient can go from tears to laughter, from silence to boisterous talking, all in a matter of minutes. A patient may deny an emotional state or feeling reaction to a situation, even with direct confrontation. Moreover, the patient's facial expression may show little response to change, although agitated and clenched body language frequently speaks volumes. Some patients sit for long periods with a blank stare. When spoken to, there seems to be a delayed reaction before the patient responds. Rumination about a variety of subjects is common.

Other personality changes involve patient judgments about critical matters, hoarding, or giving away assets. The affected individual does not seem as aware of the risks involved or the consequences of certain life decisions related to money and other assets. Not uncommonly, patients with an undiagnosed dementia appear in the psychiatrist's office seeking marital therapy because the spouse feels a husband (wife) is becoming increasingly irresponsible and not attending to previous obligations such as payment of bills.

Other factors, such as delirium, depression, and unfamiliar environments, can account for some personality changes, and these need to be accounted for before attributing them to the dementia. For example, more than a few patients in the early stage are aware that there is something wrong with their minds. When the Alzheimer's patient clutches his head, and asks "What is wrong with me," or makes statements such as "I wish I were dead" or "I want to go home," these are all poignant indications of the anguish of experiencing a world that is slipping out of view. As the disease progresses, patients become less acutely aware of most things in their world, including the meaning of their illness. Initially, however, awareness is common, and you need to monitor patients showing depressive ideation closely. Any attempt, gesture, or specific plan of suicide is cause for alarm. Antidepressant medication, carefully monitored, can provide a significantly higher quality of life for many patients in the early stage.

COMMUNICATION DIFFICULTY

Communication difficulties appear early in the disorder, occurring as one or more of the language problems identified in Table 38–8. Suggested nursing interventions are provided related to each type of deficit. Some patients handle their problem with word finding and comprehension by filling in the blanks with new data that may or may not make sense. Others become silent rather than expose their deficit. For many patients, the language deficits in dementia begin with difficulty finding the right words to express a complete thought or to describe an object.

BOX 38–5 Nursing Assessment Guide for Developing Behavioral Assessments on Dementia Patients

Category: Appearance (hygiene, physical characteristics, cleanliness, dress)

Behavioral descriptors: neat/disheveled appearance, poor/good physical hygiene, cachectic/normal body weight, erect/stooped/listing posture, weakness in arms/legs, gross/fine tremors

Category: Memory deficits (recent and remote memory, orientation, intellectual judgment, insight)

Behavioral descriptors: Memory loss (assess immediate, recent, and remote), visual/spatial skills, appropriate/inappropriate problem-solving, knowledge of current events, confabulation, presence of visual/auditory hallucinations, delusions, thought blocking, orientation to person/place/time, misinterpretation of visual/auditory/olfactory stimuli, ability to engage in tasks requiring multiple skill knowledge

Category: Personality Changes (mood, and emotions expressed)

Behavioral descriptors: Appropriate/inappropriate, bland, flat, dull, sad, fearful facial expression; labile, dull, angry, euphoric, limited, agitated, suspicious, cooperative, appropriate/inappropriate expression of feeling; personality changes noted by family; over/under reaction to situations, distractibility, appropriate/inappropriate judgment (give specific example); makes lewd remarks, exposes self, openly masturbates, touches people inappropriately

Category: Psychomotor Functioning (motor activity, human response to situation)

Behavioral descriptors: Lack of precision in voluntary movements, hyperactive, pacing, slowed movements, repetitive or nondirective gestures; disturbance in sleep patterns, difficulty walking, seizures, loses balance, night walking, aimless/goal-directed actions, sundown syndrome

Category: Communication Ability (ability to communicate verbally and in writing)

Behavioral descriptors: Delayed/blocked verbal communication, mutism, inability to grasp meaning of spoken/written word, perseveration, inability to find words, difficulty writing words and signing name

Category: Nutrition and Elimination

Behavioral descriptors: Nutrition above/below nutritional requirements; refuses food, sits and stares at food, "cheeks" food without swallowing, tries to eat inedible objects/spoiled food; difficulty with swallowing, choking; incontinence (specify bladder, bowel); smears feces, urinates/defecates in inappropriate places

TABLE 38–8 **Communication Problems and Nursing Interventions in the Early Stage**

Patient Problem	Nursing Intervention
Problem finding words	Supply missing words, name objects, post printed signs for common word objects
Difficulty with comprehension	Use simple concrete words, one thought at a time, use names instead of pronouns
Communication anxiety increases in crowds	Limit number of people present during an interview
Shortened attention span	Use short sessions rather than long ones; gauge interactions by observing patient behavior
Delayed verbal response	Allow for additional processing time. Restate message using the same words if necessary; reinforce all attempts at communication
Increasing agitation	Use eye contact, a calm reassuring voice, and patient observation to diffuse the situation; give reassurance, acceptance, and full attention to patient needs
Tells the same story repetitively	Ask the patient to expand on a small part of the story, thank the patient for sharing and move to a different topic, identify and use the underlying theme

Compounding the language problem is a concurrent reduction in the flow of ideas.

Superficial conversations usually fail to reveal thought blocking. Only when the conversation progresses to a deeper level requiring abstract thinking and complex problem-solving does the difficulty emerge. This is both good and bad. It is good in the sense that the individual responds appropriately and continues to receive the social support from others. It is bad in the sense that other people are not always aware of the patient's problems until well into the conversation, thus creating embarrassment for the patient and the involved listener, as Case Example 38–1 shows.

Case Example 38–1 Bill's Story

Bill Clarke is a dementia patient who appears friendly and physically fit. His wife took him to the podiatrist, and as he was waiting for his turn, a Red Cross worker struck up a conversation with him. "Isn't it wonderful that Sandra O'Connor was named to the Supreme Court," she said. And Bill replied, "Yes, it is wonderful. It's about time something like this happened." Encouraged by his response, the Red Cross worker said, "And isn't it terrible that Anwar Sadat was killed." To which Bill replied, "Yes, it is wonderful. It's about time something like this happened." The worker looked at him with an odd expression, as she realized that he was responding automatically but had little comprehension of the meaning of his words.

Even in the early stage, naming familiar objects (**anomia**) is a problem for many patients. The words may still be available to the patient, but their meaning undergoes subtle modification. For example, Francis Michaels had been able to remember his law case citations without prompting. In the early stages of the disease, he was able to use the cues from his wife and look up the citations to continue his law practice. His previous reputation for legal excellence and semblance of similar functioning initially prompted his clients to overlook what was increasingly obvious to his family—that Francis was no longer able to fully comprehend what he was reading. Labeling common objects, placing clothing and utensils in sequential order, periodically explaining TV commentary, and saying the name of visitors as they enter the room are all strategies to help the patient with object name recognition.

Conversation is particularly difficult for the patient if there are several people talking or the conversation requires sudden shifts to a different topic. Patients may have difficulty understanding complex statements made by others, or they may fail to comprehend issues entirely. Transitions from one subject to another are less fluid. Simple nursing actions can help the patient maintain focus on the conversation by, for example, providing logical links through words and spacing the concrete verbal, visual, and tactile prompts needed to comprehend basic messages. Using multiple communication modalities in the delivery of a message also helps patients to grasp ideas. For example, using written words or pictures to complement the spoken word, touch to emphasize a point, or looking in the direction of the object described can assist patients in continuing a social conversation.

Because long-term memory is not affected in the early stages, conversations focused on the past have meaning to both the patient and the caregiver. Patients have an easier time expressing connected thoughts about the past. Speech is more spontaneous because the patient does not have to "think" about the interrelationships in the story. Content relationships already are present and are logically assembled in long-term memory. Thus, patients find it easier to describe a past feeling from memory than to identify their present emotional state. Comprehension of verbal messages increases with the use of simple language, presenting one idea at a time, and using the same words with repetitive instructions.

PSYCHOMOTOR FUNCTIONING

When the nurse focuses on the patient's abilities rather than disabilities and designs interventions to support strengths and compensate for behavioral losses, patients often can respond on a higher level. Being able to perform simple tasks gives the patient a sense of mastery.

The ability to handle gadgets and to carry out coordinated purposeful movements, actions so automatic for most people, fade in the course of dementia, despite the patient's ownership of intact skeletal, motor, and sensory body systems. Referred to as **apraxia,** the patient's motor deficit is more apparent with new or more complex tasks and consequently may be dismissed as an unfamiliarity with the task requirements. More automatic motor activities, such as dressing, eating, and walking, show less decline until the patient has moved into the middle stages of the disease. As tasks requiring complicated purposeful movements become increasingly difficult for patients to maneuver, the patient's behavioral response turns into anger or passivity. Either response provides a dilemma. It saddens the caregiver to watch the person give up and sit with a dejected posture, uninterested and uninvolved—without hope. Handling the anger without retaliating also is difficult because of the amount of attention and repetition required for task completion. The incessant nature of the demand with such a limited outcome tries the patience of even the most dedicated caregiver.

The inability to complete simple tasks is not the fault of the patient. In the early stage, the patient sincerely wants to help but cannot complete coordinated tasks without verbal prompts and constant attention. Yet the semi-involvement and understanding of part, but not all, of the steps needed for task completion is bewildering for the family caregiver, as Case Example 38–2 illustrates.

Case Example 38–2 Betty's Story

Betty tries to do many things around the house—set the table, wash the dishes, dust the furniture, and little things like that. She is always eager to help, but she gets confused and doesn't finish anything. That's what gets me so upset. I get so frustrated sometimes that I want to lash out. For example, she will get the silverware out of the drawer, walk to the table, pick up the napkins, and walk back to the drawer with both silverware and napkins. I know that Alzheimer's is causing her to act this way, but little things happen like this every day. She seems so normal in many ways, but it's like only half of her mind is working (Cohen and Eisdorfer, 1986, p. 204).

The family needs education and emotional support to surmount these difficulties. Practical strategies help the caregiver to respond properly to the patient's constant desire to be involved and equally persistent need for supervision to complete even simple tasks. First, acknowledge the caregiver's frustration as a valid response. It is difficult for the caregiver to be patient and understanding. Explaining that the dementia patient literally is working with half a mind even though the person appears normal often helps caregivers appreciate the paradox of the situation. Moreover, these patients pick up the caregiver's anxiety, further adding to their confusion. Tasks involving multiple or concurrent steps should be avoided. Simple tasks with well-defined sequential steps are more appropriate. The caregiver can help the patient break the task into simpler steps and can "walk" him or her verbally through each step to task completion. Praise helps reduce anxiety, and modeling behaviors provide additional cues. Knowing that the *coordinating steps* function of the cerebral cortex is lost to the patient and that this type of help is essential for task completion helps with family acceptance. If the task is too difficult or is likely to create unmanageable frustration for the patient to complete, the caregiver has another option. Distraction and postponement are always useful strategies even in the early stage.

NUTRITION AND ELIMINATION

A final area of concern is the patient's nutritional status and elimination patterns. Many patients begin to have eating difficulties even in the early stage. Their table manners become lax, and sometimes they forget they have just eaten or fail to know when it is mealtime without prompting. Caregivers need to assume responsibility for ensuring adequate nutritional intake. Elimination habits are important pieces of data. Having knowledge of the patient's normal elimination patterns during the early stage helps the caregiver time bathroom breaks later on when the patient needs assistance.

FAMILY EDUCATION

In the early stage, family members provide most of the care for patients, with episodic support from the nurse and the intermittent use of adult day centers. For months, even years, patients can remain independent with minimal assistance. Most patients in the early stage can communicate their needs, at least on a superficial level, and they seem normal to others. In fact, the spouse of a dementia patient who looked older than her husband was asked by an attorney with some embarrassment, "I know this is an unusual question, but which one of you is the Alzheimer's patient?"

Education of the family begins as soon as the diagnosis is confirmed. Immediate family members play an important role in the care of the dementia patient, first as informants, then as patient advocates, and finally as the primary caregiver and patient supporter. Moreover, research shows that family members need and respond positively to education about Alzheimer's disease (Chiverton and Caine, 1989). Legal issues and care decisions related to a dementia diagnosis make it imperative that the family understand the diagnosis and its implications for care early in the course of the disease. An excellent educational resource guide is *The Thirty-Six-Hour Day*, a compilation of family experiences with the disorder at different stages, written by Rabins and Mace (1981). Although other books also offer help, this book remains the definitive resource for family caregivers.

Support groups for family members of dementia patients offer an ongoing, practical socioeducational resource—even in the early stage. They offer a safe place to explore such specific issues as:

"Should the patient stop driving?"
"Should you tell other people of the diagnosis, particularly coworkers, or adult children?"
"Should the patient wear an ID bracelet or carry a card indicating a dementia diagnosis?"
"How do I handle my spouse's sexual desires when I don't feel as though it is an adult relationship anymore?"

Coaching family members to use all of the senses and past memories in talking with patients typically helps them feel more comfortable and increases the chance of patient participation in conversation. Part of the coaching process is supportive, but it also has an educational format. Helpful guidelines to understanding the symptoms and effects of memory loss on patient behavior include the following:

- The reduced animation found in the patient's facial expression and physical movements is part of the disease process, not a reflection on the social interaction.
- There may be noticeable pauses in the conversation and a sharp reduction in spontaneous speech. Keep conversation simple and straightforward.
- The patient's speech may be difficult to understand, and it is appropriate to provide an educated guess about what the patient is trying to say.
- Overconcern about minor matters and repetition indicate a need for additional reassurances from the family caregiver.
- Touch is an important form of communication when words no longer provide connections.
- Sharing important moments from the past with the patient provides a bridge to connection even if the patient does not seem to respond.

SAFETY ISSUES

Safety issues become the responsibility of the caregiver early in the disorder. A safe environment allows the dementia patient both physical freedom and a sense of security. These patients need a physical environment that provides room to pace. It is important to avoid the use of scatter rugs that may lead to falls, to mark clearly changes in floor elevations, and to wipe up floor spills promptly because the patient will not notice these. In addition to their cognitive inability to correct their missteps, these patients are subject to the same sensory losses that make falls in the elderly more problematic.

Safety in the home is a challenge. The dementia patient typically wants to engage in normal activities but does not always register how this should be accomplished. Patients turn on the stove and forget it is on or use a sharp instrument in an inappropriate way. Simple strategies to protect the patient include cleaning up spills, keeping sharp instruments out of reach, monitoring patients who wander, taking the knobs off the stove, and locking up toxic substances. Although the temptation exists to reprimand patients in the hope of influencing future behavior, this response rarely has a productive result even though the patient may understand what the caregiver is saying. The patient's recent memory retrieval loss does not permit learning transfer to a new situation.

Interpersonal safety is a necessary requirement for effective functioning in the early stage. Dementia patients cope with their environment best when they have a consistent and predictable daily social routine. Nurses can help family members develop and maintain a daily routine that the patient can count on for security. Changes should be avoided whenever possible. When the patient's circumstances require a significant alteration, as in a move to a nursing home, including familiar objects, such as pictures, scrapbooks, religious articles, or a favorite throw, makes the transition easier.

Safety also entails taking responsibility for ensuring the safety of others who may be inadvertently endangered by the patient with memory loss. Of considerable concern is the dementia patient's wish to drive. Family members find it difficult to take this last vestige of independence away from the patient, particularly when the individual can go to familiar places without any apparent difficulty. Significant problems, however, can affect reaction time, judgment, and recent memory recall, with direct implications for driving safety (Donnelly and Karlinsky, 1990; Dubinsky et al, 1992). Disturbances in higher cortical functioning can mean that these patients forget the meaning of red or green lights or become distracted with multiple stimuli and fail to yield the right of way. Constructional difficulties may prevent them from being able to judge the distance between their car and the car ahead of them. For any or all of these reasons, dementia patients with memory dysfunctions cannot always negotiate complex driving situations. Although restricting the patient's driving is not easy, it is absolutely essential. Patients with dementia are no longer fully responsible for their actions. Consequently the caregiver, with knowledge of the disorder's effect on reasoning and constructional abilities, must assume responsibility for the patient's actions. Explaining to families that they are acting on the patient's behalf helps with guilt feelings.

CONSERVATION OF FUNCTIONAL ABILITY

Many simple nursing strategies can help patients maintain existing function for as long as possible. Each patient presents a unique blend of behaviors and attitudes, some of which are easier to handle than others in the early stage. Nursing interventions need to be flexible, geared to the individualized needs of the patient, and adapted to fluctuations in behavior. As Case Example 38–3 shows, normalizing tasks that the patient can accomplish and providing verbal or written cues help patients perform activities that otherwise would not be possible.

Case Example 38–3 Reba's Story

Reba Jordan could not remember how to make a sandwich, which distressed her greatly. Rather than simply making the sandwich herself, her daughter took all of the ingredients out of the refrigerator and placed them on the counter. Mother and daughter then proceeded to make the sandwich as a joint fun activity. The daughter named each ingredient when the time came to use it, and her mother handed it to her. The activity became a shared experience in which both could participate and enjoy their time with each other.

Previously learned and familiar material lingers and remains intact for longer periods. It follows that interventions recognizing and using patient strengths around automatic learned activities are more likely to be successful and to foster self-confidence. When the patient requires structural cues or guidance, you need to assess how much should be given and what areas the patient can handle. By providing cues and assisting only to the point that the patient can take over, the patient can stay functional for a longer period.

Early-stage dementia patients often cannot execute complex tasks requiring memory and visuospatial skills, such as dialing a telephone or making a meal unassisted. With verbal cues and minimal assistance, they can continue to perform these activities. For example, many phone systems have a built-in memory for frequently called phone numbers. A card placed next to the phone with a single digit number and the person's name can permit independent phone use, whereas trying to remember the person's phone number and dialing sequential digits is beyond the patient's cognitive capability.

Participating in activities within his or her scope of cognitive ability enhances the patient's self-esteem. Simple activities that patients in the early stage can do without significant difficulty include polishing silver, watering plants, folding laundry, washing windows, and sorting socks. Music, rhythm, and hand clapping make use of gross and fine motor abilities and generally are enjoyed by dementia patients. Such activities offer an opportunity for socialization without a heavy demand for interaction—something beyond the patient's capability. Familiar recordings such as country or religious music encourage patient participation even more because they stimulate automatic memories. Physically focused activities, such as tossing balls, Frisbees, beanbags, or balloons to others, help patients drain off excess energy and provide a social outlet.

Excessive anxiety decreases cognitive functioning in all individuals, but the dementia patient has more limited cognitive ability to work with in responding appropriately to complex life situations. Persistent worry and overconcern about simple life issues are common occurrences. Cognitively confused patients benefit from repeated orientation to their setting. Rules and unit policies should be identified in simple, easily understandable terms. Orienting cues, such as seasonal pictures, calendars, clocks, large-print signs identifying different rooms, and printed patient names, serve as important reminders to patients in the early stage. Some hospital units print the patient's name on the door in large letters. Others place a picture of the patient when he or she was younger to stimulate recognition. All of these interventions help decrease anxiety. Patience, understanding, and frequent reassurance also can help the patient cope with the issues of the moment.

JUDGMENTS AND DECISION-MAKING

Cognitive limitations also mean that the patient may exercise poor judgment or become combative when unable to meet real or perceived expectations. At the same time, caregivers need to realize that dementia patients may have "some impaired cognitive skills, but also retain some decision-making skills" (Weiler, 1994, p. 36) during the early stage. Whenever possible, these patients should be encouraged to make their own decisions. Although it is sometimes difficult to distinguish when to support and when to limit the patient's decision-making powers, choices provide a sense of purpose and feeling in control. Issues that do not compromise the safety or well-being of self and others can be left to the patient's discretion, for example, which food to eat first or where to go next.

Related to the capacity to make decisions on one's own behalf is the issue of advance directives and durable power of attorney. Legal definitions of *competency* come into play in understanding the needs of the Alzheimer's patient and the balance between the rights of the patient and the needs of the family. Issues of competency become important with the signing of legal documents, such as wills, living wills, informed consent, and power of attorney. In legal terms, *competent* is used to describe individuals who have reached the age of 18 and are able to act on their own behalf. *Incompetent* is a legal term used to describe individuals who have had their cases reviewed in a court proceeding and have been declared incompetent by the judge or jury to manage their own affairs.

A diagnosis of dementia does not automatically mean that a person is legally incompetent. In the early stages of the disease, the patient may not be fully capable of understanding or meeting all of his or her health care needs but often is capable of handling affairs with assistance. Patients are considered competent as long as they retain their decision-making capacity. Legal matters should be handled with the dementia patient during the early stages of the disorder, when the individual is still able to understand the process of decision-making involved in durable power of attorney.

Most patients and their families appreciate a frank discussion and advance directives. Open discussion gives dementia patients opportunity to ask questions and to take charge of their lives to whatever extent is possible. By including the family in the process of developing advance directives most responsive to an individual patient's needs early on, when the patient clearly expresses wishes, most family members feel more confident during the late stages.

SUPPORT FOR SOCIAL FUNCTIONING

Supporting social functional ability is an art. Because most patients with mild or moderate cognitive deficits are treated at home for financial and personal reasons, creating social occasions in the home should be a consistent effort. Most patients respond more effectively in a familiar environment, surrounded by their customary furnishings. Activities need not be elaborate or long-lived. In the home, providing simple opportunities for socialization requires only the imagination and a little time. Uncomplicated social activities provide needed stimulation for the patient. An uncomplicated game, listening to music, group exercise, going for a walk, and pointing out flowers or trees are relevant examples. Regularly receiving a greeting or a kind word is important to the patient as a human acknowledgment. It helps decrease the patient's feelings of loneliness and anxiety.

One-to-one interactions work better than group activities. Visiting with a group provides too many simultaneous demands. Moreover, people avoid dementia patients because their behavior seems eccentric. This nonacceptance heightens the sense of social isolation for the patient and supportive others in social situations.

Reeves (1993) proposes a nursing intervention designed to support the patient's individuality and use the patient's ability to remember things in the past to enhance self-esteem. It involves making a display book with the patient and family entitled "This is Your Life." The book highlights past and present family pictures displayed in chronological order. It includes data about the patient's interests, hobbies, and past achievements. Creating an individualized display book stimulates memories and reinforces the patient's sense of self. The photographs act as a stimulant to conversation about the life story and help the staff to see the patient as a real person. Additionally the nurse can encourage patients to display personal items in their rooms. Mementos provide security for the patient and serve as a topic of conversation for professional caregivers providing direct physical care. For families who visit infrequently, suggest the making of a videotape.

ADULT DAY CARE CENTERS

Intermittent and regular respite extends the family's ability to provide a meaningful environment for the patient. Support existing social skills with referrals to adult day care programs, where the patient will have multiple opportunities for socialization. Adult day care centers for the cognitively disabled are increasing in popularity as a realistic solution for mild and moderate cognitive deficits. Established in the community as an outpatient alternative to nursing home placement, some day care centers are private pay, and others are partially or wholly subsidized by public funds. The patient is brought on a regular basis to a treatment center with a structured program for patients with cognitive impairment. Appropriate stimuli provide the patient with opportunities for personal expression, exercise, and support of remaining functioning.

Adult day care programs typically operate on a half-day or full-day schedule of activities, offered every day or on selected days of the week. Participation offers several benefits. Most significantly, adult day care programs for the cognitively impaired provide structured activities specifically geared to the patient's developmental needs. Time spent away from the primary caregiver in a supervised social setting also provides respite for the caregiver, which allows for a better attitude toward the patient. Having the patient in a safe, structured, and stimulating environment relieves family anxiety about the stress of providing 24-hour care and guilt related to resentment about the unrelenting "call to care." Thus, adult day care programs allow the patient to stay at home longer, often with considerable cost savings to the family and community.

RESPITE CARE

Another form of respite care involves overnight stays in a nursing home setting or a specified block of time in which a trained caregiver comes to the home. Respite provides at least a limited time away from the patient for rest and rejuvenation. Family members use it to catch up on errands, to visit old friends, and to take vacations. You often need to remind the family of the need to take time off: "You can't give from an empty cupboard." Because many family members become so involved, it is hard for them to see the wisdom of the intervention.

MEDICAL TREATMENT

As mentioned earlier, tetrahydroaminoacridine (tacrine) is approved for use with early dementia, and some patients in the early stage benefit from antidepressant medications. The latter prove useful in clearing the cognitive symptoms associated with depression that may complicate the overall picture. Most patients do not require other psychotropic drugs during the early stage. Many need them in the middle stages to reduce agitation and induce sleep. As with all medications in the elderly, metabolic buildup should be monitored carefully.

Middle Stages of Dementia

Yi and colleagues (1994) refer to the middle stage of dementia as the dementia stage. Neurological deficits create a global cognitive impairment, extending to all aspects of self-functioning. In the middle stage, cognitive decline is more rapid and noticeable. Consequently, if the patient is examined at six-month intervals, cognitive deficits are more pronounced with each successive evaluation related particularly to deficits in analytical reasoning skills.

DISORIENTATION

Disorientation, lack of connection to time and place, becomes a consistent feature in the middle stage. Although orientation to self typically remains intact for a longer time than place and time, patients often cannot recognize themselves in the mirror (**agnosia**), or describe their relationship to significant others. Dementia patients may not know where they are and what day or time it is. Generally, they cannot tell you much about their current circumstances. Patients also experience confusion with the identity of significant people in their lives. They misidentify close relatives who come to visit. For example, the daughter of one patient on a recent visit home stated that her mother admonished her father to send "this strange young woman out of the house." She refused to accept that this was her daughter, despite her family's assurances, and kept insisting that the daughter was her father's new lover. Most patients seem clear that the primary caregiver is a significant person, although the dimension and meaning of the bonds between them cannot be retrieved. Some look on the primary caregiver's actions as intrusive or frightening. Here again, support groups can be quite helpful because identity distortion is a common experience. Other group members can help close family members process the painful fact that the father, mother, or spouse they knew no longer exists for them. A husband describes the emotional impact in the following manner (Cohen and Eisdorfer, 1986, p. 175):

I love my wife more than life itself. It hurts so much to see her wither away. She is like a burning candle which keeps sputtering. I am afraid of the day the flame dies. She and I have been able to help each other live with this thing. But I am getting tired. She is changing a great deal now and is a shell of the person I married. She is becoming a stranger to me even though I know she is my wife.... Now I have to do everything for her. I just wish there was some little thing she could do for me so I would know that the old Lupe is still there.

Another form of disorientation is the wish to be transported to a different time and place. Not uncommonly, patients ask plaintively to "go home" or mistake people in their current environment for those in their past life. Understanding that "going home" frequently refers to longing for their more emotionally satisfying past allows you to ask questions about the patient's earlier life. In many instances, this intervention not only stops the rumination momentarily, but also reduces the patients' sense of loneliness and fear by anchoring them in a safer time. Gently stroking the patient's hand or arm, reassuring patients that they are safe and you will protect them helps, as does distraction. If the patient lacks the ability to speak, the caregiver can employ touch and use a photograph, memento in the patient's room, or a family fact from the chart to encourage the patient. Patients sometimes talk as if someone important to them who has died still lives. Asking the patient to talk about significant people in his or her past is much more helpful than providing the reality orientation that the person has died. Providing the "facts of the situation" sometimes causes the patient to grieve the loss as if it is occurring in the present.

Reality validation of past life experience is far more effective than reality orientation, which serves only to confuse the patient more in some cases. When coupled with frequent environmental orientation prompts, gentle encouragement, patience, and touch, the intervention is quite effective with many middle-stage dementia patients.

SELF-CARE

Most self-care and activities of daily living are now beyond the patient's ability to complete. The coordinated efforts required for dressing, bathing, and eating do not fit together in the patient's mind. However, although the patient's mind is dementing rapidly, the patient, at least initially, can still complete activities of daily living with significant caregiver assistance. Step-by-step prompting, using the same simple words repetitively, combining the words with touch, and filling in difficult spots make patient task achievement possible. For example, touching the patient's leg and saying, "Now lift this leg and put it in the pants," provide the multisensory cues to complete a task the patient could not accomplish otherwise. You can offer similar combined cues for performance of other simple tasks, such as bathing and eating. These simple nursing actions to help patients preserve remaining function also serve to enhance the patient's self-esteem and social participation. Over time, the patient's capacity to participate diminishes, and total care is necessary. (See Box 38–6 for common symptoms in the middle stage.)

BOX 38-6 Behavior Symptoms Common in the Middle Stages of Dementia

- Trouble eating
- Childlike behavior
- Inability to perform self-care activities unassisted
- Trouble communicating and following directions
- Emotional disinhibition
- Bowel and bladder incontinence
- Wandering, so that patient cannot be left alone
- Pacing and agitation
- Visual hallucinations
- Difficulty recognizing family and friends
- Meaningless words and actions
- Catastrophic reactions
- Sundown syndrome

TABLE 38–9 **Common Behavior Management Problems with Related Nursing Strategies in the Middle Stages**

Behavior	Possible Meanings	Suggested Intervention
Wandering	Limited awareness of environmental stimuli	Redirect patient with word cues and word signs
	Boredom	Provide sensory stimulation
	Feelings of being lost	Reorient patient frequently Increase safety monitoring Use Medic-Alert bracelet
Rummaging	Lack of control over environment	Give patient something to do Use distraction (a glass of juice, a look out the window)
	Searching for a sense of security	Give reassurance Make a busy box with safe rummaging items Ask family to bring in expendable, familiar items
Incontinence	Difficulty with finding bathroom	Take patient to bathroom at frequent intervals. Praise for performance; overlook accidents
	Inability to remove clothing	Simplify clothing to facilitate removal. Use one-step orienting commands (slip pants down to your knees)
	Limited awareness of stimulus to use toilet	Change soiled or wet clothing immediately. Note normal times of elimination and toilet. Watch for possible signs (pulling at clothing, increased agitation)
Difficulty following directions	Too much sensory input	Provide step-by-step instructions; repetitively provide information on time, place, person, schedule, routine
	Complex task	Use signs, color coding, written word plus signs, calendars, large-number clocks to facilitate recognition
Profound memory loss	Cognitive impairment, anxiety, grief	Try to focus on the feelings behind the behavior and affirm these in words and actions. Note times and patterns of behaviors to detect environmental antecedents that can be modified

Distinct neurological deficits in the middle stage directly alter the functioning of many body systems. Voluntary control of physical functions diminishes, leaving the patient with loss of control first over bowels and bladder and later with the inability to swallow (**dysphagia**). Physical movements increasingly become reflexive, rather than purposeful. Although the patient's skeletal and muscular systems demonstrate normal function potential, the neurobiological connections sending messages from the brain to the muscles are permanently disconnected. Consequently the patient becomes unable to perform voluntarily even the most routine, purposeful actions. Physical impairment also may include unsteadiness in gait and a *listing* posture, with the patient's upper torso tilted toward one side when walking. Falls are common, and the patient needs careful supervision at this point in the disease.

Marked psychomotor agitation and retardation are common. Restlessness, agitation, and aimless pacing replace normal motion. Whether the nervous energy takes the form of pacing, repetitively sitting down and getting up, or following primary caregivers wherever they go, the seemingly pointless and constant pattern is unnerving and exhausting to watch. Of all the behaviors these patients demonstrate, this is one of the most troublesome. Table 38–9 provides guidelines for understanding the meaning of selected patient behaviors in the middle stage.

As the patient enters the middle stage, the level of nursing care takes a sharp shift from compensatory support to behavior management and physical intervention. Quality care of the dementia patient requires flexibility, patience, and creativity. The patient's behavioral symptoms provide steady but highly unpredictable challenges for caregiving strategies. What worked well in coping with yesterday may not work at all today. Moreover the care required characteristically is much more intense, physically draining, and never completed. The patient in the middle stage requires close supervision and assistance with most aspects of self-care, nutrition, and elimination.

COMMUNICATION

Even simple communication in the middle stage becomes more complicated as the connections involved in thought processing are increasingly extinguished. Since communication is so closely linked to emotional connections, it is your responsibility to "not let emotional ties die too far ahead of the patient . . . (and to) nurture the hope to enjoy today and tomorrow for as long as it is possible" (Cohen and Eisendorfer, 1986, p. 261). Responses tend to be in the form of one word, a yes or no answer that may or may not bear any relationship to the question. Because the patient can no longer verbally communicate personal needs or problems, you must anticipate most patient needs and respond to them with little or no patient input. From the patient's perspective, narrowed communication translates into a frightening and lonely existence. Anyone who works with these patients cannot help but wonder if the "diminished presence" is solely a function of the cognitive disorder or also a reflection of their "giving up" because they can no longer understand what is happening or communicate their needs to others.

How frustrating it must be to "be in the world, but not able to reach out and touch it." The strange communication world of the dementia patient can be conceptualized as one in which circumstance transports them to a completely unfamiliar territory. Although they look like other people in this place, they cannot understand either the language or the customs. Being unable to speak the language of the inhabitants of this foreign territory, these alien travelers cannot tell the citizens anything about their journey or that they don't know their way around. They cannot ask for directions because they don't know the words to say. Imagining the alien traveler's situation as a permanent rather than a temporary state of affairs with no hope of getting better can provide some awareness of the terror that patients with chronic cognitive disorders experience on a daily basis.

Burgener and associates (1993) suggest that "nursing staff may better attend to an individual's needs if attempts are made to find meaning in behaviors" (p. 20). Usually the behavior is a personal response to the immediate environment (for example, sensory overload or distortion of the environment). The response may signal a lack of patience or frustration on the part of the caregiver or a physiological reaction to fecal impaction, urinary retention, medication, hunger, thirst, or sleep loss. You must act as a detective in finding the hidden meaning and responding to it. Because the patient cannot verbalize the nature of the difficulty, you will need to make an educated guess about its meaning. Reframing difficult behavior in communication terms provides the caregiver with a different perspective. For example, the patient's increased agitation may signal physical distress. Combativeness during dressing may represent the patient's misinterpretation of the caregiver's actions as intrusive and potentially harmful.

AGITATION

Persistent restlessness, irritability over small things, striking out at the air, and aimless pacing are agitated behaviors common to patients in middle-stage dementia. Assessment of a physical cause for the agitation is the first approach. If there is no evidence of a physiological cause, such as fecal impaction, infection, or fatigue, survey the environment for the presence of possible irritants or sensory overload, both frequent causes. Like young children, agitation and irritability increase when the patient is tired or hungry.

The goal of nursing interventions is to minimize any factors maintaining the behavior. Simple distraction—for example, "I'd like you to show me a picture in the day room" or "I'd like you to help me set the table"—often stops the behavior, at least momentarily. Approaching the patient with a low-key, calm approach tends to soothe the patient. A snack or simple activity can distract the patient and significantly reduce tension. High-stimuli situations should be avoided, and small doses of high-potency medications can be quite effective in interrupting agitated behaviors. Stroking the patient's arm and encouraging the individual to remain seated while talking slowly in a calm voice can reduce the penetrating agitation in some patients.

SCREAMING

A variant of agitation in dementia patients is screaming and loud repetition of single words or phrases. Screaming can represent boredom, or it can be a way of getting the caregiver's attention. Loud and incessant talking, however, rattles those who hear it, and because this behavior consists often of an unintelligible shrieking sound, it is unnerving. Again it is helpful to realize that the patient typically does not scream intentionally. In fact, most patients are unaware that they are speaking or annoying others. Screaming, similar to other behaviors, is an effort to communicate. Good baseline data can assist you in providing the most effective response. By observing when the screaming occurs, for example, you might determine whether the patient is tired, hungry, or in need of attention, allowing you to respond more appropriately to the patient's underlying needs rather than to the screaming behaviors. Soft music or television sometimes quiets the patient. One interesting study (Hallberg et al, 1990) found that vocally disruptive patients received less social and more corrective communication than control patients.

EATING DIFFICULTY

Eating becomes a problem during the middle stages of dementia, manifesting itself in a variety of ways. Aesthetically, these patients typically display grossly inappropriate table manners. Eating can become a problem nutritionally for patients who overeat or undereat with little recognition of what they are doing. Progressive neurological deficits make it physiologically harder to swallow and increase the possibility of aspiration. Moreover, patients "forget" how to get food to their mouths, to chew, and to swallow. Mealtime becomes a supervised experience.

You can use a variety of strategies to encourage good eating habits. Mirroring the eating process by picking up the fork, encouraging the patient to follow suit, and providing verbal prompts such as, "John, pick up your spoon," as you mirror the action are effective in helping patients eat more easily. Reminding patients verbally to chew and to swallow also helps. Most patients need to have their food cut up, and some may need food pureed. Following small bites with a drink also helps the patient swallow. The caregiver or nurse needs to use words and careful manipulation of the food materials to help patients avoid taking in large portions without chewing or swallowing.

Dining with the dementia patient in a community dining room is a challenge. Many patients are quite disruptive, taking food from other patients' trays, pocketing food items, and shoving food in their mouths without chewing. These patients may call out or throw and push food away onto other residents' trays. Some patients eat spoiled food, stashed at an earlier time or taken from the garbage. Their cognitive and perceptual deficits make it impossible for them to recognize food as such. If you try to assist, these patients may grab at your hands or clench their jaws to prevent intake. Because many of them can no longer smell, they may not realize the food is bad. Some patients try to eat inedible materials such as styrofoam cups, plastic tableware, plants, dirt, and paper napkins. For this reason, plastic knives, forks, and spoons should not be used because some patients may bite down on the utensil and swallow it.

Simplifying the number and presentation of food items can reduce the "work" for the patient. Some patients do better having one food item at a time, rather than facing the full meal. Opening milk cartons, cutting up meat into small bite-size pieces, and presenting one eating utensil at a time seems to help focus patients on their meal. Usually, spoons work best. Alternating foods provides variety and makes undesired foods more appealing. Here you need to allow time and to practice patience because patients in the middle stage of dementia have a tendency to start and stop eating many times during a meal. This can be nerve-racking unless you understand that the behavior is not under the patient's voluntary control. If the patient seems unable to use utensils, nutritional finger foods such as cheese squares, finger sandwiches, or fruit chunks can supply needed nutrients without agitating the patient.

COMBATIVENESS

Research has demonstrated a connection between impaired cognition and aggression. Understand that aggression exhibited by dementia patients is quite different from hostile acts demonstrated by patients with functional disorders, such as antisocial personality disorder. The dementia patient has neither a deliberate wish to harm another person nor a criminal intent. Aggressive actions typically occur as brief outbursts, most often as a random response to the environment. Frequently the aggressive behavior of the Alzheimer's patient diminishes as the disease progresses because the patient becomes less involved with the environment and simultaneously more feeble.

CATASTROPHIC REACTIONS

Catastrophic reactions have some characteristics in common with combativeness, but they are less likely to be attacks on other people. More frequently, a **catastrophic reaction** resembles in form and intent the temper tantrum of a two-year-old. These behaviors represent overreactions to stimuli in the environment and typically occur as brief episodes of heightened anger and frustration. During a catastrophic reaction, the patient may strike out at the caregiver, cry, scream, and appear extremely agitated. Like a two-year-old, the dementia patient seems to have limited awareness of the consequences of the outburst or its impact on others.

Understanding that these patients have lost the capacity to express their needs in simple ways that might reduce their frustration helps you to be more compassionate. With a limited way to respond to anxiety, these patients turn to physical aggression as a way of making their needs known to others. Their immediate familiar caregiver is the recipient of the aggressive act, as with the toddler. Catastrophic reactions often occur when the caregiver is offering genuine assistance, which makes the outburst even more troubling. A possible explanation is that the caregiver's actions remind the patients of things they can no longer do for themselves.

The best treatment is prevention. Simplifying the environment helps make the situation more manageable. Many activities of daily living that precipitate a catastrophic reaction are tolerated without incident at a different time of day. Picking the most desirable time for morning care may involve moving the activity to the afternoon. Distraction is particularly effective as an intervention strategy. For example, the nurse might say, "Betty, we can come back to this, but I would like to show you (name something) over here." Touching and moving the patient to a different location also help. Involvement in other activities, particularly those containing large motor movement, divert the patient's attention and rechannel nonproductive energy. Reducing choices, eliminating or breaking down tasks that are too complex into smaller components, and responding to questions that overwhelm the patient are strategies to offset the potential for a catastrophic reaction.

SUNDOWN SYNDROME

Sundown syndrome or sundowning (Evans, 1991), describes an increased confusion and agitation noted in many dementia patients occurring during the late afternoon and early evening hours. It also has been known to occur first thing in the morning in some isolated cases. Treatment of this diurnal pattern consists of keeping the patient active during the earlier parts of the day and planning the patient's day so that stimuli are reduced during the period traditionally associated with sundowning. Medications are helpful adjuncts to treatment, but for maximum effectiveness, they need to be given at the beginning of the episode, not after the agitation has become full-blown. Administration of low doses of antipsychotic medication (haloperidol) or a benzodiazepine (lorazepam) around 4:00 p.m. helps reduce the incidence of sundowning.

EMOTIONAL DISINHIBITION

Patients with dementia sometimes exhibit inappropriate behaviors in the form of touching others in sexually inappropriate ways, disrobing in public areas, or making sexually explicit comments referred to as **emotional disinhibition**. Patients exhibiting sexual behaviors toward others, masturbating in public, or disrobing obviously cannot be permitted to do this because of the consequences to themselves and others. Handling the problem, however, is important. Understanding the patient as having the social skills of a very young child can help you respond compassionately, as Case Example 38–4 illustrates. Patients who undress may feel too warm or may simply need to go to the bathroom. Depending on the situation, you can offer the opportunity for toileting or lead the patient to a room and help with redressing.

Case Example 38–4 Jack's Story

Jack O'Donnell was in the hospital suffering from vascular dementia and a diabetic crisis. He pinched the nurse's rear end as she came closer to the bed, saying, "I've been away from home a long time." Before his illness, Jack would never have made such a comment. The nurse, recognizing emotional disinhibition as a symptom of dementia, was able to pat his arm and say to him, "It must be hard to feel like you are alone," and change the subject. Had she taken his action as a personal attack and his statement verbatim, her nonunderstanding could have worsened Jack's cognitive impairment. From that point forward, she also made sure that she was not in a position where a similar incident might occur.

SLEEP DISTURBANCES

With dementia, there is a characteristic reversal of the sleep-wake cycle so that the patient is sleepy during the day and awake at night. Many patients wake up spontaneously throughout the night and become night walkers, much to the consternation of the caregiver who must get up and make sure that the patient gets safely back to bed. When patients wander at night, they are quite likely to get into trouble, partially because of the darkened environment. Patients who climb into bed with other patients in nursing homes or stand in the doorways of other patient rooms are causes of anxiety. At home, patients may turn on the stove or attempt to leave the house. Satlin (1994) identifies sleep-wake disturbances as a major factor in many family decisions to place the patient in a nursing home.

Several nursing interventions help reduce the incidence of night walking. First, the caregiver needs to keep the patient active during the day. Engaging in simple, stimulating activities during the day helps the patient work off excess energy. Avoiding stimulant intake, such as coffee, tea, coke, or cigarettes, near bedtime and offering a small snack in the early evening help keep the patient relaxed. If diuretics are used, it is important to use them early in the day. Patients often get up to go to the bathroom at night and, once up, begin their travels. Should the patient arise during the night, you can instruct the caregiver to guide the patient to the bathroom but to limit conversation at this time. Allowing the patient to become fully alert makes it harder to get him or her back to sleep. Careful use of medication may offset negative symptoms influencing sleep onset and duration.

REPETITIVE BEHAVIORS

Repetitive behaviors that serve no functional purpose also are a persistent element of the middle stage. They are particularly distressing to the caregiver because logical responses do not stop the repetitive flow. Typical behaviors can include asking the same question or performing the same task over and over again or following the caregiver. Understanding that repetition helps create security for the dementia patient in a world that no longer makes sense helps make responding in a different way possible. Providing a supportive, nonthreatening structural environment offsets the insecurity that cognitive disorders create. Distraction, touch, calm words, ignoring the behavior, or redirecting the conversation often helps break the repetitive words momentarily.

At least equally disconcerting is the patient's need to follow the caregiver wherever the caregiver goes. As one individual expressed it, "I can't even go to the bathroom by myself. There he is, and I feel guilty shutting him out." This phenomenon, although wearing under any circumstances, becomes a little more tolerable when caregivers can realize that these patients are simply trying to maintain their bearings in an increasingly unfamiliar environment. By staying close to the familiar caregiver, the patient feels some degree of safety and security.

USE OF RESTRAINTS

Restraints are useful only as a last resort and then only for specific short periods. Each time patients are restrained, even for a good reason, they lose a part of their personal freedom and their sense of themselves as people. As the words of one patient suggest, patients with cognitive disorders do not understand the reason for restraint: "I don't know why they would want to tie me up like this," she said sobbing. "I don't even feel like a person anymore" (Rose, 1987, p. 20).

Physically, patients in restraints are more prone to develop contracture formation and decubiti because the restraints severely restrict their voluntary movements. If restraints are continued once the patient is asleep, the head of the bed should be elevated to prevent aspiration. Being restrained can increase the patient's restlessness as the patient struggles for freedom from the restraints.

Vest restraints, used in the bed or wheelchair, can help the patient maintain an upright position and prevent unnecessary falls. When physical restraints become necessary, they should be applied with compassion and with the patient's comfort in mind. When using vest restraints, also known as a posey, make sure that it is applied correctly, so that it does not constrict breathing or abdominal organs. The patient's unsteady posture makes it more difficult to use the vest restraint because many of these patients have a tendency to travel downward in their chairs, with the restraining device twisted around their upper bodies, even when the restraint is properly applied. Rose (1987) suggests the use of a "roll bar," which prevents the patient from sliding down in the chair, and a T-strap, used to help the patient remain seated in the chair without being able to topple over. Sometimes, placing the patient in a wheelchair or Gerry Chair with a posey near the nurses' station allows the patient to feel social without being tied up like an animal. The stimulation of seeing people without needing to do very much socially has a calming effect.

You cannot expect patients to react placidly when released from restraints. Bilateral wrist and ankle restraints should be used only as a last resort, for example, for intravenous infusion. They should be applied for the shortest time possible, to prevent contracture and decubiti. They need careful monitoring. Patients with this type of restraint should be turned every hour, in good body alignment. Another selective use of restraints is to provide the individual with scheduled periods of respite from the constant pacing and agitation that seem related to the disorder. (Case Example 38–5 shows how restraints can be integrated with other interventions.)

Case Example 38–5 Sara's Story

At our nursing home, Sara, one of our residents, would restlessly pace up and down the unit, wringing her hands and muttering to herself. Each time the elevator door opened, she would dash off in that direction, her swift movements denying her 80-plus years. Each time—just as she reached the opened door—an alert staff member would stop her. "Please don't do this," she'd whine. "I gotta go now. I gotta get home to my kids." The staff tried reality orientation without success. No amount of reasoning or cajoling could wrench Sara away from her vigil near the elevator. Finally, when she could not be controlled, a staff member would place a vest restraint around her chubby body and gently sit her in a chair. Sara needed to rest, but she would often forget to do so.

In assessing her case, the nurses found that Sara did not recognize her adult daughters, who visited her frequently. Rather she perceived them as teenagers who needed her at home. Imagine Sara's fear and frustration each time she was stopped at that elevator door. The staff successfully began to use techniques of active listening and therapeutic touch. She responded in a loving way to the hugs and patient listening each time she became upset about "my kids." Eventually, Sara forgot all about the elevator and began to adjust to her nursing home placement. As the need to restrain disappeared, the order for a patient control device was discontinued (Rose, 1993, p. 20).

Once patients reach the middle stage of dementia, most are no longer legally competent to handle their own affairs. If the durable power of attorney has not been established earlier, it is too late. Another legal procedure, referred to **conservatorship,** involves the court appointment of a legal guardian to handle the patient's personal affairs. The conservator has legal power over the patient's finances but none over the actual patient. To make legal decisions about the person, a guardian is needed. This person can make decisions for the patient, including nursing home placement. Guardianship is a complex legal process "through which one person or entity (guardian) acquires legal responsibility for another person (ward) who is unable to care for his or her affairs because of mental or physical incapacity. The guardian may be granted limited or (plenary) control over the ward" (Cocker and Johns, 1994, p. 25).

End Stage of Dementia

Alzheimer's disease is a terminal disorder, always ending in death. Yi and coworkers (1994) refer to the end stage as the vegetative stage. Box 38–7 presents behaviors

BOX 38–7 Symptoms in the End Stages of Dementia

- Global loss of memory, long-term as well as short-term memory
- Significant weight loss
- Verbal communication limited to guttural sounds or mutism
- Loss of voluntary bladder and bowel control
- Extreme difficulty swallowing
- Bedridden state
- Other signs of profound neurological loss, such as blindness or seizure
- Cheyne-Stokes breathing
- Fetal position
- Contractures, pressure ulcers, systemic infection, pneumonia

associated with this stage. Typically, there is a significant weight loss related to the patient's growing inability to swallow. The patient looks cachectic, with sunken facial features. Communication with the outside world ceases, although evidence suggests that the patient is still aware of the presence of the caregiver (Michaelson et al, 1987). If not bedridden, the patient has a slow and unsteady gait. Sleep patterns increase, and it is difficult to help the patient maintain any sort of mobility. Many patients assume a fetal position and have contractures caused by immobility.

Changes in respiration (Cheyne-Stokes respirations), seizures, vital signs, and decreased urine volume signal body system shutdown before death. Some patients refuse food by clenching the jaw, spitting food out, or turning the head away from the caregiver. Other patients may bite down on a spoon or fork (for this reason, plastic should not be used) or will not close the mouth and chew (Michaelson et al, 1987). Many patients enter a coma during the last few weeks or month, demonstrating twitching and seizurelike activity but little other responsiveness to the environment. Death usually occurs from secondary neurological complications of the disorder. Frequent complications include aspiration pneumonia, systemic infection associated with tissue immobility, dehydration, and starvation because the patient is no longer able to swallow.

Nursing interventions center on keeping the patient comfortable, nourished, and hydrated. Methods for providing nutritive support include spoon feeding, intravenous infusion of fluids and electrolytes, and tube feeding. Fluid intake is critical, particularly when the patient refuses food. Fruit juices seem to be better tolerated than plain water. High-protein nutritional supplements such as Ensure are regularly offered. Guidelines for stimulating oral intake are presented in Box 38–8. Regular skin care, range of motion exercises, and frequent turning of the patient help offset the effects of serious immobility. You can help family members assume partial responsibility for these activities if they are so inclined. Sometimes providing acts of comfort for their loved one is supportive to the family. Another overlooked activity is saying a meaningful good-bye, even if the patient does not seem to register it. Encourage the patient to "let go," or pray with the patient or gently stroke an exposed body part.

You can provide for the spiritual needs of the patient, by asking the family's wishes for a priest, rabbi, or minister and arranging for a visit as indicated. If the patient is to have an autopsy, the family may wish to fill out the appropriate papers beforehand because time is a critical factor in handling brain tissue examinations. Handling funeral arrangements before the actual death also is helpful for families who wish this intervention. Above all, continue to protect the dignity of the patient and family and provide for the highest quality of life possible for the patient. When the patient actually dies, you can be helpful by acknowledging the void the caregiver is likely to experience and providing referrals if needed.

BOX 38–8 Guidelines for Encouraging Eating in End-Stage Dementia

- Use the patient's name and describe what you are doing
- Give fluids slowly and allow additional time. Use words such as "swallow it now, Dan" as an extrasensory cue
- Use frequent small offerings rather than expecting the patient to take large quantities
- Provide liquids, soup, and juices. Juices and clear liquids are generally tolerated better than water
- Stroke the throat to stimulate swallowing reflexes
- Provide frequent mouth care because of mouth breathing and general dehydration. Use lemon water or treated swabs to stimulate saliva. Vaseline or other lip preparation can keep the lips moist.

▶ Check Your Reading

11. What does sundowning mean? How can the nurse reduce its effects?
12. What guidelines should the nurse follow in deciding to apply restraints to dementia patients?
13. What is the role of the nurse in the care of the patient during the end stage?

Issues for Family Members

Dementia is a story of family deprivation for many families and of courage for those who willingly accompany the patient during this part of the journey. Chronic cognitive disorders ravish the hearts of the victim's family who watch a once strong personality gradually but inevitably and completely lose its defining characteristics. The loss of a person to dementia leaves little to hold on to for security or understanding. All that is known is that dementia patients, as the family knew them, are irrevocably lost. They know that their relative will get worse and will die and that the time from diagnosis to death can last several (up to 19) years, with an average of seven or eight years. No other conclusions can be drawn. In addition to the loss of a partner, a parent, or a sibling, the diagnosis usually creates significant alterations in lifestyle and may affect financial and estate planning. A major shift in role responsibilities is unavoidable for concerned family members.

Dementia is a "family disease" in that the dementia patient loses the ability to care for self, prompting others to step in, often with significant role reversal. Caring for the patient can affect the health and well-being of those who must provide it 24 hours a day, seven days a week. Painful issues such as putting a loved one in a nursing home, quality of life, and making end-of-life decisions for the patient create stress and guilt for many family members.

Financial matters often are of considerable concern as the care of many dementia patients is not reimbursable by a significant number of private and public insurance programs. Families need help with accessing community resources and planning financial contingencies to provide for the care of their relative without impoverishing the caregiver. Support groups sponsored by the Alzheimer's Association are particularly useful informational resources in this regard.

Abuse of Dementia Patients

Dementia, for some patients, is a troubled narrative, with accounts of abuse and neglect. Some families abandon their demented relative to the ravages of the disease with little compassion or understanding. Abuse of the elderly, similar to other forms of abuse, typically occurs in secret. The reasons for abuse vary. For some, the patient's behavior is annoying. Sometimes the designated caregiver resents being given or acquiring the care responsibility and takes it out on the patient. Other families keep a dementing patient in substandard living conditions without appropriate supervision or adequate stimulation, for none other than financial reasons. The patient's social security may be the only or major source of income. Consequently the caregiver may cash the patient's check for personal use without any consideration of the patient's care needs. There are stories of patients tied to chairs, sitting in their own excrement, with little attention to their basic needs. Because the cognitively impaired are adults, those not intimately involved with them do not want to interfere, even though it is obvious that they cannot act on their own behalf.

In many instances, the patient does not suffer active abuse but rather neglect as the patient's needs increase (Abraham et al, 1994). Distant family members may be of little assistance. Because they visit infrequently, they often assume that dementia patients can act on their own behalf, even when this is not the case. Furthermore, cognitive functioning deteriorates subtly and over a significant period, so the precise time when intervention should occur, for the patient's safety, varies considerably. Neighbors are reluctant to intervene because of their relationship with the family and the possibility of jeopardizing their friend's autonomy. In many instances, the individual with dementia has lived in the neighborhood for a long time.

Suspected abuse of the dementia patient presents an ethical dilemma for the nurse. Although some states have legislation mandating the reporting of abuse and neglect of the cognitively impaired elderly, many do not. Moreover, the patient cannot verify the nurse's suspicions. In many home care situations, you may be faced with reconciling the priority of the patient's needs with the reality of the current family circumstances. For example, the possibility exists that a patient may be further harmed through retaliation from family members, particularly when the needed services are not externally available or cost too much.

Characteristics of Family Care

Families continue to assume the bulk of responsibility for the care of cognitively impaired elderly individuals, with the most common caregiver being the spouse or daughter (Bass and Noelker, 1987). Most dementia patients do not require skilled nursing care until the disease is well advanced. Even then it is not always reimbursable because so much of the care involves basic custodial functions not covered by insurance. Yet care must be given consistently because without it, the patient would not be able to perform simple activities of living. Eventually, all dementia patients symptomatically present as a danger to self, if not others. Fortunately, efforts of the Alzheimer's Association, AARP, and the Gray Panthers have resulted in laws protecting the assets of caregivers seeking to provide adequate care for a relative with dementia.

The family should be considered an integral part of the treatment team from the moment of diagnosis. Family caregivers typically are not professionally trained, yet their knowledge, particularly their intuitive knowledge of the patient, is quite sensitive and practical. The Select Committee on Aging (1988) has suggested that this informal care system consists of approximately 2 million caregivers. This number undoubtedly has escalated in the past seven years and will carry on into the 21st century, as the number of elders continues its dramatic increase. Women still constitute the largest cohort of caregivers to the frail elderly, and their needs are just beginning to emerge as the focus of research studies (Wykle, 1994).

In many cases, the primary caregiver and other family members are hidden patients (Kahana et al, 1994), with significant health care needs obscured from view by the more pressing needs of the patient. Some are related to care of the patient. Concurrently, many older caregivers have physical and emotional needs apart from their caregiving role that receive little attention because of preoccupation with their relative's profound functional disability. The multidimensional needs of caregivers are found in common concerns expressed by family members in a 10-year support group (Table 38–10). The list of concerns and level of responsibility are only the tip of the iceberg in thinking about family needs associated with dementia. In fact, Stepworth (1994) suggests that "caregivers as an aggregate are an underserved population that is at high risk for mental and physical health difficulties" (p. 7).

Referral to support groups and allowing time to work with the family around legal, medication, and behavioral issues are extremely important. Many issues that one would not ordinarily think of plague the caregiver of patients with chronic cognitive disorders. These include parental rights expected by the patient when an adult parent is no longer capable of providing care for the adolescent or young adult, how to deal with cognitive judgments and decisions that do not make sense, how to be supportive without being controlling. Friends, particularly if the dementia patient is younger (40s or 50s), might abandon the family because they simply do not know how to handle the situation. Spouses experience discomfort with the sense of no longer being married but not being divorced or widowed either. Fortunately a

TABLE 38–10 Common Concerns of Family Members Facing Dementia

Phase of Dementia	Family Concern
Early stages	Setting limits, especially with driving Having patience with the patient Handling legal and financial matters on behalf of or for the patient Social isolation Sexual requests common with marriage partners Role reversals
Middle stages	Dealing with anger and frustration, without feeling guilty Handling the patient's bowel elimination accidents Coping with the never-ending constancy of caregiving Having personal time alone or to spend with friends Coping with the constant requests for assistance Managing the patient's excessive talking, pacing, and restlessness Responding to unintelligible or difficult-to-understand communication Strains in family relationships Coping with competing demands on time Lack of assistance or appreciation from other family members (extended, immediate) Need for respite
Late stages	Nursing home and other care decisions Quality-of-life and end-of-life decisions Autopsy and funeral home decisions
After death	Restructuring a life without caregiving Finding new meanings

number of community resources are available for family members at low or no cost because of the current emphasis on dementia and family support.

Family and environmental obstacles to preserving function in the dementia patient require careful appraisal. For example, the work schedule of the designated caregiver may preclude giving the proper attention to the patient. Lack of financial resources, other family obligations, role reversals, and other conflicts have a negative impact on potential support. The patient picks up on the family tension but lacks the cognitive skills to respond appropriately. Unable to relate in words, these patients respond in the only way they can—through acting out their frustration or anxiety. Nurses can help family members understand that many of the difficult behaviors displayed by the patient are reactions to the environment. The behaviors represent an attempt to communicate even though their meaning is not readily understandable.

Knowledge deficits also can impair the family's ability to respond with the acceptance and understanding a dementia patient needs so desperately. You need to assess the family's knowledge of the disorder. The family needs instruction in the best ways to reduce negative behaviors. There seems to be a direct correlation between the patient's level of agitation and demands and the caregiver's sense of burden.

Support for expression of negative emotions and fear about the future should be ongoing. Many caregivers feel guilty because they are angry about the major disruption in their lives. Sadness about the patient's condition and the projected outcome of the disease leave many feeling helpless and ineffective. Families need to know that it is okay to feel angry and bewildered about their lives being turned upside down, with seemingly no purpose. They need reassurance that their feelings of helplessness are real but not their fault. They often need support and understanding in making difficult decisions about the dementia patient's future, without having the patient's input. Here, support groups for family members can be invaluable in helping caregivers vent frustrations, learn about the nature of the disease, and develop new ways to help their relative conserve optimal functioning.

Support Groups

Coping with the behavior of the dementing patient is a lonely process with few rewards for the caregiver. Often the caregiver does not have adequate information about a loved one's illness or what to expect. When a previously productive family member is no longer able to assume an accustomed role, life pauses as family members ponder the meaning of the disorder for continuance of family relationships. Frequently the emotional needs of the family are unspoken because of the need to focus on the enormous level of care required for the patient with a cognitive disorder. Support groups are a protected, supportive place and space in time, where the caregiver can turn for needed nurturance. Family members learn what to expect and get excellent tips on how to make things go more easily. Support groups provide a place for the caregiver to laugh (something they don't do very often) to cry, to get mad, and to get needed support to make difficult decisions. Whether the family decides to go the nursing home route or to keep the patient at home, to extend a patient's life through tube feeding or to withdraw extraordinary measures, the group supports the caregiver's right to choose.

Support groups encourage the caregiver to express feelings about the patient and the burden of caregiving in a safe environment, where people understand and accept the feelings, as Case Example 38–6 shows. Feelings of guilt, anger, and resentment are commonly experienced emotions, and it is important that the caregiver realize that they are normal responses to a highly abnormal situation. Group members also help members anticipate the next step in the dementia process, provide useful networking contacts, and sometimes swap equipment. Even if the family member normally is not a "group person," the information obtained through the support group can be quite useful. In contrast to group psychotherapy, there is no pressure on group members to participate actively. They can listen and derive significant benefits.

▶ Check Your Reading

14. In what ways are support groups helpful in the treatment of dementia patients and their families?
15. What are some of the common concerns of family caregivers at different stages of dementia?

Case Example 38–6 Jim's Story

Jim Levit cared for his wife with compassion, from the time she was diagnosed with dementia to the time of her death, 11 years later. Even when she no longer recognized him as her husband, he dressed her, fed her, took her places, and treated her with such tenderness that others used him as a role model. He took an active role in an Alzheimer's support group for caregivers and was quite an inspiration. One of the issues for Jim was that he had struck his wife in a moment of anger and frustration. To him, this incident obliterated all of his tender loving care in one instant. The support group was able to help him put his anger in perspective and to see it as unfortunate, but not the destructive event he felt guilty about in caring for his wife.

CASE STUDY: VIVIAN

Vivian, age 87, has been diagnosed with Alzheimer's disease. Her oldest daughter diagnosed with terminal cancer had been her primary caretaker, and now a shift of burden of responsibility has moved to the youngest daughter who lives in another state. Vivian spent two months living with her youngest daughter, Helen, who herself was 68 years old and suffering from gout, hypertension, and edema of the lower extremities. Helen and her husband found it extremely difficult to cope with Vivian's mental confusion and disorientation when moving about the house. During her times of confusion, Vivian would forget names and become agitated and verbally abusive. Helen noted that Vivian would turn on the stove and then forget to turn it off. Vivian remained angry and upset with her oldest daughter, stating that there was nothing wrong with her and she did not need any help.

Prior to Vivian's placement in an adult semiassistive home care setting, she was found wandering outside Helen's home. She had hidden her morning medications and dentures under a pillow. On admission she has flat affect, is sullen and withdrawn, and reports that Helen is not giving her medications.

ASSESSMENT

Assessment data are as follows:

- Decline in cognitive function
- Forgetful, memory impairment
- Impaired judgment
- Confusion

DIAGNOSIS

***DSM-IV* Diagnosis:** Dementia, Alzheimer's disease

Nursing Diagnosis: Chronic Confusion related to altered cerebral functioning as evidenced by memory loss, decline in cognitive functioning, and impaired judgment

OUTCOME IDENTIFICATION, PLANNING, AND IMPLEMENTATION

EXPECTED OUTCOME 1: By _____ the patient will function at an optimal level, given the increasing degree of memory and cognitive loss.

SHORT-TERM GOAL	NURSING INTERVENTIONS	RATIONALES
By _____ the patient will be less confused and maintain contact with reality.	1. Orient to time, place, and person. 2. Break down complex tasks (dressing, eating) into simple, individual steps.	1–2. Alzheimer's disease leads to altered cognitive function. As the disease progresses, patients are unable to recognize their limitations. Consistent orientation is needed when short-term memory is impaired.
	3. Be consistent with approach, preferable to have same staff work with patient. 4. Put calendar, clock, and activity schedule in patient's room and throughout home. 5. Use familiar objects brought in from own home environment, i.e., favorite pictures, bedspread, drapes.	3–5. Environmental stimuli are misinterpreted, leading to reality distortions along with misidentification of close relatives and poor insight. Use of own objects maintains familiarity. Sameness and repetition lessen confusion.
	6. Speak slowly and calmly (while facing person); use simple phrases and words.	6. Impaired cognitive status may make it difficult to comprehend abstract concepts or lengthy sentences. Facing person provides the maximum amount of verbal and nonverbal communication to transpire.
	7. Plan few activities in the evening when patient is more apt to become confused.	7. Sundowning (increased confusion and agitation) occurs most often in the late afternoon and early evening hours.

EXPECTED OUTCOME 2: By _____ the patient will communicate effectively with others.

SHORT-TERM GOAL	NURSING INTERVENTIONS	RATIONALES
By _____ the patient will communicate with others.	1. Encourage reminiscing and talk to patient about familiar and meaningful things.	1. Long-term memory fades slower than short-term memory. Reminiscing helps patient by distracting from present condition and allows her to reexperience the joys and accomplishments of her past.
	2. Provide group activities (e.g., singing, dancing, crafts) that are simple and familiar to perform.	2. Group activities increase socialization and minimize feelings of alienation and despair.

Nursing Diagnosis: High risk for injury related to altered cerebral functioning as evidenced by wandering and forgetting to turn off the stove.

EXPECTED OUTCOME 3: By _____ the patient will remain safe in the assistive nursing home.

SHORT-TERM GOALS	NURSING INTERVENTIONS	RATIONALES
By _____ the patient will not wander outside of the assistive home care protective boundary.	1. Check on Vivian's status at regular intervals. Set alarm doors on alert mode. 2. Spend short, frequent intervals with Vivian.	1–2. Monitoring and supervision of patient can prevent threats to safety.
	3. Play soft music on the radio.	3. Soft music provides orientation and produces a calming effect on patient.
	4. Encourage use of bathroom before retiring.	4. This may decrease need to get up in the night to use the bathroom and may prevent incontinence.

SHORT-TERM GOALS	NURSING INTERVENTIONS	RATIONALES
	5. Maintain Vivian's activity level during the day. 6. Discourage naps or keep at a minimum.	5. Regular activity maintains muscle tone and promotes a normal sleep pattern. 6. Napping can interfere with normal sleep pattern and lead to restless, wandering behavior at night.
By _____ the patient will not cook in kitchen unless assisted by staff.	1. Supervise any cooking in the kitchen. 2. May need to remove knobs from kitchen stove. 3. Cap electrical outlets.	1–3. Cognitively impaired patients are unable to make safe judgments about seemingly routine habits.

EVALUATION

Formative Evaluation: Vivian met each of the short-term goals. She was easily distracted from using the kitchen when offered craft projects of making flower arrangements. She readily communicated with her roommate and enjoyed talking about the good old times when she lived on a farm.

Summative Evaluation: Vivian achieved each of the expected outcomes. All of the expected outcomes were continued as a part of her ongoing plan of care. Over a one-month period, as Vivian became accustomed to her new setting, less wandering behavior was noted, probably due to an increase in her socialization-type activities, which she thoroughly enjoyed. Overall, she seemed to adjust to her environment. Less confusion was noted by her family when they would visit.

CONCLUSIONS

Cognitive disorders rob the minds of their victims and the hearts of their families. In the 21st century, cognitive disorders are likely to achieve an even greater research focus as the graying of America forces clinicians and researchers to grapple with their understanding and treatment.

Dementia, in many instances, is a story of family courage. Family members who assume the burden of care for dementia patients encounter personal demands that call for constant involvement and caring. The care is emotionally, physically, and often spiritually draining. Yet many families, knowing all of these contingencies, choose to care for their demented relative in a compassionate manner for the rest of the journey. They make personal sacrifices that their relative can never acknowledge. This they do on a daily basis. Their caring actions on behalf of another human being are heroic yet are inconspicuous and undervalued by society. Even the patient cannot thank them for their efforts.

KEY POINTS TO REMEMBER

- Delirium is the name given to the acute forms of cognitive disorders. The disorder represents an acute confusional state, characterized by an abrupt onset, fluctuation in level of consciousness, disorientation, and an identifiable physical cause.
- Emergency triage of the delirious patient is a first-order assessment, followed by psychiatric intervention.
- Reducing environmental stimuli, frequent orientation to surroundings, and staff attitude are important dimensions of effective care with the delirious patient.
- Dementia is a chronic cognitive disorder. The disorder represents a progressive neurologic disorder, characterized by memory loss, changes in personality, and deficits in communication and constructional ability.
- Vascular dementia presents with a stepwise progression, not the steady decline of Alzheimer's disease.
- Alzheimer's disease is basically a rule-out disorder.
- Patient history is one of the most important sources of information in Alzheimer's disease.
- Symptoms in the early stage concern memory loss, personality changes, and psychomotor deficits. They are mild, and the patient usually can function independently.
- Protecting patient dignity, preserving patient functioning, and promoting quality of life are the three goals of patient care with patients suffering from dementia.
- Care in the early stage centers on providing compensatory care for the patient and education for the family.
- In the middle stage of dementia, the primary emphasis of care is on behavior management of difficult patient behaviors associated with global neurologic deficits.
- The end stage of dementia is characterized by a global loss of function and neurologic deficits of a magnitude that eventually lead to death from primary or secondary factors. Pneumonia and systemic infection are common causes of death.

LEARNING ACTIVITIES

1. Interview a family caregiver in your community. Ask the caregiver's perspective on caring for dementia patients. Ask what has been the hardest part of the experience. What has been the most rewarding part of the experience?

2. To avoid duplication, this exercise can be done in small groups and the results shared with the larger group. Find out about the day care programs and religious and social services that caregivers can use in your community. Use the Yellow Pages, and call the different programs. Find out eligibility requirements, payment schedules, and criteria for expulsion from the program. Report on how easy it is to access these services and any other information you think might be helpful in securing appropriate services for the Alzheimer's patient and family caregivers.

3. Attend an Alzheimer's support group in your community and report on some of the concerns expressed at the meeting.

CRITICAL THINKING EXERCISE

Nurse Carlson has been the primary nurse for Mrs. Anne Holmes, an 85-year-old dementia patient, since her arrival three weeks ago at the Bailey's Nursing Home. Today, Anne has been asking frequently to "go home" to talk to her husband. Nurse Carlson is aware that Mrs. Holmes's husband died nine months ago. She approaches Mrs. Holmes and asks her to tell her about her memories with her husband.

1. What assumption(s) can you make about Nurse Carlson's understanding of patients with dementia?

2. If Nurse Carlson had used a reality orientation approach with Mrs. Holmes, what might have resulted?

3. What is an alternative to the above approaches?

The following day, Mrs. Holmes's daughter called the nurses' station to ask what people were telling her mother. She reported that her mother had just told her in their phone conversation that she and her nurse had had a wonderful talk about her husband yesterday.

1. Suggest a response to the daughter that would make sense of the situation.

2. Consider an alternative response(s) and the possible results or consequences.

3. What conclusion(s), if any, can be drawn about the daughter's behavior?

REFERENCES

Abraham, I., Fox, J., and Cohen, B. (1992). Integrating the bio into the biopsychosocial: Understanding and treating biological phenomena in psychiatric-mental health nursing. *Archives of Psychiatric Nursing, 4,* 242–259.

Abraham, I., Holroyd, S., Snustad, D., Manning, C., Brashear, H. R., Diamond, P., and Thompson-Heisterman, A. (1994). Multidisciplinary assessment of patients with Alzheimer's disease. *Nursing Clinics of North America, 29*(1), 113–127.

Abraham, I., and Neundorfer, M. (1990). A decade of progress, a future of nursing challenges. *Geriatric Nursing, 11,* 116–119.

Abraham, I., Onega, L., Chalifoux, Z., and Maes, M. J. (1994). Care environments for patients with Alzheimer's disease. *Nursing Clinics of North America, 29*(1), 157–170.

Absher, J., and Cummings, J. (1994). Cognitive and noncognitive aspects of dementia syndromes: An overview. In A. Burns and R. Levy (Eds.), *Dementia.* London: Chapman & Hall.

Alafuzoff, I. (1992). The pathology of dementias: An overview. *Acta Neurologia Scandanavia, 138* (suppl), 8.

Albert, M. S., and Lafleche, G. (1991). Neuroimaging in Alzheimer's disease. *Psychiatric Clinics of North America, 14,* 443–459.

Alexopoulos, G. S., and Abrams, R. C. (1991). Depression in Alzheimer's disease. *Psychiatric Clinics of North America, 14,* 327–340.

Alzheimer, A. (1987). About a particular case of cerebral cortex (originally published in 1907). *Journal of Alzheimer's Disease and Related Disorders Association, 1,* 7–9.

Amaducci, L., Falcini, M., and Lippi, A. (1992). Descriptive epidemiology and risk factors for Alzheimer's disease. *Acta Neurologia Scandinavia, 138:*(suppl), 21–25.

American Psychiatric Association (1994). *Diagnostic and Statistical Manual of Mental Disorders* (4th ed.). Washington, D.C.: American Psychiatric Association.

Anton, C., and Casey, D. (1994). Clinical paths at Norton Psychiatric Clinic. In P. Spath (Ed.), *Clinical Paths: Tools for Outcome Management.* Washington, D.C.: American Hospital Association.

Barnes, E., Raskind, M., Scott, M., and Murphy, C. (1981). Problems of families caring for Alzheimer's patients: Use of a support group. *Journal of the American Geriatric Society, 29,* 80–85.

Barry, P., and Moskowitz, M. (1988). The diagnosis of reversible dementia in the elderly: A critical review. *Archives of Internal Medicine, 148,* 1914–1918.

Bass, D., and Noelker, L. (1987). The influence of family caregivers on elder's use of in home services: An expanded conceptual framework. *Journal of Health and Social Behavior, 28,* 184–196.

Batt, I. (1989). Managing delirium. *Journal of Psychosocial Nursing, 27,* 22.

Beard, C., Kokmen, E., Offord, K., et al (1992). Lack of association between Alzheimer's disease and education, occupation, marital status, or living arrangement. *Neurology, 42,* 2063.

Beck, C., and Heacock, P. (1988). Nursing interventions for patients with Alzheimer's disease. *Nursing Clinics of North America, 23,* 95–124.

Bennett, D., and Evans, D. (1992). Alzheimer's disease. *Disease Monographs, 38,* 1–64.

Berrios, G. E. (1994). Dementia: Historical overview. In A. Burns and R. Levy (Eds.), *Dementia.* London: Chapman & Hall.

Blass, J., Ko, L., and Wisniewski, H. (1991). Pathology of Alzheimer's disease. *Psychiatric Clinics of North America, 14,* 387–420.

Brayne, C. (1991). The EURODEM collaborative re-analysis of case-control studies of Alzheimer's disease: Implications for public health. *International Journal of Epidemiology, 20* (suppl 2), S68.

Breitner, J., and Folstein, M. (1984). Familial Alzheimer dementia: A prevalent disorder with specific clinical features. *Psychology of Medicine, 14,* 63–80.

Burgener, S., Shimer, R., and Murrell, L. (1993). Expressions of individuality in cognitively impaired elders. *Journal of Gerontological Nursing,* 13–21.

Burns, A. (1992). Psychiatric phenomena in dementia of the Alzheimer type. *International Psychogeriatrics, 4*(suppl 1), 43–54.

Butler, R. N., et al (1994). Vascular dementia: An updated approach to patient management. *Geriatrics, 49,* 38.

Chandra, V., Kokmen, E., Schoenberg, B., et al (1989). Head trauma with loss of consciousness as a risk factor for Alzheimer's disease. *Neurology, 41,* 1576.

Chandra, V., and Schoenberg, B. (1989). Inheritance of Alzheimer's disease: Epidemiologic evidence. *Neuroepidemiology, 8,* 165–174.

Chiverton, P., and Caine, E. (1989). Education to assist spouses in coping with Alzheimer's disease—a controlled trial. *Journal of the American Geriatric Society, 37*(7), 593–598.

Chrisman, M. (1991). Agitated behavior in the cognitively impaired elderly. *Journal of Gerontological Nursing, 17*(12), 9–13.

Cohen, D., Eisdorfer, C. (1986). *The Loss of Self.* New York: NAL Penguin.

Cohen, G. D. (1990). Alzheimer's disease: Clinical update. *Hospital and Community Psychiatry, 41*, 496–497.

Cooke, K., and Gould, M. H. (1991). The health effects of aluminum: A review. *Journal of Research in Social Health, 111*(5), 163–168.

Cooper, J. (1991). Drug treatment in Alzheimer's disease. *Archives of Internal Medicine, 151*, 245–249.

Cummings, J. (1988). Intellectual impairment in Parkinson's disease. Clinical, pathologic, and biochemical correlates. *Journal of Geriatric Psychiatry Neurology, 1*, 24–36.

Danner, C., Beck, C., Heacock, P., and Modlin, T. (1993). Cognitively impaired elders: Using research findings to improve nursing care. *Journal of Gerontological Nursing, April*, 5–11.

Davidson, M., and Stern, R. (1991). The treatment of cognitive impairment in Alzheimer's disease: Beyond the cholinergic approach. *Psychiatric Clinics of North America, 14*, 461–482.

Davis, W. The status of therapy for Alzheimer's disease. *Drug Topics, 138*(9), 96.

Deutsch, L. and Rovner, B. (1991). Agitation and other noncognitive abnormalities in Alzheimer's disease. *Psychiatric Clinics of North America, 14*, 341–351.

Dickson, L., and Ranseen, J. (1990). An update on selected organic mental syndromes. *Hospital and Community Psychiatry, 41*(3), 290–300.

Dillehay, R., and Sandys, M. (1990). Caregivers for Alzheimer's patients: What we are learning from research. *International Journal of Aging and Human Development, 30*, 263–285.

Donnelly, R., and Karlinsky, H. (1990). The impact of Alzheimer's disease on driving ability: A review. *Journal of Geriatric Psychiatry and Neurology, 3*(2), 67–72.

Dubinsky, R. M., et al (1992). Driving in Alzheimer's disease. *Journal of the American Geriatric Society, 40*, 1112–1116.

Dutherie, E., and Glatt, S. (1988). Understanding and treating multi-infarct dementia. *Clinical Geriatric Medicine, 4*(4), 749–766.

Edwards, A. (1994). *When Memory Fails: Helping the Alzheimer's and Dementia Patient.* New York: Plenum Press.

Edwards, A. (1993). *Dementia: Perspectives on Individual Differences.* New York: Plenum Press.

Evans, D., Funkenstein, H., Albert, M., et al (1989). Prevalence of Alzheimer's disease in a community population of older persons: Higher than previously reported. *Journal of the American Medical Association, 262*, 2552–2556.

Evans, L. (1991). The sundown syndrome: A nursing management problem. In W. Chenitz, J. Stone, and S. Salisbury (Eds.), *Clinical Gerontological Nursing: A Guide to Advanced Practice.* Philadelphia: W.B. Saunders.

Farlow, M., et al (1992). A controlled trial of tacrine in Alzheimer's disease. *Journal of the American Medical Association, 268*, 365.

Flint, A. (1991). Delusions in dementia: A review. *Journal of Neuropsychiatry and Clinical Neuroscience, 3*, 121–130.

Folstein, M., Anthony, J., Parhad, I., et al (1985). The meaning of cognitive impairment in the elderly. *Journal of the American Geriatric Society, 33*, 228.

Foreman, M. D. (1986). Managing confusional states in hospitalized elderly: A research dilemma. *Nursing Research, 35*, 34.

Forette, F., and Boller, F. (1991). Hypertension and the risk of dementia in the elderly. *American Journal of Medicine, 90*(3A), 14S–19S.

Given, C., Collins, C., and Given, B. (1988). Sources of stress among families caring for relatives with Alzheimer's disease. *Nursing Clinics of North America, 23*, 69–82.

Gomez, G. E., and Gomez, E. A. (1987). Delirium. *Geriatric Nursing, 8*, 330–332.

Graves, A., White, E., and Koepsell, T. (1990). The association between head trauma and Alzheimer's disease. *American Journal of Epidemiology, 131*, 491–501.

Gwyther, L. (1986). Treating behavior as a symptom of illness. *Provider, 12*, 19–21.

Hall, G. R., and Buckwalter, K. C. (1987). Progressively lowered threshold: A conceptual model for care of adults with Alzheimer's disease. *Archives of Psychiatric Nursing, 1*, 389.

Hallberg, I., Luker, K., and Norberg, A. (1990). Staff interactions with vocally disruptive demented patients compared with demented controls. *Aging, 2*(2), 163–171.

Haller, E., and Binder, R. (1995). Delirium, dementia and amnestic disorders. In H. Goldman (Ed.), *Review of General Psychiatry.* Norwalk, CT: Appleton & Lange.

Hamdy, R., Turnbull, J., Clark, W., and Lancaster, M. (1994). *Alzheimer's Disease: A Handbook for Caregivers* (2nd ed.). St. Louis: C.V. Mosby.

Harvath, T., Patsdaughter, C., Bumbalo, J., and McCann, M. (1995). Dementia-related behaviors in Alzheimer's disease and AIDS. *Journal of Psychosocial Nursing, 33*(1), 35–38.

Heim, K. M. (1986). Wandering behavior. *Journal of Gerontological Nursing, 12*, 4.

High, D. M. (1992). Research with Alzheimer's disease subjects: Informed consent and proxy decision making. *Journal of the American Geriatric Society, 40*, 950–957.

Hill, C., Risby, E., and Morgan, N. (1992). Cognitive deficits in delirium: Assessment over time. *Psychopharmacology Bulletin, 28*, 401–407

Hirsh, H. (1990). Legal and ethical considerations in dealing with Alzheimer's disease. *Legal Medicine*, 261–326.

Holcomb, H., Links, J., and Smith, C. (1989). Positron emission tomography: Measuring the metabolic and neurochemical characteristics of the living human nervous system. In N. Andreason (Ed.), *Brain Imaging: Applications in Psychiatry.* Washington, D.C.: American Psychiatric Press.

Holroyd, S., and Rabins, P. (1992). Psychoactive drug use. In J. E. Morley (Ed.), *Geriatric Care.* St. Louis: Manning.

Jacques, A. (1992). *Understanding Dementia* (2nd ed.). Edinburgh: Churchill Livingstone.

Jenike, M. (1988). Psychoactive drugs in the elderly: Antidepressants. *Geriatrics, 43*, 43–47.

Johnson, L., and Keller, K. (1989). Staging Alzheimer's disease. *Geriatric Nursing, 10*(4), 196–197.

Kahana, E., Biegel, D., and Wykle, M. (Eds.) (1994). *Family Caregiving Across the Life Span.* Thousand Oaks, Calif.: Sage Publications.

Kaplan, H., and Sadock, B. (1991). *Synopsis of Psychiatry* (6th ed.). Baltimore: Williams & Wilkins.

Kaplan, H., and Sadock, B. (1993). *Pocket Handbook of Emergency Psychiatric Medicine.* Baltimore: Williams & Wilkins.

Kase, C. (1986). Multi-infarct dementia: A real entity? *Journal of the American Geriatric Society, 34*, 482–484.

Katz, I. (1993) Delirium. In D. Dunner (Ed.), *Current Psychiatric Therapy.* Philadelphia: W.B. Saunders.

Katzman, R., Aronson, M., and Fuld, P. A. (1989). Development of dementia in an 80 year old volunteer cohort. *Annals of Neurology, 25*, 317–324.

Katzman, R. (1991). Education and the prevalence of dementia and Alzheimer's disease. *Neurology, 43*, 13–20.

Katzman, R., and Jackson, J. (1991). Alzheimer's disease: Basic and clinical advances. *Journal of the American Geriatric Society, 38*, 516–525.

Keith, I. (1994). The differential diagnosis of dementia. In A. Burns and R. Levy (Eds.), *Dementia.* London: Chapman & Hall.

Keltner, N. (1994). Tacrine: A pharmacological approach to Alzheimer's disease. *Journal of Psychosocial Nursing, 32*(3), 37.

Kuhlman, G., et al (1991). Alzheimer's disease and family caregiving: Critical synthesis of the literature and research agenda. *Nursing Research, 40*, 331–337.

Lear, M. (1980). *Heartsounds.* New York: Simon and Schuster.

Lee, V. (1991). Language changes and Alzheimer's disease: A literature review. *Journal of Gerontological Nursing, 17*, 16–20.

Levine, J., and Lawlor, B. (1991). Family counseling and legal issues in Alzheimer's disease. *Psychiatric Clinics of North America, 14*, 385–386.

Li, G., Silverman, J., and Mohs, J. (1991). Clinical genetic studies of Alzheimer's disease. *Psychiatric Clinics of North America, 14*, 267–286.

Lipowski, Z. J. (1987). Delirium: Acute confusional states. *Journal of the American Medical Association, 258*, 1789–1792.

Lipowski, Z. (1990). *Delirium: Acute Confusional States.* New York: Oxford University Press.
Maas, M., and Buckwalter, K. (1991). Alzheimer's disease. *Annual Review of Nursing Research, 9,* 19–55.
Mack, A., Forman, L., Brown, R., and Frances, A. (1994). A brief history of psychiatric classification: From the ancients to DSM-IV. *Psychiatric Clinics of North America, 17*(3), 515.
Marachlewski, M. (1994). Anticholinergic syndrome. *Journal of Psychosocial Nursing, 32*(9), 22–24.
Matzo, M. (1990). Confusion in older adults: Assessment and differential diagnosis. *Nurse Practitioner, 15*(9), 32–44.
McCracken, A. (1994). Special care units: Meeting the needs of cognitively impaired patients. *Journal of Gerontological Nursing, April,* 41–44.
Michaelson, E., Norberg, A., and Norberg, B. (1987). A quality of life issue: Feeding methods for demented patients in end stage of life. *Geriatric Nursing, 8,* 69–73.
Miller, C. (1990). *Nursing Care of Older Adults: Theory and Practice.* Glenview, Ill.: Scott Foresman/Little Brown Higher Education.
Miller, C. (1995). Medications that cause cognitive impairment in older adults. *Gerontological Nursing, 16,* 47.
Nordberg, A. (1992). Biological markers and the cholinergic hypothesis in Alzheimer's disease. *Acta Neurologia Scandinavia, 138* (suppl.), 54.
O'Brien, M. D. (1994). Vascular dementia: Definitions, epidemiology and clinical features. In A. Burns and R. Levy (Eds.), *Dementia* (pp. 624–639). London: Chapman & Hall.
Rabius, P., Mace N. (1981). *The Thirty Six Hour Day.* Baltimore: Johns Hopkins University Press.
Reeves, C. (1993). Home from home: Practical aspects of caring for the confused elderly in a nursing home. In Wilcock, G. (Ed.), *The Management of Alzheimer's Disease* (pp. 133–149). Petersfield, UK: Wrightston Biomedical Publishing Ltd.
Robertson, G. S. (1982). Dealing with the brain-damaged old—dignity before sanctity. *Journal of Medical Ethics, 8,* 173–179.
Rocca, W. (1994). Frequency, distribution, and risk factors for Alzheimer's disease. *Nursing Clinics of North America, 29,* 101–111.
Rose, J. (1987). When the care plan says restrain. *Geriatric Nursing, 8,* 20–21.
Ross, C. (1991). CNS arousal systems: Possible role in delirium. *International Psychogeriatrics, 3*(2), 353–371.
Satlin, A. (1994). Sleep disturbances in dementia. *Psychiatric Annals, 24*(4), 186–191.
Schellenberg, G. D., et al (1992). Genetic linkage evidence for a familial Alzheimer's disease locus on chromosome 14. *Science, 258,* 668.
Select Committee on Aging, House of Representatives (1988). Exploding the myths: Caregiving in America. (Committee Publication No. 100-665.) Washington, D.C.: U.S. Government Printing Office.
Stepworth, D. (1994). Telephone counseling interventions with caregivers of elders. *Journal of Psychosocial Nursing, 32*(3), 7–11.
Treves, T. (1991). Epidemiology of Alzheimer's disease. *Psychiatric Clinics of North America, 14,* 251–265.
Vitiello, M., Bliwise, D., and Prinz, P. (1992). Sleep in Alzheimer's disease and the sundown syndrome. *Neurology, 42(7 suppl),* 83–93.
Weiler, K. (1994). Legal aspects of nursing documentation for the Alzheimer's patient. *Journal of Gerontological Nursing, 20* (4), 31–40.
Wilson, H., and Skodol, A. (1994). Special report: DSM-IV: Overview and examination of major changes. *Archives of Psychiatric Nursing, 8*(6), 340–347.
Wykle, M. (1994). The physical and mental health of women caregivers of older adults. *Journal of Psychosocial Nursing, 32*(3), 41–42.
Yi, E., Abraham, I., and Holroyd, S. (1994). Alzheimer's disease and nursing: New scientific and clinical insights. *Nursing Clinics of North America, 29*(1), 85–99.
Young, S., Muir-Nash, J., and Ninos, M. (1988). Managing nocturnal wandering behavior. *Journal of Gerontological Nursing, 14,* 6.
Zarit, S., Orr, N., and Zarit, J. (1985). *The Burden Victims of Alzheimer's Disease: Families under Stress.* New York: University Press.

SUGGESTED READINGS

Albert, M. S., & Lafleche, G. (1991). Neuroimaging in Alzheimer's disease. *Psychiatric Clinics of North America, 14,* 443–459.
Cohen, D., Eisendorfer, C. (1986). *The Loss of Self.* New York: NAL Penguin.
Hall, O. R., and Buckwalter, K. (1987). Progressively lowered threshold: A conceptual model for care of adults with Alzheimer's disease. *Archives of Psychiatric Nursing, 1,* 389.
Kaplan, H., and Sadock, B. (1991). *Synopsis of Psychiatry* (6th ed.). Baltimore: Williams & Wilkins.
Rabius, P., Mace, N. (1981). *The Thirty-Six Hour Day.* Baltimore: Johns Hopkins University Press.
Yi, E., Abraham, I., Halyrod, S. (1994). Alzheimers disease and nursing: New scientific and clinical insights. *Nursing Clinics of North America, 29*(1), 85–99.

UNIT VI
THE JOURNEY AND SOCIETY

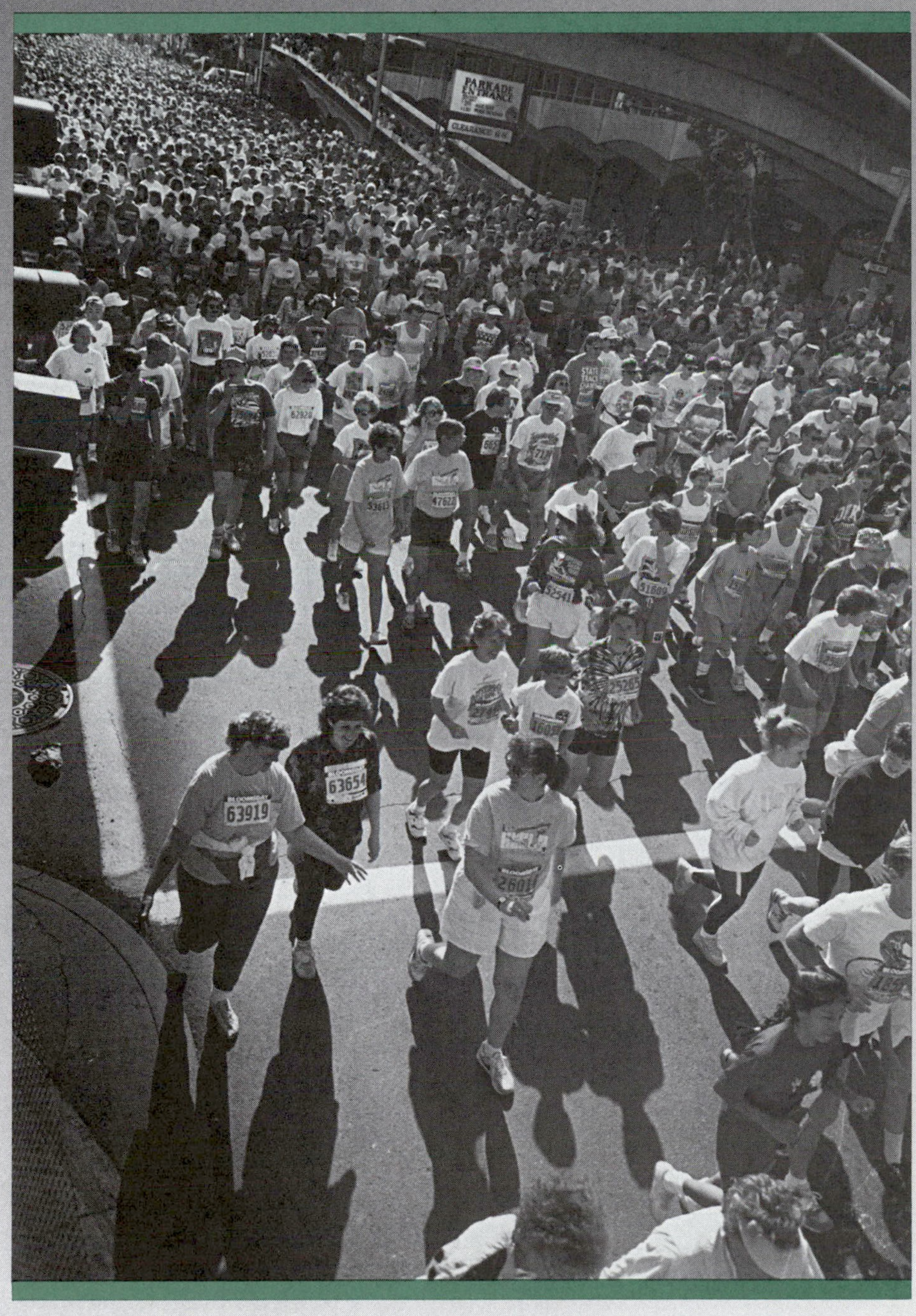

CHAPTER 39

THE JOURNEY MARKED BY HOMELESSNESS

. . . for most homeless persons and families there is no more therapeutic environment than a place of one's own—a place that is safe and warm, that allows wounds to heal, that allows you to choose your associates rather than have them thrust upon you, that gives you your own unique address, your own place in the world.

—Elliot Liebow

LEARNING OBJECTIVES

After studying this chapter, you should be able to:

1. Describe the structural and personal precipitants of homelessness.
2. Identify social and personal attitudes toward the homeless.
3. Identify populations at risk for homelessness.
4. Examine personal values and biases with regard to homeless individuals.
5. Develop an individual approach using the nursing process with homeless clients.

KEY TERMINOLOGY

Admission diversion
Deinstitutionalization
Gentrification disorder
Homelessness
Learned helplessness
Single-room occupancy unit
Social disaffiliation
Social margin
Unemployment rate

Nurses encounter the homeless in many settings including emergency departments, walk-in clinics, inpatient units, shelters, soup kitchens, and churches. Nurses may walk around the homeless as they congregate near heating grates outside a health care facility. While traveling to and from work, nurses may encounter homeless people begging for food or money. Nursing, because of its holistic focus on people, is uniquely qualified to have a major impact on the homeless. Most nurses are motivated by caring, the essential component in the roles of clinician, educator, advocate, and team member. To engage and assist the homeless, the nurse relies on the nursing process to assess real and potential problems, intervene effectively, and evaluate results.

Within the boundaries of a professional relationship, nurses are privileged to participate in clients' unique journeys. We are most effective with vulnerable clients when we establish relationships that accommodate the client's history, current life conditions, and physical, mental, and spiritual strengths and weaknesses. Remember that homelessness is the result of either chronic personal trauma or an acute personal disaster. The homeless are not faceless. Our first step in care is an appreciation of the humanity and individuality of each patient.

Robert D. is a formerly homeless man eager to share his story "so folks will know how it is." A self-aware man, his recovery program has taught him to speak unflinchingly of his struggle to conquer the self-destructive behaviors that led to his experience with homelessness.

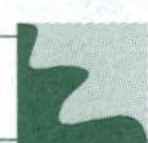

ROBERT'S STORY

I lived with my mother until I was 19 years old. We had a strong family, and I was learning to lay brick for a trade. But even then I was playing with drugs on the weekends. Not too much, never missed work, and I still had money in my pocket. But me and my friends, we were experimenting just the same.

I met my wife around the same time. She was four years older than me but had gotten married when she was 14. Because of that, she already had six little kids. My mother went through some stress because she thought it was crazy for a nineteen-year-old to take on six kids, but I loved my wife so we got together. We never actually got married—I guess you could say we were common-law married. We had two more kids of our own while we were together.

Robert's Drug Habit

I worked steady as a bricklayer for years. I'm 51 years old now, and my life didn't fall apart until seven years ago. But while I was working and raising my family, I got more and more into using drugs. I tried everything that came out a few times, but my drug of choice was heroin. They call it "drug of choice" because it's how I preferred to get high. I didn't care for cocaine, though I did snort it a couple of times. Didn't like alcohol either, but I got my wife started drinking. She wanted to be able to feel like I felt. I see now that I did her no favor, but we were stupid back then.

Seven years ago, things went bad for me. All these years, I had gotten in little scrapes with the law, but nothing too serious. I prided myself on not being willing to rip off my family to support my drug habit. Somehow, I started doing things I never thought I could do. I'd get a paycheck on Friday, shoot it up over the weekend, be broke on Monday. I was stealing things to sell to buy drugs, including stealing things from my own kids. I'm still ashamed of ripping off my son's VCR. The addiction took over my life, and I gave up everything for it. Remember, I had a steady job, nice wife, eight kids, and a home by this time. But there were dark parts of me inside that I couldn't face, so I self-medicated. I couldn't get honest, so I would get high. I was still working, but you can see I was way out of control at home. My wife and kids had a meeting. They decided that I had to get out of the house until I could get straight. It was a shock to me, but they said I could come back as soon as I was clean. If my addiction hadn't been so strong, I'm sure that it would have killed me.

So what did I do the first night? I was lost, in another world. Me, homeless? I would have said it was impossible except that it was true.

Life in a Homeless Shelter

The first night, I went to Jefferson Shelter [name changed]. It was hell when I look back—toilets not working right, rats and bugs in the building, too many guys—but I didn't have a choice. I didn't make a reservation, if you know what I mean. They put us out at seven in the morning every day, no matter what. If it was snowing, raining; you were sick; it was all too bad. I didn't know what to do those first few days—seems I wasn't working for that stretch, so I just followed the crowd. First we went to a soup kitchen and waited in a long line to get breakfast. Then after that, the men walked to a church nearby to get breakfast again. At least it was something to do. It was strange to feel like I had too much time on my hands.

I was in overnight shelters for three years while I was using heroin heavy. I look back now, and it was lost time. Can you believe I still worked? I sure didn't have any money to show for it, but I kept up my trade. While I was working one day, I hurt my back. I was laying some mortar, and I must have turned my back and then had bad pain. It was hard to walk, but believe it or not, I walked and worked. I guess the heroin did me some good!

To make a long story short, one day after my back injury, I got very sick. I was coughing and weak, so I went to the doctor at the clinic. She said I had pneumonia and needed to stay in bed to get better. The only place I could stay in bed was at the infirmary at the H.O.P.E. Shelter [name changed]. The H.O.P.E. Shelter is the Ritz of the city because you actually live there for 24 hours a day. Also, the infirmary has nurses to take care of you, and when you get better, they get you a bed upstairs in the main shelter. It was a way out of the overnight shelters, and I was so sick I needed to be taken care of. So I went to the infirmary.

The rules in the infirmary were very strict. No drugs or alcohol in the building, or you were barred for life. When I got better from my pneumonia, I stayed out three nights in a row and was discharged against my will. But by then I had been hooked up with the drug rehab program at the shelter.

Rehabilitation

The rehab program has one of the best success rates in the city. It's run by recovering alcoholics and addicts, and they don't cut you any slack. If you're not serious about recovery, they make you leave and you need to reapply to get back in. Beds are limited, so I didn't want to mess up. The inpatient program lasts a year, and then the outpatient program goes on for as long as you want. I guess I was finally sick and tired of being sick and tired, so I entered the program.

The program helped me come back to sanity. It was tough, and I went off the heroin cold turkey. I got support but also a lot of confrontation. Little by little, I got back my self-respect. I was still a homeless man, though.

I never realized that people could see you on the street and actually look through you. Man, that is cold! I was ashamed of being homeless, so I would get a defensive attitude. When I was using, I didn't care what people thought of me. When I was clean, it hurt. I felt like I was some bug that people wanted to squash.

I was clean and working my program aggressively for three years. I got promoted in the program to be hall monitor and was doing good. In the program, you can't work for a year. When it was time to go back to the world, I felt strong. I think I got cocky, though, because seven months ago, I relapsed. I overdosed on heroin and was found unconscious in the bathroom at the shelter. Not only was it humiliating, but I was barred from the shelter for life. I really blew it.

I used heroin again for two months and went back to my life in overnight shelters. But, thank God, I had folks who believed in me—my friends in the program, my doctor, and my nurses. They encouraged me to get back into recovery. Five months ago, I did. I knew I couldn't keep hiding from myself. It is hard work, but I'm trying to stay honest with myself.

I now live in an apartment with my son. I work full time, and I go to two meetings a day. I've been up and I've been down, but I see how powerful the addiction is in my life. I need to fight every day to stay clean.

Tell people that homeless folks are just folks. Some are crazy; some are high; some are just down on their luck. It's scary and lonely out there. I'm an old man, but I can truthfully say I was in bad shape when I was homeless.

I live my life day to day now. My family and I are trying to work out our differences. Seven years is a long time to be out there, you know. Did I tell you I have 20 grandkids now? I want to be a grandfather they can be proud of.

WHAT HOMELESSNESS IS

Homelessness is not a new phenomenon but a longstanding global problem that has gained increased prominence in the United States within the last 20 years. Blau (1992) identifies five major periods within the history of homelessness. The first, in the preindustrial period, is highlighted by an absolute scarcity of adequate housing. From ancient and medieval times to the early American settlers, even the fairest division of resources would have left some people unhoused.

The second period of homelessness occurred during the early industrial period, in the late 18th to early 19th centuries. Rural workers in France and England often were temporarily homeless when they journeyed to cities to find factory jobs. This transitional homelessness usually was due to lack of immediate employment, insufficient income, or paucity of housing. Though difficult, it seems to have been a sort of rite of passage for some.

The third phase of homelessness started with the colonization of the undeveloped world (Asia, South America, and Africa) and still exists today. To find work, large groups of homeless workers congregate in metropolitan areas of primitively industrialized countries. Because this system of industrialization favors cheap labor over the welfare of workers, laborers must settle for temporary and/or poorly paid jobs. Employers and governments make little investment in providing for the shelter of workers who are easily replaced by less-demanding others.

The fourth period of homelessness, coinciding with the era of modern industrialization, shifts our focus to the United States. Blau (1992) describes sharp increases in the number of homeless people during periods of unregulated capitalism (in the late 19th century as well as in the 1920s and during the Depression). These spurts of unregulated capitalism created a sharply divided economy with dramatic class and income distinctions in the population. Interestingly, homelessness essentially vanished during times of prosperity or war. Blau (1992) characterized homelessness during this phase as highly responsive to the variations in business cycles.

The fifth upsurge of homelessness started in the early 1980s with deindustrialization and a shift to a service economy. Contemporary social factors have promoted increased homelessness. These include an increase in low-paying jobs, cutbacks in low-cost housing, and reductions in social welfare programs.

The study of homelessness has been hampered by the lack of a standardized definition of the term (Bachrach, 1992). Advocates for street dwellers and shelter residents coined the word "homeless" in the late 1970s to protect undomiciled individuals from stigma and stereotyping. In 1987, the federal government defined "homelessness" as the absence of "fixed, regular, and adequate nighttime residence" or the need to use shelters, institutions, or public or private places not designed for regular sleeping accommodations as a primary nighttime residence (Stewart B. McKinney Homelessness Assistance Act of 1987). Yet homelessness is a problem more complex than the lack of a place to live (Bachrach, 1992).

Homelessness can be defined differently depending on whether the affected population is the "old homeless" or the "new homeless." The old homeless match Blau's fourth period of homelessness, during times of economic hardship. These people included tramps, hoboes, and skid row dwellers whose numbers surged during the Depression. Schubert (1935) described tramps and hoboes as young men who left home to escape economically depressed hometowns and traveled place to place to find jobs. Tramps were considered free spirits "tramping" the countryside, whereas hoboes were viewed as mobile but employable. Skid row dwellers were primarily older white alcoholic males living in run-down urban areas around railroad tracks and trucking companies. These people would find casual employment as needed and often had needs met by religious missions dedicated to the salvation and support of skid row residents. Interestingly, these people generally had some kind of stable shelter in flophouse motels, private homes, or mission dormitories. Had any of these people attempted to live in the street, they would have been taken to jail. Furthermore, skid row residents were concentrated in urban areas and were avoided and ignored (Rossi, 1990).

The face of homelessness changed in the late 1970s and early 1980s with the appearance of the "new homeless." The "new homeless" consisted of men, women, and children literally without shelter, as evidenced by the sight of people sleeping on steam grates, in abandoned cars, or cardboard boxes. Contemporary homelessness is characterized by a lack of permanent and reasonable shelter. Its precipitating factors are:

- Extreme poverty
- Social isolation
- Estrangement from family/friends networks
- Exhaustion of last-ditch resources aimed at maintaining domiciled status.

The reality of homelessness is overwhelming. Nurses function most effectively when they understand the population to be served.

▶ Check Your Reading

1. Compare and contrast the "old homeless" and the "new homeless."
2. List the five phases in the history of homelessness.
3. Define homelessness.

WHO THE HOMELESS ARE

We can no longer be lulled into the insular belief that homelessness happens only to certain groups within the population. As advocates and educators, nurses have a particular responsibility to maintain awareness of those affected by homelessness and those at risk for homelessness. Statistics prove that single men compose the largest group of homeless people in the United States. Lindblom (1991) points out that single unattached men make up approximately 70% of the adult homeless population. Similarly, Carter and colleagues (1994) found that 73% of the adult homeless patients using a free clinic in Georgia were male. Marin (1991) encouraged sensitivity to the plight of homeless men, pointing out that these men are viewed unsympathetically because of social values deriding male neediness and vulnerability. No one can dismiss the tragedy of homelessness for single men. However, they do not fit the profile of the "new homeless" because homelessness traditionally has been represented by unattached males. These people are, in a sense, remnants of the "old homeless."

The Chronic Mentally Ill

Review for yourself the number of tasks, personal encounters, and readjustments you make each day to maintain your lifestyle. Imagine being constantly challenged by a debilitating and exhausting emotional illness and having no place to call home. This is the challenge facing chronically mentally ill homeless people on a daily basis.

The numbers of the homeless mentally ill are difficult to ascertain because this population is poorly measured. Widely varying estimates of the prevalence of mental illness among the homeless range from 10% to 85% (Rossi, 1990), but most sources agree that approximately one third of the homeless population has some mental illness (Dennis et al., 1991; Federal Task Force on Homelessness and Severe Mental Illness, 1992). Mental illnesses affecting the homeless include but are not limited to schizoid personality disorder, anxiety disorders, depressive disorder, and bipolar disorder (Wallsten, 1992). The incredible stress of homelessness is in itself a predisposing factor for emotional distress.

The mentally ill generally display poor interpersonal skills, inadequate problem-solving strategies, disorganized or psychotic thinking, and a global inability to tend to their own needs. Extreme physical deprivation confounds the picture by making differentiation of psychological and somatic symptoms difficult (Bachrach, 1992). The consequence of severe mental illness can be the inability to find or maintain employment, to develop trusting relationships, to preserve housing arrangements, or to meet physical and psychological health needs (Federal Task Force on Homelessness and Severe Mental Illness, 1992). The incidence of attempted suicide is high across all groups within the adult homeless population (Interagency Council on the Homeless, 1990).

The influx of the chronically mentally ill into the homeless population generally is credited to the policy of **deinstitutionalization**. Based on a civil liberties philosophy stating that institutions provided inhumane care for the mentally ill, deinstitutionalization mandated that scores of patients be released from state mental hospitals. Advocates of deinstitutionalization believed that patients could be absorbed by community mental health centers (Bachrach, 1992). Neuroleptic medications had facilitated symptom management so the mentally ill appeared healthier. Though intended as a compassionate solution to harsh institutional conditions, deinstitutionalization released patients before adequate supports could be established in the community. Funds for state hospitals were not transferred to community mental health centers. Many patients never received a complete assessment of their needs.

Though imperfect, institutions provided structure, social context, food, clothing, and medical services to their residents. On their own, chronically mentally ill individuals have difficulty accessing bureaucratic systems. The burden of outreach and support for these patients therefore fell upon understaffed, unfunded, and unprepared community mental health clinics. These conditions have conspired to create a chaotic environment in which many chronically mentally ill patients have essentially been left to their own devices.

Deinstitutionalization also has led to **admission diversion**. Admission diversion is a gatekeeping tactic that limits access to state mental hospitals (Bachrach, 1992). Although civil rights of the mentally ill are protected, some individuals who would try to use inpatient mental health services have been discouraged from doing so. The strategy has contributed further to the number of chronically mentally ill people left homeless.

Substance Abusers

The problem of substance abuse contributes to factors that may lead to homelessness. Between 35% and 40% of the homeless are estimated to have alcohol and/or drug problems (Interagency Council on the Homeless, 1990; Fischer and Breakey, 1990; Lindblom, 1991). Alcohol abuse, drug addiction, and mental health problems also share a high coincidence. Statistics demonstrate that approximately one quarter of homeless drug and alcohol abusers have a history of mental hospital stays, and one half of the chronically mentally ill homeless abuse alcohol and/or drugs (Interagency Council of the Homeless, 1990).

Consider the impact of chemical dependence on one's life. Family and friend networks often are broken as alcohol and/or drug use becomes a prominent feature of daily existence. Individuals may display erratic, impulsive, or antisocial behavior while intoxicated or high. Fischer and Breakey (1990) found that alcoholics were more likely to come from dysfunctional families, not graduate from high school, and have fewer job skills, all of which adversely affect the capacity to find or maintain work. Those abusing illicit drugs run a high risk of arrest and legal conflicts. Not only is possession of the drug and associated paraphernalia illegal but also support of the drug habit may require further illegal activities such as drug dealing, theft, or prostitution (Fischer and Breakey, 1990).

The physical toll exacted by substance abuse is devastating. Alcoholics treated at homeless shelter medical clinics demonstrate grossly inflated incidences of liver disease, seizure disorders, hypertension, nutritional and gastrointestinal disorders, and severe trauma (Fischer and Breakey, 1990). The chemically dependent have an increased capacity for high-risk behaviors ranging from physical fights to prostitution. Unsafe sexual practices lead to increased risk of sexually transmitted disease, including exposure to HIV.

▶ Check Your Reading

4. How does chronic mental illness predispose a client to homelessness?
5. How are social ties jeopardized for homeless substance abusers?

Women

The appearance of women living in public shelters or on the streets has provided disconcerting evidence that homelessness is an increasingly universal phenomenon (Liebow, 1993). Many researchers identify women as a fast-growing subgroup among the homeless (Milburn and D'Ercole, 1991; Warren et al., 1992), but reasons for this trend are varied. The Interagency Council on the Homeless (1990) reported that women head 80% of homeless families, are younger than other homeless people, and have fewer supportive friends and relatives, lower employment rates, and less education. Eighty percent of homeless women with children belong to a minority group (Interagency Council on the Homeless, 1990). Milburn and D'Ercole (1991) list housing instability, poverty, work problems, unemployment, and victimization as primary risk factors for homelessness in women.

Poverty is a major stressor leading to female homelessness. Before losing their homes, 82% of homeless women with children lived below the poverty line (Milburn and D'Ercole, 1991). The U.S. Census Bureau defined the poverty line for 1993 as one person living on an annual income of $7,551 or a family of four living on 15,141. The daily struggle of trying to provide for one's needs as well as the needs of one's children on such meager funds is psychologically exhausting. Psychological exhaustion and crisis-oriented lifestyles are strongly associated with homeless women (Warren et al., 1992).

Vulnerability to victimization is another predominant cause of homelessness in women. Homeless women are rarely married, experience more loss of social support than homeless men, and report familial abuse (spouse or child) as a major precursor to homelessness (Milburn and D'Ercole, 1991). Experiences of abuse often lead to social isolation, which predisposes individuals to homelessness. Jackson and McSwane (1992) found that the pregnancy rate in homeless women was twice that in the domiciled population because of limited access to birth control and a high incidence of rape. Pregnancy, however, may boost the self-esteem of homeless women who feel otherwise powerless in American mainstream society.

Children

Children sadly remind us of the grim reality of poverty and homelessness. They are innocent victims, doomed to live on the street or in shelters. Shelters are large, loud, harshly lit places with little privacy and few safe places to play. It is estimated that one in five children lives in poverty (Berck, 1992) and that children compose 12% of the total homeless population (Interagency Council on the Homeless, 1990). The impact of homelessness on children is profound and long lasting (Ziesemer et al., 1994).

Children have joined the ranks of the homeless either as members of homeless families or runaways, "throwaway" children, or "unaccompanied youths." Families often become homeless as a result of eviction, parental loss of employment or benefits, or abuse in the extended family (Milburn and D'Ercole, 1991). Runaway children generally are thought to have homes they can return to if they so desire (Interagency Council on the Homeless, 1990). Most, however, cannot return home because of family conflict. "Throwaway children" are abandoned by their families because of economic hardship or parental drug addiction. Although some throwaway children are literally abandoned, others live in such deprivation that their health and welfare are seriously undermined. "Unaccompanied youths" usually are boys between the ages of 12 and 18 who have no accompanying parent and no home. These children often are failed by a shelter system that does not accept unaccompanied children and refers these youths to runaway homes where their special needs go unmet (Interagency Council on the Homeless, 1990).

Children living in poverty and hardship often are candidates for foster care. Yet foster care situations are prime launching sites into homelessness, as many children run away from foster homes before reaching "emancipation" at age 18 (Lindblom, 1991).

Infant mortality for the homeless is 25 deaths per 1000 live births, as compared with 12 deaths per 1000 births for nonhomeless babies. Homeless children are at increased risk for hunger, poor nutrition, compromised physical health, developmental delays, psychological problems, and educational underachievement (Rafferty and Shinn, 1991). They typically have immunization delays, are at increased risk for lead poisoning, and have a high incidence of iron deficiencies related to inadequate nutrition. In addition, homeless children display language delays, difficulties with personal and social tasks, shortened attention spans, depression, anxiety, behavioral problems, poor scores on standardized math and reading tests, and poor school attendance (Rafferty and Shinn, 1991; Ziesemer et al., 1994). The list of actual and potential problems for homeless children can be overwhelming. Nurses in community health, obstetrical, emergency department, mental health, and school settings are frequently the first health professionals to make contact with these children. The loss of one's home and the shock of adjusting to life in a shelter—or on the street—produces psychological trauma in all homeless people (Goodman et al., 1991). The impact of such trauma in early life has yet to be measured.

The Elderly

Estimates of the elderly homeless population range from 3% (Interagency Council on the Homeless, 1990) to 6% (Wallsten, 1992). The lower percentage of the homeless elderly may be attributed to Social Security and other entitlements that provide income to obtain some kind of housing (Interagency Council on the Homeless, 1990). Wallsten (1992) suggests, however, that the actual number of the elderly homeless is underestimated because the elderly avoid shelters where they may be mugged, treated unkindly, or referred for institutionalization. Factors specific to the elderly, such as threat of senility, the need for special transportation, and vulnerability to attack by younger people, make homelessness particularly difficult for the older person (Damrosch and Strasser, 1988).

The trauma and extraordinary stress of homelessness seem to be borne out by mortality data related to the so-called longer-term homeless. The average age of death among those enduring extended periods of homelessness is in the early 50s. According to the Interagency Council on the Homeless (1990), "Because of special available benefits, persons over 65 rarely become homeless; and because of the harsh conditions of homelessness, few long-term homeless persons ever reach 65" (p. 37).

Immigrants, Illegal Aliens, and Minorities

People living in Third World countries often will come to the United States in hopes of finding new opportunities. Unfortunately, their hopes frequently are dashed when they encounter a strange culture with an incredibly bureaucratic system. Often immigrants are simply baffled by paperwork and clearances, and illegal aliens may be innocent victims of government quotas. Employment and housing are critical problems for this group, rendering them vulnerable to abusive working conditions (if work is found) and to living with many others in inadequate housing. When multiple stresses build, the immigrant may become homeless as a casualty of an overloaded system.

Minorities in general are overrepresented in the homeless population (Burt, 1992). African-Americans consistently have composed approximately 40% of the homeless population (Interagency Council on the Homeless, 1994). In 1990, the National American Indian Housing Council estimated that 25% of the Native Americans in the United States lived in cars, makeshift shelters, tents, or substandard housing. More than 80% of homeless women with children are nonwhite (Interagency Council on the Homeless, 1990). Poverty and unequal opportunities for minorities and noncitizens are amplified in the homeless population.

▶ Check Your Reading

6. What factors make the chronically mentally ill vulnerable to homelessness?
7. How does homelessness affect children's long-range chances to succeed?
8. Why do the elderly homeless avoid public shelters?
9. List factors that make immigrants and illegal aliens vulnerable to homelessness.

AREAS OF HOMELESSNESS

The 1994 report of the Interagency Council on the Homeless lists several reasons for increased homelessness in urban areas. Cities traditionally attracted large numbers of people seeking jobs; however, the shift in the economy over the past 25 years has decreased the demand for workers and changed labor markets. The change from a manufacturing to a service economy has jeopardized the security of laborers in the cities of the northeastern and midwestern United States. Other changes leaving many workers unemployed are a shift in demand for highly skilled employees, plant closures and relocations, and the decline in the real value of the minimum wage. Because work provides both material goods and a sense of purpose to our lives, many unemployed urban dwellers have been lured to an "underground" economy associated with drugs and prostitution for income.

Homelessness in cities is a long-standing phenomenon, but the increased incidence of the rural homelessness is relatively new. Blau (1992) credits debt-saddled farms, low salaries, and shortage of housing resulting from the rural economic crunch for the surge in undomiciled rural dwellers. The Interagency Council for the Homeless (1994) stressed the toll on farming communities during the past decades. Rural areas have sustained severe economic upheaval and have lost jobs, homes, and a way of life.

Suburban areas have not felt the impact of homelessness as severely as cities and rural areas. Suburbs offer fewer public areas and often are reached only by car. As people are crowded out of cities, however, the suburbs may become a haven for the homeless.

▶ Check Your Reading

10. What are some reasons for increased homelessness in the cities?

11. How have economic changes had an impact on rural homelessness?

FACTORS LEADING TO HOMELESSNESS

Becoming homeless is a journey rather than a discrete event. The socioeconomic aspects of the journey include the withdrawal of financial support from educational/advocacy government programs, increased poverty, chronic unemployment, limited low-income housing, deinstitutionalization, and a "burn-out" syndrome in which upper- and middle-class sympathy for the homeless is waning. Personal factors such as chronic mental illness, drug and alcohol abuse, family violence, physical infirmity, estrangement from kin/friendship support systems, poor tolerance for frustration, and difficulty developing and maintaining trust also are implicated in the journey to homelessness.

Homelessness most often is caused by loss or lack of employment and independent residence and social margin. The **social margin** is composed of the group of family members, friends and associates who offer emergency assistance and support in the wake of personal disaster. Although you may wonder why anybody is homeless in America, some researchers puzzle over why all extremely poor individuals do not become homeless. Recognizing that homelessness occurs with the collision of socioeconomic and personal factors will help you understand why people travel different journeys.

Structural Causes of Homelessness

Unemployment

In 1989 the Urban Institute found that approximately 75% of homeless adults were unemployed. Rossi (1990) defined the **unemployment rate** as a measure of the percentage of people in the work force who are out of jobs, yet unemployed people not seeking employment are not counted. Defining unemployment to include only job seekers was originally a way of eliminating the retired, the disabled, and women staying at home. It was not intended to avoid counting persons out of work for long periods of time too discouraged to continue job searches. As the need for unskilled and low-skilled laborers continues to dwindle with advancing technology, many people have become "discouraged workers."

The psychological sequelae of being unemployed range from mild to crippling. Consider the benefits of employment, which Smith (1987) cites as social contacts, time structure, social status, personal identity clarification, and a regular schedule. Warr (1987) identifies nine effects of unemployment on emotional well-being (Box 39–1). Your awareness of the detrimental results of unemployment can enhance your sensitivity to the plight of the homeless unemployed.

BOX 39–1 Effects of Unemployment

1. Decreased income—the most devastating effect
2. Constricted world, with no need to go out into the world to interact
3. Loss of "traction" or momentum to achieve
4. Loss of flexibility in decision-making
5. Loss of satisfaction with new job-related skill development
6. Increasingly uncertain future
7. Discrimination experienced in society, with patient rejected more and experiencing embarrassment
8. Deterioration of quality and nature of interpersonal contacts
9. Diminished social status and position

From Warr, P. (1987). *Work, employment, and mental health.* New York: Oxford University Press, by permission of Oxford University Press.

Inadequate Low-Cost Housing

All homeless people lack a residence, even a substandard place to live. Between 1970 and 1983, an overall effort was made to renovate properties occupied by the very poor, primarily **single-room occupancy units** (SROs) (Interagency Council on the Homeless, 1990). Although often substandard, SROs offered inexpensive housing to a large segment of young and middle-aged single people ineligible for public housing or Federal housing entitlements (Interagency Council on the Homeless, 1990). The dissolution of SROs contributed significantly to homelessness.

Many SROs were destroyed or converted to other uses in an effort to revive major cities through **gentrification,** the conversion of low-cost properties to higher-rent housing. A result was the eviction of impoverished people unable to live in improved, more expensive quarters. Other low-cost housing has been lost to arson or to abandonment by investors who can invest more profitably in other real estate.

Lindblom (1991) also highlighted the deficiency of supported housing for the mentally ill, the drug or alcohol dependent, and otherwise compromised indigent people. He pointed out the difficulty of developing any new low-cost housing, especially for disadvantaged populations. Many inhabitants of upper- and middle-class neighborhoods block construction of low-cost housing in the vicinity of their homes to avoid "contamination" of the neighborhood and declines in property values. This is the so-called NIMBY ("not in my back yard") phenomenon.

Shortage of Social Services

Social service programs developed in the 1960s during the so-called War on Poverty. Programs designed to educate, train, and financially assist the poor received substantial federal and state government support. The growing economic concerns of the 1970s and 1980s, particularly the budget deficit and the focus of the Reagan administration on decreasing peoples' dependence on the government, led to widespread voter rejection of social welfare programs. Budget cutbacks caused services provided by these social welfare programs to be slashed. The federal government cut training and job program spending by 70% between 1981 and 1990. Twenty-five percent of young people have been eliminated from summer job programs. Blau (1992) notes that five programs providing income to the financially marginal—AFDC (Aid to Families with Dependent Children), Social Security, disability benefits, unemployment insurance, and food stamps—either lost funds or saw the number of recipients limited.

Income security programs awaken conflicting feelings for many people. Concern for the needy may be offset by suspicion about welfare recipients who abuse the system and by stereotypes associated with the unemployed. Racial and gender stereotypes are called into play, as are attitudes towards the aging and the young. Many social programs provide support, even if minimal, to the elderly, children, women, and minorities. Who fills in for what the government cannot provide? Advocates for the poor and homeless, churches, individuals, and service clubs contribute as they can, but needs remain overwhelming.

▶ **Check Your Reading**

12. List effects of unemployment on psychological well-being.
13. Define gentrification and explain its impact on low-cost housing resources.
14. What were the effects of budget cutbacks during the Reagan administration?

Personal Causes of Unemployment

Overwhelmed Families

The 1992 presidential campaign made much of "family values" and the devastating breakdown occurring in families. Some advocates of limiting social benefits argue that families provide the ultimate "safety net" for members lacking financial and emotional resources. If a family member is mentally ill or substance abusing, however, family resources may atrophy over time. Imagine trying to cope with a chronically schizophrenic son who responds to auditory hallucinations, speaks in neologisms, dresses bizarrely, and might disappear without warning for months at a time. A supportive family may be unduly stressed by an unexpected familial illness or loss of a job. How would you feel if you and your seventy-year-old spouse were barely making ends meet with Social Security and your daughter, her husband, and their three children needed to move in after becoming unemployed?

If intact, families of prehomeless and homeless people often are stretched to the breaking point. Not only have chronically mentally ill people been deinstitutionalized, but institutionalizing family members who need comprehensive support is now also difficult. Involuntary commitment requires a person to be harmful to self or others, and many chronically mentally ill people needing care do not meet this criterion. Inpatient substance abuse programs may have long waiting lists and often require some form of detoxification before admission. As one mother of a homeless chronically alcoholic son in Washington, D. C., said wearily, "We've run out of ideas, and we don't have enough money. It kills his father to see him like this, but it will kill me to have him home."

The family cannot be expected to take over where government policies have left huge gaps. Some families cut off contact with a troubled member to avoid being saddled with a commitment that family members cannot take on. Families that do take on their mentally ill, drug-abusing, or violent member find little community support. Programs to meet treatment needs often do not exist, and neighbors may justifiably have concerns. Expecting families to be the sole providers of economic and emotional support for family members requiring comprehensive services is unreasonable.

Reilly (1993) has researched frequently occurring patterns within families of origin of homeless individuals. A summary of dysfunctional dynamics includes physical, psychological, or sexual abuse and neglect; physical abandonment; familial alcohol and drug abuse; and isolation from communities and other family members. With this level of family distress, a homeless person has essentially no family to turn to. A family so internally broken cannot provide a haven when an individual is threatened by external stresses.

Social Disaffiliation

Social disaffiliation is estrangement from connective bonds that tie people to social support networks and provide a psychological sense of safety, security, and trust (Goodman et al., 1991). Even the threat of homelessness may precipitate actual or perceived abandonment and leave a person isolated, distrustful, and lonely.

Awareness of these dynamics should help you understand behaviors the homeless may demonstrate. Building trust with a disaffiliated client requires tremendous time and perseverance. Often, homeless individuals have been rejected as "losers" or have been blamed for their fate. These reactions from formerly supportive others reinforce feelings of isolation and hamper the homeless person's ability to form relationships (Goodman et al., 1991).

Learned Helplessness

Learned helplessness is the fixed belief that a person's actions will have no influence or impact on the course of life (Seligman, 1975). Learned helplessness is associated with profound depression and is most likely to occur when people feel personally responsible for their adverse circumstances, believe the situation to be long-term, and credit global rather than specific factors for causing their problems (Goodman et al., 1991).

The belief that one has no control over one's life may be realistic. Homelessness does attack one's sense of competence and independence. Rossi (1990) points out too that the extreme poverty that precedes homelessness is linked with depression and hopelessness, which often intensify with the deprivation of homelessness. Creating an interdependent nurse-patient relationship with someone who perceives himself or herself to be helpless is a challenge. You need to address his or her needs while simultaneously guarding against rescuing the patient and fostering passive dependence. Long-ingrained patterns require much time to change. You can provide support and hope that such growth is possible.

▶ Check Your Reading

15. What is the impact of family dysfunction on homelessness?
16. Define social disaffiliation.
17. How can learned helplessness affect the nurse-patient relationship?

ATTITUDES TOWARD THE HOMELESS

As human beings, nurses are vulnerable to preconceived ideas and attitudes about the homeless. You therefore need to clarify your own values about poverty, homelessness, mental illness, substance abuse, and other factors related to this population. If you hold a bias or unwitting prejudice, you may need to seek supervision from another nurse, to approach clients openly. As an advocate, you also will have the opportunity to assess others for preconceived ideas and attitudes.

Distancing

People who are made uncomfortable by the homeless avoid anxiety by creating interpersonal barriers. Such barriers are erected by creating and maintaining myths about the homeless and by promoting fear of personal involvement. Myths about the homeless include "They could all work if they wanted to." "They're crazy and dangerous." "I'll catch fleas if I touch one of them." "They'll drink up any money I give them anyway." You can debunk myths by educating the public about the realities of homelessness. You also should be aware of any feelings of distance from clients and seek help from colleagues in exploring those feelings.

Disgust and Disdain

Disgust and disdain for the homeless often are based on a cursory assessment. Personal hygiene may be compromised in homeless persons, but an appreciation of living conditions in shelters or on the street might foster empathy. Disdain is a contemptuous rejection of the homeless person as being unworthy of regard. Disgust and disdain are blocks to building mutual relationships and may serve a protective function for the holders of these attitudes. Your role as educator and advocate is called into service to examine and challenge these feelings.

Moral Superiority

Moral superiority goes hand in hand with fear, disgust, and a sense of one's precedence over the other. Homelessness is not a sign of personal defect or weak character. An attitude of moral superiority indicates a perception of an unequal power between people. This stance precludes honest communication, sharing, or understanding the homeless individual's circumstances. Be particularly sensitive in detecting any personal sense of moral superiority when working with the homeless.

Guilt

Guilt is a useful feeling when it motivates us to correct a wrong. If it is misdirected, however, guilt may be crippling and prevent action rather than promote it. Seeing homeless men, women, and children on the street touches a chord within us. That chord should promote responsibility rather than guilt. Taking responsibility for using our own time, money, and effort to intervene one on one is more useful than feeling a global sense of guilt about all homeless people. As an educator, you can reframe homelessness as a situation for empathy and caring rather than guilt.

Fear

Homeless people are just people like the rest of us. This knowledge should ease fears of the homeless as a group and help to challenge fear that some experience as a knee-jerk reaction. It is naive and potentially dangerous, however, to disregard fear completely. Be attentive to fear as a sign of possible peril and educate others to be respectful of those feelings. Just as people with homes can be antisocial and otherwise risky, homeless people can be dangerous as well.

▶ Check Your Reading

18. How do preconceived ideas and attitudes affect the nurse-patient relationship?

NURSING PROCESS

The nursing process offers an organized approach to working with homeless people. A sense of structure and pacing can be particularly helpful when you must practice in a potentially chaotic environment. Having a systematic guide to approaching interventions with the homeless may lessen your anxiety and communicate professional competence to the patients themselves.

ASSESSING HOMELESS PATIENTS

Because homelessness is a multidimensional state of being, assessment should be multidimensional. Physical assessment skills are put to good use as the nurse seeks to uncover any somatic deficits or dysfunction. Unusual behavior may have roots in a physical cause; for example, a confused client may be intoxicated, hypo- or hyperglycemic, or suffering from a head injury. The goal of the psychosocial assessment, however, should be to reveal and support the client's positive coping skills.

A psychosocial assessment should be approached with flexibility, sensitivity, and a willingness to go at the client's pace. Cowger (1994) has devised an assessment tool for social workers, which is easily modified for nursing (Table 39–1). Cowger states that an emphasis on the patient's dysfunction may make that the focus of the assessment, which in turn leads to self-fulfilling prophecies and increases the patient's dependence on the nurse. An assessment focused on patient strengths empowers him or her to take control of his or her life and adopt new solutions to old problems. Therefore, a nursing assessment based on identifying and maximizing patient strengths is also an initial intervention.

INTERVENTIONS FOR THE HOMELESS

Interventions for the homeless must be realistic and focused on the patient's priorities. The plan should include not just goals but also concrete steps designed to meet the objectives. For example, it's not enough to plan that a homeless patient will meet a clinic appointment. You must strategize with the patient to find transportation to the clinic, to devise a way to communicate the patient's needs to the clinic's staff (referrals or advance phone calls are helpful), and to design a plan for learning the results of the evaluation. If the clinic appointment is not a priority for the patient, it may be missed as other needs take precedence. The most effective planning is done with flexibility, patience, and a willingness to reschedule activities when necessary.

Meeting emotional and spiritual needs is more difficult than planning to meet physical needs. You may have only sporadic contact with a homeless person and lack the time to develop a long-term relationship that would allow you to respond to his or her emotional and spiritual needs. You therefore need to plan to make the most of short interactions and to communicate caring, respect, compassion, and a belief in the homeless person's innate worth and dignity.

Strategies Directed at Changing the System

Interventions include actions to address the system-wide issues that lead to homelessness and actions that directly serve the homeless person. Proactive interventions involve trying to prevent homelessness in the first place. Historically, nurses have championed the cause of the economically and socially disadvantaged through advocacy, education, and political involvement.

Advocacy means championing the cause of the homeless. Hodnicki (1990) believes that nurses, as homeless advocates, can write about health issues for community newspapers, consult with legislators on health concerns, and coordinate coalitions of public and private enterprises to support and assist the homeless. Financial contributions, volunteering in literacy programs, and voting for elected officials sympathetic to the homeless are also means of advocacy.

Education, both of self and others, is also an important strategy for change. Nurses need to learn about the problems of the homeless in their cities or towns. Where do they live? What are the problems? Where do their children go to school? What resources are available?

Nurses also need to share their knowledge about the homeless with professional associates, family, friends, and other clients. Nurses have the power to dispel many of the myths surrounding homelessness. Inaccurate information about the homeless promotes distance and blocks the development of cooperative efforts between the homeless and the domiciled to address problems.

Political involvement is a critical third strategy. Voting is an essential way to influence the political process, but nurses also need to communicate opinions and questions to legislators. Letters to legislators influence votes. Nurses need to find constructive ways to protest political decisions with which they feel dissatisfied.

Protesting homelessness is also important. People living on the streets is a national tragedy. Political involvement also may mean helping the homeless to register as voters or simply objecting to citizens being victimized. Remember that the poor feel powerless and unimportant. You need to speak for underprivileged adults and children.

STRATEGIES WITH HOMELESS PEOPLE

Direct interventions with the homeless are the basis of nurse-patient relationships in this population. Learn about the multidimensional needs of the homeless and be prepared to individualize care. The building of trust is an arduous task with the homeless, and time limits may not permit it. A long-term relationship with the patient, however, is essential for developing the patient's confidence.

Consistency is an important element in creating and sustaining trust. Remember that no matter how moving the story of the homeless person may be, you need to

TABLE 39–1 Strengths-Focused Assessment Guidelines

Guideline	Intervention/Example
Emphasize the patient's understanding of the facts	Focus the assessment on the patient's view of the situation, the meaning the patient assigns to the situation, and the patient's related feelings or emotions. For example, with a newly homeless alcoholic, tailor questions to elicit the patient's understanding of alcohol use, its relation to homelessness, and how the person feels about it.
Believe the patient	Assume the patient is trustworthy and is telling the truth. If the patient has an obvious impairment such as inebriation or psychosis, believe the patient's feeling content and reexplore the facts when symptoms are controlled.
Discover what the patient wants	Focus on what the patient wants and expects from the nurse and on what resolution the patient wants or expects in the current problem situation. For example, if a homeless patient wants the nurse to obtain free medications and sees them as a solution to depression, then the nurse can plan interventions around the patient's motivation.
Move the assessment toward personal and environmental strengths	Steer the assessment toward identifying possibilities and existing strengths rather than obstacles. A homeless patient who will accept antipsychotic medication from only one nurse can be viewed as capable of forming some trust and rapport rather than as noncompliant and uncooperative.
Do multidimensional assessment of strengths	Identify the patient's interpersonal skills, emotional strengths, ability to think clearly, and motivation. Uncover any external supports the patient may have, such as family, friends, religious affiliations, or community groups. For example, a homeless mother without a supportive family may have perseverance, intelligence, and tentative links with a church support group.
Use the assessment to discover the patient's uniqueness	Center the assessment around the patient's unique self and response to the problem. Norms are useful only in confirming that the patient is an individual. For example, if most patients are distressed by homelessness and your patient claims not to be, accept your client's novel reaction and use that for information.
Use language the patient understands	Assessments should be done in clear, self-explanatory English (or whatever language the patient best understands). The assessment must be accessible and useful for both patient and nurse. For example, write down patient statements verbatim and avoid translating them into nursing jargon.
Make assessment a mutual activity between patient and nurse	Ensure that the assessment is open and shared between patient and nurse. Allow the patient to "own" the assessment by stressing the importance of understanding the patient's wants and needs. For example, pace the assessment to allow time for the patient to ask questions, clarify feelings, and stress important points.
Reach a mutual agreement on the assessment	The nurse should do the assessment in open association with the patient. For example, write down information and share it with the patient to check accuracy and confirm goals. The patient can be given a copy of the assessment to keep.
Avoid blame and blaming	Blaming the patient for the situation is disrespectful, leads nowhere, and supports a deficit-centered style of assessment. Nurses must refrain from judging and should maintain open minds about the host of possible causes in any situation. For example, a homeless alcoholic may not view chemical dependence as detrimental. The nurse uses this as information rather blaming the patient for being homeless.

Nursing modification based on Cowger, C. D. (1994). Assessing client strengths. Clinical assessment for client empowerment. *Social Work 39* (3):262–267.

avoid making promises that are impossible to deliver. Homeless people usually can share histories replete with personal disappointments and broken promises. The nurse who is able to deliver on a promise is viewed by the homeless person as different from most other people. Promises and commitments, however, are best kept simple and limited to areas the nurse can control.

Helping people in concrete ways, developing trust,

TABLE 39–1 **Strengths-Focused Assessment Guidelines** *Continued*

Guideline	Intervention/Example
Avoid cause-and-effect thinking	Avoid cause-and-effect thinking, which leads to blaming. Don't forget that each problem is multilayered and consists of a complex set of actions and dynamics. For example, a homeless crack addict who has lost a job may have lost it because of cutbacks rather than because of addiction.
Assess, don't diagnose	Nursing diagnosis is understood as a way of labeling a deficit or dysfunction. Maintain focus on mutual exploration of the coping skills, relationship patterns, and style of negotiating the world. Nonsensical or difficult-to-understand answers will still provide information without taking away the patient's right to share a personal story in a dignified manner.

and being consistent will all help in building interpersonal bridges. These connections can help disempowered individuals see themselves as worthwhile and unique. Do not be discouraged by chronic mental illness, substance abuse, or despair. As Eleanor Roosevelt said, "It is better to light one candle than to curse the darkness." Making a difference to one person is a huge contribution.

Practical interventions are the most useful tools in relationship building. Remembering a patient's name is a small step but may have tremendous importance to someone used to being treated as invisible. Reviewing test results, setting up complicated medication regimens in individualized medicine boxes, or arranging transportation to appointments all indicate that you are invested in the patient. Even the simplest nursing tasks, if done with care and concern, may communicate greater meaning to people who feel so isolated from others.

STRATEGIES FOR SELF-CARE

An axiom in psychiatry states that the therapist can take the patient only as far as the therapist has gone. An appropriate variation of this axiom for working with the homeless might be "Nurses can care only for the homeless as well as they care for themselves." Being with the homeless is emotionally draining and often painful. You therefore must care for yourself physically, emotionally, and spiritually if you wish to continue caring for others. A support group of other nurses and professionals working with the homeless can be an important source of substance and perspective. Interventions to enhance your own self-care are also essential when working with the homeless population.

Recognizing one's own limits is very important. Homelessness is tragic, and tragedy intensified when patients stop being a faceless group and become personally familiar. Practice within appropriate personal and professional boundaries to avoid being overwhelmed and frustrated.

Another strategy for self-care is maintaining the balance between work and rest and recreation. To work with the homeless, you must feel refreshed. Recreational activities and sufficient time to relax help you maintain an even outlook.

EVALUATING INTERVENTIONS

Recognize that working with the homeless presents tremendous challenges, so that evaluation of care requires realistic expectations. Some homeless people are well motivated to change and will eagerly accept any suggestion or gesture of help. Others are noncompliant, antisocial, entrenched, actively substance abusing, or acting out. The measurement of progress may not be in achieving objective outcomes but in making infinitesimal steps in relationship-building.

Patient noncompliance may be a frequent outcome of well-planned interventions. Noncompliance may be a temporary setback or a long-established stance, but you should avoid personalizing the patient's failure to follow through. Focusing the evaluation on what the patient has achieved rather than on how the patient has failed is a helpful way to frame the final step of the nursing process. A client who takes medication once a day instead of twice a day is still halfway there.

▶ Check Your Reading

19. How is a strengths-based assessment a useful initial intervention?
20. How can you function as a homeless advocate?
21. What characteristics must you display while directly interviewing with homeless clients?

CASE STUDY: BILL

While working as a case manager in the emergency department, you are introduced to Bill, a 54-year-old male who has lived on the streets for the past five years. Prior to that time he lived with his mother who is now deceased. He is in the emergency department because he was beaten by a group of gang members. His affect is restricted, and you notice that he does not seem to trust you. When you ask Bill if he has any friends, he tells you that he does not and that he prefers to be alone. He does admit to having an older sister, Ann, but tells you he only talks to her at Christmas and is not interested in having a relationship with her. With further interviewing, you find that he has never had an intimate relationship and receives little pleasure from any hobbies or interests. He tells you that he did like working on the computer when he was living with his mother but says "I will never be able to take care of myself or have anything."

ASSESSMENT

Assessment data are as follows:

- Homeless adult male
- Multiple bruises and lacerations
- Verbalizations of inability to exert any influence in current life situation
- Restricted affect
- Mistrust of health professionals
- Receives little pleasure from social interaction
- Enjoys solitary activities

DIAGNOSIS

***DSM-IV* Diagnosis:** Schizoid personality disorder

Nursing Diagnosis: Powerlessness related to lack of support system since mother's death evidenced by reality of current living situation (homeless), verbalizations of despair and apathy

OUTCOME IDENTIFICATION, PLANNING, AND IMPLEMENTATION

EXPECTED OUTCOME 1: By discharge, the patient will be able to be an active participant in effectively managing his life.

SHORT-TERM GOAL	NURSING INTERVENTIONS	RATIONALES
By _____ the patient will participate in a decision regarding his care.	1. Encourage the patient to express needs and wants regarding care while in the hospital. 2. Allow the patient to establish self-care routines.	1–2. Providing the patient with simple choices will increase his feelings of self-control.
	3. Provide positive feedback for decisions that are made by the patient.	3. Unrealistic goals set by the patient could lead to failure and increase feelings of powerlessness.

EXPECTED OUTCOME 2: By _____ the patient will verbalize a desire to exert some control over his life.

SHORT-TERM GOAL	NURSING INTERVENTIONS	RATIONALES
By _____ the patient will request help making decisions regarding his discharge plans	1. Take time to establish a trusting relationship with the patient.	1. The patient has a long history of not trusting.
	2. Encourage the patient to consider some type of group home as a transition to living alone.	2. Attempting independent living prior to job training and necessary therapy may lead to failure.
	3. Remain a patient advocate throughout this process. 4. Tell the patient that you believe he can have a quality life and that you believe in him.	3–4. Nurses often take the place of family and friends as the sole support system for the patient.

EXPECTED OUTCOME 3: By _____ the patient will verbalize statements of hope for the future.

SHORT-TERM GOAL	NURSING INTERVENTIONS	RATIONALES
By _____ the patient will verbalize hope and meaning in his existence.	1. Encourage the patient to express negative feelings of hopelessness, despondency and alienation.	1. This allows the patient an opportunity to ventilate feelings that have been pent up for a long time.
	2. Help the patient to identify some positive aspects of his life, such as a sister who is living in the same locale and his computer skills. 3. Help the patient identify behaviors that promote hopelessness and powerlessness, such as isolation.	2–3. Feeling powerlessness does not promote an honest appraisal of one's situation.
	4. Encourage the patient to discuss how spiritual beliefs have affected him. 5. Offer to provide some spiritually based readings for the patient.	4–5. It is not unusual for homeless persons to feel abandoned by God. Finding a relationship with the God of their understanding often restores hope.

EVALUATION

Formative Evaluation Bill was able to participate in limited decision-making regarding his self-care and did ask for help from the staff in regard to living arrangements post discharge. He did acknowledge that his world fell apart after his mother died, and he acknowledged the tremendous impact of her death. He initiated a phone call to his sister and stated that he looked forward to having a relationship with her.

Summative Evaluation Bill partially met the expected outcomes. The case manager felt that Bill would need more support before he could effectively manage his life. Bill did begin to verbalize statements of hope for the future, however. He stated "I am looking forward to learning more about computers and to getting a job so I can support myself." He stated that he was never really abandoned by God and expressed a desire to attend a church service.

CONCLUSIONS

Both the journey to homelessness and the destination are complex and painful. Nurses have an important role to play in working with the homeless as clinicians, advocates, educators, and fellow human beings. The approach taken by the individual nurse must have personal meaning. This story provides one example:

It was a chilly, overcast day when the horseman spied the little sparrow lying on its back in the middle of the road. Reining in his mount, he looked down and inquired of the fragile creature, "Why are you lying upside down like that?" "I heard the heavens are going to fall today," replied the bird. The horseman laughed, "And I suppose your spindly legs can hold up the heavens?" "One does what one can," said the little sparrow.

KEY POINTS TO REMEMBER

- Homelessness results from a complex set of personal and structural factors.
- Homelessness has existed throughout history.
- A standardized definition of homelessness hampers the study of the phenomenon.
- The face of homelessness changed from tramps, hoboes, and skid row dwellers to the "new homeless" in the 1970s and 1980s.
- Deinstitutionalization is the civil rights–based action that released thousands of chronically mentally ill inpatients to community mental health centers unprepared to handle them.
- Admission diversion is a gatekeeping tactic that limits access to state mental hospitals by restricting admission criteria.
- Eighty percent of homeless families are headed by single women.
- Homeless children suffer long-term detrimental effects resulting from poor physical and mental health, inadequate nutrition, early trauma, and educational underachievement.
- "Throwaway children" are literally abandoned because of poverty and parental drug addiction.
- Alcohol is the substance most abused by the homeless population.
- Homeless substance abusers suffer from a myriad of physical illnesses that impede efforts to escape from homelessness.
- Immigrants and illegal aliens are vulnerable to homelessness because of complicated bureaucratic structures.
- Minorities are overrepresented in the homeless population.
- Homelessness primarily is still an urban problem but has appeared in rural areas because of the rural economic crunch.
- Unemployment results as a shift from a goods-based to a

service-based economy, which requires better-educated workers and eliminates less-skilled positions.

• The eradication of single-room occupancy housing units (SROs) has contributed significantly to homelessness.

• Gentrification is the destruction of low-cost properties to make room for higher-rent housing units.

• Dramatic cuts in social service programs during the Reagan administration eliminated critical economic resources for at-risk individuals who then became homeless.

• Dysfunctional family dynamics exist in the families of origin of many homeless individuals.

• Healthy families can be overwhelmed by the needs of a chronically mentally ill, unemployed, or substance-abusing member and may be unable to provide shelter and support.

• Social disaffiliation is the profound estrangement of an individual from a known social support network.

• Learned helplessness is a phenomenon in which individuals feel powerless in their own lives and become passive and indifferent as a result.

• Preconceived ideas and attitudes toward the homeless block the building of meaningful relationships.

• Nursing assessment based on identifying and maximizing the strengths of the patient is an important initial intervention.

• Planning care for the homeless must be mutually determined and reality based.

• Nursing interventions for the homeless include political, direct, and self-care strategies.

• Evaluation of nursing interventions should focus on patient success rather than on patient failure.

LEARNING ACTIVITIES

1. List any attitudes or preconceived ideas you have about the homeless as a group. Explain the experience or exposure you have had that led you to develop your attitudes or ideas.

2. Discuss your list with your classmates. How many attitudes or preconceived ideas did you identify? Did identifying your attitudes and ideas help you to view them differently? Did any other students provide feedback to challenge your attitude or preconceived idea?

3. If you were working in a homeless shelter, what would you consider important in establishing a relationship with a patient? What strategies would you employ to encourage compliance?

CRITICAL THINKING EXERCISE

Nurse Maryann Nolan works in the emergency department of the city hospital during the evening shift. In consultation with a colleague about a strategy to deal with a patient, Maryann told the story of Helen, a street woman who brought her 10-year-old son to the emergency department at least twice a week, complaining that she had to have a doctor see her son. Each time she had a different reason why her son had missed school. Sometimes it was because he had cut his finger or because he had a stomach ache or a bloody nose. At least two other nights per week, Helen would stop by the emergency department to talk to Maryann about her day.

1. What assumption can you make about Helen?

2. What is Nurse Nolan's point of view about the homeless?

3. What evidence supports your assumptions?

Maryann's colleague asked Maryann if she had ever told Helen to go to the day clinics to have her son examined. Maryann replied, "Yes, but then Helen disappeared for a month, and the next time I saw her, her son looked sick and hungry and Helen shouted at me, calling me a bouncer."

1. Make sense of the evidence.

2. What do you think Maryann is assuming about Helen and her family?

3. What are alternative explanations?

REFERENCES

Bachrach, L. (1992). What we know about homelessness among mentally ill persons: An analytical review and commentary. *Hospital and Community Psychiatry, 43* (5), 453–464.

Berck, J. (1992). No place to be: Voices of homeless children. Boston: Houghton Mifflin Company.

Blau, J. (1992). The visible poor: Homelessness in the United States. New York and Oxford: Oxford University Press.

Burt, M. (1992). *Over the edge.* New York: Russell Sage.

Carter, K. F., Green, R. D., Green, L., and Dufour, L. T. (1994). Health needs of homeless clients accessing nursing care at a free clinic. *Journal of Community Health Nursing, 11* (3), 139–147.

Cowger, C. D. (1994). Assessing client strengths: Clinical assessment for client empowerment. *Social Work, 39* (3), 262–267.

Damrosch, S., and Strasser, J. A. (1988). The homeless elderly in America. *Journal of Gerontological Nursing, 14* (10), 26–29.

Dennis, D. L., Buckner, J. C., Lipton, F. R., and Levine, I. S. (1991). A decade of research and services for homeless mentally ill persons: Where do we stand? *American Psychologist, 46* (11), 1129–1138.

Federal Task Force on Homelessness and Severe Mental Illness. (1992). *Outcasts on main street,* Washington, D. C.: Federal Task Force on Homelessness and Severe Mental Illness.

Fischer, P. J., and Breakey, W. R. (1990). The epidemiology of alcohol, drug, and mental disorders among homeless persons. *American Psychologist, 46* (11), 1115–1128.

Foscarinis, M. (1991). The politics of homelessness: A call to action. *American Psychologist, 46* (11), 1232–1238.

Goodman, L., Saxe, L., and Harvey, M. (1991). Homelessness as psychological trauma: Broadening perspectives. *American Psychologist, 46* (11), 1219–1225.

Hodnicki, D. R. (1990). Homelessness: Health-care implications. *Journal of Community Health Nursing,* 7 (2), 59–67.

Interagency Council on the Homeless. (1990). The 1990 annual report of the interagency council on the homeless. Washington, D. C.: Interagency Council on the Homeless.

Interagency Council on the Homeless. (1994). Priority: Home! The Federal plan to break the cycle of homelessness. Washington, D. C.: Interagency Council on the Homeless.

Jackson, M. P., and McSwane, D. Z. (1992). Homelessness as a determinant of health. *Public Health Nursing, 9* (3), 185–192.

Liebow, E. (1993). *Tell them who I am: The lives of homeless women.* New York: The Free Press.

Lindblom, E. (1991). Toward a comprehensive homelessness prevention strategy. Fannie Mae Annual Housing Conference, Washington, D. C., pp 1–54.

Marin, P. (1991). Why are the homeless mainly single men? *The Nation.* July 8, 46–50.

Milburn, N., and D'Ercole, A. (1991). Homeless women: Moving toward a comprehensive model. *American Psychologist, 46* (11), 1161–1169.

Rafferty, Y., and Shinn, M. (1991). The impact of homelessness on children. *American Psychologist, 46* (11), 1170–1179.

Reilly, F. (1993). Experience of family among homeless individuals. *Issues in Mental Health Nursing, 14,* 309–321.

Rossi, P. (1990). The old homeless and the new homeless in historical perspective. *American Psychologist, 45* (8), 945–959.

Schubert, H. J. P. (1935). Twenty thousand transients: A year's sample of those who apply for aid in a northern city. Buffalo, N.Y.: Emergency Relief Bureau.

Seligman, M. E. P. (1975). *Helplessness: On depression, development, and death.* San Francisco: Freeman.

Smith, R. (1987). *Unemployment and health: A disaster and challenge.* Oxford: Oxford University Press.

Urban Institute. (1991). *Policy and research report.* Washington, D. C.: Urban Institute.

Wallsten, S. M. (1992). Geriatric mental health: A portrait of homelessness. Journal of Psychosocial Nursing, *30* (9), 20–24.

Warr, P. (1987). *Work, employment, and mental health.* Oxford: Clarendon Press; New York: Oxford University Press.

Warren, B. J., Menke, E. M., Clement, J., & Wagner, J. (1992). The mental health of African-American and caucasian-American women who are homeless. *Journal of Psychosocial Nursing, 30* (11), 27–30.

Ziesemer, C., Marcoux, L., and Marwell, B. E. (1994). Homeless children: Are they different from other low income children? *Social Work, 39* (6), 658–668.

SUGGESTED READINGS

Berck, J. (1992). No place to be: Voices of homeless children. Boston: Houghton Mifflin Company.

Carter, K. F., Green, R. D., Green L., Dufour, L. T. (1994). Health needs of homeless clients accessing care at a free clinic. *Journal of Community Health Nursing, 11* (3), 139–147.

Liebow, E. (1993). *Tell them who I am. The lives of homeless women.* New York: The Free Press.

Smith, R. (1987). *Unemployment and health: A disaster and challenge.* Oxford: Oxford University Press.

CHAPTER 40

THE JOURNEY MARKED BY VIOLENCE

If a child lives with criticism, he learns to condemn.
If a child lives with hostility, he learns to fight.
If a child lives with ridicule, he learns to be shy.
If a child lives with shame, he learns to feel guilty.
If a child lives with tolerance, he learns to be patient.

—*Dorothy Law Nolte*

LEARNING OBJECTIVES

After studying this chapter, you should be able to:

1. Appreciate the scope of violence in American society.
2. Define terms such as violence, abuse, neglect, and sexual abuse.
3. Discuss some of the key characteristics of family violence and abuse.
4. Discuss the *hostage response*, which is so characteristic of victims of any interpersonal violence.
5. Describe the various types of family victimization, including sibling violence and parents as victims.
6. Discuss at least three causes of family violence.
7. Describe the perpetrator of abuse.
8. Describe the victim of abuse.
9. Describe the cycle of abuse.
10. Apply the nursing process to a case study in which spousal abuse is present.
11. Apply the nursing process to a case study in which child abuse is present.
12. Apply the nursing process to a case study in which elder abuse is present.
13. Apply the nursing process to a case study in which a psychiatric patient becomes violent.

KEY TERMINOLOGY

Abuse
Battered-child syndrome
Battering syndrome
Child abuse
Cycle of abuse
Elder abuse
Emotional abuse
Expressive violence
Hostage response
Instrumental violence
Mutual combat model
Neglect
Restraints
Seclusion
Sexual abuse
Spousal abuse
Violence
Wife-battering model

Almost daily, in newspapers, on television, and on radio, we are confronted with stories of random violence. We are horrified and frightened. We fear that we will be touched by the violence. We comfort ourselves with the thought that violence occurs "somewhere out there," somewhere we are not. In the summer of 1994, we watched the undoing of an American hero, O. J. Simpson, as he drove along the Los Angeles Freeway, a fugitive of the law and the prime suspect in the brutal murder of his wife and her male friend. We were horrified to hear the 911 recording of Nicole Simpson frantically calling the police because O. J. Simpson was breaking into her house and threatening to kill her. Americans could not comprehend that the public persona of Simpson was no more than a superficial cover for a violent, angry, and dangerous man. Read Joyce's story and think about how many other women live with violence or the threat of violence as an everyday occurrence.

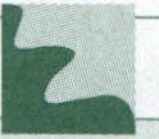

JOYCE'S STORY

I did not, and even today, do not think of my husband, Lou, as a violent man. He wouldn't always be violent when he was upset. I guess that's what unsettled me the most. I could never exactly figure what it was that would set him off. He hit me for the first time shortly after we were married. He couldn't find his cuff links. Since I unpacked everything, he tore into me. He hit me with the back of his hand and sent me across the room. He was full of apologies the next day, and more than a year went by before he hit me again. I don't really remember what set him off that time. But soon the time between the hitting was down to months, then weeks. I did everything I could think to please him. But I just couldn't think of everything. I remember once when I yelled at him, he came back at me and said, "I guess things are getting too easy around here." Then he slapped and punched me. I started to go a little crazy. I just couldn't think of everything. All the time he was around I felt like I was walking on a tightrope. Just one little slip and I knew I might get it. When he did hit me, I was relieved. At least I didn't have to be so tense anymore.

FAMILY VIOLENCE, ABUSE, AND THE JOURNEY

Joyce's denial of her husband's violence kept her in a dangerous situation. Denial prevents individuals as well as society from facing up to the truth and the need for change. Increasingly, our denial is shattered by incidents of violence that take place in schools and even in hospital settings. Across the United States, Emergency Departments are being equipped with metal detectors to search visitors and patients for weapons. Nurses in settings other than psychiatry are being trained to deal with aggressive behavior (Selby, 1992).

Violence is not limited to the random and senseless murders that occur on the streets of the United States. Violence affects families—women, children, and elders. Atrocities are committed against friends and neighbors, by someone in the family, by one or more of the persons supposed to love, protect, and cherish them. These acts of betrayal, violence, and sometimes murder usually take place in the home, the one place we should be assured a safe haven from the stresses of the world. As *Time* magazine highlighted in the cover story of the December 21, 1987 issue, for far too many Americans, "Home is where the hurt is." The violence that occurs in our homes is not a private matter to be dealt with and handled by those most intimately involved. Rather, violence is a public matter. We are all affected. When we turn away from the brokenness, pain, and suffering of others; when we allow ourselves to be immune to the screams, bruises, and cuts of a child; when we ignore the blackened eyes and the bruised belly of a pregnant woman; when we deny that elders are abused by their children—then we give tacit approval to acts of violence that are fundamentally wrong.

As Gelles and Straus (1988, p. ii) stated in their comprehensive research into intimate violence, "People are not for hitting." The victims of abuse do not need criticism or pity. What they need is the support and intervention of a society both shocked and appalled at what is transpiring behind closed doors. Our outrage must be operationalized into strategies that change attitudes encouraging violence, that offer refuge and places of healing for victims, and that offer both consequences for violent acts and treatment for abusers.

One of the difficulties in estimating the extent of family violence is in defining the term *violence*. For example, is parental spanking of a child an act of child abuse or discipline? Can a husband who forces his wife to perform oral sex be found guilty of a crime, or is he just an insensitive, mean individual? Figure 40–1 illustrates that all acts of physical and sexual violence are issues of power and control.

Terms Describing Violence

Gelles and Straus (1988) as well as others who write about family violence generally support a definition of **violence** that includes any acts (from a pinch or a slap to murder) carried out with the intention of causing physical pain or injury to another person. **Abuse** is more difficult to define. The term has been politicized, and it is not clinical or scientific. Therefore, definition of abuse varies greatly across individuals. In 1974, however, the National Center on Child Abuse and Neglect (Child Abuse Prevention and Treatment Act) defined **child abuse** as follows:

The physical or mental injury, sexual abuse, negligent treatment, or maltreatment of a child under the age of 18 by a person who is responsible for the child's welfare under circumstances which indicate that the child's health or welfare is harmed or threatened thereby.

Gil (1975) broadened this formal definition by including "any acts of commission or omission by a parent or an individual, an institution, or by society as a whole which deprive a child of equal rights and liberty, and/or interfere with or constrain the child's ability to achieve his or her optimal developmental potential." These definitions of abuse focus on children. We should not, however, be limited to children when we consider abuse. Clearly, adults can be victims of abuse as well.

The National Center on Child Abuse and Neglect introduced the concepts of mental injury, sexual abuse, and neglect as dimensions of abuse. Examining the specifics of abuse poses a formidable task. For instance, how do we define **emotional abuse?** Such things as belittling, scorning, ignoring, tearing down, harping, and criticizing are all possible forms of emotional abuse. Emotional abuse can be overt as well as subtle. Gelles and Straus (1988) report that one woman, on repeated occasions, was subjected to her husband showing her

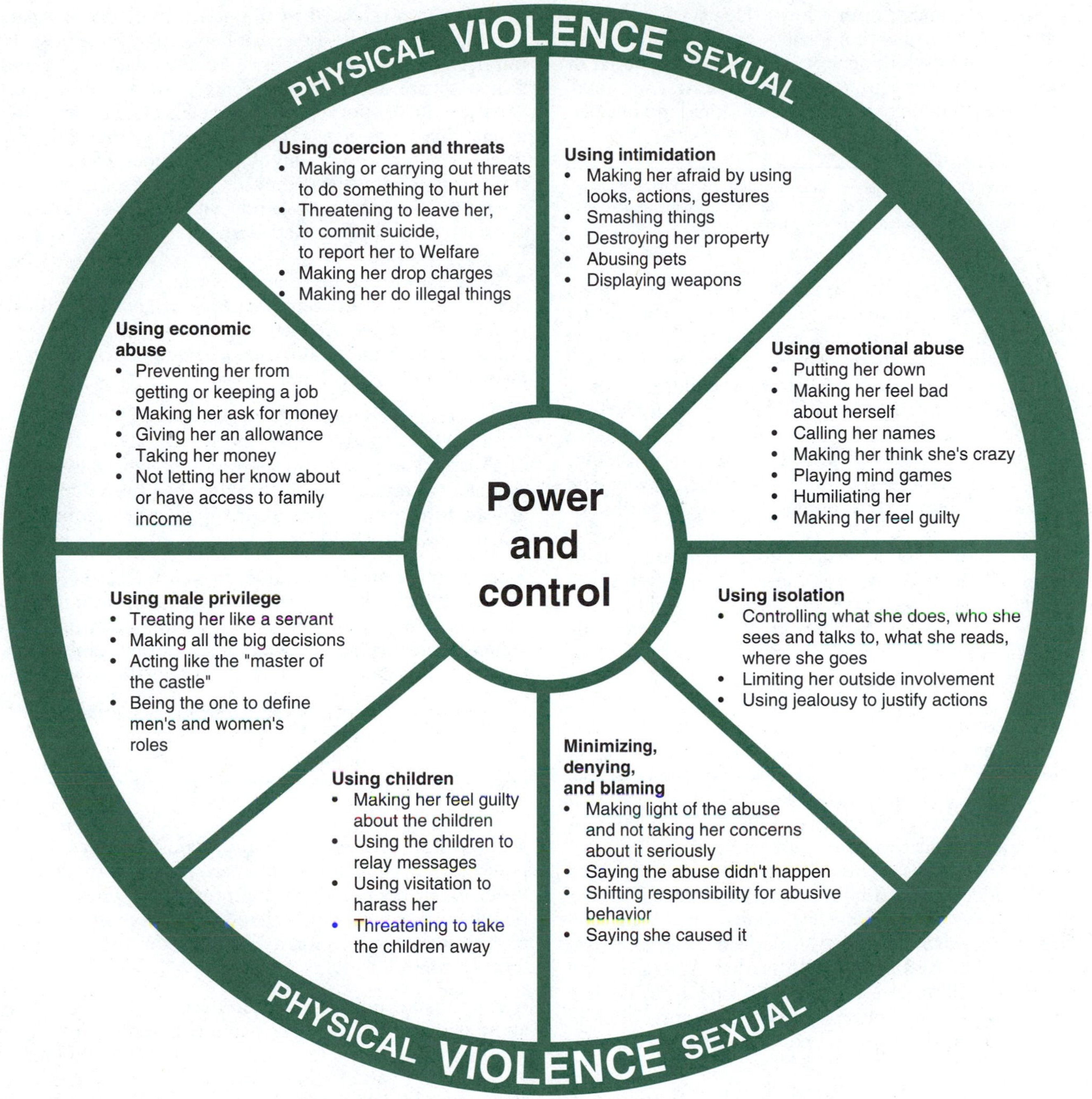

FIGURE 40–1

All acts of physical and sexual violence are issues of power and control. (Redrawn from the Domestic Abuse Intervention Project, 204 West Fourth St., Duluth, MN 55806.)

gifts he had purchased for his girlfriend. The husband told his wife that he would return home after delivering the gifts. These behaviors continued while the family was on welfare.

Repeated attacks on an individual's self-esteem can leave deep, lasting scars. Victims of physical abuse frequently say that the physical scars of family violence fade, but the pain from emotional wounds continues to fester beneath the surface forever. The signs of emotional abuse are not as easily recognized as the bruises, cuts, and scars from physical abuse. Instead, emotional abuse becomes apparent when we hear the stories of victims. Consider Tracy's comments in Case Example 40–1.

Case Example 40–1 Tracy's Story

He rarely says a kind word to me. He is always critical. The food is too cold or it's too hot. The kids are too noisy.

The house is a mess. I am a mess. He says I spend too much money and then complains that I look like I got dressed in a used-clothing store. He says I am too fat or too skinny. No matter what I do he says it isn't any good. He tells me I am lucky he married me 'cause no one else would have me.

From *Intimate violence*: The Definitive Study of the Causes and Consequences of Abuse in the American Family. Published by Simon & Schuster. Copyright © 1988 by Richard J. Gelles and Murray A. Straus.

How do we define **neglect?** Generally, neglect represents acts of omission rather than a physical act of commission. Parents may fail to provide the basic necessities for their children or on a more passive level may be emotionally unavailable to their children, leaving them as isolates in a harsh world. Acts of neglect include failing to seek and follow through with medical care for a sick child. In areas of neglect, the dilemma is whether the neglect is purposeful or comes from lack of adequate financial and material resources to care properly for children.

Finally, what about sexual abuse? Kempe and associates (1962) defined **sexual abuse** as "the involvement of dependent and developmentally immature children and adolescents in sexual activities that they do not fully comprehend, to which they are unable to give informed consent, or that violate social taboos of family roles." This definition has not been without detractors. Some say the definition is so broad as to allow social scientists to define even excessive hugging as abuse. Others would like to see sexual abuse of children limited to only forced sexual intercourse. Finekelhor and Yllo (1985) suggest that sexual abuse refers to activities involving the genitals that are for the gratification of at least one person.

Until the 1970s, sexual abuse of children remained largely hidden. Two attitudes promoted secrecy. The first was the powerful taboo against adults having sex with children that exists not only in American society, but also in others. The second attitude is that Americans are generally unwilling to discuss sexuality openly. By the late 1970s, however, an explosion of official reports of child sexual abuse caused a general concern for the welfare of children.

▶ Check Your Reading

1. Define violence.
2. Define sexual abuse.
3. Define neglect.

Extent of Violence and Abuse

National statistics provide an incomplete picture of the incidence and extent of family violence and abuse. Data from the National Crime Survey conducted by the Department of Justice, in which 60,000 households throughout the United States were surveyed, usually reflect violence that victims are willing to label as criminal and report to authorities. In addition, the Federal Bureau of Investigation (FBI) compiles data about eight categories of crimes reported to the police. Included are data regarding homicide, rape, robbery, aggravated assault, burglary, larceny, motor-vehicle theft, and arson. Crimes that originate out of family violence, such as nonaggravated assault, are not reported to the FBI, and information about the relationship between the victim and the offender is collected only for homicide. Despite the limitations of the data, they do provide some insights regarding the extent of family violence. For instance, consider the following statistics:

- About 20% of all murder victims in the United States are related to their assailants. In about one third of these situations, the victim is a woman killed by either her husband or boyfriend (*Attorney General's task force on family violence, final report*, 1984).

- Most crimes committed by relatives—57%—are committed by spouses or ex-spouses. In about 25% of situations in which the spouse or ex-spouse is the assailant, victims reported that they had been attacked at least three other times in the previous six months (Klaus & Rand, 1989).

- Between 1.8 and 2.9 million women are battered yearly. In fact, battering is the single most common cause of injury to women, exceeding mugging, motor-vehicle accidents, and occupational injuries combined (Battered Women and Criminal Justice, 1987).

- The cost of absenteeism from work as a result of assaults on women results in an economic loss to the United States of millions of dollars every year, plus many more millions spent on medical bills (Berger, 1990).

- Pregnancy offers no immunity against violence. Eight percent of all pregnant women are assaulted by their husbands or boyfriends during pregnancy. These assaults inflict both physical and psychological harm to the mother-to-be. Some also injure or kill the fetus (Koop, 1987–88).

- More than 2 million reported cases of child abuse occur at the hands of parents, grandparents, guardians, or others. In addition, there may be another 1 million cases of child abuse that go unreported. Between 2000 and 5000 children die every year as a result of their injuries (Saltman, 1986; Landes et al, 1991).

- Almost as many adolescents are mistreated as younger children. Approximately 42% of abused children are between the ages of 12 and 17 (Saltman, 1986).

- Incest—the act of sexual intercourse between closely related family members—is the most common form of adolescent sexual abuse. Incest is estimated to occur in about 14% of all families. The common perpetrators include fathers, stepfathers, uncles, and brothers. In some cases, a father sexually abuses all of his daughters throughout their preadolescent and adolescent years (Saltman, 1986).

• **Elder abuse**—the abuse of parents and grandparents by children and grandchildren—is estimated to claim between 500,000 and 1 million victims yearly. The House Select Committee on Aging estimates that only one in every six cases is reported (Saltman, 1986).

No data are available regarding the extent of emotional abuse. Survey results yielding data regarding incidence of physical abuse, however, indicate that physical and emotional abuse go hand in hand. Thus, we know that there are no fewer victims of emotional abuse than there are victims of physical abuse. The true picture may be many times that of physical violence. Little research has been done on emotional abuse, perhaps because so many of us are guilty of an occasional or even frequent verbal barrage against a loved one that the behavior is too close or too common to allow for objective study. Gelles and Straus (1988) contend that emotional abuse is not a case of "there but for the grace of God go I"; rather, it is that we know the enemy, and it is ourselves.

CHARACTERISTICS OF THE JOURNEY MARKED BY FAMILY VIOLENCE AND ABUSE

The problems of family violence and abuse are not limited to a particular socioeconomic group. Violence occurs at all levels of society and in all parts of the United States. Even the "best" families produce "victims" of violent behavior, but there are certain key characteristics of family violence.

Family violence is the only crime in which the victim always knows the identity of the offender. Moreover the perpetrators of family violence do not see their acts as crimes, nor do they see their victims as such. Family violence is usually accompanied by a certain amount of brainwashing. Abused children come to believe that they deserve the severe beatings they receive because they are bad and uncontrollable. Abused wives become convinced that they are failures in carrying out their responsibilities as wives and mothers. Sexually abused children are told that their perpetrator's actions are normal signs of affection. In truth, the victim assumes responsibility for the crime.

Responses of Victims

This assumption of responsibility, characteristic of a generalized **hostage response**, is common to victims of any form of interpersonal violence (Tilden and Shepherd, 1987; Fauman, 1982). Victims tend to blame themselves for the abuse and develop a sense of being unworthy of help, a fear of not being believed, a skepticism regarding the motivations of others, and, in the case of chronic abuse, a persistent irrational belief that each attack will be the last. Abused wives typically say, "If only I had. . . ." Children might say, "I deserved that beating to keep me in line." Sexual abuse victims are likely to think, "I must have led him on." Each of the victims harbors the hope that the abuse will stop if they act differently.

The victim feels shame, guilt, and embarrassment. These feelings form a cloak of silence that prohibits the victim from seeking outside help. Victims find it difficult to believe that outsiders could possibly understand or identify with the humiliation that is part of their lives. This appraisal of society's response increases the feelings of hopelessness and isolation experienced by victims.

The spiritual distress is almost unfathomable as the victim becomes increasingly hopeless and despairing. Some victims, seeking help from their organized faith, have experienced more blame as they are told to be "better wives" and to "forgive and forget." It becomes difficult for victims to pray and to believe in a loving and powerful God when the reality of their lives is so out of control and frightening.

Because of fears of reprisal from their abuser, victims are hesitant to seek help from the criminal justice system. In addition, victims are immobilized by the belief that they are economically and emotionally dependent on the abuser. They fear that by reporting the violence the family will be torn apart.

It is common for victims to believe that violence and abuse are natural parts of family life. The long-term effects of violence and abuse are depression, suicidal ideation, low self-esteem, and impaired relationships outside of the family. Family violence tends to be repeated and to grow worse over time. Therefore, early intervention is needed to prevent abuse from occurring and to deal with it once it has occurred.

▶ Check Your Reading

4. What are the characteristics of the hostage response?
5. What are the spiritual issues of abuse?
6. How does "brainwashing" fit in with abuse?
7. What are the usual feelings experienced by victims of abuse?
8. Why don't victims of abuse seek help from the criminal justice system?

Forms of Victimization

A common assumption is that women and children are the only victims of family violence or that if they are not the *only* victims, they are at least the most common victims. Neither of these views is correct. Hidden victims compose a significant part of the problem of family violence. The most common form of family violence is between siblings. The most overlooked may be the violence directed at parents by adolescent children. These forms of victimization have received far less attention as social problems.

Sibling Violence and Abuse

Sibling violence is not new. The Bible recounts the story of Cain and Abel, a story of intense sibling rivalry that eventually led to the death of Abel at his brother's hands. Sibling conflict is such a common aspect of family relations that many people accept it as the norm. American families have a set of expectations that maintain that "boys will be boys" and "kids will fight." These attitudes may actually encourage sibling conflict.

Most cases of sibling conflict involve slaps, pushes, kicks, bites, and punches. Significant numbers of siblings, however, face brothers or sisters who pose a more lethal threat because they have guns or knives.

Parents as Victims

Another form of abuse is physical violence perpetrated by children, usually adolescents, against their parents. This form of violence seldom comes to public attention unless the child kills or maims the parent. Parent victims find little support in the community and virtually no services to help them. Parents fear that if they reveal how they are victimized at home, they will be publicly victimized as well by being blamed for their child's behavior. They feel ashamed, guilty, and embarrassed and, as a result, suffer from anxiety and depression. Terrified of their violent children and afraid that they will be publicly blamed for their children's behavior, they remain prisoners at home. Harbin and Madden (1979) suggest that parents create a "veil of denial," which serves to give license to the child's violence and to perpetrate this form of hidden intimate violence.

Elders as Victims

"Honor thy father and thy mother," one of the Ten Commandments, has taken on greater significance with today's increasing lifespan (Janz, 1990). Yet five types of elder abuse exist:

- Physical: "I know I push her sometimes, but she is always there," a daughter explaining the repeated bruising of her mother (Landes et al, 1991).
- Financial: "My grandsons only come to see me at the beginning of the month. They take my social security check to the corner store and cash it for me. Sometimes they don't come right back, and when they do, most of the money is gone. So I have to make do for the rest of the month" (Anonymous, 1992b).
- Psychological: "My son gets so frustrated with me, I guess I move too slow for him, and I am a burden . . . but he yells at me, tells me he wishes that I would die . . . I know he doesn't mean it" (Anonymous, 1992b).
- Sexual: "It started when my grandson had to help me in the bathroom. He started to touch me . . . I didn't like it, but I was too embarrassed to say anything" (Anonymous, 1992a).
- Self-abuse or self-neglect: "She was brought to the hospital by paramedics. She was confused, dehydrated, and had a maggot-infested leg and weighed about 60 pounds. She was bruised all over her body and had a gash on her face. 'I don't want to get anyone in trouble,' she said. Efforts to find out who had done these things to her were futile. Two weeks after being brought to the hospital, she died, and her daughter could not be located" (Laudes and Foster, 1991, p. 41).

▶ Check Your Reading

9. What is sibling abuse?
10. What is the "veil of denial" that maintains the secrecy of a parent as a victim?
11. Give an example of psychological abuse directed against an elder.
12. Why don't parents who are victims get help from the community?

CAUSES OF FAMILY VIOLENCE AND ABUSE

In their seminal work on family violence, Gelles and Straus (1988) contend that people who hit family members do so because they can get away with it. This proposition is based on three beliefs. The first is that there are few, if any, costs for being violent at home. The second belief is that American society lacks effective social controls to deal with domestic violence. The third belief is that certain social and family structures reduce social controls and, in doing so, reduce the costs and increase the rewards of being violent.

Few Costs of Family Violence

Most people who abuse family members are able to control their temper when they are confronted with situations that make them angry outside the home. An abusive husband is usually not abusive to his secretary. An abusive father would not dream of hitting someone else's child who happened to annoy him. Why? These people share the unconscious knowledge that potential costs and punishments await them if they engage in violent behavior. This recognition is enough to restrain most people.

Violence that occurs within the home results in few costs for the perpetrator. The abusive husband may be encouraged by police to leave the home situation "just to cool down." The abusive father may be reported to an overwhelmed social service department that makes a cursory investigation and dismisses the charge as unfounded.

Gelles and Straus (1988) contend that the social exchange theory provides explanation for the proposition that people who hit family members do so because they can. The social exchange theory asserts that human interaction is regulated by the pursuit of rewards and the avoidance of punishments and costs. When one individual provides services to another, the other is obliged to render a reward in some way. As long as the exchange is reciprocal, the relationship continues. Without reciprocity, the interaction is broken off because the first person realizes all the costs and no benefits.

Family dynamics add an important twist to the normal assumptions of social exchange theory. With no reciprocity in the exchange of services and rewards, it is not so easy to break off interaction. Divorce is always an option but never an easy one. Divorce carries with it decisions regarding children, distribution of property, living space, and financial resources. Yet even with the difficulties in seeking a divorce, it is possible to become an ex-spouse; it is never possible to become an ex-parent. Children are seldom able to respond equitably with rewards for what parents provide. Some parents, unable to break off the relationship with their children, respond to being asked to give more with anger, frustration, and resentment. Conflict is a common response; violence may be involved. Social exchange theory suggests that people would engage in violence against family members only when the costs of violence do not outweigh the rewards. Although our society has standard costs for violence, these costs are rarely paid by those who are violent in the home.

Absence of Effective Social Controls

A number of factors contribute to the lack of consequences for the perpetrators of domestic violence. Police tend to respond slowly to calls regarding violence in the home. This tendency can be explained by three factors. First, domestic violence poses a threat to the police officer. Every year, significant numbers of officers are killed responding to domestic disturbances. Second, police officers are not traditionally rewarded for how well they handle domestic violence. Instead, rewards are given for good police work involving robberies and drug trafficking. Consequently, responding to domestic calls receives a low priority among law enforcement officers. Third, the police officer may be an abusing spouse and not inclined personally to be responsive to the needs of the victims.

Even when the police are called to a home, arrests are not common. Child abuse usually is handled as a child welfare matter and not as a criminal justice matter. In unusual cases when arrests are made, chances are that no additional costs will be paid by the abuser. The criminal justice system does not want to bear responsibility for breaking up families. Wives who press charges are frequently counseled to drop them. The argument presented to wives places them in a "no-win" situation. A representative of the court system may argue, "If we put him in jail, he'll lose his job, and you will have to go on welfare. Why don't you go home and "kiss and make up." This same line of reasoning is used when fathers batter their children. When the mother is the perpetrator of the abuse, judges are even more hesitant about placing them behind bars for fear of further damaging the children. Clearly the criminal justice system holds little threat for the person who is violent against loved ones. The lack of real cost may even encourage further violence.

Some women seek restraining orders in the hope of keeping their husbands away. All too frequently, the restraining order serves to fuel the anger and violence that the wife is trying desperately to avoid. Few other costs exist. Presumably, public knowledge of a person's violence at home could lead to a loss of social or economic status. In reality, however, such a loss seldom occurs.

Family and Social Structures That Support Violence

The social and family structures that are most important in reducing the cost of family violence include (1) social attitudes regarding family violence, (2) high value placed on the right to privacy within the home, and (3) the structural inequality that exists within the modern family.

Social Attitudes

Violence may be woven into the American character. Certainly we do not have to delve far or deep into our history to find many examples of violence. Reading a newspaper or listening to the evening news provides us with daily reminders of the violent nature of our society.

We legitimize violence. This legitimization can be seen in the public outcries for retribution in statements such as "blow them to smithereens" following public awareness of crimes committed abroad against Americans and perceived abuses of American interests. There was a great deal of support for military intervention when American hostages were taken by Iran in 1979, when Lebanese terrorists hijacked a TWA airliner in the summer of 1985, and, most recently, when Saddam Hussein moved Iranian troops into Kuwait. In a 1986 Gallup poll, more than 65% of Americans supported the death penalty as an appropriate means to punish capital offenses. Violence is common in cartoons, television shows, movies, and even in children's fairy tales and nursery rhymes.

During the 1960s, the U.S. Commission on the Causes and Prevention of Violence conducted a survey focusing on attitudes about public as well as private, or family, violence. This survey revealed the following:

- Twenty-five percent of men and 17% of women stated that there were some circumstances in which spouse-to-spouse violence was warranted and appropriate.
- Eighty-six percent of those surveyed stated that "strong discipline" was necessary in the rearing of children.
- Seventy percent of the respondents indicated that it was necessary for young boys to engage in fistfights as part of growing into manhood (Stark & McEvoy, 1970).

Fifteen years after the U.S. Commission on the Causes and Prevention of Violence survey was conducted, Gelles and Straus (1988) asked a national sample of more than 2000 subjects two questions that focused on attitudes about violence between family members. The responses revealed that 25% of wives and 33% of husbands believed that slapping between spouses was sometimes necessary, normal, and good. More than 70% of the respondents believed that slapping a 12-year-old child was necessary, normal, or good.

Parent-to-child violence is so common that most Americans consider physical discipline an essential part of parenting. In the Gelles and Straus national survey, the *absence* of physical punishment, not the hitting of children, was considered deviant.

Society closes its eyes and ears to family violence even when the violence escalates beyond what society tolerates as normal within families. Neighbors might report violence to the police but seldom become personally involved both because of fear for their own safety and because violence is a "family matter." Society tends to deny that many of the violent acts that occur between family members are "really violent." Instead the true nature of these acts is hidden behind euphemisms such as "domestic disturbance" or "family matter." Box 40–1 identifies many of the societal myths that support abuse.

Value of Privacy

Factors such as industrialization, urbanization, and modernization have caused family to evolve from a public institution to a private one. As the family became increasingly private, it also became isolated from social control. The audience for violence is typically limited to husband, wife, and one or two children. This privacy shelters offenders and victims from public eyes and social sanctions and affords a shielded setting for private violence. In families in which abuse is the norm, the abuser increasingly limits and controls the amount of time victims can socialize outside of the family. In the notorious 1987 case in which 6-year-old Lisa Steinberg was found unconscious, in the apartment of Hedda Nussbaum and Joel Steinberg, Steinberg's abuse was directed at both Lisa and Hedda. For years, he systematically cut Hedda off from all outside contacts, including her job and her family (Ferrato, 1991).

Structural Inequality of the Family

Many areas of family inequality support violent and abusive behavior. First is inequality of size. Most husbands are larger and stronger than their wives and certainly larger than their children; most mothers are larger and stronger than young children. Size is important. Surveys have shown that mothers who typically hit their children engage in less physical discipline as the children enter into adolescent years, not because of fewer conflicts between mother and child but because the adolescent's larger size poses a risk of retaliatory violence directed toward the mother.

Beyond physical inequality are social and economic inequality. Men typically enjoy greater social and economic status than do women. This greater status translates into power within the family. Husbands can hit their wives without fear of economic or social costs. Likewise, parents control the economic and social resources of their children. Wives put up with an occasional beating rather

BOX 40–1 Myths Regarding Domestic Violence and the Facts Concerning These Myths

- *Violence among family members is a private matter.* Violence is a public concern. It is costly to society in multiple ways, including lost productivity and health care costs. The long-term costs of damaged lives is unestimable.
- *The abuse cannot be that terrible, or the woman would leave.* The ties that bind women to abusive men are complex. The woman may be financially dependent on him and afraid that she will not be able to manage on her own.
- *Women who remain in abusive relationships tend to become helpless.* Sometimes abused women seem to be placating and passive toward their abuser. These behaviors must be viewed in the context of the constant fear in which the woman lives. Placating, passive behavior represents an effort to avoid future violence. Many women have the courage and will eventually to leave even though the odds are stacked against them.
- *Alcohol and drugs cause abuse.* The use of alcohol and drugs only gives the abuser an excuse for violence; they do not cause violent behavior.
- *Abuse occurs more in lower socioeconomic groups.* Battering takes place just as often among middle and upper classes. This myth is maintained by racial bias. Many women in middle and upper classes may go to greater lengths to conceal their injuries. Health care providers are less likely to suspect abuse in a middle-class or upper-class woman.
- *Batterers are uneducated men who cannot cope in the world.* Many batterers are successful professionals—physicians, attorneys, public officials, clergymen, college professors. They share a common characteristic of being unusually dependent on their partners.
- *Battered wives will never change.* Most women who leave abusive relationships are careful not to marry another batterer, if they remarry at all.
- *Battering men will never change.* Some men are shocked into confronting their problems when their partners leave them or when they serve prison sentences. Behavioral therapy can teach battering men how to express aggression appropriately and how to negotiate with rather than coerce women.
- *Families should be kept together at all costs.* Children develop severe emotional problems from living with a batterer. They improve dramatically when they are removed from the situation when their mother moves out.

Data from King, M. C., and Ryan, J. (1989). Abused women: Dispelling myths and encouraging intervention. *Nurse Practitioner, 14*(5), 47–58; and Collier, J. A. (1987). When you suspect your patient is a battered wife. *RN, May,* 22–25.

than deal with the costs of trying to survive outside the home without money, credit, or work experience. Viewing violence within an unequal family structure makes it clear that all violence is really an abuse of power in which the stronger person takes advantage of the weaker.

Wives and children have historically been regarded as the legal property of the husband and father. This view not only allowed a man's violent behavior, but also encouraged it as a way of controlling and keeping his possessions "in line." Although those laws have long since been abolished in favor of recognizing the worth of women and children, attitudes do not die just because laws change. The attitude that husbands have rights to "discipline" their wives and children and the family and social structures that support violent behavior serve to "stack the cards" against the victims of domestic violence and abuse. In no other social situation in which violence plays a factor do the victims have to weigh losing their homes and financial security against the costs of being physically assaulted.

▶ Check Your Reading

13. How does the value placed on privacy support violence?
14. How does the structural inequality of the family support violence?
15. When Gelles and Straus state that violence continues because the abusers can get away with it, what do they mean?

Characteristics of Abusers

Social and cultural factors that allow abusers to hit family members are not the total explanation for violence. Many couples never engage in violent physical exchanges; some parents abhor hitting their children. What other factors predispose some people to become violent? Some researchers have focused on the role of biology, including neurophysiology, neurotransmitters, genetics, and the presence of a psychiatric disorder. Others have focused on the personal characteristics of abusers, the role of alcohol and drugs, and abuse as mutual combat.

Biological Factors and Violence

In addition to the social factors that support violence, researchers continue to look to the brain for explanations of violent behavior. The results of biological research are not conclusive but seem to indicate a higher incidence of violence in persons with partial complex seizures. This research has focused on the role of the limbic system in episodic dyscontrol. Monroe (1985) argues for the validity of this theory by pointing out the effectiveness of anticonvulsant regimens in limiting or eliminating episodic dyscontrol (Tardiff, 1989).

Other researchers have focused attention on the role of the neurotransmitters in violent behavior. For instance, increased levels of norepinephrine and dopamine are associated with violence and aggression. Additionally, decreased levels of serotonin are associated with impulsivity.

Genetics may also play a part in violent behavior, but the research is equivocal. A number of studies of prison populations have shown a disproportionate number of XYY men, but other researchers have failed to show a relationship between this genetic abnormality and violence. Mednick and Volavka (1980) showed that a higher rate of criminal activity occurred in monozygotic twins than in dizygotic twins, but these early twin studies failed to account for the shared environmental as well as genetic heritage of the subjects. Later studies looked at subjects who had been adopted and found that the crimes of the subjects were more related to their alcohol use than their genetics, although there was support for the thesis that nonviolent petty property crime has a genetic basis (Tardiff, 1989; Schiavi et al, 1984).

Presence of Psychiatric Illness

One of the myths about psychiatric patients is that they are all wild, violent, and out of control. Although this myth is not true, some diagnoses carry an association between violence and the symptoms of the illness. For instance, Andreason and Black (1995) note that "patients with schizophrenia, mania, mental retardation, and brain disorders are more likely to become violent . . . In the hospital psychotic disorders are more likely to lead to violence than nonpsychotic disorders" (p. 521). Within the psychotic group, those driven by their delusions were more likely to commit seriously violent acts.

Patients experiencing psychotic symptoms, however, are not the only perpetrators of violence. Menuck (1984) reviewed the literature and found that borderline and antisocial personality disorders as well as childhood and adolescent diagnoses and substance abuse all correlated with increased rates of violent and assaultive behaviors.

▶ Check Your Reading

16. What is the relationship between psychiatric problems and incidents of violence?
17. How is the limbic system implicated in explanations of the cause of violence?
18. How do delusions and hallucinations relate to acts of violence?
19. What neurotransmitters are implicated in violent behavior?
20. What does research suggest regarding the role of genetics in violent behavior?

Personal Characteristics of Abusers

Personal factors such as low self-esteem, immaturity, extreme dependence, and insecurity certainly contribute to abuse. The hate-filled man releases his hostility by beating his wife. The frustrated mother lashes out at her young children. The rebellious adolescent expresses anger by beating up younger siblings. For a brief moment, the violent behavior provides the abuser with a false sense of power.

Some people hit others to relieve pent-up anger and then justify their actions as necessary. Violence is used to control. Parents use it to control children. Men use it to

BOX 40–2 Ways to Spot a Potential Batterer

There are ways to spot a potential batterer, but often we don't see the warning signs. Here is a list to watch for. Please share these characteristics with friends and family members in dating relationships

- *He comes on too strong.* Beware of the man who loves you instantly and wants to see you all the time. He is responding to his own fantasies, not the real you.
- *He has very traditional ideas about men's and women's roles.* Watch out for the man who thinks a woman should stay at home, take care of her husband, and follow orders.
- *He believes in using force or violence to solve problems.* If he overreacts to little problems, such as not being able to find a parking space, that's a bad sign. Other signals include throwing things, punching walls, and being cruel to animals when he is angry.
- *He thinks poorly of himself.* Batterers are insecure people with low self-esteem, but they may act tough to cover up these feelings of inferiority.
- *He is jealous.* He keeps tabs on you and wants to know where you are at all times. He is jealous not only of other men, but also of your friends and family.
- *He is self-centered.* The man who thinks only of fulfilling his own needs is a bad risk.
- *He has extreme highs and extreme lows in his moods.* His mood swings are like Dr. Jekyll and Mr. Hyde.
- *He blames others when things don't work out.* Anything bad that happens to him is someone else's fault. He will eventually start blaming you when things go wrong.
- *He is a product of a violent family.* Children from violent homes often grow up regarding violence as normal, acceptable behavior.
- *He behaves badly toward others.* Even if he is kind to you now, the way he functions with the rest of the world may be the way he ultimately functions with you.
- *He treats you roughly at times.* Abuse during dating is a *guarantee* of later, more violent abuse. Even playful wrestling or tickling to the point at which you're frightened or have been hurt may suggest an abusive nature. Do not think that marriage will change him for the better; it will almost certainly change him for the worse.
- *He makes you feel scared or threatened.* Are you afraid to break up with him because he might hurt you? Do you change your life to keep from making him angry? If so, you are being abused and should seek help.

control women. Some abusers beat down their victims until the victim will do anything just to prevent further violence. The measure of control gained by the abuser temporarily boosts self-esteem.

The violence may follow disappointments in the work setting. Abusive men, unable to fulfill the masculine ideals of American society and feeling desperate and hopeless about their social situation, may choose to vent their anger and frustration at their wives and children.

Men who abuse their wives often say that their violence was caused by their wive's infidelity or by threats to separate or seek a divorce. The violence is a desperate means to control the wife. The couple may be locked in a sequence of actions and reactions that lead to tragic consequences (Berger, 1990). Box 40–2 details the similarities between abusive men.

Alcohol and Drugs

Sometimes abusers use alcohol or drugs as an excuse for their violence. The truth, however, is that alcohol and drugs are only factors in abuse. Someone who is violent will be violent with or without drinking and drug use. Drinking to excess and using drugs provides a "time-out" from the rules of society and gives a convenient excuse for violent behavior.

A drunk usually denies responsibility for actions. American society feeds into that denial by offering excuses for the violence stemming from drinking. The individual was not in control, could not think rationally, and had fewer inhibitions. American culture tends to minimize aggression that comes with drunkenness.

Not only does heavy drinking afford an occasion for violence to occur, but also it can lead to problems with alcohol among women who are abused. Alcoholism among women is a growing problem, and the largest precipitating cause is believed to be spouse abuse (Berger, 1990). Box 40–3 details the myths regarding the relationship between alcohol and abuse.

Abuse as Mutual Combat

Gage's (1991) alternative view of spousal abuse suggests a continuum along which abusive relationships occur (Table 40–1). There are two continua along which violence occurs. The first is characterized by what Steinmetz and Straus call **expressive violence,** in which the goal is to cause pain or injury to the other. This type of violence is also referred to as "mutual combat or conjugal violence." The second is characterized by **instrumental violence,** in which the goal is to control the behavior of the other.

Expressive violence results from intense emotional upheaval combined with poor impulse control. Each partner plays a role (although not necessarily an equal role) in the escalation of this type of violence. Each partner feels victimized by the other. The roles of victim and perpetrator are blurred and may fluctuate with the circumstances. The partners share responsibility for the eruption of violence. This view of violence is consistent

BOX 40-3 Domestic Violence and Alcohol Abuse—Debunking the Myths

Myths	Facts
1. Battering is a direct result of alcohol abuse.	1. Battering is a socially learned behavior and is not a direct result of substance abuse.
2. Most abuse occurs at the hands of alcohol abusers.	2. Many men who batter do not abuse alcohol; many alcoholic men do not batter their female partners. Alcohol use may provide the excuse for battering; however, batterers also engage in violent behavior toward their female partners when they are cold sober.
3. Treatment for alcohol use also cures battering behavior.	3. Alcoholism and battering require separate treatment. The first priority even before treatment is protection of the woman.
4. Women who abuse alcohol are more likely to be abused.	4. Some women have alcohol abuse problems and they are also abused; other women turn to substance abuse in response to the battering.
5. A woman's substance abuse is a direct cause of violent behavior in her partner.	5. A woman's substance abuse problems in no way relate to the cause of the battering she receives.

with a **mutual combat model** because violence is not congruent with the value systems of the participants, they usually express genuine remorse after incidents of violence, and the possibility for constructive change is favorable.

Instrumental violence is used to exploit and control another person. In cases of instrumental violence, the roles of victim and perpetrator are clearly defined, and the man is almost always the perpetrator. Any expression of remorse is usually shallow and is itself a form of manipulation directed toward meeting the needs of the perpetrator rather than a genuine concern for the victim. This form of violence is consistent with the **wife-battering model**. There is usually little motivation for change when instrumental violence is the norm.

Neidig and colleagues (1984) contend that without intervention, many couples progress from the expressive to the instrumental end of the violence continuum.

Role of Religion and Spirituality in Violence

There has been no research examining the relationship between violence and spirituality or religion, but we may assume that a person who is victimized suffers spiritually.

TABLE 40–1 **Expressive Versus Instrumental Violence**

Expressive Violence	Instrumental Violence
Violence that is primarily an expression of emotion (anger, jealousy)	Violence that is used primarily as an instrument to achieve a goal
Mutual and reciprocal violence; victim and perpetrator roles not fixed	Unilateral violence; victim and perpetrator roles fixed
Violence in context of escalating conflict	Violence as deliberate effort to punish or control
Sequential, gradual, predictable progression to violence	Relatively sudden and rapid progression to violence
Mutual conflict, stress, frustration, and anger precede violent incident	Little provocation for violent incident
Genuine remorse and sorrow follow incident; violence inconsistent with values; belief that violence will be controlled	Shallow remorse and sorrow follow incident; violence consis- tent with values; feelings of resignation and hopelessness
Unpredictable; high potential for escalation and "accidental" injury	Potential for violent retaliation, homicide or suicide
Relatively benign psychological consequences	Serious psychological consequences: helplessness, depression, low self-esteem, external locus of control
Brief, skill-building therapy with couples	Long-term therapy with individuals; separation; legal sanctions
Termed *mutual combat, spouse abuse, conjugal violence*	Termed *battering*

Published in *RN.* Copyright © 1987 Medical Economics. Montvale, NJ. Reprinted by permission. Modified from Collier, J. A. (1987). When you suspect your patient is a battered wife. *RN, May,* 22–25.

For instance, the woman or child victim might wonder, "Why has God forsaken me?" "I must really deserve this treatment. Even God doesn't care about me." These feelings may be intensified if the woman is encouraged by a church member or leader to "try harder to please your husband," or is asked "what did you do to make him angry," or is counseled to "obey your husband no matter what because that is what God commands." Such advice is destructive to the woman and only adds to the pain and difficulty of her situation. Furthermore, it is a distortion of a theistic and a scriptural view of life. There is *absolutely no justification* within Scripture for a husband to beat his wife. In fact, Scripture commands husbands to love their wives as their own bodies.

In considering the spirituality of the abuser, we can only speculate that the abuser does not experience spiritual well-being. Abusing another and exerting coercive power is inconsistent with spiritual wellness and antithetical to loving others as ourselves.

▶ Check Your Reading

21. Identify three characteristics of abusive men.
22. Identify two myths regarding the role of alcohol and abuse.
23. State three ways that alcohol is linked to violence.
24. What is the difference between expressive and instrumental violence?
25. Describe the mutual combat model.

NURSING PROCESS WITH ABUSED WOMEN

The American Nurses' Association (ANA) has issued a position statement on physical violence against women, the most common form of **spousal abuse**. The ANA supports the Year 2000 Health Objectives, which cite surveillance, prevention, and intervention for violent behavior as a priority issue for the United States. The ANA's position statement is shown in Box 40–4. The following reports illustrate the problem of spousal abuse.

- Peter Martins, dancer-choreographer and artistic director of the New York City Ballet, was charged with beating his wife, the young prima donna of his company. The reason—he wanted to sleep, and she wanted to talk. To make his point, he pushed her to the floor, slapped her face, picked her up, and threw her into another room (Steinbach, 1992).
- A former Methodist minister was found liable for the nearly fatal choking of his wife. The woman, who was found unconscious on the floor of their garage, has been in a coma ever since (Berger, 1990).
- Joseph Pikul, a wealthy New York stock analyst, admitted to police that he killed his wife and said that she "deserved it" (Berger, 1990).
- The day that Lisa Steinberg was removed from the Steinberg residence for treatment of severe head trauma, Hedda Nussbaum, Lisa's adoptive mother, was pictured with a bandaged nose, puffy eyes, and bruises on her head and body. Her lips were split like a boxer's, and her nose was broken. Joel Steinberg denied ever hitting Hedda and claimed there had never been violence in their relationship (Ferrato, 1991).

ASSESSMENT

The statistics regarding the incidence of abuse toward women are frightening. In 1980, one in three women was estimated to have experienced intentional injury at the hands of a male partner (Straus et al, 1980). Moreover, many of these women were abused while pregnant. In fact, a national telephone survey of more than 6000 households revealed that the risk of pregnant women having experienced abuse during the previous year was almost 61% greater than the risk to women who were not pregnant (Straus and Gelles, 1988). Approximately 8% to 11% of pregnant women are abused during their pregnancies (Hillard, 1985; Helton et al, 1987).

Many women who are abused seek medical treatment (Moss and Taylor, 1991). Some come to Emergency Departments seeking treatment for an acute injury; others may present at medical or mental health clinics as part of scheduled or unscheduled appointments. A pregnant woman may present at an Emergency Department requesting that a nurse or physician check to see if her baby is all right. Usually the presenting complaint is not abuse. Instead the woman may present with injuries that are several days old and offer vague and incomplete histories regarding the nature of the injury. See Box 40–5 for general indicators of abuse.

It is incumbent on nurses and physicians to conduct assessments that are nonjudgmental and gentle but also direct in approach (Parker and McFarlane, 1991). Figure 40–2 displays an appropriate Abuse Assessment Screen. Figure 40–3 shows the CSR Abuse Index, and Box 40–6 includes questions for assessing emotional abuse.

The assessment is conducted in a private setting, with assurances of confidentiality. Sometimes it is essential that you intervene between the woman and her partner. The man may have accompanied her into a health facility for treatment and fully intends to stay by her side at all times. To ensure that privacy is maintained and the woman has a safety zone in which to speak outside the hearing of her partner, you may need to make a statement to the male partner such as "This part of the examination is done in private. You must remain outside." Such a statement establishes patient privacy as a protocol of the agency, maximizes the woman's opportunity to talk, and minimizes the influence exerted by the man to maintain silence regarding the abuse.

▶ Check Your Reading

26. Identify three general indicators of abuse.
27. Why is it important for the nurse to ask direct questions regarding the possibility of abuse?
28. What is the usual presenting complaint of the pregnant woman who has been abused?

BOX 40-4 Position Statement on Physical Violence Against Women

Summary: The American Nurses' Association (ANA) supports education of nurses, health care providers, and women in skills necessary for prevention of violence against women; assessment of women in health care institutions and community settings; and research on violence against women. ANA believes there is a need to increase awareness to the health problem of violence against women as well as reduce injuries and psychological misery associated with this crime. ANA believes health care professionals must be educated as to their role in the assessment, intervention, and prevention of physical violence against women. Further, ANA supports the Year 2000 Health Objectives, which cite the surveillance, prevention, and intervention for violent behavior as a priority issue for the nation.

Physical violence against women is behavior intended to inflict harm and includes slapping, kicking, choking, punching, pushing, use of objects as weapons, forced sexual activity, and injury or death from a weapon. Physical violence is by definition assault and it is a crime. Ninety-five percent of serious assaults by a spouse or intimate partner are men battering women. Abuse is the leading cause of injury to women and homicide a major cause of traumatic death to women.

Physical violence against women is pervasive and cuts across all ethnic, racial, religious, and socioeconomic groups. Based on national survey results, 1.8 million women are beaten by their husbands each year. Stated another way, one of every eight husbands assaults his wife at least once during a given year. Abuse during courtship and cohabiting relationships affects between 16% and 23% of all dating relationships. The FBI estimates that one in two women will be physically assaulted by her male partner during her lifetime. Frequently physical abuse begins during pregnancy with 25% to 30% of pregnant women reporting abuse prior to or during pregnancy. Pregnant women reporting abuse are more likely to deliver a low birth weight infant.

Injuries to women sustained from abuse include contusions, concussions, lacerations, fractures, and gun shot wounds. Emergency room records document that 22% to 35% of women presenting any complaint are there because of symptoms related to physical abuse. Some 1000 women are killed each year by their male partner, almost always following years of physical abuse. The economic costs of interpersonal violence are high, especially if a weapon is involved. The lifetime cost of firearm deaths and injuries are estimated at $23 billion in 1990 with more than 80% of the medical care costs borne by public funds. During the same year, injuries caused by interpersonal violence requiring hospitalization cost an estimated $80 billion. Because most physical violence between intimate partners goes underreported, the economic costs are grossly underrepresented.

There is a need to:

- Increase awareness and sensitivity to the health problem of physical violence against women
- Reduce intentional injuries and the associated economic costs and psychological misery
- Heighten awareness of health professionals as to their role in the assessment and intervention and prevention of physical violence against women

The American College of Obstetricians and Gynecologists, Surgeon General, and Centers for Disease Control have forwarded recommendations that all women be routinely screened for physical abuse and offered counseling, education, advocacy, and appropriate referrals. Year 2000 Health Objectives cite the surveillance, prevention, and intervention for violent behavior as a priority issue for the nation.

Therefore, the ANA supports:

- Routine education of all nurses and health care providers in the skills necessary to prevent violence against women
- Routine assessment and documentation for physical abuse of all women in any health care institution or community setting
- Targeted assessment of women at increased risk of abuse including pregnant women and women presenting in emergency rooms
- Education of all women as to the cycle of violence, the potential for homicide, and community resources for primary, secondary, and tertiary prevention and care
- Inclusion of the topic of violence against women in all undergraduate nursing curriculums
- Education of school-age children and adolescents in public schools about relationships without violence and community resources for help
- Research on violence against women, including the development and evaluation of nursing models for preventive assessment, intervention, and treatment for abused women, their children, and perpetrators of violence

Courtesy of the American Nurses' Association, Washington, D.C.

Interviewing

You may find it difficult to ask questions that allow abused women to discuss the violence openly. Many abused women have commented that when they sought treatment for their injuries, no one ever asked them if the injury was the result of abuse. Feeling ashamed and guilty, the woman is unlikely to volunteer this information unless the care provider asks for it and is willing to listen in a nonjudgmental, accepting manner. Box 40–7 includes sample assessment questions to facilitate the process.

Documentation

It is imperative that you thoroughly document the assessment process. Clinical records may be used as evidence if the woman decides to seek legal redress. Comprehensive documentation also alerts the next care provider who may intervene to deal with vague, poorly defined injuries. The use of a body map allows the specific injuries to be diagrammed and information about the injuries noted. If the woman consents, photographs are also taken. Greany (1984) suggests that the woman return the next day for more photos, so that the full extent of bruising and swelling is evident.

The pictures are signed and dated and sealed in an envelope or container with any other evidence, such as clothing. The envelope or container is stored in a safe place. The woman needs to sign a release-of-information form, so that a court may request the records. This evidence may prove useful if she attempts to substantiate charges of continued abuse. Even if she is not ready to prosecute at this time, she may be ready at a later time.

BOX 40-5 General Indicators of Abuse

- Description of how injury occurred does not fit physical evidence of injury
- Woman minimizes the frequency and seriousness of the injuries
- Woman presents for treatment one or more days after the injury
- Woman states she is accident prone
- X-rays show old and new fractures in different stages of healing
- Woman makes repeat visits with injuries becoming more severe as frequency of visits increases
- Woman accompanied by overprotective mate who does not want to allow woman to be alone with health professional
- Woman seeks treatment for miscarriage or early labor
- Woman frequently presents with somatic complaints
- Woman attempts suicide or takes drug overdose
- Patient or partner has a history of substance abuse
- Woman presents with a mental or psychiatric complaint

1. Have you ever been emotionally or physically abused by your partner or someone important to you?

   ☐ Yes ☐ No

2. Within the last year, have you been hit, slapped, kicked, or otherwise physically hurt by someone?

   ☐ Yes ☐ No

   If yes, by whom? ______________________

   Number of times ______________________

3. Since you've been pregnant, have you been hit, slapped, kicked, or otherwise physically hurt by someone?

   ☐ Yes ☐ No

   If yes, by whom? ______________________

   Number of times ______________________

   Mark the area of injury on the body map at right.

4. Within the last year, has anyone forced you to have sexual activities?

   ☐ Yes ☐ No

   If yes, who? ______________________

   Number of times ______________________

5. Are you afraid of your partner or anyone you listed above?

   ☐ Yes ☐ No

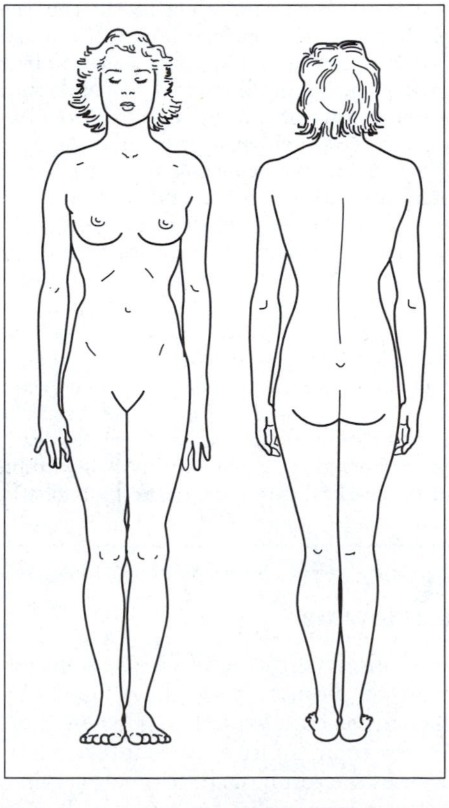

FIGURE 40-2

Abuse assessment screen. (Developed by the Nursing Research Consortium on Violence and Abuse, 1989. Redrawn from Parker, B., and MacFarlane, J. [1991]. Identifying and helping battered pregnant women. *Maternal Child Nursing* 16:162.)

DIRECTIONS: For each question, indicate the number from the designated scale that best describes your relationship with your partner.

Questions #1 to #14

3—FREQUENTLY 2—SOMETIMES 1—RARELY 0—NEVER

_______ 1. Continually monitors your time and makes you account for every minute?

_______ 2. Accuses you of having affairs with other men or acts suspicious of you?

_______ 3. Is rude to your friends?

_______ 4. Discourages you from starting friendships with other women?

_______ 5. Is critical of things such as cooking, clothes, or appearance?

_______ 6. Demands a strict account of how you spend money?

_______ 7. Moods change radically, from very calm to very angry, or vice versa?

_______ 8. Is disturbed by your working or by the thought of your working?

_______ 9. Becomes angry more easily when he drinks?

_______ 10. Pressures you for sex much more often than you like?

_______ 11. Becomes angry if you do not want to go along with his request for sex?

_______ 12. Quarrels over financial matters?

_______ 13. Quarrels about having children or raising them?

_______ 14. Strikes you with his hand or feet (slaps, punches, kicks)?

Questions #15 to #26

6—FREQUENTLY 5—SOMETIMES 4—RARELY 0—NEVER

_______ 15. Has he ever struck you with an object?

_______ 16. Has he ever threatened you with an object or weapon?

_______ 17. Has he ever threatened to kill either you or himself?

_______ 18. Does he give you visible injuries (such as welts, bruises, cuts)?

_______ 19. Have you ever had to receive first aid because his violence to you resulted in injuries?

_______ 20. Have you ever had to seek professional aid for any injury at a medical clinic, doctor's office, or hospital emergency department?

_______ 21. Has he ever hurt you sexually or made you have intercourse against your will?

_______ 22. Is he ever violent toward children?

_______ 23. Is he ever violent toward other people outside your home and family?

_______ 24. Does he ever throw objects or break things when he is angry?

_______ 25. Has he ever been in trouble with the police?

_______ 26. Have you ever called the police or tried to call them because you felt you or members of your family were in danger?

_______ TOTAL

To score responses, simply add up the points for each question. This sum is the ABUSE INDEX SCORE. To get some idea of how abusive your partner is, compare your index score with the following chart:

92–120	Dangerously abusive
35–91	Seriously abusive
13–34	Moderately abusive
0–12	Nonabusive

If at all possible, your partner should complete a CSR Abuse Index form. The difference in the results should be discussed with the program counselor. Does your partner grossly underestimate that he is abusive? If so, why?

FIGURE 40–3
The CSR Abuse Index. (From THE FAMILY SECRET by William Stacey and Anson Shupe. Copyright © 1983 by William Stacey and Anson Shupe. Reprinted by permission of Beacon Press.)

If the woman does not admit to being beaten, you cannot note abuse in the chart, but you can write, "the explanation of the patient's injuries is inappropriate," or "the patient's description of the circumstances surrounding the infliction of her injuries is inconsistent with the injury pattern" (Lake, 1982). If the woman states that her injuries were the result of abuse, it is imperative for you to document accordingly. For example, write, "patient states she was beaten up by her husband" (Moss and Taylor, 1991).

You must recognize that the abused woman may feel embarrassment, shame, and even responsibility for the abuse. The abuse victim may use denial as a coping mechanism. Even if she reports abuse, there is a tendency to minimize its frequency and severity. Hart (1988) suggests that if the woman believes that others will not define her problem as seriously as she does, minimizing the event makes her feel less alienated from others. To respond to these feelings, establish rapport through concern, interest expressed in the woman's story, and an expressed desire to assist the woman.

Determining the Woman's Safety

Initially, you are interested in determining whether the woman is safe. Keeping in mind that the frequency and severity of violence usually escalate over time, recognize that the risk for a lethal outcome is a frightening reality (Case Example 40–2). The risk of homicide is increased in the presence of the following factors:

- A handgun in the home
- Substance abuse
- Extreme jealousy
- Battering during pregnancy (Campbell, 1986; Parker & McFarlane, 1991).

The battered woman's risk of being killed by her partner is greater if she leaves him or makes it clear to him that she is ending the relationship.

BOX 40–6 Emotional Abuse Checklist

Keeping You Away from Other People

- Does your partner get angry when you talk on the phone?
- Does he open your mail?
- Does he keep you from seeing friends?
- Is he angry when you are just a little late getting home?
- Does he want you home when he is home?

Always on Your Mind

- Do you worry about what he will think about your make-up? Or how you dress?
- Do you ask him whom you can see or where you can go?
- Are you careful of what you say so that he will not get upset?
- Do you feel you are "walking on eggshells"?

Putting You Down: Humiliation

- Does he call you names like "stupid," "bitch," or "whore"?
- Does he tell you what is "wrong" with you in front of other people?
- Has he made you do things that make you feel ashamed?
- Does he say that no one else would want you or love you?

Threats

- Does he threaten to leave you?
- Has he said he will go crazy or kill himself if you leave?
- Does he say he will hit you or beat you if you don't obey?

Feeling Sick and Tired

- Does he keep you up late asking you about men in your past?
- Do you work so hard to please him that you feel worn out?
- Do you feel sick, yet you are not sure what is wrong?
- Are you unable to do things you used to do easily?

Small Demands

- Does he demand that dinner be served right on the minute?
- Does he insist that the house look just so?
- Do you have to report how you spend every dollar?

Sweet Talk and Threats

- After he has been mean, does he act sweet and loving?
- After he has hit you, does he give you a present or take you out?
- When you decide to leave, does he give you hope for change?

BOX 40-7 Sample Assessment Questions in Determining Abuse

- Has somebody hurt you?
- Are you safe at home?
- Your partner seems to frighten you. Has he hurt you?
- Can you tell me about any times during your relationship when you and your partner have had physical fights?
- Is your present relationship one in which you are hurt?
- Do you feel that your partner controls your life too much?
- The injuries that you have remind me of injuries that I have seen on other women who have been hurt or abused. Did anyone hurt you?
- It is routine for me to ask all women patients if they are presently in a relationship with someone who is abusing them. Are you in such a relationship?

Data from King, M. C., and Ryan, J. (1989). Abused women: Dispelling myths and encouraging intervention. *Nurse Practitioner, 14* (5), 47–58; and Moss, V. A., and Taylor, W. K. (1991). Domestic violence. *AORN Journal, 53* (5), 1158–1164.

As a result of research conducted after killings, several risk factors have been associated with homicides (murders) of both batterers and battered women. We cannot predict what will happen in your case. However, we would like you to be aware of the danger of homicide in situations of severe battering, and we would like you to see how many of the risk factors apply to your situation. (The "he" in the questions refers to your husband, partner, ex-husband, ex-partner, or whoever is currently physically hurting you.)

Please circle Yes or No for each question below.

1. Has the physical violence increased in frequency over the past year?	Yes	No
2. Has the physical violence increased in severity over the past year, or has a weapon or threat with a weapon been used?	Yes	No
3. Does he ever try to choke you?	Yes	No
4. Is there a gun in the house?	Yes	No
5. Has he ever forced you into sex when you did not wish to do so?	Yes	No
6. Does he use drugs ("uppers" or amphetamines, speed, angel dust, cocaine, "crack," heroin, mixtures, or other street drugs)?	Yes	No
7. Does he threaten to kill you, or do you believe he is capable of killing you?	Yes	No
8. Is he drunk every day or almost every day? (In terms of quantity of alcohol)	Yes	No
9. Does he control most of your daily activities? For instance, does he tell you who you can be friends with, how much money you can take shopping, or when you can take the car?	Yes	No
10. Have you ever been beaten by him while you were pregnant? (If never pregnant by him, check here: _______ .)	Yes	No
11. Is he violently and consistently jealous of you? (For instance, does he say, "If I can't have you, no one can.")	Yes	No
12. Have you ever threatened or tried suicide?	Yes	No
13. Has he ever threatened or tried suicide?	Yes	No
14. Is he violent toward your children?	Yes	No
15. Is he violent outside the home?	Yes	No

Total Yes answers __________

THANK YOU. PLEASE TALK TO YOUR NURSE, ADVOCATE, OR COUNSELOR ABOUT WHAT THE DANGER ASSESSMENT MEANS IN YOUR SITUATION.

FIGURE 40-4

Danger assessment. (From Campbell, J. [1986]. Nursing assessment for risk of homicide in battered women. *Advances in Nursing Science 8* (36–51), 45. Copyright © 1986 Aspen Publishers, Inc.)

Case Example 40–2 Kate's Story

Kate was hiding from her boyfriend, who'd hurt her several times. He tracked her down by tricking one of her children into giving him the address. He broke through the front door and went after Kate, shoving her against cupboards, breaking her nose, kicking and punching her, breaking her ribs, and blackening her eyes. While the boyfriend splattered Kate's blood across the kitchen, her deaf and mute daughter watched in silent terror.

From Ferrato, D. (1991). *Living with the enemy* (p. 61). New York: Aperture.

Campbell (1986) developed an instrument to use in assessing the potential for homicide (Figure 40–4). The instrument is currently being used in research to determine whether some items indicate more risk than others. Pending those findings, however, the instrument provides an objective way for the woman to evaluate her own safety.

▶ Check Your Reading

29. Identify three situations that increase the woman's risk of being murdered at the hands of her abuser.
30. What is the significance of taking pictures of the woman's injuries? Why would you want her to return the next day for more pictures?
31. If the woman's explanation of her injuries is not consistent with what you observe, how would you document this inconsistency?

Cycle of Abuse

The **cycle of abuse** usually occurs in three predictable stages. The first stage is one of *increasing tension*. The batterer becomes displeased over things that his victim has done. These things can be either real or imagined, minor or trivial. The event that precipitates an angry outburst may be that his mate burned his toast or "talked back."

The batterer reacts to this perceived insult with verbal abuse or slapping his partner. In an effort to minimize his anger, the woman may attempt to appease him or move out of his way. Her passivity actually fuels his lack of self-control. His verbal barrages last increasingly longer. The slaps get harder. He blankets her with his physical presence as he looks for signs of resistance.

The second stage occurs with an *explosion of anger*. The abuser, no longer exercising any self-control, releases his tension in an outburst of physical violence that can result in serious injury or even death. The abuser may use his fists, he may throw his mate across a room, he may burn her with cigarettes or scald her with hot liquids, he may break her arms, or he may force sexual acts on her. The form of abuse may vary, but it is always out of proportion to the woman's perceived offense.

Women who have experienced severe beatings do not always seek medical care immediately. They may try to hide the beatings and convince themselves that they are not really hurt.

The third stage, that of *loving reconciliation*, frequently referred to as the *honeymoon phase*, occurs as the abuser apologizes and makes amends. He appears to be contrite and promises that he will control himself from now on. He also believes that he has taught her such a lesson that he will never be forced to strike her again. Even in his contrite mode, he is able to blame the woman for the event.

Wanting desperately to believe that this man who presents himself as loving and contrite is really what her partner is like, the woman may decide to stay and give him another chance. She believes he loves her and needs her.

There are other reasons for taking him back. The woman may feel trapped in this relationship because of lack of a support system or lack of economic resources or job skills. She may be too ashamed to tell her family. Or she may fear retaliation from her spouse if she should leave.

Regardless of why she stays, tension starts to build once the reconciliation is over, and the cycle begins again. Figure 40–5 illustrates the cycle of violence.

Sexual Abuse

In addition to the beatings that abused women suffer, many are also subjected to rape and other forms of sexual abuse (Weingourt, 1990; Pagelow, 1982). This form of abuse is typically not reported unless the woman is specifically asked about it (Gelles, 1977) (for a discussion of rape, refer to Chapter 41).

In a study conducted by Weingourt (1990), a convenience sample of 53 women was interviewed at a major medical center in New England. The focus of the research was marital and cohabitant relationships. The women were being treated for a primary depressive or anxiety disorder; women with psychotic behavior were excluded from the study. Data were collected by a means of a semistructured interview protocol. Each woman was asked, "Have you ever felt as if you were being pressured or forced to have sexual relations with a man when you really didn't want to?"

The analysis of the 53 interviews revealed that 17 (32%) of the women had been raped by their husbands, and 16 (32%) had been raped and battered by their husbands. Two women reported being battered but not raped, and 18 denied abuse of any kind in their marital relationships. Therefore, 33 (62%) of the women being treated for depression and anxiety had been raped by their husbands. In addition, all but two of the women reported that the rape had occurred more than twice.

This study did not use a nonclinical sample, but the results can be compared with other studies that relied on nonclinical samples. Russell (1982) reported that 14% of her married sample had been raped by their spouses. Frieze (1983) reported that 34% of her sample of battered women had experienced marital rape, whereas only 7% of her nonbattered group had similar experiences.

A comparison of these results with the results of Weingourt's (1990) sample demonstrates that the incidence of marital rape in the clinical sample is at least twice as high as that of the nonclinical sample. In 33 (62%) of the interviews, the women identified marital rape. Seventeen (51%) of the women who were raped reported no other form of violence, whereas 16 (48%) reported physical and sexual abuse. This finding tends to challenge Frieze's (1983) conclusion that marital rape is typically linked with battering and tends to support Russell's (1982) conclusion that rape may be the only form of abuse experienced by women and must be separately investigated.

Weingourt's (1990) data also revealed a significant relationship between child sexual abuse and wife rape. Twenty-four women out of the 33 who had been raped reported being sexually abused as children, whereas only 8 out of the 20 nonraped wives had been sexually molested as children.

The clinical ramifications of these findings suggest that wife rape is a significant negative factor in the lives of clinically depressed and anxious women and is closely linked with a history of having child abuse. The comments made by the women indicated high levels of self-deprecation, feelings of worthlessness and helplessness, negative feelings toward men and marriage, and feelings of shame about sex (Weingourt, 1990).

▶ Check Your Reading

32. What is the cycle of abuse?
33. What happens in the honeymoon phase of the cycle of abuse?
34. What does research suggest about the relationship between depression or anxiety and sexual abuse?
35. What does research suggest regarding the relationship between child abuse and wife rape?
36. Identify three of the feelings commonly expressed by women who have been raped within their marriages.

DIAGNOSIS

The analysis of the assessment data leads to a long list of potential nursing diagnoses as well as potential *DSM-IV* diagnoses.

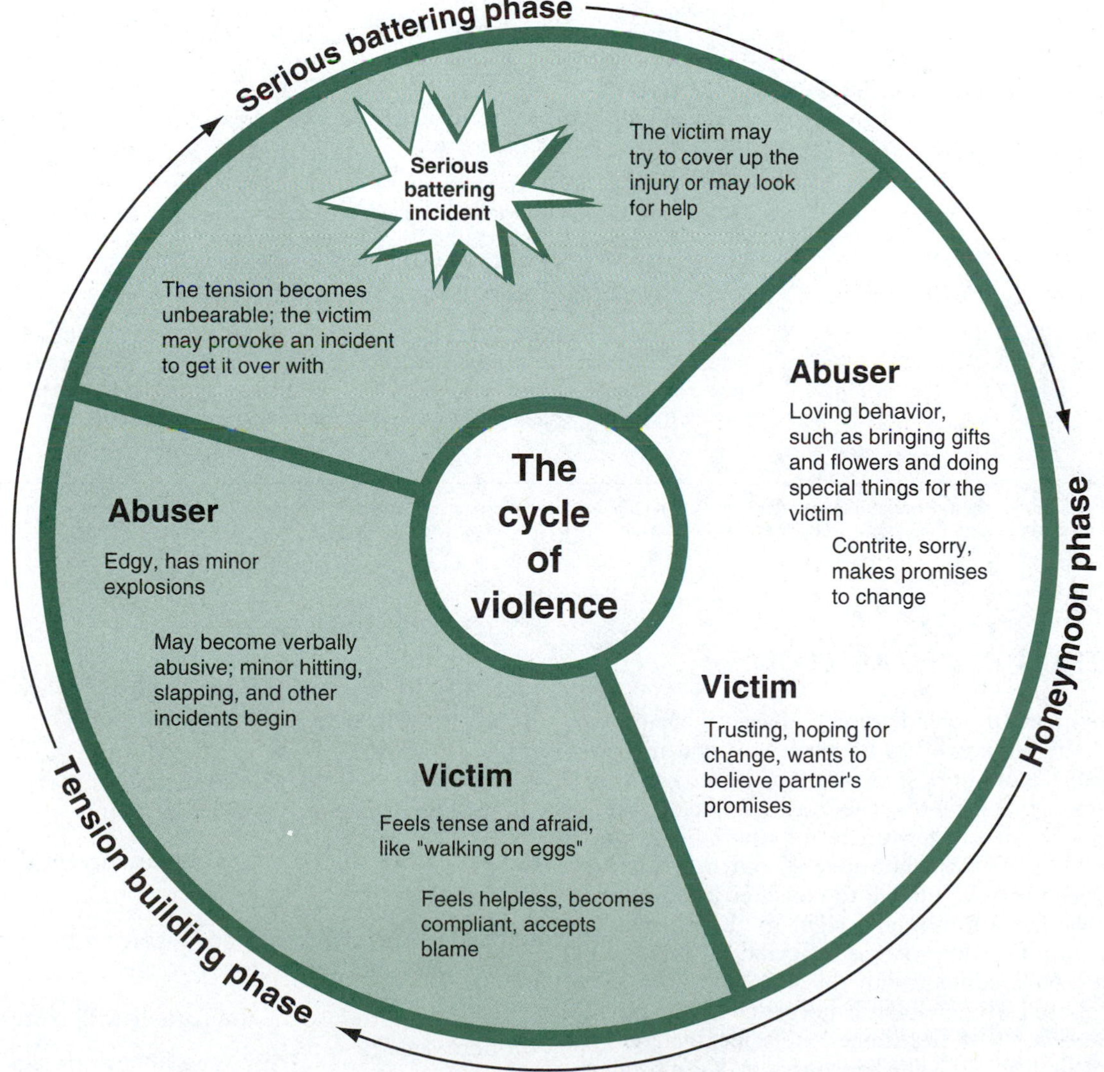

FIGURE 40–5
The cycle of violence. (Redrawn from YWCA of Annapolis and Anne Arundel County, 1517 Ritchie Hwy., Arnold, MD 21012.)

MEDICAL DIAGNOSES AND RELATED NURSING DIAGNOSES — Violence

***DSM-IV* Diagnoses**
Adjustment Disorder With Anxiety
Adjustment Disorder With Depressed Mood
Major Depressive Disorder (see Chapter 30)
Dysthymic Disorder
Generalized Anxiety Disorder (see Chapter 28)
Alcohol Dependence (see Chapter 31)
Alcohol Abuse (see Chapter 31)
Other Substance-Related Disorders (see Chapter 31)

RELATED NURSING DIAGNOSES	DEFINITION	EXAMPLE
Anxiety	A vague, uneasy feeling whose source is often nonspecific or unknown to the individual	Anxiety related to unpredictable and dangerous behavior of partner as evidenced by fearful comments
Ineffective Individual Coping	Impairment of adaptive behaviors and problem-solving abilities of a person in meeting life's demands and roles	Ineffective Individual Coping related to living in a violent situation as evidenced by use of alcohol to deal with an unbearable situation
Altered Family Processes	The state in which a family that normally functions effectively experiences a dysfunction	Altered Family Processes related to tension, fear, and violence as evidenced by acting-out behaviors of children and fear of wife
RELATED NURSING DIAGNOSES	DEFINITION	EXAMPLE
Fear	Feeling of dread related to an identifiable source, which the person validates	Fear related to constant threat of physical harm as evidenced by comments related to history of old injuries
Spiritual Distress	Disruption in the life principle, which pervades a person's entire being and which integrates and transcends one's biological and psychosocial nature	Spiritual Distress related to feelings of abandonment by God as evidenced by comments that prayers are unanswered
Hopelessness	A subjective state in which an individual sees limited or no alternatives or personal choices available and is unable to mobilize energy on own behalf	Hopelessness related to belief that cycle of abuse cannot be broken as evidenced by comments that none of the suggested measures will change current circumstances

DSM-IV diagnoses from American Psychiatric Association (1994). *Diagnostic and statistical manual of mental disorders, fourth edition.* Washington, D.C.; nursing diagnoses and definitions from North American Nursing Diagnosis Association (1994). *NANDA nursing diagnoses: Definitions and classification 1995–1996.* Philadelphia: NANDA.

OUTCOME IDENTIFICATION

The development of goals with the abused woman is a mutual, collaborative process between you and the patient. You must avoid imposing goals on the woman. For instance, you may believe that the most important objective is for the woman to terminate the relationship with her partner. This may be the expected outcome for the woman, but she may be unable to consider it. You must respect the woman's timing and right to choose what is best for her. Additionally, goals are affected by the setting in which you have contact with the woman. When you care for an abused woman in an Emergency Department, you are concerned with her immediate safety, whereas if you are working as a psychiatric nurse in a counseling relationship with an abused woman, you might focus more on the long-term psychological effects of abuse.

PLANNING

Keeping the woman's goals and the practice setting in mind, identify goals that might include the following:

- The patient will be able to identify a place of safety should she decide to leave her partner.
- The woman will be able to discuss freely the abusive incident.
- The woman will experience caring and concern from nurses and other health care providers.
- On a self-rating scale, the patient will express feelings of increased self-esteem.
- On a self-rating scale (or a standardized depression scale), the patient will rate her mood as less depressed.

- On a self-rating scale (or a standardized anxiety scale) the woman will rate her mood as less anxious.
- The woman will be able to verbalize a plan to leave her partner.
- The woman will abstain from substance abuse.
- The woman will be able to discover meaning from her experiences and experience spiritual well-being as she moves toward physical and emotional healing and wholeness.

▶ Check Your Reading

37. Identify at least two potential nursing diagnoses associated with abuse.
38. Identify two expected outcomes of working with an abused woman.
39. Identify two short-term goals for working with an abused woman.

IMPLEMENTATION

Nursing's responses to abuse are best analyzed by looking at the three levels of prevention: primary, secondary, and tertiary. Two general caveats regarding interventions, however, affect all levels of prevention. The first is the need to treat the woman with the utmost respect and dignity and avoid blaming her for what has happened. Victim blaming has been implicated in the development of the **battering syndrome** characterized by unsuccessful help seeking, vague physical complaints, and serious psychosocial problems such as substance abuse (Burgess, 1985; Kurz, 1987; Campbell and Sheridan, 1989; Flitcraft and Stark, 1989). Campbell and Sheridan warn that the women who receive negative care or are blamed for their situation are at increased risk for a number of consequences:

- Killing their abusers
- Being killed by their abusers
- Committing suicide
- Losing their unborn children

A second caveat permeating all interventions is that the woman must receive necessary information regarding local shelters and the national hotline number for shelter and battering information. This information may be essential to her own safety and that of her children when and if she decides to leave her partner.

Primary Prevention

Your nursing role is that of a community educator regarding the problems of battering, the cycle of abuse, risk factors that place a woman at risk for battering, and available community resources and services for women who are at risk or experiencing battering. Education is essential in preventing abuse. Nurses must work to heighten the public's awareness of the extent and seriousness of battering (Anderson et al, 1986).

Your educational role extends to the law enforcement and legislative communities as well. These groups must examine practices and laws that encourage or provide tacit approval or just indifference to the plight of abused women. Letter writing, petitions, and lobbying are all effective interventions to change attitudes and practices at the societal level and to increase funding for community resources to serve abused women. Nurses have been particularly effective in the areas of community education, lobbying, and national policy. For instance, Burgess (1985) has devoted her career to conducting research on violence, rape, and the science of victimology. She was appointed to serve on the 1983 U.S. Attorney General's Task Force on Family Violence.

Secondary Prevention

The second level of intervention includes all the screening activities within the community: focusing on formal abuse assessment of women who seek care in Emergency Departments; informal referrals among concerned friends and family members; and referrals for abuse by health providers in other settings, such as mental health clinics, women's health clinics, and drug treatment centers (Sabatino, 1992). Figure 40–6 provides safety planning information that you could give to a woman during a screening or counseling session. Many shelters include a 24-hour hotline, telephone or walk-in crisis counseling, and information and referral services for nonresidents of the shelter (Germain, 1984).

Tertiary Prevention

The third level of intervention usually occurs when the woman seeks medical care at an Emergency Department, a drug treatment center, physician's office or clinic, or a mental health facility. The woman's help-seeking behavior take various forms. She might seek treatment for injuries incurred during an acute battering incident, substance abuse, vague physical symptoms, or emotional difficulties.

Campbell and Sheridan (1989) identify a three-part focus for the nurse in an Emergency Department who intervenes to deal with life-threatening, health-threatening, and health-related problems. Table 40–2 identifies these problems and the appropriate interventions.

Limandri (1987) looks at the psychiatric nurse's role with the abused woman who seeks therapy. Usually the woman does not openly seek therapy to deal with the effects of abuse but presents herself with depression or extreme anxiety. You must screen the woman for abuse and respond appropriately. Curry and colleagues (1988) suggest five strategies to assist the woman, to assist her in breaking out of the cycle of abuse:

- Guiding the woman toward examining her feelings

- Helping the woman to look at her situation realistically
- Supporting the woman during the decision-making process
- Supporting the woman through any crises
- Providing the woman with the opportunities to express her anger and to work through her depression

Specific facilitative and inhibitive nursing responses are shown in Box 40–8.

Tertiary prevention also involves long-term therapy, counseling, and rehabilitation offered to battered women, their children, and the batterer. Many women and their children seek refuge in shelters, where they are assured physical safety, their basic material needs are met, and they find the much needed emotional support that allows healing to begin.

Shelters do not provide long-term solutions to the problems of abuse. They do provide a safe place for women to begin to make plans for the future. More than 50% of shelter residents return to their mates for varying lengths of time. Many women return to the shelter many times before finally deciding to leave their partner permanently (Andresen, 1985). Box 40–9 includes information given to women seeking shelter at Maryland's House of Ruth.

Shelter staff assist abused women to develop problem-solving skills. Crisis intervention is provided, and referrals are made for long-term counseling, including marital counseling. Figure 40–7 illustrates a model of nonviolence presented to residents as an alternative to the violence that has characterized their lives. Residents are encouraged to practice self-sufficient behaviors while residing in the shelter. They share in the daily chores of meal preparation, caring for children, laundry, and cleaning. Special attention is paid to the needs of children who have also been victimized either by being abused or by witnessing their mothers' abuse (Finley, 1984; Germaine, 1984; Andresen, 1985; Hollenkamp & Attala, 1986; Everett, 1990; Bennett, 1991; Humphreys, 1991).

Nurses play important roles in shelters both in salaried and volunteer positions. The nurse's role includes

- Assessing health status of the residents.
- Intervening to meet the health needs of residents.
- Developing and coordinating programs designed to address the developmental and health needs of children.

Whether you leave or stay, you will be safer if you have an escape plan

Where can you go for safety? The best choice is to the home of someone who cares for you—someone who will support you no matter what you do. This might be a good friend or a relative. If you do not have this kind of person in your life, or if it is unsafe to go there, think about a motel (if you can afford it) or a shelter for battered women.

Practice getting to a safe place from your house when you are not under stress. Plan for a quick getaway day or night. Find excuses to go outdoors that will not make your abusive partner suspicious; for example, walking the dog or taking out the garbage.

When you need to escape, pretend you are going to do one of those tasks. Once outside, just keep going. Get into the car and drive off quickly, or keep walking until you get to a phone. Call for help.

If you have children, make plans for taking them. Prepare older children to go to a neighbor's house if you cannot get away. They can call the police. Police officers may help you leave with younger children. If you must leave without the children, go back for them with the police, or pick them up at school or a babysitter's when your partner is not around.

PREPARATION

1. Identify some behaviors or circumstances leading up to an explosive situation; for example, chemical or alcohol use, stress, sex, and holidays.
2. How have you protected yourself and your children from being hurt in this past? What has worked? What has been unsafe?
3. What supports do you have available? Friends? Family? Neighbors? Church? Counselors?
4. Are you familiar with the legal protection available to you?
5. Are you familiar with medical services available to you?

SAFETY PLAN CHECKLIST

_______ 1. Access to important phone numbers—police, friends, shelters, hotline

_______ 2. Access to transportation—money for the bus, extra set of car keys, taxi phone numbers

_______ 3. Important papers organized and ready to take in the event of sudden flight—Social Security card, legal papers, food coupons, driver's license, children's birth certificates

_______ 4. Access to money—cash, checkbook, savings account number, credit cards

_______ 5. Clothes—prepacked suitcase for you and your children

FIGURE 40–6
Safety-planning information that you could give to a woman during a screening or counseling session.

TABLE 40–2 **Appropriate Interventions with an Abused Woman in an Emergency Situation**

Problems	Intervention
Life-threatening issues	
Physical injuries	Initiate body map detailing old and new injuries
	Take photographs of injuries
	Notify police if serious injury (wound from weapon, head injury) to explain options to woman
	X-ray body map of old and new fractures
Suicide risk	Psychiatric admission
	Homicide risk assessment
	Assist woman to assess her risk, explore possibility of having neighbors call police when they hear sounds of fighting. Teach woman to monitor frequency and severity of beatings. Initiate restraining order procedures. Discuss disarming gun or having police impound gun
	Make sure woman has a safe place to go
Health-threatening issues	
Sexual abuse	Allow freedom to discuss. Assure woman of normality of her response to partner's behavior. Examine for vaginal and anal injury. Assess for sexually transmitted diseases. Collect evidence of rape. Explore contraceptive concerns
Substance abuse	Discuss with woman and make appropriate referral
Depression	Refer to support group and/or mental health facility. Psychiatric admission if symptoms are severe enough or in presence of suicide intent
Health-related issues	
Low self-esteem	Help woman identify strengths. Let her know her reactions and feelings are normal. Refer to support group
Support systems	Refer to community nurse. Explore ways of expanding support system. Refer to supportive professionals
Concern for children	Explore effects of abuse on children. Explore adequacy of children's health care
Legal concerns	Explain laws related to child abuse (make sure this is done by police if present). Show woman her records. Discuss confidentiality and explain future access. Refer to police for restraining order or arrest, to legal aid for divorce.
Alternative residency (family or shelter)	Refer to shelter hotline—National Domestic Violence Hotline for shelter and battering information is 1-800-333-SAFE (7233).
	Initiate calls if woman desires
	Provide privacy and phone for woman to initiate contact
Obtaining belongings	Shelter hotline has suggestions
Transportation	Police often will help

Modified from Campbell, J. C., and Sheridan, D. J. (1989). Emergency nursing interventions with battered women. *Journal of Emergency Nursing, 15* (1), 14–15.

- Serving as a resource to shelter staff regarding access to other community services.
- Offering support and guidance to the residents.
- Serving as a health teacher on important topics such as prevention of sexually transmitted diseases, use of birth control methods, risks of cigarette smoking, nutrition, use of prescription medications, child care and development, and stress reduction.
- Serving on the advisory board of the shelter that evaluates and develops programs, reviews policies, and educates the community at large (Germain, 1984; Andresen, 1985; Hollenkamp & Attala, 1986).

Nursing faculty have used shelters as clinical placements for students. Such placements offer valuable learning experiences to nursing students and additional nursing resources to the shelter residents and staff (Finley, 1984; Everett, 1990). In other areas, nurses are managing employee assistance programs to reach out to abused nurses.

► **Check Your Reading**

40. Give at least two nursing interventions aimed at primary prevention.
41. Give at least two nursing interventions aimed at secondary prevention.
42. Give at least two nursing interventions aimed at tertiary prevention.
43. Identify at least three potential roles for nurses working in shelters for abused women.
44. What is the battering syndrome?

EVALUATION

The evaluation of nursing care is a formative and summative process. The formative evaluation is ongoing. The nurse who comes to know a woman better gains a greater appreciation of the woman's story, the processes she uses for decision-making, and the dilemmas facing her. This greater knowledge adds to the assessment and leads to mutual modification of goals, plans, and interventions.

The summative evaluation at the termination of the relationship is dictated by the mutually established goals and by the setting where relationship between the nurse and the woman occurs. For instance, it would be unrealistic for a nurse in an Emergency Department to expect to see a woman permanently leave her abusing partner. A more realistic goal would be to make sure that the woman's immediate safety is ensured. In a longer-term relationship with an abused woman, however, you might assist the woman to work toward a permanent dissolution of the abusive relationship. Andresen (1985) suggests that the woman is ready to leave her partner if the answer to the following questions is "yes":

- Has she begun to develop concrete plans about income, shelter, legal aid, and so on?
- Does she no longer worry about him but instead focuses on her own needs?
- Does she recognize abuse as a pattern rather than isolated incidents?

► **Check Your Reading**

45. What is important in a summative evaluation of nursing care for an abused woman?
46. Identify what is important in conducting a formative evaluation of the nursing care provided to an abused woman.

NURSING PROCESS WITH ABUSED CHILDREN

- Vernon. Two years old. Death is due to fractures of the ribs and multiple tears of the liver, pancreas, and mesentery. The mother and her lover are on drugs. The mother says her lover beat the child.
- Sally. Five years old. Second-degree and third-degree burns on her hands and palms. Mother says the child's father punished her for being naughty by holding her hands over the stove.
- Anne. Five years old. Dead on arrival when brought to hospital by mother and police. Death attributed to overdose of methadone. Mother admits to being an addict and says she left the drug "lying around" (Fontana, 1983, pp. 48–49).

The stories go on and on. In 1962, Kempe coined the term **battered-child syndrome** to describe the serious pattern of injuries frequently resulting in deaths in some of the children he was seeing. He undertook a nationwide survey of hospitals and law enforcement agencies in an attempt to determine how many cases of physical abuse were reported in a year. The results were published in the *Journal of the American Medical Association*. Seventy-one major hospitals had reported a total of 302 cases of the battered-child syndrome. Thirty-three of the these chil-

BOX 40-8 Facilitative and Inhibitive Nurse Responses to the Abused Woman

Facilitative Responses

- Asking woman if abuse is occurring
- Identifying behavior as abusive
- Acknowledging seriousness of abuse
- Expressing belief in woman's story
- Acknowledging that woman does not deserve the abuse
- Being directive in exploring resources
- Telling the man to stop the abuse
- Aiding woman to consider full range of available options
- Avoiding telling woman what to do
- Aiding woman to evaluate her own strengths
- Suggesting tangible resources, such as a shelter or financial aid
- Offering support groups with other abused women
- Listening actively and empathically

Inhibitive Responses

- Demonstrating anger/irritation with woman
- Blaming woman
- Advising woman to accept battering as better than nothing
- Withholding help until woman leaves abuser
- Aligning with abuser
- Not responding to abuse after disclosure
- Advising woman to leave abuser

Modified from Limandri, B. (1987). The therapeutic relationship with abused women. *Journal of Psychosocial Nursing, 25* (2), 9–16.

BOX 40-9 Maryland Legal Remedies for Battered Women

Criminal Remedies

- *Police protection:* The police must respond to domestic disturbance calls in the same manner that they respond to all other calls for assistance. Police may arrest an individual if the officer has an arrest warrant. Police may arrest on the scene without a warrant in all cases in which a crime was committed or attempted in the presence of an officer. Police may also arrest on the scene if the crime was not committed in their presence, if a weapon was used, and/or great bodily harm resulted. Police may also arrest without a warrant if the officer has probable cause to believe that the person battered the person's spouse or other individual with whom the person resides and there is evidence of physical injury and unless the person is immediately arrested the person may not be apprehended or may cause injury or damage property or tamper with or dispose of evidence, if a report is made to the police within 48 hours of the incident.
- *Police accompaniment:* The police are required by law to accompany the battered woman back to the family home to retrieve clothes and personal belongings for the immediate use of her and her children. Use of this law is technically limited to married women but is routinely extended to unmarried women. Police usually cooperate with this law, but the officer's attitude may vary.
- *Criminal prosecution:* Any battered woman can bring criminal charges against her assailant. To do so she must obtain a police report number and request a court commissioner to issue either a warrant or a summons for her violent partner. The most common disposition of criminal charges is either probation or probation before judgment. Batterers are rarely incarcerated, and this generally occurs when they have an extensive violent criminal record.

Civil Remedies

- *Protection from Domestic Violence Act:* Effective October 1, 1992, the *protection order* available to battered women has been changed. The new law in Maryland allows victims of abuse to receive protection, child support, and other financial support. The abuser can also receive counseling. *Abuse* is defined as an act that causes serious bodily harm or that places one in fear of imminent serious bodily harm. Assault and battery, sexual offenses, false imprisonment, and the abuse of a child or vulnerable adult also constitute abuse. If you have experienced any of this in your relationship with your partner, *legal protection* is available.

To be entitled to receive assistance under the new law, any one of the following must apply:

- You must be married to, separated from, or divorced from the abuser.
- If you are not married to the abuser but have a sexual relationship with him currently or in the past, you must have lived with the abuser for at least 90 days within the past year.
- You must be related to the abuser by blood, marriage, or adoption.
- You must be a parent, stepparent, child, or stepchild of the abuser and have lived with the abuser for at least 90 days within the past year.
- You must have children in common with the abuser, even if you are not married to him and don't live with him (the children must be biological or adopted).
- You must be an adult who is physically or mentally disabled (unable to provide their daily needs).
- If a child is being abused in the home, the following persons can ask the court for protection for the child: a blood relative of the child, an adoptive parent a State's Attorney, or the Department of Social Services in the county where the child lives.

There is a two-step process that you must follow to get a protection order against your abuser. You must go to the District Court or circuit court in your city or town and complete the paperwork provided by them detailing the incidence of abuse and your fear. If you are eligible for the ex-parte the judge can order protection from the abuser for up to 7 days and also give you temporary custody of the children. A hearing will then be scheduled where you and the abuser appear before a judge to state your case. It is at this time that you can receive additional protection from the abuser. The judge can order your abuser out of your home for up to 200 days. He can also order other measures to protect you and your children.

For assistance in filing an ex-parte, the House of Ruth has an advocate available at the District Court of Baltimore City, Fayette and Gay Streets, room #303 (385-2263) from 8:30 to 12:30 Monday through Friday to provide you with support and assistance in going through this process.

For more information on legal options for battered women in Maryland, call the domestic violence legal clinic at (410) 554-8463 or 554-8464.

Maryland Legal Remedies for Battered Women from House of Ruth. c/o 2201 Argonne Drive, Baltimore, MD 21218.

dren had died, and 85 had sustained permanent brain damage. Furthermore, 77 district attorneys reported encountering 447 cases of child abuse (Fontana, 1983).

Kempe's landmark research served to raise the consciousness of physicians in the United States. They began to look beyond the vague and incredulous explanations provided by parents regarding their child's injury. Physicians began to look at x-rays showing evidence of old fractures, bruises in various stages of resolution, and unexplainable scars to tell them the stories of abuse that the child was too young or too frightened to tell.

The estimated incidence of child abuse exceeds those 1962 figures by at least 5000-fold. More than 2 million cases of child abuse are reported yearly; perhaps as many as 1 million cases go unreported. The numbers are staggering and almost incomprehensible. So are the ways in which adults abuse children. Children are bashed, lashed, beaten, flayed, stomped, suffocated, strangled, gut-punched, choked with rags, beaten with cords and wires, poisoned, sliced, ripped, steamed, fried, boiled, and dismembered. Adults use every conceivable weapon, including fists, belt buckles, straps, hairbrushes, lamp cords, sticks, baseball bats, rulers, shoes and boots, lead or iron pipes, bottles, brick walls, bicycle chains, pokers, knives, scissors, chemicals, lighted cigarettes, boiling water, steaming radiators, open gas flames, and drugs (Fontana, 1983; Hyde, 1986; Forward, 1989; Landau, 1990; Fontana and Moolman, 1991; Miller, 1991).

Many children seen today are likely to have serious injuries resulting from sudden explosive acts of violence, often precipitated by the child's crying, feeding behaviors, or toilet-training problems.

▶ Check Your Reading

47. What is the battered-child syndrome?
48. Who focused the nation on the plight of abused children?

ASSESSMENT

Not all children are at equal risk for the battering syndrome. Box 40–10 shows the risk factors for child abuse. Prompt identification and assessment of the abused child is essential to intervene and prevent some of the long-term consequences of abuse. Although most abused children do not grow into delinquent adolescents or even abusive adults, the risk is considerably higher for these children. They are also at risk for school problems, psychological adjustment difficulties, failed marriages, and loss of productivity (Houck and King, 1989; Anonymous, 1992a; Anonymous, 1992b; Childs-Clarke, 1992).

Identification of the abused child begins with a

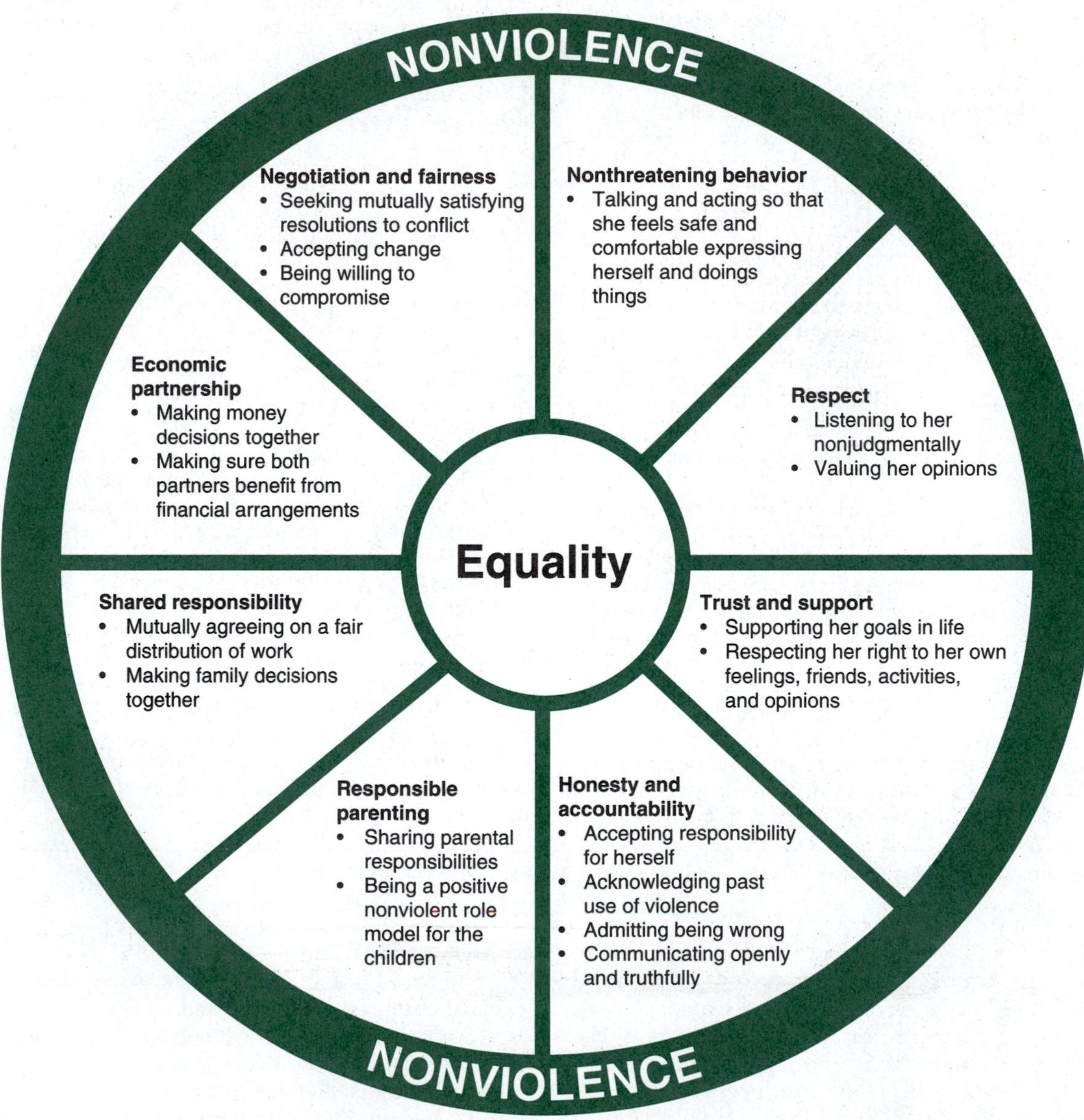

FIGURE 40–7
A model of nonviolence. (Redrawn from the Domestic Abuse Intervention Project, 204 West Fourth St., Duluth, MN 55806.)

BOX 40-10 Risk Factors for Child Abuse

- Child is physically, mentally, or emotionally impaired
- Family is experiencing high levels of stress
- One or both parents' childhood history(ies) includes substance abuse, depression, isolation, or abuse
- One or both parents use or abuse alcohol or drugs
- Society generally accepts parental right to use corporal punishment to discipline children

complete history and physical examination. During the history-taking, note whether the history seems adequate or lacking comprehensiveness. Does the history come from one of the parents? If not, where are the parents? Are there any discrepancies or contradictions in the history? Has there been a delay in seeking treatment for the child's injuries?

Parents are interviewed regarding the child's social and medical history. Do the parents report past injuries? Are their explanations believable? Are the bruises in places that are normally points of contact in a fall or accident? In some communities, hospitals are linked by a networked database that allows identification of children who have been taken to many different facilities for emergency care. If the child requires inpatient admission, the reaction of the parent(s) is carefully observed and documented.

If abuse is suspected, the parent(s) needs to be informed regarding the suspicions of the health care team. Any suspicions of child abuse *must be reported to the child protective authorities*. Reporting is not a matter of judgment or choice; it is a matter of law. Health professionals are required to report their suspicions and are protected against litigation if their suspicions are found to be ungrounded (Bliss, 1990; Binford et al, 1991).

The child(ren) should also be interviewed. The feasibility of interviewing the child depends on the child's age and physical condition. Figure 40–8 shows *the TRIADS checklist*, a useful form in assessing for child abuse (Burgess et al, 1990). This form can be used to guide the interview with the child. TRIADS is an acronym that encompasses the dimensions of child abuse:

- *T*ypes of abuse (physical, sexual, or psychological)
- *R*ole of the offender (intrafamilial or extrafamilial)
- *I*ntensity of the abuse (age when abuse began, number of times abused, and numbers of offenders involved)
- *A*utonomic response of the child (either numbness that may be manifested in depression, anger, hostility, defiance, or rebelliousness or hyperarousal manifested in night terrors, stomachaches, startle reflex, avoidance behaviors, crying, and enuresis)
- *D*uration of the abuse (over what period has abuse taken place)
- *S*tyle of the offender (whether the activities to child were blitz or spontaneous, repetitively patterned, or ritualistic and ceremonial)

Comprehensive documentation is essential in cases in which child abuse is suspected. This documentation consists of the results of the physical examination, including x-rays and other specialized tests used for dating injuries, the history and interview, and photographs taken (CIBA-GEIGY, 1991).

▶ Check Your Reading

49. What must you do if you suspect child abuse?
50. What is the TRIADS checklist?
51. Identify two future problems that abused children are at greater risk for developing.

DIAGNOSIS

The analysis of child abuse is generally done by a team of health care providers consisting of a physician, nurse, and social worker. They examine the assessment data and determine the answers to two questions:

- Is the history consistent with the observed injury(ies)?
- Could this child have received this(these) injury(ies) in the manner described?

The conclusions of this team may be presented in legal proceedings to determine whether the child should be removed from the custody of care providers.

Burgess and colleagues (1990) suggest that the analysis of the TRIADS checklist provides useful direction for intervention. For instance, if the child has been subjected to either patterned or ritualized sexual abuse, there is overwhelming arousal of the child's autonomic nervous system—so much so that the child's innate protective system is totally disrupted. The child's symptoms can be grouped under sensory, perceptual/cognitive, and interpersonal disruptions leading to the following potential nursing diagnoses:

- Sensory/Perceptual Alterations, hyperactivity, related to living in constant fear of abuse and evidenced by mother's report that child is difficult to manage and always on the "move."
- Sensory/Perceptual Alterations, nightmares, related to recurring thoughts and fears of being abused as evidenced by child's waking up during the night crying and frightened and child's verbalizations regarding content of nightmares.

- Sensory/Perceptual Alterations, startle response, related to living in constant fear of abuse as evidenced by child's quick startle response to any stimuli.
- Sensory/Perceptual Alterations, internal and external cues that produce intrusion of images and auditory and kinesthetic information, related to the trauma as evidenced by child's description of auditory and kinesthetic hallucinations.
- Altered Thought Processes related to sense of guilt and responsibility about cause, predictability, and future concerns about abuse as evidenced by child's verbalizations of personal blame.
- Powerlessness related to inability to assert and protect self and to repeated violations of personal boundaries by abuser as evidenced by child's fearfulness when anyone touches the child.
- Fear related to repeated incidents of abuse as evidenced by child's withdrawal from others.
- Altered Sexuality Patterns related to acting out actions previously directed toward self by abuser as evidenced by child's sexually precocious verbalizations and acting-out behaviors.

OUTCOME IDENTIFICATION

Some communities have done a better job than others in establishing home-based, family-centered interventions (Amundson, 1989). The expected outcomes of such home-based programs are to

- Decrease the stress in the home by providing many nontraditional child services including homemaker service, respite care, transportation, emergency child care, and vocational counseling.
- Assist the parent(s) to learn alternative coping responses to deal with children.
- Improve communication patterns and methods of problem-solving and to provide therapy for the parent(s) and child(ren).

Children removed from a home need ongoing support and therapy. Burgess and coworkers (1990) suggest that the goals of therapy include

- Desensitizing the child to the sensory and perceptual cognitive cues associated with the abuse.
- Assisting the child to master relaxation techniques to correct the sensory overload.
- Assisting the child to learn cognitive strategies to deal with the distress related to the trauma experience.
- Assisting the child to develop healthy relationships that allow the development of trust and empathy.

I. TYPE OF ABUSE

Physically Abusive Acts (check all that apply)

_______ 1. Bit, cut, punched
_______ 2. Deprived of meals
_______ 3. Physically restrained, tied up
_______ 4. Witnessing physical violence

Sexually Abusive Acts

_______ 5. Touching/fondling of breasts
_______ 6. Touching/fondling of genitals
_______ 7. Placing of finger into victim's vagina or rectum
_______ 8. Oral-genital sexual activity
_______ 9. Placement of penis into victim's vagina
_______ 10. Placement of penis into victim's rectum
_______ 11. Placement of object into victim's vagina
_______ 12. Placement of object into victim's rectum
_______ 13. Taking sexualized pictures of victim (e.g., naked)
_______ 14. Sexual acts with other victims
_______ 15. Witnessing sexual acts

Psychologically Abusive Acts and Threats

_______ 16. Being called derogatory names
_______ 17. Being told he or she was the cause of the abuse
_______ 18. Threatened not to tell about the abuse
_______ 19. Threatened he or she would be killed
_______ 20. Threatened parents would be killed
_______ 21. Threatened siblings would be killed
_______ 22. Threatened with loss of parents' love
_______ 23. Witnessing psychological abuse to others

Ritual Use of Any of the Following

_______ 24. Special table or altar
_______ 25. Sex involving unusual practices
_______ 26. Imitations and reversals of the Roman Catholic Mass
_______ 27. Excretions (e.g., semen, urine, feces, blood)
_______ 28. Circle
_______ 29. Chants or songs, especially with names of demons
_______ 30. Animals or insects
_______ 31. Robes or masks
_______ 32. Torches, candles, or darkness
_______ 33. Drugs or potions
_______ 34. Dismemberment or cannibalism

II. ROLE RELATIONSHIP OF VICTIM TO OFFENDER

_______ 35. Intrafamilial (biological)
_______ 36. Intrafamilial (step)
_______ 37. Extrafamilial, acquaintance
_______ 38. Extrafamilial, authority figure to child
_______ 39. Extrafamilial, caretaker to child
_______ 40. Extrafamilial, stranger
_______ 41. Age of offender
_______ 42. Male offender
_______ 43. Female offender

FIGURE 40–8
The TRIADS checklist for assessing child abuse. (From Burgess, A. W., Hartman, C. R., and Kelley, S. J. [1990]. The TRIADS checklist. *Journal of Psychosocial Nursing and Mental Health Services, 28* (4), 13, 14.)

III. INTENSITY OF ABUSE

________ 44. Age of victim when abuse began
________ 45. Age of victim when abuse ended
________ 46. Sex of child (M or F)
________ 47. Multiple offenders
________ 48. Multiple victims

Please estimate how many times abuse occurred.

________ 49. One time
________ 50. Five to 10 times
________ 51. 11 to 20 times
________ 52. More than 20 times

IV. AUTONOMIC RESPONSE OF THE CHILD

________ 53. Hyperaroused state (describe): ________________________________
________ 54. Numbed state (describe): ________________________________
________ 55. Frightened by threats: no somewhat very extreme
________ 56. Has continuing fears: no somewhat very extreme

V. DURATION OF ABUSE

For what length of time did the abuse occur?

________ 57. Less than 1 month
________ 58. 1 to 6 months
________ 59. 6 to 11 months
________ 60. 1 to 2 years
________ 61. 3 to 5 years
________ 62. More than 5 years

VI. STYLE OF ABUSE

________ 63. Single abusive incident: blitz
________ 64. Multiple abusive incidents: patterned
________ 65. Ritualistic abuse

FIGURE 40–8 *Continued*

PLANNING

The planning phase of care for the battered child revolves around whether the child remains in the home or not. Courts are reluctant to remove children from homes and efforts are made to keep families together.

▶ Check Your Reading

52. State one expected outcome of nursing interventions with an abused child.
53. State two short-term goals of nursing interventions with an abused child.

IMPLEMENTATION

Primary Prevention

The primary level of intervention involves increasing community sensitivity to the issue of child abuse. You might be involved in education regarding the incidence of child abuse, the long-term sequelae to child abuse, and each community member's responsibility to report suspected cases of abuse. Primary prevention includes lobbying efforts to increase funding and resources that support educational efforts in this area.

Secondary Prevention

Secondary prevention involves identifying the child at risk and referring the child for appropriate treatment. It also involves the maintenance of 24-hour hotlines that allow potential abusers to defuse their angry and violent impulses.

Tertiary Prevention

The tertiary level of prevention involves intervening with the abused child as well as with the abuser. Recognize that for the cycle of abuse to stop, both the victim and the perpetrator need help. You may work directly with the abuser to examine patterns of abuse and alternative ways of responding, or you may refer the abuser to a mental health clinic or specific therapy group designed to deal with the problems of the perpetrator of abuse (Robinson, 1982; Hunka et al, 1985; McCay and Baker, 1985; Sonkin and Durphy, 1985; Urbancic, 1987).

Abused children usually require long-term therapeutic support in the following areas:

- Providing corrective emotional experiences that allow the development of trust and empathy.
- Teaching cognitive strategies such as thought stopping, clarification, reframing beliefs, and linking stress directly to the trauma of abuse.
- Role-playing focused to teach the child to discriminate threatening exploitive behavior from safe behavior in others.
- Desensitizing to fearful involvement with others.
- Training in empathy skills.
- Teaching relaxation.
- Using psychopharmacological aids in achieving relaxation.

Hartman and Burgess (1988) suggest a model that explains how the experience of abuse is processed by the child. This model, shown in Figure 40–9, includes four phases. The first looks at the characteristics of the child before the incident occurs. The second phase examines how the child processes the experience. The third focuses on what happens when and if the child discloses the experience. The fourth phase deals with the postabuse outcome.

▶ Check Your Reading

54. State one nursing intervention aimed at primary prevention.
55. State one nursing intervention aimed at secondary prevention.
56. Identify two areas of focus in long-term therapy with abused children.

EVALUATION

The evaluation of care for the abused child focuses on both formative and summative issues. The formative outcomes include the following questions:

- Is the abuser open to receiving assistance?
- Does the abuser remain involved in a therapeutic relationship?
- Is there abatement of the abuse to the child?

The summative evaluation focuses on the following questions:

- Has the cycle of abuse been broken?
- Is the abuser seeking help to change the responses to the child?
- Is the child still being physically, emotionally, or sexually abused?
- Is there evidence that the long-term consequences to abuse are abating (e.g., the child is performing better academically and socially in the school setting, the child is no longer acting out sexually aggressive behavior, the child's delinquent behavior is decreasing, the child is able to form meaningful friendships).

▶ Check Your Reading

57. What would be included in a formative evaluation of the nursing care of an abused child?
58. What would be included in the summative evaluation of the nursing care of an abused child?
59. What behaviors would indicate that the long-term consequences of child abuse were abating?

NURSING PROCESS WITH AN ABUSED ELDER

ASSESSMENT

The five types of elder abuse are physical, psychological, sexual, financial, and self-neglect. Frequently, they are seen in Emergency Departments with injuries that do not fit the description given by the caregiver. Other times, the abuse and neglect come to the attention of neighbors or community and home care nurses who have occasion to enter the elderly person's home and observe the living conditions. Others may observe the elderly person being psychologically abused by an elderly spouse or an adult child or grandchild. Financial abuse may come to the attention of others when the elderly person is unable to pay bills or buy groceries, medication, or other necessary items (see Chapter 38).

A study conducted by Fulmer and Ashley (1989) identified nine neglect indicators that strongly suggest that an elder is being neglected:

- Poor hygiene
- Poor nutrition
- Poor skin integrity
- Contractures
- Urine burns/excoriation
- Pressure ulcers
- Dehydration

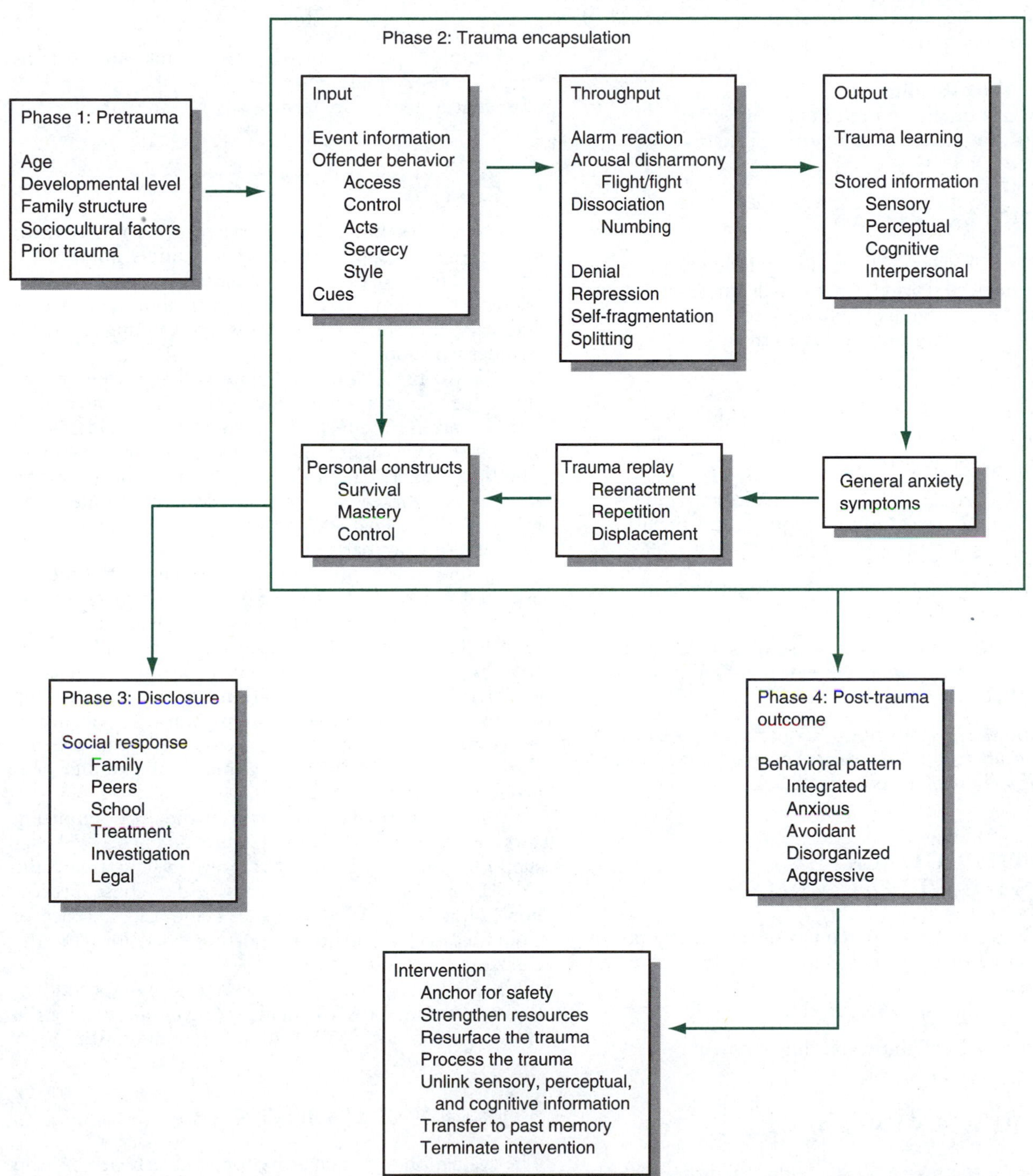

FIGURE 40–9

Information processing in victims. (Redrawn from Hartman, C. R., and Burgess, A. W., Information processing of trauma. *Journal of Interpersonal Violence, 3* [4], 443–457, copyright © 1988 by Sage Publications. Reprinted by permission of Sage Publications, Inc.)

- Impaction
- Malnutrition

Fulmer and Ashley also suggest that the decision tree in Figure 40–10 be used in deciding whether or not a particular indicator points to neglect.

▶ Check Your Reading

60. What are the five types of elder abuse?
61. Identify at least four indicators of elder abuse.

DIAGNOSIS

The analysis of data when an elderly individual is being abused or neglected leads to nursing diagnoses that cover the gamut of physical, psychological, social, and spiritual issues that nurses are responsible to treat. Possible nursing diagnoses might include

- Fluid Volume Deficit related to inadequate fluid consumption evidenced by poor skin turgor and imbalance in electrolytes.
- Colonic Constipation related to inadequate fluid intake, lack of exercise, and inadequate nutritional intake of fiber as evidenced by impaction.
- Pain related to injury sustained when pushed by son or daughter as evidenced by massive bruising on left side.
- Spiritual Distress related to sense of isolation and betrayal by son or daughter as evidenced by verbalizations that "God has forgotten me."
- Nutrition, Less Than Body Requirements, related to lack of money to buy adequate groceries as evidenced by loss of weight of 10 pounds in last two months.

OUTCOME IDENTIFICATION

There are two expected outcomes for an elderly person who is abused or neglected. These long-term goals are

- Provide for the safety of the elder.
- Break the cycle of abuse and mistreatment.

PLANNING

Short-term goals for an abused elder might include the following:

- The patient will have normal fluid and electrolyte balance.
- The patient's injuries will heal completely.
- The patient will consume adequate calories for age, body size, and energy requirements.
- The patient will feel secure in her environment.
- The patient will be free from violence.
- The patient will experience spiritual well-being.

▶ Check Your Reading

62. Identify expected outcomes of nursing interventions with an abused elder.
63. Identify two short-term goals for an abused elder.

IMPLEMENTATION

Fulmer (1989) suggests that intervention in cases in which elder abuse is suspected requires a multidisciplinary approach. This process allows a particular nurse or case manager to obtain a variety of opinions about a given case and make appropriate decisions when planning care with an elderly person.

A key consideration when intervening is whether the elderly person is in immediate danger. If so, emergency action is taken to remove the elder. Other considerations include these: Is there anyone else in the environment who is in danger? Are health care providers or protective service case workers who go into the home to intervene in danger? The goal is to protect the elderly person and anyone else from harm.

In an effort to break the cycle of abuse, the second expected outcome, consideration must be given to the *family as patient*, mandatory reporting laws, and long-term follow-up of high-risk and mistreated elders. The *family as patient* is an essential consideration. In cases of elder abuse, there is usually more than one person in the family unit in need of psychosocial or health intervention. For instance, if an elderly woman is being abused by an alcoholic daughter, both mother and daughter need treatment.

You must be familiar with mandatory reporting laws in your state. Every Congress since 1974 has supported the legislation that prevents and treats the elderly, prompting states to pass elder abuse protection statutes. By 1990, 42 states and the District of Columbia had mandatory reporting provisions for the elderly.

Box 40–11, developed by the American Association of Retired Persons (AARP), includes prevention tips for the elderly person, for families, and for communities.

EVALUATION

The evaluation of nursing care for an elderly person who has been abused or neglected includes a formative and a summative aspect. Formative evaluation is ongoing and addresses the database, nursing diagnoses, plan, and achievement of short-term goals. The formative evaluation address the following questions:

- Is the patient safe?
- Are the patient's injuries healing?

- Has a normal balance been reestablished regarding nutrition and fluid needs?
- Is the patient adequately cared for?
- Is the patient feeling secure?
- Is the patient feeling spiritually well?
- Is the patient's caregiver(s) receiving help?

The summative evaluation focuses on the safety of the elder and whether the cycle of abuse or mistreatment has ended.

▶ Check Your Reading

64. Why is a multidisciplinary approach the best when dealing with potential elder abuse?
65. Identify three questions that you would want an-

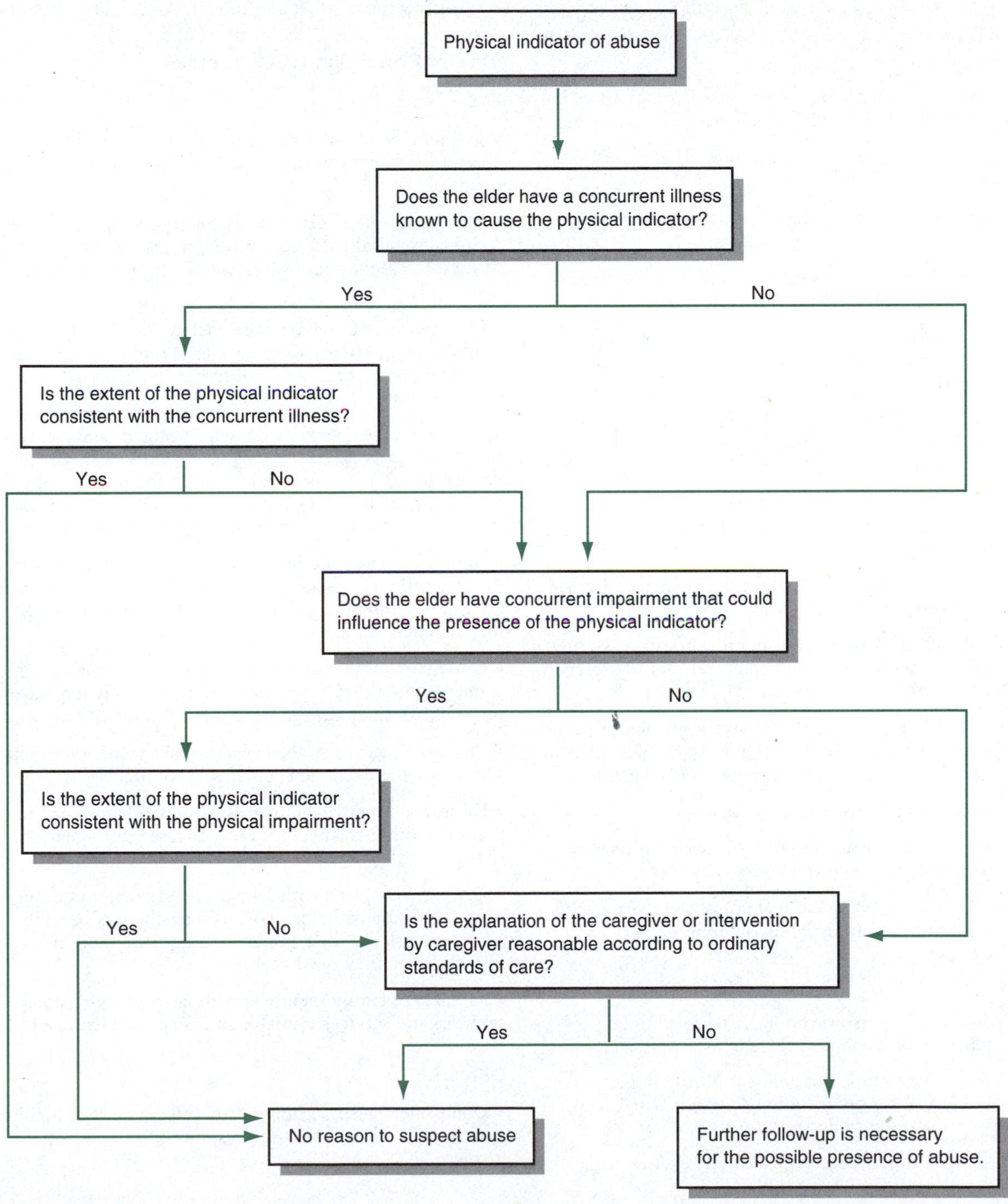

FIGURE 40–10
Clinical indicators of elder abuse. (Redrawn from Fulmer, T. T., and Aschley, J. [1989]. Clinical indicators of elder abuse. *Applied Nursing Research, 2* (4), 161–167.)

BOX 40-11 Toward Prevention: Some Do's and Don'ts

Toward Prevention . . . for Individuals

Do's

- Stay sociable as you age; maintain and increase your network of friends and acquaintances.
- Keep in contact with old friends and neighbors if you move in with a relative or to a new address.
- Develop a "buddy system" with a friend outside the home. Plan for at least a weekly contact and share openly with this person.
- Ask friends to visit you at home; even a brief visit can allow observations of your well-being.
- Accept new opportunities for activities. They can bring new friends.
- Participate in community activities as long as you are able.
- Volunteer or become a member or officer of an organization. Participate regularly.
- Have your own telephone; post and open your own mail. If your mail is being intercepted, discuss the problem with postal authorities.
- Stay organized. Keep your belongings neat and orderly. Make sure others are aware that you know where everything is kept.
- Take care of your personal needs. Keep regular medical, dental, barber, hairdresser, and other personal appointments.
- Arrange to have your social security or pension check deposited directly to a bank account.
- Get legal advice about arrangements you can make now for possible future disability, including powers-of-attorney, guardianships, or conservatorships.
- Keep records, accounts, and property available for examination by someone you trust as well as by the person you or the court has designated to manage your affairs.
- Review your will periodically.
- Give up control of your property or assets only when *you* decide you cannot manage them.
- Ask for help when you need it. Discuss your plans with your attorney, physician, or family members.

Don'ts

- Don't live with a person who has a background of violent behavior or alcohol or drug abuse.
- Don't leave your home unattended. Notify police if you are going to be away for a long period. Don't leave messages on the door while you are away.
- Don't leave cash, jewelry, or prized possessions lying about.
- Don't accept personal care in return for transfer or assignments of your property or assets unless a lawyer, advocate, or another trusted person acts as a witness to the transaction.
- Don't sign a document unless someone you trust has reviewed it.
- Don't allow anyone else to keep details of your finances or property management from you.

Toward Prevention . . . for Families

Do's

- Maintain close ties with aging relatives and friends. Keep abreast of changes in their health and ability to live independently.
- Discuss an older relative's wishes regarding health care, terminal medical care alternatives, home care in the case of incapacitation, and disposition of his or her personal assets.
- Find sources of help and use them. Chore services, housekeeping, home-delivered meals, senior recreation, day care, respite care, and transportation assistance are available in many communities.
- With the older person's consent, become familiar with his or her financial records, bank accounts, will, safe deposit boxes, insurance, debts, and sources of income before he or she becomes incapacitated. Talk and plan together now about how these affairs should be handled.
- Anticipate potential incapacitation by planning as a family who will take responsibility, such as power-of-attorney or in-home caregiving if an aging relative becomes incapacitated.
- Closely examine your family's ability to provide long-term, in-home care for a frail and increasingly dependent relative. Consider the family's physical limits.
- Plan how your own needs will be met when your responsibility for the dependent older relative increases.
- Explore alternative sources of care, including nursing homes or other relatives' homes, in case your situation changes.
- Discuss your plans with friends, neighbors, and other sources of support before your responsibilities become a burden. Ask for their understanding and emotional support—you may need them.
- Familiarize family members with emergency response agencies and services available in case of sudden need.

Don'ts

- Don't offer personal home care unless you thoroughly understand and can meet the responsibilities and costs involved.

BOX 40-11 Toward Prevention: Some Do's and Don'ts *Continued*

- Don't wait until a frail older person has moved in with you to examine his or her needs. You need to consider access, safety, containment, and special needs. (Do you need a first-floor bathroom, bedroom, or entry ramp? Will carpets or stairs become barriers? Do you need a fenced yard to prevent the loved one from wandering away? Does your kitchen allow you to prepare special diets or store medications properly? Can you move the person safely in case of fire?)
- Don't assume that poor interpersonal relationships between you or other members of the household and the older person involved will disappear.
- Don't expect irritating habits or problems such as alcohol abuse to stop or be controlled once the dependent person moves into your home.
- Don't ignore your limitations and overextend yourself. Passive neglect could result.
- Don't hamper the older person's independence or intrude unnecessarily on his or her privacy. Provide a private telephone if you can and make other changes if possible.
- Don't label your efforts a failure if home care is not possible and you must seek an alternative.

Toward Prevention . . . for Communities

Do's

- Develop new ways to provide direct assistance to caregiving families. Improve crisis response to help families that face the difficult decision to discontinue home care.
- Through public awareness programs, advocate the cause of caregiving families and the needs of victims of mistreatment.
- Ask other community groups to become more involved in aging service programs, including those at nursing homes or senior citizen housing projects. Their involvement can lead to improved facilities and services.
- Encourage both public and private employers to help caregiving families, especially those with caregivers nearing or beyond retirement age, with fixed incomes and increasing health problems.
- Publicize available support services and professionals available to caregivers, such as senior day care centers, chore services, companions, and housekeeping services. Caregivers may not know about them.
- Give public agency employees basic training in responses and case management. They can be trained to recognize some of the causes of neglect or abuse of older persons and can help in support roles.
- Provide training for community "gatekeepers" and service workers—primary care physicians, public health and social workers, law enforcement officers, transportation and utility workers, postal employees, and others—to help them recognize at-risk situations and take appropriate action.
- Expand Neighborhood Watch programs and similar community groups to include training on home care of frail elderly, identification of the signs of mistreatment, and how to provide assistance or initiate preventive actions to reduce such victimization.
- Open your eyes and ears to the possibility that mistreatment is occurring. Become aware of individuals who are at risk. Develop procedures for investigation, public education, and public support of assistance to troubled families.
- Recognize that many forms of mistreatment or abuse are crimes. Volunteers can help victims file formal complaints, seek compensation for losses, seek prosecution of guilty parties, and give the victim assistance subsequent to prosecution. Prosecution can result in sentencing, diversion, training, counseling, or other types of family assistance services as alternatives to criminal sanctions. Urge public support of agencies to provide the necessary services.

Don'ts

- Don't ignore family caregivers of dependent elderly. They are significant parts of the community. Community services can try to involve isolated people in appropriate services or self-help programs. Those at risk, or living in isolation, simply may lack knowledge or information and may welcome community outreach
- Don't assume that gerontology is a study confined to universities and hospitals. Begin to educate the entire community about aging. (This should be as common in public education as information about child care.)
- Don't sensationalize stories of abuse of older persons. Instead, try to arouse public interest in techniques and strategies to prevent abuse.
- Don't start a major intervention just because an older person is alone or is said to be eccentric. The goal is to seek the least intrusive alternative.

Adapted from AARP (1987). *Domestic mistreatment of the elderly: Towards prevention—some do's and don'ts* (Pamphlet) in Fulmer, T. T. (1989). Mistreatment of elders: Assessment, diagnosis, and intervention. *Nursing Clinics of North America, 24* (3), 707–716.

swered in evaluating the care provided to an abused elder.

NURSING PROCESS AND VIOLENT PATIENTS

As violence in society has increased, so too has violence in hospital settings (Morrison, 1993). According to Distasio (1994), 65% of psychiatric staff are assaulted by psychiatric patients. Although the prediction of violence is the focus of a great deal of psychiatric research, little progress has been made in our ability to predict who among the mentally ill will become violent. Morrison cites five myths about violence in psychiatric settings that need to be debunked (Box 40–12).

ASSESSMENT

Distasio (1994) identifies violence as a process with a preassaultive stage, when intervention is possible. Figure 40–11 illustrates the violence continuum with three basic stages: the calm, or baseline, stage; the preassaultive stage, which can last for brief periods or for more extended periods; and the violent act or the assaultive–acute excitement stage.

There are four key predictors of violence: diagnosis, history, legal status on admission, and presence or absence of dementia. The following psychiatric diagnoses are associated with violent behavior:

- Psychosis
- Bipolar disorder
- Mania
- Paranoia
- Dementia
- Substance abuse
- Personality disorders

A history of assaultive or violent behavior is an excellent predictor of future assaultive or violent behavior. When staff are aware of this aspect of the patient's history, violence is assumed to be a possibility in caring for this patient. Patients with a known history of violent behavior should never be underestimated (Tardiff, 1992).

Patients who are committed to a psychiatric facility by the court system are more prone to violent behaviors than patients who are admitted voluntarily. Involuntarily committed patients are frequently angry about having been committed, are not compliant with medications or other aspects of the treatment plan, and are usually hostile to staff members.

Patients with dementia often exhibit poor behavioral control. This dyscontrol is associated with hitting, punching, pinching, biting, and other aggressive acts. Staff caring for demented patients must exercise excellent judgment to maintain safety for themselves and others (Cahill et al, 1991).

Usually it is possible to assess behaviors that indicate that the patient's behavior is escalating. These behaviors include the following (Distasio, 1994):

- Affective changes such as labile mood swings and inappropriate reactions.
- Pressured speech, response to hallucinations, intrusiveness, negative verbalizations, muttering to self.
- Motor agitation and inability to be still, pacing.
- Sudden changes in level of consciousness, confusion, increased disorientation.
- Reddened face, flaring nostrils, clenched fists, gritted teeth, glaring, angry facial expressions.

▶ Check Your Reading

66. Identify four behaviors that should alert you of a patient's increasing agitation.

BOX 40–12 Commonly Held Myths Regarding Violence in Psychiatric Settings

- *The person with a mental illness who strikes out is viewed as out of control or impulsive.* Most incidents of violence are deliberate and chosen to get what the patient wants.
- *Using a punching bag when angry decreases aggression and violence.* Social learning theory indicates that using a punching bag reinforces the likelihood that aggression will be repeated or will escalate to actual physical violence. Patients should be encouraged to talk over their anger with those involved. Appropriate limits must be set on the patient's behavior. Patients must be held responsible for their behavior. Negotiated contracts and brief time-outs are effective strategies in dealing with violence.
- *For psychiatric nursing staff, doing a good job means helping patients regain control to ensure a safe environment.* Patients who have a coercive interactional style tend to use violence in settings where the focus is on control.
- *Aggression and violence occur when staff are inconsistent or are in conflict.* Research conducted on this relationship shows that only about 8% of patient violence is related to staff inconsistencies.
- *The clinician who is afraid is most often the victim of assault.* When studying violence, two patterns have been found for the patient's choice of victim. Either patients assaulted other men, or they assaulted vulnerable others. It is generally the staff member without peer support who is the most vulnerable. Frequently, this staff member does not support the overuse of physical restraints and is "set up" by other staff for assaults from patients.

From Morrison, E. F. (1993). Toward a better understanding of violence in psychiatric settings: Debunking the myths. *Archives of Psychiatric Nursing*, 7 (6), 328–335.

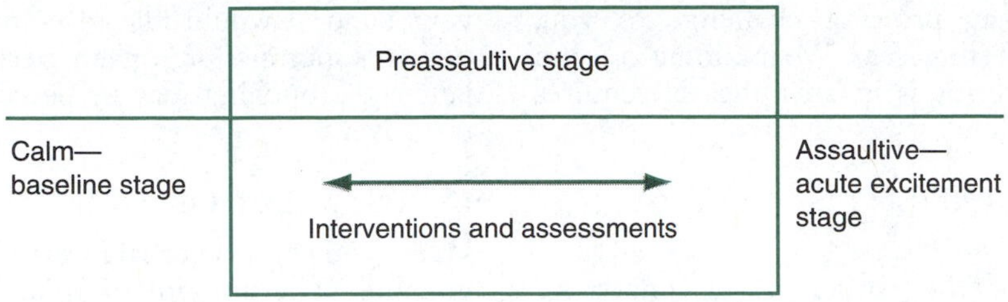

FIGURE 40–11

Violence continuum and stages. (Redrawn from Distasio, C. [1994]. Violence in health care: Institutional strategies to cope with the phenomenon. *Health Care Supervisor, 12* (4), 1–34. Copyright © 1994 Aspen Publishers, Inc.)

67. What are the four predictors of patient violence?
68. Why is it not an appropriate intervention to suggest that the patient defuse anger by using a punching bag?
69. Identify two myths that surround the issue of patient violence.

DIAGNOSIS

The nursing diagnosis most appropriate in the situation of a potentially violent patient is Risk for Injury directed at others related to having limits placed on personal behavior and evidenced by pacing, muttering obscenities, and clenched fists.

OUTCOME IDENTIFICATION

The expected outcomes of intervening with an angry and potentially explosive patient include these:

- The patient will refrain from violence.
- The patient will use nonviolent strategies to deal with anger.
- No one will get hurt.

PLANNING

The short-term goals for an angry and potentially explosive patient include the following:

- The patient will demonstrate greater calm.
- The patient's behavior will not escalate to the assaultive stage.
- The patient will experience a decrease in stress.

IMPLEMENTATION

When considering interventions to prevent or to deal with patient violence, we need to focus on the stages that occur across the violence continuum. These include the preassaultive stage, the assaultive stage, and the postassaultive stage, when the patient returns to baseline behaviors.

Preassaultive Stage of the Violence Continuum

Multiple interventions exist to deescalate violence. Staff require training in both verbal techniques of deescalation and physical techniques to restrain without harm so that they are prepared to respond to violent behavior. Appropriate training is effective in decreasing injuries to patients as well as staff (Perez, 1990; Cahill et al, 1991; Murray and Snyder, 1991; Rosenthal et al, 1992).

Verbal interventions can be effective during the escalation stage when the patient is becoming more agitated. Stevenson (1991) identified eight broad areas involved in intervention.

ANALYSIS OF PATIENT AND SITUATION

As soon as you begin to determine exactly what the patient feels is needed, you have begun to intervene. During this process, you are attempting to hear the patient's feelings and concerns. If you already know the patient well, this time initially spent listening and attending to the patient's concerns may allow you accurately to determine the problem and a suitable solution. If you do not know the patient well, your role is primarily an observer, gathering sufficient information with which to plan an intervention.

Initially, you want to encourage the patient to get to a place that is quiet and safe. Frequently, this goal can be accomplished by telling the patient that you are concerned and want to listen. The patient needs the reassurance that people are interested and willing to help. It is essential during this beginning stage to acknowledge the patient's needs regardless of whether the expressed needs are rational or irrational, possible or impossible to meet. Clearly and simply state your expectations for the patient's behavior: "I expect that you will stay in control." Offer prn medication, if it is available and appropriate.

USE OF VERBAL TECHNIQUES OF DEESCALATION

You need to be an excellent listener and able to respond to the patient in a therapeutic manner. The goal is to convey to the patient that you are calm, controlled, open, nonthreatening, and caring. You should maintain a relaxed poise. This may prove a challenge to you, especially if you are feeling fear. Maintaining a calm exterior when your interior is in an upheaval requires considerable self-discipline.

RESPECT FOR THE PATIENT'S PERSONAL SPACE

The personal space of the patient is an important consideration. If the patient is sitting, you should sit. Having your eyes on the same level as the patient's eyes decreases the sense of intimidation and gives the patient the message that you are communicating as equals. Allow the patient enough personal space, large enough so that the patient does not perceive you as intrusive but not so much that you and the patient cannot talk in a normal voice. Lanza (1988) states that persons who are poised for violence need up to four times more space than they would normally require.

The patient may invade your space with verbal abuse and use of profanity. You cannot take the patient's words personally or respond in kind. It is also important not to end the conversation because of the patient's verbal abusiveness or forbid the patient from communicating in this way. Abusive language may be the only way that the patient can express feelings.

INTERACTION WITH THE PATIENT

When you speak to the patient, your voice should be low and calm. Never respond to the patient with yelling, but continue to model controlled behavior. Using open-ended statements such as "You think people are always unkind to you?" is more effective than asking "What is wrong with you?" It is important to avoid ending statements with "okay?" This may create ambivalence in the patient and give the erroneous impression that choices exist. Your interaction with the patient should not sound punitive, threatening, accusatory, or challenging. It is better to find out what is behind the patient's feelings and behaviors.

Honestly verbalize the patient's options. Encourage the patient to assume responsibility for the choices made. This approach decreases the sense of powerlessness that often precipitates violence. Do not, however, offer options that are not possible. Discovering that you have promised something you cannot deliver only increases the patient's anger. If the patient is unable to make a choice, acknowledge the patient's decision-making difficulty: "You seem too upset to make a decision right now. I will make the decision for you now."

AWARENESS OF POSTURE AND BODY LANGUAGE

Pay attention to your posture and body language while interacting with the patient. Body language needs to be congruent with the words spoken and the tone of your voice. Slouching sometimes conveys ease and relaxation, whereas arms folded across the chest denotes being closed and unwilling to listen to another person's ideas. Sometimes a gentle touch may be helpful, *but do not touch the patient if you are unsure about its appropriateness*. It is best to ask the patient, "Would it be okay if I touched your hand? I would like to comfort you." Without the patient's permission, given verbally or through body language, touching may be perceived as threatening and intrusive.

INVESTMENT OF TIME IN THE PROCESS

When you begin a verbal intervention, have a time frame in mind. The amount of time needed varies with the patient and the particular situation—depressed, suicidal, or frightened patients may require more time; manipulative patients should be given less time. According to Stevenson (1991), eight to ten minutes is usually sufficient initially; if progress is being made, the time can be extended. Limits need to be firmly yet gently set regarding time, informing the patient that there will be no further discussion of the matter. Once these limits have been set, see that they are consistently enforced.

ATTENTION TO THE ENVIRONMENT

Not only is it important to attend to the verbal techniques of deescalation, but also the environment in which this occurs is critical. A quiet place, but one that is visible to staff, is most beneficial in helping a patient regain control. Staff should know who is working with the patient and for how long, so that uninterrupted time is allowed.

ASSURANCE OF THE NURSE'S SAFETY

If you are going to communicate in a calm manner, you must feel safe. There are some basic considerations for ensuring your safety. First, avoid wearing dangling earrings or necklaces. The patient may become focused on these, and serious injury is possible if the patient were to grab at them. If you are wearing such jewelry, take it off before going to deal with an agitated patient. Second, having enough staff for backup is essential. Although you do not want to appear overly threatening, do not handle potential violence without this backup. Only one person should talk to the patient, but staff need to maintain an unobtrusive presence in case the situation escalates.

Third, always know the layout of the area. The placement of furniture and the presence of obstacles or hazards are important to prevent injury if the patient requires **restraints**. Fourth, make sure that you are not standing directly in front of the patient or in front of the doorway; this position could be perceived as confrontational. It is better to stand off to the side and encourage the patient to have a seat.

Fifth, if you are interviewing a patient who begins to escalate, provide feedback to the patient about what you observe: "You seem to be very upset." Such an observation allows the feeling to be explored and may deescalate the situation. If the patient's behavior continues to escalate, end the interview and assure the patient that the staff will provide for the patient's as well as everyone else's safety. Sixth, avoid confrontation with the patient either through verbal means or through a "show of force" with security guards. Verbal confrontation and processing of the incident must occur when the patient is calm. The "show of force" by security guards may serve to escalate the patient's behavior; therefore, security personnel are better kept in the background until they are needed to assist (Rosenthal et al, 1992).

Assaultive Stage of the Violence Continuum

If the verbal deescalation techniques fail to calm the patient and the patient progresses to the assaultive or excitement phase, the staff must respond quickly. Generally a team approach of about five staff members is advisable, but the team may need to be larger if the patient requires it. One leader speaks to the patient and instructs members of the team.

Each team member is trained in the correct use of physical restraining maneuvers as well as the use of physical restraints. The team is organized before approaching the patient so that each team member is clear regarding individual responsibility regarding limb-securing assignments. Before approaching the patient, the team is prepared with the correct number and size of restraints and medication, if ordered. The team leader explains to the patient in a matter-of-fact manner exactly what the team is about to do and why. The team remains calm and acts to restrain the patient physically as quickly as possible and escort the patient to the seclusion room. If restraints are to be used, the patient is informed at this point of the team's intent and the reason for the team's actions. Sometimes, the patient is ready to cooperate and lies down on the bed with arms at each side. The patient is then restrained with either four-point or two-point restraints.

Once the patient is restrained, the nurse might administer an intramuscular injection of a benzodiazepine, a major tranquilizer, barbiturate, or antihistamine, depending on the physician's order. Your role in administering an intramuscular injection to an agitated patient is to provide an explanation to the patient for the medication and to make sure that the patient is properly restrained so that the medication can be safely administered. Note that chemical restraint (i.e., use of a medication to sedate a patient) is considered to be the most restrictive intervention, even more restrictive than mechanical restraints. Throughout this time, the team leader must continue to relate to the patient in a calm, steady voice, communicating decisiveness, consistency, and control.

While the patient is restrained and in **seclusion**, staff must closely monitor the patient to determine the patient's ability to reintegrate into the unit activities (Tooke, 1992). Reintegration is gradual and is geared to the patient's ability to handle increasing amounts of stimulation. If the reintegration proves to be too much for the patient, resulting in increased agitation, the patient is returned to the room or another quiet area.

Generally a structured reintegration is the best approach. For instance, reintegration can begin by reducing a patient in four-point restraints to two-point restraints. Once the patient no longer requires restraints or once the patient no longer requires the locked seclusion room, the patient may be given specified time-out periods to leave the room and move slowly into the milieu of the unit. The time-out periods are gradually increased until the patient is able to maintain control within the unit.

Postassaultive Stage of the Violence Continuum

Once the patient no longer requires seclusion and restraints, the staff should process the incident with the patient as well as among themselves. Processing with the patient is an important part of the therapeutic process. Discussing what has occurred allows the patient to learn from the situation, to identify the stressors that precipitated the out-of-control behavior, and to plan alternative ways of responding to these stressors in the future (Cahill et al, 1991).

RETURN TO BASELINE

The staff processing is critical for a number of reasons. First, a review is necessary to ensure that quality care was provided to the patient. The staff need to examine critically their responses to the patient. Questions to be answered include the following:

- Could we have done anything that would have prevented the violence?
- If the answer is yes, then what could have been done, and why wasn't it done in this situation?
- Did the team respond as a team? Were team members acting according to the policies and procedures of the unit? If not, why not?
- How do staff members feel about this patient? About this situation? Feelings of fear and anger must be discussed and handled. Otherwise the patient may be dealt with in a punitive and nontherapeutic manner. Employee morale, productivity, use of sick leave time, transfer requests, and absenteeism are all affected by patient violence, especially if a staff member has been injured. Staff members must feel supported by their peers as well as by the organizational policies and procedures established to maintain a safe environment (Murray and Snyder, 1991).
- Is there a need for additional staff education regarding how to respond to violent patients?

▶ Check Your Reading

70. Why is verbal intervention so important during the preassaultive stage of the violence continuum?
71. Why is a team approach critical when dealing with a violent patient?
72. Identify three issues that you need to consider to protect yourself when you intervene with an agitated patient.

DOCUMENTING A VIOLENT EPISODE

There are a number of areas that you must document in situations in which violence was either averted or actually occurred:

- The assessment of behaviors that occurred during the preassaultive stage.
- The nursing interventions and the patient's responses.

- An evaluation of the interventions used.
- A detailed description of the patient's behaviors during the assaultive stage.
- All nursing interventions used to defuse the crisis.
- The patient's responses to those interventions.
- How the patient was reintegrated into the unit milieu.

EVALUATION

The evaluation of the nursing care provided to a patient who is either potentially violent or who becomes violent is a critical step in the nursing process. It is necessary to evaluate the nursing staff's ability to avert violence whenever possible through deescalation techniques and to deal with violence in a manner that minimizes the chance of injury to both the patient and the staff. The evaluation is also important in determining whether factors inherent in the nurse-patient interactions or within the environment actually promote anger and violence. For instance, are staff interacting in a punitive and arbitrary manner without respect for patients' rights? When limit setting is necessary, is it done in a respectful way? Are privacy needs of patients being respected? Is the unit overcrowded? Does the unit provide a healthy balance between structured time and quiet time? An evaluation of this type provides vital information regarding the quality of care, the adequacy of unit and organizational policies regarding safety, and the need for continuing staff education related to management of aggressive behavior.

▶ Check Your Reading

73. What do you document regarding the preassaultive stage?
74. What do you document regarding the handling of a violent episode?
75. Identify two areas of information provided by the evaluation of care for a patient who became violent.
76. Why is it important to look at the environment when evaluating care for a patient who became violent?

CASE STUDY: RHONDA

Rhonda, a 27-year-old mother of three preschool children, has had frequent emergency room visits for bruises, contusions, and two broken fingers. She relates that her husband has a fiery temper just like her father's and that he gets real mad when the children don't pick up their toys and behave. Rhonda confides that she is afraid that she will take her anger out on the children. She states that out of fearing for the children's safety, she will try to divert her husband's anger at the children to her. She has voiced the desire to get out of the abusive relationship but admits having few marketable skills and that the cost of supporting three children would not allow them to survive on a minimum-wage income.

ASSESSMENT

Assessment data are as follows:

- Contusions, bruises, broken fingers
- Unsafe home environment
- Few marketable skills
- Feelings of hopelessness and powerlessness

DIAGNOSIS

***DSM-IV* Diagnosis:** Adjustment Disorder with Anxiety

Nursing Diagnosis: Powerlessness related to inability to control violent home situation as evidenced by physical injury and feelings of dissatisfaction over present life situation.

OUTCOME IDENTIFICATION, PLANNING, AND IMPLEMENTATION

EXPECTED OUTCOME 1: By _____ the patient will experience support, caring, and concern from staff and friends.

SHORT-TERM GOALS	NURSING INTERVENTIONS	RATIONALES
By _____ the patient will experience a safe, supportive environment.	1. Reassure the patient of her safety. 2. Determine and make arrangements for safety of the children. Can they stay with a relative, or does the child protective services need to be contacted? 3. Explore effects of abuse on children and adequacy of their health care.	1–2. Safety is the primary goal for both the patient and children when abuse occurs. 3. It is important to be an advocate not only for the abused mother, but also for the children.
By _____ the patient will have dealt with any life-threatening or physical injuries.	1. Take photos; initiate body map detailing old and new injuries. 2. Conduct assessment in private, being especially attentive of a nonjudgmental and gentle approach.	1. Documentation of injuries is an important legal function. The medical record may be used as evidenced in legal litigation. 2. This type of approach maintains patient's self-esteem.
By _____ the patient will experience comfort and power from other sources.	1. Encourage the patient to seek comfort from religious sources, i.e., clergy, praying. 2. Provide privacy and support for any other additional measures, such as meditation or visual imagery.	1–2. Spiritual distress is very real for the abused. Often, it becomes difficult for them to pray or feel that God is a loving, powerful force in their lives.

Nursing Diagnosis: Risk for Violence: Directed at Others related to abusive environment as evidenced by outbursts of anger from father

OUTCOME IDENTIFICATION, PLANNING, AND IMPLEMENTATION

EXPECTED OUTCOME 1: By _____ the patient will verbalize a plan to leave her partner and the abusive family situation.

SHORT-TERM GOAL	NURSING INTERVENTIONS	RATIONALES
By _____ the patient will identify two strategies to break out of the cycle of abuse.	1. Provide educational information regarding the cycle of abuse. 2. Provide numbers and addresses for local shelters and the national and local hotline numbers for shelter and battering information. 3. Provide opportunities for the patient to control decisions regarding plan of care, i.e., arrange for social work to give information about financial alternatives. 4. Encourage the patient to express feelings such as anger, depression, and anxiety.	1–2. The role of education as primary prevention is important. Awareness of risk factors, cycle of abuse, and problems associated with battering are essential to be discussed with the patient. 3. Encouraging decision-making increases the patient's self-esteem and feelings of being in control of her life situation. 4. Expression of feelings provides opportunity for the patient to come to terms with situation and work through feelings in a supportive atmosphere.

EXPECTED OUTCOME 2: By _____ the patient and her children will have a plan of safety and escape whether they leave or stay.

SHORT-TERM GOAL	NURSING INTERVENTIONS	RATIONALES
By _____ the patient will have identified the components of a safety plan checklist.	1. Administer the TRIADS checklist and the Danger Assessment.	1. Accurate assessment of the family situation is imperative for early intervention, so that both the patient and her children are assured physical safety.

SHORT-TERM GOAL	NURSING INTERVENTIONS	RATIONALES
	2. Review the components of safety planning for both the patient and her children. 3. Provide information about police protection and specific legal remedies for patient.	2–3. Safety planning includes a plan to escape and information about police and legal protection.

EVALUATION

Formative Evaluation: Rhonda was able to meet all of her short-term goals, although she had the most difficulty in determining how she was going to separate herself from her husband and manage her affairs financially. Social work was helpful in presenting information on Aid for Dependent Children and various battered women and family shelters. Her children were placed in a program that provides for long-term therapeutic support in dealing with the violent family environment.

Summative Evaluation: Rhonda achieved all of the expected outcomes, including the decision to not take herself or her children back into the abusive environment. She and her children sought protection in a battered family's shelter. With assistance from the social worker and public attorney, she brought criminal charges against her husband, which involved issuing a warrant and restraining order. Other avenues of support, which the attorney explained to her that are entitled to battered women under a new Domestic Violence Act, included financial and child support and placement of her husband into a counseling program that provides rehabilitation and services to the violent partner. Emotionally, Rhonda felt more powerful in making decisions to care for both herself and children. She told her nurse she felt like God had finally answered her prayers.

CONCLUSIONS

Violence is a growing problem in the United States. We read about it daily in our newspapers; we see the graphic pictures on the covers of popular magazines; and we are inundated with the details of drive-by shootings and other random acts of violence in our television news broadcasts. The problem is not limited to streets and ghettos but reaches into our homes. Wives are battered by husbands, children are battered by parents, and grandparents are battered by grandchildren. We should not be surprised that the violence has spilled over to health care facilities and is a major concern for health care providers in Emergency Departments as well as in psychiatric settings. Nursing's role extends beyond that of direct caregiver. Nurses have a responsibility to the community to provide education, to lobby legislators to change laws that support violence, and to lend their support to activities that reach out to the victims of violence.

KEY POINTS TO REMEMBER

- Violence includes any acts carried out with the intention of causing physical pain or injury to another person.
- Abuse is difficult to define. Gil (1975) defined it to mean any acts of commission or omission by a parent or an individual, an institution, or society as a whole that deprive a child of equal rights and liberty or interfere with or constrain the child's ability to achieve optimal developmental potential.
- Neglect represents acts of omission rather than a physical act of commission.
- Sexual abuse is the involvement of dependent and developmentally immature children and adolescents in sexual activities that they do not fully comprehend, to which they are unable to give informed consent, or that violate social taboos of family roles.
- The extent of violence in families is great. About 2 million women are abused every year; about 20% of all murder victims are related to their assailants.
- Most crimes committed by relatives are committed by spouses or ex-spouses. Pregnancy offers no immunity against violence.
- More than 2 million children are abused every year.
- About as many adolescents are mistreated as younger children.
- Incest is estimated to occur in about 14% of all families.
- Approximately 500,000 to 1 million elders are abused yearly.
- Family violence is usually accompanied by brainwashing of the victims.
- Victims frequently assume responsibility for the abuse; this process is called the hostage response.
- Victims of family abuse frequently experience shame, guilt, embarrassment, and extreme spiritual distress.
- Family violence tends to be repeated and grow worse over time.
- Other forms of victimization include sibling violence and abuse, abuse of parents by children, and elder abuse.
- Contributing causes to family violence include few costs for family violence, absence of effective social controls, inequality in

the family structure, social attitudes that support violence, value of privacy, biological factors, psychiatric illness, personal characteristics of the abuser, alcohol and drugs, and abuse as mutual combat.

• Two types of violence between spouses are instrumental violence and expressive violence.

• Sometimes abused women are further abused spiritually by people who distort Scripture and religion.

• The American Nurses' Association has taken an official position against violence.

• There are a number of assessment screens for assessing the abused woman.

• The interview of the abused woman must be gentle and direct.

• Pregnant women who have been abused generally present at Emergency Departments expressing concern over the health of the baby.

• Documentation is critical when a woman has been abused. Nursing notes may be subpoenaed if the woman presses charges against her assailant. Document all evidence of injury, use a body map to show the location of injury, and take pictures of injuries.

• It is vitally important when assessing an abused woman to determine her safety.

• The cycle of abuse includes a period of increasing tension; followed by an explosion of anger; followed by the honeymoon, or reconciliation, phase.

• Sexual abuse is another area to assess for in working with women.

• When working with an abused woman, avoid anything that sounds like blaming her for her situation.

• Primary prevention with battered women includes education of the community regarding the risks of abuse.

• Secondary prevention with battered women includes screening activities that occur within the community.

• Tertiary prevention with battered women includes emergency treatment, counseling, and the work that goes on in shelters.

• The battered-child syndrome was identified in 1962 by Kempe to describe the serious pattern of injuries frequently resulting in death in some of the children he was seeing.

• Whenever you suspect child abuse, you must report it to the child protective authorities.

• The TRIADS checklist is an excellent form for assessing child abuse.

• The interventions used in cases of child abuse also include primary, secondary, and tertiary prevention.

• Five types of elder abuse are physical, psychological, financial, sexual, and self-neglect.

• Fulmer and Ashley (1989) have identified nine neglect indicators for elder abuse: poor hygiene, poor nutrition, poor skin integrity, contractures, urine burns, pressure ulcers, dehydration, impaction, and malnutrition.

• Intervention in cases of elder abuse is best done by a multidisciplinary team that focuses on making sure the elder is safe, ensuring the environment is safe for the elder, and working with the family.

• As violence increases in society, it is also increasing in the health care system.

• Violence occurs along a continuum moving from the baseline stage, to the preassaultive stage, to the assaultive-acute excitement stage.

• Four key predictors of violence are diagnosis, history, legal status on admission, and presence or absence of dementia.

• During the preassaultive stage of violence, verbal deescalation can be effective.

• The assaultive stage requires a crisis team approach involving seclusion, mechanical restraints, and use of medication.

• During the postassaultive stage, the patient is gradually reintegrated into the unit; the incident is processed both with the patient and with the staff.

• Evaluation of the nursing care provided to a patient who became violent may suggest the need for staff continuing education and revision of unit policies and procedures.

LEARNING ACTIVITIES

1. Watch the made-for-television movie "The Burning Bed," with Farrah Fawcett. What factors supported the violence that was directed toward the character played by Fawcett? What led to her killing her spouse? What does the movie suggest to you about society's response to abused women?

2. Find out what facilities are available for abused women in your community. Take a field trip to a shelter for abused women and find out how the shelter operates. What services do they offer? Who pays for those services? Who goes there for help? What can you do to help in the problem of violence against women and children?

3. Call the child protective services and inquire about procedures for handling a report of potential child abuse.

4. Find out about the laws in your state regarding your role in reporting elder abuse.

CRITICAL THINKING EXERCISE

Bill Bains, a 35-year-old dual diagnosis patient was admitted by the court system ten days ago, following an incident in which he drove his car through the neighbor's front porch. Before the car incident, Bill had just been told by his wife that she was not interested in a man who could not keep a job. He had recently been fired from his job as assistant police chief in their small town. The staff members were concerned that Bill was suicidal and attempted to delay his discharge as long as possible. Finally, Bill's physician, Dr. Yu, suggested to him that the team would review his case and consider his discharge. Pacing the hall with his suitcase in tow, Bill waited for the team's approval of his discharge. At 10:00 A.M., Dr. Yu told Bill that the team wanted him to wait one more day.

1. What evidence might suggest Bill's potential for violence?

2. What assumption(s) do you think Bill is operating under?
3. What possible reactions might Bill have?

As Dr. Yu was informing Bill of the team's decision, Nurse Roberts was on the phone calling a code blue (a silent emergency code for an assault team). Bill turned to Dr. Yu and shouted, "You S.O.B., you lied to me!" Pushing the doctor, he bolted out of his room and yelled, "I've got to get out of here and find a job." Nurse Roberts standing near Bill's room, said to Bill, "Can you listen to what the team decided?"

1. How might Bill respond to Nurse Roberts's words?

2. Evaluate Nurse Roberts's response based on your evaluation of Bill's violence potential.

3. Consider alternate reactions; what else could happen as a result?

REFERENCES

Amundson, M. J. (1989). Family crisis care: A home-based intervention program for child abuse. *Issues in Mental Health Nursing, 10*, 285–296.

Anderson, E., McFarlane, J., and Helton, A. (1986). Community as client: A model for practice. *Nursing Outlook, 34* (5), 220–224.

Andreason, N., and Black, D. (1995). Suicide and vigilent behavior. In *Introductory textbook of psychiatry* (2nd ed.). Washington, DC: American Psychiatric Press.

Andresen, P. A. (1985). The prevention and treatment of spouse abuse: A community health perspective. *Journal of Community Health Nursing, 2*(4), 181–190.

Anonymous (1992a). The ultimate betrayal. *Nursing Times, 88* (6), 24–36.

Anonymous (1992b). Turning point. *Nursing Times, 88* (6), 29–30.

Attorney General's task force on family violence, final report (1984). Washington, D.C.: U.S. Department of Justice.

Battered Women and Criminal Justice (1987). *A report of the committee on domestic violence and incarcerated women*. Quoted in: Landes A., Foster, C. D., and Siegel, M. A. (1991). *Domestic violence: No longer behind the walls*. Wylie, Texas: Information Plus.

Bennett, L. (1991). Adolescent girls' experience of witnessing marital violence: A phenomenological study. *Journal of Advanced Nursing, 16*, 431–438.

Berger, G. (1990). *Violence and the family*. New York: Franklin Watts.

Binford, S. M., Siegel, M. A., and Landes, A. (1991). *Child abuse: Fear in the home*. Wylie, Texas: Information Plus.

Bliss, J. (1990). *Child abuse*. Vero Beach, Fla.: The Rourke Corporation.

Burgess, A. (1985). Advancing the science of victimology. *Journal of Psychosocial Nursing, 23* (1), 35–38.

Burgess, A. W., Hartman, C. R., and Kelley, S. J. (1990). Assessing child abuse: The TRIADS Checklist. *Journal of Psychosocial Nursing and Mental Health Services, 28* (4), 6–14.

Cahill, C. D., Stuart, G. W., Laraia, M. T., and Arana, G. (1991). Inpatient management of violent behavior: Nursing prevention and intervention. *Issues in Mental Health Nursing, 12*, 239–252.

Campbell, J. C. (1986). Nursing assessment for risk of homicide with battered women. *Advances in Nursing Science, 8* (4), 36–51.

Campbell, J. C., and Sheridan, D. J. (1989). Emergency nursing interventions with battered women. *Journal of Emergency Nursing, 15* (1), 12–17.

Child Abuse Prevention and Treatment Act of 1974 (PL-93-247).

Childs-Clarke, A. (1992). Treating the adult survivor. *Nursing Times, 88* (6), 27–29.

CIBA-GEIGY (1991). *Physical, sexual, and emotional abuse of children*. Summit, NJ: Medical Education Division.

Coker, L. S. (1990). A therapeutic recovery model for the female adult incest survivor. *Issues in Mental Health Nursing, 11*, 109–123.

Collier, J. A. (1987). When you suspect your patient is a battered wife. *RN, May* , 22–25.

Curry, L., Colvine, L., and Lancaster, J. (1988). Breaking the cycle of family abuse. *American Journal of Nursing, 89* (9), 1189–1190.

Distasio, C. (1994). Violence in health care: Institutional strategies to cope with the phenomenon. *Health Care Supervisor, 12* (4), 1–34.

Everett, L. W. (1990). A family violence shelter as a place for psychiatric-mental health nursing students. *Nurse Educator, 15* (3), 6–7.

Fauman, B. J. (1982). Psychiatric intervention with victims of violence. *Topics in Emergency Medicine, 3*, 85–93.

Ferrato, D. (1991). *Living with the Enemy*. New York: Aperture.

Finkelhor, D., and Yllo, K. (1985). *License to rape: Sexual abuse of wives*. New York: Holt, Rinehart & Winston.

Finley, B. (1984). The use of a battered women's shelter as a clinical agency for student learning. *Journal of Nursing Education, 23* (7), 310–313.

Flitcraft, A. H., and Stark, E. (1989). Woman battering: A prevention-oriented approach. In E. Stark and A. Flitcraft (Eds.), *Domestic violence: Survivors and their assailants*. New York: Garland Press.

Fontana, J. V. (1983). *Somewhere a child is crying*. New York: Mentor.

Fontana, V. J., and Moolman, V. (1991). *Save the family, save the child*. New York: A Dutton Book.

Forward, S. (1989). *Toxic parents*. New York: Bantam Books.

Frieze, I. H. (1983). Investigating the causes and consequences of marital rape. *Journal of Women in Culture and Society, 8*, 532–553.

Fulmer, T. T. (1989). Mistreatment of elders: Assessment, diagnosis, and intervention. *Nursing Clinics of North America, 24* (3), 707–716.

Fulmer, T. T., and Ashley, J. (1989). Clinical indicators of elder neglect. *Applied Nursing Research, 2* (4), 161–167.

Gage, R. B. (1991). Examining the dynamics of spouse abuse: An alternative view. *Nurse Practitioner, 16* (4), 11–16.

Gallup, G. (1986). 7 in 10 Favor death penalty for convicted murderers. *The Gallup Poll*.

Gelles, R. J. (1977). Power, sex and violence: The case of marital rape. *Family Coordinator, 26*, 340–347.

Gelles, R. J., and Straus, M. A. (1988). *Intimate violence*. New York: Simon & Schuster.

Germaine, C. P. (1984). Sheltering abused women: A nursing perspective. *Journal of Psychosocial Nursing, 22* (9), 24–31.

Gil, D. (1975). Unraveling child abuse. *American Journal of Orthopsychiatry, 45* (4), 346–356.

Greany, G. D. (1984). Is she a battered woman? *American Journal of Nursing, 85* (6), 725–727.

Harbin, H., and Madden, D. (1979). Battered parents: A new syndrome. *Journal of Psychiatry, 136* (10), 1288–1291.

Hart, B. (1988). Beyond the "duty to warn": A therapist's "duty to protect" battered women and children. In K. Yllo and M. Bograd (Eds.), *Feminist perspectives on wife abuse*. Newberry Park, CA: Sage.

Hartman, C. R., and Burgess, A. W. (1988). Information processing of trauma. *Journal of Interpersonal Violence, 3* (4), 443–457.

Helton, A., et al (1987). Battered and pregnant: A prevalence study. *American Journal of Public Health*, 77, 1337–1340.

Hillard, P. J. (1985). Physical abuse in pregnancy. *Obstetrics and Gynecology, 66*, 185–190.

Hollenkamp, M., and Attala, J. (1986). Meeting health needs in a crisis shelter: A challenge to nurses in the community. *Journal of Community Health Nursing, 3* (4), 201–209.

Home is where the hurt is [cover story]. *Time*, December 21, 1987.

Houck, G. M., and King, M. C. (1989). Child maltreatment: Family characteristics and developmental consequences. *Issues in Mental Health, 10*, 193–208.

Humphreys, J. (1991). Children of battered women: Worries about their mothers. *Pediatric Nursing, 17* (4), 342–354.

Hunka, C. D., O'Toole, A. W., and O'Toole, R. (1985). Self-help therapy in parents. *Journal of Psychosocial Nursing, 23* (7), 24–32.

Hyde, M. O. (1986). *Cry softly! The story of child abuse*. Philadelphia: The Westminister Press.

Janz, M. (1990). Clues to elder abuse. *Geriatric Nursing, (September/October)*, 220–222.

Kempe, C. H., Silverman, F. N., Steele, B. F., Droegmuleller, W., and Silver, H. K. (1962). The battered-child syndrome. *Journal of the American Medical Association, 181*, 105–112.

King, M. C., and Ryan, J. (1989). Abused women: Dispelling myths and encouraging intervention. *Nurse Practitioner, 14* (5), 47–58.

Klaus, P., and Rand, M. R. (1989). *Family violence. Bureau of Justice Statistics Special Report*. Washington, D.C., U.S. Department of Justice.

Koop, C. E. (1987–88). Family violence "appalling." *The Washington COFO Memo, Coalition of Family Organizations*, 7 (4), 1.

Kurz, D. (1987). Emergency department response to battered women: Resistance to medicalization. *Social Problems, 34*, 501–513.

Lake, A. (1982). New hope for battered wives. *Woman's Day, 65*, 120–123.

Landau, E. (1990). *Child abuse*. Englewood Cliffs, N.J.: Julian Messner.

Landes, A., Foster, C. D., and Siegel, M. A. (1991). *Domestic violence: No longer behind the curtains*. Wylie, TX: Information Plus.

Lanza, M. L. (1988). Factors relevant to patient assault. *Issues in Mental Health Nursing, 9*, 259–270.

Lanza, M. L., Kayne, H. L., Hicks, C., and Milner, J. (1991). Nursing staff characteristics related to patient assault. *Issues in Mental Health Nursing, 12*, 253–265.

Limaudri, B. (1987). The therapeutic relationship with abused women. *Journal of Psychosocial Nursing, 25* (2):9–16.

McCay, E., and Baker, E. (1985). Incest: A violation of trust. *The Canadian Nurse, February*, 26–28.

Menuck, M. (1983). Clinical aspects of dangerous behavior. *Journal of Psychiatry and Law, 11*, 227–304.

Miller, A. (1991). *Breaking Down the Wall of Silence*. New York: A Dutton Book.

Monroe, R. R. (1970). *Episodic behavioral disorders* (p. 25). Cambridge, MA: Harvard University Press.

Morrison, E. (1993). Toward a better understanding of violence in psychiatric settings: Debunking the myths. *Archives of General Psychiatry*, 7 (6), 328–335.

Moss, V. A., and Taylor, W. K. (1991). Domestic violence. *AORN Journal, 53* (5), 1158–1164.

Murray, M. G., and Snyder, J. C. (1991). When staff are assaulted. *Journal of Psychosocial Nursing and Mental Health Nursing, 29* (7), 24–29.

Neidig, P. H., Friedman, D. H., and Collins, B. S. (1984). *The violence continuum: A conceptual model of spouse abuse with clinical implications*. Unpublished paper. Beaufort, SC: Behavioral Science Associates Inc.

Nolte, D. L. (1992). Your child learns. *The Catholic Review, May 27*, quoted in Father Joseph Breighner's column: Giving Great Comfort (p. 15).

Pagelow, M. D. (1982). *Woman batterings: Victims and their experiences*. Beverly Hills: Sage.

Parker, B., and McFarlane, J. (1991). Identifying and helping battered pregnant women. *Maternal Child Nursing, 16*, 161–164.

Perez, L. W. (1990). Safe and sound: Orienting nurses to psychiatry. *Perspectives in Psychiatric Care, 26* (3), 7–11.

Robinson, L. (1982). Nursing therapy of an incest victim. *Issues in Mental Health Nursing, 4*, 331–342.

Rosenthal, T. L., Edwards, N. B., Rosenthal, R. H., and Ackerman, B. J. (1992). Hospital violence: Site, severity and nurses' preventive training. *Issues in Mental Health Nursing, 13*, 349–356.

Russell, D. E. H. (1982). *Rape in marriage*. New York: MacMillan.

Sabatino, F. (1992). Hospitals cope with America's new 'family value.' *Hospitals, November 5*, 24–30.

Saltman, J. (1986). *The many faces of family violence* (No. 640, p. 4). New York: Public Affairs Pamphlets.

Schiazi, R. C., et al. (1984). Sex chromosome abormalities, hormones and aggressivity. *41*, 93–99.

Selby, T. L. (1992). Nurses face growing risk of violence and abuse. *The American Nurse, April*, 3.

Sonkin, D. J., and Durphy, M. (1985). *Learning to live without violence*. San Francisco: Volcano Press.

Stark, R., and McEvoy, J. (1970). Middle-class violence. *Psychology Today, 4* (11), 52–54, 110–112.

Steinbach, A. (1992). Men about whom one can only ask, "What's to love?" *Baltimore Sun* August 9, 1992, p. F1.

Stevenson, S. (1991). Heading off violence with verbal de-escalation. *Journal of Psychosocial Nursing and Mental Health Nursing, 29* (9), 6–10.

Straus, M. A., and Gelles, R. J. (1988). Societal change and change in family violence from 1975 to 1985 as revealed by two national surveys. *Journal of Marriage and Family, 48*, 465–479.

Straus, M., et al (1980). *Behind closed doors: Violence in the American family*. New York: Anchor Books.

Tardiff, K. (1989). The current state of psychiatry in the treatment of violent patients. *Archives of General Psychiatry, 49*, 493–499.

Thobaben, M. (1993). Elder abuse. *Home Healthcare Nurse, 6* (4), 37–38.

Tilden, V. P., and Shephard, P. (1987). Battered women: The shadow side of families. *Holistic Nurse Practitioner, 1*(2), 25–32.

Tooke, S. K. (1992). Perceptions of seclusion. *Journal of Psychosocial Nursing and Mental Health Services, 30* (8), 23–26.

Urbancic, J. C. (1987). Incest trauma. *Journal of Psychosocial Nursing, 25* (7), 33–35.

U.S. House of Representatives, Select Committee on Aging. (1990). *Elder abuse: A decade of shame and inaction* (hearings). Washington, D.C.: U.S. Government Printing Office.

Weiler, K., and Buckwalter, K. C. (1992). Geriatric mental health: Abuse among the rural mentally ill. *Journal of Psychosocial Nursing, 30* (9), 32–36.

Weingourt, R. (1990). Wife rape in a sample of psychiatric patients. *Image: Journal of Nursing Scholarship, 22* (3), 144–147.

SUGGESTED READINGS

Distasio, C. (1994). Violence in health care: Institutional strategies to cope with the phenomenon. *Health Care Supervisor, 12* (4), 1–34.

Everett, L. W. (1990). A family violence shelter as a place for psychiatric-mental health nursing students. *Nurse Educator, 15* (3), 6–7.

Ferrato, D. (1991). *Living with the Enemy*. New York: Aperture.

Moss, V. A., and Taylor, W. K. (1991). Domestic violence. *AORN Journal, 53* (5), 1158–1164.

Murray, M. G., and Snyder, J. C. (1991). When staff are assaulted. *Journal of Psychosocial Nursing and Mental Health Nursing, 29* (7), 24–29.

Thobaben, M. (1993). Elder abuse. *Home Healthcare Nurse, 6* (4), 37–38.

CHAPTER 41

THE JOURNEY MARKED BY RAPE

Rape often exacts a heavy toll on its victims both physically and psychologically. Rape is generally thought to be a crime of violence motivated by aggression, not sexual impulse. However, this has not generally been accepted without controversy in that many segments of society still see rape as a sexual act—and maybe a result of carelessness or provocation. Herein lies some of the roots of stigmatization that has occurred with relation to the treatment of the rape victim. Some rape victims have said that they felt they had been "raped twice"; once by their assailant and then again by the police and health care system.

—G. Mantese

LEARNING OBJECTIVES

After studying this chapter, you should be able to:

1. Describe the types of sexual assault and identify their risk factors.
2. Describe the expected short-term and long-term reactions of victims of sexual assault.
3. Define and describe rape-trauma syndrome.
4. Describe the nurse's role with the victim of sexual assault.
5. Describe nursing research to promote the development of legislation aimed at helping victims of sexual assault.
6. Describe an innovative nurse examiner program that was developed to meet the forensic and supportive clinical needs of victims of sexual assault.
7. Identify expected outcomes and short-term goals for patients who have experienced rape.
8. Apply the nursing process to a patient situation in which Rape-Trauma Syndrome is the nursing diagnosis.

KEY TERMINOLOGY

Acute stress disorder
Attempted rape
Evidence
Posttraumatic stress disorder
Rape
Rape-trauma syndrome
Sexual coercion
Sexual contact
Sexual harassment
Sexual imposition

Rape is a devastating act with far-reaching and often long-lasting consequences. It is an act of violence in which the perpetrator violates the personhood of the survivor while exerting absolute control over her. This heinous act has been with us since the beginning of recorded history. Rape played a prominent role in Greek mythology. The Bible chronicles historical incidents of rape. More recently, during the Bosnian war, women and children were being raped as the world looked on in horror at the level of atrocities that were being committed (Weaver, 1993).

The outcomes of this violent act show similarities to the story of Persephone, which follows, who though sad and resistant to being taken by force, eventually is able to seek and receive the pity of her captor, returning to earth and the birth of spring. If only each survivor were able to recover from this trauma of rape and be reborn. But even Persephone is doomed to relive forever her journey to the dark underworld, where she had been swept away against her will to become the "mate" and thus sexual partner of the powerful male ruler of the kingdom of the dead.

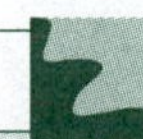

PERSEPHONE'S STORY

Persephone, young, beautiful, and innocent daughter of harvest goddess Demeter in the ancient Greek legend, wanders alone to the shade of forest trees in a meadow by the sea to pick flowers. She is suddenly swept up by the strong arm of Hades, king of the underworld, and forced to be his mate. She cries out and resists her kidnapper but is unable to escape his strong, forceful attack. Kept in the underworld against her will, she refuses to eat or drink and withers and grows very sad. Finally, Hades takes pity on her and allows her to return to her family on earth but not before she eats four pomegranate seeds. When Persephone returns to earth, the flowers sprout and spring returns. However, because she has eaten these seeds of the forbidden fruit of the underworld, she is destined always to return to Hades for four months in the year, and the season of winter is born.

The story of Persephone is an allegory shielding the reader from the true terror of the person being raped. A first person account graphically recounts the horror and powerlessness of a rape victim.

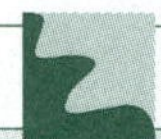

JANE'S STORY

I got raped about three years ago about this time of year. At the time I was married and living with my husband in a rather dangerous part of town. One night we had been attending a community meeting together... at the meeting I felt he was putting me down and ignoring what I had to say and so I left by myself....

I was still very angry when I left and got on the subway. I was preoccupied with my anger at my husband, and I wasn't noticing what was going on around me. So when I got off the train, I didn't notice the fact that a man—a Puerto Rican man—was following me. In the neighborhood where I was living, it was rather dark and we rarely saw any police. And I just got off the train and I was walking along with my head down and thinking and not noticing footsteps behind me until I got to my house. And I got to my house and went into the entryway. This man suddenly appeared and slipped through the door behind me and he had a gun. At that point he said (he looked sort of excitable), "Do what I tell you, I won't hurt you."

He made me leave the building and took me down the block and across the street. While he was taking me there—with this gun on me—a car passed and there were people around the block and nobody noticed anything. With this excitable man with a gun I didn't appeal to anybody in the cars or the people I saw down the block because I had no confidence that anybody would help me anyway and that people would just mind their own business. I would end up getting shot and nobody would help me if I tried to call out to somebody.

This man made me go behind a building, and as we were going behind the building, there were people in lighted apartments with windows open and I didn't call out to them. But they could hear us going around the building, but nobody noticed or nobody decided to mind anybody's else's business. And nobody came to investigate or anything.

And... um... he... um. So, the man... um. He forced me to take off my lower clothing, he forced me to have intercourse with him behind this building. Before the actual rape took place, I was frantically trying to talk him out of it by saying things. "You don't want me." Like, you know, he was white. "I'm ugly, I'm black, and you don't want me...."

After the rape I didn't feel anything, just like I was trying to think like he was thinking so that he would let me go and not kill me ... because he certainly had the power to do that... he had hurt me and he had promised he wouldn't... so, it was real weird, like he was real chummy and started talking to me, offering me a cigarette and telling me that he had just gotten out of jail and he hadn't had a woman for so long that he couldn't wait. I was acting as though I was real concerned for him because he had this gun, right?

And, okay, we were having this discussion and the chummy thing about the cigarettes afterward, but every once in a while he would say, "Are you going to tell anybody?" and he still had the gun. "You're not going to tell anybody, are you?" and like these threats in between this friendly conversation. And so I said, "No, I'm not going to tell anybody. No, I'll certainly not." I told him I wouldn't even tell my husband because my husband would kill me. And no, I wouldn't do that, I wouldn't tell anybody. And so he finally believed me and we got back onto the street and he disappeared.

Although there is certainly no "typical" rape survivor, Jane's story illustrates the surprise, shock, horror, bargaining for one's life, and potential for shame that are characteristic of the journey marked by rape. The remainder of this chapter explores not only these reactions, but also the nurse's role in caring for rape survivors, definitions of rape and related terms, incidence and demographics of rape, types of rape, the impact of nursing research, the rape-trauma syndrome, and the application of the nursing process to a patient who has been raped.

THE ROLE OF NURSES IN THE JOURNEY MARKED BY RAPE

Rape is one of the fastest-growing violent crimes reported in the United States. Victims of this crime are cared for by both psychiatric nurses and nurses in a variety of clinical settings. Rape survivors typically enter the health care delivery system through the emergency department but may also be seen in pediatric units, intensive care units, medical-surgical units, ambulatory care facilities, or psychiatric settings or in the community. Nurses may play a significant role in providing treatment for rape survivors as well as their families as they try to make sense of what has happened and attempt to get their journey back on course.

Emergency Department Nurses

The nurse in the emergency department frequently has the first caring contact with the rape survivor. The emergency department nurse is responsible for providing emotional support and physical treatment for possible sequelae of the trauma, including prophylactic treatment for potential sexually transmitted disease. The nurse also participates in ensuring the accurate collection of **evidence,** such as pictures of injuries and semen samples, which are used to prosecute the perpetrator of the crime (Holloway and Swan, 1993).

Community and Ambulatory Care Nurses

Nurses who work within the community or in ambulatory care settings often see rape survivors who are struggling to recover from the trauma. The nurse provides continued caring through counseling, support, and referral to support groups for rape survivors. It is important that nurses within all clinical settings are knowledgeable about the possible long-term psychological sequelae of the experience on the patient's journey. Nurses need to understand normal and abnormal coping patterns and to be able to teach about these issues (Ruckman, 1992). In addition, increasing public awareness of rape through community teaching activities allows nurses to become active in rape prevention and to influence public policy.

▶ Check Your Reading

1. What is unique about the emergency department nurse in relation to the rape survivor?
2. Identify two of the services provided to rape survivors by nurses working in the community and in ambulatory care settings.
3. What is the nurse's role in collecting evidence from a rape survivor?

DEFINITION OF RAPE AND RELATED TERMS

Rape is defined as sexual intercourse with a woman, without her consent, and by the use of actual physical force or the threat of such force (Mantese et al, 1991). Rape within the scope of this chapter refers to any forced sex act with lack of adult consent. In this expanded definition, men can be included as rape survivors. Precise legal definitions vary from state to state, and in some states, rape includes a variety of sex acts. Other states limit the definition of rape to forced sexual intercourse against a female not married to the abuser. These states protect the husband's legal right to have sex with his wife, no matter how forced or violent it becomes, and deny the wife the right to press charges against her spouse. Fortunately the legal climate is beginning to change.

Related to rape are other forms of sexual victimization. These are different from sexual intercourse and penetration, yet they produce common sequelae and long-lasting damage to the survivor.

For example, **attempted rape** involves force or threat of force to have sexual intercourse against the person's consent. It differs from rape only in that penetration has not occurred. Threat or actual force is present, so that the intended victim may actually fear for her life.

Sexual harassment involves nonconsensual sexual activity obtained from a person through abuse of a power relationship, such as a teacher or boss.

Sexual imposition involves the use of actual force or threat of harm to obtain sexual favors, e.g., kissing or petting.

Sexual contact involves the nonconsensual touching of the intimate body parts of the person such as breasts or buttocks.

Sexual coercion refers to ostensibly consensual intercourse that occurs subsequent to intense verbal coercion, including emotional pressure, threats to end the relationship, or false promises (Koss and Harvey, 1987).

It is likely that these different types of sexual victimization result in traumatic aftereffects, in that attitudes toward men, sexuality, and intimate relationships are influenced. The overall traumatic impact of sexual victimization depends on the survivor's past experiences, perception of the experience, and the trauma itself (Hall et al, 1993).

▶ Check Your Reading

4. Define rape.
5. Define sexual harrassment.
6. What is the difference between sexual contact and sexual coercion?

DEMOGRAPHICS OF RAPE

A "typical" rape survivor does not exist. Of the reported survivors, 93% are female, and 90% of perpetrators are male. Although one can be raped at any age (Tyra, 1993), women between the ages of 16 and 19 are at the greatest risk. It is projected that one of every six women is raped sometime in her lifetime. Nonwhite women are likely to be raped at a younger age, between ages 12 and 19, whereas white women are at highest risk between 20 and 34. As Brownmiller (1975) points out, rape can be a crime of opportunity. Women who live in urban lower-class neighborhoods having high rates of crime and juvenile delinquency are subject to the greatest risk. African-American, teenage, urban lower-class girls are the group of women who run the greatest risk of being assaulted.

Male victims of rape have great difficulty reporting the crime because of stigmatization and the fear of being ridiculed or not believed. Rapes can occur anywhere, not just in the stereotypical prisons or in isolated living situations. The motivating factor of the perpetrator, again, is not one of homosexual attack because of sexual desire resulting from deprivation but one of violence and domination. Some rapists who define themselves as heterosexual rape both men and women.

► **Check Your Reading**

7. Why are African-American, teenage, urban, lower-class girls at greatest risk for sexual assault?
8. What is the motivating factor when men rape other men?

INCIDENCE OF RAPE

Rape affects the lives of thousands of people each year. The statistics on rape in the United States alone are alarming. It has been estimated that a rape is reported every 2 to 6 minutes. The number of reported rapes increased dramatically during the 1970s, with a 59% rise from 1970 to 1977 alone. The increase of reported rapes was likely the result of a more responsive legal system as well as the establishment of rape crisis centers across the United States. Between 1978 and 1987, there was a 34.8% increase in reported cases of rape, compared with an increase of 2.8% in murders. This increase in reported rapes was higher than for any other violent crime except aggravated assault, which had a 49.6% increase (Mantese et al, 1991).

These statistics are even more alarming because only one out of every five rapes is actually reported. The most frequent reason (39%) for not reporting rape is the woman's own feelings of guilt for somehow causing the rape. Other reasons include being too embarrassed to tell anyone (35%), fear of police response (23%), and feared retribution from the assailant (19%), whose parting words often were "If you tell anyone . . . I'll rape your daughter next" or "I'll kill you the next time." Another 19% believed that reporting the rape would do no good (Ledray, 1990).

► **Check Your Reading**

9. State three reasons why women do not report being raped.
10. Identify two possible reasons why rape statistics have increased so dramatically.

TYPES OF RAPE

Marital Rape

The basis for *marital immunity* appears to have been the opinion published in 1736 by then chief justice of England, Matthew Hale. It was his view that "the husband cannot be guilty of a rape committed by himself upon his lawful wife, for by their mutual matrimonial consent and contract the wife hath given up herself in this kind unto the husband which she cannot retract" (Trevelyan, 1991, p. 40).

Clearly the law today has moved from viewing a woman as the "property" of her husband to viewing her as an equal partner in the marriage. In 1965, the Law Commission [United Kingdom] was set up by statute to promote reform of the law and pointed out that a husband's right to sexual intercourse was not now enforceable by the courts. It argued that "a woman, like a man is entitled on any particular occasion to decide whether or not to have sexual intercourse, outside or inside marriage" (Trevelyan, 1991, p. 41). A husband has no immunity from conviction for indecent assault. Therefore, a wife who has been raped by her husband can take him to court. There continues to be some differing interpretations of this law, and conflicting decisions have been rendered by different judges.

Nursing research was influential in changing the laws on marital rape in Michigan. Jacquelyn Campbell, associate professor of nursing at Wayne State University, Detroit, and Peggy Alford, a nursing doctoral student at Wayne State University, measured the physical effects of violence on women raped by their husbands. They surveyed women living in shelters in Detroit. Based on their clinical experience and earlier research, Campbell and Alford estimated that at least 500 women living in shelters had been raped by their husbands.

The results of their survey demonstrated that although vaginal intercourse was the most frequently reported type of forced sex, more than half of the women had been forced to have anal sex. Just under half had been hit, kicked, or burned during sex. More than 25% had objects inserted into them, and others reported having to endure other sexual acts of extreme degradation. Women had been threatened with violence for refusing sex, and more than one third had suffered physical beatings. More than half had been forced to have sex when ill and just under half immediately after discharge from the hospital (usually following childbirth). Of women who responded, more than half were married and the rest divorced or separated, and most said their husband thought he had a right to sex whenever he wanted it (Campbell and Alford, 1989).

These disturbing results forced the researchers to action. Campbell, along with shelter staff, wives who had been raped by their husbands, lawyers, rape victim advocates, and nurses, formed the Coalition to End Legalized Rape (CELR). Members of the coalition initially worked to have the marital rape law declared unconstitutional by the state supreme court. CELR took one case to the Michigan Supreme Court, and although the case was decided in favor of the woman, the court failed to consider the constitutionality of the law. The media coverage of this case attracted the attention of a Michigan state legislator, who drafted a bill to include marital rape in Michigan's criminal sexual conduct statute. Some women who had been raped testified at the hearings, and the nursing research of Campbell and Alford was presented for additional support.

Supporting health information was critical to the eventual passage of the bill and included evidence regarding physical problems reported by women as well as the evidence concerning damage to children who were forced to watch acts of sexual violence. On June 1, 1988, the law was changed, to include marital rape in Michigan's criminal sexual conduct statute (Trevelyan, 1991). This is an excellent example of the power that nurses can exert in the political arena by conducting nursing research in support of patients and their families. See Linda's Story (Case Example 41–1).

Case Example 41–1 Linda's Story

My husband was particularly demanding in bed. He took all his frustrations out on me. He told me to be ready for sex at any time, that's what it means to be a wife. He told me my future depended on him and that to keep him, I had better do whatever he wanted, whenever he wanted it. He would throw me down on the bed and pin my arms down. Then he would do things to me. I hated it when I responded. I felt betrayed by my own body.

From Weingourt, L. (1990). Wife rape in a sample of psychiatric patients. *Image: The Journal of Nursing Scholarship, 22*(3), 146.

In a study conducted by Weingourt (1990), a convenience sample of 53 women were interviewed at a major medical center in New England. The sample were being treated for a primary depressive or anxiety disorder; women with psychotic behavior were excluded from the study. Data were collected by means of a semistructured interview protocol. Each woman was asked, "Have you ever felt like you were being pressured or forced to have sexual relations with a man when you really didn't want to?" The focus of the research was marital and cohabitant relationships.

The analysis of the 53 interviews revealed that 17 (32%) of the women had been raped by their husbands and 16 (32%) had been raped and battered by their husbands. Two women reported being battered but not raped, and 18 denied abuse of any kind in their marital relationships. Therefore, 33 (62%) of the women being treated for depression and anxiety had been raped by their husbands. In addition, all but two of the women reported that the rape had occurred more than twice.

This study did not use a nonclinical sample. The results, however, can be compared with other studies that relied on nonclinical samples. Russell (1982) reported that 14% of her married sample had been raped by their spouses. Frieze (1983) reported that 34% of her sample of battered women had experienced marital rape, whereas only 7% of her nonbattered group had similar experiences. Weingourt's (1990) sample demonstrates that the incidence of marital rape in the clinical sample is at least twice as high as that of a nonclinical sample. In 33 (62%) of the interviews, marital rape was identified by the women. Seventeen (51%) of the women who were raped reported no other form of violence. This finding tends to challenge Frieze's (1983) conclusion that marital rape is typically linked with battering and tends to support Russell's (1982) conclusion that rape may be the only form of abuse experienced by women and must be investigated.

Weingourt's (1990) data also revealed a significant relationship between child sexual abuse and wife rape: Twenty-four women out of 33 who had been raped reported being sexually abused as children. Only 8 out of 20 nonraped wives had been sexually abused as children.

The clinical ramifications of these findings suggest that wife rape is a significant negative factor in the lives of clinically depressed and anxious women and is closely linked with a history of having been abused as a child. The comments made by women indicated high levels of self-deprecation, feelings of worthlessness and helplessness, negative feelings toward men and marriage, and feelings of shame about sex (Weingourt, 1990).

▶ Check Your Reading

11. What is marital rape?
12. What has supported marital rape as an accepted practice?
13. What is the relationship between marital rape and depression and anxiety in women?

Date or Acquaintance Rape

Growing in recognition, but still often unreported, is the phenomenon of date or acquaintance rape. Of all women raped on college campuses, 50% are raped by acquaintances. Investigations indicate that up to 78% of interviewed women had experienced some form of sexually assaultive date behavior, with 15% of the sample reporting date rape (Linton, 1987). Women rarely report rapes when they know their attackers and especially if they were on a date. *Date rape* refers to forced sexual contact within the context of what could be construed as a date or the preliminaries of what could lead to a date. Failure to report such rapes may reflect in part the cultural value that under certain circumstances it is acceptable for a man to coerce or force a woman to have sex. The rape survivor is often "blamed" by herself or others for having been provocative or even naive.

Some rape survivors continue to date the person who raped them, confusing their boyfriend's force with love and affection. Some rape survivors come from dysfunctional families and may not see forced sex as unusual. Others may have their first sexual experience this way and so have no way of knowing if this behavior is unusual or not. Rape is traumatic, whether it happens to girls, women, men, or boys, but it can be especially devastating to adolescents who are forming their own identities and sexual patterns in this developmental stage (Ellis, 1991; Kennedy, 1993; Sawyer et al, 1993).

As a result of public exposure of this problem, especially on college campuses, colleges across the United States are sponsoring antirape seminars and establishing counseling centers to raise awareness of rape as a potentially significant problem. Nurses need to be aware of this type of rape because the survivors may present for treatment in a variety of settings.

▶ Check Your Reading

14. What is date rape?
15. Why is date rape so dangerous for adolescents?

NURSING PROCESS

When the rape survivor presents for initial treatment after the trauma, she is first informed of personal rights. The nurse functions as a patient advocate to ensure that these rights are explained and supported. Box 41–1 summarizes the rights of people who have been raped.

ASSESSMENT

The assessment focuses not only on a physical examination, but also on emotional, spiritual, cognitive, and social assessment. Legal evidence is collected in addition to the routine nursing responsibilities.

Physical Assessment and Collection of Medicolegal Evidence

It is important for the nurse involved in the initial assessment following a rape to be familiar with any local reporting regulations or procedures to ensure that the examination is completed and the evidence is collected in the proper legal or forensic method. For example, in some jurisdictions, there may be state-issued *evidence collection kits* with specific procedures to be followed. The kit is used when the evidence may be used potentially to prosecute the perpetrator. These evidence collection kits ensure that certain specimens are collected uniformly from each survivor. The kits are then sealed so that all evidence will not be tampered with. The use of these kits allows for more consistency in the type of evidence collected and ensures the chain of evidence is carefully followed (Aiken, 1993).

There are five essential components that are addressed in the forensic examination by any treating facility for the rape survivor (Ledray and Arndt, 1994):

- Treatment and documentation of injuries
- Treatment and evaluation of sexually transmitted diseases
- Pregnancy risk evaluation and prevention
- Arrangements for follow-up counseling
- Collection of evidence following protocols

BOX 41–1 Rights of People Who Have Been Raped

- The right to have contact with a rape crisis advocate
- The right to decide how family or friends are notified
- The right to notify their personal physician
- The right to have gentle, sensitive treatment and confidentiality ensured
- The right to have all tests and consents explained
- The right to have follow-up referrals for counseling and, if necessary, medical treatment

BOX 41–2 Sample Assessment Questions for Rape Survivors

- "Could you describe what the attacker did to you?"
- "Were you fondled?"
- "Did the attacker perform oral sex on you? Did the attacker force you to perform oral sex?"
- "Did the attacker attempt vaginal intercourse with you? Was there penetration?"
- "Did the attacker attempt rectal intercourse with you? Was there penetration?"
- "Did the attacker experience an ejaculation? Did it happen on your body or inside of your body?"

The rape survivor receives a thorough physical assessment. Particular note is made of evidence of trauma, i.e., contusions, lacerations, and so forth. If the police were involved, they may recommend a police photographer be called for legal documentation before treatment is initiated. Vaginal, oral, and anal examinations are performed with the woman's permission to determine need for treatment and to obtain documentation for legal proceedings.

In this initial assessment, you act as patient advocate, providing privacy, supporting and explaining all aspects of this procedure, assisting with the collection of evidence, assuring the patient of safety, and recognizing the significance of all these details to the patient's journey. The evidence collection usually involves some special training because it is imperative to ensure that proper legal procedures are followed. The physical assessment must be documented carefully, to assist with possible prosecution of the perpetrator. In 53 cases associated with women pressing charges against the assailant, evidence of trauma was significantly associated with a successful prosecution (Rambow et al, 1992; Aiken, 1993).

You need to assess the type of assault, the time, place, and circumstances of the assault. Ask the patient to describe what occurred. For instance, you might gently ask the patient specifics about the attack. Box 41–2 provides sample questions that you might ask.

▶ Check Your Reading

16. What are the five essential components of the forensic examination?
17. What is included in the physical assessment of a rape survivor?
18. What is the purpose of police photographs of a rape survivor?

Assessment of Mental State

The rape survivor's mental status is assessed for cognitive, behavioral, and affective changes. The person may seem confused, may be unable to respond verbally, and may have alterations in psychomotor functioning, all of which can be normal reactions to a devastating event. Make careful note of all behaviors, emotions, and cognition, including subjective and objective data. A persistent pattern of fear and anxiety is one of the most common and well-documented reactions to sexual assault. Initial reactions during the assault itself may be predictive of later problems. Survivors almost always report fearing for their lives during a sexual assault. Being under the total domination of a threatening, unpredictable person is a terrifying experience, whether or not weapons are used or overt life-threatening statements are made (Calhoun and Atkeson, 1991; Ruckman, 1992).

In the past few years, hospitals throughout the United States have successfully developed treatment protocols specific to the rape survivor, usually emphasizing evidence collection. Hospital staff and the police have also become educated to dispel the long-held beliefs and myths about rape survivors. One of the most common myths is that the attacker was overcome with sexual desire. Sometimes myths have interfered with the survivor's receiving supportive care and the reassurance so essential during the emergency room examination and subsequent interviews (Anonymous, 1992). Box 41–3 lists the common myths about rape.

▶ Check Your Reading

19. What are some of the common feelings reported by rape survivors?
20. Name at least four myths associated with rape.

BOX 41–3 Common Myths About Rape

- Women "ask" to be raped by the provocative dress that they wear, the seductive behaviors that they display, and the places that they frequent.
- Most rapists are oversexed.
- Most rapes are committed by strangers.
- Rape is usually an impulsive act, done without planning.
- Only females get raped.
- Rape is a sexual act.
- It is dangerous for a person to try to get away from the attacker.
- Rapes usually take place in dark, secluded places.
- A healthy woman should be able to "fight off" the attack of an unarmed man.
- Only promiscuous women get raped.
- Women mean "yes" when they say "no."

Assessment of Spiritual State

Survivors of rape usually ask "why me?" In attempting to answer this question, they may conclude that they were responsible for the attack. They may accept the myths about rape as if they were truths and act on them accordingly, heaping greater pain and suffering on themselves. They may feel guilty and even sinful if they have concluded that they dressed "too flirtatiously" or were "overly friendly" or "led the attacker on." Such conclusions are, of course, erroneous because no matter how someone dresses or behaves, no one asks to be hurt or violated in the way that rape does. The feelings of guilt and perhaps sinfulness are spiritual issues. These feelings may isolate the victim from God and the loving support that a relationship with Him offers. You need to assess these spiritual concerns because significant spiritual distress could block healing.

▶ Check Your Reading

21. What is the impact of guilt on the patient's spirituality?
22. What factors would make the patient experience guilt?

Assessment of Family Response

Because the support of family and the patient's significant other can be critical to healing, you must assess their level of understanding as well as their feelings about rape. This is possible if the patient is accompanied into a treatment center by family or significant other. Observe the family or significant other with the patient to determine the feeling toward the patient. Also, ask the following questions:

"What do you understand about the crime of rape?"
"Tell me what you know about the survivor's responses to being raped?"
"Tell me what you know about the myths that surround rape?"
"How are you feeling now?"

Your observations of nonverbal behavior and the answers that the family or significant other gives provide you with a foundation from which to intervene in a supportive manner.

▶ Check your reading

23. Identify at least two reasons why the nurse assesses families or the patient's significant other in relation to their understanding of and feelings about rape.

DIAGNOSIS

The most appropriate *DSM-IV* diagnosis for a patient who has been raped is either **posttraumatic stress disorder** or **acute stress disorder,** both of which relate to anxiety- and stress-related behavioral symptoms associated with a traumatic event (see Chapter 28 for *DSM-IV* criteria for acute stress disorder). The main NANDA diagnosis for the person who has been raped is Rape-Trauma Syndrome, which describes both the acute and the long-term effects of being raped. There may be other appropriate nursing diagnoses depending on the results of the physical and mental examinations and the survivor's needs. Burgess and Holmstrom's (1974) description of the rape-trauma syndrome divides the reaction into an acute phase, lasting from a few days to several weeks, and a long-term reorganization phase, which may last for years. *DSM-IV* diagnoses for rape survivors and the related nursing diagnoses are shown in "Medical Diagnoses and Related Nursing Diagnoses."

Burgess, a professor of nursing, and Holmstrom, a professor of sociology, first coined the term rape-trauma syndrome in 1974. Their initial work analyzed the responses of 92 adult rape survivors treated at Boston City Hospital between 1972 and 1974 and identified an acute stress reaction to the life-threatening forcible rape that they had just experienced (Block, 1990). Their sample ranged in age from 17 to 73, worked at a variety of occupations, and represented a variety of ethnic classes and social backgrounds. The rape survivors ranged in physical attractiveness from plain to very pretty and were dressed in a wide range of styles. Interviews were conducted within 30 minutes after the woman had been admitted to the hospital, and telephone and in-home follow-up visits were conducted for a year (Burgess and Holmstrom, 1974).

Rape-trauma syndrome includes both the acute-phase and the long-term reorganization process that occurs as a result of forcible rape or attempted forcible rape. The behavioral, somatic, and psychological reactions are a part of a syndrome that is an acute stress reaction to a life-threatening situation.

Inherent in the definition is the concept that although rape is primarily a sexual act, it should be properly considered an act of violence with sex used as the weapon (Burgess and Holmstrom, 1974). Viewing the rape survivor as a victim of violence might lead to more compassionate, more objective, and less judgmental responses. Both health care providers and the criminal justice system stigmatize rape survivors in a manner that is not afforded any other victim of violent crime (Aguilera, 1990). It is not surprising then that the survivor of rape experiences a syndrome with specific symptoms.

▶ Check Your Reading

24. What are the two probable *DSM-IV* diagnoses for a patient who has been raped?
25. What are the two phases of the rape-trauma syndrome?
26. What are the manifestations of rape-trauma syndrome?

Disorganization (Acute) Phase

The two-phase reaction of the syndrome begins with an acute phase, in which there is a great deal of disorganization in the person's lifestyle resulting from the rape.

IMPACT REACTION

In the immediate hours following the attack, the person may experience an extremely wide range of emotions. Feelings of fear as well as shock or disbelief may predominate. In Burgess and Holmstrom's initial study (1974), two emotional styles were described:

- The *expressed* style, in which emotion was outwardly expressed through crying, smiling, sobbing, restlessness, or tenseness.
- The *controlled* style, in which feelings were not outwardly displayed, and the person appeared calm, composed, and subdued.

SOMATIC REACTIONS

In the weeks immediately following the incident, rape survivors describe a number of somatic reactions. If the person has suffered physical trauma, general soreness, bruising, and other physical complaints of injury are apparent. If the person was forced to have oral sex, irritation and trauma to the throat are frequently reported. Sleep pattern disturbances are common, with either inability to sleep or inability to fall back asleep once awakened as the reported disturbances. Rape survivors often become nauseated just thinking of the rape and frequently have decreased appetite. Gynecological symptoms are usually present, e.g., vaginal discharge, burning on urination, or itching (Burgess and Holmstrom, 1974). In general, the symptoms appear to be both directly related to the physical trauma sustained and partly generated by the emotional trauma.

EMOTIONAL REACTIONS

In the days and weeks after the rape, survivors continue to express a wide range of emotions: fear, humiliation, embarrassment, anger, and self-blame. A fear for their lives is the most pervasive emotion, which is expressed in a variety of ways. Some are hysterical and cry a great deal; others withdraw and refuse to talk with anyone. During the days and weeks that follow the original assault, rape survivors commonly experience nervousness, nightmares, inability to concentrate, startle responses, and other manifestations of anxiety. These responses tend to decrease over time, but sometimes spontaneous recovery reaches a limit beyond which there can be little improvement without professional intervention (Calhoun and Atkeson, 1991).

Depressive symptoms, including crying spells; sleep and appetite disturbances; fatigue; suicidal ideation; and feelings of guilt, worthlessness, hopelessness, and spiritual distress, are common in the first few weeks following an assault. Depression is more common in women than men, and some women may have had problems with depression before the assault. Frank and coworkers (1981) studied the relationship between past psychiatric symptoms and the woman's response to sexual assault. The researchers' results were inconclusive but suggested that women with a history of psychiatric problems, including but not limited to depression, represent a group at high risk for sexual assault or that women with a history of psychiatric

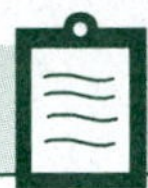

MEDICAL DIAGNOSES AND RELATED NURSING DIAGNOSES Rape

***DSM-IV* Diagnosis:** Posttraumatic Stress Disorder

Diagnostic Criteria

A. The person has been exposed to a traumatic event in which both of the following were present:
  (1) The person experienced, witnessed, or was confronted with an event or events that involved actual or threatened death or serious injury, or a threat to the physical integrity of self or others.
  (2) The person's response involved intense fear, helplessness, or horror. **Note:** In children, this may be expressed instead by disorganized or agitated behavior.

B. The traumatic event is persistently reexperienced in one (or more) of the following ways:
  (1) Recurrent and intrusive distressing recollections of the event, including images, thoughts, or perceptions. **Note:** In young children, repetitive play may occur in which themes or aspects of the trauma are expressed.
  (2) Recurrent distressing dreams of the event. **Note:** In children, there may be frightening dreams without recognizable content.
  (3) Acting or feeling as if the traumatic event were recurring (includes a sense of reliving the experience, illusions, hallucinations, and dissociative flashback episodes, including those that occur on awakening or when intoxicated). **Note:** In young children, trauma-specific reenactment may occur.
  (4) Intense psychological distress at exposure to internal or external cues that symbolize or resemble an aspect of the traumatic event.
  (5) Physiological reactivity on exposure to internal or external cues that symbolize or resemble an aspect of the traumatic event.

C. Persistent avoidance of stimuli associated with the trauma and numbing of general responsiveness (not present before the trauma), as indicated by three (or more) of the following:
  (1) Efforts to avoid thoughts, feelings, or conversations associated with the trauma.
  (2) Efforts to avoid activities, places, or people that arouse recollections of the trauma.
  (3) Inability to recall an important aspect of the trauma.
  (4) Markedly diminished interest or participation in significant activities.
  (5) Feeling of detachment or estrangement from others.
  (6) Restricted range of affect (e.g., unable to have loving feelings).
  (7) Sense of a foreshortened future (e.g., does not expect to have a career, marriage, children, or a normal life span).

D. Persistent symptoms of increased arousal (not present before the trauma), as indicated by two (or more) of the following:
  (1) Difficulty falling or staying asleep.
  (2) Irritability or outbursts of anger.
  (3) Difficulty concentrating.
  (4) Hypervigilance.
  (5) Exaggerated startle response.

E. Duration of the disturbance (symptoms in Criteria B, C, and D) is more than 1 month.

F. The disturbance causes clinically significant distress or impairment in social, occupational, or other important areas of functioning.

RELATED NURSING DIAGNOSIS	DEFINITION	EXAMPLE
Rape-Trauma Syndrome	The state in which an individual experiences a forced, violent sexual assault (vaginal or anal penetration) against his or her will and without his or her consent. The trauma syndrome that develops from this attack or attempted attack includes an acute phase of disorganization of the victim and family's lifestyle and a long-term process of reorganization of lifestyle.	Rape-Trauma Syndrome related to rape as evidenced by emotional reactions, physical trauma, genitourinary trauma, and spiritual distress.

Diagnostic Criteria from American Psychiatric Association (1994). *Diagnostic and statistical manual of mental disorders, fourth edition.* Washington, D.C.: American Psychiatric Association; nursing diagnosis and definition from North American Nursing Diagnosis Association (1994). *NANDA nursing diagnoses: Definitions and classification 1995–1996.* Philadelphia: NANDA.

problems are at risk for particularly severe reactions to sexual assault. Additionally the researchers discovered a strong relationship between certain aspects of a person's prior psychiatric history and response to rape, which suggests that although assessment of current state is important, information about the rape survivor's past psychiatric history is also valuable to the clinician. Rape survivors with a history of psychotropic drug treatment, suicidal ideation, and suicide attempts seem to be especially likely to experience a severe reaction following a rape (Frank et al, 1981).

Another common response was to seek support from family members not normally seen daily; in Burgess's study, 48 of 92 women made special trips home, which often meant traveling to another city. The women did not always tell family why they were contacting them for support, and deciding whether or not to tell family often was difficult (Burgess and Holmstrom, 1974). Continuing nightmares and dreams are especially disturbing during this phase.

Reorganization Phase

In Burgess and Holmstrom's study (1974), the coping and reorganization process began at different times for individual survivors, based somewhat on their ego strength, social support networks, and the way others treated them as victims. In Frank and coworkers' study (1981), the impact of the trauma was affected somewhat by the survivor's previous contact with mental health professionals and previous psychiatric history. In general, survivors did not experience all the same symptoms in the same sequence; what was consistent were the two phases: the acute phase of disorganization and the mild to moderate symptoms experienced in the reorganization process.

You may come in contact with rape survivors who may be in the reorganization phase in a variety of settings; for example, women may come to a community clinic seeking treatment for an apparently unrelated problem. These women may appear to have made an outward adjustment; they are back to their jobs; and relationships on the surface appear relatively "normal." This is positive and should be supported. Despite seeming outwardly adjusted, however, these women may experience a variety of subtle but troubling symptoms. Rape may have long-term effects on behavior. Survivors may have prolonged depressions and unexplained crying spells. It is not uncommon for nightmares to persist. Burgess and Holmstrom (1974) reported that nearly 50% of their sample changed residence within a relatively short period of time after the rape, generally to ensure safety and facilitate functioning in a normal style.

Some rape survivors develop new phobias as a defensive reaction to the rape. Often the link between the circumstances of the rape and the phobic behavior is clear: A woman attacked in her bed is afraid of being indoors; a woman attacked while walking to her car from the grocery store may become fearful of leaving her home to do errands. Almost all women fear being alone. A woman who has been raped by her husband has an especially difficult time in readjustment, needing to interact with her attacker and perhaps pretending to family and to herself that the rape did not occur. Often, women experience a crisis in their sexual life following a rape. Box 41–4 summarizes the responses characteristic of the two phases of rape-trauma syndrome.

BOX 41–4 Responses Characteristic of Rape-Trauma Syndrome

Acute Phase

Fear	Denial
Anger	Guilt
Anxiety	Self-blame
Tension	Embarassment
Crying	Shock or disbelief
Masked feelings	Somatic reactions
Calmness	Self-blame
Composure	

Reorganization Phase

Increased motor activity	Anxiety
Outward composure	Prolonged symptoms of depression
Denial of feelings	Phobias
Sexual problems	
Nightmares and other sleep disturbances	

▶ Check Your Reading

27. Describe the patient's behavior in the impact stage.
28. State at least four somatic concerns that are common in the acute phase of rape-trauma syndrome.
29. Describe two common emotional reactions that occur during the acute phase of rape-trauma syndrome.
30. What happens during the reorganization phase of rape-trauma syndrome?

OUTCOME IDENTIFICATION

The expected outcomes for a patient with the nursing diagnosis of Rape-Trauma Syndrome include:

- The patient will demonstrate decreased anxiety, fear, and guilt.
- The patient will experience physical healing.
- The patient will establish an adequate balance of rest, sleep, and activity.
- The patient will verbalize feelings about the rape.
- The patient will be able to find meaning in the trauma and to find spiritual comfort.
- The patient will participate in treatment programs.

PLANNING

Based on the identified expected outcomes, you and the patient, working together with the interdisciplinary team, jointly establish short-term goals, such as the following:

Expected Outcome	Short-Term Goals
1. The patient will demonstrate decreased anxiety, fear, and guilt.	The patient will verbalize feelings of anxiety, fear, and guilt.
	The patient will recognize that she did not cause the rape.
	The patient will verbalize strategies for keeping safe.
2. The patient will experience physical healing.	The patient will express the resolution of physical irritations such as sore throat, vaginal itching and burning, and bruises.
3. The patient will establish an adequate balance of rest, sleep, and activity.	The patient will sleep through the night and feel rested.
	The patient will experience decreasing frequency of nightmares.
	The patient will resume normal eating and will regain any lost weight.
4. The patient will verbalize feelings about the rape.	The patient will verbalize the details of the rape experience.
	The patient will freely express feelings about the rape experience.
5. The patient will be able to find meaning in the trauma and to find spiritual comfort.	The patient will verbalize the significance of this experience to her life's journey.
	The patient will use spiritual resources (e.g., prayer, meditation, Scripture reading, pastoral counseling) to seek comfort for the trauma.
6. The patient will participate in the treatment program.	The patient will make and keep appointments for follow-up treatment.
	The patient will follow through with treatment suggestions.

The plan takes into account whether or not the patient is in the acute disorganization phase or in the reorganization phase of rape-trauma syndrome. Progressive hospitals have planned ahead for the treatment of rape victims and have established protocols to provide care in a comprehensive, caring, sensitive manner. Such hospitals frequently have hired employees, either nurses or counselors, who are trained to meet the needs of the rape survivor.

Disorganization (Acute) Phase

The initial plan involves identifying the person who will work closely with the patient within the hospital setting. Depending on the organization system of the hospital's emergency department, either a nurse or rape crisis worker acts as patient advocate. The counselor's role varies depending on the counselor's skill and background, the philosophy of the center, and the needs of the survivor. Ideally the plan provides the woman with access to a supportive person who facilitates and guides the initial stages of her journey into the health care system. This nurse and other members of the health care team, including a physician with special training in gynecology and forensics related to the rape examination, need to establish quickly physical and mental status priorities that need immediate attention. Often the immediate care of the rape survivor falls to the generalist nurse in the emergency department who may have conflicting treatment priorities, managing a busy patient load. This person may assist in the forensic examination but does not always have the special training to provide the empathetic counseling and support that the victim needs. At the very least, this nurse can provide the privacy the rape survivor needs. This patient needs to be triaged as an emergency and taken to a private area. The patient cannot shower or douche prior to physical examination if she plans to prosecute. If oral penetration is a factor, she cannot take anything by mouth, as this also will destroy the evidence. After the physical examination, the patient should be allowed to shower. Some hospitals provide clean underwear. Prophylactic measures to prevent the possibility of pregnancy often are given.

The initial planning must also address the long-term issues that the patient will encounter in her continuing journey. Therefore, a comprehensive initial plan includes anticipatory guidance regarding the long-term consequences of rape and options to respond to these consequences.

Reorganization Phase

The long-term plan for rape survivors provides for continuing support and counseling. The time for this continuing support varies with the individual—some recover quickly, others spend years struggling to heal from the trauma inflicted by the attack. In the next section, interventions are described that address both the needs during the acute phase and the continuing need to support the victim struggling to reorganize.

▶ Check Your Reading

31. Identify at least three expected outcomes for a rape survivor.
32. Identify at least three short-term goals for nursing care of a rape survivor.
33. Identify two ways in which the initial plan differs from the long-term plan.

IMPLEMENTATION

Disorganization (Acute) Phase: Crisis Intervention

In Chapter 15, you learned about the Aguilera model of intervention known as crisis intervention. Crisis intervention is the ideal means of helping rape survivors. Rape is a sudden, overwhelming experience in which usual coping mechanisms can be inadequate. With rapid, skillful intervention, development of serious long-term disabilities may be prevented and new coping patterns may emerge that can help the individual function at a higher level of equilibrium than before the crisis (Aguilera, 1990). The nurse who encounters and intervenes with a rape survivor at any phase of disintegration or reorganization should be mindful of both crisis intervention theory and the rape-trauma syndrome. One of the most effective intervention models exists in Minneapolis, Minnesota, the Sexual Assault Resource Service (SARS). This model focuses on providing care not only during the acute phase following the rape, but also during the long-term healing process of the rape-trauma syndrome.

Reorganization Phase

A number of intervention models in the United States are devoted solely to the care of the rape survivor; these models use sexual assault nurse examiners (Jezierski, 1992; Scott, 1992).

THE SARS MODEL

SARS in Minnesota provides care to rape survivors immediately after the attack as well as follow-up care. Since September, 1977, nurses trained in both mental health and gynecology have provided primary care to rape survivors in Minneapolis through SARS, which was originally begun as a research demonstration treatment program funded through the National Institute of Mental Health. This program began as a result of concern of nurses working in the obstetrics-gynecology clinic at Hennepin County Medical Center, where rape survivors were referred for follow-up care. Before the program's inception, 75% of survivors never returned for follow-up to the clinic, a fact disturbing to the nurses who realized they were not adequately meeting their patients' needs (Ledray, 1992). Now as a result of the program's success, survivors are seen at five private hospitals as well as in the county hospital, and service has been expanded to treat males and children as well.

SARS is staffed by salaried professional nurses trained in obstetrics and mental health, who are on call 24 hours a day, 7 days a week, to see rape survivors who come to the center or who are brought to the emergency department. The SARS staff have identified seven components of care important to provide during the initial crisis period. Research conducted has confirmed that women who received this crisis support recovered more quickly than those who did not (Ledray, 1992).

Providing Emotional Support. The SARS counselors first focus on providing emotional support, as many other counselors do, offering an atmosphere of positive regard in which the rape survivor is able to express anxieties and fears freely without fear of criticism.

Responding to the Patient as Normal. The counselors respond to the patient as a normal healthy individual who is reacting to a serious life crisis, a second important component of rape counseling. The woman is reassured that her response to the rape, whether or not she fought or struggled, was the right thing to do, recognizing her survival as paramount. Rape survivors are told that their confusion and disorganization are normal responses to a traumatic event and that frequent shifts in feelings are often experienced by others after being raped.

Maintaining a Nonjudgmental Attitude. The third component is a nonjudgmental attitude on the part of the counselor. The counselor must be nonjudgmental, not only to the behavioral response of the survivor, but also in judging the event to be a "rape." Survivors have often been subject to the myths and prejudices of police and treatment staff, who may subtly or overtly convey to the woman that "she asked for it" or that the rape is "faked" to achieve some sort of secondary gain or attention. This blaming response of the caregiver can compound the survivor's response and prolong the inability to cope with the event.

Helping the Patient Regain Control. The fourth identified component is to help the patient regain control of her body, self, and situation. The physical assault of the rape results in a tremendous loss of power and control, and unfortunately, in many more traditional situations, experiences with the police, medical staff, and the courts can reinforce loss of control. Acting as a patient advocate and guide through the maze of physical examinations, treatment options, and legal alternatives, you can assist the survivor to make informed decisions and help her to regain a sense of control.

Communicating Separateness from the Event. The fifth component is to communicate to the woman that she is separate from the event; "the victim is not a raped woman; she is a woman who has been raped" (Ledray, 1990). Women who have been raped often express that they feel "dirty." Separating themselves from the event assists them in the task of regaining some self-esteem.

Helping the Patient Find Support. The sixth component involves helping the rape survivor to identify who within her social support network can handle the knowledge about the rape. Survivors are often hesitant to talk with family or friends because of feelings of guilt or embarrassment or fear of rejection. Rape survivors need to be gently supported to understand that others may respond to the rape event in a less than sensitive manner, based on their personal inability to deal with the reality of the rape.

Ensuring Personal Safety. The seventh component of rape counseling is to help the survivor identify those factors that can ensure her personal safety and make her less vulnerable. Not only are external factors relating to safety discussed, but also the fears and concerns that often continue long after the life-threatening event has occurred (Ledray, 1990). Box 41–5 provides tips for prevention of sexual assault.

BOX 41-5 Tips for Prevention of Sexual Assault

At Home

- Your obvious hiding places for keys are just as obvious to your attacker. Consider leaving a key with a trusted neighbor.
- *Everyone* should use only initials and last names on mailboxes and phone listings.
- Be prepared to enter your house without complications. Have your keys in hand when you reach the door.
- If a window or door has been forced or broken while you were absent, *do not enter*. Go to your neighbor's house and call police.
- Install the proper deadbolt locks and a door viewer, and *remember to use them.*
- Make sure that all windows are properly secured.
- Install good interior and exterior lighting for protection. Use timers for additional security while you are away.
- Instruct all family members not to answer the door automatically. Before unlocking the door, they should use the door viewer and require identification from all delivery and repair persons as well as police officers.
- Never let strangers inside your house to use the phone. Keep the door locked and offer to make the call for them. Also, remember not to reveal that you are home alone. Do not leave messages on the outside of your door advertising your absence.
- If you live in an apartment, avoid going to the basement laundry room alone.

In Your Car

- Always lock your car doors when driving or parked.
- Be mindful of suspicious activity, and always park in lighted areas.
- Always have keys in hand when entering your car.
- Do not stop for stranded motorists. Call for assistance at the nearest police station or phone booth.
- Never leave your house keys attached to car keys at service stations or parking lots.

When Walking

- If you must carry a purse, don't dangle it by your side.
- Don't carry large sums of cash or extra credit cards.
- Always be aware of your surroundings and note any suspicious characters. Try to walk with a "buddy."
- Stay in well-lighted areas and avoid short-cuts.
- If a driver stops to ask questions, avoid getting close to the car.
- If someone threatens or harasses you, attract attention to yourself by screaming, yelling, whistling or activating a hand-held siren device.
- Don't depend entirely on tear gas, pepper spray, or other sprays for protection. The wind may sabotage your defense.

FAMILY SUPPORT AND EDUCATION

The support and understanding of the patient's significant other and family is significant to the healing process. If the patient is accompanied by a family member, ask the patient's permission about whether or not she wants the family involved in the teaching and support. If the patient is agreeable, actively engage the family in the interventions. For instance, the family needs to know about:

- The myths that surround rape
- The range of normal responses to the trauma
- The characteristics of the rape-trauma syndrome
- The need for long-term support from the family and perhaps from a professional source

Some family members also may need help from a professional source to work through their own feelings about the rape.

EVALUATION

Evaluating the outcome of the nursing intervention depends on reviewing the short-term goals leading to the expected outcomes. In any crisis, the goal focuses on assisting the individual to restore equilibrium and to prevent serious long-term disability. The answers to the following questions provide important information for evaluation.

- Is the patient less anxious, fearful, and guilty?
- Have the physical injuries healed?
- Has the patient reestablished balance in rest, sleep, and activity patterns?
- Can the patient verbalize feelings about the rape?
- Is the patient able to fit the rape into the pattern of her life?
- Is the patient experiencing spiritual well-being?
- Is the patient able to use meaningful spiritual interventions for comfort?
- Has the patient participated in follow-up treatment?

The person who has been raped reaches a critical juncture in the journey of life. The assault violates the person's sense of personal safety, sexuality, and self-esteem. Effective nursing care can play a significant role in the healing of the patient who has been raped.

▶ Check Your Reading

34. What is SARS?
35. Identify at least three components of effective counseling with rape survivors.
36. Identify at least five safety practices for women that decrease the risk of being raped.
37. What is involved in family support and education?

CASE STUDY: MARY

Mary is transported by the police to the emergency department of the local hospital. The initial intake is done by a staff nurse who obtains Mary's signed authorization for treatment. A physician examines Mary's wrist and proceeds to stitch up the laceration.

You are a psychiatric liaison nurse called to the emergency department to provide support to Mary. You take Mary into a private setting, assure Mary that she is safe, and gently ask her to recount her story.

> I awoke tonight gagged, my hands pinned down by someone wearing leather gloves and holding a razor to my throat. I wasn't quite sure I was awake. The main thing I can remember wanting was the light. I was able to notice the time because I had a luminous dial watch on. I had this terrible feeling of being in the middle of a nightmare that seemed more realistic than ordinary and I couldn't make it stop. I was trying to establish if there was really a person there. When I struggled, I got my wrist cut and then I realized that I was risking my life and that I'd better hold still and let the man have intercourse with me. He was very fast. He didn't have any clothes on the bottom half of his body. He didn't say much and I couldn't see his face because he had a ski mask on. He ran out the window still not wearing any clothes. I got up and turned on the lights after I got my wrists untied. I felt numb. I tried to leave the apartment after about 45 minutes and then I realized that I didn't have any cash because the man had stolen my purse. I had a fear of going outside my building because I realized he could be nearby. I realized that the man had been in my apartment for some time and that he must have had a flashlight because he gagged me with my own dish towel. It was then that I thought to call the police, not because I had been raped but because I wanted to get out of my apartment.

Mary is tearful and anxious and states, "I feel so dirty" and "I was so scared." As you continue to spend time with Mary, you review her legal rights and assure her that throughout the examination process you will remain with her. As you talk with Mary, you are formulating the following nursing care plan.

ASSESSMENT

Assessment data are as follows:

- Laceration on wrist.
- Crying.
- Verbalization of fear of the perpetrator: "I'm so scared."
- Verbalization about the rape.
- Verbalization of self-denigrating comments: "I feel so dirty."
- Evidence of bruising on inner thighs and perineal area.

DIAGNOSIS

***DSM-IV* Diagnosis:** Posttraumatic Stress Disorder.

Nursing Diagnosis: Rape-Trauma Syndrome related to rape as evidenced by verbalizations of sexual attack, crying, anxiety, laceration on wrist, and comments about feelings of fear and self-denigration.

OUTCOME IDENTIFICATION, PLANNING, AND IMPLEMENTATION

EXPECTED OUTCOME 1: By _____ the patient will demonstrate decreased anxiety, fear, and guilt.

SHORT-TERM GOALS	NURSING INTERVENTIONS	RATIONALES
By _____ the patient will verbalize feelings of anxiety.	1. Stay with the patient. 2. Provide privacy. 3. Listen attentively to the patient's story. 4. Display empathy. 5. Explain what will happen to the patient during the medicolegal examination. 6. Obtain signed consent for the examination. 7. Document all physical and emotional data (including verbatim accounts of what the patient said). 8. Document laboratory test results and whether any pictures of the patient's injuries were taken.	1–3. Your manner conveys respect and a safe environment that allows for free expression of feelings. 4–5. Explaining what will happen decreases anticipatory anxiety and increases a sense of personal control. 6. Signed consent is part of the legal protocol. 7–8. Comprehensive documentation is needed for medical and legal follow-up.
By _____ the patient will verbalize an understanding of rape-trauma syndrome.	Explain to the patient the normal reactions of rape survivors during the acute phase as well as during the reorganization phase.	Anticipatory guidance lowers anxiety and increases a patient's sense of being in control.
By _____ the patient will verbalize strategies for keeping safe.	1. Teach the patient strategies to minimize risk at home, in her car, and on the street. 2. Provide a written teaching guide of these strategies. 3. Arrange for the patient to go home with a family member or support person.	1–3. Knowing that there are concrete steps to take to maximize safety and minimize risk gives the patient a sense of control and decreases fear and anxiety. The written guide allows the patient to review the strategies when anxiety lessens.

EXPECTED OUTCOME 2: By _____ the patient will experience decreased physical symptoms.

SHORT-TERM GOAL	NURSING INTERVENTIONS	RATIONALES
By _____ the patient will express decreased discomfort from her physical injuries.	1. Treat the patient's physical injuries. 2. Instruct the patient to manage her injuries at home.	1–2. Taking care of physical injuries validates the patient's worth, provides comfort, and allows for collection of physical evidence to be used for prosecution of the perpetrator.

EXPECTED OUTCOME 3: By _____ the patient will verbalize her feelings about the rape.

SHORT-TERM GOAL	NURSING INTERVENTIONS	RATIONALES
By _____ the patient will verbalize the details of the experience and will verbalize her feelings about the rape experience.	1. Gently inquire about what happened. 2. Encourage the patient's free expression. 3. Remain neutral and empathetic.	1–3. Verbalization decreases feelings of guilt, anxiety, and isolation and allows for validation from others that the rape was as serious as the patient perceives it to be.

EXPECTED OUTCOME 4: By _____ the patient will find meaning in the trauma and find spiritual comfort.

SHORT-TERM GOALS	NURSING INTERVENTIONS	RATIONALES
By _____ the patient will verbalize the significance of the rape on her life's journey.	1. Ask the patient what she thinks this event means to her life. 2. Explain to the patient the importance of trying to find significance in all of life's experiences, even the most painful and difficult ones.	1–2. Initially the patient may not be able to verbalize the meaning and significance of the event, but your questions will encourage her in the process of finding meaning.

SHORT-TERM GOALS	NURSING INTERVENTIONS	RATIONALES
By _____ the patient will use spiritual resources to seek comfort and to relieve the distress she is feeling.	1. Ask the patient if she has spiritual resources (such as prayer, Bible reading, and meditation) that are meaningful to her.	1. Encouraging the patient to use spiritual resources draws on an important source of strength.
	2. Ask if there is something you can do to respond to her spiritual distress (i.e., pray with or for her).	2. Offering to meet spiritual needs can be a loving and compassionate intervention to someone who is feeling traumatized and unable to meet her own spiritual needs.

EXPECTED OUTCOME 5: By _____ the patient will participate in the treatment program.

SHORT-TERM GOAL	NURSING INTERVENTIONS	RATIONALES
By _____ the patient will keep follow-up appointments.	1. Give the patient the results of her physical examination. 2. Provide information about physical and emotional follow-up. 3. Provide appointments or referrals.	1–3. These interventions encourage the patient to be part of decision-making and help the patient to deal with the long-term reorganization phase of recovery.

EVALUATION

Formative Evaluation: Mary met each of the short-term goals except that she was not able to use spiritual resources in her healing. She stated that she was just "too angry at God" for allowing the rape to happen to her and that at this time she was not ready to turn to God or anything remotely related to God.

Summative Evaluation: Mary achieved each of the expected outcomes except that she did not find meaning in her trauma or find spiritual comfort. For most of the expected outcomes, the nursing care plan was adequate, appropriate, efficient, and effective. To help Mary find meaning in her trauma and help her to find spiritual comfort, the nurse gathered additional spiritual assessment data and discovered that for some time Mary has suffered from spiritual distress related to other unresolved losses in her life. Mary says, "I know that I am going to have to deal with my anger toward God at some point . . . but I am just not ready to do it now." The nurse therefore modified the plan of care to accept Mary's feelings and to encourage her to pursue this area when she believes she is ready.

CONCLUSIONS

Rape, an act of violence, dramatically alters the survivor's journey. The attack itself frequently results in physical injury, including lacerations and bruises. The most significant impact, however, is on the emotional and spiritual aspects of the survivor's journey. As if the rape were not traumatic enough, sometimes the survivor is blamed and stigmatized by society, health care workers, the legal system, and loved ones, who hold her responsible for the rape.

Rape-Trauma Syndrome, a NANDA diagnosis describing the survivor's response to rape, identifies an acute reaction of disorganization followed by long-term reorganization. The survivor experiences a wide array of reactions that involve somatic complaints, affective lability, cognitive problems, and spiritual distress. The nurse plays an important role in responding to the rape survivor, both in the immediate aftermath of the rape and during the long-term process of healing.

KEY POINTS TO REMEMBER

- The nurse may encounter the rape survivor in a variety of health care settings and so must be knowledgeable about the possible long-term psychological sequelae of the experience. This knowledge assists in understanding normal and abnormal coping patterns, in developing appropriate teaching and support, and in making referrals.
- Although there is no "typical" rape survivor, young women between the ages of 12 and 34 are at most risk. It is estimated that one of six women is raped at one time in their lives.
- Some people assume that sexual assault is motivated by sexual desire. It isn't. It is a violent crime, a hostile attack, that attempts to hurt, humiliate, and control the victim.
- Sexual assault includes all forms of sexual contact carried out against the will and without the consent of the survivor. It can affect both men and women. These assaults can include both the actual use of force and the threat of force on the survivor or another person.
- *Date rape*, referring to forced sexual contact within the context of what could be construed as a date, is a growing problem on college campuses.

• Rape-Trauma Syndrome, as originally identified by Burgess and Holmstrom (1974) is the acute-phase and the long-term reorganization process that occurs as a result of forcible rape or attempted forcible rape. The behavioral, somatic, and psychological reactions are part of a syndrome that is an acute stress reaction to a life-threatening situation.

• The rape survivor's initial contact with the health care system may be a forensic examination. The sexual assault nurse clinician, or examiner, a specially trained nursing professional as exemplified by Ledray's program in Minneapolis (1994), can provide comprehensive care to the sexual assault survivor. In other areas, statewide protocols and evidence collection kits have been developed. The forensic examination should include treatment and documentation of injuries, treatment and evaluation of sexually transmitted diseases, pregnancy risk evaluation and prevention, crisis intervention, and arrangements for follow-up counseling. This also includes the collection of medicolegal evidence while maintaining the proper chain of evidence.

LEARNING ACTIVITIES

1. Look in your local telephone directory and see if there are any rape crisis centers in your community. If there are, call and talk to one of the counselors. Ask about the types of services that are provided. What are the major issues confronting the person who is healing from the trauma of rape?

2. Take an informal survey of your family and friends. Ask them what they think about rape. Take note of how many people's thinking is affected by myths that surround the issue of rape.

3. Call up your state legislature and ask for copies of laws pertaining to rape. Ask about your state's position on marital rape.

4. Visit the emergency department of your local hospital. Inquire regarding what services are provided for rape survivors. Do they provide rape counselors or psychiatric nurses? What procedures do they have in place to gather evidence to be used for a legal examination?

CRITICAL THINKING EXERCISE

Karen Polk, a 26-year-old paralegal, decided to work late to finish some extra work. As she was getting into her car in the parking lot at 10:00 p.m., a man with a knife told her that he would kill her if she resisted. At knifepoint Karen was raped. Bruised and frightened, she was unable to move or scream. At 11:00 p.m., a jogger saw her lying on the ground near her car and called the police. Karen was taken by the police to the emergency ward at a nearby hospital.

1. What assumptions do you have about who is to blame?

2. What evidence led you to this point of view?

3. If you were the nurse in the emergency department, what would you say to Karen?

Nurse Abbott met Karen at the door of the emergency department. She stayed with her while the doctor examined her. Nurse Abbott allowed Karen to talk as much as she needed to. As Karen talked, she shook her head saying, "I shouldn't have worked late. Please don't call my mother, she will have a heart attack." Nurse Abbott responded, "We'll do whatever is needed to keep you safe."

1. What other types of reactions would you expect to see with rape survivors?

2. Consider alternate responses that Nurse Abbott might use.

3. What conclusion(s) can you draw about Nurse Abbott's clinical abilities?

REFERENCES

Aiken, M. M. (1993). False allegation: A concept in the context of rape. *Journal of Psychosocial Nursing and Mental Health Services, 31*(11), 15–20.

Aguilera, D. (1990). *Crisis Intervention: Theory and Methodology.* St. Louis: C. V. Mosby.

Anonymous (1992). Responding to rape and sexual attack. *Nursing Standard, 5* (18), 31.

Block, A. (1990). Rape-Trauma Syndrome as scientific expert testimony. *Archives of Sexual Behavior, 19*(54), 309–323.

Brownmiller, S. (1975). *Against our will: Men, women, and rape.* New York: Simon & Shuster.

Burgess, A., and Holmstrom, L. (1974). Rape-Trauma Syndrome. *American Journal of Psychiatry, 131*(9), 981–985.

Campbell, J. C., and Alford, P. (1989). The dark consequences of marital rape. *American Journal of Nursing, 89*(7), 946–949.

Calhoun, K., and Atkeson, B. (1991). *Treatment of rape victims: Facilitating psychosocial adjustment.* New York: Pergamon Press.

Davis, L., and Brody, E. (1979). *Rape and older women: A guide to prevention and protection.* Washington, D.C.: U.S. Department of Health, Education, and Welfare, Public Health Service, NIMH.

American Psychiatric Association (1994). *Diagnostic and statistical manual of mental disorders, fourth edition.* Washington, D. C.: American Psychiatric Association.

Ellis, G. M. (1991). Acquaintance rape. *Perspectives in Psychiatric Care, 30*(1), 11–16.

Frank, E., et al (1981). Past psychiatric symptoms and the response to sexual assault. *Comprehensive Psychiatry, 22*(5), 479–487.

Frieze, I. H. (1983). Investigating the causes and consequences of marital rape. *Journal of Women in Culture and Society, 8,* 532–553.

Hall, G. C. N., Hirschman, R., Graham, J. R., and Zaragoza, M. S. (1993). *Sexual aggression: Issues in etiology, assessment, and treatment.* Bristol, Pa.: Taylor & Francis.

Holloway, M., and Swan, A. (1993). A & E Management of sexual assault. *Nursing Standard,* 7(45), 31–35.

Kennedy, P. H. (1993). Sexual abuse within adult intimate relationships. *Clinical Issues in Perinatal and Women's Health Nursing, 4*(3), 391–401.

Koss, M., and Harvey, M. (1987). *The rape victim: Clinical and community approaches to treatment.* Lexington, Mass.: Stephen Greene Press.

Jezierski, M. (1992). Sexual assault nurse examiner: A role with lifetime impact. *Journal of Emergency Nursing, 18*(2), 177–179.

Ledray, L. (1992). The sexual assault nurse clinician: A fifteen year experience in Minneapolis. *Journal of Emergency Nursing, 18*(3), 217–222.

Ledray, L. (1990). Counseling rape victims: The nursing challenge. *Perspectives in Psychiatric Care, 26*(2), 21–27.

Ledray, L., and Arndt, S. (1994). Examining the sexual assault victim: A new model for nursing care. *Journal of Psychosocial Nursing, 32*(2), 7–12.

Linton, M. A. (1987). Date rape and sexual aggression in dating situations: Incidence and risk factors. *Journal of Counseling Psychology, 34*(2), 186–196.

Mantese, G., et al (1991). Medical and legal aspects of rape and resistance. *Journal of Legal Medicine, 12,* 58–84.

McIvor, D., and Harting, C. (1990). Working with female adolescent date-rape victims. *Psychiatric Nursing, July/Aug/Sep*, 8–15.

Rambow, B., Adkinson, C., Frost, T., and Peterson, G. (1992). Female sexual assault: Medical and legal implications. *Annals of Emergency Medicine, 21*(6), 78–82.

Ruckman, L. M. (1992). Rape: How to begin the healing. *American Journal of Nursing, 92*(9), 48–51.

Russell, D. E. H. (1982). *Rape in marriage.* New York: Macmillan.

Sawyer, R. G., Desmond, S. M., and Lucke, G. M. (1993). Sexual communication and the college student: Implications for date rape. *Health Values: Achieving High Level Wellness, 17*(4), 11–20.

Scott, V. (1992). More information on SANE's in Houston . . . sexual assault nurse examiners. *Journal of Emergency Nursing, 18*(2), 95.

Tomaino, S. (1971). *Persephone: Bringer of spring.* New York: Crowell.

Trevelyan, J. (1991). Marital rape. *Nursing Times, 87*(13), 40–41.

Tyra, P. A. (1993). Older women: Victims of rape. *Journal of Gerontological Nursing, 19*(5), 36–37.

Weaver, K. (1993). A city under siege. *Nursing Standard,* 7(49), 18–20.

Weingourt, L. (1990). Wife rape in a sample of psychiatric patients. *Image: The Journal of Nursing Scholarship, 22*(3), 144–147.

William, W. (1992). The gun is always pointed: Sexual violence and Title III of the Violence Against Women Act. *Georgetown Law Journal, 80*(6), 2197–2225.

SUGGESTED READINGS

Aiken, M. M. (1993). False allegation: A concept in the context of rape. *Journal of Psychosocial Nursing and Mental Health Services, 31*(11), 15–20.

Burgess, A., and Holstrom, L. (1974). Rape trauma syndrome. *American Journal of Psychiatry, 131*(9), 981–985.

Davis, L., and Brody, E. (1979). *Rape and older women: A guide to prevention and protection.* Washington, D.C.: U.S. Department of Health, Education, and Welfare, Public Health Service, NIMH.

Ledray, L. (1990). Counseling rape victims: The nursing challenge. *Perspectives in Psychiatric Care, 26*(2), 21–27.

Ruckman, L. M. (1992). Rape: How to begin the healing. *American Journal of Nursing, 92*(9), 48–51.

CHAPTER 42

THE JOURNEY MARKED BY AIDS

AIDS does not inevitably lead to death, especially if you suppress the co-factors that support the disease. It's very important to tell this to people who are infected. Psychological factors are critical in supporting immune function. If you suppress this psychological support by telling someone he's condemned to die, your words alone will have condemned him. It simply isn't true that the virus is 100 percent fatal.

—*Luc Montagnier*

LEARNING OBJECTIVES

After studying this chapter, you should be able to:

1. Define terms such as AIDS, AIDS-dementia complex, and HIV-positive.
2. Discuss the nature of AIDS as a holistic disease.
3. Identify three psychological responses to AIDS.
4. Identify three spiritual responses to AIDS.
5. Describe compassion fatigue.
6. Discuss the significance of compassion fatigue on professionals as well as on nonprofessionals caring for people with AIDS.
7. Discuss the psychiatric sequelae of AIDS.
8. Discuss at least three strategies for differentiating depression from AIDS-dementia complex.
9. Discuss the implications of AIDS for family members.
10. Discuss the two paths available to nurses faced with the AIDS crisis.
11. Apply the nursing process to a patient with AIDS.

KEY TERMINOLOGY

Acquired immunodeficiency syndrome
AIDS
AIDS-dementia complex
Compassion fatigue
HIV
HIV-positive
Human immunodeficiency virus
"Safer" sex
"Worried well"

The journey involving **Acquired Immunodeficiency Syndrome (AIDS)** exacts a high toll from patients and caregivers alike. AIDS is a terrible disease. But it is important to keep in focus, as this chapter's initial quote exhorts us to do, that maintaining a positive outlook and hope are essential ingredients to maintaining quality of life through the journey marked by AIDS. Reading this chapter will help you to appreciate the psychological and spiritual concomitants of AIDS as well as the nature of your role in responding to these issues.

The following excerpt from *Thanksgiving: An AIDS Journal* (Cox, 1990) provides a glimpse into the inner world of Elizabeth Cox as she stood by watching and caring for her husband as he fought against AIDS.

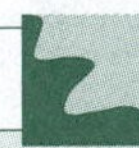

KEITH'S STORY

This morning Keith went to see Dr. Davis about the sores in his mouth. Dr. Davis said that they looked like herpes. They have been very painful and debilitating for about five days now. I am terrible with this kind of health problem when it comes to sympathy for Keith—I seem to have no patience. He is uncomfortable enough to be miserable but it isn't serious enough for me to switch into my Florence Nightingale role. Hearing Keith moan about his mouth reminds me that he is sick and that this disease isn't going away. He is too uncomfortable for me to leave Luke with him for any length of time. Lots of feelings of being trapped and I hate them.

Constantly worrying about Keith. He is so white and thin. He went off ribavirin two weeks ago because he couldn't tolerate it. He is starting a lesser dose tomorrow. The plan is two weeks on, two weeks off. I don't understand how it can be good for him if it takes away his appetite and keeps him from sleeping.

Keith is on so many drugs. Or on and off them. If they don't have to be kept in the refrigerator, Keith keeps them in a plastic cosmetics bag. Diphenhydramine, naltrexone, tetracycline, metronidazole, lidocaine, dapsone, Zovirax, triamcinolone cream, Mycelex.

Timelessness. Marooned in the present. No way of planning for the future. Like living in a vacuum. I feel it is killing us. Hot and sticky outside. Uncomfortable inside: Keith says air conditioning makes him cough and his skin itch. In any case the air conditioner in the bedroom is broken. It makes a terrible sound and blows hot air.

Time has stopped and it makes me panic. I cannot sleep. I walk into Luke's room and remember another time I felt that everything had stopped. We were waiting for Luke to be born. He was two weeks overdue. I couldn't sleep at night; I was too uncomfortable. I tossed and turned and periodically lumbered to the bathroom. I knew I was disturbing Keith, he often joked or complained about my fitfulness, but I was too miserable to care. One night Keith turned to me and said, "Would it help if I read to you?" I was touched: Keith hardly ever read. I handed him the collection of stories by Colette by my side of the bed and he took the book, sat up in bed, and read, slowly and carefully, occasionally putting his hand on my belly or stroking my hair. I don't remember the story; I remember watching him read. He finished the story at dawn. I said I still didn't feel sleepy but felt so incredibly tired. Maybe a beer would help. So we shared a beer and watched the sun come up. We held hands. It didn't matter that it was morning; we were waiting for something that transcended the limits of night and day. We watched the dawn and then fell asleep.

I am haunted by the thought that we are waiting now, waiting for something equally monumental. And now there is no pregnant belly to watch move.

Last night Keith said to me, "It is a very strong instinct, the feeling that you want to reach a resolution. Dying is a temptation. You and Luke keep reminding me that dying is not the solution ... but it never goes away."

I worry about Keith's depression. I am bitchy, angry, aggressive, hostile. But Keith seems to be beyond that. He is so angry he is silent and withdrawn. When his father was noncommittal and almost uninterested in helping us out financially (his uncle never responded), it was as if Keith had been stabbed and now he has retired to lick his wounds. But it seems to me that his wounds are not healing naturally. He is trying to heal them with determination. And it is just too exhausting.

Acquired immunodeficiency syndrome has been recognized in the United States since 1981. During that year the pattern of unexpected illness and deaths in the homosexual population was attributed to AIDS. Since then most of the research interest and monies have been focused on discovering a cure and better treatments for the disease. The focus has been on the physical aspects of the disease. Little interest has been given to the emotional, psychological, and spiritual aspects of AIDS. Yet as Dr. Montagnier's quote indicates, these issues are essential to maintaining a healthy immune system.

A shift in thinking from purely "curing" to "caring" is beginning to occur. Such a shift requires a transformation of thinking for many because the tools are no longer pharmacological preparations and miracles of medical technology, but rather are the self to communicate acceptance of the sufferer, provision of support through the dying process, education about the disease and its course, exploration of ways to improve quality if not duration of life, and existential support as the sufferer struggles to find meaning and purpose in his or her life (Belcher et al, 1989; Carson, 1989; Carson, 1990; Carson et al, 1990; Carson and Green, 1992; Carson, 1993). Caring, as described, contains both psychological and spiritual elements.

PSYCHOLOGICAL PROBLEMS ASSOCIATED WITH AIDS

The psychological problems most often associated with **HIV** (Human Immunodeficiency Virus) infection can be graphed on a continuum, moving from the problems of those whose behaviors place them at low risk for the infection to the problems of those whose behaviors are highly risky and to those who are infected. Figure 42–1 illustrates the continuum of HIV-related psychiatric problems. The first group of people with whom we are concerned have either no risk or little risk for the infection. Persons at low risk include

- Those who have been involved in monogamous relationships since 1978
- Those who have engaged only in **"safer" sex,** such as mutual masturbation and sex with condoms
- Those who are not sexually active
- Those who have *only* household, social, and/or workplace contact with HIV-infected people. People who fall into this level of risk and who have HIV-related psychosocial problems are called the **"worried well."**

The next group includes those who are at moderate risk for the infection but are presently negative for HIV. The people who fall into this risk category include

- Heterosexual with multiple sexual partners
- Health care workers with accidental needle sticks

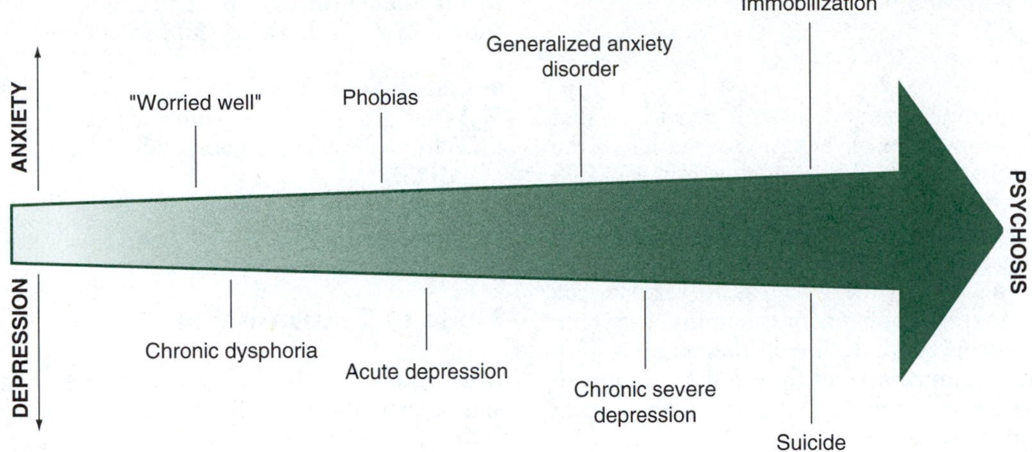

FIGURE 42–1
The continuum of HIV-related psychiatric problems. (From Ostrow, D. G. [1986]. A psychiatric overview of AIDS. *International Journal of Neuroscience, 32* [3/4], 647–659.)

or with significant exposure to blood of **HIV-positive** (serum positive for HIV) people

The third and fourth groups engage in the same high-risk behaviors; however, the third group is not infected and the fourth group is HIV-positive. These include

- Men who engage in same-sex relations
- People who use intravenous drugs and share needles
- People who engage in bisexual behavior or those with a bisexual sexual partner
- People who engage in sexual contact with an intravenous drug user
- Infants born to intravenous drug–using mothers
- Sexual partners of HIV-infected people
- Hemophiliacs
- People who received blood transfusions before 1985

The psychological reactions differ for each of these groups.

The "worried well" generally display symptoms of anxiety. They feel angry and concerned about their chances of becoming infected and may experience sexual difficulty. They may even develop symptoms similar to those of HIV-positive people (e.g., fatigue, weight loss, and diarrhea). People who are at both moderate and high risk for HIV infection but who are not infected are subject to all the concerns of the "worried well" with some significant additions. These people may experience immediate relief when the results of a blood test to determine the presence of HIV are negative. But in the face of risky behaviors, fears persist regarding the accuracy of the test and whether the inevitable has only been postponed. The person is faced with choices regarding future sexual behaviors and how to deal with sensitive issues such as practicing safer sex. They may experience guilt over former sexual practices and intravenous drug use. They fear disclosing their risk to partners who themselves are at low risk. Pathological denial is also a mechanism used by the HIV-negative person who is at risk. Such individuals block the reality of their risky behaviors and continue with such behaviors as if everything were OK (Taylor and Robertson, 1994; Wenger et al, 1994).

The psychological problems of the fourth group, those who are HIV infected, can be categorized into two types:

1. Functional, which usually involves an adjustment disorder with depression and/or anxiety as the predominant symptoms (Faulstich, 1987; Taylor & Lavallee, 1989)
2. Organic brain syndrome, which includes major depression, dementia, and delirium (Taylor and Lavallee, 1989)

The spiritual issues of AIDS, having to do with finding meaning and purpose in life, dealing with possible guilt over lifestyle choices, and resolving a relationship with God or a higher power, present concurrently with the aforementioned psychosocial and psychiatric problems (Carson, 1990; Carson and Green, 1992; Kendall, 1994).

▶ Check Your Reading

1. What are the spiritual issues of a person diagnosed with AIDS?
2. What are the three psychological reactions to AIDS?
3. Who are the "worried well"?
4. Identify three risk factors for acquiring AIDS.

AIDS: THE DISEASE

Etiology

The human immunodeficiency virus, a retrovirus that attacks specific components of the immune system, is the etiological agent of AIDS. The transmission of AIDS occurs through the exchange of body fluids, particularly blood and semen. HIV has an affinity for the T helper (T) cells and inserts its genetic material into the host chromosome. The role of the T cell is to regulate the functioning of other components of the immune system. HIV produces a progressive decline in the numbers of T cells, causing the immune system to lose the stimulus to "turn on" in response to invaders; this leaves the person susceptible to many diseases.

Solomon and colleagues (1987) strongly suggest that a complete understanding of AIDS must proceed from a perspective combining biological, psychological, and social factors. Carson (1990) suggests that the spiritual component is also essential to understanding the disease progression. In a study of 100 HIV-infected people, Carson and Green (1992) and Carson (1993) demonstrated a significant relationship between hardiness and spiritual well-being. Individuals who were both hardy and spiritually well demonstrated a high degree of participation in prayer, vitamin use, and support to other people with AIDS. This suggests that physical, psychological, social, and spiritual changes associated with AIDS may contribute to the disease's progression. The change in immunological functioning caused by HIV affects other bodily systems as well. For instance, the immunosuppression that occurs with HIV opens the door to opportunistic infections such as toxoplasmosis and to neoplasms such as Kaposi's sarcoma.

At the beginning of 1995, a cumulative number of 441,528 cases of AIDS had been diagnosed since 1981. The majority of these cases (376,889) are in men. An estimated one million Americans currently are infected with the virus but are asymptomatic. More than 3000 new cases are reported to the Centers for Disease Control (CDC) every month. Children account for 1% of the total number of cases, and over half of these children have already died. As of the beginning of 1995, 6209 cases of AIDS were reported in children younger than 13 years of age. Over 58,420 women of childbearing age presently are infected with the virus. Women represent approximately 7% to 8% of the AIDS population, with a disproportionate number of women coming from minority groups. A total of 52% of them are black, and 19% are Hispanic (Unpublished data, CDC Hotline, May, 1995).

Although in the United States the largest groups of AIDS sufferers are homosexual men and intravenous drug users, the disease does not affect only these groups. The virus does not have an affinity for individuals with a specific sexual preference; rather, it has an affinity for a specific environment in which it can best thrive. HIV is a very fragile group of cells that dies very quickly once outside of the body. It requires an extremely warm medium with a specific pH level to remain alive. It finds that medium primarily in blood and semen and, to a lesser extent, in all body fluids (Johnson, 1989).

▶ Check Your Reading

5. What group has been most affected by AIDS?
6. Why is the spiritual component important in our focus on AIDS?
7. What type of virus causes AIDS?
8. What are the three modes of HIV transmission?

Mode of Transmission

Because HIV is spread through the exchange of blood and semen, the virus is transmitted primarily through sexual activity, blood exposure, and childbirth. Although the most risky *sexual activity* is receptive anal intercourse, vaginal and oral intercourse also are risky. At present, most cases of HIV infection have occurred in men who engage in homosexual behavior. However, HIV can be transmitted through heterosexual or lesbian sexual activities.

Blood contains an even higher concentration of HIV than does semen. Intravenous drug use with needle-sharing is the most common *blood exposure* transmission. In addition, clotting factors given to hemophiliacs that were derived from blood transfusions between 1978 and 1985 have been implicated in blood exposure to HIV. Several cases have been reported of health care workers becoming infected with HIV through accidental needlestick injuries or through blood contact on nonintact skin and mucous membranes.

Perinatal transmission—transmission from mother to child occurs in utero; it is found in about 50% of all infants whose mothers are HIV infected. The CDC also has documented HIV transmission through breast milk.

Prevention

Currently no known cure exists for AIDS. Although intensive research is being directed toward the discovery of a cure, the thrust of public health programs is prevention through education. Former Surgeon General Koop was instrumental in waging an intensive AIDS education campaign aimed at all Americans but especially at those engaging in risky behaviors, such as intravenous drug use and casual and unprotected sexual contact. The educational efforts have two purposes: to provide information about methods to stop the spread of the virus, and to decrease the epidemic of fear.

Prevention can be accomplished by avoiding risky behaviors through

- Safer sex practices (e.g., the use of condoms and no exchange of body fluids)
- Disinfection of dirty needles and syringes used to inject street drugs
- For health care workers, the use of universal precautions with *all patients* including the use of barrier

methods (e.g., gloves, eye shields) to prevent contact with patient's blood and body fluids on provider's skin or mucous membranes; and *no capping* of used needles and disposal of used needles in puncture-proof containers

Education to deal with the epidemic of fear focuses on the fact that AIDS is *only* spread through exchange of blood and/or body fluids. This means that social, household, and workplace contact can continue unchanged. It is safe to talk to an HIV-infected person, hug, touch, eat meals together, and use the same bathroom facilities with no fear of contagion (Aruffo et al, 1995)

A study by Baldwin and Baldwin (1988) examined the effectiveness of AIDS education in reducing the risk-taking behavior among college students. The results of this study were not very encouraging. Although students were very knowledgeable about AIDS and a few worried about either contracting the disease or their assessment of their risk, this did not greatly motivate cautious behavior. Knowledgeable students were no more inclined to avoid risky behaviors than were less knowledgeable students. Although students with more accurate knowledge were inclined to have had fewer vaginal intercourse partners in the previous three months, the effect was small. For every point increase in knowledge score, only a 0.03 decline in the number of partners was seen. Also, having more knowledge did not reduce casual sexual relationships or increase the use of condoms.

Paradoxically, students who assessed themselves to be at risk actually increased their number of sexual partners. Students who worried about contracting the disease reported using condoms more than students who did not worry, but the worriers did not decrease the number of sexual encounters in which they engaged. In fact, the frequency of casual sexual relationships was greater in the worrying group than in the nonworrying group. Factors that correlated with more cautious behavior were gender (females were more cautious than males), the use of seat belts, and the delay of age of first sexual intercourse experience (the younger the student was when he or she became sexually active, the more partners he or she had experienced, and the more he or she engaged in casual sex).

The researchers hypothesized that some people may be greater risk-takers, whereas others are less inclined to take risks. The researchers concluded that AIDS education that focuses on cognitive-emotional factors alone is insufficient to change behavior. They suggest a much broader socialization program that aims at making young people more aware of and responsible regarding risks of social problems such as alcohol and drug abuse, unwanted pregnancies, driving without seat belts, sexually transmitted diseases, and AIDS transmission. Turner and colleagues (1988) also support the notion that effective AIDS education must address more than the cognitive domain; it must be directed to the whole person. Other, more recent, studies also have documented the inadequacy of cognitive knowledge to change behaviors (McLean et al, 1994; Ridge et al, 1994; Seal and Agostenelli, 1994).

▶ Check Your Reading

9. Describe universal precautions for health care workers.
10. Identify the two-pronged focus of public education with regard to AIDS.
11. Why is a cognitive approach to AIDS education insufficient?

PSYCHOLOGICAL, SOCIAL, AND SPIRITUAL IMPLICATIONS OF AIDS

This section deals with the psychological, social, and spiritual implications of AIDS and includes vignettes from the story of W. Carole Chenitz, a nurse who died of AIDS in February 1992. These vignettes, which are excerpts from a chapter entitled "Living with AIDS" in a book called *HIV/AIDS: A Guide to Nursing Care* (Chenitz, 1992), are a poignant window into the impact of AIDS on a woman, nurse, and mother.

The Stigma of AIDS

The reaction of society to AIDS has been so negative and fear-laden that people diagnosed as HIV-positive become the recipients of society's emotional baggage in regard to the disease. As Carole Chenitz (1992) wrote:

We were afraid that if people found out that I had AIDS, Kimberly would be ostracized by her classmates. So we decided to wait. Kim felt comfortable with this, since many of her classmates had made negative comments about gays and people with AIDS. While we were sure that the overwhelming majority of people in our community would respond with concern and compassion, we were afraid about the one or two who would react from unbridled fear.

People with AIDS can be expected to experience the same shock, denial, fear, anger, acceptance, and resignation that Kübler-Ross (1975) describes as part of the dying process (Nichols, 1983; Forstein, 1984). (See Chapter 27 for further discussion of reaction to loss.) However, the reaction to AIDS is further complicated by factors not present in other terminal illnesses. Tibesar (1986) notes that the transmissible, terminal, and stigmatizing characteristics of AIDS place an unusual burden on those afflicted. Because the disease has been linked with homosexual and intravenous drug–using behaviors, it has been approached from a moralistic view.

Kayal (1985) discusses what happens when the etiology of a disease is framed in moral language and the illness in question affects individuals who have been . . . "religiously stigmatized and legally proscribed minorities (p. 218)." The afflicted are blamed for their illness. This is exactly what has happened with AIDS.

It is worthwhile to read a quote from Kevin Cahill (1983, p. 2), an internationally known parasitologist:

When a fatal infection had struck down veterans attending an American Legion convention, health professionals across the country joined in the search for a solution. When women using tampons became ill with toxic shock syndrome, medical societies and research centers immediately focused their enormous talents on that problem. But when the victims were drug addicts, and poor Haitian refugees and homosexual men, their plight did not, somehow, seem as significant to those expected to speak for the health professions. No major research programs were announced, and until it became clear that the disease could spread to the general population through blood transfusions, organized medicine seemed a part of the conspiracy of silence.

Kayal (1985) asserts that AIDS has been so tied to a lifestyle that is viewed by many as sinful, hedonistic, or perverted that society has failed to respond to the suffering of people with AIDS. This failure to respond has characterized more than just the medical system. The response of government, families, churches, and other social institutions has been too little too late (Shilts, 1987).

The present epidemic of AIDS challenges American society to examine its attitudes about sexuality—specifically homosexuality. Some contend that AIDS is a just punishment for sexual activity that they view as immoral, and even that AIDS is God's response to immoral behavior. People who hold this view claim to know the mind of God, which may lend them a degree of credibility; however, this view increases the social alienation of people with AIDS (Kayal, 1985; Hover-Kramer, 1988). Murphy (1988) argues against the idea of AIDS being a just punishment, noting the disproportion between the impact of the activity and a "punishment" as devastating as AIDS. After all, said Murphy, if AIDS is a just punishment for a particular sexual behavior, why aren't child abusers afflicted with an even greater punishment?

Regardless of why AIDS occurred, or how or why a particular person contracted the infection, both a theistic perspective and the high standards of professional nursing call for compassion rather than judgment.

The Isolation of People with AIDS

American society is further challenged to examine persistent attitudes about the ministrations of comfort and compassion, acceptance of individual differences, and society's responsibility to deal with the suffering of its young. As Carole Chenitz (1992) wrote:

Not only did the emotional needs I had go unrecognized, but no one touched me. No one in the hospital staff took my hand, rubbed my back, gave me support, or did any of the comfort and care measures that we nurses pride ourselves on. I will never forget how I felt. . . . I was unclean, untouchable, undesirable, a patient with a disgusting disease. If you get too close, you may get it, too.

These are not challenges to be addressed easily or without pain, and their debate continues without resolution in government, schools, places of business, and families.

In her book, *AIDS: The Ultimate Challenge*, Elizabeth Kübler-Ross (1987, p. 13) speaks to the challenge facing America in the care of people with AIDS:

Since we can no longer deny that AIDS is a life threatening illness that will eventually involve millions of people and decimate large portions of our human population, it is our choice to grow and learn from it, to either help people with this dread disease or abandon them. It is our choice to live up to this ultimate challenge or to perish.

Some individuals and organizations have exemplified a positive response to the challenge of AIDS and have reached out with compassion and willingness to care for people with the disease. In San Francisco, the Shanti project is such an example. Shanti is a community organization that uses a peer counseling model to work with people with AIDS, their significant others, and family members. The counselor's job is to empathize with patients without judging them and to work collaboratively with other health care providers regarding ways to approach certain people with the disease (McCaffrey, 1987).

In some other cases, the response to the AIDS challenge has been far from compassionate. For example, in 1987, three young children living in Tampa, Florida were expelled from school, harrassed by citizen's groups and burned out of their home because they tested HIV-positive as a result of contaminated blood transfusions (Hover-Kramer, 1988).

What happens to the person with AIDS who is caught in this societal struggle? Sometimes he or she is left to deal with the illness in isolation. The homosexual person with AIDS frequently bears the brunt of society's homophobia—an irrational fear, intolerance, and dread of any person believed to be homosexual. The homosexual person with AIDS is rejected, condemned, and ostracized (Murphy, 1986). Homophobia can seriously harm a homosexual person's self-image. Murphy quotes a young gay man, who in the midst of a counseling session in which the counselor was attempting to assure the young man of God's love said, "How can God love me? I am one of His mistakes" (1986, p. 39).

The "Crisis of Knowing"

The crisis of AIDS for the person with the disease begins with the diagnosis. As Carole Chenitz (1992, p. 442) wrote:

Two years ago I donated blood during a blood drive. Ninety days later, on a cold, gray northern California day, I received a certified, registered letter. It was my day to work the evening shift, as I did every Monday. This enabled me to conduct a seminar for the nurses and to facilitate a multifamily therapy group on the substance abuse inpatient unit. The letter was from the blood bank, informing me that I was HIV-positive. My heart stopped as I read the letter. "How can this happen? There must be some mistake. Oh my God, I'm going to die!" I was scared. I felt that I had just walked through a warp in time and space. I was now on the other side of the pale seeing myself and my life as if it belonged to someone else. I felt each breath would be my last. Waves of pain, fear, and sadness washed over me. "What am I going to do? Who can I talk to? What about my children?"

For many, the diagnosis brings the knowledge that even though they feel fine, they are HIV-positive. Feeling as if he or she is carrying a time bomb ticking away the minutes and days of life, the person with AIDS is faced with questions that are not easy to answer. "How do I tell others that I am HIV-positive? What do I tell them about how I became HIV-positive?" This may mean "coming out" with honesty about a lifestyle characterized by intravenous drug use or homosexual behavior. Figure 42–2 illustrates the spectrum of social responses to AIDS.

Because these are such difficult issues to face, the initial "telling" of the diagnosis must be done by a professional knowledgeable about the course of AIDS—someone who can provide accurate information that the person can hear and comprehend. This professional must also possess counseling skills. The incidence of suicide among newly diagnosed AIDS patients is significant enough to warrant every safeguard against this happening. Perry and Markowitz (1986) report that the incidence of suicidal crisis, suicide attempts, and completed suicides is high in AIDS patients. The relative risk of suicide in the AIDS population is 66.15 times that of the general population (Marzuk et al, 1988).

For people with AIDS or those who are HIV-positive, the diagnosis precipitates a crisis of such magnitude that it can totally overwhelm their psychological defenses (Neumark, 1984). AIDS not only presents the possibility of death, but it also generates fears regarding disfigurement, changes in role, body function, and self-esteem.

The Loss of Social Support

The loss of social support is one of the many losses experienced by people with AIDS. As they become increasingly more debilitated by the disease process, they find themselves more alone in their efforts to cope. Some people with AIDS rely on denial to block the pain of confronting what their ultimate future will probably hold. Many throw themselves into a frenzy of activity as if by keeping active they can stop the disease from progressing. This denial has both healthy and unhealthy implications. It allows a semblance of hope and the ability to plan for a future that may not occur, but the denial may block the reflection about needed lifestyle changes that could result in a healthier immune system.

The Process of Dying of AIDS

Death is another issue confronting the person with AIDS. As Chenitz (1992, p. 454) wrote:

> *Like many people with AIDS, I am not afraid of death, I am afraid of dying. The dying process and how that will be handled is of great concern to me. Everyone is going to die. Death is a part of life. However, AIDS brings with it a terribly painful, often humiliating dying process and that terrifies me.*

Hinton (1972) observed that younger people have greater difficulty coping with terminal illness because the pros-

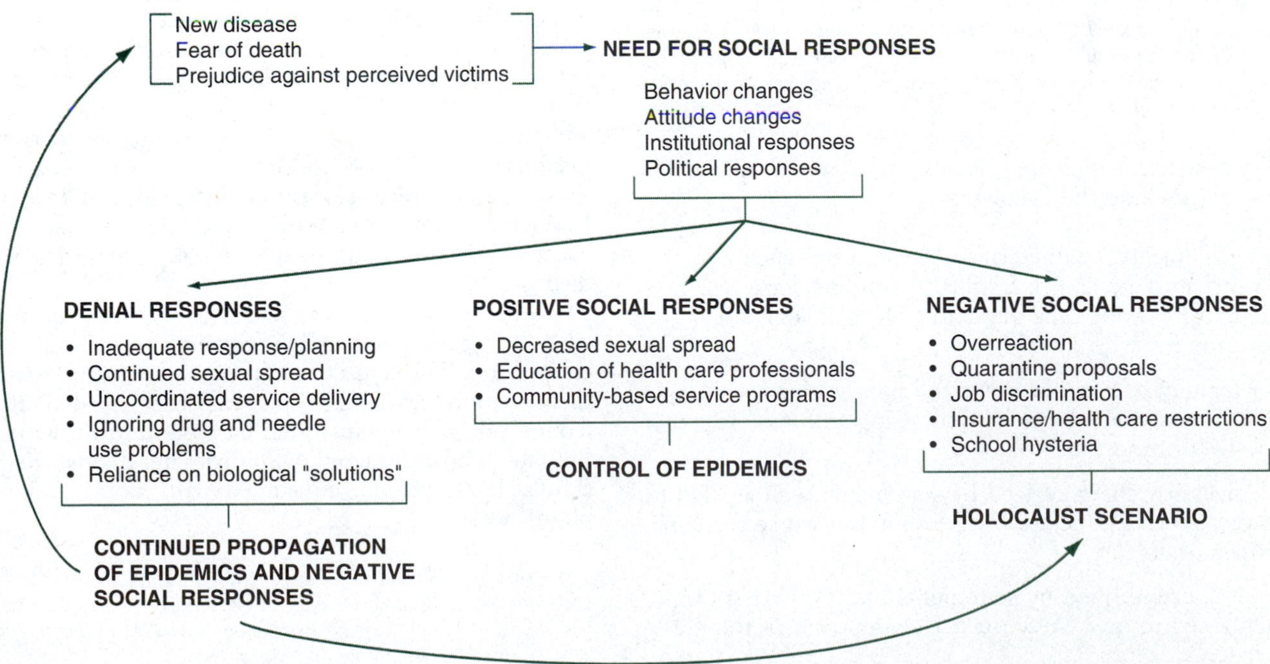

FIGURE 42–2

The spectrum of social responses to AIDS. (From Ostrow, D. G. [1988]. Models for understanding the psychiatric consequences of AIDS. In T. P. Bridge, et al. [Eds.]. *Psychological, neuropsychiatric, and substance abuse aspects of AIDS.* Vol. 44 [pp. 85–94]. New York: Raven Press.

pect of dying disrupts many hopes, plans, and expectations. Some fear leaving dependent children.

The fear of death is heightened by the exacerbations of the illness, negative reactions to the treatments, and the perception of increasing losses. For instance, a 35-year-old actor, who had suffered severe weight loss and had Kaposi's lesions on his face, was fearful of losing future auditions for television commercials. His fear was not just for the immediate loss of financial security but also for the ultimate loss of his self-image (Moynihan et al, 1987).

In discussing the impact of losses, Sister Patrice Murphy (1986, p. 39) states:

Many AIDS patients have lost or relinquished their roles as son, brother, grandchild, husband, and/or father. This illness also means that the patient is further diminished by loss of still another role such as an actor who cannot act, an artist who cannot paint, or a physician who cannot heal. If an individual cannot do the things that one identifies with the fact of being, one is no longer whole.

Existential Issues and AIDS

Tibesar (1986) notes the importance of facing existential issues as the person with AIDS increasingly contemplates his or her own death as a reality. As Carole Chenitz (1992, p. 451) wrote:

It was still a shock to me that my life was evolving this way. Initially I was too sick to think about my life and my goals. Later when my energy was so low, loss of work wasn't difficult to bear, since I couldn't do it anyway. However, the loss of who I was and what I had done my entire adult life hit after several months: I wasn't a nurse anymore. I still had a license, but I would never practice nursing again. All of the articles published, papers presented, book chapters written, grants developed, and classes taught didn't matter now. It was gone. If I were to survive, I would need to develop new skills. I would have to learn to accept my new life. I needed to learn to relax. Maybe I could salvage something from my old life, but I wasn't sure what.

These issues, which are psychosocial as well as spiritual in nature, include the following:

- Self-identity, characterized by questions such as "Who am I now? Am I still the same person even though my body fails me daily? Does anyone still love me for who I am?"
- Meaning of life, characterized by questions such as "Is there some value to my suffering and loss? Has my life been important?"
- Adversity, characterized by statements such as "Is life always so cruel? Can there be anything worse than an unfair death?"
- Fate, exemplified by statements like "Why has this happened to me? Why must I be deprived of the life I love?"
- Stigma, characterized by statements such as "Is this a punishment for being who I am?"
- Relationships, characterized by fears such as "Will my friends and family reject me? Will my lover leave me?"
- Productivity, characterized by statements such as "I've lost my job. I feel so weak, and I'm fatigued doing the slightest tasks. Am I of any use to anyone?"
- Heritage, characterized by concerns such as "What can I leave behind? How will people remember me?" (Tibesar, 1986).

Coming to grips with these existential issues frequently is complicated by unresolved conflicts and concerns over life choices, such as intravenous drug use, or guilt over sexual activities that exposed the person to HIV. Further complicating this existential quest may be low self-esteem, social isolation and alienation, and public discrimination and condemnation (Kayal, 1985; Murphy, 1986; Tibesar, 1986; Bellemare, 1988; Graydon, 1988; and Walker-Robbins and Christiana, 1989).

The spiritual issues facing the person with AIDS may be greatly affected by whether he or she is homosexual or bisexual or whether AIDS was contracted through intravenous drug use or a blood transfusion. The gay person with AIDS frequently is faced with a church that reacts by blocking the meeting of his or her existential, spiritual needs. Fortunato (1987) claims that because much of Western religion has been so terrified of sexuality in general, it is completely put off by those whose sexuality is remarkable in its difference. Gay people may need to go beyond the mainline traditional church, regardless of denomination, to seek spiritual support.

The spiritual needs of the intravenous drug user may be at the heart of his or her dependence on drugs and may partially explain the success of the many 12-step recovery programs (e.g., Narcotics Anonymous) that have at their core a reliance on a higher power to overcome the addictive behavior. Leech (1977) contends that much drug use is an attempt to fill a spiritual void regarding a sense of inner, spiritual meaning in the lives of drug users. Life seems empty, directionless, and filled with pain. Drug use may be one attempt to anesthetize a gnawing spiritual distress.

Still another spiritual scenario concerns the person who has contracted AIDS through a tainted blood transfusion. The sense of unfairness and anger regarding this situation may lead to spiritual despair and alienation from God. This is illustrated by a quote from Kimberly Bergalis, who contracted AIDS from her dentist. Bergalis (Hilts, 1991, p. 11), consumed with anger about her plight, wrote:

"My life has been sheer hell. Who do I blame? I blame Dr. Acer and every single one of you bastards. Dr. Acer was infected and had full-blown AIDS and you stood by not doing anything about it. You are all just as guilty as he was. You've ruined my life and my family's."

▶ Check Your Reading

12. What is the "crisis of knowing" for the person newly diagnosed as HIV-positive?

13. Describe at least four of the existential issues confronted by the person with AIDS.
14. Why are AIDS patients so stigmatized?

PSYCHIATRIC IMPLICATIONS OF AIDS

Depression

Given the nature of AIDS, it is no surprise that depression is a common response to the diagnosis (Flaskerud, 1987). In one study that involved a retrospective chart review of 52 hospitalized AIDS patients, 83% of the patients exhibited affective mood disturbance. Characteristically, the patients were sad and withdrawn, expressed low self-esteem and hopelessness, and displayed psychomotor retardation (Perry and Markowitz, 1986). Ostrow (1988) contends that the epidemic curve of new AIDS cases combined with the knowledge regarding the fate of most individuals with AIDS is enough to explain all behavioral responses, including depression and fear.

Etiology

The organic depression that is sometimes seen in AIDS patients may be due to brain lesions caused by the HIV infection. Pert and associates (1988) identified CD4 receptors in the limbic system structures of the brain. Since expressions of emotion are regulated in the limbic system, a limbic system infection may result in mood disturbances. This relationship between depression and neurochemical disturbances in AIDS patients is a tentative explanation open to considerably more research.

The adjustment disorder with depressed mood reported in people with AIDS also may be a response to the multiple losses they experience. Specifically, the losses associated with role, body image, and social support, coupled with fear of death and feelings of helplessness, have been implicated in the depression of the AIDS patient (Frierson and Lippmann, 1987). Untreated, this depression can further erode the patient's immune system and decrease his or her interest in engaging in health-promoting behaviors. In the opening story, Keith's journey with AIDS was punctuated with an adjustment disorder with depressive symptoms.

Treatment

Depression is treated with a variety of antidepressant medications to deal with the sadness and apathy. In addition, a psychostimulant such as methylphenidate hydrochloride (Ritalin) may be added to deal with fatigue and weakness. Supportive therapy also is used to assist the patient to deal with the many issues that seem to go hand in hand with AIDS, such as issues of loss, self-esteem, guilt, isolation, and anger (Grant, 1988).

AIDS-Dementia Complex

AIDS-dementia complex (ADC), also referred to in the American Psychiatric Association's (1994) *Diagnostic and Statistical Manual-IV (DSM-IV)* as dementia due to HIV disease, is a major complication of HIV infection occurring in 70% to 90% of all AIDS patients (McArthur et al, 1988). Symptoms of ADC may appear in the absence of other symptoms of AIDS. This fact has led researchers to consider ADC to be a direct consequence of HIV infection. Belinda Mason, a young woman who contracted AIDS through a tainted blood transfusion during emergency surgery, illustrates the impact of ADC in the following quote (Hilts, 1991, p. 11):

"Sometimes I forget what I'm saying in the middle of a sentence. I am constantly confronted with the obvious losses in my life, but one of the greatest is the diminishing of my intellect; I used to have a razor-sharp tongue and I could use my hillbilly wisdom, fly by the seat of my pants. That used to define who I was; now AIDS has consumed my identity."

Etiology

Several explanatory hypotheses regarding the etiology of ADC exist. The first has to do with how HIV gets into the brain. It has been suggested that monocytes may transport HIV into the central nervous system (Ho et al, 1987). The monocyte, a circulating white blood cell, triggers an immune response by engulfing invader cells and delivering these cells to other components of the immune system. Monocytes possess a migratory ability that allows them to travel throughout the body to remove foreign particles. When a monocyte enters a tissue, it is called a macrophage. HIV binds to the CD4 receptor found on the surface of the monocyte as well as on that of the T helper (T) cell. Unlike the T cell, however, the monocyte is not killed by the HIV and may serve as a reservoir for the virus.

Ho and colleagues (1987) report that HIV has been found in macrophages recovered from the brain tissue of persons with ADC. Monocytes have the ability to cross the blood-brain barrier and may be the transport mechanism for HIV into the central nervous system. In a more recent study (Schnittman et al, 1989), HIV could be isolated from circulating monocytes in only 2 of 14 AIDS patients. This raises another possibility that HIV is transported into the central nervous system by some other, yet unknown, mechanism.

Once HIV enters the central nervous system, the exact mechanism of inducing cognitive, behavioral, and sensorimotor changes is unknown, although several hypotheses exist. One hypothesis states that products toxic to the nervous system are released by infected monocytes. One such product is tumor necrosis factor (TNF), a protein secreted by monocytes in response to invasive stimuli. TNF mediates the inflammatory response.

Tumor necrosis factor is toxic for oligodendrocytes, cells whose role is to produce the myelin characteristic of white matter (Robbins et al, 1987). Wright and coworkers (1988) have reported that in vitro, HIV-infected monocytes spontaneously produce large amounts of TNF, which may be responsible for the white matter pallor characteristic of ADC.

Lee and colleagues (1987) hypothesize that HIV interferes with the effects of neuroleukin by competing for binding sites in the central nervous system. Neuroleukin, a substance produced in skeletal muscle, brain tissue, and bone marrow, is essential to the survival of neurons. Ho and coworkers (1987) have demonstrated that a moderate amount of structural similarity exists between HIV and neuroleukin. Lee and colleagues (1987) demonstrated that in vitro, HIV inhibits the growth of neurons cultured in neuroleukin. Competitive binding in vivo may decrease the survival time of some cells, with resultant neurological dysfunction.

Neurodiagnostic Findings

Computed tomography reveals cerebral atrophy with ventricular enlargement. MRI has been shown to be more sensitive in displaying the characteristic white matter pallor. EEGs show mild slowing of brain wave activity, but it is nonspecific (Holland and Tross, 1985). White blood cells are found in cerebrospinal fluid in 20% of ADC patients, and elevated protein levels are present in 60% of ADC patients (Gabuzda and Hirsch, 1987). McArthur and colleagues (1988) posit that the presence of HIV in the cerebrospinal fluid of most patients with ADC may serve as a marker of neurological involvement.

Symptoms

In the early stages of ADC, the symptoms are difficult to distinguish from a functional adjustment depressive reaction to a disease as terrible as AIDS. Initially, the patient may present with apathy, withdrawal, loss of interest in social activities, impaired memory, decreased ability to concentrate, decreased libido, ataxia, subtle difficulties in coordination, erratic and impulsive behavior, agitation, confusion, increased sensitivity to alcohol and prescribed medications, and hallucinations (Holland and Tross, 1985; Navia and Price, 1986). Patients may need to make lists to be able to carry out activities of daily living. They may lose their train of thought in midsentence. The changes in cognitive functioning and problem-solving affect their ability to think abstractly. They may display difficulty transferring learned information to new situations.

These patients may exhibit impaired impulse control and emotional lability, characterized by agitation, combativeness, and panic attacks. Safety and self-care issues are major nursing concerns regarding the patient with ADC.

Central nervous system abnormalities become more profound as the disease progresses. The primary symptoms are moderate to severe global cognitive impairment and psychomotor retardation. Characteristically, patients may stare vacantly, display little spontaneous verbal or motor activity, and as death approaches, lapse into a mute state. Paradoxically, some patients display the exact opposite behavior and become restless and agitated. Incontinence of urine and feces also is common (Navia and Price, 1986).

Treatment

The treatment of ADC may include the use of low-dose antipsychotics such as haloperidol (Haldol) to decrease confusion, disorganization, and agitation. Psychostimulants such as methylphenidate hydrochloride (Ritalin) and antidepressants such as fluoxetine hydrochloride (Prozac) are used to treat the fatigue, weakness, and apathy (Wolcott et al, 1985; Perry and Markowitz, 1986).

▶ Check Your Reading

15. What is AIDS-dementia complex (ADC)?
16. What does neurodiagnostic testing reveal in regard to ADC?
17. What medications are used to treat depression associated with AIDS?
18. Give two ways the cognitive functioning is impaired in ADC.

CAREGIVERS OF PEOPLE WITH AIDS

In any comprehensive discussion of AIDS, the needs of the caregivers of people with AIDS must be addressed. Just as AIDS dictates a challenging journey for the patients themselves, so the caregivers are faced with their own journey of psychological and spiritual adjustment. The initial story focusing on Elizabeth Cox's experiences illustrates the daily struggle faced by the care provider. The stigmatizing effect of AIDS on patients is also experienced by caregivers, whether they are family members, lovers, or friends. Not only are they confronted with the intense pain of their own grief but also they may be faced with society's reactions of fear, homophobia, and moral self-righteousness, as well as isolation and rejection (Piemme and Bolle, 1990; Roth et al, 1994). In addition, the caregiver frequently is dealing with his or her own feelings of shock, denial, and anger at first learning that a daughter, son, spouse, parent, lover, or friend is either homosexual, bisexual, or an intravenous drug user. Similar feelings surround the realization that the loved one has contracted the disease. Spiritually, caregivers contend with feelings about God's role in the disease, God's availability as a support, and the meaning that their loved one's illness holds for them.

The bereavement following the death of a lover from AIDS is complicated by the fact that the significance of the lost relationship is totally discounted by society. Individuals facing such loss experience feelings of isolation and disconnectedness, emotional confusion, and denial of their own vulnerability (Sowell et al, 1991). Let's look back and continue with our initial story.

BOX 42-1 Signs of Compassion Fatigue

If you experience these symptoms when caring for people with AIDS, it is time to take measures to relieve the stress in your life.

- Withdrawal from others
- Inappropriate anger, hostility, or general irritation
- Reluctance to cooperate with coworkers or to participate on the health care team
- Inability to enjoy life
- A sense of being overwhelmed by endless tasks, both at home and on the job
- Chronic fatigue
- A feeling of isolation
- A rigid approach to problems
- A constant sense of pressure
- A sense that your work has become rote, routine

Modified with permission from: Cassidy, J. (1991). Compassion fatigue. *HEALTH PROGRESS*, Jan–Feb, p. 55.

Elizabeth Cox's journey included the challenge of integrating the facts about her husband's past homosexual activity into her sense that she knew him. The diagnosis of AIDS in Keith left her shocked and dismayed but also with an overwhelming sense of betrayal. The fact of AIDS did not fit in with her knowledge of who Keith was. Fortunately for Keith, Elizabeth successfully dealt with her sense of betrayal. Her decision to stand by Keith's side as he battled AIDS was supported by the love she had for him. However, she still struggled with how to tell people about what was wrong with Keith, who to tell, and then how to deal with the reactions of others once they were told. Spiritually, Elizabeth found meaning and purpose in her journey through the writing of her journal, which she hoped would help others faced with a similar walk.

In addition to the psychological and spiritual adjustments that can be overwhelming to the caregiver, the whole spectrum of physical care also must be dealt with. AIDS in its full-blown stage is a debilitating disease that wastes once-robust bodies with relentless diarrhea and vomiting, unsightly lesions, cognitive deficits, and overwhelming weakness. Many of those who die with AIDS are young. This fact holds a special poignancy for caregivers. The care requirements of such a disease are demanding (Hays et al, 1994).

Nurses who provide much of the hospital-based care for AIDS patients are not immune to the demands of the caring role. In a survey conducted by *Nursing 88* (Brennan, 1988) of 346 nurses from 15 institutions, their responses reflected how AIDS had spread over the preceding five years—1983 to 1988. On the average, respondents had cared for a total of 44 people with AIDS. However, most of the nurses reported having cared for over half that number in 1987 and 1988. At the time of the survey, most of the nurses were caring for at least 10 AIDS patients.

When asked how they felt about caring for AIDS patients, 73% of the nurses responded that they were concerned for their own safety. About half (47%) reported feeling frustrated at their patients' poor prognoses. Others (19%) reported feeling angry about having to care for people with AIDS. Their anger was directed at the disease itself, hospital and government authorities, and the patients, some of whom the nurses held responsible for their illness.

When asked about their families' reactions to their caring for people with AIDS, 80% responded that their relatives were concerned about their (the nurses') safety. The responses to the query "What is your overall reaction to caring for PWA's?" were mixed. Many (41%) expressed ambivalence; over one third of the nurses disliked caring for AIDS patients, either moderately (23%) or intensely (14%). However, some nurses responded that they enjoyed taking care of people with AIDS, moderately (10%) or very much (11%). These nurses identified the work as challenging and rewarding. One nurse said, "If nurses don't take care of the AIDS patients, who will (p. 63)?"

Nurses and other caregivers are subject to what Poliandro (1991) calls **compassion fatigue.** This is a result of chronic stress and occurs before burnout. The signs of compassion fatigue are shown in Box 42–1. The needs of the patients are so great that the caregiver may find that increasingly the needs of the patient come first and his or her own needs come last. Poliandro suggests four rules for caregivers for preventing compassion fatigue (Box 42–2).

Support groups, where caregivers can vent their feelings associated with the caregiving role, provide a mechanism for preventing physical and emotional ex-

BOX 42-2 Rules for Preventing Compassion Fatigue

- Give to yourself just as you take care of others.
- Allow yourself to feel good about what you do. Feeling good about yourself makes you a more effective caregiver.
- It is part of your professional duty to see to your own daily replenishment.
- Set realistic limits for yourself and others. This ensures that you will be able to continue to care for others.

Modified with permission from: Cassidy, J. (1991). Compassion fatigue. *HEALTH PROGRESS*, Jan–Feb, p. 54.

haustion. These groups have proved beneficial to nurses as well as to nonprofessional caregivers. The caregiver is allowed to talk about feelings of frustration, of being overwhelmed, of the difficulty in maintaining the semblance of being "strong and in control," and of the pain of loss. The group is usually structured in a way that the caregiver receives affirmation, suggestions for dealing with concrete problems, a sense of connectedness with caregivers who are struggling with similar issues, and encouragement to care for and nurture self (Scanlon and Packard, 1991).

▶ **Check Your Reading**

19. What is compassion fatigue?
20. Give three characteristics of compassion fatigue.
21. Give two strategies for prevention of compassion fatigue.

NURSING AND AIDS

The nursing profession is faced with its own journey in dealing with AIDS. Nurses are part of society as a whole and as such are subject to the same fears and stereotypes as others. What sets nurses apart is the expectation, society's and their own, not only that they will provide care but also that they will care. The AIDS journey for nursing offers a path of avoidance and a path of care. The path of avoidance is taken by nurses who would rather not confront AIDS. This is exemplified in Chenitz's (1992, p. 445) observation of nursing care during her first admission for pneumocystis pneumonia:

That is, they cared more about whether all of the rules were complied with, whether I had the blanket I needed when I rang the call bell, whether my bed was neat and clean, whether I had the oxygen at the proper setting, and not at all about how I was. I was a case, not a person. Shocked and emotionally distraught about my AIDS diagnosis, this dispassionate care fed my sense of unreality. I was in a living nightmare.

As time goes on and the number of AIDS patients increases, the path of avoidance will become increasingly more difficult to choose.

The path of care includes research, education, and direct care; many nurses have chosen to walk this path. A review of nursing literature for the period of 1987 to 1995 reveals over 700 articles on AIDS. These articles, focusing on research, education, and care issues, reflect the commitment of nursing to take this journey. In a 1991 article appearing in the *American Journal of Nursing*, Meyer states that "HIV disease has challenged nurses' competence, courage, and compassion—and they've risen to meet that challenge." Many nurses have confronted their own fears and anxieties and have decided to rise above their feelings to care for people with AIDS. Nursing stands in the forefront in the care of people with AIDS. The disease is one that places high demands for compassionate and skilled care (Peloquin, 1990). The nurse, armed with a holistic approach to patient care, is the best equipped of the health team members to respond to these demands. The following quote from Chenitz (1992, p. 440) illustrates the impact that a caring approach can have on the person with AIDS:

All the nurses on this unit were like that (compassionate). They loved being nurses, and they defined nursing as caring, compassionate, loving, nonjudgmental care. They cleaned, bathed, touched, started IV's, helped me to the commode and gave me medicine with great efficiency, but what really mattered is that they did it with compassion. I felt my sense of dignity return, the dignity I felt in their care. The unit was a healing place where I knew I would live and be okay. I got a glimmer that there is life after AIDS.

Psychiatric Nursing and AIDS

Psychiatric nurses are involved in the care of AIDS patients in many service settings. Nurses who function in a psychiatric consultation-liaison capacity are confronted with the demands of AIDS in general inpatient units where patients are treated for the opportunistic infections that are the hallmark of AIDS. Psychiatric nurses also are confronted with caring for people with AIDS in psychiatric inpatient units, community mental health centers, and the home. Both physical and psychiatric care is being provided in all of these arenas. A brief description of the nurse's role in each of these settings is followed by an examination of the nursing process with AIDS patients.

Psychiatric Consultation-Liaison Nursing and AIDS

Again, let's focus on the initial story.

Keith fell ill on a trip to England and was hospitalized for treatment of *Pneumocystis carinii* pneumonia. Although no psychiatric consultation-liaison nurse was available, a staff counselor worked with Keith and his wife, attempting to support them as they dealt with the magnitude and terror associated with the diagnosis.

In the United States, providing support could very well be the role of the psychiatric consultation-liaison nurse who is part of the support system when a patient first receives the diagnosis of AIDS. The role draws on knowledge of crisis intervention to help the patient and/or family in practical problem-solving and decision-making (Grant, 1988).

The psychiatric consultation-liaison nurse may be part of the discharge planning team and, as such, needs to be familiar with community resources. For instance, the nurse may provide information related to the availability of support groups, self-help groups, counseling about financial, legal, and social matters, psychiatric counseling, and buddy systems, in which individuals in the community assist with shopping, transportation, and other necessities of life.

The psychiatric consultation-liaison nurse may be part of nursing's initial assessment of organic mental disorders and may be the stimulus for an in-depth neuropsychiatric evaluation. Perry and Markowitz (1986) reported that in several studies, a review of nursing notes in both medical and psychiatric settings revealed that nurses documented discrete neuropsychological symptoms such as "unable to remember my name" or "somewhat disoriented" yet made no request for neurological or psychiatric evaluations. Perry and Markowitz concluded that nurses' lack of knowledge regarding the neuropsychiatric complications of AIDS led them to attribute unusual behaviors to hostility and psychopathology.

Another aspect of the psychiatric consultation-liaison nurse's role in working with AIDS patients is to assist the medical nurses to cope with their own feelings about this type of care. A psychiatric consultation-liaison nurse might conduct a staff support group in which nurses can ventilate their feelings. Still another role involves supporting the family, friends, and significant others who are faced with their own grief.

Psychiatric Inpatient Nursing and AIDS

The most common psychiatric problems associated with AIDS—adjustment disorder with depression as the major symptom and an organic mental disorder—already have been discussed. However, these diagnoses could quite possibly lead to an inpatient psychiatric stay. The presence of a person with AIDS on an inpatient psychiatric unit presents nursing with new challenges.

For instance, a psychotic patient who has an AIDS-related syndrome raises some really tough nursing issues. Simple procedures such as using universal precautions become complex and time consuming with a psychotic patient. How do you explain wearing gloves to a psychotic patient, who may already be dealing with delusional and hallucinatory ideation regarding feelings of guilt, worthlessness, and shame? Whenever nursing staff members implement universal precautions, they must provide a clear explanation to each patient. They must assess each patient thereafter for countertherapeutic effects. They also must intervene therapeutically to minimize anxiety and other feelings triggered by universal precautions.

Polk-Walker (1989) discusses a case scenario that illustrates the problems of treating a patient who is both psychotic and diagnosed with AIDS (Case Example 42–1). This example raises issues concerning safety as well as resource allocation. Psychiatric facilities may be faced with making decisions regarding the needs of many patients versus the needs of a few. In the future, AIDS patients may find that admission to a psychiatric unit is difficult and that early transfers or discharges become the norm.

Case Example 42–1 Sherri's Story

Sherri is a young intravenous drug abuser who was transferred to a psychiatric hospital from a local hospital, where she had just given birth. In addition to being HIV-positive, Sherri was paranoid and verbally and physically assaultive at the time of admission. She was placed in a single room with private bathroom facilities. However, she was allowed to freely walk the unit. Although universal body fluid precautions were standard hospital procedure, the staff could not maintain the isolation of Sherri's body fluids because she continually removed her sanitary napkin and sat in patient chairs, thereby contaminating patient-care areas. Various options, including seclusion, were discussed and dismissed. The treatment team decided to place this patient on one-to-one supervision for the remainder of her hospital stay. However, the use of one-to-one intervention represented a significant expenditure of nursing resources. In addition, the one-to-one intervention exacerbated the patient's paranoia, requiring more intensive psychotherapeutic intervention.

The inpatient psychiatric nurse must confront other issues as well. For instance, ethical concerns regarding who should receive information regarding the patient's HIV antibody status become very important. The rights of the patient to confidentiality versus the need to know by other patients, staff members, and medical facilities must be examined. The doctor is allowed to disclose information regarding a patient's positive antibody test to the rest of the staff because the entire staff is considered one treatment unit. However, the disclosure of AIDS antibody testing to outpatient facilities is not clear (Binder, 1987).

Binder (1987) cites two examples that vividly illustrate the ethical and legal quagmire surrounding the issue of confidentiality with AIDS patients. The first case involved a 22-year-old with a diagnosis of paranoid schizophrenia who suddenly bit a patient who was HIV-positive. In the second case, a 23-year-old bisexual man was admitted for depression and suicidal ideation and requested an HIV antibody screening. The test result was positive yet he refused to tell his girlfriend with whom he was having an active sexual relationship. In both of these cases, the law protected the patient's right to confidentiality. However, according to the Tarasoff decision, clinicians are required to warn potential victims of violence (Kadzielski, 1991). The question that arises is whether the Tarasoff decision be extended to cover other types of life-threatening risks (see Chapter 5).

Community Mental Health Nursing and AIDS

People with AIDS receive most of their care outside of hospitals. This fact, coupled with the devastating emotional toll exacted by the disease on patients, family members, and caregivers, creates a tremendous vacuum of need that can be filled with the services of community mental health nurses. The interventions most likely to be provided include crisis intervention; support and bereavement groups; individual, family, couples, and group psychotherapy; case management; and community education and consultation (Knox, 1989).

The recognition of HIV as a community mental health problem has stimulated the development of training programs designed to prepare community mental health professionals to deal with the problems associated with HIV. The training programs usually target the needs of individual patients with AIDS as well as strategies for safeguarding the community's health in relation to HIV (Knox and Gaies, 1990).

Psychiatric Home Care and AIDS

Increasingly, people with AIDS are receiving skilled nursing care in their homes. Economics is one of the primary driving forces that support this move. In the first study on costs of the care of people with AIDS, the CDC (Centers for Disease Control, 1986) estimates of cost were approximately $150,000 per patient. This estimate was determined from inpatient costs. In 1989, estimates were between $23,000 and $55,000 for the cost of AIDS health care (AIDS Alert). These conservative estimates were based on home care, community support, outpatient therapies, and hospice care, with little emphasis on inpatient care. Neither of these studies included the costs of zidovudine (azidothymidine [AZT]) or aerosolized pentamidine for treatment of *Pneumocystis carinii* pneumonia (Rothstein, 1989). The most recent (1992) estimates of the cost of care cite the following figures (unpublished data, Centers for Disease Control, May, 1995):

- An average of $38,300 for yearly care for a patient with full-blown AIDS
- An average of $102,000 for lifetime care for a patient with AIDS
- An average of $10,000 yearly for a patient who is HIV-positive

Although these estimates lack precision, they clearly indicate that the most cost-effective method of treatment is community and home based.

Most of home care to the person with AIDS is provided by medical-surgical and hospice nurses. However, as more home care agencies develop a psychiatric service component, increasingly the psychiatric home care nurse also is involved in this care. The psychiatric home care nurse is confronted not only with the patient's feelings of depression, social isolation, stigmatization, helplessness, and grieving but also with the caregiver's similar feelings that must be dealt with to teach that person how to care for the person with AIDS. People with AIDS who display the neuopsychiatric complications associated with AIDS-dementia complex present safety and support challenges to nurses as well as to nonprofessional care providers.

Although home care is preferable to inpatient care, it is not without difficulties (Carney, 1990). These difficulties range from social to medical to personal, and they have an additive impact on the patient's feelings of depression. The social difficulties revolve around returning to a community setting where neighbors, acquaintances, landlords, and others are terrified of the disease and therefore terrified of association with the person with AIDS. Consequently, many people with AIDS have encountered housing problems when fearful landlords initiated eviction proceedings based on vague pretexts.

As a result of rejection by family and friends, the person with AIDS may be alone at home without any support except that offered by home care staff. Families and friends do not always rally around to offer love and support to the person with AIDS. It seems that in periods of crisis, families either pull together or become more alienated. Many families who have a son or daughter with AIDS are confronted with the dual realizations that their loved one engaged in either a homosexual or an intravenous drug–using lifestyle and that their loved one is dying. Adjustments to these facts may prove too much for the coping abilities of families, and they may retreat from contact with the person with AIDS.

Some communities have intricate social support systems in place to assist the person with AIDS in meeting many daily needs. The psychiatric home care nurse must be knowledgeable about the available community services. For instance, in San Francisco a group of volunteers delivers meals to homebound people with AIDS who are too weak to prepare their own meals. Baltimore has a volunteer "buddy" system, in which the person with AIDS is assisted with transportation, obtaining housing, clothing, food, and other necessities of life. Other communities have little social support available to the person with AIDS.

▶ Check Your Reading

22. What are the two paths available to nurses facing the crisis of AIDS?
23. Give an example of an appropriate nursing intervention for a psychiatric consultation-liaison nurse.
24. Give an example of an appropriate nursing intervention for an inpatient psychiatric nurse.
25. Give an example of an appropriate nursing intervention for a community mental health nurse.

NURSING PROCESS

The nursing process is applied to the care of the person with AIDS in a fashion similar to the care of other patients.

ASSESSMENT

The assessment of the person with AIDS uses the strategies suggested in Chapter 13 for evaluating mental status. Specific assessment skills focus on determining the degree of depression. For instance, you might use a standardized depression scale, such as the Montgomery-Asburg Depression Scale, for this purpose. Slowed cognitive and sensorimotor functions are revealed with neuropsychological tests. For instance, the Mini–Mental State Examination would be used as part of a dementia assessment providing specifics regarding short-term memory, attention, and fine motor skills. Patients with AIDS-dementia complex (ADC) perform poorly on tests that require rapid fine motor movements, sustained attention and concentration, and cognitive flexibility. Grant (1988) reports the need for a thorough mental status examination with special attention to performance in serial sevens and other tasks requiring sequencing. Asking patients to repeat a list of numbers provides information regarding short-term memory. Individuals with unaffected cognition can remember five to seven numbers. Scores of four or less suggest memory impairment and a need to provide the patient with verbal and/or written cues to assist in the completion of routine tasks. Because anxiety and educational level can affect patients' performance on this test, the results must be interpreted with caution.

Gait ataxia or slowing of rapid movements may be one of the clearest signs of neurological damage, especially in the early stages of ADC. Swanson and coworkers (1990) suggest the need for close observation of patients during day-to-day care. For instance, suspected sensory deficit should be further assessed by asking the patient to identify numbers "written" on his or her fingertips with a capped pen while his or her eyes are closed. If the patient is unable to do this accurately, this suggests the need to attend to safety issues. For instance, it becomes essential for someone to check the water temperature before a patient bathes or showers.

Swanson and coworkers (1990) have identified strategies to assess for upper extremity functioning. Patients can be asked to alternately supinate and pronate their hands. If a patient has difficulty initiating this movement, frontal lobe damage is suggested. Clumsiness or inability to maintain the movements may suggest basal ganglia damage. Upper extremity motor deficits may benefit from assistive devices from occupational therapy.

Abstract thinking, a higher neuropsychological function, can be assessed by asking patients to explain the meaning of common proverbs, such as "People who live in glass houses shouldn't throw stones." The inability to explain the proverb or the provision of a literal, concrete answer may indicate the patient's impaired ability to abstract. This limits the patient's ability to learn new behaviors, such as practicing safer sex, and to problem-solve. Problem-solving ability can be evaluated by providing a patient with a hypothetical situation, such as "What would you do if you were in a theater and saw a fire?"

Swanson and coworkers (1990) report that asymptomatic patients perform better on tests of memory, motor coordination, and general intellectual functioning than do patients who have progressed farther in the disease process. For example, a patient who had progressed to full-blown AIDS could not remember short word lists, was unable to solve problems, and was unable to insert pegs into holes.

Differentiating Depression from Dementia

The differentiation between depression and ADC is not an obvious one; however, because the treatment is different it is an important distinction to make. Both psychiatric complications are behaviorally displayed through apathy and psychomotor retardation. Depressed individuals usually express feelings of hopelessness and worthlessness during interviews. They may admit to suicidal ideation. They usually present with a sad and morose affect. These behaviors are not typical of the ADC patient.

Further differentiation can be made through neuropsychological tests that distinguish between depression and dementia. Individuals with dementia experience difficulty in drawing; this is not true of the depressed person. Asking patients to draw simple figures such as squares or triangles may be very telling in determining whether the patient is depressed or not. Another test to differentiate depression from dementia involves asking patients to generate a list of words beginning with a specific letter of the alphabet. Demented persons will be unable to produce more than a few words, whereas this task will pose no challenge to the depressed individual (Swanson et al, 1990).

Assessment of Coping

Van Servellen and colleagues (1989) have developed a Coping Assessment Profile (CAP) to help nurses focus on how the HIV-positive patient is coping with the crisis of the diagnosis. The CAP consists of both a patient self-assessment (CAP-A) and a nurse assessment (CAP-B). The CAP-A provides important information in diagnosing the adaptive and maladaptive responses of patients to AIDS. The CAP-B integrates knowledge gained from the patient with the nurse's judgments about the patient.

▶ Check Your Reading

26. Give two ways to differentiate between depression and ADC.
27. Why would you use a standardized assessment scale such as the Montgomery-Asburg Depression Scale?
28. What information would the Mini–Mental State Examination provide?
29. What could you use to assess coping ability?

DIAGNOSIS

The analysis of the assessment data leads to decisions regarding the nature of the patient's problems and provides direction for your interventions. For example, Jim is newly diagnosed with AIDS. He has *Pneumocystis carinii* pneumonia. He is devastated with the diagnosis and very despondent. He states that he wishes he were dead and he is sure that AIDS is a punishment from God for his homosexual lifestyle. Jim comments that everyone has deserted him except his significant other. Jim's family has totally disowned him. Part of the assessment involved administering the Montgomery-Asburg Depression Scale. Jim received a score of 44 of

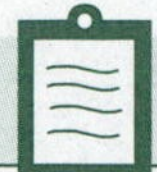

MEDICAL DIAGNOSES AND RELATED NURSING DIAGNOSES AIDS

DSM-IV Diagnosis: Adjustment Disorder

Diagnostic Criteria

A. The development of emotional or behavioral symptoms in response to identifiable stressor(s) occurring within 3 months of the onset of the stressor(s).

B. These symptoms or behaviors are clinically significant as evidenced by either of the following:
(1) Marked distress that is in excess of what would be expected from exposure to the stressor
(2) Significant impairment in social or occupational (academic) functioning

C. The stress-related disturbance does not meet the criteria for another specific Axis I disorder and is not merely an exacerbation of a preexisting Axis I or Axis II disorder.

D. The symptoms do not represent Bereavement.

E. Once the stressor (or its consequences) has terminated, the symptoms do not persist for more than an additional 6 months.

Specify if:

Acute: If the disturbance lasts less than 6 months

Chronic: If the disturbance lasts for 6 months or longer

Adjustment Disorders are coded based on the subtype, which is selected according to the predominant symptoms. The specific stressor(s) can be specified on Axis IV.

309.0 With Depressed Mood
309.24 With Anxiety
309.28 With Mixed Anxiety and Depressed Mood
309.3 With Disturbance of Conduct
309.4 With Mixed Disturbance of Emotions and Conduct
309.9 Unspecified

RELATED NURSING DIAGNOSES	DEFINITION	EXAMPLE
Risk for Violence: Self-Directed	A state in which a person experiences behaviors that can be physically harmful to the self	Risk for Violence: Self-Directed related to feelings of hopelessness secondary to diagnosis of AIDS, as evidenced by suicidal ideation
Ineffective Individual Coping	Impairment of adaptive behaviors and problem-solving abilities of a person in meeting life's demands and roles	Ineffective Individual Coping related to new diagnosis of AIDS, as evidenced by verbalizations of hopelessness and suicidal ideation
Spiritual Distress	Disruption in the life principle that pervades a person's entire being and that integrates and transcends one's biological and psychological nature	Spiritual Distress related to feelings of guilt about lifestyle as evidenced by verbalizations that God will punish him
Hopelessness	A subjective state in which a person sees limited or no alternatives or personal choices available and is unable to mobilize energy on own behalf	Hopelessness related to belief that the person has no reason for living once diagnosed with AIDS, as evidenced by suicidal ideation
Anticipatory Grieving	Intellectual and emotional responses and behaviors by which people work through the process of modifying self-concept based on the perception of potential loss	Anticipatory grieving related to awareness of many losses associated with diagnosis of AIDS, as evidenced by sad affect and verbalization that he has lost so much already

Diagnostic Criteria from American Psychiatric Association: *Diagnostic and statistical manual of mental disorders, fourth edition.* Washington, D.C.: American Psychiatric Association, 1994; nursing diagnoses and definitions from North American Nursing Diagnosis Association. (1994). *NANDA nursing diagnoses: Definitions and classification 1995–1996.* Philadelphia: NANDA.

a possible 60 on the Montgomery-Asburg Depression Scale, indicating serious depression. His score of 29 on the Mini–Mental State Examination indicates no cognitive deficit. This data, combined with observations of sad affect, verbalizations of hopelessness, psychomotor retardation, Jim's isolation from his family, his sense of guilt, and suicidal ideation point to the medical and nursing diagnoses shown in "Medical Diagnoses and Related Nursing Diagnoses: AIDS."

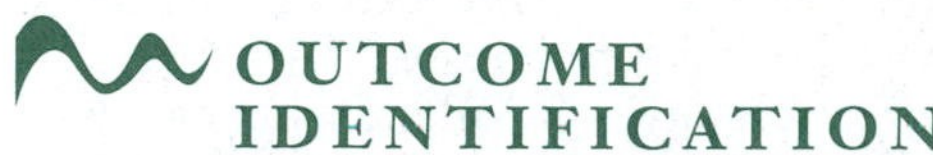

OUTCOME IDENTIFICATION

The expected outcomes for a patient such as Jim diagnosed with AIDS might include:

- The patient will remain free from harm.
- The patient will demonstrate effective coping skills in dealing with the diagnosis of AIDS.

- The patient will resolve his guilt feelings and experience the forgiveness of God.
- The patient will express hope in being able to find meaning in the remainder of his life.
- The patient will resolve the grief feelings associated with his many actual and anticipated losses.

PLANNING

The plan for Jim involves carrying out any medically ordered treatment and establishing goals that improve his coping, relieve his sense of spiritual distress, reduce his hopelessness, and support him in his grieving. Appropriate short-term goals include:

Expected Outcomes	Short-Term Goals
The patient will remain free from harm.	1. Within two weeks of taking antidepressant medication, the patient will have an improvement in his score on the Montgomery-Asburg Scale.
	2. After attending two medication group sessions, Jim will state the major action of his antidepressant medication, and at least four side effects and strategies for managing them.
	3. After participating in individual psychotherapy, Jim will exhibit a brightening in his mood, as evidenced by smiling, spontaneous verbalizations, attention to appearance, and a statement that he has no suicidal ideation.
The patient will demonstrate effective coping skills in dealing with the diagnosis of AIDS.	1. After participating in individual psychotherapy, Jim will express hope and, through self-appraisal, will evaluate his mood to be improved.
	2. After participating in individual psychotherapy, Jim will state a willingness to participate in AIDS support groups as a way to bolster his own coping skills.
The patient will resolve his guilt feelings and experience the forgiveness of God.	As a result of talking to the nurse and clergy about his feelings of spiritual distress, Jim will verbalize a feeling of peace about this issue and a sense of meaning and order to the experience.
The patient will express hope in being able to find meaning in the remainder of his life.	After participating in several educational groups addressing the issue of living with AIDS, Jim will verbalize that life can still have significance—in fact, even more significance—with a diagnosis of AIDS.
The patient will resolve the grief feelings associated with his many actual and anticipated losses.	After participating in an educational group emphasizing strategies for coping with AIDS, Jim will express knowledge about the grieving process and greater confidence in his ability to deal with the losses related to AIDS.

IMPLEMENTATION

Implementation of nursing care for the person with AIDS must be truly holistic. As Chenitz (1992) wrote:

> *Compassion, assurance, and competence is what I need from health care providers. You have not failed me if I die. You have failed me if I die alone, frightened, in pain or distress. It is enlightened help with the dying that I need. I want help to maintain my dignity, keep me pain free, and allow my family and friends to be there. Too often today this type of treatment is not available. Why not? This is nursing care, and for this we are responsible.*

Examining the issues of implementation involved in Jim's care includes specific interventions such as:

- Administering the antidepressant medication
- Assigning Jim to a medication teaching group
- Assigning Jim to a nurse psychotherapist with whom he will meet for individual sessions
- Assigning Jim to an AIDS educational group
- Contacting a clergy person of Jim's choice, or if Jim has no preference, contacting the clergy person assigned to the institution where Jim is admitted
- Ensuring that Jim's individual treatment plan includes spiritual interventions such as talking about Jim's guilt and his feelings that God will punish him, assisting Jim to create some order and meaning out of his present situation, possibly praying with Jim, and informing him about chapel services.

More important than the specific interventions used with Jim is the overall quality of the relationships that are developed with Jim. He cries out for acceptance, affirmation, and reassurance that hope exists and that he is worthy of such hope. These needs cannot be met in the mechanized or rote manner implied in a step-by-step list of interventions but in relationships in which Jim's basic sense of worth is unconditionally affirmed without judgment or qualification (Carson, 1990; Carson, et al, 1990).

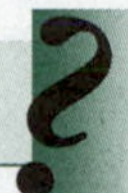

WHAT SOCIETY NEEDS TO KNOW AIDS

What type of contact is OK and safe in caring for a person with AIDS?

The HIV infection most often is transmitted through intimate sexual contact; however, contact with blood and other body fluids may result in transmission of the infection. Authorities say that casual, nonintimate contact is safe. Studies have been conducted of noninfected people who share household utensils, towels, linens, and toilet facilities with infected people, and the noninfected people show no evidence of HIV transmission. Authorities also say that it is highly improbable that AIDS can be transmitted by an insect bite. Touching the person with AIDS on the arm or hand and avoiding the use of unnecessary protective clothing are important ways of expressing your care. It is important to remember that AIDS is a largely preventable disease because of its mode of viral transmission and the fragile nature of the virus. Although abstinence from sexual intercourse is the only certain way of preventing the transmission of AIDS, the consistent use of latex condoms and a spermicide containing nonoxynol 9 can significantly reduce the likelihood of HIV transmission. Education about safe health practices is important for both patient and family.

The person with AIDS is immunosuppressed and is at increased risk of developing opportunistic infections. People with normally benign infections such as colds or flu should therefore temporarily avoid contact with the person with AIDS. Intermittent acute infections interspersed with periods of wellness characterize the course of AIDS.

What community resources are available for people with AIDS?

The following is a partial list of community resources:

- Public Health Service AIDS Hotline: 800-342-AIDS
- American Public Health Association *Special Initiatives on AIDS* series: American Public Health Association Publication Sales, Department 5037, Washington, D.C. 20061–5037
- National Gay Task Force Crisis Line: 800-221-9044

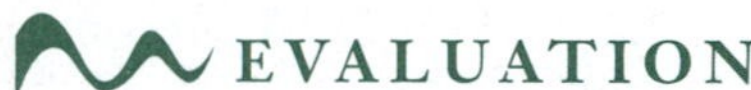

EVALUATION

The care of a patient diagnosed with AIDS such as Jim requires ongoing evaluation. This formative evaluation looks at the patient's day-to-day responses to the nursing interventions and identifies any new assessment data as well as any additional nursing diagnoses not identified in the initial plan of care.

The summative evaluation of care is specified in the expected outcomes and the short-term goals. If the criteria for goal achievement are not met, the data are reexamined to determine the answers to questions such as:

- Was the assessment adequate?
- Does additional assessment data need to be incorporated?
- Were the goals appropriate?
- Was the intervention appropriate?
- Was the specified time frame for achieving the goal appropriate?

The answers to these questions give direction to possible modifications of the plan of care.

CASE STUDY: TONY

Tony is a 25-year-old homosexual man who was diagnosed as being HIV-positive a year ago. At that time, he was spending many of his free evenings in gay bars. Since his diagnosis, he has stopped going to gay bars and has tended to spend his free time watching television or taking his dog Sparky for walks in the park. Tony is employed as an assistant grocery store manager and is well liked by his employees. Recently, however, he has missed work because of infections associated with AIDS. His coworkers suspect the diagnosis and are beginning to avoid him. Tony feels isolated and extremely lonely. His family members, who live in another state, are not aware of his diagnosis, sexual orientation, or lifestyle.

ASSESSMENT

Assessment data are as follows:

- Feeling isolated and lonely
- Increasing work absences
- Cut off from family both emotionally and geographically
- Deteriorating medical condition

DIAGNOSIS

***DSM-IV* Diagnosis:** Adjustment Disorder with depressive symptoms and AIDS

Nursing Diagnosis: Anticipatory Grieving related to decreased quality of life and near-certain death as evidenced by loss of health status and awareness of losses associated with AIDS

OUTCOME IDENTIFICATION, PLANNING, AND IMPLEMENTATION

EXPECTED OUTCOME 1: By _____ the patient will express his feelings, concerns, and fears about having AIDS.

SHORT-TERM GOAL	NURSING INTERVENTIONS	RATIONALES
By _____ the patient will express his grief to the health care team.	1. Provide and support anticipatory grief responses. 2. Acknowledge the stage of grief Tony is experiencing (denial, anger, bargaining, depression, or acceptance).	1–2. Grief is a normal response to all types of loss. Strong feelings are evoked when dealing with issues of AIDS and death.
	3. Listen to Tony's perceptions about his diagnosis of AIDS by using therapeutic communication skills, active listening, silence, and acknowledgment.	3. Any type of meaningful loss (e.g., loss of parent, body part, role, or functioning) will precipitate a reaction that will follow the general stages or patterns of the grief response.

EXPECTED OUTCOME 2: By _____ the patient will make decisions about his care and the near-certain loss of his life.

SHORT-TERM GOAL	NURSING INTERVENTIONS	RATIONALES
By _____ the patient will examine the loss within a spiritual context.	1. Help Tony to identify those aspects of AIDS that he can control—informed consent, advanced directives—and those specific aspects that are distressing and uncontrollable. 2. Keep Tony informed of his condition, of prescribed treatments, medications, and therapies, and of test results.	1–2. The diagnosis of AIDS can strip the patient of a sense of meaning and purpose in life. A disease with a grave prognosis, AIDS challenges coping and adaptive behavior. Being informed and educated about the disease helps patients to cope.

Nursing Diagnosis: Social Isolation related to lack of family support and to the stigma and societal nonacceptance and fear of the disease as evidenced by changes in work friendships.

OUTCOME IDENTIFICATION, PLANNING, AND IMPLEMENTATION

EXPECTED OUTCOME 1: By _____ the patient will explore contact with and seek assistance from family, friends, clergy, and community resources.

SHORT-TERM GOALS	NURSING INTERVENTIONS	RATIONALES
By _____ the patient will verbalize his fears of rejection related to telling his parents about his illness.	1. Support Tony in all endeavors to initiate contact with family and friends. 2. Provide education about AIDS to Tony's family and friends.	1. Support encourages the patient to verbalize needs and initiate actions. 2. Often, people withdraw out of fear of contracting AIDS from the patient. Education assists in alleviating this ignorance and reduces the fear of transmission.

SHORT-TERM GOALS	NURSING INTERVENTIONS	RATIONALES
By _____ the patient will identify behaviors that increase meaningful relationships.	1. Introduce Tony to the various types of support and outreach groups for people with AIDS. 2. Ask Tony whether he participates in, or is interested in participating in, a religious group or activity; if so, contact an appropriate group or institution that has programs supportive of people with AIDS.	1–2. Community support through self-help groups and religious institutions can help patients cope with not only emotional and social issues but also spiritual issues.

EVALUATION

Formative Evaluation: Tony met each of the short-term goals. In therapy, Tony was encouraged to express his feelings and to take as much time as needed to forgive himself for not taking appropriate precautions to avoid contracting and transmitting AIDS, so that he could move on. Tony also talked with other homosexual patients who were cut off from their families, and this helped him considerably in dealing with his emotional pain and fears of reaching out and asking for help. Tony had a great deal of difficulty in calling his parents to tell them of his diagnosis. When he did tell them about the diagnosis, they asked about how he contracted the disease. After years of keeping his sexual orientation a secret from his family, Tony finally admitted to them that he lived a homosexual lifestyle. To his utter surprise, Tony's parents said that they loved him unconditionally, regardless of his lifestyle. Tony told them how ashamed he felt about not taking precautions to protect himself during sexual relations.

Summative Evaluation: Tony met each of the expected outcomes, except for showing interest in religious activities; Tony said that he wasn't ready to deal with "all that stuff." The staff respected his wishes. Tony did, however, reach out to a local AIDS support group and attended meetings regularly after discharge. The staff arranged for a member of the support group to visit Tony prior to discharge to establish a support network. Tony did finally call his parents, and to his surprise they caught the next flight to be with him. Tony stated that in his meetings with his parents, he felt accepted and loved for who he is.

CONCLUSIONS

Increasingly, the care of the person with AIDS is extending into the psychiatric arena. AIDS is a terrible disease that exacts an enormous psychological and spiritual toll on people with AIDS, families, caregivers, and others. The disease taxes coping responses to the limit—and beyond. The level of support required to assist patients and others who deal with AIDS demands skilled interventions and an integrated team effort among mental health professionals, including psychiatric nurses.

The crisis initiated by an HIV-related infection is of such magnitude as to lead people to commit suicide at alarming rates. The existential and spiritual crisis that follows the diagnosis of AIDS can strip the person of a sense of meaning, purpose, and worth, or the spiritual comfort that is possible with a relationship to God, leaving the person spiritually and emotionally naked and vulnerable.

The psychiatric problems of adjustment disorder with depressed mood, AIDS-related dementia (dementia due to HIV disease), and major depressive episode necessitate active treatment and are not illnesses that can be managed by the patient alone or by a single caregiver, no matter how concerned and involved he or she is.

Psychiatric nurses therefore have a major role to play in the care of the person with AIDS. Psychiatric nurses encounter these patients in the general hospital population, in psychiatric units, in the community, and in the home. In all of these sites, the nursing process provides the framework for approaching care in a systematic manner; the interventions of crisis intervention, psychological and spiritual support, and education are the tools needed to assist the person with AIDS in coping with the disease.

KEY POINTS TO REMEMBER

- AIDS is a terrible disease; it affects individuals in a holistic manner.
- The psychological reactions to AIDS vary from those who are the "worried well" to those with psychiatric disorders like major depression.
- The spiritual implications of AIDS include feelings of guilt for lifestyle choices; a sense of hopelessness and despair; existential crises; and alienation from God.
- AIDS has been recognized since 1981.
- Since 1981 almost a half million cases of full-blown AIDS have been reported.
- Most cases of AIDS are among homosexual and bisexual men and intravenous drug users. However, the incidence of cases among women and children is increasing.
- AIDS is preventable through sexual abstinence, practicing

safer sex practices, avoiding intravenous drug use or avoiding sharing needles, and avoiding the exchange of body fluids.

- AIDS is not spread through casual contact.
- The most common psychiatric sequelae of AIDS are adjustment disorder with either feelings of depression or anxiety, major depression, and AIDS-dementia complex.
- AIDS patients endure isolation, stigma, and feelings of worthlessness.
- Caregivers of AIDS patients can experience compassion fatigue.
- Assessment of an AIDS patient differentiates between depression and dementia.
- The nursing process offers a systematic way to provide holistic care for people with AIDS.

LEARNING ACTIVITIES

1. Read an excerpt from Elizabeth Cox's book *Thanksgiving: An AIDS Journal.* Write your reflections in your journal. If you were in Elizabeth's place, how do you think that you would react?

2. Find out what supports are available for AIDS patients in your community and your state.

3. The following diseases are either caused or exacerbated by lifestyle choices:

   AIDS
   Herpes
   Congestive heart failure
   Diabetes
   Substance abuse disorder

Why is it that some of these diseases provoke stigma and moral indignation and others do not?

4. Reflect on your thoughts, feelings, and attitudes about AIDS. Would your responses facilitate or hinder your caring for a patient with AIDS?

5. What does the following statement mean to you: "Rather than consider AIDS a terrible physical disease, it has been couched in terms of immorality and religious imperatives."

CRITICAL THINKING EXERCISE

Roy Jefferson, a 29-year-old AIDS patient was admitted to the inpatient psychiatric unit with extreme anxiety and depression following a doctor's appointment where he learned that his T cells were dangerously low. Roy, since being diagnosed as being HIV-positive four years ago, had turned his life around. No longer sexually active, he had stopped abusing drugs and was experiencing relatively good health. Part of his rehabilitation included being a spokesman for a local AIDS association to educate others about the disease.

1. What assumptions do you have about people who are HIV-positive?

2. Consider the psychiatric nurse's role in comparison to the role of the nurse in another setting.

3. What effect might your assumptions have on your clinical comfort with AIDS patients?

Following an interview with Roy, Bruce, a nursing student, informed his teacher that he had asked Roy to speak to the group of student nurses about his course of illness. The teacher wanted to know the purpose of the meeting and was told that it was an intervention strategy to allow Roy to resume a previous level of functioning.

1. What assumptions can you make about Bruce's point of view concerning AIDS patients?

2. How would you check your assumptions?

3. Consider alternate interventions.

REFERENCES

AIDS Epidemic causes financial drain on return in hospitals. (1989). *AIDS Alert, 4* (9), 152.

Aruffo, J. F., Thompson, R. G., Gottlieb, A. A., and Dobbins, W. N. (1995). An AIDS training program for rural mental health providers. *Psychiatric Services, 46* (1), 79–81.

American Psychiatric Association. (1994). *Diagnostic and Statistical Manual of Mental Disorders, Fourth Edition.* Washington, D.C.: American Psychiatric Association.

Baldwin, J. D., and Baldwin, J. I. (1988). Factors affecting AIDS-related sexual risk-taking behavior among college students. *The Journal of Sex Research, 25* (2), 181–196.

Belcher, A., Dettmore, D., and Holzmer, S. (1989). Spirituality and sense of well-being in persons with AIDS. *Holistic Nursing Practice, 3* (4), 16–25.

Bellemare, D. (1988). AIDS: The challenge to pastoral care. *Journal of Palliative Care, 4* (4), 58–60.

Binder, R. (1987). AIDS antibody tests on inpatient psychiatric units. *American Journal of Psychiatry, 144* (2), 176–180.

Brennan, L., et al. (1988). The battle against AIDS: A report from the nursing front. *Nursing '88, 18* (4), 60–67.

Cahill, K. (1983). *The AIDS epidemic* (p. 2). New York: St Martin's Press.

Carney, K. L. (1990). AIDS care comes home. *Home Healthcare Nurse, 8* (2), 32–37.

Carson, V. (1989). *Spiritual dimensions of nursing practice.* Philadelphia: W. B. Saunders.

Carson, V. (1990). Spirituality and spiritual direction: Important issues to the person with AIDS. *The Journal of Christian Healing, 12* (3), 3–7.

Carson, V., Soeken, K. L., Shanty, J., and Terry, L. (1990). Hope and spiritual well-being: Essentials for living with AIDS. *Perspectives in Psychiatric Care, 26* (2), 28–34.

Carson, V., and Green, H. (1992). The relationship of spiritual well-being and hardiness in the AIDS patient. *Journal of Professional Nursing, 8* (4), 209–220.

Carson, V. (1993). Prayer, meditation, exercise, and vitamin use: Behaviors of the hardy individual who is HIV+, diagnosed with ARC or AIDS. *Journal of the Association of Nurses in AIDS Care, 4* (3), 18–28.

Chenitz, W. C. (1992). Living with AIDS. In J. H. Flaskerud, and P. J. Ungvarski (Eds.), *HIV/AIDS: A guide to nursing care* (pp. 440–460). Philadelphia: W. B. Saunders.

Cox, E. (1990). *Thanksgiving: An AIDS journal.* New York: Harper & Row.

Faulstich, M. (1987). Psychiatric aspects of AIDS. *American Journal of Psychiatry, 144* (5), 551–556.

Flaskerud, J. H. (1989). *AIDS/HIV infection: A reference guide for nursing professionals.* Philadelphia: W. B. Saunders.

Forstein, M. (1984). The psychosocial impact of the acquired immunodeficiency syndrome. *Seminars in Oncology, 11* (1), 77–82.

Fortunato, J. (1987). *AIDS: The spiritual dilemma.* San Francisco: Harper & Row.

Frierson, R. L., and Lippmann, S. B. (1987). Psychological implications of AIDS. *American Family Practitioner, 35,* 109–116.

Gabuzda, D. H., and Hirsch, M. D. (1987). Neurological manifestations of infection with human immunodeficiency virus. *Annals of Internal Medicine, 107,* 383–391.

Grant, S. M. (1988). The hospitalized AIDS patient and the psychiatric liaison nurse. *Archives of Psychiatric Nursing, 2* (1), 35–39.

Graydon, D. N. (1988). AIDS: Observations of a hospital chaplain. *Journal of Palliative Care, 8* (4), 66–69.

Hannon, S. (1990). Adaptable nursing care plan for AIDS patients at home. *AIDS Patient Care,* (4), 23–30.

Hays, R. B., Magee, R. H., and Chauncey, S. (1994). *AIDS Care, 6* (4), 393–397.

Hilts, P. J. (1991). Patient's letter begs Bush to fight stigma of AIDS. *The Sun,* August 4, 1991, 1A, 11A.

Hinton, J. (1972). *Dying.* Baltimore: Penguin Books.

Ho, D. D., Pomerantz, R. J., and Kaplan, J. C. (1987). Pathogenesis of infection with human immunodeficiency virus. *New England Journal of Medicine, 317,* 278–286.

Holland, J., and Tross, S. (1985). The psychosocial and neuropsychiatric sequelae of the Acquired Immunodeficiency Syndrome and related disorders. *Annals of Internal Medicine, 103,* 765–767.

Hover-Kramer, D. (1988). AIDS: A holistice perspective. *Journal of Holistic Nursing, 6* (1), 7–10.

Johnson, L. T. (1989). AIDS update: Home care's challenge. *Caring, 8* (3), 24–28.

Kadzielski, M. (1991). Recent cases interpret the Tarasoff duty to warn. *Health Progress, 2,* 15, 16.

Kayal, P. M. (1985). "Morals," medicine, and the AIDS epidemic. *Journal of Religion and Health, 24* (3), 218–237.

Kendall, J. (1994). Wellness spirituality in homosexual men with HIV infection. *Journal of the Association of Nurses in AIDS Care, 5* (4), 28–34.

Knox, M. D. (1989). Community mental health's role in the AIDS crisis. *Community Mental Health Journal, 25,* 185–196.

Knox, M. D., and Gaies, J. S. (1990). The HIV tutorial for community mental health professionals. *Community Mental Health Journal, 26* (6), 559–566.

Kübler-Ross, E. (1975). *Death—The final stage of growth.* Englewood Cliffs, NJ: Prentice-Hall.

Kübler-Ross, E. (1987). *AIDS: The ultimate challenge.* New York: Macmillan.

Lee, M. R., Ho D. D., and Gurney, M. E. (1987). Functional interaction and partial homology between the human immunodefiency virus and neuroleukin. *Science, 237,* 1047–1051.

Leech, K. (1977). *Soul friend.* San Francisco: Harper & Row.

Marzuk, P., Tierney, H., Tardiff, K., et al. (1988). Increased risk of suicide in persons with AIDS. *JAMA, 259* (9), 1333–1337.

McArthur, J. C., Cohen, B. A., Farzedegan, H., Cornblath, D. R., Selnes, O. A., Ostrow, D., et al. (1988). Cerebrospinal fluid abnormalities in homosexual men with and without neuropsychiatric findings. *Annals of Neurology, 23* [supplement], S34–S37.

McCaffrey, E. A. (1987). Counseling AIDS patients. *AIDS Patient Care, 1* (2), 26–28.

McLean, J., Bouton, M., Brookes, M., Lakhani, D., Fitzpatrick, R., Dawson, J., McKechnie, R., and Hart, G. (1994). Regular partners and risky behavior: Why do gay men have unprotected intercourse? *AIDS Care, 6* (3), 331–341.

Meyer, C. (1991). Nursing and AIDS: A decade of caring. *AJN, 91* (12), 26–31.

Moynihan, R. T., Christ, G. H., and Gallo-Silver, L. (1987). Psychosocial, spiritual, and bereavement issues in the treatment of terminally ill people with AIDS. Conference proceedings from a North American Conference of "Care of Terminally Ill Persons with AIDS". April 8–10, 1987, Ottawa, Canada.

Murphy, P. (1986). Pastoral care and persons with AIDS. *The American Journal of Hospice Care,* (March/April), 38–40.

Murphy, T. (1988). Is AIDS a just punishment? *Journal of Medical Ethics, 14,* 154–160.

Navia B., and Price, R. (1986). Dementia complicating AIDS. *Psychiatric Annals, 16,* 158–166.

Neumark, D. (1984). Review of a support group for patients with AIDS. *Topics in Clinical Nursing, 6* (2) 38–44.

Nichols, S. (1983). Psychiatric aspects of AIDS. *Psychosomatics, 24,* 1083–1089.

Ostrow, D. G. (1988). Models for understanding the psychiatric consequences of AIDS. In T. P. Bridge, et al (Eds.), *Psychological, neuropsychiatric, and substance abuse aspects of AIDS* (pp. 85–94). Vol. 44, New York: Raven Press.

Peloquin, S. M. (1990). AIDS: Toward a compassionate response. *The American Journal of Occupational Therapy, 44* (3), 271–278.

Perry, S., and Markowitz, J. (1986). Psychiatric interventions for AIDS-spectrum disorders. *Hospital and Community Psychiatry, 37,* 1001–1006.

Pert, C. B., Ruff, M. R, Ruscetti, F., Ferrar, W., and Hill, J. (1988). HIV receptors in the brain and peptide that block viral activity. In T. Peter Bridge, et al. *Psychological, neuropsychiatric and substance abuse aspects of AIDS* (pp. 73–83). New York: Raven Press.

Piemme, J. A., and Bolle, J. L. (1990). Coping with grief in response to caring for persons with AIDS. *The American Journal of Occupational Therapy, 44* (3), 266–269.

Poliandro, E. (1991). Compassion fatigue. *Health Progress,* January–February, 54–55, 64.

Polk-Walker, G. C. (1989). Treatment of AIDS in a psychiatric setting. *Perspectives in Psychiatric Care, 25* (2), 9–13.

Ridge, D. T., Plummer, D. C., and Minichiello, V. (1994). Young gay men and HIV: Running the risk? *AIDS Care, 6* (4), 371–378.

Robbins, D. S., Shirazi, Y., Drysdale, B., Lieberman, A., Shin, H. S., and Shin, M. (1987). Production of cytotoxic factor for oligodendrocytes by stimulated astrocytes. *Journal of Immunology, 8,* 2593–2597.

Roth, J., Siegel, R., and Black S. (1994). Identifying the mental health needs of children living in families with AIDS or HIV infection. *Community Mental Health, 30* (6), 581–593.

Rothstein, M. (1989). Medical screening: AIDS, rights and health care costs. *National Forum, 69* (4), 7–10.

Scanlon, C., and Packard, M. (1991). Seeing to one's self. *Health Progress,* January–February, 50–53.

Schnittman, S. M., Psallidopoulos, M. C., Lande, H. C., Thompson, L., Baselor, M., Massari, F., et al. (1989). The reservoir for HIV-1 in human peripheral blood is a T cell that maintains expression of CD4. *Science, 245,* 305–308.

Seal, D. W., and Agostenelli, G. (1994). Individual differences associated with high-risk sexual behavior: Implications for intervention programmes. *AIDS Care, 6* (4), 393–397.

Shilts, R. (1987). *And the band played on: Politics, people, and the AIDS epidemic.* New York: St. Martin's Press.

Solomon, G. F., Temoshok, L., O'Leary, M., and Zich, J. (1987). A psycho-neuroimmunological perspective on AIDS research: Questions, preliminary findings, and suggestions. *Journal of Applied Psychology, 17* (3), 286–308.

Sowell, R. L., Bramlett, M. H., Gueldner, S. H., Gritzmacher, D., and Martin, G. (1991). The lived experience of survival and bereavement following the death of a lover from AIDS. *IMAGE: Journal of Nursing Scholarship, 23* (2), 89–94.

Swanson, B., Cronin-Stubbs, D., and Colletti, M. A. (1990). Dementia & depression in persons with AIDS: Causes and care. *Journal of Psychosocial Nursing, 28* (10), 33–39.

Taylor, I., and Robertson, A. (1994). The health needs of gay men: A discussion of the literature and implications for nursing. *Journal of Advanced Nursing, 20.*

Taylor, K., and Lavallee, D. (1989). Neuropsychiatric management of AIDS. In *AIDS Reference Guide* (pp. 1–6). Atlantic Information Services.

Tibesar, L. J. (1986). Pastoral care: Helping patients on an inward journey. *Health Progress, 67* (4), 41–47.

Turner, N. H., Mclaughlin, J., and Shrum, J. C. (1988). AIDS education: Process, content, and strategies. *Health Values, 12* (3), 6–12.

Van Servellen, G., Nyamathi, A. M., and Mannion, W. (1989). Coping with a crisis: Evaluating psychological risks of patients with AIDS. *Journal of Psychosocial Nursing,* 27 (12), 16–21.

Walker-Robbins, C. G., and Christiana, N. M. (1989). The spiritual needs of persons with AIDS. *Family Community Health, 12* (2), 43–51.

Wenger, N. S., Kusseling, F. S., Beck, K., and Shapiro, M. F. (1994). *AIDS Care, 6* (4), 399–405.

Wolcott, D., Fawzy, F., and Pasnau, R. (1985). Acquired Immune Deficiency Syndrome (AIDS) and consultation-liaison psychiatry. *General Hospital Psychiatry*, 7, 280–292.

Wright, S. C., Jewett, A., Mitsuyasu, R., and Bonavida, B. (1988). Spontaneous cytotoxicity and tumor necrosis factor production by peripheral blood monocytes from AIDS patients. *Journal of Immunology, 141*, 99–104.

SUGGESTED READINGS

Carson, V. (1990). Spirituality and spiritual direction: Important issues to the person with AIDS. *The Journal of Christian Healing, 12* (3), 3–7.

Carson, V., Soeken, K. L., Shanty, J., and Terry, L. (1990). Hope and spiritual well-being: Essentials for living with AIDS. *Perspectives in Psychiatric Care, 26* (2), 28–34.

Carson, V., and Green, H. (1992). The relationship of spiritual well-being and hardiness in the AIDS patient. *Journal of Professional Nursing, 8* (4), 209–220.

Carson, V. (1993). Prayer, meditation, exercise, and vitamin use: Behaviors of the hardy individual who is HIV+, diagnosed with ARC or AIDS. *Journal of the Association of Nurses in AIDS Care, 4* (3), 18–28.

Chenitz, W. C. (1992). Living with AIDS. In J. H. Flaskerud, and P. J. Ungvarski (Eds.), *HIV/AIDS: A guide to nursing care* (pp. 440–460). Philadelphia: W. B. Saunders.

Cox, E. (1990). *Thanksgiving: An AIDS journal.* New York: Harper & Row.

CHAPTER 43

THE JOURNEY THROUGH COMMUNITY MENTAL HEALTH CARE

We must delight in each other, make others' conditions our own, rejoice together, mourn together, labor and suffer together, always having before our eyes our community as members of the same body.

—*John Winthrop, first governor of the Massachusetts Bay Colony, speaking in 1630*

LEARNING OBJECTIVES

After studying this chapter, you should be able to:

1. Discuss at least three events that influenced the development of community mental health care.

2. Describe the group of chronically mentally ill served by community mental health care.

3. Define the terms institutionalization, deinstitutionalization, revolving door cycle, and catchment area.

4. Discuss at least three of the housing options available to the chronically mentally ill.

5. Define and give examples of primary, secondary, and tertiary prevention.

6. Describe the services that are available to meet the needs of the individual mental health patient within the community.

7. Apply the nursing process when the focus of community mental health care is on the community and when the focus is on the individual or family.

KEY TERMINOLOGY

Catchment area
Chronically mentally ill
Community mental health centers
Congregate housing
Day treatment
Deinstitutionalization
Institutionalization
Mobile treatment unit
Primary prevention
Remotivation therapy
Revolving door cycle
Secondary prevention
Seriously and persistently mentally ill
Sheltered housing
Single-room occupancy
Tertiary prevention

In the following story you are introduced to Dymphna, the legendary princess who was killed by her father in the forests outside of Gheel, Belgium. The legend of Dymphna has dramatically influenced the history of Gheel, a community (like the one envisioned by John Winthrop) that makes the conditions of others its own. The care offered at Gheel serves as an exemplar of what was intended to occur in the United States with the advent of community mental health care. Individuals suffering from psychiatric and emotional illnesses would no longer be warehoused in large, unwieldly bureaucratic state institutions but instead cared for in the least restrictive environment and in the most loving and familylike setting possible. Sometimes when we look at what presently exists in community mental health care we see large numbers of the chronically mentally ill for the most part abandoned by society. They may be left to wander the streets in search of food and shelter—basic rights that many Americans take for granted. Such a picture makes us recognize how far short we are of reaching the ideal of a community that cares about and provides for its least fortunate members. We could easily become discouraged. In a society that places such a high value on rugged individualism, any efforts that counteract social isolation and encourage interdependence of community members is to be encouraged (Peck, 1987).

In this chapter, we explore the concept, history, and significance of community mental health care, who receives community-based psychiatric services, what services are offered, the role of nursing, an evaluation of community mental health care, and a discussion of its future directions. First, let's look at the story of Dymphna.

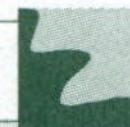

DYMPHNA'S STORY

As legend has it, Dymphna, a beautiful Irish princess, seeking refuge from the incestuous demands of her demented father, escaped to the forests surrounding present-day Gheel, Belgium. Her father pursued her relentlessly, and when he finally found her he killed her in the forests where she had sought a safe haven (Dolan et al, 1983).

After her death and burial, people began to attribute miraculous cures to this saintly young girl. The most dramatic cures were said to occur at Dymphna's tomb and were of those who were mentally ill and mentally retarded.

Dymphna's Fame Spreads

Dymphna's fame spread far and wide. More and more people, expecting to receive healing, came and brought their relatives, especially children. Over time, a shrine was built, and later a church was constructed, where pilgrims came to worship and to pray for a cure.

The Community Gets Involved

Soon these structures could not contain the numbers of pilgrims who arrived at Gheel. A building adjoining the church was used to house the pilgrims, although it too proved too small to house them adequately. The women of Gheel responded by opening their homes to accommodate the large numbers of mentally ill and mentally retarded guests who arrived at Gheel. These women and their families became skilled at caring for these foster members who entered their homes.

The Government Gets Involved

As early as the 15th century, the Municipal Board of Gheel enacted regulations that prevented potential abuses of these faithful and expectant pilgrims. These regulations were modified and updated, so that even today the community continues to refine its special ministry of caring for the mentally ill.

Arriving at Gheel Today

When a mentally ill person arrives at Gheel today, he or she is taken to the "infirmary," or general hospital, where he or she is observed and evaluated. Before a placement is made with a foster family, a comprehensive plan is developed. To ensure that the patient is adjusting to his or her new environment, psychiatrists and psychiatric nurses make home visits.

The Gheel Difference

Patients under mental health care in Gheel receive the best of community care. They reside within loving families. They interact with normal people. They are linked with meaningful volunteer activities fitted to their own capabilities. They participate in the entertainment that is available to all the citizens of Gheel.

Between 1926 and 1950, the Gheel community accepted 8358 patients. Of these patients, 2197 (26%) either received a cure or recovered sufficiently to return to their families (Dolan et al, 1983). In 1957, almost 2000 of Gheel's 6000 families accepted patients into their homes.

An Institutional Town

Today, Gheel is considered an institutional town that receives patients from around the world. The town places patients under the spiritual care of St. Dymphna and under the mortal care of her 20th century counterparts. This unique community of health professionals and caring laypeople provides love, compassion, and—most of all—*care* for the benefit of needy people.

Why is community mental health care in Gheel so successful? According to Shapiro, who has studied the unique healing environment that is Gheel, the answer is nothing miraculous. The difference is caring. "... Treatment is not the question," he said. "What is at issue is the care of these people" (Goldin, 1971, p. 400).

THE ADVENT OF COMMUNITY MENTAL HEALTH CARE

Before 1963, community mental health care was nonexistent in the United States. Severely impaired patients were admitted to psychiatric hospitals, where they frequently remained the rest of their lives, forlorn, forgotten, and forsaken by family, professionals, and society. The act of admission to a psychiatric hospital was viewed as the end of the road, the last stop for dealing with chronic, seemingly intractable problems. In the 1950s, psychiatry was revolutionized with the discovery of the phenothiazine drugs (e.g., chlorpromazine [Thorazine]). The effects of these drugs were nothing less than miraculous because they eliminated or ameliorated the most bizarre of psychiatric symptoms. Suddenly, discharge became not only a possibility, but also a reality for many patients. Even though patients were dramatically improved, however, they were not ready to reenter the community, nor was the community prepared to receive them. Many heretofore unexamined issues became major hurdles blocking discharge. For many patients, there was no family waiting with open arms, so other living arrangements had to be made. For other patients, although they were improved, they still exhibited behaviors that interfered with social interactions. Still other patients, accustomed to having needs met and decisions made by the institution, lacked the ability to function without institutional support, and therefore discharge occurred from the state institution to a smaller institution, such as a nursing home or a group home. The condition of these patients led to the recognition of **institutionalization,** a condition characterized by impaired social interactions, decision-making, and independent living skills resulting from long-term care in an institutional setting.

As more and more patients readied for discharge, the need for supportive services in the community became increasingly apparent. As awareness of this need grew among mental health professionals and the lay public, so also grew the awareness that the community was lacking these supportive services.

Concurrent with these changes, there were legislative mandates that focused psychiatry toward the community. In 1955, the Mental Health Survey Act was enacted by Congress that created the Joint Commission on Mental Illness and Health. This group was charged with analyzing the needs and resources of the mentally ill in the United States and making recommendations to Congress for a national mental health program (Krauss & Slavinsky, 1982). In 1961, the Joint Commission on Mental Illness and Health published its report, which recommended that treatment of the mentally ill be moved from state hospitals to the community. The process of **deinstitutionalization** was underway. The goal of the deinstitutionalization movement was a 50% reduction in the number of patients cared for in state hospitals over a two-decade time span (Minkoff, 1978).

The conclusions of the commission that set in motion what is considered to be the *third revolution* in psychiatry (the first was the provision of treatment for the mentally ill rather than incarceration; the second was the emphasis on intrapsychic causes of mental illness), that of the community mental health care movement, are summarized in the following quote from the Joint Commission on Mental Illness and Health (1961):

> *The objective of modern treatment of persons with mental illness is to enable the patient to maintain himself in the community in a normal manner. To do so, it is necessary (1) to save the patient from debilitating effects of institutionalization, (2) to return him to home and community life as soon as possible, and (3) thereafter, to maintain him in the community as long as possible. Therefore, aftercare and rehabilitation are essential parts of all service to mental patients, and the various methods of achieving rehabilitation should be integrated in all forms of services, among them day hospitals, night hospitals, aftercare clinics, public health nursing services, foster family care, convalescent nursing homes, rehabilitation centers, work services, and expatient groups.*

In 1963, the U.S. government appropriated $150 million to fund **community mental health centers** through the Mental Retardation Facilities and Community Mental Health Centers Construction Act (PL88-164; frequently referred to as the Community Mental Health Act). This money was to be matched by state funds over a three-year period and used for the construction of comprehensive community mental health centers. For states to qualify for federal funding, they were required to provide five essential services: inpatient care, outpatient care, partial hospitalization, emergency care, and consultation and education. Each center would continue to receive federal funding in decreasing amounts over an eight-year period. The expectation was that after eight years, financial support of the centers would come from state and local funds and fees generated from services offered. In 1965, federal funding was extended through 1968.

Before the system had a chance to get firmly established, while the available community resources were in the infancy stage of development, hospitals began to discharge large numbers of patients. Communities were unprepared to receive these patients—the system was fragile and incomplete. Financial support was lacking, housing and treatment facilities were scarce, and community attitudes were inhospitable to the patients who were discharged. Psychiatric patients were feared, mocked, generally misunderstood, and stigmatized for conditions that they had little or no control over. Proposals for housing facilities in residential neighborhoods met with outcries of indignation, alarm, and fear from residents. Communities felt that they had become "dumping grounds" for the large psychiatric hospitals. Patients, largely unwelcomed and rebuffed, found that life outside the hospital was frightening and unappealing. They found themselves caught up in a **revolving door cycle** of short inpatient stay, rapid discharge, and eventual repeat admissions. Attempts to smooth the transition from hospital to community were blocked by inadequate community resources. Many advocates for the rights of the mentally ill argued in the 1960s and even now that the needs of the chronically mentally ill were better served within the walls of the large state institutions (Case Example 43–1).

Case Example 43–1 Mary's Story

I had been working as a registered nurse in a state mental hospital for several years when the first community mental health center was constructed in my area. I was so excited—both for my patients and myself. I believed that this was a new opportunity for them as well as me. Many of the folks that I worked with seemed capable of functioning in the outside world. And for me, working in the community seemed to offer a chance to practice nursing the way I thought it should be done. It didn't take me long to get on the community bandwagon where I have been for many years. I was right about opportunity—but I never dreamed of all the roadblocks that had to be overcome. Community has more frustrations than I ever dreamed of. So many people are really ignorant about patients and treat them horribly. And there has never been enough resources—not just money—all resources are scarce. Yet in spite of this I still believe we need to care for people in the midst of our communities. Now I see myself as a crusader for the rights of the mental patient in the community. There are times when I think it's only my lone voice speaking out. But I'll keep doing it—probably as long as I'm able.

▶ Check Your Reading

1. Define institutionalization and deinstitutionalization.
2. What is meant by the revolving door cycle?

3. What happened legislatively in the 1960s that led to advent of community mental health care?
4. Why is community mental health care referred to as the third revolution in psychiatry?

Moving Forward in the 1970s

The funding for community mental health programs was extended once again in 1970. At this time, Congress, in response to the Joint Commission on the Mental Health of Children, which cited inadequate services for young people, specifically earmarked money to serve youth. In addition, funding was added for drug and alcohol services.

By 1975, the U.S. government amended its original 1963 law (Community Mental Health Center Amendment PL94-63) and specified that community mental health centers must provide 12 services to qualify for federal monies. In addition to the original five services, the following were required: specialized services for children and the elderly, screening, aftercare, transitional housing, drug abuse services, and alcoholism treatment (United States Congress, Public Law 94-63).

By the beginning of the 1970s, it was clear that there were real problems in the community mental health care movement. Among these problems was the fact that many states and local governments were not able to match federal funds. Other community mental health centers, located in rural or poverty-stricken areas, were unable to generate the necessary fees to be self-sufficient. Important services that generated little or no income, such as public education and consultation, began to suffer.

In 1977, President Jimmy Carter mandated a major reassessment of mental health needs. He established a 20-member President's Commission on Mental Health that included a nurse, Martha Mitchell, who was the Chairperson of the American Nurses' Association Division on Psychiatric and Mental Health Nursing Practice. In 1978, the *Report to the President of the President's Commission on Mental Health* was published and focused on strengthening the community mental health care system as the foundation for the mental health system. This would involve improving community support systems, continuing the phase-out of large public hospitals, establishing a center with a focus on primary prevention within the National Institute of Mental Health, and improving the delivery of services to underserved and high-risk populations. The report also advocated other major changes in the delivery of mental health care. These suggestions included

- Establishing national health insurance that included coverage for mental health.
- Encouraging private insurance carriers to include mental health coverage (including outpatient care) in their packages.
- Providing funding to increase the number of mental health professionals, especially those who work with children, elderly, and minorities.
- Developing advocacy programs for the chronically mentally ill.
- Protecting the rights of all persons in need of mental health services.
- Increasing support for research related to mental health and illness.
- Providing public health education to increase the public's understanding of mental health and illness.
- Centralizing the evaluation efforts of governmental agencies.

Hadley (1978) cited this commission and their report as the first official high-level document to recognize the professional contributions of nurses to mental health care.

Losing Ground in the 1980s

In 1980, the Community Mental Health Systems Act was passed. It was designed to implement the recommendations of the president's commission and to coordinate the two-tiered mental health system that had evolved since the original 1963 legislation that mandated the establishment of community mental health centers. The most severely disabled of the chronically mentally ill still resided within state institutions, and those less disabled used the services of the community mental health centers. There was virtually no coordination between these two systems. Consequently, patients "fell through the cracks" so to speak because of the lack of continuity and communication between the two tiers.

The programs authorized by this legislation were to be implemented in 1982, but before this could occur there was a significant retrenchment by the federal government in terms of its responsibilities in the area of mental health. The 97th Congress essentially repealed the 1980 Community Mental Health Systems Act with the passage of the Reagan administration's Omnibus Budget Reconciliation Act (PL97-35). This bill moved the authority and administration of mental health programs from the National Institute of Mental Health to the individual states. Each state received a block grant to cover alcohol, drug abuse, and mental health services. As of 1984, federal funding for community mental health care and other mental health care delivery programs was terminated. Community mental health centers are now mandated to provide only five essential services: outpatient care, partial hospitalization, 24-hour hospitalization and emergency care, consultation and education, and screening services. The continued existence of community mental health centers depends on state support, private funding, and ability to earn revenue.

▶ Check Your Reading

5. Cite two pieces of legislation in the 1970s that supported the community mental health care movement.
6. What are the five essential services that community mental health centers must provide?

7. How did the Omnibus Bill of 1980 affect community mental health?
8. How did former President Carter support the community mental health care movement?

Doing More with Less in the 1990s

It is clear as the 1990s continue to unfold that we can no longer rely on the federal government to provide more funding. The political climate seems to support "smaller" rather than "bigger" when it comes to programs directed to meeting human needs. With so many programs competing for limited funds, the challenge of the mental health care system is to realize the promise of community mental health care by doing more with less. The trend is to move increasingly toward managed care (Grob, 1994).

Drolen (1990) warns that community mental health care seems to be focusing on the importance of an "aggressive, entrepreneurial management style with an emphasis on efficiency and accountability" (p. 548). This emphasis traditionally occurs when resources decline. As Drolen points out, however, there is danger in this simplistic approach, especially when it is applied to human services organizations. When administration clamps down, work often suffers from poor morale, inflexibility, and increased tension among staff. Drolen (1990) suggests that when it is essential to husband resources, administrators would be wise to examine what factors facilitate an innovative climate.

THE POPULATION SERVED BY COMMUNITY MENTAL HEALTH CARE

Primarily, community mental health care serves the needs of the **chronically mentally ill,** also called the **seriously and persistently mentally ill.** Bachrach (1979) defined this group as follows: "Those individuals who are, have been, or might have been but for the deinstitutionalization movement on the rolls of the long-term mental institutions, especially state hospitals." The DSM-IV defines the chronically mentally ill as people who are continuously ill for two years.

Who Are the Chronically Mentally Ill?

The chronically mentally ill are a diverse group with a variety of diagnoses, including schizophrenia; major affective disorders; and organic disorders secondary to trauma, disease, or substance abuse. They include the chronically mentally ill elderly, who may reside independently with supportive family nearby or with a supportive network of caring people that might include the landlord, the mailman, the local grocer, and others who look out for the welfare of the individual (Buckwalter and Light, 1989). Some of the elderly chronically mentally ill live with family and friends; some live in supervised housing, such as foster care or nursing homes (Richter, 1990). Those individuals with schizophrenia may hold jobs in the community during periods when symptoms are in remission; those with residual symptoms that interfere with their functional capacity rely on disability checks and sporadic employment. They also may reside in foster or group homes. Some seek shelter in decrepit urban hotels, whereas others take to the street and end up in shelters for the homeless. Some of those with severe mental illness reside inappropriately in prisons. Many have complicating patterns of substance abuse. For some, substance abuse is a primary problem. For others, substance abuse may be an attempt to self-medicate to ease the pain of a difficult life (Bostelman et al, 1994; Conway et al, 1994).

The group of chronically mentally ill range in age from the very young, who have never experienced long-term institutionalization, to the very old, who suffer from deinstitutionalization. All experience problems of being emotionally and mentally disabled and must live with the stigma of mental illness. Sheets and coworkers (1982) identified three subgroups among the young chronically mentally ill, those from 18 to 30 years of age. There is a high-functioning group, a passively accepting (low energy, low demand) group, and those who actively deny that they have mental illness (high energy, high demand sub-group). Those who aggressively deny the reality of their illness have the most difficulty accepting any help, including supervised housing. They prefer the independence of hotels and the streets. Those who choose to live with limited interpersonal contact may withdraw, may neglect themselves, may stop taking their medications, and are especially vulnerable to exploitation of others. There has been reported success in working with these patients to persuade them to accept help within the community mental health care system, even to accepting residential living arrangements (Cutler, 1986). Table 43–1 provides a profile of the three subgroups of young adult chronically mentally ill patients. Case Example 43–2 illustrates the characteristics of a young adult chronically mentally ill patient.

Case Example 43–2 Sarah's Story

My name is Sarah. I've been sick for a long time. I have been in every big mental hospital in my state. Once I ran away and I was put in a hospital in another state. My family came and got me. They put me on medication that I don't like and give me shock treatments. Sometimes I think I'm a human guinea pig. I'm living in a hotel now. My family don't see me too much—I think they feel fed up with me. But I do okay. Sometimes I go to the shelter for meals. Sometimes I don't eat. I go to the clinic for a shot of Prolixin [fluphenazine] every two weeks. I hate it, but I hate being in the big hospitals more. I have some friends. We hang out on the streets. Sometimes we drink together. Sometimes the police pick us up for being noisy. But I think they pick us up because they know we're crazy.

TABLE 43–1 **Profile of the Three Subgroups of Young Adult Chronically Mentally Ill Patients**

Low-Energy, Low-Demand Subgroup	High-Energy, High-Demand Subgroup	High-Functioning Subgroup
Sees self as patient	Chooses agency to get what they want	Generally higher socioeconomic status and better appearance
Does poorly, even in remission	Functional abilities and interests fluctuate	New to mental health system
Becomes attached to program and program locations	"Give me what I want or stay out of my life" attitude toward mental health system	Resists mental health involvement; wants control over life
Probably became a patient in adolescence	Low frustration tolerance, acting out, encounters with the law	Interested in learning about disorders and ways to stay well
Passive, poorly motivated	Frequently evicted, mobile	Wants to avoid being identified as a mental patient
Accepts mental health services	Expects to be self-reliant	
Appears burned out at an early age	Includes revolving door people and street people	

▶ **Check Your Reading**

9. What are the characteristics of the chronically mentally ill?
10. List two types of housing used by the chronically mentally ill?.
11. How are the young chronically mentally ill different from those that are elderly?
12. What is another name for the chronically mentally ill?

What Are the Needs of the Chronically Mentally Ill?

Krauss (1980) identified a number of needs for which the chronically mentally ill require care:

- Basic life necessities
- A sense that life is meaningful
- Access to medications
- Support for family members
- Integrated nursing, medical, and social services

Each of these is discussed.

Basic Life Necessities. Included in basic life necessities are items such as food, clothing, both permanent and temporary housing, income maintenance, health care, and legal protection. Many of the chronically mentally ill are without these basic items.

A Sense That Life Is Meaningful. A sense that life is meaningful is an essential need for community adjustment, yet it is often denied to the patient because they are discriminated against in their efforts to obtain employment as well as participate in recreational and other social activities. A sense that life is meaningful can be met through social and vocational rehabilitation that allows them to be employed in a gainful occupation (Birks, 1987).

Resocialization and sheltered workshops also provide for time structuring and meaningful activities (Janssen and Giberson, 1988). Leisure and recreational activities are important to provide a healthy balance in life. Spiritual activities allow patients to connect not only with their God, but also with the meaning of their own lives in a broader context. Participation in peer support and former-patient groups also provides patients with the sense that their own suffering makes some sort of sense. As they are able to draw from their experiences to assist others similarly afflicted, they may be able to make sense out of life. Box 43–1 shows the five basic steps of **remotivation therapy.** Box 43–2 illustrates a sample session of remotivation therapy.

Access to Medication. Access to medication is essential. This includes not only availability of reasonably priced medications, but also ongoing support for motivation to comply with the medication regimen, continual reassessment of dosage requirements and side effects, and active coordination with other aspects of treatment (Soumerai et al, 1994).

Support for Family Members. Support for family members is critical in maintaining an important element of the patient's support network. The burden of caregiving on the family can be quite high (Adams, 1994). They benefit tremendously from encouragement, affirmation, education about their loved one's illness, and a collaborative attitude on the part of care providers that values and considers their opinions regarding what is in the best interests of the patient.

Integrated Nursing, Medical, and Social Services. Integrated nursing, medical, and social services are a tremendous need for the chronically mentally ill. For the

BOX 43-1 Five Basic Steps of Remotivation Therapy

Step 1: Climate of acceptance (approximately 5 minutes)
Purpose: To provide a nonthreatening atmosphere in which the leader and participants can establish relationships and feel relaxed.

Step 2: Creating a bridge to reality (approximately 15 minutes)
Purpose: To create a bridge to reality by presenting poetry or songs to the group that would apply to the theme of the session topic. This step should help to stimulate the patients to think of realistic topics that they may want to share with the group.

Step 3: Sharing the world we live in (approximately 15 minutes)
Purpose: This step should further develop the topic of the remotivation session. Group discussion should be stimulated through the use of visual/audio aids and other physical props. Stimulation of the clients' senses should be promoted during this step by having them see, hear, touch, or taste something objective in the world.

Step 4: An appreciation of the work of the world (approximately 20 minutes)
Purpose: This step in remotivation encourages the clients to think about work in the world as it relates to the topic of discussion. Work in the world discussions also attempt to promote individual discussions about their past job experiences. Practical application of a job-related task may be encouraged for each individual.

Step 5: Climate of appreciation (approximately 5 minutes)
Purpose: This step terminates the group session. Each member is given appreciation for participating in the group. Anticipation for the next meeting is generated.

From Janssen, J. A., and Giberson, D. L. (1988). Remotivation therapy. *Journal of Gerontological Nursing, 34* (6), 31–34.

BOX 43-2 Sample Session of Remotivation Therapy

Theme for Session 4: Bodies of Water

Step 1: Climate of acceptance
On arrival to the group, the leaders personally welcomed each participant. After the leaders introduced themselves, each group member made a self-introduction. The leader used a calendar to orient the members to the date and time of the current remotivation session. The theme for session 4 was introduced by the leader as "bodies of water—rivers, lakes, and oceans." All group members had some familiarity with bodies of water because of their residence in Seattle.

Step 2: Creating a bridge to reality
The world globe was used as a visual aid to stimulate discussion on bodies of water. The leader asked questions, for example, "How are bodies of water formed from glaciers?" Pictures of glaciers, rivers, and lakes were shown.

The leaders read poems about tide pools, sea shells, and fishing written by anonymous grade school children. Discussion was stimulated by the leader asking, "What can we do at the ocean?" Visual aids and physical props were provided for direct sensory stimulation. Some examples of these aids and props included (a) different types of sea shells, (b) fishing tackle and bait, (c) suntan lotion, (d) sunning hat, and (e) sunglasses.

A poem by an anonymous author about fishing was read to the group. This was followed by recorded music with lyrics about fishing experiences.

Step 3: Sharing the world we live in
Group discussion focused on jobs related to bodies of water. Topics participants discussed in regard to self or others included crabbing, clamming, shrimping, and fishing. Visual aids were provided to stimulate further discussions on past related experiences involving bodies of water. Pictures of river-rafting, canoeing, scuba diving, and sailing were shared.

Step 4: An appreciation of the work of the world
This time was used for the members to think about work in relation to others. More experiences in past related work roles were discussed as well as hobbies and pastimes. The group then participated in singing a familiar, oldstanding song, "Love Letters in the Sand," written in 1931 by J. Fred Coots and revived in 1957 when sung by Pat Boone.

Step 5: Climate of appreciation
The group members were thanked individually by the leaders for coming to the group and sharing their experiences. The following remotivation session theme and meeting date were announced before terminating the session.

Group Response to Session 4
Most members of the group appeared to enjoy discussing their experiences in relation to bodies of water. Many members recalled fishing and boating experiences. Other members expressed interest in this topic by their nonverbal participation in touching and smelling some physical props and observation of visual aids. All but two participants touched the sea shells and smelled the fish eggs. One lady in the group stood up and modeled the sunning hat and glasses, while a man demonstrated how to reel in line on a fishing pole. Several participants remarked on how beautiful the pictures of the glaciers were. All but a couple of group members sang to the recorded lyrics on fishing. One member stood up and danced to the music, while many others clapped to her movements.

From Janssen, J. A., and Giberson, D. L. (1988). Remotivation therapy. *Journal of Gerontological Nursing, 34* (6), 31–34.

chronically mentally ill to negotiate the maze of services necessary to facilitate community tenure, the system must do all that it can to facilitate this process. The intent is not to see how clever the patient is in negotiating the crooked path of a cumbersome bureaucracy but to make the path of care so clear that patients do not become frustrated before they even attempt the journey.

Additional Needs. In addition to the needs identified by Krauss, chronically mentally ill patients have a great need for care, concern, and acceptance for who they are and at whatever their level of functioning is (Chafetz, 1988; Krauss, 1989b; Dalgard et al, 1995). This means that care providers must be cognizant of the nature of chronicity, which is characterized by exacerbations and remissions, periods of apparent equanimity punctuated by major setbacks (Beebe, 1990). This awareness must translate into patience, gentle encouragement, a willingness to help the patient pick the pieces up and begin again, and an acceptance that the patient's level of functioning may be very impaired. Appropriate goals and interventions must begin where the patient is "at" and not where the care provider wishes the patient to be (Case Example 43–3).

Case Example 43–3 Amanda's Story

Amanda had been in and out of mental hospitals for years. For a short time, she lived with her sister, a situation that caused Amanda great anxiety. When Amanda was anxious, she made a strange barking noise that made her sound like a seal. She also focused on strange somatic complaints, like having "pus run down my throat." While at her sister's house, Amanda became completely nonfunctional, staying in bed all the time and finding it impossible to communicate without making the "seal" sound. The sister's tolerance for this behavior wore down, and she placed Amanda in a boarding home. Amanda received psychiatric follow-up at a community mental health center. When she was initially placed in the boarding home her nurse therapist worked with the care provider to establish appropriate goals for Amanda's care. It was clear that one of Amanda's needs was for increased diversional activities. Yet her level of functioning was so low that any aggressive effort to involve her in diversional activities precipitated her barking noises and somatic complaints. It was clear that Amanda was very anxious and that she coped with her anxiety by retreating. The nurse helped the care provider arrive at a plan that seemed a bit unorthodox. Instead of focusing on keeping Amanda out of bed, the care provider gave her permission to go back to bed when she felt the need to do so. Amanda was required to tend to her personal needs and join the other residents for meals. After about a week, Amanda stopped making the barking noises. Receiving permission to retreat from others when she felt the need seemed to lessen her anxiety and allowed her to interact even more, but more at her own speed.

Certainly it is not possible for one service to meet all of these needs. In fact, many of these needs may have to be coordinated by the community mental health nurse who assists the patient in accessing a network of both professional and natural helpers. The professional helpers might include the following:

- Public welfare agencies
- A general hospital
- Mental health centers
- Courts
- Schools
- Churches
- Charitable organizations
- Child guidance centers
- Nursing homes
- Social service organizations
- Emergency/crisis services

The natural informal helpers might include the following:

- Family
- Friends
- Neighbors
- Neighborhood organizations
- Voluntary organizations
- Self-help groups
- Clergy
- Teachers
- Police
- Pharmacists
- Gas and electric person
- Landlord
- Anyone else who is interested and able to assist the patient

▶ Check Your Reading

13. What are the five needs of the chronically mentally ill?
14. Give one example of the need for access to medications; to housing.
15. Name at least three professional helpers and three natural helpers.
16. Provide a rationale for family support as one of the needs of the chronically mentally ill.

THE PHILOSOPHY OF COMMUNITY MENTAL HEALTH CARE

A Focus on the Community and on the Individual

The philosophy of community mental health care contains a two-pronged focus. The first is to consider the community as patient and attempt to ameliorate situations in the community that detract from optimal mental health and could conceivably lead to mental illness. This focus results in educational and consultation programs.

The second focus is to consider the individual within the community as patient. To serve the individual, a full range of comprehensive services are provided. These include

- Outpatient care.
- Partial hospitalization.
- 24-hour hospitalization and emergency care.
- Screening services.

Other services may also be available, including those designed to meet the needs of children, adolescents, and elderly; alcohol and drug abuse services; and transitional services.

The community is defined in terms of a **catchment area,** which is a city or several rural communities whose total population ranges from 75,000 to 200,000 residents. The intent of this approach is to divide the larger population into manageable segments for the delivery of mental health services. Ideally the system is small enough to allow collaboration among the components of the system.

Care That Is Continuous and Comprehensive

The stated goals of community mental health care are to provide care that is continuous and comprehensive. In an editorial written by Krauss (1989a), she argues that of all the disciplines involved in community mental health care, the nurse is the best prepared to offer to the chronically mentally ill the "c's" of:

Care
Comprehensiveness
Continuity

Krauss (1989a) asserts that nursing is prepared to care "through the power of privileged intimacy and with the authority of our roles as clinician, teacher, advocate, and reformer of the health care system" (p. 59).

The goal of providing care that is continuous means that if patients are receiving care from different parts of the system, the providers are assuming responsibility for monitoring that care and assisting the patient in moving through the system. Ideally, there is a communication interface between programs so that patients do not feel that they are left to fend for themselves but rather that the road has been paved for them as they obtain a variety of needed services. Moving through the system should be smooth and appear seamless. Unfortunately, community mental health care has a long way to go before realizing the goal of providing continuity of care.

The goal of providing comprehensive care recognizes that the population of chronically mentally ill have complex and multifaceted medical, nursing, and social needs, and each of these needs must be met in an integrated approach that is continually mindful of the holistic nature of the individual patient.

▶ Check Your Reading

17. Define catchment area.
18. List two goals of community mental health care.
19. What is the two-pronged focus in community mental health care?
20. List at least three services that must be available to provide comprehensive care to the individual.

THE SERVICES PROVIDED IN COMMUNITY MENTAL HEALTH CARE

A variety of services are made available to patients as part of community mental health care. Not all of these services are available in every community.

Types of Community Mental Health Services

Community Mental Health Centers. These centers are staffed by a variety of mental health professionals who provide individual, group, and family therapy to community residents. These services may be offered by a psychiatric nurse, a social worker, a psychologist, a mental health paraprofessional, or a psychiatrist.

Alternative Living Arrangements. These arangements vary from the least restrictive to very restrictive. An example of an arrangement with little restrictions is a family placement. Some patients reside in **single-room occupancy**, in which they rent a room from a landlord. In this arrangement, they may share meals with other residents in the house, or they make seek food at restaurants, soup kitchens, and shelters. **Sheltered housing** or **congregate housing** also allows the patient a good deal of freedom. In this arrangement, the patient has a separate apartment and receives support in meal preparation, housekeeping chores, and errands. Other patients may need closer supervision and require placement in a group home or a foster care home. Still others requiring 24-hour supervision and skilled nursing care may need a nursing home environment. Ideally the housing placement takes into consideration patients' strengths and abilities for independent living, their ability to live safely, their ability to make decisions in their own best interest, and their requirement for supervision, and matches them with housing that allows them to be in a safe, healthy environment in which maximum independence is possible.

Support Groups. These groups are self-help groups whose focus is to assist individuals, families, or communities. Their purpose may be to help individuals maintain their health, such as Alcoholics Anonymous or Narcotics Anonymous. Others provide support to individuals and families who are dealing with a particular stress, such as the groups for families of AIDS patients. Some groups such as "Seasons"—a Support Group for the Survivors of Suicide actually help restore mental health by bringing people together who have suffered similar tragedies. Groups exist whose primary focus is to reform the mental health system. These groups are frequently composed of former patients, their family members, and mental health professionals. Other groups define their goals to change a particular aspect of community life. An example of this type of group is Mothers Against Drunk Drivers (MADD).

Day Treatment Centers. **Day treatment** centers are set up to provide for meaningful social interaction, time structuring, and participation in recreational and learning activities to individuals who might otherwise be isolated or who lack the ability to structure their time independently. The day treatment centers also provide respite for family care providers who benefit by having their loved one go to another facility to spend a portion of their time.

Mobile Treatment Teams. **Mobile treatment units** consist of teams of professionals who go into the community to provide care. This type of service is appropriate for patients who are unable to comply with clinic appointments and medication regimens as well as for crisis intervention (see Chapter 15). The treatment is basically delivered to the patient where they reside. This approach requires familiarity with the patient's usual patterns of behavior, a willingness to track patients who may not be in their residence but instead be in a favorite neighborhood haunt, and a flexible approach on the part of the provider.

Community Services. These are services that contribute to the mental health of a community. They may include direct intervention with an individual, such as a rape crisis center or Meals-on-Wheels. The focus may be on the family, as in family recreation centers; day care centers for children, the disabled, and the elderly; or shelters for victims of domestic violence. The community itself may be the focus of a group. The police and fire departments, public parks, social service departments, and educational groups are all examples of groups that serve the needs of the entire community (Case Example 43–4).

Case Example 43–4 William's Story

William, an elderly man diagnosed with chronic schizophrenia, missed his clinic appointments on a regular basis. In fact, the only thing that the staff could depend on about William was that he was usually not compliant with appointments or medication. After many hospitalizations, William was referred to the mobile treatment team. One of the nurses would track him down in his neighborhood. His favorite "hangout" was a social club for men down the street from William's boarding home. Usually when the nurse found William he would be laughing, happy, and generally enjoying life—always apologetic that the nurse had to come find him. But once he was found, William was more than willing to step into a backroom in the social club and get his injection of Prolixin. By many people's standards, William was irresponsible and barely functional. But a successful plan of treatment had been developed that accommodated William's lifestyle and provided interventions that were useful to him.

▶ Check Your Reading

21. What is congregate housing?
22. What is a single-room occupancy?
23. List two examples of support groups.
24. What is a mobile treatment team?

Providers of Community Mental Health Services

A variety of health care professionals deliver care within the community. These include community mental health nurses, psychiatrists, psychologists, social workers, recreational and physical therapists, and pharmacists. In addition, the patient may receive care from mental health paraprofessionals who lack academic preparation but have life experiences, good interpersonal and communication skills, and common sense to draw on. These workers may be supervised by a mental health professional such as the nurse. The patient may also interact with government workers, religious leaders, educators, and a variety of others who in some way support the patient. Family members, neighbors, and employers often play crucial roles in the patient's ability to do well within the community.

THE ROLE OF NURSING IN COMMUNITY MENTAL HEALTH CARE

Nurses with various levels of academic preparation, ranging from diploma or associate degree all the way to doctorate, practice within the community setting. Professional responsibilities are directly influenced by education, experience, licensure, and certification (Berns and Hamilton, 1981).

Focus on Prevention

The principles of primary, secondary, and tertiary prevention are essential to community psychiatric work. These three principles provide direction for interventions carried out by nurses within the community setting.

Primary Prevention

In **primary prevention,** the nurse focuses on preventing new occurrences of mental illness. To implement this role, the nurse develops interventions and programs that eliminate stresses that lead to or aggravate existing mental disorders. Examples include the following:

- Teaching parenting and sibling classes to assist new parents with a new or expanding family.
- Offering support to self-help groups.
- Providing mental health consultation to schools, businesses, and other community agencies.
- Advocating within the political arena for the rights of the mentally ill.

Box 43–3 describes a number of suicide prevention programs in which psychiatric nurses play an important role in primary prevention.

Secondary Prevention

Secondary prevention involves treatment of a diagnosed disorder within a given individual and case finding and referrals to decrease the incidence of mental disorders. Nursing interventions that exemplify secondary prevention include the following:

- Psychotherapy for individuals, families, and groups.
- Crisis intervention, including hotline counseling.
- Emergency mental health services.
- Counseling for women who have been raped.
- Support for victims of violence.

Tertiary Prevention

Tertiary prevention involves rehabilitative services for patients who have been diagnosed with a mental disorder. Discharge planning is an example of a nursing intervention directed at tertiary prevention. Assisting the patient in making the transition between hospital and place of residence is another. Still others include making appropriate referrals to aftercare services or self-help groups, teaching patients about medication management, and acting as a patient's advocate.

BOX 43–3 Suicide Prevention Programs in Which Psychiatric Nurses Play an Important Role in Primary Prevention

- *The Adolescent Suicide Awareness Program* in New Jersey provides a continuous program focusing on intervention with school staff, parents, and students. The program is coordinated by the community mental health center and the school. The focus is on increasing awareness among teachers, parents, and students regarding depression, suicide warning signs, methods of helping the suicidal person, and community referral resources.
- *The Fairfax County (VA) Public Schools* developed a program with help of school staff, nurses, social workers, guidance counselors, and school psychologists. Parents, police, and other mental health professionals have also been involved. The program involves teacher training, parent education, and student support.
- *The Cherry Creek (Colorado) Schools* provide crisis training for school psychologists, nurses, counselors, and social workers. Parents, teachers, and other school personnel are taught to recognize students at risk. The school curriculum includes a suicide prevention component.
- *The San Mateo (California) Schools* make resources available to high-risk students. Teachers, nurses, and counselors are trained to identify and intervene with adolescent depression and suicidal behavior. Student programs include an educational component, workshops, and peer counseling.

Information from Puskar, K., Lamb, J., and Norton, M. (1990). Adolescent mental health: Collaboration among psychiatric mental health nurses and school nurses. *Journal of School Health, 60* (2), 69–71.

▶ Check Your Reading

25. Define primary prevention; give an example.
26. Define secondary prevention; give an example.
27. Define tertiary prevention; give an example.
28. What type of intervention is a crisis hotline?

Use of the Nursing Process

Although there are many mental health professionals who may work with a patient, the nurse occupies a unique position. Traditionally, nursing has concerned itself with the needs of the downtrodden, the underdogs, the forsaken of society. Certainly the chronically mentally ill fit this description. Nursing possesses a holistic view that recognizes the interaction among body, mind, and spirit and focuses on the nurse-patient relationship as the vehicle through which change occurs. In addition to focus on the individual, nurses possess skills related to effective community work as well as family intervention. They are accustomed to interfacing with a variety of disciplines, and according to Worley and Albanese (1989), nurses probably have the greatest ease and skill at crossing boundaries between lay and professional groups and marshalling resources. Nurses are oriented to assisting patients to move from a dependent state to a relatively independent state of self-care (Morrison et al, 1985). These skills are essential to assisting the chronically mentally ill to meet the multifaceted problems and needs that they confront.

In community mental health care, as in other areas of nursing, you rely on the nursing process to gain an understanding of the patient, to diagnose the patient's needs, to determine appropriate outcomes, to plan effective and appropriate interventions, and to evaluate the results of the interventions. The one area that sets community mental health care apart is that sometimes the patient is an individual or family, and sometimes the patient is the community. The following discussion leads you through the application of the nursing process in the community setting.

NURSING PROCESS: COMMUNITY AS PATIENT

ASSESSMENT

You may focus a community assessment in a number of different ways. For instance, you might be interested in gauging community acceptance of a mental health initiative. The following questions are appropriate to this type of assessment:

- Do you believe that former patients of mental hospitals are able to function well in your community?
- Would you have any objections if an organization that you belonged to accepted a former mental patient as a member?
- What would your feelings be if a former mental patient moved next door to you?
- Do you think you could ever become friends with a former mental patient?
- What would your feelings be about having a halfway house for mentally ill people located in your neighborhood? Next door to you?
- Would you offer a former mental patient assistance in obtaining a job at your place of employment?
- Do you think you would participate or support in some other way programs in your neighborhood designed to help the mentally ill person?

DIAGNOSIS

The analysis of these answers leads to nursing diagnoses for the community, such as

- Knowledge Deficit related to lack of understanding of the characteristics of the chronically mentally ill.
- Anxiety related to misinformation about the chronically mentally ill.
- Ineffective Community Coping related to the high stress level associated with perceptions of the chronically mentally ill.

OUTCOME IDENTIFICATION

The expected outcomes for a community might be

- After presentation of educational talks and materials, a random posttest of the community will show significantly greater understanding of the characteristics of the chronically mentally ill.
- The response to the posttest questions measuring affective and attitudinal issues will show a significant change toward greater acceptance and more positive feelings.
- Plans for the development and enhancement of existing resources and programs to meet the needs of the chronically mentally ill will come from the community.

PLANNING

The plan that is developed to achieve these expected outcomes might rely heavily on education. The nurse, as program coordinator, might target public forums such as schools, clinics, churches, and neighborhood recreation centers and health fairs as sites to begin education of the community. Possible short-term goals for such a plan might include the following:

Expected Outcome	Short-Term Goals
1. After presentation of educational talks and materials, a random posttest of the community will show significantly greater understanding of the characteristics of the chronically mentally ill.	Community members will participate in a variety of educational programs offered throughout the community. Community members will take a pre-posttest to measure their level of knowledge about the chronically mentally ill.
2. The response to the posttest questions measuring affective and attitudinal issues will show a significant change toward greater acceptance and more positive feelings.	Community members will take a pre-posttest to measure their attitudes toward the chronically mentally ill.

3. Plans for the development and enhancement of existing resources and programs to meet the needs of the chronically mentally ill will come from the community.	Community members will participate in small focus groups to identify existing resources and programs within their community. Community members will participate in small focus groups to plan what resources are needed to support the chronically mentally ill. Community members will participate in small focus groups to plan how to develop the needed resources and programs to support the chronically mentally ill.

IMPLEMENTATION

The interventions to support this plan might include

- Developing a brochure outlining the achievements of many who are chronically mentally ill.
- Developing a slide and lecture presentation depicting the mentally ill in productive occupations contributing to the health of the community.
- Focusing on the spiritual benefits of caring for and being tolerant of those who are less fortunate than ourselves.
- Explaining the economic benefits that a community receives when it cares for its own and does not send the mentally ill off to a state institution.

The interventions are limited only by the creativity and resources of those presenting such an educational program.

EVALUATION

A project of this magnitude requires ongoing or formative evaluation. Issues that must be evaluated include but are not limited to the following:

- Is the community assessment comprehensive enough? Are there areas that have not been explored?
- Is the planned teaching approach at an appropriate level for the community?
- Are the teaching materials effective?
- Are facilities available to offer the programs?
- Are community members adequately informed regarding the upcoming educational programs?

The summative evaluation of this particular approach is specified in the objectives. There are other ways, however, to gauge effectiveness of a program. For instance, if a halfway house opened in a particular neighborhood, observations about how former patients were treated when they went for walks and frequented stores and other neighborhood establishments would be subjective data to support or refute the success of a community-based intervention.

In addition to using the nursing process to help a community become more accepting of the chronically mentally ill, you might be interested in assessing the presence of a particular community need, such as dealing with substance abuse (Wetherill et al, 1987). Such data would form the basis of future community programs. Case Example 43–5 demonstrates how a psychiatric nurse, Britt Finley, used the nursing process in the development of a community substance abuse prevention program in Montana.

Case Example 43–5 Britt Finley's Story

Psychiatric nurse Britt Finley sought to develop a community substance abuse prevention program in Montana. She used the nursing process to develop a program that tackled alcohol abuse on several fronts simultaneously: schools, law enforcement agencies, parents, and health professionals.

To develop the program, Finley began by conducting a thorough *assessment*. She examined statistics related to the consumption of alcoholic substances in the community then compared the data to national norms from several sources, including the Centers for Disease Control.

In the *diagnosis* step, Finley analyzed the data and came to the conclusion that the community was at substantial risk for health-related problems stemming from alcohol abuse. Finley therefore identified the following nursing diagnosis:

> Ineffective Community Coping related to excessive consumption of alcoholic substances as evidenced by statistics demonstrating an incidence higher than the national norm for alcohol-related illnesses and alcohol-related accidents.

The *outcome identification* step yielded the following expected outcome:

> There will be evidence of a significant decrease in the purchase and consumption of alcoholic substances.

The *planning* step involved the participation of community leaders, who devised short-term goals. Those goals included:

- Parents, teachers, and students will be educated about alcohol.
- Chapters of Alcoholics Anonymous and Students Against Drunk Driving will be established.

- Police will consistently enforce the minimum drinking age of 19 years of age.
- The drinking age will be increased.
- A statewide school policy will be instituted prohibiting drinking at extracurricular functions.
- Employee assistance programs will be established at major employment sites.
- In-service educational sessions will be provided for nursing and medical personnel to increase awareness of the problem.

In the *implementation* step, Finley used the following interventions: networking with concerned people, "spreading the word" about the dangers of alcohol, and widening the scope of people who were involved in making a commitment to the problem.

The *evaluation* step involved the use of a number of different approaches, including the following:

- Surveying grade school and high school teachers to determine their perceptions of the extent of the problem.
- Examining statistics on alcohol-related traffic injuries.
- Examining student drinking patterns.

By each of these measures, the efficacy of the program was clear.

Information from Finley, B. (1989). The role of the psychiatric nurse in a community substance abuse prevention program. *Nursing Clinics of North America, 24* (4), 121–136.

▶ Check Your Reading

29. Give three examples of questions that could be used to assess a community's acceptance of a mental health initiative.
30. Give an example of a nursing diagnosis that might be applicable to a community preparing for a mental health initiative.
31. Cite one expected outcome for a community preparing for a mental health initiative.
32. Cite at least two strategies that might be used in working with a community to prepare the community for a mental health initiative.

NURSING PROCESS: INDIVIDUAL OR FAMILY AS PATIENT

ASSESSMENT

To assess the individual or family within the community, examine how well the patient's basic needs are being met. As we saw earlier, the basic needs of the chronically mentally ill include basic life necessities; a sense that life is meaningful; access to medication; support for family members; integrated nursing, medical, and social services; and other needs. By observing and interviewing, you can assess how well each of these needs is being met (Table 43–2).

DIAGNOSIS

Based on the results of the assessment, analyze the data and identify appropriate nursing diagnoses for problems in each basic community need. Possible nursing diagnoses for the person with problems in the area of *basic life necessities* are as follows:

- Bathing/Hygiene Self-Care Deficit related to low level of motivation.
- Altered Nutrition: Less than Body Requirements related to homelessness.
- Sleep Pattern Disturbance related to unstable living arrangements.
- Dressing/Grooming Self-Care Deficit related to low level of motivation.

Possible nursing diagnoses for the person with a deficient *sense that life is meaningful* are as follows:

- Spiritual Distress related to conflict about God's role in permitting illness.
- Diversional Activity Deficit related to inability to structure time.
- Social Isolation related to lack of social skills.

Nursing diagnoses for the person with problems of *access to medication* might be as follows:

- Knowledge Deficit related to effects of medication, side effects of medication, and how to obtain financial aid to purchase medications.
- Noncompliance related to taking medication as prescribed.

Nursing diagnoses for the person with problems in relation to *support for family members* might be as follows:

- Altered Thought Processes related to noncompliance with antipsychotic medication regimen.
- Self-Concept Deficit: Chronic Low Self-Esteem related to repeated rejections by family, friends, and acquaintances.
- Coping: Ineffective Individual related to changes in living arrangements, interpersonal difficulties, and the stress of daily living.

TABLE 43–2 **Assessment of the Chronically Mentally Ill Individual or Family**

Basic Need	Observation	Interview
Basic life necessities: areas such as nutrition, clothing, temporary and permanent housing, income, legal protection, and health care	The extent to which the patient is able to perform basic hygiene and activities of daily living Level of energy and motivation General assessment of health status	What arrangements have you made to obtain daily meals? Describe a typical day's diet. Tell me about the place where you live. Who manages your living quarters? Cleaning? Laundry? What arrangements have you made to handle money? What is your source of income? How do you pay bills? Where do you go to see a doctor? What kind of doctor do you usually see? What symptoms make you go to see a doctor? Do you work? Tell me about your job. The people you work with. Your boss.
A sense that life is meaningful: areas such as structuring of time, diversional activities, a sense of purpose, support system, use of spiritual resources	The extent to which the patient can structure time, plan activities that she enjoys The degree of social isolation (use the nurse-patient relationship as a barometer of the patient's social competence) Verbalizations that indicate either hopelessness and a sense of despair or a feeling that life has some purpose Verbalizations that indicate that the patient is engaging in some enjoyable or purposeful activities	How do you spend your time every day? Do you think what you do makes a difference to anyone else? Do you think that you matter to anyone else? Tell me about something you do that gives you pleasure. What kind of spiritual or religious activities do you participate in? Does anyone depend on you? If so, tell me about that relationship. Do you work? What do you do?
Access to medication: whether the patient is on medication, what kind of medication, the presence of side effects, the patient's knowledge of the drug, the availability of the drug, compliance with the medication regimen	The extent to which the patient's behavior indicates effectiveness of the drug The extent to which the patient's behavior indicates the presence of side effects The number of doses left of the drug; does this correspond with the amount that should be remaining if the patient were compliant? Verbalizations that indicate an appropriate degree of understanding and compliance	Tell me about the medications you are taking. What are they? When are you supposed to take them? How much are you supposed to take? What effect does the medication have on you? Describe any problems you have run into while taking this medication. Tell me about the side effects of the medication. Are there any precautions you should be aware of when taking this medication? Are you attending the medication clinic? Where do you get your prescriptions filled? Do you have any difficulties with getting the prescriptions filled?

Table continued on following page

Nursing diagnoses for the person with needs for *integrated nursing, medical, and social services* might be as follows:

- Anxiety related to inability to negotiate the community mental health system.
- Decisional Conflict related to which health-related services to access.
- Knowledge Deficit related to how to access transportation to the clinic.

TABLE 43–2 **Assessment of the Chronically Mentally Ill Individual or Family** *Continued*

Basic Need	Observation	Interview
Support for family members: areas that are indicative of the patient's ego functioning, sense of self-esteem, and interpersonal relationships; the family's needs related to coping with the patient	The patient's general affect: does the patient appear depressed, angry, anxious?	Do you feel that you are "together"? If not, how do you feel?
	Verbalizations that indicate that the patient "feels bad" about himself	How would you describe your adjustment in the community? Boarding home? Family's home?
	Verbalizations that indicate fear of making decisions	Do you feel satisfied with the progress you are making? If not, tell me what you would like to change.
	Verbalizations that indicate interpersonal problems	Tell me about the people you spend your time with. What kind of relationships do you have? Are you satisfied with them? If not, what would you change?
	Family member's affect and general response to the patient; does the family member appear angry or "fed up"? Does the family member act impatient or disdainful toward the patient?	What problems are you (family member) experiencing on a day-to-day basis with . . . . ?
		Are you (family member) able to arrange time away from the patient so that you get a break?
		How do you help the patient to feel that she is okay?
Integrated nursing, medical, and social services: needs for community services, availability of a support person to assist with transportation and other needs	The extent to which the patient is able to access community services independently	Who helps you to make appointments and get to them?
	Behaviors that indicate that other services are needed (e.g., Alcoholics Anonymous and adult day care)	What community service do you use in addition to this clinic?
	Verbalizations indicative of a patient's sense of being overwhelmed in attempts to negotiate the health care and social service system	How would you go about getting information about . . . (whatever community service is needed)?
		What would you think if I made a referral to . . . . ?
		What do you know about . . . (appropriate community resources)?
		Who assists you in dealing with . . . (e.g., medical assistance, renewal of your pharmacy assistance card, access to other social programs)?
		Are you (family member) involved in any type of community support groups?

OUTCOME IDENTIFICATION

The expected outcomes for an individual or family receiving community mental health care for problems with *basic life necessities* might be as follows:

- The patient will demonstrate appropriate bathing and hygiene skills by the end of the fourth week.
- The patient will access sheltered housing within one week.
- The patient will sleep at least seven hours a night within two weeks.
- The patient will eat three meals a day by the end of one week.

The expected outcomes for a patient with a deficient *sense that life is meaningful* might be as follows:

- The patient will discuss spiritual conflicts with nurse therapist and be able to come to resolution on this issue.

- The patient will attend an adult day care center at least three times a week.
- The patient will demonstrate appropriate ways to initiate a conversation within three weeks.

The expected outcomes for a patient with problems of *access to medication* might be as follows:

- The patient will be knowledgeable about his or her medications.
- The patient will take all medications as prescribed within two weeks.

The expected outcomes for a patient needing *support for family members* might be as follows:

- The patient will verbalize at least one positive quality about self by the end of the third week of therapy.
- The patient will demonstrate that he or she has learned new responses for coping with interpersonal conflict.
- The patient will demonstrate deep breathing exercises as a means of dealing with situational stress.

For the patient needing *integrated nursing, social, and medical services,* expected outcomes might be as follows:

- The patient will use the available support system to access health care appointments.
- The patient will demonstrate the ability to make appropriate appointments and follow through with those appointments.

PLANNING

During the planning step, identify short-term goals aimed at achieving the expected outcomes that you identified previously. For the patient with problems with *basic life necessities,* short-term goals might be as follows:

Expected Outcome	Short-Term Goals
The patient will demonstrate appropriate bathing and hygiene skills by the end of the fourth week.	1. The patient will talk about reasons for not bathing and taking care of self. 2. The patient will state at least three benefits that accompany bathing and good hygiene. 3. The patient will wash his or her clothes. 4. The patient will brush his or her teeth. 5. The patient will bathe.
The patient will access sheltered housing within one week.	1. The patient will state the benefits of being in sheltered housing. 2. The patient will complete an application to enter sheltered housing.
The patient will sleep at least seven hours a night within two weeks.	1. The patient will state three strategies to facilitate a good night's rest. 2. The patient will use at least one of newly acquired skills before going to sleep.
The patient will eat three meals a day by the end of one week.	1. The patient will state the benefits of eating a balanced diet. 2. The patient will state two resources where he or she can obtain a healthy diet.

For the patient with a deficient *sense that life is meaningful,* short-term goals might be as follows:

Expected Outcome	Short-Term Goals
The patient will discuss spiritual conflicts with the nurse therapist and be able to come to resolution on this issue.	1. The patient will talk about his or her spiritual beliefs. 2. The patient will discuss his or her views on God's role in this illness.
The patient will attend an adult day care center at least three times a week.	1. The patient will visit an adult day treatment center. 2. The patient will agree to "try out" the center for a day to see if it works.
The patient will demonstrate appropriate ways to initiate a conversation within three weeks.	1. The patient will participate in social activities at the adult day treatment center. 2. The patient will practice initiating a conversation with a nurse.

For the patient with a need for *access to medication,* short-term goals might be as follows:

Expected Outcome	Short-Term Goals
The patient will be knowledgeable about his or her medications.	1. The patient will state the reason for taking the medications. 2. The patient will state at least three side effects of the medications and how to deal with them.

Expected Outcome	Short-Term Goals
The patient will take all medi cations as prescribed within two weeks.	1. The patient will state the schedule for taking medications.
	2. The patient will state the benefits of taking medications.
	3. The patient will set up a weekly compliance medication pack according to his or her schedule for taking medications.

For the patient needing *support for family members*, short-term goals might be as follows:

Expected Outcome	Short-Term Goals
The patient will verbalize at least one positive quality about self by the end of the third week of therapy.	1. The patient will do a sentence completion exercise: "My best qualities are ____________________ ____________________."
	2. The patient will discuss the feelings involved in performing this assignment.
The patient will demonstrate that he or she has learned new responses for coping with interpersonal conflict.	1. The patient will identify two areas of interpersonal conflict.
	2. The patient will discuss his or her present responses to conflict.
	3. The patient will evaluate present responses to conflict.
	4. The patient will discuss how he or she would like conflicts to be resolved.
	5. The patient will discuss three ways to resolve conflict differently.
The patient will demonstrate deep breathing exercises as a means of dealing with situational stress.	1. The patient will identify two sources of situational stress.
	2. The patient will identify his or her current responses to this stress.
	3. The patient will identify how he or she would like to respond to stress.
	4. The patient will demonstrate the technique of deep breathing and relaxation as a strategy for dealing with situational stress.

For those patients needing *integrated nursing, social, and medical services*, short-term goals might be as follows:

Expected Outcome	Short-Term Goals
The patient will use the available support system to access health care appointments.	1. The patient will identify resources in the community that might be beneficial to him or her.
	2. The patient will initiate contact with one community agency.
The patient will demonstrate the ability to make appropriate appointments and follow through with those appointments.	1. The patient will state one reason for keeping follow-up mental health appointments.
	2. The patient will call the community agency for a follow-up appointment.

IMPLEMENTATION

The interventions used by the community mental health nurse are directed toward the patient as well as the community. The patient-focused interventions fall into four categories:

Teaching
Consulting
Providing therapy
Case management

The community-focused interventions include the following:

Networking
Crossing boundaries between the professional and lay communities
Advocating

Teaching

According to Manderino and Bzdek (1987), psychiatric nurses are in an excellent position to teach the patient as well as the family and community as a whole about

- Medication issues.
- Stress management.
- Illness.
- The components of mental health.
- Effective communication and interpersonal relationships.
- Parenting.
- Accessing other health and social services.
- Suicide awareness.
- Drug and alcohol prevention.

- Social skills and other issues that have an impact on the mental health of the individual as well as the larger group.

Case Management

Case management is a modality of care that holds promise in the management of the multifaceted and complex needs of the chronically mentally ill. Ideally the case manager

- Assesses patient needs.
- Compiles a plan for service.
- Links patients with needed services.
- Monitors the quality and appropriateness of services.
- Advocates for the chronically mentally ill.

Unfortunately the funding has continued to be inadequate, and case managers find themselves overworked, poorly paid, and unable to change the system (Mechanic, 1986; Worley et al, 1990; Ruffolo and Nichols, 1994; Higgins, 1994). See Chapter 44 for a discussion of specific models of case management.

Consulting

The consultant role allows you to offer mental health services to agencies within the community such as schools, churches, or businesses. For instance, you might consult on the development of a suicide prevention program for the local school system or the development of a stress management course for local business groups.

Providing Therapy

In the role of therapist, you are concerned with both the individual and the family and may provide the appropriate therapy. For the most part, the therapy offered to the chronically mentally ill and their families is of a supportive nature in which the goals are symptom management, relationship building, and ego strengthening. An evaluation is made regarding whether individual or group therapy is the most appropriate modality for a particular patient. For instance, Beth, a 19-year-old chronic schizophrenic, had a great deal of difficulty tolerating the one-to-one relationship with her nurse. Beth was initially placed in a small group with the intention of developing such a relationship between her and the nurse therapist (Abbondanza et al, 1994; Shea et al, 1994).

Part of the therapy role involves continual assessment regarding changes in the patient's life that might be linked to symptomatic exacerbation. Many times, patients fail to report changes because they do not see the connection between stress and symptoms. A therapist who seeks this type of information is in a position to intervene and to provide anticipatory guidance that may be the difference between the patient coping or "falling apart." John's story provides a good example (Case Example 43–6). Therapy skills are also directed at relieving the burden of caregiving felt by the family (Maurin and Boyd, 1990).

Case Example 43–6 John's Story

John had been seeing a nurse every two weeks for about a year. On the last visit, the nurse observed that John seemed more scattered in his thinking. He was disheveled in his appearance, and he reported a return of the "voices" that had plagued him intermittently for years. Gentle questioning revealed that John was having difficulty with a fellow tenant who was stealing from him. The nurse asked whether John would like her to talk to the manager of the boarding home where he lived. John agreed that this might help. The nurse made a visit to John's home to discuss the problem with the manager. Together, the nurse, manager, and John were able to work out an arrangement to secure John's personal belongings in an effort to cut down on the thievery. On the following visit to the community center, John was back to his "old self."

Networking

This intervention is one in which you coordinate services on behalf of patients who need them and try to create services where there are none (Krauss and Slavinsky, 1982). Worley and Albanese (1989) report great success at tapping the private sector for resources for the chronically mentally ill that were previously unconsidered.

Crossing Boundaries

Nurses seem to have the ability to cross the boundaries between the lay and professional communities to marshal resources and to communicate the needs of disadvantaged groups.

Advocating

The psychiatric nurse can and should be an advocate for the needs of the chronically mentally ill. In an editorial, Krauss (1989b) bemoans the fact that nurses' advocacy attempts are frequently behind the scenes, focused only on the nurse's individual caseload of patients, and go unnoticed. Krauss recommends that we take our role of advocates and extend it aggressively in the policy-making arena, where we can have an impact on the system as a whole.

EVALUATION

Evaluation criteria measure the extent to which the nurse's interventions are able to support a mentally ill individual's capacity to remain functional and autonomous in the community.

▶ Check Your Reading

33. Cite three patient-focused interventions.
34. What is meant by networking?
35. What is case management?
36. What does being an advocate entail?

THE SUCCESS OF COMMUNITY MENTAL HEALTH CARE

Community mental health care has not always lived up to the expectations to improve the quality of life for the severely mentally ill or to counteract isolation and social disabilities resulting from institutionalization (Worley and Lowery, 1988). Sometimes community mental health care works, and other times it falls short of its goals. Some charge that patients are inappropriately discharged; the services are fragmented and sporadic; families assume an inordinate burden of the care; there is minimal cost savings; patients are sometimes abandoned and enter the ranks of the mentally ill homeless; and there is an increased likelihood of readmission (Sharfstein, 1984). Others assert that these reported failings of the system are inaccurate assumptions. In a study conducted by Solomon and coworkers (1986), 59 patients were interviewed about their hospital and community experiences. This study demonstrated that the majority of patients were connected with an aftercare agency, and although there appears to be some duplication of services, it is necessary to help the patient gain access to the services. In addition, the study indicated that services offered are not adequate in intensity or appropriate in nature to assist in meaningful rehabilitation and that the system is not unified in a systematic way that allows various subsystems offering services to coordinate efforts to ensure that the patient's total needs are met.

Over the last three decades, since the passage of community mental health care legislation, a large network of community mental health centers has developed nationwide. In addition, there have been research projects designed and implemented to evaluate various approaches to this type of care. For instance, in the early 1970s, Stein and Test, working at Mendota State Hospital in Madison, Wisconsin, developed a community model that they called *training in community living*. This model was designed to address three characteristics that had been identified in patients who made tenuous adjustments to community life. According to Stein and Test (1980), these disabling characteristics included

- A limited repertoire of coping behaviors to deal with the stresses of life.
- Powerful dependency needs.
- The capacity to develop severe psychiatric symptoms when confronted with mild to moderate degrees of stress.

The training in community living program included 24-hour support for patients. Visits were made to patients in the community; links were forged with family, landlords, neighbors, police, and other community members who could have an impact on the adjustment of the patient. Other services included

- Medication monitoring.
- Providing transportation to clinic visits.
- Going into the community to find out why patients have not kept appointments.
- Seeking guardianship to monitor finances.
- Facilitating housing placement as well as vocational rehabilitation and job placement.

The training in community living research project produced two major findings: (1) that hospitalization of the chronically mentally ill could be dramatically reduced and (2) that patients in such a system were less symptomatic, felt greater satisfaction with life, and made better social and work adjustments than patients treated with a traditional model (Test et al, 1985). The training in community living research has been replicated many times with similar findings.

In the 1980s, the National Institute of Mental Health targeted monies for research and programs specifically to deal with the needs of the chronically mentally ill, an underserved population. In 1982, the National Institute of Mental Health published their report concerning the *community support programs*, which on close examination includes the elements described in the training in community living approach. These programs are becoming the cornerstone on which the national mental health policy for the chronically mentally ill is built (Reinke and Greenley, 1986; Morrissey et al, 1994). The community support programs follow one of three models:

1. The caseworker model, which emphasizes assisting patients with the skills necessary for day-to-day living and problem-solving.
2. The paraprofessional extender model, which uses the services of nonprofessionals to provide care to patients in rural settings.
3. The team model, in which staff members share responsibility for all patients (see Chapter 44 for a more detailed discussion of these three models).

The caseworker model has proven to be the most efficient at serving a larger number of patients at the least cost (Reinke and Greenley, 1986). Continued research has demonstrated the effectiveness of community support programs in treating the chronically mentally ill (Turner and Tenhoor, 1978; Turner and Shifren, 1979). Based on the evidence that supports the effectiveness of community support programs we might expect that they would enjoy widespread implementation. This has not proven to be the case, however (Brekke, 1988).

Bachrach (1980, 1982) argues that community support programs have not made a major impact on the care of the chronically mentally ill, and she asserts that the programs may be successful only in certain situations and may not be generalizable. In fact, evidence supports the notion that the model programs work best in small or midsize cities and are ineffective in large urban areas. To address this problem, the Robert Wood Johnson Foundation launched the Program on Chronic Mental Illness in 1985. This program provides grants and assistance to nine cities across the United States in their efforts to improve services to persons who are chronically mentally ill.

To receive the funding, each city was required to submit a plan that included a centralized mental health system and focused on continuity of care, full range of services, a housing plan, and new sources of financing. Cities chosen for participation included Austin, Texas; Baltimore; Charlotte, North Carolina; Cincinnati, Ohio; Columbus, Ohio; Denver; Honolulu; Philadelphia; and Toledo, Ohio. Funding from the Robert Wood Johnson Foundation extended until December 1991, when the participating cities were expected to take over the financial management of their newly developed system of care. The evaluation of the Robert Wood Johnson initiative, which is still underway, is providing additional information and direction for systematic implementation of community mental health care in large urban settings (Bentley, 1994; Morrissey et al, 1994).

▶ Check Your Reading

37. What was the training in community living project?
38. What is the Robert Wood Johnson initiative?
39. What is the most cost-effective model of the three case management models used?
40. What is the paraprofessional extender model of case management?

FUTURE DIRECTIONS FOR COMMUNITY MENTAL HEALTH CARE

One of the major innovations of the 1990s will most likely be an involvement of recipients of services in the planning efforts (Chamberlin and Rogers, 1990). The prime motivation for this change comes from former-patient organizations that have been organizing since the early 1970s. Former patients have traditionally joined these groups as a way of reclaiming their voice and being heard by a system that has considered them incapable of defining their own needs. Included among the goals of the former-patient groups is to influence public policy about implementing mental health programs. These groups (which include diverse local, regional, and national organizations) have influenced the passage of legislation such as Public Law 99-660. This law requires the participation of various constituencies including families, patients, and professionals in the planning of a community-based system of mental health care. This may provide the modality for former patients and their families to promote their vision regarding how care should and should not be given to people who suffer with mental illnesses.

Chamberlin and Rogers (1990) observed that it is fashionable to refer to patients as *consumers*, a term that many former-patients find objectionable. Consumer implies choice and power, a misnomer considering that patients in the mental health system are captive populations who have little choice regarding the services or the providers selected.

Another change that may be in the offing in the 1990s is the possibility that in many states the large psychiatric hospitals will be closed entirely. Vermont is currently implementing a plan that will close down the state hospital without abandoning people to the streets or to shelters (Carling et al, 1987).

Still another change gaining popularity in the 1990s is the movement toward self-help programs, which are user-run programs that serve as drop-in centers and provide peer case management. Such services provide former patients with a feeling that they can make a difference to someone else, that they can give as well as receive, and that their lives have meaning (Gyulay et al, 1994).

Nurses are in strategic positions to influence mental health care in this decade. They have proven to be cost-effective providers to the chronically mentally ill, whose nursing needs are complex and multifaceted. Traditionally, they have held a view of patients that includes a holistic approach to assessing needs, recognition of the patient's and family's need for care, and a respect for the patient's autonomy that encourages self-direction. These views provide nursing with a vantage point to advocate for change within the health care system and within the community. Such advocacy could influence reform within the system and lessen responses within the community that stigmatize and discriminate against people with psychiatric histories. Fox and Chamberlain (1988) suggest that nurses should be prepared specifically to deal with the needs of the chronically mentally ill patient. It remains to be seen whether nursing realizes its potential as an agent of change in the community mental health care movement.

▶ Check Your Reading

41. Why do former patients object to being called consumers?
42. What is the anticipated impact of the former-patient support groups on the community mental health care movement?
43. What benefits accompany the self-help groups that have gained popularity in the 1990s?
44. Give two reasons why nurses are in strategic positions to influence mental health care in the 1990s.

CONCLUSIONS

Today the concept of community mental health care is an important force in psychiatric care; it is alive and still struggling for the best method of implementation. Thirty years ago, state hospitals cared for more than 50% of all psychiatric patients.

Today, with more than 2.5 million severely mentally ill in the United States, only about 10% are cared for in state hospitals. The pattern of psychiatric care in the 1990s is brief hospitalization during the acute phase of an illness and rapid return to community living. Usually only the most dysfunctional people and those who pose a serious threat to themselves and others reside in long-term psychiatric facilities. Clearly, we have a long way to go before the chronically mentally ill receive the kind of community care described in Dymphna's story and envisioned by John Winthrop.

KEY POINTS TO REMEMBER

- Before 1963, community mental health care was nonexistent.
- Institutionalization refers to the process of becoming dependent on an institution for care and decision-making.
- Deinstitutionalization refers to the process of preparing patients who have spent a great deal of time within the walls of an institution for life in the world.
- Community mental health care is sometimes referred to as the third revolution in psychiatry.
- Funding for community mental health care is subject to the views of Congress and has never been sufficient for the needs of the mentally ill.
- Community mental health care serves the needs of the chronically mentally ill, also referred to as the seriously and persistently mentally ill.
- The chronically mentally ill are a diverse group made up of people of all ages with many different psychiatric diagnoses.
- The needs of the chronic mentally ill include the need for basic life necessities; a sense that life is meaningful; access to medication; support for family members; and integrated nursing, medical, and social services.
- Community mental health care focuses on the community as well as the individual or family.
- A catchment area is a city or several rural communities whose total population ranges from 75,000 to 200,000 residents.
- The goal of community mental health care is to provide care that is continuous and comprehensive.
- The services offered by community mental health care include community mental health centers; availability of a variety of living arrangements, including single-room occupancy and sheltered or congregate housing; support groups; day treatment centers; mobile treatment teams; and community services.
- Nurses focus on primary, secondary, and tertiary prevention in the community setting.
- The nursing process can be applied to a community as a whole or to an individual or family within the community.
- The interventions used by the community mental health nurse include teaching, case managing, consulting, providing therapy, networking, crossing boundaries to forge linkages, and advocating.
- Community mental health care has never met the initial expectations that greeted its inception in the 1960s. It still remains, however, a viable option in the continuum of psychiatric services.
- Future directions in community mental health care will include more participation in the planning and development of programs by families and former patients.

LEARNING ACTIVITIES

1. Conduct an informal survey in your community. Ask your family and neighbors how they would react to having a halfway house for the chronically mentally ill established in their community.
2. Find out where the nearest community mental health center is in your area. Call to find out what services are offered to patients.
3. Call the mental health association in your community. Ask if there are any self-help groups in your area. If there are, what services do they provide?
4. Visit a day treatment center. What types of patients use the center? What services are offered?

CRITICAL THINKING EXERCISE

Penny Johnson, a 27-year-old drug abuser, attends a women's group led by the psychiatric nurse specialist Mrs. Hargood every Monday and Thursday in the partial hospitalization program. During group, she expresses great concern that her 4-year-old daughter's father has just been released from jail and wants to live with her. She thinks he is still taking drugs.

1. What assumptions do you think Penny is operating under?
2. How could Mrs. Hargood check these assumptions out by some simple inquiry?
3. Suggest a response to Penny's concern(s).

Jerome, an elderly patient who walked Penny home every day, told the group that he had a gun and would shoot "this guy" if he ever came around to bother Penny.

1. What assumptions might Jerome have about his relationship with Penny?
2. Consider the nurse's legal responsibility to report this threat.
3. What other evidence is needed to draw a conclusion about the situation?

REFERENCES

Abbondanza, D. M., Puskar, K. R., Wilkinson, B., Welch, C., Rudert, S., and Gallippi, B. (1994). Psychiatric mental health nursing in a biopsychosocial era. *Perspectives in Psychiatric Care, 30* (3), 21–25.

Adams, T. (1994). The emotional experience of caregivers to relatives who are chronically confused—implications for community mental health nursing. *International Journal of Nursing Studies, 31* (6), 545–553.

Bachrach, L. L. (1979). Planning mental health services for the chronically ill patient. *Hospital and Community Psychiatry, 30,* 387–392.

Bachrach, L. L. (1980). Overview: Model programs for chronically ill mental patients. *American Journal of Psychiatry, 137,* 1023–1031.

Bachrach, L. L. (1982). Assessment of outcomes in community support systems: Results, problems, and limitations. *Schizophrenia Bulletin, 8,* 39–60.

Beebe, L. H. (1990). Reframe your outlook on recidivism. *Journal of Psychosocial Nursing, 28* (9), 31–33.

Bentley, K. J. (1994). Supports for community-based mental health care: An optimistic review of federal legislation. *Health Social Work, 19* (4), 288–294.

Berns, J. S., and Hamilton, M. S. (1981). Nursing role in community mental health. In L. L. Jarvis (Ed.), *Community health nursing: keeping the public healthy* (p. 328). Philadelphia: F. A. Davis.

Birks, T. (1987). Community care for the chronically mentally ill. *New Zealand Nursing Journal, 12,* 20–22.

Bostelman, S., Callan, M., Rolincik, L. C., Gantt, M. Herink, M., King, J., Massey, M. K., Morehouse, D., Sopata, T., and Turner, J. (1994). *Public Health Report, 109* (2), 153–157.

Brekke, J. S. (1988). What do we really know about community support programs? Strategies for better monitoring. *Hospital and Community Psychiatry, 39* (9), 946–952.

Buckwalter, K. C., and Light, E. (1989). New directions of psychiatric mental health nurses: The chronically mentally ill elderly. *Archives of Psychiatric Nursing, 3* (1), 53–54.

Carling, P. J., Miller, S., Daniels, L., and Randolph, F. (1987). Operating a state mental health system without a state hospital: The Vermont feasibility study. *Hospital and Community Psychiatry, 38,* 617–623.

Chafetz, L. (1988). Recidivist clients: A review of pilot data. *Archives of Psychiatric Nursing, 2* (1), 14–20.

Chamberlin, J., and Rogers, J. A. (1990). Planning a community-based mental health system. *American Psychologist, 45* (11), 1241–1244.

Conway, A. S., Melzer, D., and Hale, A. S. (1994). The outcome of targeting community mental health services: Evidence from the West Lambeth schizophrenia cohort. *British Medical Journal, 308* (6929), 627–630.

Cutler, D. L. (1986). Community residential options for the chronically mentally ill. *Community Mental Health Journal, 22* (1), 61–72.

Dalgard, O. S., Bjork, S., and Tambs, K. (1995). Social support, negative life events and mental health. *British Journal of Psychiatry, 166* (1), 29–34.

Dolan, J. A., Fitzpatrick, M. L., and Herrmann, E. K. (1983). *Nursing in society: A historical perspective.* Philadelphia: W. B. Saunders.

Drolen, C. S. (1990). Current community mental health center operations: Entrepreneurship or business as usual? *Community Mental Health Journal, 26* (6), 547–558.

Finley, B. (1989). The role of the psychiatric nurse in a community substance abuse prevention program. *Nursing Clinics of North America, 24* (1), 121–136.

Fox, J. C., and Chamberlain, J. (1988). Preparing nurses to work with the chronically mentally ill. *Community Mental Health Journal, 24* (4), 296–309.

Goldin, G. (1971). A painting in Gheel. *Journal of the History of Medicine and Allied Sciences, 26* (4), 400–412.

Grob, G. N. (1994). Government and mental health policy: A structural analysis. *Milbank Quarterly, 72* (3), 471–500.

Gyulay, R., Mound, B., and Flanagan, E. (1994). Mental health consumers as public educators: A qualitative study. *Canadian Journal of Nursing Research, 26* (2), 29–42.

Hadley, R. (1978). President's commission sets national mental health goals. *American Nurse, 10* (1).

Higgins, R. (1994). Implementing case management in mental health services. *Journal of Nurse Management, 2* (1), 25–30.

Janssen, J. A., and Giberson, D. L. (1988). Remotivation therapy. *Journal of Gerontological Nursing, 14* (6), 31–34.

Joint Commission on Mental Illness and Health (1961). *Action for mental health.* New York: Basic Books.

Krauss, J. B. (1980). The chronically psychiatric patient in the community—a model of care. *Nursing Outlook, May,* 308–314.

Krauss, J. (1989a). The three Cs and the chronically mentally ill. *Archives of Psychiatric Nursing, 3* (2), 59–60.

Krauss, J. (1989b). New conceptions of care, community, and chronic illness. *Archieves of Psychiatric Nursing, 3* (5), 281–287.

Krauss, J., and Slavinsky, A. (1982). *The chronically ill psychiatric patient and the community* (pp. 76, 78). Boston: Blackwell.

Manderino, M. A., and Bzdek, V. M. (1987). Social skill building with chronically ill patients. *Journal of Psychosocial Nursing and Mental Health Services, 25* (9), 18–23.

Maurin, J. T., and Boyd, C. B. (1990). Burden of mental illness on the family: A critical review. *Archives of Psychiatric Nursing, 4* (2), 99–107.

McLaughlin, J. S. (1981). Towards a theoretical model of community health programs. *Advances in Nursing Science, 5,* 7–28.

Mechanic, D. (1986). The challenge of chronic mental illness: A retrospective and prospective view. *Hospital and Community Psychiatry, 37,* 891–896.

Minkoff, K. (1978). A map of chronically mental patients. In J. Talbot (Ed.), *The chronically Mental Patient* (pp. 11–73). Washington, D.C.: American Psychiatric Association.

Morrison, E., Fisher, L. Y., Wilson, H. S., and Underwood, P. (1985). The nursing adaptation evaluation (NSGAE): A proposed axis VI of DSM-III. *Journal of Psychosocial Nursing and Mental Health Services, 23* (8), 10–13.

Morrissey, J. P., Calloway, M., Bartko, W. T., Ridgely, M. S., Goldman, H. H., and Paulson, R. I. (1994). Local mental health authorities and service system change: Evidence from the Robert Wood Johnson program on chronic mental illness. *Milbank Quarterly, 72* (1), 49–80.

Peck, M. S. (1987). *The different drum: Community making and peace.* New York: Simon & Shuster.

Puskar, K., Lamb, J., and Norton, M. (1990). Adolescent mental health: Collaboration among psychiatric mental health nurses and school nurses. *Journal of School Health, 60* (2), 69–71.

Reinke, B., and Greenley, J. R. (1986). Organizational analysis of three community support program models. *Hospital and Community Psychiatry, 37* (6), 624–629.

Report to the President of the President's Commission on Mental Health (1978). Vol. 1. Washington, D.C.: U.S. Government Printing Office.

Richter, J. M. (1990). Social support: The chronically mentally ill institutionalized elderly. *Journal of Gerontological Nursing, 16* (8), 32–35.

Ruffolo, M. C., and Nichols, N. (1994). Satisfaction and role performance of case managers in the mental health system. *Journal of Case Management, 3* (1), 36–42.

Sharfstein, S. S. (1984). Sociopolitical issues affecting patients with chronic schizophrenia. In A. S. Bellack (Ed.), *Schizophrenia: Treatment, management, and rehabilitation.* Orlando, FL: Grune & Stratton.

Shea, D. G., Streit, A., and Smyer, M. A. (1994). Determinants of the use of specialist mental health services by nursing home residents. *Health Service Research, 29* (2), 169–185.

Sheets, J. L., Prevost, J. A., and Reihman, J. (1982). Young adult chronically mentally ill patients: Three hypothesized subgroups. *Hospital and Community Psychiatry, 33* (3), 197–203.

Shore, M. F., and Cohen, M. D. (1990). The Robert Wood Johnson Foundation Program on Chronic Mental Illness: An overview. *Hospital and Community Psychiatry, 41* (41), 1212–1216.

Solomon, P., Gordon, B., and Davis, J. M. (1986). Reconceptualizing assumptions about community mental health. *Hospital and Community Psychiatry, 37* (7), 708–712.

Soumerai, S. B., McLaughlin, T. J., Ross-Degnan, D., Casteris, C. S., and Bollini, P. (1994). Effects of a limit on Medicaid drug-reimbursement benefits on the use of psychotropic agents and acute mental health services by patients with schizophrenia. *New England Journal of Medicine, 331* (10), 650–655.

Stein, L. I., and Test, M. A. (1980). An alternative to mental hospital treatment: Conceptual model, treatment program and clinical evaluation. *Archives of General Psychiatry, 37,* 392–397.

Test, M. A., Knoedler, W. H., and Allness, D. J. (1985). The long-term treatment of young schizophrenics in a community support program. In *The training in community living model: A decade of experience.* New Directions for Mental Health Services, no. 26. San Francisco: Jossey-Bass.

Turner, J. C., and Shifren, I. (1979). Community support systems: How comprehensive? New Directions for Mental Health Services, no. 2, San Francisco: Jossey-Bass.

Turner, J. C., and Tenhoor, W. J. (1978). The NIMH community support program: Pilot approach to a needed reform. *Schizophrenia Bulletin, 8,* 39–60.

United States Congress Public Law 94-63, Title 3 Community Mental Health Centers Amendment Packet A. Section 201 (b) (1) (c). July 29, 1975.

Wetherill, J., Kelly, T., and Hore, B. (1987). The role of the community psychiatric nurse in improving treatment compliance in alcoholics. *Journal of Advanced Nursing, 12,* 707–711.

Winthrop, J. (1965). *Puritan political ideas, 1558–1794* (E. S. Morgan, Ed.) (p. 92). Indianapolis: Bobbs-Merrill.

Worley, N. K., and Albanese, N. (1989). Independent living for the chronically mentally ill. *Journal of Psychosocial Nursing and Mental Health Services, 27* (9), 18–23.

Worley, N. K., Drago, L., and Hadley, T. (1990). Improving the physical health-mental health interface for the chronically mentally ill: Could nurse case managers make a difference? *Archives of Psychiatric Nursing, 4* (2), 108–113.

Worley, N. K. and Lowery, B. J. (1988). Deinstitutionalization: Could the process have been better for patients? *Archives of Psychiatric Nursing, 2* (3), 126–133.

SUGGESTED READINGS

Abbondanza, D. M., Puskar, K. R., Wilkinson, B., Welch, C., Rudert, S., and Gallippi, B. (1994). Psychiatric mental health nursing in a biopsychosocial era. *Perspectives in Psychiatric Care, 30* (3), 21–25.

Adams, T. (1994). The emotional experience of caregivers to relatives who are chronically confused—implications for community mental health nursing. *International Journal of Nursing Studies, 31* (6), 545–553.

Gyulay, R., Mound, B., and Flanagan, E. (1994). Mental health consumers as public educators: A qualitative study. *Canadian Journal of Nursing Research, 26* (2), 29–42.

Higgins, R. (1994). Implementing case management in mental health services. *Journal of Nurse Management, 2* (1), 25–30.

CHAPTER 44

THE JOURNEY THROUGH HOME MENTAL HEALTH CARE

No matter how dreary and grey our homes are, we people of flesh and blood would rather live there than in any other country, be it ever so beautiful. There is no place like home.

—*Dorothy, speaking to the Scarecrow in* The Wizard of Oz

LEARNING OBJECTIVES

After studying this chapter, you should be able to:

1. Discuss the three factors that are influencing the growth of psychiatric home care.
2. Discuss the impact of Medicare legislation on the home care industry.
3. Define psychiatric home care as a bridge to the community and an anchor to help patients remain there.
4. Discuss Bay Area Health Care's model of psychiatric home care.
5. Discuss the sources of reimbursement for psychiatric home care.
6. Discuss Medicare's criteria for determining whether patients will receive psychiatric home care.
7. Discuss the services provided to patients and families through psychiatric home care.
8. Apply the nursing process to psychiatric home care.

KEY TERMINOLOGY

Case management
Homebound status
Psychiatric home care
Skilled nursing services

Psychiatric home health care is a relatively new phenomenon in a burgeoning home health care industry. The provision of nursing services within the home has expanded tremendously in the last decade. Care is offered to all age groups, from infants being monitored for sleep-apnea disturbance, to new mothers for assessment of their postpartum recovery and support in initiating breast-feeding, to AIDS patients requiring administration of an intravenous antibiotic, to geriatric patients receiving physical therapy following a cerebrovascular accident. The inclusion of psychiatric patients among those receiving care reflects three national trends that are affecting home health care.

First, there is increased public awareness of the benefits of home health care, with more individuals and families demanding that care be provided in the comforts of their homes. The National Alliance for the Mentally Ill (NAMI) has exerted tremendous influence and pressure regarding the need to support the mentally ill in the least restrictive settings. Second, the population needing home health services, specifically the dependent elderly, is growing dramatically (Daubert, 1987; Burbach et al, 1988; Eliopoulos, 1991, 1993). Third, cost containment pressures have led to patients being discharged "quicker and sicker." Psychiatric home care is a cost-effective alternative to inpatient treatment and offers the continued, necessary stabilization to patients who are discharged from psychiatric inpatient facilities.

Let's take a look at Dorothy's story to remind us of the importance of home.

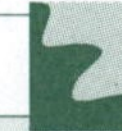

DOROTHY'S STORY

The Wizard of Oz, the story of Dorothy, the little girl from Kansas who found herself in a strange and wonderful land, has become a classic of American fantasy. Long loved by children, the book is also well established in the hearts of adults. In Dorothy's journey to reach Oz, she travels with her dog Toto and her strange new friends, the Scarecrow, the Tin Woodsman, and the Cowardly Lion. This unusual cadre of traveling companions encounters adventures that would test the courage, cleverness, and fortitude of the bravest. As they quest toward Oz, each in search of a personal treasure, they learn that the important things in life are found in relationships and commitments. The Scarecrow longs for a brain, yet he doesn't recognize how clever he is in protecting Dorothy and the rest. The Cowardly Lion believes that because he feels fear, he lacks courage. He doesn't recognize the courage and bravery that he has displayed even in the face of fear. The Tin Woodsman wants a heart, yet fails to recognize that through his caring, concern, and compassion he already possesses the qualities of a heart. For Dorothy, her single-minded goal is to return to Kansas, to her Aunt Em and Uncle Henry and to the gray bleak farm that Dorothy knew as home. Dorothy learns that her heart's desire is really in her own backyard.

What does Dorothy's story teach us? Surely, *The Wizard of Oz* can be read just as a delightful fairy tale with no deeper meanings ascribed to it. Yet the story does invite us to look beyond to explore the meaning of each traveler's quest. The Scarecrow's desire for a brain encourages reflection on the importance of cognitive processes to learning and discovery. The Cowardly Lion's search for courage leads us to look at what qualities strengthen people and give them resolve in the face of adversity. The Tin Woodsman's quest for a heart reminds us of the symbolic importance of the heart as the seat of feelings and emotions. Finally, Dorothy's yearning to return home awakens in many individuals a longing for the attributes associated with home—a loving family, safety and refuge from the outside world, and the comfort of being surrounded by the familiar and known. These are significant and basic human longings, sometimes experienced even when the objective evidence denies that home is wonderful.

Dorothy's yearning to go home speaks to us about the importance of delivering health care in the home as opposed to an institutional setting. People desire to be home. Surrounded by family and possessions that create a sense of comfort, the individual may respond to health care interventions with a more peaceful spirit and greater willingness of mind and body.

This chapter explores psychiatric home care by looking at:

- The historical background to psychiatric home care.
- A definition of psychiatric home care.
- The Bay Area Health Care model of psychiatric home care.
- Criteria to receive this type of care.
- Reimbursement for these services.
- Qualifications of nurses who provide psychiatric home care.
- The kinds of services included.
- The application of the nursing process to psychiatric home care.

HISTORICAL BACKGROUND

In the early recordings of home health care, there is a noticeable lack of reference to any specific focus on psychiatric problems. There is evidence, however, that nurses acted out the supportive, counseling, and teaching roles that are as much a part of psychiatric nursing as they are medical-surgical or maternal-child nursing. It is hard to imagine working with new mothers, infants, and children, the focus of much home nursing at the turn of the century, and not providing a great deal of emotional, spiritual, and perhaps even psychiatric support (Mundinger, 1983; Spiegel, 1983).

Home Health Services After World War II

In 1947, the first hospital-based home care program was founded by Bluestone at Montefiore Hospital in New York City. This program was developed to shorten the hospital stays of patients with chronic illnesses. A team approach was used to plan acute care that could be delivered in the home setting. Thus, the concept of convalescent home care was initiated. The program was not limited to the poor or elderly. As this program evolved, it expanded to include nutrition, x-ray and laboratory services, and home health aide services. There was also an emphasis on coordinating community resources that could provide chore services and homemakers (MacNamara, 1982). Psychiatric services were still not primary home health care services but were met incidentally as other patient needs were addressed.

Influence of Medicare/Medicaid Legislation

With the passage of the Medicare and Medicaid legislation in 1965, the home health care industry underwent a dramatic transformation. It changed from a service provided primarily by visiting nurse associations to elderly patients who required some nursing care and health aide assistance to a comprehensive package of health care services provided by proprietary agencies. Before Medicare legislation, payment came from Welfare or personal payment based on a sliding scale and subsidized by charity.

Medicare mandated that the physician rather than the nurse direct all home health care services. With the physician as the director of the home health care team, the service approach moved away from caring and supportive roles and embraced the medical model of treating and eradicating diseases. In the post-Medicare transformed thinking, home health care was more narrowly defined.

Eligibility for Medicare reimbursement was based on the three criteria:

• The patient's acute care needs.

• The patient's homebound status.

• The patient's need for skilled care, medically directed by a nurse or other professional under the orders of a physician.

The Medicare influences on home health care overlooked the need for preventive and health-promoting services and ignored the clear need of homebound patients for continued support. Those who made policy seemed unaware of the range of health needs of patients in the home setting (Neiman et al, 1986). The assumption was made that discharge from an acute care setting meant that the patient was ready to resume, without assistance, activities such as meal preparation, shopping, cleaning, laundry, and so forth. Health promotion, health teaching, and holistic family care are nonreimbursable services under Medicare and Medicaid. These services, still considered part of home health care, were assumed by public health agencies without charge through their nurses. Also, agency nurses who had a personal commitment to holistic care continued to provide this type of care but billed Medicare only for the skilled services.

The structure of home health care agencies also changed with the passage of Medicare legislation. For home care agencies to be certified for Medicare reimbursement, they were required to provide at least one health-related service in addition to nursing. Agencies could choose to include physical, occupational, or speech therapy; social services; or home health aide services. In 1966, there were 1163 agencies. Of this number, only 250 met the Medicare requirements. Immediately following the passage of Medicare, many of the smaller voluntary agencies went out of business because they could not provide the comprehensive services required. This void was filled with a burgeoning growth in proprietary agencies, public home health agencies, and hospital-based agencies. By 1976, the number of agencies had increased by 71% to about 430, with the most pronounced growth in hospital-based agencies. Currently, there are more than 10,000 Medicare-certified home health agencies.

In 1979, psychiatric home care was added to Medicare benefits. At this time, neither the Health Care Financing Administration nor the Medicare intermediaries know how many agencies are actually providing psychiatric home care.

▶ Check Your Reading

1. Identify two ways in which Medicare legislation changed the home care industry.
2. What are the three influences that are driving the growth of psychiatric home care?
3. What areas of care were overlooked by the Medicare legislation?

PSYCHIATRIC HOME CARE DEFINED

Psychiatric home care is a bridge to patients who are transitioning from a setting of greater restriction to their homes, which are the least restrictive, as well as an anchor to assist patients to remain in their homes. Psychiatric home care provides **skilled nursing services** to patients with primary psychiatric disorders or secondary emotional problems. According to Thobaben (1989), the overall goals of psychiatric home health care are to:

• Improve the quality of life.

• Prevent unnecessary hospitalizations.

• Facilitate more rapid discharges from an acute care setting.

• Maximize the potential of patients to live in their own homes.

The specific goals include (Minnesota Community Health Services, 1981; Davis, 1987; Pelletier, 1988; Newton and Brauer, 1989; Thobaben, 1989; Carson, 1994a, b, c, d, 1995):

• Teaching coping skills to patients and family members.

• Offering respite to families and responsible caretakers from the demands of caring for psychiatrically impaired people.

• Teaching patients and families about the psychiatric illness, medications, strategies to stay well, and interpersonal and communication strategies.

• Teaching patients appropriate social interaction skills, the importance of structuring time, and the need to be involved in healthy diversional activities.

• Linking the patient to other community-based health and social services.

• Helping the patient to achieve spiritual well-being by finding meaning and purpose in the present situation and by assisting the patient in accessing spiritual resources within the environment.

• Acting as a resource to the nonpsychiatric medical community by defining mental health needs.

• Linking with nursing schools to provide educational experiences to nursing students.

These goals are accomplished through an effective, coordinated home care system and a system that values a holistic approach to patient care.

▶ Check Your Reading

4. Define psychiatric home care.
5. What are the overall goals of psychiatric home care?
6. State at least four of the specific goals of psychiatric home care.

BAY AREA HEALTH CARE'S MODEL OF PSYCHIATRIC HOME CARE

On the surface, psychiatric home care is very eclectic. Although psychiatric nurses draw on crisis intervention, as noted by Duffy and colleagues (1993), there are a number of other psychiatric intervention models that are also helpful, including psychoeducation; interpersonal, cognitive, supportive, family, individual, and brief therapy; psychiatric rehabilitation; and behavioral modification. It should be noted, however, that even though various therapeutic models are useful, psychotherapy is not the primary focus of psychiatric home care. There are two reasons for this: First, many of the patients are the persistently and seriously mentally ill, who have experienced an acute exacerbation of their illness and are not candidates for traditional therapy. Second, the length of stay is often too short to conduct anything but supportive psychotherapy focusing on improving problem-solving skills, strengthening ego boundaries, and enhancing self-concept.

In addition, the psychiatric home care nurse must also be cognizant of public health concepts of primary, secondary, and tertiary prevention. Finally, the role of case manager, with its inherent responsibilities for forming linkages between the patient and needed community services, is a vital component of the role of the psychiatric home care nurse.

The Bay Area Health Care model of psychiatric home care provides coherence, direction, and vision to services. The symbol of a home is used to conceptualize the model (Carson, 1994a, 1995) (Figure 44–1).

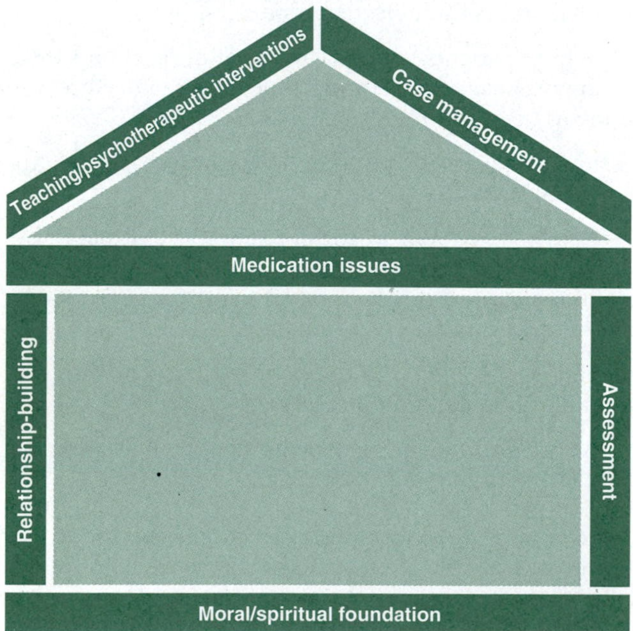

FIGURE 44–1
The symbol of a home used to conceptualize Bay Area Health Care's Psychiatric Home Care Model. (Redrawn from Carson, V. B., et al. [1994]. *Psychiatric home care manual.* Baltimore: Bay Area Health Care.)

The Foundation of the House: A Moral/Spiritual Base

The foundation of the house is a moral/spiritual one. Moral and spiritual interventions involve the realm of valuing and respecting the integrity of the individual. Nurses must exhibit the moral qualities of trust, gratitude, loyalty, devotion, and most of all respect for the patient. The nurse is resolute in standing by the patient and willing to tolerate a certain degree of moral failure in the patient. This moral/spiritual foundation is the basis for the care provided. By the time most psychiatric patients are in a position to receive home care services, they have already suffered the stings and barbs of a society that ostracizes them, treats them as subhuman, blames them for their illnesses, and offers little in the way of support and understanding. Approaching patients from a moral/spiritual foundation conveys an attitude of respect, recognizes them as people of worth and dignity, shows a desire to hear their stories and a willingness to help them find meaning in their suffering, recognizes that they have strengths as well as disabilities, and conveys a deep appreciation for them as individuals.

Pellegrino's (1985) description of care as having three levels is relevant to understanding this moral-spiritual foundation (Figure 44–2). Pellegrino describes the first level of care as involving doing for another what they cannot do for themselves. This entails assisting the patient with all of the activities of daily living that are compromised by illness or disability, such as physical needs of feeding, bathing, and clothing. Home care provides this type of service through the work of home care aides. Many psychiatric illnesses leave patients feeling demoralized and without energy to take care of their bodies, and they need assistance in this area.

This brings us to the second level of care, which is concerned with skilled medical and nursing care through which professionals "carry out all the necessary procedures, personal and technical, with conscientious detail" (Pellegrino, 1985, p. 12). For the psychiatric nurse, these skills include assessing the patient and family, teaching, using psychotherapeutic techniques to facilitate patient change, managing medication, and supervising the patient's care in a holistic fashion.

The third level of care, according to Pellegrino (1985), means to be in the service of the whole individual. This includes sustaining the patient's physical, emotional, and spiritual life by promoting health, relieving suffering, and helping the patient to find meaning in and through suffering. It means to be present to the patient and to offer emotional and spiritual assistance (Carson, 1994e). This third type of care, which is what the Bay Area Health Care model is built on, is not something that Medicare requires, and it is not a reimbursable skill. The model affirms, however, that offering skilled interventions without dedication and care is insufficient for any patient, most especially for the psychiatric patient.

▶ Check Your Reading

7. What are the three levels of care described by Pellegrino?

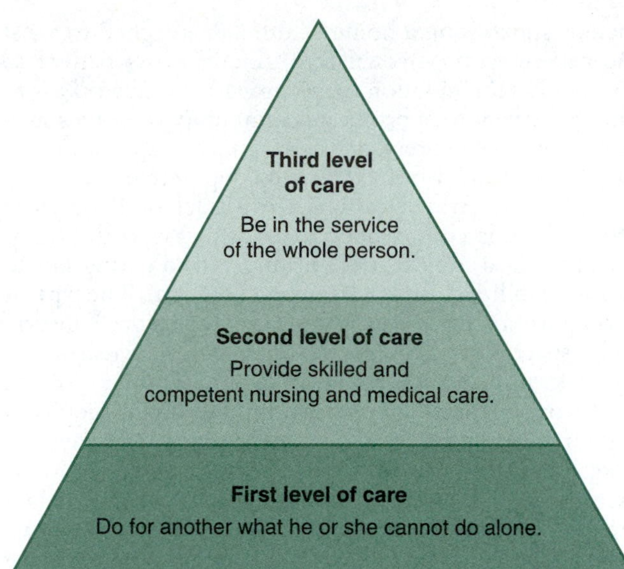

FIGURE 44–2
Pellegrino's three levels of home care. (Based on information in Pellegrino, E. [1985]). The caring ethic: The relation of physician to patient. In A. H. Bishop, & J. R. Scudder [Eds.]. *Caring, curing, coping: Nurse, physician, patient relationships* [pp. 8–30]. Tuscaloosa, AL: University of Alabama Press.)

8. State one reason why a moral/spiritual foundation is so important to psychiatric home care.

The Walls of the House: Assessment and Relationship-Building

The walls of the house are made up of assessment skills and relationship-building. These walls provide the necessary supports to all other psychotherapeutic interventions. Without a comprehensive assessment and a thorough knowledge of the patient's journey, nurses are working blindfolded. The assessment is ongoing but begins with a comprehensive review of psychiatric issues such as a mental status examination (including the use of standardized assessment tools such as the mini-mental examination, Montgomery-Asburg Depression Inventory, Young Mania Scale, Sheehan Anxiety Scale, and the AIMS Scale for Tardive Dyskinesia); activities of daily living such as eating, elimination, sleep, recreation, and work; medication issues; psychiatric follow-up issues; relationship issues focusing on what kinds of supports the patient has among family, friends, neighbors, and through a place of worship; and spiritual issues such as the importance of God, the meaning of the illness to the patient, and whether the patient seeks solace from religious beliefs or practices.

Concurrent to the assessment process is the work of relationship-building, which forms the second wall of the psychiatric home care model. Without a relationship built on trust, caring, compassion, empathy, hopefulness, and a sense of humor, no effective teaching or case management can take place. The nurse uses verbal and nonverbal communication techniques to convey a genuine interest in the patient, to discern what the patient would like to accomplish through the relationship, to clarify the boundaries of the relationship, and to affirm the patient as a person of worth. Trust is built not only through the nurse's commitment to follow through on promises made, but also through the nurse's consistent responses and careful listening. The nurse is sensitive to timing issues, taking care not to rush the patient into a relationship before the patient is ready.

The Second Floor of the House: Medication Issues

The second floor of the psychiatric home care model, supported by the walls of assessment and relationship, is made up of all the issues surrounding medications. One of the primary reasons that psychiatric patients get caught in a cycle of discharge and readmission is that they have difficulty adhering to a long-term medication regimen. Many patients do not even get their initial prescription filled after they are discharged from an inpatient facility. The nurse determines whether the patient has a supply of medication(s), understands the reason for taking medication(s), is taking medication(s) according to schedule, and is experiencing side effects and, if so, which ones.

Medication issues are a major challenge for the nurse and patient to tackle mutually. Because there are many reasons that patients resist taking medications, there is no one right way to solve the dilemmas surrounding medication useage. For some patients, the side effects are almost as bad as the illness. For others, remembering to take their medications is an issue. Other patients cannot accept having a chronic illness. Some lack understanding about the reasons for taking the medications. Others deny that they have a psychiatric illness. Still others cannot afford to get the prescriptions filled.

The solutions to these issues must be tailored to the individual patient. Whatever the solution, the underlying message communicated to the patient is that the nurse respects the patient's concerns and choices. Some patients find that using a compliance pack helps them to follow a medication schedule. For other patients, juggling the times certain medications are taken to minimize the side effects (e.g., taking sedating medications at night; taking medications that cause nervousness in the morning; taking medications that cause nausea with meals) helps them to take their medications. For other patients, the nurse advocates the patient's concerns with the prescribing psychiatrist in an effort to modify the medication regimen. Teaching about the major effects and side effects of medications is an empowering technique for still other patients (Witt, 1981; Davidhizar and McBride, 1985; Brown et al, 1987; Collins-Colon, 1990).

▶ Check Your Reading

9. What are the skills that define the walls of the model?
10. Why are medication issues so important for the nurse to address in psychiatric home care?

11. State two elements that go into relationship-building.
12. State at least three reasons that patients do not take psychiatric medications as directed.

The Roof on the House: Teaching/Psychotherapeutic Interventions and Case Management

The two sides of the roof of the psychiatric home care model are made up of teaching/psychotherapeutic interventions and case management. Teaching is a broad concept in psychiatric home care that subsumes many therapy issues. Medicare values and reimburses teaching as a skilled intervention; teaching is concrete and results in measurable outcomes. Medicare reviewers look less favorably on therapy, unless the therapeutic skill is well defined and the outcomes are clearly explicated. The Bay Area Health Care Model of Psychiatric Home Care has taken almost all therapy issues that the nurse might engage in and translated them into teaching terms. For instance, nurses teach about the causes of depression; the physical, cognitive, interpersonal, and spiritual effects of depression; the relationship of guilt to depression; and cognitive strategies for dealing with depression, such as thought stopping and the use of personal affirmations. The same teaching approach is used for informing the patient about anxiety and stress, schizophrenia, and grief (Frisch, 1993; Kelley and Lehman, 1993).

Psychiatric patients may need help in negotiating the health care system to make and keep follow-up appointments or in developing a workable budget for managing their money. Some patients are lacking in social skills and may experience severe difficulty getting along with others and developing a support system. The nurse may assist the patient to learn skills of social interaction through role-playing and practice sessions. Many patients are unable to structure their time, so they do nothing meaningful or productive. The nurse might focus on teaching about the value of structure and how to establish it and might assist the patient to work out a schedule of daily activities. Incorporated into these teaching strategies are a variety of therapy approaches, including supportive, cognitive, behavioral, and interpersonal therapy, but regardless of the approach, the outcomes are specific and measurable (Klebanoff and Casler, 1986; Lesseig, 1987).

The second side of the roof of the psychiatric home care model is made up of **case management.** Because psychiatric illnesses affect patients physically, cognitively, interpersonally, socially, spiritually, and emotionally, the impact is far reaching. All areas of life are usually affected. Patients seldom present with uncomplicated needs but rather with an array of tangled life affairs that leaves them feeling scattered, disorganized, and disconnected. The psychiatric nurse works with the patient to introduce order into chaos and to forge the links that connect or reconnect the patient to the community. The better these connections are made, the more successful the patient will be at staying out of the hospital. Case management may include supervising a home health aide assigned to assist the patient with personal care, referring the patient to vocational rehabilitation, working with social workers to link the patient to appropriate community resources such as psychosocial centers, and setting up transportation for the patient to and from follow-up appointments.

The Bay Area Health Care Model of Psychiatric Home Care is comprehensive. In contrast to the traditional medical model, it is not directed to curing but to caring, stabilizing, and maximizing potential. The patient is supported with a foundation of compassion, concern, and respect. Care is planned involving skilled assessment and a loving, therapeutic relationship. The roof of the house is supported by assisting the patient acquire a greater understanding of and compliance with medication. The roof of care is built with teaching and case management. The finished structure leaves the patient more organized, knowledgeable about his or her own health care concerns, better linked to a community of supportive resources, and feeling cared about as an individual.

▶ Check Your Reading

13. Give two examples of teaching interventions.
14. What is the role of case management in psychiatric home care?
15. What types of therapy are integrated into the Bay Area Health Care's model of psychiatric home care?

MEDICARE CRITERIA FOR RECEIVING PSYCHIATRIC HOME CARE

Presently, Medicare reimburses 100% for home care services. Under Medicare, the services provided to patients receiving home health care are viewed as intermittent and transitional rather than continuous or long-term. To receive psychiatric home care under Medicare, the patient must meet four criteria. First, the patient must be certified as homebound by a physician. Second, the patient must have a psychiatric diagnosis. Third, the patient must require the skills of a psychiatric nurse. Fourth, the patient must be under the care of a psychiatrist. Each of these criteria is discussed.

The Person Must Be Homebound

Homebound Status means that the patient's condition generally precludes them from leaving home without significant assistance from another person, and therefore the patient rarely leaves home (Eggland, 1987; Carson 1994a). The homebound status of a psychiatric patient is determined either by the degree of disability associated with the patient's psychiatric condition or by any concomitant physical limitations experienced by the patient. Box 44–1 lists examples of patient conditions that might be grounds for considering a person psychiatrically homebound.

BOX 44–1 Examples of Patient Conditions That Might Be Grounds for Considering a Person Psychiatrically Homebound

- Confusion, disorientation, and poor judgment
- Psychomotor retardation caused by severe depression
- Altered perception or cognition
- Altered thought processes
- Risk for self-harm
- Vulnerability in the community
- Poor impulse control
- Requirement of 24-hour supervision
- Impairment in social interactions
- Excessive fear or anxiety
- Agoraphobia
- Need for assistive devices (e.g., cane, walker, wheelchair) for mobility
- Inability to leave home independently
- Inability to leave home without taxing effort
- Dependence on assistance from others for leaving home

The Person Must Have a Psychiatric Diagnosis

The patient must have a recognized *DSM-IV* diagnosis to receive psychiatric home care. The *DSM-IV* diagnoses and diagnostic categories most commonly encountered in psychiatric home care are listed in Box 44–2.

The Person Must Require the Skills of a Psychiatric Nurse

Medicare states that services provided to patients require the skills of a "psychiatrically trained nurse who has special training and/or experience beyond the standard curriculum for an R.N." (Health Care Financing Administration, 1989). Such special training or experience includes the following (Transmittal letter from Independence Blue Cross and Blue Shield, 1993):

- A master's degree in psychiatric nursing or community health nursing
- A bachelor's degree in nursing, with one year of adult or geriatric psychiatric experience
- A diploma or associate degree in nursing, with two years of adult or geriatric psychiatric experience

The Plan of Care Must Be Directed by a Psychiatrist

Presently, Medicare requires that the services of the psychiatric nurse must be provided under a plan of care established and reviewed by a psychiatrist (p. 15.2, Medicare Home Health Agency Manual, HCFA Pub. 11). This last criterion has been challenged by psychiatric home care programs across the United States for a number of reasons: First, most elderly patients never see a psychiatrist for treatment of depression or anxiety, but rather they receive treatment from their general practitioners or family practice physicians. Medicare's requirement that the plan of care be directed by a psychiatrist limits access to psychiatric home care by patients who chose to see a physician other than a psychiatrist. Second, in some areas of the United States, there are no psychiatrists available to provide care to patients. Third, this is the only specialty for which Medicare requires a physician specialist to oversee the plan of care.

Because of these reasons, the Health Care Financing Administration, which controls Medicare, has ruled that the criterion requiring a psychiatrist to oversee the plan of care will eventually be eliminated (*Federal Register*, 1994; *NAHC Report*, 1995).

Case Example 44–1 illustrates the type of care that could be provided during psychiatric home care visits. In the example, Frances' homebound status was related to her psychological inability to leave home and to access psychiatric follow-up care as well as to her impaired mobility. Frances had a psychiatric diagnosis of depression. Furthermore, she required the skills of a psychiatric nurse who understood her diagnosis, her medications,

BOX 44–2 *DSM-IV* Diagnoses and Diagnostic Categories Most Commonly Encountered in Psychiatric Home Care

Axis I Diagnoses

- Schizophrenia and other psychotic disorders
- Affective disorders
- Anxiety disorders
- Dual diagnoses (used for patients who have a psychiatric diagnosis in addition to a substance abuse problem)
- Early-onset dementia
- Substance-related disorders
- Dissociative disorders

Axis II Diagnoses

- Personality disorders
- Mental retardation

and the needs that Frances presented. Finally, her plan of treatment was ordered by the psychiatrist in the inpatient unit.

Case Example 44–1 Story of Frances

I had been admitted to a psychiatric hospital from a medical hospital where I was recuperating from a fall I had taken out on the street. My doctor noticed that I was depressed and asked me if I would be willing to go to a place where I could get treatment. I said yes. I stayed at the psychiatric hospital for a month.

The people were grand! They made me feel taken care of. I was so tired and worn down from running back and forth to the nursing home to see my husband, that I needed to be taken care of.

When they told me I was ready to go home, I was excited and scared at the same time. I couldn't wait to be back in my own home with my own things. But, to tell you the truth I was worried that I wouldn't be able to make it. I knew that I felt better, but would I still feel okay when I went back to my apartment? I'd be alone a lot. I still wasn't walking too good. What if I fell again? Well, to make a long story short, the hospital staff asked if I minded if they referred me to a psychiatric home health nurse. Boy, was I relieved! I knew that I wouldn't be entirely on my own.

My nurse visited me two days after I came home. We hit it off right away. The first visit she asked a lot of questions. Trying to get to know me, she said. I was happy when she told me her visits would be covered by my Medicare. Then we talked about what we both saw as my needs. I told her I needed help telling my husband that I could no longer be at his beck and call. In fact, I needed help telling anyone no. She said she could help me with that, and she thought that I needed some teaching about my medication, how to worry less, and how to use the resources that were available to me in my senior apartment house.

At first she came three times a week. Over a three-month span of time, she eventually dropped her visits back to once a week. At first those visits were a life line to me. A major step happened one month after she started coming. She was at the apartment when my husband called from the nursing home demanding that I drop everything and bring him money. I had already taken him money two days before. Well, I took a deep breath and told him that I couldn't do this, that he would have to make do with the money that I had already given him, and that I would come back at the end of the week. This was what I had practiced with my nurse. My heart was beating fast, but did I feel good when I stood up for myself. Over the next two months I noticed that I was actin' kinda bossy sometimes, but my nurse said it was a good bossiness. She said I was being assertive. I started going to bingo once a week and gossiping in the lobby with some of my friends. One day my nurse visited and noticed that I had gone to the beauty parlor in the building and gotten my hair and nails done. She told me how pleased she was with all the progress I was making. She said that she had a feeling that I was ready to move on without her services. I hated to see her go, but she was right. I wonder if I would have done as good if she didn't visit. I'll never know, but I'm sure glad that she came.

▶ Check Your Reading

16. Define homebound status.
17. What are the four criteria that must be met for a patient to be eligible for psychiatric home care under Medicare?
18. Discuss two of the arguments made against the requirement that a psychiatric plan of care be ordered by a psychiatrist.
19. What qualifications does Medicare require for psychiatric nurses?

THE CRITERIA OF OTHER PAYERS FOR RECEIVING PSYCHIATRIC HOME CARE

In addition to Medicare, there are other payers who reimburse for psychiatric home care. Although some states have eliminated their Medicaid benefits for home care, patients who receive Federal Medicaid are still eligible for this service. Federal Medicaid follows similar criteria in determining eligibility for services as well as qualifications for nurse providers. There can be differences across states, however, in how these criteria are interpreted.

Funding is also available from the Veterans Administration (VA). The VA's guidelines governing eligibility for services and qualifications of psychiatric nurses are also similar to those spelled out by Medicare. Each VA field office must be contacted, however, to verify approval for psychiatric home health care before initiating the service.

Managed care companies are increasingly looking to psychiatric home care as a way of cutting the health care costs of patients who have traditionally been high users of psychiatric services. The primary criterion used by these companies in deciding to use psychiatric home care is whether or not psychiatric home care services might eliminate or reduce expensive hospitalizations. The one requirement made by most managed care companies is that the nurses delivering the services be certified clinical specialists in psychiatric nursing.

Commercial insurance companies are sometimes willing to use part of a patient's inpatient psychiatric benefit to pay for psychiatric home care. Again, their criteria for flexing benefits is similar to that of the managed care companies; they must be convinced that the patient will benefit from care in a less costly setting. Some commercial insurers, however, are resistant to reimbursing for psychiatric home care. In response to this resistance and in recognition that insurance companies reimburse (either partially or completely) for the services of a psychiatric nurse who is certified as a clinical specialist, some home health care agencies have set up professional organizations for their psychiatric nurse providers and allow the practitioners to bill the private insurance companies (Thobaben, 1989).

Psychiatric home health care services are also available to patients who can and are willing to pay for the service. Service is usually initiated by obtaining a contract signed by the patient indicating the patient's willingness to assume the cost of skilled nursing visits.

▶ **Check Your Reading**

20. What is the expectation of managed care companies in making referrals for psychiatric home care?
21. What are the Medicaid criteria for receiving psychiatric home care?

POPULATIONS SERVED BY PSYCHIATRIC HOME CARE

The population using psychiatric home health care is varied in age and needs, and as such the services offered must be equally broad in coverage. These services include not only the direct nursing care of a psychiatric nurse, but also access to medical nursing skills; dental care; pharmaceutical services; social services; physical, speech, and occupational therapies; laboratory testing; nutrition advice; homemaker or home health aide services; provision for durable medical equipment and supplies; chore services; and transportation (Warhola, 1980; Holland, 1993).

The Elderly

The bulk of all home care referrals including psychiatric are for the elderly. In the last two decades, the over-65 age population has increased more than twice as fast as those who are younger than 65 (Rice and Feldman, 1983; Research News, 1984; Eliopoulos, 1991, 1993). As people live longer, their use of health services increases as they contend with the demands and limitations imposed by chronic illnesses. It is estimated that more than 80% of the elderly have chronic diseases, and at least 50% of this number suffer physical and social limitations as a result of their chronic illnesses. Many of these individuals face multiple hospitalizations to deal with exacerbations of chronic conditions. It is not surprising then that this population with its heightened need for acute care services would also be the primary beneficiary of all types of home health care services, including psychiatric services (Crawford, 1987).

A major concern of the elderly, expressed by Frances in Case Example 44–1, is that they will lose the ability to cope with their conditions within the comforts of their homes and be forced into institutions. Bakken (1983) contends that this fear could be alleviated by providing the elderly with the kinds of supports available through home health care. Such support allows the elderly to continue to derive a sense of meaning and purpose from their lives even though their activities may become increasingly more restricted.

Patients with Acute Disorders

Another group benefiting from psychiatric home health services are those patients who have been treated in an acute care facility. Many of these patients, no longer requiring the 24-hour supervision of a hospital, are still in need of intense monitoring once they return to their homes. They may be seen by a psychiatric nurse on a daily basis to assist them in making the transition between hospital and home (Case Example 44–2).

Case Example 44–2 Mrs. Clark's Story

Mrs. Clark underwent cardiac bypass surgery. After surgery, she developed major depression. While still in the hospital, Mrs. Clark was started on fluoxetine (Prozac), an antidepressant. At the time of discharge, she was still very sad and not motivated to engage in the cardiac rehabilitation program offered by the hospital. A psychiatric home health nurse began working with her to

- Help her resolve her feelings of sadness and despair.
- Facilitate Mrs. Clark's integration of this experience into the totality of her life story.
- Support her in her rehabilitation program.
- Monitor Mrs. Clark's compliance with and response to the Prozac.

Initially, Mrs. Clark was seen by the nurse three times a week with visits gradually tapering down to once every other week. At the end of four months, Mrs. Clark was discharged from home health care, fully engaged in her cardiac rehabilitation, actively participating in a local senior center, and completely free of her depression.

The Seriously and Persistently Mentally Ill

The seriously and persistently mentally ill, also referred to as the chronically mentally ill, represent another group who benefit from home health care services. Many in this group fall into the "revolving door" cycle of hospital to home to hospital to home. Research has demonstrated for this group that home health care decreases the total number of hospital days and presumably improves the quality of their adjustment to the home and community (Weisbrod et al, 1980; Stein and Diamond, 1985; Sandrick, 1986; Goering et al, 1988; Raschko, 1988;

Wasylenski et al, 1985; Dickstein et al, 1988; Bush et al, 1990). Other studies have documented the cost-effectiveness of home versus hospital psychiatric care (Fenton et al, 1979, 1982; Braun et al, 1981). Rusch (1986) reports on a successful program that involved establishing a central department for home health services within the structure of a hospital. The purpose was to provide continuity of care between the inpatient unit and the patient and his or her family (Case Example 44–3).

Case Example 44–3 The Story of Edgar James

Edgar James, a 72-year-old treated repeatedly for acute episodes of chronic paranoid schizophrenia, provides an example of a patient with a chronic illness who benefited from psychiatric home health care. Mr. James' admissions always followed a similar pattern. His wife and son would obtain an emergency petition for his involuntary admission. The precipitating behavior usually involved a threat of physical harm made by Mr. James to his family. After a brief stay where he would be stabilized, he was always returned to his family. Once out of the hospital, he would continue to take his medication for a month or two and then abruptly stop. After this scenario had been repeated five times, the hospital staff referred Mr. James for psychiatric home care. The psychiatric home care nurse assessed that the primary needs centered around encouraging medication care compliance and psychiatric follow-up, increasing Mr. James' involvement in diversional activities, and teaching the family coping strategies. Home health care continued for six months. At the end of this time, Mr. James was still out of the hospital, involved in an adult day treatment center three times a week, compliant with taking his medications, and getting along fairly well with his wife and son. In addition, his network of family support was expressing a sense of their own importance to the welfare of Mr. James as a result of the nurse's focus of providing them support.

Patients with AIDS

A relatively new group of home health care patients are those with AIDS, who require not only intensive medical supervision, but also psychiatric therapy as they deal with AIDS-related psychiatric problems (Barrick, 1988) (Case Example 44–4).

Case Example 44–4 Tony's Story

During his fourth admission for treatment of *Pneumocystis carinii* pneumonia, the nursing staff noted that there were pronounced behavioral and cognitive changes in Tony. He was forgetful and irritable, displayed emotional lability, and expressed a sense of profound sadness not only over his impending death, but also over his sense that he "counted for nothing." On one occasion, he angrily threw his telephone on the floor when he could not remember how to dial a friend's number. After a thorough neurological evaluation, the medical staff determined that Tony was suffering from AIDS-related dementia and depression. Discharge planning included referral for psychiatric home health care. The nurse who visited Tony identified several needs, including monitoring Tony's safety and his ability to comply with his medication regimen; working with his significant other to ensure that Tony's environment was safe given his deteriorating cognitive capabilities; assisting Tony to find meaning and value in his life; and helping the significant other who was Tony's primary caregiver to continue responding to Tony in the most helpful and loving manner. This care continued for three months, at which time Tony was readmitted with another bout of *Pneumocystis carinii* pneumonia. Tony did not survive this admission. Tony's caregiver, however, expressed gratitude to the psychiatric nurse for assisting him in making Tony's last days of life meaningful.

Children and Adolescents

Children and adolescents are a small but growing number of home health care recipients. They are seen in their homes for the purposes of continued individual therapy as well as for assisting families to deal with problematic behaviors in the real-life environment of home. Usually when children and adolescents require acute care treatment for psychiatric problems the hospital stay is kept as brief as possible. The stay may not provide the family enough time to learn workable strategies for dealing with difficult behaviors. Psychiatric nursing visits allow the nurse to work directly with the family to develop communication and behavioral techniques that will be effective within their life situations and to assist the family to discover a sense of meaning and significance in their parenting efforts.

▶ Check Your Reading

22. What is a major concern of the elderly?
23. Give one reason for providing psychiatric home care to children and their families.
24. What are the benefits of psychiatric home care for the seriously and persistently mentally ill?

NURSING PROCESS

The psychiatric nurse uses the nursing process to collect data, to assess and analyze the patient's needs, to plan mutually with the patient or family or significant other what needs will be addressed and how, and to evaluate the effectiveness and appropriateness of the plan. The steps of the process are the same even though the setting may be different as well as your approach. Within the hospital, your role is one of greater authority and control, whereas in the home, you are the patient's guest. This may influence how an assessment is performed and the manner in which treatment recommendations are made. The home setting requires that you innovate and display greater flexibility to be able to work in what is an atypical clinical setting. For instance, the patient's home may be crowded, dirty, noisy, and full of interruptions. These are situations that you may not be able to change but must work around. The following discussion proceeds through the steps of the nursing process to show what can be done as part of psychiatric home health care.

ASSESSMENT

Assessment focuses on mental status, family dynamics, social support, home environment, functional status, safety, and physical needs.

Assessment of Mental Status

The mental status of the patient includes orientation, recent and remote memory, general fund of knowledge, attention and concentration, ability to abstract, judgment, insight, presence of a thought disorder, and suicidal/homicidal ideation or intent (see Chapter 13 for specifics related to assessment). In addition, you must be able to assess the lethality of a patient's suicidal status and be able to determine whether the patient is at high or low risk (Casserta, 1993; Rice, 1993). See Chapter 36 for specifics related to lethality assessment. Case Example 44–5 gives the story of Mr. Kramer, a patient at risk for suicide.

Case Example 44–5 Mr. Kramer's Story

Mr. Kramer, who had a recent cerebrovascular accident, was receiving several skilled services: A registered nurse came three times a week to change a leg wound dressing; a physical therapist also came three times a week to assist Mr. Kramer in ambulating; and a psychiatric nurse visited once a week because Mr. Kramer was depressed. In addition, Mr. Kramer received the services of a home health aide five times a week to assist him in meeting hygiene needs and performing activities of daily living. During one of the psychiatric nurse's visits, Mr. Kramer said that he wished he were dead. The nurse questioned Mr. Kramer to determine the lethality of his suicidal thoughts. He stated he had a plan. He would take all his medications. The psychiatric nurse initiated a contract with Mr. Kramer in which he agreed that he would not harm himself until the nurse visited again and that if he felt strongly that he could not keep the contract he would call the nurse. Because Mr. Kramer was wheelchair bound, he had limited access to his medications. So the nurse prepared the day's dosage of medications and placed all drugs on an upper shelf out of the patient's reach. In addition, the nurse contacted the psychiatrist, asked for and received an order to increase the psychiatric visits to once a day for two weeks, and also increased Mr. Kramer's Prozac from 20 to 40 mg every day. With more intensive psychotherapy, Mr. Kramer's suicidal ideation began to recede and his depression began to lift.

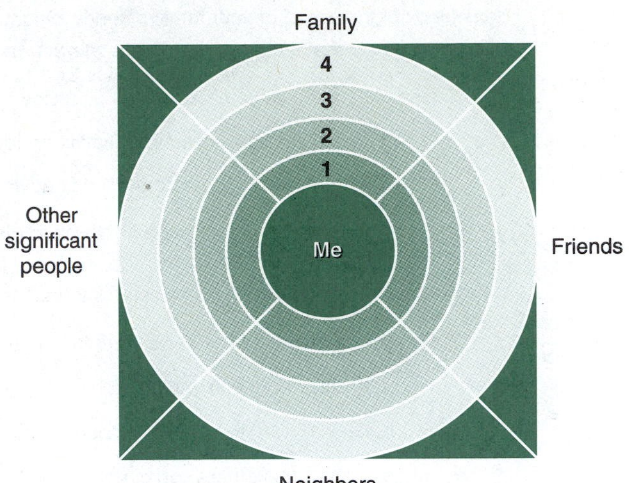

FIGURE 44–3
A social network map. (From Biegel, D. E., Shore, B. K., and Gordon, E. [1984]. *Building support networks for the elderly: Theory and applications.* [p. 29]. Beverly Hills: Sage.)

Assessment of Family Dynamics

Providing care within the home setting allows you to develop a collaborative relationship with the family. To capitalize on this collaborative opportunity, it is essential that you possess an understanding of the many, varied ways that families respond (Soreff, 1983).

Assessment of Social Support

People who have adequate social support systems are able to deal with stress in a more constructive fashion. Social support seems to benefit people in two ways. The first is through a buffering effect that reduces the stress of a crisis. The second is through a direct effect in which self-esteem and confidence are increased when a person is a member of a socially cohesive group (Crawford, 1987). Who is available to assist the patient with activities of daily living? With finances? With emotional support? With companionship? With transportation?

The construction of a social network map (Figure 44–3) facilitates the clinical assessment of social support. This method has been recommended by many experts who have written about strategies to develop support (Pender, 1982; Maguire, 1983; Biegel et al, 1984). The map is divided into three concentric circles in which patients are asked to write the initials of relatives, friends, neighbors, and important others. Patients begin near the center with the initials of those who are closest to them

Please look at the "map" of your family, friends, neighbors, and other people who are important to you as I ask you some questions about the ways that the people you have listed may help you.

1. Does anyone give you information or advice? ☐ Yes ☐ No
   a. If yes, who gives you information or advice? ____________
   b. Do you want more information or advice? ☐ Yes ☐ No
   c. Do you give information or advice to others? ☐ Yes ☐ No

   If yes, to whom do you give information or advice? ____________
2. Can you count on others to be there for you when you need them? ☐ Yes ☐ No
   a. If yes, whom can you count on? ____________
   b. Do you want to be able to count on others more than you do? ☐ Yes ☐ No
   c. Do you feel others can count on you? ☐ Yes ☐ No

   If yes, who can count on you? ____________
3. Do others help you get out of the dumps when you feel down? ☐ Yes ☐ No
   a. If yes, who helps you? ____________
   b. Do you want more help to get out of the dumps when you feel down? ☐ Yes ☐ No
   c. Do you help others get out of the dumps when they feel down? ☐ Yes ☐ No

   If yes, whom do you help? ____________
4. Do others let you know that they care about you? ☐ Yes ☐ No
   a. If yes, who lets you know that they care about you? ____________
   b. Do you need more help from others in letting you know they care about you? ☐ Yes ☐ No
   c. Do you let others know you care about them? ☐ Yes ☐ No

   If yes, whom do you help? ____________
5. Do others help you with everyday things such as household chores, shopping, or transportation? ☐ Yes ☐ No
   a. If yes, who helps you with everyday things, and how do they help you? ____________
   b. Do you need more help with everyday things? ☐ Yes ☐ No

   If yes, what kinds of help do you need? ____________
   c. Do you help others with everyday things such as household chores, shopping, or transportation? ☐ Yes ☐ No

   If yes, whom do you help, and how? ____________

FIGURE 44–4

A questionnaire for assessing the need for social support. (From Biegel, D. E., Shore, B. K., and Gordon, E. [1984]. *Building support networks for the elderly: Theory and applications* [p. 29]. Beverly Hills: Sage.)

and then move outward with the initials of those they are not close to. After completing the initials of those involved in the support network, patients draw lines to connect the initials of all those who know each other. This task can be completed by the patient alone or by the nurse and patient.

The map serves as a database to determine the composition of the patient's support network. You use this information to help the patient identify who provides what kind of support and who might be involved to provide additional support. Figure 44–4 provides questions to assist you in assessing social support. For instance, it is customarily assumed that support is provided primarily from women. Stoller (1990), however, reports that men also function in the caregiver role. Although their assistance is generally intermittent and limited to specific tasks, viewing male relatives and neighbors as potential helpers may expand the supportive network.

Assessment of Home Environment

The home environment allows you the opportunity to assess the patient's actual ability to perform daily chores. Although the ability to perform tasks generally corresponds to the severity of cognitive impairment documented in testing, occasionally there may be a discrepancy between these areas (Weintraub et al, 1982; Weintraub and Mesulam, 1985). For instance, an elderly person who is depressed may lack the motivation necessary to perform daily chores even though the individual performed normally in the context of the structured, supportive testing environment. Formal testing of cognitive functioning sheds little light on exactly how real-life activities are impaired. For example, a patient's inability to dress herself may be related to apathy, a spatial defect, or the inability to sequence the necessary steps. Your assessment of the nature of the impairment has important implications for management.

Assessment for Safety Issues

A natural extension of assessment of the patient's functional abilities has to do with whether the patient is safe to live at home alone. If the answer is no, there are options other than institutionalization that are worth exploring. Home sharing is an option that has been documented as a way to help elderly individuals remain in their homes (Danigelis and Fengler, 1990). Home sharing has been done as a way of easing the financial burdens of maintaining a home, acquiring help with the housekeeping chores, and easing the loneliness of countless hours spent in solitude. When the safety of the patient becomes an issue, the patient might be willing to exchange room, board, and a small weekly stipend paid to a caregiver in return for round-the-clock personal care services. This arrangement might seem more palatable than a boarding home or nursing home placement.

Assessment of Physical Needs

Another area that you assess is the patient's physical needs. If the patient is recovering from a cerebrovascular accident, the services of a medical nurse, a physical therapist, and a home health aide may all be warranted. If this is the case, write an order for these services, which is reviewed and signed by the referring physician (Case Example 44–6).

Case Example 44–6 The Story of Enrique Conches

Enrique Conches was referred for psychiatric home health visits because he was depressed with multiple physical problems. Included among his medical concerns were left-sided weakness from a previous cerebrovascular accident, legal blindness from diabetic retinopathy, a history of cardiac bypass surgery, the fear of impending gastrointestinal surgery, and chronic back pain. When the nurse performed the assessment, he discovered that Mr. Conches had fallen from his wheelchair twice in the last two weeks. Following his stroke, Mr. Conches had never received physical therapy and did not know safe transfer techniques. In addition, his knowledge regarding the management of his diabetes was inadequate. Given these data, the psychiatric nurse ordered the additional services of a physical therapist to work with the patient to ensure safety in transferring techniques and a medical nurse to teach the patient about diabetes, insulin administration, and adherence to a diabetic diet. By recognizing there were needs other than psychiatric and seeking out the appropriate resources, the psychiatric nurse ensured comprehensive care for Mr. Conches. This also freed the psychiatric nurse to focus on the issues that contributed to Mr. Conche's depression.

▶ Check Your Reading

25. Name at least three areas assessed by the psychiatric home care nurse.
26. Why is an in-home assessment of functional status valuable?
27. What does a social support map demonstrate?

DIAGNOSIS

The analysis of data focuses on the interactions that occur among the patient's unique psychiatric symptoms, environmental and social factors, and family dynamics and leads to the formulation of nursing diagnoses. Because of the multiplicity of patient situations that are encountered in psychiatric home care, the possible nursing diagnoses run the gamut of the NANDA taxonomy.

OUTCOME IDENTIFICATION

Again, because of the limitless patient situations encountered in psychiatric home care, the possible expected outcomes are limitless. The following, however, are selected general outcomes that could be individualized to specific patients:

- The patient will demonstrate a reduction in psychiatric symptoms by the termination of psychiatric home care.

- The patient will demonstrate greater functional abilities at the termination of psychiatric home care.
- The patient will consistently access psychiatric follow-up care.
- The patient will demonstrate an increase in medication knowledge as evidenced by a grade of at least 75% on a medication posttest.
- The patient will demonstrate at least five new coping skills to deal with psychiatric illness.

PLANNING

In developing a care plan, you must know or have access to information regarding available community services and be able to access these for the patient. Whenever it is appropriate, engage the patient and family or significant other in the planning process. This results in establishing a plan of care that includes short-term goals, determining rehabilitation potential and discharge plans, and writing nursing orders that are then reviewed and signed by the referring physician.

IMPLEMENTATION

The interventions used by the psychiatric home care nurse generally fall into four categories: continued assessment, teaching, psychotherapeutic skills, and case management. Implicit in each of these interventions is your ability to use communication skills to develop a meaningful relationship with the patient and family or significant other. You must be able to synthesize understandings of the patient's psychiatric and emotional disability, medication effects, and family dynamics. In addition, you must be able to respond appropriately to specific behavioral manifestations of the patient's illness, such as the physical, emotional, and spiritual expressions of depression. You must be able to respond effectively to a crisis situation such as that occurring when a patient is verbally or physically assaultive. Box 44–3 summarizes nursing interventions commonly used in psychiatric home care.

Continued Assessment

Continued assessment is essential with each visit. You must be attuned to even the slightest changes in the patient's behavior. These changes may indicate improvement and progress, or they may be an indication of regression and a need for more intensive evaluation, perhaps by a psychiatrist. For example, the fact that a patient smiles may seem insignificant. If the patient has been guarded and obsessed with paranoid ideation, however, a smile may indicate that the patient is beginning to engage in a relationship. In another situation, an elderly depressed patient has been treated with various drugs to assist him with his feelings of

BOX 44-3 Nursing Interventions Commonly Used in Psychiatric Home Care

Continual Assessment of:

- Medication compliance
- Medication side effects
- Mental status
- Nutrition/hydration
- Sleep pattern

Teaching About:

- New medication regimens
- Coping patterns related to whatever issues the patient is confronting
- Activities of daily living to meet basic needs
- Communication skills
- Signs and symptoms of exacerbations of illness
- Access to medical follow-up

Applying Psychotherapeutic Skills to:

- Improve self-concept
- Decrease fear
- Decrease anxiety
- Decrease hopelessness
- Increase motivation
- Increase spiritual well-being
- Decrease eating pattern disturbances
- Decrease sleep pattern disturbances
- Increase social interaction
- Increase diversional activities

Case Management to:

- Manage and evaluate care on a regular basis
- Coordinate unskilled services
- Coordinate skilled services
- Coordinate community resources

hopelessness. He also experiences alterations in his sleep pattern, occasionally awakening from 1 to 3 A.M. After being started on Prozac, the nurse discovers that the patient's wakefulness is occurring every night resulting in feelings of exhaustion. In addition, his once healthy appetite has been diminished considerably. The nurse recognizes these behaviors as untoward side effects related to Prozac administration. Her assessment convinces the psychiatrist to discontinue the Prozac and start the patient on a small dose of thioridazine (Mellaril). Within two days, the problems of wakefulness and decreased appetite disappear.

Teaching

Teaching is another intervention that is performed by the psychiatric home care nurse. There are many areas of patient need that might benefit from instruction. Box 44–4 lists possible areas of knowledge deficit in psychiatric home care that you might consider addressing.

BOX 44-4 Possible Areas of Knowledge Deficit in Psychiatric Home Care

- Signs and symptoms of illness
- Medications: uses, side effects, how to take
- Communication skills
- Access to community resources, including spiritual supports
- Stress reduction techniques
- Assertiveness techniques

Application of Psychotherapeutic Skills

Basic strategies are employed in the same manner as in inpatient and outpatient settings, the only difference being the modifications needed in the home environment.

Psychotherapeutic skills often applied in psychiatric home care include

- Behavior modification
- Cognitive reframing
- Communication and interpersonal skills
- Therapeutic use of self
- Problem-solving training
- Assertiveness training

Case Management

Case management is increasingly viewed as an intervention model that has the potential to offset the problems of fragmentation and escalating costs associated with health care. Psychiatric patients whose needs are complex and whose problems are severe and persistent are good candidates for the case management approach (Maurin, 1990). Included in this group are the elderly, those with psychological or emotional disabilities, and AIDS patients.

One of the main goals of case management is to deliver quality, comprehensive care while containing costs. This is accomplished through the coordination efforts of the case manager, who connects with other providers, communicates the treatment plan in its entirety, advocates for the patient, and monitors the effects of various interventions. These coordination efforts are designed to minimize duplication of services, avert potential crises, ensure that the least cost-restrictive setting is used for care, and result in a significant cost savings (ANA, 1988).

Maurin (1990) reviewed the literature related to case management and concluded that the research presents mixed results as to the cost benefits derived from case management. Borland and coworkers (1989) contend, however, that it is difficult to compare the results of various case management studies because of the lack of control over intervening variables. These variables include the following:

- The availability of services to the control group in the environment varied (in some communities there is an abundant selection of services).
- Research methodologies differed.
- The characteristics of patients selected in different studies makes comparison difficult.
- There are wide variations in the operational definition of the term *case management.*

Maurin (1990) asserts that at this point the only safe conclusion that we can come to in relation to case management is that it allows treatment-resistant, chronically mentally ill patients to remain at home and in the community for extended periods of time at no more cost than standard treatment.

One of the major issues related to case management is the lack of agreement about who is capable of being a case manager. The literature reports a broad range of personnel as capable of managing a case, from paraprofessionals to psychiatrists. This broad range greatly complicates outcome studies that look at the effectiveness of the case management model. We would expect wide variations in assessment and intervention ability depending on the knowledge, skill, and professional preparation of the case manager. To date, none of the research has explored whether there is a difference in outcome depending on whether the case manager is a psychiatrist, a psychiatric nurse, or a paraprofessional. This is a question that needs to be addressed in future research.

When home care is paid for by Medicare and Medicaid, there is always a professional who acts as the case manager. Reinke and Greenley (1986) refer to this as the caseworker model of case management. The professional might be and usually is a nurse. A physical therapist or an occupational therapist, however, might also act as case managers. The benefits of a caseworker model of case management are twofold. (1) The nurse who is managing the case is directly involved in the patient's care, and (2) this involvement gives the nurse intimate knowledge of what additional services and skills might benefit the patient. The disadvantage of this model is that many of the tasks performed by the case manager, such as telephone referrals, verbal and written communication of the treatment plan, and coordination of appointments, may out of necessity occur outside of the patient visit. Under Medicare and Medicaid, only direct care costs are billable. Therefore, case management may demand tremendous amounts of the nurse's time, which is nonreimbursable. Borland and associates (1989) documented the morale problem and burnout that occurs with this model. They reviewed a five-year project in which only the project psychiatrist remained the full five years. The turnover for case managers occurred on the average of every two to three years. Case Example 44–7 tells Lizzie's story, an example of the caseworker model of case management.

Case Example 44–7 Lizzie's Story

Lizzie, a frail elderly woman diagnosed with chronic schizophrenia, was referred for psychiatric home care for evaluation of her living environment and her ability to maintain herself independently in the community. She had been seen by the psychiatrist at the senior center at the request of the social services department of the city. Lizzie lived in what was considered a project apartment, or housing for the poor of the city. Her apartment was filthy and overrun with roaches. Lizzie wore layers of clothing, usually consisting of several dresses, at least two sweaters, and stockings rolled down around her ankles. Her most distinguishing feature, though, was a matted braid of hair that extended all the way down her back. The braid weighed several pounds and by Lizzie's admission might have insects in it. Yet, for all this apparent disarray in her life, there was a core of healthy functioning in Lizzie. She managed to pay her bills on time; she shopped every other day searching for the best bargains in food; she made attempts at housekeeping and sewing; she decorated her apartment at holidays; and she had accumulated at least $25,000 in a savings account. The nurse who worked with her determined that Lizzie's living environment posed a health hazard to her as well as to other tenants. The nurse determined that Lizzie's greatest need was not for psychotherapy but for a supportive relationship that would assist Lizzie in making a major move in her life. The nurse, acting as case manager, made arrangements for Lizzie to be shown an available apartment in a nearby senior high rise. The apartment manager, however, refused to allow Lizzie to move in as long as she had her long braid. The manager claimed, and rightly so, that Lizzie's hair posed a health hazard. Working with Lizzie, the nurse was able to help Lizzie make the decision to have her hair cut. Social service arranged to take Lizzie to a beautician, but only after the nurse agreed to check Lizzie's hair for head lice. The nurse also worked with social service so they would help Lizzie with the financial aspects of the move and the practical aspects of packing her belongings. A home health care aide was installed to aid Lizzie with the physical packing. A homemaker came in to assist Lizzie to clean up her apartment before she left. The nurse maintained weekly visits to help Lizzie deal with the emotional tension of having to move from a place where she had lived for over 20 years. The nurse continued to visit Lizzie every week for several weeks after she moved into her new apartment to ensure that Lizzie made a good adjustment.

Reinke and Greenley (1986) describe two other models of case management. One is the paraprofessional-extender, and the other is the team model. Dana Home Care, a for-profit, private-pay agency, operating out of Chicago, uses the paraprofessional-extender model in psychiatric home health (Newton and Brauer, 1989). The agency uses specially trained and supervised paraprofessional in-home caregivers to provide patient care. For patients who require 24-hour care, Dana uses a team of three to six caregivers. The most experienced caregiver acts as the team leader. The team is supervised by a senior staff member who is usually a social worker. The social worker assumes responsibility for making case management decisions; coordinating care; communicating with family, physician, and others; leading team meetings; and supervising the caregivers. In this model, there is a need for careful training and supervision, and a great deal of time and energy are devoted to maintain good communication and coordination among staff.

The team model is one in which all team members are expected to engage in all functions with all patients (Maurin, 1990). Medication dispensing, which is regulated by law, is the only exception to this policy. Staff workers are not encouraged to develop individual attachments to patients, and lines of role differentiation become blurred. The team participates in daily patient case reviews to discuss the patient's status. Everyone is expected to participate in the planning and monitoring for each patient. Staff are seen as interchangeable, which allows for shifting of responsibilities and workload during times of crisis. The intense team interaction seems to build morale. This model, however, requires the most effort to maintain internal communication and coordination among the team members. In addition, by blurring role distinctions, the unique skills of individual team members may be underused. Although this model is used in community mental health centers, there is no report of its application to psychiatric home care.

▶ Check Your Reading

28. Describe the case worker model of case management.
29. State three general outcome indicators for psychiatric home care.
30. Discuss the continued assessment intervention.

31. Identify at least two psychotherapeutic interventions used in psychiatric home care.

EVALUATION

The process of evaluation is as critical in home health as in any other setting, and it depends on excellent documentation by you. The nursing notes are reviewed not only by the agency's own quality improvement staff, but also periodically by the payor (e.g., Medicare or Medicaid). Decisions regarding reimbursement are made based on the quality of documentation provided by the nurse. Every note must tell a story that includes facts such as what skilled intervention was performed, the patient's response to the intervention, what progress has been made and what is still to be accomplished, and an evaluation of the goals for that particular visit. Payors such as Medicare and Medicaid hire registered nurses as chart reviewers. Usually these reviewers are not psychiatric nurses. Therefore, notes must make it absolutely clear that the nursing interventions were skilled ones. Nursing progress notes are written after every visit and provide formative evaluation. There are periodic summative evaluations done as well, generally at monthly intervals, where the nurse summarizes the patient's initial condition, what progress has been made, and future goals. Discharge occurs when the goals have been achieved, the patient has reached the maximum benefit from services, or the patient is rehospitalized. At this time, the nurse writes a final summary note. These notes provide a broad basis of evaluation. For instance, the quality of an individual patient's care can be evaluated as well as the provider's performance. Reviewing many charts provides a method of evaluating the quality of care provided by an agency. From these reviews, modifications are made in care plans, policies and procedures, and programs are developed for necessary staff development (Hughes, 1987).

▶ Check Your Reading

32. Who reviews the psychiatric nurse's documentation?
33. Discuss two purposes served by reviewing documentation.

CONCLUSIONS

Psychiatric home care is a fairly new approach to treating psychiatric patients. This is a promising treatment modality that recognizes that patients frequently do better when they remain within the comforts of their own homes. It also recognizes that psychiatric home care is effective as a cost containment measure.

Psychiatric home care is likely to become increasingly more important as a primary treatment approach for the chronically mentally ill in a cost-cutting, resource driven health care system. The primary difference in providing psychiatric care in the patient's home lies in the amount of autonomy the nurse has in the home. Psychiatric home health care supports the patient's ability to remain functional in the comfort of their own homes and allows the nurse a unique opportunity to understand and treat patients realistically in the context of their own natural environment.

KEY POINTS TO REMEMBER

- Psychiatric home care is a relatively new phenomenon in the health care industry.
- Psychiatric home care is growing because of increased consumer demand, growth in the population needing the service, and cost containment pressures.
- Medicare and Medicaid legislation changed home care from a nursing model to a physician model with emphasis on curing rather than caring and sustaining.
- Psychiatric home care has been reimbursable under Medicare since 1979.
- Psychiatric home care can be defined as a bridge to transition patients from a more restrictive setting to the least restrictive settings, which are their homes, as well as an anchor to help maintain patients in their homes.
- The overall goals of psychiatric home care are to improve quality of life, prevent unnecessary hospitalizations, and maximize patients' potential to live in their own homes.
- Bay Area Health Care's model of psychiatric home care has six components: the foundation is a moral/spiritual one; the walls are made up of assessment and relationship-building skills; the second floor is made up of medication issues; and the roof is constructed of teaching/psychotherapeutic interventions and case management.
- Medicare requires that patients receiving psychiatric home care are homebound, have a psychiatric diagnosis, require the skills of a psychiatric nurse, and be under the care of a psychiatrist.
- Homebound status means that the patient's condition generally precludes them from leaving home without significant assistance from another person, and therefore the patient rarely leaves home.
- Psychiatric home care is appropriate for the elderly, patients with acute disorders, the seriously and persistently mentally ill, children and adolescents, and AIDS patients.
- The psychiatric home care nurse assesses mental status, family dynamics, social support, home environment, safety, functional status, and physical needs of the patient.
- The psychiatric home care patient could receive multiple NANDA diagnoses.
- Outcomes for the psychiatric home care patient are specific and measurable.
- Implementation includes continued assessment, teaching, psychotherapeutic skills, and case management.
- Case management can follow one of three models: the case worker model, the paraprofessional extender model, and the team model.
- Evaluation involves a careful review of documentation.

LEARNING ACTIVITIES

1. As you participate in your psychiatric nursing experiences, take note of the discharge planning that is done for each patient. Is anyone referred for psychiatric home care? Could any patient benefit from psychiatric home care services?

2. Call several home care agencies in your area to determine whether they offer psychiatric services. If they do not, ask them why they do not.

3. What benefits do you think that at-home care provides that inpatient care does not?

4. What situations do you think require an inpatient stay?

5. See if you can arrange a buddy visit with a psychiatric home care nurse. If you are able to do this, compare the role of the psychiatric home care nurse to the inpatient psychiatric nurse.

CRITICAL THINKING EXERCISE

Mary Clark, a psychiatric nurse clinical specialist used to work as the nurse manager on the inpatient psychiatric unit. Six months ago, she started her job as psychiatric consultant for home health care. Today she just received a call to evaluate the suicidal risk and possible hospitalization of Mr. Jenner. Mr. Jenner, 64 years old, has had a history of depression and suicide attempts since he was diagnosed with prostate cancer 18 months ago. In the first year of his illness, he had three inpatient admissions. Since Mary has been seeing him, he had maintained a moderate level of functioning without being hospitalized.

1. Is there evidence to suggest that home health care can deter inpatient hospitalizations?

2. What evidence is needed to conclude that psychiatric home health care is effective?

3. What evidence will Mary look for to determine the extent of the suicidal risk?

Mary was greeted at the door by Mrs. Jenner when she arrived. Mrs. Jenner quickly took Mary into the bathroom. Mr. Jenner was sitting on a stool with his head in his hands crying. Mary noticed fresh blood on his left wrist that had smeared on his forehead.

1. What assumptions can Mary make about Mr. Jenner?

2. Consider alternative possibilities.

3. What conclusions can you draw from this evidence?

REFERENCES

American Nurses' Association (1988). *Nursing case management.* Kansas City, MO: American Nurses' Association.

Bakken, K. L. (1983). Integrated health care: The whole person in community. *Nursing Economics, 1* (2), 178–180.

Barrick, B. (1988). Caring for AIDS patients. *Nursing, 88* (11), 50–59.

Baum, L. F. (1982). *The wizard of Oz.* New York: Puffin Books.

Biegel, D. E., et al (1984). *Building support networks for the elderly: Theory and applications.* Beverly Hills, Calif.: Sage.

Borland, A., McRae, J., and Lycan, C. (1989). Outcomes of five years of continuous intensive case management. *Hospital and Community Psychiatry, 40* (4), 411–418.

Braun, P., et al (1981). Overview: Deinstitutionalization of psychiatric patients: A critical review of outcome studies. *American Journal of Psychiatry, 138,* 736–739.

Brown, C. S., et al (1987). Association between type of medication, instruction, and patient's knowledge, side effects, and compliance. *Hospital and Community Psychiatry, 38* (1), 55–60.

Burbach, C. A., et al (1988). Community and home health nursing: Keeping the concepts clear. *Nursing and Health Care, 9*(2), 96–100.

Bush, C. T., et al (1990). Operation outreach: Intensive case management for severely psychiatrically disabled adults. *Hospital and Community Psychiatry, 41* (6), 647–649.

Carson, V. B., et al (1994a). *Bay Area psychiatric home care manual.* Baltimore: Bay Area Health Care.

Carson, V. B. (1994b). Doing psych, but talking med-surg language. *Caring, 13* (6), 32–41.

Carson, V. B. (1994c). Spiritual care of Evelyn. *Caring, 13* (12), 27–29.

Carson, V. (1994d). Spirituality and depression: An important relationship. *Smooth Sailing: DRADA Newsletter, January,* 3–4.

Carson, V. B. (1994e). Caring: The rediscovery of our nursing roots. *Perspectives in Psychiatric Care, 30* (2), 4–6.

Carson, V. B. (1995). Bay Area Health Care model of psychiatric home care. *Home Healthcare Nurse, 13* (4), 26–32.

Casserta, J. E. (1993). The mind-body connection. *Home Healthcare Nurse, 11* (2), 6.

Collins-Colon, T. (1990). Do it yourself medication management for community based clients. *Journal of Psychosocial Nursing and Mental Health Services, 28* (6), 25–27.

Crawford, G. (1987). Support networks and health related changes in the elderly: Theory based nursing strategies. *Family and Community Health, 10* (2), 39–48.

Danigelis, N. L., and Fengler, A. P. (1990). Homesharing: How social exchange helps elderly live at home. *Gerontologist, 30* (2), 162–170.

Daubert, E. (1987). Strategic planning in home care. *American Journal of Nursing, 87* (9), 1161–1163.

Davidhizar, R. E., & McBride, A. B. (1985). Teaching the client with schizophrenia about medication. *Patient Education and Counseling,* 7 (2), 233–255.

Davis, E. J. (1987). Home care—what is needed? *Public Health Nursing, 4* (2), 82–83.

Dickstein, D., et al (1988). Reducing treatment costs in a community support program. *Hospital and Community Psychiatry, 39* (10), 1033–1035.

Duffy, J., Miller, M., and Parlocha, P. (1993). Psychiatric home care. *Home Healthcare Nurse, 11* (2), 22–28.

Eggland, E. T. (1987). Home health care. *Nursing 87, 10,* 75–80.

Eliopoulos, C. (1991). Development tasks of aging. In *Long-Term Educator* (Vol. 1, Lesson 6). Glen Arm, Md.: Health Education Network.

Eliopoulos, C. (1993). *Gerontological Nursing* (3rd ed.). Philadelphia: J. B. Lippincott.

Federal Register, December 20, 1994. *59* (243), 65486.

Fenton, F. R., et al (1979). A comparative trial of home and hospital psychiatric care. *Archives of General Psychiatry, 36* (9), 1073–1079.

Fenton, F. R., et al (1982). A comparative trial of home and hospital psychiatric treatment: Financial costs. *Canadian Journal of Psychiatry,* 27 (4), 177–187.

Frisch, N. (1993). Home care nursing and psychosocial-emotional needs of clients. *Home Healthcare Nurse, 11* (2), 64–65, 70.

Goering, P. N., et al (1988). What difference does case management make? *Hospital and Community Psychiatry, 39* (3), 272–276.

Harris, M. D. (1993). Psychiatric evaluation and therapy. *Home Healthcare Nurse, 11* (2), 66–67.

Health Care Financing Administration (1979). *Hm11: Medicare home health agency manual,* Transmittal 114, Section 204.6.
Holland, L. (1993). Mental health supportive home care aides. *Caring Magazine, April,* 44–48.
Hughes, F. (1987). Quality assurance in home care services. *Nursing Management, 18* (12), 33–36.
Kelley, J. H., and Lehman, L. (1993). Assessment of anxiety, depression and suspiciousness in the home care setting. *Home Healthcare Nurse, 11* (2), 16–20.
Klebanoff, N., and Casler, B. (1986). The psychosocial clinical nurse specialist: An untapped resource for home care. *Home Healthcare Nurse, 4,* 36–40.
Lehman, L., and Kelley, J. H. (1993). Nursing interventions for anxiety, depression, and suspiciousness in the home care setting. *Home Healthcare Nurse, 11* (3), 35–40.
Lesseig, D. (1987). Home care for psych problems. *American Journal of Nursing, 10,* 1317–1320.
Lundberg, C. J. (1984). Home health care: A logical extension of hospital services. *Topics in Health Care Financing, 10* (3), 22–33.
MacNamara, E. (1982). Home care: Hospitals rediscover comprehensive home care. *Hospitals, 16* (21), 60–66.
Maguire, L. (1983). *Understanding social networks.* Beverly Hills, Calif.: Sage.
Maurin, J. T. (1990). Case management: Caring for psychiatric clients. *Journal of Psychosocial Nursing and Mental Health Services, 28* (7), 6–12.
Medicare home health agency manual (1989). HCFA Pub. 11; 04-89; Rev. 222; Retrieval Title: P11R222.
Minnesota Community Health Services, Office of Community Development (1981). *Home care guidelines.* Minneapolis, Minn.: Minnesota Department of Health.
Mundinger, M. (1983). *Home care controversy: Too little, too late, too costly.* Rockville, Md.: Aspen Systems.
NAHC Report, January 1995.
Neiman, E., et al (1986). Bridging the gap: Hospital to home in a changing health care environment. *Emphases on Nursing, 2,* 35.
Newton, N. A., and Brauer, W. F. (1989). In-home mental health services. *Caring, 8* (6), 16–19.
Pellegrino, E. (1985). The caring ethic: The relation of physician to patient. In A. H. Bishop and J. R. Scudder (Eds.), *Caring, curing, coping: Nurse, physician, patient relationships* (pp. 8–30). Tuscaloosa, AL: University of Alabama Press.
Pelletier, L. R. (1988). Psychiatric home care. *Journal of Psychosocial Nursing and Mental Health Services, 26* (3), 22–27.
Pender, N. J. (1982). *Health promotion in nursing practice.* Norwalk, Conn.: Appleton-Century-Crofts.
Raschko, R. (1988). Assertive at-home case management for impaired elderly persons. *Hospital and Community Psychiatry, 39* (11), 1201–1202.
Reinke, B., and Greenley, J. R. (1986). Organizational analysis of three community support program models. *Hospital and Community Psychiatry, 37* (6), 624–629.
Research News: Studies on elderly show need for home care (1984). *Caring, 3* (5), 11–13.
Rice, D. P., and Feldman, J. J. (1983). Living longer in the United States: Demographic changes and health needs of the elderly. *Milbank Memorial Fund Quarterly, 6,* 362–395.
Rice, R. (1993). Suicidal thoughts and ideation. *Home Healthcare Nurse, 11* (3), 67.
Rusch, S. C. (1986). Continuity of care: From hospital unit into home. *Nursing Management, 17* (12), 39–41.
Sandrick, K. (1986). Home care: Cutting health care's safety net. *Hospitals, 5,* 48–52.
Soreff, S. M. (1983). New directions and added dimensions in home psychiatric treatment. *American Journal of Psychiatry, 140* (9), 1213–1216.
Spiegel, A. D. (1983). *Home health care: Home birthing to hospice care.* Owings Mills, Md.: National Health Publishing.
Stein, L. I., and Diamond, R. J. (1985). A program for difficult-to-treat patients. *New Directions for Mental Health Services, 26,* 29–39.
Stoller, E. P. (1990). Males as helpers: The role of sons, relatives and friends. *Gerontologist, 30* (2), 228–235.
Thobaben, M. (1989). Developing a psychiatric nursing home health service. *Caring, 8* (6), 10–14.
Transmittal letter from Independence Blue Cross and Blue Shield, Medicare Intermediary. (1993).
Warhola, C. (1980). Planning for home health services—a resource handbook. (D.H.H.S. Pub. No. [HRA] 80-14017.) Washington, D.C.: U.S. Government Printing Office.
Wasylenki, D. A., et al (1985). Impact of a case manager program on psychiatric aftercare. *Journal of Nervous and Mental Disease, 173* (5), 303–308.
Weintraub, S., and Mesulam, M. M. (1985). Mental state assessment of young and elderly adults in behavioral neurology. In M. M. Mesulam (Ed.), *Principles of behavioral neurology.* Philadelphia: F. A. Davis.
Weintraub, S., et al (1982). Daily living activities in the assessment of dementia. In S. Corkin, K. L. Davis, J. H. Growdon, E. Usdin, and R. J. Wurtman (Eds.), *Alzheimer's disease: A report of progress in research.* New York: Raven Press.
Weisbrod, B. A., et al (1980). Alternative to mental hospital treatment. *Archives of General Psychiatry, 37,* 400–405.
Witt, R. (1981). Medication compliance among discharged psychiatric patients. *Issues in Mental Health Nursing, 3* (4), 305–317.

SUGGESTED READINGS

Carson, V. B. (1994b). Doing psych, but talking med-surg language. *Caring, 13* (6), 32–41.
Carson, V. B. (1994c). Spiritual care of Evelyn. *Caring, 13* (12), 27–29.
Casserta, J. E. (1993). The mind-body connection. *Home Healthcare Nurse, 11* (2), 6.
Duffy, J., Miller, M., and Parlocha, P. (1993). Psychiatric home care. *Home Healthcare Nurse, 11* (2), 22–28.
Kelley, J. H., and Lehman, L. (1993). Assessment of anxiety, depression and suspiciousness in the home care setting. *Home Healthcare Nurse, 11* (2), 16–20.
Lehman, L., and Kelley, J. H. (1993). Nursing interventions for anxiety, depression, and suspiciousness in the home care setting. *Home Healthcare Nurse, 11* (3), 35–40.
Rice, R. (1993). Suicidal thoughts and ideation. *Home Healthcare Nurse, 11* (3), 67.

UNIT VII
IMPROVING THE JOURNEY

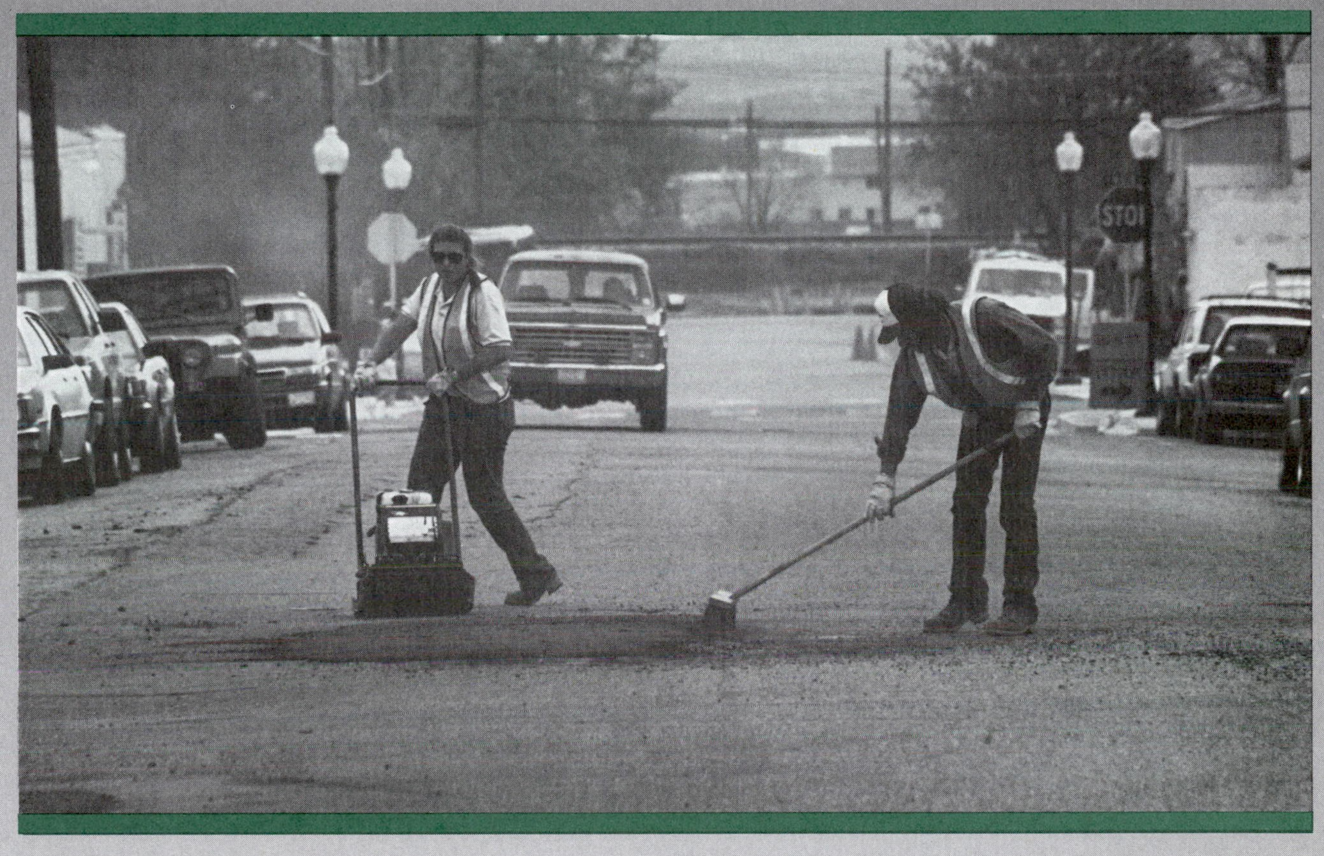

CHAPTER 45

TOTAL QUALITY MANAGEMENT

Quality is never an accident; it is always the result of high intention, sincere effort, intelligent direction and skillful execution. It represents the wise choice of many alternatives.

—John Ruskin

LEARNING OBJECTIVES

After studying this chapter, you should be able to:

1. Distinguish between total quality management and quality assurance.
2. Explain the process of continuous quality improvement.
3. List the components of organizational assessment.
4. Describe the nurse's role in continuous quality improvement.
5. Describe the patient's role in a health care setting implementing continuous quality improvement.

KEY TERMINOLOGY

Benchmarking
Brainstorming
Cause-and-effect diagram
Clinical indicator
Clinical pathway
Collaborative practice
Continuous quality improvement (CQI)
Critical path
Decision matrix
Flow charting
Multivoting
Pareto diagram
Quality assurance (QA)
Strategic planning
Total quality management (TQM)

Hospitals are required to have a **total quality management (TQM)** program to satisfy the Joint Commission on the Accreditation of Healthcare Organizations (JCAHO) and other regulatory agencies that monitor and evaluate the quality of services. But traditional **quality assurance (QA)** programs have provided little help to staff confronted with internal and external problems that create roadblocks and barriers to quality treatment. Patients with chronic mental illness often seem trapped in a "revolving-door" syndrome that creates feelings of disillusionment and powerlessness in the staff. Staff become frustrated by their inability to help the patient get better, stay better, and improve the quality of life.

An increasing emphasis on TQM focuses on management accountability, teamwork, continuous improvements in work processes, customer orientation, and statistical analysis. **Continuous quality improvement (CQI)** incorporates the philosophy of TQM and is evolving as the foundation for quality management (Zonsius, Klingelsmith & Murphy, 1995). This trend toward TQM/CQI is not going away. You need to understand this trend so that you can be a full participant in the process. Instead of focusing on individual staff performance and interventions, typical of a QA model, CQI depends on a systems approach. The patient's treatment needs are viewed as an ongoing process, not a narrow distinction between inpatient or outpatient services. The patient is also viewed as a consumer. The system's response to patient needs and expectations is reviewed.

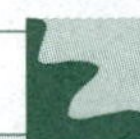

JEAN'S STORY

Pat sat in the staff lounge reviewing the quarterly quality assurance report that she had prepared for the nursing staff meeting. As the nursing quality assurance representative for psychiatry, Pat had spent considerable time monitoring the important aspects of nursing care that the unit's head nurse, Karen, and she had identified. Although Karen and Pat had included some generic screens that all nursing units monitored, they had tried to identify aspects of nursing care that they thought were particularly important in psychiatry and had significant impact on the patient's treatment.

Important aspects of care for which all of the nursing units had developed indicators included nursing assessments, medication administration, patient education, patient safety, management of violent behavior, and discharge planning. For the psychiatric unit, Karen and Pat had developed additional indicators: the use of locked-door seclusion or restraint, therapy groups, documentation of response to prn medication, and therapeutic leaves of absence. Whenever she presented the results of her monitoring to the staff, however, Pat heard complaints that the monitoring focused on finding problems or on documentation that everyone knew had to be done. Staff complained that monitoring didn't help deal with the day-to-day issues that really affected patient care.

Bill's Complaints

Pat looked up as the door to the lounge opened and Bill, the assistant head nurse, came in. "Hi, Bill. How are you doing?" she asked.

"Terrible," Bill groaned. "Guess who's back?"

"Who?"

"Jean Smith! I just finished doing another admission assessment. She was discharged last Tuesday, and she's already back in. I wish we could send her somewhere else. The police brought her into the ER about two hours ago on an emergency petition. It's the same old story. What are you doing?" he asked looking over her shoulder at the report. "Uh-oh. QA again. What are we doing wrong now? Don't you ever get tired of looking at all those charts just so you can tell us that somebody forgot to write a temporary leave of absence return note or put down a patient's sexual orientation on the admission assessment?"

"Come on, Bill," Pat protested. "QA helps us solve problems and provide better care. It's not just a matter of finding fault. We try to make improvements that will help everybody."

Jean's Continuing Problems

"Improvements," Bill snorted. "You mean that you keep changing the forms so that the staff are constantly making mistakes because they're not familiar with the form. Or you create additional paperwork so we have less time to spend with patients. How has the QA program helped Jean or any of the other patients on the unit? I just spent an hour with her. Jean has been drinking again and threatened her boyfriend with a knife. She's got a black eye and several other bruises. The neighbors called the police because she and her boyfriend really got into it. The police reported that Jean threatened to kill herself after they arrived, so they brought her into the ER. For the past hour, she's been sobbing and asking why we don't just let her die. She claims that the landlord is poisoning her with gas fumes. The landlord is threatening to evict her because she and her boyfriend are constantly fighting and he's getting noise complaints from the other neighbors."

"Has she been taking her medications or attending the partial hospitalization program (PHP)?" Pat asked.

"Oh, no! After all the time that we spent talking to her last time she was here about taking her medications and working to get her into the partial hospitalization program (PHP), she hasn't followed through on anything. She said she didn't have any money to get the prescriptions filled, and she couldn't get to PHP because the weather has been cold and rainy. Now she's complaining that the voices have been real bad and they're telling her that she's a bad person and should die. Come on, Pat. For Jean, the hospital is a revolving door. Your QA program hasn't done anything about the multiple hospitalizations that Jean and so many other patients have. What impact has all this QA had on her mental illness or her substance abuse?"

"Well, she looked better the last time she was on the unit. The social worker told me that Jean's considering going into supervised housing, and Dr. Grant has been talking to her about taking Prolixin Decanoate [fluphenazine decanoate] so it will be easier for her to comply with her medications. You can't say that Jean hasn't made any progress despite all of her readmissions," Pat replied.

"Pat, I'm glad to see you're still optimistic, but let's be realistic," Bill said. "Jean was physically and sexually abused as a kid. She's 44 now and has been in and out of psych hospitals and alcohol or drug programs since the age of 16. She has diabetes that is frequently out of control, and she smokes two packs of cigarettes a day. Jean comes into the hospital when she's in crisis but rarely follows up with her medication or outpatient therapy after discharge. On the unit, she's usually cantankerous and argues with the nursing staff about the no-smoking rules and her diet. She's had several serious suicide attempts.She has overdosed three times that I know of on her medications and alcohol, and she's slashed her wrists in the past. She's always creating trouble between the staff and other patients, but whenever we try to set limits, Dr. Grant complains that we're being hard on her. We'll all agree in team meeting that she will be discharged if she doesn't follow the unit rules, but whenever we try to follow through, Dr. Grant will say that she deserves another chance. QA fixes the little problems but doesn't touch the real issues," Bill complained.

TOTAL QUALITY MANAGEMENT AS A TEAM EFFORT

Jean's story describes the all-too-frequent plight of patients with a psychiatric illness as well as the feelings of frustration of the staff working with them. Many nurses, when confronted with TQM, react with the same level of frustration expressed by Bill. They view QA activities as having limited value.

Integrating QA with CQI, however, requires a complete understanding of both. Nursing and other disciplines must adjust their thinking to make the integration of the two concepts beneficial and effective in improving the care provided the psychiatric patient. They must move from retrospective to concurrent review, from

BOX 45-1 The Initiation of Quality Assurance

1910	Dr. Abraham Flexner conducted a study that focused concern on the quality of medical education and helped eliminate "diploma mills"
1913	The American College of Surgeons, established as an accrediting body, developed minimum standards for medical education and performance
1950	The American College of Surgeons was replaced by the Joint Commission on the Accreditation of Healthcare Organizations, the accrediting body responsible for evaluating quality in health care

an individual to a team approach, with continuous improvements focused on work processes, customer orientation, and statistical analysis.

Psychiatry has long used the multidisciplinary approach to treatment planning. Treatment teams regularly include the psychiatrist, a nurse, a social worker, and a recreation or occupational therapist. In some cases, psychologists or other professionals participate in treatment planning and therapy. Treatment teams have resulted in greater coordination and integration of patient care on inpatient units, but these teams have usually limited participation and input from crisis intervention services counselors, outpatient therapists, social workers, group home supervisors, and others who have a significant role in the patient's treatment.

A number of other hospital departments affect both the cost of services provided and the quality of the patient's journey. The availability of medical records can facilitate emergency services, admission procedures, and greater integration and coordination of services between different levels of care. Delays in obtaining laboratory results or consultations can result in longer patient stays with increased costs. If the physician prescribes medications not included on the pharmacy formulary, there may be delays in obtaining the medication, or the physician may need to substitute other, less effective medications. Scheduling problems in ambulatory services can prevent patients from following through with outpatient care and cause patient dissatisfaction. Billing problems can mean delays in the payment for the hospital services and generate patient complaints. Resolution of these kinds of problems requires problem-solving teams with members from all departments and services.

▶ Check Your Reading

1. What is one difference between a QA and a CQI approach?
2. Name at least one driving force behind the TQM/CQI movement.
3. In what ways does the traditional multidisciplinary psychiatric team need to change to incorporate a CQI approach fully?

FROM QUALITY ASSURANCE TO TOTAL QUALITY MANAGEMENT

Historical Influences

The quest for quality in health care has been evolving over a number of decades. Historically, physicians functioned independently, and it was the individual practitioner's responsibility first "to do no harm," as stated in the Hippocratic oath, and to provide the best care possible. With the development of hospitals and the emergence of nursing, medical specialty practices, and ancillary health care services, the responsibility and accountability for "quality" health care came to include a variety of providers and the institutions in which health care professionals worked. Box 45–1 provides a historical summary.

Legal and Regulatory Actions

Legal and regulatory actions also spurred the demand for health care organizations to assess the quality of care provided and develop standards. Between 1950 and 1990, several significant court decisions expanded hospital responsibility and oversight for monitoring the activities of physicians and other staff. In 1955, *Leneris v. Haas* established hospital liability for employees and agent acts. In 1965, hospital liability for the quality of care provided by physicians was established in *Darling v. Charleston Community Memorial Hospital.* The hospital's duty to protect patients from malpractice with "known or should have known" responsibility was established in 1973 by the case of *Gonzales v. Nork and Mercy Hospital.* Hospital corporate liability was further expanded in 1982 by the decision in the case *Elam v. College Park Hospital.* This decision required hospitals to provide peer review to identify substandard practices.

Federal regulation of hospitals was significantly increased by the Social Security Act of 1965, which created Medicare and Medicaid and established conditions of participation for hospitals. In 1972, amendments to the Social Security Act required professional standards review organizations and QA standards for health care providers. Further amendments to Title VI of Social Security, the enactment of the Consolidated Omnibus Budget Reconciliation Act (COBRA) in 1985, and the Omnibus Budget Reconciliation Acts of 1986, 1987, 1989, and 1990 expanded the demand for hospital monitoring and evaluation of the quality, efficiency, and costs of care.

Joint Commission on the Accreditation of Healthcare Organizations

In 1972, the JCAHO published a manual on hospital accreditation, and the American Hospital Association developed a patient bill of rights and a QA program for medical care in hospitals. In 1975, JCAHO published the Quality of Professional Services standard. This was replaced in 1979 with a chapter on QA.

Focus on Inspection and Individual Performance

Initially the focus of professional, accrediting, and regulatory groups was on inspection and individual performance to improve the quality of care. The approach was problem-oriented and focused on minimizing "bad outcomes" and meeting minimal standards. As health care costs began to spiral upward, however, increasing attention focused on cost containment and improved efficiency in health care.

The Ten-Step Process

During the 1980s, the JCAHO moved from a problem-focused approach to systematic monitoring and evaluation. To facilitate this process, the Joint Commission published the *Ten-Step Model for the Monitoring and Evaluation Process* in 1985. The model was modified in 1991 to incorporate the CQI approach. Box 45–2 lists the ten steps.

This ten-step process is used to identify patterns of care that do not meet the established standards and need improvement. The highest priority for monitoring and evaluation are high-volume, high-risk, or problem-prone aspects of care. Data are collected over a series of cases or events. Data are then analyzed to identify specific patterns or trends that indicate a need for improvement. When the threshold, a preestablished level, is reached, a more intensive evaluation is triggered.

BOX 45–2 Ten-step Model for the Monitoring and Evaluation Process

1. Assign responsibility
2. Delineate the scope of care and service
3. Identify important aspects of care and service
4. Identify indicators
5. Establish thresholds for evaluation
6. Collect and organize data
7. Initiate evaluation
8. Take action to improve care
9. Assess the effectiveness of actions taken and maintain the gain
10. Communicate results to affected individuals and groups

The weakness in the earlier monitoring and evaluation approach was that it followed the organizational structure and focused on intradepartmental issues rather than patient care improvement. Problems related to the integration of services from a number of departments and services often require interdepartmental analysis and problem-solving.

Traditional Nursing Approaches to Quality Assurance

Nursing has traditionally focused on aspects of nursing care such as the quality and timeliness of nursing assessments, nursing care plans, and specific nursing interventions (e.g., use of locked-door seclusion and restraints, prn medication, and medication errors). Although these are important aspects of care, many critical issues related to patient care would be ignored or evaluated narrowly. The goal is to focus on processes and integration of services.

In Jean's story, focusing only on traditional nursing care limits the impact on the course of her illness or treatment. The problem of multiple hospitalizations needs to be assessed by the entire treatment team, which includes the psychiatrist, nursing staff, social worker, recreational or occupational therapist, and others. It also requires close coordination among crisis intervention services, inpatient staff, and outpatient providers.

In traditional nursing QA, the full spectrum of services and the flow of patient care are not addressed. Only those processes and interventions within nursing's scope of concern are considered. The quality improvement approach encourages interdisciplinary analysis and problem-solving without assignment of blame to specific disciplines or individuals. The result is a more holistic approach to patient care.

▶ Check Your Reading

4. Describe nursing's traditional approach to QA.
5. Identify two legal issues that have affected QA.
6. Name at least four steps in the Joint Commission's ten-step process.
7. The ten-step process represented a change in the JCAHO's approach to monitoring quality. What was the change?

History of Continuous Quality Improvement

The movement from quality control to QA and now to CQI began in industry. In the 1920s and 1930s, American manufacturing and engineering industries began to implement quality control groups. The greatest effort,

BOX 45-3 Deming's 14 Points of Quality Improvement

1. Create and publish to all employees a statement of the aims and purposes of the company or other organization. The management must demonstrate constant commitment to this statement
2. Learn the new philosophy—top management and everybody
3. Understand the purpose of inspection, for improvement of processes and reduction of cost
4. End the practice of rewarding business based on price tag alone
5. Improve constantly and forever the system of production and service
6. Institute training
7. Teach and institute leadership
8. Drive out fear. Create trust. Create a climate for innovation
9. Optimize toward the aims and purposes of the company the efforts of teams, groups, staff areas
10. Eliminate exhortations for the work force

11a. Eliminate numerical quotas for production. Instead, learn and institute methods for improvement

11b. Eliminate management by objective. Instead, learn the capabilities of processes and how to improve them

12. Remove barriers that rob people of pride of workmanship
13. Encourage education and self-improvement for everyone
14. Take action to accomplish the transformation

however, took place in Japan after the World War II. Japan was faced with severe economic problems and realized that it would be necessary to improve the quality of its products if the nation was to be become a leader in the world markets.

Impact of Deming and Juran on Continuous Quality Improvement

Two of the leading experts on quality control, W. Edwards Deming and Joseph Juran, worked with Japanese companies to develop strategies for improving the quality of products and services. They recognized the need for a management approach to quality improvement and the need to involve staff at all levels in the quality improvement process. Deming and Juran built on the theoretical work done in the 1920s by the Bell Telephone Laboratories quality engineering group. Walter Shewhart, a member of this group, had identified the need for statistical analysis in evaluating quality. Shewhart recognized that some minor variation in quality would always occur over time. The real issue, Shewhart proposed, is to determine when this variation is statistically significant (Juran, 1988).

Applying this principle, Deming studied the Japanese approach to industrial application of quality improvement and developed his famous 14 points of quality improvement shown in Box 45–3. Deming stressed that it is important for managers to understand that most people want to do a good job and that most quality problems are systems problems unrelated to individual performance. Resolving systems problems requires a coordinated management approach and teamwork. Rather than focusing on finding the "bad apples," it is important to develop the overall competency of all employees.

Definition of Quality

Deming, Juran, and other leaders in the quest for quality recognized the importance of defining terms, particularly *quality*. They noted that people often have a fuzzy idea of quality, although many claim that they "know it when they see it." A typical problem is that personal definitions vary. Hospital administrators may look at services provided, census reports, financial statements, physician satisfaction, and patient complaints to develop a definition of quality. Physicians may judge quality according to the types of medical equipment and facilities available; working relationships with hospital administrators, nurses, and other personnel; the reliability and response time for obtaining laboratory results; the drugs in the pharmacy's formulary; and patient responses to the treatment provided. Nurses may define quality according to their working conditions and relationships with other staff, cleanliness of the units, time spent in direct patient care, and practice standards. Patients may define quality according to their improved health; treatment by physicians, nurses, and other hospital staff; ease of registration; respect for confidentiality; the hospital menu; and billing problems.

Juran (1988) notes that quality has multiple meanings but cites two critical definitions: "[Q]uality is product satisfaction" and "quality is freedom from deficiencies." Crosby (1979) defined quality as conforming to requirements and focused on lack of defects. Deming (1986, p. 5) stated that "quality should be aimed at the needs of the consumer, present and future." Organizations need to recognize that they have both internal and external customers and that these customers are integral to defining quality. Internal customers are departments or individuals dependent on the services provided or processes performed by another department. All the leaders in the quality revolution agree that it is the responsibility of management to define quality and to ensure that all employees know that definition.

The quality control models of the 1920s and 1930s all focused on inspection. Deming, Juran, and Crosby all noted that quality control built in an expectation that a given percentage of work was going to be defective. Quality improvement focuses on minimizing variation. Crosby (1984, p. 73) noted that "[t]he system for causing quality is prevention, not appraisal." Deming and Juran realized that there were no quick fixes or overnight solutions to quality problems.

Implementation of a quality improvement program takes years, not weeks or months. Organizations must make a long-term commitment to quality. The first step is to recognize your customers and their needs. Once an organization has identified current and potential customers, internal and external, a mission statement can be developed and planning begun.

▶ **Check Your Reading**

8. What was Deming's contribution to the development of CQI?
9. How did Juran define quality?
10. Identify at least five of the steps in Deming's 14 points of quality improvement.

CONCEPTS OF CONTINUOUS QUALITY IMPROVEMENT AND HEALTH CARE

The implementation of a CQI program requires a systematic approach on the part of the organization.

Mission, Goals, Objectives, and Philosophy

The first step for an organization moving toward a program of CQI involves the development of a mission statement and a philosophy to guide to its future and goals and objectives to guide its daily operations. Therefore, the mission, goals, and objectives, and philosophy should reflect

- The purpose of the organization (i.e., to provide quality patient care services).
- Its commitment to quality improvement (as reflected by definition and as evidenced at all levels).
- A system of values and beliefs that ensures quality improvement (excellence through standards of practice and performance).
- A patient care delivery system conducive to quality improvement (e.g., primary nursing, case management, collaborative practice).
- A system to quantify results.

These strategic components must also strongly emphasize

- The organizational commitment and leadership as essential components in CQI.
- The organization's shared purpose in CQI.
- The organization's focus on customers in CQI.
- The organization's long-term commitment to CQI.

The organizational commitment to CQI, however, must be operationalized throughout the organization.

Strategic Planning

Like all organizations, health care organizations must have some guiding force that gets them from point A to point B. Most organizations, including health care, call this guiding force **strategic planning.** Strategic planning helps all involved look at the future three to five years in advance using current and projected environmental changes and trends. It is within this strategic plan that the foundation for quality improvement is laid.

To develop a strategic plan, however, the organization must first complete an organizational assessment (see Box 45–4). Once the assessment has been completed, the organization can develop service features that respond to customers' needs and processes to provide these services. These plans can then be operationalized.

CQI places great emphasis on planning for quality and the need for continuous feedback so corrections can be made. The Deming quality cycle (1989) (Fig. 45–1) emphasizes the ongoing nature of this process. Activities included under the *planning* portion of the cycle are determining improvement goals and targets and determining methods of reaching these goals. The *do* portion of the cycle includes providing education and training and implementing work. *Study* refers to reviewing the results and evaluating the effects of implementation. *Act* requires that appropriate action be taken. CQI is based on the continuous cycle of these four processes.

BOX 45–4 Steps in the Organizational Assessment Process

- Identify customers
- Determine needs, wants, and expectations
- Assess organizational strengths, weaknesses, opportunities, and threats (SWOT analysis)
- Develop hypotheses about how to satisfy customers' desires

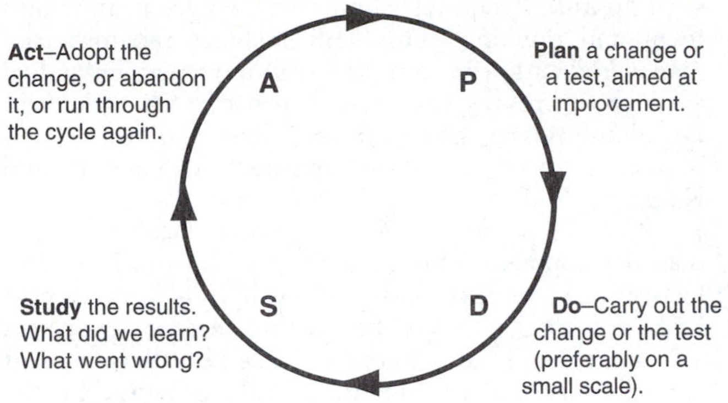

Act–Adopt the change, or abandon it, or run through the cycle again.
A
P
Plan a change or a test, aimed at improvement.
Study the results. What did we learn? What went wrong?
S
D
Do–Carry out the change or the test (preferably on a small scale).

FIGURE 45–1

The Deming quality cycle. (Redrawn from *The new economics for industry, government, education* by W. Edwards Deming by permission of MIT and The W. Edwards Deming Institute. Published by MIT, Center for Advanced Engineering Study, Cambridge, MA 02139. Copyright 1993 by The W. Edwards Deming Institute.

Benchmarking Performance

Another feature of quality management is **benchmarking.** Fortuna and Vazari (1990, p. 50) note that "[b]enchmarking is the process of continually comparing a company's performance on critical customer requirements against the best in the industry (direct competitors) or the class (companies recognized for superiority in performing certain functions) in order to determine which areas should be targeted for improvement." Garvin (1988, p. 31) reported that analysis of survey data on customer reactions to a given company and its competitors' products was organized around four basic questions:

- Is the competition better? If so, by how much?
- Why are they better?
- What can we learn from them?
- How can we apply what we have learned to our business?

In health care, management can use the principles of benchmarking to compare their organization to similar health care organizations, focusing on such outcomes as cost, length of stay, mortality rates, readmission rates, and patient satisfaction. Using benchmarking in Jean's case would help to review successful treatment modalities used in other similar facilities. The CQI leader might look at how leading competitors handle recidivism in noncompliant patients.

Establishing Quality Councils and Quality Teams

The quality council has the task of identifying the specific needs for improvement—the quality projects. For each project, a quality team or circle has responsibility for resolving the problem successfully. The members of the team may be drawn from all levels of the management hierarchy and from different departments or levels of care. The team collects data, diagnoses the causes of the problems, stimulates the development and implementation of remedies, and establishes controls to "hold" the gains.

Developing a quality team in Jean's case might be helpful in identifying key factors that affect her noncompliance and keep her coming back to the hospital. The team might be composed of the inpatient treatment team (physician, nurse, counselor, social worker). In Jean's case, the team might bring in people outside the organization (with her consent) who will be involved in her care after discharge.

The quality team might determine that Jean would be more likely to comply with her medication regimen if she had a home visit by a psychiatric home care nurse for the first three days after discharge. The team might also identify some of the stressors that trigger crisis in Jean's life and—in conjunction with a significant other and the home care nurse—develop a plan to diminish these.

Collecting and Organizing Data

Tools used by quality teams help them analyze problems, set priorities, facilitate decision-making, generate solutions, and document progress. These techniques are defined in Table 45–1.

In Jean's case, **flow charting,** displaying the process from admission to discharge to readmission, might reveal some important information about where the system may be breaking down. It might indeed show that problems occurring within the first three days after discharge lead to noncompliance. It might also show that support is adequate, but structure is insufficient. The idea is that looking at the process in its entirety can provide valuable information that would otherwise not be brought forth.

Once members of the quality team identify Jean's potential problems through problem analysis, they use the **brainstorming** process to generate some ideas, prioritize the ideas through the **multivoting** process, and develop a flow chart that will display the entire process. They can then use a **cause-and-effect diagram** or **Pareto diagram** to identify factors contributing to the problem or causing a certain effect (e.g., noncompliance, substance abuse, recidivism). Once Jean's team has decided on the root cause of a problem, a **decision matrix** can help determine the best solution. A decision matrix allows the team to list all the pertinent criteria and then evaluate different alternatives according to specified criteria. This effort helps the team select the best "solution."

Statistical Analysis and Display of Data

Recognizing that some variation in quality is inevitable, Shewhart proposed that it is necessary to be able to determine when variation is significant (Juran, 1988). CQI is the process of minimizing variation and increasing conformance to standards. To assess and evaluate the data collected in the monitoring and evaluation process, team members must have a basic understanding of statistical concepts, such as sampling techniques, validity, reliability, sensitivity, the nature of variables, frequency distributions, and standard deviation. It is also important to become familiar with some of the types of graphic displays used to communicate results. These include pie charts, bar charts, histograms, scatter diagrams, cumulative frequency curves, and frequency distributions.

▶ Check Your Reading

11. What are the six concepts of CQI?
12. List three of the tools used to collect data in a CQI system.
13. Define benchmarking.
14. Give one reason why strategic planning is essential.
15. What is the function of a quality council?

ROLE OF NURSING IN THE CONTINUOUS QUALITY IMPROVEMENT PROCESS

The primary role of nursing in the CQI process is to help provide an environment that facilitates the *paradigm shift* necessary for the movement from a QA to CQI process. Moving from the traditional QA approach to CQI approach requires significant changes in nursing's focus and thinking. This shift includes moving from managerial authority to participation; from an individual to a collective responsibility approach, from rigid to flexible objectives, and from traditional monitoring and evaluation to continuous improvement (McLaughlin and Kaluzny, 1990).

Nursing practice must concentrate less on individual development and responsibility and more on collective development and responsibility. Nurses must look at practice as it fits within certain processes and understand how nursing processes affect patient care delivery and the quality of care provided by the system.

To understand how quality improvement differs from QA, imagine that Jean becomes verbally abusive toward other patients and staff as a result of her paranoia. The unit is short staffed because one nurse called in sick and a second nurse was delayed by a minor car accident on her way to work. One staff replacement has been located but has not arrived on the unit yet. Another patient has just been placed on suicide precautions, and one staff nurse has been assigned to monitor him continuously.

Jean continues to escalate and threatens to hit a peer. A decision is made to place her in locked-door seclusion. She refuses to cooperate with the request to go quietly to the seclusion room and is becoming increasingly

TABLE 45–1 **Continuous Quality Improvement Tools**

Term	Definition
Brainstorming	Method used to generate ideas without criticism or judgment. Team members are asked quickly to list or call out all the ideas that they think of, related to a specific problem or topic, without filtering or evaluating the ideas
Multivoting	Used once the brainstorming has been completed to determine whether all or only a few of the ideas noted will be explored. Multivoting is a process of setting priorities or narrowing the field of possibilities
Idea logs	Logs of good ideas that surface but may not be relevant to the task at hand. Use of the log prevents the team from being distracted from its main task, yet allows the group to return to that idea at a later time
Storyboards	Graphic representations of proposals or process stories. Storyboards have frequently been used in marketing and advertising to present ideas. Quality teams can use storyboards to document and communicate the activities and progress of the group
Flow charts	Graphic displays of all the steps and decision points in a process that help a team see the "big picture"
Cause-and-effect diagrams	Representations of the various factors that might contribute to a problem
Pareto diagrams	Diagrams using the Pareto principle, that in any group of things that contribute to a common effect, a relatively few contributors account for most of the effect. These diagrams help the team members to focus on the "vital few" rather than the "trivial many." They help identify those factors most significant in causing a certain effect
Decision matrix	A listing of all pertinent criteria followed by an evaluation of different alternatives according to specified criteria

BOX 45–5 JCAHO Revised Standards Concepts

- A hospital can improve patient care quality—that is, increase the probability of desired outcomes, including patient satisfaction—by assessing and improving those governance, managerial, clinical, and support processes that most affect patient outcomes
- Some of these processes are carried out by medical, nursing, and other clinicians; some by governing body members; some by managers; and some by support personnel. Some are carried out jointly by more than one of these groups
- Whether carried out by one or more groups, the processes must be coordinated and integrated. Coordination and integration require the attention of the managerial and clinical leaders of the hospital
- Most governance, managerial, medical, nursing, and other clinical and support staff are both motivated and competent to carry out the process well. Therefore, the opportunities to improve the process—and, thus, improve patient outcomes—are much more frequent than are mistakes and errors. Consequently, without shirking its responsibility to address serious problems involving deficits in knowledge or skills, the hospital's principal goal should be to help everyone improve the process in which he or she is involved

threatening. Only three staff members are available for a take down, but they proceed anyway. Jean struggles. One of the staff members is kicked and falls. The staff finally manages to get Jean to the seclusion room, where she is medicated per physician order.

The nurse who fell is now complaining that her back hurts. She is sent to employee health, where it is determined that she will be unable to return to work, and she is referred to her private physician.

The traditional, individual (detect and correct) focus would result in staff interrogation and assignment of blame. Using the CQI (improve and prevent) approach would change the focus from the individual to the process. Here the CQI focus would be on examining staffing patterns, intervention techniques, aggressive behavior management, and changes to allow the system to respond better. CQI concentrates on changing the *system* so that the conditions likely to result in problems are less likely to occur. This process treats the root cause of the problem rather than a symptom. This approach, however, runs counter to the prevailing assumption in health care that a problem is a result of one individual's error rather than of the larger structure or system within which the individual functions (McLaughlin and Kaluzny, 1990).

Nursing, as an integral part of the hospital, must develop a culture and environment conducive to developing CQI programs that fit these standards. The JCAHO revised standards are based on the concepts shown in Box 45–5. For nursing a new culture requires the following processes:

- Strategic planning
- Collaborative practice
- Identification of important aspects of care
- Indicators and standards of excellence through performance

Planning and Collaboration

In strategic planning, nursing executive leadership becomes instrumental in the success of a nursing CQI process. The first step involves ensuring that all CQI initiatives are based on the organization's strategic plan, mission, goals and objectives, and philosophy (Figure 45–2). The nursing administration commitment to the CQI process must reflect

- A pursuit toward meeting the nursing quality goal.
- Demonstrated commitment to CQI principles.
- A rigorous training program for all employees.
- An environment conducive to teamwork, creativity, and risk-taking.

The second process for creating a nursing CQI program is **collaborative practice.** Here all involved in a specific process work together as a multifunctional team to improve the quality of care provided the patient. Collaboration could potentially include housekeeping, dietary, radiology, medicine, nursing, and other functions. As indicated by the potential composition of a team, team members need not be from the clinical arena only. Collaboration is understood to imply that the individuals share a common goal and desire to affect the situation at hand positively. Without collaboration, traditional boundaries and barriers are not successfully overcome, and the ability to study processes and systems diminishes.

Collaboration has been shown to improve patient care and enhance patient outcomes. Yet despite its known value, collaboration remains difficult to promote among health care providers. Some resist its integration into their practices, thinking that it is "easier to do it myself." Still, CQI can be achieved only through successful collaboration. (See also Chapter 46.)

Collaboration has not been the traditional method of communicating patient care needs between nurses and physicians. Physicians have traditionally assumed the power in any decision-making process regarding patient care and patient outcomes. In the past, decisions regarding the patient's care were solely the responsibility of the physician. Trueman (1981, p. 70) states:

> The power of decision-making concerning every aspect of the patient's care was vested in the physician. Input from the realm of nursing was nonexistent. Physicians gave orders and nursing carried them out.

The shift in attitudes has been brought on in many ways by a change in the patient population (more in formed patients), a change in the focus of patient care (shorter hospitalization and more outpatient care), and a change in the educational level of the nurse. These trends must continue for collaborative practice to be successful. Continued collaboration will depend on

- All health team members being clear about their professional focus and the extent of their contribution.
- All health team members being be able to accept and respect the contributions of others.
- All health team members being willing to make and implement decisions together.
- Nurses being clinically skilled in their practice.

Such skill development and validation in psychiatric nursing can be ensured by the development of clinical standards of practice (see Chapter 4). Collaboration is never easy, but the benefits in patient outcome and staff development almost always exceed the effort.

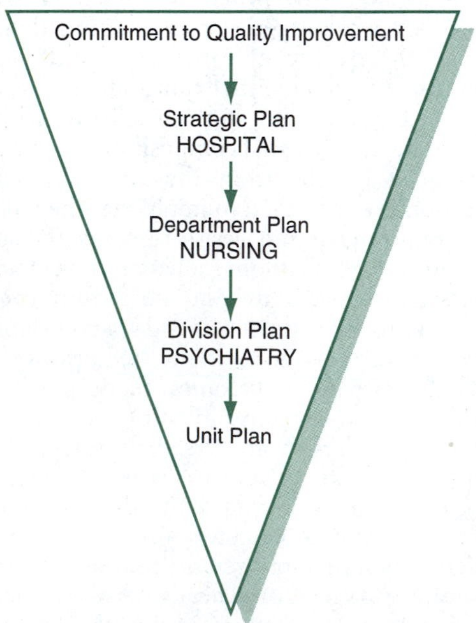

FIGURE 45–2
The flow of quality improvement, from commitment to unit plan.

Monitoring and Evaluating Care and Service

Important aspects of care and service are those with the highest priority and greatest significance in determining outcomes. The JCAHO guidelines recommend that organizations concentrate on aspects of care or service that are high volume, high risk, or problem prone. Fauman (1990, p. 80) notes that determining which aspects of psychiatric care to monitor and how to monitor them has proved difficult for many clinicians. Difficulties exist in

- Determining which aspects of care and service are most important.
- Determining ways to measure and quantify clinical aspects of care.
- Determining appropriate indicators to monitor these aspects of care and service.
- Allocating the time and resources required for monitoring.
- Trying to change treatment outcomes when many factors over which clinicians have limited or no control influence the outcomes.

Brainstorming can facilitate the selection of important aspects of care and service. Once a number of ideas have been generated, the members of the quality team can use multivoting to select those activities on which they will concentrate their efforts. Defining the activities in behavioral terms helps the team quantify and measure them. Schroeder and Katz (1992) reported on sets of universal and specialty aspects of care identified at the Third Annual Conference on Nursing Quality Assurance. Some of the universal aspects of care most applicable to nursing were as follows:

- Knowledge deficit
- Hygiene
- Safety
- Psychosocial issues/emotional support
- Patient/family education
- Medication administration
- Patient satisfaction
- Management of violent behavior

Aspects of care identified by the mental health nursing group included the following:

- Therapeutic groups
- Hallucination/psychosis
- Multidisciplinary treatment
- Withdrawal

- Electroconvulsive therapy
- Suicide precautions

Some additional aspects of care pertinent to psychiatry are discharge planning; crisis management of ambulatory patients; and special treatment procedures such as seclusion, restraints, and patient rights.

Standards of Care and Practice

For each identified aspect of care or practice, it is important to determine standards. Kirk and Hoesing (1991, p. 64) state that standards are needed to

- Provide direction.
- Reach agreement on expectations.
- Monitor and evaluate results. Did results meet the standard, not meet the standard, or exceed the standard?
- Guide organizations, people, and patients to obtain optimal results.

Some standards are established by external organizations such as the JCAHO, the Health Care Financing Administration (HCFA), federal and state regulatory organizations, the American Nurses' Association, specialty boards, and licensing or certification groups. Internally, standards can be developed by a department or a discipline.

Considerable attention is currently focused on clinical practice guidelines. These are valuable in facilitating health care delivery and improving patient outcomes. Guidelines or standards of practice represent appropriate evaluation and treatment based on the state-of-the-art in medicine and nursing. Standards of care or practice allow us to compare an organization to the state-of-the-art in medicine and nursing. These standards change as knowledge and technology increase. In 1989, the American Medical Association established the Practice Parameters Partnership and the Practice Parameters Forum to address the development of practice parameters by physician groups.

The American Nurses' Association published the first Standards of Psychiatric and Mental Health Nursing in 1973. These were revised in 1982 and again in 1994. Valentine and coworkers (1990) noted that physician and nursing groups have had different approaches to standards. They stress the need for physicians and nurses to work together to develop collaborative practice standards to facilitate more cohesive patient care and better treatment outcomes.

Clinical Indicators

JCAHO has defined a **clinical indicator** as a quantitative measure that can be used to monitor and evaluate the quality of important aspects of care and practice (JCAHO, 1995). Indicators serve as screens that identify or direct attention to specific performance issues that require more intense review (see Box 45–6).

BOX 45–6 Indicators

For each indicator, it is necessary to

- Define all terms that may be ambiguous or require clarification for collection purposes
- Indicate whether it is a sentinel event or a rate-based indicator. All sentinel events require further investigation, but rate-based indicators require further assessment only if the occurrence rate shows a significant trend, exceeds predetermined thresholds, or differs substantially from benchmarks. Examples of sentinel events in psychiatry are patient self-injury, suicide, or use of seclusion or restraints. Some rate-based indicators are AMAs (against medical advice), elopements, and transfers to medicine
- State whether the indicator addresses a process or an outcome of care or service
- Provide a rationale for the use of the indicator
- Provide a description of indicator population
- List the specific data elements that will be collected
- Describe underlying factors that may influence the indicator's rate or activity
- Reference the indicator to existing databases

One important aspect of care identified in psychiatry is the use of special treatment procedures. The standard is that designated special treatment procedures require clinical justification. Using standards of care and standards of practice, we can now develop an indicator for the use of seclusion (Box 45–7 lists data elements that we might examine for this indicator.) By collecting data on all occurrences of seclusion, we could then determine if all the applicable standards of care and practice are being maintained. We could also compare our rates of seclusion to the rates in comparable facilities. Using the same process, we could continue to develop indicators for other important aspects of care.

Reporting of Data

In developing a monitoring system, the quality team must agree on the information needed and on the frequency of data collection. Data may be available through medical records, management information systems, logs, or other databases. Use of computer systems facilitates the collection, organization, and display of data. Automation may also be more cost-effective in the long-term. Adequate sample sizes are determined through statistical methods. The data should be organized in a manner that facilitates display and communication of the results. Specific attention is paid to trends or patterns in the data. The quality team analyzes the data to identify any potential for improvement. If so, the quality team facilitates the development and implementation of a plan to improve the process or service. Follow-up is then required to maintain the gains and to assess the effectiveness of actions.

Diagnosis-Specific Criteria and Critical Paths

Critical paths, or **clinical pathways,** are diagnosis-specific or procedure-specific guidelines for the management and treatment of patients. For each diagnosis, expectations of types of services and timeliness of services are being developed. The guidelines identify key functions and services needed and time frames for these activities. For example, a critical path for a diagnosis of bipolar disorder, mixed state, would establish for each day of hospitalization the services and activities expected to take place. (See also Chapter 46.)

The American Psychological Association and the American Psychosocial Association are currently developing critical path material to facilitate utilization review and quality improvement. Overall, psychiatry has lagged behind other specialty areas in the development of critical paths because of the greater differences in treatment response for patients with the same diagnosis. Variation in treatment response for conditions such as total hip replacement, for example, are more limited.

BOX 45-7 Possible Data Elements for Seclusion as a Clinical Indicator

- The rationale for using seclusion is clearly stated in the record
- Seclusion was used to prevent patient from injuring self or others or to prevent serious disruption to the therapeutic environment
- The rationale for use of seclusion addresses the inadequacy of less restrictive techniques
- There is a written order for restraint or seclusion that is time limited and does not exceed 24 hours
- Clinical assessment of the patient before and during the period of seclusion is documented in the record
- A physician's oral order is obtained within 1 hour if seclusion is implemented on an emergency basis by nursing staff
- prn orders are not used to authorize the use of seclusion
- Patient is observed at least every 15 minutes, and observations of behavior are documented in the record
- The door to the seclusion room is opened at least once an hour, and the patient is checked and offered use of the toilet

Keyes and Moynihan (1992), however, report progress. They reviewed a CHAMPUS Mental Health Services Demonstration project that focused on developing, assessing, and refining quality-of-care criteria. This project developed level-of-care criteria and milestones for mental health services. Using DSM, participants developed diagnosis-specific criteria for depressive disorders. Clinical paths can also be developed for specific treatment protocols. Figure 45–3 is an example of an inpatient lithium plan of care.

As diagnostic and treatment procedures become more refined, the use of critical paths will increase in psychiatry. We will be able to assess and evaluate variations from clinical guidelines and treatment outcomes more effectively.

Patient Response and Outcomes

Increasing attention is being paid to treatment outcomes in psychiatry, particularly with the expansion of managed care. Psychiatric services are being forced to define their treatment goals and interventions better to achieve these goals. Goals need to be defined in behavioral terms, and psychiatry programs must be able to demonstrate effectiveness in the utilization management of services and the achievement of positive patient outcomes based on these goals.

One way to demonstrate quality and effectiveness of services is to monitor whether or not critical treatment objectives are achieved. Quality teams can focus on analysis of the treatment process to develop critical paths and outcome data that are valid and reliable. Assessing the quality of services means focusing on patient response and outcomes. Documenting clinical outcomes provides a way of monitoring results. Using the assessments and treatment plans, we can review the problems, goals, and interventions to evaluate patient outcomes.

Wells (1992) described a documentation strategy to facilitate charting of clinical progress and outcomes. The clinical outcome assessment documentation (COAD) system communicates the plan of care, expedites charting, and facilitates documentation of the patient's progress toward outcome-oriented goals. Wells developed a flow sheet of routine categories of care that eliminated documentation of treatments and activities unless they were abnormal. Normal parameters are given for each treatment or activity, and documentation of response is not required unless it falls outside the normal parameters. Other systems, such as the problem-intervention-evaluation (PIE) system, which combines the care plan with the progress notes (Siegrist et al, 1985), can also facilitate assessment and evaluation of treatment outcomes.

Decision Analysis

Traditionally, health care organizations have used hierarchical decision models based on hospital structure organized around functional areas or disciplines. Fargason and Haddock (1992) discuss the need to move to cross-functional, integrative team decision-making as part of

IMPRINT WITH PATIENT CHARGE PLATE

THE UNION MEMORIAL HOSPITAL
NURSING SERVICE DEPARTMENT
INITIATION OF INPATIENT LITHIUM
PLAN OF CARE

EXPECTED LOS ______________ DAYS
(LOS DEPENDENT ON DIAGNOSIS)
DATE POC REVIEWED BY MD ______________

DATE	DAY 1	DAY 2	DAY 3	DAY 4	DAY 5	DAY 6	DAY 7	DAY 8
CONSULTS	Med consult if indicated. Consider diet consult.			Check lithium results				
TESTS	Thyroid function test, BUN, serum creat. (or within 7 days pre-adm.). Baseline pregnancy test if indicated. Consider 24-hr urine for creat. clear.		Lithium level (± q2–3 days) ————	————	————	————	————	————
ACTIVITY	Dependent on condition. ————	————	————	————	————	————	————	————
TREATMENTS	Baseline VS, wt. I&O. ————	————	————	————	————	————	————	————
	Assess for lithium toxicity (nausea, vomiting diarrhea, tremors, muscle twitching, edema) & therapeutic effects qd. ————	————	————	————	————	————	————	————
MEDS	Lithium (dose per MD order). ————	————	————	————	————	————	————	————
			Reevaluate for ↑ + q 3 days. ————	————	————	————	————	————
DIET	Maintain pre-hosp. diet unless contraindicated. ————	————	————	————	————	————	————	————
	Maintain adeq. fluid intake (min. 32 oz/day). ————	————	————	————	————	————	————	————

FIGURE 45–3
An example of a clinical path, or clinical pathway. (Courtesy of The Union Memorial Hospital, Baltimore, Maryland.)

Illustration continued on following page

IMPRINT WITH PATIENT CHARGE PLATE

THE UNION MEMORIAL HOSPITAL
NURSING SERVICE DEPARTMENT
INITIATION OF INPATIENT LITHIUM
PLAN OF CARE

EXPECTED LOS ____________ DAYS
(LOS DEPENDENT ON DIAGNOSIS)
DATE POC REVIEWED BY MD ____________

DATE	DAY 1	DAY 2	DAY 3	DAY 4	DAY 5	DAY 6	DAY 7	DAY 8
DISCHARGE PLANNING	Assess for compliance/discharge needs/referrals.	Initiate/implement discharge plan. Refer to PHP, OPD, HHC, NBC if indicated.						On disch.: Follow-up evaluate discharge plan
TEACHING	Basline med. teaching	Offer lithium teaching booklet. Refer to med/illness teaching group.	Reinforce med/illness teaching qd (reason, dosage, time, side effects). Teach warning signs of illness qd. Teach expected results of med qd (mild transient edema, inc. urination).					

ADMISSION DATE ____________ DAYS IN ROUTINE BED ____________ DISCHARGE DATE ____________ DAYS IN ICU ____________

FIGURE 45–3 *Continued*

the transition to a CQI system. Quality teams need to include all areas or disciplines involved in a given process or provision of a service. These teams need to be empowered to participate in the decision-making processes that affect their projects.

The process of integrative decision-making requires education and training of participants. It also requires the support of administration. Managers may fear that this process will undermine their authority, but they need to be trained to recognize how this process actually facilitates their ability to resolve problems that affect their areas but fall outside their purview. They need to recognize that the barriers between departments are one of the primary causes of system problems.

Quality teams also need to use decision analysis in assessing and evaluating treatment processes and outcomes. Coleman (1989) described diagnostic probabilities for patients with suicidal ideation. Coleman (1989, p. 389) stated that decisional analysis can improve indicator development because it can assist in determining which decisions are most likely to be appropriate, thereby making indicators based on those decisions more likely to be valid and useful. Participation in the quality improvement process requires that all employees, regardless of discipline or area, be trained in problem-solving and decision-making.

▶ Check Your Reading

16. What is collaborative practice?
17. Define critical pathway.
18. What role do standards of practice play in a CQI model?

PATIENT SATISFACTION VERSUS PATIENT NEEDS

The transition from traditional QA to CQI made including the patient in care a necessity rather than an option. Patients are no longer willing to accept the services provided them without questions. The patient is demanding quality care delivered in a cost-effective manner. Patient satisfaction is directly proportional to the organization's ability to meet the needs, wants, and desires of the patient.

Patient satisfaction traditionally has all too often been focused on the patient's assessment of services provided, but these determinations were often made without the input of the patient. In the past, health care organizations frequently developed patient care services goals without ever asking patients what was important to them. Today, health care organizations have changed their focus to one of patient involvement, as dictated by the new philosophy of CQI. Patient-provider interactions now play an important part in the patient's perception of the services. Services provided must be based on the premise that the demand depends on the provider satisfying the patient. Patient dissatisfaction encourages the patient to seek the same services from another provider. Perception is important, for the patient's perception of having needs, wants, and desires met results in patient satisfaction. "The patient's perception in the actual production process is paramount in most health care services. The patient must participate in the delivery of care, cooperating with even the most painful of procedures" (Wilson, 1991, p. 11).

The process of assessing patient's needs, wants, and desires and incorporating these into the organization's quality improvement plan depend on several components according to Black (1992, p. 320):

- A commitment to addressing patient satisfaction issues at all levels of the organization
- Monitoring and analyzing trends of patient complaints
- Incorporation of patient satisfaction and dissatisfaction as a component of the QA or quality improvement program
- Development of and continuing maintenance of a "guest relations"–type program
- Active solicitation of patient opinions and perceptions

Organizational Commitment

Organizational commitment to patient satisfaction must be reflected in the organization's strategic plan and operationalized throughout the organization at all levels. It must be reflected in each department's mission, vision, philosophy, goals, and objectives. The nursing division quality improvement plan must include a commitment to meeting the needs, wants, and desires of its patients.

Monitoring and Analyzing Trends

Monitoring patient complaints is paramount in the process continuously to improve patient care. The level of patient satisfaction is frequently reflected in the complaints voiced by the patient or the patient's family. This monitoring device has become so important that many regulatory and licensing agencies have enacted legal requirements that an individual be specifically identified and dedicated to this function in both psychiatry and medicine. Analyzing trends in patients' complaints allows for changes in the systems that will be responsive to meeting patient needs and improving patient satisfaction.

Focus on Satisfaction and Dissatisfaction

Traditional QA programs have been designed to detect and correct patient problems; in other words, the focus has been on dissatisfaction. The quality improvement model implies an organization should look at both: "It is just as important to look at patient satisfaction as at patient dissatisfaction" (Black, 1992, p. 321). Black suggests acknowledging and incorporating into an overall

BOX 45-8 Laws and Standards Upholding Patients' Rights

1973	The American Hospital Association issued a patients' Bill of Rights
1976	The American Nurses' Association defined the nurse's professional responsibility to ensure and uphold patients' rights in the Code for Nurses
1980	Congress passed the Mental Health Systems Act (MHSA), which created rights for the mentally ill
1983	The JCAHO developed policy statements on the rights of the mentally ill

improvement plan compliments in the form of verbal praise, written letters, telephone calls, and so forth. Studying and duplicating satisfiers can only enhance an organization's ability to meet the needs, wants, and desires of its patients. Incorporating such items in the CQI plan also helps identify positive outcomes.

Guest Relations

The business industry incorporated the concept of guest relations many years ago and found it to be effective in increasing customer satisfaction. Health care is now beginning to incorporate guest relations in its strategic plan. The guest relations concept can be operationalized, for instance, in a "patient-first" program. Patient-first programs usually emphasize behaviors such as caring and compassion, courtesy, respect, dignity, and "the patient is always right." This area has become so important that organizations are incorporating the concept into job descriptions and performance standards.

Guest relations programs are important because patients frequently use the "halo effect" when rating hospital services; for example, the nurse is not caring and compassionate; therefore, the hospital is not caring and compassionate. Because this effect happens all too frequently, employees must be aware of guest relations.

Patient Feedback

Health care providers have traditionally failed to place enough emphasis on the impact of patients' perceptions on their level of satisfaction. Therefore, organizations have been remiss in developing effective patient feedback systems. Feedback systems are essential if organizations are to develop services responsive to patient needs. Feedback systems allow an organization to

- Determine what is important to the patient.
- Determine if the organization is meeting patient needs.
- Determine how to improve services presently provided.
- Communicate to the patient, and say "thanks" for the feedback.

Many methods have been used to assess patient satisfaction and obtain patient feedback in general. These include suggestion boxes, patient surveys such as Gallup polls, informal interviews by senior management, and interviews at the time of discharge. Organizations have employed individuals to filter complaints as well as feedback. In some organizations, these individuals are referred to as patient representatives and in others as patient advocates. The titles are not important, but their roles are.

Patients' Rights

One of the most important rights that any individual has is the right to receive quality medical care regardless of race, creed, nationality, economic status, or illness. Unfortunately, obtaining this right has been a long struggle for many. To ensure that all individuals are treated ethically in relation to the majority, civil laws have been enacted to ensure further that the rights of all individuals are protected.

Health care rights have always been somewhat controversial, however, especially in mental health. Yet in recent years, special attention has been focused on the rights of the mentally ill. Many federal, state, local, professional, and health regulatory agencies and organizations have enacted laws and standards that help ensure that the rights of the mentally ill are upheld (Box 45–8). In 1973, the American Hospital Association issued a patients' Bill of Rights, which has been used

BOX 45-9 JCAHO Patients' Rights

- The right of the patient to the hospital's reasonable response to his or her request and needs for treatment or services, within the hospital's capacity, its stated mission, and applicable law and regulations
- The right of the patient to considerate and respectful care
- The right of the patient, in collaboration with his or her physician, to make decisions involving his or her health care
- The right of the patient to information, at the time of admission, about the hospital's mechanism for the initiation, review, and, when possible, resolution of patient complaints concerning the quality of care
- The right of the patient to the information necessary to enable him or her to make treatment decisions that reflect his or her wishes

in many hospitals throughout the United States. In 1980, Congress passed the Mental Health Systems Act (MHSA), which created rights for the mentally ill. In 1983, the JCAHO developed policy statements on the rights of the mentally ill. The importance of patients' rights and the protection of those rights are also found in the Code for Nurses (American Nurses' Association, 1985). This code explicitly defines your professional responsibility to ensure and uphold these rights (see Chapter 5).

The JCAHO dedicated an entire section of the Accreditation Manuals for Hospitals (1995) to patient rights. This section of the manual stresses that organizational policies and procedures must describe the mechanisms by which the patient's rights are protected and exercised (JCAHO, 1995). Box 45–9 lists patient rights.

Local organizations such as Community Mental Health Centers, in conjunction with federal and state agencies, have developed standards that ensure that the rights of mentally ill patients are not violated. These organizations have become the gatekeepers, ensuring quality health care. Their mission is to develop standards that ensure the mentally ill not only have access to health care, but also have access to "quality" health care. The standards ensure that when access is denied or the quality is less than expected, patients have a mechanism by which to address their concerns without repercussions.

Any quality improvement program developed in psychiatry, like any other discipline, must take into account the rights of the mentally ill patient, especially the right to quality care. Involving the patient in care and assessing the needs, wants, and desires of the patient are important in implementing a process that ensures these needs will be met.

▶ Check Your Reading

19. Why is patient involvement a necessity in a CQI model?
20. Give one reason why it is important to monitor and analyze trends in patient complaints.
21. Give two reasons why patient feedback systems are important.
22. What is the most important right that any patient has?

CONCLUSIONS

The health care environment is changing at a rapid pace. To facilitate the patient's journey, health care organizations must develop systems that provide and ensure continuous quality improvement and quality assessment. This system must be based on

- Staff involvement at all levels.
- A focus on prevention instead of detection.
- Organizational and leadership commitment to quality improvement.
- A collective rather than an individual approach.
- An emphasis on customer satisfaction.

Developing a system based on these components will ensure an environment conducive to the transition from traditional QA to CQI. The most important point to remember, however, is that CQI must be a systematic team approach that includes the patient. There's no magic, just commitment.

KEY POINTS TO REMEMBER

- The trend in monitoring services is from a quality assurance model, which emphasizes detection, to a continuous quality improvement model, which emphasizes prevention.
- The movement began in industry and then moved to health care.
- CQI includes a concurrent review, a shift from an individual to a team approach, with continuous improvements focused on work processes, customer orientation, and statistical analysis.
- The movement to a CQI model was influenced by legislative and regulatory issues, JCAHO, and the work of industry giants Deming and Juran.
- The processes of CQI include establishment of a mission, philosophy, goals, and objectives; strategic planning; benchmarking performance indicators; establishing quality councils and teams; collecting and organizing data; and statistical analysis and data display.
- Nursing's role in establishing a CQI program involves providing an environment that facilitates a change in thinking from a QA to a CQI approach.
- Nursing must put into place the following processes: strategic planning, collaborative practice, identification of important aspects of care, and identification of indicators and standards through performance.
- Patient satisfaction and dissatisfaction are important indicators in a CQI program.
- Organizations must have a commitment to patient satisfaction. They must monitor and analyze trends in patient complaints as well as patient satisfaction. They must provide training in guest relations, seek patient feedback, and honor patient rights.

LEARNING ACTIVITIES

1. Using several of the CQI tools, apply them to a problem that you experience as a student.
2. Define quality and identify what is important to you in providing quality care. Compare your criteria with those of other students.

3. Interview three to four people who are currently patients or who have been patients in the last six months. Ask them to evaluate their care. What reasons do they give for their evaluation?

CRITICAL THINKING EXERCISE

Consider the following passage about quality assurance: "The hospital is required to have a QA program to satisfy . . . regulatory agencies that the quality of services is continuously monitored and evaluated. But traditional QA programs have provided little help to staff confronted with internal and external system problems that create roadblocks . . . to quality treatment. Patients with chronic mental illness often seem trapped in a revolving door syndrome that creates feelings of disillusionment and powerlessness on behalf of the staff. There is an increasing focus . . . on quality assessment . . . that is not going away, and nurses need to understand to be full participants in the process. Instead of focusing on individual staff performance and interventions, a systems approach is needed. The patient's treatment needs to be viewed as an ongoing process rather than focusing narrowly on inpatient or outpatient services."

1. What is the point of view of the authors about the current method of QA?

2. What assumption(s) are the authors making?

3. What inferences can you draw about the authors' statements about QA?

The authors continue to say the following: "The new approach is one of analyzing system problems . . . using concepts from traditional QA and integrating them with concepts from CQI. Nursing . . . must experience a paradigm shift . . . to make the integration of the two concepts beneficial and effective in improving the care provided the psychiatric patient. It . . . requires a shift . . . to concurrent review and continuous problem solving."

1. Do the authors paint a clear picture of the proposed new method of QA?

2. What evidence is offered to support the argument for a new QA?

3. What conclusions, if any, can be drawn about the authors' belief in QA?

REFERENCES

American Nurses' Association (1985). *Code for nurses with interpretive statements.* Washington, D.C.: American Nurses' Association.

Andrews, S. L. (1991). Q.A. vs. Q.I.: The changing role of quality in health care. *Journal of Quality Assurance, 13*(1), 14–15, 38.

Black, M. K. (1992). The consumer: Product of our efforts. In C. G. Meisenheimer (Ed.), *Improving quality: A guide to effective program.* Rockville, MD: Aspen Publishers.

Brown, J. A. (1992). *The quality management professional's study guide.* Pasadena, CA: Managed Care Consultants.

Brown-Stewart, P. (1991). Enhancing collaboration—a beginning. *Nursing Quality Connection, September,* 7.

Coleman, R. L. (1989). The use of decision analysis in quality assessment. *Quality Review Bulletin, 15*(12), 383–391.

Crosby, P. B. (1979). *Quality is free.* New York: McGraw-Hill.

Crosby, P. B. (1984). *Quality without tears.* New York: McGraw-Hill.

D'Arco, S. H., and Hargreaves, M. (1995). Needlestick injuries: A multidisciplinary concern. *Nursing Clinics of North America, 30*(1), 61–76.

Deming, W. E. (1986). *Out of the crisis.* Cambridge: Massachusetts Institute of Technology.

Fargason, C. A., and Haddock, C. C. (1992). Cross-functional integrative team decision-making: Essential for effective QI in health care. *Quality Review Bulletin, 18*(5), 157–163.

Fauman, M. A. (1990). Monitoring the quality of psychiatric care. *Psychiatric Clinics of North America, 13*(1), 73–88.

Field, M. J., and Lohr, K. N. (1992). Guidelines for clinical practice: From development to use (p. 8). *Institute of Medicine, Committee on Clinical Practice Guidelines,* Washington, D.C.: National Academy Press.

Fortuna, R. M., and Vazari, H. K. (1990). Orchestrating change: Policy deployment. In E. C. Huge (Ed.), *Total quality: An executive's guide for the 1990's.* Homewood, IL: Dow Jones-Irwin.

Joint Commission on the Accreditation of Healthcare Organizations (1989). Characteristics of clinical indicators. *Quality Review Bulletin, 15*(11), 330–339.

Joint Commission on the Accreditation of Healthcare Organizations (1991). *Using CQI Approaches to Monitor, Evaluate, and Improve Quality.* Oakbrook Terrace, Ill.: JCAHO.

Joint Commission on Accreditation of Healthcare Organizations (1995). *1995 Accreditation Manual for Healthcare.* Oakbrook Terrace, Ill.: JCAHO.

Juran, J. M. (1988). *Juran on planning for quality.* New York: The Free Press.

Keyes, M. A., and Moynihan, C. (1992). Developing, assessing, and refining quality of care criteria for a CHAMPUS mental health services demonstration. *Quality Review Bulletin, 17*(10), 331–339.

Kirk, R., and Hoesing, H. (1991). *The Nurses' Guide to Common Sense Quality Management.* West Dundee, IL: S-N Publications, Inc.

Lehmann, R. (1989). Forum on clinical indicator development: A discussion of the use and development of indicators. *Quality Review Bulletin, 15*(7), 223–227.

McLaughlin, C. P., and Kaluzny, A. D. (1990). Total quality management in health: Making it work. *Health Care Management Review, 15*(3), 7–14.

Mittman, B. S., Tonesk, X., and Jacobson, P. D. (1992). Implementing clinical practice guidelines: Social influence strategies and practitioner behavior change. *Quality Review Bulletin, 18*(2), 413–422.

Schroeder, P. (1991). Successful collaboration—learning the rules. *Nursing Quality Connection, July,* 1, 4.

Schroeder, P. (1992). Quality improvement: Evolution or revolution. *Nursing Quality Connection.*

Schroeder, P., and Katz, J. (1992). Seeking consensus on important aspects of nursing care. *Quality Review Bulletin, 18*(2), 63–65.

Siegiest, L. M., Dettor, R. E., and Stocks, B. (1985). The PIE systems: Complete planning and documentation of nursing care. *Quality Review Bulletin, 11*(6), 186–189.

Trueman, M. S. (1981). Collaboration: A right and responsibility of professional practice. *Critical Care Nurse, 2*(1), 70–71.

Valentine, N. M., Verkey, M., Hrendert, E., and Kayne, P. (1990). A collaborative approach to clinical standards development: Psychiatry and psychiatric nursing in a changing world. *Psychiatric Clinics of North America, 13*(1), 171–185.

Walton, M. (1990). *Deming management at work.* New York: G. P. Putnam.

Wells, P. (1992). COAD charting: Using the quality improvement process to meet the new JCAHO nursing standards. *Journal of Healthcare Quality, 14*(2), 34–37.

Wilson, C. K. (1991). A climate for excellence—an impossible dream? In P. Schroeder (Ed.), *The encyclopedia of nursing care quality—issues and strategies for quality care.* Rockville, MD: Aspen Publishers.

Zonsius Klingelsmith, M., and Murphy, M. (1995). Use of total quality management sparks staff nurse participation in continuous quality improvement. *Nursing Clinics of North America, 30*(1), 1–12.

SUGGESTED READINGS

Brown-Stewart, P. (1991). Enhancing collaboration—a beginning. *Nursing Quality Connection, September,* 7.

D'Arco, S. H., and Hargreaves, M. (1995). Needlestick injuries: A multidisciplinary concern. *Nursing Clinics of North America, 30* (1), 61–76.

Kirk, R., and Hoesing, H. (1991). *The nurses' guide to common sense quality management.* West Dundee, IL: S-N Publications, Inc.

Zonsius Klingelsmith, M., and Murphy, M. (1995). Use of total quality management sparks staff nurse participation in continuous quality improvement. *Nursing Clinics of North America, 30* (1), 1–12.

CHAPTER 46

RESEARCH AND THE FUTURE OF PRACTICE

As you go the way of life,
You will see a great chasm.
Jump.
It is not as wide as you think.
—Joseph Campbell

LEARNING OBJECTIVES

After studying this chapter, you should be able to:

1. Specify the relevance of research as an integral part of quality psychiatric nursing practice.
2. Describe recent concerns in psychiatric nursing related to current research and changes in the health care delivery system occasioned by resource-driven health care.
3. Identify two types of research methodologies relevant for psychiatric nursing.
4. Describe the role of the nurse in research.
5. Describe the role of the nurse as clinician.
6. Discuss the trend toward interdisciplinary management of mental health care.
7. Identify critical pathways as an interdisciplinary methodology in psychiatric nursing.

KEY TERMINOLOGY

Audit trail
Bracketing
Clinical decision-making trees
Collaborative models
Critical pathways
Deductive reasoning
Fittingness
Grounded theory
Inductive reasoning
Informational privacy
Informed consent
Intersubjective recognizability
Purposive sample
Qualitative research
Quantitative research
Triangulation
Truth-telling

The reader of this text has been guided on a journey through states, moods, treatment approaches, and detours from the normal. With this chapter, the journey ends but, ironically, it also offers the promise of a new beginning.

Psychiatric nurses now have an opportunity to make a difference in an unsettling, resource-driven health care system. The journey of psychiatric nursing in the 21st century will be researched based, with an emphasis on emerging biological developments in the neurosciences. Sophisticated technology is providing perspectives on mental illness. Increasingly, we are learning that psychiatric illness is largely determined by biochemical dysfunctions of the brain. Pinpointing structural and functional differences in the brain, made possible through imaging techniques, has reframed our understanding of the etiology of mental illness.

As the focus of psychiatric care changes from mind to brain, long-term psychosocial treatment of chronically ill patients is no longer available. These therapies are being replaced with medication, managed care, and psychosocial intervention limited by third-party reimbursement schedules. While acknowledging the important role of neuropsychology in the development of mental illness care, nurses need to become strong advocates for treating the psychosocial human side of mental illness and striking the needed holistic and integrated balance of mind-body-spirit in understanding and treating the individual with mental illness. Armed with knowledge and the promise of discovery through research, we may return to our patients, see them in a new way, and deal with their problems more effectively.

In 1993, five nursing theorists (King, Leininger, Parse, Peplau, and Rogers) participated as panelists in a Biennial Nurse Theorist Conference. Their topic was the "future of professional nursing in the next century." Hildegard Peplau's remarks describe the dilemma facing the nursing profession at the turn of the century. She effectively captures the reasons why psychiatric nurses need to find their voices as researchers and as members of interdisciplinary committees in the current health care arena. Returning to a historical perspective, she sets the tone for the direction of professional nursing.

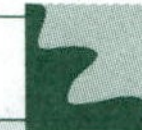

HILDEGARD PEPLAU'S STORY

In the 1940s and 1950s I was a member of many important governmental committees which made decisions about government money and where it should go in terms of training grants and research grants and things like that. Additionally, I also was on some World Health Organization consultations in the same vein, and inevitably these committees or meetings were interdisciplinary. The one thing that I observed fairly early on was that as nurses we were coming pretty much empty-handed. When it came to talking about what it was that we did, we could always come up with an activity. We could say, we make beds, and we pass out medicine, and we take temperatures. So we could say what we *did* but not what we *knew* or *understood* or what the phenomena of nursing were. What were the kinds of phenomena patients presented to nurses about which they were supposed to be knowledgeable and about which they were supposed to provide a beneficial service? When those kinds of questions were raised, we began to stretch it and blow it up and make it up as we went along. I can tick off some of the nurse leaders who along with me would get together afterward and discuss how we did that day. Had we persuaded the boys that we really had this body of knowledge, which was called nursing knowledge, which, of course, at this point we didn't have?

Remember, in the United States we didn't even have a nursing journal until 1952, and then they had to beat the bushes to get articles for it because there was so little research being conducted. That situation has changed. We have a lot of information, a lot of research results and theory development. We have the international theory conferences on a biennial basis now, so that we have many ways to say what it is that nurses know. So when we get into an interdisciplinary meeting we don't come empty-handed. But it would be a grave mistake to say that we know all that we must know or that we must stop the development of finding out more in order to get in and work with the disciplines in terms of what we should do, which is the main point of interdisciplinary work in treatment centers, unless you are going to be involved in doing the research for them. If you go empty-handed to the interdisciplinary team, you go gravely disadvantaged, and you are then very vulnerable to being put in the position of handmaiden instead of colleague.

Story by Hildegard Peplau, from Huch, M. (1995). Nursing and the next millennium. *Nursing Science Quarterly, 8* (1), 40–41.

IDENTIFYING THE PROBLEM

Knowledge and Research

Knowledge is power. But what do we know about the knowledge that we need to succeed in psychiatric nursing in the year 2000? Psychiatric knowledge is both like and unlike the data that underpin quality nursing care in other clinical areas. While knowledge is generally conceptualized in the sciences (and in other clinical practice areas) as a body of demonstrated facts that, taken together, constitute a theory of how things actually are, in psychiatry, knowledge has historically been viewed in a less "scientific" manner. Certain arenas, for example the biological, which seek answers to behavioral phenomena in the physiological and chemical realms, use a structured and traditional research approach to the investigation of problems. But many of our everyday interactions with patients are based on information that has been passed on to us by practitioners who have observed behavior over time, tried interventions to see what would happen, and have found that a particular conclusion is meaningful. Some of those individuals have developed sufficient insight to allow them to develop a partial or entire theory of behavior and have therefore been able to posit profitable interventions based on that theory.

How is this important knowledge passed on from one generation of practitioners to the next? On one level, the answer is obvious; we learn from our teachers, read from printed texts, prepare and share articles in journals with our colleagues, and interact at conferences and seminars specifically designed to increase the transfer of knowledge throughout the community of interest. But these approaches are not foolproof, and we cannot take in all the information with which we are confronted. We will need a variety of research methodologies to ensure the transmission of knowledge in its broadest sense.

Changes in the Health Care Delivery System

There is little question that the therapeutic pathways of psychiatric nursing care will look quite different in the 21st century. The nation's health care delivery system is in a state of chaos, the full dimensions of which are not understood currently. The problems are monumental and complex. The solutions will not be easy. First, the system simply has less money to pay for mental health treatment of behaviors that compromise an individual's ability to negotiate the journey successfully, particularly for the poor and chronically ill (Lowery, 1992). This problem creates ethical issues about access to care. Efforts to reduce health care costs while providing universal access to health care have forced the nation to make health care reform a priority. Whatever form it takes, the health care delivery system will be reconceptualized. Therefore, we need to take a fresh look at the role nurses might play in its development. The dilemma faced by nurses in the 1990s revolves around "overwhelming demands for more service from fewer professionals, all in the presence of increasingly technological practice demands" (Barnum, 1994, p. 400).

As a stop-gap measure that shows every indication of becoming a permanent reality, insurance companies are employing clinicians who have never evaluated the individual patient or considered the person-environment fit as a factor in clinical decisions. These clinicians, rather than the professionals actually treating the patient, often determine the length and type of treatment a psychiatric patient needs. The implications of this change have been shortened inpatient stays, the shift from caring for serious mental illness in the hospital to care in the community, and interdisciplinary models of health care delivery. In the process of a profound "paradigm shift" in nursing care for the mentally ill, Zwerdling (1994, p. 422) cautions that "We must develop new adaptive skills or we will become further impaired. Much of our confusion and anxiety as a society stems from the fact that our identity has changed and we do not yet recognize who we are."

DEVELOPING SOLUTIONS

Nursing leaders such as Peplau, Paterson, Zdrad, and Parse have developed conceptual models and nursing theory relevant to psychiatric nursing practice. Other theoretical insights are drawn from the social and biological sciences. But as we approach the 21st century, we must be willing to explore new frontiers of knowledge and skill in collaborating with other health professionals and health care consumers. Peplau argues that "The 21st century is quite likely to be the century of the professional nurse" (Huch, 1995, p. 40). This will be true only if nurses take advantage of the opportunity offered by changes in the health care delivery system.

Psychiatric knowledge is gained through formal research, and psychiatric nurses will need to develop research protocols to augment practical clinical experience passed from practitioner to practitioner. Integrating new knowledge with current values and standards allows us to place its parts into a meaningful whole. We need to be able to look at the materials passed on to us and understand how the originators of these ideas thought. We need to consider how their thinking related to that of others working in the same field and what elements of the knowledge base we can identify with, build on, and incorporate into our own practice.

Why is research so important to nursing? As Virginia Henderson has so eloquently stated, "A profession is known and judged by its literature" (Henderson, 1990). The printed word (books and journals) provides access to new knowledge, which in turn is the first step in the process of transforming practice.

If psychiatric nurses wish to be recognized for what they do, they must be willing to reflect on their interactions with patients and to communicate their clinically based research findings orally and in writing. Without a research base that psychiatric nurses can claim as their own, the voices of those closest to the patient remain unheard. Without a clear and united voice as professionals, nurses cannot hope to be recognized as peers in health care. Research that integrates ideas from different disciplines can help advance models that will make a difference in health care delivery in a time of tightened resources.

Research findings and generalizations are important for making critical clinical judgments and affecting policy decisions. It is not the findings of a single study or even a body of related studies that directly affect policy. Rather, it is the concepts and theoretical perspectives developed through social science research that permeate every aspect of policy-making. As a body of knowledge emerges, it accumulates and combines with data derived from other sources to define and redefine issues. Solid research acts as a supportive rationale for recommending certain policies over others. In doing research, the nurse may assume the combined role of researcher, teacher, and advocate in developing interdisciplinary health care policies that directly and indirectly affect nursing care.

The Nurse as Researcher

How important is it that every member of a given discipline do research? In 1932, Ortega y Gasset stated that

> *Science is rarely advanced by what is known in current jargon as a "breakthrough," rather does our increasing knowledge depend on the activity of thousands of our colleagues throughout the world who add small points to what will eventually become a splendid picture much in the same way the Pointillistes built up their extremely beautiful canvasses . . .*

Every practicing nurse has a part to play in nursing research, whether as an investigator, user of the outcomes, data collector, or someone identifying problem areas requiring research (Case Example 46–1). Nurses require advanced graduate education to develop an appropriate research design and conduct a relevant data analysis. All nurses, however, can read a research article that identifies a problem judged amenable to clinical research or look at findings of a research study and determine implications for practice. Good research studies have relevance, a practical focus that permits them to be realistically implemented, and writing that is clear but not overly technical.

Case Example 46–1 Verna's Story

My own journey in nursing is shaped by what I believe is a calling to incorporate spirituality in all that I do. To this end, I have dedicated my teaching, writing, clinical, and research efforts to understanding and applying spiritual concepts. The following abstract summarizes a study of AIDS patients that I conducted in 1990. The findings have implications not only for nurses working with AIDS patients but also for nurses working with other chronic, stigmatizing illnesses:

Literature on long-term survivors with AIDS is replete with anecdotal evidence linking survival to such things as (1) holding a positive attitude toward the illness; (2) participating in health-promoting behaviors; (3) engaging in spiritual activities; and (4) taking part in AIDS-related activities. To determine whether there is quantitative research support for this anecdotal evidence, 100 subjects who were HIV+ diagnosed with either ARC or AIDS completed Kobasa's Personal Views Survey (hardiness measure) and responded to questions regarding perceptions of their spiritual, emotional, and physical health; participation in spiritual activities; participation in selected health-promoting behaviors; and participation in AIDS-related activities. The results demonstrated positive relationships between hardiness and perception of physical, emotional, and spiritual health; participation in prayer and meditation; and participation in exercise and the use of special diets (Carson, 1993).

This study simply demonstrates relationships—our journey needs to take us beyond this. We need to study what spiritual interventions are effective and in what ways they are effective. We also need to explore these issues for the psychiatric patient for whom spirituality is frequently the most healing factor in the journey.

Story by Verna Benner Carson.

In clinical practice situations in which research is carried out, the nurse most often is involved as a data collector or as the one who performs the research protocol under the direction of the principal investigator. Therefore, although not the initiator of research, the nurse is essential in ensuring that the data are accurate and the study is valid. If for any reason, data are inaccurately measured or not recorded properly, a specimen is lost, or a part of the protocol missed, the mistake needs to be honestly and quickly reported so that the error can be incorporated in the analysis. Otherwise the validity of the study stands in jeopardy.

Staff nurses also may play a primary role in identifying research questions. The clinically based nurse who works with the mentally ill on a daily basis probably has more opportunity to identify questions related to patient care than do researchers, who traditionally work in nonclinical settings. That nurse is constantly asking about the significance of a patient behavior, the best response in a particular situation, or the basis for using one treatment approach rather than another. Any of these reflections may yield productive research questions that could have a significant impact on the diagnosis and treatment of psychiatric symptoms.

The staff nurse also facilitates others' research. The nurse can act as a role model for others in the carefulness and seriousness with which one approaches data collection. Nurses sometimes have opportunities in their own institutions and at external research conferences to attend meetings at which the results of research are reported. These conferences offer the chance to participate in discussions about the implementation of research findings and, most valuable of all, to work with members of other disciplines caring for the mentally ill. Psychiatry is more advanced than any other discipline in understanding that its subject matter is interdisciplinary and that most of the work done in the psychiatric setting can be accomplished by a variety of specially trained health professionals.

By taking a more active role in the research process, the nurse can assume responsibility for enhancing research protocols. An energetic investment in research carries with it not only a better understanding of mental illness and how its deviations twist and torture so many lives but also the responsibility to search vigorously for the answers that will allow us to diminish suffering. By valuing the research process and participating in that process, we can offer other human travelers the possibility of fuller and happier lives.

Associated Legal and Ethical Responsibilities

In addition to assuming greater responsibility for the actual conduct of research, nurses often need to be advocates and teachers in implementing their legal and ethical responsibilities in the research process. As the person most often present in the patient's therapeutic environment, the nurse plays an important role in protecting the patient's right to self-determination in matters of informational privacy, informed consent, and truth-telling. Managing this role becomes a truly awesome responsibility when a patient lacks the cognitive ability to understand fully the nature of consent.

Informational Privacy

Informational privacy is a term describing a person's right to have full control over any personal information used in research studies. Scanlon and Fibison (1995) identify the key elements associated with informational privacy in Box 46–1. Nurses have an added obligation to make sure that mentally ill patients' right to informational privacy is honored. Patients frequently are neither aware

BOX 46–1 Key Elements of Informational Privacy

- Only relevant personal information should be collected.
- Rationale for collecting the information should exist.
- Informed consent must be obtained before disclosure of information to others.
- Information gathered for one purpose should not be used for another purpose without informed consent from the patient.

From Scanlon, C., and Fibison, W. (1995). *Managing genetic information: Implications for nursing practice.* Washington, D.C.: American Nurses' Association.

of potential difficulties nor able to act fully on their own behalf. The nurse must ensure that

- The patient understands the type of information sought and agrees to it
- The patient is given the opportunity to correct errors in the data
- The data are reported on a group rather than on an individual basis
- Nothing of a personal nature that could result in harm to or discrimination against a patient is disclosed

Issues regarding storage of information, access to it or to the patient by people other than the investigator, and procedures for ensuring the anonymity also need to receive attention. Having well-defined policies and procedures for protecting the patient's right to informational privacy helps prevent inopportune disclosure.

Informed Consent

Informed consent is another legal and ethical concern with mentally ill patients. Although health care providers in all research settings are charged with full disclosure of facts and potential risks of engaging in the study before a patient signs the consent form, the decision-making abilities of the mentally ill often are not fully intact. Consequently, the nurse may need to consider carefully the words used to convey the information needed for informed consent so that the patient readily and completely understands. Often more than one session is needed. In the case of an incompetent patient, the person acting on the patient's behalf or designated as the patient's guardian must have the complete information needed for informed consent that the patient normally would receive.

Informed consent involves the presentation of the data in Box 46–2, with sufficient opportunity for the person to ask questions and to have them honestly answered before making a decision about engaging in a study. Furthermore, the person must retain the option to withdraw from study participation without penalty at any time. *Documentation* of informed consent usually is a requirement for conducting research. The form for consent is submitted for review as part of the research proposal to the Institutional Review Board for Human Subjects before research begins.

Truth-telling

Truth-telling is providing a person with full disclosure of all known facts related to the research upon request during and after research completion. However, information management of research outcomes can have a number of implications for the patient, and some of these can be quite disturbing. Although nurses have an obligation to inform patients of sensitive information upon request, Scanlon and Fibison (1995) note that this requirement can create a dilemma for the nurse as part of the interdisciplinary health care team.

The nurse may at times be confronted with conflicts in the area of truth-telling, in part because the nurse does not interact with the client in isolation, but rather as a part of a team. A patient may ask the nurse directly for information that someone else has decided the patient should not have. This experience of being "caught in the middle" can be very stressful for the nurse and can compromise professional integrity. Nurses should seek opportunities within the team to arrive at more honest and direct ways of managing information (Scanlon and Fibison, 1995).

As research becomes a more integral part of clinical practice in psychiatric nursing, nurses will increasingly need to attend to all the human details of research protocols consistently and carefully.

Research Models in the 21st Century

Psychiatric nursing students must become acquainted with the types, goals, and purposes of research methodologies used in psychiatric nursing. Research models used in psychiatric nursing in the next century will be more resource driven and biologically based than they have been to date. Funding for psychiatric research will focus on multidisciplinary empirical studies related to health

BOX 46–2 Essential Information Required for Informed Consent

- Purpose of the study
- Benefits and risks of participation
- Measures to ensure confidentiality
- Withdrawal from the study
- Third-party access to research information
- Publication of research findings
- Secondary use of individual data by the same investigator in other subsequent studies

care delivery systems, biochemical links between neurotransmitters and behavior, and outcome-oriented clinical studies of behavior (McKeon, 1990).

The neurosciences are likely to become increasingly important as an essential framework for considering the etiology of major mental disorders. This development has implications for prevention and treatment. McBride (1990) calls for a reintegration of neurological nursing and psychiatric nursing because of a joint interest in understanding central nervous system impairment and ways to treat it. She cites "Austin's research [1989] on childhood epilepsy with its emphasis on understanding seizure control *and* the attitude-adjustment link" (p. 24).

The last decade has produced significant research findings related to abnormalities in the brain structure and function in patients suffering from major mood disorders, schizophrenia, and Alzheimer's disease (Bornstein et al, 1993; Blanchard and Neale, 1994; and Keefe, 1995). Brain imaging allows clinical researchers to study the complex relation between neuropsychological function and brain structure as the brain interacts with patterns of electrical activity. Keefe (1995) conducted an extensive review of the literature for all research articles since 1991, focusing on a neurobiological assessment of psychiatric patients. In addition to providing objective data about neurological deficits responsible for patient behaviors, Keefe argues that neurophysiological data can be used to

- Predict the course of psychiatric illness
- Reduce the diagnostic heterogeneity within disorders and thus improve diagnostic classifications
- Aid in the development of treatment options
- Create individualized management of patient care

One of the most interesting findings in Keefe's review was the report that cognitive deficits were the single most important predictor of hospital admission, even more important than diagnosis. Cognitive deficits also may precede and predict the onset of schizophrenia and Alzheimer's disease.

Although objective physiological studies of brain functioning are important, we need qualitative studies to balance them with the patient's subjective perceptions of the journey with mental illness as a possible handicap. McBride (1990) identifies three general areas of research emphasis in psychiatric nursing in the 1990s (Box 46–3). Comprehensive clinical nursing practice research will require the use of both quantitative and qualitative research approaches.

BOX 46–3 Areas of Research Emphasis in Psychiatric Nursing Defined by the National Institute of Mental Health's Task Force on Nursing

- Fostering mental health, preventing mental illness, and improving the understanding, treatment, and rehabilitation of the mentally ill
- Facilitating care of people who are acutely or chronically mentally ill
- Improving the delivery of mental health nursing services

Quantitative Research Methods

The rational scientific model is perhaps the most common and well established model of clinical research in psychiatric nursing. Tanner et al (1993) note that "the rational tradition, represented by Descartes and Spinoza, holds that all knowledge can be expressed in self-evident propositions or consequences" (p. 273). The type of knowledge acquired from **quantitative research** represents decontextualized data-based information that is particularly useful in comparing treatment approaches and developing appropriate medication protocols. Quantitative studies require deductive reasoning skills. Findings derive from empirically based quantitative data analyses. **Deductive reasoning** skills include the development of hypotheses related to the purposes of the study, the testing of these hypotheses through established research methods, and the drawing of conclusions that can be generalized to similar populations. Quantitative researchers depend on explicit numbers and facts to explain their findings. They use pencil and paper instruments to measure objective change. For example, pre- and post-tests measure how much patients have learned from a psychoeducation class.

Researchers in a quantitative study try to maintain an objective distance from their subjects, frequently never personally meeting them. Random sampling and strict attention to statistical detail help ensure the researcher's objectivity. Statistical analyses help identify patient problems and issues and provide explicit support for different treatment options in the care of a patient suffering from mental illness.

The advantages of using quantitative studies are many. Well-designed deductive studies can be replicated by other researchers. Quantitative data provide the concrete numerical information needed to support external funding of research projects and treatment protocols. Objective data about the efficacy of treatment related to days lost from work, cost of care, length of time in the hospital, and so on provide the rationale for making needed changes in the delivery of psychiatric nursing care.

Qualitative Research Methods

Qualitative research, also used in psychiatric nursing, is sometimes referred to as a phenomenological approach. With this methodology, the researcher uses **inductive reasoning,** drawing from descriptions of individual experience to create a narrative about its meaning. Drew (1993, p. 345) posits that, "the human sciences have begun to use the phenomenological approach in research because it honors human experience, keeping it intact and in context with descriptions that ultimately draw us close to each other, connecting us to one another and validating our experience." This relational methodology is particularly consistent with Peplau's (1952) observation that the nurse-patient relationship represents the crux of psychiatric nursing. Parse's (1995) development of qualitative methodology illuminates concepts important to clinical nursing practice.

Qualitative methodologies take a holistic approach to the study of phenomena and seek to look effectively at the whole person, not just at discrete variables—at the unspoken meanings as well as the articulated facts. Through qualitative methodologies it becomes possible to describe human concerns, meanings, and practices through shared language about happenings in everyday clinical practice (Tanner et al, 1993).

Qualitative research considers the subject's views as the key element in understanding human reality. Thus the data are always contextually bound. Understanding does not flow from a simple quantitative assessment of the individual's social or psychological reality. For example, with a qualitative approach, the researcher would ask the subject to describe his or her social support system. By contrast, empirical research would use a written instrument such as the Norbeck Social Support Scale to measure the individual's level of social support. The information from each would be important. They might complement each other, but the reported findings are likely to be quite different in many ways.

Dialogue with subjects helps develop a mutual understanding of human processes. The researcher asks selected subjects to describe an action or experience in their own words. The interview process is collaborative and informal. Storytelling helps the researcher and informant construct a joint reality, which the researcher then seeks to interpret within the subject's contextual framework. Rather than beginning with established hypotheses and proving their validity, qualitative methodologies seek to describe experiences and to generate hypotheses through logical inference. Qualitative research calls for the careful description of the phenomena and amplification until all possible explanations are exhausted and meaning can be described.

Embedded in a phenomenological methodology is the concept of "the lived experience," a recognition that the contexts of human behavior differ and so do behavioral frameworks for understanding. **Grounded theory** uses data to explore social processes in human interaction. Its purpose is to "elicit meaning in a given situation and to develop reality-based theory (Field and Morse, 1985, p. 122). Qualitative methods charge the researcher to develop alternative thought processes of simultaneous discovery in data analysis and reflective introspection about meaning. As one graduate student suggests, "Studying the lived experience of another human being is a discovery: there are multiple truths and realities. The journey of uncovering meanings has been compared to peeling away the layers of an onion. One must peel away the layers to get to the core" (May, 1995).

An inductive reasoning process forms the basis of inquiry. The researcher strives to capture another person's experiences and to incorporate their common meanings into distinct themes. The search for truth about the phenomena lies not in the facts but in the participant's experience. Synthesized meanings drawn from a person's story allow practitioners a fresh opportunity to view life experiences from a different perspective.

Qualitative research is time consuming, and the researcher must stop, truly look, and listen for deeper meanings. With qualitative research, the data come alive with the actual words of the participants, spoken in their own voices, and deeply connected with their personal experience. It is, as Munhall and Boyd (1993) suggests, a unique opportunity "to understand the sense that a given situation bears for a person . . . to grasp something of that person's reality—to see what is true from his or her point of view" (p. 74).

The goal of qualitative research is to provide depth and breadth about the phenomena under study. Concerned less about replicability of results, the researcher seeks to resonate with the reader, creating a recognizability about the subject's experiences, strengthened by descriptions in the participant's own words.

Qualitative researchers use a **purposive sample** rather than the randomly selected sample population that is recommended in quantitative studies. A purposive sample derives from a specific population that best represents the phenomena under investigation. It should be diverse enough to include all possible stakeholders. Failure to broaden the sample population is sometimes referred to as elite bias, confined to a very select population that does not represent the full picture. The reader is asked to judge the diversity and appropriateness of the sample.

Qualitative studies require the researcher's active participation in data collection. In a sense, the investigator and the study participants become coparticipants in executing the research process. Because this method requires such a close relationship with the data and the study participants, bias is always a risk. The researcher needs to enter the research arena with the eyes of a newborn baby, seeing the event for the first time. Obviously, this approach is not truly possible, so a research technique referred to as **bracketing** assists the investigator in this process. Bracketing is a cognitive strategy for identifying and temporarily suspending judgment related to personal assumptions, values, beliefs, cultural attitudes, personal perspectives, previous knowledge, and experience with the phenomena. The researcher maintains constant awareness of personal feelings and subjective reflections about the reporting process experienced during data collection. These techniques allow the investigator to "see" and "hear" the voices of another and to learn from them without superimposed ideas of what the experience is really like for each individual.

The researcher collects data through semistructured interviews, direct observation, field notes, debriefings, video or audio tapes, journals, and diaries. Usually, multiple sources of data collection—second interviews, participant observation, and transcription of taped interviews—

are used. The investigator typically keeps ongoing field notes to develop key concepts and direct questions in later interviews. Qualitative studies tend to be conducted in the informant's natural settings with the focus on each individual's subjective life experience.

Once data collection is complete, the researcher begins an exhaustive analysis of the data, clustering relevant data into separate categories with related themes and interpretative statements. Further questions may be generated to explicate the phenomena. Interviewing and data analysis continue until no new information can be obtained from the study participants or the data analysis. The study findings are described as basic categories, themes, or synthesized essences. Including direct excerpts from the interviews lends further support for the conclusions that the researchers draw from the data.

Lack of scientific rigor is often a concern with qualitative studies. In qualitative studies, credibility rather than a statistical formula is used to judge internal validity. The research attains credibility through the development of an audit trail, intersubjective recognizability, and description of the researcher's own behavior and experiences (bracketing). First, the researcher describes the data analysis in an **audit trail,** which details the steps used to interpret the data. The audit trail allows the reader to evaluate the study and its fittingness in explaining the phenomena. The audit trail thus helps ensure the reliability of the data. **Intersubjective recognizability** is a way to develop the validity of the data. Subjects are asked to corroborate the findings and to suggest changes that would make the findings clearer or more comprehensive.

In quantitative studies, threats to external validity are evaluated related to real-life study conditions that are not similar for all groups; however, in qualitative studies, external validity is evaluated in a different way. Qualitative studies regard **fittingness** as the criterion by which to judge external validity. Such studies focus on two questions: Do the findings fit the experiences of the participants? and do the findings have meaning and usefulness with other similar populations? Threats to fit include (1) researcher overinvolvement with the participants, (2) bias in sampling, causing too little diversity in the sample population, and (3) "holistic fallacy" in which a general conclusion is drawn in error (Sandelowski, 1986). For example, it was originally thought that all swans were white until a black swan was observed in France. This single exception forced theorists to conclude that a holistic fallacy related to the singular color of swans had been made.

Triangulation

Triangulation refers to the use of multiple methods, both quantitative and qualitative, to gather research data. For example, the researcher might use observation, written assessment tests, and structured interviews to obtain information about a person's depression. Triangulation is particularly useful in complex studies with many possible or interacting variables. When multiple methods of analysis are used, it is critical to compare and contrast the findings and offer explanations for unexpected or conflicting results.

Models for Disseminating Research Findings

Models for Transmitting Research Knowledge

The printed word (books and journals), serves the important function of providing access to new knowledge: the first step in the process of translating new knowledge into practice. In fact, a field of study has developed that explores the relationship between the producer of new information, the user (an individual or organization), strategies for disseminating the information, and the role of a knowledge broker. It has been called technology transfer, research dissemination, research utilization, and, more recently, knowledge exchange.

This field of study is of special concern to the nursing profession for a number of reasons. One major reason is that the practice of nursing is highly influenced by ongoing research that addresses better ways to provide care or to understand normal and disease processes; thus, researchers and educators are interested in knowing how best to share this information with clinicians. Another reason is that we, as nurses, are very interested in the process of change. Much of our practice is related to teaching. We teach patients and families about their disease and about illness prevention for the purpose of getting them to change or modify their health practices. This, too, is a form of knowledge dissemination. So, nurse educators, researchers, and clinicians should all have an investment in understanding how people learn new ways of doing something. Knowledge utilization is believed to occur in the following ways:

1. Knowledge enters awareness and is judged on its own merits and against other information and factors (e.g., political, organizational, socioeconomic, and personal beliefs and attitudes).
2. It is implemented by the potential user (usually on a tentative basis).
3. It enters into general practice or policy.
4. It is integrated into an ongoing program so that its original identifying characteristics are no longer discernible (institutionalization) (Rogers and Shoemaker, 1971; and Zaltman et al, 1973).

Over the past 30 years, different models have been proposed to explain how knowledge moves from the researcher to the clinicians or policy makers and is used to change beliefs, practice, and/or policy. Three major theoretical models have been used in nursing.

THE RATIONAL LINEAR MODEL

The rational linear model is perhaps the most common and well established model of knowledge utilization. It is based on the notion that one set of activities will naturally lead to another. This model, as described in Havelock's

(1969) linkage model, Rogers' (1962) communication process model, and Bennis and colleagues' (1969) empirical-rational strategies model, assumes a linear transfer from knowledge producer to knowledge user in the following sequence: (1) a need is identified, (2) relevant information is presented, and (3) the information is used. An assumption is made that both researchers and users behave rationally and in predictable ways; thus, if relevant, understandable information is given, even from a remote resource person, chances are that it will result in a decision to use it or not use it and eventual confirmation.

Although the belief that new knowledge occurs in an orderly process from research to development to use is now seen as a much too simplistic approach and as an incomplete picture, it still represents the major view of how research utilization occurs. The pre- and post-tests used in nursing schools to measure how much students have learned and in clinical practice to ascertain if patients have learned what the nurse has "taught" them exemplify this approach.

The major problems with this model are related to the assumption that the receiver of the information is a passive recipient who will take in the new information wholesale and relate it back in the same form. The term *instrumental utilization* is used to describe the process whereby the subjects can cite and document the specific way in which knowledge is being used for decision-making or problem-solving purposes. But, in reality, it is more common that the new information has *conceptual utilization*, which refers to influencing a decision-maker's thinking about the issue without putting information to any specific, documentable use; e.g., "I did this because of what I learned in the workshop." This approach expands the way in which change can be measured to include indirect measures, such as noting what the person pays attention to in practice, or how goals are set.

THE USER-ORIENTED MODEL

In this model, the user is primary and initiates use of information to interact with some decision or problem. The Zaltman, Duncan, and Holbek (1973) model, the Havelock and Havelock (1973) model, and Wiess' (1977) problem-solving model all emphasize the user system and its involvement in working out strategies of information utilization.

The basic notion underlying this model is a belief that change is a planned process with identifiable strategies that result in a predetermined goal. Heavy emphasis is placed on the role of the change agent in working with the user in defining and addressing the problem and in identifying sets of environmental conditions (workplace) necessary for acceptance of new ideas, as listed below:

1. *Interpersonal contact:* To get an innovation used in a new setting, direct personal contact must occur between those who have had experience with the new innovation and those who will be implementing it.
2. *Planning and conceptual foresight:* A carefully thought out plan for how the innovation will be used in the new workplace is needed.
3. *Outside consultation on the change process:* This helps in designing the change effort and provides some objectivity about the course of action needed.
4. *User-oriented transformation of information:* The clearer the information, the greater the likelihood of its use. The key issues are "Does it work?" "How?" and "What changes are needed to make it work in my organization?"
5. *Individual and organization championship:* The innovation's chances for successful adoption are much greater if influential staff members and organizational leaders express enthusiasm for its adoption. Change is more likely in small organizations or in midsize or larger organizations with new or recent changes in leadership.
6. *Potential user involvement:* Anyone who must live with the results of an organizational change will feel more ownership of the new program if he or she is involved in the planning and adoption of that innovation (Havelock and Havelock, 1973; Zaltman et al, 1973; Backer, 1991).

The major problem with this model is that it assumes that the users have a clear idea of the goals, acceptable alternatives, and the type of information that is relevant to their needs. In truth, rarely are decisions the result of clear-cut choices and cooperative actions. More often they are formed from conflicts among individuals based on differences in interests, objectives, and perceptions (Weiss, 1977).

This model has been used in nursing to design two very important research utilization projects: the Western Interstate Commission for Higher Education (WICHE) project and the Michigan Conduct and Utilization of Research in Nursing (CURN) project. In each of these projects, nurses were asked to define a nursing problem, seek out research and critically evaluate its quality and usability, and then apply the principles of planned change to introduce the research findings into practice.

Based on their experience with this project, the WICHE staff made a strong recommendation to nursing. They suggested that the responsibility for reviewing, analyzing, and collating nursing research applicable to practice is the responsibility of the nursing profession, not of the individual nurse. This includes publishing research findings in such a way that their applicability to practice is obvious, and the use of knowledge brokers who are adept at presenting research in a "down-to-earth" style.

THE INTERACTIVE MODEL

The third model, which reflects current trends in thinking, is the interactive model. It assumes that the user, the research information, and the situational context all have an influence on knowledge utilization. In describing this model, Larsen (1980) notes that research findings and generalizations are used to produce an effect when presented in the context of related research, beliefs, and political realities, all of which are relevant to the user. It is not the findings of a single study, nor even of a body of related studies, that directly affect policy; rather, it is the concepts and theoretical perspectives that social science research has engendered that permeate the policy-making process. Rarely can people cite a finding of a single research study that changed their behavior. Instead, the process works in the following manner: As a body of knowledge emerges, it accumulates and combines with data derived from other sources to define or redefine issues. Nurses, like others, often fall prey to having a very restricted frame of reference and do not read journals outside their own discipline. This severely restricts the knowledge base from which they are working and results in repeating studies without any gain in understanding. But the major issue still remains, "When research findings are solid, how do you get policy makers or administrators to use research?"

APPLICATION: BRIDGING THE RESEARCH-PRACTICE GAP

The division between social scientists and decision makers is usually characterized by the former being unrealistic and living in ivory towers and the latter as only being interested in practical solutions and economics. But when Weiss and Weiss (1981) asked researchers and administrators in mental health to identify what factors made social research useful for public policy, the results were surprising. Both groups agreed that the research studies must have relevance, be able to be implemented, and be written in clear and not overly technical language. But they differed most with social scientists in overestimating the role of personal politics and underestimating the importance of the scientific merit of the research. They also differed in their view of what "use of research" meant.

Decision makers stated that they rarely used research in its pure form, but used it to bring new ideas to public attention, for framing or conceptualizing a problem, for keeping up with professional developments, for gaining information about what other agencies do, for legitimizing budget allocations, for attacking established policies, or for lobbying for new programs.

Social scientists, not seeing direct applications of their research, believed that the reason was that decision makers required (1) explicit recommendations with direct implications for a course of action, (2) a practical focus, or (3) that it was not compatible with the political views of the policy maker.

The findings of this study underscore the fact that research utilization occurs through multiple channels and that it is a progressive relationship rather than a linear cause-effect. This principle should also be kept in mind in evaluating the effectiveness of any nursing teaching project: The use of new information is not a linear process and therefore simple pre- and post-test strategies may not capture new learning.

The interactive model, then, can be used to examine the complexity of the process whereby research is translated into public policy. The translation into use is not an orderly set of interconnections, but is influenced by the potential user's experience, political sense, pressure, social technologies, and judgment (Weiss, 1977).

A major opportunity to help bridge the gap between research and clinical practice occurred with the establishment of the National Center for Nursing Research at the National Institutes of Health.

The National Center for Nursing Research holds special promise for increasing research efforts critical to nursing practice and research initiatives in the 21st century. Planned initiatives at the National Center for Nursing Research are presented in Box 46–4.

Two other resources for enhancing clinical effectiveness through research methods are the NIH consensus development conferences and the Agency for Health Care Policy and Research.

NIH CONSENSUS DEVELOPMENT CONFERENCES

Since 1977, the Office of Medical Applications of Research of the National Institutes of Health has sponsored consensus development conferences, topics for which may be proposed by any individual or group (National Institutes of Health, 1993). Topics are selected that have wide public health importance; are associated with controversy or unresolved issues that could be addressed in such a conference; are adequately defined and have available a sufficient base of scientifically derived information to allow reasonable resolution of questions; and which are amenable to clarification on technical grounds, rather than on the subjectivity of panelists. Experts are called together in a public forum, and the selected issue is addressed in intensive sessions. The report that results from such a conference is widely disseminated and constitutes the unified view of a panel of experts who understand the issues before them and who have examined, discussed, and spoken with regard to the scientific data available to them on those issues. The final publication is of enormous assistance to the larger community that seeks to understand the research questions associated with the particular area of focus and to move research findings into practice. Reports of concensus conferences on topics of particular interest to psychiatric nurses have focused on pharmacological prevention of recurrences of mood disorders, electroconvulsive therapy, the utility of therapeutic plasmapheresis for neurological disorders, the treatment of behavioral problems in persons with developmental disabilities, depression in later life, panic, and sleep disorders in older people (National Institutes of Health, 1984, 1985, 1986, 1989, 1990, 1991).

CLINICAL PRACTICE GUIDELINES

In 1989, legislation established the Agency for Health Care Policy and Research. Within that agency, the Office of the Forum for Quality and Effectiveness in Health Care has an important responsibility for supporting the development of performance measures, standards of quality, and medical review criteria for use by health care practitioners and others in reviewing health care quality and services. One of the important approaches used by this office has become the development of clinical practice guidelines. Such guidelines, which reflect standards for practice, are essential if we are to measure the quality of work provided by clinicians. Like the NIH Consensus Conference, experts are brought together to address the specific subject area. Unlike the NIH Consensus Conference, however, the resulting document is extensive in its review of the disease and the research related to it and is specific with regard to the manner in which individuals presenting with the condition should be treated. To date, the office has published guidelines in only one area directly related to psychiatry, "Depression in Primary Care" (Agency for Health Care Policy and Research, 1993). Because these clinical guidelines will be important in the evaluation of all disciplines working with depressed individuals, it is important that the psychiatric nurse be familiar with them and with subsequent sets of guidelines that are issued by this office.

▶ Check Your Reading

1. How does the nurse protect the patient's right to self-determination through the principles of informational privacy and informed consent?
2. How would you describe the differences between quantitative and qualitative research methodologies?
3. Why is research so important to the development of psychiatric nursing and the role of the nurse in the 21st century?
4. Why does Peplau refer to the 21st century as the century of the nurse?

BOX 46-4 Planned Initiatives at the National Center for Nursing Research

Development of a research agenda identifying research initiatives that combine scientific rigor with societal relevance

Targeting nursing research priorities determined by the nursing scientific community as most likely to influence nursing practice

Funding research programs capable of generating multiple interlocking studies that build on and support one another

Developing a cohort of nurse scientists through postdoctoral and individual career development study opportunities for midcareer and senior-level nursing scientists

Generating strategies to enhance interdisciplinary collaboration and cofunding of interdisciplinary research projects

Establishing an intramural research program at the National Center for Nursing Research at the NIH, related to both basic and clinical research initiatives

The Nurse as Clinician

The journey of health care in the future will be collaborative, with patient and professional travelers embarking on a jointly traveled interdisciplinary path. **Collaborative models** of care make the patient a partner in the treatment process. Instead of viewing the individual components of health care delivery separately, collaborative models use an integrated approach to identify critical treatment outcomes and determine the treatment process required to meet those outcomes. Key to a collaborative model is the organization, coordination, and integration of all health-related activities into a comprehensive, holistic treatment approach.

To facilitate the journey, interdisciplinary health care teams will make the necessary "travel arrangements." Written interdisciplinary clinical care plans, referred to as **critical pathways, clinical decision-making trees,** or care mapping will direct travelers toward the desired destination and will document their progress. As health care accountability becomes more and more of an issue, interdisciplinary case management of symptoms and integrated reporting mechanisms are likely to replace discipline-specific treatment protocols and reporting measures.

Role of Case Management in Collaborative Models

Psychiatric nurses have a unique opportunity to develop their role as case manager into a "power position" in the health care system (see Chapter 43). As Barnum (1994, p. 401) points out, "The power of the case manager is stronger than that of any other player in the field because (1) it mediates cross-professional goals, and (2) the goals it mediates direct the dollars." Case management paradigms support a collaborative interdisciplinary health care model with a "new" emphasis on "care and doing *with* the person rather than cure and doing *to* the person" (Phillips, 1995, p. 4). Case management legitimizes the nurse's caring role in psychiatric nursing, prompting greater ownership of caring that nurses have always provided patients. Shared responsibility in health care decision-making will make outcome research and the development of interdisciplinary collaborative models a prominent feature of mental health care as we enter the next century.

Critical Pathways

Health care delivery in times of scarce resources typically involves task orientation provided by multiple caregivers (Barnum, 1994). An integrated approach to documentation of care and outcome achievement is thus critical. The nursing process undoubtedly will be a fundamental component in some form of the "new" interdisciplinary approach to documentation, but a restructured way of ordering patient care is inevitable. The critical path method of tracking progress toward goal achievement is one such method. Originally developed in the 1950s to increase cost-efficient practice in industry, the critical path method increasingly is being incorporated to guide and document the patient's care, both in the hospital and in the community. It directs cost-effective use of personnel in implementing care and in the critical evaluation of patient outcomes.

Each critical pathway represents a detailed written care plan for all levels of patient care related to a particular medical diagnosis. It identifies every aspect of the patient's care and defines who is accountable for the care, when the care will be delivered, and how. The plan includes the coordination of all patient activities. It specifies time estimates for procedures, tests, and treatment completion. Patient activities are ordered sequentially, and the plan identifies potential problems that might arise. This information becomes a part of a flow chart that provides a graphic representation of the interdisciplinary health care prescribed for the patient.

The development and use of critical pathways to plan and organize patient care have several advantages. First, the method, when properly implemented, promotes a more coordinated approach to health care delivery and results in reduced hospital and patient costs. Collaboration about the disorder and choices about intervention lead to greater consistency of approach among diverse practitioners. Developing the critical pathway forces different disciplines to discuss their differences and overlap in function. The result is an expedient care plan that all disciplines own and agree to implement.

A critical pathway can be used as an education tool. It provides specific data related to diagnostic tests and mandates preparation to meet critical pathway requirements. The written flow chart provides concrete information for the patient and for family members interested in learning about patient care needs.

A caution is needed about critical pathways, care maps, and clinical decision-making trees as a format to direct and evaluate patient care outcomes. The quality of the plan as the medium for communication about patient care ultimately "depends upon an interdisciplinary and collaborative approach among health care providers in identifying practice patterns to assure appropriate and timely delivery of patient care" (Metcalf, 1991, p. 25). To be acknowledged as equal members of the health care team, nurses must maintain comprehensive up-to-date knowledge about the nature and treatment of mental illness. They must be articulate and willing to share professional insights, taking a leadership role in the development of research questions and other activities that demonstrate clinical competence. The danger is that clinical pathways will mechanize health care treatment, leaving little room for individualized patient needs and unique human responses. Nurses need to make sure that this does not happen.

Advanced-Practice Nursing

The dramatic shift in the health care delivery system from a medical/nursing model to a collaborative model concerned with holistic care and an integrated continuum of service options will require significant upgrading of the future role of the psychiatric nurse. At every level of debate about health care in the 21st century, the term *interdisciplinary team* emerges. For example, the Pew commission advocates a stronger teamwork approach in health care, with integrated practice across health disciplines (McEwen, 1994). The advanced-practice nurse in the psychiatric field can play a significant role in charting the course of mental health care delivery.

To meet the challenges of the 21st century, the profession will have to consider how to increase the number of advanced-practice nurses and how to use their independent and interdependent functions in the service of the discipline. Smith (1995, p. 2) describes the advanced-practice nurse as "expert at focusing on the whole client within the context of her/his significant environment, mobilizing person-family-community strengths and resources for health and healing, exploring person-family-community health-related experiences, cocreating environments that can support health and healing processes, and engaging in caring relationships that foster health and healing." Advanced-practice nurses in all clinical specialties will need to be mentors to their colleagues, develop realistic research agendas, and manage initiatives that integrate research findings into clinical practice.

▶ Check Your Reading

5. What do we mean by collaborative models of health care delivery?
6. How do critical pathways enhance and support the design and goals of collaborative models?

CONCLUSIONS

In a poignant discourse entitled "Into the 21st Century," Margaret Newman (1994, p. 45) notes that the next century will be a time of opportunity and challenge. She suggests that

What we need is the commitment to act. It is a time for a parting with the past. It is time to replace the anchor of the past with the pull of the future. We are in the process of creating a shared vision. In order to do so, it is necessary to connect all parts of the system, to integrate the similar and the dissimilar unleashing the power of creativity. The future vision draws from the past, but is not held back by it. How do we do this? Jose Arguelles says stand in the center of your truth.

The full truth in psychiatric nursing is just beginning to emerge, and many research questions remain to be explored. How do mind-body-spirit interactions influence one another? Which psychiatric interventions are most effective with different subpopulations? What nursing concepts are most relevant to the care of the psychiatric patient (for example, caring, belonging, social support, self-esteem)? Do certain physical, demographic, and environmental factors place some people at risk for developing a mental disorder? What constitutes a caring interaction from the nurse's perspective? from the patient's perspective? What sources of social support does the psychiatric patient perceive as helpful? Do particular educational experiences encourage student nurses to select psychiatric nursing as a career? These are only a few of the research areas needed to support clinical practice in psychiatric nursing.

Collaborative models of health care delivery offer nurses an opportunity to become central figures with a clearly articulated function as case managers in a restructured health care delivery system. This role has the potential for providing better access to health care and more cost-efficient care for people suffering from mental illness.

Newman (1994) proposes that "The power of the future pull is in knowing your purpose and vision and in bringing about circumstances in which *everyone can win*" (p. 45). Supporting the inner truth of psychiatric nursing through research will be the challenge for nurses in the 21st century. Developing a health care arena in which all members of the interdisciplinary health team are respected, where everyone—including the patient—can win, needs to become the explicit caring commitment in 21st-century psychiatric nursing.

KEY POINTS TO REMEMBER

- The journey of psychiatric nursing in the 21st century will be researched based, with an emphasis on emerging biological developments in the neurosciences.
- Sophisticated technology provides a perspective of mental illness as biologically based.
- Psychiatric nurses must be willing to explore new frontiers of knowledge and skill in collaborating with other health professionals and patients.
- A profession is known and judged by its literature.
- Good research studies have relevance, a practical focus that permits them to be realistically implemented. They need to be written in clear but not overly technical language.
- Every practicing nurse has a part to play in nursing research, whether as an investigator, a user of the research outcomes, a data collector, or as someone who identifies problems requiring research.
- Nurses have legal and ethical responsibilities in the research process.
- In the next century, the model of health care delivery in psychiatric nursing will be more resource driven and biologically based than has been the case to date.
- The neurosciences are likely to become increasingly important as an essential framework for considering the etiology of major mental disorders.
- Quantitative research represents a decontextualized data-based type of information useful in comparing treatment approaches and developing appropriate medication protocols.
- Qualitative research uses inductive reasoning, drawing from descriptions of individual experience to create a narrative about its meaning.
- An interdisciplinary health team needs an integrated approach to documentation of care. Outcome achievement and critical pathways serve this purpose.
- Advanced-practice nurses in the psychiatric field will need to take leadership roles in mentoring their colleagues, developing realistic research agendas, and managing initiatives that integrate research findings into clinical practice.

LEARNING ACTIVITIES

1. Think about a problem or an issue you have observed on the psychiatric unit or during a home visit with a mentally ill patient. Identify a research question you might want to ask about this problem or issue. Defend your rationale for choosing it. Specify the methodology you think would best address your research question.

2. Attend a meeting of an interdisciplinary planning team and obtain the following information:

- Meeting leader (from what discipline)
- Disciplines represented
- Conflicts and resolution
- Formal and informal power structures
- Sources of tension
- Whether the client and family members participate in decisions regarding care

Describe your impression of the ability of the team to work together and make suggestions for improvement (McEwen, 1994).

3. Plan a critical pathway for a patient on your unit. Develop the corresponding flow chart. Include all diagnostic tests and treatments, describing the schedule and preparation needed to complete the critical pathway standards. Use the flow chart to plan and document care of the selected patient. In class, discuss any problems you encountered in using the critical path method.

CRITICAL THINKING EXERCISE

Professor Toman was completing an exit interview with a graduating senior. During the interview, the student was asked to evaluate her research course. Her response was, "I'd rather have a longer practicum experience instead of the research course. I don't see the relevance of it. Besides, I'm not going to graduate school and I'll never need it."

1. What assumptions is the senior making about research?

2. What other evidence is needed to determine Professor Toman's point of view?

3. What would you like to say to this student?

The following passage is the chapter author's point of view concerning the clinically based nurse's need for knowing research: "The nurse who is clinically based and who works with the mentally ill on a daily basis probably has more opportunity to identify questions about nursing practice than any of her peers who work in nonclinical situations. That nurse is constantly asking herself what is going on in a particular situation, what the significance of patient behavior might be, or how one might best respond in a particular situation."

1. What is the point of view expressed in this quote?

2. Compare this point of view to that of the nursing student quoted earlier.

3. Based on your educational experiences, provide an argument for one or both of these positions.

REFERENCES

Backer, T. E. (1991). Knowledge utilization: The third wave. *Knowledge: Creation, Diffusion, Utilization, 12*(3), 225–240.

Barnum, B. (1994). Realities in nursing practice: A strategic view. *Nursing and Health Care, 15* (8), 400–405.

Bennis, W., Bennek, Chin R. (1969). *The planning of change.* New York: Holt, Rinehart and Winston.

Blanchard, J., and Neale, J. (1994). The neuropsychological signature of schizophrenia: Generalized or differential deficit? *American Journal of Psychiatry, 151,* 40–48.

Bornstein, R., Schwarzkopf, Olson, S., and Nasrallah, H. (1993). Third ventricle enlargement and neurophysiological deficit in schizophrenia. *Biological Psychiatry, 31,* 954–961.

Campbell, J. (1991). In D. Osborn (Ed.), *Reflections on the art of living: A Joseph Campbell companion.* New York: HarperCollins.

Carson, V. B. (1993). Prayer, meditation, exercise and special diets: Behavior of the hardy person who is HIV+, diagnosed with ARC or AIDS. *Journal of the Association of Nurses in AIDS Care, 4* (3), 18–24.

Dickens, C. (1906). *A tale of two cities.* London: J. Sen & Sons. [Reprinted 1979.]

Field, P., and Morse, J. (1985). *Nursing research: The application of qualitative approaches.* London: Crown Helm.

Guiliamo, K., and Poirier, C. (1991). Nursing care management: Critical pathways to desirable outcomes. *Nursing Management, 22* (3), 52–55.

Havelock, R., and Havelock, M. (1973). *Training change agents.* Ann Arbor: Institute for Social Research, University of Michigan.

Huch, M. (1995). Nursing and the next millennium. *Nursing Science Quarterly, 8* (1), 38–44.

Keefe, R. (1995). The contribution of neuropsychology to psychiatry. *American Journal of Psychiatry, 152* (1), 6–13.

Lowery, B. (1992). Psychiatric nursing in the 1990's and beyond. *Journal of Psychosocial Nursing, 30* (1), 7–13.

May, A. (1995). Class assignment. [Unpublished data]. Baltimore: University of Maryland, School of Nursing.

McBride, A. (1990). Psychiatric nursing in the 1990s. *Archives of Psychiatric Nursing, IV* (1), 21–27.

McEwen, M. (1994). Promoting interdisciplinary collaboration. *Nursing and Health Care, 15* (6), 304–307.

McKeon, K. (1990). Introduction: A future perspective on psychiatric mental health nursing. *Archives of Psychiatric Nursing, IV* (1), 19, 20.

Metcalf, E. M. (1991). The orthopedic critical path. *Orthopedic Nursing, 10* (6), 25–31.

Munhall, P. L., and Boyd, C. O. (1993). *Nursing research: A qualitative perspective.* New York: National League for Nursing Press.

Newman, M. (1994). Into the 21st century. *Nursing Science Quarterly,* 7 (1), 44, 45.

Ortega Y Gasset, J. (1985). *The revolt of the masses.* South Bend, IN: University of Notre Dame Press.

Peplau, H. Quoted in Huch, M. (1995). Nursing and the next millennium. *Nursing Science Quarterly, 8* (1), 40–41.

Phillips, J. (1995). Nursing theory based research for advanced nursing practice. *Advances in Nursing Science, 8* (1), 4, 5.

Rogers, E. (1962). *Diffusion of innovations.* New York: The Free Press.

Rogers, E. and Shoemaker, F. (1971). *Communication of innovations.* New York: The Free Press.

Sandelowski, M. (1986). The problem of rigor in qualitative research. *Advances in Nursing Science, 8* (3), 27–37.

Scanlon, C., and Fibison, W. (1995). *Managing genetic information: Implications for nursing practice.* Washington, D.C.: American Nurses' Association.

Smith, M. (1995). The core of advanced practice nursing. *Nursing Science Quarterly, 8* (1), 2, 3.

Tanner, C., Benner, P., Chesla, C., and Gordon, D. (1993). The phenomonology of knowing the patient. *Image, 25* (4), 273–280.

Van Manen, M. (1990). *Researching lived experience.* Albany, NY: State University of New York.

Weiss, C. (1977). *Using social research in public policy making.* Lexington, MA: Lexington Books.

Weiss, J., and Weiss, C. (1981). Social scientists and decision makers look at the usefulness of mental health research. *American Psychologist, 36,* 837–847.

Zaltman, G., Duncan, R., and Holbek, J. (1973). *Innovations and organizations.* New York: Wiley & Sons.

Zwerdling, M. (1994). Nursing care for the societal client in the year 2000. *Nursing and Health Care, 15* (8), 422–424.

SUGGESTED READINGS

Guiliamo, K., and Poirier, C. (1991). Nursing care management: Critical pathways to desirable outcomes. *Nursing Management, 22* (3), 52–55.

Huch, M. (1995). Nursing and the next millennium. *Nursing Science Quarterly, 8* (1), 38–44.

McBride, A. (1990). Psychiatric nursing in the 1990s. *Archives of Psychiatric Nursing, IV* (1), 21–27.

McEwen, M. (1994). Promoting interdisciplinary collaboration. *Nursing and Health Care, 15* (6), 304–307.

Newman, M. (1994). Into the 21st century. *Nursing Science Quarterly,* 7 (1), 44, 45.

Van Manen, M. (1990). *Researching lived experience.* Albany, NY: State University of New York.

APPENDIX I

STANDARDIZED RATING SCALES

Sheehan Patient Rated Anxiety Scale

Scoring and Interpretation

Assign a value of 0 to the first answer column ("Not at all"), 1 to the second column, 2 to the third, and so on. Scores above 30 are usually considered abnormal and scores above 80 are severe. The mean score in panic disorder and agoraphobia is 57 ± 20. The goal of treatment is to bring the score below 10.

CP93-0327 (C1.VP)

Project ID	Investigator ID	Today's Date: Month	Day	Year	Visit	Patient ID	Birth Date: Month	Day	Year
0–9	0–9	Jan, Feb, Mar, Apr, May, Jun, Jul, Aug, Sep, Oct, Nov, Dec	0–3 / 0–9	0–9	s, b, w, 1–9 / 0–9	0–9	Jan, Feb, Mar, Apr, May, Jun, Jul, Aug, Sep, Oct, Nov, Dec	0–3 / 0–9	0–9

Form # 22.1

Page # 1 of 3

Investigator's Initials X

Patient's Initials X

SHEEHAN PATIENT RATED ANXIETY SCALE

INSTRUCTIONS: Below is a list of problems and complaints that people sometimes have. Part 1 asks about how you have felt during THE PAST WEEK; Part 2 asks about how you feel RIGHT NOW. Mark only one box for each problem, and do not skip any items.

PART 1--DURING THE PAST WEEK, HOW MUCH DID YOU SUFFER FROM . . .	Not At All	A Little	Moderately	Markedly	Extremely
1. Difficulty in getting your breath, smothering, or overbreathing.	▭	▭	▭	▭	▭
2. Choking sensation or lump in throat.	▭	▭	▭	▭	▭
3. Skipping, racing, or pounding of your heart.	▭	▭	▭	▭	▭
4. Chest pain, pressure, or discomfort.	▭	▭	▭	▭	▭
5. Bouts of excessive sweating.	▭	▭	▭	▭	▭
6. Faintness, lightheadedness, or dizzy spells.	▭	▭	▭	▭	▭
7. Sensation of rubbery or "jelly" legs.	▭	▭	▭	▭	▭
8. Feeling off balance or unsteady like you might fall.	▭	▭	▭	▭	▭
9. Nausea or stomach problems.	▭	▭	▭	▭	▭
10. Feeling that things around you are strange, unreal, foggy, or detached from you.	▭	▭	▭	▭	▭
11. Feeling outside or detached from part or all of your body, or a floating feeling.	▭	▭	▭	▭	▭
12. Tingling or numbness in parts of your body.	▭	▭	▭	▭	▭
13. Hot flashes or cold chills.	▭	▭	▭	▭	▭
14. Shaking or trembling.	▭	▭	▭	▭	▭

← Changes: date & initial in box at left in line with the change.

CONTINUED ON BACK

Form # 22.1	Page # 2 of 3	DO NOT WRITE IN THIS AREA

SHEEHAN CLINICIAN RATED ANXIETY SCALE - Part 1 (Continued)

DURING THE PAST WEEK, HOW MUCH DID YOU SUFFER FROM . . .	Not At All	A Little	Moderately	Markedly	Extremely
15. Having a fear that you are dying or that something terrible is about to happen.	▭	▭	▭	▭	▭
16. Feeling you are losing control or going insane.	▭	▭	▭	▭	▭
17. SITUATIONAL ANXIETY ATTACK Sudden anxiety attacks with 4 or more of the symptoms listed previously that occur when you are in or about to go into a situation that is likely, from your experience, to bring on an attack.	▭	▭	▭	▭	▭
18. UNEXPECTED ANXIETY ATTACK Sudden unexpected anxiety attacks with 4 or more symptoms (listed previously) that occur with little or no provocation (i.e., when you are NOT in a situation that is likely, from your experience, to bring on an attack).	▭	▭	▭	▭	▭
19. UNEXPECTED LIMITED SYMPTOM ATTACK Sudden unexpected spells with only one or two symptoms (listed previously) that occur with little or no provocation (i.e., when you are NOT in a situation that is likely, from your experience, to bring on an attack).	▭	▭	▭	▭	▭
20. ANTICIPATORY ANXIETY EPISODE Anxiety episodes that build up as you anticipate doing something that is likely, from your experience, to bring on anxiety that is more intense than most people experience in such situations.	▭	▭	▭	▭	▭
21. Avoiding situations because they frighten you.	▭	▭	▭	▭	▭
22. Being dependent on others.	▭	▭	▭	▭	▭
23. Tension and inability to relax.	▭	▭	▭	▭	▭
24. Anxiety, nervousness, restlessness.	▭	▭	▭	▭	▭
25. Spells of increased sensitivity to sound, light, or touch.	▭	▭	▭	▭	▭
26. Attacks of diarrhea.	▭	▭	▭	▭	▭
27. Worrying about your health too much.	▭	▭	▭	▭	▭
28. Feeling tired, weak, and exhausted easily.	▭	▭	▭	▭	▭
29. Headaches or pains in neck or head.	▭	▭	▭	▭	▭
30. Difficulty in falling asleep.	▭	▭	▭	▭	▭
31. Waking in the middle of the night, or restless sleep.	▭	▭	▭	▭	▭

CONTINUED ON NEXT PAGE

Changes: date & initial in box at right in line with the change. →

CP93-0327 Page 3 (C1.VP)

Project ID	Investigator ID	Today's Date: Month	Day	Year	Visit	Patient ID	Birth Date: Month	Day	Year
		Jan					Jan		
		Feb					Feb		
0 0 0 0	0 0 0 0	Mar	0 0	0 0	S 0 0	0 0 0 0 0 0	Mar	0 0	0 0
1 1 1 1	1 1 1 1	Apr	1 1	1 1	B 1 1	1 1 1 1 1 1	Apr	1 1	1 1
2 2 2 2	2 2 2 2	May	2 2	2 2	W 2 2	2 2 2 2 2 2	May	2 2	2 2
3 3 3 3	3 3 3 3	Jun	3 3	3 3	T 3 3	3 3 3 3 3 3	Jun	3 3	3 3
4 4 4 4	4 4 4 4	Jul	4	4 4	L 4 4	4 4 4 4 4 4	Jul	4	4 4
5 5 5 5	5 5 5 5	Aug	5	5 5	5 5	5 5 5 5 5 5	Aug	5	5 5
6 6 6 6	6 6 6 6	Sep	6	6 6	6 6	6 6 6 6 6 6	Sep	6	6 6
7 7 7 7	7 7 7 7	Oct	7	7 7	7 7	7 7 7 7 7 7	Oct	7	7 7
8 8 8 8	8 8 8 8	Nov	8	8 8	8 8	8 8 8 8 8 8	Nov	8	8 8
9 9 9 9	9 9 9 9	Dec	9	9 9	9 9	9 9 9 9 9 9	Dec	9	9 9

Form # 22.1

Page # 3 of 3

Investigator's Initials X

Patient's Initials X

SHEEHAN PATIENT RATED ANXIETY SCALE - (cont'd.)

PART 1 (continued) -- DURING THE PAST WEEK . . .	Not At All	A Little	Moderately	Markedly	Extremely
32. Unexpected waves of depression occuring with little or no provocation.	▭	▭	▭	▭	▭
33. Emotions and moods going up and down a lot in response to changes around you.	▭	▭	▭	▭	▭
34. Recurrent and persistent ideas, thoughts, impulses, or images that are intrusive, unwanted, senseless, or repugnant.	▭	▭	▭	▭	▭
35. Having to repeat the same action in a ritual, e.g., checking, washing, counting repeatedly, when it's not really necessary.	▭	▭	▭	▭	▭

PART 2 -- RIGHT NOW, AT THIS MOMENT . . .	Not At All	A Little	Moderately	Markedly	Extremely
1. Mouth drier than usual.	▭	▭	▭	▭	▭
2. Worried, preoccupied.	▭	▭	▭	▭	▭
3. Nervous, jittery, anxious, restless.	▭	▭	▭	▭	▭
4. Afraid, fearful.	▭	▭	▭	▭	▭
5. Tense, "uptight."	▭	▭	▭	▭	▭
6. Shaky inside or out.	▭	▭	▭	▭	▭
7. Fluttery stomach.	▭	▭	▭	▭	▭
8. Warm all over.	▭	▭	▭	▭	▭
9. Sweaty palms.	▭	▭	▭	▭	▭
10. Rapid or heavy heart beat.	▭	▭	▭	▭	▭
11. Tremor of hands or legs.	▭	▭	▭	▭	▭

← Changes: date & initial in box at left in line with the change.

Courtesy of David V. Sheehan, M.D., University of South Florida, Institute for Research in Psychiatry, Tampa, Florida.

Zung Self-Rating Depression Scale

The Measurement of Depression
William W. K. Zung, MD

A self-rating depression scale (SDS) for the quantitative measurement of depression as an emotional disorder based upon an operational definition was first published in 1965.[1] This was followed by a series of reports that described its validity and reliability on the basis of investigations performed in the United States as well as in other countries throughout the world.[2–5]

Although devised for use in psychiatric research, the scale readily lends itself to use in the general practice of medicine in which most depressions are first encountered. The use of the SDS in a variety of patients with physical complaints with no apparent organic basis may uncover and measure depression in the so-called masked depressions. This saves valuable time for the doctor and the patient, since the unmasking of the patient's depression by the doctor is the first necessary step toward treatment.

HOW TO USE THE SELF-RATING DEPRESSION SCALE

Depression is defined operationally as a syndrome comprised of coexisting signs and symptoms that signify the presence of pathologic disturbances or changes in four areas: somatic, psychologic, psychomotor, and mood (see Table 1).

The SDS comprises a list of 20 items. Each item relates to a specific characteristic of depression. The 20 items together comprehensively delineate the depressive disorders as they are widely recognized. Opposite the statements are four columns headed: *None or a Little of the Time*, *Some of the Time*, *Good Part of the Time*, and *Most or All of the Time*.

For each item, the patient is asked to put a check mark in the box according to how it relates to his/her feelings within a specified time period: "during the past week." Although some depressed patients orally volunteer little information, most will readily cooperate when asked to check the scale if told that this will help the doctor know more about them.

To obtain the patient's depression rating, the completed scale is placed under the transparent overlay for scoring, and the indicated value for each item is written in the margin and totaled. This raw score is then converted to an SDS Index based on 100 (Table 2). The SDS Index is a total indication of "How depressed is this patient?" in terms of the operational definition and is expressed as a percentage. Thus, an SDS score of 65 may be interpreted to mean that the patient demonstrates 65% of the depression measurable by the scale.

Individual item scores tell us what specific sign or symptom the patient is manifesting, whereas aggregate scores of several items tell us in what area(s) the patient is having the most difficulty. For example, items 1 and 3 refer to affect; items 2 and 4 through 10 measure physiologic disturbances; items 12 and 13 measure psychomotor disturbance, and items 11 and 14 through 20 measure psychologic disturbances.

The statements in the scale are worded in the everyday language of the patient. Questions about how to complete the scale usually indicate the patient's desire to cooperate with the physician. For example, a patient may ask how to check Item 5 because he or she is on a diet and therefore should not be eating as much. In this case, the patient is asked to answer as if he or she were not on a diet.

After the patient has filled out the scale, take a moment to check that all statements have been answered.

INTERPRETATION OF SDS RATINGS IN DEPRESSION AND OTHER EMOTIONAL DISORDERS

"Depression" as a word can be used to describe: (1) an affect that is a subjective feeling tone of short duration, (2) a mood that is a state sustained over a longer period

TABLE 2 **Conversion of Raw Scores to SDS Index**

$$\left(\text{Index} = \frac{\text{Raw Score Total}}{\text{Maximum Score of 80}} \times 100\right)$$

Raw Score	**SDS Index**	Raw Score	**SDS Index**	Raw Score	**SDs Index**
20	**25**	40	**50**	60	**75**
21	**26**	41	**51**	61	**76**
22	**28**	42	**53**	62	**78**
23	**29**	43	**54**	63	**79**
24	**30**	44	**55**	64	**80**
25	**31**	45	**56**	65	**81**
26	**33**	46	**58**	66	**83**
27	**34**	47	**59**	67	**84**
28	**35**	48	**60**	68	**85**
29	**36**	49	**61**	69	**86**
30	**38**	50	**63**	70	**88**
31	**39**	51	**64**	71	**89**
32	**40**	52	**65**	72	**90**
33	**41**	53	**66**	73	**91**
34	**43**	54	**68**	74	**92**
35	**44**	55	**69**	75	**94**
36	**45**	56	**70**	76	**95**
37	**46**	57	**71**	77	**96**
38	**48**	58	**73**	78	**98**
39	**49**	59	**74**	79	**99**
				80	**100**

TABLE I

Symptoms of Depressive Disorder	SDS Items	Item Number
I. Pervasive affective disturbance		
1. Depressed, sad, downhearted, low, and blue	I feel downhearted, blue, and sad	(1)
2. Tearful	I have crying spells, or feel like it	(3)
II. Physiologic disturbances		
1. Diurnal variation: exaggeration of symptoms in the AM and some relief as the day goes on	Morning is when I feel the *best*	(2)
2. Sleep: characteristically early or frequent waking	I have trouble sleeping through the night	(4)
3. Appetite: decreased food intake	I eat as *much* as I used to	(5)
4. Weight loss: associated with decreased food intake or increased metabolism and decreased rest	I notice that I am losing weight	(7)
5. Sex: decreased libido	I *enjoy* looking at, talking to, and being with attractive women/men	(6)
6. Gastrointestinal: constipation	I have trouble with constipation	(8)
7. Cardiovascular: tachycardia	My heart beats faster than usual	(9)
8. Musculoskeletal: increased and unexplainable fatigue	I get tired for no reason	(10)
III. Psychomotor disturbances		
1. Agitation	I am restless and can't keep still	(13)
2. Retardation	I find it *easy* to do the things I used to do	(12)
IV. Psychologic disturbances		
1. Confusion	My mind is as *clear* as it used to be	(11)
2. Emptiness	My life is pretty *full*	(18)
3. Hopelessness	I feel *hopeful* about the future	(14)
4. Indecisiveness	I find it *easy* to make decisions	(16)
5. Irritability	I am more irritable than usual	(15)
6. Dissatisfaction	I *still* enjoy the things I used to do	(20)
7. Personal devaluation	I feel that I am *useful and needed*	(17)
8. Suicidal rumination	I feel that others would be better off if I were dead	(19)

of time, (3) an emotion that comprises feeling tones along with objective indications, and (4) a disorder that has characteristic symptom clusters and complexes of signs and symptoms. The SDS is intended to rate depression as a disorder. However, the SDS is not intended to differentiate the different types of depression. It serves rather to quantitatively measure the intensity of depression, regardless of the diagnostic label used.[6]

Certain safeguards are incorporated in the construction of this rating scale. The patient is unable to discern a trend in answers because half of the statements are worded symptomatically positive and half are worded symptomatically negative. For example, Item 1, "I feel downhearted, blue, and sad," is a positive statement. Item 2, "Morning is when I feel the best," is a negative statement reflecting the opposite of the way most depressed patients feel (worse in the morning). Negatively worded items are identified by asterisks on the transparent overlay, and the key words of the negative item appear in italics in Table 1. In addition, an even rather than an odd number of columns is used to offset any possibility of a patient's checking middle columns in order to appear "average."

By combining results from several studies, the SDS Index can be interpreted as follows:

SDS Index	Equivalent Clinical Global Impressions
Below 50	Within normal range, no psychopathology
50–59	Presence of minimal to mild depression
60–69	Presence of moderate to marked depression
70 and over	Presence of severe to extreme depression

The above interpretations are based on data that compare depressed versus nondepressed patients as well as depressed patients versus normal subjects in the 20- to 64-year-old range. High scores are not in themselves diagnostic but indicate the presence of symptoms that may be of clinical significance.

Results from several studies have shown that there is usually some depressive symptomatology present in almost all of the psychiatric disorders. Patients may have several diagnoses: headache AND depression, schizophrenia AND depression, diabetes AND depression. Thus, a primary diagnosis other than depression does not eliminate the possibility that the patient is also depressed. If the SDS Index is above 50, the patient may need treatment for the depression in addition to treatment for the primary diagnosis.

Zung Self-Report Inventory

Name ______________________

Age _______ Sex _______ Date ___________

	None OR a Little of the Time	Some of the Time	Good Part of the Time	Most OR All of the Time	
1. I feel downhearted, blue, and sad					
2. Morning is when I feel the best					
3. I have crying spells or feel like it					
4. I have trouble sleeping through the night					
5. I eat as much as I used to					
6. I enjoy associating with attractive men/women					
7. I notice that I am losing weight					
8. I have trouble with constipation					
9. My heart beats faster than usual					
10. I get tired for no reason					
11. My mind is as clear as it used to be					
12. I find it easy to do the things I used to do					
13. I am restless and can't keep still					
14. I feel hopeful about the future					
15. I am more irritable than usual					
16. I find it easy to make decisions					
17. I feel that I am useful and needed					
18. My life is pretty full					
19. I feel I would be better off dead					
20. I still enjoy the things I used to do					

SDS Raw Score __________

SDS Index __________

DIAGNOSTIC CRITERIA FOR DEPRESSIVE DISORDERS AND THEIR RELATION TO SDS ITEMS

The SDS items in Table 1 are not in the same order as in the SDS scale but are listed opposite corresponding symptoms of depression organized into: (I) pervasive affective, (II) physiologic, (III) psychomotor, and (IV) psychologic disturbances.

In the items, words that appear in italics reflect the opposite of what most patients complain of. As stated earlier, these words have been converted from symptomatically positive to symptomatically negative statements to prevent the patient from discerning the pattern of his/her answers.

[1]Zung WWK: A self-rating depression scale, *Arch Gen Psychiatry* 1965; 12:63–70.

[2]Zung WWK: Evaluating treatment methods for depressive disorders. *Am J Psychiatry* 1958; 124 (suppl):40–48.

[3]Zung WWK: A cross-cultural survey of symptoms in depression. *Am J Psychiatry* 1989; 128:116–121.

[4]Zung WWK, Wonnacott TH: Treatment prediction in depression using a self-rating scale. *Biol Psychiatry* 1970; 2:321–329.

[5]Zung WWK: A cross-cultural survey of depressive-symptomatology in normal adults. *J Cross-Cult Psychol* 1972; 3:177–183.

[6]Zung WWK: From art to science: The diagnosis and treatment of depression, *Arch Gen Psychiatry* 1973; 29:328–337.

Name ______________________
Age ________ Sex ________ Date ________

	None OR a Little of the Time	Some of the Time	Good Part of the Time	Most OR All of the Time	
1. I feel downhearted, blue and sad	1	2	3	4	4
2. Morning is when I feel the best*	4	3	2	1	3
3. I have crying spells or feel like it	1	2	3	4	3
4. I have trouble sleeping through the night	1	2	3	4	3
5. I eat as much as I used to*	4	3	2	1	2
6. I enjoy looking at, talking to, and being with attractive men/women*	4	3	2	1	2
7. I notice that I am losing weight	1	2	3	4	2
8. I have trouble with constipation	1	2	3	4	1
9. My heart beats faster than usual	1	2	3	4	3
10. I get tired for no reason	1	2	3	4	3
11. My mind is as clear as it used to be*	4	3	2	1	2
12. I find it easy to do the things I used to do*	4	3	2	1	4
13. I am restless and can't keep still	1	2	3	4	3
14. I feel hopeful about the future*	4	3	2	1	3
15. I am more irritable than usual	1	2	3	4	3
16. I find it easy to make decisions*	4	3	2	1	3
17. I feel that I am useful and needed*	4	3	2	1	3
18. My life is pretty full*	4	3	2	1	3
19. I feel that others would be better off if I were dead	1	2	3	4	1
20. I still enjoy the things I used to do*	4	3	2	1	4

(Key for Scoring. Do Not Remove.)

SDS Raw Score 55

SDS Index 69

Yale-Brown Obsessive Compulsive Scale

Patient's name ____________________ Date of 1st report ____________________

Therapy ____________________ Date of this report ____________________

Instructions: Complete Y-BOCS Symptom Checklist (flip side) before administering Y-BOCS (below). In administering Y-BOCS, make specific reference to patient's principal obsessions and compulsions.

	None	Mild	Moderate	Severe	Extreme
1. TIME SPENT ON OBSESSIONS	0	1	2	3	4
2. INTERFERENCE FROM OBSESSIONS	0	1	2	3	4
3. DISTRESS OF OBESSIONS	0	1	2	3	4
	Definitely resists				Completely yields
4. RESISTANCE	0	1	2	3	4
	Complete control	Much control	Moderate control	Little control	No control
5. CONTROL OVER OBSESSIONS	0	1	2	3	4

OBSESSION SUBTOTAL (Items 1–5) ________

	None	Mild	Moderate	Severe	Extreme
6. TIME SPENT ON COMPULSIONS	0	1	2	3	4
7. INTERFERENCE FROM COMPULSIONS	0	1	2	3	4
8. DISTRESS OF COMPULSIONS	0	1	2	3	4
	Definitely resists				Completely yields
9. RESISTANCE	0	1	2	3	4
	Complete control	Much control	Moderate control	Little control	No control
10. CONTROL OVER COMPULSIONS	0	1	2	3	4

COMPULSION SUBTOTAL (Items 6–10) ________

TOTAL Y-BOCS SCORE (Items 1–10) ________

Abridged from Goodman, W. K., Price, L., Rasmussen, S. A., et al. (1988). Yale-Brown obsessive-compulsive scale: Validity. In *New research abstracts.* 141st Annual Meeting of the American Psychiatric Association. Washington, D.C.: American Psychiatric Association. Full scale is available from Wayne K. Goodman, M.D., University of Florida College of Medicine.

Y-BOCS Symptom Checklist

Instructions: Generate a *Target Symptoms List* from the attached *Y-BOCS Symptom Checklist* by asking the patient about specific obsessions and compulsions. Check all that apply. Distinguish between current and past symptoms. Mark principal symptoms with a "p." These will form the basis of the *Target Symptoms List*. Items marked * may or may not be OCD phenomena.

AGGRESSIVE OBSESSIONS

Current Past

____ ____ Fear might harm self
____ ____ Fear might harm others
____ ____ Violent or horrific images
____ ____ Fear of blurting out obscenities or insults
____ ____ Fear of doing something else embarrassing*
____ ____ Fear will act on unwanted impulses (e.g., to stab friend)
____ ____ Fear will steal things
____ ____ Fear will harm others because not careful enough (e.g., hit/run motor vehicle accident)
____ ____ Fear will be responsible for something else terrible happening (e.g., fire, burglary)
____ ____ Other ____________________

CONTAMINATION OBSESSIONS

____ ____ Concerns or disgust with bodily waste or secretions (e.g., urine, feces, saliva)
____ ____ Concern with dirt or germs
____ ____ Excessive concern with environmental contaminants (e.g., asbestos, radiation, toxic waste)
____ ____ Excessive concern with household items (e.g., cleansers, solvents)
____ ____ Excessive concern with animals (e.g., insects)
____ ____ Bothered by sticky substances or residues
____ ____ Concerned will get ill because of contaminant
____ ____ Concerned will get others ill by spreading contaminant (Aggressive)
____ ____ No concern with consequences of contamination other than how it might feel
____ ____ Other ____________________

SEXUAL OBSESSIONS

____ ____ Forbidden or perverse sexual thoughts, images, or impulses
____ ____ Content involves children or incest
____ ____ Content involves homosexuality*
____ ____ Sexual behavior towards others (Aggressive)*
____ ____ Other ____________________

HOARDING/SAVING OBSESSIONS

(Distinguish from hobbies and concern with objects of monetary or sentimental value)

____ ____ ____________________

RELIGIOUS OBSESSIONS (Scrupulosity)

____ ____ Concerned with sacrilege and blasphemy
____ ____ Excess concern with right/wrong, morality
____ ____ Other ____________________

OBSESSION WITH NEED FOR SYMMETRY OR EXACTNESS

____ ____ Accompanied by magical thinking (e.g., concerned that another will have accident unless things are in the right place)
____ ____ Not accompanied by magical thinking

MISCELLANEOUS OBSESSIONS

____ ____ Need to know or remember
____ ____ Fear of saying certain things
____ ____ Fear of not saying just the right thing
____ ____ Fear of losing things
____ ____ Intrusive (nonviolent) images
____ ____ Intrusive nonsense sounds, words, or music
____ ____ Bothered by certain sounds/noises*
____ ____ Lucky/unlucky numbers
____ ____ Colors with special significance
____ ____ Superstitious fears

SOMATIC OBSESSIONS

Current Past

____ ____ Concern with illness or disease*
____ ____ Excessive concern with body part or aspect of appearance (e.g., dysmorphophobia)*
____ ____ Other ____________________

CLEANING/WASHING COMPULSIONS

____ ____ Excessive or ritualized handwashing
____ ____ Excessive or ritualized showering, bathing, toothbrushing, grooming, or toilet routine
____ ____ Involves cleaning of household items or other inanimate objects
____ ____ Other measures to prevent or remove contact with contaminants
____ ____ Other ____________________

CHECKING COMPULSIONS

____ ____ Checking locks, stove, appliances, etc.
____ ____ Checking that did not/will not harm others
____ ____ Checing that did not/will not harm self
____ ____ Checking that nothing terrible did/will happen
____ ____ Checking that did not make mistake
____ ____ Checking tied to somatic obsessions
____ ____ Other ____________________

REPEATING RITUALS

____ ____ Rereading or rewriting
____ ____ Need to repeat routine activities (e.g., in/out door, up/down from chair)
____ ____ Other ____________________

COUNTING COMPULSIONS

____ ____ ____________________

ORDERING/ARRANGING COMPULSIONS

____ ____ ____________________

HOARDING/COLLECTING COMPULSIONS

(Distinguish from hobbies and concern with objects of monetary or sentimental value (e.g., carefully reads junk mail, piles up old newspapers, sorts through garbage, collects useless objects)

____ ____ ____________________

MISCELLANEOUS COMPULSIONS

____ ____ Mental rituals (other than checking/counting)
____ ____ Excessive listmaking
____ ____ Need to tell, ask, or confess
____ ____ Need to touch, tap, or rub*
____ ____ Rituals involving blinking or staring*
____ ____ Measures (not checking) to prevent: harm to self ____; harm to others ____; terrible consequences ____
____ ____ Ritualized eating behaviors*
____ ____ Superstitious behaviors
____ ____ Trichotillomania*
____ ____ Other self-damaging or self-mutilating behaviors*
____ ____ Other ____________________

Mania Rating Scale

Guide for Scoring Items—The purpose of each item is to rate the severity of that abnormality in the patient. When several keys are given for a particular grade of severity, the presence of only one is required to qualify for that rating.

The keys provided are guides. One can ignore the keys if that is necessary to indicate severity, although this should be the exception rather than the rule.

Scoring between the points given (whole or half points) is possible and encouraged after experience with the scale is acquired. This is particularly useful when severity of a particular item in a patient does not follow the progression indicated by the keys.

1. *Elevated Mood*
   0. Absent
   1. Mildly or possibly increased on questioning
   2. Definite subjective elevation; optimistic, self-confident; cheerful; appropriate to content
   3. Elevated, inappropriate to content; humorous
   4. Euphoric; inappropriate laughter; singing

2. *Increased Motor Activity—Energy*
   0. Absent
   1. Subjectively increased
   2. Animated; gestures increased
   3. Excessive energy; hyperactive at times; restless (can be calmed)
   4. Motor excitement; continuous hyperactivity (cannot be calmed)

3. *Sexual Interest*
   0. Normal; not increased
   1. Mildly or possibly increased
   2. Definite subjective increase on questioning
   3. Spontaneous sexual content; elaborates on sexual matters; hypersexual by self-report
   4. Overt sexual acts (toward patients, staff, or interviewer)

4. *Sleep*
   0. Reports no decrease in sleep
   1. Sleeping less than normal amount by up to one hour
   2. Sleeping less than normal by more than one hour
   3. Reports decreased need for sleep
   4. Denies need for sleep

5. *Irritability*
   0. Absent
   2. Subjectively increased
   4. Irritable at times during interview; recent episodes of anger or annoyance on ward
   6. Frequently irritable during interview; short, curt throughout
   8. Hostile, uncooperative; interview impossible

6. *Speech (Rate and Amount)*
   0. No increase
   2. Feels talkative
   4. Increased rate or amount at times, verbose at times
   6. Push; consistently increased rate and amount; difficult to interrupt
   8. Pressured; uninterruptible, continuous speech

7. *Language-Thought Disorder*
   0. Absent
   1. Circumstantial; mild distractibility; quick thoughts
   2. Distractible; loses goal of thought; changes topics frequently; racing thoughts
   3. Flight of ideas; tangentiality; difficult to follow; rhyming, echolalia
   4. Incoherent; communication impossible

8. *Content*
   0. Normal
   2. Questionable plans, new interests
   4. Special projects; hyperreligious
   6. Grandiose or paranoid ideas; ideas of reference
   8. Delusions; hallucinations

9. *Disruptive-Aggressive Behavior*
   0. Absent, cooperative
   2. Sarcastic; loud at times, guarded
   4. Demanding; threats on ward
   6. Threatens interviewer; shouting; interview difficult
   8. Assaultive; destructive; interview impossible

10. *Appearance*
    0. Appropriate dress and grooming
    1. Minimally unkempt
    2. Poorly groomed; moderately disheveled; overdressed
    3. Disheveled; partly clothed; garish make-up
    4. Completely unkempt; decorated; bizarre garb

11. *Insight*
    0. Present; admits illness; agrees with need for treatment
    1. Possibly ill
    2. Admits behaviour change, but denies illness
    3. Admits possible change in behaviour, but denies illness
    4. Denies any behaviour change

From Young, R. C., Biggs, J. T., Ziegler, V. E., and Meyer, D. A. (1978). A rating scale for mania: Reliability, validity and sensitivity. *British Journal of Psychiatry, 133*, 429–435.

Abnormal Involuntary Movement Scale

Patient identification ______________________________ Date ______________

Rated by ____

Either before or after completing the examination procedure, observe the patient unobtrusively at rest (e.g., in waiting room).

The chair to be used in this examination should be a hard, firm one without arms.

After observing the patient, he/she may be rated on a scale of 0 (none), 1 (minimal), 2 (mild), 3 (moderate), and 4 (severe) according to the severity of symptoms.

Ask the patient whether there is anything in his/her mouth (i.e., gum, candy, etc) and if there is to remove it.

Ask patient about the *current* condition of his/her teeth. Ask patient if he/she wears dentures. Do teeth or dentures bother patient *now?*

Ask patient whether he/she notices any movement in mouth, face, hands or feet. If yes, ask to describe and to what extent they *currently* bother patient or interfere with his/her activities.

0	1	2	3	4	
0	1	2	3	4	Have patient sit in chair with hands on knees, legs slightly apart and feet flat on floor. (Look at entire body for movements while in this position.)
0	1	2	3	4	Ask patient to sit with hands hanging unsupported. If male, between legs, if female and wearing a dress, hanging over knees. (Observe hands and other body areas.)
0	1	2	3	4	Ask patient to open mouth. (Observe tongue at rest within mouth.) Do this twice.
0	1	2	3	4	Ask patient to protrude tongue. (Observe abnormalities of tongue movement.) Do this twice.
0	1	2	3	4	Ask the patient to tap thumb with each finger as rapidly as possible for 10–15 seconds; separately with right hand, then with left hand. (Observe facial and leg movements.)
0	1	2	3	4	Flex and extend patient's left and right arms. (One at a time.)
0	1	2	3	4	Ask patient to stand up. (Observe in profile. Observe all body areas again, hips included.)
0	1	2	3	4	*Ask patient to extend both arms outstretched in front with palms down. (Observe trunk, legs and mouth.)
0	1	2	3	4	*Have patient walk a few paces, turn and walk back to chair. (Observe hands and gait.) Do this twice.

*Activated movements.

From National Institute of Mental Health. (1976). Abnormal involuntary movement scale. In Guci, W. (Ed.). *The ECDEU assessment manual,* pp. 534–537. Rockville, MD: US Department of Health, Education and Welfare.

Brief Psychiatric Rating Scale

(Overall and Gorham)

Instructions: *Insert General Scoring Sheet and Code 01 Under Sheet Number.*

This form consists of 18 symptom constructs, each to be rated on a 7–point scale of severity ranging from "not present" to "extremely severe." If a specific symptom is not rated, mark "0" = Not Assessed.

Mark the column headed by the term which best describes the patient's present condition.

USE A NO. 2 LEAD PENCIL. BE SURE TO MAKE MARKS HEAVY AND DARK. ERASE COMPLETELY ANY MARKS YOU WISH TO CHANGE.

NOT ASSESSED	NOT PRESENT	VERY MILD	MILD	MODERATE	MODERATELY SEVERE	SEVERE	EXTREMELY SEVERE
0	1	2	3	4	5	6	7

Mark on right half of scoring sheet on row specified

		ROW NO.
1. SOMATIC CONCERN	Degree of concern over present bodily health. Rate the degree to which physical health is perceived as a problem by the patient, whether complaints have a realistic basis or not.	1
2. ANXIETY	Worry, fear, or over-concern for present or future. Rate solely on the basis of verbal report of patient's own subjective experiences. Do not infer anxiety from physical signs or from neurotic defense mechanisms.	2
3. EMOTIONAL WITHDRAWAL	Deficiency in relating to the interviewer and to the interviewer situation. Rate only the degree to which the patient gives the impression of failing to be in emotional contact with other people in the interview situation.	3
4. CONCEPTUAL DISORGANIZATION	Degree to which the thought processes are confused, disconnected or disorganized. Rate on the basis of integration of the verbal products of the patient; do not rate on the basis of patient's subjective impression of his own level of functioning.	4
5. GUILT FEELINGS	Over-concern or remorse for past behavior. Rate on the basis of the patient's subjective experiences of guilt as evidenced by verbal report with appropriate affect; do not infer guilt feelings from depression, anxiety or neurotic defenses.	5
6. TENSION	Physical and motor manifestations of tension, "nervousness," and heightened activation level. Tension should be rated solely on the basis of physical signs and motor behavior and not on the basis of subjective experiences of tension reported by the patient.	6
7. MANNERISMS AND POSTURING	Unusual and unnatural motor behavior, the type of motor behavior which causes certain mental patients to stand out in a crowd of normal people. Rate only abnormality of movements; do not rate simple heightened motor activity here.	7
8. GRANDIOSITY	Exaggerated self-opinion, conviction of unusual ability or powers. Rate only on the basis of patient's statements about himself or self-in-relation-to-others, not on the basis of his demeanor in the interview situation.	8
9. DEPRESSIVE MOOD	Despondency in mood, sadness. Rate only degree of despondency; do not rate on the basis of inferences concerning depression based upon general retardation and somatic complaints.	9

Continue marking on right half of scoring sheet on row specified

		ROW NO.
10. HOSTILITY	Animosity, contempt, belligerence, disdain for other people outside the interview situation. Rate solely on the basis of the verbal report of feelings and actions of the patient toward others; do not infer hostility from neurotic defenses, anxiety nor somatic complaints. *(Rate attitude toward interviewer under "uncooperativeness.")*	10
11. SUSPICIOUSNESS	Belief *(delusional or otherwise)* that others have now, or have had in the past, malicious or discriminatory intent toward the patient. On the basis of verbal report, rate only those suspicions which are currently held whether they concern past or present circumstances.	11
12. HALLUCINATORY BEHAVIOR	Perceptions without normal external stimulus correspondence. Rate only those experiences which are reported to have occurred within the last week and which are described as distinctly different from the thought and imagery processes of normal people.	12
13. MOTOR RETARDATION	Reduction in energy level evidenced in slowed movements. Rate on the basis of observed behavior of the patient only; do not rate on basis of patient's subjective impression of own energy level.	13
14. UNCOOPERATIVENESS	Evidence of resistance, unfriendliness, resentment, and lack of readiness to cooperate with the interviewer. Rate only on the basis of the patient's attitude and responses to the interviewer and the interview situation; do not rate on basis of reported resentment or uncooperativeness outside the interview situation.	14
15. UNUSUAL THOUGHT CONTENT	Unusual, odd, strange, or bizarre thought content. Rate here the degree of unusualness, not the degree of disorganization of thought processes.	15
16. BLUNTED AFFECT	Reduced emotional tone, apparent lack of normal feeling or involvement.	16
17. EXCITEMENT	Heightened emotional tone, agitation, increased reactivity.	17
18. DISORIENTATION	Confusion or lack of proper association for person, place or time.	18

Global Assessment of Functioning Scale*

Consider psychological, social, and occupational functioning on a hypothetical continuum of mental health–illness. Do not include impairment in functioning due to physical (or environmental) limitations.

Code	(**Note:** Use intermediate codes when appropriate, e.g., 45, 68, 72.)
100–91	**Superior functioning in a wide range of activities, life's problems never seem to get out of hand, is sought out by others because of his or her many positive qualities. No symptoms.**
90–81	**Absent or minimal symptoms** (e.g., mild anxiety before an exam), **good functioning in all areas, interested and involved in a wide range of activities, socially effective, generally satisfied with life, no more than everyday problems or concerns** (e.g., an occasional argument with family members).
80–71	**If symptoms are present, they are transient and expectable reactions to psychosocial stressors** (e.g., difficulty concentrating after family argument); **no more than slight impairment in social, occupational, or school functioning** (e.g., temporarily falling behind in schoolwork).
70–61	**Some mild symptoms** (e.g., depressed mood and mild insomnia) **OR some difficulty in social, occupational, or school functioning** (e.g., occasional truancy, or theft within the household), **but generally functioning pretty well, has some meaningful interpersonal relationships.**
60–51	**Moderate symptoms** (e.g., flat affect and circumstantial speech, occasional panic attacks) **OR moderate dfficulty in social, occupational, or school functioning** (e.g., few friends, conflicts with peers or coworkers).
50–41	**Serious symptoms** (e.g., suicidal ideation, severe obsessional rituals, frequent shoplifting) **OR any serious impairment in social, occupational, or school functioning** (e.g., no friends, unable to keep a job).
40–31	**Some impairment in reality testing or communcation** (e.g., speech is at times illogical, obscure, or irrelevant) **OR major impairment in several areas, such as work or school, family relations, judgment, thinking, or mood** (e.g., depressed man avoids friends, neglects family, and is unable to work; child frequently beats up younger children, is defiant at home, and is failing at school).
30–21	**Behavior is considerably influenced by delusions or hallucinations OR serious impairment in communication or judgment** (e.g., sometimes incoherent, acts grossly inappropriately, suicidal preoccupation) **OR inability to function in almost all areas** (e.g., stays in bed all day; no job, home, or friends).
20–11	**Some danger of hurting self or others** (e.g., suicide attempts without clear expectation of death; frequently violent; manic excitement) **OR occasionally fails to maintain minimal personal hygiene** (e.g., smears feces) **OR gross impairment in communication** (e.g., largely incoherent or mute).
10–1	**Persistent danger of severely hurting self or others** (e.g., recurrent violence) **OR persistent inability to maintain minimal personal hygiene OR serious suicidal act with clear expectation of death.**
0	Inadequate information.

*The rating of overall psychological functioning on a scale of 0–100 was operationalized by Luborsky in the Health-Sickness Rating Scale (Luborsky L: "Clinicians' Judgments of Mental Health." *Archives of General Psychiatry* 7:407–417, 1962). Spitzer and colleagues developed a revision of the Health-Sickness Rating Scale called the Global Assessment Scale (GAS) (Endicott J, Spitzer RL, Fleiss JL, Cohen J: "The Global Assessment Scale: A Procedure for Measuring Overall Severity of Psychiatric Disturbance." *Archives of General Psychiatry* 33:766–771, 1976). A modified version of the GAS was included in *DSM-III-R* as the Global Assessment of Functioning (GAF) Scale.

From American Psychiatric Association. (1994). *Diagnostic and statistical manual of mental disorders, fourth edition.* Washington, D.C., American Psychiatric Association.

Mini-Mental State Examination

Patient ____________________

Examiner ____________________

Date ____________________

Maximum Score	Score	
		Orientation
5	____	What is the (year) (season) (date) (day) (month)?
5	____	Where are we: (state) (county) (town) (hospital) (floor)?
		Registration
3	____	Name 3 objects: 1 second to say each. Then ask the patient all 3 after you have said them. Give 1 point for each correct answer. Then repeat them until he learns all 3. Count trials and record.
		Trials ______
		Attention and Calculation
5	____	Serial 7's. 1 point for each correct. Stop after 5 answers. Alternatively spell "world" backwards.
		Recall
3	____	Ask for the 3 objects repeated above. Give 1 point for each correct.
		Language
9	____	Name a pencil and watch (2 points).
		Repeat the following "No ifs, ands, or buts." (1 point). Follow a 3-stage command: "Take a paper in your right hand, fold it in half, and put it on the floor." (3 points). Read and obey the following: Close your eyes (1 point). Write a sentence (1 point). Copy a design (1 point).

Total Score ______

Assess level of consciousness along a continuum

Alert	Drowsy	Stupor	Coma

Instructions for Administration of Mini-Mental State Examination Orientation

1. Ask for the date. Then ask specifically for part omitted (e.g., "Can you also tell me what season it is?"). One point for each correct.
2. Ask in turn "Can you tell me the name of this hospital?" (town, county, etc.). One point for each correct.

Registration

1. Ask the patient if you may test his memory. Then say the name of 3 unrelated objects, clearly and slowly, about 1 second for each. After having said all 3, ask him to repeat them. This first repetition determines his score (0–3), but keep saying them until he can repeat all 3, up to 6 trials. If he does not eventually learn all 3, recall cannot be meaningfully tested.

Attention and Calculation

1. Ask the patient to begin with 100 and count backwards by 7. Stop after 5 subtractions (93, 86, 79, 72, 65). Score the total number of correct answers.
2. If the patient cannot or will not perform this task, ask him to spell the word "world" backwards. The score is the number of letters in correct order (e.g., DLROW = 5; DLORW = 3).

Recall

1. Ask the patient if he can recall the 3 words you previously asked him to remember. Score 0–3.

Language

1. Naming: Show the patient a wrist watch and ask him what it is. Repeat for pencil. Score 0–2.
2. Repetition: Ask the patient to repeat the sentence after you. Allow only one trial. Score 0 or 1.
3. 3-Stage command: Give the patient a piece of plain blank paper and repeat the command. Score 1 point for each part correctly executed.
4. Reading: On a blank piece of paper print the sentence "Close your eyes," in letters large enough for the patient to see clearly. Ask him to read it and do what it says. Score 1 point only if he actually closes his eyes.
5. Writing: Give the patient a blank piece of paper and ask him to write a sentence for you. Do not dictate a sentence; it is to be written spontaneously. It must contain a subject and a verb and be sensible. Correct grammar and punctuation are not necessary.
6. Copying: On a clean piece of paper, draw intersecting pentagons, each side about 1 inch, and ask him to copy it exactly as it is. All 10 angles must be present, and 2 must intersect to score 1 point. Tremor and rotation are ignored.

Scoring:

Children's Psychiatric Rating Scale

Instructions: *Insert General Scoring Sheet, Form 50, and Code 01 under Sheet Number.*

Rate the first 28 items exclusively on the basis of direct observation during the interview.

Rate the last 34 items (29–63) on the basis of the child's verbal report of occurrence at the time of the interview or during the past seven days. Do not use any other data but that obtained in the interview with the child.

Mark all rows consecutively—do not skip any rows. Each row is numbered on the scoring sheet and also on the page with the item to facilitate marking on the correct row.

USE A NO. 2 PENCIL. BE SURE TO MAKE MARKS HEAVY AND DARK. ERASE COMPLETELY ANY MARKS YOU WISH TO CHANGE.

NOT ASSESSED	NOT PRESENT	VERY MILD	MILD	MODERATE	MODERATELY SEVERE	SEVERE	EXTREMELY SEVERE

Mark on right half of scoring sheet on row specified — ROW NO.

1. TENSION (*Do not include fidgetiness*) 1

Musculature appears taut, strained, or tense. Fingers clothing, clenches jaws, grips arms of chair, hands tremulous.

2. UNDERPRODUCTIVE SPEECH (*Rate amount of speech only, not rate or relevance*) 2

Fails to answer questions, monosyllabic, has to be pushed to get an answer, doesn't elaborate, blocked.

3. FIDGETINESS (*Do not include tics*) 3

Wriggles, squirms, moves or shifts restlessly in chair.

4. HYPERACTIVITY 4

Has difficulty sitting in chair, gets up, moves fast, vigorously, impulsive bursts of locomotion. Exclude slow ambling even if constant. In rating degree of overactivity, consider the ease with which the hyperactivity can be controlled.

5. HYPOACTIVITY 5

Few or no spontaneous movements. Sluggish. Movements are slowed, feeble, or labored. Requires prompting for initiation of motor movements. Long latencies of appropriate motor behavior.

6. DISTRACTIBILITY 6

Distracted by usually minor, irrelevant stimuli. Shifts from one topic to another. Interrupts thought or action abruptly.

7. ABNORMAL OBJECT RELATIONSHIPS 7

Autistic use of objects with disregard for usual function. Stereotyped and repetitive sequences or fragments of play. Aimless behavior without organizing goal idea.

8. WITHDRAWAL 8

Oblivious to examiner, preoccupied. Facial expression and behavior do not respond directly to examiner. Attention focus is oblique and vague in direction, with avoidance of eye contact. Responses are very delayed and require forceful stimuli. *(The fact that the child may have peculiar interest in examiner, such as obsessive interest in parts of body or clothing does not preclude a rating of withdrawal.)*

9. OVERCOMPLIANT 9

Goes along with whatever examiner says in a passive fashion, even contradicting self. Does not assert self in a reasonable manner.

10. NEGATIVE, UNCOOPERATIVE 10

Active opposition and resistance to examiner's initiative *(differs from withdrawal and oblique avoidance)*. Guarded, evasive replies, teasing, manipulative or hostile refusal to cooperate. Child may remain silent in passive-aggressive fashion.

11. ANGRY AFFECT 11

Irritable, touchy, erupts easily—shouts, screams at examiner, overtly and directly hostile.

NOT ASSESSED	NOT PRESENT	VERY MILD	MILD	MODERATE	MODERATELY SEVERE	SEVERE	EXTREMELY SEVERE

Continue marking on right half of scoring sheet on row specified — ROW NO.

12. SILLY AFFECT 12

Clowning, inappropriately giddy, playful, silly behavior.

13. CONFUSION 13

Confused, bewildered, perplexed in behavior or verbal expression.

14. DISORIENTATION 14

Child is unaware of identity of surroundings after being told where he is. Not aware of time discriminations. Doesn't know age or surname.

15. CLINGING BEHAVIOR 15

Clinging, in physical and verbal behavior with the examiner. Seeks physical contact; demands constant direction.

16. UNSPONTANEOUS RELATION TO EXAMINER 16

Responds to examiner, but does not initiate social or verbal overtures nor sustain conversation once begun. Lacks spontaneity. Restricted.

17. SUSPICIOUS AFFECT 17

Expresses concern about the intent of the examination. Questions instructions and good will of interviewer.

18. DEPRESSED DEMEANOR 18

Exhibits a dejection, depression in mood. Looks sad. Seems to be in a state of painful dejection.

19. BLUNTED AFFECT 19

Restricted range and intensity of emotional expressions; blank or fixed facial expression, monotonous voice.

20. LABILITY OF AFFECT 20

Can suddenly vary from calm or silly to sullen mood, to screaming, crying, loud complaining.

21. PRESSURE OF SPEECH 21

Speech is hurried, accelerated, pushed, difficult to interrupt.

22. LEVEL OF SPEECH DEVELOPMENT (*Do not include diction, rate of speech, or relevance of speech*) 22

From age-appropriate (1) to severely retarded (7) speech development. Using your clinical judgment of verbal I.Q., estimate the level of speech development (in percent) in relation to verbal I.Q.

1 = Over 90%
2 = 76–90%
3 = 61–75%
4 = 46–60%
5 = 31–45%
6 = 15–30%
7 = Less than 15%

23. STUTTERING 23

24. LOW VOICE 24

Voice weak, mumbling, whispering, almost inaudible.

25. LOUD VOICE 25

Voice loud, boisterous, shouting.

Continue marking on right half of scoring sheet on row specified	ROW NO.
26. MISPRONUNCIATIONS Lisping, mispronounces letters such as r, s, l. Unclear speech.	26
27. OTHER SPEECH DEVIANCE Echolalia; questionlike melody; neologisms; sentences fragmented, unusual syntax.	27
28. RHYTHMIC MOTIONS (STEREOTYPE) Rocking, whirling, head-banging; rolling; repetitive jumping; hand movements, athetoid, twiddling; arm-flapping.	28
RATE THE FOLLOWING 34 ITEMS ON THE BASIS OF THE CHILD'S VERBAL REPORT OF OCCURRENCE AT THE TIME OF THE INTERVIEW OR DURING THE PAST 7 DAYS. DO NOT USE ANY OTHER DATA BUT THAT OBTAINED IN INTERVIEW WITH THE CHILD.	
29. EXPRESSED FEELINGS OF INFERIORITY Describes feelings of inadequacy, inferiority; self-deprecating, self-belittling.	29
30. EXPRESSED FEELINGS OF GRANDIOSITY Exaggerates own value, boasting. Unduly pleased with own achievement. Says he is much better than others. Distorted sense of own capacity.	30
31. PHYSICAL COMPLAINTS Somatic complaints of headaches, stomach aches, dizziness, not feeling well *(do not include fatigue).*	31
32. OBESITY Judge from child's appearance from normal physical appearance to severe obesity.	32
33. OTHER EATING PROBLEMS Picky, fussy, many dislikes, extremely restricted diet, peculiar food tastes.	33
34. SEPARATION ANXIETY Ease with which child separates from mother or other significant people. Extent of observed or reported anxiety (by child) experienced by child when separated from mother or other significant people.	34
35. DEPRESSION Admits feeling sad, lonely, feels like crying, expresses a despondent or despairing attitude. Difficulty in anticipating success and enjoyment.	35
36. EUPHORIA—ELATION States he feels terrific, great; elevation of mood, hypomanic state. "This is the best of all possible worlds." Feels elated and wonderful. Nothing is impossible.	36

	ROW NO.
When you have completed this page (item 41), turn all pages on this side and continue with text (item 42) on page RI	
37. LACK OF ENERGY States he feels sluggish, fatigued. Everything is too much. Weary and feels unable to make slightest effort. *(Do not infer from motor retardation or expressed indifference.)*	37
38. PREOCCUPATION WITH TOPICS OF ANXIETY Says he has nervous or scary feelings, concerns, apprehension, fears. Says he worries about failure or other mishaps, thinks about something happening to self or parents—illness, injury, death, loss or separation.	38
39. PREOCCUPATION WITH DEPRESSIVE TOPICS Preoccupied with feelings of inadequacy and inferiority. Expresses feeling that nothing can turn out all right. Preoccupied with feelings of uselessness, futility, and possibly guilt. Suicidal preoccupation.	39
40. SUICIDAL ATTEMPTS 0 = Not assessed 1 = None 2 = Suicidal threat 3 = One minor gesture without danger 4 = A couple or several minor gestures without danger 5 = Dangerous gesture 6 = Infliction of life-threatening damage to self 7 = Several life-threatening attempts	40
41. FEARS AND PHOBIAS Irrational morbid fears of specific objects, person, or situations, which, if extreme, lead to avoidance behavior. Rate 6 or 7 only when fear is so severe it leads to phobic avoidance.	41

ROW NO.	*Mark on left half of scoring sheet on row specified*
1	**42. COMPULSIVE ACTS** Acts or "habits" that are regarded as unreasonable by the child, such as counting, checking, rituals, excessive orderliness and cleanliness.
2	**43. NERVOUS HABITS AND MANNERISMS** Stereotyped movements; rituals that are not perceived as irrational. Facial tics or mannerisms. Biting nails, fingers, cuticles. Sucking of objects or body parts *(thumb, fingers, hair, etc.)*; picking on skin, scabs, nose, twisting hair.
3	**44. OBSESSIVE THINKING** Inability to "turn off" repetitive thought. Preoccupation, ruminations about abstract problems or personal matters.
4	**45. SOLITARY INTERESTS** Interested in activities that require little if any peer interaction, such as stamp-collecting, movie-going, reading, school work, solitary activities.
5	**46. LACK OF PEER INTERACTION** Isolated from other children. Has no friends or cannot name current close friend or describe participation in play with peers. Lacks interest in peers.
6	**47. GANG ACTIVITY** Joins in antisocial activities along with a group of children *(fighting, trouble-making, stealing)* as a cooperating group against others.
7	**48. FIGHTING WITH PEERS** Says he frequently gets into fights—beats up other kids or gets beaten up. Says he has a bad temper.
8	**49. BULLY** Says he's always the leader, winner; or says he teases, bullies children; pushes children around; threatens them.
9	**50. TEMPER OUTBURSTS** Admits to feeling angry, irritable, touchy, admits he has a temper.
10	**51. SCAPEGOAT** Says he's picked on, teased, left out or pushed around, and bullied by other children. May be called "sissy" or "baby."
11	**52. LYING** Contradicts self in ways indicative of effort to hide the truth. Reports telling tall stories, fibs, or admits he's accused of telling lies.
12	**53. EXPLOITATIVE RELATIONSHIPS** Interested in other people insofar as he can get something out of it. Callous and calculating in interpersonal activities.

ROW NO.	*Continue marking on left half of scoring sheet on row specified*
13	**54. INABILITY TO FALL ASLEEP** Child reports a long time to fall asleep after going to bed. 1 = Not present; 5 = 46 to 60 min. 2 = 10 to 15 min.; 6 = 60 to 90 min. 3 = 16 to 30 min.; 7 = Over 90 min. 4 = 31 to 45 min.
14	**55. OTHER SLEEP DIFFICULTIES** Nightmares, early-morning awakening, sleep-walking, interrupted sleep.
15	**56. BEDWETTING** Rating is for frequency of bedwetting for past 7 nights 1 = None; 5 = 4 times 2 = One time; 6 = 5 times 3 = 2 times; 7 = 6 to 7 times 4 = 3 times
16	**57. IDEAS OF REFERENCE** People are looking at him, following him, staring, etc. Malevolent intent is not necessary but may occur.
17	**58. PERSECUTORY** Feels people have it in for him, try to hurt him. In the extreme rating, the thinking has a delusional quality, in that the belief is impervious to change, rational arguments, or corrective experiences.
18	**59. OTHER THINKING DISORDERS** Irrelevant speech; or incoherent speech; or loose associations.
19	**60. DELUSIONS** Delusional beliefs or convictions besides paranoia (58), i.e., believes has introjected persons or objects in his body, has a mission; is some other person or character, has unusual powers; is guilty of some event.
20	**61. HALLUCINATIONS** The overall rating is a frequency rating reflecting the constancy of the experience: 1 = Not present; 5 = 4 to 5 times 2 = Once; 6 = 5 to 6 times 3 = 2 times; 7 = Daily recurrent phenomenon 4 = 3 times
21	**62. PECULIAR FANTASIES** Morbid or bizarre fantasies and preoccupations, peculiar body sensations, disturbances of body image experiences *(not figure drawings)*; preoccupation with flying, supernatural influences, sadism, masochism.
22	**63. LACK OF INSIGHT** Is convinced of the reality of hallucinations or fantasies.

The Children's Psychiatric Rating Scale (CPRS) is an original scale constructed by members of the Pediatric Psychopharmacology Workshop. It is a comprehensive scale that endeavors to assess the broad spectrum of psychopathology within this age group. As a consequence, items of the CPRS will have varying degrees of relevance when assessing a circumscribed diagnostic group. The CPRS is formatted for use with the General Scoring Sheet and contains 63 items. A 7-point scale derived from the Adult Brief Psychiatric Rating Scale is employed. The CPRS should be regarded as experimental. Standardization procedures will be undertaken as soon as sufficient data are accumulated.

APPLICABILITY For children to age 15.

UTILIZATION Once at pretreatment; at least one posttreatment assessment. Additional ratings are at the discretion of the investigator.

TIME SPAN RATED The first 28 items are rated on the basis of direct observation of behavior during the interview. The last 34 items are rated on the basis of the child's report of occurrence during the interview or within the past week.

CARD FORMAT—ITEMS

CARD 01 = (19×, 41I1)

Item	Column	Item	Column	Item	Column	Item	Column
1	20	11	30	21	40	31	50
2	21	12	31	22	41	32	51
3	22	13	32	23	42	33	52
4	23	14	33	24	43	34	53
5	24	15	34	25	44	35	54
6	25	16	35	26	45	36	55
7	26	17	36	27	46	37	56
8	27	18	37	28	47	38	57
9	28	19	38	29	48	39	58
10	29	20	39	30	49	40	59
						41	60

CARD 02 = (19×, 22I1)

Item	Column	Item	Column	Item	Column	Item	Column
42	20	47	25	52	30	57	35
43	21	48	26	53	31	58	36
44	22	49	27	54	32	59	37
45	23	50	28	55	33	60	38
46	24	51	29	56	34	61	39
						62	40
						63	41

CARD FORMAT—CLUSTERS

CARD 51 = (19×, 9F6.2)
(Code "5" in Column 18 indicates a card containing factors, clusters, or other grouped scores.)

Cluster	Column	Cluster	Column
I	20–25	VI	50–55
II	26–31	VII	56–61
III	32–37	VIII	62–67
IV	38–43	IX	68–73
V	44–49		

CARD 52 = (19×, 6F6.2,F4.0)

Cluster	Column	Cluster	Column
X	20–25	XIII	38–43
XI	26–31	XIV	44–49
XII	32–37	XV	50–55
		Total Score	56–59

Cluster score = $\frac{\text{Sum of composite items}}{\text{Number of composite items}}$ **Cluster score range = 1–7**

Total score = Sum of all items **Total score range = 63–441**

CLUSTER COMPOSITION—As a means of data reduction, the clusters have been empirically derived for use in statistical analyses. It is planned to undertake psychometric analyses of the CPRS when sufficient data are accumulated.

I. Psychotic
- 2. Underproductive speech
- 7. Abnormal object relationships
- 19. Blunted affect
- 27. Other speech deviance
- 28. Rhythmic motions (stereotypic)
- 57. Ideas of reference

II. Hostile—Uncooperative
- 10. Negative, uncooperative
- 11. Angry affect
- 17. Suspicious affect
- 50. Temper outbursts

III. Hyperactive
- 3. Fidgetiness
- 4. Hyperactivity
- 6. Distractibility
- 20. Lability of affect

IV. Anxiety
- 1. Tension
- 15. Clinging
- 34. Separation anxiety
- 38. Preoccupation—anxiety
- 41. Fears and phobias

V. Thought disturbance
- 58. Persecutory ideation
- 59. Other thinking disturbances
- 60. Delusions
- 62. Peculiar fantasies
- 63. Lack of insight

VI. Neurotic
- 31. Physical complaints
- 42. Compulsive acts
- 43. Nervous habits
- 44. Obsessive thinking

VII. Depression
- 5. Hypoactivity
- 18. Depressed demeanor
- 24. Low voice
- 29. Expressed feelings of inferiority
- 35. Depression
- 37. Lack of energy
- 39. Preoccupation with depressive topics
- 40. Suicidal attempts

VIII. Excited mood
- 12. Silly affect
- 21. Pressure of speech
- 25. Loud voice
- 30. Expressed feelings of grandiosity
- 36. Euphoria—elation

IX. Withdrawal
- 8. Withdrawal
- 9. Overcompliant
- 16. Unspontaneous relation to examiner
- 45. Solitary interests
- 46. Lack of peer interaction
- 51. Scapegoat

X. Antisocial
- 47. Gang activity
- 48. Fighting with peers
- 49. Bully
- 52. Lying
- 53. Exploitative relationships

XI. Organic
- 13. Confusion
- 14. Disorientation

XII. Speech disturbance
- 22. Level of speech development
- 23. Stuttering
- 26. Mispronunciations

XIII. Sleep disturbance
- 54. Inability to fall asleep
- 55. Other sleep difficulties

XIV. Eating disturbance
- 32. Obesity
- 33. Other eating problem

XV. Enuresis
- 56. Bedwetting

SPECIAL INSTRUCTIONS—Cues for rating as well as specific instructions for each item are printed on the scale. Strict adherence to these instructions is required of all raters.

Item 22—Level of speech development. This item may be confusing. The rater is asked to judge whether the level of speech development is appropriate to the child's verbal I.Q. For example, response position 4 is read as level of speech development is only 46 to 60% of Verbal I.Q.; position 2 as level of speech development is 76 to 90% of Verbal I.Q.

Item 56—Bedwetting and Item 61. Hallucinations. Remember that these items (as with all items from 29 to 63) refer to the past 7 days.

DOCUMENTATION

a. Raw score printout
b. Cluster score printout
c. Means and standard deviations for cluster scores
d. Cross tabulations
e. Variance analyses

From National Institute of Mental Health. (1976). Abnormal involuntary movement scale. In Guci, W. (Ed.). *The ECDEU assessment manual*, pp. 124–129. Rockville, MD: US Department of Health, Education and Welfare.

The Michigan Alcoholism Screening Test (MAST)

POINTS		
2	(*1.)	Do you feel you are a normal drinker?
2	2.	Have you ever awakened the morning after some drinking the night before and found that you could not remember part of the evening before?
1	3.	Does your wife (or parents) ever worry or complain about your drinking?
2	*4.	Can you stop drinking without a struggle after one or two drinks?
1	5.	Do you ever feel bad about your drinking?
2	(*6.)	Do friends or relatives think you are a normal drinker?
0	7.	Do you ever try to limit your drinking to certain times of the day or to certain places?
2	*8.	Are you always able to stop drinking when you want to?
5	(9).	Have you ever attended a meeting of Alcoholics Anonymous (AA)?
1	10.	Have you gotten into fights when drinking?
2	11.	Has drinking ever created problems with you and your wife?
2	12.	Has your wife (or other family member) ever gone to anyone for help about your drinking?
2	(13.)	Have you ever lost friends or girlfriends/boyfriends because of your drinking?
2	(14.)	Have you ever gotten into trouble at work because of drinking?
2	15.	Have you ever lost a job because of drinking?
2	(16.)	Have you ever neglected your obligations, your family, or your work for two or more days in a row because you were drinking?
1	17.	Do you ever drink before noon?
2	18.	Have you ever been told you have liver trouble? Cirrhosis?
2	(19.)	Have you ever had delirium tremens (DTs), severe shaking, heard voices, or seen things that weren't really there after heavy drinking?
5	(20.)	Have you ever gone to anyone for help about your drinking?
5	(21.)	Have you ever been in a hospital because of your drinking?
2	22.	Have you ever been a patient in a psychiatric hospital or on a psychiatric ward of a general hospital where drinking was part of the problem?
2	23.	Have you ever been seen at a psychiatric or mental health clinic, or gone to a doctor, social worker, or clergyman for help with an emotional problem in which drinking has played a part?
2	24.	Have you ever been arrested, even for a few hours, because of drunk behavior?
2	(25.)	Have you ever been arrested for drunk driving or driving after drinking?

* Negative responses are alcoholic responses.
( ) Indicates questions included in the Brief MAST.
– Indicates questions included in the SMAST (a shortened version of the MAST with good reliability).
Scoring: A score of three points or less is considered nonalcoholic; four points is suggestive of alcoholism; a score of five points or more indicates alcoholism.

APPENDIX 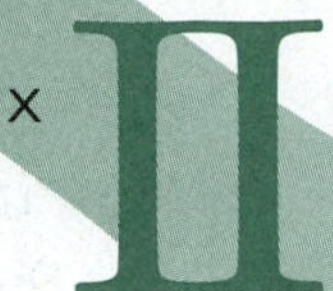

DSM-IV CLASSIFICATION

NOS = Not Otherwise Specified.

An *x* appearing in a diagnostic code indicates that a specific code number is required.

An ellipsis (. . .) is used in the names of certain disorders to indicate that the name of a specific mental disorder or general medical condition should be inserted when recording the name (e.g., 293.0 Delirium due to Hypothyroidism).

Numbers in parentheses are page numbers.*

If criteria are currently met, one of the following severity specifiers may be noted after the diagnosis:

Mild
Moderate
Severe

If criteria are no longer met, one of the following specifiers may be noted:

In Partial Remission
In Full Remission
Prior History

Disorders Usually First Diagnosed in Infancy, Childhood, or Adolescence (37)

MENTAL RETARDATION (39)
Note: *These are coded on Axis II.*

317 Mild Mental Retardation (41)
318.0 Moderate Mental Retardation (41)
318.1 Severe Mental Retardation (41)
318.2 Profound Mental Retardation (41)
319 Mental Retardation. Severity Unspecified (42)

LEARNING DISORDERS (46)

315.00 Reading Disorder (48)
315.1 Mathematics Disorder (50)
315.2 Disorder of Written Expression (51)
315.9 Learning Disorder NOS (53)

MOTOR SKILLS DISORDER

315.4 Developmental Coordination Disorder (53)

COMMUNICATION DISORDERS (55)

315.31 Expressive Language Disorder (55)
315.31 Mixed Receptive-Expressive Language Disorder (58)
315.39 Phonological Disorder (61)
307.0 Stuttering (63)
307.9 Communication Disorder NOS (65)

* Refers to page numbers in *DSM-IV.*

PERVASIVE DEVELOPMENTAL DISORDERS (65)

299.00 Autistic Disorder (66)
299.80 Rett's Disorder (71)
299.10 Childhood Distintegrative Disorder (73)
299.80 Asperger's Disorder (75)
299.80 Pervasive Developmental Disorder NOS (77)

ATTENTION-DEFICIT AND DISRUPTIVE BEHAVIOR DISORDERS (78)

314.xx Attention-Deficit/Hyperactivity Disorder (78)
.01 Combined Type
.00 Predominantly Inattentive Type
.01 Predominantly Hyperactive-Impulsive Type
314.9 Attention-Deficit/Hyperactivity Disorder NOS (85)
312.8 Conduct Disorder (85)
Specify type: Childhood-Onset Type/Adolescent-Onset Type
313.81 Oppositional Defiant Disorder (91)
312.9 Disruptive Behavior Disorder NOS (94)

FEEDING AND EATING DISORDERS OF INFANCY OR EARLY CHILDHOOD (94)

307.52 Pica (95)
307.53 Rumination Disorder (96)
307.59 Feeding Disorder of Infancy or Early Childhood (98)

TIC DISORDERS (100)

307.23 Tourette's Disorder (101)
307.22 Chronic Motor or Vocal Tic Disorder (103)
307.21 Transient Tic Disorder (104)
Specify if: Single Episode/Recurrent
307.20 Tic Disorder NOS (105)

ELIMINATION DISORDERS (106)

—.– Encopresis (106)
787.6 With Constipation and Overflow Incontinence
307.7 Without Constipation and Overflow Incontinence
307.6 Enuresis (Not Due to a General Medical Condition) (108)
Specify type: Nocturnal Only/Diurnal Only/Nocturnal and Diurnal

OTHER DISORDERS OF INFANCY, CHILDHOOD, OR ADOLESCENCE

309.21 Separation Anxiety Disorder (110)
Specify if: Early Onset
313.23 Selective Mutism (114)
313.89 Reactive Attachment Disorder of Infancy or Early Childhood (116)
Specify type: Inhibited Type/Disinhibited Type

307.3 Stereotypic Movement Disorder (118)
Specify if: With Self-Injurious Behavior

313.9 Disorder of Infancy, Childhood, or Adolescence NOS (121)

Delirium, Dementia, and Amnestic and Other Cognitive Disorders (123)

DELIRIUM (124)

293.0 Delirium Due to . . . *[Indicate the General Medical Condition]* (127)

—.– Substance Intoxication Delirium (129) *(refer to Substance-Related Disorders for substance-specific codes)*

—.– Substance Withdrawal Delirium (129) *(refer to Substance-Related Disorders for substance-specific codes)*

—.– Delirium Due to Multiple Etiologies *(code each of the specific etiologies)* (132)

780.09 Delirium NOS (133)

DEMENTIA (133)

290.xx Dementia of the Alzheimer's Type, With Early Onset *(also code 331.0 Alzheimer's disease on Axis III)* (139)
- .10 Uncomplicated
- .11 With Delirium
- .12 With Delusions
- .13 With Depressed Mood

Specify if: With Behavioral Disturbance

290.xx Dementia of the Alzheimer's Type, With Late Onset *(also code 331.0 Alzheimer's disease on Axis III)* (139)
- .0 Uncomplicated
- .3 With Delirium
- .20 With Delusions
- .21 With Depressed Mood

Specify if: With Behavioral Disturbance

290.xx Vascular Dementia (143)
- .40 Uncomplicated
- .41 With Delirium
- .42 With Delusions
- .43 With Depressed Mood

Specify if: With Behavioral Disturbance

294.9 Dementia Due to HIV Disease *(also code 043.1 HIV infection affecting central nervous system on Axis III)* (148)

294.1 Dementia Due to Head Trauma *(also code 854.00 head injury on Axis III)* (148)

294.1 Dementia Due to Parkinson's Disease *(also code 332.0 Parkinson's disease on Axis III)* (148)

294.1 Dementia Due to Huntington's Disease *(also code 333.4 Huntington's disease on Axis III)* (149)

290.10 Dementia Due to Pick's Disease *(also code 331.1 Pick's disease on Axis III)* (149)

290.10 Dementia Due to Creutzfeldt-Jakob Disease *(also code 046.1 Creutzfeldt-Jakob disease on Axis III)* (150)

294.1 Dementia Due to . . . *[Indicate the General Medical Condition not listed above] (also code the general medical condition on Axis III)* (151)

—.– Substance-Induced Persisting Dementia *(refer to Substance-Related Disorders for substance-specific codes)* (152)

—.– Dementia Due to Multiple Etiologies *(code each of the specific etiologies)* (154)

294.8 Dementia NOS (155)

AMNESTIC DISORDERS (156)

294.0 Amnestic Disorder Due to . . . *[Indicate the General Medical Condition]* (158)
Specify if: Transient/Chronic

—.– Substance-Induced Persisting Amnestic Disorder *(refer to Substance-Related Disorders for substance-specific codes)* (161)

294.8 Amnestic Disorders NOS (163)

OTHER COGNITIVE DISORDERS (163)

294.9 Cognitive Disorder NOS (163)

Mental Disorders Due to a General Medical Condition Not Elsewhere Classified (165)

293.89 Catatonic Disorder Due to . . . *[Indicate the General Medical Condition]* (169)

310.1 Personality Change Due to . . . *[Indicate the General Medical Condition]* (171)
Specify type: Labile Type/Disinhibited Type/Aggressive Type/Apathetic Type/Paranoid Type/Other Type/Combined Type/Unspecified Type

293.9 Mental Disorder NOS Due to . . . *[Indicate the General Medical Condition]* (174)

Substance-Related Disorders (175)

[a]*The following specifiers may be applied to Substance Dependence:*

With Physiological Dependence/Without Physiological Dependence

Early Full Remission/Early Partial Remission
Sustained Full Remission/Sustained Partial Remission
On Agonist Therapy/In a Controlled Environment

The following specifiers apply to Substance-Induced Disorders as noted:
[I]With Onset During Intoxication/[W]With Onset During Withdrawal

ALCOHOL-RELATED DISORDERS (194)

Alcohol Use Disorders

303.90 Alcohol Dependence[a] (195)

305.00 Alcohol Abuse (196)

Alcohol-Induced Disorders

303.00 Alcohol Intoxication (196)

291.8 Alcohol Withdrawal (197)
Specify if: With Perceptual Disturbances

291.0 Alcohol Intoxication Delirium (129)

291.0 Alcohol Withdrawal Delirium (129)

291.2 Alcohol-Induced Persisting Dementia (152)

291.1 Alcohol-Induced Persisting Amnestic Disorder (161)

291.x Alcohol-Induced Psychotic Disorder (310)

.5 With Delusions[I,W]

.3 With Hallucinations[I,W]

291.8 Alcohol-Induced Mood Disorder[I,W] (370)

291.8 Alcohol-Induced Anxiety Disorder[I,W] (439)

291.8 Alcohol-Induced Sexual Dysfunction[I] (519)

291.8 Alcohol-Induced Sleep Disorder[I,W] (601)

291.9 Alcohol-Related Disorder NOS (240)

AMPHETAMINE (OR AMPHETAMINE-LIKE)–RELATED DISORDERS (204)

Amphetamine Use Disorders

304.40 Amphetamine Dependence[a] (206)

305.70 Amphetamine Abuse (206)

Amphetamine-Induced Disorders

292.89 Amphetamine Intoxication (207)
Specify if: With Perceptual Disturbances

292.0 Amphetamine Withdrawal (208)

292.81 Amphetamine Intoxication Delirium (129)

292.xx Amphetamine-Induced Psychotic Disorder (310)

.11 With Delusions[I]

.12 With Hallucinations[I]

292.84 Amphetamine-Induced Mood Disorder[I,W] (370)

292.89 Amphetamine-Induced Anxiety Disorder[I] (439)

292.89 Amphetamine-Induced Sexual Dysfunction[I] (519)

292.89 Amphetamine-Induced Sleep Disorder[I,W] (601)

292.9 Amphetamine-Related Disorder NOS (211)

CAFFEINE-RELATED DISORDERS (212)

Caffeine-Induced Disorders

305.90 Caffeine Intoxication (212)

292.89 Caffeine-Induced Anxiety Disorder[I] (439)

292.89 Caffeine-Induced Sleep Disorder[I] (601)

292.9 Caffeine-Related Disorder NOS (215)

CANNABIS-RELATED DISORDERS (215)

Cannabis Use Disorders

304.30 Cannabis Dependence[a] (216)

305.20 Cannabis Abuse (217)

Cannabis-Induced Disorders

292.89 Cannabis Intoxication (217)
Specify if: With Perceptual Disturbances

292.81 Cannabis Intoxication Delirium (129)

292.xx Cannabis-Induced Psychotic Disorder (310)

.11 With Delusions[I]

.12 With Hallucinations[I]

292.89 Cannabis-Induced Anxiety Disorder[I] (439)

292.9 Cannabis-Related Disorder NOS (221)

COCAINE-RELATED DISORDERS (221)

Cocaine Use Disorders

304.20 Cocaine Dependence[a] (222)

305.60 Cocaine Abuse (223)

Cocaine-Induced Disorders

292.89 Cocaine Intoxication (223)
Specify if: With Perceptual Disturbances

292.0 Cocaine Withdrawal (225)

292.81 Cocaine Intoxication Delirium (129)

292.xx Cocaine-Induced Psychotic Disorder (310)

.11 With Delusions[I]

.12 With Hallucinations[I]

292.84 Cocaine-Induced Mood Disorder[I,W] (370)

292.89 Cocaine-Induced Anxiety Disorder[I,W] (439)

292.89 Cocaine-Induced Sexual Dysfunction[I] (519)

292.89 Cocaine-Induced Sleep Disorder[I,W] (601)

292.9 Cocaine-Related Disorder NOS (229)

HALLUCINOGEN-RELATED DISORDERS (229)

Hallucinogen Use Disorders

304.50 Hallucinogen Dependence[a] (230)

305.30 Hallucinogen Abuse (231)

Hallucinogen-Induced Disorders

292.89 Hallucinogen Intoxication (232)

292.89 Hallucinogen Persisting Perception Disorder (Flashbacks) (233)

292.81 Hallucinogen Intoxication Delirium (129)

292.xx Hallucinogen-Induced Psychotic Disorder (310)

.11 With Delusions[I]

.12 With Hallucinations[I]

292.84 Hallucinogen-Induced Mood Disorder[I] (370)

292.89 Hallucinogen-Induced Anxiety Disorder[I] (439)

292.9 Hallucinogen-Related Disorder NOS (236)

INHALANT-RELATED DISORDERS (236)

Inhalant Use Disorders

304.60 Inhalant Dependence[a] (238)

305.90 Inhalant Abuse (238)

Inhalant-Induced Disorders

292.89 Inhalant Intoxication (239)

292.81 Inhalant Intoxication Delirium (129)

292.82 Inhalant-Induced Persisting Dementia (152)

292.xx Inhalant-Induced Psychotic Disorder (310)

.11 With Delusions[I]

.12 With Hallucinations[I]

292.84 Inhalant-Induced Mood Disorder[I] (370)

292.89 Inhalant-Induced Anxiety Disorder[I] (439)

292.9 Inhalant-Related Disorder NOS (242)

NICOTINE-RELATED DISORDERS (242)

Nicotine Use Disorder

305.10 Nicotine Dependence[a] (243)

Nicotine-Induced Disorder

292.0 Nicotine Withdrawal (244)

292.9 Nicotine-Related Disorder NOS (247)

OPIOID-RELATED DISORDERS (247)

Opioid Use Disorders

304.00 Opioid Dependence[a] (248)

305.50 Opioid Abuse (249)

Opioid-Induced Disorders

292.89 Opioid Intoxication (249)
Specify if: With Perceptual Disturbances

292.0 Opioid Withdrawal (250)

292.81 Opioid Intoxication Delirium (129)

292.xx Opioid-Induced Psychotic Disorder (310)

.11 With Delusions[I]

.12 With Hallucinations[I]

292.84 Opioid-Induced Mood Disorder[I] (370)

292.89 Opioid-Induced Sexual Dysfunction[I] (519)

292.89 Opioid-Induced Sleep Disorder[I,W] (601)

292.9 Opioid-Related Disorder NOS (255)

PHENCYCLIDINE (OR PHENCYCLIDINE-LIKE)–RELATED DISORDERS (255)

Phencyclidine Use Disorders

304.90 Phencyclidine Dependence[a] (256)

305.90 Phencyclidine Abuse (257)

Phencyclidine-Induced Disorders

292.89 Phencyclidine Intoxication (257)
Specify if: With Perceptual Disturbances

292.81 Phencyclidine Intoxication Delirium (129)

292.xx Phencyclidine-Induced Psychotic Disorder (310)

.11 With Delusions[I]

.12 With Hallucinations[I]

292.84 Phencyclidine-Induced Mood Disorder[I] (370)

292.89 Phencyclidine-Induced Anxiety Disorder[I] (439)

292.9 Phencyclidine-Related Disorder NOS (261)

SEDATIVE-, HYPNOTIC-, OR ANXIOLYTIC-RELATED DISORDERS (261)

Sedative, Hypnotic, or Anxiolytic Use Disorders

304.10 Sedative, Hypnotic, or Anxiolytic Dependence[a] (262)

305.40 Sedative, Hypnotic, or Anxiolytic Abuse (263)

Sedative-, Hypnotic-, or Anxiolytic-Induced Disorders

292.89 Sedative, Hypnotic, or Anxiolytic Intoxication (263)

292.0 Sedative, Hypnotic, or Anxiolytic Withdrawal (264)
Specify if: With Perceptual Disturbances

292.81 Sedative, Hypnotic, or Anxiolytic Intoxication Delirium (129)

292.81 Sedative, Hypnotic, or Anxiolytic Withdrawal Delirium (129)

292.82 Sedative-, Hypnotic-, or Anxiolytic-Induced Persisting Dementia (152

292.83 Sedative-, Hypnotic-, or Anxiolytic-Induced Persisting Amnestic Disorder (161)

292.xx Sedative-, Hypnotic-, or Anxiolytic-Induced Psychotic Disorder (310)

.11 With Delusions[I,W]

.12 With Hallucinations[I,W]

292.84 Sedative-, Hypnotic-, or Anxiolytic-Induced Mood Disorder[I,W] (370)

292.89 Sedative-, Hypnotic-, or Anxiolytic-Induced Anxiety Disorder[W] (439)

292.89 Sedative-, Hypnotic-, or Anxiolytic-Induced Sexual Dysfunction[I] (519)

292.89 Sedative-, Hypnotic-, or Anxiolytic-Induced Sleep Disorder[I,W] (601)

292.9 Sedative-, Hypnotic-, or Anxiolytic-Related Disorder NOS (269)

POLYSUBSTANCE-RELATED DISORDER

304.80 Polysubstance Dependence[a] (270)

OTHER (OR UNKNOWN) SUBSTANCE–RELATED DISORDERS (270)

Other (or Unknown) Substance Use Disorders

304.90 Other (or Unknown) Substance Dependence[a] (176)

305.90 Other (or Unknown) Substance Abuse (182)

Other (or Unknown) Substance–Induced Disorders

292.89 Other (or Unknown) Substance Intoxication (183)
Specify if: With Perceptual Disturbances

292.0 Other (or Unknown) Substance Withdrawal (184)
Specify if: With Perceptual Disturbances

292.81 Other (or Unknown) Substance–Induced Delirium (129)

292.82 Other (or Unknown) Substance–Induced Persisting Dementia (152)

292.83 Other (or Unknown) Substance–Induced Persisting Amnestic Disorder (161)

292.xx Other (or Unknown) Substance–Induced Psychotic Disorder (310)

.11 With Delusions[I,W]

.12 With Hallucinations[I,W]

292.84 Other (or Unknown) Substance–Induced Mood Disorder[I,W] (370)

292.89 Other (or Unknown) Substance–Induced Anxiety Disorder[I,W] (439)

292.89 Other (or Unknown) Substance–Induced Sexual Dysfunction[I] (519)

292.89 Other (or Unknown) Substance–Induced Sleep Disorder[I,W] (601)

292.9 Other (or Unknown) Substance–Related Disorder NOS (272)

Schizophrenia and Other Psychotic Disorders (273)

295.xx Schizophrenia (274)

The following Classification of Longitudinal Course applies to all subtypes of Schizophrenia:

Episodic With Interepisode Residual Symptoms (*specify if:* With Prominent Negative Symptoms)/Episodic with No Interepisode Residual Symptoms/Continuous (*specify if:* With Prominent Negative Symptoms)
Single Episode In Partial Remission (*specify if:* With Prominent Negative Symptoms)/Single Episode In Full Remission
Other or Unspecified Pattern

.30 Paranoid Type (287)

.10 Disorganized Type (287)

.20 Catatonic Type (288)

.90 Undifferentiated Type (289)

.60 Residual Type (289)

295.40 Schizophreniform Disorder (290)
Specify if: Without Good Prognostic Features/With Good Prognostic Features

295.70 Schizoaffective Disorder (292)
Specify type: Bipolar Type/Depressive Type

297.1 Delusional Disorder (296)
Specify type: Erotomanic Type/Grandiose Type/Jealous Type/Persecutory Type/Somatic Type/Mixed Type/Unspecified Type

298.8 Brief Psychotic Disorder (302)
Specify if: With Marked Stressor(s)/Without Marked Stressor(s)/With Postpartum Onset

297.3 Shared Psychotic Disorder (305)

293.xx Psychotic Disorder Due to . . . *[Indicate the General Medical Condition]* (306)

.81 With Delusions

.82 With Hallucinations

—.– Substance-Induced Psychotic Disorder *(refer to Substance-Related Disorders for substance-specific codes)* (310)
Specify if: With Onset During Intoxication/With Onset During Withdrawal

298.9 Psychotic Disorder NOS (315)

Mood Disorders (317)

Code current state of Major Depressive Disorder or Bipolar I Disorder in fifth digit:

1 = Mild
2 = Moderate
3 = Severe Without Psychotic Features
4 = Severe With Psychotic Features
Specify: Mood-Congruent Psychotic Features/Mood-Incongruent Psychotic Features
5 = In Partial Remission
6 = In Full Remission
0 = Unspecified

The following specifiers apply (for current or most recent episode) to Mood Disorders as noted:
[a]Severity/Psychotic/Remission Specifiers/[b]Chronic/[c]With Catatonic Features/[d]With Melancholic Features/[e]With Atypical Features/[f]With Postpartum Onset

The following specifiers apply to Mood Disorders as noted:
[g]With or Without Full Interepisode Recovery/[h]With Seasonal Pattern/[i]With Rapid Cycling

DEPRESSIVE DISORDERS

296.xx Major Depressive Disorder (339)

.2x Single Episode[a,b,c,d,e,f]

.3x Recurrent[a,b,c,d,e,f,g,h]

300.4 Dysthymic Disorder (345)
Specify if: Early Onset/Late Onset
Specify: With Atypical Features

311 Depressive Disorder NOS (350)

BIPOLAR DISORDERS

296.xx Bipolar I Disorder (350)
 .0x Single Manic Episode[a,c,f]
 Specify if: Mixed
 .40 Most Recent Episode Hypomanic[g,h,i]
 .4x Most Recent Episode Manic[a,c,f,g,h,i]
 .6x Most Recent Episode Mixed[a,c,f,g,h,i]
 .5x Most Recent Episode Depressed[a,b,c,d,e,f,g,h,i]
 .7 Most Recent Episode Unspecified[g,h,i]
296.89 Bipolar II Disorder[a,b,c,d,e,f,g,h,i] (359)
 Specify (current or most recent episode): Hypomanic/Depressed
301.13 Cyclothymic Disorder (363)
296.80 Bipolar Disorder NOS (366)
293.83 Mood Disorder Due to . . . *[Indicate the General Medical Condition]* (366)
 Specify type: With Depressive Features/With Major Depressive–Like Episode/With Manic Features/With Mixed Features
—.– Substance-Induced Mood Disorder *(refer to Substance-Related Disorders for substance-specific codes)* (370)
 Specify type: With Depressive Features/With Manic Features/With Mixed Features
 Specify if: With Onset During Intoxication/With Onset During Withdrawal
296.90 Mood Disorder NOS (375)

Anxiety Disorders (393)

300.01 Panic Disorder Without Agoraphobia (397)
300.21 Panic Disorder With Agoraphobia (397)
300.22 Agoraphobia Without History of Panic Disorder (403)
300.29 Specific Phobia (405)
 Specify type: Animal Type/Natural Environment Type/Blood-Injection-Injury Type/Situational Type/Other Type
300.23 Social Phobia (411)
 Specify if: Generalized
300.3 Obsessive-Compulsive Disorder (417)
 Specify if: With Poor Insight
309.81 Posttraumatic Stress Disorder (424)
 Specify if: Acute/Chronic
 Specify if: With Delayed Onset
308.3 Acute Stress Disorder (429)
300.02 Generalized Anxiety Disorder (432)
293.89 Anxiety Disorder Due to . . . *[Indicate the General Medical Condition]* (436)
 Specify if: With Generalized Anxiety/With Panic Attacks/With Obsessive-Compulsive Symptoms
—.– Substance-Induced Anxiety Disorder *(refer to Substance-Related Disorders for substance-specific codes)* (439)
 Specify if: With Generalized Anxiety/With Panic Attacks/With Obsessive-Compulsive Symptoms/With Phobic Symptoms
 Specify if: With Onset During Intoxication/With Onset During Withdrawal
300.00 Anxiety Disorder NOS (444)

Somatoform Disorders (445)

300.81 Somatization Disorder (446)
300.81 Undifferentiated Somatoform Disorder (450)
300.11 Conversion Disorder (452)
 Specify type: With Motor Symptom or Deficit/With Sensory Symptom or Deficit With Seizures or Convulsions/With Mixed Presentation
307.xx Pain Disorder (458)
 .80 Associated With Psychological Factors
 .89 Associated With Both Psychological Factors and a General Medical Condition
 Specify if: Acute/Chronic
300.7 Hypochondriasis (462)
 Specify if: With Poor Insight
300.7 Body Dysmorphic Disorder (466)
300.81 Somatoform Disorder NOS (468)

Factitious Disorders (471)

300.xx Factitious Disorder (471)
 .16 With Predominantly Psychological Signs and Symptoms
 .19 With Predominantly Physical Signs and Symptoms
 .19 With Combined Psychological and Physical Signs and Symptoms
300.19 Factitious Disorder NOS (475)

Dissociative Disorders (477)

300.12 Dissociative Amnesia (478)
300.13 Dissociative Fugue (481)
300.14 Dissociative Identity Disorder (484)
300.6 Depersonalization Disorder (488)
300.15 Dissociative Disorder NOS (490)

Sexual and Gender Identity Disorders (493)

SEXUAL DYSFUNCTIONS (493)
The following specifiers apply to all primary Sexual Dysfunctions:

Lifelong Type/Acquired Type
Generalized Type/Situational Type
Due to Psychological Factors/Due to Combined Factors

Sexual Desire Disorders

302.71 Hypoactive Sexual Desire Disorder (496)

302.79 Sexual Aversion Disorder (499)

Sexual Arousal Disorders

302.72 Female Sexual Arousal Disorder (500)

302.72 Male Erectile Disorder (502)

Orgasmic Disorders

302.73 Female Orgasmic Disorder (505)

302.74 Male Orgasmic Disorder (507)

302.75 Premature Ejaculation (509)

Sexual Pain Disorders

302.76 Dyspareunia (Not Due to a General Medical Condition) (511)

306.51 Vaginismus (Not Due to a General Medical Condition) (513)

Sexual Dysfunction Due to a General Medical Condition (515)

625.8 Female Hypoactive Sexual Desire Disorder Due to . . . *[Indicate the General Medical Condition]* (515)

608.89 Male Hypoactive Sexual Desire Disorder Due to . . . *[Indicate the General Medical Condition]* (515)

607.84 Male Erectile Disorder Due to . . . *[Indicate the General Medical Condition]* (515)

625.0 Female Dyspareunia Due to . . . *[Indicate the General Medical Condition]* (515)

608.89 Male Dyspareunia Due to . . . *[Indicate the General Medical Condition]* (515)

625.8 Other Female Sexual Dysfunction Due to . . . *[Indicate the General Medical Condition]* (515)

608.89 Other Male Sexual Dysfunction Due to . . . *[Indicate the General Medical Condition]* (515)

—.– Substance-Induced Sexual Dysfunction *(refer to Substance-Related Disorders for substance-specific codes)* (519)
Specify if: With Impaired Desire/With Impaired Arousal/With Impaired Orgasm/With Sexual Pain
Specify if: With Onset During Intoxication

302.70 Sexual Dysfunction NOS (522)

PARAPHILIAS (522)

302.4 Exhibitionism (525)

302.81 Fetishism (526)

302.89 Frotteurism (527)

302.2 Pedophilia (527)
Specify if: Sexually Attracted to Males/Sexually Attracted to Females/Sexually Attracted to Both
Specify if: Limited to Incest
Specify type: Exclusive Type/Nonexclusive Type

302.83 Sexual Masochism (529)

302.84 Sexual Sadism (530)

302.3 Transvestic Fetishism (530)
Specify if: With Gender Dysphoria

302.82 Voyeurism (532)

302.9 Paraphilia NOS (532)

GENDER IDENTITY DISORDERS (532)

302.xx Gender Identity Disorder (532)

.6 in Children

.85 in Adolescents or Adults
Specify if: Sexually Attracted to Males/Sexually Attracted to Females/Sexually Attracted to Both/Sexually Attracted to Neither

302.6 Gender Identity Disorder NOS (538)

302.9 Sexual Disorder NOS (538)

Eating Disorders (539)

307.1 Anorexia Nervosa (539)
Specify type: Restricting Type; Binge-Eating/Purging Type

307.51 Bulimia Nervosa (545)
Specify type: Purging Type/Nonpurging Type

307.50 Eating Disorder NOS (550)

Sleep Disorders (551)

PRIMARY SLEEP DISORDERS (553)

Dyssomnias (553)

307.42 Primary Insomnia (553)

307.44 Primary Hypersomnia (557)
Specify if: Recurrent

347 Narcolepsy (562)

780.59 Breathing-Related Sleep Disorder (567)

307.45 Circadian Rhythm Sleep Disorder (573)
Specify type: Delayed Sleep Phase Type/Jet Lag Type/Shift Work Type/Unspecified Type

307.47 Dyssomnia NOS (579)

Parasomnias (579)

307.47 Nightmare Disorder (580)

307.46 Sleep Terror Disorder (583)

307.46 Sleepwalking Disorder (587)

307.47 Parasomnia NOS (592)

SLEEP DISORDERS RELATED TO ANOTHER MENTAL DISORDER (592)

307.42 Insomnia Related to . . . *[Indicate the Axis I or Axis II Disorder]* (592)

307.44 Hypersomnia Related to . . . *[Indicate the Axis I or Axis II Disorder]* (592)

OTHER SLEEP DISORDERS

780.xx Sleep Disorder Due to . . . *[Indicate the General Medical Condition]* (597)

- .52 Insomnia Type
- .54 Hypersomnia Type
- .59 Parasomnia Type
- .59 Mixed Type

——.– Substance-Induced Sleep Disorder *(refer to Substance-Related Disorders for substance-specific codes)* (601)
Specify type: Insomnia Type/Hypersomnia Type/Parasomnia Type/Mixed Type
Specify if: With Onset During Intoxication/With Onset During Withdrawal

Impulse-Control Disorders Not Elsewhere Classified (609)

312.34 Intermittent Explosive Disorder (609)

312.32 Kleptomania (612)

312.33 Pyromania (614)

312.31 Pathological Gambling (615)

312.39 Trichotillomania (618)

312.30 Impulse-Control Disorder NOS (621)

Adjustment Disorders (623)

309.xx Adjustment Disorder (623)

- .0 With Depressed Mood
- .24 With Anxiety
- .28 With Mixed Anxiety and Depressed Mood
- .3 With Disturbance of Conduct
- .4 With Mixed Disturbance of Emotions and Conduct
- .9 Unspecified

Specify if: Acute/Chronic

Personality Disorders (629)

Note: *These are coded on Axis II.*

301.0 Paranoid Personality Disorder (634)

301.20 Schizoid Personality Disorder (638)

301.22 Schizotypal Personality Disorder (641)

301.7 Antisocial Personality Disorder (645)

301.83 Borderline Personality Disorder (650)

301.50 Histrionic Personality Disorder (655)

301.81 Narcissistic Personality Disorder (658)

301.82 Avoidant Personality Disorder (662)

301.6 Dependent Personality Disorder (665)

301.4 Obsessive-Compulsive Personality Disorder (669)

301.9 Personality Disorder NOS (673)

Other Conditions That May Be a Focus of Clinical Attention (675)

PSYCHOLOGICAL FACTORS AFFECTING MEDICAL CONDITION (675)

316 . . . *[Specified Psychological Factor]* Affecting . . . *[Indicate the General Medical Condition]* (675)
Choose name based on nature of factors:
Mental Disorder Affecting Medical Condition
Psychological Symptoms Affecting Medical Condition
Personality Traits or Coping Style Affecting Medical Condition
Maladaptive Health Behaviors Affecting Medical Condition
Stress-Related Physiological Response Affecting Medical Condition
Other or Unspecified Psychological Factors Affecting Medical Condition

MEDICATION-INDUCED MOVEMENT DISORDERS (678)

332.1 Neuroleptic-Induced Parkinsonism (679)

333.92 Neuroleptic Malignant Syndrome (679)

333.7 Neuroleptic-Induced Acute Dystonia (679)

333.99 Neuroleptic-Induced Acute Akathisia (679)

333.82 Neuroleptic-Induced Tardive Dyskinesia (679)

333.1 Medication-Induced Postural Tremor (680)

333.90 Medication-Induced Movement Disorder NOS (680)

OTHER MEDICATION-INDUCED DISORDER

995.2 Adverse Effects of Medication NOS (680)

RELATIONAL PROBLEMS (680)

V61.9 Relational Problem Related to a Mental Disorder or General Medical Condition (681)

V61.20	Parent-Child Relational Problem (681)
V61.1	Partner Relational Problem (681)
V61.8	Sibling Relational Problem (681)
V62.81	Relational Problem NOS (681)

PROBLEMS RELATED TO ABUSE OR NEGLECT (682)

V61.21	Physical Abuse of Child (682) *(code 995.5 if focus of attention is on victim)*
V61.21	Sexual Abuse of Child (682) *(code 995.5 if focus of attention is on victim)*
V61.21	Neglect of Child (682) *(code 995.5 if focus of attention is on victim)*
V61.1	Physical Abuse of Adult (682) *(code 995.81 if focus of attention is on victim)*
V61.1	Sexual Abuse of Adult (682) *(code 995.81 if focus of attention is on victim)*

ADDITIONAL CONDITIONS THAT MAY BE A FOCUS OF CLINICAL ATTENTION (683)

V15.81	Noncompliance With Treatment (683)
V65.2	Malingering (683)
V71.01	Adult Antisocial Behavior (683)
V71.02	Child or Adolescent Antisocial Behavior (684)
V62.89	Borderline Intellectual Functioning (684) **Note:** *This is coded on Axis II.*
780.9	Age-Related Cognitive Decline (684)
V62.82	Bereavement (684)
V62.3	Academic Problem (685)
V62.2	Occupational Problem (685)
313.82	Identity Problem (685)
V62.89	Religious or Spiritual Problem (685)
V62.4	Acculturation Problem (685)
V62.89	Phase of Life Problem (685)

Additional Codes

300.9	Unspecified Mental Disorder (nonpsychotic) (687)
V71.09	No Diagnosis or Condition on Axis I (687)
799.9	Diagnosis or Condition Deferred on Axis I (687)
V71.09	No Diagnosis on Axis II (687)
799.9	Diagnosis Deferred on Axis II (687)

Multiaxial System

Axis I	Clinical Disorders Other Conditions That May Be a Focus of Clinical Attention
Axis II	Personality Disorders Mental Retardation
Axis III	General Medical Conditions
Axis IV	Psychosocial and Environmental Problems
Axis V	Global Assessment of Functioning

From American Psychiatric Association. *Diagnostic and Statistical Manual of Mental Disorders, Fourth Edition.* Washington, D.C., American Psychiatric Association, 1994.

ANSWERS TO *CHECK YOUR READING* QUESTIONS

CHAPTER 1

1. A world view is a way of looking at the big picture of life and making sense of it, organizing our experiences in a meaningful way and drawing conclusions about the significance of these experiences to our lives.
2. A theistic world view is one that involves spirituality.
3. The basic beliefs of a theistic world view are (1) that a loving and benevolent creator God exists, (2) that we are created in God's image, (3) that God loves us, (4) that our actions toward each other should reflect God's love, (5) that hope of change always exists, and (6) that we are holistic beings with integrated physical, emotional, and spiritual dimensions.
4. A theistic world view stresses forgiveness and treating people with kindness, patience, gentleness, and forbearance.
5. A theistic world view tells us that patients are people who have rich life experiences to share with us who just happen to manifest a particular psychiatric symptom.
6. We need to know patients from physical, social, emotional, and spiritual perspectives because these understandings are all essential to piecing together the patient's story.
7. The difference between the terms *patient* and *client* is that *client* means someone who is dependent on another for protection, whereas *patient* means one who suffers and forbears, which seems more accurate when describing the person in need of psychiatric services.
8. The three concentric circles represents a model of human beings and best describes the interaction of body, mind, and spirit.
9. The innermost circle refers to the spirit—the part of the person that pervades all other dimensions—and within this spiritual center lies the potential for consciousness of and relatedness to God.
10. The model illustrates the interactive aspects of the dimensions of human beings by showing the outside influences, such as social support, loving family and friends, the help of God, and material resources that strengthen the person.
11. The Stallwood and Stoll model has implications for psychiatric nursing because it considers the human as a dynamic whole and not as separate dimensions; the model deals with the mind, the body, and the spirit.
12. A focus on brain physiology "fits in" with a theistic world view in that it should be included in a holistic perspective because imbalances in brain physiology cause vulnerabilities or predispositions to certain illnesses.
13. A theistic world view suggests that our interventions with psychiatric patients should be holistic and should include the patient's spiritual concerns, including values, sense of purpose and meaning in life, and relationship to the transcendent.
14. The acronym BASIC-IS stands for behaviors, affective processes, sensations, images, cognitions, interpersonal relationships, and spirituality.
15. Two nonreligious world views are behaviorism and humanism.
16. Humanism affects psychiatric nursing because this world view extols the value and importance of the human being.
17. Behaviorism contributes to psychiatric nursing because we study behavior (believing that all behavior is meaningful), and we sometimes draw on techniques to change behavior.
18. Existentialism emphasizes the importance of the person's story and how the person makes decisions when faced with choices. These are essential in psychiatric nursing to understand and assist patients.
19. Monism is a world view that suggests a basic oneness of being and that the transcendent force in the universe is not a personal god but rather a universal energy force. Pantheism is a world view that suggests that everything is the same; that there is no difference between what exists in the world and the universal energy; and that all peoples and things share in the divine energy source and essentially all are God. Polytheism is a world view that suggests that many gods are present in the universe.
20. Monism and pantheism are similar in that they value relativism rather than absolutes and emphasize striving for balance within individual lives and the eradication of self. Polytheism involves sacrifices made to appease the gods or to appeal to the gods for special favors.
21. Two of the issues facing you as a nursing student entering a psychiatric nursing rotation for the first time are (1) anxiety about the new situations you will encounter, and (2) threats to your role as a nurse.
22. Two situations that may pose a threat to your role as a nurse are (1) a lack of professional attire, and (2) a lack of structure.
23. Two common fears that you may experience as a nursing student are that (1) you may have preconceived ideas about what a psychiatric hospital is like, and (2) you may have a loved one with a psychiatric illness.
24. Three strategies that you can use to cope with the anxiety that you might feel as a novice in psychiatric nursing are (1) to increase your self-awareness (e.g., by journaling, meditation, prayer, periods of quiet solitude, sharing in groups or individual clinical supervision sessions, and completing process recordings); (2) to read the patient's chart before meeting him or her to lessen your anxiety and to help to structure your time; and (3) to evaluate your own approach and modify it if your patient is not cooperating.
25. Cost of involvement is the impact that care of patients has on the individual nurse, which perhaps causes the nurse pain, sorrow, anger, or frustration. Implicit in this is the need for the nurse to take care of himself or herself in terms of body, mind, and spirit.

CHAPTER 2

1. In early history, people attributed the cause of mental illness to supernatural forces. Evil spirits, punishment from the gods, or possession by the devil or demons was seen as the cause of diseases, including the mental diseases.
2. The earliest "psychiatrists" were witch doctors or medicine men.
3. Hippocrates believed that depression was caused by an excess of black bile.
4. Philippe Pinel was credited with risking his career in medicine and perhaps his own life when he released patients from chains and restraints in Bicêtre mental hospital and also at the women's asylum at Salpêtrière.
5. William Tuke established the York Retreat, which exemplified the humanitarian approach to the mentally ill—the basis of Pinel's actions. Tuke and his fellow Quaker colleagues believed that treating people with kindness in a pleasant environment could help them to recover. This was considered one of the precursors to the modern-day milieu (environment) therapy.
6. America's first trained psychiatric nurse was Linda Richards (1891–1930).
7. The first psychiatric training school in the United States was established by Linda Richards, Dr. Edward A. Cowles, and Mary Palmer and was called the McLean Training School for Nurses (located at the McLean Asylum).
8. The first psychiatric nursing textbook was *Nursing Mental Diseases* by Harriet Bailey, B.S., R.N. This book was published in 1920 by Macmillan.
9. The first professor of psychiatric nursing was Euphemia "Effie" Jane Taylor (1874–1970). She was designated "Professor of Nursing" in 1926.
10. Clifford Beers, a crusader for the mentally ill, wrote his autobiography, *A Mind That Found Itself* (1908), in which he describes his experiences as a patient with a mental illness.
11. Emil Kraepelin's major contributions to psychiatry were his observations and descriptions of mental illness, particularly the mood disorders.
12. Dorothea Lynde Dix was a crusader during the Civil War (1861–1865), in which she volunteered her services as a nurse.
13. Benjamin Rush (1745–1813) is attributed with inventing the "tranquilizing chair," in which patients were restrained with their heads covered.

14. Dr. Harry Stack Sullivan (1892–1949) is credited with his theory of the significance of interpersonal relationships in his Interpersonal Theory of Psychiatry.
15. Dr. Hildegard Peplau wrote *Interpersonal Relations in Nursing* (1952), which translated Dr. Sullivan's interpersonal perspective into a language that nurses could understand and utilize in their practice.
16. "Bedlam" is famous as a lunatic asylum (formerly known as Bethlehem Hospital in London). This facility was founded in the 16th century, but by the 18th century it had become notorious for the deterioration of its care of the mentally ill.
17. Pennsylvania Hospital in Philadelphia was founded as a result of the efforts of Benjamin Franklin.
18. Gheel, Belgium is famous for its community in which mentally ill people reside in the family homes of residents. They maintain some semblance of a "normal" life while regularly seeing a psychiatrist.
19. Two alternative settings for psychiatric care outside of the inpatient unit are (1) mobile treatment teams, and (2) psychiatric home care in the patient's own home.
20. World Wars I and II influenced the treatment of mental illness by exposing the prevalence of mental illness, especially among the population of age for induction into military service. Draftees who became ill during active duty in World War I tended to be diagnosed as having "shell shock"; in World War II, draftees were said to develop "combat exhaustion."
21. During wartime, conscientious objectors served their equivalent of military service in some form of public service—many in large public psychiatric hospitals.
22. The impact of *The Shame of the States* (written by Albert Deutsch in 1948) was that it exposed the existing conditions in psychiatric hospitals and heightened the awareness of the public.
23. The National Mental Health Act was passed in 1946. Its purpose was to improve the mental health of Americans. Its impact on issues of mental health was that funds were established for the training of personnel in psychiatry, nursing, clinical psychology, and social work. Furthermore, the National Institute of Mental Health was established in 1946 for research into the causes and treatment of mental illness.
24. The Hill-Burton Bill of 1946 provided federal funding to the states for the purpose of surveying health needs and planning and constructing hospitals and other health centers.
25. The purpose of the Community Mental Health Act of 1963 was to facilitate the treatment of people with mental illness within their communities.
26. The Americans with Disabilities Act of 1990 protects people with disabilities (including those with a mental illness) from discrimination.
27. The first antipsychotic drug was chlorpromazine.
28. ECT (electroconvulsive therapy, also known as electroshock therapy) is used particularly for those suffering from depression.
29. The doctors who invented ECT were Italian.
30. Lithium is a drug used to control mood swings.
31. Deinstitutionalization has had an impact on state mental hospitals in that it drastically reduced the number of people hospitalized.
32. The impact of deinstitutionalization on communities was that many of the mentally ill now live on the streets of our nation. Torrey reported that one third of the homeless are mentally ill, and many have no caregivers.
33. The use of psychiatric medications had an impact on the practice of psychiatric nursing in that for the first time many patients were able to engage in interpersonal relationships with psychiatrists, nurses, and others; also, these medications expanded the responsibilities and activities of the psychiatric nurse.
34. The movie "Psychiatric Nursing: The Nurse-Patient Relationship" is about a withdrawn patient, "Trudy" (portrayed by a nursing student), who benefits from the nurse-patient relationship. The nurse also benefits from the recording and analysis of her nurse-patient interactions.
35. The first university program in psychiatric nursing was established at the Catholic University of America in 1943.
36. *Essentials of Psychiatric Nursing* was written by Dorothy Mereness.
37. The two levels of certification established by the American Nurses' Association Certification Program (1979) are the generalist and the clinical specialist.
38. NAMI stands for the National Alliance for the Mentally Ill, which was founded in 1979 and brought families together for needed support.
39. The 1990s were declared the "Decade of the Brain" by President George Bush.
40. The goals of Healthy People 2000 that are appropriate for psychiatric nursing are those associated with psychiatric nursing practice. These include a 10% reduction in suicide rates; an 18% reduction in adverse effects of stress; a 15% reduction in homicide rates; and a 10% decrease in assault injuries.
41. The acronym PET stands for positron emission tomography; the acronym MRI stands for magnetic resonance imaging.

CHAPTER 3

1. The *DSM-IV* is the *Diagnostic and Statistical Manual of Mental Disorders, fourth edition.* It describes 300 mental disorders and contains not only nomenclature but also the numerical codes for each of the disorders.
2. As a psychiatric nurse, you need to understand and be able to use the *DSM-IV* because insurance companies use the *DSM-IV* to determine reimbursement for psychiatric services. Furthermore, the *DSM-IV* represents the language of psychiatry, and if you are to communicate with other mental health care providers, you must be able to speak and understand this language.
3. The *ICD-9-CM* is the *Clinical Modification of the International Classification of Diseases—the Ninth Revision*, published by the World Health Organization. This manual provides a classification of diseases for use in coding morbidity and mortality data for statistical purposes.
4. As a psychiatric nurse, you need to understand and be able to use the *ICD-9-CM* because it is used in clinical situations to index hospital records by disease and procedure. Also, the codes and terms provided in the *DSM-IV* are fully compatible with the *ICD-9-CM*, in which names of diseases and codes are used to designate Axis III in the multiaxial system of the *DSM-IV.*
5. The multiaxial system of diagnosis is retained in the *DSM-IV.* It has five axes and contains nomenclature and also the numerical codes for each of the disorders.
6. The five axes are Axis I, in which the clinician reports "clinical disorders" and "other conditions that may be a focus of clinical attention"; Axis II, in which the clinician reports personality disorders and mental retardation; Axis III, in which the clinician reports "general medical conditions"; Axis IV, in which "psychosocial and environmental problems" are reported; and Axis V, in which the clinician reports on a "global assessment of functioning."
7. The Community Mental Health Legislation of 1963 launched a major shift in the delivery of care, as well as in attitudes toward the mentally ill. The shift in delivery of care was from large state hospitals to community mental health centers. However, fear and stigma impaired efforts to promote attitudes of acceptance and support.
8. In 1981, the federal government began to reverse its position on the public approach to the mentally ill. Congress, at President Reagan's request, repealed the earlier community mental health legislation that had mandated 12 essential services. The mandated services were reduced to five, and no funds were to be used for inpatient care. This represented a major departure from the 1963 Community Mental Health Act. Homelessness, drug abuse, and crime increased after these changes.
9. The Sherman R. McKinney Homeless Assistance Act was passed in the late 1980s, with the intent of solving the problem of the homeless mentally ill. It did not achieve its intended purpose; in 1992 an estimated 160,000 persons with mental illnesses were still living on the streets. The act did not provide for prevention of

homelessness among the domiciled mentally ill or for stabilizing mentally ill people in permanent housing.

10. Nursing's Agenda for Healthcare Reform (1991) covers the following areas: (1) primary care mental health services, (2) managed care, (3) universal access to a basic mental health benefit package, and (4) structure and financing of the public mental health system for continuous care.
11. The "right to treatment" focuses on the issue of a patient's right to receive adequate treatment. This states that a patient being confined without treatment is tantamount to incarceration. The court affirmed that the purpose of involuntary hospitalization was treatment, not punishment; if the patient did not receive this treatment, the patient could be transferred, released, or even awarded damages for his or her period of confinement. In 1972, the court defined criteria for adequate treatment in three areas: (1) physical and psychological environments that are humane, (2) sufficient numbers of qualified staff members able to administer adequate treatment, and (3) individualized treatment plans.
12. The "right to treatment in the least restrictive setting" produced strict standards for determination of dangerousness to self or others, which is the criterion for an involuntary admission. For the mental health care system, this means that patients could be transferred to the community, even if the transfer involved creating alternative facilities. In some instances, the results have been inhumane, with mentally ill people living in unsafe and unclean housing and receiving no treatment.
13. The social problem that is directly linked to the Community Mental Health Act of 1963 is that a large number of patients had no families at all or none who would welcome them into their homes. As a result of this false assumption of the community mental health movement, many of the chronic mentally ill became homeless on the streets of our cities. Communities have not provided adequate housing, health care, or social support.
14. The mid-1960s through mid-1970s were characterized as the era of the "baby boomer generation" and the decade of change. The baby boomer generation questioned values, structure, and religion, and the whole fabric of American culture was the focus of their examination and rejection. They constituted an activist group that organized antiwar rallies and marches to challenge American involvement in the Vietnam War, they took over draft offices and burned draft records, they held peaceful sit-ins to protest the rules of campus life, they experimented with drugs, they questioned sexual mores and supported sexual freedom, and they questioned racial as well as gender discrimination. The Community Mental Health legislation of 1963 generated positive excitement and anticipation in this generation.

    The mid-1970s to mid-1980s were characterized by resignation, disillusionment, and depression. This period was the decade of entrenchment. The realization that perhaps the problems of the mentally ill were bigger than the country was willing to tackle began to infiltrate public policy.

    The 1980s were characterized by materialism and self-focus and the decade of the self. The 1990s were characterized by doing more with less and finding creative solutions to devastating problems, one of which is the problem of the homeless.
15. The drug problem had an impact on the mental health system in that many chemically dependent people eluded the grasp of the mental health system or became patients only when in crisis. They represent a challenge to mental health providers because they do not respond well to established treatments and protocols; thus, nurses require great patience and ingenuity when dealing with these patients.
16. The "graying of America" has affected the mental health system because as people live longer, their use of health services, including mental health services, increases as they contend with the demands and limitations imposed by chronic illnesses. Many of these people require multiple hospitalizations to deal with exacerbations of chronic illness. Many psychiatric nurses specialize in psychogeriatric nursing to provide care to these older people.
17. "Dual diagnosis" refers to the condition of an increasing number of young adults who have both chronic mental illnesses and substance abuse problems. Such patients are very difficult to treat and pose great challenges to psychiatric nurses.
18. The relationship between unemployment and mental health problems is that the increased numbers of unemployed Americans placed greater demands on the mental health system. We see the devastating effects of job loss on human behavior, family functioning, and social and emotional well-being.
19. Over the last 30 years, since the population has increased and people have not had the means to pay for care in private mental hospitals, most of those who developed mental illnesses went to state hospitals. Financial support for these hospitals was rarely enough to support adequate care. Some hospitals had large appropriations to provide therapies such as occupational therapy, hydrotherapy, and electroconvulsive therapy to selected patients; others could barely supply adequate diets and clean, comfortable surroundings.
20. Medicare (federal insurance for those 65 years of age or older or for those disabled) and Medicaid (federal insurance for those who are judged to be in the lowest socioeconomic group) became available in 1965. The quality of care in the psychiatric hospitals was expected to improve. Medicare covered active treatment of patients over 65 years of age for a limited time, but it did not cover custodial care. Medicaid covered adult inpatient care under specified circumstances. State hospitals saw the Medicare and Medicaid programs as sources of additional funds; however, rather than use this influx of federal monies to improve care, states frequently responded with significant decreases in state appropriations.
21. The purpose of health maintenance organizations (HMOs) is to manage care (an approach involving close monitoring of the use of health care benefits) to provide preventive and remedial care at a lower cost than other types of health service organizations. Usually, they place severe limitations on mental health services, and those with serious, long-term mental illnesses are refused treatment.
22. The decrease in available funds for training purposes has meant that fewer psychiatric nurses have advanced preparation in the field.
23. Mental health parity involves the elimination of insurance discrimination against people seeking men- tal health care and the achievement of parity with the coverage accorded other illnesses.
24. The purpose of inpatient psychiatric treatment is (1) the restoration of patients to health so they can leave the hospital at the earliest possible moment short of success and (2) sufficient functional improvement so that patients can live as nearly normal lives as possible in the institutional setting.
25. A forensic unit is used for people accused of crimes who are found not guilty by reason of insanity but are deemed by the courts to be too dangerous to others to be released. These units also are used for people convicted of crimes who develop symptoms of psychiatric disorders after they have been convicted.
26. Two types of specialty units for the treatment of psychiatric problems are detoxification units and forensic units.
27. A residential treatment center is used for children and adolescents with behavioral and emotional problems who cannot be effectively managed in their homes. It offers these children affirmation and hope and helps them see alternatives.
28. Certified specialists in psychiatric mental health nursing have entered the private practice of psychotherapy.
29. The role of a psychiatric nurse in a community mental health center often involves administrative, case management, and therapeutic assignments. Many are expert at providing individual, group, and family therapy as well as managing a therapeutic milieu.
30. One change in the health care system that has encouraged the development of psychiatric home care programs is that Medicare authorized payment for psychiatric home care services in 1975.

CHAPTER 4

1. Direct care involves the actions that you as a nurse carry out for a particular patient and family.
2. Indirect care encompasses all the patient-related activities performed by someone other than you but supervised by you.
3. The role of manager of the environment recognizes your ability to negotiate environmental issues and to teach patients and families to do the same.
4. In your role as teacher, you might teach self-care and assist the patient and family to attain greater facility at living with the effects of mental illness.
5. A continuum of care requires a seamless transition of care to prevent the patient and family from "falling through the cracks" of the health care system.
6. Being a patient advocate involves three roles: educating patients about their rights and responsibilities, negotiating for mental health services, and influencing legislation on local, state, national, and international levels.
7. Two examples of psychiatric nursing functions that are part of preventive care are (1) providing information about mental health issues (e.g., facilitative communication skills, parenting, stress reduction principles of mental health, and sex education) and (2) affecting societal changes that have an impact on mental health (e.g., improved living conditions, greater access to affordable housing, and better education).
8. Primary care is preventive care. It precedes disease and is applied to the healthy population. Secondary care involves nursing activities directed at reducing actual illness by early detection and treatment of the problem. Tertiary care involves nursing activities that focus on reducing the residual impairment or disability resulting from an illness.
9. Entering a partnership with the patient and family on their journey involves the role that focuses the nurse on the patient and family's story. This role allows you to choose the personal gifts and professional skills that will assist the patient and family to divert the journey to one of greater health and improved functioning.
10. The two levels of expertise within psychiatric-mental health clinical practice are the basic-level psychiatric-mental health nurse with a baccalaureate degree and the advanced-level psychiatric-mental health nurse with a Master's degree.
11. At the basic level of practice, a baccalaureate degree in nursing and demonstrated clinical skills are required.
12. At the advanced level, a Master's degree is required at a minimum, and the nurse is nationally certified as a clinical specialist in psychiatric and mental health nursing. This nurse has a greater depth of knowledge of theory and practice, has supervised clinical practice, and has competence in advanced clinical nursing skills.
13. The basic-level psychiatric-mental health nurse describes the psychiatric nurse who is a licensed registered nurse (RN) with a baccalaureate degree in nursing and demonstrated clinical skills within the specialty that exceed those of a beginning RN or a novice in the specialty. The practice path chosen is characterized by direct care.
14. Three indirect care roles performed by the certified specialist are teaching, consulting, and administering and conducting research.
15. Peer review involves the quality assurance monitoring of the practice of other nurses to maintain quality of care.
16. Accountability means being responsible both personally and publicly for the quality of care one delivers.
17. Continuing education is important as a requisite for staying clinically competent and for growing professionally as knowledge expands and is incorporated into the field of practice.
18. As a community participant, you assume responsibility to assist others in acquiring knowledge and skills through formal and informal teaching, through sharing clinical observations and interpretations with colleagues and other professionals, and through encouraging others to continue to seek out knowledge.
19. A collaborator is a nurse who recognizes that nursing is only one component of the health care team. You must work with other team members to ensure that patients receive the highest quality of care possible.
20. Networking includes developing a group of associates whose skills, talents, knowledge, and influence may enhance your own goals.
21. Lobbying is a strategy used to influence policy decisions by influencing the policy makers.
22. Two levels of research participation for the psychiatric-mental health nurse involve participating in studies designed by other nurses or health professionals, and acting as principal investigator in conducting research.
23. Stewardship involves good management of time and talents, of the material resources of the agencies for which the nurses work, and of the insurance and personal resources of the patients and families for whom they care.
24. Stress is part of both the direct as well as the indirect care roles. Stress can affect physical and mental health when you are called on daily to give comfort, solace, and support, even when your own resources for doing so are depleted.
25. Burnout is exhaustion of physical and emotional strength.
26. Burnout is a spiritual issue for nurses whose inner spirit is assaulted and whose life feels fragmented.
27. Three strategies to deal with burnout are changing the external environment in which you practice, establishing an interpersonally supportive environment, and being educated about ways to deal with conflict, to negotiate, and to manage change.

CHAPTER 5

1. The two main ethical principles operating in a theistic world view are justice and love.
2. The eight ethical principles are justice, love, beneficence, nonmaleficence, autonomy, paternalism, veracity, and fidelity.
3. Justice is the distributive principle concerned with the equitable treatment and fair handling of people.
4. An example of the principle of justice in the care of people with mental illness is as follows: If you have agreed to serve a second dinner to one patient who has a particularly hearty appetite that day, it would be *unjust* to deny a dessert to another patient with an equally hearty appetite that day.
5. Love, when applied in ethical dilemmas, has to do with a self-giving and sacrificial attitude. In this context, love is an overall moral principle, all-inclusive and exceptionless, and is not dependent on reciprocal admiration.
6. As ethical principles, justice and love subsume all the other principles from a theistic world view.
7. Beneficence operates whenever you engage in making decisions for persons who are incompetent and do not have the facilities to decide for themselves. Beneficence is active in promoting good, preventing harm, and removing evil.
8. Nonmaleficence means that no harm or risk of harm may be inflicted on another.
9. An example of violation of beneficence is when you do not actively thwart harmful actions that could lead to suicide or homicide. An example of violation of nonmaleficence is when you display sarcasm or irritation, belittle a patient, show unpleasant feelings to others, or use patients to meet your own needs. A violation of nonmaleficence then means that one does not take responsibility for one's actions, thoughts, feelings, and personal behavior.
10. Autonomy means choosing freely and living with the consequences of the choice.
11. When you respect the patient's autonomy, one conflict that might arise is that the patient's choice might not be one that you would have made. For instance, a mother might decide not to sign for permission to give an adolescent a psychotropic medication.
12. Paternalism is based on the belief that the knowledge and education

of the professional authorizes him or her to make decisions for the good of the patient, irrespective of the patient's wishes.

13. Veracity refers to telling the truth, an obligation that is sometimes difficult to meet in the health care setting.
14. Paternalism is the preferred principle when the purpose is to maintain the life of the person and when the actions are consistently done on behalf of the person.
15. One example is when a patient might ask you if you think that if they take their medicine they won't have their psychiatric symptoms any more.
16. Fidelity is faithfulness to obligations, duties, or observances; it is keeping promises and is akin to veracity.
17. Fidelity plays a part in team work on a unit, in that it is vital in establishing trustworthy relationships with patients and staff members.
18. It would be difficult to tell the patient the truth when you fear that your response may threaten your relationship with the patient.
19. The three levels of decision-making as described by Kohlberg are the preconventional level, the conventional level, and the postconventional level.
20. Gilligan's theory differs from Kohlberg's in that Gilligan challenged Kohlberg's assumption that justice and moral rights are the highest form of moral development. She asserted that females tend to focus on conflicting personal responsibilities rather than on conflicting rights and justice.
21. The requirements for informed consent involve a choice (1) based on understanding the situation, the outcome, the alternatives, the risks, and benefits; (2) made freely without inducement, force, or any other kind of coercion; and (3) made by a competent person who fully comprehends all the information being given.
22. Informed consent involves the patient's understanding of the situation. It is a process during which the patient may change his or her mind, ask more questions, or need someone to listen as the meaning of a decision or condition is explored.
23. The risk in giving the patient advice is that certain factors create a subtly coercive environment when advice is given, with the core issue being power and the misuse of it.
24. Robert objected to Wanda's receiving ECT because he thought that Wanda was responding to treatment, and he had questions about her ability to freely give informed consent.
25. You can talk with your supervisor, clinical specialist, clinical ethicist, and/or patient advocate when faced with an ethical dilemma to assist in developing appropriate strategies in responding to the dilemma.
26. We are using the principle of paternalism when we use manipulation to convince a patient to take medication.
27. Psychosis can interfere with the patient's ability to recognize that he or she needs medication.
28. When new graduates leave the school environment, they encounter legal accountability for their actions as well as for actions delegated to unlicensed assistive personnel; an increase in the number and acuity of patients being served; and an awareness of the need for additional growth in knowledge base necessitated by choosing a particular setting and population with which to work.
29. The new graduate enters the work world feeling prepared to handle most situations. If you are practicing ethically you must understand that no "ideal" exists; however, you must not tolerate abuses in the name of "reality." You must therefore be reality based but strive for an ideal vision.
30. One conflict in which you must make a choice between the good of the individual and the good of the staff pertains to the current social issue of smoking.
31. The guiding principle when a conflict arises between the individual's and group's needs is to try to affirm the rights of the individual and group within the context of their responsibilities.
32. The most restrictive form of constraint is chemical (medication).
33. The crux of the behavior control issue is accountability; the person who controls the behavior is accountable for it. Behind the issue of accountability is the question of control.
34. Two types of coercive behavioral controls are seclusion and restraint.
35. Voluntary treatment is when the person chooses treatment, enters into an active decision-making process with the treatment team, and works to achieve treatment goals.
36. Before an involuntary admission can occur, the clinicians must determine the need for treatment based on imminent danger of the person to self and/or others or on the person's inability to take care of basic human needs.
37. Three types of information included in each state's nurse practice act are the process to obtain licensure and practice within the state, the definition of the educational requirements for entry into practice, and the definition of the scope of practice for each level of nursing practice.
38. The purpose of the nurse practice acts in each state is to establish boundaries within which the nurse must practice.
39. Two examples of behaviors that a person with undefined or loose boundaries might display are intruding into others' personal space by standing too close and moving too quickly toward others.
40. A person with very rigid boundaries may need an unusually large amount of personal space.
41. Four rights of psychiatric patients are to wear one's own clothes, to keep and use one's own personal possessions, to keep and spend a reasonable sum of one's own money, and to refuse convulsive or other forms of shock therapy or psychosurgery.
42. The purpose of the ANA *Code for Nurses* is to establish baseline performance expectations for all registered nurses without exception.
43. Keeping information confidential means that intimate communications are handled with the utmost respect and shared only with members of the health care team who need to know.
44. Two examples of conflicts that arise from the issue of confidentiality are when the patient's friends ask how the patient is faring on a unit at the hospital, and when a child wants a specific example (including defining characteristics) of how the nurse or patient helped somebody that day.
45. The implication of the Tarasoff decision is that it is the therapist's duty to use reasonable care to protect a known, intended victim of a patient's threats by either warning the prospective victim or by taking other reasonable steps under the circumstances (but the extent of this duty to warn and how it may be discharged varies from one state to another).
46. A therapeutic alliance is one in which the therapist is obliged to try to reach the patient and to make a healthy connection with the patient that is helpful and encouraging.
47. The purpose of advocacy is to protect the patient's rights and interests.

CHAPTER 6

1. Theory reflects the personal journey of the theorist, in that each theory represents an intricate tapestry, the threads of which reflect not only the theorist's careful thinking about the phenomena but also his or her rich personal history. Theory reflects the author's formative life experiences as well as his or her professional reflections.
2. Current understandings of psychiatric mental health emerged originally from the writings of ancient Greek scholars.
3. Wundt and James marked the journey of psychology as a profession, in that Wundt established modern psychology as a science and created the important link between experimental and social psychology, while James spearheaded the development of psychology as a professional discipline in America.
4. Psychoanalytic theory principles influenced an assessment of a psychiatric patient in that the structure and function of the personality was examined systematically in terms of the id, ego, and superego.
5. Carl Jung's most important contribution to the study of personality

is that he developed his own method of psychoanalysis called analytical psychology. He developed the notion of the collective unconscious, consisting of peoples' cultural and ethnic heritage.

6. Sullivan's interpersonal theory challenges the ideas of the psychoanalytic model, in that Sullivan proposed that personality cannot be studied apart from the social and cultural influences on behavior.
7. Erikson's theory remains relevant today because he provides a useful framework for understanding developmental aspects of human behavior throughout the lifespan.
8. Humanistic theory enhances the personal journey of the patient because it emphasizes a person's capacity for self-actualization. Humanists seek to understand behavior from the patient's perspective, as he or she subjectively experiences it.
9. Humanistic and existential models diverge from each other, in that existential models focus on taking responsibility, personal freedom, authenticity, anxiety, meaning, and death. Humanistic and existential models parallel each other, in that they both arose in protest to the psychoanalytic school of thought.
10. Behavioral models consider personality as what people do rather than who they are; they propose that personality consists of learned behaviors. Social learning models, however, integrate both environmental conditions and personal attributes.
11. A respondent conditioning strategy involves a subject who is basically a passive agent. Respondents are responses that result from specific, identifiable stimuli. An operant conditioning strategy, on the other hand, refers to the manipulation of selected reinforcers to elicit and strengthen desired behavioral reinforcers. The patient thus takes an active role in performing a behavior (discharges an operant) and receives a consequence (reinforcer) as a result of performing a behavior.
12. The value of behavioral models for psychiatric nursing is that in psychiatric settings, behavioral models can be used to manage problem behaviors and modify behavior in a particular environment.
13. You should be concerned with nursing theory because nursing theories represent a number of world views about the discipline of nursing and its particular domain of knowledge. Nursing theories lay out the domain of the profession, establish the boundaries of nursing practice, provide a basis for research, and serve as a guide for curriculum development.
14. The structure of nursing knowledge proceeds from the general to the more specific in a structural hierarchy that begins with a metaparadigm, develops conceptual models, and completes its structural mission with the construction of theories that can be tested empirically.
15. A "caring" relationship in psychiatric nursing involves a caring mode of interaction with patients that contains existential or spiritual significance. In this relationship, you value feelings, intuition, and other forms of subjective participation in the client's world.
16. Hildegard Peplau's contribution to psychiatric nursing is that she was the first nurse to identify psychiatric nursing both as an essential element of general nursing and as a specialty area that embraces specific governing principles. She identified ways in which the nurse makes specialized use of a professional relationship to identify and therapeutically intervene in psychosocial nursing problems. She presented her classic theory of interpersonal nursing, which became the accepted foundation of psychiatric nursing practice.

CHAPTER 7

1. Psychobiology is the study of the biochemical foundations of thought, mood, affect, emotion, and behavior.
2. Asclepiades first described light treatment for depression.
3. The behaviorists hoped to map the general laws governing human behavior.
4. Neuroscience encompasses a set of related disciplines that share the common goal of understanding the relationship between brain structure and function and human thoughts, feelings, and behavior.
5. Genetic and molecular biological studies of neuroreceptors provide new areas of research that have a direct impact on psychiatry.
6. White matter is made up of myelinated (insulated) cells, whereas gray matter consists of unmyelinated (uninsulated) cells.
7. The right and left hemispheres are attached to each other by the corpus callosum.
8. Afferent tracts travel to the brain, while efferent tracts travel away from it.
9. The frontal lobe involves motor control. The parietal lobe involves sensations from the arms and legs and receives information about various sensory bodily sensations and synthesizes and elaborates sensory impulses. The occipital lobe receives and sends out information and contains the primary visual receptive area. The temporal lobe receives auditory impulses, stores memory patterns for symbolic sounds, receives and transmits gustatory impulses, and receives and transmits olfactory input.
10. The somatosensory area receives sensations from the arms and legs; it receives information about various body sensations and synthesizes and elaborates sensory impulses.
11. Disruption in the occipital lobe may lead to illusions and hallucinations.
12. The function of the structures of the diencephalon is to serve as the relay stations between lower brain centers and the higher cortical centers.
13. The role of the thalamus is to modulate emotions and behavior.
14. The hypothalamus regulates hormonal function.
15. The brain stem regulates the activities of the heart, lungs, and other vital organs.
16. The cerebellum is a major modulator of movement.
17. The role of the limbic system is to modulate emotions, and it plays a role in the development of mental illnesses.
18. Some types of mood disorders may be associated with hyperarousal in the hypothalamic pituitary adrenal axis.
19. Schizophrenia is associated with dysfunction of the basal ganglia.
20. The ventricular system is of interest to neuroscientists because ventricular enlargement provides a useful index of brain atrophy or shrinkage. The ventricles are major landmarks that can be seen clearly with computed tomography, and ventricular enlargement has been noted in some patients with schizophrenia and dementia.
21. The cell body is the main work center of the neuron—it sends out tiny fingers of branching fibers called "dendrites" (treelike structures), which form a treelike web around the cell body and greatly increase its ability to receive information, allowing other cells to communicate either to the cell body or to the dendrites. The axon is a long, tubular projection sent out from the cell body to communicate with other neurons.
22. During an action potential, the positively charged sodium ions flow in and trigger a large positive charge inside the cell.
23. The function of the neurotransmitters is to release neurochemicals into the synaptic cleft, and these neurochemicals interact directly with receptor molecules in the postsynaptic membrane.
24. Anticholinergic effects are interactions that occur when some drugs used to treat depression and schizophrenia inhibit the acetylcholine system.
25. Dopamine is the neurotransmitter involved with the development of schizophrenia.
26. Norepinephrine and serotonin are implicated in the development of depression.
27. The sensory area collects information on bodily sensations, such as heat, cold, pain, and pressure or touch.
28. Damage to Broca's area leads to difficulty in speaking fluently.
29. Wernicke's area permits recognition of language in auditory form.
30. Frontal lobe dysfunction is suggested in schizophrenia.
31. The command center of the neuroendocrine system lies in the hypothalamus.
32. Changes in appetite, sleep regulation, and adaptability to stress and change are consistent with neuroendocrine abnormalities.
33. CT scans use x-ray beams through the body to construct the image.
34. In examining schizophrenia, structural brain pathology and various types of schizophrenic symptoms are being correlated.

35. Compared with CT scans, magnetic resonance imaging produces images of extremely high resolution with clear differentiation between small gray and white matter structures, and the scanning procedures involve no risk because no radiation is used.
36. Patients suffering from autism and schizophrenia may have a "hypofrontal" pattern while at rest.
37. SQUID has been utilized to delineate brain areas associated with the acquisition and utilization of different types of knowledge.
38. People with major depression experience an abnormality of cortisol production.
39. Challenge tests are being used to identify panic disorders.
40. MHPG measures the breakdown of norepinephrine.
41. Patients with temporal lobe epilepsy resemble patients with obsessive-compulsive disorder.
42. The drug clozapine has been effective in the treatment of the negative symptoms of schizophrenia.
43. A higher incidence of schizophrenia is seen in monozygotic twins than in dizygotic twins.
44. The viral theory of the etiology of schizophrenia is supported by a viruslike agent found in the cerebrospinal fluid of some schizophrenics and by the observation that more schizophrenics are born daily during the winter when viral diseases are more prevalent.
45. Inherent cycles of depression, the pronounced abnormalities in rest-activity cycle, the length and timing of sleep stages, and the clinical responsiveness of experimental alterations in circadian organization are all factors in mood disorders that point to changes in circadian rhythms.
46. The gradual worsening of episodes over time and the decreasing amount of time between episodes are symptoms of mood disorders that support a kindling-sensitization model of etiology.
47. One way antianxiety drugs work is to enhance the effect of the GABA system in the brain.
48. Patients with panic disorders share some biochemical similarities with patients with depression.

CHAPTER 8

1. The transition from a novice nurse to an expert requires time, experience, and risk-taking. The nurse must trust in his or her limited theory-based abilities and be willing to share his or her humanness to facilitate connectedness with others.
2. To use the self therapeutically, you need to explore the personal self and then use that awareness to help understand each person's uniqueness.
3. You should know yourself and understand your uniqueness before your professional self can emerge and you can "connect" with another human being.
4. Two of the initial concerns of students beginning a psychiatric clinical experience are fears about personal safety and concern about perceived inadequacies in communicating with patients.
5. Two common fears of patients as they reveal themselves to nurses is that they may be seen as weak and ineffective and that they may find that no one understands them.
6. The self is "the part of the human being that knows himself [herself] as 'I.' It is the thinking, knowing, feeling part of the human organism which deals with the world" (Robinson, 1974).
7. The self differs from the self-concept in that the self is made up of both physical and psychological characteristics and includes both conscious and unconscious components, whereas *self-concept* is the term given to the part of the self that deals only with conscious awareness.
8. Self-esteem is a person's own judgment of his or her own worth.
9. The dimensions of self-concept are physical, psychological, social, and spiritual. They characterize the inner state of a person and allow him or her to relate to the environment in a very unique way.
10. The wider the gap between the self-concept and the ideal self, the lower the level of self-esteem.
11. Body image is the picture that each of us creates concerning our physical self.
12. Body space refers to the personal body space required by each physical self and is the amount of distance that most people are comfortable with in different social settings.
13. The four "body spaces" are intimate distance (3 to 18 inches), personal distance (1½ to 4 feet), social distance (4 to 12 feet), and public interaction distance (10 to 12 feet).
14. Culture influences the physical self, in that people reflecting the desired cultural norm often feel good about the self, whereas those who are different from what is desired may feel inferior and unattractive.
15. Two examples of developmental processes that affect the physical self are loss of baby teeth, and the changes that occur with pregnancy.
16. Personal identity is composed of perceptual, cognitive, and emotional images that we have of ourselves. Taken together, these images form a unified sense of who we are.
17. Perception is the experience of sensing, interpreting, and comprehending the world in which we live. Perception is basically how we make sense out of what we experience.
18. Our perceptual processes develop in relationship with our parents and continue to be modified by relationships and experiences with others.
19. Perception relates to the self-concept, in that with healthy development, the self-concept corresponds closely with confirmed, factual perceptions, and with less than healthy development, the self-concept is hemmed in by unresolved conflicts and misinformation.
20. Someone is "reality oriented" when the inner reality is close to the external reality (i.e., the person is "grounded" in reality).
21. Piaget defines intelligence as a dynamic trait that is always related to a person's adaptation to the environment under the existing circumstances.
22. According to Piaget, four stages of development occur: the sensorimotor stage, preoperational thinking, concrete operations, and formal operations.
23. *Assimilation* refers to the way a person responds to the environment based on existing schemata; no cognitive growth occurs with assimilation since experiences are continually assimilated into existing cognitive structures. *Accommodation* provides for modification of existing cognitive structures. *Disequilibration* refers to cognitive and affective discord.
24. Two influences on the cognitive process are physiological and psychological structures, since alteration in either can affect cognitive functioning.
25. *Self-efficacy* is our ability to perform certain tasks based on what we know. *Perceived self-efficacy* may or may not correspond with reality, meaning that we may believe that we are more or less capable than the facts of our actual performance would indicate.
26. *Global self-esteem* is the measure of how much we like and approve of our perceived self as a whole. *Specific self-esteem* is the measure of how much we like and approve of a certain part of ourselves.
27. *Self-confidence* is the feeling that one is a competent person with the ability to accomplish things. *Self-respect* is the feeling that what one is doing or has done is right according to the value system held.
28. For self-esteem, the following traits are necessary: a sense of significance, a sense of competence, a sense of connectedness to others balanced by a sense of separateness from them, a sense of realism about self and the world, and a coherent set of ethics and values.
29. The emotional or affective self consists of the spontaneous feelings that we experience in response to life.
30. Positive self-esteem enables us to meet life's demands with a sense of confidence.
31. A role is a socially expected behavior pattern associated with a person's function in various social groups (e.g., student, friend, or boss) and is very much influenced by the culture in which the person is raised.

32. Role conflict may occur at any time when different expectations place people in situations in which they have to choose one role function to the detriment of another.
33. Sibling position influences roles in a family.
34. Gender identity, or sex role, is the expectation of appropriate male and female behavior found in the attitudes and beliefs of a particular society.
35. An example of an *ascribed* role is family position. An example of an *assumed* (or chosen) role is the social or public self, which represents the way that we are known by others.
36. The spiritual self functions to help the person connect with God, find meaning, and make sense from life's circumstances.
37. The universal aspect of the spiritual self involves beliefs about the universe, our place in it, and feelings of transcendence, joy, hope, and love.
38. Different world views shape the spiritual self.
39. Morality develops within the spiritual self out of the earliest interaction between the child and parents and/or significant others. The spiritual self is the seat of morality. The child learns which behaviors are acceptable and which are not.
40. A certain level of cognitive development and emotional maturity are requisite for dealing with the tough questions that accompany spiritual growth.
41. Basic needs are important for mental health because these needs must be satisfied for physiological and psychological homeostasis to be maintained. Physiological needs are the most basic and include the need for food, water, and air.
42. If a person fails to accomplish a major developmental task, he or she cannot successfully move on to the next challenge or phase without experiencing some degree of intrapsychic conflict.
43. The degree of mental illness lies on a continuum and involves the amount of difficulty a person experiences in coping with daily living. The quality of relationships with self, others, the environment, and God determine where the person is along the continuum.
44. Mental health is characterized as a dynamic state in which thought, feeling, and behavior are age appropriate and congruent with local and cultural norms.
45. Personality consists of all the behavioral traits and attitudinal characteristics by which we are recognized as individuals. Personality reflects a lasting pattern of behavior that is conscious and unconscious and reflects a means of adapting to a particular environment and its cultural, ethnic, and community standards.

CHAPTER 9

1. Three attributes of successful travelers are that they are survivors, hardy, and resilient.
2. Three characteristics of "triumphant survivors" are that they manage to stay active through times of trouble, live each day moment by moment, and proceed with a sheer determination to get to the next step.
3. The three components of hardiness are a composite of control, commitment, and challenge.
4. Resilience consists of five themes: equanimity, perseverance, self-reliance, meaningfulness, and existential aloneness.
5. You can help your patients develop their personal strengths by helping them to overcome loss and grief, empowerment, and instilling hope.
6. Bailey's six stages in the "journey of grief" are loss, protest, searching, despair, reorganization, and reinvestment.
7. Empowerment means that patients take as much responsibility as they can handle comfortably and accept changes in themselves and their circumstance. Acceptance, responsibility, and trust are the basic concepts involved.
8. Hope can be defined as "the turning point that must be followed by a willingness to act" (Deegan, 1988) and as "an expectation of goal attainment modified by the importance of the goal and the probability of attaining it" (Stotland, 1992).
9. Humor typically is used during each stage of recovery from substance abuse by alleviating stress and feelings of anger, anxiety, frustration, and tension.
10. Social support can be a cushion for both patients and their families who are dealing with mental illness. A support system can enhance recovery by providing feedback about themselves and validation of their expectations about others (Caplan, 1979).
11. You can strengthen the spirituality of patients and their families by supporting the use of coping strategies such as prayer, listening to music, reminiscence, devotional reading, church attendance, physical exercise, and journaling.
12. A danger of the nurse's being first born or a "big brother" or "big sister" is that this stance can hinder the nurse-patient relationship. Nurses in this position can overfunction for patients and may inadvertently stifle patients' efforts to accomplish actions on their own.
13. An authoritarian management style can result from a health care system that requires you to "do more with less."
14. This management style can lead to serious tension and morale problems that are conducive to acting-out behaviors and power struggles by patients as well as by staff members.

CHAPTER 10

1. *Communication* is defined as an interactional process that occurs between people and involves cognitive and emotional connections with others. *Communication* also is defined as a learned process and as a complex phenomenon that takes place on many different levels. Several different types of communication are verbal communication, metacommunication, and nonverbal communication.
2. Effective communicators demonstrate self-awareness and awareness of the needs of others in the communication. They give simple, clear messages that are appropriate to the situation and responsive to the needs of others. They recognize that timing is a critical element in successful communication and frequently validate that the receiver has heard the message as the sender intended it.
3. A good psychosocial assessment depends on the skillful use of communication strategies through which patients are able to tell their story. Therapeutic communication strategies enhance the quality of the patient's journey by providing a means of understanding his or her suffering and developing the most appropriate ways to assist him or her. The accuracy of the nurse's understanding affects the quality of the assessment data and related nursing interventions.
4. Clear communication is important in psychiatric nursing because messages give evidence of confirming the other person and respecting that person's values.
5. Therapeutic communication is a special form of communication that has a health-related purpose. The focus is on the needs of the patient, and it occurs within designated time frames, terminating when therapeutic goals are achieved.
6. Therapeutic conversations differ from social conversations, in that reaching another human being through a therapeutic conversation involves not simply talking to the other about a problem or need, but actually being with the other in understanding and resolving the barriers to successful realization of the journey's potential.

7. Linear models of communication are simple and straightforward models involving a sender, a message, and a receiver, focusing on the structure of the communication process. Circular models broaden the process of communication to include internal and external factors that represent revolving communication patterns with feedback loops, affecting the communication of both parties. Cognitive processing models assert that people develop their own models of the world based on a combination of sensory inputs and on the way that they interpret them.
8. Types of communication are identified in terms of verbal, nonverbal, and metacommunication.
9. Active listening is purposeful and focused. It requires disciplined attention involving making sense of a person's message and attaching meaning.
10. *Restatement* could be used as a mirroring strategy in which you replay all or part of the patient's message exactly as stated for emphasis or clarity. *Paraphrasing* could be used to broaden the scope of the patient's comment and to develop a shared meaning of the content. *Reflection* is used when your listening response focuses on the feelings verbally present in the patient's message or on the underlying feeling implied in the statement. Its purpose is to help the patient focus on the feelings experienced in relation to a situation. *Clarification* is used as a listening response that directly asks for information not contained in the patient's statement. This brings the patient's dialogue into sharper focus. *Silence* is used to allow the patient additional time in the interaction to think about what has been said without an intrusive comment; thus, the patient has more of a chance for further elaboration. *Summarizing* can be used at the end of a therapeutic conversation to review important points.
11. You would use silence as a therapeutic listening response by waiting for a few seconds, rather than moving directly to the next question, so that the patient has a chance to elaborate further and give a more thoughtful response. For the elderly and for culturally diverse patients, silence provides additional time for them to process information.
12. *Mirroring* is a communication strategy in which you reflect, through words, behaviors observed in the patient that the patient might not otherwise notice. *Redirecting* is a communication strategy in which you refocus the patient from a tangential train of thought to a more precise discussion of the topic at hand. *Reframing* is a communication strategy that offers a different interpretation of the patient's situation. Modifying the meaning of a situation allows for more options for changing behavior.
13. Humor is appropriate to ease an overly intense moment, put situations into perspective, and share connected moments. Humor cuts through defensiveness and can provide new insights. Timing is important. Also, before using humor, you should be aware of the patient's normal response patterns and current mood; humor requires a certain amount of flexible thinking that not all patients possess. Finally, humor should focus on events, circumstances, or situations rather than on the personal characteristics of the patient.
14. You would use feedback as a verbal intervention strategy with a mentally ill patient to develop a realistic appraisal of his or her situation and the role he or she plays in maintaining or changing it.
15. Hallucinations, illusions, and delusions are barriers to communication. *Hallucinations* are sensory experiences that have no discernible external stimulus and are usually vivid and intrusive. *Illusions* are misperceptions of visual or auditory external stimuli. *Delusions* are fixed erroneous beliefs that cannot be corrected by logical argument.
16. You would respond to a patient who is having a hallucination by stating that you do not hear or see what the patient is experiencing but that you can acknowledge that it is bothering the patient. You would respond to a patient who is having an illusion by touching the patient's arm gently, orienting the patient to where he or she is, and refocusing the conversation without discounting the patient's communication. You would respond to a patient having a delusion by decoding the underlying dynamics and by helping the patient focus on the emotional dynamics of her or his delusional thinking without a direct challenge to its validity.
17. You create barriers in the communication process by worrying about whether you will say the right thing and anticipating how the patient is likely to respond.
18. You could focus feedback on behaviors rather than on the person by using descriptive statements that make the person take responsibility if he or she wants to achieve a different consequence. The link between cause and effect occurs, with the nurse suggesting an alternative solution.

CHAPTER 11

1. The process of "taming" and the therapeutic relationship with a mentally ill patient have in common an interpersonal process by which one person struggles to know and accept the other as "unique in all the world," a relationship process by which people connect with each other in meaningful ways.
2. The fundamental characteristics of a therapeutic relationship make the relationship safe for patients by providing a defined structure and focus on the patient related to meeting defined health goals.
3. Social and therapeutic relationships differ in their purpose, focus, responsibility, degree of self-exposure, and level of personal involvement.
4. You can make the therapeutic relationship a healing pathway for the patient to feel valued as a worthwhile human being through respect, acceptance, empathy, and genuineness. You must earn the patient's trust before the patient will be able to take advantage of the help offered.
5. The primary value for the psychiatric field of Peplau's interpersonal theory of nursing lies in her descriptions of the type of relationship desired in psychiatric nursing and in careful descriptions of the developmental stages of the therapeutic relationship (orientation, working, and resolution phases). These phases still serve as the matrix for understanding relationships in psychiatric nursing.
6. Carl Rogers views the patient as a person in the "here and now." Rogers focuses on how the patient feels he or she is subjectively experienced by the helping person in the relationship.
7. Martin Buber's model emphasizes the need for the nurse-patient relationship to be one of equal and respectful partnership in an I-thou relationship.
8. Boundaries facilitate the goals of the therapeutic relationship by aiding in establishing the patient as separate from the nurse and the nurse as neither controlling nor controllable by the patient.
9. Caring and mutuality are related in the nurse-patient relationship, in that they both involve a human relationship between the nurse and the patient in which the patient is viewed as a person first and as a patient second.
10. Authenticity is integrated into a nurse-patient relationship and means being real with the patient, not hiding behind the mask of professionalism. Your natural feelings and attitudes are brought into the relationship.
11. Reciprocal trust is an essential characteristic of the nurse-patient relationship, in that trust involves a patient's inner confidence that a helping person respects, understands, and responds fairly to him or her. Trust is a mutual process. It begins with your confidence in your skills and includes the firm belief that the patient is capable of changing his or her behavior.
12. Consistency is important in the development of trust. Structural consistency means that the nurse organizes the relationship around the health-related needs of the patient and does not deviate from helping the patient achieve identified goals. Attitudinal consistency relates to your understanding of the professional role and to equity in patient care.
13. During the preinteraction phase, identify professional goals, establish the physical setting, and work through arrangements with other members of the interdisciplinary health care team.
14. During the orientation phase, establish a working alliance with the

patient and gain enough relevant assessment data to begin the development of a care plan.

15. The function of the therapeutic contract is to support the aims of the relationship and concretely spell out the role expectations and goals. The use of a therapeutic contract places the responsibility directly on the patient for taking actions related to goal achievement. You would use the therapeutic contract in the clinical area with patients who are acting out or experiencing impulse control. The contract serves as an integral part of the nursing care plan.
16. The working phase is divided into two components: the identification phase, in which the patient explores the nature of the problem and its associated feelings, and the exploitation phase, in which the patient maximizes use of all appropriate resources to resolve the problem.
17. In the exploitation phase, you can provide feedback to the patient and can validate the legitimacy of the feelings. You can help patients to use their inner resources to affect desired behavioral change. Thus, patients can gradually assume greater mastery for creating their own life experiences.
18. During the termination phase, you may see a number of regressive behaviors, including a return of symptoms, anger, and withdrawal and a minimizing of the relationship.
19. The best approach to handling the issue of gift-giving is to turn down a material gift while at the same time acknowledging the value of all that you have received from the client, thus reinforcing the worth of the client and of the relationship that you shared.
20. The phases of the nurse-patient relationship parallel those of the nursing process, in that the identification segment of the working phase parallels the outcome identification and planning steps of the nursing process, the exploitation phase relates to the implementation step of the nursing process, and the termination phase of the relationship parallels the evaluation phase of the nursing process.
21. Transference refers to the emergence of strong feelings and behavioral attitudes during the course of the relationship when they occur in the patient; in countertransference, these feelings occur in the nurse.
22. Transference and countertransference are related to each other, in that they both continually shape one another in a specific pattern of reciprocal mutual influence.

CHAPTER 12

1. The purpose of the nursing process is to provide a systematic and individualized method of fulfilling the goals of nursing: to help the patient to promote and maximize her or his level of health, to maintain the highest level of functioning, and to prevent illness and the sequelae of illness.
2. The nursing process is related to problem-solving, in that to carry out the nursing process, you must be able to think critically.
3. The steps of the nursing process are assessment, diagnosis, outcome identification, planning, implementation, and evaluation.
4. The authoritative statement on nursing practice is *Standards of Clinical Nursing Practice*, published by the American Nurses' Association; this publication provides generic standards for all nurses.
5. *Standards of Psychiatric-Mental Health Clinical Nursing Practice* identifies specific interventions appropriate to the basic-level practitioner and to the certified specialist.
6. The 1994 publication *Standards of Care* for psychiatric nurses relates to the nursing process, in that it specifies the role of the psychiatric nurse in carrying out the six-step nursing process. The standards delineate both basic and advanced nursing practice.
7. During the assessment phase, your focus is on data collection and on developing a database for determining the direction of care for the patient. A comprehensive and holistic data collection is made.
8. The patient is the primary source for data collection.
9. The quality of assessment can be enhanced by obtaining additional information from family members, friends, significant others, health team members, records, and the results of various tests and laboratory procedures.
10. The psychological assessment includes descriptions of behaviors, information about the patient's coping skills and emotions, and information about the patient's growth and development.
11. Nursing diagnoses are clinical judgments about individual, family, or community responses to actual and potential health problems.
12. Nursing diagnoses are derived from nursing problems and patterns of behavior, and they often flow from medical diagnoses.
13. The steps in logical decision-making are to identify the patient's behavioral, biological, psychosocial, and spiritual responses to stress; to categorize the data into functional groups; to identify missing data and any incongruencies; to identify any patterns; to compare the data to theoretical information, norms, and standards; to identify basic needs and concerns, taking into account the patient's strengths and limitations; to identify any causal relationships; and to identify the applicable nursing diagnoses.
14. The North American Nursing Diagnosis Association (NANDA) develops the approved list of nursing diagnoses.
15. The nursing diagnosis statement consists of the health problem, the etiological or contributing factors, and the defining characteristics.
16. Nursing diagnoses and the psychiatric diagnoses in the *DSM-IV* are related, in that they identify many patterns of behavior that provide clues to specific and appropriate nursing diagnoses.
17. The purpose of nursing outcomes is to formulate a plan of care using defined criteria for measurement.
18. The criteria for writing an expected outcome are that it must be patient centered, singular, observable, measurable, time limited, mutual, and realistic.
19. It is advisable to organize the expected outcomes into a series of short-term goals that lead to the fulfillment of the longer-term expected outcome.
20. Nursing interventions might be categorized in a plan of nursing care according to the types of interventions allowed by your level of practice.
21. The interventions available to you as a psychiatric nurse at the basic level of practice include counseling, milieu therapy, self-care, psychobiology, health teaching, case management, and health maintenance and health promotion.
22. Counseling involves the use of communication and interviewing.
23. The focus of milieu therapy is the therapeutic use of the environment.
24. Self-care interventions are aimed at maintaining and improving the person's functional status.
25. Psychobiological interventions involve monitoring the effects of psychotropic medications.
26. Health teaching is directed at meeting the nursing diagnosis of Knowledge Deficit.
27. Case management interventions include negotiating for services on behalf of patients, maintaining relationships with agencies and health care providers, and providing services that meet patient needs.
28. Health promotion and health maintenance include a broader community perspective.
29. A formative evaluation includes reassessment of all aspects of the nursing process as you are implementing care to analyze the patient's responses.
30. A summative evaluation is one in which you make a concluding statement about the entire nurse-patient journey. It includes information from the formative evaluation as well as recommendations for future nursing care, as appropriate.
31. Both are essential for excellent nursing care because the formative evaluation covers all aspects of the nursing process as you provide care, whereas the summative evaluation draws conclusions about the effectiveness of the entire nurse-patient interaction. Thus, the two evaluations provide valuable information.
32. Documentation is essential to the successful planning and implementation of nursing care.

33. The APIE method consists of assessment, planning, interventions, and evaluation.
34. The basis of the problem-oriented method is a list of problems.
35. SOAPIE stands for *s*ubjective data, *o*bjective data, *a*ssessed information, *p*lan, *i*nterventions, and *e*valuation.
36. Focused charting uses the *DAR* format, documenting data, nursing actions, and patient responses as a means of providing a specified focus.
37. Agencies review nursing documentation for reimbursement purposes and for quality improvement purposes.

CHAPTER 13

1. The three primary goals of the nursing assessment interview are to establish the foundation for nursing diagnosis, to develop the nursing care plan, and to begin the therapeutic relationship.
2. The seven aspects to evaluate in the rehabilitation model for nursing are intake of air, food, and fluid; elimination; maintenance of temperature and hygiene; balance between solitude and social activity; balance between rest and activity; prevention of hazards to life and functions; and promotion of normalcy.
3. The two main functions of the nursing database are to provide objective details about patient problems and strengths and to identify subjective nurse-patient reactions during the interview.
4. The nurse must be explicit about subjective impressions when interviewing the psychiatric patient to prevent personal reactions from interfering with an accurate description of the patient.
5. Three ways to reduce your subjectivity in the assessment interview are to use structured questions, to observe, and to use standardized rating scales.
6. Barker's five stages of the assessment interview are (1) identification of the problem from the patient's perspective, including how he or she feels about the problem, how it affects his or her relations with others, and whether it is inside of his or her head or his or her body; (2) measurement—a focus on the frequency of the problem behavior and the intensity of the patient's feelings about it; (3) clarification—asking about the effect of various situations or people on the problem behavior; (4) seeking the patient's explanation; and (5) variation—looking for the patient's view of any patterns for his or her feelings and thoughts about the problem.
7. The two techniques you can use to demonstrate respect for the patient are listening attentively and accepting the patient's report in a nonjudgmental way.
8. The four therapeutic factors that begin in the assessment interview are (1) providing information about the setting and admission procedures to reduce the patient's anxiety about the unknown; (2) letting the patient know that he or she is not the only person with that particular problem to bring out the factor of universality (i.e., other people have felt or believed the same thing); (3) reducing the patient's feelings of anxiety and isolation to encourage the patient's sense of hope and positive expectations of treatment; and (4) communicating that the patient will be actively involved in decisions about care to reinforce the sense of responsibility of self.
9. Three advantages of standardized rating scales are that results of a standardized test enhance the data collection, adding another observation to the baseline that lends itself to future comparisons; that test results may be used by the treatment team to individualize a treatment plan, incorporating starting scores and improvement in scores as measurable goals; and that because you may have the opportunity to participate in formal research, it is important to be familiar with valid and reliable tools.
10. The six steps of the nursing process, as defined by the American Nurses' Association, are assessment, diagnosis, outcome identification, planning, implementation, and evaluation.
11. The three significant principles guiding the nursing assessment are that on admission to psychiatric care, the highest priority is placed on evaluation of the patient's safety; that you must tailor the interview to the patient's immediate condition, prioritizing the questions to gain the most information possible at that time; and that data collection must be ongoing to complete the original database as soon as it is feasible.
12. Routine vital signs may be the first clue about a concurrent physical problem that the patient may not be aware of or able to verbalize clearly.
13. Record the patient's perceptions of the problem, because the patient's perceptions are the key to planning appropriate early interventions, and acceptance of his or her viewpoint engages him or her in planning for his or her own care.
14. A medication history documents the names, dosages, and therapeutic effects of all psychotropic medications; a full description of any side effects or allergic reactions; and a description of any prescription or over-the-counter medications taken for concurrent health problems.
15. The primary reason for relapse in psychiatric patients is noncompliance with medications.
16. You need to be able to carefully explain each descriptive term so that you can record the patient's exact words and actions that lead to selection of a particular term.
17. The Mini-Mental State Examination may be used as an effective screening tool in identifying cognitive impairments, especially in the elderly.
18. Specific information gathered about hallucinations includes the type of perception, how long it has been present, when it started, how much the patient believes it is real, the major emotional theme, the presence of any commands and the patient's response, and the coping strategies that the patient uses to control the hallucinations.
19. Two risk factors that may be identified during the physical assessment are risk for human immunodeficiency virus (HIV) infection and past or current physical or sexual abuse.
20. Three reasons to complete the sociocultural assessment are to understand the whole person, to develop realistic treatment goals, and to clarify the presence or absence of the support system that is relevant for successful discharge planning.
21. The biggest risk if the patient's culture clashes with the treatment plan is that he or she is at increased risk for premature withdrawal from care or treatment failure.
22. Although similarity between the patient and therapist may make the therapist more of a role model to the patient, it does not necessarily improve the patient's general level of functioning. Patient-therapist congruence in defining the problems and setting treatment goals is more important than matching their sociocultural backgrounds.
23. The significant risk factor that can be identified during the spiritual assessment is that specific religious beliefs may be directly linked to the patient's view of the cause of the illness and the direction for treatment.

CHAPTER 14

1. Culture is the pattern of beliefs, food, dress, music, and traditions that gives a group its distinctiveness.
2. External influences in the forms of economic conditions, media influences, war, famine, and political upheavals can change cultures.
3. Stereotypes perpetuate "isms" about a person or a group of people by labeling them, thus hiding individual identity, values, aspirations, and achievements and resulting in rigid preconceptions.
4. Stereotyping exists in relation to race, sex, religion, and culture.

5. The levels of prejudice can vary in intensity—sometimes it can be subtle, sometimes overt—and it can lead to violence in societies with a low tolerance for persons with mental illness, especially during great upheavals, such as war and famine.
6. The mentally ill are targets of prejudice and are depersonalized and dehumanized. They are considered "incurable and dangerous" and "to blame for their condition." Discrimination exists in employment, promotion, and professional or political careers. Also, cases of physical attack and extermination have been documented during times of war and famine.
7. The levels of racism include prejudice, institutional racism, individual orientations to racism, reactions of those affected by racism, and symbolic racism.
8. Racism might interfere with psychiatric nursing through cultural differences in the manifestations of distress and in the way in which such manifestations are interpreted.
9. Ethnocentrism is making one's own world view the center or focal point for decisions and judging it as superior to others.
10. The implication of ethnocentrism when providing nursing care to those whose culture is different from your own is that you may not recognize the inherent bias of your ethnocentric viewpoint.
11. Ethnic identity encompasses the perception and inner sense of affiliation with a group that shares a racial, national, linguistic, or cultural background. It provides the security of knowing that one belongs, a stirring in the soul, and a sense of roots.
12. Ethnicity is linked to a person's social identity and includes history, language, and religion. It describes a self-awareness possessed by the person(s) to whom the terms are ascribed.
13. Variations in transcultural identification can lead to conflicts for people and families regarding whether to acculturate their children and grandchildren into the dominant culture, thus fostering acceptance, or to nurture ethnic pride in their descendants.
14. Three losses that occur with transcultural identification are loss of one's country, culture, and family traditions.
15. Assessment and diagnosis are important considerations in a discussion of ethnic competence because diagnosis creates labels and can mitigate against delivering nursing care that includes a cultural care perspective; furthermore, extensive knowledge of different assessment approaches as well as face-to-face interactions with people from different cultures is required.
16. Ethnic competence means acting in a manner congruent with the behavior and expectations of a particular culture.
17. Culture-bound syndromes raise the issues about the differential contribution of biological and cultural factors in the etiology and shaping of mental disorders.
18. Three culture-bound syndromes are old hag, a culture-bound syndrome found in Newfoundland; koro, found in Chinese communities in Britain; and jiryan, found commonly in Pakistan.
19. The concept of the appointment time may vary depending on the culture and its definition of being on time or late. This means that you as the nurse must be aware that if you want a patient from a certain culture to keep an appointment by American time standards, you may need to ask the patient to come earlier; that is, if the actual appointment is meant for 2:00 p.m., the patient should be asked to come at 1:00 p.m.
20. Acquaintance time is the period needed by the patient and family to "size up" the professional providing health care service. Bearing this in mind, you should use acquaintance time not only for dialogue but also for validating cultural concepts about mental health, mental illness, and traditional treatment. You then can familiarize the patient with American standards of mental health care.
21. Asians are usually very sensitive to each other's personal space and have definite rules concerning physical contact. Conversation is held at a distance of 5 to 6 feet from the other person. West Indians maintain very little space between friends when communicating.
22. Regarding cultural views of touch, contact between males and females in Arab culture is prohibited, whereas in Latin America, physical contact may extend to a kiss on the female's hand.
23. Voice tone and gestures differ across cultural groups. For example, in American culture, speaking distinctly in a well-moderated and self-controlled tone is the desirable norm, but a cool, logical approach to conversation may be regarded by Middle Easterners with suspicion. Regarding gestures, the Arab is encouraged from childhood to express his or her feelings without inhibition, while throughout much of Asia, respect and communication are enhanced by speaking politely and softly.
24. A patient from a geographical region where nurses wear uniforms might have difficulty relating to an American nurse in an institution that no longer requires uniforms.
25. It is important to know different terms of address in different cultures because this can enhance communication with a patient.
26. Throughout much of Asia, mental health problems are viewed as imbalances in the body, whereas in Africa and much of the Caribbean, mental illness is viewed as suffering from a spell.
27. An example of how religion affects people across cultures is that some fervent Catholics rely on God's greatness and prayers to help them through a crisis, whereas Buddhists accept suffering as a reality of life.
28. Because mental illness creates a sense of shame for the Irish-American patient and family, a pervasive sense of guilt and intrapunitiveness often is experienced by an Irish patient when mental illness occurs. A family might hide a mental problem in a loved one by keeping the person confined to one part of the house and might seek divine intervention for a cure through prayer. University graduates are more willing to seek professional help when problems occur.
29. The role of religion (predominantly Catholicism) in the life of many Irish-Americans is to offer hope, but it demands commitment. The hopeful message of Catholicism focuses on love and forgiveness and is helpful to the patient trying to overcome mental illness. The church is a refuge for sinners, a comfort to the afflicted, and a source of spiritual nourishment.
30. For Italian Americans, although strong family ties can reinforce good mental health, family bonds that are tenuous, critical, or hostile can contribute to depression.
31. The Jewish community has developed a strong ethnic self-consciousness as well as elaborate support systems to address the needs of its members, including those with mental illness. This network is important for meeting a Jewish patient's needs.
32. A cultural broker might be useful for an African because this person has ascribed or achieved acceptance in two distinct cultures and, as such, facilitates a bond with the minority patient and enhances the patient's ability to operate in the dominant culture.
33. Trust is important to African-Americans because their culture teaches that a person should not share personal information with outsiders.
34. Three qualities that Hispanic Americans look for in a mental health professional are formal friendliness (personalismo), warmth and concern (simpatía), and respect for the person and culture (respeto).
35. The core belief of espiritismo is the soul voyaging, altered states of consciousness, and the presence of spirit-beings who can enter into a person's body.
36. In Hinduism, depression might be understood, according to the law of Karma, as an atonement for some misdeeds in life.
37. Whereas Buddhism talks about abandoning the self, the Western psychiatric emphasis is on self-worth and self-acceptance.
38. Although individualism is encouraged among Americans, Japanese-Americans are expected to conform to family expectations and community norms. Therefore, they frown on individualism, even today.
39. The Filipino extended family, in response to mental illness, can help by listening and giving guidance to help resolve a psychological conflict. Beliefs in the preservation of the family name and in the power of prayer are strong behavioral determinants.
40. "Chit chat" with a Native American patient might only increase his or her anxiety, since this culture discourages small talk and emphasizes symbols and periods of silence.
41. In the Flathead Indian culture, depression and consequent drinking may have positive connotations because heart and spirit are central to an understanding of Flathead life. Life for them is characterized not only by close ties of kinship and friendship but also by feelings of loneliness, of being uncared for, of having nothing, or of fears of being abandoned. Depression can thus be a positive expression of belonging in this milieu.
42. Within the Flathead Indian culture, drinking is seen as a positive expression of sociality, a reaffirmation of the bonds of friendship and kinship. If a person does not drink, this may be interpreted as a slight against family and friends.

43. A sweat lodge is a symbol of Native American religion and identity and is used by all North American tribes. It combines ancient ritual and incantations to promote healing, and its common purpose is to bring a person closer to the elemental forces of life and to express unity between all humans, animals, the earth, and the physical forces in the universe.
44. The role of the shaman in Native American cultures is to control the spirits through ritual, magic, incantations, sacred objects, or herbal remedies.
45. Someone from the Caribbean might explain mental illness by stating that the spirits have taken control or that God has destined them for great power.
46. The family of a West Indian patient remains the key element in helping the patient explore emotional problems and in engaging him or her in treatment.

CHAPTER 15

1. Crisis represents an interruption in the human journey by emotional disequilibrium, cognitive disorientation, and a perceived inability to use previous problem-solving skills. Thus, people in crisis experience the confusion and emotional pain of the event as an overpowering life experience.
2. A theoretical framework is useful in a crisis situation for evaluating the impact of the crisis event in functional terms (e.g., the Aguilera/Messick model).
3. Caplan's model focuses on problem-centered intervention and the need for community-based intervention for basically healthy people in active crisis. Caplan stresses the need for reexamination of what is useful in our lives and what is useless in light of the crisis and for restructuring of outmoded beliefs and actions.
4. Erikson's model could be used to help a patient in crisis by identifying situational stressors that occur during different stages of life and by understanding common situations that occur during transitional stages (e.g., marriage, the first pregnancy, retirement). As a nurse, you can help people anticipate developmental passages and provide help to those people and their families with psychosocial needs.
5. The Aguilera/Messick model is useful in crisis intervention as an assessment framework for evaluating the impact of a crisis event in functional terms. It also serves as a nursing theory–based guidepost for identifying where the intervention needs to focus.
6. A crisis state refers to a personal response—physical, emotional, spiritual, and behavioral—to an important, often negative, situation (e.g., loss of an important relationship). Elements of a crisis state are interactive and involve a critical stressor, a vulnerable state, failure of normal problem-solving methods, lack of social supports, and intolerable tension.
7. Knowledge of risk factors is helpful in organizing an immediate situation into workable terms and in assisting the patient to generate creative alternatives in a difficult situation. To direct the patient effectively, you must have a general understanding of the nature of the crisis state and the progressive steps involved in crisis intervention.
8. A situational crisis occurs unpredictably, whereas a maturational crisis is identifiable in relation to predictable stages of human development.
9. The assessment phase in crisis intervention differs from that in other types of therapeutic relationships, in that it is more immediately and closely associated with crisis resolution. The assessment and intervention are joined together from the very beginning.
10. When planning care for patients in crisis, consider the nature of the crisis and its meaning to the patient, including evaluation of risk related to self-harm or harm to or from others. Initially, do a triage assessment for medical and psychiatric emergency, engage the patient in the treatment process, and develop a comprehensive database that will serve as the foundation for planning and intervention. When planning care for patients, also make a realistic assessment of the crisis event, coping resources, and sources of personal support.
11. You might use a patient's strengths in crisis intervention by pointing them out to the patient. Asking questions about how the patient dealt with previous stresses helps him or her to recall past mastery of difficult times, and recognition of previous achievements helps sustain motivation when current outcomes are uncertain. Credit for managing small tasks in the immediate situation and taking initial steps toward problem-solving encourages the patient to take the "next best step."
12. Normalizing feelings means that you assure the patient that crisis precipitates a wide range of reactions. This knowledge can be very consoling to the person experiencing these feelings.
13. A nursing note for a patient in crisis should be accurate and complete and should contain the date and time of admission, interview notes containing a precise description of the patient, an initial treatment plan, behavioral notes, treatment recommendations, and behavioral responses. Notations should be made regarding physician and family notifications with name, date, time, and response included. Rationale for exceptions to regular protocols should be made. Dialogue with the patient regarding the nature of the discussion, the patient's response, behaviors noted, and the time and date of departure should be recorded. Information also should include the names of the physician, social worker, family members who were notified, and the time, date, and their response. The note should clearly state whether the patient left against medical advice, what instructions were given, if any, and further treatment or referrals suggested.
14. Mobile crisis units are forms of preventive psychiatry, in that they function as an outreach mechanism for people who might not seek treatment on their own initiative. By providing immediate support, reinforcing family strategies, and referring to the appropriate support services, an acute crisis can be reduced.
15. Factors to consider in a patient referral include knowledge of relevant referral sources and how to access them, patient readiness and ability, and coordination of efforts if more than one agency is involved.
16. It is important for you to engage in a critical stress debriefing with other nurses following a crisis incident to help you understand what happened from a "big picture" perspective, to provide you with a safe place to ventilate feelings, to assist you in differentiating between the things that can and cannot be controlled related to resource allocation, and ultimately to reduce the tension to a workable level and restore you to precrisis functioning.

CHAPTER 16

1. Ancient people believed that emotions were controlled by the lunar cycles (hence the term *lunacy* to describe mental illness).
2. St. Augustine changed thinking about emotions by describing the feelings, conflicts, and anguish of a person and stressing the importance of psychological self-understanding as the pathway to changing behaviors.

3. The id consists of instincts (related to pleasure and aggression) that are largely unconscious and drive the individual to get what he or she wants.
4. The ego involves reality and the need to behave appropriately.
5. The superego helps to keep the primitive impulses of the id in check, involves values and morals, and often helps the ego or conscious mind to self-perform in a healthy manner.
6. It is important for the therapist to remain neutral during the transference process as the patient reveals memories to allow him or her to experience any conflicts, through the transference, in a different and more healthy way than in the childhood experience. Because the therapist does not react in the way that a caretaker does, the patient is free to respond in a different manner.
7. Psychoanalysis and psychoanalytic psychotherapy are long term because they require deep exploration of the mind. The patient may need to go to therapy once or twice a week, possibly lasting from 6 months to 3 years.
8. Early insurance policies gave unlimited coverage for long-term therapy; however, in the 1970s and 1980s, health care costs rose, and insurance companies began to put limits on the amount of therapy that a person could have. These companies were unwilling to pay for open-ended therapy and forced therapists to think about how to help patients in shorter periods.
9. The psychoanalytic therapist believes in a long-term approach to therapy, during which the patient's early childhood memories are analyzed so he or she can change his or her personality characteristics.
10. The psychodynamic short-term therapist believes that the unconscious plays a role in the emotions and that past events as well as genetics and present reality influence current behavior. He or she assesses patient problems utilizing Freud's theories but does not have the goal of childhood memory exploration for the purpose of personality change. The goal is to help the patient with "here and now" issues based on the patient's biological, psychological, social, cultural, and spiritual presence. The short-term therapist views the patient as basically well but at a point in life when new behaviors need to be learned.
11. A utilization manager is hired by the insurance company to review the therapy and progress of the patient. He or she often is found in the inpatient setting evaluating treatment and often limiting the number of days that will be reimbursed for that particular admission.
12. The focus of an inpatient hospitalization involves stabilization of acute symptoms rather than long-term issues underlying the acute episode.
13. The four areas important for discharge planning are medication compliance, symptom recognition and management, relapse prevention, and planning for follow-up treatment.
14. The short-term therapist might teach the patient about what he or she is experiencing. With knowledge of the patient's history and the current problem, the short-term therapist helps the patient define goals for treatment and the approximate length of time to reach these goals. The therapist presents ideas for change, with the expectation that the patient is motivated and will utilize these ideas outside the therapy session.
15. The psychodynamic short-term therapist views the patient as basically well but at a point in life when new behaviors need to be learned. The therapeutic approach emphasizes the positive aspects that a person brings to therapy, facilitates the development of a working partnership between the nurse and the patient, helps the patient to develop future-oriented positively worded goals, and identifies actions necessary for reaching those goals.
16. During a first interview, you should convey respect for the relationship and set the tone and the boundaries for how the therapy is to proceed. After listening initially to the patient's presenting problem and gathering enough information on the patient's history, explain the patient's role in the therapy.
17. Assessment should cover the patient's presenting problem and his or her psychiatric, medical, developmental, family, and abuse or trauma history, as well as information regarding his or her sleep, nutrition, exercise, strengths, uplifts, and friendships.
18. Written exercises are useful during analysis and planning because they are designed to help the patient observe himself or herself and the environment in which he or she becomes most anxious.
19. In long-term therapy, transference behavior and feelings are important for the patient to work through childhood experiences and influences. In short-term therapy, transference is important to consider if the patient is resisting doing any work outside the therapy session. Countertransference refers to your responses to or feelings toward the patient. It is important that if you start to notice that you feel indifferent, bored, irritable, or sad toward the patient, you should be aware that these behaviors and feelings often are signals of countertransference and need to be discussed with another clinician so that they do not get in the way of patient care.
20. Two techniques often used in cognitive therapy are training patients to recognize automatic thoughts and exploring alternative ways to think.
21. Cognitive distortions exist when a patient who is depressed interprets events around him or her as negative, dangerous, and burdensome. The patient interprets his or her relationship to these events as hopeless, undesirable, and worthless and expects only unpleasant events in the future. These cognitive distortions become the patient's way of interpreting the world and thus become the first thoughts that come to mind as he or she perceives events of the day. These first thoughts are automatic and continual.
22. Two components of cognitive distortions are arbitrary inference and selective abstraction.
23. Automatic thinking schema are basic attitudes about self, such as being stupid or unworthy, that have been learned in childhood and have been fueled and supported by the cognitive distortions. These schema also can be explored in helping the patient to formulate more healthy perceptions and thoughts.
24. As a therapist, you become a sort of role model or parent figure for the patient in a supportive and understanding manner. As such, you help the patient to maintain the best level of functioning.
25. In supportive therapy, use knowledge of the patient's interpersonal skills, problem-solving ability, affect regulation, and impulse control to help him or her understand current problems and handle those problems rather than waiting for the patient to gain insight or to complete homework assignments. You may use some cognitive therapy to help the patient see certain situations differently, or you may utilize some behavior therapy techniques to help the patient deal more effectively with a certain situation.
26. To benefit from supportive psychotherapy, the patient needs to have had other successful relationships in life. The length of time spent in supportive psychotherapy is almost completely determined by the patient's situation.

CHAPTER 17

1. The early models of group psychotherapy are similar, in that the focus is on the group and that within the group, members affirm each other's humanness and learn to resolve behavioral problems, with an emphasis on peer relationships as a supportive structure. The groups differ from one another in terms of having a broader or narrower focus; for example, some focus on patients with a particular disease, some focus on children and adolescents, and others focus on the group as a social field.
2. Public awareness of group psychotherapy as a form of treatment for people with emotional problems developed during World War II. A significant number of war-related psychiatric casualties and a limited number of psychiatrists to treat military personnel caused group psychotherapy to become the primary treatment for mental illness in the military.
3. Group therapy helped bring about a behavioral change in people by

using peer relationships as a supportive structure to enhance the healthy parts of a person rather than the illness aspects.

4. The size of the group affects interaction. Large groups limit the amount of interaction that can take place. Smaller groups (e.g., six to eight members) permit sufficient interpersonal space for intimate sharing. Groups that are too small create an emotional intensity or the formation of subgroups, both of which are difficult to regulate.
5. Time boundaries are important, in that meetings should begin and end on time; otherwise members may become fidgety, and explorations in the last few minutes of the group are impossible because selected individuals have left the group (at least psychologically).
6. Inpatient and outpatient groups differ in several ways. Group membership in inpatient groups tends to be more diverse. It reflects the current population rather than a deliberate attempt to match treatment with patient needs. A qualitative difference also exists in the level of interpersonal analysis. Outpatient groups typically last over a greater time span (minimum of 8 to 12 weeks). Inpatient groups, because of short-term stays, do not deal in the same depth with long-standing interpersonal communication styles.
7. Curative factors contribute to the improvement of a patient's condition. They constitute a function of the actions of the group therapist, the other group members, and the patient himself or herself.
8. Task and maintenance role functions work together to support group goals by producing an intellectually stimulating and emotionally satisfying capacity to achieve desired outcomes.
9. The necessary substitute for elements of successful coleadership are an equal peer relationship with two professional leaders assuming shared responsibility for the conduct of the group. Coleaders need to be philosophically in agreement with norms of openness, honesty, and respect for each others' opinions.
10. "Group think" describes a mindless group decision-making process in which the value of group membership becomes so important that opposing opinions or conflicting values and ideas are suppressed in favor of group harmony and consensus. It is potentially dangerous when a group bands together in rationalizing decisions that are morally wrong or that could adversely affect a given population without their input (e.g., the group beliefs of the Nazis).
11. In psychodrama, the patient (protagonist) is brought directly into the situation as an active participant. The director coordinates the process so that the group of patients receives maximum benefit. Other group members act as auxiliary egos or play the roles of significant others with whom relationships are being explored. A double is used when the protagonist has difficulty expressing feelings about all or part of the situation.
12. The group leader has to modify group formats for the chronically mentally ill because these patients usually need more flexible group boundaries regarding attendance. Many need more reminders to attend. The leader also must be more proactive, eliciting comments from patients and making the linkages. Direct instructions must be given by the leader on how to respond.
13. A reminiscence group for the elderly matches their stage in life in terms of integrity versus despair. The group focuses on the patient's perceptions of significant life events occurring throughout the lifespan.

CHAPTER 18

1. Classical conditioning uses cues to stimulate desired behavioral change. During a cueing process, generalization takes place, whereby the patient responds to similar stimuli in the same way. Operant conditioning is built on the principles of classical conditioning and refers to voluntary (operant) behavior. The focus is on controlling behavior by reinforcement, extinction, and punishment. Strengthening can occur as a reward (positive reinforcement) or as the removal of a negative contingency (negative reinforcement).
2. Behavioral learning is regularly used in daily life in the ways people learn in school and develop stereotypes about the way things should be from the media.
3. It is important to precisely define target behaviors that contribute to the development of maladaptive interpersonal relationships because these behaviors form the baseline for measuring progression toward goal achievement.
4. In targeting behaviors, consider behaviors that interfere with the patient's functioning and are amenable to change. You might use patient self-report, direct observation of patient behaviors, ratings of others, administration of appropriate tests to target behaviors, or a combination of these. Problem behaviors are identified as discrete actions that are counted precisely over an identified period and recorded or graphed. The specific needs of the patient and the patient's capabilities will dictate which sources of assessment data are most relevant.
5. The Premack Principle is sometimes referred to as "Grandma's rule." In some situations, a more preferred activity can serve as a reinforcer for a less preferred activity. When you apply it, you must remember that the low-frequency behavior must occur first. The principle is often applied in everyday life; for example, a parent may tell a child that he or she must eat everything on his or her plate before getting dessert or that he or she must clean his or her room before going to the zoo.
6. Different types of reinforcers affect behavior because they have meaning to the patient. The choice of the most appropriate reinforcer depends on both the patient's preferences and the situation. You should choose reinforcers that are present naturally in the real world and are desired by the patient. They allow the patient to experience positive and negative reinforcement in real situations.
7. Negative reinforcement involves a consequence that strengthens desired behavior by removing an aversive stimulus. Extinction is a behavioral strategy to decrease the frequency of an undesirable behavior by ignoring it. Positive reinforcement is rewarding with a desired consequence (e.g., praise) after the desired behavior. Punishment reinforces behavior through disapproving and nonconfirmation.
8. Three basic tools of behavioral therapy are shaping, chaining, and fading.
9. Chaining might be more appropriate for patients with lower levels of functioning.
10. Token economies are used in many settings; tokens or other symbolic rewards are awarded for demonstration of appropriate (desired) behavior. The tokens have no value in and of themselves but can be used to obtain specified rewards such as tangible goods, activities, or privileges.
11. A socially competent person can get and maintain the attention of others and use others as resources in socially acceptable ways, express affection and hostility to others, lead and follow peers, compete with others, and express pride in something that he or she has done. This person also has several nonsocial abilities such as linguistic competence, executive abilities, and the ability to attend to two things at once. A socially incompetent person lacks most of these characteristics, is unable to function smoothly in society, and has feelings of low self-esteem, isolation, and anger.
12. Cognitive theory has been integrated with behaviorism through observational learning and the taking of a cognitive/problem-solving approach, in which interpersonal and problem-solving skills are taught.
13. Aversive reinforcers are likely to be used to treat such behaviors as alcoholism, sexual deviation, shoplifting, hallucinations, violent and aggressive behavior, and self-mutilation.
14. Behavioral strategies (e.g., biofeedback, desensitization, guided mastery, and applied relaxation) are tools for engaging the patient's participation in his or her own successful self-management.
15. Behavioral techniques have been applied to preventive psychiatry in preventive activities, such as the community mobilization against substance abuse and in behavior modification programs using cognitive educational techniques for addictive conditions and chronic disease control.

CHAPTER 19

1. In 1843, Dorothea Dix advocated for improved conditions for the incarcerated insane.
2. The Community Mental Health Act of 1963 contributed to a rising interest in milieu therapy.
3. Two assumptions of milieu therapy are that the therapeutic relationship is worthy of respect and that patient ego strengths can be built upon.
4. With regard to dependence, the patient can identify when and where help is needed; such a patient is more functional than the patient who is unable to recognize the need for assistance. It is important to support the patient while he or she is gaining this awareness, which is necessary for his or her coping and adaptation.
5. A holding environment is one that provides consistency, caring, and object consistency, thus facilitating growth, intimacy, and possibly use of higher defenses.
6. Mechanical restraints are used only in conjunction with one-to-one staffing, verbal intervention, and pharmacological intervention, if ordered, to minimize the time a patient is restrained.
7. The concept of treatment continuum is important in caring for the seriously and persistently mentally ill because these people often need treatment for extended periods in several settings along the continuum.
8. Three phases of the treatment continuum are acute, transitional, and follow-up.
9. Five factors to be considered for milieu therapy in short-term inpatient units are a focus on the crisis that led to hospitalization, provision for a holding environment, integration of the social and emotional context, provision for an aftercare plan that is consistent with patient needs and resources, and graduated therapy.
10. The phases of graduated therapy are orientation, engagement, education, and understanding.
11. Mobile treatment is a community treatment modality that provides clinical services to seriously and persistently mentally ill patients in patient homes, in neutral settings, or wherever the patient can be engaged.
12. Considerations for the outpatient clinic milieu are access to services, safety of the environment, barriers to care, and managing the interactions within the clinic setting.
13. Limit-setting may be used by the nurse in each of the community settings. Clearly articulate the rationale for limits. Staff use verbal deescalation techniques, removal of oneself from harm, and law enforcement, if necessary. Emergency petition for psychiatric evaluation may be used within the laws of the state if the patient shows potential harm to himself or herself or to others and is unwilling to follow treatment recommendations.
14. The level of milieu therapy is on a continuum parallel to the level of residential services, extending from the most restrictive-supportive to the least restrictive-supportive. A patient may receive one level of treatment services and another level of residential services. Because treatment is generally more costly than residential services, higher levels of treatment generally would be only used on a short-term basis.
15. A crisis unit is generally an extension of a residential program where 24-hour staff coverage is provided by paraprofessionals who provide a supportive, low-stress environment. The goal is to prevent hospitalization and to stabilize the patient.
16. Adult psychiatric foster care provides care for psychiatric patients who have been released from state hospitals after long stays. It often works well for the elderly psychiatric patient.

CHAPTER 20

1. Using a family focus in their care, nurses can work as nurse generalists as well as nurse specialists. A nurse prepares to be a family therapist after formal instruction and clinical supervision in family therapy. He or she must have an advanced practice degree and have a broader understanding of the patient as a member of the family system.
2. At least three family forms common in the United States (other than the traditional nuclear family) are gay couples with children, single-parent families, and people living alone or with others without being married.
3. With recent demographic trends, one of the implications for you as a nurse as you offer health care to families is that family configurations and needs are quite different today than in previous times and and must be taken into consideration. A comprehensive family assessment identifies strengths that can be useful in the plan of care.
4. A family is a group of people related by blood, marriage, or emotional ties who define themselves as a unit and cooperate to accomplish the normal tasks of daily life. In terms of emerging family trends, family forms in today's society have become increasingly diverse.
5. We can look at individual family members; however, a systems way of looking at an emotional problem takes into account how the family works together and how the whole of the parts are greater and different than the separate pieces.
6. When boundaries are closed and impermeable, the system is shut off from information, resources, and sources of support. The level of anxiety tends to increase, and the patterns of interaction within the system are intensified. When boundaries are open and permeable, information flows in and out, leading to open, healthier systems.
7. Boundaries around and between subsystems should be age appropriate; for example, a 13-year-old boy does not belong in a parental subsystem but instead should be acting like an adolescent in the family power structure. It would be inappropriate for a child to take on a parental role.
8. Four dimensions of healthy communication are openness, honesty, clarity, and congruency.
9. Some family roles that detract from open communication are placater, computer, distracter, or blamer.
10. Family secrets affect families because communication is shut down and anxious behavior is intensified around similar incidents. Family myths, which are longtime beliefs, shape a family's interactions with each other and the outside world.
11. The result of the multigenerational transmission process is that a level of emotional health is transmitted to the next generation, and this level of health is influenced by the degree of fusion that one has with one's parents.
12. According to Duval, the Blount family is in stage 4—family with school-aged children. At this stage, you would expect the family to let the son go to sports and Boy Scouts, to go to church as a family, and to create a meaningful family life.
13. A pileup of events can affect a family by depleting the family's resources. Thus, the family will experience greater difficulty adjusting to a present crisis. Families that are exposed to stress over long periods end in a situation of maladaptation and function less well over time.
14. Five characteristics of functional families involve flexible roles, permeable boundaries, clear role definition and appropriate rules, open systems, and healthy communication. In dysfunctional families, boundaries are too rigid or diffuse, and all variables and patterns become fixed and less able to be adapted.
15. Family therapy first began to appear in the 1950s. The focus changed from treating individual patients to treating the family group, and family therapy became a profession in its own right. It has become a modality with many different approaches.
16. The national professional association of family therapists is the American Association for Marriage and Family Therapy (AAMFT). It specifies curriculum and training requirements for clinical members and approves supervisors, credentials members, and accredits approved training centers. It also helps its members to

define the extent of their practice, deals with ethical issues, and supports its credentialed members who are dealing with legal and ethical concerns.

17. Psychoeducation differs from family therapy, in that it provides information and training about a specific area of family life; it provides information and support to families dealing with a specific stress or crisis; and it provides prevention and enrichment (e.g., premarital counseling). Family therapy on the other hand, offers a broader view of the problem.
18. Three goals of marital therapy are to build an effective communication system, to learn to use conflict constructively, and to emphasize the series of tasks and adjustments to new situations that make up married life.
19. The triangle becomes the basic building block of interpersonal relationships, with a close side, a distant side, and a side where tension or conflict occurs between the two people. In a marriage, for example, tension lies in the struggle between togetherness and separateness, and typically the twosome will attempt to manage the tension by triangling in a third person (thus forming a triangle). When tension increases, people in a triangle find it difficult to manage tension, and this can escalate, with people acting automatically to each other rather than dealing thoughtfully with the issue at hand.
20. Emotional cut-off is a way of handling tension in a family by separating self from the process.
21. "Differentiation of self" refers to the degree to which a person can separate thought from feeling. A person with a high degree of differentiation of self will react with a high degree of thought and less emotional reactivity.
22. Societal regression suggests crowding and environmental pressures that are more likely to push levels of differentiation down rather than up. As a society becomes more populated with more people responding automatically, more individual dysfunction and social irresponsibility occurs.
23. Individuals taking an "I stand" have a high level of differentiation. A society with more people having a higher level of differentiation would take a position and effectively enforce the consequences. The key to managing triangles is not to avoid them but to learn to manage and retain a self within them (i.e., detriangling, which requires that people remain connected with others while defining a self or starting an "I position").
24. Sibling position suggests that people develop certain personality characteristics related to their position in their family of origin. Birth order and gender within one's family of origin are the two main variables that influence behavior.
25. Multigenerational transmission process suggests that a level of emotional health is transmitted or passed down to the next generation.
26. A genogram is a format for drawing a family tree that records information about family members and their relationships for at least three generations. It makes it easier for a clinician to think about the family members, patterns, and significant events that are important in the family's care.
27. A genogram is used as an assessment tool throughout the contact with the family as a therapeutic tool to help individuals to see family processes more clearly. It also is used as a process of collecting and recording information so that the interviewer and family can connect in a personal but emotionally safe way.
28. The genogram has three functions: mapping the family structure, recording family information, and delineating family relationships.
29. Goals for family therapy must be specific and communicated to all and should include long- and short-term outcomes. Choosing priorities is a mutual process in which you and the family agree on the goals.
30. In family therapy, the evaluation takes place with each interaction between you and the family. It involves an examination of goals, of effect on the "sick member" and on each other member, and of effect on subsystems and on the whole family.
31. Three principles of family intervention are that families naturally have resistance to change, that a change in one part of the system will affect the entire system, and that the more important a family member is to the family functioning, the more impact a change in that member will have on the family.

CHAPTER 21

1. Taoism teaches that the reality of existence is in us and that we are one with all that is around us. It teaches a respect for the life force of nature and emphasizes that we should recognize a oneness of ourselves with the universe.
2. Ch'i (or yin and yang) is the creative energy or life force to change.
3. Taoism states that health is the balance achieved for healing of mind, body, and spirit. It involves a balance between good and evil and love and fear. Taoism focuses on understanding imbalances.
4. Traditional Chinese medicine is based on Taoist natural philosophy, and its goal is to promote harmony (health), or order, out of chaos (illness). It is a vast system of medicine based on many concepts, laws, and principles of energy movement within the body.
5. The five elements in traditional Chinese medicine are wood, fire, earth, metal, and water.
6. Yin and yang, or life force, is the concrete expression of the Taoist concept of Ch'i, a two-part force with each part complementary to the other and neither part more important than the other.
7. In traditional Chinese medicine, the transition of the five elements reflects the human condition of transformation. In this system, transformation is the essence of healing.
8. Two of the goals of healing from an Eastern world view are to be in harmony with one's environment and all of creation in mind, body, and spirit and to reawaken the spirit to its possibilities.
9. Two of the principles of healing from an Eastern world view are that all nature tends toward order and harmony and that all living systems are interdependent.
10. The stages of healing from an Eastern world view are awakening, intentionality and focus, commitment, transformation, attainment, and empowerment.
11. *Energetics* refers to a view of functional energetic systems and their interrelation, which portrays the body as a microcosm of the forces of the universe, with humans situated between heaven and earth.
12. Practitioners of acupuncture believe that energy courses through humans in precise meridians. They believe that this energy is flowing, dynamic, observable, and measurable, and that its transition affects the balance of health.
13. A unique aspect of acupuncture is that the practitioner provides hands-on patient care 100% of the time during acupuncture therapy.
14. Imagery is "the mind thinking in pictures."
15. The purpose of imagery is to visualize not only what is real but also what one wants to become real. The idea is that our mental pictures actually change reality.
16. Therapeutic touch is described as a "conscious, intentional therapy" and is without a basis in established religion.
17. The purpose of therapeutic touch is to use oneself (i.e., one's own localized energy field) as an instrument to help whatever areas within the patient's field that have become obstructed and disordered by disease.
18. The spiritual basis of therapeutic touch is that it involves use of oneself as an instrument to heal. The belief is that we are all healers and that a life force is present in all of us that we can manipulate to balance all levels of mind, body, and spirit.
19. Therapeutic massage is a systematic manipulation of soft body tissue by movements such as rubbing, kneading, pressing, rolling, slapping, and tapping.
20. It has been used to improve immune function in people with human immunodeficiency virus, and it may open energy channels, releasing a blocked life force, to promote relaxation.

21. The Eastern spiritual explanation of the effectiveness of therapeutic massage is that the massage practitioner becomes attuned to the life force as he or she reads the symptoms of imbalance (e.g., muscle spasms, fatigue, and depression) and validates with the patient the changes resulting from therapy.
22. A biochemical explanation of the effectiveness of therapeutic massage is that the patient interprets the actions of the practitioner as loving and caring. Biochemical changes result, leading to feelings of calm and peace.
23. *Bioenergy*, another name for the life force or Ch'i, is a force that can be manifested in physical or emotional planes.
24. Transcendental meditation is a process whereby a person strives to experience pure consciousness, or oneness, with the universal energy force.
25. The purpose of transcendental meditation is to encourage people to focus less on the material and more on the immaterial energy force.
26. The purpose of bioenergetics is to release physical tensions, which allows the expression of repressed feelings and eventual resolution of conflict.
27. The Maharishi-Mahesh Yogi's purpose of spreading the technique of transcendental meditation was to eliminate social problems as people focused more on the spiritual world and less on the material world.
28. Biofeedback teaches the patient to bring under conscious voluntary control functions such as respiratory rate, heart rate, blood pressure, and skin temperature and thus to relieve some physiological problems.
29. Four conditions in which biofeedback could be used are to relieve migraine headaches, stuttering, insomnia, and chronic pain.
30. Two of the electronic instruments used in biofeedback are an electroencephalogram (EEG) and a thermistor to measure skin temperature.
31. The four steps used in biofeedback are to become aware of the functioning associated with the targeted symptom, to learn to recognize internal changes associated with the targeted symptom, to learn to voluntarily alter those internal changes, and to become motivated to learn this control.

CHAPTER 22

1. Patient education is a process of deliberately creating cognitive, affective, behavioral, and/or psychomotor changes.
2. Health education involves the dissemination of information to foster a state of well-being of mind and body so the patient can strive toward achieving the highest level of functioning.
3. Learning occurs in various ways and in numerous situations. Active learning involves the investment of time and energy in activities that lead to the acquisition of the desired knowledge and skills. Passive learning occurs when the learner is expected to absorb or internalize information that is conveyed by others without active participation.
4. The basis for behavioral learning theory is the stimulus-response patterns of conditioning and reinforcement.
5. The phases of psychosocial learning theory are the "unfreezing" phase, in which the person must recognize the need to learn and be willing to work toward the goal of learning; the "moving" phase, in which the person must actively engage in learning new behaviors and testing them; and the "refreezing" phase, in which the behaviors are solidified, new patterns are adopted, and the behavior is learned and integrated.
6. The cognitive learning theory involves the development of insights or understanding of the meaning of situations that provide impetus to change behavior.
7. The social cognitive learning theory (developed by Bandura) is based on the proposition that a person responds to the world with information, values, attitudes, and standards of behavior that are learned from observing others. The observations are encoded, and the information is stored mentally to serve as a guide for all future learning.
8. Self-efficacy is the belief that a person can carry out certain behaviors. It is based on the patient's perspective of ability and evolves out of the person's past experience, attitudes about learning, the situation, the social context, and expectations for self and others.
9. Perception influences learning, in that the learning process is stimulated by the person's perception of a problem, usually arising out of some unmet need. For a person to be motivated to learn new behaviors that influence health status, the person must perceive a risk for developing a problem or situation that will be of sufficient severity to warrant engaging in the learning process.
10. Motivation is the willingness to take action (to learn something) because of the perceived existence, susceptibility, and severity of the problem. The person then searches for some effective way to resolve the situation and to take action.
11. The different methods for accessing information depend on major sensory functions: visual, auditory, kinesthetic, and olfactory or gustatory modes. People use different strategies to learn. In some situations, modeling may work best; in some cases, trial and error may be used; and in others, problem-solving is the preferred strategy.
12. It is advisable to progress from simple to complex to enhance the efficiency and effectiveness of the learning process.
13. Piaget's stages of cognitive development are sensorimotor (0 to 2 years), preoperational intuitive (4 to 7 years), concrete operations (7 to 11 years), and formal operations (11 to 15 years).
14. Two characteristics of adult learners are that they use reasoning and reflectively critique situations and that most have many other responsibilities and thus time constraints impinge on the learning process.
15. Adult learners are accountable for their own learning.
16. Readiness is evidence of motivation at any point.
17. Readiness and motivation have an impact on learning because internal motivation (self-directed by the patient) lasts longer than external motivation. If the learner's internal motivations are reaffirmed, this strengthens the learning process and the interaction between the learner and the instructor.
18. A learning style is the manner in which an individual perceives and processes information in a learning situation.
19. The four learning styles identified by Kolb are convergent, divergent, assimilation, and accommodation.
20. Assessment for learning includes assessing the person's readiness to learn, his or her learning needs, and his or her preferred learning style. It is necessary to identify potential obstacles to the educational endeavor, including psychosocial factors, past experiences, and environmental factors.
21. An objective is a behavioral statement that guides the learning process and establishes the parameters for evaluating the success of the learning.
22. An objective states the expected specific behaviors of the patient, the situation of conditions surrounding performance, and criteria for measuring acceptable performance.
23. We often arrive at goals for teaching by expanding the knowledge base of an individual and/or family members. The goals may focus on developmental issues, legal aspects, coping, rehabilitation, self-care, or compliance with treatment regimens. The goals are reached after identification of alternative concerns and any potential restraining factors so that a clear agreement can be made with the learner as to the focus of the educational endeavor.
24. Five different teaching strategies are individual lecture/explanations, individual discussion, demonstration/return demonstration, workbooks, and group lecture.
25. The purpose of journal writing is to provide learners with a chance to express their thoughts and feelings on various topics, to provide a way to explore how their lives are being affected, and to enhance personal understanding of a situation.
26. Role-playing is used in patient education to provide a purposeful simulation of a life event in which patients participate and learn from structured situations.

27. The benefits of an individual lecture include providing didactic explanations and the opportunity to transmit information, as well as a chance to explore understanding and provide reinforcement, especially if linked with a discussion.
28. One constraint of a group lecture is that teaching the class is likely to take longer than interacting with a single person.
29. Two methods of evaluating the effectiveness of patient education are to review each objective for the criteria for measurement (best done on an individual basis) and to check the learner's retention and understanding of information that has been presented by means of a well-constructed test.
30. Demonstration and return demonstration are used when a patient has to learn some new procedure involving psychomotor skills. The learner can explore, experience mistakes, and rectify them in learning the correct performance of the procedures.
31. A workbook would be used in patient education as a teaching tool in much the same way as self-study instruction, or it may be used to reinforce information presented in other ways. It allows the learner to systematically review or apply information.
32. If family members are educated about the patient's illness, this information allows them to develop reasonable and realistic expectations.
33. The biopsychosocial-spiritual model is unique, in that this model encompasses biological, psychological, and sociological theories. The spiritual component makes the model more holistic.
34. The patient's illness acts as a constraining variable in teaching, in that the characteristics of the person suffering from a mental illness have an impact on the educational endeavor and its content. Generally, education is delayed until the psychotic symptoms are no longer a problem.
35. Three common questions posed by family members are "What is 'wrong' and what caused it?"; "What treatment is available, who can do it and what else can be done?"; and "Will the patient get better?"
36. Three broad content areas that would most likely be included in patient/family education are information about different diagnoses, associated symptoms and probable causes, and treatment options.
37. The three themes that are woven throughout the teaching sessions are control of illness versus cure, balance between rights and responsibilities, and illness-monitoring techniques.
38. The specific content areas presented in patient/family education include definition of mental illness, aspects of different diagnoses, explanation of symptoms, causes of mental illness, treatment options, medication management, coping and stress management, communication and relationship skills, and support systems.
39. Families are taught about the rights and responsibilities of family members in various relationships to the patient.
40. The family's role in management of illness involves monitoring the progress of treatment and encouraging the learning of skills in maintaining a therapeutic living environment (e.g., knowledge of medication management, promotion of a healthy lifestyle, and coping and stress management techniques for the caregiver).

CHAPTER 23

1. Neurotransmitters are stored in the nerve terminal within vesicles, which are tiny packets present in the axon terminal. Each neurotransmitter contains a large number of transmitter-filled vesicles.
2. When a transmitter binds to its receptor on a postsynaptic neuron, the binding initiates a series of events that result either in excitation or inhibition of the postsynaptic neuron.
3. An agonist is a drug that causes receptor activation when it binds to a receptor. An antagonist (or blocking agent) is a drug that prevents receptor activation as a result of receptor binding.
4. A drug that blocks transmitter reuptake causes the concentration of transmitter in the synaptic gap to rise, thus intensifying transmission.
5. The major indication for use of antipsychotic drugs is schizophrenia.
6. Antipsychotic drugs are thought to relieve symptoms of schizophrenia by blocking dopamine receptors in the mesolimbic and mesocortical areas of the brain. Antipsychotic drugs take several weeks to produce a full therapeutic response.
7. There are three types of early extrapyramidal reactions: parkinsonism, acute dystonia, and akathisia. Parkinsonism is treated with anticholinergic drugs (e.g., benztropine) and amantadine. Acute dystonia is treated with anticholinergic drugs. Akathisia is treated with anticholinergic drugs, beta blockers, and benzodiazepines. Tardive dyskinesia (TD) is the most troubling of the extrapyramidal reactions. It is characterized by involuntary choreoathetoid (twitching, writhing, wormlike) movements of the tongue and face. Over time, TD produces involuntary movements of the limbs, toes, fingers, and trunk. No reliable means of treatment has been found.
8. Early extrapyramidal reactions are more likely with high-potency agents, whereas anticholinergic effects, hypotension, and sedation are more likely with the low-potency agents.
9. Neuroleptic malignant syndrome is a rare but serious reaction that carries a 4% risk of mortality. Primary symptoms are "lead-pipe" rigidity, fever, sweating, and autonomic instability, manifested as dysrhythmias and fluctuations in blood pressure. Level of consciousness may rise and fall, the patient may appear confused or mute, and seizures or coma may develop. Death can result from respiratory failure.
10. Agranulocytosis is the major adverse effect of clozapine. A few deaths have occurred with the drug despite weekly hematological monitoring. Because of this danger, weekly hematological monitoring is mandatory, and treatment should be stopped if the total white blood cell count falls below $1500/mm^3$ or if the granulocyte count falls below $1500/mm^3$. Clozapine produces little or no extrapyramidal effect.
11. Antidepressant drugs do not relieve symptoms immediately. Initial responses take from one to three weeks to develop. One or two months may be needed before a maximal response is achieved.
12. The most common adverse effects of the tricyclic antidepressants are orthostatic hypotension, sedation, and anticholinergic effects.
13. The most serious adverse effect of the tricyclic antidepressants is cardiac toxicity.
14. Tyramine-containing foods are dangerous for patients taking MAOIs because they can cause a life-threatening hypertensive crisis.
15. The principal advantage of SSRIs over tricyclic antidepressants is that these new drugs are as effective as the tricyclic antidepressants, cause fewer side effects, and are safer when taken in overdosage.
16. Lithium can provide symptomatic control during both the manic phase and the depressed phase of bipolar disorder; furthermore, when taken prophylactically, lithium can reduce the frequency and severity of recurrent manic and depressive episodes.
17. Lithium blood levels are monitored because this drug has a low therapeutic index, and toxicity is a concern.
18. Lithium levels must be kept below 1.5 mEq/l; levels greater than this can produce significant toxicity.
19. Sodium depletion will decrease renal excretion of lithium, thus causing the drug to accumulate, resulting in toxicity. Sodium levels should therefore remain normal.
20. Carbamazepine (Tegretol) and valproic acid (Depakene, Depakote) have been used on an investigational basis to treat manic-depressive illness. These drugs represent an alternative to lithium for patients who fail to respond to lithium or who find its side effects intolerable.
21. Benzodiazepines are preferred to barbiturates and other general CNS depressants for treating anxiety because they are much safer and have a lower potential for abuse.
22. Although physical dependence can occur with benzodiazepines, symptoms of withdrawal are usually mild. However, with some patients, withdrawal symptoms can be severe.
23. Buspirone differs from benzodiazepines in four important ways: it does not cause sedation, it has no abuse potential, it does not potentiate the effects of CNS depressants, and its antianxiety effects are delayed.
24. For situational anxiety, treatment should be short term if drugs are used. To determine the need for continued therapy, patients should be reevaluated regularly. In some cases, use of an "on-off" dosing schedule may be helpful (e.g., with treatment interrupted periodically every six to eight weeks).

CHAPTER 24

1. Freud's developmental stages are the oral phase (0 to 18 months), the anal phase (18 to 36 months), the Oedipal phase (4 to 6 years), the latency phase (6 or 7 to 10 or 11 years), and the genital phase (12 to 20 years).
2. Play is important because it can serve as a window into the child's life for assessment and treatment purposes.
3. Erikson proposed that maturation involves the mastery of a series of basic developmental crises across the lifespan.
4. Kohlberg's theory outlined distinct stages in the development of moral reasoning that follow a progression (the preconventional phase, the conventional phase, and the postconventional phase).
5. The three phases of adolescence are early adolescence, corresponding to the beginning of physical maturation and the development of primary and secondary sex characteristics; middle adolescence, marked by the struggle for independence, often involving an uncomfortable degree of defiance and limit testing; and late adolescence, in which some stability has been attained in peer relationships, academic and leisure interests, and financial responsibility.
6. The most significant consideration in understanding *the child* is that he or she can be the best teacher when the subject is himself or herself; *the family* in terms of isolation from any real sense of community and enjoyment of one another; *the outside world* in terms of education and relationships at school; friends; and community activities.
7. Nurses need to consider models other than the middle-class nuclear family when evaluating family functioning because this type of family is not representative of all people.
8. Friends are important because self-evaluation and evaluation of others, attachment and loyalty, and attribution of qualities evolve primarily through the peer culture.
9. Nurses need to be aware of community resources because the more the nurse knows about them, the more helpful he or she can be to parents who may themselves feel disconnected and alone.
10. A feature of transference that is unique to children is that transference in the strictest sense cannot occur because children are generally still living with their parents and have a primary relationship with them.
11. Countertransference is when the nurse projects strong feelings stirred up in him or her (e.g., feelings of hostility, destructiveness, aggression, excitement, seductiveness) onto the client. These feelings arise from the nurse's own unresolved issues from his or her own adolescence.
12. Three manifestations of countertransference are a noticeable increase in anxiety, a sudden rush of any strong emotion, and a persistent feeling of dislike for a child or parent.
13. Four examples of coping mechanisms and the developmental phase(s) to which each is appropriate are denial (0 to 5 years), projection (3 to 15 years), intellectualization (3 years to adulthood), and altruism (adulthood).
14. As many as 13% of children are believed to have a psychiatric disturbance.
15. Six risk factors associated with mental illness in children and adolescents are poverty, neglect and abuse, exposure to violence, parental psychopathology, medical illness and disability, and divorce.
16. The factor most strongly correlated is poverty.
17. After parental divorce, a child must acknowledge the reality of the marital rupture, disengage from parental conflict and distress, resume customary pursuits, and resolve losses.
18. A child who lives in a violent household is more likely to have difficulties in the security of attachment, control of aggression, mood, self-esteem and social performance, academic performance, and juvenile crime.
19. Poverty is a risk factor for children because it makes it more likely that a child will be deprived of optimal nutrition and stimulation, exposed to environmental dangers, given inadequate health care, poorly educated, and cut off from a rich cultural heritage and opportunities for creative expression.
20. Neglect is described by the American Humane Association as "the deprivation of necessities" such as food, clothes, health care, education, and responsible supervision.
21. As part of the physical examination, the nurse assesses any unusual observations (e.g., abnormal head circumference, bruises, or abdominal distention), asymmetries, delays in coordination or speech, and visual difficulties.
22. One example that shows important features of a play assessment is observation of a child whose play behavior is solitary, repetitive, and lacking in imagination and narrative line. You should assess play for content, anxiety, imagination, narrative line, persistence, reciprocity, and adherence to rules.
23. Four areas of assessment are attachment/separation, sexuality, moral development, and spiritual development.
24. The most significant risk factor for a potentially suicidal child is current suicidal ideation, particularly in the presence of a lethal plan.
25. A spiritual assessment is included because it gives the nurse an understanding of a person's values.
26. Most children's psychiatric disorders are different from medical diseases because the diagnoses are based on a cluster of attributes or behaviors.
27. A child with ADHD shows a persistent pattern of inattention and/or hyperactivity or impulsivity.
28. An adolescent with a disruptive behavior disorder might be given the nursing diagnosis of Risk for Violence or Ineffective Family Coping: Compromised.
29. An example of an unrealistic worry one might see in an overanxious child is excessive and unrealistic worry about separation from the child's major attachment figures lasting at least four weeks.
30. Exposure involves intentionally confronting the child with provocative stimuli. Response prevention is when one does not allow the compulsion.
31. Two symptoms of PTSD in children are recurrent recollections of the event and disturbing dreams.
32. Anorexia involves a refusal to maintain minimum weight normal for height and age, intense fear of becoming fat, a distorted body image, and, in females, the absence of at least three consecutive postmenarchal menstrual cycles. Bulimia is defined as episodes of binge eating alternating with extreme weight loss measures (e.g., self-induced vomiting or use of laxatives). Both anorexia and bulimia involve a feeling of being out of control and anxiety about body appearances. Both can lead to significant medical problems if carried to an extreme.
33. Pica is defined as the ingestion of nonnutritive substances over a period of one month or more.
34. Gender identity disorder is characterized by a persistent wish to be or a belief that one is of the opposite gender. It should be clearly distinguished from sexual orientation, which simply indicates preference for homosexual, heterosexual, or bisexual activity.
35. Tourette's disorder involves motor and vocal tics that have occurred in the chronically affected individual for over one year.
36. A treatment plan for nocturnal enuresis could involve medication and the "bell-and-pad" system, which involves an alarm triggered by the child voiding. This allows immediate clean-up to be started, and the child is rewarded for progress.
37. Functional encopresis is fecal incontinence with the repeated passage of feces in inappropriate places (e.g., clothing or floor).
38. The five broad categories of developmental disorders are mental retardation, learning disorders, motor skills disorder, communication disorder, and pervasive developmental disorder.
39. Learning disabilities have been listed as a major risk factor in developing serious behavior problems and have been correlated with diagnoses of conduct disorder and borderline personality disorder in adolescents.
40. Four possible signs of depression in children are sadness, irritability, changes in appetite, and sleep disturbances.
41. Two nursing diagnoses for an adolescent with a major depressive disorder are Impaired Adjustment and Sleep Pattern Disturbance.
42. The most commonly missed pediatric diagnosis is substance abuse.
43. Two expected outcomes for Jordi are that he will demonstrate improved social skills and will employ more adaptive coping skills when frightened, upset, or angry.
44. As a nurse, you should not "humor" a patient by temporarily going along with a delusion because you must not collude with the patient's distorted perceptions (instead, reassure the patient of his or her safety by describing the real context that he or she is in, using simple, concrete terms).

45. To practice individual psychotherapy, the nurse is required to have a Master's degree.
46. It is important not to allow a child to hurt the therapist because this is likely to disrupt the treatment seriously and can terrify the child.
47. It is important for a child's family to be involved in treatment to achieve any long-term therapeutic gains because behavior management works to change the behaviors of the child by first changing the behaviors of the managers.
48. Behavior management techniques involve the parents being responsible for making decisions about what choices the children can make, the family agreeing on a simple set of rules based on safety and respect for one another, the family agreeing on a set of consequences for breaking the rules, the family agreeing on a set of rewards for following the rules, and the parents keeping in mind that all behavior is a form of communication—the goal being to help the child recognize this and find acceptable ways of expressing feelings.
49. The fundamental belief of the British group-as-a-whole school is that the group itself must be seen as the patient—as an entity greater than the sum of its individual parts.
50. Child psychiatric treatment is provided in various settings, including inpatient hospitalization (being the most restrictive modality) for evaluation and treatment of the most seriously disturbed children, residential treatment programs (which provide structured living and education to children who have been unable to function adaptively at home), partial hospitalization and day treatment programs (helping the patient to maintain sufficient self-control to live at home), and home-based services.
51. The well-functioning therapeutic milieu provides containment, structure, support, involvement, and validation.

CHAPTER 25

1. Adults in their 20s focus on meeting society's expectations and are concerned with establishing a career, choosing a life mate, and selecting a mentor. Adults in their 50s focus more inward, seeking meaning in life and redirecting their energy.
2. The midlife crisis is a normal psychosocial event characterized by emotional upheaval, often resulting in a life that has more personal meaning. It is influenced by physical, social, and psychological factors needing attention in midlife.
3. Social changes in the last 35 years have altered our understanding of adult human development. The role of women has changed dramatically (affecting family and work life), and the roles of men also have changed. Greater flexibility of social roles allows men and women a broader sense of identity.
4. Vertical and horizontal stressors are directly related to mental health issues in early and middle adulthood. Vertical stressors are carried from generation to generation in the forms of beliefs, values, and modes of conduct. Horizontal stressors occur as normative, expected, or unexpected life events.
5. The "sandwich generation" is composed of the people caught between two generations (children and aging parents), both of which require different types of care.
6. Education can be considered as a primary means of preventive psychiatry by reducing risk behaviors associated with mental illness and by promoting protective factors to enhance emotional health and well-being.
7. Support groups are used as a tool to promote mental health by providing emotional respite, practical advice, and direction for adult travelers.

CHAPTER 26

1. It is significant to subcategorize the elderly population because each subgroup has unique needs.
2. Differences exist between the sexes and races. Women outlive men, resulting in a decrease in the ratio of males to females over the years. Life expectancy has shown a steady increase for the white population, a substantial decrease for black males, and, to a lesser extent, a decrease for black females.
3. The developmental tasks of late life are coping with losses and changes, establishing meaningful roles, exercising independence and control, and finding meaning in life.
4. You can facilitate reminiscence by asking memory-provoking questions, showing sincere interest and listening when patients talk about the past, and accepting and validating feelings.
5. Major changes in mental function with age are slower retrieval of information that is not used daily, increased ease of distraction by stimuli, and decreased vigilance performance.
6. An older patient can exhibit subtle cues of depression, including slower movements and stooped posture; changes in sleep, appetite, elimination, and activity; low mood, unclear thinking, and vegetative symptoms; somatic complaints; and poor grooming and dress habits.
7. Physical care considerations for the older depressed patient include food and fluid intake, bowel elimination, and quality and quantity of sleep.
8. Delirium is an acute impairment in cerebral circulation that consequently disturbs cognition. Dementia is a general, progressive, irreversible deterioration in cognitive function. Although delirium and dementia both demonstrate altered cognition and abnormal behaviors, the patient with delirium describes an abrupt onset of symptoms, whereas the patient with dementia indicates subtle, progressive development of symptoms over a long period. Some altered level of consciousness occurs with delirium, whereas patients with dementia show no change in level of consciousness.
9. Patients with sundowner's syndrome display symptoms of disorientation, agitation, and wandering as the sun goes down in the evening.
10. Anxiety is often undetected in older adults because the elderly tend to present somatic complaints that confuse the diagnosis.
11. Older schizophrenics avoid seeking medical care because they are less aware of physical illness or can derive secondary gains by causing or complicating physical health problems.
12. Some basic measures to promote mental health in old age are the development of meaningful roles and interests, methods to manage stress effectively, good communication skills, and problem-solving capabilities.
13. Some precautions that must be taken to assure an accurate mental status assessment are to check for fluid and electrolyte imbalances, hyper- or hypoglycemia, hypoxia, dehydration, hypotension, anemia, and adverse drug reactions. A thorough physical evaluation and a thorough health history should accompany every mental health assessment.
14. The validity of data obtained during an interview with the older person may be influenced by the overwhelming number of activities faced and anxiety evoked after admission to a health care facility. Repeated assessments are necessary if impaired cognition is observed during the initial assessment. Symptoms and observations noted should be put in proper perspective before drawing conclusions about the older person's mental status.

CHAPTER 27

1. Loss is an event that involves the involuntary separation from something we have possessed and perhaps treasured. It requires that we give up that which is familiar, comfortable, and personal.
2. Grieving is a necessary process for all of the losses we face. This process involves recovering from the pain of loss, healing oneself, and moving forward with one's life.
3. The length and intensity of grieving depend on the amount of investment we have had in a person, object, project, or pursuit we lost. The greater the investment, the greater will be the sense of loss when it is gone. Significant losses are grieved intensely and for a longer period.
4. Three pioneers who did clinical work in the areas of grieving and loss are Eric Lindemann, George Engel, and John Bowlby.
5. In the 1980s and 1990s, research was done on the course of the mourning process, the experiences of bereaved parents, and the increasing prevalence of complicated mourning. Research also has focused on dying infants and children, parenting the child with a life-threatening illness, survival guilt in both bereaved parents and in those escaping natural disasters, and bereavement guilt after a suicide occurs.
6. Some losses felt during young adulthood involve the giving up of self-focused and personal pursuits to embrace corporate ideals, marital decisions, or business partnerships. We lose that which is solely "mine" to acquire that which is "ours."
7. Some disadvantages of using repression as a means of coping with loss are that the painful memories do not disappear but are rather stored in the subconscious to be dealt with later. Stored grief and loss have a cumulative effect and increase a person's vulnerability to experience a major grief reaction, triggered at some later time.
8. The *DSM-IV* differentiates a normal grief reaction from a major depressive episode as follows: "Normal" grief reactions affect the feelings, behaviors, thought patterns, and physical well-being of a person, but symptoms lose their intensity as time passes. A person suffering from a major depressive episode is likely to experience increased stresses, much guilt about actions taken or not taken on behalf of the deceased, extreme feelings of worthlessness, a period of prolonged and marked functional impairment, psychomotor retardation, and thoughts of death. The premorbid relationship with the deceased may have been marked by anger, ambivalence, or dependence.
9. People with mental illness are vulnerable to the same loss issues as emotionally sound people; however, the psychiatric patient also experiences losses directly related to having a form of mental illness. These include loss of job or career because of unstable mental health, loss of financial well-being due to bills for treatment or the inability to work, loss of friends as a result of frequent relapses or the difficulties of entering into meaningful relationships, and loss of rootedness and a place called "home" as a result of the tendency to disengage from reality and the flow of human life. Other losses include loss of purpose and direction in life, loss of meaning for one's life, loss of health and wholeness, loss of hope, and loss of a grasp of what is real and true.
10. People grieve in different ways and at different rates. People usually grieve most intensely during the first months after their loss. By the end of the first year, persons who allowed the grieving to occur and who have had no complicating circumstances surrounding their grief process may be near to some point of resolution.
11. The initial reaction to loss according to Kubler-Ross is that of denial. The initial reaction according to Engel is shock and disbelief. According to Westberg, the initial reaction is a state of shock. Therefore, shock, disbelief, and the tendency to deny what has happened are initial responses to having experienced a significant loss.
12. Two tasks of grieving are acceptance of the reality of the loss and experiencing the pain of the loss.
13. Normal grieving has three distinct phases. The initial one is marked by feelings of dismay and disbelief that may last for hours, days, or weeks. This is followed by the long period (months to a year or so) of deep sadness with its difficulties in concentrating, making decisions, and remembering. Somatic symptoms can develop, leading to concerns about failing health. Crying and some degree of social isolation may be common during this time. The long midphase of grieving is followed by new strength for coping, a returning sense of well-being, and an increasing degree of purpose and meaning for one's life. During this last phase, more emotional energy becomes available for meeting responsibilities, facing challenges, and accepting new undertakings.
14. Three categories of complicated grieving are absent grief (prolonged denial and psychic numbing), delayed grief (postponement of grieving for weeks, months, or years), and chronic grief (a persistent pattern of grieving that tends to be exaggerated and does not reach resolution).
15. Children grieve differently from adults. Their reactions are a direct reflection of the responses and actions of the adults around them. They come to understand that death involves leaving and separation. They consider how they might have caused what has happened. Children 3 to 6 years of age feel the separation from a parent and will desire to undo this loss. Children 6 to 9 years of age begin to realize that death is permanent, and they have a lot of questions. Children 10 to 12 years of age realize that death can come to anyone at any time. Adolescents may vacillate between having a mature attitude and a very childlike attitude toward death. They have a tendency to want to defy death or to remain immune to it.
16. Four obstacles to grieving are fear of struggling with the pain of loss; lack of commitment to the long process involved in grieving; lack of support from extended family members, religious support persons, and a religious belief system; social norms that sanction certain losses or that dictate the "proper manner" of grieving for men and women.
17. Significant losses in the life of the psychiatric patient may trigger intense feelings of shame, self-blame, diminished worth, or a more negative self-concept. Grieving may lead the psychiatric patient to become psychotic, immersed in depression, or out of touch with reality of the loss. Feelings of loss are intense when the lost person is the one on whom the patient depended for support, care, or supervision. These circumstances must be addressed before grieving can proceed to a point of resolution.
18. It is more difficult for couples to cope with and grieve the loss of a child if they begin to blame each other for the loss. This can easily lead to marital strife, making coping with the loss much more difficult.
19. Coping mechanisms are learned patterns of behavior that permit us to deal with stressful situations or crisis moments.
20. Expected outcome in working with a patient with a nursing diagnosis of dysfunctional grieving is that the patient will display behaviors indicative of successful grieving (e.g., reengaging in life's personal pursuits, resuming self-care and self-enhancement activities, demonstrating behaviors that are indicative of spiritual well-being, and reconnecting with one's support system).
21. Four interventions that you would use with the grieving adult are to reach out and give the person permission to grieve; determine which tasks of grieving are accomplished and which are incomplete; let genuine concern and caring show; and hold out the expectation that grief work will terminate at some point.
22. Four interventions that could be used with children are to talk with openness and honesty about death, to assure them of their safety and physical well-being and of being loved, to include the child in the rituals of mourning, and to help the child to remember the deceased through pictures, stories, and shared memories.

CHAPTER 28

1. Anxiety is the feeling of alertness and concern that prepares the person to take action of some kind. Anxiety in normal proportions is a trigger that is helpful to growth.
2. "Normal" anxiety is short term and of low to moderate intensity. Abnormal anxiety balloons to greater proportions and is sometimes transformed into crippling physical or psychological symptoms.
3. Anxiety is often treated with anxiolytics.
4. The prime regulators of anxiety are the monoamine and GABA receptors.
5. Monoamine neurotransmitters are found in blood vessels, the heart, and lung tissue.
6. A definite anatomical pathway through the limbic system underlies the experience of anxiety. The first limbic system pathway involves endocrine function regulation. The second limbic pathway involves memory and evaluation of sensory information. The third limbic pathway sends signals from the cortex to the lower limbic structures.
7. Norepinephrine may be responsible for the amplification of anxiety. GABA is thought to affect the modulation of sleep, the decreasing of muscle tone, and the reduction of anxiety.
8. The therapeutic effects of anxiolytic drugs on anxiety occur through the decrease of activity of serotonin or the enhancement of GABA.
9. According to Freud, anxiety is caused by a failure to work through repressed painful memories, impulses, or thoughts.
10. The behaviorists believe that anxiety is the outcome of conditioning and is a learned response.
11. Biofeedback treatment relates to anxiety being a conditioned response, in that the patient is taught to regulate various physiological processes that cause his or her symptoms.
12. A stress response is a prolonged psychophysiological reaction whose initial phase manifests itself through perceived anxiety. Stress is the broader response of which anxiety is one dimension.
13. Stressors are person-specific because of individual interpretation. Major stressors are illness, accidents, and catastrophic events.
14. In the immediate stress response, the autonomic nervous system is activated after the individual perceives a threat or taxing demand from the environment. The body prepares for "flight or fight." The effects of sympathetic stimulation occur in two or three seconds and last between 5 and 10 minutes. The characteristics are perspiration, tremulousness, and rapid pulse and breathing.
15. The intermediate stress response occurs within two to three minutes after the presentation of the stressor.
16. The long-term response involves the endocrine system and elevates blood pressure and alters the breakdown of fats and proteins for energy.
17. In mild anxiety, the person is aware and able to problem-solve. In moderate anxiety, tension and fear are felt, and a greater increase in the physical symptoms such as blood pressure and heart rate occurs. The person has a sense of helplessness but also an ability to increase a focus in one area and to shut out irrelevant data. In severe anxiety, the physical symptoms are exaggerated, and the person is obviously distressed. The person has a fear of losing control and greatly diminished perception. In panic levels of anxiety, physical arousal continues and the person is emotionally overwhelmed. He or she only responds to internal distress and feels as if he or she is going to die.
18. Coping mechanisms are conscious voluntary behaviors to alter the experience and reduce anxiety (e.g., distraction, avoidance, and seeking information). Defense mechanisms are preconscious and unconscious processes used to alter anxiety.
19. People think more clearly during mild anxiety.
20. People begin to experience physiological responses during moderate anxiety.
21. It is possible to use guided imagery during moderate anxiety.
22. Guided imagery involves the patient being in a quiet, calm environment free from distractions. The patient closes his or her eyes and imagines and describes a peaceful place. Gradually, the patient's focus on the stressful event is weakened, resulting in a temporary decrease of anxiety.
23. The distracting techniques that may facilitate lowering anxiety are teaching breathing and relaxation exercises and using play therapy with dolls, puppets, and games.
24. Generalized anxiety disorder is unrealistic or excessive anxiety and worry about two or more life circumstances.
25. Adult children of alcoholics may be particularly vulnerable to severe anxiety disorders such as generalized anxiety disorder. Studies have identified divorce, separation, spousal abuse, and poor parental modeling as common stressors.
26. The benzodiazepines alleviate anxiety by facilitating the inhibitory actions of the neurotransmitter GABA in the brain.
27. Buspirone has the advantage over the benzodiazepines of treating anxiety due to its low abuse and dependence profile.
28. A panic disorder is characterized by discrete periods of intense fear or discomfort that are recurrent.
29. Agoraphobia is the fear of being in places or situations from which escape might be difficult or embarrassing or in which help might not be available in the event of an attack of anxiety. Agoraphobic situations include being in a crowd, standing in a waiting line, or certain aspects of travel.
30. Most patients who experience a panic attack erroneously conclude that they are going crazy and fear doing something uncontrolled during the attack. They have a feeling of impending doom.
31. The most effective medication in the treatment of panic attacks is imipramine, a tricyclic antidepressant.
32. An obsession is a persistent thought, idea, impulse, or even image experienced as intrusive and senseless.
33. A compulsion is repetitive behavior that follows an obsession. The behavior is performed in a particular order and is designed to neutralize or prevent some dreaded situation or event.
34. The drug treatment of choice for OCD is clomipramine (Anafranil), a tricyclic antidepressant.
35. As a nurse, you would teach a patient engaged in excessive hand-washing to safeguard his or her skin with special preparations that will replace the natural oils that are being removed in washing.
36. The symptoms of posttraumatic stress disorder are recurrent flashbacks and dreams of the event and attempts to avoid thoughts, feelings, activities, people, and places associated with the event. The person may experience difficulty sleeping, inability to feel loving feelings, irritability, difficulty concentrating, hypervigilance, and inability to recall specific aspects of the trauma.
37. The patient must have experienced an acute trauma that interrupts his or her ability to process information.
38. A phobia is an irrational fear.
39. A social phobia is a profound and enduring fear of social or performance situations where embarrassment could occur. Specific phobia includes severe fear of clearly identifiable objects or situations.
40. Social phobias are treated effectively with beta blockers, including propranolol, metoprolol, or atenolol.
41. The behavioral patterns commonly used to cope with anxiety are an adaptive growth-producing behavior that incorporates problem-solving and uses anxiety to learn positive adaptive behaviors, withdrawal and avoidance, acting-out, and somatization.
42. Of those behavior patterns, only adaptive growth-producing behavior is adaptive.
43. You should ask a person for information on his or her childhood, family issues, marital issues, sleep problems, somatic complaints, drug and alcohol use, current medications, prior psychiatric illnesses, social and occupational functioning, and relationship with his or her personal god.
44. The standardized anxiety rating scales that are used to evaluate anxiety are the Anxiety Disorders Interview Schedule–Revised (ADIS-R) and the Sheehan Patient-Rated Anxiety Scale.
45. Four nursing diagnoses are Ineffective Individual Coping, Post-Trauma Response, Social Isolation, and High-Risk for Self-Directed Violence.
46. One expected outcome for Ineffective Individual Coping is that the patient will demonstrate alternative ways of coping with stress. An expected outcome for Post-Trauma Response is that the patient will begin the grieving process. An expected outcome for Social Isolation is that the patient will participate in social exchange. An expected outcome of High Risk for Self-Directed Violence is that the patient will not experience behaviors that are physically harmful.
47. Three of the content areas that would be covered in an inpatient

group focused on stress and coping are safety of the patient, decreasing anxiety, and teaching patients to use controlled breathing to relieve anxiety.

48. Homework assignments are given to patients participating in a group on stress and anxiety to help patients relate their own problems to the theoretical material presented.
49. If you are assigned to a patient who suffers from both extreme anxiety and a substance abuse problem, you should know where that patient is at all times and what he or she is doing during the shift.
50. The tenets of rational-emotive therapy are that a person's emotions and behaviors are not caused by events that happen to him or her but by the beliefs that he or she holds about the events. To change this, one must dispute the "irrational beliefs" that cause the disturbance.
51. Flooding involves the presentation of high-intensity aversive anxiety-producing stimuli, either in imagery or in vivo without relaxation or pause until the anxiety is extinguished. It would be used as a behavioral therapy to desensitize the patient.
52. The treatment goal for a patient who suffers from OCD is to reduce anxiety and to learn to delay ritualistic behavior.
53. Suicidality is a risk for a patient suffering from OCD because if one belongs to a family in which other members carry the same diagnosis, experience of these problems and anticipation of the future based on observations of older family members with unremitting OCD is very difficult to bear.

CHAPTER 29

1. The perceptual experiences of a schizophrenic are similar to a peak experience, in that the senses become sharper; however, the schizophrenic is also unable to filter anything out, and the senses are flooded with stimuli.
2. A thought disorder occurs when the person who is receiving all the input (i.e., sensory stimuli, thoughts, emotions, memories, and ideas) is unable to automatically sort the information into a pattern of coherent thought that allows for logical responses.
3. The limbic system is thought to be the area of the brain that is defective in filtering sensory stimuli.
4. The schizophrenic patient poses a challenge to the psychiatric nurse, in that the nurse must reach out without being threatening and must be natural and honest while maintaining a professional role.
5. You assess whether or not a person is experiencing hallucinations by asking the patient about hallucinations and by observing behaviors that might indicate that the patient is neither responding or attending to internal stimuli. You ask the patient to describe experiences and note the degree to which this description differs from your perception of the environment.
6. Two historical examples of how schizophrenia was viewed are that until the 18th century, people with mental disorders were hidden rather than treated because many people believed that insanity resulted from possession by the devil or evil spirits and that as early as 1400 B.C., schizophrenia was described in Hindu literature as being brought on "by devils."
7. It is difficult to diagnose schizophrenia on the basis of psychotic symptoms alone because symptoms can be caused by metabolic abnormalities as well as by other neurological diseases.
8. It is important to differentiate schizophrenia from another disorder that might produce similar psychiatric symptoms because the diagnosis determines the type of treatment.
9. Kraepelin attempted to identify the syndrome of schizophrenia. He classified psychoses into dementia praecox and manic-depressive psychosis, recognizing their similarities and lack of external causes.
10. The four "As" are affect, association, autism, and ambivalence.
11. The front-rank symptoms of schizophrenia (as described by Schneider) are the hearing of one's thoughts spoken aloud, auditory hallucinations that comment on the patient's behavior, somatic hallucinations, the experience of having one's thoughts controlled, the spreading of one's thoughts to others, delusions, and the experience of having one's actions controlled or influenced from the outside.
12. The second-rank symptoms include other forms of hallucinations, depression, euphoria, and perplexity as disorders of affect and emotional blunting.
13. The purpose of IPSS was to obtain new knowledge about the epidemiology of schizophrenia.
14. The 12-point diagnostic system was derived from the work of the IPSS. This system standardized the diagnosis of schizophrenia across nine cultures.
15. The *DSM-IV* addresses the course of the illness by dividing it into five subcategories: subchronic, chronic, subchronic with acute exacerbation, chronic with acute exacerbation, and remission.
16. The *DSM-IV* identifies five types of schizophrenia: catatonic, disorganized, paranoid, undifferentiated, and residual.
17. Some established facts about schizophrenia are that schizophrenia is a brain disease, that the limbic system and its connections are primarily affected, that schizophrenia often runs in families, and that the brain damage may occur very early in life.
18. Schizophrenia is no longer considered a "functional" disorder because the brains of persons who have schizophrenia are different from those of persons who do not have the disease.
19. MRIs and CT scans have demonstrated the following abnormalities: enlargement of the lateral ventricles or the third ventricles, atrophy of a portion of the cerebellum, abnormalities in brain density, increased markings on the surface of the brain suggesting loss of brain tissue, and abnormalities in brain symmetry.
20. Twin studies demonstrated anatomical changes in the brains of schizophrenic twins. The fact that the twins could be differentiated on the basis of structural differences probably meant that the cause of the underlying neuropathological process was at least partially not genetic.
21. The two major cautions when interpreting from studies are that a "biological abnormality" is, at most, a correlation and should not be assumed to be a causal factor and that it often is difficult to determine whether the abnormality is related to the disease process itself or to treatment, especially with antipsychotic medication.
22. In humans, diseases of the limbic system are likely to produce schizophreniclike symptoms. Many researchers believe that the primary brain lesion may be in the limbic system.
23. Researchers are cautious about concluding that the limbic system is the site of the primary cause for schizophrenia because the fact that pathology has been identified in this area does not mean that the primary area of pathology has been defined. Furthermore, a single pathological process in the brain can cause a wide range of phenomena in different patients, and a single specific abnormality in the brain can have many different etiologies.
24. It generally is acknowledged that schizophrenics inherit a genetic vulnerability to the disease rather than the disease itself. Relatives of schizophrenics have a greater chance of developing the disease than does the general population.
25. The data suggest that schizotypal and paranoid personality disorders are genetically related to schizophrenia.
26. People with schizophrenia appear to have excessive levels of dopamine.
27. Observations suggest that schizophrenic psychoses sometimes occur in relation to infective illness. Crow has found that the cerebrospinal fluid of one third of patients with schizophrenia has viral-like activity, suggesting the presence of a virus.
28. Boyd and colleagues found evidence that schizophrenics are more likely to be born in the winter than in other seasons. If a seasonal factor damages the central nervous system during fetal development and predisposes the fetus to later development of schizophrenia or other major mental illness, we might expect to find the subgroup of

schizophrenics exposed to that seasonal factor to be different from other schizophrenics.

29. Sullivan concluded that anxiety caused the disintegration of ego function seen in schizophrenia.
30. Bateson's and Sullivan's work came to signify "blaming" the family for the schizophrenic's illness. Thus, the families had to undergo increased shame, stress, stigma, and guilt, and the families began to mistrust health care practitioners.
31. The stress-vulnerability model of schizophrenia identifies personal and environmental factors that contribute to relapse or minimize schizophrenic symptoms. The model attempts to identify people who may be more vulnerable to developing this disorder.
32. Biological vulnerability factors are factors that may inhibit the person's ability to cope with even minor stressors, and stressful family relationships may be potentiators of the disorder.
33. Personal vulnerability factors are brain biochemistry (dopaminergic dysfunction), dysfunction in attention and information processing, autonomic nervous system hyperactivity, and certain personality traits.
34. A positive symptom is present in the schizophrenic but absent in normal people. Three examples are hallucinations, delusions, and thinking disorders, such as loose associations.
35. A negative symptom is an altered emotional response that responds less successfully to medication. Two examples are apathy and social withdrawal.
36. Both illusions and hallucinations are positive symptoms. Illusions occur when the patient misperceives or exaggerates stimuli in the environment. Hallucinations are sensory experiences of perceptions without corresponding stimuli in the environment.
37. A delusion is a false fixed belief that cannot be corrected by reasoning.
38. Ideas of reference are delusional ideas wherein schizophrenic people believe that the actions of others are directed toward them.
39. Two explanations are that researchers believe that this withdrawal may be a reaction to overstimulation, an adaptive response to a world that the person experiences is too full of stimuli and too complex; and that withdrawal may be a response to understimulation.
40. The family assessment includes any history of mental illness in the patient's family, especially schizophrenia, mood disorders, or substance abuse; family communication patterns; the patient's environment; and family stress and cohesion.
41. Families have most difficulty dealing with chronic schizophrenia in a family member, which creates long-term stress in the family, particularly psychological stress.
42. In regard to spiritual or religious issues, you assess whether the patient experiences delusions or hallucinations with religious content.
43. Two findings are that schizophrenics who have a religious foundation have fewer exacerbations of the illness and spend less time hospitalized.
44. The usual age of onset for schizophrenia is during adolescence or early adulthood.
45. The young adults who are chronic schizophrenics are more visible today and are not confined to institutions as they were years ago. Young schizophrenic adults today hope to be rid of their symptoms and lead a normal life.
46. A good outcome is predicted if the patient was considered relatively normal before getting sick. If as a child the patient was able to make friends with others, did not have major problems with delinquency, and achieved successfully in school according to intelligence level, his or her outcome is likely to be good.
47. Sensory deficits, specifically deafness, may be a general risk factor for the development of hallucinations and delusions in later life.
48. The diagnosis of a dementing illness such as Alzheimer's disease makes differential diagnosis for schizophrenia very difficult.
49. In the prodromal phase, a clear deterioration from the previous level of functioning occurs. This may be marked by social withdrawal, poor hygiene, blunted affect, perceptual changes, and changes in usual interests and energy. The active phase has symptoms like hallucinations, delusions, and formal thought disorder that persist for at least one week, unless they are successfully treated. A residual phase usually follows the active phase and is similar to the prodromal phase, except that affective blunting and problems in role functioning are more prominent.
50. Five of Frese's suggestions to schizophrenics for staying well are that education about the illness is vitally important; that medications usually are necessary to stabilize the biochemical imbalance in the brain; that delusional thinking can be very seductive, so each person needs to identify how delusions are patterned; that denial is part of the illness and must be addressed early; and that circumstantiality, or the tendency to stray from a train of thought, is common, so patients need to teach themselves to stay on target in conversations.
51. Schizophrenics at greatest risk for suicide are those who have a relapsing course of illness, good insight, and a poor response to medication. They live in social isolation, feel helpless about the future, and perceive gross discrepancies between their earlier achievements and their current level of function.
52. Confrontational drug treatment programs with strong emphasis on dramatic confrontation may produce too much anxiety; thus, a different approach is required.
53. Substance abuse has been identified as a source of vulnerability and a cause for relapse for schizophrenic patients; however, the use of illicit substances does not produce schizophrenia.
54. Medical diagnoses are descriptive, so that a minimum number of symptoms meeting a minimum level of severity lead to a medical diagnosis. Nursing diagnoses, in contrast, describe the quality, content, or context of the patient's health concern and its relationship to contributing factors.
55. Two nursing diagnoses for a schizophrenic patient are Alterations in Perception and Alteration in Thought Processes.
56. Two aspects of the nurse's role in discharge planning are assessing factors related to the precipitating crisis and relapse, with the purpose of formulating the discharge plan, and establishing a working relationship with the patient and family.
57. Community living options are an important consideration in discharge planning for schizophrenics because periods of hospitalization are shorter today and dependence on a wide assortment of aftercare and rehabilitation services has increased, with large numbers of psychiatrically impaired persons returning to their families.
58. Antipsychotic treatment is used to enable the patient to exert self-control, to relieve specific symptoms of psychosis, and to improve the patient's self-care ability.
59. Antiparkinsonian drugs are used to treat tremors and akathisia caused by antipsychotic drugs.
60. The benefits of teaching patients and families to identify the early signs of illness exacerbation are that these signs will facilitate efforts to initiate restabilization. Furthermore, by helping the family and the patient to identify the individual pattern and to notify the outpatient therapist as soon as possible, a relapse can be prevented.
61. Prodromes can be treated with neuroleptics and increased psychosocial support.
62. Supportive counseling focuses on strengths, increasing coping and problem-solving skills, offering affirmation, long-term concern, hopefulness, and commitment.
63. Insight-oriented therapy is inappropriate for the schizophrenic because it is too stressful and because the illness is biologically based.
64. Two purposes of family education regarding schizophrenics are to increase the stability and predictability of family life by decreasing the family's guilt and anxiety and to increase self-confidence.
65. Two topics covered in a psychoeducational group are schizophrenia and medication side effects and communication.
66. An effective treatment program for dually diagnosed patients is directed toward both conditions. You may need to function more as a coach to the patient in a nonjudgmental relationship and extinguish maladaptive ones, with emphasis on the positive steps that the patient has made.
67. A group psychoeducational approach for the dually diagnosed patient is to combine education and support about schizophrenia and the complications of substance abuse. Group support may help the patient to make a behavioral change and may help to reduce loneliness and provide concrete encouragement, not only for the patient but also for his or her family.

68. It is essential to provide spiritual interventions in the care of the schizophrenic because this component focuses on the meaning of the illness in the patient as well as the patient's relationship with God.
69. During the evaluation process, one should recognize that schizophrenia is a chronic illness; therefore, an exacerbation of the illness should not be viewed as a treatment failure, since chronic illnesses are episodic, with remissions and exacerbations.

CHAPTER 30

1. The symptoms of depression include feelings of unbearable sadness or irritability, despair, and hopelessness. People with depression frequently desire suicide and may have disturbances in emotional, cognitive, behavioral, somatic, and spiritual dimensions.
2. The symptoms of mania include excitement, elation, or extreme irritability. People with mania have disturbances in emotional, cognitive, behavioral, somatic, and spiritual dimensions.
3. Mood refers to a person's pervasive feeling state.
4. *Affect* refers to the feelings that are reflected on our faces, in our expressions, and by our demeanor.
5. The central issue is whether the patient is experiencing a persistent change in mood, self-attitude, and vital sense.
6. Bipolar I disorder is a major mood disorder characterized by major depression and mania or hypomania. It requires one or more episodes of mania. Bipolar II disorder requires the presence of a major depressive episode accompanied by at least one hypomanic episode. The presence of a manic episode or a mixed episode excludes the diagnosis of bipolar II disorder.
7. A seasonal affective pattern describes a variation of mood disorder typically characterized by depression occurring in the fall and winter and normal moods in the spring and summer.
8. Rapid cycling is characterized by four episodes of a mood disturbance occurring in the previous 12 months and meeting the criteria for major de pressive disorder, manic episode, mixed episode, or hypomanic episodes.
9. Research shows a relationship between sleep and mood, in that one of the hallmarks of major depression is sleep disturbance.
10. Three drugs implicated in causing depression are steroids, oral contraceptives, and sedatives and minor tranquilizers.
11. According to psychoanalytical theory, depression is caused by anger turned inward after a real or perceived loss.
12. According to the cognitive model, people with depression think and process information in negative ways. This thinking develops over time as the person experiences stress in life. Early stress seems to shape the development of cognitive patterns in a negative self-referring manner.
13. According to the interpersonal model, a relationship exists between depression and current interpersonal functioning. Multiple interpersonal factors that are important in the development of depression are unsatisfactory early interpersonal experiences, stresses in current interpersonal relationships, and lack of supportive relationships.
14. Five areas to assess in a patient with a mood disorder are the patient's feelings, attitudes, and knowledge about the illness; the degree and intensity of suicidal thinking and the potential risk for suicide; the family's feelings, attitudes, and knowledge about the illness; issues of powerlessness; and spiritual concerns such as hopelessness.
15. Three negative feelings expressed by patients suffering from mood disorders are shame, humiliation, and denial.
16. In regard to suicide risk, you assess whether or not the patient is currently suicidal, if he or she has a plan, and the lethality of the plan.
17. Powerlessness is an important issue because when illness develops, the sense of control over one's life may be threatened. People's responses to the stress of illness depend on personal characteristics and social resources.
18. Five nursing diagnoses that might be appropriate for a depressed patient are Risk for Self-Directed Violence, Self-Esteem Disturbance, Powerlessness, Spiritual Distress, and Social Isolation. Five nursing diagnoses that might be appropriate for a manic patient are Risk for Injury, Risk for Violence: Self-Directed or Directed at Others, Altered Nutrition: Less Than Body Requirements, Sensory/Perceptual Alterations, and Sleep Pattern Disturbance.
19. Three expected outcomes for a patient with depression are that the patient will remain free from self-inflicted harm, be free of psychotic symptoms, and demonstrate functional behavior in activities of daily living. Three expected outcomes for the patient with mania are that the patient will remain free from self-inflicted harm; be free of restlessness, hyperactivity, and agitation; and demonstrate behaviors indicating feelings of self-worth.
20. Three short-term goals for a patient with depression are that the patient will be free of self-inflicted harm; be oriented to person, place, and time; and express feelings.
21. In the role of counselor, you would teach a person alternative ways to handle stress, explore how the illness affects the person's life, deal with the issue of denial, provide a safe place to express feelings of anger and shame and to work toward acceptance, and educate about the illness and its medical basis.
22. You would teach the patient and/or family about the causes, characteristics, and appropriate treatments for the mood disorders.
23. You collaborate with the patient and family by assisting family members to know how to help the patient and how to pull together. You affirm family efforts on behalf of the patient, make suggestions for their continued well-being, provide information so that family members can be more effective, and invite them to collaborate in planning the patient's care.
24. Empowerment is a social process of recognizing, promoting, and enhancing people's abilities to meet their own needs, solve their own problems, and mobilize necessary resources to take control of their own lives.
25. You can facilitate empowerment through knowledge, confidence, and communication skills.
26. You can facilitate spiritual growth in a patient by encouraging and supporting his or her faith and convictions about life and God and the will to live.
27. The nurse can collaborate with support groups by making referrals, serving on professional advisory boards, serving as a consultant to existing groups, and initiating and working in the development of new mutual help groups.
28. Before a patient receives ECT, your role is to teach the patient and family about the risks and benefits of ECT, to offer handouts that might include a guide to ECT, and to encourage the exchange of information between patients and family members about their experiences with ECT.
29. In a formative evaluation, you would review whether the patient remained safe or made suicide attempts and, if so, how the plan needs to be modified; whether the patient "connected" with a caring professional; whether the patient reestablished balance in eating, sleeping, and activity; whether the patient feels better; whether the patient verbalizes understanding of medication and illness issues; whether the patient is participating in therapy and if the family is involved in care; and whether the patient has begun to address the spiritual components of the illness.
30. In a summative evaluation, it would be important to consider issues such as discharge planning, referral to a support group, continuation of therapy, and the patient's ability to establish realistic goals.

CHAPTER 31

1. Drug abuse and chemical dependency differ, in that the former represents a voluntary behavior and the latter does not.
2. The historical context of substance use disorders provides the background to understand the multifaceted nature of substance use disorders.
3. Genetic factors contribute to the development of alcoholism, but their precise levels and influence differ related to gender, age of onset, and severity of the disorder. More evidence of genetic contributions has been found with males and in early-onset and severe drinking patterns.
4. The distinguishing characteristics of substance dependence vary with the agent involved. Physical and psychological dependence are both important to the understanding of substance use disorders. People who are considered to have a substance use dependency are sometimes called chemically dependent.
5. Alcohol compromises a person's life journey through its physical and psychological effects. Alcoholism is the third leading cause of death, and cirrhosis, its most common sequela, is the fifth cause of death in the United States. Physically, chronic alcoholism affects every organ in the body. At toxic levels, psychological symptoms include marked alterations in sensory perceptions. Chronic alcohol use can cause irreversible brain damage. Alcoholism also can disrupt family, social, and work relationships.
6. Cocaine addiction is difficult to treat because of its "reinforcing" properties. Cocaine is known as one of the most powerful reinforcers and habit-forming drugs. Patients experiencing withdrawal complain of craving as one of the main symptoms. With cocaine, psychological dependence is associated with the reinforcing property of craving, whereby the person experiences an insatiable compulsive desire for more cocaine.
7. The implications for women who have a substance use disorder are that they often have secondary social problems; a higher incidence of abuse, incest, and exploitation has been reported among these women. These women are more likely to become prostitutes when they have a chemical dependency, and this increases their risk of getting AIDS and other sexually transmitted diseases. Treatment issues are also more complicated because physicians tend to overlook substance use disorders as a primary diagnosis in women.
8. Substance use affects pregnancy, in that all psychoactive drugs cross the placenta, and most are capable of causing serious teratogenic effects in the fetus. In the United States, approximately 2.6 million of the babies born each year will have had exposure to alcohol, and 1 baby in 100 will demonstrate clinical teratogenic effects. Heavy drinking increases the risk of miscarriage and stillbirth. Excessive alcohol consumption can lead to the development of fetal alcohol syndrome in the newborn infant. Regular cocaine use contributes to abruptio placentae, miscarriage, and premature birth. Opiates compromise infant birth and cause withdrawal symptoms in the newborn.
9. Important considerations in the nursing care of adolescents with substance use disorders are that developmental arrest occurs with psychoactive disorders at the point when chemical dependency begins, and psychosocial skills fall behind when the adolescent stops maturing developmentally. These adolescents can eventually become unemployed high school dropouts with easy access to drugs, higher levels of stress, and lower conformity to social norms.

CHAPTER 32

1. Three behaviors necessary to a healthy personality are to balance work and play, to identify "self" as the total of strengths and weaknesses, and to express spirituality.
2. The autistic phase of development is that during which the neonate (1 to 2 months old) was encased in a self-absorbed barrier with no recognition of others.
3. Mahler and associates identified the rapprochement subphase as an important stage in the development of borderline personality disorder because the mother is either too emotionally distant from the child or clings excessively to a child who needs to explore the environment.
4. Biological tests have been applied to people with personality disorders. The current focus is on cognitive-perceptual organization, affective regulation, impulse control, and anxiety or social inhibition as well as on genetic studies and research on the role of neurotransmitters in personality disorders.
5. Stanley and Stanley noted changes in both pre- and postsynaptic serotonergic binding sites in people who were examined after suicide.
6. A person must demonstrate this pattern to have a personality disorder (as defined in *DSM-IV*). The person who demonstrates a long-term pattern of thoughts and behaviors that vary markedly from the expectations of their culture may have a personality disorder.
7. Three behavioral or thought patterns exhibited by patients with personality disorder are related to cognition or thought pattern—the person has different ways of perceiving and interpreting self, others, and events in the environment; to affect—the person displays a range, intensity, lability, and appropriateness of emotional response different from those in the same cultural group; and to interpersonal functioning—people with a personality disorder experience more difficulty socializing and maintaining friendships, work relationships, and marital relationships than others in the cultural group.
8. Someone with a schizotypal personality might be considered odd because cognitive and/or perceptual distortions and eccentricities are apparent in his or her behavior, and the person has ideas of reference.
9. Someone with a paranoid personality disorder displays a pattern of distrust and suspiciousness of others, beginning by early adulthood.
10. Someone with a schizoid personality disorder has a pervasive pattern of detachment from social relationships and a restricted range of expression of emotions, particularly in interpersonal settings, beginning by early adulthood.
11. Someone with an antisocial personality disorder has a pervasive pattern of disregard for and violation of the rights of others. The person with a borderline personality disorder has a pervasive pattern of unstable interpersonal relationships, difficulty defining self and determining self-image, labile affect and/or mood, and marked impulsive behavior, beginning by early adulthood.
12. Someone with a borderline personality disorder is often evaluated in the emergency department for suicidal ideation and/or gestures and self-mutilating behavior.
13. One characteristic of the avoidant personality disorder is avoidance of any occupational activities involving significant interpersonal contact. One characteristic of the dependent personality disorder is difficulty initiating projects or doing things independently. One characteristic of the obsessive-compulsive personality disorder is preoccupation with details, rules, lists, organization, or schedules to the extent that the major reason for an activity is lost.
14. You could ask the patient whether he or she has different views of the world than most people and, if so, to describe them.
15. You could determine that the patient demonstrates an enduring pattern of inflexible behavior by evaluating whether the patterns of relating, emotions, behavior and thought occurred over time and were a stable part of the patient's responses to the world.
16. An example of an assessment question that you might ask to determine the quality of a patient's relationships is "Tell me about your relationships with others."
17. One expected outcome for Joanne is that she will recognize what behaviors are evidence of defensive coping and begin to identify a pattern of that behavior. An expected outcome for Martin is that he

will be able to identify when he is critical of himself and others. With this information, he can begin to determine the cause of the criticism and plan other ways to solve the problems that elicited the critical behavior.

18. One must note that the patient with a personality disorder has behaviors that are stable and of long duration and, consequently, hard to modify. Treatment is slow, and you must be patient.
19. An example of counseling as a nursing intervention is assisting the patient to interpret the environmental stimuli in the therapy room.
20. Limit-setting can encourage patient learning by assisting the patient to explore a lifelong behavioral pattern.

CHAPTER 33

1. The term "dissociation" was first coined by Pierre Janet.
2. Freud described dissociation as a type of repression employed in the excision of threatening or unacceptable mental contents from conscious awareness.
3. An example of a minor dissociation associated with normal life is daydreaming.
4. The Dissociative Experiences Scale (DES) is used to determine the degree of dissociation used by a particular individual.
5. Two psychiatric illnesses that may include dissociative experiences are anxiety and substance abuse disorders.
6. The five hallmark symptoms of dissociative disorders are amnesia, derealization, depersonalization, identity confusion, and identity alteration.
7. The major symptom of amnesia is memory loss related to personal data or events occurring during a specific period or even a loss of all past memories. Derealization occurs when objects in the external world take on a quality of unreality and estrangement. Thus, familiar people and places are perceived as unfamiliar and unreal. Depersonalization is an alteration in the perception or experience of the self; one's usual sense of relatedness to the rest of the world is temporarily lost or changed. With identity confusion, a subjective sense of conflict, puzzlement, or uncertainty occurs in relation to one's identity, usually accompanied by significant distress. Identity alteration is an organized shift in one's personality, including the way one relates to others, character traits, knowledge, and preferences. It occurs without the individual's awareness.
8. Dissociative amnesia pertains to a person suffering from the sudden inability to access information that already has been stored in his or her memory bank. Dissociative fugue is when a person wanders, sometimes far from home, and may assume a completely new identity for an indefinite period of time. The patient is unaware of having forgotten anything. Depersonalization disorder is characterized by a recurrent or persistent change in the quality of self-awareness. One's own sense of reality may be temporarily lost. Dissociative identity disorder is characterized by the existence of two or more personality states that can take full control of the person's behavior, accompanied by an inability to remember significant personal information. Dissociative disorders not otherwise specified constitute a dissociation syndrome that does not meet the criteria for the other types.
9. The most controversial of all psychiatric disorders is the dissociative identity disorder (previously known as multiple personality disorder).
10. Assess for dissociative symptoms, assess the patient's perception of reality, collect subjective and objective data, and perform a careful physical assessment.
11. Two nursing diagnoses appropriate to a patient with a dissociative disorder are ineffective individual coping and altered role performance.
12. The primary expected outcome for a patient with a dissociative disorder is that he or she will develop new, more adaptive ways of coping with stress.
13. Two interventions that can be used with a patient with a dissociative disorder are to initiate and develop a trusting relationship with the patient and to help the patient determine what is real and what is not.

CHAPTER 34

1. Sex refers to whether the person is anatomically male or female.
2. Sexual identity is the identification of oneself as being male or female, the process of developing social traits of masculinity or femininity, and the unfolding of the socially appropriate eroticism. Gender identity is the earliest acquisition of the basic sense of maleness or femaleness, which occurs normally during the first 18 months of life.
3. A person is gender dysphoric if he or she has a sense of discomfort because he or she feels his or her sex and gender differ.
4. Gender refers to the person's psychological reaction to or sense of being male or female.
5. The desire phase is characterized by the desire for sexual activity. It is the period during which sexual tension rises from the preceding level of sexual desire to the relatively high sexual tension levels that merge into the following plateau phase.
6. During orgasm, sexual tension is produced by a combination of mental activity and erotic stimulation of erogenous areas. It may be described as a neurophysiological event with accompanying release of erotic tension. In women, a sudden surge of sexual tension and an equally sudden release of sexual tension occur. In men, pooling of seminal fluid in the proximal urethra is caused by contractions of the prostate, seminal vesicles, and vas deferens, followed by a sensation of ejaculatory inevitability.
7. The plateau phase is a waiting period between the development of sexual excitement and the onset of orgasm. It is characterized by increases in muscle tone, heart rate, blood pressure, and respiratory rate, and a sex flush.
8. During the desire phase, dysfunctions that can occur are hypoactive sexual desire disorder, sexual aversion disorder, female sexual arousal disorder, and male erectile disorder.
9. Three causes of erectile dysfunction (impotence) are prescribed or illicit drug use, acute or chronic medical illness, and structural defects of the genitalia and hormonal disturbances.
10. Impotence refers to an erectile dysfunction due to difficulty achieving and maintaining an erection. It may be caused by medical illness, surgery, injury, anatomical defects, acute infection, medication side effects, and psychological causes. Infertility is caused by the sperm cells being unviable and by their inability to reach and penetrate the ovum.
11. Erectile dysfunction is typically associated with feelings of discomfort.
12. Three medical conditions associated with impotence are diabetes, hypertension, and cardiac disease.
13. Primary anorgasmia is when the patient has never experienced orgasm, either during intercourse of adequate duration or during masturbation.
14. Secondary anorgasmia (called situational anorgasmia) occurs if the patient had reported anorgasmia only during the time of a depression or in relation to the physiological effects of a substance or a general medical condition.

15. The most common cause of primary anorgasmia is sexual abuse.
16. The interventions used to treat anorgasmia are behavior modification and sex education.
17. A paraphilia is a repetitive or preferred sexual fantasy or behavior that involves the preference for use of a nonhuman object, repetitive sexual activity with humans involving real or simulated suffering or humiliation, and repetitive sexual activity with nonconsenting partners.
18. Three types of paraphilias are exhibitionism, fetishism, and frotteurism.
19. Two possible etiological explanations for the paraphilias are abnormalities in the limbic system and temporal lobes of the brain and abnormal levels of androgens.
20. When the etiology is considered to be physiological, treatment for the paraphilias might include blocking or decreasing the level of circulating androgens or treating with an antidepressant (e.g., fluoxetine [Prozac]) or a mood stabilizer (e.g., lithium).
21. Two characteristics of childhood gender identity disorder are a repeatedly stated desire to be, or insistence that he or she is, the opposite sex and a strong preference for playmates of the opposite sex.
22. Two characteristics of adolescent gender identity disorder are a desire to live or be treated as the opposite sex and the conviction that he or she has the typical feelings and reactions of the opposite sex.
23. Two characteristics of adult gender identity disorder are that the person has persistent discomfort with his or her sex and frequently masquerades as the opposite sex.
24. Obligatory homosexuality is when erotic and sexual desires are uniformly directed toward members of the same sex.
25. In situational homosexuality, erotic and sexual desire are directed toward members of the same sex only in certain situations, such as long-term confinement in same-sex institutions like prisons.
26. The biological theory of homosexuality is that homosexual orientation may be inherited genetically.
27. According to Bieber, the mother dominates both father and son; is overprotective, possessive, and seductive in her interactions with her son; and is demeaning toward the father.
28. The usual goals of treatment when homosexuals seek therapy are to help patients to deal with the social stigma associated with homosexual behavior, exploring psychological conflicts, helping patients foster healthy relationships, teaching patients how to avoid infection with the human immunodeficiency virus and other sexually transmitted organisms, and generally facilitating the efforts of patients to live emotionally satisfying lives.
29. The connection between head trauma and sexual problems is that patients who have experienced head trauma with damage to the frontal lobe of the brain may display symptoms of promiscuity, poor judgment, inability to recognize triggers that set off sexual desires, and poor impulse control.
30. With psychotic behavior, sexual functioning may be adversely affected. This is especially true for schizophrenic patients who have difficulty coping with stress, a decrease in reality-based orientation to the world, and defense mechanisms that lead to withdrawn behavior.
31. Klinefelter's syndrome is a condition found on genetic examination, in which the patient has an extra X chromosome in his genetic make-up. This produces a situation in which a male displays immature physical sex characteristics and psychological symptoms.
32. The setting for a sexual assessment is one that allows for privacy and an absence of distractions. The interview is free from personal biases and judgmental attitudes.
33. One nursing diagnosis for a sexual dysfunction is Sexual Dysfunction Related to Marital Problems evidenced in painful intercourse and inability to have orgasm.
34. Medroxyprogesterone acetate (Depo-Provera) is used with sexual disorders such as pedophilia to decrease sexual urges and assist in controlling the offending sexual behavior.
35. Two interventions used with patients with sexual disorders are milieu therapy and psychotherapy.

CHAPTER 35

1. Three characteristics of anorexia nervosa are refusal to eat, emaciation, and amenorrhea.
2. Three roles that food plays in our lives are to provide nutrition, to reward achievement and punish misbehaviors, and to provide a feeling of comfort, support, and love.
3. Bulimia nervosa is characterized by repeated episodes of binging and purging.
4. A binge eating disorder is characterized by excessive intake of calories.
5. Anorexia nervosa is a potentially life-threatening illness in which young adolescents literally starve themselves to death. Anorexia nervosa has a mortality rate of 5% to 18%. Bulimia nervosa is also associated with life-threatening consequences, such as severe electrolyte imbalances including hypokalemia, which can lead to cardiac arrhythmias and cardiac arrest.
6. The hypothesized role of serotonin in anorexia nervosa is that serotonin inhibits food intake and acts as a satiety agent. Some evidence supports a link between genetics and eating disorders.
7. Twin studies demonstrate a higher incidence of eating disorders in monozygotic twins than in dizygotic twins. Mothers and sisters of anorexics have a higher incidence of anorexia than sisters of controls.
8. Psychological issues that may be part of the picture in the development of eating disorders are the issues of self-esteem and perfectionism. The psychological characteristics of an anorexic are that she or he is well behaved, eager to please, not consciously willing to be singled out for attention, and a perfectionist; that she or he has poor self-image; that she or he is dependent on the opinions of others; and that she or he is dependent. People with bulimia often feel tense and anxious before they binge. Bulimia has been seen in combination with borderline personality disorder. People with binge-eating disorder use food as a substitute for relationships that are not working or do not exist and attain some sense of comfort from gorging food.
9. Spiritual issues play into the etiology of eating disorders, in that for some anorexics, religious influences may accentuate their drive to be perfect. The anorexic may rationalize her behavior as a spiritual act of devotion. The bulimic patient's superstitious and insecure thinking spills over into her view of spirituality and has been equated in some patients with a spiritual cleansing of evil. Compulsive overeaters use eating as a coping mechanism to deal with the emptiness or absence of a spiritual reality in their lives.
10. Family issues in eating disorders include the fact that mother-daughter and parental relationships and the role that the eating-disordered person plays in the family have an impact on the development and maintenance of the eating disorder.
11. The anorexic patient frequently has hypotension.
12. Two areas in which anorexics and bulimics differ are that the anorexic tends to use greater denial than the bulimic—not only denying hunger but also denying that he or she has a problem at all—while the bulimic usually is aware of her or his problem and is distressed about it and that the family environment of the anorexic is more controlled, rigid, and marked by less overt discord, whereas the family environment of the bulimic is marked by conflict and chaos, with violence and substance abuse being the norm.
13. You would want to know the bulimic's pattern of eating; where she or he eats; whether she or he engages in binge-purge cycles of eating and, if so, how she or he feels about this pattern; where she or he binges; whether she or he purges; whether she or he eats, binges, and purges in secret; whether the patient fasts; how often she or he engages in these behaviors; and whether she or he takes amphetamines, diet pills, or caffeine pills to lose weight.
14. Society's message is that "you can never be too thin," and this can impact on people with eating disorders.

15. One expected outcome for a patient with an eating disorder is that the patient will express an accurate appraisal of body size and body weight.
16. One short-term goal to support the expected outcome is that the patient will eat a balanced diet.
17. Two physical symptoms that would lead to inpatient treatment of an anorexic are heart rate less than 40 beats per minute and weight loss greater than 30% of body weight over 3 months. Two psychiatric symptoms are severe depression and high risk for suicide.
18. One benefit of outpatient therapy for a patient with an eating disorder is that this environment is the least restrictive.
19. One nursing diagnosis that might be applied to a patient with an eating disorder is Altered Nutrition: Less than Body Requirements.
20. Two intervention strategies are behavior modification and family therapy.
21. One psychotropic medication used in the treatment of anorexia is fluoxetine (Prozac), an antidepressant.
22. The goal of family therapy is to transform the issue of an anorexic patient to that of a dysfunctional family.

CHAPTER 36

1. Life balance refers to the interaction among the physical, psychological, social, and spiritual variables in each of our lives that keep us feeling well and that allow us to believe that life is generally good.
2. Indirect self-destructive behavior refers to activities that are potentially detrimental to a person's physical, psychological, social, and spiritual well-being. These behaviors may result in death but without the person's conscious intent or awareness.
3. Indirect self-destructive behavior differs from direct self-destructive behavior in that indirect behavior arises without the person being aware of what he or she is doing, whereas with direct behavior, the person has an awareness of the desired outcome.
4. Suicidal behavior is direct self-destructive behavior for the expressed purpose of killing oneself. However, indirect self-destructive behaviors also may result in death.
5. The eighth cause of death in the United States is suicide.
6. Women tend to make more suicide gestures than men.
7. Single white men are at highest risk for completing suicide.
8. You need to do a suicide assessment on a patient diagnosed with schizophrenia because many of these patients experience hopelessness about the chronicity of their illness and do not always communicate their suicidal intent or plan.
9. Depression, delusions, guilt, paranoid thoughts, and social withdrawal, along with bipolar disorder, schizophrenia, and substance disorders result in a high risk for completed suicide.
10. Some patients self-mutilate because they have a history of being neglected and sexually and physically abused as children.
11. "Aggression turned inward" provides a way of understanding suicide, in that the person may turn aggression against the self rather than on the person for whom it was intended.
12. The social and cultural context in which a person lives contributes to an understanding of suicide behavior, in that the person is integrally linked to the quality of community life. In an egotistical suicide, a person's ties to the community are too loose or tenuous, and the person does not respond to the usual social constraints on behavior. In an anomic suicide, the person experiences the aloneness or estrangement that comes as a result of a precipitous deterioration in his or her relationship with society. In a fatalistic suicide, the person feels that he or she is excessively regulated. In altruistic suicide, rules or customs demand suicide under certain situations.
13. The "spirit of life" is the life essence. According to Frankl, it is intricately tied to meaning and purpose in life, as well as to hope. Frankl claims that when people find life meaningless and without purpose, they have no reason to live.
14. If a risk is present in the physical domain, you would ask a patient about his or her thoughts about the illness and the impact that the illness has on his or her life. You would ask the patient to describe the pain and state whether the pain is more difficult to handle at certain times. You would also ask if the patient has noticed changes in his or her concentration, appetite, energy level, interest in sex, or need for sleep.
15. In the emotional domain, questions about feelings of despair and hopelessness are expressed through a suicide plan.
16. In the cognitive domain, it is important to determine how often the patient thinks about suicide or a suicide plan. You should ask if the patient is preoccupied with himself or herself, what is the patient's view of the problems that are overwhelming him or her, and whether the patient has insight into the problem areas of his or her behavior. You also could ask if the patient's judgment is clouded with intrusive thoughts of suicide and if he or she focuses on negative themes to the exclusion of other, more positive, thoughts.
17. In the social domain, it is important to determine the patient's level of suicidal ideation because often people who are suicidal feel a lack of social support.
18. Three indicators present when a patient has severe thoughts of suicide are intense anger, devastating depression, and profound feelings of hopelessness and loss of life's meaning and purpose.
19. A nursing diagnosis that might be appropriate for a patient who has threatened to slash his or her wrists is Risk for Violence: Self-Directed.
20. Two expected outcomes for the patient who is at risk for self-mutilation or suicide are that the patient will remain free from self-harm while maintaining the highest degree of autonomy that is possible and that the patient will not exhibit suicidal or self-mutilative behaviors.
21. A short-term goal for a patient whose expected outcome is that he or she "will remain free from self-harm while maintaining the highest degree of autonomy possible" is that the patient will sign a no-harm contract.
22. The indications for hospitalization for a patient with suicidal ideas are that the patient is unable to make future plans or engage in problem-solving, including not being able to effectively structure time for meaningful activity.
23. It is appropriate to utilize checks every 15 minutes to ensure patient safety if the patient demonstrates less lethal thoughts of suicide with no explicit plan and is still able to engage in problem-solving. The patient signs a no-harm contract.
24. It is appropriate to place a patient on one-to-one supervision if the patient has a suicide plan, has been thinking about a note that he or she wants to leave behind, has a means to carry out the suicide plan, has no plans for the future, and is hesitant to write a no-harm contract or will not sign a no-harm contract.
25. You can avoid being "drained" by patients who are suicidal and who self-mutilate by attending a staff meeting to discuss each patient's care and the feelings of staff members about the behavior. You can also maintain a positive life balance by integrating work, play, spiritual beliefs, and exercise.
26. It is appropriate to evaluate the nursing care of a patient who is suicidal or self-mutilating in a formative evaluation to provide information about the patient's progress, deficiencies, and reasons for not having benefited from the implementation of the plan. The evaluation of care for a patient with suicidal ideation should be done on an ongoing routine basis to decrease mistakes or omissions made due to predictions of the patient's behavior based on your emotional response to the behavior.
27. This evaluation should take place daily, and be communicated during change of shift report.
28. When the nursing interventions are not helping the patient achieve the desired outcomes, a peer review by a nurse who is interested in the patient's problem may be helpful. Also, a review of current literature can assist in planning and implementing nursing care.

CHAPTER 37

1. The theory of homeostasis views the body as a self-regulating machine designed to remain in balance through internal feedback.
2. Selye described the general adaptation syndrome, which involves adrenal gland enlargement, thymus involution, and gastrointestinal ulceration as a triad of pathological consequences of prolonged stress.
3. Factors within the individual that interact to either decrease or increase responsivity to stress involve age, sex, socioeconomic status, occupation, education, and fitness.
4. The mediating factors that either diminish or attenuate responsivity to stress are coping (diminishes the person's responsiveness to stress) and conflict (attenuates the person's responsiveness to stress).
5. The assessment includes the use of psychometric instruments to answer specific questions about the psychological status of the patient and to quantify the client's health status and allow for objective comparison with other clients.
6. The Life Experience Survey is used to evaluate a person's assessment of life stresses experienced during the preceding year.
7. The Minnesota Multiphasic Personality Inventory is a 566-item true-false questionnaire with 10 basic clinical scales. It is the most thoroughly researched personality instrument available.
8. The two components of the Spiritual Well-Being Scale are the Religious Well-Being (RWB) and the Existential Well-Being (EWB) subscales. The RWB measures the individual's well-being in relationship to God. The EWB measures the individual's well-being in relation to a personal sense of life's meaning and significance.
9. Depression often accompanies lower back pain because of the physical pain and because of limitations in activities of daily living.
10. Cognitive-behavioral treatments include biofeedback, relaxation, exercise, and diet. Those techniques can be used to help decrease anxiety and muscle spasm.
11. Chronic pelvic pain is nonmenstrual pelvic pain of greater than six months' duration and may be intermittent or continuous.
12. Two of the psychiatric disorders that are commonly associated with chronic pelvic pain are depression and somatization.
13. The psychological treatment for chronic pelvic pain includes stress management, relaxation, cognitive therapy, spiritual support, and sexual education.
14. Two of the symptoms of IBS are abdominal pain relieved with a bowel movement and abdominal pain associated with a change in either the frequency or texture of the stool. These symptoms must be present for at least three months.
15. Psychological stress plays a role in the etiology and recurrence of IBS, in that people who experience IBS and psychological symptoms are more likely to consult a health care provider than are patients with IBS symptoms only.
16. Two of the treatment approaches used with IBS patients are insight-oriented psychotherapy, and relaxation-based stress management training.
17. The theory of hyperreactivity states that excessive reactivity in blood pressure to all environmental stimuli initiates and maintains essential hypertension.
18. Anger (suppressed and expressed) is positively related to hypertension.
19. Speech is also related to increased blood pressure reactivity and/or hypertension.
20. Two of the behavioral and psychological approaches to the treatment of hypertension are psychotherapy and biofeedback.
21. Two precipitants of migraine headaches are stress and certain foods and alcohol.
22. Levels of serotonin fall during a migraine. This causes constriction of large vessels in the external carotid tree and dilatation of small vessels.
23. Levels of norepinephrine rise during a migraine, causing vasoconstriction in the peripheral vascular bed.
24. The most widely used nonpharmacological treatment for migraine headaches is relaxation training, combined with thermal biofeedback.
25. Two foods that are associated with migraines are hard cheeses (high in tyramine) and chocolate (containing phenylethylamine).
26. Temporomandibular joint syndrome (TMJ) is chronic or intermittent pain in the face, neck, and/or ears, which is the result of a problem in the mandibular joint, caused by a variety of muscular, nerve, and orthodontic problems.
27. Stress leads to clenching the jaw and "grinding" the teeth and has been found to be the origin of some of the pain associated with TMJ.
28. Two of the treatment approaches used with TMJ involve resting the joint and relaxing the muscles through the use of local heat and nonsteroidal antiinflammatory and muscle-relaxing drugs.
29. La belle indifference refers to calmness and relative lack of concern in a person with a conversion disorder.
30. A conversion disorder is the presentation of an alteration or loss of a sensory-motor function that is not the result of a physiological disorder.
31. The characteristics of a somatoform disorder are disorders in which the individual presents with physical symptoms, suggesting physiological etiology. They are classified as psychiatric disorders.
32. Body dysmorphic disorder (dysmorphophobia) is the preoccupation with an imagined flaw in appearance in a normal-appearing person.
33. Three areas to assess in patients with psychopathological illnesses are physiological problems, psychosocial problems, and spiritual problems.

CHAPTER 38

1. Wernicke's aphasia (also called receptive aphasia) involves damage to the left temporal lobe, causing a person's inability to understand language and to use words in a meaningful way. Broca's aphasia involves damage to the left frontal lobe, resulting in an impaired use of expressive language. A person with this problem struggles to form words without much success.
2. Dementia is considered a syndrome because it describes chronic cognitive disorders with multiple etiologies (cognitive disorders are not thought of as a syndrome rather than as a specific disease).
3. The *DSM-IV* now classifies acute and chronic cognitive disorders, each as a unit, with delirium and dementia due to multiple etiologies. This is important to mental health nursing, as these disorders are classified as an explicit syndrome of behaviors rather than as a single disease.
4. The common characteristics of delirium are reduced level of consciousness, perceptual disturbances, disturbance of sleep-wake cycle with insomnia or daytime sleepiness; increased or decreased psychomotor activity; disorientation to time, place, or person; memory impairment; disorganized thinking; reduced ability to maintain attention to external stimuli; hallucinations; and illusions.
5. An accurate diagnosis is important because it can mean the difference between life and death.
6. As a nurse, you would try to contain the patient's anxiety by maintaining a nonanxious presence and a consistent approach. You should use a minimum of simple, concrete words spoken in a calm, low, but authoritative voice. The patient needs clear boundaries, reduced environmental stimuli, minimized perceptual distortions, and medication (if the patient is out of control). Eliminate causal factors and manage aggressive behavior.
7. The medication most useful for delirium is a high-potency neuroleptic, such as haloperidol, to reduce tension. This drug has fewer sedative, cardiotoxic, hypotensive, and anticholinergic effects and is less likely to decrease the seizure threshold.
8. The first nursing action in the treatment of delirium is to stabilize the patient medically. Nursing interventions are oriented toward

behavior and symptom reduction, once the patient's physical condition is secure.

9. In contrast to delirium, which responds to treatment, dementia is a degenerative neurological disorder that invariably worsens and always ends in death. Dementia has a slow, insidious onset, with gradual deterioration of cognitive, mental, and physical neurological systems. Delirium represents acute forms of cognitive disorders characterized by abrupt onset, fluctuation in level of consciousness, disorientation, and an identifiable physical cause.
10. Vascular dementia presents with a stepwise progression—not the steady decline of Alzheimer's disease. The onset of vascular dementia is more abrupt, and the patient displays a fluctuating course of symptom development.
11. Sundowning describes increased confusion and agitation noted in many dementia patients occurring during the late afternoon and early evening hours. You can reduce its effects by keeping the patient active during the earlier day so that stimuli are reduced during the period traditionally associated with sundowning. Medications are helpful adjuncts to treatment and should be given at the beginning of the episode for maximum effectiveness.
12. Restraints are used only as a last resort and only for specific short periods. Each time patients are restrained, they lose a part of their personal freedom and their sense of themselves as people. Patients do not understand the reason for the restraint. Patients in restraints are more prone to develop contracture formation and decubiti. Restraints can be used selectively to provide the patient with scheduled periods of respite from the constant pacing and agitation related to dementia.
13. Your role in the care of the patient during the end stage of dementia centers on keeping the patient comfortable, nourished, and hydrated.
14. Support groups are helpful in the treatment of dementia patients and their families because they are a protected, supportive place and time in which the caregiver can receive needed nurturance. Family members learn what things to expect and excellent tips on how to make things go more easily. The group supports the caregiver's right to express feelings about the patient and the burden of caregiving in a safe environment where people understand and accept the feelings.
15. Some common concerns of family caregivers at different stages of dementia involve end-of-life decisions, financial matters, quality of life, access to community resources, and behavior management.

CHAPTER 39

1. The "old homeless" include tramps, hoboes, and skid row dwellers who left home as young men to escape economically depressed hometowns and who traveled around to find jobs. The "new homeless" consist of men, women, and children without shelter who sleep on steam grates, in abandoned cars, or in cardboard boxes.
2. The five phases in the history of homelessness are the preindustrial period, the early industrial period, the period beginning with the colonization of the undeveloped world that still exists today, the era of modern industrialization, and deindustrialization and a shift to a service economy.
3. Homelessness, not having a permanent home, results from a complex set of personal and structural factors. It has existed throughout history. Homelessness can be defined differently depending on whether the affected populations are the "old homeless" or the "new homeless."
4. Chronic mental illness predisposes a client to homelessness because of deinstitutionalization. Many chronically mentally ill patients were essentially abandoned to their own devices and became homeless.
5. Social ties are jeopardized for homeless substance abusers because family and friend networks are often broken as alcohol and/or drug use becomes a prominent feature of daily existence.
6. The chronically mentally ill are vulnerable to homelessness because they display poor interpersonal skills, inadequate problem-solving strategies, disorganized thinking, and an inability to tend to their own needs. They are unable to find or maintain employment, form trusting relationships, or preserve housing arrangements.
7. Homelessness affects children's long-range chances to succeed because they are doomed to live on the street or in shelters. The impact is profound and long-lasting. Some "throwaway" children are abandoned and live in such deprivation that their health and welfare are seriously undermined. Homeless children are at increased risk for hunger, poor nutrition, developmental delays, psychiatric problems, and educational underachievement.
8. The elderly homeless avoid public shelters because they may be mugged, treated unkindly, or referred to institutions.
9. Immigrants and illegal aliens are vulnerable to homelessness because multiple stresses build, and the immigrant becomes a casualty of an overloaded system. Minorities in general are overrepresented in the homeless population. Employment and housing are critical problems for this group.
10. Increased homelessness occurs in the cities because cities traditionally attracted large numbers of people seeking jobs. Many workers have become unemployed due to changes in the economy.
11. Economic changes have had an impact on rural homelessness due to debt-saddled farms, low salaries, and a shortage of housing.
12. Unemployment has mild to crippling psychological effects on emotional well-being in terms of decreased income, constricted world with no need to go out into the world to interact, loss of "traction" or momentum to achieve, loss of flexibility in decision-making, increasingly uncertain future, discrimination experienced in society with the person rejected more and more, deterioration of quality and nature of interpersonal contacts, and diminished social status and position.
13. Gentrification is the conversion of low-cost properties to higher-rent housing. A result is the eviction of impoverished people who are unable to live in the more expensive, improved quarters.
14. The effects of budget cutbacks during the Reagan administration caused social welfare programs to be slashed. Aid to Families with Dependent Children (AFDC), Social Security, disability benefits, unemployment insurance, and food stamps either lost funds or had a reduced number of recipients.
15. The impact of family dysfunction and distress to a homeless person is that he or she essentially has no family to turn to. A dysfunctional family cannot provide a haven when an individual is threatened by external stresses.
16. Social disaffiliation is estrangement from connective bonds that tie individuals to social support networks and provide a psychological sense of safety, security, and trust.
17. Learned helplessness can affect the nurse-patient relationship, in that the nurse must address needs while simultaneously guarding against rescuing the patient and fostering passive dependence.
18. Preconceived ideas and attitudes can affect the nurse-patient relationship. If you hold a bias or unwitting prejudice, you will affect the relationship. This bias may take the form of distancing, disgust and disdain, moral superiority, guilt, and fear.
19. A strengths-based assessment is a useful initial intervention because it is focused on the patient's strengths to take control of his or her life and adopt new solutions to old problems. It identifies and maximizes the patient's strengths.
20. As a nurse, you can function as an advocate for the homeless by proactive interventions, such as trying to prevent homelessness and championing the cause of the homeless. You can write on health issues for newspapers, consult with legislators on health concerns, and coordinate coalitions of public and private enterprises to support and assist the homeless.
21. While interviewing clients, plan to make the most of short interactions and communicate caring, respect, and a belief in the homeless person's innate worth and dignity.

CHAPTER 40

1. Violence includes any acts (from a punch or a slap to murder) carried out with the intention of causing physical pain or injury to another person.
2. Sexual abuse is defined by Kempe as the involvement of dependent and developmentally immature children and adolescents in sexual activities that they do not fully comprehend, to which they are unable to give informed consent, or that violate social taboos of family roles.
3. Neglect represents acts of omission rather than a physical act of commission.
4. In the hostage response, victims tend to blame themselves for the abuse and to develop a sense of being unworthy of help, a fear of not being believed, skepticism, and, in the case of chronic abuse, a persistent irrational belief that each attack will be the last.
5. The spiritual issue of abuse is that the spiritual distress is almost unfathomable as the victim becomes increasingly hopeless and despairing.
6. "Brainwashing" fits in with abuse in that it is common for victims to believe that violence and abuse are natural parts of family life.
7. Victims of abuse feel spiritual distress, hopelessness, shame, guilt, and embarrassment and find it difficult to believe that outsiders could understand or identify with the humiliation that is part of their lives.
8. Victims of abuse often do not seek help from the criminal justice system because of fears of reprisal from their abuser.
9. Sibling abuse is when brothers or sisters pose a threat to one another.
10. Parents create a "veil of denial" that gives license to the child's violence and perpetuates this form of hidden intimate violence.
11. An example of psychological abuse directed against an elder is when a son yells at his elderly father and verbally abuses him.
12. Parents who are victims do not get help from the community because this form of violence seldom comes to public attention, and if it does, the victims may be blamed for their child's behavior.
13. The value placed on privacy supports violence, in that this privacy shelters offenders and the family becomes isolated from social control.
14. The structural inequality of the family supports violence because of the inequality of size—most husbands are larger and stronger than their wives and children, and most mothers are larger and stronger than their younger children. Social and economic inequality also can occur, in that men typically enjoy greater social and economic status than do women, which translates into power within the family.
15. Violence continues because the costs of violence do not outweigh the rewards. The costs are rarely paid by those who are violent in the home.
16. It is a myth that psychiatric patients are all wild, violent, and out of control. Some diagnoses do carry an association between violence and symptoms of the illness. Within the psychotic group in one study, those driven by their delusions were more likely to commit seriously violent acts.
17. Research has focused on the role of the limbic system in episodic dysfunction.
18. Delusions and hallucinations can drive people to commit violent acts.
19. Increased levels of norepinephrine and dopamine are associated with violence and aggression.
20. Genetics may play a part in violent behavior, but the research is equivocal. A number of studies of prison populations have shown a disproportionate number of XYY men; however, other researchers have failed to show a relationship between genetics and violence.
21. Three characteristics of abusive men are low self-esteem, immaturity, and insecurity.
22. Two myths regarding the role of alcohol in abuse are that the use of alcohol and drugs only give the abuser an excuse for violence and that they do not cause violent behavior. However, someone who is violent will be violent with or without drinking and drug abuse.
23. Alcohol is linked to violence in that men living with women who have alcohol abuse problems often try to justify their violence as a way to control them when they are drunk; men who batter frequently use alcohol abuse as an excuse for their violence; and alcoholism and battering share some similar characteristics, including that both may be passed from one generation to another, both involve denial or minimization of the problem, and both involve isolation of the family.
24. In expressive violence, the goal is to cause pain or injury to the other. In instrumental violence, the goal is to control the behavior of the other.
25. In the mutual comfort model, the partners share responsibility for the eruption of violence.
26. Three general indicators of abuse are when a woman minimizes the frequency and seriousness of the injuries, when a woman states that she is accident prone, and when radiographs show old and new fractures in different stages of healing.
27. It is important to ask direct questions regarding the possibility of abuse because usually the presenting complaint is not abuse, and the woman may present with injuries that are several days old and offer a vague and incomplete history regarding the nature of the injury. The woman may feel too ashamed and guilty to volunteer this information unless asked.
28. The usual presenting complaint of the pregnant woman is usually not abuse, but rather that the woman wants to see if her baby is all right.
29. Three situations that increase the woman's risk of being murdered at the hands of the abuser are a handgun in the home, substance abuse, and extreme jealousy.
30. The woman should return the next day to have more photographs taken, so that the full extent of the bruising and swelling will be evident. The pictures are signed, dated, and sealed in an envelope with other evidence and may be used later as evidence in court.
31. If the woman's explanation of her injuries is not consistent with what you observe, you can document that "the explanation of the patient's injuries is inappropriate."
32. Abuse usually occurs in a three-stage cycle. In the first stage, tension increases. The second stage occurs with an expression of anger. In the third stage, loving reconciliation (the honeymoon phase) occurs. The cycle begins again once tension starts to build.
33. In the honeymoon phase of the cycle, the abuser apologizes and makes amends. He appears contrite and promises to control himself from now on.
34. Findings suggest that a relationship exists between clinical depression or anxiety and sexual abuse. The women have negative feelings toward men and marriage and feelings of worthlessness and shame about sex.
35. Research suggests that wife rape is a significant negative factor in the lives of clinically depressed, anxious women and is closely linked with a history of child abuse. In one study, 24 of 33 women who were raped had been abused sexually as children.
36. Women who have been raped within their marriages feel worthless and helpless and feel shame about sex.
37. Two potential nursing diagnoses associated with abuse are Ineffective Individual Coping and Hopelessness.
38. Two expected outcomes of working with an abused woman are that on a self-rating scale, the patient will express feelings of increased self-esteem and that on a standardized self-rating depression scale, the patient will rate her mood as less depressed.
39. Two short-term goals for working with an abused woman are that the woman will experience caring and concern from nurses and other health care providers and that the patient will identify a place of safety.
40. Two nursing interventions aimed at primary prevention are education to prevent abuse and work to increase the public's awareness of the extent and seriousness of the battering.
41. Two nursing interventions aimed at secondary prevention are screening activities in the community and safety planning information that could be given to a woman during a screening or counseling session.
42. Two nursing interventions aimed at tertiary prevention to deal with life-threatening, health-threatening, and health-related problems are to initiate a body map detailing old and new injuries and to help the woman to identify her strengths and refer her to a support group.
43. Three potential roles for nurses working in shelters for abused

women are assessing health status of the residents, intervening to meet the health needs of residents, and offering support and guidance to the residents.

44. The battering syndrome is characterized by unsuccessful help-seeking, vague physical complaints, and serious psychosocial problems, such as substance abuse.
45. In a summative evaluation of nursing care for an abused woman, it is important to recognize that mutually established goals agreed on by the nurse and the patient dictate the outcome.
46. It is important to gain more knowledge about the woman and the dilemmas facing her to mutually modify goals, plans, and interventions.
47. The battered child syndrome describes the serious pattern of injuries that often result in deaths in some children.
48. Dr. C. Henry Kempe of the University of Colorado focused the nation on the plight of abused children.
49. If you suspect child abuse, you must report it to the child protective authorities.
50. The TRIADS checklist is a useful form for assessing for child abuse.
51. Two future problems that abused children are at greater risk for developing as they grow up are social problems and failed marriages.
52. One expected outcome of nursing interventions with an abused child is to decrease the stress in the home by providing many nontraditional child services, including homemaker service, respite care, transportation, emergency child care, and vocational counseling.
53. Two short-term goals of nursing interventions with an abused child are to desensitize the child to the sensory and perceptual cognitive cues associated with the abuse and to assist the child in mastering relaxation techniques to correct the sensory overload.
54. One nursing intervention aimed at primary prevention is to lobby for increased funding and resources that support educational efforts in the area.
55. One nursing intervention aimed at secondary prevention is to maintain 24-hour hotlines that allow potential abusers to defuse their angry and violent impulses.
56. Two areas of focus in long-term therapy with abused children are providing corrective emotional experiences that allow the development of trust and empathy and teaching cognitive strategies such as thought-stopping, clarification, reframing beliefs, and linking stress directly to the trauma.
57. A formative evaluation of the nursing care of an abused child would include an inquiry into whether the abuser remained involved in a therapeutic relationship.
58. The summative evaluation would include checking for evidence that the long-term consequences to abuse are abating.
59. Indications that the long-term consequences of child abuse are abating are that the child is performing better academically and socially in school, the child is no longer acting out sexually, the child's delinquent behavior is decreasing, and the child is able to form meaningful friendships.
60. The five types of elder abuse are physical, psychological, sexual, financial, and self-neglect.
61. Four indicators of elder abuse are that the patient may be seen in the emergency department with injuries that do not fit the description given by the caretaker, that neighbors or community and home care nurses might observe the living conditions, that the elderly person might be psychologically abused by an elderly spouse or an adult child or grandchild, and that financial abuse may come to the attention of others when the elderly person is unable to pay the bills or buy groceries, medication, or other necessary items.
62. An expected outcome of nursing interventions with an abused elder is to provide for his or her safety.
63. Two short-term goals for an abused elder are that the patient will have normal fluid and electrolyte balance and that the patient's injuries will heal completely.
64. A multidisciplinary approach is the best one when dealing with potential elder abuse because this allows a particular nurse or case manager to obtain a variety of opinions about a given case and make appropriate decisions when planning care with an elderly person.
65. Three questions that you would want answered in evaluating the care provided to an abused elder are "Is the patient safe?", "Are the patient's injuries healing?", and "Is the patient feeling secure?"
66. Four behaviors that should alert you of a patient's increasing agitation are affective changes, such as labile mood swings and inappropriate reactions; pressured speech, response to hallucinations, intrusiveness, negative verbalizations, and muttering to self; motor agitation and inability to be still; and sudden changes in level of consciousness, confusion, and increased disorientation.
67. Four predictors of patient violence are diagnosis, history, legal status on admission, and presence or absence of dementia.
68. It is not an appropriate intervention to suggest that the patient defuse anger by using a punching bag because this will escalate rather than deescalate violence.
69. Two myths that surround the issue of patient violence are that violence among family members is a private matter and that alcohol and drugs cause abuse.
70. Verbal intervention is important during the preassaultive stage of the violence continuum to deescalate violence without harm and decrease the patient's level of agitation.
71. A team approach is critical when dealing with a violent patient because the staff must respond quickly, and to avoid injury, they must be organized before approaching the patient so that each team member is clear regarding individual responsibility regarding limb-securing assignments.
72. Three issues that you need to consider to protect yourself when you intervene with an agitated patient are to avoid wearing dangling earrings or necklaces to avoid serious injury if the patient tries to grab them, to have enough staff for backup, and to always know the layout of the area to prevent injury if the patient requires restraints.
73. Regarding the preassaultive stage, you document an assessment of behaviors that occurred.
74. Regarding the handling of a violent episode, you document the nursing interventions used and the patient's responses.
75. Two areas of information provided by the evaluation of care for a patient who became violent are the nursing staff's ability to avert violence whenever possible through deescalation techniques and to deal with violence in a manner that minimizes the chance of injury to both the patient and the staff.
76. It is important to look at the environment when evaluating care for a patient who became violent because factors in the environment might actually promote anger and violence (e.g., overcrowding or lack of privacy).

CHAPTER 41

1. The emergency department nurse plays a significant role in providing treatment for rape survivors and their families. The nurse often has the first caring contact with the rape survivor and is responsible for providing emotional support and physical treatment for possible sequelae of the trauma.
2. In the community and in ambulatory care settings, the nurse provides continued caring through counseling, support, and referral to support groups for rape victims, and also provides community teaching activities.
3. The nurse ensures the accurate collecting of evidence from a rape victim, such as pictures of injuries and semen samples, which are used to prosecute the perpetrator of the crime.
4. Rape is defined as sexual intercourse with a woman without her consent and by the use of actual physical force.
5. Sexual harassment involves nonconsensual sexual activity advances, jokes, or comments obtained from a victim through abuse of a power position, such as teacher or boss.
6. Sexual contact involves the nonconsensual touching of the intimate body parts of the victim, such as breasts or buttocks. Sexual coercion refers to consensual intercourse that occurs subsequent to intense

verbal coercion, including emotional pressure, threats to end the relationship, or false promises.

7. Rape is a crime of opportunity. African-American teenaged, urban, lower-class girls are at greatest risk for sexual assault because they often live in urban lower-class neighborhoods with high rates of crime and juvenile delinquency.
8. When men rape other men, the motivating factor is violence and domination.
9. Women sometimes do not report being raped because they feel guilty for somehow causing the rape, they are too embarrassed to tell anyone, and they fear retribution from the assailant.
10. Rape statistics have increased dramatically, possibly due to a more responsive legal system as well as to the establishment of rape crisis centers across the United States.
11. Marital rape is when a married woman is forced against her will to have a sexual relationship with her husband.
12. Up to 1965, the law stated that a husband could not be guilty of rape when it was committed by himself against his lawful wife because sex was part of the marriage contract.
13. Weingourt revealed that 62% of the women being treated for depression and anxiety had been raped by their husbands.
14. Date rape is forced sexual contact within the context of what could be construed as a date or during other social situations involving acquaintances.
15. Date rape is dangerous for adolescents because they are forming their own identities and sexual patterns in this developmental stage.
16. The five essential components of the forensic examination are treatment and documentation of injuries, treatment and evaluation of sexually transmitted diseases, pregnancy risk evaluation and prevention, arrangements for follow-up counseling, and collection of evidence following protocols.
17. The physical assessment of a rape victim is thorough and involves documentation of evidence. Vaginal, oral, and anal examinations are performed, with the victim's permission, to determine need for treatment of the rape and to obtain documentation for legal proceedings.
18. Police photographs of a rape victim are used for legal documentation purposes before treatment is initiated.
19. Rape victims may feel persistent fear and anxiety. They may seem confused, unable to respond verbally, and may have alterations in psychomotor functioning.
20. One of the most common myths is that the attacker was overcome with sexual desire. Other myths are that most rapists are oversexed, that most rapes are committed by strangers, that only females get raped, and that rapes usually take place in dark, secluded places.
21. The impact of guilt may isolate the victim from God and the loving support that a relationship with God offers. Spiritual distress could therefore block healing.
22. The victim could experience guilt if she believed she dressed "too flirtatiously" or was "overly friendly" or "led the attacker on."
23. As a nurse, you assess families and/or the patient's significant other in relation to their understanding of and feelings about rape because the support of family and the patient's significant other can be critical to healing.
24. Two possible *DSM-IV* diagnoses for a patient who has been raped are Rape-Trauma Syndrome and Posttraumatic Stress Disorder.
25. Two phases of the rape-trauma syndrome are the acute phase and the long-term reorganization phase.
26. The manifestations of rape-trauma syndrome involve behavioral, somatic, and psychological reactions, which are part of an acute stress reaction to a life-threatening situation.
27. In the impact stage, the victim may experience a wide range of emotions. Feelings of fear as well as shock or disbelief may predominate.
28. Four somatic concerns that are common in the acute phase of rape-trauma syndrome are as follows: if the victim has suffered physical trauma, then general soreness, bruising, and other physical complaints of injury are apparent; if the victim was forced to have oral sex, irritation and trauma to the throat are frequently reported; sleep pattern disturbances are common, with the patient reporting either inability to sleep or inability to fall back to sleep once awakened; and victims often become nauseated thinking of the rape and often have decreased appetite.
29. Two common emotional reactions that occur during the acute phase of rape-trauma syndrome are that in the days and weeks after the rape, victims continue to express a wide range of emotions, including anger and self-blame, and that some are hysterical and cry a great deal.
30. During the reorganization phase of rape-trauma syndrome, the patient may appear to have made an outward adjustment; the person may resume work, and relationships may appear relatively normal on the surface.
31. Three expected outcomes for a rape victim are that the patient will demonstrate decreased anxiety, fear, and guilt; that the patient will experience physical healing; and that the patient will verbalize feelings about the rape.
32. Three short-term goals for nursing care of a rape victim are that the patient will verbalize feelings of anxiety, fear, and guilt; that the patient will recognize that she did not cause the rape; and that the patient will verbalize strategies for keeping safe.
33. The initial plan differs from the long-term plan. In the initial plan, the victim is given access to a supportive person who can facilitate and guide the initial stages of her journey into the health care system. It also includes anticipatory guidance regarding options to respond to these consequences. The long-term plan provides for continuing support and counseling. The time for this continued support varies with the individual victim.
34. SARS is the Sexual Assault Resource Service, an intervention model that exists in Minneapolis, Minnesota. This model focuses on providing care not only during the acute phase but also during the long-term healing process.
35. Effective counseling with rape victims involves providing emotional support, maintaining a nonjudgmental attitude, and helping the victim to regain control.
36. Five safety practices for women that decrease the risk of being raped are using only initials of last names on mailboxes and phone listings, being prepared to enter the house without complications (having keys in hand when reaching the door), installing the proper deadbolt locks and a door viewer and remembering to use them, ensuring that all windows are properly secured, and installing good interior and exterior lighting for protection and using timers for additional security while away.
37. Family support and education involve your teaching the family about myths that surround rape, the range of normal responses to the trauma, the characteristics of rape-trauma syndrome, and the need for long-term support from the family and perhaps from a professional source.

CHAPTER 42

1. The spiritual issues of a person diagnosed with AIDS have to do with finding meaning and purpose in life, dealing with possible guilt over lifestyle choices, and resolving a relationship with God or a higher power.
2. The three psychological reactions to AIDS are psychosis, depression, and anxiety.
3. The "worried well" are individuals at risk for HIV infection who are not infected. These people generally display symptoms of anxiety, and they feel angry about their chances of becoming infected.
4. Three risk factors for acquiring AIDS are heterosexual sex with multiple partners, accidental needle sticks or significant blood exposure to HIV-positive patients in a health care setting, and intravenous drug use involving shared needles.
5. The population groups that have been most affected by AIDS consist of homosexual men and IV drug users.

6. The spiritual component is important in our focus in AIDS to understand the disease progression. A significant relationship exists between hardiness and spiritual well-being.
7. AIDS is caused by the human immunodeficiency virus (HIV), which is a retrovirus that attacks specific components of the immune system.
8. The three modes of HIV transmission are through blood exposure, sexual behavior, and perinatal transmission.
9. Universal precautions include use of barrier methods to prevent contact with patients' blood and body fluids on the health care provider's skin or mucous membranes, no capping of used needles, and disposal of used needles in a puncture-proof container.
10. Public education focuses on providing information about methods to stop the spread of the virus and to decrease the epidemic of fear.
11. A cognitive approach to AIDS education is insufficient to change behaviors because it addresses only one domain and not the whole person.
12. The crisis of knowing begins with the diagnosis, which brings the knowledge that even though one feels fine, one is HIV positive.
13. Four existential issues confronted by the person with AIDS are self-identity, meaning of life, fate, and stigma.
14. Patients with AIDS are stigmatized because the reaction of society to AIDS is very negative and fear laden due to the fact that AIDS is a transmissible and eventually terminal illness.
15. ADC refers to AIDS-dementia complex (referred to in *DSM-IV* as Dementia due to HIV Disease), which is a major complication of HIV infection.
16. Neurodiagnostic testing reveals white blood cells in the cerebrospinal fluid in 20% of patients with ADC, elevated protein levels in 60% of patients with ADC, and the presence of HIV in the cerebrospinal fluid of most patients with ADC.
17. A variety of antidepressants are used to treat depression in patients with AIDS. In addition, a psychostimulant such as Ritalin may be added to deal with fatigue and weakness.
18. Cognitive functioning is impaired in ADC, in that problem-solving is disturbed and patients have difficulty transferring learned information to new situations. As death approaches, they lapse into a mute state.
19. Compassion fatigue is a result of chronic stress and occurs before burnout.
20. Three characteristics of compassion fatigue are withdrawal from others, inability to enjoy life, and chronic fatigue.
21. Two strategies to prevent compassion fatigue are to allow yourself to feel good about what you do, and to tend to your own daily replenishment.
22. Nurses can face two paths: the path of avoidance and the path of care.
23. An appropriate nursing intervention for a psychiatric-consultant liaison nurse is that of crisis intervention to help the patient and/or family in practical problem-solving and decision-making.
24. An appropriate nursing intervention for an inpatient psychiatric nurse is to intervene therapeutically to minimize anxiety and other feelings triggered by universal precautions.
25. An appropriate nursing intervention for a community mental health nurse is holding support and bereavement group meetings.
26. One way to differentiate between depression and ADC is that depressed patients usually express feelings of hopelessness and worthlessness during interviews and may admit to suicidal ideation, whereas these behaviors are not typical of the patient with ADC. Also, people with dementia may have trouble drawing, whereas those with depression don't have this difficulty.
27. You would use a standardized assessment scale such as the Montgomery-Asberg Scale to determine the degree of depression present in a patient.
28. The Mini-Mental State Examination provides specific information regarding short-term memory, attention, and fine motor skills.
29. You could use the Coping Assessment Profile (CAP) to assess coping ability and adaptive and maladaptive responses of patients to AIDS.

CHAPTER 43

1. Institutionalization is a condition characterized by impaired social interactions, decision-making, and independent living skills, resulting from long-term care in an institutional setting. Deinstitutionalization is a process whereby treatment of the mentally ill is moved from state hospitals to the community.
2. The revolving door cycle is one of short inpatient stay, rapid discharge, and eventual repeat admissions.
3. In 1961, the Joint Commission on Mental Illness and Health published its report that recommended that treatment of the mentally ill be moved from state hospitals to the community. This led to the advent of community mental health with the help of federal government funding.
4. Community mental health is referred to as the "third revolution" in psychiatry. The first conclusion made by the Joint Commission on Mental Illness and Health was the provision of treatment for the mentally ill rather than incarceration, and the second conclusion was the emphasis on intrapsychic causes of mental illness.
5. Two pieces of legislation in the 1970s that supported the community mental health movement were the Community Mental Health Center Amendment PL94-63 and the United States Congress Public Law 94-63.
6. The five essential services that community mental health centers must provide are inpatient care, outpatient care, partial hospitalization, emergency care, and consultation and education.
7. The Omnibus Bill of 1980 affected community mental health by moving the authority and administration of mental health programs from NIMH to the individual states, which each received a block grant to cover alcohol abuse, drug abuse, and mental health services.
8. Former President Carter supported the community mental health movement by establishing a 20-member President's Commission on Mental Health. The committee's report focused on strengthening the community mental health system.
9. The chronically mentally ill are a diverse group with a variety of diagnoses including schizophrenia, major affective disorders, and organic disorders secondary to trauma, disease, or substance abuse.
10. Two types of housing used by the CMI are foster care and nursing homes.
11. Young CMIs differ from those who are elderly, in that young CMIs (from 18 to 30 years of age) are broken into three subgroups (a highly functioning group; a passively accepting group; and those who actively deny that they have a mental illness).
12. Another name for the CMI is the seriously and persistently mentally ill.
13. The five needs of the CMI are basic life necessities; a sense that life is meaningful; access to medications; support for family members; and integrated nursing, medical, and social services.
14. An example of the need for access to medications is that medication be not only available at reasonable prices but also that ongoing support is provided for motivation to comply with the medical regimen. Furthermore, in terms of housing, basic life necessities include permanent and temporary housing.
15. Three professional helpers are public welfare agencies, a general hospital, and churches. Three natural helpers are family, friends, and neighbors.
16. Support for family members is critical in maintaining an important element of the patient's support network, especially as the burden of caregiving on the family can be quite high.
17. A catchment area is a city or several rural communities whose total population ranges from 75,000 to 200,000 residents.
18. The goals of community mental health are to provide care that is continuous and comprehensive.
19. The two-pronged focus in community health is to consider the community as patient and attempt to improve conditions in the community and to consider the individual within the community as patient.
20. To provide comprehensive care to the patient, the following services

must be available: outpatient care, partial hospitalization, 24-hour hospitalization and emergency care, and screening services.

21. Congregate housing is sheltered housing that allows the patient a good deal of freedom.
22. An SRO is single-room occupancy where patients rent a room from a landlord.
23. Two examples of support groups are Alcoholics Anonymous and Narcotics Anonymous.
24. A mobile treatment team is a team of professionals who go into the community to provide care.
25. In primary prevention the focus is on preventing new occurrences of mental illness (e.g., offering support to self-help groups).
26. Secondary prevention involves treatment of a diagnosed disorder within a given patient and case finding and referrals to decrease the incidence of mental disorders (e.g., emergency mental health services).
27. Tertiary prevention involves rehabilitative services for patients who have been diagnosed with a mental disorder (e.g., discharge planning).
28. A crisis hot line is an example of a nursing intervention that exemplifies a secondary prevention.
29. Three examples of questions that could be used to assess a community's acceptance of a mental health initiative are "Do you believe that former patients of mental hospitals are able to function well in your community?" "Do you think that you could ever become friends with a former mental patient?" and "Would you offer a former mental patient assistance in obtaining a job at your place of employment?"
30. A nursing diagnosis that might be applicable to a community preparing for a mental health initiative is Knowledge Deficit related to lack of understanding of the characteristics of the chronically mentally ill.
31. One expected outcome for a community preparing for a mental health initiative is that plans for the development and enhancement of existing resources and programs to meet the needs of the chronically mentally ill will come from the community.
32. Two strategies that might be used in working with a community to prepare it for a mental health initiative are that you, as program coordinator, might target public forums such as schools, clinics, churches, neighborhood recreation centers, and health fairs as sites to begin education of the community.
33. Three patient-focused interventions are teaching, case management, and consulting.
34. Networking is an intervention in which you coordinate services on behalf of patients who need them and try to create services where none exist.
35. Case management is management of the multifaceted and complex needs of the CMI, which includes assessing patient needs, compiling a plan for service, linking patients with needed services, monitoring the quality and appropriateness of services, and advocating for the mentally ill.
36. An advocate fights for the needs of the CMI. This may be done behind the scenes or more aggressively in the policy-making arena where you can have an impact on the system as a whole.
37. The training in community living project was a model designed to address three characteristics (i.e., a limited repertoire of coping behaviors to deal with the stresses of life, powerful dependency needs, and the capacity to develop severe psychiatric symptoms when confronted with mild to moderate degrees of stress) that had been identified in patients who had made tenuous adjustments to community life.
38. The Robert Wood Johnson initiative is a program that provides grants and assistance to nine cities in the United States in their efforts to improve services to persons who are chronically mentally ill.
39. The most cost-effective model is the caseworker model.
40. The paraprofessional extender model of case management utilizes the services of nonprofessionals to provide care to patients in rural settings.
41. Former patients object to being called consumers because the term implies choice and power, which is a misnomer, considering that patients in the mental health system are captive populations with little choice regarding the services or the providers selected.
42. The anticipated impact of the former-patient support groups in the CMH movement is to influence public policy with regard to implementing mental health programs.
43. The benefits are that former patients are provided with a feeling that they can make a difference to someone else, they can give as well as receive, and their lives have meaning.
44. As a nurse, you are in a strategic position to influence mental health care in the 1990s because you have a vantage point to advocate for change within the health care system and within the community. Such advocacy could influence reform within the system and reduce stigmatization and discrimination against people with psychotic histories.

CHAPTER 44

1. Medicare legislation has changed the home care industry by moving away from caring and supportive roles and embracing a medical model of treating and eradicating disease and overlooking the need for preventive and health-promoting services.
2. Three influences that are driving the growth of psychiatric home care are increased public demand, an increase in the population needing psychiatric home care, and cost containment pressures.
3. Medicare legislation overlooked the need for preventive and health-promoting services and ignored the clear need of homebound patients for continued support.
4. Psychiatric home care is defined as a bridge to patients who are transitioning from a setting of greater restriction to their homes, which are the least restrictive. Home care also acts as an anchor to assist patients to remain in their homes.
5. The overall goals of psychiatric home care are to improve the quality of life, prevent unnecessary hospitalization, facilitate more rapid discharges from an acute care setting, and maximize the potential of patients to live in their own homes.
6. The specific goals of psychiatric home care are teaching coping skills to patients and family members; offering respite to families and responsible caretakers from the demands of caring for psychiatrically impaired people; teaching patients and families about the psychiatric illness, medications, strategies to stay well, and interpersonal and communication strategies; and teaching patients appropriate social interaction skills, the importance of structuring time, and the need to be involved in healthy diversional activities.
7. The three levels of care described by Pellegrino are doing for another what he or she cannot do alone, providing skilled and competent nursing and medical care, and being in the service of the whole person.
8. One reason why a moral/spiritual foundation is so important to psychiatric home care is that this foundation conveys an attitude of respect, recognizes patients as people of worth and dignity, and conveys a deep appreciation for them as individuals. The integrity of the person is respected and valued.
9. The skills that define the walls of the model are assessment skills, relationship-building, teaching, psychotherapeutic intervention, case management, and medication issues.
10. Medication issues are important to address in psychiatric home care because psychiatric patients have difficulty adhering to a long-term medication regimen. You can help the patient to solve the dilemmas surrounding medication usage so that he or she will avoid getting caught in the discharge and readmission process due to nonadherence to a drug regimen.
11. Two elements that go into relationship-building are affirming the patient as a person of self-worth and clarifying the boundaries of the relationship.
12. Three reasons why patients do not take psychiatric medications as

directed are that for some patients, the side effects are almost as bad as the illness; that remembering to take medications is an issue for some; and that some lack understanding about the reasons for taking the medications.
13. Two examples of teaching interventions are teaching about the causes of depression and teaching about the physical, cognitive, interpersonal, and spiritual effects of depression.
14. Your role as a case manager in psychiatric home care is to work with the patient to introduce order into chaos and to forge links that connect or reconnect the patient to the community.
15. The Bay Area Health Care model involves a skilled assessment and a loving, therapeutic relationship. Almost all therapy issues the nurse might engage in are translated into teaching terms.
16. *Homebound status* means that the patient's condition generally precludes him or her from leaving home without significant assistance from another person; thus, the patient rarely leaves home.
17. A person is eligible for psychiatric home care if the following criteria are met: the patient must be certified as homebound by a physician; the patient must have a psychiatric diagnosis; the patient must require the skills of a psychiatric nurse; and the patient must be under the care of a psychiatrist.
18. Two arguments made against the requirement that a psychiatric plan of care be ordered by a psychiatrist are that most elderly patients never see a psychiatrist for treatment of depression and/or anxiety but instead they receive treatment from their general practitioners and that some areas in the country have no psychiatrists available to provide care to patients.
19. Psychiatric nurses must have a Master's degree in psychiatric nursing or community health nursing, a bachelor's degree in nursing with one year of adult or geriatric psychiatric experience, and a diploma or associate degree in nursing with two years of adult or geriatric psychiatric experience.
20. The expectation of managed care companies in making referrals for psychiatric home care is that the nurses delivering services be certified clinical specialists in psychiatric nursing.
21. The Medicaid criteria for receiving psychiatric home care are similar to those laid down by Medicare for determining eligibility for services as well as qualifications for nurse providers; however, some differences occur across states in how these criteria are interpreted.
22. A major concern for the elderly is that they will lose the ability to cope with their conditions within the comfort of their homes and be forced into institutions.
23. One reason for providing psychiatric home care to children and their families is to develop communication and behavioral techniques that will be effective within their life situation and to assist the family to discover a sense of meaning and significance in their parenting efforts.
24. The benefits of psychiatric home care for the seriously and persistently mentally ill are that home health care decreases the total number of hospital stays and presumably improves the quality of their adjustment to the home and community.
25. Three areas assessed by the psychiatric home care nurse are mental status, family dynamics, and home environment.
26. An in-home assessment of functional status is valuable to assess the patient's actual ability to perform daily chores.
27. A social support map serves as a database to determine the composition of the patient's support network. It can help to identify the kind of support available and who might be involved to provide additional support.
28. The case worker model of case management is one in which a professional (usually a nurse) acts as case manager. The nurse who is managing the case is directly involved in the patient's care. This involvement gives the nurse intimate knowledge of what additional services and skills might benefit the patient.
29. Three general outcome indicators for psychiatric home care are that the patient will consistently access psychiatric follow-up care, that the patient will demonstrate greater functional abilities at the end of psychiatric home care, and that the patient will demonstrate at least five new coping skills to deal with psychiatric illness.
30. The continued assessment intervention is one in which the nurse must be attuned to even the slightest changes in the patient's behavior. These changes may indicate improvement or they may indicate regression and a need for more intensive evaluation, perhaps by a psychiatrist.
31. Two psychiatric interventions used in psychiatric home care are behavior modification and cognitive reframing.
32. The home health agency's own quality improvement staff members review documentation. The payor (e.g., Medicare or Medicaid) periodically reviews the documentation.
33. Two purposes served by reviewing documentation are to provide a method of evaluating the quality of care provided by the agency and to evaluate the provider's performance.

CHAPTER 45

1. One difference between QA and CQI approaches is that instead of focusing on individual staff performance and interventions, typical of a QA model, CQI depends on a systems approach.
2. One driving force behind the TMI/CQI movement is that the patient's treatment needs to be viewed as an ongoing process, and the patient needs to be viewed as a consumer.
3. The traditional multidisciplinary psychiatric team needs to change by adopting problem-solving teams with members from all departments and services (not only from the traditional team).
4. Nursing's traditional approach to QA has focused on aspects of nursing care such as quality and timeliness of nursing assessments, nursing care plans, and specific nursing interventions.
5. Two legal issues that have affected QA are the quality of care provided and standards of practice and care.
6. Four steps in the Joint Commission's ten-step process are to assign responsibility, to delineate the scope of care and service, to identify important aspects of care and service, and to identify indicators.
7. A change was made to incorporate the continuous quality improvement approach, a more systematic monitoring and evaluation process.
8. Deming's contribution to the development of CQI was that he recognized the need for a management approach to quality improvement and the need to involve staff at all levels in the quality improvement process. He stressed that managers should understand that most people want to do a good job.
9. Juran defined quality as "product satisfaction" and "freedom from deficiencies."
10. Five steps in Deming's 14 points of quality management are to institute training; to teach and institute leadership; to drive out fear, create trust, and create a climate for innovation; to eliminate exhortations for the work force; and to eliminate management by objective.
11. The six concepts of CQI are developing a mission, goals, objectives, and a philosophy; strategic planning; benchmarking performance; establishing a quality council of quality teams; collecting and organizing data; and analyzing statistics and displaying data.
12. Three tools used to collect data in a CQI system are brainstorming, multivoting, and flow charting.
13. Benchmarking is the process of continually comparing a company's performance on critical customer requirements against the best in the industry or the class to determine which areas should be targeted for improvement.
14. One reason that strategic planning is essential is that health care organizations must have some guiding force that gets them from point A to point B; furthermore, strategic planning helps all involved to look at the future three to five years in advance to lay the foundations for quality improvement.
15. A quality council has the task of identifying the specific needs for improvement (i.e., the quality projects).
16. Collaborative practice means that everyone involved in a specific

process should work together as a multifunctional team to improve the quality of care provided to the patient.

17. A critical pathway provides guidelines for the management and treatment of patients through diagnostic-specific or procedure-specific guidelines.
18. In a CQI model, standards of practice are very important to determine standards needed to provide direction; to reach agreement on expectations; to monitor and evaluate results; and to guide organizations, people, and patients to obtain optimal outcomes.
19. Patient involvement is a necessity in a CQI model because patients are no longer willing to accept the services provided them without questions. Patient satisfaction is directly proportional to the organization's ability to meet the needs, wants, and desires of the patient.
20. It is important to monitor and analyze trends in patient satisfaction to continuously improve patient care.
21. Patient feedback systems are important because they allow the organization to determine what is important to the patient and they determine if the organization is meeting patient needs.
22. The most important right that any patient has is the right to receive quality medical care regardless of race, creed, nationality, economic status, or illness.

CHAPTER 46

1. As a nurse, you protect the patient's right to self-determination through the principles of informational privacy and informed consent by ensuring that the patient understands the information sought and agrees to it, that the patient is given the chance to correct errors in the data, that the data are reported in a group rather than individually, and that nothing of a personal nature that could result in harm to or discriminate against a patient is disclosed.
2. Quantitative research uses deductive reasoning processes and findings are derived from empirically based quantitative data analyses. Qualitative research uses inductive reasoning, drawing from descriptions of individual experience to create a narrative about its meaning.
3. Research is very important to the development of psychiatric nursing in the 21st century because emphasis will be on research and on emerging biological developments in the neurosciences. Psychiatric nurses must be willing to explore new frontiers of knowledge and to communicate their clinically based research findings orally and in writing. Research that integrates ideas from different disciplines can help to advance models that will make a difference to health care delivery.
4. When Peplau refers to the 21st century as the century of the nurse, she means that psychiatric nurses must be willing to explore new frontiers of knowledge and skill in collaborating with other health professionals and health care consumers. Nurses must take advantage of the opportunity offered by changes in the health care delivery system for the 21st century to be the century of the professional nurse.
5. Collaborative models of health care delivery make the patient a partner in the treatment process, and an integrated approach is used to identify critical treatment outcomes and determine the treatment process required to meet those outcomes. Organization, coordination, and integration of all health-related activities into a comprehensive, holistic treatment approach are key aspects in this model.
6. Critical pathways promote a more coordinated, collaborative approach to health care delivery and result in reduced hospital and patient costs. Developing the critical pathway forces different disciplines to discuss their differences and overlap in functions, the result being an expedient care plan.

INDEX

Note: Page numbers in *italic* type indicate figures; page numbers followed by t indicate tables, those followed by b indicate boxes.

AAMFT (American Association for Marriage and Family Therapy), 470
ABC-X (Crisis) Model of Family Coping, 468
Abnormal Involuntary Movement Scale, 1218
Absolute thinking, 207t
Abstraction, selective, 376
Abuse. See also *Abuser(s).*
  assessment of, 297
    in psychodynamic short-term therapy, 374
  definition of, 1040
  determination of, 1055b
  emotional, 1040–1042, 1044, 1054, 1054b
  extent of, 1042–1043
  indicators of, 1052b
  of children. See *Child abuse.*
  of dementia patients, 1012
  of elders. See *Elder abuse.*
  of self, 930–931
    among elders, 1044
  prevention of, 1072b-1073b
  sexual. See *Sexual abuse.*
    substance. See *Substance abuse.*
Abuser(s), 1047–1050
  biological factors in, 1047
  mental illness among, 1047
  personal characteristics of, 1047–1048
  siblings as, 1043–1044
  signs of, 1048b
  substance abuse among, 1048, 1049
Acceptance, unconditional, in therapeutic relationships, 242–243
Accommodation, 160
  as learning style, 509
Accountability, 60–62, 80
  for behavior control, 81
"Acetaldehyde syndrome," 808
Acetophenazine (Tindal), 527t
Acetylcholine, 137
  in Alzheimer's disease, 994
  mood disorders and, 145
ACME (Association of Couples of Marital Enrichment), 471
ACOAs (adult children of alcoholics),
  treatment for, 831–832, 831b
  vulnerability of, to anxiety disorders, 699
Acquaintance rape, 1089
Acquaintance times, across cultures, 310
Acquired immunodeficiency syndrome (AIDS), 1103–1122
  caregivers for, 1112–1114
  dementia in. See *AIDS-dementia complex (ADC).*
Acquired immunodeficiency syndrome (AIDS) *(Continued)*
  depression in, 1111
  diagnosis of, 1108–1109, *1109*
  dying from, process of, 1109–1110
  etiology of, 1106
  evaluation in, 1119
  existential issues in, 1110
  home care for, 1160
  isolation due to, 1108
  nursing for, 1114–1116
    psychiatric, 1114–1116
  nursing process for, 1116–1122
    assessment in, 1116–1117
      depression and, differentiating from dementia, 1117
      of coping, 1117
    case study of, 1120–1122
    diagnosis in, 1117–1118
    evaluation in, 1120
    implementation in, 1119
    outcome identification in, 1118–1119
    planning in, 1119
  prevention of, 1106–1107
  psychological problems associated with, 1104–1105, *1105*
  social support and, loss of, 1109
  societal information about, 1120
  spread of, substance abuse related to, 827, 828b
  stigma of, 1107–1108
  transmission of, 1106
Action for Mental Health, 21–22
Action potentials, 135, *136*
Action-oriented models, for group psychotherapy, 391
Active learning, 505
Active listening, 211–216
  characteristics of, 212–213
  clarifying for, 215, 217t
  minimum encouragers for, 213
  paraphrasing for, 214–215, 217t
  questions for, 213–214
  reflecting for, 215, 217t
  restating for, 214, 217t
  silence for, 215–216, 217t
  summarizing for, 216, 217t
  validating for, 216
Activity(ies), assessment of, in eating disorders, 915
  for milieu therapy, 452, 457, 460
Activity groups, 415
Actualizing tendency, 109–110
Acupuncture, 491–492, 492t
Adapin (doxepin), 537t
  dosage of, 540t
Adaptation model, data collection using, 285
Adaptive model, of substance abuse, 799
Adaptors, 200
ADC. See *AIDS-dementia complex (ADC).*
Addiction(s). See also *Substance abuse;* specific substances.
  definition of, 798
ADHD (attention-deficit hyperactivity disorder), 589–590, 591–592
ADIS-R (Anxiety Disorders Interview Schedule-Revised), 707
Adjourning (termination) phase, of group development, 399
Adjustment disorder, in acquired immunodeficiency syndrome, 1118
  nursing process for, case study of, 1120–1122
  with anxiety, case study of, 1078–1080
Admiralty Island, 318
Admission diversion, 1026
Adolescent(s), body consciousness of, 157
  gender identity disorders in, 598, 892–893
  grief in, 674
  group psychotherapy for, 387, 416–417
  home care for, 1160
  losses of, 665
  normal development of, 575–576
  sexual development of, 882t
  spiritual development of, 588t
  substance abuse by, 825–826
Adoption studies, of mood disorders, 768
β-Adrenergic blocking agent(s), for anxiety, 555
Adult(s), 617–640. See also *Elderly people.*
  development of, 618–622
    Erikson's theory of, 620
    gender differences in, 619
    Gilligan's theory of, 622
    Jung's theory of, 619–620
    Levinson's theory of, 620–621, *621*
    promoting character, 634
    sexual, 882t
    social changes affecting. See *Adult(s), social change(s) affecting.*
  during 50s, 625–626
  during 40s, generational responsibilities of, 625
    menopause and, 625

Adult(s) *(Continued)*
during 30s, 623–625
life goals of, 623–624
midlife crisis of, 624–625
during 20s, 622–623
empowerment of, 635
health education for, 634
lifelong learning and, 632
future of, 632–633
losses of, 665
maturity of, measures of, 626
nursing diagnoses for, 628
nursing process with, case study of, 636–639
preventive mental health for, technology in, 635
self-actualization of, 626
social change(s) affecting, 628–632
aging parents as, 631
development linked to, 633
dual careers as, 629
empty nest as, 631
ending relationships as, 630
in family structures, 629
infertility as, 629–630
unemployment as, 631–632
social support for, 635–636
stressors for, 626–628, *627*
values clarification for, 634–635
young, schizophrenia in, 742
Adult children of alcoholics (ACOAs), treatment for, 831–832, 831b
vulnerability of, to anxiety disorders, 699
Adult day care. See *Day treatment.*
Adult learning, 508
Adult Nurse Practitioners, 47
Adult psychiatric foster care settings, milieu therapy in, 459–460
Adult state, in transactional communication model, 205
Adulthood, novice, 622
Advanced practice registered nurse(s), 59, 1204
Advice, precautions against giving, 78, 224t, 225
Advisory Council on the Cost and Treatment of Serious Mental Illness, 44
Advocacy, 85, 87. See also *National Alliance for the Mentally Ill (NAMI).*
for homeless people, 1032
in community mental health care, 1145
in therapeutic relationships, 240–241
influence on mental health care, 26
nurse's role in, 57
Affect, definition of, 761
flat, 296t
in personality disorders, 844
in schizophrenia, 729
inappropriate, 296t
labile, 296t
Affective domain, 510
Affective self, 161–162
African American(s), communication among, 314
culture-bound mental illness among, 211t
homelessness among, 1028
hypertension among, 957
substance abuse among, 825
Aftercare, for substance abuse, 822–823
Age. See also specific age groups.
developmental stages related to, 575t
suicide related to, 929t
Ageism, 305
Agency for Health Care Policy and Research, 1202–1203
Aggressors, in psychotherapy groups, 408t
Aging. See also *Elderly people.*
body consciousness and, 157
developmental theories of, 649b
of population, 43
Agitation, in Alzheimer's disease, middle stages of, 1007
Agnosia, in Alzheimer's disease, middle stages of, 1005
Agonists, 525
Agoraphobia, 699
Agranulocytosis, antipsychotic agents causing, 531
clozapine causing, 532
Agraphia, 990t
Aguilera, Donna, crisis intervention model of, 332–333, *334*
AIDS. See *Acquired immunodeficiency syndrome (AIDS).*
AIDS: The Ultimate Challenge (Kübler-Ross), 1108
AIDS-dementia complex (ADC), 992, 1111–1112
assessment of, 1117
differentiating depression from, 1117
etiology of, 1111–1112
neurodiagnostic findings in, 1112
symptoms of, 1112
treatment of, 1112
Akathisia, 528, 529, 529t, 990t
Al-Anon, 604
Alcohol, 497
early understanding of, 794, 795
in migraine headaches, 960
Alcohol abuse, 805–809, *807*. See also *Adult children of alcoholics (ACOAs).*
alcohol toxicity and, 808, 808t
among disadvantaged people, 825
among homeless people, 1026–1027
among Native Americans, 319
as medical disorder, 795
case study of, 832–836
codependency and, 797
comorbidity of, 809
diagnosis of, 807–808
domestic violence and, 1049b
societal information about, 820, 822b
symptoms of, physical, 807, 807b
psychological, 807
teratogenic effects of, 826, 827t
treatment of, Alcoholics Anonymous in, 396, 797, 819, 823, 1136
Disulfiram for, 808
federal guidelines for, 797
withdrawal in, 808, 808t
Alcoholics Anonymous, 396, 797, 823, 1136
12 steps of, 819b
Alcohol-induced persistent amnestic disorder, 808, 992
Alexithymia, 930
Alford, Peggy, 1088
Aliens, illegal, homeless, 1028
ALI/LifeSkills Program, 181
Alliance for the Mentally Ill, 44
Almshouses, 19
Aloneness, existential, 178–179
Alprazolam (Xanax), dosage of, 552t
for panic attacks, 551
Altruism, in group psychotherapy, 402–403
Altruistic community, 341
Altruistic egoism, for stress management, 66
Altruistic suicide, 932
Aluminum, in Alzheimer's disease, 994
Alzheimer, Alois, 979
Alzheimer's disease, 979, 989–990, 990t. See also *Dementia.*
behavioral assessment in, 999
brain in, 980, 981, 989
causes of, 993–994
comorbidity of, with Down's syndrome, 994
early stages of, 996–1004
adult day care centers for, 1004
appearance in, 998
behavior patterns in, 998
cognitive limitations in, 1003–1004
communication problems in, 999–1001, 1000t
differential diagnosis of, 997t, 997–998, 999
elimination in, 1001
family concerns in, 1013t
family education about, 1001–1002
functional ability in, conservation of, 1002–1003
memory deficits in, 998
nutrition in, 1001
personality changes in, 998–999
psychomotor functioning in, 1001
psychopharmacological treatment of, 1004
respite care during, 1004
safety issues in, 1002
social functioning in, supporting, 1004
end stage of, 1010–1011
eating in, encouraging, 1011
symptoms in, 1010
families of patients with, education for, 1001–1002
support for, 1001
incidence and prevalence of, 993
middle stages of, 1004–1010
agitation in, 1007
behavioral symptoms of, 1005, 1006t
catastrophic reactions in, 1008
combativeness in, 1008
communication problems in, 1007
disorientation in, 1005
eating problems in, 1007–1008
emotional disinhibition in, 1009
family concerns in, 1013t
repetitive behaviors in, 1009
restraints in, 1009–1010
screaming in, 1007
self-care in, 1005–1007, 1006t
sleep disturbances in, 1009
sundown syndrome in, 1008–1009
nursing process for, case study of, 1014–1017
patient care in, 994t, 994–996
for early stages. See *Alzheimer's disease, early stages of.*
for end stage, 1010–1011
for middle stages. See *Alzheimer's disease, middle stages of.*
psychiatric assessment in, 997t
Amaranth, 497
Ambivalence, in schizophrenia, 730
Amerasian Homecoming Act of 1987, 316
American Association for Marriage and Family Therapy (AAMFT), 470
American Association of Marriage Counselors, 471
American College of Surgeons, 1177
American Group Psychotherapy Association, 387, 416–417
American Hospital Association, patients' Bill of Rights of, 83, 84, 86, 1190–1191
American Indians. See *Native American(s).*

American Journal of Nursing, establishment of, 18
American Medical Association, Practice Parameters Forum established by, 1185
Practice Parameters Partnership established by, 1185
American Nurses' Association (ANA), 25, 53, 1185
Certification program of, 26
Code for Nurses of, 83–84
Code of Ethics of, 25
crisis intervention defined by, 345
on milieu therapy, 445
on patient education, 504
on spousal abuse, 1050, 1051
psychiatric mental health nursing defined by, 54, 286
standards of, for mental health clinical nursing practice, 25, 54, 55b, 60, 266–267, 267, 273, 285, 288, 1185
for substance abuse treatment, 797
Statement on Psychiatric Nursing of, 25
Statement on Psychiatric-Mental Health Clinical Nursing Practice of, 447
American Psychiatric Nurses Association (APNA), 25, 26
American Psychological Association, 1186, *1187–1188*
American Psychosocial Association, 1186, *1187–1188*
American Society for Group Psychotherapy and Psychodrama, 387
Americans with Disabilities Act of 1990, 22–23
Amino acids, 497–498
Amitriptyline (Elavil; Endep), 537t, 540
dosage of, 540t
for children, 595t
for posttraumatic stress disorder, 704–705
Amnesia, anterograde, benzodiazepines causing, 551
continuous, 868
dissociative, 867–868, 872
in dissociative disorders, 866, 866t
persistent, alcohol-induced, 808, 992
psychogenic, 863–864
Amok, 309
Amoxapine (Asendin), 537t, 545
dosage of, 540t
Amphetamines, abuse of, 812–813
Amygdala, anxiety and, 693
ANA. See *American Nurses' Association (ANA).*
Anafranil (clomipramine), for children, 596t
for obsessive-compulsive disorder, 702, 716
Anal retentive people, 102
Anal stage, 102, 103t
Analytical psychology, 104
Angel dust (phencyclidine), abuse of, 810
psychosis induced by, 744
Anger, family interventions for, 344t
grief and, 179
in bipolar disorders, 771–772
in group psychotherapy, 400
Angular gyrus, 138–139
Anima, 104
Animus, 104
Anomia, 990t
in Alzheimer's disease, early stages of, 1000
Anomic suicide, 932
Anorexia nervosa, 910, 910t, 911b, 916
case study of, 921–923
causes of, 911–914
comorbidity of, 914
Anorexia nervosa *(Continued)*
in children, 594, 600
patient information about, 920
psychological characteristics of, 915b
Anorgasmia, 887–890
Antabuse (disulfiram), 808
Antagonists, 525
Antecedents, of behavior, 421, 429–430
Anterograde amnesia, in dissociative disorders, 866t
Antianxiety agent(s), 549–555, 692. See also specific drugs and drug types.
nursing process for treatment with, 563–567
assessment in, 563
diagnosis in, 563
implementation in, 563
outcome identification in, 563
planning in, 563, *565*
Anticholinergic agent(s). See also specific drugs.
drug interactions of, 531, 539, 548
for schizophrenia, 747
Anticholinergic effect(s), 137
antipsychotic agents causing, 530
tricyclic antidepressants causing, 538, 539
Anticonvulsant agent(s), for children, 597t
Anti-Crime Bill of 1994, 435–436
Antidepressant agent(s), 535–545. See also specific drugs.
for AIDS-dementia complex, 1112
for children, 595t–597t
for eating disorders, 919
monoamine oxidase inhibitors as. See *Monoamine oxidase inhibitor(s) (MAOIs).*
nursing process for treatment with, 563–567
assessment in, 563
diagnosis in, 563
implementation in, 563
outcome identification in, 563
planning in, 563, *564–567*
selective serotonin re-uptake inhibitors as. See *Selective serotonin re-uptake inhibitor(s) (SSRIs).*
tricyclic, 536–540
action of, 537, 537t
administration routes for, 540
adverse effects of, 537t, 538–539
dosage of, 539–540, 540t
drug interactions of, 539, 543
for children, 595t–596t
for panic disorder, 700
pharmacokinetics of, 537
selection of, 540
therapeutic uses of, 538
toxicity of, 539
Antihistamines, for children, 597t
Antihypertensive agent(s), drug interactions of, 543
for children, 599t
Antilocution, 306
Antimanic agent(s). See also specific drugs.
for children, 599t
Antioxidants, 498
Antiparkinsonian agent(s), for schizophrenia, 747
Antipsychotic agent(s), 526–535. See also specific drugs.
action of, 733–734
administration routes for, 534–535
in initial therapy, 535
in maintenance therapy, 535
promoting compliance and, 535
Antipsychotic agent(s) *(Continued)*
atypical, 531–533
contraindications to, 533
for AIDS-dementia complex, 1112
for bipolar disorder, 546, 546t, 547
for children, 598t–599t
for schizophrenia, 528, 533–534, 747
dosing for, 534
drug selection for, 533–534, 534t
positive symptoms of, 737
preadministration assessment for, 533
high potency, 526, 527t
low potency, 526, 527t
nursing process for treatment with, 555–563
assessment in, 555, 556, 562
diagnosis in, 556, 562
evaluation in, 556, *560–562*
implementation in, 556, 562–563
outcome identification in, 556, 562
planning in, 556, *557–559*, 562–563
toxicity of, 531
traditional, 526–531
action of, 526, 528
adverse effects of, 526, 528–531
classification of, 526, 527t
dependence on, 531
depot preparations of, 531, 532t
drug interactions of, 531
therapeutic uses of, 528
Antisocial personality disorder, 845, 847
Anxiety, 691. See also *Anxiety disorder(s); Fear(s); Phobia(s); Stress.*
as communication barrier, 224
decreasing, 714
family interventions for, 344t
Freud's view of, 100
in children, 590, 593–594
in delirium, containing, 986
in elderly people, 652
in existential models, 110
in family therapy, 474
mild, 695, 695t
moderate, 695, 695t, 696
of nurses, 6
patient information about, 693
severe, 695t, 695–696
speech patterns and, 201
stress related to, 695t, 695–698
Sullivan's theory of, 105
symptoms of, 692
theories of, 693–694
behavioral, 694
psychobiological, 693–694
psychodynamic, 694
treatment of, 554
for generalized anxiety, 554
for situational anxiety, 554
nursing strategies for, 696
psychopharmacological, 551, 552t, 554–555. See also *Antianxiety agent(s);* specific drugs and drug types.
Anxiety disorder(s), 691–722. See also *Obsessive-compulsive disorder (OCD); Panic disorder; Phobia(s); Posttraumatic stress disorder (PTSD).*
causes of, 145–146
genetic, 146
neurochemical, 146
generalized. See *Generalized anxiety disorder (GAD).*
nursing process for, 706–711
assessment in, 706–707
case study of, 716–722
diagnosis in, 707, 708–712

Anxiety disorder(s) *(Continued)*
implementation in, 713–716
outcome identification in, 707, 713
planning in, 707, 713
Anxiety Disorders Interview Schedule-Revised (ADIS-R), 707
Anxiety gradient, in interpersonal nursing, 119
Anxiolytic(s). See *Antianxiety agent(s);* specific drugs and drug types.
Aphasia, 981, 990, 990t
APIE method, 276
APNA (American Psychiatric Nurses Association), 25, 26
Approach, consistency in, trust and, 245
Apraxia, 990t
in Alzheimer's disease, early stages of, 1001
Arbitrary inference, 376
Archetypes, 104
Archives of Psychiatric Nursing, 26
Aristotle, 94–95, 96t
Arousal, sexual, dysfunction of, 886–887
Art, of nursing, assessment and, 285–286
"ARTWorks paradigm," 181
Asclepiades, 128
Ascribed roles, 163
Asendin (amoxapine), 537t, 545
dosage of, 540t
Asians, 315–318
communication among, 316
culture-bound mental illness among, 211t
mind-body-spirit therapies of. See *Mind-body-spirit therapy(ies), Eastern.*
Asides, in psychodrama, 413t
Asklepios, 14
Asperger's disorder, in children, 603
Assault, 77
Assessment, 283–299
art of nursing and, 285–286
beginning, 287–288
chief complaint in, 289, 295
cognitive, 295, 297
in mental retardation, 601, 602
of suicidal patients, 936
data collection for, 285
during therapeutic relationship, 249–250
using behavior modification principles, 285
using Gordon's functional health patterns, 285
using Orem's model, 285
using Roy's model, 285
data for, validation of, 250
emotional, 295, 296t
of suicidal patients, 935–936
findings of, terminology for, 296t
focus of, 285
for acquired immunodeficiency syndrome, 1116–1117
depression in, differentiation dementia from, 1117
of coping, 1117
for antidepressant, mood stabilizer, and antianxiety agent treatment, 563
for antipsychotic treatment, 555, 556, 562
for anxiety disorders, 706–707
for behavioral therapy, 424
multiple sources of, 426–427
for child abuse, 1064–1065, *1066–1067*
for community mental health care, community-focused, 1138
individual- or family-focused, 1140, 1141t–1142t
Assessment *(Continued)*
for crises, 345
for dissociative disorders, 871
for eating disorders. See *Eating disorder(s), assessment of.*
for elder abuse, 1068, 1070, *1071*
for family therapy, 476–479
during interview, 477–478
tools for, *478,* 478–479, *479,* 480
for grief, 677, 678
for group psychotherapy, 396–397
for home care. See *Home care, nursing process for.*
for mood disorders, 770–773
of family feelings, attitudes, and knowledge, 772–773
of patient feelings, attitudes, and knowledge, 770–772
for patient education, 509–510
for personality disorders, 851, 852
for psychophysiological disorders, 969
for rape. See *Rape, nursing process for.*
for schizophrenia. See *Schizophrenia, assessment in.*
for sexual disorders. See *Sexual disorder(s), assessment of.*
for spousal abuse. See *Spousal abuse, of women, assessment of.*
for substance abuse, 816, *817,* 818
for suicide potential. See *Suicide, potential for, assessment of.*
for violent patients, 1074–1075, *1075*
guidelines for, 353b
in Bay Area Health Care model, 1155
in nursing process, 268
medication history in, 289, 295
of children. See *Child(ren), assessment of.*
of elderly people. See *Elderly people, assessment of.*
of homeless people, 1032, 1033t–1034t
other health team members in, 299
patient identification in, 289
patient perceptions in, 286–287
philosophical, 298–299
physical. See *Physical assessment.*
Psychiatric Nursing Assessment Tool for, 289, *290–294*
psychiatric treatment history in, 295
psychophysiological, 951–953
psychometric instruments in, 951–953
stress response measures in, 953
secondary sources for, 299
self-awareness for, 286, *287*
sociocultural, 297–298
spiritual. See *Spiritual assessment.*
standardized scales for. See *Standardized rating scale(s).*
standards of, 288
subjective reactions in, 299
Assimilation, 160
as learning style, 509
Association(s), loose, 296t
in schizophrenia, 729
simple, 423
Association of Couples of Marital Enrichment (ACME), 471
Assumed roles, 163
Asylums, 19
Ataxia, 990t
in AIDS dementia complex, 992
Ativan (lorazepam), dosage of, 552t
for delirium, 986
Attachment, of children, assessment of, 585
Attainment stage, of healing, 491
Attendants, as treatment team members, 63t
Attention, for active listening, 212
social learning theory of, 114
Attention-deficit hyperactivity disorder (ADHD), 589–590, 591–592
Attitude consistency, trust and, 245
Audit trail, 1200
Auditory hallucinations, 223, 738t
Aura, with migraine headaches, 959
Authenticity, in therapeutic relationships, 244
Autism, in children, 603
in schizophrenia, 729–730
Autistic phase, in object relation theory, 843
Automatic thinking schema, 377
Autonomy, as ethical guide, 74
Autonomy versus shame and doubt stage, 103t, 107, 167t
stressors during, 333t
Aventyl. See *Nortriptyline (Aventyl; Pamelor).*
Aversive reinforcement, 429
in behavioral therapy, 436–437
Avoidance, prejudice and, 306
Avoidance training, 437
Avoidant personality disorder, 848, 849
Avoiders, in psychotherapy groups, 408t
Awakening stage, of healing, 491
Awareness, conscious, 104
in grieving process, 669
of others' needs, for effective communication, 195–196
of self. See *Self-awareness.*
of stress, 65
Axons, 135, *135*

Back pain. See *Low back pain.*
Bailey, Harriet, 18
Bain, Alexander, 97
Balance, for stress management, 65, 65b
Balancing factors, 332–333
Bales, Robert, 388
Bandura, Albert, social learning theory of. See *Social learning theory(ies).*
Barbiturate(s), abuse of, 796, 809–810
teratogenic effects of, 827t
Basal ganglia, 132, 134, 139
"Basic assumptions," Bion's concept of, 389
Basic trust versus mistrust stage, 103t, 107
BASIC-ID approach, 5
BASIC-IS approach, 5
Battered women, Maryland legal remedies for, 1063b
Battered-child syndrome, 1062–1063. See also *Child abuse.*
Batterer, potential, 1048b
Battering syndrome, 1059. See also *Family violence; Spousal abuse.*
Battery, 77
Bay Area Health Care model, of home care, *1154,* 1154–1156
assessment and relation-building in, 1155
moral/spiritual base of, 1154, *1155*
patient education in, 1156
psychopharmacological treatment in, 1155
psychotherapy in, 1156
BDI (Beck Depression Inventory), in psychophysiological disorders, 952
Beck Depression Inventory (BDI), in psychophysiological disorders, 952
Beer, interaction with monoamine oxidase inhibitors, 543t
Beers, Clifford, *16,* 16–17

Behavior(s), antecedents of, 421, 429–430
caring, 238b, 241
changes in, reinforcing, in crisis intervention, 357–358
consequences of, 421
control of, ethics of, 81
in alcoholism, 807
nursing, associated with empathy, 244b
problem, definition of, 424–425
targeting, for behavioral therapy, 425–426, 425b
Behavior modification, 112
for eating disorders, 919
principles of, data collection using, 285
Behavioral contracting, 430–431, *431*
Behavioral disorders. See *Personality disorder(s).*
Behavioral learning, 112
Behavioral theory(ies), 5, 111–114, 129
learning, 505, 505t
of anxiety, 694
generalized, 698
of Bandura, 113–114
of Pavlov, 111–112
of Skinner, *112*, 112–113
of Watson, 112
Behavioral therapy, 379, 421–440
application of, 424–434
antecedents in, 429–430
assessment for, 424
behavioral contracting for, 430–431, *431*
cueing for, 432–433
distraction for, 433
extinction in, 429
flooding for, 432
multiple data sources for, 426–427
negative reinforcement in, 429
nursing diagnoses for, 427
outcome identification for, 427
planning for, 427
positive reinforcement in, 428–429
Premack principle in, 428
problem behavior definition in, 424–425
punishment in, 429
reinforcement schedules for, 430, 430t
reinforcer identification for, 428
response prevention for, 432
sample care plan for, 433–434
shaping for, 431–432
substitute gratification for, 433
targeting behaviors in, 425–426
types of reinforcers for, 428
aversive reinforcers in, 436–437
cognitive behavioral models for, 436
for obsessive-compulsive disorder, 702
for substance abuse, 821
preventive, 439
self-management using, 437–439
biofeedback for, 437
desensitization for, 437–438
guided mastery for, 438
relaxation for, 438–439
social skills training based on, 435–436
theoretical bases of, 422–424
classical conditioning as, 423, 424
operant conditioning as, 423–424
simple association as, 423
token economies based on, 434–435
Behaviorism, 5, 129
Being needs, 108
Bell Telephone Laboratories, 1179
Bell-and-pad system, for enuresis, 599–600
Belonging needs, 166
Benadryl (diphenhydramine), for children, 597t
Benchmarking, 1181
Bender, Lauretta, 24
Beneficence, 73
Benner, Pat, 151
Benzisoxazoles, for children, 599t
Benzodiazepine(s), 549–553. See also specific drugs.
abuse of, 796, 809
action of, 550
administration routes for, 552–553
adverse effects of, 551–552
contraindications to, 551–552
dependence on, 552
dosage of, 552
drug interactions of, 552
pharmacokinetics of, 550–551
pharmacologic effects of, 550
receptors for, anxiety disorders and, 146
teratogenic effects of, 827t
therapeutic uses of, 551
for akathisia, 529
for anxiety, 554, 699
for bipolar disorder, 546, 546t, 547
tolerance to, 552
toxicity of, 553
Bereavement. See *Grief; Loss(es).*
Bereavement overload, 664
Bergalis, Kimberly, 1110
Bernade, Claude, 951
Berne, Eric, 101
Bethlehem Hospital, 19, *20*
Bias, Len, 814
Bill of Rights for patients, 84, 85b, 86b–87b, 1190–1191
Binge eating disorder, 910t
causes of, 911–914
comorbidity of, 914
Bini, Lucio, 23
Binswanger's disease, 992
Bioenergetics, 495
Biofeedback, 437, 495–496
for migraine headaches, 960
Biological interventions, 273
influence on mental health care, 23
Biological psychology, 127–146
history of, 128–130
early, 128–129
in early 20th century, 129
in United States, 129–130
laboratory tests and, 140–142
brain imaging, 141
neurochemical, 142
neuroanatomy and. See *Brain; Neuroanatomy.*
neurophysiology and. See *Neurophysiology.*
of causes of mental illness. See *Mental illness, causes of.*
Biological theory(ies), 114–115. See also *Brain; Genetics; Neurotransmitter(s).*
of anxiety, 693–694
of substance abuse, *795*, 795–796, 799
legal interpretations of, 795–796, 796t
Biological vulnerability, to schizophrenia, 735
The Biology of Mental Disorders, 44
Bion, Wilfred, 388–389
Biopsychosocial-spiritual model, for patient education, 515–516
Bipolar disorder, 545–546, 760, 763
clinical manifestations of, 545–546
comorbidity of, with Huntington's disease, 767
definition of, 765t
diagnosis of, 777
family's feelings about, 772–773
Bipolar disorder (*Continued*)
feelings in, 771–772
in children, 604
not otherwise specified, definition of, 765t
treatment of, psychopharmacological, 528, 538, 546t, 546–549, 548t. See also specific drugs and drug types.
Birth order, 163
Bisexuals, 881
Black, Kathleen, 22, 24
Black Americans. See *African American(s).*
Blackouts, definition of, 798
in alcoholism, 807
Blended family, 465t
Bleuler, Eugene, 129
on schizophrenia, 729–730, 729b
Block grants, 44
Blockers, in psychotherapy groups, 408t
Blocking, 296t
Blood, acquired immunodeficiency syndrome transmission by, 1106
Blood pressure. See *Hypertension; Hypotension.*
B-motives, 108
Boat people, 316
Body dysmorphic disorder, 962–963, 968t
Body image, 156–158
during developmental stages, 156–158
Body language, 199–200
with violent patients, 1076
Body Mind Energetics (Seem), 491
"Body spaces," 156, *157*
Borderline personality disorder, 845–847, 848
case study of, 856–860
Boundary(ies), cultural concepts of, 311
in families, 482
in systems, 466
in therapeutic relationships, 239–240, 240b
of violent patients, respect for, 1076
personal, legal issues regarding, 82–83, 83b
violation of, in groups, 416
Bourne, Ansel, 868
Bowen, Murray, 473
family therapy model of, 473–476
Bowlby, John, 663
Bracketing, 1199
Brain, 130–136
imaging of, 130, 141
in Alzheimer's disease, 980, 981, 989
in anxiety, 693–694
lesions in, dementia due to, 991–992
neurotransmitters in, 137b
normal function of, 980
physiology of, theistic view of, 4–5
structure of, changes in, in schizophrenia, 141, 143–144, 731–733
in substance abuse, 800
macrostructure and, 130–135, *131*
inner, 133–135, *134*
of surface, 130–132, *132*, *133*
microstructure and, *135*, 135–136, *136*
trauma to, sexual problems resulting from, 894
The Brain: The Last Frontier (Restak), 694
Brain stem, 132
in cognitive disorders, 981
Brainstorming, 254
by quality teams, 1181, 1182t, 1184
Breathing, controlled, 714b
Breuer, Josef, 99
Brewer's yeast, 497
Brief Psychiatric Rating Scale, 1219
Brief therapy. See *Psychodynamic therapy, short-term.*
Briggs, Katherine, 169

British Group-Analytic Society, 388
Broca, Paul, 981
Broca's aphasia, 981
Broca's area, 129, 131, 138
Bromocriptine, for neuroleptic malignant syndrome, 530
Browne, Esther Louise, 53
Bryant, Jane, 53
Buber, Martin, 110
Buckwheat, 497
Buddhism, 317
Budget Reconciliation Act of 1981, 42
Bulimia nervosa, 910, 910t, 917
  causes of, 911–914
  comorbidity of, 914
  in children, 594, 600
  patient information about, 920
  psychological characteristics of, 915b
Bupropion (Wellbutrin), 537t, 545
  dosage of, 540t
  for children, 597t
Burdett, Henry, 444
Burnout, among nurses, *64*, 64–67
  strategies for dealing with, *65*, 65–67
Bush, George, 27
BuSpar. See *Buspirone (BuSpar).*
Buspirone (BuSpar), 553–554
  action of, 553
  adverse effects of, 553
  dosage of, 552t
  drug interactions of, 553
  for anxiety, 554–555, 699
  therapeutic uses of, 553
  tolerance, dependence, and abuse of, 553–554
Butler, Robert, 305
Butyrophenones, 526, 527t
  for children, 598t

Cade, John, 546
Caffeine, 496, 814
  anxiety and, 701
  vasopressive action of, 543t
CAGE Questionnaire, 808
Cahill, Kevin, 1107–1108
Cambodian refugees, 316
Campbell, Jacquelyn, 1088
Camphill communities, 602–603
Cannabis, abuse of, 810–811
  early understanding of, 795
CAP (Coping Assessment Profile), 1117
Caplan, Gerald, crisis intervention model of, 331
Carbamazepine (Tegretol), for bipolar disorder, 546, 549
  for children, 597t
Cardiotoxic action(s), of tricyclic antidepressants, 538, 539
Cardiovascular system, aging of, 647t
Care, as ethical guide, 77
  continuum of, nurse as provider of, 57
  direct and indirect, 54, 56
  managed, 45–46
    home care funding under, 1158
  perspective of, Gilligan's theory of, 75–77, *76*
Care mapping, for collaborative models, of care, 1203–1204
Care of the Soul (Moore), 492
Care plan(s). See *Nursing care plan(s).*
Caregiver(s), for acquired immunodeficiency syndrome patients, 1112–1114
  for dementia patients, family members as, 1012–1013
Caregiver(s), for acquired immunodeficiency syndrome patients *(Continued)*
  for elderly people, children as, 625, 631
Caring behavior(s), in therapeutic relationships, 238b, 241
Caring model(s), 118
Carphologia, 990t
Carroll, Lewis, 192
Carson's Psychiatric Care Plan, 276, *277–278*
Carter, Jimmy, 22, 1130
Case management, 274
  in community mental health care, 1145
  in home care, 1156, 1165–1166
Catapres (clonidine), for children, 599t
  for narcotic abuse, 812
Catastrophic reactions, in Alzheimer's disease, middle stages of, 1008
Catatonic schizophrenia, 732t
Catchment area, 1134
Catecholamine hypothesis, of depression, 144
Cathartic method, 99, 102
  in group psychotherapy, 400
Catholic University of America, 26
Catholicism, among Filipinos, 318
  among Irish Americans, 313
  among Italian Americans, 313
Caudate nucleus(i), 133, 134
Cause-and-effect diagrams, 1181, 1182t
Celestial Interlude (Haun), 588–589
CELR (Coalition to End Legalized Rape), 1088
Central nervous system. See also *Brain.*
  depression of, benzodiazepines causing, 551
  stimulation of, by monoamine oxidase inhibitors, 542
Centrax (prazepam), dosage of, 552t
Cerebellum, *131*, 132
Cerebral cortex, in cognitive disorders, 980–981
Cerebral hemispheres, 130, 132
Cerebrovascular accident, comorbidity of, with depression, 767–768
Cerletti, Ugo, 23
Certified Specialist in Psychiatric and Mental Health Nursing (R.N., C.S.), 59
Chaining, 432
Character development, promoting, 634
Charcot, Jean-Martin, 16, 99
Charles Marie, Sister, 19
Chemical abuse. See *Substance abuse;* specific substances.
Chemical restraints, 81
Chenitz, W. Carole, 1107, 1108, 1109, 1110, 1114, 1119
Ch'i, 488
Chief complaint, in assessment, 289, 295
Child(ren), 573–609. See also *Adolescent(s).*
  abuse of. See *Child abuse; Family violence.*
  acquired immunodeficiency syndrome in, 1106
  acute stress disorder in, 594
  adult, of alcoholics, treatment for, 831–832
    vulnerability of, to anxiety disorders, 699
  AIDS in, 827, 828
  anorexia nervosa in, 594, 600
  Asperger's disorder in, 603
  assessment of, 582–589, *583*
    mental status examination in, 584
    of attachment/separation, 585
    of moral development, 586–587
    of play, 584–585
    of sexuality, 585–586
    of spiritual development, 587–589, 588t
    of suicide potential, 589
    physical, 582, 584
Child(ren) *(Continued)*
  attention-deficit hyperactivity disorder in, 589–590, 591–592
  autism in, 603
  bipolar disorder in, 604
  bulimia nervosa in, 594, 600
  communication disorders in, 603
  community of, 577
  conduct disorder in, 590, 591–592
  coping mechanisms of, 579, 579t
  depression in, 603–604
  development of, normal, 574–576, 575t
    sexual, 882t
  Education of the Handicapped Act Amendments of 1986 and, 40
  empty nest and, 631
  encopresis in, 600
  enuresis in, 599–600, 602
  families of, 576–577. See also *Family(ies); Parent(s).*
    family therapy with, 606
  friends of, 577
  gender identity disorders in, 597–598, 892–893
  grief of, 674
  group psychotherapy for, 387, 416–417
  home care for, 1160
  homelessness among, 1027–1028
  inability to have, 629–630
  individual psychotherapy with, 605–606
  integrative disorder in, 603
  learning disorders in, 603
  losses of, 665
  medication use in, 608b
  mental illness in, abuse as risk factor for, 580
    divorce as risk factor for, 581–582
    epidemiology of, 579
    medical illness and disability as risk factors for, 581
    neglect as risk factor for, 580
    parental psychopathology as risk factor for, 581
    poverty as risk factor for, 579–580
    violence as risk factor for, 580–581
  mental retardation in, 601–603
  motor skills disorders in, 603
  nursing process with, 582–612
    assessment in. See *Child(ren), assessment of.*
    case study of, 609–612
    diagnosis in, 589–604. See also specific diagnoses under *Child(ren).*
    evaluation in, 608–609
    implementation in, 605–608
    outcome identification in, 604
    planning in, 604–605
  obesity in, 595–596
  obsessive-compulsive disorder in, 593–594
  of chemically dependent parents, treatment for, 830–831
  oppositional defiant disorder in, 590
  overanxious disorder of childhood in, 593
  pervasive developmental disorder, not otherwise specified in, 603
  pica in, 594
  posttraumatic stress disorder in, 594
  psychopharmacological treatment of, 595t–599t, 608
  racial, ethnic, and cultural differences among, 578
  Rett's disorder in, 603
  rumination disorder in, 595
  schizophrenia in, 604
  school and, 577
  separation anxiety disorder in, 590, 593
  substance abuse in, 604

Child(ren) *(Continued)*
therapeutic relationships with, 578–579
countertransference in, 578–579
transference in, 578
Tourette's syndrome in, 598–599, 601
treatment settings for, 606–608, *607*
violence of, toward parents, 1044
Child abuse, 1040. See also *Family violence.*
family structural inequality causing, 1046, 1047
mental illness related to, 580
nursing process for, 1062–1068
assessment in, 1064–1065, *1066–1067*
diagnosis in, 1065–1066
evaluation in, 1068
implementation in, 1067–1068
outcome identification in, 1066
planning in, 1067
prevention of, 1067–1068
primary, 1067
secondary, 1067
tertiary, 1067–1068, *1069*
reporting, 1065
risk factors for, 1065b
wife rape related to, 1089
Child state, in transactional communication model, 205
Childhood disintegrative disorder, 603
Children's and Communities Mental Health Systems Improvement Act of 1990, 40
Children's Psychiatric Rating Scale (CPRS), 1222–1227
Chinese people, 317
traditional medicine of, 488–489, *489*
Chlordiazepoxide (Librium), dosage of, 552t
for withdrawal symptoms, 809
Chlorpromazine (Ormazine; Thorazine), 526, 527t
development of, 23
fact sheet for, *557*
for children, 598t
Chlorprothixene (Taractan), 527t
Chocolate, vasopressive action of, 543t
Choice(s), empowerment and, 182
for stress management, 65–66
Chromosomal abnormalities, sexual problems resulting from, 894
Chronically mentally ill patient(s), 1131
community mental health care for. See *Community mental health care.*
group psychotherapy for, 409–410
home care for, 1159–1160
Cibalith-S. See *Lithium (Cibalith-S; Eskalith; Eskalith CR; Lithane; Lithaboid; Lithonate; Lithotabs.)*
Cingulate gyrus, 133, 134, 139
anxiety and, 693
Circadian rhythm hypothesis, of mood disorders, 145, 766
Circular communication models, 204–205, *205*
Circumstantiality, 296t
Clarifying, 215, 217t
Classical conditioning, 112, 423
therapeutic applications of, 424b
Clement, J. A., 6
Clinical decision-making trees, for collaborative models, of care, 1203–1204
Clinical indicators, 1183, 1183b, 1184b, *1185, 1186*
Clinical Modification of the World Health Organization's International Classification of Diseases–The Ninth Revision (ICD-9-CM), 33, *36*, 36–37
Clinical nurse specialist (CNS), 59
Clinical Nursing Note form, 276
Clinical outcome assessment documentation (COAD), 1186
Clinical pathways, 1186, *1187–1188*
for collaborative models, of care, 1203–1204
Clinical practice guidelines, 1202–1203
Clinical psychologists, as treatment team members, 63t
Clomipramine (Anafranil), for children, 596t
for obsessive-compulsive disorder, 702, 716
Clonazepam (Klonopin), for children, 597t
Clonidine (Catapres), for children, 599t
for narcotic abuse, 812
Clorazepate (Gen-Xene; Tranxene), dosage of, 552t
Closed-ended questions, 214
Clozapine (Clozaril), 532
contraindications to, 533
fact sheet for, *558*
for children, 599t
for schizophrenia, 534
Cluster A personality disorders, 844–845
Cluster B personality disorders, 845–848
Cluster C personality disorders, 845, 848, 850–851
CMASA (Community Mobilization Against Substance Abuse), 439
CMH (community mental health) centers, 20, 22, 47, 1129, 1134
federal funding for, termination of, 22, 39–40
CNS (clinical nurse specialist), 59
Coaching, in therapeutic communication, *221*, 221–222
COAD (clinical outcome assessment documentation), 1186
Coalition to End Legalized Rape (CELR), 1088
COBRA (Consolidated Omnibus Budget Reconciliation Act) of 1985, 1177
Cocaine, abuse of, 813–814
societal information about, 820
early understanding of, 794–795
teratogenic effects of, 826, 827t
Cocaine Anonymous, 823
Cocaine blues, 813
Codependency, 828–829, *829*
Coercive behavior, 81
Cognex (tetrahydroaminoacridine), abuse of, 810–811
for Alzheimer's disease, 994
Cognitive assessment, 295, 297
in mental retardation, 601, 602
of suicidal patients, 936
Cognitive behavioral groups, 409, 410
Cognitive disorder(s), 977–1017
acute. See *Delirium.*
causes of, 980–982
cerebral, 980–981
limbic, 981
multiple, 981–982
chronic. See *Dementia.*
DSM-IV categorization of, changes in, 980
historical background of, 979–980
Cognitive distortion(s), 206–207, 207t
clarifying, in crisis intervention, 356
disputing, 207–208
in cognitive psychotherapy, 376–379, *377*, *378*, 378t
Cognitive domain, 510, 511b
Cognitive function, in Alzheimer's disease, early stages of, 1003–1004
Cognitive function, in Alzheimer's disease *Continued*
in mental retardation, 34
in children, 601–603
in personality disorders, 844
of elderly people, assessing, 654–655
Cognitive learning theory(ies), 505, 505t
social, 505t, 505–506
Cognitive model(s), of communication, 205–208
behavioral, 206, 207t, 208
neurolinguistic programming, 266
of mood disorders, 769
Cognitive process(es), 155, 160–161
development of, 160, 160t
evaluative aspect of, 161
influences on, 160–161
Sullivan's theory of, 106
Cognitive restructuring, for anxiety disorders, 715–716
Cognitive therapy, 376–379, *377*, *378*, 378t
for anxiety disorders, 715–716
for low back pain, 954
for mood disorders, 776, 778
Cohabitation, 465t
Cohesion, of families, in schizophrenia, 740
of psychotherapy groups, 392, 400–401
Coleadership, of psychotherapy groups, 405–406
Collaboration, 62–63, 63t
American Nurses' Association Code for Nurses on, 84
Collaborative model(s), of care, 1203–1204
case management in, 1203
critical pathways in, 1203–1204
for advanced-practice nursing, 1204
Collaborative practice, 1183
Collective unconscious, 104
Color, cultural concepts of, 311
"Combat exhaustion," 21
Combativeness. See also *Violence.*
in Alzheimer's disease, middle stages of, 1008
Commercial insurance companies, 45
home care funding under, 1158
Commitment stage, of healing, 491
Commune, 465t
Communication, 191–226
among African Americans, 314b
among Asian Americans, 316b
among European Americans, 313b
among Hispanic Americans, 315b
among Native Americans, 319b
among Pacific Island peoples, 318b
among West Indian peoples, 321b
as learned process, 193
as "point of intersection," 192
components of, 193
confidentiality and, 200–201
confirming, 201–202, 203t, 238
cross-cultural, 322
disconfirming, 238–239
effective, 195–197
appropriate messages for, 196
awareness of others' needs for, 195–196
clear messages for, 196
flexible communication style for, 196
requesting validation for, 196
self-awareness for, 195
suggestions for, 322b
timing for, 196
functions of, 192–195
"being with" others as, 194–195
connecting as, 192–194, *193*
responses as, 195
sharing meaning as, 195

Communication (*Continued*)
in families. See *Family(ies), communication in.*
in milieu therapy, 452, 453, 455, 457, 460
in psychotherapy groups. See *Group psychotherapy, communication in.*
metacommunication and, 195–196, 197, 201, 202t
nonverbal. See *Nonverbal communication.*
social, therapeutic communication compared with, 208t
therapeutic. See *Therapeutic communication.*
verbal, *197*, 197–198
message confusion in, 197–198
Communication disorder(s), aphasia as, 981, 990, 990t
in Alzheimer's disease, early stages of, 999–1001, 1000t
middle stages of, 1007
in children, 603
Communication therapy, with families, 474t
Community, altruistic, 341
as patient. See *Community mental health care, community-focused.*
nurse as participant in, 62
of children, 577
suicide related to, 932
Community crises, 341
Community Mental Health Act of 1963, 20, 37, 39–40, 42, 444, 1129, 1130
rescinding of, 39–40
Community mental health care, 1127–1148
community-focused, 1134
nursing process for, 1138–1140
assessment in, 1138
diagnosis in, 1138
evaluation in, 1139–1140
implementation in, 1139
outcome identification in, 1138
planning in, 1138–1139
course of, 1130–1131
family-focused. See *Community mental health care, individual- or family-focused.*
for anxiety disorders, 715–716
for chronically mentally ill, 1136
future of, 1147
impetus for, 1128–1130
individual- or family-focused, nursing process for, 1140–1146
assessment in, 1140, 1141t–1142t
diagnosis in, 1140–1141
evaluation in, 1145–1146
implementation in, 1144–1145
outcome identification in, 1142–1143
planning in, 1143–1144
milieu therapy in. See *Milieu therapy, in community treatment settings.*
nursing role in, 1136–1138
in prevention, 1137
nursing process for, 1137–1138
philosophy of, 1135
population served by, 1131–1134
identification of, 1131, 1132t
needs of, 1132–1134
service providers for, 1136
services provided by, 1135–1136
success of, 1146–1147
Community Mental Health Center Amendment of 1975, 22
Community mental health (CMH) centers, 20, 22, 47, 1129, 1134
federal funding for, termination of, 22, 39–40
Community Mental Health Systems Act of 1980, 22, 1130
Community Mobilization Against Substance Abuse (CMASA), 439
Community services, needed by mentally ill patients, 45b
Community-living programs, for schizophrenic patients, 745
Compassion fatigue, 1113–1114, 1113b
Competence, ethnic, 308–309
Competency, in Alzheimer's disease, early stages of, 1003–1004
Completed suicide, 928
Compliance, with psychopharmacological treatment, promoting, 535, 546
Complicated grieving, 663
Compound family, 465t
Comprehensive Drug Abuse Prevention and Control Act of 1970, 796
Compulsion(s), 296t, 701–702. See also *Obsessive-compulsive disorder (OCD).*
in obsessive-compulsive personality disorder, 850–851
Computed tomography (CT), 141
Conceptual models, 116
Conceptual utilization, 1201
Concern, detached, for stress management, 66
Concrete operational stage, 160, 160t
Concreteness, difficulty with, in schizophrenia, 739
Concretization, in psychodrama, 413t
Conditioning. See also *Classical conditioning; Operant conditioning.*
respondent, 112
operant conditioning versus, *112*
Conduct and Utilization of Research in Nursing (CURN) project, 1201
Conduct disorders, in children, 590, 591–592
in parents, children's disturbances related to, 581
Confabulation, 296t
Confidentiality, 200–201
American Nurses' Association Code for Nurses on, 83–84
in group psychotherapy, 395
minors and, 201
of psychotherapy, 373
therapeutic relationship and, 85, 87b
Confirming communication, 201–202, 203t, 238
Conflict(s), cultural, of refugees, 308
in families, 475
in psychotherapy groups, 409
Confrontation, in group psychotherapy, 392
in therapeutic communication, 217
Confucianism, 317
Congregate housing, 1134
Conjoint family therapy, 473
Connotation, 198
Conscience, 101
Conscientious objectors, public service performed by, 21
Conscious awareness, 104
Conscious mind, 100
Consciousness, identity, 332
of God, 164–165
Consent, informed. See *Informed consent.*
Consequence(s), of behavior, 421
Conservative Jews, 313, 314
Conservatorship, 1010
Consistency, trust and, 245
Consolidated Omnibus Budget Reconciliation Act (COBRA) of 1985, 1177
Constructional difficulty, 990t
Consultation, in community mental health care, 1145
Containment, in milieu therapy, 448
Contiguity, 423
Continuing education, 62
Continuous amnesia, 868
Continuous quality improvement (CQI), 1175
benchmarking for, 1181
data collection and organization for, 1181, 1182t
data display for, 1182
flow of, *1184*
historical background of, 1178–1180
Deming's and Juran's impact on, 1179
integrating with quality assurance, 1176–1177
mission, goals, objectives, and philosophy of, 1180
nursing role in, 1182–1189
in monitoring and evaluating care and service, 1184–1189
clinical indicators for, 1185, 1186
decision analysis for, 1186, 1189
diagnosis-specific criteria and critical paths for, 1186, *1187–1188*
patient response and outcomes for, 1186
reporting data for, 1185–1186
standards of care and practice for, 1185
in planning and collaboration, 1183–1184, *1184*
patient focus of, 1189–1191
guest relations and, 1190
organizational commitment for, 1189
patient feedback and, 1190
patients' rights and, 1190–1191
satisfaction and, 1189–1190
trend monitoring and analysis for, 1189
quality controls and quality teams for, 1181
statistical analysis for, 1181–1182
strategic planning for, 1180, *1181*
Continuous reinforcement, 430, 430t
Continuum of care, nurse as provider of, 57
Contract(s), behavioral, 430–431, *431*
group, 394
no-harm, 938, 939, *939*
no-suicide, 81
therapeutic, 250–251, *251*
Control, abuse and, 1040, *1041*
Controlled breathing, 714b
Controlled Substance Act of 1970, 796
Conventional level, of moral development, 75
Convergent learning style, 509
Conversion disorder, 963–964, 968t
Coordinator, nurse as, 57
Coping, by acquired immunodeficiency syndrome patients, assessment of, 1117
by family, 468
developmental stages related to, 166, *168*
failure of, crisis state development and, 337
of children, 579, 579t
pattern of, 166–167, 169
recovery from substance abuse and, 184t
skills for, promoting, in milieu therapy, 446–447
with anxiety, 696
with losses, 676–677, 677b
Coping Assessment Profile (CAP), 1117
Coprophilia, 891t
Corpus callosum, 133
Corpus stratum, 133
Corrective life experiences, 606

Cost(s). See also *Funding.*
of acquired immunodeficiency syndrome care, 1116
of family violence, 1042
of mental illness, 44
mood disorders and, 763
Counseling, 273. See also *Psychotherapy.*
for personality disorders, 852, 854, 855
supportive, for schizophrenia, 748–749
Counseling and Psychotherapy (Rogers), 109
Countertransference, 103, 256, 257
in psychodynamic short-term therapy, 376
with children, 578–579
Couples therapy, 473
Covenant, 87
Covert sensitization, for sexual disorders, 900
Cowles, Edward A., 18
CPRS (Children's Psychiatric Rating Scale), 1222–1227
CQI. See *Continuous quality improvement (CQI).*
Crack cocaine, abuse of, 813–814
Craving, for abused substances, 801
Creative arts therapists, as treatment team members, 63t
Creutzfeldt-Jakob disease, 990–991
Crisis(es), as opportunity, for change, 340
definition of, 329, 334–335
developmental (maturational), 343, 345
midlife, 620, 624
patients in, 354b
personal loss causing, 331
precipitating event for, determining, 352, 353
psychosocial, 107
situational, 341–343
community, 341
disasters as, 341
family, 342–343, 344t
personal, 341–342, 342b
underlying suicide attempt, identifying, 939
Crisis intervention, 329, 345–359
caring for oneself during, 361–362
critical incident debriefing following, 361–362
definition of, 345
in disasters, 359–360
orientation phase of, 345–353
assessment in, 345
database development during, 352–353
medical condition in, 346
patient engagement in, 350–352
recognizing repeaters and, 352
suicide risk in, 346–347
violent potential in, 347–350, 348t–350t
psychiatric emergency services for, 361
termination phase of, 358–359
evaluation during, 358
identifying need for further treatment during, 358–359
record-keeping during, 359
referrals during, 359
theoretical perspectives on, 331–334
of Aguilera, 332–333, *334*
of Caplan, 331
of Erikson, 331–332, 333t
of Lindemann, 331
working phase of, 354–358
diagnosis, outcome identification, and planning during, 354–355
implementation during, 355–358
Crisis (ABC-X) Model of Family Coping, 468
Crisis sequence, 341
Crisis state, 335–336, 336b
factor(s) contributing to, 336–338
failure of coping strategies as, 337
hazardous events as, 336
intolerable tension as, 337
lack of social support as, 337–338
vulnerability as, 336–337
risk factor(s) for, concurrent stressors as, 339
physical and emotional depletion as, 340
prior stressors as, *339*, 339–340
prolonged stress as, 340
"unacceptable" stressors as, 338–339
Crisis units, milieu therapy in, 459
Critical incident debriefing, 361–362
Critical pathways, 1186, *1187–1188*
for collaborative models, of care, 1203–1204
Critical stressors, 334
Critical theory, of family, 576
Cross-gender identification, 892–893
Cross-tolerance, 801
definition of, 798
Crystallized intelligence, 993
CT (computed tomography), 141
Cueing, 423, 432–433
Cultural conflicts, of refugees, 308
Culture, 303–323. See also specific cultural groups.
African-American, 211t, 314
Chinese, 317
communication and, 322
definition of, 305
ethnic competence and, 308–309
ethnic identity and, 307
ethnocentrism and, 307
Filipino, 318
Hispanic-American, 211t, 314–315
Indian, 315–316
Inuit, 320
Irish-American, 312–313
Italian-American, 313
Japanese, 317–318
Jewish, 313–314
Native-American, 318–320
of children, 578
of Pacific Island peoples, 318
perceptions related to, of color, 311
of decision makers, 312
of dress, 311
of gestures, 311
of mental illness, 312
of physical self, 156
of space, 311
of time, 310
of voice tone, 311
of words, 311
prejudice and, 306
race and, 306
racism and, 306–307
religion and, 312
sociocultural assessment and, 297–298
Southeast-Asian, 316–317
stereotyping and, 305–306
substance abuse related to, 824–825
terms of address and, 311–312
therapeutic communication and, 210–211, 211t
touch and, 311
transcultural identification and, 307–308
transcultural nursing and, 305
West Indian, 321–322
Culture shock, 308
Culture-bound syndromes, 211t, 309, 316
Cummings, Harry, 77
Curative factors, in group psychotherapy. See *Group psychotherapy, curative factor(s) in.*
CURN (Conduct and Utilization of Research in Nursing) project, 1201
Cushing's disease, mood disorders related to, 768
Cycle of abuse, 1056, *1057*
Cyclothymia, 763
Cyclothymic disorder, definition of, 765t

Dairy products, 497
interaction with monoamine oxidase inhibitors, 543t
Dantrolene, for neuroleptic malignant syndrome, 530
DARE format, 276
Darling v. Charleston Community Memorial Hospital, 1177
Darwin, Charles, 95–96
Data collection, for assessment. See *Assessment, data collection for.*
Data collection tools, 285
Date rape, 1089
Davis, Mary E. P., 18
Day treatment, for Alzheimer's patients, in early stages, 1004
for children, 607
for chronically mentally ill, 1136
milieu therapy in, 456
of substance abuse, nursing actions for, 820t
setting for, 47
Death. See also *Grief; Grieving process; Homicide; Loss(es); Suicide.*
from acquired immunodeficiency syndrome, dying process and, 1109–1110
of spouse, 630
"Decade of the Brain," 27
Decision analysis, 1186, 1189
Decision makers, cultural concepts of, 312
Decision matrices, 1181, 1182t
Decision-making trees, for collaborative models, of care, 1203–1204
Decoding, of messages, 202–204
Deductive reasoning, 1198
Defense(s), supporting, in crisis intervention, 357
Defense mechanisms, against anxiety, 696, 697b
Deficiency needs, 108
Deinstitutionalization, 23, 39, 1128–1129
homelessness related to, 1026
Delirium, 982–989, 983b
causes of, 980–982, 985t
differential diagnosis of, 984t
drug-induced, mechanisms of, 984t
family information about, 985
follow-up care for, 987
in elderly people, 650–651
nursing care for, 982–987
anxiety containment in, 986
case study of, 987–989
diagnosis in, 982–985, 984t, 985t
eliminating causative factors in, 986–987
emergency triage in, 982
medications in, 986
minimizing perceptual distortions in, 986
minimizing stimuli in, 986
patient care guidelines for, 985–987
with patient aggression, 987
Delirium tremens, 808

Delivery, depression following, 766
Delusion(s), 223–224, 296t
  in schizophrenia, 738–739, 744t
    of grandeur, 738, 744t
    paranoid, 738, 744t
Dementia, 989–1018, 997b, 998b, 1004b, 1009b, 1010b
  brain lesions causing, 991–992
    foci of, 991
  causes of, 980–982, 993–994
  common features of, 988b
  differential diagnosis of, 984t
  early stages of. See also *Alzheimer's disease, early stages of.*
    family concerns in, 1013t
  end stage of, eating in, encouraging, 1011
    family concerns in, 1013t
  family information about, 996
  family issues regarding, 1011–1012, 1013t
    abuse as, 1012
    caregiving as, 1012–1013
  historical background of, 979–980
  in AIDS. See *AIDS-dementia complex (ADC).*
  in alcohol-induced persisting amnestic disorders, 992
  in Alzheimer's disease. See *Alzheimer's disease.*
  in depression, 993
  in elderly people, 650, 651, 993. See also *Alzheimer's disease.*
  in multiple sclerosis, 993
  in normal-pressure hydrocephalus, 992
  in Parkinson's disease, 992–993
  incidence and prevalence of, 993
  Lewy body, 991
  middle stages of. See also *Alzheimer's disease, middle stages of.*
    family concerns in, 1013t
  multi-infarct, 991
  neurological deficits in, terminology for, 990t
  nursing process for, case study of, 1014–1017
  patient abuse in, 1012
  patient care in, 994t, 994–996
    for early stages. See *Alzheimer's disease, early stages of.*
    for end stage, 1010–1011
    for middle stages. See *Alzheimer's disease, middle stages of.*
    functional status in, preserving, 995
    patient's dignity in, protecting, 995
    quality of life in, promoting, 995–996
  primary, 989–991. See also *Alzheimer's disease.*
    Creutzfeldt-Jakob disease as, 990–991
    Pick's disease as, 990
  support groups for, 1013–1014
  vascular, 991–992
    with extrapyramidal symptoms, 991
    comorbidity of, with bipolar disorder, 767
Dementia praecox, 729. See also *Schizophrenia.*
Demerol (meperidine), drug interactions of, 543
Demi, Alice Sterner, 663
Deming, W. Edwards, 1179
Deming cycle, 1180, *1181*
Democratic principles, 80–81
Demonstration, for patient education, 512–513
Dendrites, 135, *135*
Denial, as defense mechanism, 697
  family interventions for, 344t
  in mood disorders, 771
Denotation, 198
Depakene (valproic acid), for bipolar disorder, 546, 549
  for children, 597t
Depakote (valproic acid), for bipolar disorder, 546, 549
  for children, 597t
Department of Defense Authorization Bill of 1990, 40
Dependence, 799
  on drugs, 800–802
    definition of, 800
    on antipsychotic agents, 531
    on benzodiazepines, 552
    physical, 800–801
      definition of, 798
    psychological, 801–802
      definition of, 798
Dependency, Bion's concept of, 389
Dependent personality disorder, 850
Depersonalization, in dissociative disorders, 866–867
Depersonalization disorder, 868–869
  case study of, 874–876
Depo-Provera (medroxyprogesterone acetate), for sexual disorders, 900
D-E-P-O-R-D model, 883, *883*
Depressant agent(s). See also specific drugs.
  as controlled substances, 796, 796t
  drug interactions of, 531, 539, 552
Depression, 759. See also *Bipolar disorder; Mood disorder(s).*
  among Native Americans, 319
  causes of, 34
    catecholamine hypothesis of, 144
  comorbidity of, with cerebrovascular accident, 767–768
    with eating disorders, 914
    with Parkinson's disease, 767
  definition of, 761, 765t
  dementia in, 993
  drugs causing, 767t
  expected outcomes for, 778b
  facial expressions in, 199–200
  family interventions for, 344t
  grief compared with, 673, 673t
  in acquired immunodeficiency syndrome, 1111
    differentiating dementia from, 1117
    etiology of, 1111
    treatment of, 1111
  in bipolar disorder, 546
  in children, 603–604
  in elderly people, 649–650
  in mother, children's disturbances related to, 581
  indicators of, 770b
  integrated model of, *769*, 769–770
  major. See *Major depression.*
  neuroendocrine tests in, 142, 144
  norepinephrine and, 142, 144–145
  not otherwise specified, definition of, 765t
  postpartum, 766
  rape causing, 1092
  risk factors for, 766b
  short-term goals for, 779b
  sleep disorders associated with, 142
  societal information about, 780
  treatment of, psychopharmacological, 538, 541. See also *Antidepressant agent(s);* specific drugs.
Derealization, in dissociative disorders, 866t, 868
Dereflection, 111
Dermatologic effects, of antipsychotic agents, 530–531
DES (Dissociative Experiences Scale), 865, 1209–1210
Descartes, Rene, 95, 160, 951
Desensitization therapy, 437–438
  for obsessive-compulsive disorder, 702
Desipramine (Norpramin; Pertofrane), 537t
  dosage of, 540t
Desire, sexual, 883–884
    disorders of, 884, 885
Despair, grief and, 179
Desyrel (trazodone), 537t, 544–545
  dosage of, 540t
Detached concern, for stress management, 66
Detention, involuntary, 82b
Detoxification, 801
  definition of, 798
Deutsch, Albert, 21
Developmental (maturational) crises, 343, 345
Developmental disorders, in children, 601–603
Developmental eras, 620–621
Developmental history, in psychodynamic short-term therapy, 374
Developmental stage(s), age related to, 575t
  body consciousness related to, 156–158
  coping related to, 166, *168*
  Erikson's theory of, 106–108, 166, 167, 649
    during adulthood, 620
    Freud's theory compared with, 103t
    hierarchy of needs related to, *168*
    relevance to nursing, 107–108
  Freud's theory of, 101–102
    Erikson's theory compared with, 103t
  Piaget's theory of, 160, 160t
  spiritual development and, 588t
Developmental tasks, 166
  of elderly people, 648, 649
  of family, 468
Dexamethasone suppression test (DST), 142
Dexedrine (dextroamphetamine sulfate), for children, 595t
Dextroamphetamine sulfate (Dexedrine), for children, 595t
Dhat syndrome, 309
Diagnosis(es), dual, 43
    with alcoholism, 809
  in nursing process. See *Nursing diagnosis(es).*
Diagnostic and Statistical Manual of Mental Disorders-IV (DSM-IV), 33, 36, *36*, 37, *38*, 268
  AIDS-dementia complex in, 1111
  anxiety in, categories of, 698
  classifications of, 1229–1237
  cognitive disorders in, 980
  dissociative disorders in, 867
  home care diagnoses and, 1157
  mood disorders in, 765
  nursing diagnoses related to, 271
  on grieving, 665–666
  on schizophrenia, 731, 732t
  paraphilias in, 890, 891t
  personality disorders in, 842, 844–851
  phobias in, 706
  posttraumatic stress disorder in, 703
  religious and spiritual problems in, 741
  sexual desire disorders in, 884, 885
  somatoform disorders in, 961–967
  substance abuse in, 798, 803, 804
Dialogue, for active listening, 212–213
Diaphoresis, tricyclic antidepressants causing, 538

Diaries, in psychophysiological disorders, 953
Diazepam (Valium), 549
  dosage of, 552t
  for bipolar disorder, 547
  for children, 597t
  for withdrawal symptoms, 809
  neurotransmitter action and, 136
Dibenzodiazepines, for children, 599t
Dibenzoxazepines, 527t
Dichotomous thinking, 207t
Dickens, Charles, 632–633
DID (dissociative identity disorder), 869–870
Diencephalon, 132
Diets, Bob, 666
Differentiation, level of, of family, 468
Differentiation subphase, in object relation theory, 843
Dignity, protecting, in dementia, 995
Dihydroindolones, 527t
Dilantin (phenytoin), for children, 597t
Diphenhydramine (Benadryl), for children, 597t
Direct care, 54, 56
Direct self-destructive behavior, 928
Disability, mental illness and, in children, 581
Disadvantaged people. See *Poverty.*
Disaster(s), 341
  crisis intervention in, 359–360
  posttraumatic stress disorder following, 703
Disbelief, in grieving process, 669
Discharge planning, 284
  nurse's role in, 745
Discipline (professional), 115
Disconfirming communication, 238–239
Discrimination (of stimuli), 423
Discrimination (racial and ethnic), 306
Discriminative stimulus, 112–113
Disdain, toward homeless people, 1031
Disease Concept of Alcoholism (Jellinek), 795
Disease model, of substance abuse, 799
Diseases of the Mind (Rush), 14
Disenfranchised grieving, 675
Disequilibration, 160
Disgust, toward homeless people, 1031
Disorganized schizophrenia, 732t
Disorientation, in Alzheimer's disease, middle stages of, 1005
  in delirium, 982
Displacement, as defense mechanism, 697
Disruptive behaviors, of children, 579
Dissociation continuum, 864–865
Dissociative amnesia, 867–868, 872
Dissociative disorder(s), 863–877
  amnestic, 867–868, 872
  cause of, 867
  depersonalization, 868–869
    case study of, 874–876
  dissociation concept and, 864
  dissociation continuum and, 864–865
  fugue as, 868
  not otherwise specified, 870
  nursing process for, 871–876
    assessment in, 871
    diagnosis in, 871, 872
    outcome identification in, 873
  of identity, 869–870
  planning in, 873
    case study of, 874–876
    evaluation in, 874
  societal information about, 869
  symptoms of, 866–867, 870b
Dissociative Experiences Scale (DES), 865, 1209–1210
Dissociative fugue, 868
Dissociative identity disorder (DID), 869–870
Distance/pursuit, in families, 475
Distancing, from homeless people, 1031
Distraction, 433
Distress, spiritual, 165
Distrust, family interventions for, 344t
Disulfiram (Antabuse), 808
Diuretics, drug interactions of, 548
Divergent learning style, 509
Divorce, 624, 630
  mental illness and, in children, 581–582
Divorce therapy, 472
Dix, Dorothea Lynde, 15, *16*, 20, 444
Dixon v. Weinberger, 41
Dizygotic twins, 144
D-motives, 108
D.N.Sc. (Doctor of Nursing Science), 59
Doble abrazo, 311
Doctor of Nursing Science (D.N.Sc.), 59
Doctor of Philosophy (Ph.D.), 59
Documentation. See also *Record-keeping.*
  for charting clinical progress and outcomes, 1186
  in nursing process, 276, *277–279*
  of abuse, of women, 1051–1052, 1054
  of violent episodes, 1077–1078
Domestic violence. See *Abuse; Child abuse; Elder abuse; Family violence; Sexual abuse; Spousal abuse.*
Dopamine, 136, 137
  in abusers, 1047
  in personality development, 844
  in substance abuse, 799
Dopamine beta-hydroxylase, 136
Dopamine hypothesis, of schizophrenia, 143, 733–734
Dopaminergic system, *138*
Double binds, schizophrenia related to, 734
Doubling, in psychodrama, 413t
Down's syndrome, comorbidity of, with Alzheimer's disease, 994
Doxepin (Adapin; Sinequan), 537t
  dosage of, 540t
Dreams, in psychoanalytic psychotherapy, 369
Dress, cultural concepts of, 311
Drug(s). See also *Psychopharmacologic treatment;* specific drugs and drug types.
  addiction to. See also *Substance abuse;* specific substances.
    definition of, 798
  body consciousness and, 158
  delirium induced by, mechanisms of, 984t
  development of, 23
  interactions with foods, 496
    monoamine oxidase inhibitors and, 542, 543t
  mood disorders caused by, 767
  neurotransmitter action and, 136
  of elderly people, assessing, 653–654
  sexual function disturbances due to, 897t
  use of, in children, 608b
  withdrawal from. See *Withdrawal, from drugs.*
Drug and Alcohol Nurses Association, 797
Drug diversion, 713, 714
DSM-IV. See Diagnostic and Statistical Manual of Mental Disorders-IV (DSM-IV).
DST (dexamethasone suppression test), 142
Dual diagnosis(es), 43
  with alcoholism, 809
Dual-career families, 629
Dulaney, Peggy, 53
Dumas, Rhetaugh, 53
Dura mater, 130
Durable power of attorney, 996
Dyad family, 465t
The Dynamic Nurse-Patient Relationship: Function, Process and Principles (Orlando), 24
Dynamism, 105
Dysarthria, 990t
Dyspareunia, 884
Dysphagia, 990t
  in Alzheimer's disease, middle stages of, 1006
Dysrhythmias, tricyclic antidepressants causing, 539
Dysthymia, 761
Dysthymic disorder, definition of, 765t
  in children, 604
Dystonia, acute, antipsychotic agents causing, 528, 529t

Early adolescence, 575
Eating, assessment of, in eating disorders, 914–915
  problems with, in Alzheimer's disease, middle stages of, 1007–1008
    in children, 594–596, 600
Eating disorder(s), 909–924. See also *Anorexia nervosa; Binge eating disorder; Bulimia nervosa.*
  assessment of, 914–915
    family, 915
    physical, 914–915
    psychological, 915
    sociocultural, 915
    spiritual, 915
  causes of, 911–914
    biological, 911–912
    psychological, 912–913
    sociocultural, 913
    spiritual, 914
  comorbidity of, 914
  family information about, 919–920
  historical background of, 910–911
  in children, 594–596, 600
  nursing process for, 914–923
    assessment in. See *Eating disorder(s), assessment of.*
    case study of, 921–923
    diagnosis in, 916–917
    evaluation in, 921
    implementation in, 918–921
    outcome identification in, 916
    planning in, 916–918
  patient information about, 919–920
Echolalia, 296t, 990t
Echopraxia, 296t
ECT (electroconvulsive therapy), 23, 496, 785, 786t
  ethics of, 78–79
Education. See also *Family education; Patient education.*
  continuing, 62
  learning and, 504–505
  of adults, 632–633, 632b
Education of the Handicapped Act Amendments of 1986, 40
Educational groups, 387, 391t, 393, 415–417
EEG (electroencephalography), 142
  for biofeedback, 496
Efforts, acknowledging, in crisis intervention, 358
Ego, 101
The Ego and the Mechanisms of Defense (Anna Freud), 579

Ego integrity versus despair stage. See *Integrity versus despair stage.*
Ego psychology, 106–108
Ego theory, of Erikson, 106–108
Ego-dystonic experiences, 868
Ego-ideal, 101
Egoism, altruistic, for stress management, 66
Egotistical suicide, 932
"Eight Stages of Man," 166, 167
Ejaculation, premature, 885
Elam v. College Park Hospital, 1177
Elavil. See *Amitriptyline (Elavil; Endep).*
Elder abuse, 1044
  definition of, 1043
  nursing process for, 1068–1074
    assessment in, 1068, 1070, *1071*
    diagnosis in, 1070
    evaluation in, 1070, 1071, 1074
    implementation in, 1070, 1072–1073
    outcome identification in, 1070
    planning in, 1070
  prevention of, do's and don'ts for, 1081–1083
Elderly people, 645–659
  abuse of. See *Elder abuse.*
  ageism and, 305
  age-related changes in, 647t, 647–648
  anxiety in, 652
  assessment of, 653–655
    interviewing in, 653
    of cognitive function, 654–655
    of medications, 653–654
    of mental status, 653
  caregivers for, children as, 625, 631
  decision makers for, cultural concepts of, 312
  delirium in, 650–651
  dementia in, 650, 651. See also *Alzheimer's disease.*
  depression in, 649–650
  developmental tasks of, 648, 649
  groups for, 413–415
    reality orientation, 414
    reminiscence, 413–414
    remotivation, 414–415, 415t
  home care for, 1159
  homeless, 1028
  illness in, 648b
  life expectancy for, 646, 646t
  living arrangements of, 646, 646t
  losses experienced by, 665
  normal mental health of, 648–649
  nursing process with, 653–656
    assessment in. See *Elderly people, assessment of.*
    case study of, 656–658
    diagnosis in, 655
    evaluation in, 655–656
    implementation in, 655
    outcome identification in, 655
    planning in, 655
  old-old, 646
  promoting mental health of, 652–653
    losses and, dealing with, 652–653
    physical problem identification and treatment for, 652
  schizophrenia in, 652, 742
  sexual development during, 882t
  substance abuse among, 826–827
  suicide among, 650
  sundowners' syndrome in, 651, 1008–1009
  terms of address for, cultural concepts of, 311–312
  young-old, 646
Electra complex, 102
Electric shock, for behavioral therapy, 437
Electroconvulsive therapy (ECT), 23, 496, 785, 786t
  ethics of, 78–79
Electroencephalography (EEG), 142
  for biofeedback, 496
Electromyography (EMG), for biofeedback, 496
Elimination. See also *Incontinence.*
  assessment of, in eating disorders, 915
  in Alzheimer's disease, early stages of, 1001
Elopement, of patients, 713–714
Embedded self, 622
Emblems, 200
Emergency department, milieu therapy in, 452–453
  nurse's role in, 56b
EMG (electromyography), for biofeedback, 496
Emotional abuse, 1040–1042, 1054b
  of elders, 1044
  of spouse, 1054
Emotional assessment, 295, 296t
  of suicidal patients, 935–936
Emotional cutoff, in families, 475–476
Emotional depletion, as risk factor, for crisis state development, 340
Emotional disinhibition, 981
  in Alzheimer's disease, middle stages of, 1009
Emotional processes, 155
Emotional reactions, to rape, 1092, 1094
Empathy, in therapeutic relationships, 243, 244b
Empowerment, *181,* 181–182
  in mood disorders, 782, *783*
  in therapeutic relationships, 243
  of adult children of alcoholics, 831
Empowerment stage, of healing, 491
Empowerment treatment model, 182
Empty nest, 631
Enabling behaviors, 829
Encoding, of messages, 202
Encopresis, in children, 600
Encounter groups, 416
Endep. See *Amitriptyline (Elavil; Endep).*
Endocrine system. See *Hormones; Neuroendocrine system.*
Endogenous opioids, in eating disorders, 911–912
Energetics, 491
Engagement (forming) phase, of group development, 397–398
    communication patterns during, 397–398
    leadership tasks during, 397
Engel, George, on grief, 663, 669
Enuresis, in children, 599–600, 602
Environment(s), for group psychotherapy, 393–394
  for home care, assessment of, 1163
  for milieu therapy, 448, 452, 453, 454, 455, 456–457, 460
  for therapeutic communication, 209–210
  for therapeutic relationship, 246
  for violent patients, 1076
  holding, 448
  nurse as manager of, 56
  safety of, in milieu therapy, 446
  stimuli in, reducing, in delirium, 986
  structuring, in crisis intervention, 355–356
Epinephrine, in panic disorders, 146
Equanimity, 178–179
Equilibration, 160
Erectile disorders, 886–887
Erikson, Erik, 106
  developmental stages of. See *Developmental stage(s), Erikson's theory of.*
Erogenous zones, 101
Erotomania, in schizophrenia, 744t
Esalan, 416
Eskalith. See *Lithium (Cibalith-S; Eskalith; Eskalith CR; Lithane; Lithaboid; Lithonate; Lithotabs.)*
Eskalith CR. See *Lithium (Cibalith-S; Eskalith; Eskalith CR; Lithane; Lithaboid; Lithonate; Lithotabs.)*
Eskimos, 320
Espiritismo, 321
Essentials of Psychiatric Nursing (Taylor), 26
Esteem needs, 166
Estrogen, sexual desire and, 884
Ethical dilemma(s), 72, 77–81
  behavior control as, 81
  electroconvulsive therapy as, 78–79
  group versus individual as, 80–81
  ideals versus reality of practice as, 79–80
  informed consent as, 77–78
  refusal of treatment as, 79
Ethics, 62, 71–81. See also *Patient(s), rights of.*
  guide(s) for, autonomy as, 74
    beneficence as, 73
    fidelity as, 75
    justice as, 72–73
    love as, 73
    nonmaleficence as, 73–74
    paternalism as, 74
    veracity as, 74
  of research. See *Research.*
  theoretical perspectives on, 75–77, *76*
Ethnic competence, 308–309
Ethnic identity, 307
Ethnicity. See also specific ethnic groups.
  of children, 578
  suicide related to, 929
Ethnocentrism, 307
European Americans, 312–313
  communication among, 316
Euthymia, 761, *762*
Evidence collection kits, for rape victims, 1090
Excitement, sexual, 884–885, 885t
Exercise, 498
  assessment of, in psychodynamic short-term therapy, 374
Exhibitionism, 891t
Existential aloneness, 178–179
Existential factors, in group psychotherapy, 404–405
Existential theory(ies), 5, 110–111
  of Frankl, 111
  of Glasser, 111
  therapeutic relationships based on, 238–239, *239*
Expected outcome(s), 272. See also *Outcome(s), identification of.*
  in nursing process, 272
    identifying. See *Outcome(s), identification of.*
  of therapeutic relationships, coordinating goals with, 247
    identifying, 252–253
  writing, 272
Experiential techniques, for family therapy, 474t
  for groups, 388
Experimental psychology, origins of, 97

Expressive violence, 1048–1049
Extended family, 465t
Extermination, 306
Externalizing behaviors, 579
Extinction, 423, 429
Extrapyramidal reactions, 526, 528–530, 529t
Extrapyramidal system, 134
Extroversion, 105
Eye contact, 200
  culture and, 210–211, 211t

Facial expressions, 199–200
Fact phase, of critical incident debriefing, 361–362
Fading, 432
Faith. See *Spiritual* entries.
False inferences, in therapeutic communication, 224t, 225
False reassurance, in therapeutic communication, 224t, 225
Familiarization, in milieu therapy, 452, 453, 455, 457, 460
Families Anonymous, 604
Family(ies), 464–470
  advocacy by, influence on mental health care, 26
  as systems, 465–466
  assessment of, for home care, 1161
    in eating disorders, 915
    instruments in, 480b
  children and, 576–577
    abuse of. See *Child abuse; Family violence.*
  codependency in, 797, 828–829, *829*
  communication in, 466–467
    in schizophrenia, 740
    mood disorders related to, 769
    schizophrenia and, 740
    substance abuse and, 830
  crises of, 342–343
    interventions for, 344t
  critical theory of, 576
  demographic trends in, 465b
  dual-career, 629
  eating disorders related to, 912
    family assessment in, 915
  education of. See *Family education.*
  elder abuse in. See *Elder abuse.*
  enabling behaviors in, 829
  forms of, 464–465, 465t
  functional, characteristics of, 469b
  functioning of, 468–470
  gay, 465t
  information for. See also *Family education.*
    about delirium, 985
    about dementia, 996
    about eating disorders, 919–920
    about schizophrenia, 749
    about 12-step programs, 824
  of Alzheimer's disease patients. See *Alzheimer's disease.*
  of chronically mentally ill, support for, 1132
  of mood disorder patients, assessment of, 772–773
    collaboration with, 781–782
  of rape victims, response of, assessment of, 1091
    support and education for, 1097
  of schizophrenic patients, assessment of, 740–741
    high expressed emotion in, 736
    psychoeducation groups for, 749–750
  overwhelmed, homelessness due to, 1030
Family(ies) *Continued*
  recapitulation of, in group psychotherapy, 404
  roles in, 162–163, 466
  schizophrenia related to, 734–735
  "sick member" of, evaluation of therapy's effect on, 482–483
  structure of, changes in, 629
    inequality of, violence due to, 1046–1047
  substance abuse in, as family disease, 828
    recovery from, 829–832
  time and, 467–468
  violence in. See *Child abuse; Family violence; Spousal abuse.*
Family coping theory, 468
Family education, about Alzheimer's disease, 1001–1002
  about mood disorders, 779–780
  about rape, 1097
  about schizophrenia, 749–750
  concerning mental illness, 516b
  content for, 518–519
  in community mental health care, 1144–1145
Family history, in psychodynamic short-term therapy, 374
Family myths, 466
Family Process, 470
Family secrets, 466
Family therapy, 470–485
  conjoint, 473b
  couples, 473b
  divorce, 472
  for eating disorders, 919–920
  for substance abuse, 830
  historical background of, 470
  individual, 473b
  marital, 471–472
  models of, 473, 474t
  multiple-family, 473b
  multiple-impact, 473b
  network, 473b
  nursing process for, 476–484
    assessment in, 476–479
    diagnosis in, 479–480, 481b
    outcome identification in, 480
    planning in, 480–483
  patients' questions about, 472
  psychoeducation in, 470–471
  with children, 606
Family violence, 1039–1080
  alcohol abuse and, 1049b
  by siblings, 1043–1044
  cause(s) of, 1044–1047
    costs and, lack of, 1044–1045
    family privacy as, 1046
    social attitudes as, 1045–1046
    social controls and, absence of, 1045
    structural inequality as, 1046–1047
  continuum of, 1049t
  extent of, 1042–1043
  individuals committing. See *Abuser(s).*
  myths regarding, 1046b
  religion and spirituality in, 1049–1050
  terminology for, 1040–1042
  toward elders. See *Elder abuse.*
  toward parents, 1044
  toward spouse. See *Spousal abuse.*
  victims' responses to, 1043
FAS (fetal alcohol syndrome), 826, 827t
Fatalistic suicide, 932
Fava beans, vasopressive action of, 543t
Fear(s). See also *Anxiety; Anxiety disorder(s); Panic; Panic attacks; Phobia(s).*
Fear(s) (*Continued*)
  desensitization for, 437–438
  family interventions for, 344t
  in bipolar disorders, 772
  in mood disorders, 771
  of homeless people, 1031
  of homosexuals, 1108
  of nurses. See *Nurse(s), fears of.*
Fecal incontinence, in children, 600
Federal funding, for mental health programs, termination of, 39–40
Feedback, from patients, in continuous quality improvement, 1190
  in group psychotherapy, 406
  in therapeutic communication, 218
  in therapeutic relationships, 242, 255
Feedback loops, neuroendocrine, 139
Feeding disorders. See *Eating; Eating disorder(s).*
Females. See *Gender* entries; *Sexual* entries; *Sexuality; Women.*
Fertility, 887
Fetal alcohol syndrome (FAS), 826, 827t
Fetishism, 891t
Fiber, dietary, 498
Fidelity, as ethical guide, 75
Fiefel, Herman, 664
Field Theory in Social Science (Lewin), 388
Fight or flight response, 694, 951
  Bion's concept of, 389
Filipinos, 318
Financial abuse, of elders, 1044
FIRO (Fundamental Interpersonal Relations Orientation), 388
First aid, psychological, do's and don'ts of, 359
First-rank symptoms, of schizophrenia, 730
Fish, interaction with monoamine oxidase inhibitors, 543t
Fittingness, 1200
Fitzpatrick, Joyce, 26
Fitzsimmons, Laura, 24
Flashbacks, 796
  definition of, 798
Flexner, Abraham, 25, 1177
Flight of ideas, 296t
Floccillation, 990t
Flooding, 432
Flow charting, 1181
Flumazenil (Romazicon), for benzodiazepine overdose, 553
Fluoxetine (Prozac), 537t, 543–544
  action of, 544
  adverse effects of, 544
  dosage and administration of, 544
  dosage of, 540t
  drug interactions of, 544
  pharmacokinetics of, 544
  therapeutic uses of, 544
    for AIDS-dementia complex, 1112
    for children, 596t
    for eating disorders, 911, 919
Fluphenazine (Permitil; Prolixin), 527t, 531, 532t
  fact sheet for, *559*
Fluvoxamine (Luvox), 537t, 544
  dosage of, 540t
Focus, for active listening, 212
  of assessment, 285
  of social versus therapeutic relationships, 233
Focused questions, 214

Folk healing, among Hispanic Americans, 315
among Inuit peoples, 320
among Native Americans, 319–320
among Southeast Asians, 317
among West Indian peoples, 321
Food(s), in migraine headaches, 960
in nutritional therapies, 496–498
interactions with medications, 496
monoamine oxidase inhibitors and, 542, 543t, 700
role in people's lives, 909–910
Food additives, 497
Fordyce, Edna, 12–13
Forehand, Jennie, 184
Forensic units, 47
Formal operations stage, 160, 160t
Formal thought disorder, in schizophrenia, 727–728, 729, 739
interventions for, 747
nursing diagnosis of, 744t
Formative evaluation, 274
Formication, 990t
Forming (engagement) phase, of group development, 397–398
communication patterns during, 397–398
leadership tasks during, 397
Fornix, 133
Forward movement, 192
Foulkes, S. H., 388
Frankfurt School, 576
Frankl, Viktor, 13, 111, 498
logotherapy of, 111
Franklin, Benjamin, 19
Free association, 102
Free will, for stress management, 66
Freud, Anna, 106, 575, 578, 579
Freud, Sigmund, 16, 94, 99, 104, 106, 129, 368–369
on anorexia, 911
on anxiety, 694
on cocaine, 794–795
on dissociation, 864
on grief, 662
on homosexuality, 893
Freudian theory, 99–104
Erikson's theory compared with, 103t
of developmental stages, 101–102
of dissociation, 864
of mood disorders, 768–769
of personality dynamics, 99–100
of personality structure, 100–101
psychoanalytic techniques of, 102–103, 368–370, 369t
relevance to nursing, 103–104
Friends Asylum, 444
Friendships, of children, 577
From Novice to Expert: Excellence and Power in Clinical Nursing Practice (Benner), 151
Fromm-Reichman, Frieda, 24
Frontal lobes, 131, *132*, 134, 139
Frotteurism, 891t
Fruits, 497
interaction of, with monoamine oxidase inhibitors, 543t
Fugue, dissociative, 868
Functional health patterns, data collection using, 285
Functional similarity, of group members, 392
Fundamental Interpersonal Relations Orientation (FIRO), 388
Funding, 43–46
before insurance, 43–44
current state of, 44–46
Funding (*Continued*)
direct reimbursement for advanced-practice psychiatric-mental health nurses and, 46
federal, termination of, 22, 39–40
for professional training, 46
health maintenance organizations as source of, 45
insurance as source of. See *Insurance.*
managed care and, 45–46
mental health parity and, 45

GABA. See *Gamma-aminobutyric acid (GABA).*
GAD. See *Generalized anxiety disorder (GAD).*
Gain, primary and secondary, 964
Galactorrhea, antipsychotic agents causing, 531
Galvanometer, for biofeedback, 496
Gamma-aminobutyric acid (GABA), in anxiety, 146, 693–694
in mood disorders, 145
in panic disorder, 700
potentiation of, by benzodiazepines, 550
receptor for, 136
GAP (Group for the Advancement of Psychiatry), 470
GAS (general adaptation syndrome), psychophysiological disorders related to, 951, *952*
Gastrointestinal system. See also *Irritable bowel syndrome (IBS).*
aging of, 647t
Gay family, 465t
Gender. See also *Men; Sexual* entries; *Sexuality; Women.*
definition of, 881
Gender difference(s), in adult development, 619
in orgasm, 885–886
in socialization, 76
in suicide rates, 929
Gender dysphoria, definition of, 881
Gender identity, 163
definition of, 881
disorders of, 892–893
in children, 597–598
Gender role(s), 163
among Hispanic Americans, 315
General adaptation syndrome (GAS), psychophysiological disorders related to, 951, *952*
Generalization, 423
Generalized (global) amnesia, in dissociative disorders, 866t, 867
Generalized anxiety disorder (GAD), 698–699
etiology of, 698–699
nursing implications of, 699
treatment of, 554, 699
Generativity versus self-absorption stage, 103t, 107, 167t, 620
stressors during, 333t
Generic support, in disasters, 359–360
Genetics, of abusers, 1047
of Alzheimer's disease, 994
of anxiety disorders, 146
of eating disorders, 911
of mood disorders, 145, 768
of panic disorder, 700
of personality development, 843–844
of schizophrenia, 144, 733
of substance abuse, 799–800
Genital stage, 102, 103t, 575
Genitourinary system, aging of, 647t
Genograms, 473, *478*, 478–479, *479*, 830
Gentrification, homelessness related to, 1029
Genuineness, in therapeutic relationships, 244
Gen-Xene (clorazepate), dosage of, 552t
Geropsychiatry, 59
Gestures, 200
cultural concepts of, 311
Gheel community, 20, 1127
A Gift of Hope: How to Survive Our Tragedies (Veninga), 670, 670t
Gilligan, Carol, adult development theory of, 622
Ginseng, vasopressive action of, 543t
Glasser, William, reality therapy of, 111
Glial cells, 135
Global (generalized) amnesia, in dissociative disorders, 866t, 867
Global Assessment of Functioning Scale, 1220
Global memory loss, 990
Global physical movements, 200
Gluten, 497
Goal(s). See also *Outcome(s), identification of.*
for behavioral therapy, 427
for crisis intervention, 355
for family therapy, 480
evaluation of, 482
for stress management, 66
for therapeutic relationship, 246
coordinating with outcomes, 247
planning, 252–253
sharing with health care team, 247
group, in group psychotherapy, 391
of adults, during 30s, 623–624
God-consciousness, 164–165
Gogh, Vincent van, 760
Goiter, lithium causing, 548
Gonzales v. Nork and Mercy Hospital, 1177
Good Grief (Westberg), 669
"Good works," as therapy, 498–499
Goodrich, Annie W., 18, 19
Government Hospital for the Insane, 15
Grains, 497
Grandiose delusions, in schizophrenia, 738, 744t
Gratification, substitute, 433
Gray matter, 130
Greek theories, 94–95, 96t
biopsychological, 128
Grief, 668–677. See also *Grieving process.*
absent, 672
Bowlby's perspective on, 663
chronic, 673
complicated, 663, 664b
converted, 673
coping with, 676–677
definition of, 662
delayed, 672–673
disenfranchised, 675
distorted, 673
Engel's perspective on, 663
family interventions for, 344t
Freud's perspective on, 662
Lindemann's perspective on, 662–663, 663b
normal versus pathological, 663, 664t
over acquired immunodeficiency syndrome victims, 1112
Parkes's perspective on, 663
patient information about, 671
Rando's perspective on, 663, 664

Grief (*Continued*)
reactions to, 672b
stages of, *179*, 179–181, *180*
Volkan's perspective on, 663, 664t
Grieving patients, nursing interventions for, 680b-681b
Grieving process, complicated, 664b, 672–673
depression compared with, 673, 673t
in children, 674
length of, 668–669
normal, phases of, 671–672
obstacles to, 674–675
of psychiatric patients, 675–676
stages of, 669–670
of Engel, 669
of Kübler-Ross, 669
of Veninga, 670, 670t
of Westberg, 669–670
tasks of, 670–671, 670b
GRISS Questionnaire, 896
Grounded theory, 1199
Group(s), individual versus, 80–81
psychotherapy. See *Group psychotherapy.*
support. See *Support group(s).*
Group Analytic Psychotherapy: Method and Principles (Foulkes), 388
Group as a whole model, 389
"Group assumptions," 389
Group contracts, 394
Group dynamics, 388
Group for the Advancement of Psychiatry (GAP), 470
Group marriage, 465t
Group psychotherapy, 385–417, 391t
activity, 391t, 415
boundary violations in, 416
cognitive behavioral, 409, 410
communication in, 392
during forming phase, 397–398
problem(s) of, 408–409
member conflicts as, 409
monopolizing as, 409
scapegoating as, 408–409
curative factor(s) in, 399–405
altruism as, 402–403
catharsis as, 400
cohesion as, 400–401
existential, 404–405
group think as, 401, 402t
guidance as, 404
hope as, 403
identification as, 403–404
interpersonal learning as, 403
recapitulation of primary family as, 404
salience of, 405
self-understanding as, 401–402
universality as, 402
development of, 386–390
during World War II, 388
educational, 391t, 393, 415–416
experiential techniques in, 388
for children and adolescents, 387
for chronically mentally ill, 409–410
for elderly patients. See *Elderly people, groups for.*
for families. See also *Family therapy.*
of schizophrenic patients, 749–750
group contracts in, 394
group(s) for, culture of, establishing, 406
development of, 395–399
adjourning phase of, 399
engagement (forming) phase of, 397–398
Group psychotherapy *Continued*
norming phase of, 398
performing (working) phase of, 398–399
preinteraction phase of, 396–397
transition (storming) phase of, 398
effective versus ineffective, 400b
norms of, 394–395
group-specific, 395
universal, 394–395
patient selection for, 392–393
size of, 393
types of, 391
here-and-now group interactions in, 388
human potential, 393
human relations, 388–389, 416
inpatient, 389
outpatient therapy versus, 395–396
interpersonal model of, 390, 393
leader function(s) in, 405–407, 407b
during forming phase, 397
feedback as, 406
group culture establishment as, 406
here-and-now approach as, 406–407
with coleadership, 405–406
meeting frequency for, 393–394
member functions in, 407–408, 408t
psychodrama, 387–388, 412–413
closure for, 413
warm-up for, 412–413
psychodynamic, 393
psychoeducational, 387, 391t, 415–417
for families, of schizophrenic patients, 749–750
purpose of, 391
record-keeping for, 416–417
reminiscence, 393, 413-414, 414b
resocialization, 393
self-help, 410–412, 411t
setting for, 394
support, 391t
tasks of, 391–392
Group Psychotherapy (Yalom), 390
Group therapy, for substance abuse, 821
with children, 606
Group think, 401, 402t
Guest relations, in continuous quality improvement, 1190
Guidance, in group psychotherapy, 404
Guided imagery, for relaxation, 696b
Guided mastery, 438
Guilt, about homelessness, 1031
family interventions for, 344t
in group psychotherapy, 400
Gull, William, 911
Gustatory hallucinations, 738t
Gynecomastia, antipsychotic agents causing, 531

Halazepam (Paxipam), dosage of, 552t
Hale, Matthew, 1088
Halfway houses, for substance abuse, 822
Hallucination(s), 223
in delirium, 982
in schizophrenia, 738, 738t
interventions for, 747
patient interviewing and, 295, 297
Hallucinogenic agent(s), abuse of, 796, 810
as controlled substances, 796, 796t
Haloperidol (Haldol), 526, 527t, 531, 532t
for bipolar disorder, 547
for children, 598t
for delirium, 986
Hampton, Isabel Adams (Robb), 25
Hardiness, 177–178
Hardnett, Linda G., 307
Harrison Narcotic Act of 1914, 795
Hashish, abuse of, 810–811
Hazardous events, crisis state development and, 336
HCFA (Health Care Financing Administration), 44, 1153, 1157, 1185
Head trauma, sexual problems resulting from, 894
Headaches. See *Migraine headache(s).*
Healing, Eastern view of, 490–491
folk. See *Folk healing.*
Health and Hospitals Corporation, 45
Health care delivery system, changes in, 1194–1195
constraints imposed by, dealing with, 186–187
Health Care Financing Administration (HCFA), 44, 1153, 1157, 1185
Health education, 273–274, 505
about acquired immunodeficiency syndrome, 1107
for adults, 634
for personality disorders, 852, 854, 855
Health maintenance, 274
Health maintenance organizations (HMOs), 45
Health People 2000, 27
Health promotion, 274
of mental health, for elderly people, 652–653
Health team(s), data collected by, for assessment, 299
for milieu therapy, 448
interdisciplinary, 1204
members of, 63t
sharing goals with, 247
Heart rate, in panic disorder, 700
Heartsounds (Lear and Lear), 982
Helping encounter, 231. See also *Therapeutic relationship(s).*
Helplessness, feelings of, in crisis intervention, 356
learned, 115
homelessness due to, 1030–1031
mood disorders related to, 769
Hemingway, Ernest, 760
Hemlock Society, 928
Henderson, Virginia, 116, 1195
Heparin locks, misuse of, 713, 714
Hepatitis, with narcotic abuse, 811–812
Herbal remedies, 492t
Here-and-now group interactions, 388, 406–407
Heroin, abuse of, 811–812
societal information about, 820
Heterosexual identity, 881
5-HIAA (5-hydroxyindoleacetic acid), 844
mood disorders and, 145
Hierarchy, of family, 466
of needs, *108*, 108–109, 109t, 166
Erikson's developmental tasks related to, *168*
relevance to nursing, 109
High expressed emotion, in family, of schizophrenic patients, 736
Higher cortical functions, 132
Hill-Burton Bill of 1946, 21
Hindbrain, 132
Hinduism, 315
Hippocampus, anxiety and, 693
Hippocrates, 14, 94, 95, 96t, 128, 979

Hispanic(s), 314–315
  communication among, 315
  culture-bound mental illness among, 211t
Histrionic personality disorder, 847, 849
HIV. See *Acquired immunodeficiency syndrome (AIDS); Human immunodeficiency virus (HIV).*
HIV/AIDS: A Guide to Nursing Care (Chenitz), 1107
HMOs (health maintenance organizations), 45
Holding environment, 448
Holism, 3
Home care, 48, 1151–1167
  case management in, 1165–1166
  definition of, 1153
  for acquired immunodeficiency syndrome patients, 1116, 1160
  for acute disorders, 1159
  for children and adolescents, 1160
  for chronically mentally ill, 1159–1160
  for elderly people, 1159
  historical background of, 1152–1153
  insurance coverage for, commercial insurance criteria for, 1158–1159
    Medicaid criteria for, 1158
    Medicare criteria for, 1156–1158
  managed care criteria for, 1158
  milieu therapy in, 456
  model for, *1154*, 1154–1156
  nursing process for, 1160–1167
    assessment in, 1161–1163
      continued, 1164–1165
      for safety, 1163
      of family dynamics, 1161
      of home environment, 1163
      of mental status, 1161
      of physical needs, 1163
      of social support, *1161*, 1161–1163, *1162*
    diagnosis in, 1163
    evaluation in, 1167
    implementation in, 1164–1167, 1164b
    outcome identification in, 1163–1164
    planning in, 1164
  psychotherapy in, 1165b
  teaching in, 1165
  Veterans Administration criteria for, 1158
Homebound status, 1156, 1157b
Homeless people, attitudes toward, 1031
  children as, 1027–1028
  elderly, 1028
  geographic location of, 1028
  illegal aliens as, 1028
  immigrants as, 1028
  McKinney Homeless Assistance Act and, 40
  mental illness among, 1026
  minorities as, 1028
  nursing process for, 1031–1036
    assessment in, 1032, 1033t–1034t
    case study of, 1034–1036
    intervention in, 1032–1034
  substance abuse among, 1026–1027
  women as, 1027
Homelessness, 80, 1023–1034
  causes of, 1029–1031
    learned helplessness as, 1030–1031
    personal, 1030
    social disaffiliation as, 1030
    structural, 1029–1030
  definition of, 1025
  historical background of, 1025
  increase in, 43
Homeostasis theory, 951
Homicide. See also *Violence.*
  risk of, 1054
    assessment of, 295b
Homophobia, 1108
Homosexuality, 893
  acquired immunodeficiency syndrome related to, 1106
  homophobia and, 1108
  homosexual identity in, 881
  in children, 597–598
Homovanillic acid, in personality development, 844
Hope, family interventions for, 344t
  fostering, 182–183
    for stress management, 66–67
    in crisis intervention, 352
    in group psychotherapy, 403
Horizontal stressors, 627
Hormones, 139, *140*. See also *Neuroendocrine system.*
  sexual desire and, 883–884
Horowitz, Mardi, 704
Hospital(s). See also *Inpatient treatment.*
  day, 47
  deinstitutionalization and, 23, 39, 1026, 1128–1129
  18th- and 19th-century, 14, 15, 19, 20
  functions of, 46
  general, psychiatric units within, 47
  nurses' accountability to, 62
  private, 46
  public, 46
  specialized, 46–47
  specialized units within, 47
  Veterans Administration, 44
Hospital Survey and Construction Act of 1946, 21
Hostage response, 1043
Hostility. See also *Violence.*
  family interventions for, 344t
Housing, for chronically mentally ill, 1135–1136
  low-cost, shortage of, homelessness related to, 1029
Howe, James, 26
Howe, John, 23
Hughes Act of 1970, 797
Hull, Clark, 129
Human functioning, theistic model of, 4, *4*
Human immunodeficiency virus (HIV). See also *Acquired immunodeficiency syndrome (AIDS).*
  assessing risk of, 297
Human potential encounter groups, 393
Human relations groups, 416
Human sexual response cycle. See *Sexual response cycle.*
Humanistic theory(ies), 5, 108–110
  of Maslow, *108*, 108–109, 109t
  of Rogers, 109–110
Humiliation, feelings of, in mood disorders, 771
Humor, for survivorship, 183–184, 184t
  in therapeutic communication, 220–221
Huntington's disease (chorea), 134, 991
  comorbidity of, with bipolar disorder, 767
Huxley, Aldous, 727
Hydrocephalus, normal-pressure, dementia associated with, 992
Hydrotherapy, 496
5-Hydroxyindoleacetic acid (5-HIAA), 844
  mood disorders and, 145
Hyperreactivity theory, of hypertension, 957
Hypertension, 957–958, 958b
  causes of, 957–958
    physiological, 957–958
      monoamine oxidase inhibitors as, 542, 543t
    psychological and social, 958
  treatment of, 958
    psychopharmacological, 543, 599t
Hypochondriasis, 964–965, 968t
Hypofrontal pattern, 141
Hypomania, 763
  definition of, 764t
  tricyclic antidepressants causing, 539
Hypotension, orthostatic, antipsychotic agents causing, 530
Hypothalamic-pituitary-adrenal axis, mood disorders and, 139
Hypothalamus, 132, 134, 139
  anxiety and, 693
Hysteria, 99
  among Inuit peoples, 320

IBS. See *Irritable bowel syndrome (IBS).*
ICD-9-CM (Clinical Modification of the World Health Organization's International Classification of Diseases–The Ninth Revision (ICD-9-CM)), 33, *36*, 36–37
Id, 100–101
Idea(s), flight of, 296t
  of reference, 296t
    in schizophrenia, 739, 744t
IDEA (Individuals with Disabilities Education Act), 40
Idea logs, 1182t
Ideal self, 155
Identification, in group psychotherapy, 403–404
  projective, 256
  transcultural, 307–308
  with patients, nurses' fear of, 7
Identity, ethnic, 307
  gender, 163
    definition of, 881
    disorders of, 892–893
      in adolescents, 597–598, 892–893
      in children, 597–598
  sexual, definition of, 881
Identity alteration, in dissociative disorders, 867
Identity confusion, in dissociative disorders, 867
Identity consciousness, 332
Identity disorder, dissociative, 869–870
Identity versus identity diffusion stage, 103t, 107, 167t
"If Hair Makes Me Black, I Must Be Purple," 307
Illegal aliens, homeless, 1028
Illusions, 223, 296t
  in schizophrenia, 737–738
Illustrators, 200
Imagery, Eastern, 492, 493
  guided, for relaxation, 696b
Imipramine (Tofranil), 537t, 540
  dosage of, 539, 540t
  for children, 595t
  for panic disorder, 146, 700
  for posttraumatic stress disorder, 705
Immigrant(s), adjustment of, 308
  homeless, 1028
  Southeast Asian, 316–317

Impact, period of, 341
Impact reaction, to rape, 1092
Implementation, for acquired immunodeficiency syndrome, 1119
 for antidepressant, mood stabilizer, and antianxiety agent treatment, 563
 for antipsychotic treatment, 556, 562–563
 for child abuse, 1067–1068
 for community mental health care, community-focused, 1139
  individual- or family-focused, 1144–1145
 for eating disorders, 918–921
 for elder abuse, 1070, 1072–1073
 for elderly people, 655
 for grieving patients, 679, 680, 681
 for home care, 1164–1167
 for mood disorders, 774–785
 for patient education, 511–513
 for personality disorders, 852, 853t–854t, 854–855
 for psychophysiological disorders, 970
 for rape, 1096–1097
 for schizophrenia, 747–750
 for sexual disorders, 900, *902*
 for spousal abuse, 1059–1062
 for suicidal patients, 938–940
 for violent patients, 1075
 in nursing process, 273–276. See also specific interventions.
 in psychodynamic short-term therapy, 375–376
 with children, 1067–1068
Impotence, 886–887
Impulse control, in personality disorders, 844
Incest, 1042
 disclosure of, facilitating, 889b
Income security programs, 1030
Incompetence, in Alzheimer's disease, early stages of, 1003–1004
Incontinence, fecal, in children, 600
 in Alzheimer's disease, middle stages of, 1006t
 urinary, in children, 599–600, 602
Indirect care, 54, 56
Indirect self-destructive behavior, 928
Individual, group versus, 80–81
Individual family therapy, 473
Individual psychotherapy, 367–382
 behavioral, 379
 cognitive, 376–378, *377*, *378*, 378t
 historical background of, 368
 long-term, 370–371, 372t, 373t
 psychoanalytic, 368–370, 369t
 short-term, 371–381
  psychodynamic model for. See *Psychodynamic therapy, short-term.*
 supportive, 379–380, 380t
 with children, 605–606
Individuals with Disabilities Education Act (IDEA), 40
Inductive reasoning, 1198
Industry versus inferiority stage, 103t, 107, 167t
 stressors during, 333t
Inexact labeling, 376
Infant mortality, among homeless people, 1027
Inferences, arbitrary, 376
 false, in therapeutic communication, 224t, 225
Infertility, 629–630
Information, for families. See *Family(ies), information for; Family education.*
Information, for families (*Continued*)
 for patients. See *Patient(s), information for; Patient education.*
 in therapeutic communication, 222
Informational privacy, 1196–1197, 1197b
Informed consent, ethics of, 77–78
 for psychotherapy, 373
 for research, 1197, 1197b
Initiative versus guilt stage, 103t, 107, 167t
 stressors during, 333t
Injury, nurses' fear of, 6–7
Inpatient treatment, crisis-oriented, for schizophrenic patients, 745, 747
 economics of, 370–371
 for eating disorders, 919
 group psychotherapy as, 389
  outpatient therapy versus, 395–396
 milieu therapy in. See *Milieu therapy, inpatient.*
 of children, 606, *607*
 of substance abuse, nursing actions for, 820t
An Inquiry Into the Effects of Ardent Spirits Upon the Human Body and Mind, With an Account of the Means of Preventing and of the Remedies for Curing Them (Rush), 795
Insecure attachment, 585
Insight, in psychoanalytic psychotherapy, 369
Insomnia, treatment of, psychopharmacological, 551
Institutional racism, 306
Institutionalization, 1129
Instrumental utilization, 1201
Instrumental violence, 1048, 1049, 1049t
Insurance, Medicaid, 44, 1177
  home care funding under, 1152, 1153, 1165, 1166
  reducing expenses of, 45
 Medicare, 44, 1177
  home care funding under, 48, 1152–1153, 1165, 1166
   criteria for, 1156–1158
 parity of, 45
 private, 45
  home care funding under, 1158–1159
 treatment duration and, 370–371
Integrated services, for chronically mentally ill, 1132, 1134
Integrity versus despair stage, 103t, 107, 167t, 620
 stressors during, 333t
Integumentary system, aging of, 647t
Intelligence, crystallized, 993
Intelligence quotient (IQ), 602
Intentionality and focus stage, of healing, 491
Interactive model, for transmitting research knowledge, 1201–1202
Interbrain, 132
Interdisciplinary teams, 1204
International Classification of Diseases–The Ninth Revision (ICD-9-CM), 33, *36*, 36–37
International Pilot Study of Schizophrenia (IPSS), 730–731
International Society for Psychiatric Consultative-Liaison Nurses (ISPCLN), 53
Interpersonal Aspects of Nursing (Travelbee), 24
Interpersonal model(s), for group psychotherapy, 390, 391
 learning in, 403
 psychodynamic, of Sullivan, 105–106
Interpersonal nursing, 24
 theory of, 118–119
Interpersonal psychotherapy, for mood disorders, 769, 776, 778–779
 group, 390, 391
  group size for, 393
  learning in, 403
Interpersonal Relations in Nursing (Peplau), 19, 24
Interpersonal relationship(s), 232–234. See also *Therapeutic relationship(s).*
 ending, 630
 in personality disorders, 844
 mental health and, 232
 mental illness and, 232–233
 of adults, during 30s, 624
 psychiatric treatment and, 233
 social relationships compared with, 233–234, 235t
  common elements and, 233
  differences and, 233–234
Interpersonal theory(ies), 118–119
 of Orlando, 110
 of Peplau, 106, 118–119, 445
  therapeutic relationships based on, 237–238
Interpersonal Theory of Nursing (Peplau), 118
Interpersonal Theory of Psychiatry, 19
Intersubjective recognizability, 1200
Intervention(s), 270. See also specific interventions.
 categories of, 272–273
 for homeless people, 1032–1034
 selection of, 273
 theistic model of, 5
Intimacy versus isolation stage, 103t, 107, 167t, 620
 stressors during, 333t
Intoxication, 801
Introjection, as defense mechanism, 697
Introversion, 105
Inuit peoples, 320
Involuntary detention, 82b
Involvement, in milieu therapy, 448
IPSS (International Pilot Study of Schizophrenia), 730–731
IQ (intelligence quotient), 602
Irish people, 312–313
 substance abuse among, 824
Irritable bowel syndrome (IBS), 956–957, 957b
 physiological basis of, 956
 psychological and spiritual responses to, 956
 treatment of, 957
Isocarboxazid (Marplan), 537t, 541
 dosage of, 540t
Isolation, of acquired immunodeficiency syndrome victims, 1108
 social, of refugees, 308
ISPCLN (International Society for Psychiatric Consultative-Liaison Nurses), 53
Italian Americans, 313
I-Thou relationship, 110
 therapeutic relationships based on, 238–239, *239*

James, William, 96, 97–99, 98t, 619
Janet, Pierre, 864, 911
Japanese people, 317–318
JCAHO. See *Joint Commission on Accreditation of Healthcare Organizations (JCAHO).*
Jenkins Type A Scale, in psychophysiological disorders, 953

Jewish Americans, 313–314
Jiryan, 309
Johnson, Betty Sue, 53
Johnson, Dorothea, 116
theory of, 117t
Joint Commission on Accreditation of Healthcare Organizations (JCAHO), 1185
criteria of, for therapeutic inpatient environment, 450, 451b
on patients' rights, 1188-1189, 1188b
quality assurance and, 1177–1178
inspection and individual performance focus for, 1178
ten-step process for, 1178
revised standards of, 1181b, 1183
Joint Commission on Mental Illness and Health, 21–22, 1129
Joint Commission on the Mental Health of Children, 22, 1130
Jokers, in psychotherapy groups, 408t
Jones, Maxwell, 389, 444, 445
Journal of Psychiatric Nursing, 26
Journal of Psychosocial Nursing and Mental Health Services, 26
Journey to Eden (Vonnegut), 726, 727, 737
Judd, Lewis L., 27
Judicial decisions, regarding quality of care, 1177
regarding right to treatment, 41
Jung, Carl, 104
theory of, 104–105
of adult development, 619–620
of personality structure, 104–105
relevance to nursing, 105
Juran, Joseph, 1179
Justice, 72–73
as ethical guide, 77

Kennedy, John F., 22
Kevorkian, Jack, 928
Kindling and behavioral sensitization hypothesis, of mood disorders, 145, 194
Kindling effect, 801
definition of, 798
Kinesics, 199–200
King, Imogene, 116
Kinnel, Galway, 386
Klismaphilia, 891t
Klonopin (clonazepam), for children, 597t
Kohlberg, Lawrence, 75
Koop, C. Everett, 1106
Koro, 309, 316
Korsakoff's syndrome, 808, 992
Kraepelin, Emil, 16, 129
on mood disorders, 761
on schizophrenia, 729
Krieger, Dolores, 493, 494
Kübler-Ross, Elisabeth, on acquired immunodeficiency syndrome, 1108
on grief, 669

La belle indifference, 963–964
Labeling, 305–306
inexact, 376
Laboratory test(s), 140–142
brain imaging, 141
neurochemical, 142
Lactate, in anxiety disorders, 146, 700
Lactation, benzodiazepines during, 552
lithium during, 548

Language function, 129
aphasia and, 981, 990, 990t
Broca's area in, 129, 131, 138
Wernicke's area in, 129, 132, 138, 139
Language system, 129, 131, 132, 138–139
Laotian refugees, 316
L'Arche movement, 750
Lasegue, Charles, 911
Latah, 309
Late adolescence, 575
Latency stage, 102, 103t, 575
"Laying on of hands," 493–494
Lazarus's Multimodal Therapy, 5
Leader, in group psychotherapy. See *Group psychotherapy, leader function(s) in.*
LEARN model, 204
Learned helplessness, 115
homelessness due to, 1030–1031
in mood disorders, 769
Learning, 504–509. See also *Education; Family education; Patient education; Psychoeducation.*
active, 505
adult, 508
behavioral, 112
disorders of, in children, 603
during adulthood, 632
education and, 504–505
levels of, 507
motivation for, 507, 508–509
needs for, assessment of, 509
objectives in, terms for, 510b
observational, 436b
of communication, 193
passive, 505
principles of, 506–508, 506b, 507b
readiness for, 508
assessment of, 509
social. See *Social learning theory(ies).*
theories of, 505–506
behavioral, 505, 505t
cognitive, 505, 505t
psychosocial, 505, 505t
social cognitive, 505t, 505–506
variables limiting, 516
vicarious, 113
Learning style, assessment of, 509
Least restrictive setting, right to treatment in, judicial decisions concerning, 41
Lecture, for patient education, 512
Legal issues, 81–83. See also *Patient(s), rights of.*
boundary issues as, 82–83, 83b
in involuntary detention, 82b
in research. See *Research.*
judicial decisions on, regarding quality of care, 1177
regarding right to treatment, 41
state nurse practice acts as, 82
voluntary versus involuntary treatment as, 81–82
Legislation. See *Public policy.*
Leininger, Madeline, 26, 116
theory of, 117t
Leneris v. Haas, 1177
Lenticular nuclei, 133
Leonard, Robert, 53
LES (Life Experience Survey), in psychophysiological disorders, 952
Lesbians, 881
Lethality, level of, 928, 935–936
determining, 938–939, *939*
Level systems, in milieu therapy, 448
Levine, Myra, 116

Levinson, Daniel, adult development theory of, 620–621, *621*
Levodopa, drug interactions of, 531
Lewin, Kurt, 388
Lewis, Garland K., 24
Lewy body dementia, 991
Libido, 99
Librium (chlordiazepoxide), dosage of, 552t
for withdrawal symptoms, 809
Life After Loss (Diets), 666
Life balance, 927
Life Experience Survey (LES), in psychophysiological disorders, 952
Life force, in Taoism, 488
Limbic system, 133–134, *134*
anxiety related to, 693
cognitive disorders related to, 981
mood disorders related to, 145
schizophrenia related to, 733
Limit setting, in milieu therapy, 452, 453, 455, 457–458, 460
in therapeutic communication, 217
Lindemann, Eric, crisis intervention model of, 331
on grief, 662–663, 663b
Linear communication models, 202–204, *204*
Listening, therapeutic (active). See *Active listening.*
Liston, Mary F., 22
Lithane. See *Lithium (Cibalith-S; Eskalith; Eskalith CR; Lithane; Lithaboid; Lithonate; Lithotabs.)*
Lithium (Cibalith-S; Eskalith; Eskalith CR; Lithane; Lithobid; Lithonate; Lithotabs), 546–548
action of, 547
adverse effects of, 547–548, 547t
contraindications to, 548
cost savings with, 23
dosage of, 548–549
drug interactions of, 548
fact sheet for, *566–567*
pharmacokinetics, 546–547
preparations of, 548, 549t
therapeutic uses of, 547
for children, 599t
nursing process for, 563–567
assessment in, 563
diagnosis in, 563
implementation in, 563
outcome identification in, 563
planning in, 563, *566–567*
Living arrangements, for chronically mentally ill, 1135–1136
Living Through Personal Crisis (Stearns), 671
Living wills, 996
Lobbying, 62–63
Lobes, of brain, 130–132, *132, 133, 134*, 139
Lobotomy, prefrontal, 139
Localized amnesia, in dissociative disorders, 866t
Logotherapy, 111
Longitudinal course specifiers, in mood disorders, 766
Long-term memory, 139
Long-term therapy, 370–371, 372t, 373t
Loose associations, 296t
in schizophrenia, 729
Lorazepam (Ativan), dosage of, 552t
for delirium, 986
Loss(es), 661–686
assumptions about, 662b
coping with, 665–666, *667*, 676–677
definition of, 662

Loss(es) *(Continued)*
grief due to. See *Grief; Grieving process.*
in life cycle, 664–665
nursing process for, 677–685
assessment in, 677, 678
case study of, 681–685
diagnosis in, 678
evaluation in, 679, 681
implementation in, 679, 680, 681
outcome identification in, 678
planning in, 678–679
of children, 665
of elderly people, 652–653
personal, 666b
psychiatric patients' responses to, 667–668
unsanctioned, grieving over, 674–675
Loss inventory, 666
Loss time line, 666, 667
Love, as ethical guide, 73
needs for, 166
Low back pain, 953–954, 954b
diagnoses for, 954
psychological and spiritual responses to, 954
source of, 953, 953b
treatment of, 954
Lowell, Robert, 772
Lower nerve knots, 132
Loxapine (Loxitane), 527t
Loxitane (loxapine), 527t
LSD (lysergic acid diethylamide), 794
Ludiomil (maprotiline), 537t, 545
dosage of, 540t
Luvox (fluvoxamine), 537t, 544
dosage of, 540t
Lyceum, 94
Lysergic acid diethylamide (LSD), 794

MAA (mutual assistance associations), 316
McGill Pain Questionnaire, in psychophysiological disorders, 953
McKinney Homeless Assistance Act, 40
McLean Asylum, 18
McLean Training School for Nurses, 18
Macrophages, in acquired immunodeficiency syndrome, 1111
MADD (Mothers Against Drunk Drivers), 1136
Magnetic resonance imaging (MRI), 141
Magnification, 207t, 376
Mahler, Margaret, 843–844
Main, Thomas, 445
Maintenance role functions, of psychotherapy group members, 407
Major depression, nursing process for, case study of, 786–790
characteristics of, 536
definition of, 764t, 765t
diagnosis of, 775–776
in children, 604
pathogenesis of, 536
suicide potential associated with, 929–930
case study of, 941–944
treatment of, psychopharmacological, 536, 544. See also *Antidepressant agent(s);* specific drugs.
psychotherapy for, 536
Males. See *Gender* entries; *Men; Parent(s); Sexual* entries; *Sexuality.*
Mammillary bodies, 133
Managed care, 45–46
home care funding under, 1158
Mania, 759, 764–765
definition of, 764t
expected outcomes for, 778b
in bipolar disorder, 545–546
indicators of, 771b
patient information about, 780
short-term goals for, 779b
treatment of. See *Antimanic agent(s);* specific drugs.
Mania Rating Scale, 1217
Manic-depressive illness. See *Bipolar disorder.*
Man's Search for Meaning (Frankl), 498
MAOIs. See *Monoamine oxidase inhibitor(s) (MAOIs).*
Maprotiline (Ludiomil), 537t, 545
dosage of, 540t
Marijuana, abuse of, 810–811
Marital enrichment programs, 471–472
Marital therapy, 471–472, 473
Marplan (isocarboxazid), 537t, 541
dosage of, 540t
Marriage, 624. See also *Divorce; Family(ies); Spousal abuse.*
Martins, Peter, 1050
Maslow, Abraham, 108
hierarchy of needs of, *108*, 108–109, 109t, 166
Erikson's developmental tasks related to, *168*
relevance to nursing, 109
Masochism, 891t
Mason, Belinda, 1111
Massage, therapeutic, 494
MAST Alcohol Screening Guide, 808
Maturational (developmental) crises, 343, 345
Maturity, measures of, 626b
May, Rollo, 400
Meaning, in experiences, 155
need for, 232
of languages, 198
sharing, 195
The Meaning of Death (Fiefel), 664
"Meaning questions," 77–78
Meaningfulness, 178–179
for chronically mentally ill, 1132
Measurement unit, for problem behavior, 425
Meats, interaction with monoamine oxidase inhibitors, 543t
Medicaid, 44, 1177
home care funding under, 1152, 1153, 1165, 1166
reducing expenses of, 45
Medical condition, in crisis intervention, 346
Medical history, in psychodynamic short-term therapy, 373–374
Medical illness, comorbidity of, with mental illness, in children, 581
with mood disorders, 762–763
in elderly people, identifying and treating, 652
presentation of, 647–648
Medical model. See *Biological theory(ies).*
Medicare, 44, 1177
home care funding under, 48, 1152–1153, 1165, 1166
criteria for, 1156–1158
Medication(s). See *Drug(s); Psychopharmacologic treatment;* specific drugs and drug types.
Medication history, 289, 295
Meditation, 498
transcendental, 495
Medroxyprogesterone acetate (Depo-Provera), for sexual disorders, 900
Mellaril (thioridazine), 527t
for children, 598t
Memory, 139
deficits of. See also *Amnesia.*
global, 990
in Alzheimer's disease, early stages of, 998
middle stages of, 1006t
long-term, 139
short-term, 139
Men. See also *Gender* entries; *Parent(s); Sexual* entries; *Sexuality.*
abuse of, spousal, 1048–1049, 1049t
acquired immunodeficiency syndrome in, 1106
adult development of, 620–621, *621*
grieving by, 674, 675t
impotence in, 886–887
orgasms in, 886
sexual desire in, 883–884
social changes affecting, 628–633
Menninger, William C., 19, 21
Menopause, 625
Mental health, continuum with mental illness, 167, *169*
interpersonal relationships and, 232
nursing diagnoses related to, 628b
of elderly people, 648–649
promoting, 652–653
preventive. See *Preventive mental health.*
Mental health nursing. See *Psychiatric–mental health nursing.*
Mental Health Survey Act of 1955, 1129
Mental Health Systems Act of 1980, 83, 84, 85b, 1191
Mental health/human services workers, as treatment team members, 63t
Mental hospitals. See *Hospital(s).*
Mental Hygiene Movement, 16
Mental illness. See also specific psychiatric disorders.
among abusers, 1047
among homeless people, 1026
causes of, 34, 142–146. See also specific disorders.
chronic, community mental health care for. See *Community mental health care.*
communication problems associated with, 193–194, 202t
continuum of mental health and, 167, *169*
cultural perceptions of, 312
culture-bound, 211t
family history of, in schizophrenia, 740
grieving and, 675–676
hardiness and, 178
in children. See *Child(ren).*
interpersonal relationships and, 232–233
losses and, 667–668
myths and realities of, 34
patient education about, 515, 516b, 517b–518b
speech patterns in, 201, 202t
stigma associated with, 39
symptom(s) of, suicide as, 929–930
Mental retardation, 34
in children, 601–603
Mental Retardation Facilities and Community Mental Health Centers Construction Act of 1963, 22, 1129
Mental status assessment, for home care, 1161
in crisis intervention, 346
Mini-Mental State Examination for, 295, 1116–1117, 1221
of children, 584

Mental status assessment, for home care (*Continued*)
  of elderly people, 653
  of rape victims, 1091
Meperidine (Demerol), drug interactions of, 543
Mesoridazine (Serentil), 527t
Message, in communication, 202
Metacommunication, 195–196, 197, 201, 202t
Metaparadigm, 116
Metaphors, in therapeutic communication, 220
Methadone, for narcotic abuse, 812, 812t
Methoxyhydroxyphenylglycol (MHPG) excretion, in depression, 142, 144
Methylphenidate (Ritalin), for AIDS-dementia complex, 1112
  for children, 595t
  for depression, in acquired immunodeficiency syndrome, 1111
Meyer, Adolph, 16, 17
Meyer, Mary, 16
MHPG (methoxyhydroxyphenylglycol) excretion, in depression, 142, 144
Middle adolescence, 575
Midlife crisis, 620, 624
Migraine headache(s), 958–960, 960b
  classification of, 959
  mechanism of, 959–960
  precipitants of, 959
  symptoms of, 958–959
  treatment of, 960
Miles, Margaret Shandor, on grief, 663
Milieu, 443
Milieu therapy, 273, 443–460
  assumptions of, 445–446
  environment for, 448–449
  for personality disorders, 854
  goals of, 446–447
  Gunderson's component(s) of, *447*, 447–448
    containment as, 448
    involvement as, 448
    structure as, 447–448
    support as, 448
    validation as, 448
  historical background of, 444–445, *445*
  in community treatment settings, 455–458
    day treatment programs and, 456
    mobile, 456
    outpatient clinics and, 456–458
    psychiatric home care and, 456
    residential, *458*, 458–460
      crisis units and, 459
      foster care and, 459–460
  inpatient, 450–455
    emergency departments and, 452–453
    for children, 606, *607*
    locked, 450, 452
    long-term, 454–455
    short-term, 453–454, *455*
  phases of, 450, *450*
  settings for, 449–460
    continuum of, *449*, 449–450, *450*
    issues related to, 450
  standards for, of American Nurses' Association, 447
  therapeutic community compared with, 445
A Mind that Found Itself (Beers), 16, 17
Mind-body-spirit therapy(ies), 487–499
  Eastern, 488–496
    acupuncture as, 491–492, 492t
    bioenergetics as, 495
Mind-body-spirit therapy(ies) (*Continued*)
    biofeedback as, 495–496
    healing in, view of, 490–491
    imagery as, 492, 493
    relaxation as, 495
    Taoism as, 488
    therapeutic massage as, 494
    therapeutic touch as, 493–494
    traditional Chinese medicine as, 488–489, *489*
    transcendental meditation as, 495
  Western, 496–499
    doing "good works" as, 498–499
    hydrotherapy as, 496
    meditation as, 498
    nutritional, 496–498
    prayer as, 498
    religious practices as, 498
Minerals, 497
Mini–Mental State Examination (MMSE), 295, 1116–1117, 1221
Minimization, 207t, 376
Minimum encouragers, 213
Minnesota model, for substance abuse treatment, 818–819
Minnesota Multiphasic Personality Inventory (MMPI), in psychophysiological disorders, 952–953
Minorities. See also specific groups.
  homelessness among, 1028
Minors, confidentiality and, 201
Mirroring, in psychodrama, 413t
  in therapeutic communication, 221
Misinformation, American Nurses' Association Code for Nurses on, 84
Misunderstandings, in verbal communication, 197–198
Mitchell, Martha, 22, 1130
Mixed episodes, 765–766
  definition of, 764t
MMPI (Minnesota Multiphasic Personality Inventory), in psychophysiological disorders, 952–953
MMSE (Mini–Mental State Examination), 295, 1116–1117, 1221
Moban (molindone), 527t
Mobile treatment, for chronically mentally ill, 1136
  milieu therapy in, 456
Model communities, for mentally retarded children, 602–603
Modeling, Bandura's theory of, 113–114
  for shaping, 431–432
  in therapeutic communication, 219
Modified Anxiety Scale, 707
Molindone (Moban), 527t
Monism, 5
Monitoring, of care and service. See *Continuous quality improvement (CQI).*
Moniz, Egas, 139
Monoamine oxidase, 136
Monoamine oxidase inhibitor(s) (MAOIs), 540–543. See also specific drugs.
  action of, 537t, 541, *541*
  adverse effects of, 537t, 542
  dosage of, 540t
  drug interactions of, 539, 542–543, 700
  food interactions of, 700
  therapeutic uses of, 541–542
    for children, 596t
    for panic disorder, 700
    for posttraumatic stress disorder, 705
Monocytes, in acquired immunodeficiency syndrome, 1111
Monopolizing, in psychotherapy groups, 409
Monozygotic twins, 144
Montgomery-Asburg Depression Scale, 1116
Mood, definition of, 761
Mood disorder(s), 759–790. See also *Bipolar disorder; Depression; Major depression; Mania.*
  causes of, 144–145, 767–770
    catecholamine hypothesis of, 144
    circadian rhythm hypothesis of, 145, 766
    endocrinological, 768
    genetic, 145, 768
    kindling and behavioral sensitization hypothesis of, 145, 194
    neurochemical, 144–145
    neuroendocrine, 139, 145
    neuronal, 767–768
    pharmacological, 767, 767t
    psychodynamic, 768–770, *769*
    sleep deprivation as, 767
  comorbidity of, 762–763
    with medical conditions, 762–763
    with other psychiatric disorders, 762
  costs of, 763
  definitions of, 763, *764*, 765t
  nurse as collaborator in, with patient and family, 781–782
  nursing process for, 770–790
    assessment in, 770–773
    case study of, 786–790
    diagnosis in, 773–774, 775–777
    evaluation in, 785–786
    implementation in, 774–785
    outcome identification in, 774, 778, 779
    planning in, 774, 779
  patient information about, 772
  symptoms of, 763–765, 766
  terms describing, 761, *762*
  variations in, 765–766
Moore, Thomas, 492
Moos Ward Atmosphere Scale, 450
Moral anxiety, 100
Moral development, Kohlberg's theory of, 75
  of children, assessment of, 586–587
Moral dilemma, 80
Moral distress, 79, 80
Moral interventions, 444
  in Bay Area Health Care model, 1154
Moral superiority, toward homeless people, 1031
Moral uncertainty, 80
Morality, 165
Moralizing, in therapeutic communication, 224t, 225–226
Moreno, Joseph L., 387–388
Morphine, early understanding of, 795
Morton, Richard, 910–911
Mothers Against Drunk Drivers (MADD), 1136
Motivation, for learning, 507, 508–509
  of patient, 223
  social learning theory and, 114
Motor area, 131
Motor homunculus, 131, *133*
Motor reproduction, social learning theory and, 114
Motor skills disorders, in children, 603
Motor strip, 137
Mourning. See *Grief; Grieving process.*
Mourning and Melancholia (Sigmund Freud), 662
Moxibustion, 491
MRI (magnetic resonance imaging), 141
Multigenerational transmission, 467

Multi-infarct dementia, 991
Multiple personality disorders, 867, 869–870
Multiple sclerosis, dementia in, 993
Multiple-family group therapy, 473
Multiple-impact therapy, 473
Multivoting, 1181, 1182t
Murder, 1042. See also *Violence.*
risk of, 1054
assessment of, 295
Murphy, Marion, 53
Murphy, Michael, 416
Murphy, Patrice, 1110
Musculoskeletal system, aging of, 647t
Muslims, 318
Mutilation, of self, 930–931
Mutism, 990t
Mutual assistance associations (MAAs), 316
Mutual combat model, of spouse abuse, 1048–1049, 1049t
Mutual help groups. See *Support group(s).*
Mutuality, in interpersonal nursing, 119
in therapeutic relationships, 241–242, 242b
Myers, Isabel Briggs, 169
Myers-Briggs Personality Inventory Rating Scale, 169
Myers-Briggs Temperament Scales, 105
Myers-Briggs Type Indicator, 169
Myofascial syndrome, 954
Myths, family, 466

Naloxone, for self-mutilation, 931
NAMI (National Alliance for the Mentally Ill), 26, 1151
as support, 185
psychoeducation provided by, 471
NANDA (North American Nursing Diagnosis Association), 268, 269b–270b. See also *Nursing diagnosis(es).*
Nar-Anon, 604
Narcissistic personality disorder, 847–848
Narcotic analgesics, abuse of, 811–812
as controlled substances, 796, 796t
teratogenic effects of, 826, 827t
Narcotics Anonymous, 797, 823–824, 1136
Nardil. See *Phenelzine (Nardil).*
National Alliance for the Mentally Ill (NAMI), 26b, 1151
as support, 185
psychoeducation provided by, 471
National Center for Nursing Research, 1203b
National Institute of Alcohol Abuse and Alcoholism, 797
National Institute of Mental Health (NIMH), 22, 1130
Advisory Council on the Cost and Treatment of Serious Mental Illness of, 44
establishment of, 21
funding from, for training, 46
National Institute of Alcohol Abuse and Alcoholism of, 797
Office of Alternative Medicine of, 494
National Institutes of Health (NIH), Office of Medical Applications of Research of, 1202
National League for Nursing (NLN), 25
National Mental Health Act of 1946, 21, 37
National Mental Health Act of 1955, 21–22
National Nurses Society on Addictions, 797
National Training Laboratories (NTL), 388
Native American(s), 318–320
communication among, 319
Native American(s) *(Continued)*
homelessness among, 1028
"peyote button" use by, 794
substance abuse among, 825
The Nature of Prejudice (Allport), 306
The Nature of Soul (Plato), 94
Navane (thiothixene), 527t
for children, 598t
Necessary Losses (Viorst), 164
Necrophilia, 891t
Need(s), being, 108
belonging, 166
deficiency, 108
esteem, 166
hierarchy of, *108*, 108–109, 109t, 166
Erikson's developmental tasks related to, *168*
relevance to nursing, 109
love, 166
of chronically mentally ill, 1132–1134
physiological, 166
providing for, in milieu therapy, 446
safety, 166
self-actualization, 108–109, 109t, 166
Sullivan's theory of, 105
Negative reinforcement, 429
Negative symptoms, of schizophrenia, 144, 528, 533, 737, 739–740
Neglect, definition of, 1042
of children, mental illness and, 580
of dementia patients, 1012
Negotiating, empowerment and, 182
Neologisms, 296t
in schizophrenia, 739
Network therapy, 473
Networking, 62
in community mental health care, 1145
Neuman, Betty M., 26, 116
theory of, 117t
Neural factors, in migraine headaches, 959
Neuritic plaques, 989
Neuroanatomy, 129, 130–137. See also *Brain; Neurotransmitter(s).*
Neurochemical tests, 142
Neurochemistry, 129
Neuroendocrine system, 129, 139, *140*. See also *Hormones.*
aging of, 647t
effects on, of antipsychotic agents, 531
mood disorders and, 145, 768
tests of, 142
Neurofibrillary tangles, 989
Neuroleptic(s). See *Antipsychotic agent(s).*
Neuroleptic malignant syndrome (NMS), 530
Neuroleukin, in acquired immunodeficiency syndrome, 1112
Neurolinguistic programming, 205–206, 206b
Neurological system, aging of, 647t
Neuron(s), *135*, 135–136, *136*
neurotransmitters and, 135–137, *138*
Neuropharmacology, 129
Neurophysiology, 129, 137–140
of frontal system, 139
of language system, 138–139
of memory system, 139
of neuroendocrine system, 139, *140*
of sensory system, 137–138
Neuroscience, 129
Neuroses in the Sun (McCartney), 321
Neurotic anxiety, 100
Neurotransmitter(s), 135–137, *138*. See also specific neurotransmitters.
action of, termination of, drug effects on, 526
anxiety related to, 693–694
Neurotransmitter(s) *(Continued)*
drug depletion of, mood disorders caused by, 767, 768
in abusers, 1047
in brain, 137b
in eating disorders, 911
in migraine headaches, 959
in panic disorder, 700
in personality development, 844
in substance abuse, 800
in suicidal patient, 931
in synaptic transmission, 525
mood disorders related to, 142, 144–145
receptor binding of, drug effects on, 525
release of, drug effects on, 525
reuptake of, 525
storage of, drug effects on, 525
synthesis of, drug effects on, 525
New Hope, 636
Newman, Betty, 92–93
Newman Systems Model, 92–93
Niacin, 498
Nichols, Charles H., 15
Nicotine, 814
Nightingale, Florence, 93, 116
NIH (National Institutes of Health), Office of Medical Applications of Research of, 1202
NIMH. See *National Institute of Mental Health (NIMH).*
NLN (National League for Nursing), 25
NMS (neuroleptic malignant syndrome), 530
"Noah's Ark" phenomenon, 392
Node of Ranvier, 135
No-harm contracts, 938, 939, *939*
No-kin family, 465t
Nonmaleficence, 73–74
Nonnormative events, 468
Nonverbal communication, 197, 198–200
body language as, 199–200
gestures as, 200
global physical movements as, 200
personal space and, 200
physical appearance as, 199
Nonviolence, model of, 1060, *1064*
Noradrenaline. See *Norepinephrine.*
Noradrenergic system, 137
Norepinephrine, 136, 137
depression and, 142, 144–145
in abusers, 1047
in migraine headaches, 959
in panic disorder, 700
Norepinephrine system, *138*
Norm(s), of groups, 394–395
group-specific, 395
universal, 394–395
Normal-pressure hydrocephalus, dementia associated with, 992
Normative events, 468
Norming phase, of group development, 398
Norpramin (desipramine), 537t
dosage of, 540t
for children, 595t
Norris, Catherine, 52
North American Nursing Diagnosis Association (NANDA), 268, 269b–270b. See also *Nursing diagnosis(es).*
Nortriptyline (Aventyl; Pamelor), 537t
dosage of, 540t
fact sheet for, *563*
for children, 595t
No-suicide contract, 81
Notes on Nursing (Nightingale), 93, 116
Novice adulthood, 622

NTL (National Training Laboratories), 388
Nuclear family, 465t
Nurse(s), anxiety of, 6
as clinicians, 1203–1204
advanced-practice, 1204
case management role for, 1203
critical pathways for, 1203–1204
as collaborators, in mood disorders, 781–782
as counselors. See *Counseling; Psychotherapy.*
as parent surrogates, 577
as researchers, 1195–1196. See also *Research.*
as teachers. See *Family education; Health education; Patient education; Psychoeducation groups.*
attributes typical of, 186
burnout among, *64*, 64–67
strategies for dealing with, *65*, 65–67
communication barriers within, 224t, 224–226
competence of, American Nurses' Association Code for Nurses on, 84
costs to, of psychiatric nursing involvement, 7
countertransference of, 103, 256, 257
in psychodynamic short-term therapy, 376
with children, 578–579
direct reimbursement for, 46
fears of, of identifying with patients, 7
of injury and injuring patients, 6–7
of rejection by patients, 7
frustrations of, over inability to change patients, 7
impaired, American Nurses' Association Code for Nurses on, 84
in community mental health centers, 47
in crisis intervention, 361–362
in private practice, 48
responses of, to acquired immunodeficiency syndrome patients, 1113–1114
to personality disorders, 855–856
to sexual issues, 895–896
to suicidal patients, 939–940
roles of. See also *Nursing role(s); Practice role(s).*
threats to, 6–7
self-awareness of, need for, 6
strengths of, developing, 186–187
attributes typical of nurses and, 186
dealing with health care system constraints and, 186–187
Nurse practice acts, 82
Nurse-Patient Communication (Lewis), 24
Nurse-patient relationship. See also *Therapeutic relationship(s).*
influence on mental health care, 23–25
Nurse-Patient Relationships in Psychiatry (Render), 12
Nursing. See also *Psychiatric–mental health nursing.*
art of, need for attention to, 285–286
assessment of, aspects of, 582b
interpersonal, 24
professionalization of, influence on mental health care, 25–26
stress associated with, *64*, 64–67
strategies for dealing with, *65*, 65–67
transcultural, 305
Nursing behavior, associated with empathy, 244b
Nursing care plan(s), 273, 274, 275b
for behavioral therapy, 433–434
for patient education, *514–515*
for substance abuse, acute phase treatment of, 816, *817*
in crisis intervention, 355
Nursing diagnosis(es), 268–272, 269–270
components of, 271b
DSM-IV and, 271
for acquired immunodeficiency syndrome, 1117–1118
for adults, 628
for altered thought processes, 744t
for Alzheimer's disease, 997t, 997–998, 999
for antidepressant, mood stabilizer, and antianxiety agent treatment, 563
for antipsychotic treatment, 556, 562
for anxiety disorders, 707, 708–712
for behavioral therapy, 427
for bereavement, 666
for child abuse, 1065–1066
for children, 589–604. See also specific diagnoses under *Child(ren).*
for community mental health care, community-focused, 1138
individual- or family-focused, 1140–1141
for crisis intervention, 354
for delirium, 982–985, 984t, 985t
for dissociative disorders, 871, 872
for eating disorders, 916–917
for elder abuse, 1070
for elderly people, 655
for family therapy, 479–480, 481
for grieving patients, 678
for home care, 1163
for mood disorders, 773–774, 775–777
for paraphilias, 892
for patient education, 510
for personality disorders, 846–850, 851
for psychophysiological disorders, 962–967, 969
for rape, 1091–1094
for schizophrenia, 744, 744t, 745, 746
for sexual disorders, 898
for somatoform disorders, 962–967
for spousal abuse, 1057, 1058
for stress, 707, 708–712
for substance abuse, 803, 805
for suicidal patients, 937
for violent patients, 1075
formulating, 250
prioritization of, 271
interpersonal, 480b
specific to family functioning, 479, 480, 481
Nursing Ethics (Hampton), 25
Nursing journals, 18, 26
Nursing Mental Diseases (Bailey), 18
Nursing process, 265–280, *266*. See also under specific disorders and interventions.
assessment in, 268. See also *Assessment.*
diagnosis in, 268–272. See also *Nursing diagnosis(es).*
documentation in, 276, *277–279*
evaluation in, 274, 275
implementation in, 273–276. See also *Implementation;* specific interventions.
advanced practice, 273–274
basic practice, 273–274
outcome identification in, 272. See also *Outcome(s), identification of.*
planning in, 272–273. See also *Planning.*
problem-solving principles used in, 267t
purpose of, 266
Nursing role(s). See also *Practice role(s).*
in acquired immunodeficiency syndrome, 1114–1116
for home care, 1116
of community mental health nurses, 1115–1116
of psychiatric consultation-liaison nurses, 1114–1115
of psychiatric inpatient nurses, 1115
in community mental health care, 1136–1138
for acquired immunodeficiency syndrome, 1115–1116
nursing process for, 1137–1138
prevention as, 1137
in community treatment settings, 459–460
in continuous quality improvement. See *Continuous quality improvement (CQI), nursing role in.*
in schizophrenia, 728
Nursing theory(ies), 115–119, 117t
caring in, 118
definition of, 116
early, 116
evolution of, 116, 118
relationship, 118–119
therapeutic relationships based on, 237–238
value of, 115–116
Nursing's Plan to Provide Essential Mental Health Services (Krauss), 40–41
Nussbaum, Hedda, 1050
Nut(s), 497
Nutrition. See also *Eating; Eating disorder(s); Food(s).*
assessment of, in psychodynamic short-term therapy, 374
for anxiety disorders, 715
in Alzheimer's disease, early stages of, 1001
Nutritional therapy, 496–498

Obesity, in children, 595–596
Object(s), transitional, in object relation theory, 843
Object constancy, in object relation theory, 843
Object relation theory, 843–844
Objective(s), for patient education, 510
Objective anxiety, 100
Objective data, for dissociative disorders, 871
Observational learning, 436b
Obsession(s), 296t, 701
Obsessive-compulsive disorder (OCD), 701–702
comorbidity of, with mood disorders, 762
etiology of, 702
flooding for, 432
in children, 593–594
nursing implications of, 702
patient information about, 703
treatment of, 702, 716
Obsessive-compulsive personality disorder, 850–851
Occipital lobe, 131–132, *132*
Occupational therapists, as treatment team members, 63t
OCD. See *Obsessive-compulsive disorder (OCD).*
Oedipus complex, 102, 103t
Office of Alternative Medicine, 494
Office of Medical Applications of Research, 1202
Old hag, 309

Old-old, 646
Olfactory hallucinations, 738t
Olfactory tubercle, 133
Omnibus Budget Reconciliation Act of 1982, 22, 1130
Omnibus Budget Reconciliation Act of 1986, 1177
Omnibus Budget Reconciliation Act of 1987, 1177
Omnibus Budget Reconciliation Act of 1989, 1177
Omnibus Budget Reconciliation Act of 1990, 1177
Opara, Royce, 523–524
Open Gates, 54, 56
Open-ended questions, 214
Operant conditioning, 113, 423–424
  respondent conditioning versus, *112*
  therapeutic applications of, 424b. See also *Behavior modification.*
Opioids. See also *Narcotic analgesics.*
  endogenous, in eating disorders, 911–912
Oppositional defiant disorder, in children, 590
Optic chiasm, 133
Optic tract, 133
Oral stage, 101–102, 103t
Orem, Dorothy, 116
  rehabilitation model of, 117t
    data collection using, 285
Organic brain syndrome, 980, 980b
Organismic theory, of adult development, 619
Orgasm, 885–886, 887t
  disorders of, 887–890
Orientation phase. See *Crisis intervention, working phase of; Therapeutic relationship(s), orientation phase of.*
The Origin of the Species (Darwin), 95
Orlando, Ida Jean, 24, 26
  theory of, 119
Ormazine. See *Chlorpromazine (Ormazine; Thorazine).*
Orthodox Jews, 313, 314
Orthomolecular therapy, 497–498
Orthostatic hypotension, antipsychotic agents causing, 530
  monoamine oxidase inhibitors causing, 542
  tricyclic antidepressants causing, 538
Outcome(s), expected. See *Expected outcome(s).*
  identification of, for acquired immunodeficiency syndrome, 1118–1119
    for antidepressant, mood stabilizer, and antianxiety agent treatment, 563
    for antipsychotic treatment, 556, 562
    for anxiety disorders, 707
    for behavioral therapy, 427
    for child abuse, 1066
    for community mental health care, community-focused, 1138
      individual- or family-focused, 1142–1143
    for dissociative disorders, 873
    for eating disorders, 916
    for elder abuse, 1070
    for elderly people, 655
    for family therapy, 480
    for grieving patients, 678
    for home care, 1163–1164
    for mood disorders, 774, 778, 779
    for patient education, 510, 511
    for personality disorders, 851
    for psychophysiological disorders, 969
    for rape, 1094
Outcome(s), expected (*Continued*)
    for schizophrenia, 745
    for sexual disorders, 898–899
    for spousal abuse, 1058
    for substance abuse, 818
    for suicidal patients, 937
    for therapeutic relationships, 252–253
    for violent patients, 1075
    with children, 604
Outpatient treatment, 47. See also *Community mental health care;* specific settings.
  for eating disorders, 919
  milieu therapy in, 456–458
Overanxious disorder of childhood, 593
Overdose, definition of, 798
Overeating. See *Binge eating disorder; Eating disorder(s).*
Overgeneralization, 376
Overresponsibility/underresponsibility, in families, 475
Oxazepam (Serax), dosage of, 552t

Pacific Island peoples, 318
  communication among, 318
Pain, chronic, case study of, 971–972
  in back. See *Low back pain.*
  in headache. See *Migraine headache(s).*
  in temporomandibular disorder, 960–961
  pelvic. See *Pelvic pain, chronic.*
Pain disorder, 966–967, 968t
Pain Drawings, in psychophysiological disorders, 953
Pairing, Bion's concept of, 389
Palmer, Mary, 18
Palmer, Sophia, 18
Pamelor. See *Nortriptyline (Aventyl; Pamelor).*
Panic, 695t, 695–696
Panic attacks, patient information about, 697
  treatment of, 551
Panic disorder, 699–701
  etiology of, 700
  lactate and, 146
  nursing implications of, 700–701
  relaxation training for, 438–439
  treatment of, 700
    psychopharmacological, 538
    symptom reinterpretation as, 700
  with agoraphobia, 699
  without agoraphobia, diagnosis of, 708
Pantheism, 5
Pantothenic acid, 497
Paradoxical intention, 111
Paradoxical psychological effects, benzodiazepines causing, 551
Paranoid delusions, in schizophrenia, 738, 744t
Paranoid personality disorder, 733, 845
Paranoid schizophrenia, 732t
  case study of, 751–754
Paraphasia, 990t
Paraphilia(s), 890–892, 891t
  causes of, 890–892
  treatment of, 891–892
Paraphrasing, 214–215, 217t
Parataxic thinking, 106
Parent(s). See also *Family(ies).*
  chemically dependent, children of, treatment for, 830–831
  conduct disorders in, children's disturbances related to, 581
  depression in, children's disturbances related to, 581
Parent(s) (*Continued*)
  elderly, caring for, 625, 631
  schizophrenogenic, 734
  surrogates for, nurses as, 577
  violence toward, from children, 1044
Parent Effectiveness Training, 471
Parent state, in transactional communication model, 205
Pareto diagrams, 1181, 1182t
Parietal cortex, 137
Parietal lobe, 131, *132*
Parkes, Murray, on grief, 663
Parkinsonism, 528, 529, 529t
Parkinson's disease, 134
  comorbidity of, with depression, 767
  dementia in, 992–993
Parnate (tranylcypromine), 537t, 541
  dosage of, 540t
  for children, 596t
Paroxetine (Paxil), 537t, 544
  dosage of, 540t
  for children, 596t
Parse, Rosemarie Rizzo, 116
  theory of, 117t
Partial hospitalization, for children, 607
Partialism, 891t
Participant observers, 106, 118, 192
Participation, empowerment and, 182
Passages (Sheehy), 163
Passive learning, 505
Paternalism, 74
Patient(s), accountability to, of nurses, 62
  as therapeutic communication focus, 209
  engaging, in crisis intervention, 350–352
  fear of injuring, 6–7
  grieving, 680b–681b
  identification of, 289
  identification with, nurses' fear of, 7
  inability to change, nurses' frustration over, 7
  information for. See also *Patient education.*
    about anxiety, 693
    about eating disorders, 919–920
    about grief, 671
    about mania, 780
    about mood disorders, 772
    about obsessive-compulsive disorder, 703
    about panic attacks, 697
    about posttraumatic stress disorder, 705
    about schizophrenia, 748
    elements of offering, 222b
  participation of, 119
  perceptions of, in assessment, 286–287
  personal strengths and resources of, 255b
  rejection by, nurses' fear of, 7
  rights of, 83–84, 85b
    codes of, 83–87
    in continuous quality improvement, 1188–1189, 1188b
    to treatment, judicial decisions concerning, 41
  satisfaction of, in continuous quality improvement, 1189–1191
  selection of, for group psychotherapy, 392–393
  treatment refusal by, as ethical dilemma, 79
  understanding of, informed consent and, 77
  validation of, 119
Patient chart, reading, decisions about, 6
Patient education, 503–519, 505
  about anxiety disorders, 714–715
  about mental illness, 515, 516b, 517b–518b
  about mood disorders, 779–780
  about schizophrenia, 747–748

Patient education (*Continued*)
about sex, 890
biopsychosocial-spiritual model for, 515–516
content for, 516–518
broad, 516
detailed, 517–518
in Bay Area Health Care model, 1156
in community mental health care, 1144–1145
in home care, 1165
learning and. See *Learning.*
nursing process for, 509–514
assessment in, 509–510
diagnosis in, 510
evaluation in, 513–514, *514–515*
implementation in, 511–513
outcome identification in, 510, 511
planning in, 510–511, *512*
variables limiting learning and, 516
Patient Perception of Ward Scale, 450
Patient-centered model, therapeutic relationships based on, 238b
Patterson, Josephine G., 26
Pavlov, Ivan, 111
theory of, 111–112
Paxil (paroxetine), 537t, 544
dosage of, 540t
for children, 596t
Paxipam (halazepam), dosage of, 552t
PCP (phencyclidine), abuse of, 810
psychosis induced by, 744
PDD-NOS (pervasive developmental disorder, not otherwise specified), 603
Pedophilia, 891t
Peer review, 60, 61, *61*
Pelvic pain, chronic, 954–956, 955b
diagnosis of, 955
nature of, 955
psychological and spiritual responses to, 955
treatment of, 955–956
Pennsylvania Hospital, 19
Peoplemaking (Satir), 161
Peplau, Hildegard E., 13, 19, 24b, 26, 116, 1194
interpersonal theory of, 106, 118–119, 445
therapeutic relationships based on, 237–238
on accountability, 60–61
Perception(s), 155, 158–159
development of, 159
distortions of, reducing, in delirium, 986
in schizophrenia, normal versus enhanced, 726–727
of patient, in assessment, 286–287
self-concept and, 159
Performing (working) phase, of group development, 398–399
Permitil (fluphenazine), 527t, 531, 532t
fact sheet for, *559*
Perphenazine (Trilafon), 527t
for children, 598t
Persecution, delusions of, in schizophrenia, 738, 744t
Perseverance, 178–179
Perseveration, 296t
Persistently mentally ill. See *Chronically mentally ill patient(s).*
Persona, 104
Personal boundaries, 200
legal issues regarding, 82–83, 83b
Personal crises, 341–342, 342b
Personal identity, 158. See also *Psychological self.*
Personal involvement, in social versus therapeutic relationships, 234
Personal loss, 666b
Personal strengths. See *Nurse(s), strengths of; Strength(s).*
Personal unconscious, 104
Personal vulnerability, to schizophrenia, 736
Personality, 156
development of, 169–170, 842–844
biological perspective on, 843–844
genetics in, 843–844
neurotransmitters in, 844
Mahler's perspective on, 842–843
Freudian theory of, 99–101
dynamics and, 99–100
structure and, 100–101
healthy, 842
in Alzheimer's disease, early stages of, 998–999
Jung's theory of, 104
multiple personality disorder and, 867, 869–870
of abusers, 1047–1048
split, 34
Personality disorder(s), 841–861
antisocial, 845, 847
avoidant, 848, 849
borderline, 845–847, 848
case study of, 856–860
cluster A, 844–845
cluster B, 845–848
cluster C, 845, 848, 850–851
definition of, 842
dependent, 850
diagnostic criteria for, 844
histrionic, 847, 849
narcissistic, 847–848
nursing process for, 851–860
assessment in, 851, 852b
case study of, 856–860
diagnosis in, 851
evaluation in, 855
implementation in, 852, 853t–854t, 854–855, 855b
outcome identification in, 851
planning in, 851–852
obsessive-compulsive, 850–851
paranoid, 733, 845
schizoid, 845
case study of, 1034–1036
schizotypal, 733, 845, 846
Perspective of care, Gilligan's theory of, 75–77, *76*
Perspectives of Psychiatric Care, 26
Pertofrane (desipramine), 537t
dosage of, 540t
Pervasive developmental disorder, not otherwise specified (PDD-NOS), 603
PET (positron emission tomography), 141
in panic disorder, 700
"Peyote buttons," 794
Phallic stage, 102, 103t
Phasic relatedness, in interpersonal nursing, 119
Ph.D. (Doctor of Philosophy), 59
Phencyclidine (angel dust; PCP), abuse of, 810
psychosis induced by, 744
Phenelzine (Nardil), 537t, 541
dosage of, 540t
fact sheet for, *565*
for children, 596t
Phenobarbital, for children, 597t
Phenothiazines, 526, 527t
for children, 598t
Phenylalanine, 497–498
Phenytoin (Dilantin), for children, 597t
Philosophical assessment, 298–299, 298b
Phobia(s), 706
relaxation training for, 438–439
social, 706
diagnosis of, 709
specific, 706
Physical appearance, information provided by, 199
Physical assessment, 297
for home care, 1163
in eating disorders, 914–915
of children, 582, 584
of rape victims, 1090–1091
of suicidal patients, 933–935
Physical attack, prejudice and, 306
Physical dependence, 800–801
definition of, 798
Physical depletion, as risk factor, for crisis state development, 340
Physical environment. See *Environment(s).*
Physical factors, in suicide, 931
Physical illness, in elderly, 648b
Physical restraints. See *Restraint(s).*
Physical self, 155, 156–158
"body spaces" and, 156, *157*
consciousness of, developmental stages and, 156–158
culture and, 156
differences in, 156
similarities in, 156
Physiognomy, 491
Physiological needs, 166
Piaget, Jean, 160
cognitive development theory of, 160, 160t
Piblokto, 309
Pica, in children, 594
Pick's disease, 990
PIE (problem-intervention-evaluation) system, 1186
Pikul, Joseph, 1050
Pileup, of demands, 468
Pimozide, 527t
Pineal gland, 133
Pinel, Phillippe, 14, 20, 444
Piriformis syndrome, 954
Pituitary gland, 134
Planning, for acquired immunodeficiency syndrome, 1119
for antidepressant, mood stabilizer, and antianxiety agent treatment, 563, *564–567*
for antipsychotic treatment, 556, *557–559*, 562–563
for anxiety disorders, 707, 713
for child abuse, 1067
for community mental health care, community-focused, 1138–1139
individual- or family-focused, 1143–1144
for continuous quality improvement, 1183–1184, *1184*
for discharge, 284
nurse's role in, 745
for dissociative disorders, 873
for eating disorders, 916–918
for elder abuse, 1070
for elderly people, 655
for family therapy, 480–483
evaluation and, 482–483
implementation and, 480–482
termination and, 483
for grieving patients, 678–679
for home care, 1164
for mood disorders, 774, 779

Planning, for acquired immunodeficiency syndrome (*Continued*)
for patient education, 510–511, *512*
for personality disorders, 851–852
for psychophysiological disorders, 969
for rape, 1095
for schizophrenia, 745, 747
for sexual disorders, 899
for spousal abuse, 1058–1059
for substance abuse, 818–819, *819*, 820t
for suicidal patients, 937–938
for violent patients, 1075
in nursing process, 272–273
strategic, for continuous quality improvement, 1180, *1181*
with children, 604–605
Plaques, neuritic, 989
Plasticity, of brain, 980
Plateau phase, of sexual response cycle, 885, 886
Plato, 94, 96t
Play, aspects of, 584b
assessment of, 584–585
Pleasure principle, 100
PNOSS (Psychiatric Nurses' Occupational Stress Scale), 64
Poe, Edgar Allan, 726, 738, 760
Polytheism, 5–6
Polyuria, lithium causing, 548
POR (problem-oriented record) documentation, 276
Positive connectedness, 237–238
Positive regard, 110
Positive reinforcement, 428–429
Positive symptoms, of schizophrenia, 144, 528, 533, 727–728, 729, 737–740
Positron emission tomography (PET), 141
in panic disorder, 700
Possession syndrome, 316
Postconventional level, of moral development, 75
Posterior facet syndrome, 954
Postpartum depressive pattern, 766
Posttraumatic period, 341
Posttraumatic stress disorder (PTSD), 702–706
etiology of, 704, 704t
in children, 594
in rape victims, 1091–1092, 1093
nursing process for, case study of, 1098–1100
nursing implications of, 706
nursing process for, case study of, 716–722
patient information about, 705
treatment of, 704–706
Potentiation, definition of, 798
Poverty, among children, mental illness and, 579–580
female homelessness related to, 1027
substance abuse related to, 825
Power, abuse and, 1040, *1041*
advice-giving and, 78
Power of attorney, durable, 996
Powerlessness, in mood disorders, assessment of, 773
recognizing, 351–352
Practice, ideals of, reality versus, 79–80
path(s) for, 58–60
Psychiatric–Mental Health Advanced Practice Registered Nurse as, 58–60, *60*
Psychiatric–Mental Health Registered Nurse as, 58, 59
private, 48
Practice Parameters Forum, 1185
Practice Parameters Partnership, 1185
Practice role(s), 53–58, *56*
as advocate, 57
as champion of preventive care, 57
as coordinator of care, 57
as manager of environment, 56
as partner with patient and family, 58
as provider of continuum of care, 57
as provider of direct and indirect care, 54, 56
as teacher, 56–57
in emergency department, 56
Practicing subphase, in object relation theory, 843
Pratt, Enoch, 20
Pratt, Joseph, 387
Prayer, 498
Prazepam (Centrax), dosage of, 552t
Preconscious, 100
Preconventional level, of moral development, 75
Prefrontal lobotomy, 139
Pregnancy, abuse during, 1042
acquired immunodeficiency syndrome transmission during, 1106
benzodiazepines during, 551–552
body consciousness during, 157
lithium during, 548
substance abuse during, 826, 827, 827t, 828b
Preinteraction phase. See also *Therapeutic relationship(s), preinteraction phase of.*
of group development, 396–397
Prejudice, 306
Premack, David, 428
Premack principle, 428
Premature ejaculation, 885
Preoperational stage, 160, 160t
Presenting problem, assessment of, in psychodynamic short-term therapy, 373
President's Commission on Mental Health, 22, 1130
Preventive mental health, behavioral strategies in, 439
care for, levels of, 57
nurse's role in, 57
for adults, 633–636
character development in, 634
education in, 634
empowerment in, 635
social support in, 635–636
technology in, 635
values clarification in, 634–635
Primary care, 57
Primary gain, 964
Primary prevention, of mental illness, 1137
Primary processes, 100–101
Principles of Psychology (James), 97
Prioritization, of nursing diagnoses, 271
Privacy, informational, 1196–1197, 1197b
valuation of, family violence due to, 1046
Private hospitals, 46
Private practice, 48
Problem behavior, definition of, 424–425
Problem definition, in crisis intervention, 352–353
Problem-intervention-evaluation (PIE) system, 1186
Problem-oriented record (POR) documentation, 276
Problem-solving approach, for developing solutions, in therapeutic relationships, 253–255
for social skills training, 435–436
in nursing process, 267t
Prodrome, of migraine headaches, 958–959
Professional attire, lack of, 6
Professional training, funding for, 46
Professionalization, of nursing, influence on mental health care, 25–26
Progress notes, confidentiality and, 201
Progressive relaxation, 714b
Prohibition, 795
Projection, as defense mechanism, 697
in alcoholism, 807
in families, 475
Projective identification, 256
Prolixin (fluphenazine), 527t, 531, 532t
fact sheet for, *559*
Propranolol, for anxiety, 555
Protaxic thinking, 106
Protest, grief and, 179
Protestantism, among Filipinos, 318
Protriptyline (Vivactil), 537t
dosage of, 540t
Proxemics, 200
Prozac. See *Fluoxetine (Prozac).*
Pseudodementia, 993
Psychiatric aides (attendants; technicians), as treatment team members, 63t
Psychiatric assessment, in Alzheimer's disease, 997t
Psychiatric consultation-liaison nurse, 58
Psychiatric emergency services, 361
Psychiatric history, in psychodynamic short-term therapy, 373
Psychiatric home care. See *Home care.*
Psychiatric Nurses' Occupational Stress Scale (PNOSS), 64
"Psychiatric Nursing: The Nurse-Patient Relationship" (film), 24–25
Psychiatric Nursing Assessment Tool, 289, *290–294*
Psychiatric Nursing Clinical Note, 276, *279*
Psychiatric social workers, as treatment team members, 63t
Psychiatric units, within general hospitals, 47
Psychiatric–Mental Health Advanced Practice Registered Nurse, 58–60, *60*
Psychiatric–mental health nursing, ANA standards of, 55b
confidentiality in, 87b
definition of, 54
history of, 11–28
ancient, 14
chronology of significant events in, 27–28
"Decade of the Brain" and, 27
deinstitutionalization's influence on, 23
during 18th, 19th, and 20th centuries, 14–19
family advocacy's influence on, 26
first and second World War influences on, 21
interpersonal relationships' influence on, 23–25
litigation influencing, 21–23
of mental health care settings, 19–20, *20, 21*
of professionalization, 25–26
psychobiological treatment's influence on, 23
phenomena of concern to, 54b
Psychiatric–Mental Health Registered Nurse (R.N., C.), 58, 59
Psychiatrist(s), as home care plan directors, 1157–1158
as treatment team members, 63t
Psychic determinism, 99
Psychic secretions, 111–112

Psychoactive substance(s), 793
abuse of. See *Substance abuse;* specific substances.
definition of, 797–798, 798
early understanding of, 794–795
Psychoanalytic psychotherapy, 368–369, 368–370, 369t
techniques of, 102–103
U.S. espousal of, 129
with families, 474t
Psychoanalytic theory. See *Freudian theory.*
Psychobiology, 128. See also *Biological* entries.
Psychodrama, 387–388, 412–413, 413t
closure for, 413
warm-up for, 412–413
Psychodynamic theory(ies), 99–105
interpersonal, of Sullivan, 105–106
of anxiety, 694
generalized, 698
of group psychotherapy, 391
of Jung, 104–105
of mood disorders, 768–770, *769*
of Sigmund Freud. See *Freudian theory.*
Psychodynamic therapy, group, 391
size of, 393
short-term, 371–376, 372t, 373t
analysis and planning in, 374–375
assessment in, 373–374
first interview in, 372–373
implementation in, 375–376
Psychoeducation, in family therapy, 470–471
Psychoeducation groups, 387, 391t, 415–417
for families, of schizophrenic patients, 749–750
Psychogenic amnesia, 863–864
Psychogeriatric units, 47
Psychological assessment, in eating disorders, 915
of suicidal patients, 935–936
Psychological changes, age-related, 647t
Psychological dependence, 801–802
definition of, 798
Psychological factor(s), in acquired immunodeficiency syndrome, 1104–1105, *1105*
in eating disorders, 912–913
in hypertension, 958
in low back pain, 954
in suicide, 931–932
Psychological self, 155, *158*, 158–162
cognitive. See *Cognitive process(es).*
emotional, 161–162
perceptual, 158–159
perceptual development and, 159
Psychological theory(ies), early, 96–99, 98t
of James, 97–98, 98t
of Wundt, 96–97, 98t
therapeutic relationships based on, 238
Psychology: The Briefer Course (James), 97
Psychomotor domain, 510
Psychomotor functioning, in Alzheimer's disease, early stages of, 1001
Psychopharmacologic treatment, 114. See also *Psychotherapeutic agent(s);* specific drugs and drug types.
for AIDS-dementia complex, 1112
for Alzheimer's disease, early stages of, 1004
for anxiety, 699
for chronically mentally ill, 1132
for delirium, 986
for depression, in acquired immunodeficiency syndrome, 1111
Psychopharmacologic treatment (*Continued*)
for eating disorders, 919
for low back pain, 954
for mood disorders, 784–785
for obsessive-compulsive disorder, 702
for pelvic pain, 955
for personality disorders, 855
for posttraumatic stress disorder, 704–705
for schizophrenia, 747
for sexual disorders, 900
in Bay Area Health Care model, 1155
in milieu therapy, 448
in psychodynamic short-term therapy, 375
medication history for, 289, 295
medication teaching for, for anxiety disorders, 715
of children, 595t–599t, 608
Psychophysiological assessment, 951–953
psychometric instruments in, 951–953
stress response measures in, 953
Psychophysiological disorder(s), 949–972. See also specific disorders.
diagnosis of, 951–952
psychometric instruments for, 951–952
stress response measures in, 953
nursing process for, 969–972
assessment in, 969
case study of, 971–972
diagnosis in, 969
evaluation in, 970
implementation in, 970
outcome identification in, 969
planning in, 969
theoretical perspectives on, 951
homeostatic, 951
mechanistic, 951
stress and, 951, *952*
Psychosexual disorders. See *Sexual disorder(s);* specific disorders.
Psychosexual stages of development. See *Developmental stage(s).*
Psychosis(es). See also *Bipolar disorder; Schizophrenia.*
drug-induced, 744
personal space and, 200
sexual problems resulting from, 894–895
vocalizations and, 201
Psychosocial and environmental problems, examples of, 37b
Psychosocial crisis, 107
Psychosocial learning theory, 505, 505t
Psychotherapeutic agent(s), 496, 523–568. See also specific drugs and drug types.
action of, on synaptic transmission, 524–526, *525*
Psychotherapy, definition of, 367
economics and, 370–371
for irritable bowel syndrome, 957
for mood disorders, 774–779
cognitive, 776, 778
interpersonal, 776, 778–779
supportive, 775–776
for obsessive-compulsive disorder, 702
for pelvic pain, 955–956
for posttraumatic stress disorder, 705–706, 706–707
group. See *Group psychotherapy.*
historical background of, 368
in Bay Area Health Care model, 1156
in community mental health care, 1145
in home care, 1165
individual. See *Individual psychotherapy.*
inpatient. See *Inpatient treatment.*
Psychotherapy, definition of (*Continued*)
outpatient. See *Community mental health care; Outpatient treatment.*
private practice in, 48
psychoanalytic. See *Psychoanalytic psychotherapy.*
supportive, 379–380, 380t
for mood disorders, 775–776
for schizophrenia, 748–749
therapeutic relationship in. See *Therapeutic relationship(s).*
Psychotropic medication(s), 496, 523–568. See also specific drugs and drug types.
action of, 524–526
on synaptic transmission, 524–526, *525*
PTSD. See *Posttraumatic stress disorder (PTSD).*
Public mental hospitals, 19, 46
deinstitutionalization and, 23
Public policy, 37, *39*, 39–41
Action for Mental Health and, 21–22
Amerasian Homecoming Act of 1987 and, 316
Americans with Disabilities Act of 1990 and, 22–23
Anti-Crime Bill of 1994 and, 435–436
Budget Reconciliation Act of 1981 and, 42
Children's and Communities Mental Health Systems Improvement Act of 1990 and, 40
Community Mental Health Act of 1963 and, 20, 37, 39–40, 42, 444, 1129, 1130
rescinding of, 39–40
Community Mental Health Center Amendment of 1975 and, 22
community mental health centers and. See *Community mental health (CMH) centers.*
Community Mental Health Systems Act of 1980 and, 22, 1130
Comprehensive Drug Abuse Prevention and Control Act of 1970 and, 796
Consolidated Omnibus Budget Reconciliation Act (COBRA) of 1985 and, 1177
Department of Defense Authorization Bill of 1990 and, 40
Education of the Handicapped Act Amendments of 1986 and, 40
Harrison Narcotic Act of 1914 and, 795
Hill-Burton Bill of 1946 and, 21
homelessness related to, 1029–1030
Hospital Survey and Construction Act of 1946 and, 21
Hughes Act of 1970 and, 797
Joint Commission on Mental Illness and Health and, 21–22
Joint Commission on the Mental Health of Children and, 22
McKinney Homeless Assistance Act and, 40
Mental Health Survey Act of 1955 and, 1129
Mental Health Systems Act of 1980 and, 83, 84, 1191
Mental Retardation Facilities and Community Mental Health Centers Construction Act of 1963 and, 22, 1129
National Institute of Mental Health and, 21, 22
National Mental Health Act of 1946 and, 21, 37

National Mental Health Act of 1946 and *Continued*
National Mental Health Act of 1955 and, 21–22
Nursing's Plan to Provide Essential Mental Health Services and, 40–41
Omnibus Budget Reconciliation Acts and, 22, 1130, 1177
on alcohol abuse treatment, 797
on community mental health care, 1129, 1130
on rape, 1088–1089
on substance abuse, 797
on suicide, 928
President's Commission on Mental Health and, 22
Prohibition and, 795
regarding quality of care, 1177
Report to the President of the President's Commission on Mental Health and, 22
Social Security Act of 1965 and, 1177
toward homeless people, 1032
Pulmonary system, aging of, 647t
Pulse diagnosis, 489
Punishment, 429
in behavioral therapy, 436–437
Purpose, in experiences, 155
Purposive sample, 1199

QA. See *Quality assurance (QA).*
QI (Quality Improvement). See also *Continuous quality improvement (CQI).*
documentation for, 276
Qualitative research, 1198–1200
Quality, definition of, 1179–1180
Quality assurance (QA), 1175, 1175b. See also *Continuous quality improvement (CQI); Total quality management (TQM).*
integrating with continuous quality improvement, 1176–1177, 1176b, 1177b
traditional nursing approaches to, 1178
Quality councils, 1181
Quality Improvement (QI). See also *Continuous quality improvement (CQI).*
documentation for, 276
Quality of life, promoting, in dementia, 995–996
Quality team(s), 1181, 1189
Quantitative research models, 1198
Questions, for active listening, 213–214
"meaning," 77–78
opportunity for, in milieu therapy, 452, 453, 455, 458
Quinoa, 497

Race, 306. See also specific racial groups.
of children, 578
Racism, 306–307
suicide related to, 932
Rando, Theresa, on grief, 663, 664
Rape, 1085–1100
date or acquaintance, 1089
definition of, 1087
demographics of, 1087–1088
incidence of, 1088
marital, 1088–1089
myths about, 1091b
nurse's role in, 1086–1087
in community and ambulatory care, 1087
in emergency department, 1087
Rape (*Continued*)
nursing process for, 1090–1100
assessment in, 1090–1091
of family response, 1091
of mental state, 1091
of spiritual state, 1091
physical, 1090
questions for, 1090
case study of, 1098–1100
diagnosis in, 1091–1094
during disorganization (acute) phase, 1092, 1094
during reorganization phase, 1094
during reorganization phase, 1096–1097
evaluation in, 1097–1098
implementation in, 1096–1097
during disorganization (acute) phase, 1096
outcome identification in, 1094
planning in, 1095
during disorganization (acute) phase, 1095
during reorganization phase, 1095
prevention of, 1097b
terminology for, 1087
victims of, rights of, 1090b
Rape-trauma syndrome, 1092, 1094b
disorganization (acute) phase of, 1092, 1094, 1095, 1096
emotional reactions during, 1092, 1094
impact reaction during, 1092
somatic reactions during, 1092
reorganization phase of, 1094, 1095, 1096–1097
Rapid cycling, in mood disorders, 766
Rapport, developing, 248–249
Rapprochement subphase, in object relation theory, 843
Rational linear model, for transmitting research knowledge, 1200–1201
Rationalization, in alcoholism, 807
Reaction formation, as defense mechanism, 697
Reaction phase, of critical incident debriefing, 362
Readiness, for learning, 508
assessment of, 509
Reagan, Ronald, 39
Reality orientation groups, 414
Reality testing, 101
Reality therapy, 111
Reasoning, deductive, 1198
inductive, 1198
Reassurance, false, in therapeutic communication, 224t, 225
Receiver, of message, 202
Recognition seekers, in psychotherapy groups, 408t
Recoil, period of, 341
Reconstituted family, 465t
Record-keeping. See also *Documentation.*
for group psychotherapy, 416–417
in crisis intervention, 359
Recovery, 177
definition of, 798
from substance abuse, 800, 802
family in, 829–832
societal information about, 820
Recreational therapists, as treatment team members, 63t
Redirecting, in therapeutic communication, 218–219
Reentry phase, of critical incident debriefing, 362
Referrals, 258
for mood disorders, 782–784
in crisis intervention, 359
Reflecting, 215, 217t
Reflex action, 100
Reform Jews, 314
Reframing, assumptions underlying, 206b
in therapeutic communication, 219–220
Refugees, adjustment of, 308
Southeast Asian, 316–317
Regression, as defense mechanism, 697
Regulators, 200
Rehabilitation model, data collection using, 285
Reimbursement. See *Funding.*
Reinforcement, 112, 423
aversive, 429
in behavioral therapy, 436–437
continuous, 430, 430t
for behavioral therapy. See *Behavioral therapy.*
for token economy, 434–435
negative, 429
of self, 113
positive reinforcement and, 428–429
Premack principle and, 428
punishment and, 429
reinforcer identification and, 428
social, 428b
types of, 428
Reinforcement schedules, 430, 430t
Reinforcer(s), 113, 428
Reinforcing properties, definition of, 798
of abused substances, 800, 801–802
Reinvestment, grief and, 180
Rejection, nurses' fear of, 7
Relapse, definition of, 798
in substance abuse, 800
prevention of, 802
Relationship(s). See *Interpersonal relationship(s); Social relationship(s); Therapeutic communication; Therapeutic relationship(s).*
Relationship theory(ies), 118–119
of Orlando, 110
of Peplau, 106, 118–119, 445
therapeutic relationships based on, 237–238
Relaxation, 495
for migraine headaches, 960
progressive, 714b
teaching, 438–439
using guided imagery, 696b
Reliability, trust and, 245
Religion(s). See also *Spiritual* entries; specific religions.
among Chinese people, 317
among Filipinos, 318
among Hispanic Americans, 315
among Indian peoples, 315
among Irish Americans, 313
among Italian Americans, 313
among Japanese people, 317–318
among Jewish Americans, 313–314
among Native Americans, 320
among Southeast Asians, 317
among West Indian peoples, 321
cultural concepts of, 312
grieving and, 676
lack of, as obstacle to grieving, 674
Religious hallucinations, 738
Religious practices, as therapy, 498

Remarriage, 624
Reminiscence groups, 393, 413–414, 414b
Remorse, family interventions for, 344t
Remote memory, in Alzheimer's disease, early stages of, 998
Remotivation therapy, 1132, 1133b
groups for, 414–415, 415t
Renal toxicity, of lithium, 548
Render, Helena, 24
Reno, Janet, 436
Renouvier, Charles, 97
Reorganization, grief and, 180
Repetitive behaviors, in Alzheimer's disease, middle stages of, 1009
Report to the President of the President's Commission on Mental Health, 22, 1130
Repression, as defense mechanism, 697
Research, 1193–1203
dissemination of, application and, 1202, 1203
clinical practice guidelines for, 1202–1203
models for, 1200–1204
interactive, 1201–1202
linear, rational, 1200–1201
user-oriented, 1201
NIH consensus development conferences for, 1202
health care delivery system changes related to, 1194–1195
knowledge and, 1194
legal and ethical issue(s) in, 1196–1197
informational privacy as, 1196–1197
informed consent as, 1197
truth-telling as, 1197
model(s) for, 1197–1200
qualitative, 1198–1200
quantitative, 1198
triangulation in, 1200
nurses' role on, 63
nursing role in, 1195–1196
Residential treatment, 47
for anxiety disorders, 713–715
for children, 606–607
milieu therapy in, 459
Residential/therapeutic community, 458, *458*
Residual schizophrenia, 533, 732t, 743
Resilience, 178–179
Resistance, 223
in psychotherapy groups, 397
working through, 255–256
Resocialization groups, 393
Resolution phase, of sexual response cycle, 886
Resource(s), nurses as stewards of, 63–64
questions to ask about, 255
Respiratory depression, anterograde, 551
Respite care, for Alzheimer's patients, in early stages, 1004
Respondent conditioning, 112
operant conditioning versus, *112*
Response(s), 423
Response prevention, 432
Responsibility, communication and, 195
in existential models, 110
in reality therapy, 111
in social versus therapeutic relationships, 233–234
of therapeutic communication, 209
Restating, 214, 217t
Restitution, in grieving process, 669
Restraint(s), chemical, 81
for Alzheimer's patients, in middle stages, 1009–1010
Restraint(s), chemical (*Continued*)
for violent patients, 1076, 1077
in crisis intervention, 348–349, 350b
in milieu therapy, 449
Retention, social learning theory and, 114
Retrograde amnesia, in dissociative disorders, 866t
Rett's disorder, in children, 603
Return demonstration, for patient education, 513
Reuptake, of neurotransmitters, 525
Revolving door cycle, 1129
Richards, Linda, *17*, 17–18
Riggs, Austin, 444
Risperidone (Risperdal), 533
for children, 599t
for schizophrenia, 534
Ritalin. See *Methylphenidate (Ritalin).*
R.N., C. (Psychiatric–Mental Health Registered Nurse), 58, 59
R.N., C.S. (Certified Specialist in Psychiatric and Mental Health Nursing), 59
Robb, Isabel Hampton, 25
Robinson, Lisa, 52–53
Rogers, Carl, 109, 214, 388
person-centered model of, 109–110
relevance to nursing, 110
Rogers, Martha, 116
Role(s), assessment of, 165b
gender, 163
among Hispanic Americans, 315
in family, 162–163, 466
of nurses. See *Nursing role(s); Practice role(s).*
social self and, 162–164
Role responsibilities, in therapeutic relationship, 248
Role reversals, in psychodrama, 413t
Role-playing, in therapeutic communication, 219
Romazicon (flumazenil), for benzodiazepine overdose, 553
Roosevelt, Eleanor, 1033–1034
Rouse v. Cameron, 41
Roy, Callista, 116
Rule-out disorder, Alzheimer's disease as, 997
Rules(s), of family, 466
Rumination disorder, in children, 595
Rummaging, in Alzheimer's disease, middle stages of, 1006t
Runaway children, 1027
Rush, Benjamin, 14, 795

Sacroiliac syndrome, 954
SAD (seasonal affective disorder), 145, 766
Sadism, 891t
"Safer" sex, 1104
Safety, assessment of, for home care, 1163
in milieu therapy, 446
needs for, 166
of abused women, determining, 1054, *1055*, 1056
of Alzheimer's patients, in early stages, 1002
of nurse, with violent patients, 1076–1077
of patients, with anxiety disorders, 713–714
of rape victims, 1096, 1097
St. Augustine, 368
St. Vitus' dance, 134, 991
comorbidity of, with bipolar disorder, 767
Saint Elizabeth's Hospital, 15
"Saint Francis and the Snow" (Kinnel), 386
Sandwich generation, 631
Santayana, George, 13
SARS (Sexual Assault Resource Service) model, 1096
Satiation, 423
Satir, Virginia, 161
Sausages, interaction with monoamine oxidase inhibitors, 543t
Scapegoating, in psychotherapy groups, 408–409
Scatologia, telephone, 891t
Schedule of Recent Experiences (Holmes and Rahe), *339*, 339–340
Schema, 160
Schizoaffective disorder, 731
Schizoid personality disorder, 845
case study of, 1034–1036
Schizophrenia, 725–754
active, 742–743
acute, 533
among Indian peoples, 316
assessment in, 737–744
of clinical signs and symptoms, 737–740
of family environment, 740–741
of spiritual and religious issues, 741
of variability, over lifetime, 741–744
Bleuler's perspective on, 729–730, 729b
catatonic, 732t
causes of, 143–144, 731–736
dopamine hypothesis of, 143, 733–734
familial, 734–735
genetic, 144, 733
limbic, 733
neurochemical, 143
stress-vulnerability model of, *735*, 735–736
structural, 141, 143–144, 731–733
viral, 144, 734
comorbidity of, with substance abuse, 743–744, 750
course of, 732t, 742–743
diagnosis of, 730–731, 731b, 732t
disorganized, 732t
DSM-IV diagnosis of, 731, 732t
established facts about, 733b
facial expressions in, 199
family information about, 749
in children, 604
in elderly people, 652, 742
in young adults, 742
international pilot study of, 730–731
Kraepelin's perspective on, 729
language disorders in, 139
long-term course of, 533
normal versus enhanced perceptions in, 726–727
nurse's role in, 728
nursing process for, 736–754
assessment in. See *Schizophrenia, assessment in.*
case study of, 751–754
diagnosis in, 744, 744t, 745, 746
evaluation in, 750–751
implementation in, 747–750
outcome identification in, 745
planning in, 745, 747
onset of, age of, 741–742
paranoid, 732t
case study of, 751–754
patient education in, 747–748
patient information about, 748
residual, 533, 732t, 743
sensory alterations in, 727–728
suicide related to, 930

Schizophrenia (*Continued*)
symptoms of, 737–740
first- and second-rank, 730
negative, 144, 528, 533, 737, 739–740
positive, 144, 528, 533, 727–728, 729, 737–740
residual, 533, 732t, 743
teaching patients to identify and manage, 747–748
treatment of, dopamine transmission and, 137
psychopharmacological, 528. See also *Antipsychotic agent(s);* specific drugs.
undifferentiated, 732t
Schizophrenogenic mothers, 734
Schizotypal personality disorder, 733, 845, 846
School, 577
Schumann, Robert, 760
Schwann cells, 135
Screaming, in Alzheimer's disease, middle stages of, 1007
Searching, grief and, 179
Seasonal affective disorder (SAD), 145, 766
Seasonal factor, in schizophrenia, 734
The Seasons of a Man's Life (Levinson), 620
Seclusion, in crisis intervention, 348–349, 350b
Secondary gain, 964
Secondary prevention, 57
of mental illness, 1137
Secondary psychological processes, 101
Secondary sources, for assessment, 299
Second-rank symptoms, of schizophrenia, 730
Secrets, family, 466
Secularism, 5
Secure attachment, 585
Security needs, Sullivan's theory of, 105
Sedation, antipsychotic agents causing, 530
tricyclic antidepressants causing, 538
Seeds, 497
Seizure(s), antipsychotic agents causing, 530
clozapine causing, 532
in abusers, 1047
tricyclic antidepressants causing, 538
Selective abstraction, 376
Selective (systematized) amnesia, in dissociative disorders, 866t
Selective serotonin re-uptake inhibitor(s) (SSRIs), 543–544. See also specific drugs.
action of, 537t
adverse effects of, 537t
dosage of, 540t
for eating disorders, 911
for personality disorders, 855
Self, 154–165. See also *Self-concept.*
altered sense of, in schizophrenia, 738t
awareness of. See *Self-awareness.*
definition of, during 30s, 624–625
development of, 155
differentiation of, in family therapy, 474
embedded, 622
ideal, 155
in dissociative disorders, 865
Jung's theory of, 105
knowledge of, 154
physical. See *Physical self.*
psychological. See *Cognitive process(es); Psychological self.*
Rogers' theory of, 109
social, 155, 162–164
family role and, 162–163
gender identity and, 163
Self (*Continued*)
spiritual. See *Spiritual self.*
Sullivan's theory of, 105–106
therapeutic use of, 236
Self-abuse, 930–931
among elders, 1044
Self-actualization, 108–109, 109t
during adulthood, 626
needs for, 166b
Self-attitude, in mood disorders, 763–764
Self-awareness, 154b
for assessment, 286, *287*
for effective communication, 195
for therapeutic communication, 224
in therapeutic relationships, 236–237, 237b, 238b, 254
of nurse, need for, 6
sexual, questions to encourage, 880b
Self-care, 56, 273
in Alzheimer's disease, middle stages of, 1005–1007, 1006t
of homeless people, promoting, 1034
Self-concept, 154–155
development of, 155
perceptual processes and, 159
Self-confessors, in psychotherapy groups, 408t
Self-confidence, 161
Self-counseling, in psychodrama, 413t
Self-destructive behavior, direct, 928. See also *Suicide.*
indirect, 928
Self-diagnosis, of substance abuse, 819–821
Self-discipline, in reality therapy, 111
Self-disclosure, in social versus therapeutic relationships, 234
in therapeutic communication, 209
Self-efficacy, 161
Bandura's theory of, 114
cognitive learning theory of, 506
vulnerability and, 337
Self-esteem, 155, 161–162
high vs. low, 162b
Self-help groups. See *Support group(s).*
Self-management, behavioral strategies for. See *Behavioral therapy, self-management using.*
Self-Rating Depression Scale, 1210, 1211t, 1212t, 1212–1214
Self-realization, Jung's theory of, 105
Self-reflection, questions for, 238b
Self-reinforcement, 113
Self-reliance, 178–179
Self-respect, 161
Self-roles, of psychotherapy group members, 407–408, 408t
Self-understanding, in group psychotherapy, 401–402
Sender, of message, 202
Sensitivity groups, 416
Sensitization, covert, for sexual disorders, 900
Sensorimotor stage, 160, 160t
Sensory system, 137–138
aging of, 647t
Separation anxiety, in children, 590, 593
losses and, 663
Separation-individuation phase, in object relation theory, 843
Septal nucleus(i), 134
Septum pellucidum, 133
Serax (oxazepam), dosage of, 552t
Serentil (mesoridazine), 527t
Seriously mentally ill. See *Chronically mentally ill patient(s); Community mental health care.*
Serotonergic system, 137, *138*
Serotonin, 137. See also *Selective serotonin re-uptake inhibitors (SSRIs).*
in eating disorders, 911
in migraine headaches, 959
in panic disorder, 700
in personality development, 844
in suicide, 931
mood disorders and, 145
SERPN (Society for Education and Research in Psychiatric–Mental Health Nursing), 25
Sertraline (Zoloft), 537t, 544
dosage of, 540t
for children, 596t
Setting(s). See *Environment(s); Treatment setting(s).*
Sex. See also *Gender* entries; *Sexual* entries; *Sexuality; Women.*
definition of, 881
Sex education, 890
Sexual abuse. See also *Incest; Rape.*
assessing for, 297
definition of, 1042
of children, 1042
mental illness and, 580
of elders, 1044
of spouse, 1056–1057
Sexual activity, acquired immunodeficiency syndrome transmission by, 1106
"safer," 1104
Sexual Assault Resource Service (SARS) model, 1096
Sexual development, 881–882, 882t
Sexual disorder(s), 886–890, 890–906
antipsychotic agents causing, 530
assessment of, 896–898
do's and don't's for, 901t
facilitative statements for, 900t
guidelines for, 896–897, 897t
interview process in, 897–898, 898t, 899, 900t, 901t
settings for, 897
chromosomal abnormalities causing, 894
head trauma causing, 894
nurse's response to, 895–896
nursing process for, 896–906
assessment in. See *Sexual disorder(s), assessment of.*
case study of, 902–906
diagnosis in, 898
implementation in, 900, *902*
outcome identification in, 898–899
planning in, 899
of arousal, 886–887
of gender identity, 892–893
of orgasm, 887–890
paraphilias as, 901t, 901–902
causes of, 890–891
treatment of, 891–892
psychosis causing, 894–895
terminology for, 881
Sexual feelings, in schizophrenia, 727
Sexual identity, definition of, 881
Sexual neurosis, 316
Sexual response cycle, 882–886, *883*
desire phase of, 883–884, 885
excitement phase of, 884–885, 885t
orgasm phase of, 885–886, 887t
plateau phase of, 885, 886b
resolution phase of, 886
Sexual tension, 885
Sexuality, concerns about, cues indicating, 899b

Sexuality, concerns about, cues indicating (*Continued*)
definition of, 882
of children, assessment of, 585–586
self-awareness of, questions to encourage, 880
slang expressions related to, 898t
societal attitudes toward, 1108
Shadow, in Jung's theory, 104
Shame, feelings of, in mood disorders, 771
The Shame of the States (Deutsch), 21
Shanti project, 1108
Shaping, 113, 431–432, 432b
Sheehan Patient-Rated Anxiety Scale, 707, 1207–1208
"Shell shock," 21
Sheltered housing, 1134
Sheppard, Moses, 20
Sheppard and Enoch Pratt Hospital, 20, *21*
Sheppard Asylum, 20
Shetler, Charles, 26
Shetler, Harriet, 26
Shewhart, Walter, 1179
Shintoism, 317–318
Shock, family interventions for, 344t
in grieving process, 669
Short-term memory, 139
in Alzheimer's disease, early stages of, 998
Short-term therapy. See *Psychodynamic therapy, short-term.*
Sibling(s), of schizophrenic patients, 734–735
violence by, 1043–1044
Sibling position, 163, 476
Silence, in therapeutic communication, 215–216, 217t
Simon, Hermann, 444
Simple association, 423
Simpson, Nicole, 1039
Simpson, O.J., 1039
Sinequan (doxepin), 537t
dosage of, 540t
Single adults, 465t
Single parent family, 465t
Single-room occupancy units (SROs), 1134
shortage of, homelessness related to, 1029
Sire, James, 160
Situational anxiety, treatment of, 554
Situational crises. See *Crisis(es), situational.*
Skilled nursing services, in home care, 1153, 1157
Skinner, B. F., 111, 112, 129
theory of, *112*, 112–113
relevance to nursing, 113
Skipper, James, 53
Slavson, Samuel R., 387, 416–417
Sleep, assessment of, in psychodynamic short-term therapy, 374
brain during, electrical activity of, 142
deprivation of, mood disorders related to, 767
disturbances of, in Alzheimer's disease, middle stages of, 1009
treatment of, psychopharmacological, 551
mood disorders related to, 145
Smith, Dorothy Hoskins, 414
The Snake Pit (Ward), 21
SOAPIE format, 276
Social assessment, of suicidal patients, 936
Social disaffiliation, homelessness due to, 1030
Social factors, in suicide, 932
Social functioning, in Alzheimer's disease, early stages of, 1004
Social Interaction and Patient Care, 53
Social isolation, of refugees, 308
Social learning theory(ies), 113–114
cognitive, 505t, 505–506
of modeling, 113–114
of self-efficacy, 114
relevance to nursing, 114
Social Learning Theory (Bandura), 113
Social margin, 1029
Social phobia, 706
diagnosis of, 709
Social reinforcement, 428b
Social relationship(s). See also *Interpersonal relationship(s).*
therapeutic relationships compared with, 233–234, 235t
common elements and, 233
differences and, 233–234
Social responses, in therapeutic communication, 224t, 226
Social roles, of adults, social changes affecting. See *Adult(s), social change(s) affecting.*
Social Security Act of 1965, 1177
Social self, 155, 162–164
family role and, 162–163
gender identity and, 163
Social services, shortage of, homelessness related to, 1029–1030
Social skills, development of, for substance abuse treatment, 821–822
training in, 410b, 435–436
Social support. See *Support(s).*
Social Support Questionnaire (SSQ-6), in psychophysiological disorders, 953
Social workers, as treatment team members, 63t
Social-cognitive theory, 436
Socialization, gender differences in, 76
Societal regression, 476
Society, as obstacle to grieving, 674
attitudes of, toward family violence, 1045–1046
toward homeless people, 1031
toward sexuality, 1108
changes in, adult development related to. See *Adult(s), social change(s) affecting.*
impact on mental health care, *42*, 42–43
aging of population and, 43
dual diagnoses and, 43
during 1960s, 42
during 1970s, 42
during 1980s, 42
during 1990s, 42
homelessness and, 43
unemployment and, 43
information for, about acquired immunodeficiency syndrome, 1120
about depression, 780
about dissociative disorders, 869
about substance abuse, 820
nurses' accountability to, 62
Society for Education and Research in Psychiatric–Mental Health Nursing (SERPN), 25
Sociocultural factors. See also *Culture;* specific cultural groups.
assessment of, 297–298, 915
in eating disorders, 913, 915
Socrates, 94, 96t, 368
Socratic questioning, 94
Soliloquy, in psychodrama, 413t
Solvents, volatile, abuse of, 815
Somatic hallucinations, 738t
Somatic reactions, to rape, 1092
Somatization disorder, 965–966, 968t
Somatoform disorder(s), 961–969, 962b
body dysmorphic disorder as, 962–963, 968t
conversion disorder as, 963–964, 968t
hypochondriasis as, 964–965, 968t
not otherwise specified, 967, 968t
pain disorder as, 966–967, 968t
somatization disorder as, 965–966, 968t
treatment of, 968
undifferentiated, 967, 968t
Somatosensory area, 131, 137–138
Soranus, 729
Southeast Asians, 316–317
Space. See also *Boundary(ies).*
cultural concepts of, 311
Specific phobia, 706
Speech patterns, mental illness and, 201, 202t
Spielberger State Anxiety Scale, 707
Spiritual assessment, 298–299, 298b
for eating disorders, 915
for mood disorders, 773
for rape victims, 1091
for schizophrenia, 741
for suicide potential, 936–937
Spiritual development, of children, assessment of, 587–589, 588t
Spiritual distress, 165
Spiritual factor(s), in eating disorders, 914
in hypertension, 958
in low back pain, 954
in patient education, 515–516
in suicide, 932
Spiritual intervention(s), 185–186, 920–921. See also *Mind-body-spirit therapy(ies).*
for eating disorders, 920–921
for low back pain, 954
for mood disorders, 782, *784*
for pelvic pain, 955–956
for schizophrenia, 750
in Bay Area Health Care model, 1154
Spiritual self, 155, 164–165
development of, 165
God-consciousness and, 164–165
morality and, 165
spiritual distress and, 165
Spiritual Well-Being Scale, in psychophysiological disorders, 953
Spirituality, 3. See also *Theistic model(s).*
in family therapy, 476
supporting, in milieu therapy, 447
Split personality, 34
Splitting, in borderline personality disorder, 846–847
Spousal abuse. See also *Family violence.*
cycle of, 1056, *1057*
emotional, 1054
family structural inequality causing, 1046–1047
mutual, 1048–1049, 1049t
of men, 1048–1049, 1049t
of women, assessment of, 1050–1057, *1052*, *1053*
cycle of abuse in, 1056, *1057*
documentation of, 1051–1052, 1054
interviewing in, 1051, 1055
safety determination in, 1054, *1055*, 1056
sexual abuse in, 1056–1057
indicators of, 1052
legal remedies for, in Maryland, 1063b
nursing process for, 1050–1062, 1062b
assessment in. See *Spousal abuse, of women, assessment of.*

Spousal abuse (*Continued*)
case study of, 1078–1080
diagnosis in, 1057, 1058
evaluation in, 1062
facilitative and inhibitive responses in, 1062
implementation in, 1059–1062
outcome identification in, 1058
planning in, 1058–1059
potential batterer in, 1048b
prevention of, primary, 1059
secondary, 1059, *1060*
tertiary, 1059–1061, 1061t, 1062, *1064*
sexual, 1056–1057, 1088–1089
Spouse, death of, 630
SQUID (superconducting quantum interference device), 141
SROs (single-room occupancy units), 1134
shortage of, homelessness related to, 1029
SSQ-6 (Social Support Questionnaire), in psychophysiological disorders, 953
SSRIs. See *Selective serotonin re-uptake inhibitor(s) (SSRIs).*
STAI (State-Trait Anxiety Scale), in psychophysiological disorders, 951
Stallwood, Jean, 4
Standard(s). See also *American Nurses' Association (ANA).*
in continuous quality improvement, 1185
professional, 60–62, *61*
Standards of Care and, 54, 56
Standards of Clinical Nursing Practice and, 266–267
on patient education, 504
Standards of Psychiatric and Mental Health Nursing and, 1185
Standards of Psychiatric–Mental Health Clinical Nursing Practice and, 267, 273, 285, 288
Standardized rating scale(s), 288, 288t, 1207–1227
Abnormal Involuntary Movement Scale as, 1218
Brief Psychiatric Rating Scale as, 1219
Children's Psychiatric Rating Scale as, 1222–1227
Dissociative Experiences Scale as, 865, 1209–1210
Global Assessment of Functioning Scale as, 1220
Mania Rating Scale as, 1217
Mini–Mental State Examination as, 295, 1116–1117, 1221
Sheehan Patient-Rated Anxiety Scale as, 707, 1207–1208
Yale-Brown Obsessive-Compulsive Scale as, 1215
Yale-Brown Obsessive-Compulsive Symptom Checklist as, 1216
Zung Self-Rating Depression Scale as, 1210, 1211t, 1212t, 1212–1214
Stanford-Binet test, 601
Starvation, in eating disorders, 912
State Boards of Nursing, private practice regulation by, 48
State nurse practice acts, 82
Statement on Psychiatric–Mental Health Clinical Nursing Practice, 447
State-Trait Anxiety Scale (STAI), in psychophysiological disorders, 951
Statistical analysis, for continuous quality improvement, 1181–1182
Status inconsistency, of refugees, 308
Stearns, Ann, 671
Steinberg, Joel, 1050
Steinberg, Lisa, 1050
Stelazine (trifluoperazine), 527t
Stephen Ministry, 13
Step-parent family, 465t
Stereotype(s), 305–306
Stewart R. McKinney Homeless Assistance Act, 40
Stigma, of acquired immunodeficiency syndrome, 1107–1108
of mental illness, 39
Stimulant agent(s), 496. See also specific drugs.
as controlled substances, 796, 796t
for children, 595t
Stimulus, 423
Stoll, Ruth, 4
Storming (transition) phase, of group development, 398
Storyboards, 1182t
Strategic family therapy, 474t
Strategic planning, for continuous quality improvement, 1180, *1181*
Stream of consciousness method, 99
Strength(s), of families, 482
of patients, assessment of, for homeless people, 1032, 1033t–1034t
in crisis intervention, 353
in psychodynamic short-term therapy, 374
developing, 179–186
addressing spiritual losses and, 185–186
empowerment for, *181*, 181–182
humor for, 183–184, 184t
instilling hope for, 182–183
overcoming grief and loss for, *179*, 179–181, *180*
social support for, 184–185
hardiness as, 177–178
in milieu therapy, 446
questions to ask about, 255
reinforcing, in crisis intervention, 356
in therapeutic communication, 217
resilience as, 178–179
survivorship as, 177
Stress, 694–698. See also *Posttraumatic stress disorder (PTSD).*
anxiety related to, 695t, 695–698
general adaptation syndrome related to, 951, *952*
immediate response to, 694
in families, in schizophrenia, 740
intermediate response to, 694
long-term response to, 694–695
normal response to, phases of, 704t
nursing diagnoses for, 707, 708–712
of nursing, *64*, 64–67
strategies for dealing with, *65*, 65–67
pathological response to, phases of, 704, 704t
prolonged, as risk factor, for crisis state development, 340
psychophysiological disorders related to, 951, *952*
Stress disorder, acute, diagnosis of, 710
in children, 594
in rape victims, 1091–1092
posttraumatic. See *Posttraumatic stress disorder (PTSD).*
Stress response measures, in psychophysiological disorders, 953
Stressor(s), concurrent, as risk factors, for crisis state development, 339
critical, 334
during adulthood, 626–628, *627*
horizontal, 627
prior, as risk factors, for crisis state development, *339*, 339–340
"unacceptable," as risk factors, for crisis state development, 338–339
vertical, 627
Stress-vulnerability model, of schizophrenia, *735*, 735–736
Stroke, comorbidity of, with depression, 767–768
Structural consistency, trust and, 245
Structural family therapy, 474t
Structure, in milieu therapy, 446, 447–448
lack of, in psychiatric nursing, 6
Subjective data, for dissociative disorders, 871
Subjective reactions, in assessment, 299
Subjective Units of Distress Scale (SUDS), 432, 438
Substance abuse, 793–836. See also specific substances.
acquired immunodeficiency syndrome related to, 1106
among abusive people, 1048, 1049
among homeless people, 1026–1027
among nurses, American Nurses' Association Code for Nurses on, 84
anxiety with, 713–714
as medical disorder, *795*, 795–796
legal interpretations of, 795–796, 796t
comorbidity of, 43
with schizophrenia, 743–744, 750
definition of, 797–799
development of, 802–803
diagnosis of, 803–815
differential classification for, 805–815
DSM-IV classifications for, 803, 804
nursing diagnoses for, 803, 805, 805b
in children, 604
nursing process for, 815–836
assessment in, 816, *817*, 818
case study of, 832–836
evaluation in, 824–832
implementation in, 819–824
in acute phase, 815–816, 816t
outcome identification in, 818
planning in, 818–819, *819*, 820t
psychoactive substances and, 793–795, 800–802
brain changes caused by, 800
classification of, 806b
dependence on, 800–802
early understanding of, 794–795
synthetic, 796
variable effects of, 800
recovery from, 802
coping functions in, 184t
humor used in, 183–184, 184t
relapse prevention for, 802
self-diagnosis of, 819–821
societal information about, 820
suicide related to, 930
terminology for, 798–799, 798b
theoretical models of, 799–800
treatment of, focus of, 797
vulnerability to, 824–828
cultural differences in, 824–825
of adolescents, 825–826
of AIDS patients, 827, 828
of elderly people, 826–827
of fetuses, 826, 827t
of women, 825

Substance abuse disorder, definition of, 798
Substantia nigra, 134
Substitute gratification, 433
Subsystems, 466
  family therapy and, evaluation of effect of, 483
SUDS (Subjective Units of Distress Scale), 432, 438
Sugar, 496–497
Suicidal ideation, 928, 936
  clues to, 934, 935b
  patients with, talking to, 936, 937b
Suicide, 926–945
  altruistic, 932
  anomic, 932
  as symptom of psychiatric illness, 929–930
  causes of, 931–933
    physical, 931
    psychological, 931–932
    social, 932
    spiritual, 932
  completed, 928
  dynamics of, 933
  egotistical, 932
  epidemiology of, 928
  fatalistic, 932
  myths and realities of, 930t
  nursing process for, 933–944
    assessment in. See *Suicide, potential for, assessment of.*
  potential for, assessment of, 295b, 933–937
    cognitive domain in, 936
    emotional domain in, 935–936
    in children, 589
    in mood disorders, 772
    level of lethality in, 939b
    physical domain in, 933–935
    questions to ask in, 934, 935b
    severity index for, 933, 934, *935*
    social domain in, 936
    spiritual domain in, 936–937
    clues to, 934, 935b
    crisis underlying, identifying, 939
    high-risk groups for, 933, 934b
    in crisis intervention, 346–347
    in depression, 538
    in elderly people, 650
    in mood disorders, 763
    losses related to, 676
    nursing process for, case study of, 941–944
      diagnosis in, 937
      evaluation in, 940–941
      implementation in, 938–940
      outcome identification in, 937
      planning in, 937–938
    patient protection and, 781
  prevalence of, 929, 929t
  terminology related to, 928
  threats of, as emergencies, 938
    lethality of, level of, 928, 935–936, 938–939, *939*
Suicide attempts, 928
Suicide gestures, 928
Suicide prevention programs, 1137
Suicide watches, 938–939
Sullivan, Harry Stack, 13, 19, 24, 444, 470
    interpersonal theory of, 105–106
      relevance to nursing, 106
      self-system and, 105–106
Summative evaluation, 274
Sundowners' syndrome, 651, 1008–1009
Superconducting quantum interference device (SQUID), 141
Superego, 101
Superstitions, among West Indian peoples, 321
Support(s), as balancing factor, 333
  assessment of, for home care, *1161*, 1161–1163, *1162*
    in psychodynamic short-term therapy, 374
  engaging, 184–185
  for acquired immunodeficiency syndrome patients, 1116
  for adults, 635–636
  for Alzheimer's patients, early stages of, 1004
  for families, of Alzheimer's disease patients, 1001
    of chronically mentally ill, 1132
    of rape victims, 1097
  for rape victims, 1096
  for substance abuse recovery, 823
  for suicidal patients, 939
  generic, in disasters, 359–360
  in milieu therapy, 448, 453
  lack of, crisis state development and, 337–338
    in acquired immunodeficiency syndrome, 1109
Support group(s), 185, 410–412, 411t
  for adults, 635–636
  for Alzheimer's patients' families, 1013–1014
  for chronically mentally ill, 1136
  for families, of schizophrenic patients, 750
  for mood disorders, 783–784
  for substance abuse, 823–824
Support Group for the Survivors of Suicide, 1136
Supporting, empowerment and, 182
Supportive psychotherapy, 379–380, 380t
  for mood disorders, 775–776
  for schizophrenia, 748–749
Suppression, as defense mechanism, 697
Surmontil (trimipramine), 537t
  dosage of, 540t
Surviving Mental Illness (Hatfield), 177
Survivorship, 177
Swenson, Edna, 13
Sybil (Schreiber), 869
Symbiotic phase, in object relation theory, 843
Symbolic racism, 306
Symbolism, difficulty with, in schizophrenia, 739
Sympathomimetic agent(s), direct-acting, drug interactions of, 539
  indirect-acting, drug interactions of, 539, 542
Symptom Check List 90, in psychophysiological disorders, 952
Symptom specificity theory, of hypertension, 957–958
Synapse, 135, *136*
Synaptic transmission, 524–526
  drug effects on, 525–526
  steps in, 203, *525*
Syntaxic thinking, 106
System of Interaction Process Analysis (Bales), 388
Systematized (selective) amnesia, in dissociative disorders, 866t

Tabula rasa, 94
Tacrine (tetrahydroaminoacridine), abuse of, 810–811
  for Alzheimer's disease, 994
Tactile hallucinations, 738t
A Tale of Two Cities (Dickens), 632–633
"Taming" process, 252
Tangentiality, 296t
Taoism, 317, 488
Taractan (chlorprothixene), 527t
Tarasoff v. the Regents of the University of California, 85
Tardive dyskinesia, 136, 528, 529t, 529–530
Task(s), developmental, 166
    of elderly people, 648, 649
    of family, 468
  of psychotherapy groups, 391
Task role functions, of psychotherapy group members, 407
Tavistock Institute of Human Relations, 388–389
Taylor, Euphemia Jane, 16, *18*, 18–19
Teacher(s), nurses as, 56–57
Teaching phase, of critical incident debriefing, 362
Teaching techniques, 512b
Team(s). See *Health team(s); Quality team(s).*
Team approach, for milieu therapy, 448
Technicians, as treatment team members, 63t
Tegreton. See *Carbamazepine (Tegretol).*
Telencephalon, 132
Telephone scatologia, 891t
"The Tell-Tale Heart" (Poe), 726
Temporal lobe, 132, *132*
Temporomandibular disorder (TMD), 960–961, 961b
Tension. See also *Stress.*
  intolerable, crisis state development and, 337
  sexual, 885
Teratogenetic effects, of lithium, 548
  of psychoactive substances, 826, 827t
Termination phase. See also *Therapeutic relationship(s), termination phase of.*
  in crisis intervention. See *Crisis intervention, working phase of.*
  of family therapy, 483
  of group development, 399
  with children, 609
Terms of address, cultural concepts of, 311–312
Tertiary prevention, 57
  of mental illness, 1137
Testing behaviors, in therapeutic relationships, 248–249
Testosterone, sexual desire and, 883–884
Tetrahydroaminoacridine (Cognex; tacrine; THA), for Alzheimer's disease, 994
Tetrahydrocannabinol (THC), abuse of, 810–811
THA (tetrahydroaminoacridine), abuse of, 810–811
  for Alzheimer's disease, 994
Thalamus, 132, 133, 134
  anxiety and, 693
Thanatos, 99
Thanksgiving: An AIDS Journal (Cox), 1103
Theism, 3
Theistic model(s), 3–6
  of brain physiology, 4–5
  of human functioning, 4, *4*
  of intervention, 5
  of people and patients, 3–4
Theory(ies), 91–120. See also specific theories and types of theories.
  blending of, 115
  definition of, 93
  early Greek contributions to, 94–95, 96t
  early scientists' contributions to, 95–96
  nursing. See *Nursing theory(ies).*
  psychological, early, 96–99, 98t

Therapeutic alliance, 85
Therapeutic communication, 202–226
  barriers to, 223–226
    nursing interventions to minimize, 226
    within nurse, 224t, 224–226
    within patient, 223–224
  definition of, 208, 208t
  factors affecting, 209–211
    cultural, 210–211, 211t
    environmental, 209–210
  focus of, 209
  purpose of, 208–209
  responsibility of, 209
  self-disclosure in, 209
  social communication compared with, 208t
  strategy(ies) for, 211–222
    active listening as. See *Active listening.*
    coaching as, *221*, 221–222
    confronting as, 217
    constructive feedback as, 218
    humor as, 220–221
    information as, 222
    limit setting as, 217–218
    metaphors as, 220
    mirroring as, 221
    modeling as, 219
    redirecting as, 218–219
    reframing as, 219–220
    reinforcing strengths as, 217
  theoretical models of, 202–208
    circular, 204–205, *205*
    cognitive processing, 205–208
    linear, 202–204, *204*
Therapeutic community(ies), 389
  for substance abuse, 822
  milieu therapy compared with, 445
Therapeutic Community (Jones), 445
Therapeutic contracts, 250–251, *251*
Therapeutic listening. See *Active listening.*
Therapeutic massage, 494
Therapeutic milieu, 443
Therapeutic relationship(s), 85, 87–88, 234–260
  advocacy and, 85, 87
  conceptual components of, 239–246
    advocacy as, 240–241
    authenticity as, 244
    boundaries as, 239–240, 240b
    caring as, 238b, 241
    empathy as, 243, 244b
    empowerment as, 243
    mutuality as, 241–242, 242b
    trust as, 244–245, 245b
    unconditional acceptance as, 242–243
  confidentiality in, 85, 87
  countertransference in, with children, 578–579
  definition of, 234–236
  frameworks for, 237–239
    existential, 238–239, *239*
    nursing, 237–238
    psychological, 238
  in Bay Area Health Care model, 1155
  orientation phase of, 247–251, 247b
    collecting assessment data during, 249–250
    developing rapport during, 248–249
    developing therapeutic contracts during, 250–251, *251*
    encountering the patient during, 247–248
    establishing relationship as safe harbor during, 247
    formulating diagnoses during, 250
    validating assessment data during, 250
Therapeutic relationship(s) (*Continued*)
  preinteraction phase of, 246–247, 246b
    coordinating goals with expected outcomes during, 247
    creating supportive environment during, 246
    goal setting during, 246
    sharing goals with health care team during, 247
    timing details during, 246
  self in, use of, 236
  self-awareness in, 154b, 236–237, 237b, 238b, 254
  termination phase of, 257–260
    dealing with termination during, 258–260
    evaluation during, 258
    referrals during, 258
    tasks of, 258b
  therapeutic alliance and, 85
  transference in, with children, 578
  with children, 578–579
    countertransference in, 578–579
    transference in, 578
  working phase of, 251–257, 252b
    implementing interventions during, 257
    outcome identification and goal planning during, 252–253
    resistance during, 255–256
    solution development during, 253–255, 253b
    transference during, 255, 256–257
Therapeutic touch, 493–494
Thermistor, for biofeedback, 496
Thioridazine (Mellaril), 527t
  for children, 598t
Thiothixene (Navane), 527t
  for children, 598t
Thioxanthenes, 527t
  for children, 598t
The Thirty-Six-Hour Day (Rabins and Mace), 1002
Thomas Aquinas, St., 928
Thorazine. See *Chlorpromazine (Ormazine; Thorazine).*
Thought blocking, in schizophrenia, 729, 739
Thought broadcasting, in schizophrenia, 744t
Thought disorder, diagnosis related to, 745b
Thought meter, 97
Thought phase, of critical incident debriefing, 361–362
Thought processes, altered, 747b
Threats, Tarasoff decision and, 85
The Three Faces of Eve (Thigpen and Cleckley), 869
Three generational family, 465t
Through the Looking Glass (Carroll), 192
"Throwaway children," 1027
Tic disorders, in children, 598–599, 601
Tiffany, Francis, 15
Time, cultural concepts of, 310
  families and, 467–468
  following losses, 666, 667
  therapeutic communication and, 210
  with violent patients, 1076
"Time outs," 429
Timing, for effective communication, 196
  for therapeutic relationship, 246
  of group psychotherapy meetings, 393–394
Tindal (acetophenazine), 527t
TMD (temporomandibular disorder), 960–961
TNF (tumor necrosis factor), in acquired immunodeficiency syndrome, 1111–1112
Toddlerhood, body consciousness during, 156–157
Tofranil. See *Imipramine (Tofranil).*
Token economy, 434–435, 435b
Tolerance, 800, 801
  definition of, 798
  to benzodiazepines, 552
Tolman, Walter, 476
Torrey, E. Fuller, 26
Torrey, Elizabeth Bixler, 24
Total quality management (TQM), 1175–1191. See also *Continuous quality improvement (CQI).*
  as team effort, 1176–1177
  for Joint Commission on Accreditation of Healthcare Organizations accreditation, 1177–1178
  historical background of, 1177–1180
  legal and regulatory influences on, 1177
Touch, cultural concepts of, 311
  therapeutic, 493–494
Tourette's syndrome, in children, 598–599, 601
  treatment of, psychopharmacological, 528
Toxicity, 801
  lithium, 547–548, 547b
TQM. See *Total quality management (TQM).*
Tranquilizer(s). See *Antianxiety agent(s);* specific drugs and drug types.
Tranquilizer chair, 14, *15*
Transactional communication models, 204–205, *205*
Transcendental meditation, 495
Transcultural identification, 307–308
Transcultural nursing, 305
Transference, 103
  by children, 578
  in group psychotherapy, 404
  in psychoanalytic psychotherapy, 369
  working through, 255, 256–257
Transformation stage, of healing, 491
Transition (storming) phase, of group development, 398
Transitional objects, in object relation theory, 843
Transitional periods, in adult development, 621
Transsexualism, definition of, 881
Transvestic fetishism, 891t
Tranxene (clorazepate), dosage of, 552t
Tranylcypromine (Parnate), 537t, 541
  dosage of, 540t
  for children, 596t
Trauma. See also *Posttraumatic stress disorder (PTSD).*
  assessment of, in psychodynamic short-term therapy, 374
  to head, sexual problems resulting from, 894
Travelbee, Joyce, 12, 24, 26
Trazodone (Desyrel), 537t, 544–545
  dosage of, 540t
Treatment(s). See also *Care; Community mental health care; Inpatient treatment;* specific treatment modalities and settings.
  history of, 295
  identifying need for, in crisis intervention, 358–359
  interpersonal relationships and, 233
  involuntary, 82
  refusal of, as ethical dilemma, 79
  right to, judicial decisions concerning, 41
  voluntary, 81–82

Treatment outcomes, in continuous quality improvement, 1186
Treatment setting(s), 46–48. See also *Environment(s);* specific settings, i.e., *Hospital(s).*
  for children, 606–608, *607*
Treatment team(s). See *Health team(s).*
Tremor, lithium causing, 548
Trenton State Hospital, 15
TRIADS system, 297, 1065, *1066–1067*
Triage, in delirium, 982
Triangle, in family therapy, 474–475, *475*
Triangulation, 1200
Tricyclic antidepressant agent(s). See *Antidepressant agent(s), tricyclic.*
Trifluoperazine (Stelazine), 527t
Triflupromazine (Vesprin), 527t
Trilafon (terphenazine), 527t
  for children, 598t
Trimipramine (Surmontil), 537t
  dosage of, 540t
Trotter, Thomas, 795
Trust, in therapeutic relationships, 244–245
  lack of, family interventions for, 344t
Trust versus mistrust stage, 103t, 107, 167t
  stressors during, 333t
Truthfulness, in group psychotherapy, 402
Truth-telling, in research, 1197
Tuke, William, 14, 20
Tumor necrosis factor (TNF), in acquired immunodeficiency syndrome, 1111–1112
Twelve-step programs, patient and family information about, 824
Twin studies, of anxiety disorders, 146
  of mood disorders, 145, 768
  of schizophrenia, 144
Tyramine, interaction with monoamine oxidase inhibitors, 542, 543t

"Unaccompanied youths," 1027
Unconditional acceptance, 110
  in therapeutic relationships, 242–243
Unconscious, 100
  collective, 104
  personal, 104
Uncus, 133
Undifferentiated schizophrenia, 732t
Undifferentiated somatoform disorder, 967, 968t
Undoing, as defense mechanism, 697
Unemployment, 631–632
  effects of, 1029b
  homelessness related to, 1029
  increase in, 43
Unemployment rate, 1029
Uniqueness, in interpersonal nursing, 119
Universal access, 73
Universality, in group psychotherapy, 402
Urinary incontinence, in children, 599–600, 602
Urophilia, 891t
User-oriented model, for transmitting research knowledge, 1201

VA (Veterans Administration), home care funding under, 1158
  hospitals of, 44
Vaginismus, 884
Validation, asking for, for effective communication, 196
  for active listening, 216
Validation, asking for, for effective communication (*Continued*)
  in milieu therapy, 448
  of assessment data, 250
  of patient, 119
Valium. See *Diazepam (Valium).*
Valproic acid (Depakene; Depakote), for bipolar disorder, 546, 549
  for children, 597t
Value(s), clarification of, 634–635
Value judgments, in therapeutic communication, 224t, 225–226
Vanier, Jean, 750
Variable interval schedule, 430, 430t
Variable ratio schedule, 430, 430t
Vascular dementia, 991–992
Vascular factors, in migraine headaches, 959
VBR (ventricular-brain ratio), 141
Vegetables, 497
  interaction with monoamine oxidase inhibitors, 543t
Ventilation, encouraging, in crisis intervention, 356
Ventricles, of brain, 134–135
  in schizophrenia, 143–144, 731
  size of, 141
Ventricular-brain ratio (VBR), 141
Veracity, as ethical guide, 74
Verb(s), associated with neurolinguistic programming, 206b
Verbal communication, *197*, 197–198
  message confusion in, 197–198
Verbal intervention, for milieu therapy, 448
Vertical stressors, 627
Vesprin (triflupromazine), 527t
Veterans Administration (VA), home care funding under, 1158
  hospitals of, 44
Vicarious learning, 113
Victim(s), information processing in, 1068, *1069*
Victimization, feelings of, in crisis intervention, 356
  female homelessness related to, 1027
Vineland Adaptive Behavior Scales, 602
Violence, 34. See also *Suicide.*
  against children. See *Child abuse; Family violence.*
  against spouse. See *Family violence; Spousal abuse.*
  against women, 1051b
  assaultive stage of, 1077
  children's exposure to, mental illness and, 580–581
  definition of, 1040
  expressive, 1048–1049, 1049t
  in Alzheimer's disease, middle stages of, 1008
  in delirium, managing, 987
  in families. See *Abuse; Child abuse; Elder abuse; Family violence; Sexual abuse; Spousal abuse.*
  in psychiatric settings, 1074b
  instrumental, 1048, 1049, 1049t
  myths about, 1074
  nursing process for, 1074–1078
    assessment in, 1074–1075, *1075*
    diagnosis in, 1075
    evaluation in, 1078
    implementation in, 1075–1078
    outcome identification in, 1075
    planning in, 1075
  postassaultive stage of, 1077–1078
    documentation in, 1077–1078
Violence (*Continued*)
  potential for, in crisis intervention, 347–350
    indicators of, 348t
    interventions for, 348–350, 349t, 350t
  power and control and, 1040, *1041*
  preassaultive stage of, 1075–1077
    analysis in, of patient and situation, 1075
    deescalation in, verbal techniques for, 1075–1076
    environment and, 1076
    interacting with patient during, 1076
    patient's personal space in, respect for, 1076
    posture and body language during, 1076
    safety and, of nurse, 1076–1077
    time frame for, 1076
  prejudice and, 306
  prevention of, 1072b–1073b
    behavioral therapy for, 435–436
Viorst, Judith, 164
Viral illness, Alzheimer's disease caused by, 994
  schizophrenia caused by, 144, 734
Visual Analogue Scales, in psychophysiological disorders, 953
Visual area, 138
Visual hallucinations, 738t
Vital sense, in mood disorders, 763–764
Vital signs, in eating disorders, 914
Vitamins, 497, 498
Vivactil (protriptyline), 537t
  dosage of, 540t
Vocalizations, 201
Voice tone, cultural concepts of, 311
Volatile solvents, abuse of, 815
Voluntary repetition, 98
Voluntary treatment, 81–82
Vonnegut, Mark, 726, 727, 737
Voyeurism, 891t
Vulnerability, biological, to schizophrenia, 735
  crisis state development and, 336–337
  personal, to schizophrenia, 736

Wandering, in Alzheimer's disease, middle stages of, 1006t
Ward, Mary Jane, 21
Washington Home for the Treatment of Alcohol Abuse, 795
Washoe Medical Center, 181
Watson, Jean, 116
  theory of, 117t
Watson, John B., 111, 112, 129
Way Station, 458–459
Wechsler Intelligence Scale for Children, Revised (WISC-R), 601
Weiss, Olga, 24
Wellbutrin (bupropion), 537t, 545
  dosage of, 540t
  for children, 597t
Wernicke, Carl, 981
Wernicke's aphasia, 981
Wernicke's area, 129, 132, 138, 139
Wernicke's encephalopathy, 808
West Indian peoples, 321–322
  communication among, 321
Western Interstate Commission for Higher Education (WICHE) project, 1201
What Every Parent Should Know (Gordon), 439
Wheat, 497
When Rabbit Howls (Chase), 869–870

White matter, 130
WHO (World Health Organization), International Pilot Study of Schizophrenia conducted by, 730–731
WICHE (Western Interstate Commission for Higher Education) project, 1201
Widowhood, 630
Wife-battering model, of spouse abuse, 1049
Will, Gwen Tudor, 24
Windigo psychosis, 309
Wine, interaction with monoamine oxidase inhibitors, 543t
WISC-R (Wechsler Intelligence Scale for Children, Revised), 601
Withdrawal, from drugs, 801
  definition of, 798
  from alcohol, 808
  from benzodiazepines, 809
  from cocaine, 814
  from narcotics, 812
  from nicotine, 814
 in therapeutic relationships, 256
Women. See also *Gender* entries; *Parent(s); Pregnancy; Sexual* entries; *Sexuality.*
 abuse of. See *Abuse; Family violence; Spousal abuse.*
 acquired immunodeficiency syndrome in, 1106
 adult development of, 622
 anorgasmia in, 887–890
 battered, Maryland legal remedies for, 1063b
 depression in, following delivery, 766
 eating disorders in, 910
 homelessness among, 1027
Women (*Continued*)
 menopause and, 625
 orgasms in, 885–886
 rape of. See *Rape.*
 sexual desire in, 884
 social changes affecting, 628–633
 substance abuse among, 825
 violence against, 1051b
Women's liberation movement, gender role changes due to, 163
Woolf, Virginia, 760
Word(s), cultural concepts of, 311
Word salad, in schizophrenia, 739
Worden, Art, 59
Work, lack of, 43, 631–632
  homelessness related to, 1029
Working phase. See also *Therapeutic relationship(s), working phase of.*
 of crisis intervention, 354–358
  diagnosis, outcome identification, and planning during, 354–355
  implementation during, 355–358
 of group development, 398–399
World Health Organization (WHO), International Pilot Study of Schizophrenia conducted by, 730–731
World views, 3–6
 spiritual self and, 164–165
 theistic, 3. See also *Theistic model(s).*
World War I, influence on mental health care, 21
World War II, group psychotherapy during, 388
 influence on mental health care, 21
"Worried well," 1104
Wundt, Wilhelm, 96–97, 98t
Wyatt v. Stickney, 41

Xanax (alprazolam), dosage of, 552t
 for panic attacks, 551

Yale-Brown Obsessive-Compulsive Scale, 1215
Yale-Brown Obsessive-Compulsive Symptom Checklist, 1216
Yalom, Irving, 390
Yang, 488
Yeast, interaction with monoamine oxidase inhibitors, 543t
Yin, 488
Yogi, Maharishi-Mahesh, 495
York Retreat, 14, 444
Young, Rae Jean, 93
Young-old, 646

Zderad, Loretta T., 26
 theory of, 117t
Zoloft (sertraline), 537t, 544
 dosage of, 540t
 for children, 596t
Zoophilia, 891t
Zung Self-Rating Depression Scale, 1210, 1211t, 1212t, 1212–1214